Robbins
PATHOLOGIC BASIS OF DISEASE

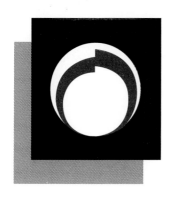

Robbins
PATHOLOGIC BASIS OF DISEASE

5th Edition

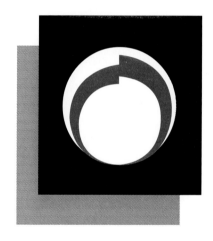

Ramzi S. Cotran, M.D.

Frank Burr Mallory Professor of Pathology
Harvard Medical School
Chairman, Departments of Pathology
Brigham and Women's Hospital
The Children's Hospital
Boston, Massachusetts

Vinay Kumar, M.D.

Vernie A. Stembridge Chair in Pathology
The University of Texas
Southwestern Medical School
Dallas, Texas

Stanley L. Robbins, M.D.

Visiting Professor of Pathology
Harvard Medical School
Senior Pathologist
Brigham and Women's Hospital
Boston, Massachusetts

Managing Editor

Frederick J. Schoen, M.D., Ph.D.

Associate Professor of Pathology
Harvard Medical School
Vice-Chairman, Department of Pathology
Brigham and Women's Hospital
Boston, Massachusetts

W.B. SAUNDERS COMPANY
A Division of Harcourt Brace & Company
Philadelphia   London   Toronto   Montreal   Sydney   Tokyo

W.B. SAUNDERS COMPANY
A Division of
Harcourt Brace & Company

The Curtis Center
Independence Square West
Philadelphia, Pennsylvania 19106

Library of Congress Cataloging-in-Publication Data

Cotran, Ramzi S.
Robbins pathologic basis of disease. —5th ed. / Ramzi S. Cotran,
Stanley L. Robbins, Vinay Kumar.
    p.   cm.
  Includes bibliographical references and index.
ISBN 0-7216-5032-5
1. Pathology. I. Robbins, Stanley L. (Stanley Leonard).
  II. Kumar, Vinay. III. Title. IV. Title: Pathologic basis of disease.
  [DNLM: 1. Pathology. QZ 4 C845r 1994]
RB111.R62 1994
616.07—dc20
DNLM/DLC   94-2629

Robbins Pathologic Basis of Disease, 5th edition   ISBN 0-7216-5032-5

Printed in the United States of America.

Last digit is the print number: 9   8   7   6   5   4

To
Kerstin
To
Raminder
and to
Elly
with love

Contributors

Douglas C. Anthony, M.D., Ph.D.
Assistant Professor of Pathology, Harvard Medical School; Director of Neuropathology, The Children's Hospital; Neuropathologist, Brigham and Women's Hospital, Boston, Massachusetts

James M. Crawford, M.D., Ph.D.
Assistant Professor of Pathology, Harvard Medical School; Pathologist, Brigham and Women's Hospital, Boston, Massachusetts

Christopher P. Crum, M.D.
Associate Professor of Pathology, Harvard Medical School; Director, Division of Women's and Perinatal Pathology, Brigham and Women's Hospital, Boston, Massachusetts

Umberto De Girolami, M.D.
Associate Professor of Pathology, Harvard Medical School; Neuropathologist, Brigham and Women's Hospital and The Children's Hospital, Boston, Massachusetts

Matthew P. Frosch, M.D., Ph.D.
Instructor in Pathology, Harvard Medical School; Associate Pathologist, Brigham and Women's Hospital; Consultant in Pathology, Children's Hospital, Boston, Massachusetts

Lester Kobzik, M.D.
Assistant Professor, Harvard Medical School, Harvard School of Public Health; Pathologist, Brigham and Women's Hospital, Boston, Massachusetts

Martin C. Mihm, Jr., M.D.
Professor of Pathology and Chief of Dermatology and Dermatopathology, Albany Medical College, Albany, New York

George F. Murphy, M.D.
Herman Beerman Professor of Dermatology, Professor of Pathology, University of Pennsylvania School of Medicine; Director of Dermatopathology Training, Hospital of the University of Pennsylvania, Philadelphia, Pennsylvania

Andrew E. Rosenberg, M.D.
Assistant Professor of Pathology, Harvard Medical School; Associate Pathologist, Massachusetts General Hospital, Boston, Massachusetts

John Samuelson, M.D., Ph.D.
Associate Professor, Department of Tropical Public Health, Harvard School of Public Health, Boston, Massachusetts

Frederick J. Schoen, M.D., Ph.D.
Associate Professor of Pathology, Lawrence J. Henderson Associate Professor of Health Sciences and Technology, Harvard Medical School; Vice-Chairman, Department of Pathology, Brigham and Women's Hospital, Boston, Massachusetts

Deborah Schofield, M.D.
Assistant Professor of Pathology, Harvard Medical School and The Children's Hospital, Boston, Massachusetts

Franz von Lichtenberg, M.D.
Professor of Pathology Emeritus, Harvard Medical School; Senior Pathologist, Brigham and Women's Hospital, Boston, Massachusetts

Preface

Once again, we are launching a new edition of this book—the fifth. In the five years since the previous edition, spectacular advances have been made in many areas of the science and practice of pathology—particularly in our understanding of the molecular and genetic origins of many diseases and in the application of modern techniques to diagnostic pathology. Although these have necessitated extensive revisions, our goals remain essentially the same.

- To integrate into the discussion of pathologic processes and disorders the newest established information available—morphologic, molecular, and genetic. This, we hope, will make the understanding of disease as up-to-date as possible and will facilitate the application of optimal diagnostic modalities and therapeutic interventions.
- To organize the presentations into logical and uniform approaches, thereby facilitating readability, comprehension, and learning.
- Not to permit the book to become larger and more cumbersome, and yet to provide adequate discussion of the significant lesions, processes, and disorders, allotting space in proportion to their clinical and biologic importance.
- To place great emphasis on clarity of writing and good usage of language in the recognition that struggling to comprehend is time-consuming and wearisome and gets in the way of the learning process.
- To make this first and foremost a student text (useful to students throughout their four years of medical school and into their residencies) but, at the same time, to provide sufficient detail and depth to meet the needs of more advanced readers.

We hope that we have, at least in some measure, achieved these goals; any shortcomings are surely not for lack of trying.

Although the newer body of knowledge has required extensive rewriting, the basic organization remains largely unchanged. The chapters on general principles and processes such as cell injury and inflammation are confined to the first third of the text, while the remainder of the book is concerned with the disorders of various organs and systems. Every chapter has been carefully updated with "state-of-the-art" material, and many have been largely rewritten. A new chapter on normal and abnormal cell growth has been added to the discussion of general pathology, stimulated by the explosion of new information. In systemic pathology emphasis has been placed on the origins of functional and structural changes (etiology and pathogenesis), but the essential morphology, highlighted by a pink background, has been carefully preserved. Whenever appropriate, newer morphologic techniques relevant to the identification of particular lesions or tumors have been incorporated. The clinical significance of the morphologic and molecular changes has been integrated throughout the text.

Particularly newsworthy in this edition is the extensive revision of the illustrative material. Fully half of the photographs have been replaced, and many of these replacements are in color. A large number of new diagrams and charts have also been incorporated where they can illuminate the text. We hope that this new infusion not only reinforces the textual matter but also makes the reading more pleasurable.

A liberal but judicious number of references are incorporated into the writing to provide source material for those who wish to pursue subjects of their own interest. Great effort was made in selecting these references for their quality, authenticity, and completeness. While most are recent— indeed some appeared in 1994, the year of publication of this text— older classics have been retained precisely because they are "classic."

The same three authors of previous editions prepared most of the chapters themselves, but reviewed, edited, and critiqued all of them. They were measurably helped by the advice and reviews of many experts who were sought out to ensure the accuracy, completeness, and authenticity of areas of their expertise, as detailed in the acknowledgments section.

We hope that we have succeeded in transmitting to the readers of this text the beauty and excitement of our expanding knowledge of the nature of many diseases and have stimulated them to learn more about the pathologic basis of disease.

Acknowledgments

Thanks and gratitude are owed to many kind individuals for their help in various ways in the completion of this edition. Without such help, this book would indeed be poorer.

First among those to whom we are indebted is Dr. Frederick J. Schoen, our Managing Editor, who not only contributed several chapters (as is shown in the Table of Contents) but also made scientific contributions to numerous areas of this text and served as the monitor of the ebb and flow of materials between W.B. Saunders Company and the authors.

We owe a great debt to our editorial personal assistants, Margarita Rosado, Julie Smith, Cathleen Quade, Claudia Davis, Beverly Shackelford, Debbie Watts, and Marilyn Gibson. Their efforts maintained the progress of the work and ultimately put the book together.

Several colleagues have added to the luster of this book by contributing chapters or segments of chapters. Their particular contributions are acknowledged in the Table of Contents or in the chapters themselves, and so it suffices here to note our gratitude to them for their willingness to lend their names and their expertise to this edition. Our thanks also to Drs. Daniel Albert, Yogeshwar Dayal, Theodore Dryja, Ronald DeLellis, and James Morris, contributors to the previous edition whose efforts are still felt in this edition.

Many experts made their contributions to the quality of the writing by providing oversight and critiques in their special areas of interest. We particularly thank Drs. M.A. Venkatachalam and Maximillian Buja (Cell Injury); Donald Ingber, Anindya Dutta, and Nelson Fausto (Cell Growth); Tucker Collins and Charles Serhan (Inflammation); Nancy Schneider (Genetic Disorders); Abul Abbas (Diseases of Immunity); Frank Vuitch and Adi Gazdar (Neoplasia, and The Lung); Arlene Sharpe and Jeffrey Joseph (Infectious Diseases); Frank Castronova (Radiation Injury); George Katsas (Forensic Pathology); Fred Bieber, George Mutter, Drucilla Roberts, and Laurie Suton (Pediatric Diseases); William Edwards (Congenital Heart Disease); Richard Mitchell and Gayle Winters (The Heart); Robert McKenna and Jose Hernandez (White Cells); Jerry Trier (Gastrointestinal Diseases); Martin Carey and David Cohen (The Liver); David Sacks (Diabetes); Helmut Rennke (Kidney Diseases); Christopher Corless (The Lower Urinary Tract); David Genest (Female Genital Tract); Susan Lester (The Breast); Mary Sunday and Michael Teitell (Endocrine Diseases); and T. Bouldin, R. Hevner, S. Mirra, and F. S. Vogel (Peripheral Nerve and Skeletal Muscle; The Central Nervous System). Such excellence as the book may have is owed in part to them, any errors are ours.

We owe thanks to many, many members of the staffs of the Brigham and Women's Hospital, The Children's Hospital, and the University of Texas Southwestern Medical School in Dallas, as well as other colleagues and friends who have added to this book by providing us with prize photographic and graphic gems. Most have been acknowledged with their contributions, but in addition, we wish to single out a few for special gratitude: Drs. Ramon Blanco, Brad Brimhall, Edmund Cibas, Christopher Corless, Paul Duray, Robert Ehrmann, Scott Granter, Prabodh Gupta, Herbert Hagler, W. Hardy Hendren, Jose Hernandez, Jeffrey Joseph, Nancy Joste, George Katsas, Madeleine Kraus, Robert McKenna, and Catherine McLachlin; Mr. Anthony Merola; Drs. Marisa Nucci, Helmut Rennke, Birgitta Schmidt, Joseph Semple, and John Sexton; Ms. Beni Stewart; and Drs. Vijay Tonk, Jerrold Turner, and Trace Worrell. To all our deepest thanks.

We are also indebted to our publisher, W.B. Saunders Company, for its tolerance of our many requests and especially for its commitment to this book and its authors. Particularly deserving of our thanks are Ms. Kim Kist, Ms. Gina Scala, Mr. Richard Zorab, Mr. David Prout, and Mr. Lewis Reines, President of W.B. Saunders, for his enthusiasm for this project, and especially Ms. Carolyn Naylor, who was a tower of strength in pulling the pieces together and an unfailing source of cheerfulness and encouragement. Undoubtedly there are many other "unsung heroes" who should be recognized for their contributions, particularly in the Illustration Department—to all of them we say thanks and ask forgiveness for their not being individually singled out.

Once again we acknowledge our wives, Kerstin Cotran, Raminder Kumar, and Elly Robbins, and wish them to know that our thanks are not merely "pro forma," they are sincerely offered and well deserved.

And finally each of us wishes to "doff his hat" to his coauthors for their unstinting efforts to make this book the best possible, for their willingness to accept the advice of the others, and for their faith in our joint effort. We began the writing years ago as good friends, and we completed it as even better friends.

RSC
VK
SLR

Contents

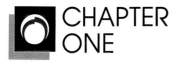

Cellular Injury and Cellular Death

INTRODUCTION TO PATHOLOGY

Pathology literally is the study (*logos*) of suffering (*pathos*). More specifically, it is a bridging discipline involving both basic science and clinical practice and is devoted to the study of the structural and functional changes in cells, tissues, and organs that underlie "dis-eases." By the use of molecular, microbiologic, immunologic, and morphologic techniques, pathology attempts to explain the "whys" and "wherefores" of the signs and symptoms manifested by patients while providing a sound foundation for rational clinical care and therapy.

Traditionally, the study of pathology is divided into general pathology and special or systemic pathology. The former is concerned with the basic reactions of cells and tissues to abnormal stimuli that underlie all diseases. The latter examines the specific responses of specialized organs and tissues to more or less well-defined stimuli. In this book, we shall first cover the principles of general pa-

thology and then proceed to specific disease processes as they affect particular organs or systems.

The four aspects of a disease process that form the core of pathology are (1) its cause (etiology), (2) the mechanisms of its development (pathogenesis), (3) the structural alterations induced in the cells and organs of the body (morphologic changes), and (4) the functional consequences of the morphologic changes (clinical significance).

1. *Etiology or cause.* The concept that certain abnormal symptoms or diseases are "caused" is as ancient as recorded history. For the Acadians (2500 B.C.), if someone became ill, it was the patient's own fault (for having sinned) or the makings of outside agents, such as bad smells, cold, evil spirits, or gods.[1] In modern terms, there are the two major classes of etiologic factors: intrinsic or genetic and acquired (e.g., infectious, nutritional, chemical, physical). Knowledge or discovery of the primary cause remains the backbone on which a diagnosis can be made, a disease understood, or a treatment developed. The concept, however, of one etiologic agent to one disease—developed

from the study of infections or single gene disorders—is no longer sufficient. Genetic factors are clearly involved in some of the common environmentally induced maladies, such as atherosclerosis and cancer, and the environment may also have profound influences on certain genetic diseases.

2. *Pathogenesis.* Pathogenesis refers to the sequence of events in the response of the cells or tissues to the etiologic agent, from the initial stimulus to the ultimate expression of the disease. The study of pathogenesis remains one of the main domains of pathology. Even when the initial infectious or molecular cause is known, it is many steps removed from the expression of the disease. For example, to understand cystic fibrosis is to know not only the defective gene and gene product but also the biochemical, immunologic, and morphologic events leading to the formation of cysts and fibrosis in the lung, pancreas, and other organs.

3. *Morphologic changes.* The morphologic changes refer to the structural alterations in cells or tissues that are either characteristic of the disease or diagnostic of the etiologic process.

4. *Functional derangements and clinical significance.* The nature of the morphologic changes and their distribution in different organs or tissues influence normal function and determine the clinical features (symptoms and signs), course, and prognosis of the disease.

Virtually all forms of organ injury start with molecular or structural alterations in *cells*, a concept first put forth in the 19th century by Rudolf Virchow, known as the "father" of modern pathology. We therefore begin our consideration of pathology with the study of the origins, molecular mechanisms, and structural changes of cell injury. Yet different cells in tissues constantly interact with each other, and an elaborate system of *extracellular matrix* is necessary for the integrity of organs. Cell-cell and cell-matrix interactions contribute significantly to the response to injury, leading collectively to *tissue* and *organ injury*, which are as important as cell injury in defining the morphologic and clinical patterns of disease.[2]

DEFINITIONS

The normal cell is confined to a fairly narrow range of function and structure by its genetic programs of metabolism, differentiation, and specialization; by constraints of neighboring cells; and by the availability of metabolic substrates. It is nevertheless able to handle normal physiologic demands—so-called *normal homeostasis.* Somewhat more excessive physiologic stresses or some pathologic stimuli may bring about a number of physiologic and morphologic *cellular adaptations,* in which a new but altered steady state is achieved, preserving the viability of the cell and modulating its function as a response to such stimuli. For example, the bulging muscles of the bodybuilders engaged in "pumping iron" result from cellular adaptations, the increase in muscle mass reflecting the increase in size of the individual muscle fibers. The workload is thus shared by a greater mass of cellular components, and each muscle fiber is spared excess work and so escapes injury. The enlarged muscle cell achieves a new equilibrium, permitting it to survive at a higher level of activity. This adaptive response is called *hypertrophy.* Conversely, *atrophy* is an adaptive response in which there is a decrease in the size and function of cells. Other cell adaptations occur and are considered in Chapter 2.

If the limits of adaptive response to a stimulus are exceeded, or in certain instances when adaptation is not possible, a sequence of events follows, loosely termed *cell injury.* Cell injury is *reversible* up to a certain point, but if the stimulus persists or is severe enough from the beginning, the cell reaches the point of no return and suffers *irreversible cell injury* and *cell death.* For example, if the blood supply to a segment of the heart is cut off for 10 to 15 minutes and is then restored, the myocardial cells experience injury but can recover and function normally. If blood flow is not restored until 1 hour later, however, irreversible injury ensues, and many myocardial fibers die. *Adaptation, reversible injury, irreversible injury,* and *cell death* can be considered states of progressive encroachment on the cell's normal function and structure (Fig. 1–1).

Cell death, the ultimate result of cell injury, is one of the most crucial events in pathology, affecting every cell type and being the major consequence of ischemia (lack of blood flow), infection, toxins, and immune reactions. In addition, it is critical during normal embryogenesis, lymphoid tissue development, and hormonally induced involution and is the aim of cancer radiotherapy and chemotherapy. There are two morphologic patterns of cell death, *necrosis* and *apoptosis. Necrosis* or *coagulation necrosis* is the more common type of cell death after exogenous stimuli, occurring after such stresses as ischemia and chemical injury, and is manifested by severe cell swelling or cell rupture, denaturation and coagulation of cytoplasmic proteins, and breakdown of cell organelles. *Apoptosis* is a more regulated event. It is designed for the normal elimination of unwanted cell populations during embryogenesis and in various physiologic processes. It also occurs, however, under pathologic conditions, in which it is sometimes accompanied by necrosis. Its chief morphologic features are chromatin condensation and fragmentation. Although the mechanisms of necrosis and apoptosis differ, as we shall see, there is overlap between these two processes.

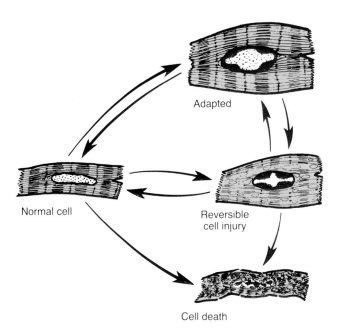

Figure 1–1. The relationships among normal, adapted, reversibly injured, and dead myocardial cells. The cellular adaptation depicted here is hypertrophy, and the type of cellular injury is ischemic necrosis.

The cellular changes described—reversible and irreversible cell injury leading to *necrosis* or *apoptosis*—are morphologic patterns of *acute cell injury* induced by various stimuli. Three other groups of morphologic alterations are described in this chapter (Table 1–1): *subcellular alterations*, which occur largely as a response to more chronic or persistent injurious stimuli; *intracellular accumulations* of a number of substances—lipids, carbohydrates, and proteins—which occur as a result of derangements in cell metabolism or excessive storage; and *pathologic calcification*, a common consequence of cell and tissue injury.

The following section considers first the broad categories of stresses and noxious influences that induce injury and then discusses the various types of cell injury separately.

Table 1–1. CELLULAR RESPONSES TO INJURY

Cellular Adaptations
    Atrophy, hypertrophy, hyperplasia, metaplasia (Chapter 2)
Acute Cell Injury
    Reversible injury
    Cell death
        Necrosis
        Apoptosis
Subcellular Alterations and Cell Inclusions
Intracellular Accumulations
Pathologic Calcification

CAUSES OF CELL INJURY

The causes of reversible cell injury and cell death range from the external gross physical violence of an automobile accident to internal endogenous causes, such as a subtle genetic lack of a vital enzyme that impairs normal metabolic function. Most adverse influences can be grouped into the following broad categories.

HYPOXIA. Hypoxia, an extremely important and common cause of cell injury and cell death, impinges on aerobic oxidative respiration. Loss of blood supply *(ischemia)*, which occurs when arterial flow is impeded by arteriosclerosis or by thrombi, is the most common cause of hypoxia. Another cause is inadequate oxygenation of the blood due to cardiorespiratory failure. Loss of the oxygen-carrying *capacity* of the blood, as in anemia or carbon monoxide poisoning (producing a stable carbon monoxyhemoglobin that blocks oxygen carriage), is a third, less frequent basis of oxygen deprivation. Depending on the severity of the hypoxic state, cells may adapt, undergo injury, or die. For example, if the femoral artery is narrowed, the skeletal muscle cells of the leg may shrink in size (atrophy). This reduction in cell mass achieves a balance between metabolic needs and the available oxygen supply. More severe hypoxia induces injury and cell death.

PHYSICAL AGENTS. Physical agents include mechanical trauma, extremes of temperature (burns and deep cold), sudden changes in atmospheric pressure, radiation, and electric shock (see Chapter 9, Environmental and Nutritional Diseases).

CHEMICAL AGENTS AND DRUGS. The list of chemicals that may produce cell injury defies compilation. Simple chemicals such as glucose or salt in hypertonic concentrations may cause cell injury directly or by deranging electrolyte homeostasis of cells. Even oxygen, in high concentrations, is severely toxic. Trace amounts of agents known as *poisons*, such as arsenic, cyanide, or mercuric salts, may destroy sufficient numbers of cells within minutes to hours to cause death. Other substances, however, are our daily companions: environmental and air pollutants, insecticides, and herbicides; industrial and occupational hazards, such as carbon monoxide and asbestos; social stimuli, such as alcohol and narcotic drugs; and the ever-increasing variety of therapeutic drugs.

INFECTIOUS AGENTS. These agents range from the submicroscopic viruses to the large tapeworms. In between are the rickettsiae, bacteria, fungi, and higher forms of parasites. The ways by which this heterogeneous group of biologic agents cause injury are diverse and are discussed in greater detail in Chapter 8 (Infectious Diseases).

IMMUNOLOGIC REACTIONS. These may be life-saving or lethal. Although the immune system serves in the defense against biologic agents, immune reactions may, in fact, cause cell injury. The anaphylactic reaction to a foreign protein or a drug is a prime example, and reactions to endogenous self-antigens are thought to be responsible for a number of so-called autoimmune diseases (see Chapter 6).

GENETIC DERANGEMENTS. Genetic defects as causes of cellular injury are of major interest to biologists today (see Chapter 5). The genetic injury may result in as gross a defect as the congenital malformations associated with Down syndrome or in subtle alterations in the coding of hemoglobin responsible for the production of hemoglobin S in sickle cell anemia. The many inborn errors of metabolism arising from enzymic abnormalities, usually an enzyme lack, are excellent examples of cell damage due to subtle alterations at the level of DNA.

NUTRITIONAL IMBALANCES. Even today nutritional imbalances continue to be major causes of cell injury. Protein-calorie deficiencies cause an appalling number of deaths, chiefly among underprivileged populations. Deficiencies of specific vitamins are found throughout the world (see Chapter 9). Ironically, nutritional excesses have also become important causes of cell injury. Excesses of lipids predispose to atherosclerosis, and obesity is an extraordinary manifestation of the overloading of some cells in the body with fats. Atherosclerosis is virtually endemic in the United States, and obesity is rampant.

CELL INJURY AND NECROSIS

GENERAL MECHANISMS

The molecular mechanisms responsible for cell injury leading to necrotic cell death are complex. As we have seen, injury to cells has many causes, and probably there is no common final pathway of cell death. There are, however, a number of considerations that are useful to remember.

- Although it is not always possible to determine the precise biochemical site of action of an injurious agent, four intracellular systems are particularly vulnerable: (1) *maintenance of the integrity of cell membranes*, on which the ionic and osmotic homeostasis of the cell and its organelles depends; (2) *aerobic respiration* involving oxidative phosphorylation and production of adenosine triphosphate (ATP); (3) *synthesis of enzymatic and structural proteins*; and (4) *preservation of the integrity of the genetic apparatus* of the cell.

- *The structural and biochemical elements of the cell are so closely inter-related that whatever the precise point of initial attack, injury at one locus leads to wide-ranging secondary effects.* For example, impairment of aerobic respiration disrupts the energy-dependent membrane sodium pump that maintains the ionic and fluid balance of the cell, resulting in alterations in the intracellular content of ions and water.

- *The morphologic changes of cell injury become apparent only after some critical biochemical system within the cell has been deranged.* As would be expected, the morphologic manifestations of lethal damage take more time to develop than those of reversible damage. For example, cell swelling is a reversible morphologic change, and this may occur in a matter of minutes. Unmistakable light microscopic changes of cell death, however, do not occur in the myocardium until 10 to 12 hours after total ischemia, yet we know that irreversible injury occurs within 20 to 60 minutes. Obviously, ultrastructural alterations are visible earlier than light microscopic changes.

- *Reactions of the cell to injurious stimuli depend on the type of injury, its duration, and its severity.* Thus, small doses of a chemical toxin or ischemia of short duration may induce reversible injury, whereas large doses of the same toxin or more prolonged ischemia might result either in instantaneous cell death or in slow, irreversible injury leading in time to cell death.

- *The type, state, and adaptability of the injured cell also determine the consequences of cell injury.* The cell's nutritional and hormonal status and its metabolic needs are important in its response to injury. How vulnerable is a cell, for example, to loss of blood supply and hypoxia? The striated muscle cell in the leg can be placed entirely at rest when deprived of its blood supply; not so, the striated muscle of the heart. Exposure of two individuals to identical concentrations of a toxin, such as carbon tetrachloride, may be without effect in one and may produce cell death in the other. This may be due, as we shall see, to the amounts of hepatic enzymes that convert carbon tetrachloride to toxic by-products.

With certain injurious agents, the mechanisms and loci of attack are well defined. Many toxins, for example, cause cell injury by interfering with endogenous substrates or enzymes. Particularly vulnerable are glycolysis, the citric acid cycle, and oxidative phosphorylation in mitochondrial inner membranes. Cyanide, for example, inactivates cytochrome oxidase, and fluoroacetate interferes with the citric acid cycle, both resulting in ATP depletion. Certain anaerobic bacteria, such as *Clostridium perfringens*, elaborate phospholipases, which attack phospholipids in cell membranes.

As we shall see, however, there are four com-

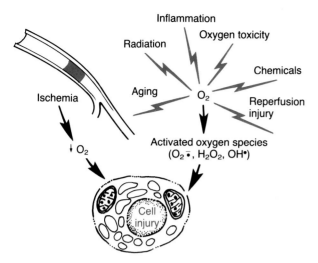

Figure 1–2. The critical role of oxygen in cell injury. Ischemia causes cell injury by reducing cellular oxygen supplies, whereas other stimuli, such as radiation, induce damage via toxic activated oxygen species.

mon biochemical themes that appear to be important in the mediation of cell injury and cell death, *whatever the inciting agent*. These include the following:

- *Oxygen and oxygen-derived free radicals* (Fig. 1–2). Lack of oxygen underlies the pathogenesis of cell injury in ischemia. It is also clear that partially reduced activated oxygen species are important mediators of cell death in many pathologic conditions. These free radicals cause lipid peroxidation and have other deleterious effects on cell structure, as we shall see.
- *Intracellular calcium and loss of calcium homeostasis.* Cytosolic free calcium is maintained at extremely low concentrations (less than 0.1 μM) compared with extracellular levels of 1.3 mM, and most intracellular calcium is sequestered in mitochondria and endoplasmic reticulum. Such gradients are modulated by membrane-associated, energy-dependent Ca^{++}, Mg^{++}-ATPases. Ischemia and certain toxins cause an early increase in cytosolic calcium concentration, owing to the net influx of Ca^{++} across the plasma membrane and the release of Ca^{++} from mitochondria and endoplasmic reticulum. Sustained rises in cell Ca^{++} subsequently result from nonspecific increases in membrane permeability. Increased Ca^{++} in turn activates a number of enzymes, with potential deleterious cellular effects. The enzymes known to be activated by calcium include *phospholipases* (thus promoting membrane damage), *proteases* (which break down both membrane and cytoskeletal proteins), *ATPases*

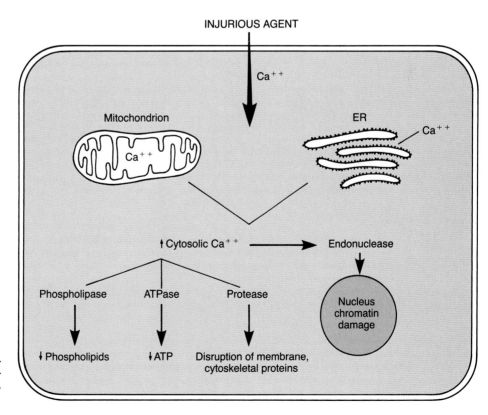

Figure 1–3. Sources and consequences of increased cytosolic calcium in cell injury. ER = endoplasmic reticulum.

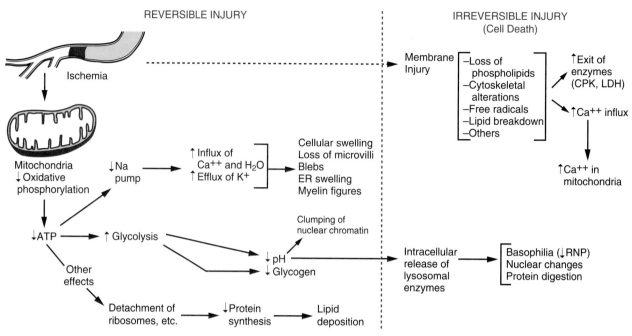

Figure 1-4. Postulated sequence of events in ischemic injury. Note that although reduced oxidative phosphorylation and ATP levels have a central role, ischemia can cause direct membrane damage.

(thereby hastening ATP depletion), and *endonucleases* (which are associated with chromatin fragmentation) (Fig. 1-3). Although it is clear that injured cells accumulate calcium and that calcium is a mediator of many of the events of cell injury, considerable controversy exists as to whether it is necessarily the proximate cause of irreversible cell injury.

- *ATP depletion.* Loss of mitochondrial pyridine nucleotides, and consequent ATP depletion, and decreased ATP synthesis are common consequences of both ischemic and toxic injury. High-energy phosphate in the form of ATP is required for many synthetic and degradative processes within the cell. These include membrane transport, protein synthesis, lipogenesis, and the deacylation-reacylation reactions necessary for phospholipid turnover. There is ample evidence that ATP depletion plays a role in the loss of the integrity of the plasma membrane that characterizes cell death.
- *Defects in membrane permeability.* Early loss of selective membrane permeability leading ultimately to overt membrane damage is a consistent feature of all forms of cell injury. Such defects may be the result of a series of events involving ATP depletion, and calcium modulated activation of phospholipases, as is discussed in detail later. The plasma membrane, however, can also be damaged directly by certain bacterial toxins, viral proteins, lytic complement components, products of cytolytic lymphocytes (perforins), and a number of physical and chemical agents.

Having briefly reviewed these general mechanisms, we now concentrate on three common forms of cell injury: (1) ischemic and hypoxic injury; (2) injury induced by free radicals, including activated oxygen species; and (3) some types of toxic injury.

ISCHEMIC AND HYPOXIC INJURY

Sequence of Events and Ultrastructural Changes

The sequence of morphologic and biochemical changes following acute hypoxic injury has been studied extensively in humans, in experimental animals, and in culture systems,[2-4] and reasonable schemes concerning the mechanisms underlying these changes have emerged (Fig. 1-4). A useful model for hypoxic injury has been occlusion of one of the main coronary arteries and examination of the cardiac muscle in the areas supplied by the artery.

REVERSIBLE CELL INJURY. *The first point of attack of hypoxia is the cell's aerobic respiration, that is, oxidative phosphorylation by mitochondria.*[5] As the oxygen tension within the cell decreases, there is loss of oxidative phosphorylation, and the generation of ATP slows down or stops. This loss of ATP—the energy source—has widespread effects on many systems within the cell. Heart muscle, for example, ceases to contract within 60 seconds of coronary occlusion. (Note, however, that noncontractility does not mean cell death.) The decrease in cellular ATP and associated increase in adenosine monophosphate (AMP) stimulate phosphofructokinase and phosphorylase activities. This results in an increased rate of *anaerobic glycolysis* designed to maintain the cell's energy sources by generating ATP from glycogen. Glycogen is thus rapidly depleted. ATP is also generated anaerobically from creatine phosphate, through the action of the enzyme *creatine kinase.* Glycolysis results in the accumulation of lactic acid and inorganic phosphates from the hydrolysis of phosphate esters. *This reduces the intracellular pH.* At this early period, there is also *early clumping of nuclear chromatin,* apparently caused by the reduced pH.

ATP depletion is primarily responsible for *acute cellular swelling* (cellular edema) (Fig. 1–5), one of the earliest events in ischemic injury. This is caused by an impairment of cell volume regulation by the plasma membrane. Recall that mammalian cells possess a high intracellular osmotic colloidal pressure, exerted by a greater intracellular than extracellular concentration of protein. To balance this, sodium is maintained at a lower intracellular than extracellular concentration by an energy-dependent sodium pump (ouabain-sensitive Na^+ K^+-ATPase), which also keeps the concentration of potassium significantly higher intracellularly than extracellularly. *Failure of this active transport, owing to diminished ATP concentration and enhanced ATPase activity, causes sodium to accumulate intracellularly with diffusion of potassium out of the cell.* The net gain of solute is accompanied by an isosmotic gain of water, cell swelling, and *dilation of the endoplasmic reticulum.* A second mechanism for cell swelling in ischemia is the increased intracellular osmotic load engendered by the accumulation of catabolites, such as inorganic phosphates, lactate, and purine nucleosides. In polarized epithelia, such as those in proximal tubules of the kidney, loss of polarity in the distribution of membrane enzymes occurs early during ischemia, accounting for early changes in transport by such cells.[6]

The next phenomenon to occur is *detachment of ribosomes from the granular endoplasmic reticulum* and *dissociation of polysomes into monosomes,* probably owing to disruption of the energy-dependent interactions between the membranes of the endoplasmic reticulum and its ribosomes. If hypoxia continues, other alterations take place and, again, are reflections of increased membrane permeability and diminished mitochondrial function. *Blebs* may form at the cell surface (Fig. 1–6; see Fig. 1–5), and cells that possess microvilli (e.g., proximal tubular epithelial cells) begin to lose their normal microvillous structure. "Myelin figures," derived from plasma as well as organellar

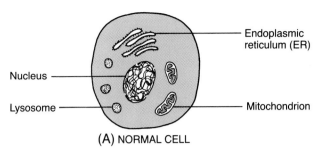

(A) NORMAL CELL

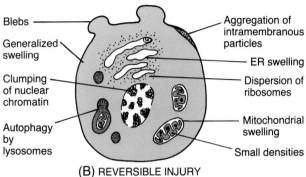

(B) REVERSIBLE INJURY

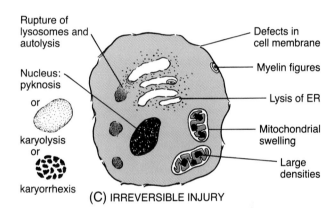

(C) IRREVERSIBLE INJURY

Figure 1–5. Schematic representation of a normal cell (A) and the ultrastructural changes in reversible (B) and irreversible (C) cell injury (see text).

membranes, may be seen within the cytoplasm or extracellularly. They are thought to result from dissociation of lipoproteins with unmasking of phosphatide groups, promoting the uptake and intercalation of water between the lamellar stacks of membranes. At this time, the mitochondria are usually swollen, owing to loss of volume control by these organelles; the endoplasmic reticulum remains dilated; and the entire cell is markedly swollen, with increased concentrations of water, sodium, and chloride and a decreased concentration of potassium. Up to a certain point, *all of these disturbances are reversible if oxygenation is restored.*

IRREVERSIBLE INJURY. If ischemia persists, irreversible injury ensues. As will be detailed later, *there is no universally accepted biochemical explanation for*

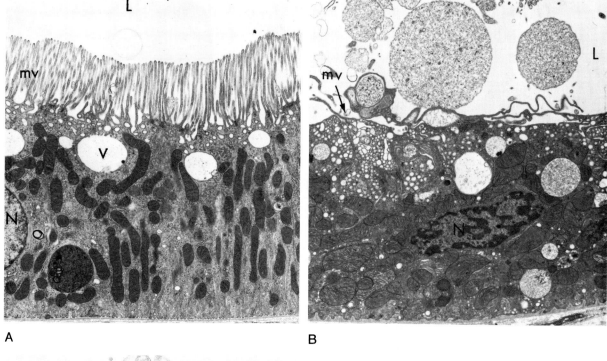

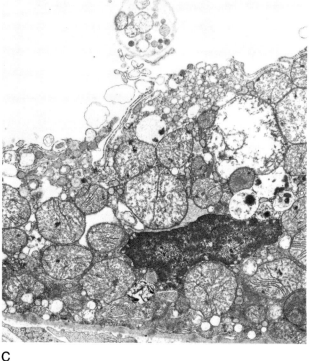

Figure 1–6. *A*, Electron micrograph of normal epithelial cell of proximal kidney tubule. Note abundant microvilli (mv) lining the lumen (L). N = nucleus; V = apical vacuoles (which are normal structures in this cell type). *B*, Epithelial cell of the proximal tubule showing reversible ischemic changes. The microvilli (mv) are lost and have been incorporated in apical cytoplasm; blebs have formed and are extruded in the lumen (L). Mitochondria are slightly dilated. (Compare with *A*.) *C*, Proximal tubular cell showing irreversible ischemic injury. Note the markedly swollen mitochondria containing amorphous densities, disrupted cell membranes, and dense pyknotic nucleus. (Courtesy of Dr. M.A. Venkatachalam.)

the transition from reversible injury to cell death. Irreversible injury, however, is associated morphologically with severe vacuolization of the mitochondria (see Figs. 1–5 and 1–6C) including their cristae, extensive damage to plasma membranes, and swelling of lysosomes. *Large, flocculent, amorphous densities develop in the mitochondrial matrix* (Fig. 1–6C). In the myocardium, these are indications of irreversible injury and can be seen as early as 30 to 40 minutes after ischemia. Massive influx

of calcium into the cell then occurs, particularly if the ischemic zone is reperfused. There is continued loss of proteins, enzymes, coenzymes, and ribonucleic acids from the hyperpermeable membranes. The cells may also leak metabolites, which are vital for the reconstitution of ATP, thus further depleting net intracellular high-energy phosphates.

At this stage, *injury to the lysosomal membranes occurs, followed by leakage of their enzymes into the cytoplasm and activation of their acid hy-*

drolases. Lysosomes contain RNAases, DNAases, proteases, phosphatases, glucosidases, and cathepsins. Activation of these enzymes leads to enzymatic digestion of cell components evidenced by loss of ribonucleoprotein, deoxyribonucleoprotein, and glycogen and the various *nuclear changes* described later. Although these changes have been traditionally ascribed to falling pH, more recent studies suggest that the early fall in pH is followed by a shift to neutral or even alkaline pH as irreversible injury proceeds. Indeed, acidosis protects against lethal injury in many models of ischemia and reperfusion, but the mechanisms are unclear.[7]

Following cell death, cell components are progressively degraded, and there is widespread leakage of cellular enzymes into the extracellular space and, conversely, entry of extracellular macromolecules from the interstitial space into the dying cells. Finally, the dead cell may become replaced by large masses composed of phospholipids in the form of myelin figures. These are then either phagocytosed by other cells or degraded further into fatty acids. *Calcification* of such fatty acid residues may occur with the formation of calcium soaps.

At this point in the story, we should note that leakage of intracellular enzymes across the abnormally permeable plasma membrane, and into the serum, provides important clinical parameters of cell death. Cardiac muscle, for example, contains glutamic-oxaloacetic transaminase (GOT), pyruvic transaminases, lactic dehydrogenase (LDH), and creatine kinase (CK). Elevated serum levels of such enzymes, and particularly the isoenzymes specific for heart muscle (e.g., CK-MB), are valuable clinical criteria of myocardial infarction, a locus of cell death in heart muscle.

Mechanisms of Irreversible Injury

The sequence of events for hypoxia was described as a continuum from its initiation to the ultimate digestion of the lethally injured cell by lysosomal enzymes. But at what stage did the cell actually die? And what is the critical biochemical event responsible for the "point of no return"? The duration of hypoxia necessary to induce irreversible cell injury varies considerably according to the cell type and the nutritional and hormonal status of the animal. In the liver, between 1 and 2 hours of ischemia are required to produce irreversible damage to liver cells. In the brain, neurons suffer irreversible damage after 3 to 5 minutes. The state of nutrition of the cell is also important. Liver cells of rats fed a normal diet contain abundant glycogen and have a higher potential for survival after ischemia than do the liver cells of starved rats.

What then are the critical events for lethal hypoxic injury? Two phenomena consistently characterize irreversibility. The first is the *inability to reverse mitochondrial dysfunction* on reperfusion or reoxygenation leading to ATP depletion, and the second is the development of *profound disturbances in membrane function.*

ATP depletion clearly contributes to the functional and structural consequences of ischemia, as described earlier (see Fig. 1–3). Indeed, infusion of ATP-rich solutions protects against ischemic injury in some experimental models.[8] In the myocardium, the marked depletion of ATP is closely related to the development of lethal injury. However, it has been possible experimentally to dissociate ATP depletion from the inevitability of cell death. It is now thought that the role of ATP depletion in irreversibility is its contribution to the second critical event in ischemia—cell membrane damage.

A great deal of evidence indicates that cell membrane damage is a central factor in the pathogenesis of irreversible cell injury. Loss of volume regulation, increased permeability to extracellular molecules, and demonstrable plasma membrane ultrastructural defects occur in the earliest stages of irreversible injury.

Several biochemical mechanisms may contribute to such membrane damage (Fig. 1–7).[4,9]

1. *Progressive loss of phospholipids.* In some ischemic tissues (e.g., liver), irreversible ischemic injury is associated with a marked decrease in the content of membrane phospholipids.[10] Normally the turnover of membrane phospholipids is coupled to their resynthesis. Degradation of membrane phospholipids involves the action of endogenous *phospholipases (PLA$_2$),* whose activation is calcium dependent. One explanation for phospholipid loss is increased phospholipid degradation due to activation of endogenous phospholipases (see Fig. 1–7). Increased cytosolic calcium concentration induced by ischemia, as well as Ca^{++}-independent factors, contributes to such phospholipase activation. Progressive phospholipid loss can also occur owing to *decreased reacylation* or *de novo synthesis* of phospholipids because these reactions involve ATP-dependent steps as well as appropriate substrate availability (see Fig. 1–7).[11]

2. *Cytoskeletal abnormalities.* Cytoskeletal filaments serve as anchors connecting the plasma membranes to the cell interior. Activation of proteases by increased cytosolic calcium may cause damage to the cytoskeleton. In the presence of cell swelling, this damage results in detachment of the cell membrane from the cytoskeleton, rendering the membrane susceptible to stretching and rupture. This has been postulated as a mechanism for membrane damage in ischemic myocardium, and indeed there is evidence of increased degradation of the intermediate filament protein *vinculin* in ischemic hearts.[12]

3. *Reactive oxygen species.* As is discussed in detail later, partially reduced oxygen free radicals are highly toxic molecules that cause injury to cell

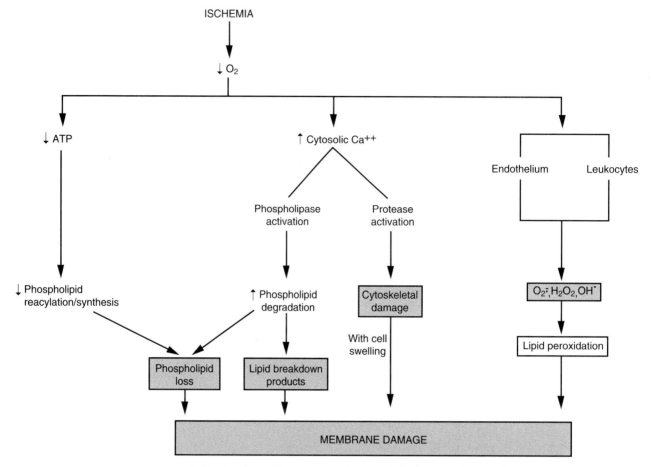

Figure 1–7. Mechanisms of membrane damage in ischemia. *(See text.)*

membranes and other cell constituents. Such free radicals are present at very low levels in myocardium during ischemia, but there is an increase in free radical production *on restoration of blood flow.* Reperfusion results in a paradoxic effect: an *increase* in damage called *reperfusion injury.* This injury can be reduced by antioxidants in some models of ischemia. Although reactive oxygen species in postischemic tissue can be derived from incomplete reduction of oxygen by mitochondria and production of superoxide ion by xanthine oxidase (from vascular endothelium), it is thought that most toxic oxygen species are *produced by polymorphonuclear leukocytes that infiltrate the site of ischemia during reperfusion.*[13] It must be emphasized that if reperfusion does not occur, lethal ischemic cell injury still eventually ensues, but toxic oxygen species are probably not involved under these conditions.

4. *Lipid breakdown products.* These include unesterified free fatty acids, acyl carnitine, and lysophospholipids, catabolic products that are known to accumulate in ischemic cells as a result of phospholipid degradation. They have a detergent effect on membranes. They also either insert into the lipid bilayer of the membrane or exchange with membrane phospholipids, potentially causing

changes in permeability and electrophysiologic alterations.

5. *Loss of intracellular amino acids.* Addition of certain amino acids, principally glycine and L-alanine, protects hypoxic cells from irreversible membrane damage *in vitro,* suggesting that loss of such amino acids—which occurs in hypoxia—predisposes to membrane structural injury.[15] The mechanisms of protection by glycine are, however, unclear.

Whatever the mechanism(s) of membrane injury, the resultant loss of membrane integrity causes further influx of calcium from the extracellular space. When, in addition, the ischemic tissue is reperfused to some extent, as may occur *in vivo,* the scene is set for massive influx of calcium. Calcium is taken up avidly by mitochondria after reoxygenation and permanently poisons them, inhibits cellular enzymes, denatures proteins, and causes the cytologic alterations characteristic of coagulative necrosis.[16]

It is evident that the molecular events that determine irreversible cell damage are complex. Indeed, it is likely that several mechanisms, acting at more than one locus, underlie cell death. *For now it must suffice to say that hypoxia affects oxi-*

dative phosphorylation and hence the synthesis of vital ATP supplies, that membrane damage is critical to the development of lethal cell injury, and that calcium is an important mediator of the biochemical and morphologic alterations leading to cell death.

FREE RADICAL–INDUCED CELL INJURY

One important mechanism of membrane damage, already alluded to in the discussion of reperfusion injury, is injury induced by free radicals, particularly by activated oxygen species. It is a final common pathway of cell injury in such varied processes as chemical and radiation injury, oxygen and other gaseous toxicity, cellular aging, microbial killing by phagocytic cells, inflammatory damage, tumor destruction by macrophages, and others (see Fig. 1–2).[17, 18]

Free radicals are chemical species that have a single unpaired electron in an outer orbital. In such a state, the radical is extremely reactive and unstable and enters into reactions with inorganic or organic chemicals—proteins, lipids, carbohydrates—particularly with key molecules in membranes and nucleic acids. Moreover, free radicals initiate autocatalytic reactions whereby molecules with which they react are themselves converted into free radicals to propagate the chain of damage.

Free radicals may be *initiated* within cells (1) by the absorption of radiant energy (e.g., ultraviolet light, x-rays); (2) by endogenous, usually oxidative, reactions that occur during normal metabolic processes; or (3) by enzymic metabolism of exogenous chemicals or drugs (e.g., $CCl_3^{\bullet}$, a product of CCl_4). An unpaired electron can be associated with almost any atom, but oxygen, carbon and nitrogen-centered free radicals are of greatest biologic relevance.

As should be well known, *oxygen* normally undergoes a four-electron reduction to H_2O, catalyzed by cytochrome oxidase. The presence of intracellular oxygen, however, also allows the inadvertent production of partially reduced toxic intermediate oxygen species. The three most important such species are *superoxide* $(O_2^{\bullet-})$, *hydrogen peroxide* (H_2O_2), and *hydroxyl ions* $(OH^{\bullet})$. These can be produced by the activity of a variety of oxidative enzymes, in different sites of the cell—cytosol, mitochondria, lysosomes, peroxisomes, and plasma membrane (Fig. 1–8).

Superoxide is generated either directly during auto-oxidation in mitochondria or enzymatically by cytoplasmic enzymes, such as xanthine oxidase, cytochrome P-450, and other oxidases.

$$O_2 \xrightarrow{\text{oxidase}} O_2^{\bullet-}$$

Once produced, $O_2^{\bullet-}$ can be inactivated either spontaneously or, more rapidly, by the enzyme superoxide dismutase (SOD), forming H_2O_2.

$$O_2^{\bullet-} + O_2^{\bullet-} + 2H^+ \xrightarrow{\text{SOD}} H_2O_2 + O_2$$

Hydrogen peroxide is produced either by the dismutation of $O_2^{\bullet-}$ as just explained or directly by oxidases present in peroxisomes—the catalase-containing organelles present in many organs (see Fig. 1–8).

Hydroxyl radicals are generated (1) by the hydrolysis of water caused by *ionizing radiation*

$$H_2O \longrightarrow H^{\bullet} + OH^{\bullet}$$

or (2) by interaction with transitional metals (e.g., iron, copper) in the Fenton reaction

$$Fe^{++} + H_2O_2 \longrightarrow Fe^{+++} + OH^{\bullet} + OH^-$$

or (3) through the Haber-Weiss reaction:

$$H_2O_2 + O_2^{\bullet-} \longrightarrow OH^{\bullet} + OH^- + O_2$$

Iron is particularly important in toxic oxygen injury. Most of free iron is in the ferric (Fe^{+++}) form and has to be reduced to the ferrous (Fe^{++}) form to be active in the Fenton reaction. This reduction can be enhanced by superoxide, *and thus sources of iron and superoxide are required for maximal oxidative cell damage.*

An example of *carbon*-centered free radical reaction is the enzymic induced conversion of carbon tetrachloride, leading to a toxic radical:

$$CCl_4 + \bar{e} \longrightarrow CCl_3^{\bullet} + Cl^-$$

Nitric oxide (NO), an important chemical mediator, described in Chapter 3, can act as a free radical and can also be converted to highly reactive peroxynitrite anion $(ONOO^-)$ as well as $NO_2^{\bullet}$ and NO_3^-.

$$NO^{\bullet} + O_2^{\bullet-} \longrightarrow ONOO^- + H^+$$

$$\Updownarrow$$

$$OH^{\bullet} + NO_2^{\bullet} \rightleftharpoons ONOOH \longrightarrow NO_3^-$$

The effects of these reactive species are wide-ranging, but four reactions are particularly relevant to cell injury.

1. *Lipid peroxidation of membranes.* Free radicals in the presence of oxygen may cause peroxidation of lipids within plasma and organellar membranes. Unsaturated fatty acids of membrane lipids possess double bonds between some of the carbon atoms. Such bonds are vulnerable to attack by oxy-

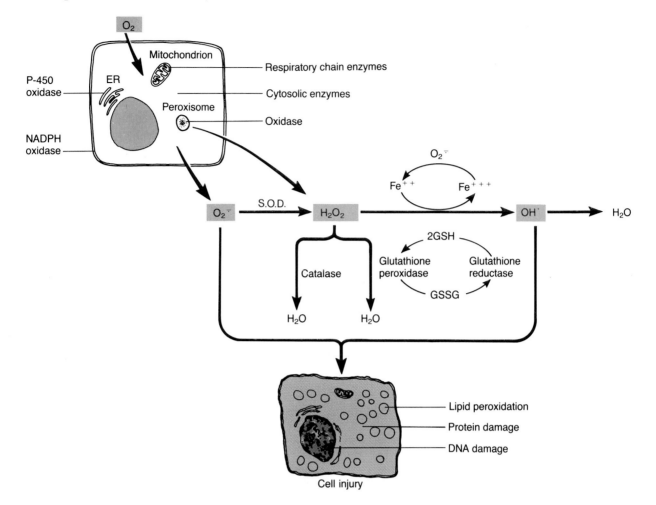

Figure 1–8. Formation of reactive oxygen species and antioxidant mechanisms in biologic systems. O_2 is converted to superoxide (O_2^-) by oxidative enzymes in the ER, mitochondria, plasma membrane, peroxisomes, and cytosol. O_2^- is converted to H_2O_2 by dismutation and thence to $OH^•$ by the Cu^{++}/Fe^{++} catalyzed Fenton reaction. H_2O_2 is also derived directly from oxidases in peroxisomes. Not shown is another potentially injurious radical, singlet oxygen. Resultant free radical damage to lipid (peroxidation), proteins, and DNA leads to various forms of cell injury. Note that superoxide catalyzes the reduction of Fe^{+++} to Fe^{++}, thus enhancing $OH^•$ generation by the Fenton reaction. The major antioxidant enzymes are SOD, catalase, and glutathione peroxidase.

gen-derived free radicals, particularly by $OH^•$.[19] The lipid-radical interactions yield peroxides, which are themselves reactive species, initiating the subsequent reduction of another fatty acid. An autocatalytic chain reaction ensues (called *propagation*), resulting in extensive membrane, organellar, and cellular damage.

   2. *Oxidative modification of proteins.* Free radicals promote sulfhydryl mediated cross-linking of such labile amino acids as methionine, histidine, cystine, and lysine as well as cause fragmentation of polypeptide chains. Oxidative modification enhances degradation of critical enzymes by cytosolic neutral proteases,[20] raising havoc throughout the cell.

   3. *Lesions in deoxyribonucleic acid (DNA).* Reactions with thymine in DNA produce single-strand breaks in DNA, and such DNA damage has been implicated both in cell killing and in eventual ma-

lignant transformation of cells. Mitochondrial DNA is also affected.

   Once free radicals are formed, how does the body get rid of them? They may spontaneously decay. Superoxide, for example, is unstable and decays spontaneously into oxygen and hydrogen peroxide. There are, however, several nonenzymatic and enzymatic systems that contribute to *termination* or inactivation of free radical reactions. These include the following:

- Endogenous or exogenous *antioxidants*, which either block the initiation of free radical formation or inactivate (e.g., scavenge) free radicals. Examples are *vitamin E; sulfhydryl-containing compounds, such as cysteine and glutathione; and serum proteins, such as albumin, ceruloplasmin, and transferrin.* Transferrin is thought to act as an antioxidant by binding free iron, which, as we have seen, can catalyze free radical formation.

- *Enzymes.* These include the following:

  - *Superoxide dismutase,* which converts superoxide to H_2O_2.
  - *Catalase,* present in peroxisomes, which decomposes H_2O_2

$$2 H_2O_2 \longrightarrow O_2 + 2 H_2O$$

  - *Glutathione peroxidase,* which catalyzes the ability of reduced glutathione (GSH) to release hydrogen from $-SH$ to a hydroxyl radical or to H_2O_2.

$$2 OH^\bullet + 2GSH \longrightarrow 2 H_2O + GSSG$$

or

$$H_2O_2 + 2GSH \longrightarrow 2 H_2O + GSSG$$

In many pathologic processes, the final effects induced by free radicals depend on the net balance between free radical formation and termination. As stated earlier, free radicals are now thought to be involved in many pathologic and physiologic processes, to be reviewed throughout this book. We now discuss certain forms of chemical injury because the toxicity of several chemicals and drugs can be attributed either to conversion of these chemicals to free radicals or to the formation of oxygen-derived metabolites.

Chemical Injury

Chemicals induce cell injury by one of two general mechanisms:

- Some chemicals, mostly water-soluble chemicals, can act *directly* by combining with some critical molecular component or cellular organelle. For example, in *mercuric chloride poisoning,* mercury binds to the sulfhydryl groups of the cell membrane and other proteins, causing increased membrane permeability and inhibition of ATP-ase-dependent transport. In such instances, the greatest damage is usually to the cells that use, absorb, excrete, or concentrate the chemicals—in the case of mercuric chloride, the cells of the gastrointestinal tract and kidney. *Cyanide* directly poisons mitochondrial enzymes. Many antineoplastic chemotherapeutic agents and antibiotic drugs also induce cell damage by direct cytotoxic effects.
- Most other chemicals, particularly lipid-soluble toxins, are not biologically active but must be converted to reactive toxic metabolites, which then act on target cells. Although these metabolites might cause membrane damage and cell in-

jury by *direct covalent binding* to membrane protein and lipids, by far the most important mechanism of membrane injury involves the formation of *reactive free radicals* and subsequent lipid peroxidation.[21]

One enzyme system that is critical in the metabolism of toxins is the *P-450 mixed function oxidase* in the endoplasmic reticulum of the liver and other organs. This enzyme is involved in the pathogenesis of two well-characterized models of chemical injury in the liver: carbon tetrachloride and acetaminophen.

Carbon tetrachloride (CCl_4) is used widely in the dry-cleaning industry. The toxic effect of CCl_4 is due to its conversion by P-450 to the *highly reactive toxic free radical* $CCl_3^\bullet$ ($CCl_4 + e \longrightarrow CCl_3^\bullet + Cl^-$). The $CCl_3^\bullet$ initiates lipid peroxidation, as has been described for hydroxyl radicals. The free radicals produced locally cause auto-oxidation of the polyenic fatty acids present within the membrane phospholipids. There, oxidative decomposition of the lipid is initiated, and organic peroxides are formed after reacting with oxygen (lipid peroxidation). This *reaction is autocatalytic* in that new radicals are formed from the peroxide radicals themselves. Thus, rapid breakdown of the struc-

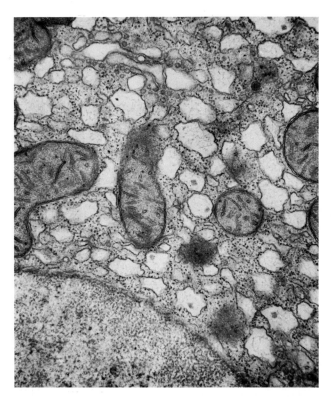

Figure 1-9. Rat liver cell 4 hours after carbon tetrachloride intoxication; with swelling of endoplasmic reticulum and shedding of ribosomes. At this stage, mitochondria are unaltered. (Courtesy of Dr. O. Iseri.)

CCl₄ in liver cells

↓ SER

CCl₃

↓ Microsomal polyenoic fatty acid

Lipid radicals

↓ + O₂

LIPID PEROXIDATION

Autocatalytic
spread
along microsomal
membrane

Membrane damage to RER   Release of products of
                                lipid peroxidation

↓   ↓

Polysome detachment   Damage to plasma membrane

↓   ↓

                                ↑ Permeability to Na⁺, H₂O, Ca⁺⁺

↓   ↓

↓ Lipid acceptor   Cell swelling
protein synthesis

↓   ↓

                                Massive influx of Ca⁺⁺

↓   ↓

Fatty liver   Inactivation of mitochondria,
                                cell enzymes, and denaturation
                                of proteins

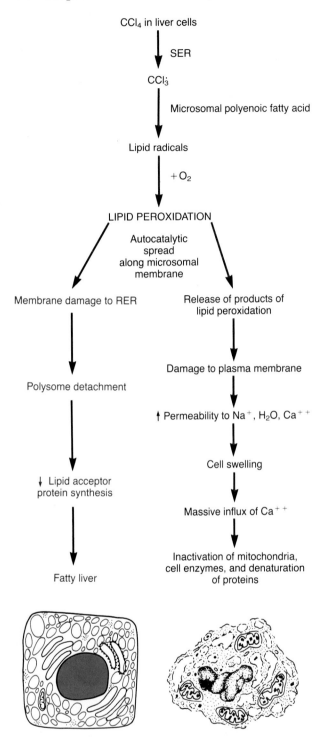

Figure 1–10. Sequence of events leading to fatty change and cell necrosis in CCl₄ toxicity. RER = rough endoplasmic reticulum; SER = smooth endoplasmic reticulum.

ture and function of the endoplasmic reticulum is due to decomposition of the lipid. *It is no surprise, therefore, that CCl₄-induced liver cell injury is both severe and extremely rapid in onset.* Within less than 30 minutes, there is a decline in hepatic protein synthesis and within 2 hours, swelling of

smooth endoplasmic reticulum (SER) and dissociation of ribosomes from the rough endoplasmic reticulum (RER) (Fig. 1–9). Accumulation of lipid then ensues, owing to the inability of cells to synthesize lipoprotein from triglycerides and "lipid acceptor protein." This leads to the fatty liver (described later) of CCl₄ poisoning. Mitochondrial injury then occurs, and this is followed by progressive swelling of the cells owing to increased permeability of the plasma membrane. Plasma membrane damage is thought to be caused by relatively stable fatty aldehydes, which are produced by lipid peroxidation in the SER but are able to act at distant sites. This is followed by massive influx of calcium and cell death (Fig. 1–10).

Acetaminophen (Tylenol), a commonly used analgesic drug, is detoxified in the liver through sulfation and glucuronidation, and small amounts are converted by cytochrome P-450–catalyzed oxidation to an electrophilic, highly toxic metabolite. This metabolite itself is detoxified by interaction with reduced glutathione (GSH). When large doses of the drug are ingested, GSH is depleted, and thus the toxic metabolites accumulate in the cell, destroy nucleophilic macromolecules, and covalently bind (arylate) proteins and nucleic acids. The decrease in GSH concentration, coupled with covalent binding of toxic metabolites, increases drug toxicity, resulting in massive liver cell necrosis, usually 3 to 5 days after the ingestion of toxic doses. This hepatotoxicity correlates with lipid peroxidation and can be reduced by administration of antioxidants, suggesting that the oxidative damage may be more important than covalent binding in the ultimate toxicity of the drug.[22]

MORPHOLOGY OF REVERSIBLE CELL INJURY AND NECROSIS

Reversible Injury

In classic pathology, the morphologic changes resulting from nonlethal injury to cells were termed degenerations, but today they are more simply designated *reversible injuries.* Two patterns can be recognized under the light microscope: *cellular swelling* and *fatty change.* Cellular swelling appears whenever cells are incapable of maintaining ionic and fluid homeostasis; its pathogenesis has been described earlier. *Fatty change* may be another indicator of reversible cell injury. It is manifested by the appearance of small or large lipid vacuoles in the cytoplasm and occurs in hypoxic and various forms of toxic injury. It is principally encountered in cells involved in and dependent on fat metabolism, such as the hepatocyte and myocardial cell. Fatty change in the liver can also be a manifestation of metabolic derangements and is described later in this chapter as a form of intracellular accumulation.

> **MORPHOLOGY. Cellular swelling** is the first manifestation of almost all forms of injury to cells: It is a difficult morphologic change to appreciate with the light microscope; it may be more apparent at the level of the whole organ. When it affects all cells in an organ, it causes some pallor, increased turgor, and increase in weight of the organ. Microscopically, enlargement of cells is most often discernible by compression of the microvasculature of the organ as, for example, the hepatic sinusoids and the capillary network within the renal cortex.
>
> If water continues to accumulate within cells, small clear vacuoles appear within the cytoplasm. These vacuoles represent distended and pinched-off or sequestered segments of the endoplasmic reticulum. This pattern of nonlethal injury is sometimes called **"hydropic change"** or **"vacuolar degeneration."** Swelling of cells is reversible.
>
> The ultrastructural changes of reversible cell injury previously described (see Figs. 1–5 and 1–6) include (1) **plasma membrane alterations,** such as blebbing, blunting, and distortion of microvilli; creation of myelin figures; and loosening of intercellular attachments; (2) **mitochondrial changes,** including swelling, rarefaction, and the appearance of small phospholipid-rich amorphous densities; (3) **dilatation of the endoplasmic reticulum** with detachment and disaggregation of polysomes; and (4) **nucleolar** alterations, with disaggregation of granular and fibrillar elements.

Necrosis

Necrosis, one of the two morphologic expressions of cell death (the second being apoptosis), refers to a spectrum of morphologic changes that follow cell death in living tissue, largely resulting from the progressive degradative action of enzymes on the lethally injured cell.[23] Cells placed immediately in fixative are dead but not necrotic. Two essentially concurrent processes bring about the changes of necrosis: (1) enzymic digestion of the cell and (2) denaturation of proteins. The catalytic enzymes are derived either from the lysosomes of the dead cells, in which case the enzymic digestion is referred to as *autolysis,* or from the lysosomes of immigrant leukocytes, termed *heterolysis.* Depending on whether denaturation of proteins or enzymic digestion is ascendant, one of two patterns of cell necrosis develops. In the former instance, *coagulative necrosis* develops. In the latter, progressive catalysis of cell structures leads to so-called *liquefactive necrosis.* Both of these processes require hours to develop, and so there would be no

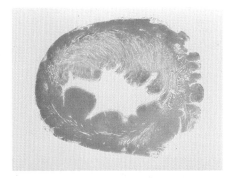
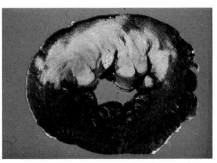

Figure 1–11. Histologic section of heart stained with H&E *(top)* and gross section *(bottom)* stained with a chemical reaction for lactic dehydrogenase (the triphenyltetrazolium chloride (TTC) reaction), 6 hours after coronary occlusion. The histologic section shows only edema between myocardial fibers, but the enzyme stain shows clear-cut loss of enzyme—which stains red in the TTC reaction—from the area of infarction. (Courtesy of Dr. Michael Fishbein.)

detectable changes in cells if, for example, a myocardial infarct caused sudden death. The only telling evidence might be occlusion of a coronary artery. The earliest histologic evidence of myocardial necrosis does not become manifest until 8 to 12 hours later, but loss of enzymes (e.g., LDH) from necrotic muscle can be detected grossly or microscopically by 4 to 6 hours (Fig. 1–11).

> **MORPHOLOGY.** The necrotic cells show increased eosinophilia, attributable in part to loss of the normal basophilia imparted by the RNA in the cytoplasm and in part to the increased binding of eosin to denatured intracytoplasmic proteins (Fig. 1–12). The cell may have a more glassy homogeneous appearance than that of normal cells, mainly as a result of the loss of glycogen particles. When enzymes have digested the cytoplasmic organelles, the cytoplasm becomes vacuolated and appears moth-eaten. Finally, calcification of the dead cells may occur. By electron microscopy, necrotic cells are characterized by overt discontinuities in plasma and organelle membranes, marked dilation of mitochondria with the appearance of large amorphous densities, intracytoplasmic myelin figures, amorphous osmiophilic debris, and aggregates of

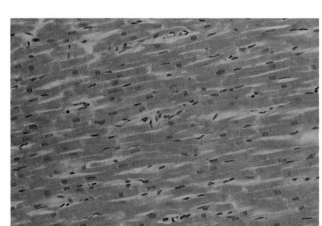
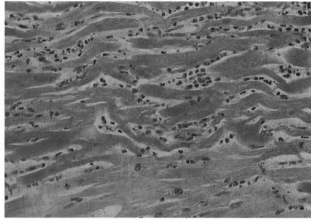

A   B

Figure 1–12. *A,* Normal myocardium. *B,* Myocardium with coagulation necrosis (upper two-thirds of figure), showing strongly eosinophilic anucleate myocardial fibers. Leukocytes in the interstitium are an early reaction to necrotic muscle. Compare with *A* and with normal fibers in the lower part of the figure.

fluffy material probably representing denatured protein (see Fig. 1–6C).

Nuclear changes appear in the form of one of three patterns (see Fig. 1–5C). The basophilia of the chromatin may fade **(karyolysis),** a change that presumably reflects DNAse activity. A second pattern is **pyknosis,** characterized by nuclear shrinkage and increased basophilia. Here the DNA apparently condenses into a solid, shrunken basophilic mass. In the third pattern, known as **karyorrhexis,** the pyknotic or partially pyknotic nucleus undergoes fragmentation. With the passage of time (a day or two), the nucleus in the necrotic cell totally disappears.

Once the necrotic cells have undergone the early alterations described above the mass of necrotic cells may have several morphologic patterns: **coagulative necrosis, liquefactive necrosis,** or, in special circumstances, **caseous necrosis and fat necrosis.**

Coagulative necrosis implies preservation of the basic outline of the coagulated cell for a span of at least some days. Presumably, the injury or the subsequent increasing intracellular acidosis denatures not only structural proteins but also enzymic proteins and so blocks the proteolysis of the cell. **The process of coagulative necrosis is characteristic of hypoxic death of cells in all tissues save the brain.** The myocardial infarct is a prime example, characterized by coagulated, anucleate cells (see Fig. 1–12). Ultimately, the necrotic myocardial cells are removed by fragmentation and phagocytosis of the cellular debris by scavenger white cells and by the action of proteolytic lysosomal enzymes brought in by the immigrant white cells.

Liquefactive necrosis resulting from autolysis or heterolysis is mainly characteristic of focal bacterial infections because bacteria constitute powerful stimuli to the accumulation of white cells (Fig. 1–

13). For obscure reasons, hypoxic death of cells within the central nervous system often evokes liquefactive necrosis. Although **gangrenous necrosis** in reality does not represent a distinctive pattern of cell death, the term is still commonly used in surgical clinical practice. It is usually applied to a limb, generally the lower leg, which has lost its blood supply and has undergone coagulation necrosis. When bacterial infection is superimposed, coagulative necrosis is modified by the liquefactive action of the bacteria and the attracted leukocytes (so-called wet gangrene).

Caseous necrosis, a distinctive form of coagulative necrosis, is encountered most often in foci of tuberculous infection. The term "caseous" is derived from the gross appearance (white and cheesy) of the area of necrosis (Fig. 1–14). Histologically, the necrotic focus appears as amorphous granular debris seemingly composed of frag-

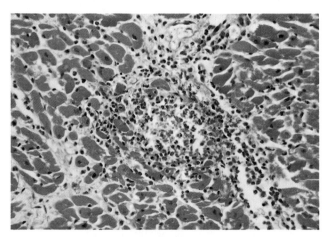

Figure 1–13. Liquefaction necrosis of a focus in the myocardium caused by fungal infection. The focus is filled with white cells, creating a myocardial abscess.

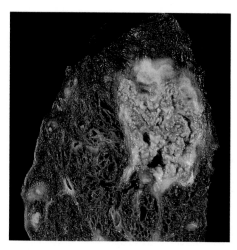

Figure 1–14. A tuberculous lung with large area of caseous necrosis. The caseous debris is yellow-white and cheesy.

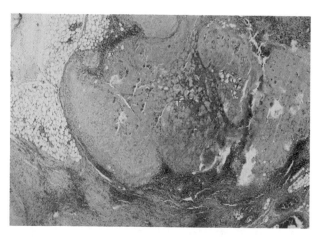

Figure 1–15. A circumscribed focus of enzymatic necrosis of fat. Normal fat is seen in the upper left corner. The necrotic area shows shadowy outlines of fat cells surrounded by a zone of inflammation (blue).

mented, coagulated cells enclosed within a distinctive inflammatory border known as a granulomatous reaction (see Chapter 3). It is important to be able to recognize this morphologic pattern because it is evoked by only a limited number of agents. Among these, tuberculosis is pre-eminent, as discussed in greater detail in Chapter 8.

Enzymic fat necrosis is a term that is well fixed in medical parlance but does not in reality denote a specific pattern of necrosis. Rather, it is descriptive of **focal areas of destruction of fat resulting from abnormal release of activated pancreatic lipases into the substance of the pancreas and the peritoneal cavity.** This occurs in the uncommon but calamitous abdominal emergency known as "acute pancreatic necrosis." In this condition, discussed more completely in Chapter 19, activated pancreatic enzymes escape from acinar cells and ducts; the activated enzymes liquefy fat cell membranes, and the activated lipases split the triglyceride esters contained within fat cells. The released fatty acids combine with calcium to produce grossly visible chalky white areas, which enable the surgeon and the pathologist to identify this disease on inspection of involved fat depots. Histologically, the necrosis takes the form of foci of shadowy outlines of necrotic fat cells, with basophilic calcium deposits, surrounded by an inflammatory reaction (Fig. 1–15).

Ultimately, in the living patient, most necrotic cells and their debris disappear by a combined process of enzymic digestion and fragmentation, with phagocytosis of the particulate debris by leukocytes. If necrotic cells and cellular debris are not promptly destroyed and reabsorbed, they tend to attract calcium salts and other minerals and to become calcified. This phenomenon, so-called *dystrophic calcification*, is considered later.

APOPTOSIS

This morphologic pattern of cell death has long been recognized by pathologists, but only recently has it been appreciated as a distinctive and important mode of cell injury, which should be differentiated from the common coagulative necrosis (Fig. 1–16 and Table 1–2). Its designation as apoptosis, introduced in 1972 (from the Greek for "falling off"),[24] survived more than 15 years of dormancy, and today it is one of the most vigorously investigated processes in biology.[25-27]

Apoptosis is thought to be responsible for numerous physiologic and pathologic events including the following:[25]

- *The programmed destruction of cells during embryogenesis* (including implantation, organogenesis, developmental involution) and *metamorphosis*. Although apoptosis is a morphologic event, which may not always underlie the functionally defined "programmed cell death" of embryogenesis, the terms are currently used synonymously by most workers.
- *Hormone-dependent involution in the adult,* such as endometrial cell breakdown during the menstrual cycle, ovarian follicular atresia in the menopause, and the regression of the lactating breast after weaning.
- *Cell deletion in proliferating cell populations,* such as intestinal crypt epithelia.
- *Cell death in tumors,* most frequently during regression but also in tumors with active cell growth.
- *Death of immune cells,* both B and T lymphocytes after cytokine depletion, as well as deletion of autoreactive T cells in the developing thymus.[28] (See Chapter 6.)
- *Pathologic atrophy of hormone-dependent tissues,*

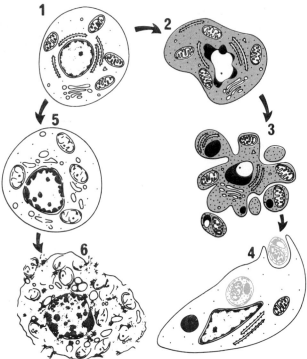

Figure 1–16. Diagram illustrating the sequential ultrastructural changes in apoptosis *(right)* and necrosis *(left)*. A normal cell is shown at 1. The onset of apoptosis (2) is heralded by compaction and segregation of chromatin against the nuclear envelope and condensation of the cytoplasm. Rapid progression of the process (3) is associated with nuclear fragmentation and marked convolution of the cellular surface with the development of protuberances. The latter then separate to produce membrane-bound apoptotic bodies, which are phagocytosed and digested by adjacent cells (4). Signs of necrosis include (5) clumping of chromatin into ill-defined masses, gross swelling of organelles, the appearance of flocculent densities in the matrix of mitochondria, and later (6) membrane damage. (With permission from Kerr, J.F.R., and Harmon, B.V.: Definition and incidence of apoptosis: A historical perspective. *In* Tomei, L.D., and Cope, F.O. (eds.): Apoptosis: The Molecular Basis of Cell Death. Cold Spring Harbor, NY, Cold Spring Harbor Laboratory Press, 1991, p.7.)

Table 1–2. FEATURES OF NECROSIS VERSUS APOPTOSIS

	NECROSIS	APOPTOSIS
Stimuli	Hypoxia, toxins	Physiologic and pathologic
Histology	Cellular swelling Coagulation necrosis Disruption of organelles	Single cells Chromatin condensation Apoptotic bodies
DNA breakdown Mechanisms	Random, diffuse ATP depletion Membrane injury Free radical damage	Internucleosomal Gene activation Endonuclease
Tissue reaction	Inflammation	No inflammation Phagocytosis of apoptotic bodies

MORPHOLOGY. The following morphologic features, best seen with the electron microscope, characterize cells undergoing apoptosis:[29]

1. ***Cell shrinkage.*** The cell is smaller in size; the cytoplasm is dense; and the organelles, although relatively normal, are more tightly packed.

2. ***Chromatin condensation.*** This is the most characteristic feature of apoptosis. The chromatin aggregates peripherally, under the nuclear membrane, into well-delimited dense masses of various shapes and sizes (Fig. 1–17). The nucleus itself may break up, producing two or more fragments.

3. ***Formation of cytoplasmic blebs and apoptotic bodies.*** The apoptotic cell first shows extensive surface blebbing, then undergoes fragmentation into a number of membrane-bound **apoptotic bodies** composed of cytoplasm and tightly packed organelles, with or without a nuclear fragment.

4. ***Phagocytosis of apoptotic cells or bodies*** by adjacent healthy cells, either parenchymal cells or macrophages. The apoptotic bodies are rapidly degraded within lysosomes, and the adjacent cells migrate or proliferate to replace the space occupied by the now deleted apoptotic cell.

Histologically, in tissues stained with hematoxylin and eosin, apoptosis involves single cells or small clusters of cells. The apoptotic cell appears as a round or oval mass of intensely eosinophilic cytoplasm with dense nuclear chromatin fragments (Fig. 1–18). Because the cell shrinkage and formation of apoptotic bodies are rapid, however, and the fragments are quickly phagocytosed, degraded, or extruded into the lumen, **considerable apoptosis may occur in tissues before it becomes apparent in histologic sections.** In addition, **apoptosis—in contrast to necrosis—does not**

such as prostatic atrophy after castration and loss of lymphocytes in the thymus after glucocorticoid administration.

• *Pathologic atrophy in parenchymal organs after duct obstruction,* such as occurs in the pancreas, parotid gland, and kidney.

• *Cell death induced by cytotoxic T cells,* such as in cellular immune rejection and graft-versus-host disease.

• *Cell injury in certain viral diseases,* as for example in viral hepatitis, in which apoptotic cell fragments in the liver are known as Councilman bodies.

• *Cell death produced by a variety of injurious stimuli* that are capable of producing necrosis, but when given in low doses—including mild thermal injury, radiation, cytotoxic anticancer drugs, and possibly hypoxia—induce apoptosis.

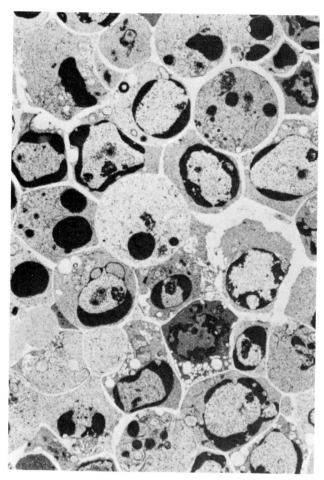

Figure 1-17. Apoptotic bodies in lymphoma cells. Some nuclear fragments show peripheral crescents of compacted chromatin, whereas others are uniformly dense. (With permission from Kerr, J.F.R., and Harmon B.V.: Definition and incidence of apoptosis: A historical perspective. *In* Tomei, L.D., and Cope, F.O. (eds.): Apoptosis: The Molecular Basis of Cell Death. Cold Spring Harbor, NY, Cold Spring Harbor Laboratory Press, 1991, pp. 5-29.)

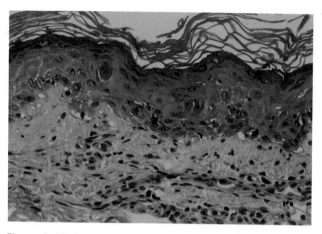

Figure 1-18. Apoptosis in the skin in an immune-mediated reaction. The apoptotic cells are visible in the epidermis with intensely eosinophilic cytoplasm and small, dense nuclei. H&E stain. (Courtesy of Dr. Scott Granter.)

elicit inflammation, making it even more difficult to detect histologically.

MECHANISMS

In examining the diverse conditions in which apoptosis occurs, it is clear that apoptosis can be triggered by the addition or withdrawal of hormones or other trophic factors and that there is a coordinated but often inverse relationship between cell growth and apoptosis. Indeed, as we shall see in the discussion of cell growth (see Chapter 2) and neoplasia (see Chapter 7), apoptosis is important in the regulation of normal cell population density,[30] and suppression of cell death by apoptosis may be a determinant of the growth of cancer.[26] In addition, apoptosis may be one mechanism of deleting abnormal cells or cells that have been damaged by toxins, radiation injury, or other stimuli.

The pathways by which apoptosis is induced clearly vary, depending on stimulus and cell type, and the sequence of events that result in the ultimate cellular changes is far from clear. A number of mechanisms, however, appear to be established, and various clues derived from models of apoptosis suggest the scenario depicted in Figure 1-19.

- The mechanism underlying the characteristic *chromatin condensation* has been studied extensively. This change is associated with cleavage of nuclear DNA occurring at the linker regions between nucleosomes, to produce a series of fragments that are multiples of 180 to 200 base pair lengths. Such fragments give a characteristic ladder pattern for apoptotic cells by gel electrophoresis (Fig. 1-20). This pattern contrasts with the diffuse smear pattern of random DNA breakdown that occurs in necrosis. This *internucleosomal DNA fragmentation* is mediated by a calcium-sensitive *endonuclease*. The endonuclease is present constitutively in some cell types (e.g., thymocytes), where it is activated by a rise of free cytosolic calcium, whereas in others the enzyme is induced transcriptionally before the onset of apoptosis. It is not established, however, that the endonuclease-induced DNA fragmentation itself causes the chromatin condensation.[31]
- The alterations in cell volume and shape have been ascribed in part to the induction, within apoptotic cells, of transglutaminase activity. This enzyme causes extensive cross-linking of cytoplasmic proteins, forming a shell under the plasma membrane similar to that of keratinized squamous cells.
- The *phagocytosis* of apoptotic bodies by macrophages and other cell types is mediated by receptors on these cells, which bind and engulf the

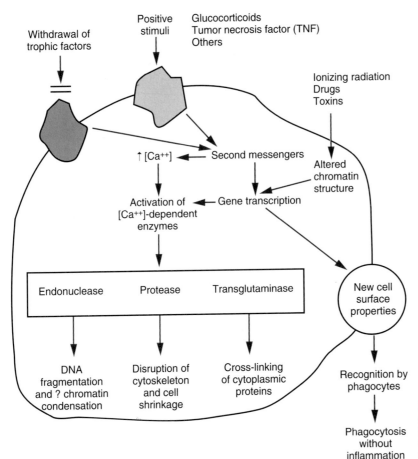

Figure 1-19. Mechanisms in apoptosis. (Redrawn with permission from Carson, D.A., and Ribeiro, J.M.: Apoptosis and disease. Lancet 341:1252, 1993 © by the Lancet Ltd. 1993.)

apoptotic cells. One such receptor on the macrophage is the *vitronectin receptor*, a beta₃-integrin that mediates phagocytosis of apoptotic neutrophils.

- *One important feature of apoptosis is its dependence in many* (but not all) *instances on gene activation and new protein synthesis.*[32] A number of genes can be induced by stimuli causing apoptosis, such as heat-shock proteins and proto-oncogenes, but these genes are not directly related to the triggering of apoptosis. Apoptosis-specific genes that stimulate *(ced-3,4)* or inhibit *(ced-9)* cell death have been identified in the development of the nematode *C. elegans*[33] and mammalian homologs are being described. For example, *ced-9* is homologous to *bcl-2*, described below.[34]

- Certain genes involved in growth and in the causation of cancer (oncogenes and suppressor genes) play a regulatory role in the induction of apoptosis. These include the *bcl-2* oncogene, which inhibits apoptosis induced by hormones and cytokines and thus extends cell survival;[35] the c-*myc* oncogene, whose protein product can stimulate either apoptosis or (in the presence of other survival signals such as *bcl-2*) cell growth;[36] and *p53*, which normally stimulates apoptosis, but, when mutated or absent (as it is in certain

cancers), favors cell survival. It appears that p53 is required for the apoptosis following DNA damage by irradiation, while apoptosis induced by glucocorticoids or aging is p53 independent.[37] (See also Chapter 7.)

It should be emphasized that in many models of apoptosis, new gene expression is not required, and indeed inhibition of gene expression *causes* apoptosis. One explanation for such a phenomenon is that apoptosis is normally held in abeyance by an inhibitor, which has a significantly shorter half-life than those of the proteins that cause apoptosis, and thus inhibition of protein synthesis would lead to rapid decline of such inhibitor and release of the apoptosis-inducing program.[28]

To summarize, apoptosis is a distinctive form of cell death manifested by characteristic chromatin condensation and DNA fragmentation, whose function is the deletion of cells in normal development, organogenesis, immune function, and tissue growth, but which can also be induced by pathologic stimuli. Some of the known effector mechanisms include endonuclease activation, stimulated by increased cytosolic calcium, which causes the DNA fragmentation; transglutaminase activation, which partly accounts for the shape and volume changes; and receptor-me-

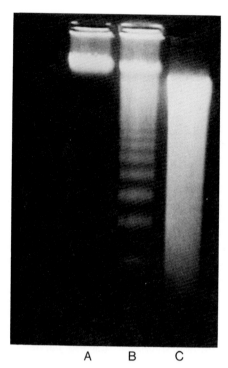

Figure 1-20. Agarose gel electrophoresis of DNA extracted from culture cells. Ethidium bromide stain; photographed under UV illumination. *Lane A,* Control culture. *Lane B,* Culture showing extensive apoptosis; note characteristic ladder pattern of DNA fragment induced by heat. *Lane C,* Culture showing massive necrosis; note diffuse smearing of DNA. (With permission from Kerr, J.F.R., and Harmon, B.V.: Definition and incidence of apoptosis: A historical perspective. *In* Tomei, L.D., and Cope, F.O. (eds.): Apoptosis: The Molecular Basis of Cell Death. Cold Spring Harbor, NY, Cold Spring Harbor Laboratory Press, 1991, p. 13.)

diated phagocytosis of apoptotic bodies. In some instances, gene transcription and protein synthesis are required for the induction of apoptosis, and the process is regulated by a set of genes that are involved in normal cell growth and differentiation.

STRESS (HEAT-SHOCK) PROTEINS AND CELL INJURY

One of the most highly conserved responses in biology is the induction of stress proteins by potentially injurious stimuli.[38] Initially called heat-shock proteins (HSP) because they were described in fruit fly larvae after slight elevations of temperature, these molecules appear to be essential to cell survival in all species subjected to injury. In mammalian cells, they are induced by a variety of physical and chemical agents and by ischemia.

Heat-shock proteins are present constitutively in normal cells, where they play an important role in normal cell metabolism. Two families of such proteins, called *Hsp70* and *Hsp60* (also called chaperones, or chaperonins) are intimately involved in intracellular protein folding and translocation as well as targeting of proteins to their final destination.[39] Another, ubiquitin, is a small (± 8 kd) heat-shock protein that is critical to *protein degradation* because intracellular proteins destined to be degraded are first covalently modified by conjugation with ubiquitin. Thus in stress, it is thought that the chaperonins "rescue" unfolded or aggregated polypeptides, and ubiquitin facilitates the degradation of proteins denatured beyond repair, thus protecting the cell from further injury.

Although experimental proof of this scenario in mammalian tissues is still lacking, heat-shock proteins have been shown to be induced in myocardial and neuronal ischemic injury.[40] The heat shock response appears to limit tissue necrosis in ischemia-reperfusion injury in rabbit hearts.[41] The capacity of certain areas in the nervous system to survive an ischemic attack is also correlated with the increased expression of stress proteins. Finally, the toxicity of certain drugs, such as Adriamycin, appears to be related, at least in part, to inhibition of heat-shock proteins.

SUBCELLULAR ALTERATIONS IN CELL INJURY

To this point in the chapter, the focus has been on the cell as a unit. Certain conditions, however, are associated with rather distinctive alterations in cell organelles or cytoskeleton. Some of these alterations coexist with those described for acute lethal injury; others represent more chronic forms of cell injury, and still others are adaptive responses that involve specific cellular organelles. Here we touch on only some of the more common or interesting of these reactions.

LYSOSOMES: HETEROPHAGY AND AUTOPHAGY

As should be well known, lysosomes contain a variety of hydrolytic enzymes, including acid phosphatase, glucuronidase, sulfatase, ribonuclease, collagenase, and so on. These enzymes are synthesized in the RER and then packaged into vesicles in the Golgi apparatus (Fig. 1-21). At this stage they are called *primary lysosomes.* Primary lysosomes fuse with membrane-bound vacuoles that contain material to be digested (the latter called *phagosomes*), forming *secondary lysosomes* or *phagolysosomes.*

Lysosomes are involved in the breakdown of phagocytosed material in one of two ways (see Fig. 1-21).

HETEROPHAGY. In this phenomenon, materials from the external environment are taken up through the process of *endocytosis.* Uptake of par-

HETEROPHAGY   AUTOPHAGY

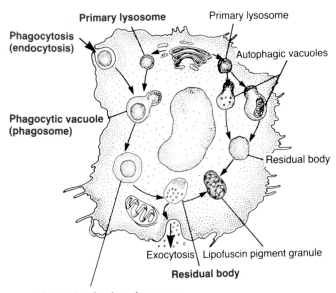

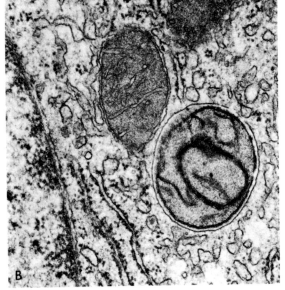

Figure 1–21. A, Schematic representation of autophagy (right) and heterophagy (left). (Redrawn from Fawcett, D.W.: A Textbook of Histology, 11th ed. Philadelphia, W.B. Saunders Co., 1986, p. 17.) B, Electron micrograph of an autolysosome containing a degenerating mitochondrion and amorphous material.

ticulate matter is known as *phagocytosis,* and that of soluble smaller macromolecules as *pinocytosis.* Heterophagy is most common in the "professional" phagocytes, such as neutrophils and macrophages. Examples of heterophagocytosis include the uptake and digestion of bacteria by neutrophilic leukocytes and the removal of apoptotic cells and bodies by macrophages. Fusion of the phagocytic vacuole with a lysosome then occurs, with eventual digestion of the engulfed material.

AUTOPHAGY. In this process, intracellular organelles and portions of cytosol are first sequestered from the cytoplasm in an *autophagic vacuole* formed from ribosome-free regions of the RER, which then fuses with pre-existing primary lysosomes or Golgi elements to form an *autophagolysosome.*[42] Autophagy is a common phenomenon involved in the removal of damaged organelles during cell injury and the cellular remodeling of differentiation and is particularly pronounced in cells undergoing atrophy induced by nutrient deprivation or hormonal involution.

The enzymes in the lysosomes are capable of breaking down most proteins and carbohydrates, but some lipids remain undigested. Lysosomes with undigested debris may persist within cells as *residual bodies* or may be extruded. *Lipofuscin pigment* granules represent undigested material that results from intracellular lipid peroxidation. Certain indigestible pigments, such as carbon particles inhaled from the atmosphere or inoculated pigment in tattoos, can persist in phagolysosomes of macrophages for decades.

Lysosomes are also wastebaskets in which cells sequester abnormal substances when these cannot be adequately metabolized. Hereditary *lysosomal storage disorders,* marked by deficiencies of enzymes that degrade various macromolecules, cause abnormal amounts of these compounds to be sequestered in the lysosomes of cells all over the body, particularly neurons, leading to severe abnormalities. These are discussed in detail in Chapter 5. Certain drugs, such as the antiarrhythmic drug amiodarone, become trapped and bind to phospholipids within the lysosome, rendering them resistant to breakdown. The resultant disorder is called *acquired* or *iatrogenic storage disease.*

INDUCTION (HYPERTROPHY) OF SMOOTH ENDOPLASMIC RETICULUM

It is known that protracted human use of barbiturates leads to a state of increased tolerance, so repeated doses lead to progressively shorter time spans of sleep. The patients have thus "adapted" to the medication. This adaptation is due to induction of an increased volume (hypertrophy) of the SER of hepatocytes (Fig. 1–22). Barbiturates are detoxified in the liver by oxidative demethylation, which involves the P-450–centered, mixed-function oxidase system found in the SER.[43] The barbiturates stimulate *(induce)* the synthesis of more enzymes as well as more SER. In this manner, the cell is better able to detoxify the drugs and so adapt to its altered environment. The mixed-func-

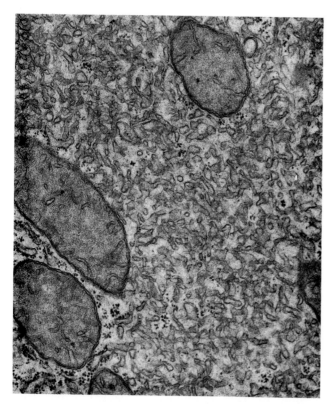

Figure 1–22. Electron micrograph of liver from phenobarbital-treated rat showing marked increase in smooth ER. (Reproduced with permission from Jones, A.L., and Fawcett, D.W.: Hypertrophy of the agranular endoplasmic reticulum in hamster liver induced by phenobarbital. *Journal of Histochemistry & Cytochemistry* 14:215, 1966. Courtesy of Dr. Fawcett.)

tion oxidase system of the SER is also involved in the metabolism of other exogenous compounds—carcinogenic hydrocarbons, steroids, carbon tetrachloride, alcohol, insecticides, and others. It is noteworthy that cells adapted to one drug have increased capacity to detoxify other drugs handled by the system or endogenous metabolic products, such as bilirubin and bile acids.

MITOCHONDRIAL ALTERATIONS

We have seen that mitochondrial dysfunction plays an important role in acute cell injury. In addition, various alterations in the number, size, and shape of mitochondria occur in some pathologic conditions. For example, in cell hypertrophy and atrophy, there is an increase and a decrease, respectively, in the number of mitochondria in cells. Mitochondria may assume extremely large and abnormal shapes (megamitochondria). These can be seen in the liver in alcoholic liver disease and in certain nutritional deficiencies (Fig. 1–23). In certain inherited metabolic diseases of skeletal mus-

cle, the *mitochondrial myopathies*, defects in mitochondrial metabolism are associated with increased numbers of mitochondria that often are unusually large, have abnormal cristae, and contain crystalloids. In addition, certain tumors (found in salivary glands, thyroid, parathyroids, and kidneys) called "oncocytomas" consist of cells with abundant enlarged mitochondria, giving the cell a distinctly eosinophilic appearance.

CYTOSKELETAL ABNORMALITIES

Abnormalities of the cytoskeleton underlie a variety of pathologic states. The *cytoskeleton* consists of microtubules (20 to 25 nm in diameter), thin actin filaments (6 to 8 nm), thick myosin filaments (15 nm), and various classes of intermediate filaments (10 nm). Several other nonpolymerized and nonfilamentous forms of contractile proteins also exist. Cytoskeletal abnormalities may be reflected by (1) defects in cell function, such as cell locomotion and intracellular organelle movements, or (2) in some instances by intracellular accumulations of fibrillar material. Only a few examples are cited.

Functioning myofilaments and microtubules are essential for various stages of leukocyte migration and phagocytosis, and functional deficiencies of the cytoskeleton appear to underlie certain defects in leukocyte movement toward an injurious stimulus (chemotaxis; see Chapter 3) or the ability of such cells to perform phagocytosis adequately. For example, a defect of microtubule polymeri-

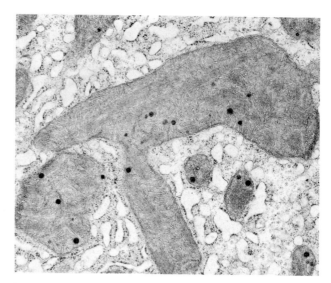

Figure 1–23. Enlarged, abnormally shaped mitochondria from liver of patient with alcoholic cirrhosis. Note also crystalline formations in mitochondria.

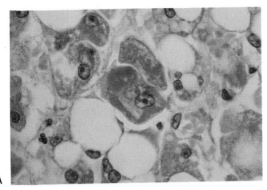

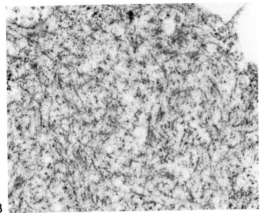

Figure 1–24. *A,* The liver of alcohol abuse (chronic alcoholism). Hyaline inclusions in hepatic parenchymal cell in center appear as eosinophilic networks disposed about the nuclei. *B,* Electron micrograph of alcoholic hyalin. The material is composed of intermediate (prekeratin) filaments and an amorphous matrix.

INTRACELLULAR ACCUMULATIONS

One of the cellular manifestations of metabolic derangements in pathology is the accumulation of abnormal amounts of various substances. The stockpiled substances fall into three categories: (1) *a normal cellular constituent* accumulated in excess, such as water, lipid, protein, and carbohydrates; (2) *an abnormal substance,* either exogenous, such as a mineral, or a product of abnormal metabolism; and (3) *a pigment* or an infectious product. These substances may accumulate either transiently or permanently, and they may be harmless to the cells, but on occasion they are severely toxic. The substance may be located in either the cytoplasm (frequently within lysosomes) or the nucleus. In some instances, the cell may be producing the abnormal substance, and in others it may be merely storing products of pathologic processes occurring elsewhere in the body. The intracellular accumulation of *fluid* is most commonly a reflection of acute cell injury and cellular swelling, as previously discussed.

Many processes result in abnormal intracellular accumulations in non-neoplastic cells, but most can be divided into three general types (Fig. 1–25).

1. *A normal endogenous substance is produced at a normal or increased rate, but the rate of metabolism is inadequate to remove it.* An example of this type of process is *fatty change* in the liver due to intracellular accumulation of triglycerides.

2. *A normal or abnormal endogenous substance accumulates because it cannot be metabolized or is deposited intracellularly in an amorphous or filamentous form.* One important cause is a genetic enzymatic defect in a specific metabolic pathway, so that some particular metabolite cannot be used. The resulting diseases are referred to as *storage diseases* (discussed in Chapter 5).

3. *An abnormal exogenous substance is deposited* and accumulates because the cell has neither the enzymic machinery to degrade the substance nor the ability to transport it to other sites. Accumulations of carbon particles and such nonmetabolizable chemicals as silica particles are examples of this type of alteration. Viral inclusions also fall into this category and are discussed in Chapter 8.

Whatever the nature and origin of the intracellular accumulation, it implies the storage of some product by individual cells. If the overload is due to a systemic derangement and can be brought under control, the accumulation is reversible. On the other hand, in genetic storage diseases, accumulation is progressive, and the cells may become so overloaded as to cause secondary injury, leading in some instances to death of the tissue and the patient.

zation in the *Chédiak-Higashi syndrome* causes delayed or decreased fusion of lysosomes with phagosomes in leukocytes and thus impairs phagocytosis of bacteria. Large abnormal lysosomes appear in the cytoplasm of leukocytes. Some drugs, such as cytochalasin B, inhibit microfilament function and thus affect phagocytosis. Defects in the organization of microtubules can inhibit sperm motility, causing male sterility, and at the same time can immobilize the cilia of respiratory epithelium, causing interference with the ability of this epithelium to clear inhaled bacteria, leading to bronchiectasis (the *immotile cilia syndrome*).

Accumulations of intermediate filaments may be seen in certain types of cell injury. For example, the *Mallory body,* or "alcoholic hyalin," is an eosinophilic intracytoplasmic inclusion in liver cells that is characteristic of alcoholic liver disease but seen in many other conditions as well. Such inclusions are now known to be composed largely of intermediate filaments of predominantly *prekeratin* (Fig. 1–24). The *neurofibrillary tangle* found in the brain in Alzheimer's disease contains microtubule-associated proteins and neurofilaments, a reflection of a disrupted neuronal cytoskeleton.

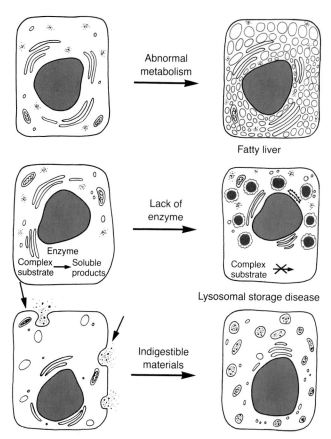

Figure 1–25. The general mechanisms of intracellular accumulation: (1) abnormal metabolism, as in fatty change in the liver; (2) deficiency of critical enzymes that prevent breakdown of substrates—which accumulate in lysosomes, as in lysosomal storage diseases; and (3) inability to degrade phagocytosed particles, as in hemosiderosis and carbon pigment accumulation.

LIPIDS

All major classes of lipids can accumulate in cells: triglycerides, cholesterol/cholesterol esters, and phospholipids. Phospholipids, as we have seen, are components of the myelin figures found in necrotic cells. In addition, abnormal complexes of lipids and carbohydrates accumulate in certain genetic storage diseases, such as the mucopolysaccharidoses and Gaucher's disease (see Chapter 5). Here we shall concentrate on triglyceride and cholesterol accumulations.

Steatosis (Fatty Change)

The terms *steatosis* and *fatty change* describe abnormal accumulations of *triglycerides* within parenchymal cells. Fatty change is often seen in the liver because it is the major organ involved in fat metabolism, but it also occurs in heart, muscle, and kidney. The causes of steatosis include toxins, pro-

tein malnutrition, diabetes mellitus, obesity, and anoxia. *In industrialized nations, by far the most common cause of significant fatty change in the liver (fatty liver) is alcohol abuse.*[45]

Different mechanisms account for triglyceride accumulation in the liver. As should be well known, lipids are transported to the liver from adipose tissue and from the diet. From adipose tissue, lipids are released and transported as free acids and from the diet either as chylomicra or as free fatty acids. Free fatty acids enter the liver cell, and most are esterified to triglycerides. Some are converted to cholesterol, incorporated into phospholipids, or oxidized in mitochondria into ketone bodies. Some fatty acids are synthesized from acetate within the liver proper. To be secreted by the liver, intracellular triglyceride must be complexed with specific apoprotein molecules called "lipid acceptor proteins" to form lipoproteins.

Excess accumulation of triglycerides within the liver may result from defects in any one of the events in the sequence from fatty acid entry to lipoprotein exit (Fig. 1–26). A number of such defects are induced by alcohol, a hepatotoxin that alters mitochondrial and microsomal functions. CCl_4 and protein malnutrition act by decreasing synthesis of lipid acceptor proteins. Anoxia inhibits fatty acid oxidation. Starvation increases adipose tissue mobilization and thus triglyceride synthesis. Acute fatty liver of pregnancy and Reye's syndrome are some-

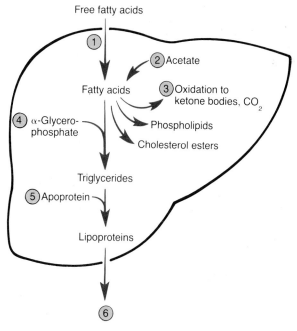

Figure 1–26. Possible mechanisms in the pathogenesis of fatty liver. The illustration depicts the uptake and metabolism of fatty acids by the liver, formation of triglycerides, and secretion of lipoproteins. Defects in any of the six numbered steps can lead to accumulation of triglycerides and fatty liver.

times fatal but fortunately rare conditions in which a defect in mitochondrial oxidation is suspected (see also Chapter 18).

The significance of fatty change depends on the cause and severity of the accumulation. When mild, it may have no effect on cellular function. More severe fatty change may impair cellular function, but unless some vital intracellular process is irreversibly impaired (e.g., in CCl_4 poisoning), fatty change *per se* is reversible. As a severe form of injury fatty change may be a harbinger of cell death, *but it should be emphasized that cells may die without undergoing fatty change.*

MORPHOLOGY. Fatty change is most often seen in the liver and heart.

In all organs, fatty change appears as clear vacuoles within parenchymal cells. Intracellular accumulations of water or polysaccharides (e.g., glycogen) may also produce clear vacuoles, and it becomes necessary to resort to special techniques to distinguish these three types of clear vacuoles. The identification of lipids requires the avoidance of fat solvents commonly used in paraffin embedding for routine hematoxylin and eosin stains. To identify the fat, it is necessary to prepare frozen tissue sections of either fresh or aqueous formalin-fixed tissues. The sections may then be stained with Sudan IV or Oil Red-O, both of which impart an orange-red color to the contained lipids. The PAS reaction is commonly employed to identify glycogen, although it is by no means specific. When neither fat nor polysaccharide can be demonstrated within a clear vacuole, it is presumed to contain water or fluid with a low protein content.

LIVER. In the liver, mild fatty change may not affect the gross appearance. With progressive accumulation, the organ enlarges and becomes increasingly yellow until, in extreme instances, the liver may weigh 3 to 6 kg and be transformed into a bright yellow, soft, greasy organ.

Fatty change begins with the development of minute, membrane-bound inclusions (liposomes) closely applied to the endoplasmic reticulum. It is first manifested light microscopically by the appearance of small fat vacuoles in the cytoplasm around the nucleus. As the process progresses, the vacuoles coalesce, creating cleared spaces that displace the nucleus to the periphery of the cell (Fig. 1–27). Occasionally, contiguous cells rupture, and the enclosed fat globules coalesce, producing so-called fatty cysts.

HEART. Lipid, as a neutral fat, is sometimes found in heart muscle in the form of small droplets. It occurs in two patterns. In one, prolonged moderate hypoxia, such as that produced by profound anemia, causes intracellular deposits of fat, which create grossly apparent bands of yellowed myocardium alternating with bands of darker, red-brown, uninvolved myocardium (tigered effect). In the other pattern of fatty change produced by more profound hypoxia or some forms of myocarditis (e.g., diphtheritic), the myocardial cells are uniformly affected.

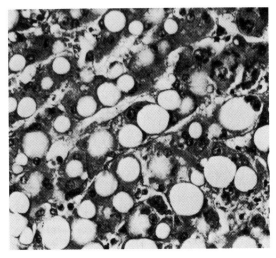

Figure 1–27. High-power detail of marked fatty change of liver. The variability in size of vacuoles is evident. In some cells, the well-preserved nucleus is squeezed into the displaced rim of cytoplasm about the fat vacuole.

Cholesterol and Cholesterol Esters

The cellular metabolism of cholesterol (discussed in detail in Chapter 5) is tightly regulated such that most cells use cholesterol for the synthesis of cell membranes without intracellular accumulation of cholesterol or cholesterol esters. However, accumulations, manifested histologically by intracellular vacuoles, are seen in several pathologic processes (Fig. 1–28).

- *Atherosclerosis.* In atherosclerotic plaques, smooth muscle cells and macrophages within the intimal layer of the aorta and large arteries are filled with lipid vacuoles, most of which are made up of cholesterol and cholesterol esters. Such cells appear foamy, and aggregates of them in the intima produce the yellow cholesterol-laden atheromas characteristic of this serious disorder. Some of these fat-laden cells rupture, releasing lipids into the extracellular space. The mechanisms of cholesterol accumulation in both cell types in atherosclerosis are discussed in detail in Chapter 11. The extracellular cholesterol esters may crystallize in the shape of long needles, producing quite distinctive clefts in tissue sections.
- *Xanthomas.* Intracellular accumulation of cholesterol within macrophages is also characteristic of acquired and hereditary hyperlipidemic states. Clusters of foamy cells are found in the subepithelial connective tissue of the skin and in ten-

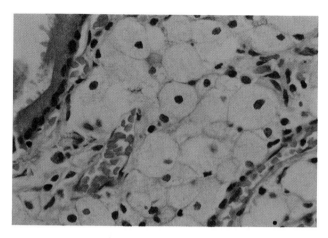

Figure 1–28. Cholesterol-laden macrophage (foam cell) from a focus of gallbladder cholesterolosis. The gallbladder mucosa is in the upper left.

dons producing tumorous masses known as xanthomas.

- *Inflammation and necrosis.* Foamy macrophages are frequently found at sites of cell injury and inflammation, owing to phagocytosis of cholesterol from the membranes of injured cells, including parenchymal cells, leukocytes, and erythrocytes. Phospholipids and myelin figures are also found in inflammatory foci. When abundant, the cholesterol-laden macrophages impart a yellowish discoloration to such inflammatory foci.
- *Cholesterolosis.* This refers to the focal accumulations of cholesterol-laden macrophages in the lamina propria of the gallbladder. The mechanism of accumulation is unknown (Fig. 1–28).

Stromal Infiltration of Fat or Fatty Ingrowth

This is a form of *accumulation of lipids that has a mechanism and connotation completely different from those of intracellular fatty accumulation.* It is discussed at this time merely to differentiate it from the condition described as fatty change. Fatty ingrowth refers to the accumulation of lipids *within stromal connective tissue cells.*

> **MORPHOLOGY.** Fatty ingrowth is most commonly encountered in the heart and pancreas, where adult adipose cells appear within the connective tissue stroma. The stromal adipose tissue does not damage the adjacent myocardial cells. In the pancreas, the fat is found in the connective tissue septa of the pancreatic lobules.

As far as is known, stromal infiltration of fat rarely affects cardiac or pancreatic function.

PROTEINS

Excesses of proteins within the cells sufficient to cause morphologically visible accumulation are less common than accumulation of lipids. They usually appear as rounded, eosinophilic droplets, vacuoles, or masses. Accumulation of filamentous proteins has already been alluded to in the discussion of cytoskeletal alterations. Examples of intracellular protein accumulations include the following:

- *Reabsorption droplets in proximal renal tubules.* This is seen in renal diseases associated with protein loss in the urine (proteinuria). If a protein leaks across the glomerular filter, it passes into the proximal tubule, where it is reabsorbed by the epithelial cell through pinocytosis. Pinocytotic vesicles fuse with lysosomes to produce phagolysosomes, which appear as pink hyaline droplets within the cytoplasm of the tubular cell (Fig. 1–29).
- *Immunoglobulin in plasma cells.* The endoplasmic reticulum of plasma cells engaged in active synthesis of immunoglobulins may become hugely distended, producing large, homogeneous eosinophilic inclusions called *Russell bodies.*
- *Alpha$_1$-antitrypsin (AAT) in liver cells.* In AAT deficiency, the enzyme accumulates in the *endoplasmic reticulum of the liver* in the form of globular eosinophilic inclusions. Here, the defect is attributed to a single genetic amino acid substitution in the enzyme, resulting in defects of folding and transport across the cytoplasm (see Chapter 18).

GLYCOGEN

Excessive intracellular deposits of glycogen are seen in patients with an abnormality in either glucose or glycogen metabolism. Whatever the clinical setting, the glycogen masses appear as clear vacuoles within the cytoplasm. Glycogen is best pre-

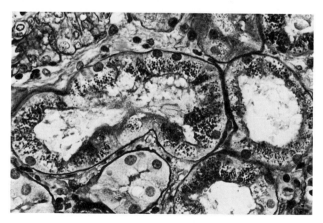

Figure 1–29. Hyaline droplets (dark-staining) in the renal tubular epithelium.

served in nonaqueous fixatives; for its localization, tissues are best fixed in absolute alcohol. Staining with Best's carmine or the PAS reaction imparts a rose-to-violet color to the glycogen, and diastase digestion of a parallel section before staining serves as a further control by hydrolyzing the glycogen.

Diabetes mellitus is the prime example of a disorder of glucose metabolism. In this disease, glycogen is found in the epithelial cells of the distal portions of the proximal convoluted tubules and sometimes in the descending loop of Henle as well as within liver cells, beta cells of the islets of Langerhans, and heart muscle cells.

Glycogen also accumulates within the cells in a group of closely related disorders, all genetic, collectively referred to as the *glycogen storage diseases,* or *glycogenoses* (see Chapter 5). In these diseases, some abnormal or normal form of glycogen cannot be metabolized. These diseases represent instances in which massive stockpiling of substances within cells causes secondary injury and cell death.

PIGMENTS

Pigments are colored substances, some of which are normal constituents of cells (e.g., melanin), whereas others are abnormal and collect in cells only under special circumstances.[46] Pigments can be either exogenous, coming from outside the body, or endogenous, synthesized within the body itself.

The most common *exogenous pigment* is *carbon* or *coal dust,* which is a virtually ubiquitous air pollutant of urban life. When inhaled, it is picked up by macrophages within the alveoli and is then transported through lymphatic channels to the regional lymph nodes in the tracheobronchial region. Accumulations of this pigment blacken the tissues of the lungs *(anthracosis)* and the involved lymph nodes. In coal miners and those living in heavily polluted environments, the aggregates of carbon dust may induce a fibroblastic reaction or even emphysema and thus cause a serious lung disease known as *coal worker's pneumoconiosis* (see Chapter 17). *Tattooing* is a form of localized, exogenous pigmentation of the skin. The pigments inoculated are phagocytized by dermal macrophages, in which they reside for the remainder of the life of the embellished. Although the pigments do not evoke any inflammatory response, they have a distressing habit of persisting as a reminder of bygone follies.

Endogenous pigments include lipofuscin, melanin, and certain derivatives of hemoglobin.

Lipofuscin is an insoluble pigment, also known as lipochrome and "wear-and-tear" or aging pigment.[47] Lipofuscin is composed of polymers of lipids and phospholipids complexed with protein, *suggesting that it is derived through lipid peroxidation of polyunsaturated lipids of subcellular membranes.* Lipofuscin is not injurious to the cell or its functions. Its importance lies in its being the telltale sign of free radical injury and lipid peroxidation. The term is derived from the Latin (*fuscus* = brown), thus brown lipid. In tissue sections, it appears as a yellow-brown, finely granular intracytoplasmic, often perinuclear pigment. It is seen in cells undergoing slow, regressive changes and is particularly prominent in the liver and heart of aging patients or patients with severe malnutrition and cancer cachexia. It is usually accompanied by organ shrinkage *(brown atrophy).* On electron microscopy, the granules are highly electron dense, often have membranous structures in their midst, and are usually in a perinuclear location (Fig. 1–30).

Melanin (derived from the Greek word *melas,* meaning black) is an endogenous, non–hemoglobin-derived, brown-black pigment formed when the enzyme tyrosinase catalyzes the oxidation of tyrosine to dihydroxyphenylalanine in melanocytes. It is discussed further in Chapter 26. For all practical purposes, melanin is the *only endogenous brown-black pigment.* The only other that could be considered in this category is homogentisic acid, a black pigment that occurs in patients with *alkaptonuria,* a rare metabolic disease. Here the pigment is deposited in the skin, connective tissue, and cartilage, and the pigmentation is known as ochronosis.

Hemosiderin is a hemoglobin-derived, golden-yellow to brown, granular or crystalline pigment in which form iron is stored in cells. Iron metabolism and the synthesis of ferritin and hemosiderin are considered in detail in Chapter 13. Suffice it to say here that iron is normally carried by transport proteins, transferrins. In cells, it is normally stored in association with a protein, apoferritin, to form ferritin micelles. Ferritin is a constituent of many cell types under normal conditions. *When there is a local or systemic excess of iron, ferritin forms hemosiderin granules,* which are easily seen with the light microscope. Thus, hemosiderin pigment represents aggregates of ferritin micelles. Under normal conditions, small amounts of hemosiderin can be seen in the mononuclear phagocytes of the bone marrow, spleen, and liver, all actively engaged in red cell breakdown.

Excesses of iron cause hemosiderin to accumulate within cells, either as a localized process or as a systemic derangement. *Local excesses* of iron and hemosiderin result from gross hemorrhages or the myriad minute hemorrhages that accompany severe vascular congestion. The best example of localized hemosiderosis is the common bruise. Following local hemorrhage, the area is at first red-blue. With lysis of the erythrocytes, the hemoglobin

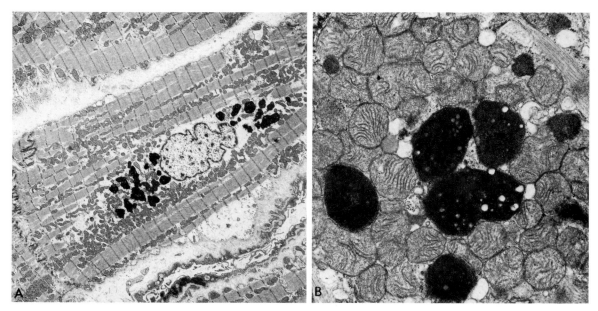

Figure 1–30. Lipofuscin. Lipofuscin granules in myocardial fiber. *A,* Low magnification, showing perin',clear localization. *B,* Electron-dense bodies are composed of lipid-protein complexes.

eventually undergoes transformation to hemosiderin. Macrophages take part in this process by phagocytizing the red cell debris, and then lysosomal enzymes eventually convert the hemoglobin, through a sequence of pigments, into hemosiderin. The play of colors through which the bruise passes reflects these transformations. The original red-blue color of hemoglobin is transformed to varying shades of green-blue, comprising the local formation of biliverdin (green bile), then bilirubin (red bile), and thereafter the iron moiety of hemoglobin is deposited as golden-yellow hemosiderin.

Whenever there are causes for *systemic overload of iron,* hemosiderin is deposited in many organs and tissues, a condition called *hemosiderosis.* It is seen with (1) increased absorption of dietary iron, (2) impaired utilization of iron, (3) hemolytic anemias, and (4) transfusions because the transfused red cells constitute an exogenous load of iron. These conditions are discussed in Chapter 18.

MORPHOLOGY. The pigment appears as a coarse, golden, granular pigment lying within the cell's cytoplasm. When the basic cause is the localized breakdown of red cells, the pigmentation is found at first in the reticuloendothelial cells in the area. In systemic hemosiderosis, it is found at first in the mononuclear phagocytes of the liver, bone marrow, spleen, and lymph nodes and in scattered macrophages throughout other organs such as the skin, pancreas, and kidneys. With progressive accumulation, parenchymal cells throughout the body (principally in the liver, pancreas, heart, and endocrine organs) become pigmented. Iron can be visualized in tissues by the Prussian blue histochemical reaction, in which colorless potassium ferrocyanide is converted by iron to blue-black ferric ferrocyanide (Fig. 1–31).

In most instances of systemic hemosiderosis, the pigment does not damage the parenchymal cells or impair organ function. The more extreme accumulation of iron, however, in a disease called *hemochromatosis* is associated with liver and pancreatic damage, resulting in liver fibrosis, heart failure, and diabetes mellitus (see Chapter 18).

Bilirubin is the normal major pigment found in bile. It is derived from hemoglobin but contains no iron. Its normal formation and excretion are vital to health, and jaundice is a common clinical disorder due to excesses of this pigment within cells and tissues. Bilirubin metabolism and jaundice are discussed in Chapter 18.

Bilirubin pigment within cells and tissues is visible morphologically only when the patient is rather severely jaundiced for some period of time. Even though this pigment is distributed throughout all tissues and fluids of the body, the *accumulations are most evident in the liver and kidneys.* In the liver, particularly with diseases caused by obstruction of the outflow of bile (e.g., cancers of the common bile duct and head of the pancreas), bilirubin is encountered within bile sinusoids, Kupffer's cells, and hepatocytes. *In all these sites, it appears as a mucoid, green-brown to black, amorphous, globular deposit.* In advanced cases of such obstructive jaundice, the aggregates of pigment may be quite large, creating so-called bile lakes.

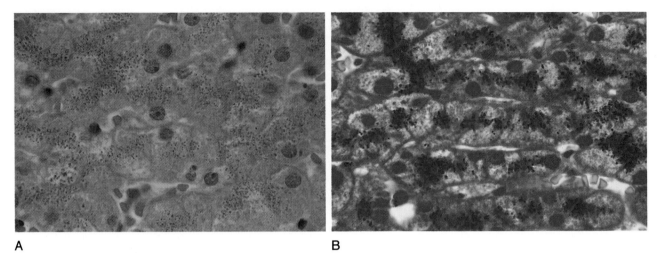

A   B

Figure 1–31. Hemosiderin granules in liver cells. *A,* H&E section, showing golden-brown, finely granular pigment. *B,* Prussian blue reaction, specific for iron.

These may cause necrosis of hepatocytes in the focal area. Bilirubin pigment is encountered in the renal tubular epithelial cells in various forms of jaundice.

PATHOLOGIC CALCIFICATION

Pathologic calcification implies the abnormal deposition of calcium salts, together with smaller amounts of iron, magnesium, and other mineral salts. It is a common process occurring in a variety of pathologic conditions.[48] There are two forms of pathologic calcification. When the deposition occurs in nonviable or dying tissues, it is known as *dystrophic calcification;* it occurs despite normal serum levels of calcium and in the absence of derangements in calcium metabolism. In contrast, the deposition of calcium salts in vital tissues is known as *metastatic calcification,* and it almost always reflects some derangement in calcium metabolism, leading to hypercalcemia.

DYSTROPHIC CALCIFICATION

This alteration is encountered in areas of necrosis, whether they are of coagulative, caseous, or liquefactive type and also in foci of enzymic necrosis of fat. Calcification is almost inevitable in the atheromas of advanced atherosclerosis, which, as will be seen, are focal intimal injuries in the aorta and larger arteries characterized by the accumulation of lipids. It also commonly develops in aging or damaged heart valves, further hampering their function (Fig. 1–32). Whatever the site of deposition, the calcium salts appear macroscopically as

fine, white granules or clumps, often felt as gritty deposits. Sometimes, a tuberculous lymph node is virtually converted to stone.

MORPHOLOGY. Histologically, with the usual hematoxylin and eosin stain, the calcium salts have a basophilic, amorphous granular, sometimes clumped appearance. They can be **intracellular, extracellular,** or **in both locations.** In the course of time, **heterotopic** bone may be formed in the focus of calcification. On occasion, single necrotic

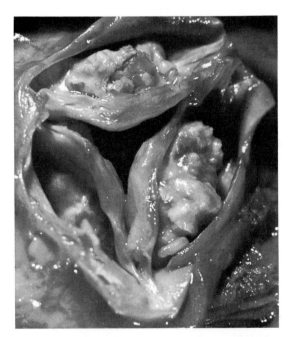

Figure 1–32. A view looking down onto the unopened aortic valve in a heart with calcific aortic stenosis. The semilunar cusps are thickened and fibrotic. Behind each leaflet are seen irregular masses of piled-up dystrophic calcification.

cells may constitute seed crystals that become encrusted by the mineral deposits. The progressive acquisition of outer layers may create lamellated configurations called **psammoma bodies** because of their resemblance to grains of sand. Some types of papillary cancers (e.g., thyroid) are apt to develop psammoma bodies. Strange concretions emerge when calcium iron salts gather about long slender spicules of asbestos in the lung, creating exotic, beaded dumbbell forms.

In the pathogenesis of dystrophic calcification the final common pathway is the formation of crystalline calcium phosphate mineral in the form of an apatite similar to the hydroxyapatite of bone.[49] The process has two major phases: *initiation* (or *nucleation*) and *propagation;* both can occur intracellularly and extracellularly. Initiation in *extracellular* sites occurs in membrane-bound *vesicles,* about 200 nm in diameter; in cartilage and bone, they are known as *matrix vesicles,* and in pathologic calcification, they are derived from degenerating or aging cells. It is thought that calcium is concentrated in these vesicles by its affinity for acidic phospholipids, and phosphates accumulate possibly as a result of the action of membrane-bound phosphatases. Initiation of *intracellular calcification* occurs in the *mitochondria* of dead or dying cells that accumulate calcium, as described earlier.

After mineral initiation in either location, *propagation* of crystal formation occurs, dependent on the concentration of Ca^{++} and PO_4 in the extracellular spaces, the presence of mineral inhibitors, and the presence of collagen and other proteins. *Osteopontin,* an acidic, calcium-binding phosphoprotein with high affinity to hydroxyapatite — and known to be involved in bone mineralization — is abundant in dystrophic calcification, at least in arteries and kidney.[49] Collagen itself enhances the rate of crystal growth.

Although dystrophic calcification may be simply a telltale sign of previous cell injury, it is often a cause of organ dysfunction. Such is the case in calcific valvular disease and atherosclerosis, as will become clear in further discussion of these diseases.

METASTATIC CALCIFICATION

This alteration may occur in normal tissues whenever there is hypercalcemia. Hypercalcemia also accentuates dystrophic calcification. The causes of hypercalcemia include hyperparathyroidism, vitamin D intoxication, systemic sarcoidosis, milk-alkali syndrome, hyperthyroidism, idiopathic hypercalcemia of infancy, Addison's disease (adrenocortical insufficiency), increased bone catabolism associated with disseminated bone tumors (e.g., multiple myeloma and metastatic cancer) and leukemia, and decreased bone formation as occurs in immobilization. Hypercalcemia also arises in some instances of advanced renal failure with phosphate retention, leading to secondary hyperparathyroidism.

Metastatic calcification may occur widely throughout the body but principally affects the interstitial tissues of the blood vessels, kidneys, lungs, and gastric mucosa. In all these sites, the calcium salts morphologically resemble those described in dystrophic calcification. Thus, they may occur as noncrystalline amorphous deposits or, at other times, as hydroxyapatite crystals. Metastatic calcification appears to begin also in mitochondria except in kidney tubules, where it develops in the basement membranes, probably in relation to extracellular vesicles budding from the epithelial cells.

In general, the mineral salts cause no clinical dysfunction, but, on occasion, massive involvement of the lungs produces remarkable x-ray films and respiratory deficits. Massive deposits in the kidney (nephrocalcinosis) may in time cause renal damage.

HYALINE CHANGE

The term "hyaline" is widely used as a descriptive histologic term rather than a specific marker for cell injury. *It usually refers to an alteration within cells or in the extracellular space, which gives a homogeneous, glassy, pink appearance in routine histologic sections stained with hematoxylin and eosin.* This tinctorial change is produced by a variety of alterations and does not represent a specific pattern of accumulation. Intracellular accumulations of protein, described earlier (reabsorption droplets, Russell bodies, Mallory alcoholic hyalin), are examples of intracellular hyaline deposits.

Extracellular hyalin has been somewhat more difficult to analyze. Collagenous fibrous tissue in old scars may appear hyalinized, but the physiochemical mechanism underlying this change is not clear. In long-standing hypertension and diabetes mellitus, the walls of arterioles, especially in the kidney, become hyalinized, owing to extravasated plasma protein and deposition of basement membrane material. With hematoxylin and eosin stains, the protein *amyloid* (discussed in Chapter 6) also has a hyaline appearance. This is a very specific fibrillar protein, however, with characteristic biochemical composition. Amyloid can be clearly identified by its special staining characteristics with the Congo red stain, with which it appears red and shows bipolar refringence. Thus, although the term "hyaline" is convenient to use, it is important to recognize the multitude of mechanisms that produce this change and the implications of the alteration when it is seen in different pathologic conditions.

Before concluding this discussion of cell injury and various cellular changes, we must turn to a consideration of cellular aging, which also results in cellular deterioration.

CELLULAR AGING

Despite its universality, aging is difficult to define. Shakespeare probably characterized it best in his elegant description of the seven ages of man. It begins at the moment of conception, involves the differentiation and maturation of the organism and its cells, at some variable point in time leads to the progressive loss of functional capacity characteristic of senescence, and ends in death.

With age, there are physiologic and structural alterations in almost all organ systems. Aging in individuals is affected to a great extent by genetic factors, diet, social conditions, and the occurrence of age-related diseases, such as atherosclerosis, diabetes, and osteoarthritis. In addition, there is good evidence that aging-induced alterations in cells are an important component of the aging of the organism. Here we discuss cellular aging because it could represent the progressive accumulation over the years of sublethal injury that may lead to cell death or at least to the diminished capacity of the cell to respond to injury.

A number of cell functions decline progressively with age. Oxidative phosphorylation by mitochondria is reduced, as is DNA and RNA synthesis of structural and enzymatic proteins and of cell receptors. Senescent cells have a decreased capacity for uptake of nutrients and for repair of chromosomal damage. The morphologic alterations in aging cells include irregular and abnormally lobed nuclei, pleomorphic vacuolated mitochondria, decreased endoplasmic reticulum, and distorted Golgi apparatus. Concomitantly, there is a steady accumulation of the pigment lipofuscin, which, as described previously, represents a product of lipid peroxidation.

Although a number of theories have been proposed, it is now clear that cell aging is multifactorial. It involves an *endogenous* molecular program of cellular senescence as well as continuous exposure throughout life to adverse *exogenous* influences, leading to progressive encroachment on the cell's survivability (so-called wear and tear).[50] In this scenario, molecular injury to cells exceeds their repair capacity, thus accelerating the aging process. We shall first review the process of *cellular senescence* and then the currently known molecular causes of cellular wear and tear.

The phenomenon of *cellular senescence in vitro* has been extensively studied since the original observations of Hayflick that normal human diploid fibroblasts in culture have a finite life span—they stop dividing and become senescent after about 50 doublings.[51] In contrast, cells from patients with progeria or Werner syndrome, who show premature aging, have a markedly reduced *in vitro* life span, whereas cancer cells proliferate indefinitely and are immortal (Fig. 1–33). The cause of such replicative senescence is unclear. The activation of senescence-specific genes (on chromosome 1 and 4); altered or loss of growth regulator genes (e.g., c-fos and the *Rb gene*, described in Chapter 2); induction of growth inhibitors in senescent cells; and a variety of other genetic mechanisms have been proposed.[52] One hypothesis for these gene defects is chromosomal *telomeric shortening*.[52] Telomeres are critical in stabilizing the terminal portions of chromosomes and anchoring them to the nuclear matrix. Telomeres are reduced in length in late passage cultures and in cultures of patients with increased age. They are longest in sperm and longer in fetal than in adult cells—their *de novo* synthesis is regulated by the enzyme telomerase, and there is a correlation between telomere length and telomerase content. It has thus been proposed that loss of DNA from the ends of the chromosome with telomere shortening leads to the deletion of essential genes, with consequent limiting of the life span.

More is known about acquired defects in aging cells. A favored theory for cells aging invokes the progressive effects of *free radical damage* throughout life.[53] This damage can occur by repeated environmental exposure to such influences as ionizing radiation or progressive reduction of antioxidant defense mechanisms (e.g., vitamin E, glutathione peroxidase) or both. The accumulation of *lipofuscin* is consistent with free radical damage, but the pigment itself is not toxic to cells. In addition to lipid

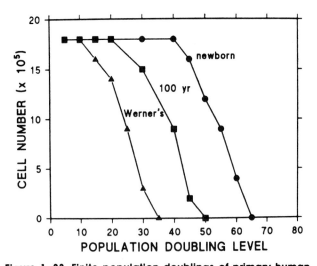

Figure 1–33. Finite population doublings of primary human fibroblasts derived from a newborn, a 100-year-old person, and a 20-year-old patient with Werner's syndrome. The ability of cells to grow to a confluent monolayer (top) declines with increasing population doubling level. (From Dice, J.F.: Cellular and molecular mechanisms of aging. Physiol. Rev. 73:150, 1993.)

peroxidation, free radicals induce nucleic acid damage. Indeed, it has been estimated that reduced oxygen species are responsible for some 10,000 DNA base modifications per cell per day, eventually exceeding the known DNA repair mechanisms.[20] Not only nuclear but also mitochondrial DNA mutations can be induced by free radicals, and mitochondrial DNA mutations and deletions increase dramatically with age. Oxygen free radicals also catalyze the oxidative modification of proteins, including enzymes, rendering them degradable by cytosolic neutral or alkaline proteases, further affecting cell function.[20]

Post-translational modifications of intracellular and extracellular proteins, which are known to occur with age, underlie some of the morphologic and functional changes in cell aging. One modification that has received attention is *nonenzymatic glycosylation of proteins*, leading to the formation of advanced glycosylation end products capable of cross-linking adjacent proteins.[54] There is a significant increase in such products with age, and, as we shall see, there is evidence that they play a role in the pathogenesis of the microvascular lesions of diabetes mellitus (see Chapter 19). Age-related glycosylation of lens proteins underlies senile cataracts.

Finally, there is evidence of *alterations in the induction of heat-shock proteins*, particularly Hsp70 *in vitro* in senescent cells and *in vivo* in experimental animals with age.[56] Because the heat-shock response is an important defense mechanism against a variety of stresses, its loss with age may decrease cell survival.

Much more might be said about the mechanisms responsible for the cell alterations that occur in cell aging, but it suffices here to say that some of these mechanisms are probably programmed and relatively unique events involving the proliferation and differentiation of cells, and others are the consequence of progressive environmental injury, overwhelming the cell's defense mechanisms. Oxidative free radical damage, post-translational modification of proteins, and alterations in the heat-shock response are possible molecular determinants of these exogenous structural and functional cell derangements.

CONCLUSION

It is apparent that the various forms of cellular derangements described cover a wide spectrum, ranging from the reversible and irreversible forms of acute cell injury, to the regulated type of cell death represented by apoptosis, to the pathologic alterations in cell organelles, to the less ominous forms of intracellular accumulations, including pigmentations. Reference will be made to all these alterations throughout this book because all organ injury and ultimately all clinical disease arise from derangements in cell structure and function.

1. Majno, G.: The Healing Hand: Man and Wound in the Ancient World. Boston, Harvard University Press, 1975, p. 43.
2. Szabo, S., and Kovacs, K.: Causes and mechanisms of cell and tissue injury in endocrine glands. In Kovacs, K., and Asa, S.L. (eds.): Functional Endocrine Pathology. Oxford, Blackwell Scientific Publications, 1992, pp. 914–933.
3. Mergner, W.J., et al. (eds.): Cell Death: Mechanisms of Acute and Lethal Cell Injury, Vol. 1. New York, Field and Wood Medical Publishers, 1990.
4. Buja, L.M., et al.: Apoptosis and necrosis: Basic types and mechanisms of cell death. Arch. Pathol. Lab. Med. 117:1208, 1993.
5. Reimer, K.A., and Ideker, R.E.: Myocardial ischemia and infarction. Hum. Pathol. 18:462, 1987.
6. Molitoris, B.A.: Ischemia-induced loss of polarity: Potential role of the actin cytoskeleton. Am. J. Physiol. 260:769, 1991.
7. Lemasters, J.J., et al.: Reperfusion injury to heart and liver cells: Protection by acidosis during ischemia and a "pH paradox" after reperfusion. In Hochachka, P.W., et al. (eds): Surviving Hypoxia: Mechanisms of Control and Adaptation. Boca Raton, FL, CRC Press, 1993, pp. 495–507.
8. Venkatachalam, M.A., et al.: Salvage of ischemia cells by impermeant solute and ATP. Lab. Invest. 49:1, 1983.
9. Bonventre, J.: Mechanisms of ischemic renal failure. Kidney Int. 43:1160, 1993.
10. Chien, K.R., et al.: Phospholipid alterations in canine ischemic myocardium: Temporal and topographical correlations with Tc-99m-PPi accumulation and an in vitro sarcolemmal Ca²⁺ permeability defect. Circ. Res. 48:711, 1981.
11. Das, D. K., et al.: Role of membrane phospholipids in myocardial injury induced by ischemia and reperfusion. Am. J. Physiol. 251:H71, 1986.
12. Armstrong, S.C., and Ganote, C. E.: Flow cytometric analysis of isolated rat cardiomyocytes: Vinculin and tubulin fluorescence during metabolic inhibition and ischemia. J. Mol. Cell. Cardiol. 24:149, 1992.
13. Menger, M.D., et al.: Microvascular ischemia/reperfusion injury in striated muscle: Significance of reflow paradox. Am. J. Physiol. 263:H1901, 1992.
14. Venkatachalam, M.A., et al.: Energy thresholds that determine membrane integrity and injury in a renal epithelial cell line (LLC-PK₁). J. Clin. Invest. 81:745, 1988.
15. Venkatachalam, M.A., and Weinberg, J.: Structural effects of intracellular amino acids during ATP depletion. In Hochachka, P.W., et al. (eds.): Surviving Hypoxia: Mechanisms of Control and Adaptation. Boca Raton, FL, CRC Press, 1993, pp. 473–491.
16. Farber, J.: Membrane injury and calcium homeostasis in the pathogenesis of coagulative necrosis. Lab. Invest. 47:114, 1982.
17. Borg, D.C.: Oxygen free radicals and tissue injury. In Tarr, M., and Samson, F. (eds.): Oxygen Free Radicals in Tissue Damage. Boston, Birkhauser, 1993, pp. 12–53.
18. Moslen, M.T.: Protection against free radical–mediated tissue injury. In Moslen, M. T., and Smith, C.V. (eds.): Free Radical Mechanisms of Tissue Injury. Boca Raton, FL, CRC Press, 1992, pp. 203–215.
19. Farber, J., et al.: The mechanisms of cell injury by activated oxygen species. Lab. Invest. 62:670, 1990.
20. Stadtman, E.R.: Protein oxidation and aging. Science 257:1220, 1992.
21. Farber, J.: Xenobiotics, drug metabolism, and liver injury. In Farber, E., et al. (eds.): Pathogenesis of Liver Diseases. Baltimore, Williams & Wilkins, 1987.
22. Nakae, D., et al.: Liposome-encapsulated superoxide dis-

mutase prevents liver necrosis induced by acetaminophen. Am. J. Pathol. *136*:787, 1990.

23. Majno, G., et al.: Cellular death and necrosis: Chemical, physical, and morphologic changes in rat liver. Virchows Arch. *333*:421, 1960.
24. Kerr, J.F., et al.: Apoptosis: A basic biological phenomenon with wide-ranging implications in tissue kinetics. Br. J. Cancer *26*:239, 1972.
25. Kerr, J.F.R., and Harmon, B.V.: Definition and incidence of apoptosis: A historical perspective. *In* Tomei, L.D., and Cope, F.O. (eds.): Apoptosis: The Molecular Basis of Cell Death. Cold Spring Harbor, NY, Cold Spring Harbor Laboratory Press, 1991.
26. Carson, D.A., and Ribeiro, J.M.: Apoptosis and disease. Lancet *341*:1251, 1993.
27. Gerschenson, L.E., and Rotello, R.J.: Apoptosis: A different type of cell death. FASEB J. *6*:2450, 1992.
28. Cohen, J.J., and Duke, R.C.: Apoptosis and programmed cell death in immunity. Annu. Rev. Immunol. *10*:267, 1992.
29. Wyllie, A.H., et al.: Cell death: The significance of apoptosis. Int. Rev. Cytol. *68*:251, 1980.
30. Wyllie, A.H.: Apoptosis and the regulation of cell numbers in normal and neoplastic tissues: An overview. Cancer Metastasis Rev. *11*:95, 1992.
31. Sun, D.Y., et al.: Separate metabolic pathways leading to DNA fragmentation and apoptotic chromatin condensation. J. Exp. Med. *179*:559, 1994.
32. Vaux, D.: Towards an understanding of the molecular mechanisms of physiological cell death. Proc. Natl. Acad. Sci. *90*:786, 1993.
33. Hengartner, M.O., et al.: *Caenorhabditis elegans* gene ced-9 protects cells from programmed cell death. Nature *356*:494, 1992.
34. Hengartner, M.O., and Horvitz, H.R.: *C. elegans* survival gene ced-9 encodes a functional homolog of the proto-oncogene bcl-2. Cell *76*:665, 1994.
35. Korsmeyer, S.J.: Bcl-2: An antidote of programmed cell death. Cancer Surv. *15*:105, 1992.
36. Bissonette, R.P., et al.: Apoptotic cell death induced by c-myc is inhibited by bcl-2. Nature *359*:552, 1992.
37. Lane, D.P.: A death in the life of p53. Nature *362*:786, 1993.
38. Welch, W.J.: Mammalian stress response: Cell physiology, structure/function of stress proteins, and implications for medicine and disease. Physiol. Rev. *72*:1063, 1992.
39. Craig, E.A.: Chaperones: Helpers along the pathways to protein folding. Science *260*:1902, 1993.
40. Knowlton, A.A., et al.: Rapid expression of heat shock protein in the rabbit after brief cardiac ischemia. J. Clin. Invest. *87*:139, 1991.
41. Cunie, R.W., et al.: Heat-shock response and limitation of tissue necrosis during occlusion/reperfusion in rabbit hearts. Circulation *87*:2023, 1993.
42. Dunn, W.A.: Studies on the mechanisms of autophagy. J. Cell Biol. *110*:1923, 1990.
43. Jones, A.L., and Fawcett, D.W.: Hypertrophy of the agranular endoplasmic reticulum in hamster liver induced by phenobarbital. J. Histochem. Cytochem. *14*:215, 1966.
44. Kachi, K., et al.: Synthesis of Mallory body, intermediate filament, and microfilament proteins in liver cell primary cultures. Lab. Invest. *68*:71, 1993.
45. Lee, R.J. (ed.): Fatty change and steatohepatitis. *In* Diagnostic Liver Pathology. St. Louis, Mosby-YearBook, 1994, pp. 167–194.
46. Wolman, M.: Pigments in Pathology. New York, Academic Press, 1969.
47. Sohal, R.S. (ed.): Age Pigments. New York, Elsevier North-Holland Biomedical Press, 1981.
48. Schoen, F.J., et al.: Calcification: Pathology, mechanisms, and strategies of prevention. J. Biomed. Mater. Res. *22*:A1, 1988.
49. Giachelli, C.M.: Osteopontin is elevated during intima formation in rat arteries and is a novel component of human atherosclerotic plaques. J. Clin. Invest. *92*:1686, 1993.
50. Martin, G.R., et al.: Aging—causes and defenses. Annu. Rev. Med. *44*:419, 1993.
51. Hayflick, L., and Moorhead, P.S.: The serial cultivation of human diploid cell strains. Exp. Cell Res. *25*:585, 1961.
52. Cristofalo, V.J., and Pignolo, R.J.: Replicative senescence of human cells in culture. Physiol. Rev. *73*:617, 1993.
53a. Broccoli, D., and Cooke, H.: Aging, healing, and telomeres. Am. J. Hum. Genet. *52*:657, 1993.
53b. Vaziri, R., et al.: Loss of telomeric DNA during aging. Am. J. Hum. Genet. *52*:661, 1993.
54. Yu, B.P.: Oxidative damage by free radicals and lipid peroxidation in aging. *In* Yu, B.P. (ed.): Free Radicals in Aging. Boca Raton, FL: CRC Press, 1993, pp. 57–88.
55. Bucala, R., and Cerami, A.: Advanced glycosylation: Chemistry, biology, and implications for diabetes and aging. Adv. Pharmacol. *23*:1, 1992.
56. Blake, M.J., et al.: Stress-induced heat shock protein 70 expression in adrenal cortex: An adrenocorticotropic hormone–sensitive, age-dependent response. Proc. Natl. Acad. Sci. U.S.A. *88*:9873, 1991.

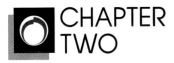

Cellular Growth and Differentiation: Normal Regulation and Adaptations

CONTROL OF CELL
GROWTH
CELL CYCLE AND TYPES OF
CELLS
MOLECULAR EVENTS IN CELL
GROWTH

GROWTH INHIBITION
GROWTH FACTORS
EXTRACELLULAR MATRIX
AND CELL-MATRIX
INTERACTIONS

CELLULAR ADAPTATIONS
OF GROWTH AND
DIFFERENTIATION
HYPERPLASIA

HYPERTROPHY
ATROPHY
METAPLASIA

The body's ability to replace injured or dead cells is critical to survival. Indeed, a variety of injurious agents—at the same time that they create havoc within the cell—set in motion a series of events that serve not only to contain the damage but also to prepare the nonlethally injured cells for the replication necessary to replace the dead cells. We have seen, for example, how the heat-shock response protects intracellular proteins, and how the initiation of apoptosis may delete cells bearing damaged DNA (which may be potentially harmful to the organism). Injurious stimuli, as we shall see, also trigger the activation of genes, such as c-*fos*, c-*jun*, and c-*myc*, that are involved in cell replication.

Repair of tissues involves two distinct processes: (1) *regeneration*, denoting the replacement of injured cells by cells of the same type, sometimes leaving no residual trace of the previous injury, and (2) *replacement by connective tissue*, or *fibroplasia*, which leaves a permanent scar. In most instances, both processes contribute to repair. In addition, both regeneration and fibroplasia are determined by essentially similar mechanisms involving cell migration, proliferation, and differentiation as well as cell-matrix interactions. The latter are particularly important. The orderly regeneration of the epithelial tissue of the skin and viscera requires the presence of the basement membrane (BM). This specialized extracellular matrix (ECM) functions as an extracellular scaffold for accurate regeneration of pre-existing structures. Maintenance of BM integrity provides for the specificity of cell type and polarity and influences cell migration, growth, and differentiation.

In adult tissues, the size of a population of cells is determined by the rates of cell proliferation, differentiation, and death by apoptosis.[1] Figure 2–1 depicts these relationships and shows that increased cell numbers may result from either increased proliferation or decreased cell death. The impact of *differentiation* depends on the circumstance under which it occurs. The progeny of stem cells in the bone marrow, for example, may divide several times but eventually become terminally differentiated and cannot multiply further. On the other hand, replication of differentiated cells occurs in certain adult tissues; for example, after partial hepatectomy, liver cell division continues until the signals for such division are abrogated.

35

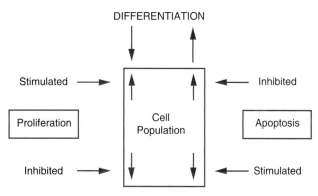

Figure 2–1. Control of cell populations. Cell numbers can be altered by increased or decreased apoptosis and changing rates of proliferation and differentiation. (Redrawn from McCarthy, N.J., Smith, C.A., and Williams, G.T.: Apoptosis in the development of the immune system: Growth factors, clonal selection, and bcl-2. Cancer Metastasis Rev. 11:157, 1992.)

Apoptosis, as we have reviewed in Chapter 1, is induced by a variety of injurious stimuli and is controlled by a number of genes.

In this chapter we shall review the mechanisms involved in the regulation of normal cell growth and the maintenance of normal cell populations and differentiation. Such mechanisms are critical to understanding the important process of wound healing (Chapter 3), and neoplasia (Chapter 7). In addition, we shall consider the adaptive changes in cell growth and differentiation that are particularly important in pathologic states. These include *hyperplasia* (increase in cell number), *hypertrophy* (increase in cell size), *atrophy* (decrease in cell size), and *metaplasia* (change in cell type).

CONTROL OF CELL GROWTH

Injury, cell death, and mechanical deformation of tissues all can stimulate cell proliferation; however, it is now clear that cell replication is controlled largely by chemical factors in the microenvironment, which either stimulate or inhibit cell proliferation. An excess of stimulators or a deficiency of inhibitors leads to net growth and, in the case of cancer, uncontrolled growth. Growth can be accomplished by shortening the cell cycle, but *the most important factors are those that recruit G_0 cells into the cell cycle.*[2]

CELL CYCLE AND TYPES OF CELLS

The cells of the body are divided into three groups on the basis of their proliferative capacity and their relationship to the cell cycle (Fig. 2–2).

1. *Continuously dividing cells* (also called *labile cells*) follow the cell cycle from one mitosis to the next and continue to proliferate throughout life, replacing cells that are continuously being destroyed. Tissues that contain labile cells include surface epithelia, such as stratified squamous surfaces of the skin, oral cavity, vagina, and cervix; the lining mucosa of all the excretory ducts of the glands of the body (e.g., salivary glands, pancreas, biliary tract); the columnar epithelium of the gastrointestinal tract and uterus; and the transitional epithelium of the urinary tract and cells of the bone marrow and hematopoietic tissues. In most of these tissues, regeneration is derived from a population of *stem cells*, which have an unlimited capacity to proliferate and whose progeny may undergo various streams of differentiation.

2. *Quiescent* (or *stable*) *cells* normally demonstrate a low level of replication; however, these cells can undergo rapid division in response to stimuli and are thus capable of reconstituting the tissue of origin. They are considered to be in G_0 but can be stimulated into G_1. In this category are the parenchymal cells of virtually all the glandular organs of the body, such as the liver, kidneys, and pancreas; mesenchymal cells, such as fibroblasts and smooth muscle; and vascular endothelial cells. The regenerative capacity of stable cells is best exemplified by the ability of the liver to regenerate after hepatectomy and following toxic, viral, or chemical injury.

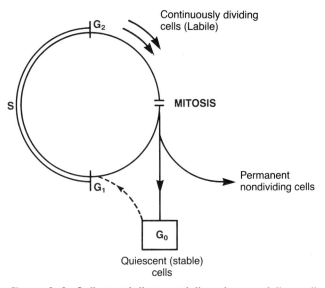

Figure 2–2. Cell populations and the phases of the cell cycle. Continuously dividing cells (labile cells) go around the cell cycle from one mitosis to the next. Nondividing cells have left the cycle and are destined to die without dividing again. Quiescent G_0 cells are neither cycling nor dying and can be induced to re-enter the cycle by an appropriate stimulus. (Modified and reprinted with permission from Baserga, R.: The cell cycle. The New England Journal of Medicine 304:453, 1981.)

Although labile and stable cells are capable of regeneration, it does not necessarily follow that there will be restitution of normal structure. *The underlying supporting stroma of the parenchymal cells—particularly, the basement membrane—is necessary for organized regeneration, forming a "scaffold" for the replicating parenchymal cells.* When BMs are disrupted, cells may proliferate in a haphazard fashion and produce disorganized masses of cells bearing no resemblance to the original arrangement. To use the liver as an example, the hepatitis virus destroys parenchymal cells without injuring the more resistant connective tissue cells, or framework, of the liver lobule. Thus, after viral hepatitis, regeneration of liver cells may completely reconstitute the liver lobule. By contrast, a liver abscess that destroys hepatocytes and the connective tissue framework is followed by scarring.

The *connective tissue and mesenchymal cells* (fibroblasts, endothelial cells, smooth muscle cells, chondrocytes, and osteocytes) are quiescent in adult mammals. However, all proliferate in response to injury, and fibroblasts in particular proliferate widely, constituting the connective tissue response to inflammation (see section on wound healing, Chapter 3.)

3. *Nondividing (permanent) cells* have left the cell cycle and cannot undergo mitotic division in postnatal life. To this group belong the nerve cells and the skeletal and cardiac muscle cells. *Neurons* destroyed in the central nervous system (CNS) are permanently lost. They are replaced by the proliferation of the CNS supportive elements, the glial cells. The situation is somewhat more complicated with respect to the neurons of the peripheral nerves, as detailed in Chapter 29. *Skeletal muscle* does have some regenerative capacity, and most of the regeneration appears to occur from transformation of the satellite cells found attached to the endomysial sheaths. If the ends of severed muscle fibers are closely juxtaposed, muscle regeneration in mammals can be excellent, but this is a condition that can rarely be attained under practical conditions. As to *cardiac muscle*, it is fair to state that if cardiac muscle has regenerative capacity, it is limited, and most large injuries to the heart are followed by connective tissue scarring. Certainly, scarring follows the all too common myocardial infarction in humans.

MOLECULAR EVENTS IN CELL GROWTH

Although many chemical substances can affect cell growth, the most important are *polypeptide growth factors* present in serum or produced by cells. Some of these substances are *competence factors,* which do not stimulate deoxyribonucleic acid (DNA) synthesis but render cells in G_0 or G_1 competent to do so; others are *progression factors,* which stimulate DNA synthesis in competent cells.[3] Most growth factors also influence a great number of other cell functions, and many initiate cell migration, differentiation, and tissue remodeling and may be involved in various stages of wound healing.

The explosion in our understanding of the molecular events that lead to cell proliferation has stemmed largely from the discovery that oncogenes (genes that are involved in cancer formation) are highly homologous to cellular genes involved in normal growth control (proto-oncogenes). Oncogenes are discussed in detail in the chapter on neoplasia (see Chapter 7). Here we shall review the chain of molecular events that leads to cell division and focus on those proteins that participate in the control of cell growth and that may be involved in oncogenesis.

LIGAND-RECEPTOR BINDING. Cell growth is initiated by the binding of a putative growth factor (ligand) to specific receptors either at the cell surface or inside the cell. Most of the growth factors have receptors on the plasma membrane, but steroid receptors are intracellular, interacting with lipophilic ligands that cross the cell membrane to interact with the receptor in the nucleus or cytoplasm.

GROWTH FACTOR RECEPTOR ACTIVATION. Most growth factor receptors (e.g., epidermal growth factor [EGF] and platelet-derived growth factor [PDGF] receptors) are equipped with intrinsic protein tyrosine kinase activity, which is activated after ligand binding. Such receptor kinases have a large glycosylated extracellular ligand–binding domain, a single hydrophobic transmembrane region, and a cytoplasmic domain that contains the tyrosine kinase activity. Ligand binding induces a conformational alteration of the extracellular domain, which in turn induces dimerization of receptors. It is thought that this dimerization, by allowing interactions between adjacent cytoplasmic domains, leads to activation (phosphorylation) of the kinase[4] (Fig. 2–4).

Other transmembrane growth factor receptors that do not possess endogenous kinase activity recruit intracellular protein kinases to the cell periphery. *The net result in either case is activation of a protein phosphorylation cascade, which stimulates quiescent cells to enter the growth cycle.*

SIGNAL TRANSDUCTION AND SECOND MESSENGERS. Tyrosine kinases are essential for signal transduction, *and thus phosphorylation of tyrosine residues on one or more target proteins is a critical event in the transfer of extracellular signals to cell proliferation.*[5] A series of proteins strategically located on or close to the inner surface of the cell membrane play a role in such signaling. The

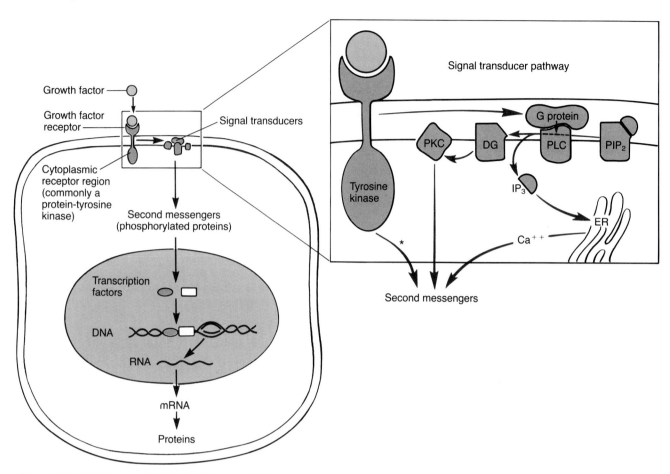

Figure 2–3. Cellular events initiated by growth factors shown here for platelet-derived growth factor (PDGF) (see text). The inset on the right illustrates some of the events in signal transduction. Certain growth factor receptors do not possess tyrosine kinase activity, as shown here, but recruit protein kinases (PKC) to the cell periphery. The events relating to *ras* protein activation are shown in Figure 2–5.

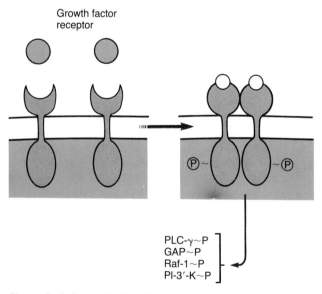

Figure 2–4. A mechanism for receptor tyrosine kinase activation. Engagement of PDGF receptor by PDGF causes a conformational alteration in its extracellular domain, in turn inducing dimerization of receptors and activation of the kinase by tyrosine phosphorylation.

initial activation of these signaling proteins appears to result from the binding of specific domains (called (SH2), for *src* homology) to the phosphotyrosine of the activated receptor.[6] The signaling proteins include the following:

- *Phospholipase C-γ.* This enzyme catalyzes the degradation of phosphatidylinositol-4,5-biphosphate (PIP_2), resulting in the generation of two second messengers: inositol-1,4,5-triphosphate (IP_3), which releases intracellular calcium stores, and diacylglycerol (DAG).[10] DAG, in turn, activates protein kinase C (PKC), a member of a family of serine threonine kinases that are bound to the plasma membrane and are thus in the same perimembrane region as the kinases of the receptors (see Fig. 2–3).
- *GTP-binding proteins.* These are the well-known G proteins and the *ras family of proteins.* They function by coupling the extracellular signals to cellular effectors (such as phospholipase). Normally, *ras* proteins are present in an *inactive GDP-binding form.* This is converted to the *active GTP-binding form* by a protein complex

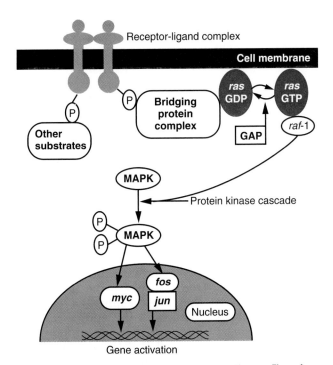

Figure 2–5. The *ras* signal transduction pathway. The phosphorylated receptor tyrosine kinase binds to a bridging protein complex which converts inactive *ras* GDP to active *ras* GTP. The *ras* GTP activates *raf*-1, which in turn phosphorylates a series of other mitogen-induced protein kinases (MAPKs), leading to activation of nuclear transcription factors. GAP, also phosphorylated by receptor-ligand binding, counteracts *ras* activation.

TRANSCRIPTION FACTORS. The precise method by which the signals for mitosis are transferred across the cytoplasm is unknown, but the cascade of MAP kinases[12] as well as a variety of second messengers (CA^{2+}, calmodulin) eventually transmit the growth signal to the nucleus, where a large number of cellular genes are induced.[13] These have been divided into *early growth-regulated genes* (e.g., c-*fos*, c-*jun*, and c-*myc*), whose mRNAs increase well before mid-G_1 of the cell cycle and which are induced *in the absence of protein synthesis;* and *late growth-regulated genes*, whose mRNAs start to increase in mid-G_1, or even at the G_1-G_s boundary and which are dependent on protein synthesis. It should be emphasized that not only growth factors but also a variety of other injurious stimuli (e.g., ischemia, irradiation, chemicals) activate the immediate early response genes. Among the growth-regulated genes are a number of proto-oncogenes in which mutations may be associated with malignant transformation. Some, such as *myc*, *fos*, and *jun*, code for transcription factors and are involved in the regulation of DNA synthesis and, possibly, cell division. The importance of these proto-oncogenes in normal cell growth is well exemplified by their expression during liver regeneration after partial hepatectomy in rats, as we shall see. Their role in oncogenesis is discussed in Chapter 7.

Cell Cycle and Cyclins

Thus far we have discussed the cellular events initiated by growth factor stimulation, but what precisely are the signals that trigger the orchestrated events that lead to cell division? The evidence is now clear that these processes are controlled by changes in the intracellular concentration and activity of a group of proteins called *cyclins*, which form a complex with a constitutively present protein kinase called cdc2 or p34^{cdc2}.[14] The cyclin-kinase complexes phosphorylate a number of substrate proteins involved in DNA replication, formation of mitotic spindle, and other events in the cell cycle. Levels of G_1 *cyclins* (cyclins D_1, E) rise sharply before entry of the cell into the S phase, and the G_1 cyclin–cdc2 complexes trigger DNA replication.[15] During the G_2 phase (Fig. 2–6) genes for a different set of cyclins called G_2 or *B cyclins* are induced. The phosphorylated cdc2–cyclin B complex is the active kinase that induces mitosis, and a number of kinases and phosphatases contribute to its activation (see Fig. 2–6). Following cell division the B cyclins are degraded, and in the presence of a stimulus the daughter cells start a new cell cycle again. Some of the oncogenes, such as *bcl1*,[16] and antioncogenes, such as *Rb* gene and possibly p53, act in the cyclin pathway to control cell growth[17] (see Chapter 7).

To summarize, polypeptide growth factors bind to and activate their receptors, many of which pos-

which forms a bridge between the receptor phosphotyrosine and *ras*[7] (Fig. 2–5). Activation of *ras* is counteracted by another protein, GAP (GTPase-activating protein), which augments the GTPase activity of *ras* and thus switches *ras* to the inactive GDP form.[9] Activated *ras*, in turn, phosphorylates a cascade of cytoplasmic enzymes, called mitogen-activated protein kinases (MAPKs), culminating in the activation of transcription factors important for cell division (see Fig. 2–5).[8] Thus, *ras* plays a central role in signal transduction leading to mitogenesis, and it is not surprising that about one-third of all human cancers contain mutated versions of the *ras* proteins, as will be explained in Chapter 7.

- *Raf-1*. This is a serine threonine kinase that is activated by growth factors. *Raf-1* itself is activated by *ras*, and in turn activates the rest of the MAPK.

Protein phosphorylation is counteracted by a number of *cellular phosphatases*, which are receiving increased attention as regulators of cell growth, either by balancing the action of kinases, thus acting as growth inhibitors, or by direct effects on protein substrates important in mitogenesis (see later, in the section on cell cycle, and Fig. 2–6).

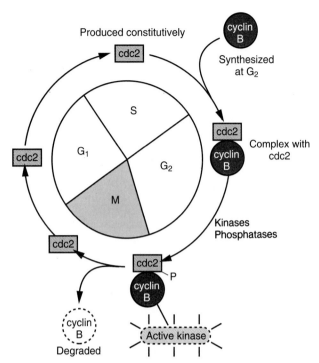

Figure 2–6. Mitotic activation of cdc2 by cyclin B (G₂ cyclin). Similar reactions regulate cyclin A/cdc2 activation. (Courtesy of Dr. Anindya Dutta.)

sess tyrosine kinase activity. The activation phosphorylates several substrates that are involved in signal transduction and the generation of second messengers, including ras proteins, phospholipase C-γ, and raf-1. A cascade of kinases, in turn, transmit the signals to the nucleus, where activation of transcription factors leads to the initiation of DNA synthesis and, ultimately, cell division. This process of cell cycling is tuned by a family of proteins, appropriately called cyclins, that complex with cdc kinases to phosphorylate the substrate proteins involved in mitosis.

GROWTH INHIBITION

The other side of the coin in cellular growth control is growth inhibition. The existence of growth inhibitory signals that maintain the integrity of a tissue has been suspected for decades from observations that populations of cells in culture or *in vivo* can limit one another's growth. *Contact inhibition* of growth in confluent cultures is one such manifestation of growth inhibition. There is also *in vivo* evidence for growth suppression. After partial hepatectomy, for example, cells stop multiplying when the liver has attained its normal preoperative size and configuration, suggesting the action of an inhibitory signal. The recent discovery that loss of tumor suppressor genes (or antioncogenes) occurs in certain cancers suggests that such

genes encode components of some cellular inhibitory pathway. Growth inhibition, like growth stimulation, apparently utilizes polypeptide factors and signal transducers, including cell surface receptors, cytoplasmic second messengers, and transcription regulators. Few of these mechanisms have been well described, although work with tumor suppressor genes gives some clues (see Chapter 7). Polypeptide factors that act as growth inhibitors are transforming growth factor-beta (TGF-β), tumor necrosis factor (TNF), and the cytokine interferon-beta. Insoluble extracellular matrix molecules may also serve to suppress cell responsiveness to soluble mitogens in the local tissue microenvironment. All these factors are described later.

Finally, it should be mentioned that these two pathways—growth inhibition and growth stimulation—almost certainly intertwine along their intracellular routes. One example is the interaction of the product of the tumor suppressor gene of neurofibromatosis type 1 with the normal *ras* p21 protein, serving to inactivate the p21 protein (see Chapter 7). You will recall that the *ras* protein is involved in signal transduction after stimulation by growth factors.

GROWTH FACTORS

Having reviewed the molecular events in cell growth, we can now turn to a description of polypeptide growth factors (Table 2–1).[18] Some of the

Table 2–1. GROWTH FACTORS

EPIDERMAL GROWTH FACTOR FAMILY (EGF)
  EGF
  Transforming growth factor α
PLATELET-DERIVED GROWTH FACTOR (PDGF)
FIBROBLAST GROWTH FACTOR
  Basic
  Acidic
TRANSFORMING GROWTH FACTOR β (TGF) FAMILY
  TGF isoforms
INSULIN-LIKE GROWTH FACTORS (IGF)
  IGF-1
  IGF-2
VASOPERMEABILITY FACTOR (VPF)
  (Endothelial cell–derived growth factor (ECGF))
HEPATIC GROWTH FACTOR (Scatter factor)
MYELOID COLONY-STIMULATING FACTORS (CSFs)
  Granulocyte-macrophage CSF (GM-CSF)
  Granulocyte CSF (G-CSF)
  Macrophage CSF (M-CSF)
ERYTHROPOIETIN
CYTOKINES
  Interleukins
  Tumor necrosis factor (TNF)
  Interferons
NERVE GROWTH FACTOR (NGF)

growth factors act on a variety of cell types, whereas others have relatively specific targets. Growth factors also have effects on cell locomotion, contractility, and differentiation—effects that may be as important to repair and wound healing as the growth-promoting effects.

Growth factors act by endocrine, paracrine, or autocrine signaling. Paracrine stimulation is most common in connective tissue repair by healing wounds, in which a factor produced by one cell type has its growth effect on adjacent cells, usually of a different cell type (e.g., macrophage-derived growth factors acting on fibroblasts). Many cells, however, have receptors for their endogenously produced growth factors (autocrine stimulation), a process that plays a role in compensatory epithelial hyperplasia (e.g., hepatic regeneration) and, particularly, in tumors.

Table 2–1 lists the most important groups of growth factors. Here we shall review only those that have broad targets and seem to be involved in general pathologic processes. More specific growth factors will be alluded to in other sections of the book.

1. *Epidermal growth factor (EGF)/transforming growth factor-alpha (TGF-α)*. EGF was first discovered by its ability to cause precocious tooth eruption and eyelid opening in newborn mice.[19] EGF is mitogenic for a variety of epithelial cells and fibroblasts *in vitro* and causes hepatic cell division *in vivo*. It stimulates cell division by binding to specific tyrosine kinase receptors on the cell membrane, followed by the events described earlier. The EGF receptor is c-*erb* B1.[20] EGF is widely distributed in tissue secretions and fluids, such as saliva, urine, and intestinal contents.

TGF-α was initially extracted from sarcoma virus–transformed cells and was thought to be involved in transformation of normal cells to cancer. TFG-α has extensive homology with EGF, binds to the EFG receptor, and produces most of the biologic activities of EGF.

2. *Platelet-derived growth factor (PDGF)*. This is a highly cationic protein (of approximately 30,000 daltons) composed of two chains (A and B). PDGF is stored in the platelet alpha granules and released on platelet activation.[5] It can also be produced by activated macrophages, endothelial and smooth muscle cells, and a variety of tumor cells. PDGF causes both migration and proliferation of fibroblasts, smooth muscle cells, and monocytes and has other proinflammatory properties as well. It binds to two types of specific receptors (α and β) that have protein kinase activity.

3. *Fibroblast growth factors (FGFs)*. First described as fibroblast mitogens extracted from bovine brain and pituitary, basic and acidic FGF (β-FGF, α-FGF) represent a family of polypeptide factors that have many activities in addition to growth stimulation.[21] Basic FGF, in particular, has *the ability to induce all the steps necessary for new blood vessel formation (angiogenesis)*, both *in vivo* and *in vitro* (see Chapter 3). FGFs have strong affinity for heparin (heparin-binding growth factors) and other anionic molecules and bind avidly to BMs. *Basic FGF* is present in the extracts of many organs and is elaborated by activated macrophages, whereas *acidic FGF* is confined to neural tissue.

4. *TGF-β and related growth factors*. TFG-β belongs to a family of homologous polypeptides that includes three isoforms of mammalian TFG-β (TGF-β-1–3) and factors of such wide-ranging functions as bone morphogenetic protein (BMP) and Müllerian inhibitory factor.[22] TFG-β-1 is the most widespread in distribution in mammals. TFG-β has varied and often conflicting effects. It is a *growth inhibitor* to most epithelial cell types in culture. Its effects on fibroblasts and smooth muscle cell proliferation are variable. In low concentrations, it induces the synthesis and secretion of PDGF and is thus indirectly mitogenic. In high concentrations, it is growth inhibitory, owing to its ability to inhibit the expression of PDGF receptors. TFG-β also stimulates fibroblast chemotaxis and the production of collagen and fibronectin by cells, at the same time inhibiting collagen degradation by decreasing proteases and increasing protease inhibitors (see Chapter 3). *All these effects favor fibrogenesis*, and indeed there is increasing evidence that TGF-β is involved in the development of fibrosis in a variety of chronic inflammatory conditions.[24] TFG-β is produced by different cell types, including platelets, endothelial cells, T cells, and macrophages.

5. *Cytokines*. Many of these are growth factors, and indeed there is so much overlap between these two groups of mediators as to make distinctions between them tenuous. *Interleukin-1 (IL-1)* and *TNF*, for example, are mitogenic and chemotactic for fibroblasts, and they stimulate the synthesis of both collagen and collagenase by fibroblasts. They are known as the *fibrogenic cytokines*.

EXTRACELLULAR MATRIX AND CELL-MATRIX INTERACTIONS

Cells grow, move, and differentiate in intimate contact with the extracellular matrix, and there is

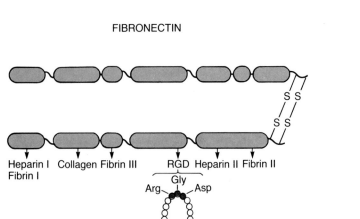

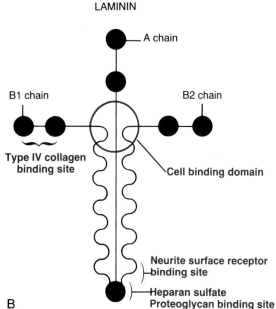

Figure 2–7. The fibronectin molecule (A) consists of a dimer held by S—S bonds. Note the various domains that bind to extracellular matrices and the cell-binding domain containing an Arg-Gly-Asp sequence. The cross-shaped laminin (B) molecule spans BMs and has ECM and cell-binding domains. (B Reproduced, with permission, from The Annual Review of Cell Biology, Vol. 3 © 1987 by Annual Reviews Inc.)

overwhelming evidence that the matrix critically influences these cell functions.[25]

The ECM, which forms a significant proportion of the volume of any tissue, consists of *fibrous structural proteins* and an interstitial matrix composed of *adhesive glycoproteins* embedded in a gel of proteoglycans and glycosaminoglycans.[26] The fibrous structural proteins are the collagens and elastin. The interstitial matrix is organized as a basement membrane (BM) around epithelial, endothelial, and smooth muscle cells. Besides its well-known function of providing turgor to soft tissues and rigidity to skeletal tissues, ECM and, particularly, the BM provide a substratum where cells can adhere, migrate, and proliferate and directly influence the form and function of cells.

COLLAGEN. *The collagens* are composed of a triple helix of three polypeptide alpha chains, having a gly-x-y repeating sequence. About 30 distinct alpha chains form approximately 15 distinct collagen types. Some collagen types form fibrils (e.g., the interstitial or fibrillar collagens, types I, III, and V), whereas others (e.g., type IV) are nonfibrillar and are components of BMs. The interstitial collagens form a major proportion of the connective tissue in healing wounds, and particularly in scars. These collagens as well as elastin will be discussed further separately in the section on wound healing (Chapter 3).

ADHESIVE GLYCOPROTEINS. These are structurally diverse proteins whose major property is their ability to bind with other ECM components, on the

one hand, and to specific integral cell membrane proteins on the other. *They thus link ECM components to one another and to cells.* They include fibronectin, laminin, thrombospondin, tenascin, and others, but here we shall discuss only the first two (Fig. 2–7).

Fibronectin is a large (400 kd) multifunctional glycoprotein consisting of two chains held together by disulfide bonds (see Fig. 2–7A).[27] Associated with cell surfaces, BMs, and pericellular matrices, fibronectin is produced by fibroblasts, monocytes, endothelial cells, and other cells. Fibronectin binds to a number of other ECM components (including collagen, fibrin, heparin, and proteoglycans) via specific domains and to cells via *integrin receptors.* Integrins are transmembrane glycoproteins made up of alpha and beta chains whose intracellular domains interact, *in areas of focal adhesion,* with elements of the cytoskeleton (e.g., talin, vinculin, alpha-actinin, actin), to signal cell attachment, locomotion, or differentiation.[28] Their extracellular domains bind to fibronectin by recognizing the specific amino acid sequence of the tripeptide arginine-glycine-aspartic acid (RGD), a sequence that is thought to play a key role in cell adhesion (see Fig. 2–7A). One scenario for such interactions in the focal adhesion complex is shown in Figure 2–8B. Thus, fibronectin is thought to be directly involved in attachment, spreading, and migration of cells. In addition, it serves to enhance the sensitivity of certain cells, such as capillary endothelial cells, to the proliferative effects of growth factors.

Laminin is the most abundant glycoprotein in

BMs. It is a large (800 to 1000 kd) cross-shaped structure that spans the BM and binds, on the one hand, with specific receptors on the surface of cells and, on the other, with matrix components such as collagen type IV and heparan sulfate. Laminin is also believed to mediate cell attachment to connective tissue substrates; in culture, it alters the growth, survival, morphology, differentiation, and motility of various cell types. In endothelial cell cultures exposed to FGF, laminin causes alignment of endothelial cells and subsequent capillary tube formation, a most critical event in angiogenesis. Other ECMs can also induce capillary tube formation.

The molecular pathways that link extracellular matrix proteins to the control of cell growth and differentiation are less clear than those that are involved in cell stimulation by growth factors, described earlier. It is likely, however, that receptors for growth factors and different ECM molecules may share common intracellular signaling mecha-

nisms.[29] For example, adhesion to fibronectin stimulates PIP_2 synthesis in cells (PIP_2, as you recall, is hydrolyzed to IP_3 and DAG by phospholipase C-γ); (see Fig. 2–3) and also enhances PIP_2 hydrolysis in response to growth factors.[30]

PROTEOGLYCANS. These compose the third component of the ECM. Proteoglycans consist of glycosaminoglycans (e.g., dermatan sulfate and heparan sulfate) linked covalently to a protein core. Glycosaminoglycans without a protein core, such as hyaluronic acid, can also be found in tissues. They have diverse roles in regulating connective tissue structure and permeability. Proteoglycans can also be integral membrane proteins and are thus modulators of cell growth and differentiation. For example, *syndecan*, an integral membrane glycoprotein, binds collagen, fibronectin, thrombospondin, and basic fibroblast growth factor. It associates with actin cytoskeleton and has been shown to maintain the morphology of epithelial sheets.[31]

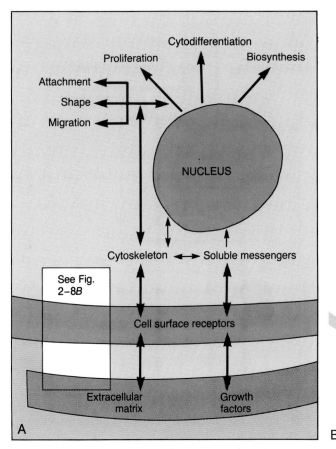

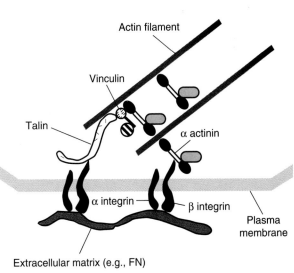

Figure 2–8. *A*, Schema of possible mechanisms by which extracellular matrix (ECM) and growth factors influence cell shape, motility, and growth. Receptors for ECM, such as the integrins — which recognize the RGD sequence — interact with various proteins of the cytoskeleton at focal adhesions and initiate the production of diffusible second messengers, which act on both nucleus and cytoplasm to cause the cell responses, as illustrated. Cell surface receptors to growth factors also initiate second messengers, which modulate cell growth, locomotion, and differentiation. (Redrawn from Madri, J., et al.: *In* Simionescu, N., and Simionescu, M. (eds.): Endothelial Cell Biology. New York, Plenum Publishing, 1988.) *B*, One scenario for the molecular interactions in a focal adhesion complex. Note that integrins join the ECM to contractile elements (actin) via a variety of cytoskeletal proteins. (Courtesy of Dr. Donald Ingber, Harvard Medical School.)

To summarize, cell growth and differentiation involve at least two groups of signals, one soluble and the other insoluble. Soluble molecules are largely polypeptide growth factors and growth inhibitors. Insoluble factors are the ECMs, such as laminin, fibronectin, collagens, and proteoglycans, and these usually act in concert as regulators of cell growth and differentiation. Figure 2–8 is a model of the interactions between growth factors, ECM, and cell responses.

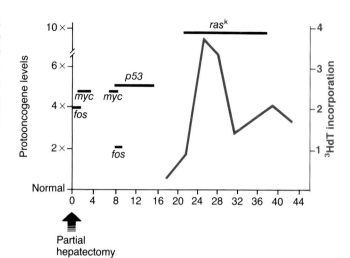

Figure 2–9. Expression of proto-oncogenes after partial hepatectomy and its relation to DNA synthesis by hepatocytes, shown here by the level of 3H-thymidine incorporation. Note that there is induction of *fos, myc,* and p53 prior to the onset of DNA synthesis. During the S phase, *ras*^κ peaks. (Courtesy of Dr. Nelson Fausto, Brown University, Providence, RI.)

CELLULAR ADAPTATIONS OF GROWTH AND DIFFERENTIATION

As explained earlier, cells must constantly adapt, even under normal conditions, to changes in their environment. These *physiologic adaptations* usually represent responses of cells to normal stimulation by hormones or endogenous chemical substances —for example, as in the enlargement of the breast and induction of lactation by pregnancy. *Pathologic adaptations* may share the same underlying mechanisms, but they provide the cells with the ability to survive in their environment and perhaps escape injury. Cellular adaptation, then, is a state that lies intermediate between the normal, unstressed cell and the injured, overstressed cell.

There are numerous types of cellular adaptations. Some involve *up- or down-regulation of specific cellular receptors* involved in metabolism of certain components—for example, in the regulation of cell surface receptors involved in the uptake and degradation of low-density lipoproteins (LDL) (see Chapter 5). Others are associated with the *induction of new protein synthesis by the target cell*, as in the heat-shock response. Other adaptations involve a switch by cells from producing one type of a family of proteins to another or markedly overproducing one protein; such is the case in cells producing various types of collagens and ECM proteins in chronic inflammation and fibrosis (see Chapter 3). These adaptations then involve all steps of cellular metabolism of proteins—*receptor binding, signal transduction, transcription, translation*, or *regulation of protein packaging and release*.

In this section we consider some common adaptive changes in cell growth, size, and differentiation that underlie many pathologic processes.

HYPERPLASIA

Hyperplasia constitutes an increase in the number of cells in an organ or tissue, which may then have increased volume. Hypertrophy (increase in cell size) and hyperplasia are closely related and often develop concurrently. Hypertrophy does not involve cell division, but hyperplasia takes place if the cellular population is capable of synthesizing DNA, thus permitting mitotic division.

Hyperplasia can be *physiologic* or *pathologic*.

PHYSIOLOGIC HYPERPLASIA. This can be divided into (1) *hormonal hyperplasia*, best exemplified by the proliferation of the glandular epithelium of the female breast at puberty and during pregnancy, and the physiologic hyperplasia that occurs in the pregnant uterus; and (2) *compensatory hyperplasia*, for example, the hyperplasia that occurs when a portion of the liver is removed (partial hepatectomy). The ancient Greeks knew of the capacity of the liver to regenerate. According to the myth, Prometheus was chained to a mountain, and his liver was daily devoured by a vulture, only to regenerate anew every night.

The experimental model of partial hepatectomy has been especially useful in examining mechanisms of compensatory hyperplasia. In the normal mature liver, only 0.5 to 1.0% of cells are undergoing DNA replication. An increase in the number of DNA-synthesizing cells begins as early as 12 hours after hepatectomy and peaks between 1 and 2 days later, when about 10% of all cells may be involved in DNA synthesis (Fig. 2–9). Initiation of cell growth is associated with specific and sequential increases in the expression of proto-oncogenes (e.g., c-*fos*, c-*myc*, c-*ras*) involved in cell proliferation (see Fig. 2–9). Subsequently, DNA synthesis declines, and by the time the liver mass is restored (at 1 to 2 weeks), the liver cells become quiescent again.

There is substantial evidence that cell proliferation in this setting is dependent on the action of

PARTIAL HEPATECTOMY

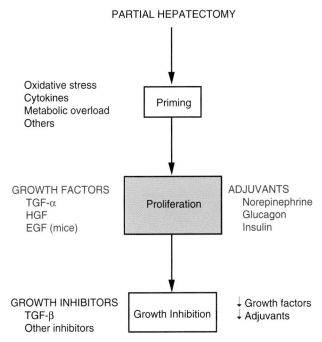

Oxidative stress
Cytokines
Metabolic overload
Others

Priming

GROWTH FACTORS
TGF-α
HGF
EGF (mice)

Proliferation

ADJUVANTS
Norepinephrine
Glucagon
Insulin

GROWTH INHIBITORS
TGF-β
Other inhibitors

Growth Inhibition

↓ Growth factors
↓ Adjuvants

Figure 2–10. Postulated sequence of events in the compensatory hyperplasia following partial hepatectomy.

polypeptide growth factors.[32] Two growth factors seem to be the most critical: *TFG-α and hepatocyte growth factor (HGF). TFG-α* is mitogenic for hepatocytes in culture, and its expression is markedly increased in remnant hepatic cells 4 to 24 hours after partial hepatectomy. *Hepatic growth factor (HGF),*[33] initially identified in the serum of hepatectomized rats as a potent mitogen for cultured hepatocytes,[34] is produced in the liver by nonparenchymal cells and by mesenchymal cells in many organs. These growth factors, however, do not seem to be sufficient to induce proliferation in normal liver cells *in vivo,* and it has been proposed that an initial "priming" signal to the remnant hepatic cells is necessary for the full effect of these mitogens[32] (Fig. 2–10). Such priming signals may include metabolic overload secondary to the hepatectomy, cytokines (e.g., TNF) or oxidative stress, as these are known to activate such early growth response genes as c-*fos,* c-*jun,* and c-*myc.* In addition, certain hormones, such as insulin, glucagon, and norepinephrine, whose blood levels are also increased following hepatectomy, may function as adjuvants for cell proliferation. Cessation of cell growth, after the liver mass has been restored, appears to be caused by *growth inhibitors* produced in the liver itself. One of these inhibitors is TGF-β, which is produced by nonparenchymal cells of the liver.

In addition to proliferating differentiated hepatocytes, adult livers contain a small population of *stem cells* located in the junction between hepatocytes and the smallest segments of the biliary tree. Such stem cells do not play a major role in the compensatory hyperplasia following hepatectomy but give rise to the proliferating "oval cells" that arise after some forms of toxic liver injury.[36]

PATHOLOGIC HYPERPLASIA. Most forms of *pathologic hyperplasia are instances of excessive hormonal stimulation or are the effects of growth factors on target cells. An example of hormonally induced hyperplasia is hyperplasia of the endometrium.* After a normal menstrual period, there is a rapid burst of proliferative activity, which might be viewed as reparative proliferation or physiologic hyperplasia in the endometrium. As is well known, this proliferation is potentiated by pituitary hormones and ovarian estrogen. It is brought to a halt by the rising levels of progesterone, usually about 10 to 14 days before the anticipated menstrual period. In some instances, however, the balance between estrogen and progesterone is disturbed. This results in absolute or relative increases in the amount of estrogen, or both, with consequent hyperplasia of the endometrial glands. Although this form of hyperplasia is a common cause of abnormal menstrual bleeding, the hyperplastic process remains controlled nonetheless: if the estrogenic stimulation abates, the hyperplasia disappears. Thus, it responds to regular growth control of cells. As will be discussed in the chapter on neoplasia, it is this response to normal regulatory control mechanisms that differentiates benign pathologic hyperplasias from cancer. However, it should be stressed here that *pathologic hyperplasia constitutes a fertile soil in which cancerous proliferation may eventually arise.* Thus, patients with hyperplasia of the endometrium are at increased risk for developing endometrial cancer (see Chapter 23).

Hyperplasia is also an important response of connective tissue cells in wound healing, in which proliferating fibroblasts and blood vessels aid in repair. Under these circumstances growth factors are responsible for the hyperplasia. Stimulation by growth factors is also involved in the hyperplasia that is associated with certain *virus infections,* such as papillomaviruses, causing skin warts. These warts are composed largely of masses of hyperplastic epithelium.

HYPERTROPHY

Hypertrophy refers to an increase in the size of cells and, with such change, an increase in the size of the organ. Thus, the hypertrophied organ has no new cells, just larger cells. The increased size of the cells is due not to an increased intake of fluid, called cellular swelling or edema, but to the synthesis of more structural components.

Hypertrophy can be *physiologic* or *pathologic* and is caused by increased functional demand or by specific hormonal stimulation. The physiologic growth of the uterus during pregnancy involves

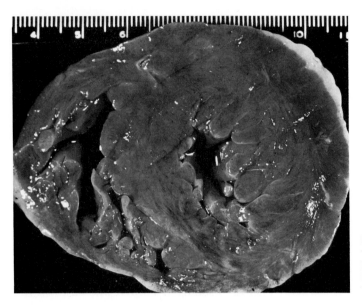

Figure 2–11. Cross-section of a heart with marked left ventricular hypertrophy. The left ventricular wall *(right)* is over 2 cm in thickness (normal = 1 to 1.5 cm). In the interventricular septum, the mottled, dark area is a focus of fresh ischemic necrosis (myocardial infarct).

both hypertrophy and hyperplasia. The cellular hypertrophy is stimulated by estrogenic hormones through smooth muscle estrogen receptors, which allow for interactions of the hormones with nuclear DNA, eventually resulting in increased synthesis of smooth muscle proteins and an increase in cell size. This is then physiologic hypertrophy effected by hormonal stimulation. Hypertrophy as an adaptive response is exemplified by muscular enlargement. The striated muscle cells in both the heart and skeletal muscles are most capable of hypertrophy, perhaps because they cannot adapt to increased metabolic demands by mitotic division and formation of more cells to share the work.

The environmental change that produces hypertrophy of striated muscle appears mainly to be increased workload. In the heart, the most common stimulus is chronic hemodynamic overload, due either to hypertension or to faulty valves (Fig. 2–11). In skeletal muscles, it is heavy work. Synthesis of more proteins and filaments occurs, achieving a balance between the demand and the cell's functional capacity. The greater number of myofilaments permits an increased workload with a level of metabolic activity per unit volume of cell not different from that borne by the normal cell. Thus the draft horse readily pulls the load that would break the back of a pony.

Not only the size but also the phenotype of the individual myocytes is altered in hypertrophy (Fig. 2–12).[37] In volume overload, for example, there is a switch of contractile proteins to fetal or neonatal forms. For example, there is activation of the beta-myosin heavy chain (β-MHC) and repression of the α-MHC gene, as well as switching from alpha cardiac to alpha skeletal isoactin genes — both of these alterations result in slower velocity of contraction in the hypertrophied fibers. A number of other genes are also activated during hypertrophy, including some of the early growth regula-

tion genes,[38] heat-shock response genes, growth factor genes (TFG-β), and the gene for atrial natriuretic factor (ANF), a peptide hormone that by regulating blood pressure and causing salt secretion by the kidney serves to reduce hemodynamic load.[39]

But what are the triggers for hypertrophy and for these changes in gene expression? In the heart there are at least two groups of signals: *mechanical triggers,* such as stretch, and *trophic triggers,* such as polypeptide growth factors and vasoactive agents (angiotensin II, alpha-adrenergic agonists).[40]

Whatever the exact mechanism of hypertrophy, it eventually reaches a limit beyond which enlargement of muscle mass is no longer able to compensate for the increased burden, and cardiac failure ensues. At this stage, a number of "degenerative" changes occur in the myocardial fibers, of which the most important are lysis and loss of myofibrillar contractile elements. The limiting factors for continued hypertrophy and the causes of the cardiac dysfunction are poorly understood; they may be due to limitation of the vascular supply to the enlarged fibers, diminished oxidative capabilities of mitochondria, alterations in protein synthesis and degradation, or cytoskeletal alterations.[41]

Although hypertrophy and hyperplasia are two distinct processes, frequently both occur together, and they may well be triggered by the same mechanism. Estrogen-induced growth in the uterus involves both increased DNA synthesis and enlargement of smooth muscle and epithelium. In certain instances, however, even cells capable of dividing, such as renal epithelial cells, undergo hypertrophy but not hyperplasia. Growth inhibitors, such as TGF-β, may be involved in this phenomenon. In *nondividing cells* (e.g., myocardial fibers), only hypertrophy occurs. Nuclei in such cells have a much higher DNA content than that of normal myocar-

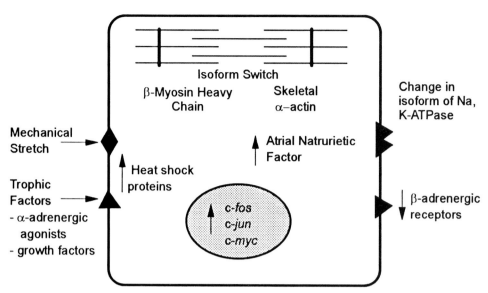

Figure 2–12. Phenotypic changes in hypertrophy, shown here in myocardial fibers subjected to hemodynamic overload. (Modified and redrawn with permission of the publisher by Dr. C. McLachlin from Boheler, K.R., and Schwartz, K.: Gene expression in cardiac hypertrophy. Trends Cardiovasc. Med. 2:176, 1992. Copyright 1992 by Elsevier Science Inc.)

dial cells, probably because the cells arrest in the G_2 phase of the cell cycle without undergoing mitosis.

ATROPHY

Shrinkage in the size of the cell by loss of cell substance is known as atrophy. It represents a form of adaptive response. When a sufficient number of cells are involved, the entire tissue or organ diminishes in size or becomes atrophic.

The causes of atrophy are the following:

1. Decreased workload
2. Loss of innervation
3. Diminished blood supply
4. Inadequate nutrition
5. Loss of endocrine stimulation
6. Aging

When a limb is immobolized in a plaster cast, or when muscles become paralyzed from loss of innervation as in poliomyelitis, atrophy of muscle ensues. In late adult life, the brain undergoes progressive atrophy, presumably as atherosclerosis narrows its blood supply (Fig. 2–13), and the sex glands shrink with depletion of endocrine stimulation. Some of these stimuli are physiologic (e.g., the loss of endocrine stimulation following the menopause), whereas others are clearly pathologic (e.g., loss of nerves). However, the fundamental cellular change is identical in all, representing a retreat by the cell to a smaller size at which survival is still possible. By bringing into balance cell volume and lower levels of blood supply, nutrition, or trophic stimulation, a new equilibrium is achieved. Although *atrophic cells may have diminished function, they are not dead.* However, apop-

tosis may be induced by the same signals that cause atrophy and thus may contribute to loss of organ mass. For example, as described earlier, apoptosis contributes to the regression of endocrine organs after hormone withdrawal and the shrinkage of secretory glands after obstruction of their ducts.

Atrophy represents a reduction in the structural components of the cell. The cell contains fewer mitochondria and myofilaments and a lesser amount of endoplasmic reticulum. The biochemical mechanisms responsible for atrophy are incompletely understood, but it must be stressed that there is a finely regulated balance between protein synthesis and degradation in normal cells, and either decreased synthesis or increased catabolism, or both, may cause atrophy. Hormones, particularly insulin, thyroid hormones, glucocorticoids, and prostaglandins, influence such protein turnover. Thus, only slight increases of degradation over a long period of time may result in atrophy, as seems to occur in some muscle dystrophies. Intracytoplasmic *nonlysosomal proteinases* play a role in such protein degradation. The heat-shock proteins, and particularly ubiquitin, are also involved.

In many situations atrophy is also accompanied by marked increases in the number of *autophagic vacuoles.* As stated earlier, these are membrane-bound vacuoles within the cell that contain fragments of cell components (e.g., mitochondria, endoplasmic reticulum), which are destined for destruction, and into which the lysosomes discharge their hydrolytic contents. The cellular components are then digested. The formation of autophagic vacuoles can be surprisingly rapid. For example, in experimental occlusion of the portal venous blood supply to the liver lobe, large numbers of autophagic vacuoles are formed within 5 to 10 minutes after the blood supply is occluded.

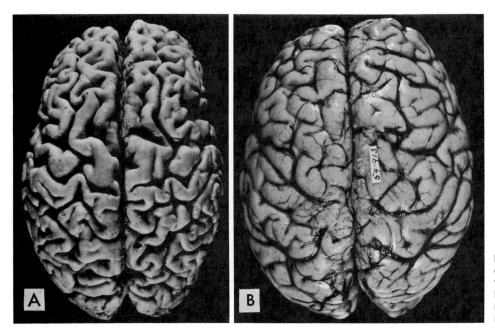

Figure 2-13. *A*, Physiologic atrophy of the brain in an 82-year-old male. The meninges have been stripped. *B*, Normal brain of 36-year-old male.

Some of the cell debris within the autophagic vacuole may resist digestion and persist as membrane-bound *residual bodies* that may remain as a sarcophagus in the cytoplasm. An example of such residual bodies is the *lipofuscin granules*, discussed earlier. When present in sufficient amounts, they impart a *brown discoloration* to the tissue (brown atrophy).

Obviously, atrophy may progress to the point at which cells are injured and die. If the blood supply is inadequate even to maintain the life of shrunken cells, injury and cell death may supervene. The atrophic tissue may then be replaced by fatty ingrowth.

METAPLASIA

Metaplasia is a reversible change in which one adult cell type (epithelial or mesenchymal) is replaced by another adult cell type. It, too, may represent an adaptive substitution of cells more sensitive to stress by cell types better able to withstand the adverse environment.

The most common adaptive metaplasia is *columnar* to *squamous*, as occurs in the respiratory tract in response to chronic irritation. In the habitual cigarette smoker, the normal columnar ciliated epithelial cells of the trachea and bronchi are often replaced focally or widely by stratified squamous epithelial cells. Stones in the excretory ducts of the salivary glands, pancreas, or bile ducts may cause replacement of the normal secretory columnar epithelium by nonfunctioning stratified squamous epithelium (Fig. 2–14). A deficiency of vitamin A (retinoic acid) induces squamous metaplasia in the

respiratory epithelium, and vitamin A excess *suppresses* keratinization.

In all these instances, the more rugged stratified squamous epithelium is able to survive under circumstances in which the more fragile specialized epithelium most likely would have succumbed. Although the squamous metaplastic cells in the respiratory tract, for example, are capable of

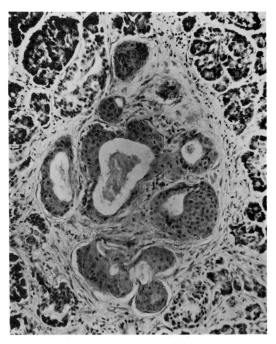

Figure 2-14. Metaplastic transformation of adult columnar epithelial cells to adult stratified squamous cells in pancreatic ducts.

surviving, an important protective mechanism—mucus secretion—is lost. Thus, epithelial metaplasia is a two-edged sword and, in most circumstances, represents an undesirable change. *Moreover, the influences that predispose to such metaplasia, if persistent, may induce cancer transformation in metaplastic epithelium.* Thus, the common form of cancer in the respiratory tract is composed of squamous cells. However, metaplasia from squamous to columnar type may also occur, as in Barrett's esophagitis in which the squamous esophageal epithelium is replaced by gastric columnar cells (see Chapter 17). The resulting cancers that may arise are glandular (adeno) carcinomas.

Metaplasia may also occur in mesenchymal cells but less clearly as an adaptive response. Fibrous connective tissue cells may become transformed to osteoblasts or chondroblasts to produce bone or cartilage where it is normally not encountered. This occurs particularly in foci of injury, but occasionally with no cause.

Metaplasia is thought to arise from genetic reprogramming of stem cells that are known to exist in most epithelia, or of undifferentiated mesenchymal cells present in connective tissue. Chemicals, vitamins, or growth factors most likely play a role in such metaplasias. Retinoids, for example, derived from retinoic acid (vitamin A) are known to be regulators of cell growth and differentiation, particularly in embryogenesis.[42] Bone morphogenetic factors (of the TGF-β-1 family) cause osseous differentiation both *in vivo* and *in vitro*. Certain cytostatic drugs cause a disruption of DNA methylation patterns and can transform mesenchymal cells from one type (fibroblast) to another (muscle, cartilage). The current explosion of work on tissue-specific and differentiation genes is bound to help clarify some of the elusive instances of metaplasias in tissues.

1. McCarthy, N.J., et al.: Apoptosis in the development of the immune system: Growth factors, clonal selection, and *bcl-2*. Cancer Metastasis Rev. *11*:157, 1992.
2. Baserga, R.: The Biology of Cell Reproduction. Cambridge, MA, Harvard University Press, 1985.
3. Morgan, C.J., and Pledger, J.W.: Fibroblast proliferation. *In* Cohen, I.K., Diegelmann, R.F., and Lindblad, W.J. (ed.): Wound Healing: Biochemical and Clinical Aspects. Philadelphia, W.B. Saunders Co., 1992, pp. 76–83.
4. Schlessinger, J., and Ullrich, A.: Growth factor signaling and receptor tyrosine kinases. Neuron *9*:383, 1992.
5. Heldin, C.H., and Westermark, B.: Platelet-derived growth factor and autocrine mechanisms of oncogenic processes. Crit. Rev. Oncog. *2*:109, 1991.
6. Pawson, T., and Gish, G.D.: SH$_2$ and SH$_3$ domains. Cell *71*:359, 1992.
7. Feig, L.A.: The many roads that lead to *ras*. Science *200*:767, 1993.
8. Marx, J.: Forging a path to the nucleus. Science *260*:1588, 1993.
9. Wang, A.J., and Croce, C.M.: Oncogenesis and signal transduction. Hosp. Pract. *28*:7, 1993.
10. Berridge, M.J.: Inositol triphosphate and calcium signalling. Nature *361*:315, 1992.
11. Fischer, E.H., et al.: Protein tyrosine phosphatases: A diverse family of intracellular and transmembrane enzymes. Science *253*:401, 1991.
12. Lange-Carter, C.A., et al.: A divergence in the MAP kinase regulatory network defined by MEK kinase and *raf*. Science *260*:315, 1993.
13. Feramisco, J.R., and Watterson, M.D. (eds.): Cell Regulation. Curr. Opin. Cell Biol. *5*:239, 1993.
14. Hunt, T., and Kirchner, M.: Cell multiplication. Curr. Opin. Cell Biol. *5*:163, 1993.
15. Scherr, C.J.: Mammalian G$_1$ cyclins. Cell *73*:1059, 1993.
16. Marx, J.: How cells cycle toward cancer. Science *263*:319, 1994.
17. Wiman, K.G.: The retinoblastoma gene: Role in cell cycle control and cell differentiation. FASEB J. *7*:841, 1993.
18. Gross, M., and Dexter, M.: Growth factors in development, transformation, and tumorigenesis. Cell *64*:271, 1991.
19. Cohen, S.: Isolation of a mouse submaxillary gland protein accelerating incisor eruption and eyelid opening in a newborn animal. J. Biol. Chem. *237*:1555, 1962.
20. Carpenter, G., and Cohen, S.: Epidermal growth factor. J. Biol. Chem. *265*:7709, 1990.
21. Klagsbrun, M., and Dluz, S.: Smooth muscle cell and endothelial cell growth factors. Trends Cardiovasc. Med. *3*:213, 1993.
22. Roberts, A.B., and Sporn, M.D.: The transforming growth factor B's. *In* The Handbook of Experimental Pharmacology. Heidelberg, Springer-Verlag, 1990, pp. 419–472.
23. Barnard, J.A., et al.: The cell biology of transforming growth factor beta. Biochem. Biophys. Acta *1032*:79, 1990.
24. Border, W.A., and Ruoslahti, E.: Transforming growth factor in disease: The dark side of tissue repair. J. Clin. Invest. *90*:1, 1992.
25. Brichmeier, W.: Molecular aspects of epithelial mesenchymal interactions. Annu. Rev. Cell Biol. 9, 1993.
26. Hay, E.D. (ed.): The Cell Biology of the Extracellular Matrix, 2nd ed. New York, Plenum Press, 1992.
27. Schwarzbauer, J.E.: Fibronectin: From gene to protein. Curr. Opin. Cell Biol. *3*:780, 1992.
28. Burridge, K., *et al.*: Focal adhesions: Transmembrane junctions between the extracellular matrix and the cytoskeleton. Annu. Rev. Cell Biol. *4*:487, 1988.
29. Ingber, D.E., and Folkman, J.: How does extracellular matrix control capillary morphogenesis? Cell *58*:803, 1989.
30. NcNamee, H.P., et al.: Adhesion to fibronectin stimulates inositol lipid synthesis and enhances PDGF-induced inositol lipid breakdown. J. Cell Biol. *121*:673, 1993.
31. Bernfield, M., et al.: Biology of the syndecans: A family of transmembrane heparan sulfate proteoglycans. Annu. Rev. Cell Biol. *8*:365, 1992.
32. Fausto, N., and Webber, E.M.: Liver regeneration. *In* Arias, I.M., et al. (eds.): The Liver: Biology and Pathobiology, 3rd ed. New York, Raven Press, 1993.
33. Matsumoto, K., and Nakamura, T.: Hepatocyte growth factor: Molecular structure, roles in liver regeneration, and other biological functions. Crit. Rev. Oncog. *3*:27, 1992.
34. Michaelopoulos, G.K., and Zarnegar, R.: Hepatocyte growth factor. Hepatology *15*:149, 1992.
35. Appasamy, R., et al.: Hepatocyte growth factor, blood clearance, organ uptake, and biliary excretion in normal and partially hepatectomized rats. Lab. Invest. *68*:270, 1993.
36. Fausto, N.: Liver stem cells. *In* Arias, I.M., et al. (eds.): The Liver: Biology and Pathobiology, 3rd, ed. New York, Raven Press, 1993.
37. Schwartz, K., et al.: Switches in cardiac muscle gene expression as a result of pressure and volume overload. Am. J. Physiol. *252*:R364, 1992.
38. Robbins, R., and Swain, J.L.: C-*myc* protooncogene modulates cardiac hypertrophic growth in transgenic mice. Am. J. Physiol. *262*:H590, 1992.
39. Saito, Y., et al.: Augmented expression of atrial natriuret-

ic polypeptide gene in ventricle of human failing heart, J. Clin. Invest. *83*:298, 1989.

40. Boheler, K.R., and Schwartz, K.: Gene expression in cardiac hypertrophy. Trends Cardiovasc. Med. *2*:176, 1992.

41. Tsatsui, T., et al.: Cytoskeletal role in the contractile dys-

function of hypertrophied myocardium. Science *260*:682, 1993.

42. Tabin, C.J.: Retinoids, homeoboxes, and growth factors: Toward molecular models for limb development. Cell *66*:199, 1991.

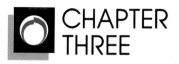

CHAPTER THREE

Inflammation and Repair

In Chapter 1 we saw how various exogenous and endogenous stimuli can cause cell injury. These same stimuli also can provoke a *complex reaction in the vascularized connective tissue* called inflammation. Invertebrates with no vascular system, single-celled organisms, and multicellular parasites all have their own responses to local injury. These include phagocytosis of the injurious agent; entrapment of the irritant by specialized cells (hemocytes), which then ingest it; and neutralization of noxious stimuli by hypertrophy of the cell or one of its organelles.[1] All these reactions have been retained in evolution, but what characterizes the inflammatory process in higher forms is *the reaction of blood vessels, leading to the accumulation of fluid and leukocytes in extravascular tissues.*

The inflammatory response is closely intertwined with the process of repair. Inflammation serves to destroy, dilute, or wall off the injurious agent, but it, in turn, sets into motion a series of events that, as far as possible, heal and reconstitute the damaged tissue. Repair begins during the early phases of inflammation but reaches completion usually after the injurious influence has been neutralized. During repair, the injured tissue is replaced by *regeneration* of native parenchymal cells, or by filling of the defect with fibroblastic tissue *(scarring),* or most commonly by a combination of these two processes.

Inflammation is fundamentally a protective response whose ultimate goal is to rid the organism of both the initial cause of cell injury (e.g., microbes, toxins) and the consequences of such injury, the necrotic cells and tissues. Without inflammation, infections would go unchecked, wounds would never heal, and injured organs might remain permanent festering sores. *However, inflammation and repair may be potentially harmful.* Inflammatory reactions, for example, underlie life-threatening hypersensitivity reactions to insect bites, drugs, and toxins as well as some of the common chronic diseases of modern times, such as rheumatoid arthritis, atherosclerosis, and lung fibrosis. Repair by fibrosis may lead to disfiguring scars or fibrous bands that cause intestinal obstruction or limit the mobility of joints. For this reason our pharmacies abound with "anti-inflammatory drugs," which

51

CONNECTIVE TISSUE   VESSELS   CONNECTIVE TISSUE
MATRIX   CELLS

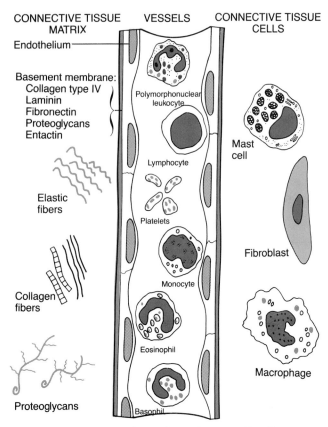

Endothelium

Basement membrane:
  Collagen type IV
  Laminin
  Fibronectin
  Proteoglycans
  Entactin

Polymorphonuclear
leukocyte

Mast
cell

Lymphocyte

Elastic
fibers

Platelets

Fibroblast

Collagen
fibers

Monocyte

Eosinophil

Macrophage

Proteoglycans

Basophil

Figure 3–1. Intravascular cells and connective tissue matrix and cells involved in the inflammatory response.

ideally would enhance the salutary effects of inflammation yet control its harmful sequelae.

The inflammatory response occurs in the vascularized connective tissue, including plasma, circulating cells, blood vessels, and cellular and extracellular constituents of connective tissue (Fig. 3–1). The circulating cells include *neutrophils, monocytes, eosinophils, lymphocytes, basophils,* and *platelets.* The connective tissue cells are the *mast cells,* which intimately surround *blood vessels;* the connective tissue *fibroblasts;* and occasional *resident macrophages* and *lymphocytes.* The extracellular matrix (ECM), as described in Chapter 2, consists of the structural fibrous proteins *(collagen, elastin),* the adhesive glycoproteins *(fibronectin, laminin, nonfibrillar collagen, entactin, tenascin,* and others), and proteoglycans. The basement membrane is a specialized component of the ECM consisting of adhesive glycoproteins and proteoglycans.

Inflammation is divided into acute and chronic patterns. *Acute inflammation* is of relatively short duration, lasting for minutes, several hours, or a few days, and its main characteristics are the exudation of fluid and plasma proteins (edema) and the emigration of leukocytes, predominantly neutrophils. *Chronic inflammation,* on the other hand, is of longer duration and is associated histologically with the presence of lymphocytes and macro-

phages and with the proliferation of blood vessels and connective tissue. Many factors modify the course and histologic appearance of both acute and chronic inflammation, and these will become apparent later in this chapter.

The vascular and cellular responses of both acute and chronic inflammation are mediated by chemical factors derived from plasma or cells and triggered by the inflammatory stimulus. Such mediators, acting singly, in combinations, or in sequence, then *amplify* the inflammatory response and influence its evolution. But it must be remembered that necrotic cells or tissues themsevles—whatever the cause of cell death—can also trigger the elaboration of inflammatory mediators. Such is the case with the acute inflammation following myocardial infarction. Inflammation is *terminated* when the injurious stimulus is removed and the mediators are either dissipated or inhibited.

In this chapter we shall first describe the sequence of events in acute inflammation, as well as the structural and molecular mechanisms underlying them, and then review the various classes of specific mediators that contribute to these events. This will be followed by a discussion of chronic inflammation and then repair, with emphasis on *wound healing* as a classic example of repair. But inflammation has a rich history, intimately linked to the history of wars, wounds, and infections, and we shall first touch on some of the historical highlights in our understanding of this fascinating process.[1,2]

HISTORICAL HIGHLIGHTS

Though they were described in an Egyptian papyrus (3000 BC), *Celsus,* a Roman writer of the first century A.D., first listed the four cardinal signs of inflammation: *rubor, tumor, calor,* and *dolor* (redness, swelling, heat, and pain). A fifth clinical sign, loss of function *(functio laesa),* was later added by Virchow. In 1793, the Scottish surgeon *John Hunter* noted what is now considered an obvious fact: that inflammation is not a disease but a nonspecific response that has a "salutary" effect on its host.[3] *Julius Cohnheim* (1839–1884) first used the microscope to observe inflamed blood vessels in thin, transparent membranes, such as the mesentery and tongue of the frog. Noting the initial changes in blood flow, the subsequent edema due to increased vascular permeability, and the characteristic leukocyte emigration, he wrote descriptions that can hardly be improved on.[4]

The Russian biologist *Elie Metchnikoff* discovered the process of *phagocytosis* by observing the ingestion of rose thorns by amebocytes of starfish larvae and of bacteria by mammalian leukocytes (1882).[5] He concluded that the purpose of inflammation was to bring phagocytic cells to the injured area to engulf invading bacteria. At that time, Metchnikoff contradicted the prevailing theory that the purpose of inflammation was to bring in factors from the serum to neutralize the infectious agents. It soon became clear that both cellular (phagocytes) and serum factors (antibodies) were critical to the defense against micro-organisms, and in recognition of this both Metchnikoff and Paul Ehrlich (who developed the humoral theory) shared the Nobel Price in 1908.

To these names must be added that of *Sir Thomas Lewis*, who, on the basis of simple experiments involving the inflammatory response in skin, established the *concept that chemical substances, such as histamine locally induced by injury, mediate the vascular changes of inflammation.* This fundamental concept underlies the important discoveries of *chemical mediators* of inflammation and the potential to use anti-inflammatory agents.

ACUTE INFLAMMATION

Acute inflammation is the immediate and early response to an injurious agent. Since the two major defensive components against microbes—antibodies and leukocytes—are normally carried in the bloodstream, it is not surprising that vascular phenomena play a major role in acute inflammation. Therefore, acute inflammation has three major components: *(1) alterations in vascular caliber that lead to an increase in blood flow, (2) structural changes in the microvasculature that permit the plasma proteins and leukocytes to leave the circulation, and (3) emigration of the leukocytes from the microcirculation and their accumulation in the focus of injury.*

Certain terms must be defined before we describe specific features of inflammation. The escape of fluid, proteins, and blood cells from the vascular system into the interstitial tissue or body cavities is known as *exudation.* An *exudate* is an inflammatory extravascular fluid that has a high protein concentration, much cellular debris, and a specific gravity above 1.020. It implies significant alteration in the normal permeability of small blood vessels in the area of injury. In contrast, a *transudate* is a fluid with low protein content (most of which is albumin) and a specific gravity of less than 1.012. It is essentially an ultrafiltrate of blood plasma and results from hydrostatic imbalance across the vascular endothelium. In this situation, the permeability of the endothelium is normal. *Edema* denotes an excess of fluid in the interstitial or serous cavities; it can be either an exudate or a transudate. *Pus*, a *purulent exudate*, is an inflammatory exudate rich in leukocytes (mostly neutrophils) and parenchymal cell debris.

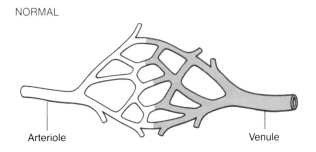

NORMAL

Arteriole   Venule

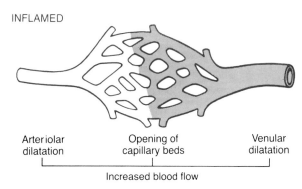

INFLAMED

Arteriolar   Opening of   Venular
dilatation   capillary beds   dilatation

Increased blood flow

Figure 3–2. Alterations in blood flow associated with inflammation.

Alterations in blood flow associated with inflammation.

VASCULAR CHANGES

Changes in Vascular Flow and Caliber

Changes in vascular flow and caliber begin very early after injury and develop at varying rates, depending on the severity of the injury. The changes occur in the following order:

- Following an inconstant and transient vasoconstriction of arterioles, lasting a few seconds, *vasodilatation* occurs. This first involves the arterioles and then results in opening of new capillary beds in the area. Thus comes about *increased blood flow*, which is the cause of the heat and the redness (Fig. 3–2). How long vasodilatation lasts depends on the stimulus; it is followed by the next event:

- *Slowing of the circulation.* This is brought about by *increased permeability of the microvasculature,* with the outpouring of protein-rich fluid into the extravascular tissues. The latter results in concentration of red cells in small vessels and increased viscosity of the blood, reflected by the presence of dilated small vessels packed with red cells—termed *stasis.*

- As stasis develops one begins to see peripheral orientation of leukocytes, principally neutrophils, along the vascular endothelium, a process called *leukocytic margination.* Leukocytes then stick to the endothelium, at first transiently (rolling), then more avidly, and soon afterward they migrate through the vascular wall into the interstitial tissue, in processes that will be discussed presently.

The time scale of these events is variable. With mild stimuli the stages of stasis may not become apparent until 15 to 30 minutes have elapsed, whereas with severe injury, stasis may occur in but a few minutes.

Increased Vascular Permeability (Vascular Leakage)

Increased vascular permeability leading to the escape of a protein-rich fluid (exudate) into the interstitium *is the hallmark of acute inflammation.* The loss of protein-rich fluid from the plasma reduces the intravascular osmotic pressure and in-

creases the osmotic pressure of the interstitial fluid. Together with the increased hydrostatic pressure due to vasodilatation, this leads to a marked *outflow* of fluid and its accumulation in the interstitial tissue (Fig. 3–3). This net increase of extravascular fluid is *edema.*

Normal fluid exchange and microvascular permeability are critically dependent on an intact en-

Figure 3–3. Blood pressure and plasma colloid osmotic forces in normal and inflamed microcirculation. *A,* Normal hydrostatic pressure of about 32 mm Hg at arterial end of capillary and 12 mm Hg at venous end. Mean capillary pressure equals colloid osmotic pressure *(horizontal line).* *B,* Acute inflammation. Mean capillary pressure is increased because of arteriolar dilatation, while osmotic pressure is reduced because of protein leakage across venule. Result is net excess of extravasated fluid. (Redrawn with permission from Wright, G.P.: An Introduction to Pathology, 3rd ed. London, Longmans, Green and Co., 1958.)

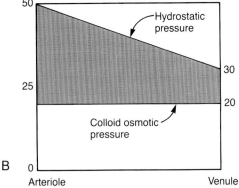

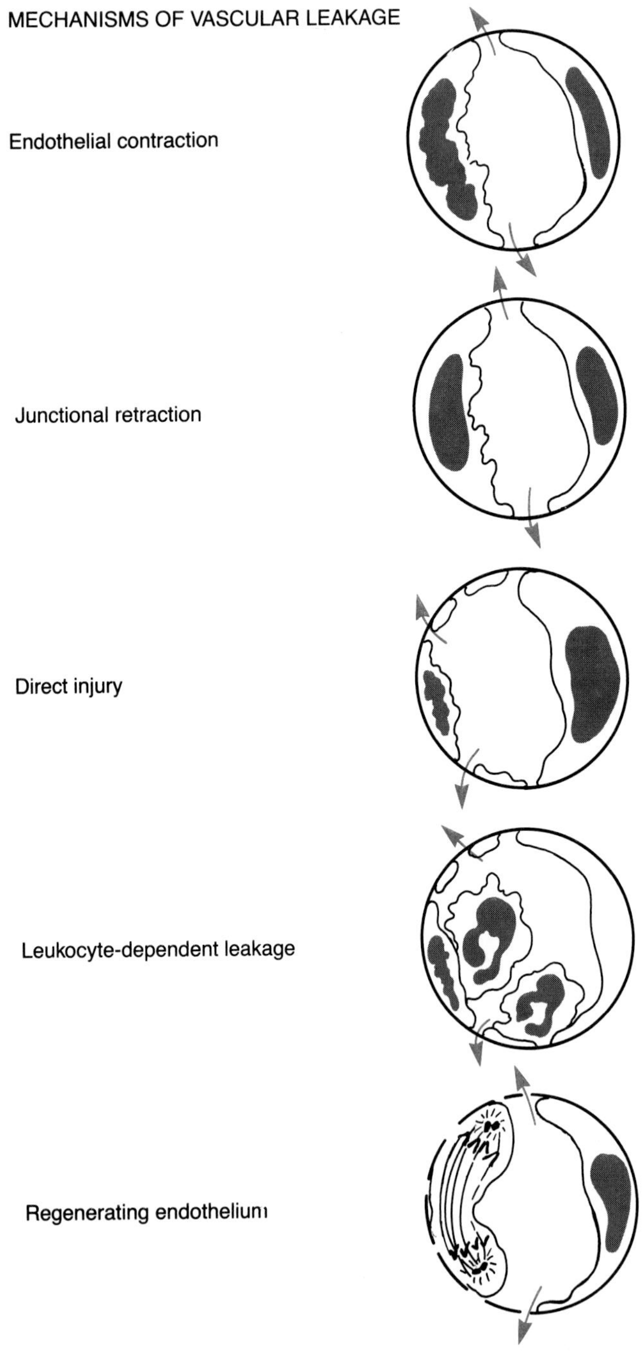

MECHANISMS OF VASCULAR LEAKAGE

Endothelial contraction

Junctional retraction

Direct injury

Leukocyte-dependent leakage

Regenerating endothelium

Figure 3–4. Diagrammatic representation of the five mechanisms of increased vascular permeability in inflammation (see text).

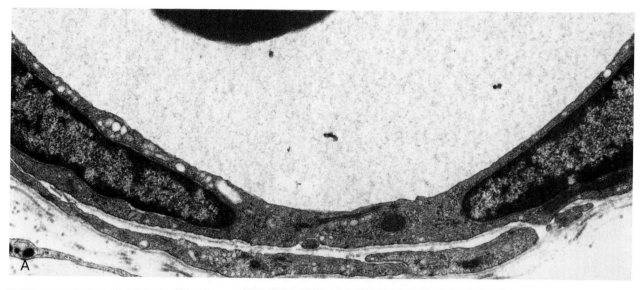

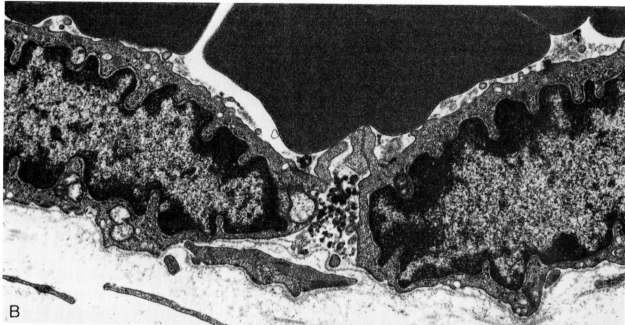

Figure 3–5. *A*, Electron micrograph of wall of normal venule, showing closed intercellular junction and flattened endothelial cells. *B*, Venule after injection of a histamine-type mediator, showing an intercellular gap through which injected black carbon particles have leaked. Note that the cells have bulged into the lumen and their nuclei show many indentations, suggesting contraction. (With permission from Joris, I.J., et al.: The mechanism of vascular leakage induced by leukotriene E₄. Am. J. Pathol. *126*:19, 1987.)

dothelium. How then does the endothelium become leaky in inflammation? At least five mechanisms are known (Fig. 3–4).[7]

1. *Endothelial cell contraction, leading to the formation of widened intercellular junctions, or intercellular gaps* (Fig. 3–5).[8] This is by far the most common mechanism of vascular leakage and is elicited by histamine, bradykinin, leukotrienes, and many other classes of chemical mediators. This type of vascular leakage occurs rapidly after exposure to the mediator and is usually reversible and

short-lived (15 to 30 minutes); it is thus known as the *immediate transient response.*

Classically, this type of leakage affects only venules 20 to 60 μm in diameter, leaving capillaries and arterioles unaffected (Fig. 3–6). The precise reason for this restriction to venules is uncertain but may be related to a greater density of receptors to the putative mediator in venular endothelium. Parenthetically, many of the later leukocyte events in inflammation—adhesion and emigration—also occur predominantly in the venules in most organs.

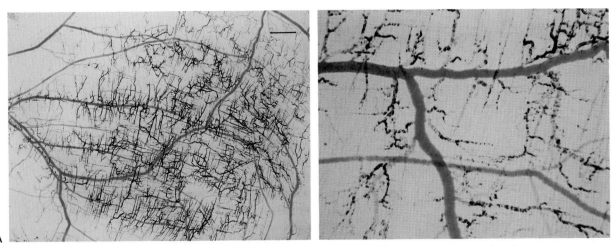

Figure 3–6. *A* and *B,* Vascular leakage as induced by most chemical mediators. This is a laminar muscle of the rat (cremaster), fixed, cleared in glycerin, and examined unstained by transillumination. One hour prior to sacrifice, brady- kinin was injected over this muscle, and colloidal carbon was given intravenously; bradykinin caused small gaps to appear between endothelial cells in some vessels. Plasma, loaded with carbon, escaped, but most of the carbon particles were retained by the basement membrane of the leaking vessels, with the result that these became "labeled" in black. *Note that not all the vessels leak*—only the venules. In *B,* a higher power, the capillary network is very faintly visible in the background. (Courtesy of Dr. Guido Majno.)

2. *Cytoskeletal and junctional reorganization (endothelial retraction).* An apparently different mechanism of *reversible* intercellular leakage, re- sulting in interendothelial gaps, can be induced *in vitro* by cytokine mediators, such as interleukin-1 (IL-1), tumor necrosis factor (TNF), and inter- feron-gamma (IFN-γ).[9] These cytokines cause a structural reorganization of the cytoskeleton, such that endothelial cells retract from one another along their junctions, leading to endothelial dis- continuities. In contrast to the histamine effect, the response is somewhat delayed (4 to 6 hours) and long-lived (24 hours or more). How frequently this mechanism accounts for vascular leakage *in vivo* is still uncertain.

3. *Direct endothelial injury, resulting in endo- thelial cell necrosis and detachment.* This effect is usually encountered in necrotizing injuries and is due to direct damage to the endothelium by the injurious stimulus, as for example by severe burns or lytic bacterial infections. In most instances leak- age starts immediately after injury and is sustained at a high level for several hours until the damaged vessels are thrombosed or repaired. The reaction is known as the *immediate sustained response. All levels of the microcirculation are affected, including venules, capillaries, and arterioles.* Endothelial cell detachment is often associated with platelet adhe- sion and thrombosis.

Delayed prolonged leakage is a curious but rel- atively common type of increased permeability that *begins after a delay of 2 to 12 hours, lasts for several hours or even days, and involves venules as well as capillaries.* Such leakage is caused, for ex- ample, by mild-to-moderate thermal injury, X- or

ultraviolet radiation, and certain bacterial toxins. The late-appearing sunburn is a good example of a delayed reaction. The mechanism for such leakage is unclear. It may result from the direct effect of the injurious agent, leading to delayed cell damage (perhaps by apoptosis), or the effect of cytokines causing endothelial retraction, as described earlier.

4. *Leukocyte-mediated endothelial injury.* Leu- kocytes adhere to endothelium relatively early in inflammation. As we shall see, such leukocytes may be activated in the process, releasing toxic oxygen species and proteolytic enzymes, which then cause endothelial injury or detachment—resulting in in- creased permeability.

5. *Leakage from regenerating capillaries.* As described later in this chapter, during repair, en- dothelial cells proliferate and form new blood ves- sels *(angiogenesis).* These capillary sprouts remain leaky until the endothelial cells differentiate and form intercellular junctions, accounting for the edema characteristic of healing inflammation.

Increased transcytosis via vesicles and vacuoles across the cytoplasm is another potential mecha- nism of increased permeability and has been dem- onstrated in blood vessels within tumors.[9a]

It should be noted that although these mecha- nisms are separable, all may play a role in response to one stimulus. For example, in various stages of a thermal burn, leakage results from chemically me- diated endothelial contraction as well as direct and leukocyte-dependent injury—and from regenerat- ing capillaries when the injury heals. This accounts for the life-threatening loss of fluid in severely burned patients.

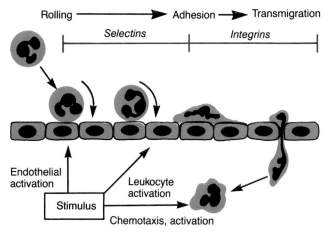

Figure 3–7. Sequence of leukocytic events in inflammation. The leukocytes first *roll*, then arrest and adhere to endothelium, then transmigrate through an intercellular junction, pierce the basement membrane, and migrate toward chemoattractants emanating from the source of injury. The roles of selectins, activating agents, and integrins are also shown. (Modified and redrawn from Travis, J.T.: Biotech gets a grip on cell adhesion. Science 26:906, 1993.)

CELLULAR EVENTS: LEUKOCYTE EXTRAVASATION AND PHAGOCYTOSIS

A critical function of inflammation is the delivery of leukocytes to the site of injury. Leukocytes ingest offending agents, kill bacteria and other microbes, and degrade necrotic tissue and foreign antigens. Unfortunately, leukocytes may also prolong inflammation and induce tissue damage by releasing enzymes, chemical mediators, and toxic oxygen radicals.

The sequence of events in the journey of leukocytes from the lumen to the interstitial tissue, called extravasation, can be divided into the following steps: (1) in the lumen: margination, rolling, and adhesion; (2) transmigration across the endothelium (also called diapedesis); and (3) migration in interstitial tissues toward a chemotactic stimulus (Fig. 3–7).

In normally flowing blood, erythrocytes and leukocytes are confined to a central axial column, leaving a cell-poor layer of plasma in contact with endothelium. As blood flow slows early in inflammation (as a result of the increased vascular permeability), white cells fall out of the central column and assume a peripheral position along the endothelial surface. This initial process, called *margination*, is caused largely by changes in hemodynamic conditions engendered by low and slow blood circulation. Subsequently, individual and then rows of leukocytes tumble slowly along the endothelium and adhere transiently (a process called *rolling*), finally coming to rest at some point where they adhere firmly (resembling "pebbles or

marbles over which a stream runs without disturbing them"). In time, the endothelium can be virtually lined by white cells, an appearance called *"pavementing."* Following firm adhesion, leukocytes insert pseudopods into the junctions between the endothelial cells, squeeze through interendothelial junctions, and assume a position between the endothelial cell and the basement membrane. Eventually they traverse the basement membrane and escape into the extravascular space. Neutrophils, monocytes, lymphocytes, eosinophils, and basophils all use the same pathway. We shall now examine the molecular mechanisms of each of the steps.

Adhesion and Transmigration

It is now clear that leukocyte adhesion and transmigration are determined largely by the binding of complementary adhesion molecules on the leukocyte and endothelial surfaces (like a key and lock), and that chemical mediators—chemoattractants and certain cytokines—affect these processes by modulating the surface expression or avidity of such adhesion molecules.[6,10]

The adhesion receptors involved belong to three molecular families—the *selectins*, the *immunoglobulins*, and the *integrins*. The most important of these are shown in Table 3–1.[11]

Selectins, so-called because they are characterized by an extracellular N-terminal domain related to sugar-binding mammalian lectins, consist of E-selectin (also known as ELAM-1) that is confined to endothelium; P-selectin (also called GMP140), present in endothelium and platelets; and L-selectin (also called LAM-1), which decorates most leukocyte types. P and E selectins bind, through their lectin domain, to sialylated forms of oligosaccharides (e.g., sialylated Lewis X), which themselves are covalently bound to various cell surface glycoproteins. L-selectin binds to mucin-like glycoproteins (GlyCAM-1 and CD34).

The *immunoglobulin* family molecules include two *endothelial* adhesion molecules: ICAM-1 (intercellular adhesion molecule 1) and VCAM-1 (vascular cell adhesion molecule 1), and both interact with *integrins* found on leukocytes. (You may recall from Chapter 2 that integrins are transmembrane-adhesive heterodimeric glycoproteins, made up of alpha and beta chains that also function as receptors for the extracellular matrix [ECM].) The principal integrin receptors for ICAM-1 are the β_2 integrins LFA-1 and MAC-1 (CD11a/CD18 and CD11b/CD18), and that for VCAM-1 is the β_1 integrin VLA-4 ($\alpha_4\beta_1$ integrin).

But how are these molecules modulated to induce adhesion in inflammation? There are a number of mechanisms, dependent on the duration of

Table 3-1. LEUKOCYTE–ENDOTHELIAL ADHESION MOLECULES

ENDOTHELIAL MOLECULE	Family	LEUKOCYTE RECEPTOR	Family	Distribution
E-selectin (ELAM-1)	Selectin	Sialyl-Le^x Glycoprotein	Oligosaccharides	Neutrophils T cells Monocytes
P-selectin (GMP-140)	Selectin	Sialyl-Le^x Glycoprotein	Oligosaccharides	Neutrophils Monocytes
ICAM-1	Immunoglobulin	LFA-1 Mac-1	β_2 integrin	All leukocytes
VCAM-1	Immunoglobulin	VLA-4	β_1 integrin	Lymphocytes Monocytes Basophils Eosinophils
LAM-1 Ligand(s) (GlyCam-1; CD34)	Mucin-like glycoproteins	L-selectin (LAM-1)	Selectin	Neutrophils Lymphocytes Monocytes

Modified and used with permission from Briscoe, D.M., and Cotran, R.S.: Role of leukocyte–endothelial cell adhesion molecules in renal inflammation: In vitro and in vivo studies. Kidney Int. 42:S-28, 1993.

inflammation, the type of inflammatory stimulus, and blood flow conditions (Fig. 3–8).

1. *Redistribution of adhesion molecules to the cell surface* (Fig. 3–8A). P-selectin, for example, is normally present in the membrane of specific intracytoplasmic endothelial granules, called Weibel-Palade bodies. On stimulation by mediators such as histamine, thrombin, and platelet-activating factor (PAF), P-selectin is rapidly redistributed to the cell surface, where it can bind the leukocytes.[12] This process occurs within minutes in flowing blood and serves to deliver preformed adhesion molecules in short order to the surface. Studies suggest that this process may be particularly important in early leukocyte *rolling* on endothelium.

2. *Induction of adhesion molecules on endothelium.* Some inflammatory mediators, and particularly cytokines (IL-1 and TNF), induce the synthesis and surface expression of endothelial adhesion molecules (Fig. 3–8B). This process requires new protein synthesis and begins usually after a delay of some 1 or 2 hours.[13] E-selectin, for example, which is not present in normal endothelium, is induced by IL-1 and TNF, maximally after 4 to 6 hours and mediates the adhesion of neutrophils by binding to its receptor sialylated Lewis X. The same cytokines also increase the expression of ICAM-1 and VCAM-1, which are present at low levels in normal endothelium.

3. *Increased avidity of binding* (Fig. 3–8C). This mechanism is most relevant to the binding of integrins. For example, LFA-1 is normally present on leukocytes—neutrophils, monocytes, and lymphocytes—but does not adhere to its ligand ICAM-1 on endothelium. When neutrophils are activated by chemotactic agents or other stimuli, the LFA-1 is converted from a state of low- to high-affinity binding toward ICAM-1, owing to a confor-

mational change in the molecule. During inflammation, the increased affinity of LFA-1 on the activated leukocyte, coupled with the increased ICAM-1 expression on endothelium induced by cytokines, sets the stage for strong LFA-1/ICAM-1 binding. In the low-flow conditions generated by stasis, the LFA-1/ICAM-1 interaction causes *firm adhesion* to the endothelium and appears also to be necessary for the subsequent *transmigration* across the endothelium.

Based on such studies, a currently popular scenario for neutrophil adhesion and transmigration in acute inflammation postulates the following steps (Fig. 3–9):[15] (1) First, there is initial rapid and relatively loose adhesion that accounts for *rolling*, involving mainly the naturally occurring P- and L-selectins, and, in cytokine-induced endothelium, E-selectin; (2) the leukocytes are then activated, by agents made by endothelium or other cells or emanating from the site of injury, to increase the avidity of their integrins (as in Fig. 3–8C); (3) they then bind stably to endothelium, largely through the β_2 integrin–ICAM-1 pathway, and undergo transmigration. Neutrophils, monocytes, eosinophils, and various types of lymphocytes use different (but overlapping) molecules for adhesion, and their adhesivity can be modulated by the state of activation of the leukocyte and endothelium.[16]

The most telling proof of the importance of adhesion molecules is the existence of clinical genetic deficiencies in the leukocyte adhesion proteins, which are characterized by impaired leukocyte adhesion and recurrent bacterial infections. In *leukocyte adhesion deficiency type 1*, patients have a defect in the biosynthesis of the β_2 chain shared by LFA-1 and Mac-1 integrins.[17] *Leukocyte adhesion deficiency type 2* is caused by absence of sialyl-Lewis X, the ligand for E-selectin, due to a generalized defect in fucose metabolism.[18] In addi-

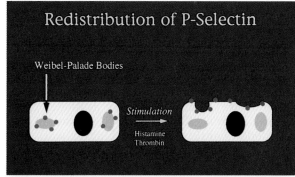

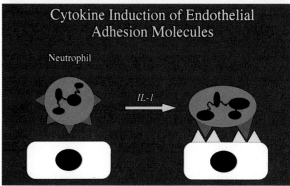

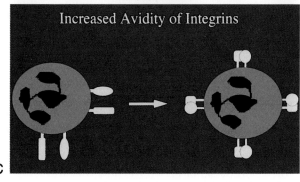

Figure 3-8. Three mechanisms of mediating leukocyte endothelial adhesion. A, Redistribution of P-selectin. B, Cytokine activation of endothelium. C, Increased binding avidity of integrins (see text). (Courtesy of Dr. Madeleine Kraus.)

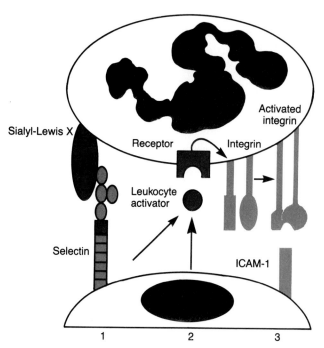

Figure 3-9. Steps in endothelial-neutrophil recognition: (1) initial adhesion via selectins; (2) activation of leukocytes by mediators, or by step 1, causing increased avidity of integrin; and (3) firm adhesion/transmigration via integrin/ICAM-1.

tion, antibodies to adhesion molecules abrogate leukocyte extravasation in experimental models of acute inflammation,[19] and transgenic mice deficient in these molecules show a compromise in leukocyte rolling and extravasation.[20]

As described earlier (see Fig. 3-7), transmigration of all leukocyte types occurs along the intercellular junctions. Certain homophilic adhesion molecules (i.e., adhesion molecules that bind to each other) present in the intercellular junction of endothelium may be involved. One of these is a member of the immunoglobulin gene superfamily called *PECAM-1* (platelet endothelial cell adhesion molecule) or CD31.[21] Antibodies to this molecule inhibit transmigration *in vitro*. In passing, it should be noted that *leukocyte diapedesis, like increased vascular permeability, occurs predominantly in the venules* (except in the lungs, where it also occurs in capillaries). After traversing the endothelial junctions, leukocytes are transiently retarded in their journey by the continuous basement membrane but eventually pierce it, probably by secreting collagenases that degrade the basement membrane.

The type of emigrating leukocyte varies with the age of the inflammatory lesion and with the type of stimulus. In most forms of acute inflammation, *neutrophils predominate in the inflammatory infiltrate during the first 6 to 24 hours, and then are replaced by monocytes in 24 to 48 hours* (Fig. 3-10). The sequence can best be explained by the activation of different adhesion molecule pairs and of chemotactic factors in different phases of inflammation. In addition, short-lived neutrophils disintegrate and disappear after 24 to 48 hours, whereas monocytes survive longer. However, there are exceptions to this pattern of cellular exudation. In certain infections, for example those produced by Pseudomonas organisms, neutrophils predominate over 2 to 4 days; in viral infections, lymphocytes may be the first cells to arrive; in some hypersensitivity reactions, eosinophilic granulocytes may be the main cell type.

Chemotaxis and Leukocyte Activation

Following extravasation, leukocytes emigrate in tissues toward the site of injury by a process called

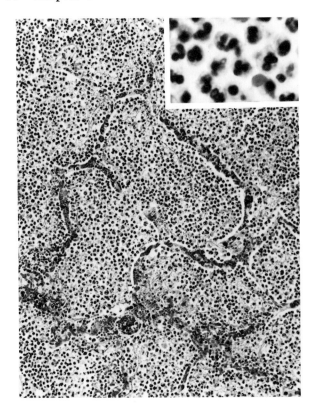

Figure 3–10. Photomicrograph of an acutely inflamed lung (pneumonia) showing emigration of inflammatory cells into the alveoli. Most of the cells in the exudate are neutrophils *(inset)*.

chemotaxis, defined most simply as locomotion oriented along a chemical gradient. All granulocytes, monocytes, and, to a lesser extent, lymphocytes respond to chemotactic stimuli with varying rates of speed.

Both exogenous and endogenous substances can act as chemoattractants. The most common exogenous agents are *bacterial products.* Some of these are peptides that possess an N-formyl-methionine terminal amino acid. Others are lipid in nature. Endogenous chemical mediators, which will be detailed later, include (1) *components of the complement system,* particularly C5a, (2) *products of the lipoxygenase pathway,* mainly leukotriene B_4 (LTB_4), and (3) *cytokines,* particularly those of the IL-8 family.

But how does the leukocyte "see" (or "smell") the chemotactic agents, and how do these substances induce directed cell movement? Although not all the answers are known, several important steps and second messengers are recognized (Fig. 3–11).[22] Binding of chemotactic agents to specific receptors on the cell membranes of leukocytes results in activation of phospholipase C (mediated by unique G-proteins), leading to the hydrolysis of phosphatidylinositol-4,5-biphosphate (PIP_2), to inositol-1,4,5-triphosphate (IP_3) and diacylglycerol (DAG), and the release of calcium, first from intra-

cellular stores and subsequently from the influx of extracellular calcium. It is the increased cytosolic calcium that triggers the assembly of contractile elements responsible for cell movement.

The leukocyte moves by extending a pseudopod (lamellipod) that pulls the remainder of the cell in the direction of extension, just as an automobile with front-wheel drive is pulled by the wheels in front (Fig. 3–12). The interior of the pseudopod consists of a branching network of filaments composed of *actin* as well as the contractile protein *myosin.* Locomotion involves rapid assembly of actin monomers into linear polymers at the pseudopod's leading edge, cross-linking of filaments, followed by disassembly of such filaments away from the leading edge.[23] These complex events are controlled by the effects of calcium ions and phosphoinositols on a number of actin-regulating proteins, such as *actin binding protein (filamin), gelsolin, profilin,* and *calmodulin.* Precisely how myosin interacts with actin in the pseudopod to produce contraction is unclear.

In addition to stimulating locomotion, many chemotactic factors, particularly in high concentrations, induce other responses in the leukocytes, referred to under the rubric of *leukocyte activation* (see Fig. 3–11). Such responses, which can also be induced by phagocytosis and antigen-antibody complexes, include the following:

- *Production of arachidonic acid metabolites* from phospholipids, due to activation of phospholipase A_2 by DAG and increased intracellular calcium.
- *Degranulation and secretion of lysosomal enzymes, and activation of the oxidative burst* (see discussion under phagocytosis). These two processes are induced by DAG-mediated activation of protein kinase. Activation of intracellular phospholipase D by the increased calcium influx contributes to the sustained DAG accumulation.
- *Modulation of leukocyte adhesion molecules.* Certain chemoattractants cause increased surface expression and, as stated earlier, increased adhesive avidity of the LFA-1 integrin, allowing firm adhesion of activated neutrophils to ICAM-1 on endothelium. In contrast, neutrophils shed L-selectin from their surface, making them less adhesive to the L-selectin ligand on endothelium.

A newly appreciated phenomenon in leukocyte activation is *priming,* denoting an increased rate and extent of leukocyte activation by exposure to a mediator that itself causes little activation. The cytokine TNF, in particular, markedly increases leukocyte activation by other chemotactic agents, accounting for its powerful *in vivo* effects, described later in this chapter.

Phagocytosis

Phagocytosis and the release of enzymes by neutrophils and macrophages constitute two of the

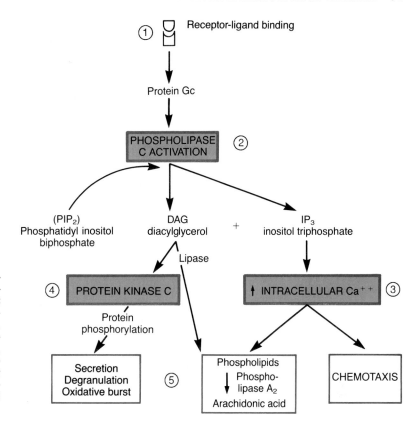

Figure 3-11. Biochemical events in leukocyte activation. The key events are (1) receptor-ligand binding, (2) phospholipase-C activation, (3) increased intracellular calcium, and (4) activation of protein kinase C. The biologic activities (5) resulting from leukocyte activation include chemotaxis, elaboration of arachidonic acid metabolites, secretion, and degranulation. Not shown is phospholipase D activation by increased Ca^{++}, which increases DAG and amplifies protein kinase C activation.

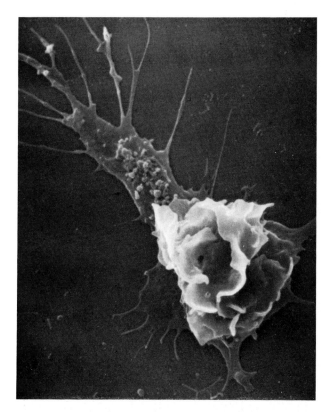

Figure 3-12. Scanning electron micrograph of a moving leukocyte in culture showing a pseudopod *(upper left)* and a trailing tail. (Courtesy of Dr. Morris J. Karnovsky, Harvard Medical School, Boston.)

major benefits derived from the accumulation of leukocytes at the inflammatory focus. Phagocytosis involves three distinct but inter-related steps (Fig. 3-13A): *recognition* and *attachment* of the particle to be ingested by the leukocyte; its *engulfment*, with subsequent formation of a phagocytic vacuole; and *killing* or *degradation* of the ingested material.[24]

RECOGNITION AND ATTACHMENT. On occasion neutrophils and macrophages recognize and engulf bacteria or extraneous matter (e.g., latex beads) in the absence of serum. Most microorganisms, however, are not recognized until they are coated by naturally occurring factors called *opsonins*, which bind to specific receptors on the leukocytes. The two major opsonins are (1) the *Fc fragment of immunoglobulin G (IgG)*, presumably naturally occurring antibody against the ingested particle; and (2) *C3b*, the so-called "opsonic fragment of C3" (and its stable form *C3bi*), generated by activation of complement by immune or nonimmune mechanisms, as described later. The corresponding receptors on leukocytes are FcγR which recognize the Fc fragment of IgG, and *complement receptors 1, 2, and 3 (CR1, 2, 3)*, which interact with C3b and C3bi. *CR3*, which recognizes C3bi, is a particularly important receptor; it is identical with the β_2 integrin–Mac-1, which, as you recall, is involved in adhesion to endothelium. It binds certain bacteria by recognizing bacterial lipopolysaccharides (LPS), without the intervention of antibody or complement, accounting for so-called *nonopsonic phagocy-*

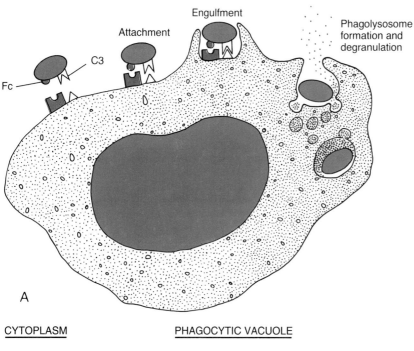

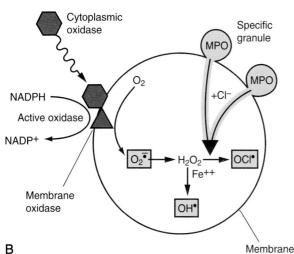

Figure 3–13. *A,* Phagocytosis of a particle (e.g., bacterium) involves attachment and binding of Fc and C3b to receptors on the leukocyte membrane, engulfment, and fusion of granules *(in red)* with phagocytic vacuoles, followed by degranulation. Note that during phagocytosis, granule contents may be released extracellularly. *B,* Summary of oxygen-dependent bactericidal mechanisms within phagocytic vacuole, as described in text.

tosis. CR3 also binds the ECM components fibronectin and laminin.

ENGULFMENT. Binding of the opsonized particle to the FcγR is sufficient to trigger engulfment, which is markedly enhanced in the presence of CRs. However, binding to the C3 receptors alone requires activation of such receptors before engulfment occurs. Such activation is accomplished by simultaneous binding to extracellular fibronectin and laminin or by certain cytokines. During engulfment, extensions of the cytoplasm (pseudopods) flow around the object to be engulfed, eventually resulting in complete enclosure of the particle within a phagosome created by the cytoplasmic membrane of the cell. The limiting membrane of this phagocytic vacuole then fuses with the limiting membrane of a lysosomal granule, resulting in discharge of the granule's contents into the phagolysosome (see Fig. 3–13A). In the course of this action, the neutrophil and the monocyte become progressively degranulated.

Many of the biochemical events involved in phagocytosis and degranulation are similar to those described for chemotaxis (see Fig. 3–11). The process is associated with receptor-ligand binding, phospholipase C activation, DAG and IP_3 production, protein kinase C activation, and increased concentration of cytosolic calcium, the latter two acting as second messengers to initiate the cellular events.

KILLING OR DEGRADATION. The ultimate step in phagocytosis of bacteria is killing and degradation. *Bacterial killing is accomplished largely by oxygen-dependent mechanisms* (see Fig. 3–13B).[25] Phagocytosis stimulates a burst in oxygen consumption, glycogenolysis, increased glucose oxidation via the hexose-monophosphate shunt, and production of reactive oxygen metabolites.

The generation of oxygen metabolites is due to the rapid activation of an oxidase (NADPH oxidase), which oxidizes NADPH (reduced nicotinamide-adenine dinucleotide phosphate) and, in the process, reduces oxygen to superoxide ion (O_2^-).

$$2O_2 + NADPH \xrightarrow{\text{oxidase}} 2O_2^- + NADP^+ + H^+$$

Superoxide is then converted into H_2O_2, mostly by spontaneous dismutation ($O_2^- + 2H^+ \longrightarrow H_2O_2$). The NADPH oxidase is a complex enzyme system consisting of *cytosolic* phosphoproteins and *membrane* cytochrome protein components (cytochrome b-558). Activation of the oxidase requires translocation of the cytosolic components to interact with the fixed cytochrome on the membrane or, when the membrane is invaginated, in the phagolysosome (see Fig. 3–13*B*). Thus, the *hydrogen peroxide is produced within the lysosome.*

The quantities of H_2O_2 produced in the phagolysosome are insufficient to induce effective killing of bacteria. However, the azurophilic granules of neutrophils contain the enzyme *myeloperoxidase* (MPO), which, in the presence of a halide such as Cl^-, converts H_2O_2 to $HOCl^{\bullet}$. The latter is an antimicrobial agent that destroys bacteria by *halogenation* (in which the halide is bound covalently to cellular constituents) or by oxidation of proteins and lipids (lipid peroxidation). A similar mechanism is also effective against fungi, viruses, protozoa, and helminths. Most of the H_2O_2 is eventually broken down by catalase into H_2O and O_2, and some is destroyed by the action of glutathione oxidase.

Although the H_2O_2-MPO-halide system is the most efficient bactericidal system in neutrophils, MPO-deficient leukocytes are capable of killing bacteria (albeit more slowly than control cells), by virtue of the formation of superoxide, hydroxyl radicals, and singlet-oxygen (see Fig. 3–13).

The importance of oxygen-dependent bacterial mechanisms is shown by the existence of a group of congenital disorders in bacterial killing called *chronic granulomatous disease (CGD)*, which make patients susceptible to recurrent bacterial infection.[26] CGD results from *inherited defects in the genes encoding the several components of NADPH oxidase*, which generates superoxide. The most common variants are an *X-linked defect* in one of the subunits of the membrane-bound cytochrome and an *autosomal recessive* defect in gene encoding one of the cytoplasmic components.

Bacterial killing can also occur in the absence of an oxidative burst, by substances in the leukocyte granules. These include *bactericidal permeability increasing protein* (BPI), a highly cationic granule-associated protein that causes phospholipase activation, phospholipid degradation, and increased permeability in the outer membrane of the micro-organisms; *lysozyme*, which hydrolyzes the muramic acid–N-acetyl-glucosamine bond, found in the glycopeptide coat of all bacteria; *lactoferrin*, an iron-binding protein present in specific granules; *major basic protein* (MBP), a cationic protein of eosinophils, which has limited bactericidal activity but is cytotoxic to many parasites; and *defensins*, cationic arginine-rich granule peptides that are cytotoxic to microbes (and certain mammalian cells).[27]

Following killing, acid hydrolases found in azurophil granules degrade the bacteria within phagolysosomes. The pH of the phagolysosome drops to between 4 and 5 after phagocytosis, this being the optimal pH for the action of these enzymes.

Release of Leukocyte Products

The membrane perturbations that occur in neutrophils and monocytes during chemotaxis and phagocytosis result in the release of products not only within the phagolysosome but also potentially into the extracellular space. The most important of these substances are (1) *lysosomal enzymes*, present in the neutrophil granules, (2) *oxygen-derived active metabolites*, detailed earlier; and (3) *products of arachidonic acid metabolism*, including prostaglandins and leukotrienes. These products are powerful mediators of endothelial injury and tissue damage and amplify the effects of the initial inflammatory stimulus. Thus, if persistent and unchecked, the leukocytic infiltrate itself becomes the offender, and indeed leukocyte-dependent tissue injury underlies many human diseases, such as rheumatoid arthritis and certain forms of chronic lung disease. This will become evident in the discussion of chronic inflammation.

The ways by which lysosomal granules and enzymes are secreted are diverse. Release may occur if the phagocytic vacuole remains transiently open to the outside before complete closure of the phagolysosome (*regurgitation during feeding*). In cells exposed to potentially ingestible materials, such as immune complexes, on flat surfaces (e.g., glomerular basement membrane), attachment of immune complexes to the leukocyte triggers membrane movement, but, because of the flat surface, phagocytosis does not occur, and lysosomal enzymes are released into the medium (*frustrated phagocytosis*). *Cytotoxic release* occurs after phagocytosis of potentially membranolytic substances, such as urate crystals. In addition, there is some evidence that certain granules, particularly the specific granules of neutrophils, may be directly secreted by *exocytosis*.[28]

Table 3-2. DEFECTS IN LEUKOCYTE FUNCTIONS

DISEASE	DEFECT
Genetic	
Leukocyte adhesion deficiency 1	Beta chain of CD11/CD18 integrins
Leukocyte adhesion deficiency 2	Sialylated oligosaccharide (receptor for selectin)
Neutrophil specific granule deficiency	Absence of neutrophil specific granules Defective chemotaxis
Chronic granulomatous disease	Decreased oxidative burst
X-linked	NADPH oxidase (membrane component)
Autosomal recessive	NADPH oxidase (cytoplasmic component)
Myeloperoxidase deficiency	Absent MPO-H_2O_2 system
Chédiak-Higashi syndrome	Multiple defects
Acquired	
Thermal injury, diabetes, malignancy, sepsis, immunodeficiencies	Chemotaxis
Hemodialysis, diabetes mellitus	Adhesion
Leukemia, anemia, sepsis, diabetes, neonates, malnutrition	Phagocytosis and microbicidal activity

Modified from Gallin, J.I. (ed): Disorders of phagocytic cells. *In* Inflammation: Basic Principles and Clinical Correlates, 2nd ed. New York, Raven Press, 1992, pp. 860 and 861.

Defects in Leukocyte Function

From the preceding discussion it is obvious that leukocytes play a cardinal role in host defense. Not surprisingly, therefore, defects in leukocyte function, both genetic and acquired, lead to increased vulnerability to infections (Table 3-2).[26] Impairments of virtually every phase of leukocyte function—from adherence to vascular endothelium to microbicidal activity—have been identified. We have described, for example, the genetic deficiencies in leukocyte adhesion molecules (LAD types 1 and 2) and in NADPH oxidase (CGD). Another is the *Chédiak-Higashi syndrome*, an autosomal recessive disorder characterized by neutropenia, defective degranulation, and delayed microbial killing. The neutrophils and other leukocytes have *giant granules*, resulting from fusion of predominantly azurophilic granules, which can be readily appreciated in peripheral blood smears. The molecular basis of this disease is unknown, but defects in microtubule function are suspected. Although individually rare, these genetic disorders underscore the importance of the complex series of leukocyte events that must occur *in vivo* following invasion by microorganisms.

SUMMARY OF THE ACUTE INFLAMMATORY RESPONSE

At this point it would be profitable to review the events in acute inflammation discussed so far. The vascular phenomena are characterized by increased blood flow to the injured area, resulting mainly from arteriolar dilatation and opening of capillary beds. Increased vascular permeability results in the accumulation of protein-rich extravascular fluid, which forms the exudate. Plasma proteins leave the vessels, most commonly through widened interendothelial cell junctions of the venules or by direct endothelial cell injury. The leukocytes, initially predominantly neutrophils, adhere to the endothelium via adhesion molecules, transmigrate across the endothelium, and migrate to the site of injury under the influence of chemotactic agents. Phagocytosis of the offending agent follows, which may lead to the death of the microorganism. During chemotaxis and phagocytosis, activated leukocytes may release toxic metabolites and proteases extracellularly, potentially causing tissue damage.

CHEMICAL MEDIATORS OF INFLAMMATION

Having described the events in acute inflammation, we can now turn to a discussion of the chemical mediators that account for the events. So many mediators have been identified that we are confronted with an embarrassment of riches. While the multitude may have survival value for the organism (and also for investigators searching for mediators and pharmaceutical companies for new drugs), they are most difficult for students to remember. Here we review general principles and highlight some of the more important mediators.

- *Mediators originate either from plasma or from cells* (Fig. 3–14). Plasma-derived mediators (e.g., complement) are present in plasma in *precursor forms* that *must be activated*, usually by a series of proteolytic cleavages, to acquire their biologic properties. Cell-derived mediators are normally *sequestered in intracellular granules* (e.g., histamine in mast cell granules) that need to be secreted or *are synthesized de novo* (e.g., prostaglandins) in response to a stimulus. The major cellular sources are platelets, neutrophils, monocytes/macrophages, and mast cells.
- Most mediators perform their biologic activity by initially *binding to specific receptors on target cells.* Some, however, have direct enzymatic activity (e.g., lysosomal proteases) or mediate oxidative damage (e.g., oxygen metabolites).
- *A chemical mediator can stimulate the release of mediators by target cells themselves.* These sec-

CHEMICAL MEDIATORS

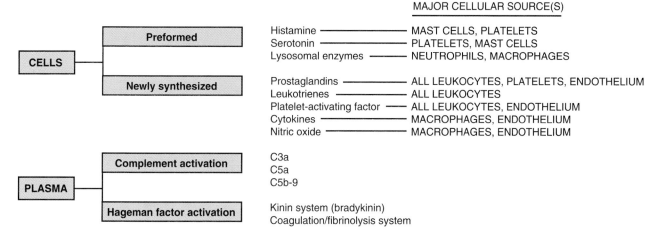

Figure 3–14. Chemical mediators of inflammation.

ondary mediators may be identical or similar to the initial mediators but may also have opposing activities. They provide mechanisms for amplifying—or in certain instances counteracting—the initial mediator action.

- Mediators can act on one or few target cell types, have widespread targets, or may even have differing effects, depending on cell and tissue types.
- *Once activated and released from the cell, most of these mediators are short-lived.* They quickly decay (e.g., arachidonic acid metabolites) or are inactivated by enzymes (e.g., kininase inactivates bradykinin), or they are otherwise scavenged (antioxidants scavenge toxic oxygen metabolites) or inhibited (e.g., complement inhibitors). There is thus a system of checks and balances in the regulation of mediator actions.
- *Most mediators may have harmful effects.* We shall now discuss the specific mediators.

VASOACTIVE AMINES

HISTAMINE. *Histamine* is widely distributed in tissues, the richest source being the mast cells that are normally present in the connective tissue adjacent to blood vessels (Fig. 3–15). It is also found in blood basophils and platelets. Preformed histamine is present in mast cell granules and is released by mast cell degranulation in response to a variety of stimuli: (1) physical injury such as trauma, cold, or heat; (2) immune reactions involving binding of antibodies to mast cells (see Chapter 6); (3) fragments of complement called anaphylatoxins (C3a and C5a); (4) histamine-releasing proteins derived from leukocytes; (5) neuropeptides (e.g., substance P); and (6) cytokines (IL-1, IL-8).

In humans, histamine causes dilatation of the arterioles and increases vascular permeability of the venules (it, however, *constricts* large arteries).

It is considered to be the principal mediator of the immediate phase of increased vascular permeability, causing venular endothelial contraction and widening of the interendothelial cell junctions, as we have seen. It acts on the microcirculation mainly via H_1 receptors.

SEROTONIN. *Serotonin* (5-hydroxytryptamine) is a second preformed vasoactive mediator with actions similar to those of histamine. It is present in platelets and enterochromaffin cells, and in mast cells in rodents but not humans.

Release of serotonin (and histamine) from *platelets* is stimulated when platelets aggregate after contact with collagen, thrombin, adenosine diphosphate (ADP), and antigen-antibody complexes. Platelet aggregation and release are also stimulated by platelet-activating factor (PAF) de-

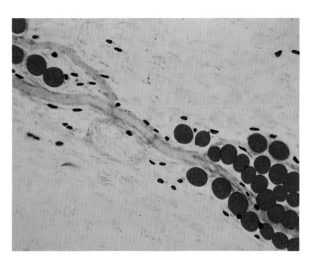

Figure 3–15. A flat spread of omentum showing mast cells *(dark blue)* around blood vessels and in the interstitial tissue. Stained with metachromatic stain to identify the mast cell granules. The red structures are fat globules stained with fat stain. (Courtesy of Dr. G. Majno.)

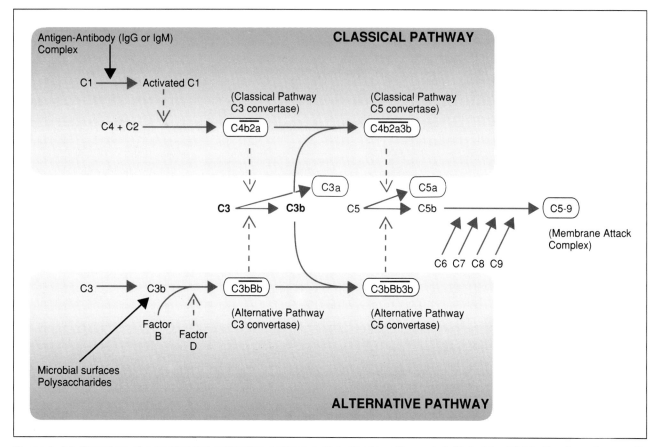

Figure 3-16. Overview of complement activation pathways. The classic pathway is initiated by C1 binding to antigen-antibody complexes, and the alternative pathway is initiated by C3b binding to various activating surfaces, such as microbial cell walls. The C3b involved in alternative pathway initiation may be generated in several ways, including spontaneously, by the classic pathway, or by the alternative pathway itself (see text). Both pathways converge and lead to the formation of inflammatory complement mediators (C3a and C5a) and the membrane attack complex. In this figure, bars over the letter designations of complement components indicate enzymatically active forms, and dashed lines indicate proteolytic activities of various components. (Modified from Abbas, A.K., et al.: Cellular and Molecular Immunology, 2nd ed. Philadelphia, W.B. Saunders Co., 1994.)

rived from mast cells during IgE-mediated reactions. In this way the platelet release reaction results in increased permeability during immunologic reactions. As will be discussed later, PAF itself has many inflammatory properties.

PLASMA PROTEASES

A variety of phenomena in the inflammatory response are mediated by three inter-related plasma-derived factors: the complement, kinin, and clotting systems (Figs. 3–16 and 3–17).

The Complement System

The complement system consists of 20 component proteins (together with their cleavage products), which are found in greatest concentration in plasma. This system functions in immunity for defense against microbial agents, culminating in lysing microbes by the so-called membrane attack complex (MAC). In the process, a number of complement components are elaborated that cause increased vascular permeability, chemotaxis, and opsonization (see Fig. 3–16).

Complement components present as inactive forms in plasma are numbered C1 through C9. Although it is not our intention to go into the detailed sequence of the activation of the "complement cascade," a brief review of the salient features will be helpful. The most critical step in the elaboration of the biologic functions of complement is the activation of the third component, C3. Cleavage of C3 can occur by the so-called *classical pathway*, which is triggered by fixation of C1 to antibody (IgM or IgG) combined with antigen, or through the *alternative pathway*, which can be triggered by microbial surfaces (e.g., endotoxins), aggregated IgA, complex polysaccharides, endotoxins, cobra venom, and so forth. The alternative pathway involves the participation of a distinct set of serum components called the properdin system (properdin [P], factors B and D). Whichever pathway is involved, *C3 convertase* splits C3 into two critical fragments—C3a, which is released, and C3b. C3b then binds to the fragments to form

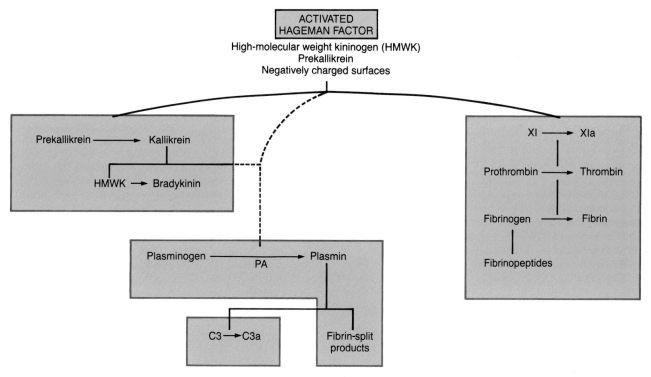

Figure 3–17. Inter-relations between the four plasma mediator systems. Interrupted lines indicate that the pathway may not be physiologically important. PA = plasminogen activator.

C5 convertase, which interacts with C5 to release C5a and initiate the assembly of the membrane attack complex (C5-C9). MAC causes lysis by initial hydrophobic binding to the lipid bilayer of target cells, eventually forming transmembrane channels.

Complement derived factors affect a variety of phenomena in acute inflammation:

- *Vascular phenomena. C3a, C5a,* and, to a small extent, *C4a* (called anaphylatoxins) are the split products of the corresponding complement components (see Fig. 3–16). They increase vascular permeability and cause vasodilatation mainly by releasing histamine from mast cells. C5a also activates the lipoxygenase pathway of arachidonic acid (AA) metabolism in neutrophils and monocytes, causing further release of inflammatory mediators.
- *Leukocyte adhesion, chemotaxis, and activation. C5a* is a powerful chemotactic agent for neutrophils, monocytes, eosinophils, and basophils. It also increases the adhesion of leukocytes to endothelium by activating the leukocytes and increasing the avidity of surface integrins to their endothelial ligand. C5a is rapidly converted in human serum to *C5a des Arg,* which is also chemotactic in the presence of a serum polypeptide called *cochemotaxin.*
- *Phagocytosis.* C3b and C3b$_i$, when fixed to the bacterial cell wall, act as an opsonin and favor phagocytosis by neutrophils and macrophages, which bear cell surface receptors for C3b.

Among the complement components, C3 and C5 are the most important inflammatory mediators. Their significance is further enhanced by the fact that, in addition to the mechanisms discussed above, C3 and C5 can be activated by several proteolytic enzymes present within the inflammatory exudate. These include plasmin and lysosomal enzymes released from neutrophils (see discussion later in this chapter). Thus, the chemotactic effect of complement and the complement-activating effects of neutrophils can set up a self-perpetuating cycle of neutrophil emigration.

The Kinin System

The kinin system is directly triggered by contact (surface) activation of Hageman factor (factor XII of the intrinsic clotting pathway) described below and in Chapter 4 (see Fig. 3–17). The kinin system results in the ultimate release of the vasoactive nonapeptide *bradykinin,* a potent agent that increases vascular permeability. *Bradykinin also causes contraction of smooth muscle, dilation of blood vessels, and pain when injected into the skin.* The cascade that eventually produces kinin is shown in Figure 3–17. It is triggered, as noted, by activation of Hageman factor by contact with negatively charged surfaces, such as collagen and basement membranes. A fragment of factor XII (prekallikrein activator, or factor XIIa) is produced, and this converts plasma prekallikrein into an active proteolytic form, the enzyme *kallikrein.* The latter cleaves a plasma-glycoprotein precursor, *high-molecular-weight kininogen (HMWK),* to produce *bradykinin* (HMWK also acts as a cofactor or catalyst in the activation of Hageman factor). The action of bradykinin is short-lived because it is quickly inactivated by an enzyme called *kininase. Of importance is that kallikrein itself is a potent activator of Hageman factor, allowing for autocatalytic amplification of the initial stimulus.* Kallikrein has chemotactic activity, and it also directly converts C5 to C5a.

The Clotting System

The clotting system (see also Chapter 4) is a series of plasma proteins that can also be activated by Hageman factor (see Fig. 3–17). The final step of the cascade is the conversion of fibrinogen to fibrin by the action of thrombin. During this conversion, *fibrinopeptides* are formed, which induce increased vascular permeability and chemotactic activity for leukocytes. *Thrombin* also has inflammatory properties, including causing increased leukocyte adhesion and fibroblast proliferation (see Chapter 4, Fig. 4–4).

The *fibrinolytic system* contributes to the vascular phenomena of inflammation in several ways, (Fig. 3–17). Plasminogen activator (released from endothelium, leukocytes, and other tissues) cleaves plasminogen, a plasma protein that binds to the evolving fibrin clot to generate *plasmin,* a multifunctional protease. (Kallikrein and activated Hageman factor can also convert plasminogen to plasmin *in vitro,* but the physiologic relevance of this is uncertain.) Plasmin is important in lysing fibrin clots, but in the context of inflammation it also cleaves C3 to produce C3 fragments, and it degrades fibrin to form "fibrin split products," which may have permeability-inducing properties.

From this discussion of the complex mediators generated by the kinin, complement, and clotting systems, a few general conclusions can be drawn:

- *Bradykinin, C3a, and C5a (as mediators of increased vascular permeability), and C5a (as the mediator of chemotaxis),* and *thrombin* (which has effects on many cell types) are the most likely to be important *in vivo.*
- *C3 and C5* can be generated by three different groups of influences: (a) classic immunologic reactions; (b) alternative complement pathway activation; and (c) agents with little immunologic specificity, such as bacterial products, plasmin, kallikrein, and some serine proteases found in normal tissue.
- *Activated Hageman factor (factor XIIa)* initiates the clotting, kinin and possibly the fibrinolytic systems. Some of the products of this initiation —particularly kallikrein—can, by feedback, activate Hageman factor, resulting in profound amplification of the effects of the initial contact.

ARACHIDONIC ACID (AA) METABOLITES: PROSTAGLANDINS AND LEUKOTRIENES (EICOSANOIDS)

Products derived from the metabolism of AA (called eicosanoids) affect a variety of biologic processes, including inflammation and hemostasis. They are best thought of as *autocoids,* or local short-range hormones, which are formed rapidly, exert their effects locally, and then either decay spontaneously or are destroyed enzymatically.

Arachidonic acid (AA) is a 20-carbon polyunsaturated fatty acid (5,8,11,14-eicosatetraenoic acid) that is derived directly from dietary sources or by conversion from the essential fatty acid *linoleic acid.* It does not occur free in the cell but is normally esterified in membrane phospholipids, particularly in the carbon 2 position of phosphatidylcholine and phosphatidylinositol. It is released from phospholipids through the activation of cellular phospholipases by mechanical, chemical, and physical stimuli or by other mediators (e.g., C5a). AA metabolism proceeds along one of two major pathways (Fig. 3–18) named after the enzymes that initiate the reactions.

- The *cyclooxgenase pathway* leads to the generation of *prostaglandins.* These include PGE_2, PGD_2, $PGF_{2\alpha}$, PGI_2 (prostacyclin), and thromboxane (TxA_2), each of which is derived by the action of a specific enzyme. Some of these enzymes have restricted tissue distribution. For example, platelets contain the enzyme thromboxane synthetase, and hence TxA_2 is the major product in these cells. TxA_2, a potent platelet-aggregating agent and vasoconstrictor, is itself unstable and rapidly converted to its inactive form TxB_2. Vascular endothelium, on the other hand, lacks thromboxane synthetase but posseses prostacyclin synthetase, which leads to the formation of prostacyclin (PGI_2) and its stable end product $PGF_{1\alpha}$. Prostacyclin is a vasodilator and a potent inhibitor of platelet aggregation. The opposing roles of TxA_2 and PGI_2 in hemostasis are further discussed in Chapter 4. PGD_2 is the major metabolite of the cyclooxygenase pathway in mast cells; along with PGE_2 and PGF_2 (which are more widely distributed) it causes vasodilatation and potentiates edema formation. Aspirin and nonsteroidal anti-inflammatory agents, such as indomethacin, inhibit cyclooxygenase and thus inhibit prostaglandin synthesis. Lipoxygenase, however, is not affected by these anti-inflammatory agents.
- In the *lipoxygenase pathway,* 5-lipoxygenase is the predominant enzyme in neutrophils, and the

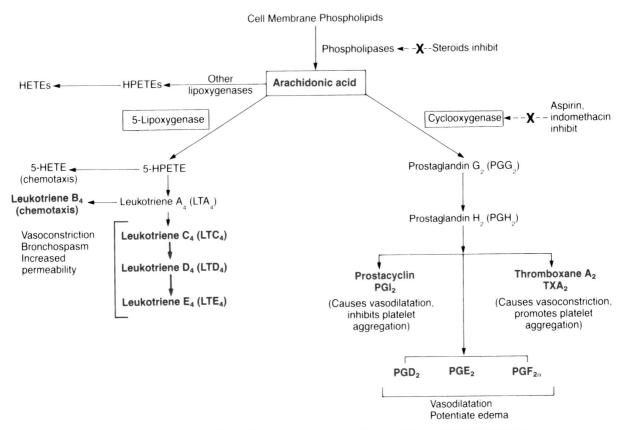

Figure 3–18. Generation of arachidonic acid metabolites and their roles in inflammation.

metabolites derived by its actions are the best characterized. The main product, 5-HETE, which is chemotactic for neutrophils, is converted into a family of compounds collectively called *leukotrienes*. LTB$_4$ is a potent chemotactic agent and causes aggregation of neutrophils. LTC$_4$, LTD$_4$, and LTE$_4$ cause vasoconstriction, bronchospasm, and increased vascular permeability. Neutrophils also produce trihydroxymetabolites of AA called *lipoxins*.[32] Lipoxins have both anti- and proinflammatory effects, and their role *in vivo* is currently being pursued.

Eicosanoids can mediate virtually every step of acute inflammation (Table 3–3).

- *Prostaglandin E and prostacyclin* are important mediators of inflammatory vasodilation. They also markedly potentiate the permeability-increasing and chemotactic effects of other mediators.

- *The cysteinyl-containing leukotrienes C$_4$, D$_4$, and E$_4$* cause intense vasoconstriction and increase vascular permeability. The vascular leakage, as with histamine, is restricted to venules. They are also potent bronchoconstrictors.

- *Leukotriene B$_4$* causes aggregation and adhesion of leukocytes to venular endothelium and is a powerful chemotactic agent. Some of the other products of lipoxygenase metabolism, such as HETE, are also chemotactic.

- *The prostaglandins* are also involved in the pathogenesis of *fever* and *pain* in inflammation. PGE$_2$ causes a marked increase in pain produced by intradermal injection of suboptimal concentrations of histamine and bradykinin and interacts with cytokines in causing fever during infections, as described later in this chapter.

- Eicosanoids can be found in inflammatory exudates, and agents that suppress cyclooxygenase (aspirin, indomethacin) also suppress inflammation *in vivo*. Glucocorticoids, which are powerful anti-inflammatory agents, may act at least in part by inducing the synthesis of a protein that inhibits phospholipase A$_2$.

- Finally, variations in AA metabolism may account for some of the beneficial effects of *fish oil*. Diets rich in fish oil contain essential fatty acids of the

Table 3–3. INFLAMMATORY ACTIONS OF EICOSANOIDS

ACTION	METABOLITE
Vasoconstriction	Thromboxane A$_2$, leukotrienes C$_4$, D$_4$, E$_4$
Vasodilatation	PGI$_2$, PGE$_1$, PGE$_2$, PGD$_2$
Increased vascular permeability	Leukotrienes C$_4$, D$_4$, E$_4$
Chemotaxis	Leukotriene B$_4$, HETE

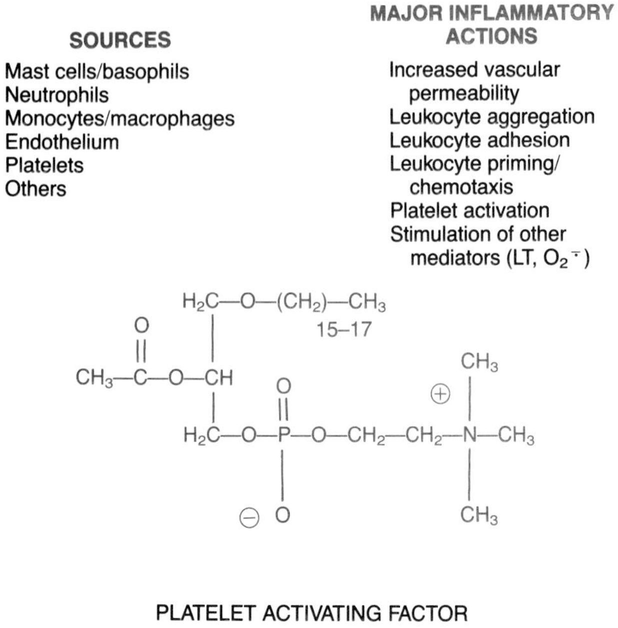

SOURCES	MAJOR INFLAMMATORY ACTIONS
Mast cells/basophils	Increased vascular permeability
Neutrophils	Leukocyte aggregation
Monocytes/macrophages	Leukocyte adhesion
Endothelium	Leukocyte priming/ chemotaxis
Platelets	Platelet activation
Others	Stimulation of other mediators (LT, O_2^-)

$$H_2C-O-(CH_2)-CH_3 \quad 15-17$$

PLATELET ACTIVATING FACTOR

Figure 3–19. Structure, sources, and main inflammatory actions of PAF. LT = leukotrienes.

ω 3 variety (e.g., *linolenic acid*) rather than ω 2 linoleic acid found in most animal or vegetable fat. The ω 3 fatty acids serve as poor substrates for conversion to active metabolites of the cyclooxygenase and, particularly, the lipoxygenase series. Such diets inhibit platelet aggregation and thrombosis and prevent certain inflammatory processes.

PLATELET-ACTIVATING FACTOR

Platelet-activating factor (PAF) is another phospholipid-derived mediator.[34] Its name comes from its initial discovery as a factor derived from antigen-stimulated IgE-sensitized basophils, which causes platelet aggregation and release but is now known to have multiple inflammatory effects. Chemically, it is an acetyl glycerol ether phosphocholine and it is synthesized from membrane phospholipids by activation of phospholipases (PLA_2) (Fig. 3–19). In addition to platelet stimulation, PAF causes vasoconstriction and bronchoconstriction, and at extremely low concentrations it induces vasodilation and increased venular permeability with a potency 100 to 10,000 times greater than that of histamine. PAF also causes increased leukocyte adhesion to endothelium (by enhancing leukocyte integrin binding), chemotaxis, degranulation, and the oxidative burst. Thus, PAF can elicit most of the cardinal features of inflammation. A variety of cell types, including basophils, neutrophils, monocytes, and endothelial cells, can elaborate PAF, in both secreted and cell-bound forms.

PAF acts directly on target cells via specific receptors, but it also boosts the synthesis of other mediators, particularly eicosanoids, by leukocytes and other cells. A role for PAF *in vivo* is supported by the ability of synthetic PAF antagonists to inhibit inflammation in some experimental models.

CYTOKINES

Cytokines are polypeptides produced by many cell types (but principally activated lymphocytes and macrophages) that modulate the function of other cell types. Long known to be involved in cellular immune responses (see Chapter 6), these products have additional effects that play important roles in the inflammatory response.[35] The main cytokines that mediate inflammation are IL-1, TNF (α and β), and the IL-8 family.

IL-1 and *TNF* share many biologic properties. IL-1 and TNF-α are produced by activated macrophages, TNF-β by activated T cells, and IL-1 by many other cell types as well. Their secretion can be stimulated by endotoxin, immune complexes, toxins, physical injury, and a variety of inflammatory processes. Like growth factors, they induce their effects in three ways: they can act on the same cell that produces them (an *autocrine* effect), on cells in the immediate vicinity (as in lymph nodes and joint spaces; a *paracrine* effect); or systemically, as with any other hormone (*endocrine* effect). Their most important actions in inflammation are their effects on endothelium, leukocytes, and fibroblasts, and induction of the systemic acute-phase reactions (Fig. 3–20). The latter are relevant to the process of repair and are described in Chapter 2 and later in this chapter. In endothe-

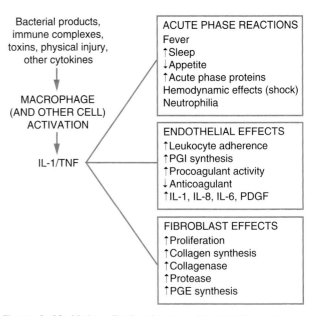

Figure 3–20. Major effects of interleukin-1 (IL-1) and tumor necrosis factor (TNF) in inflammation.

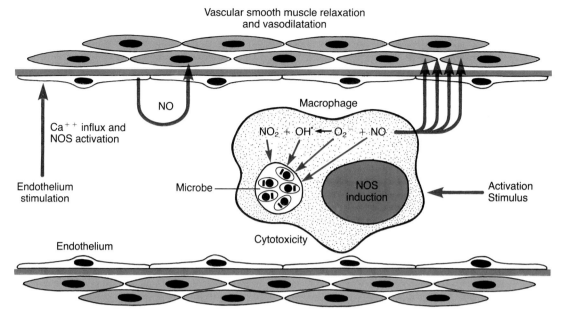

Figure 3–21. Two types of NO synthesis in endothelium *(left)* and macrophages *(right)*. NO causes vasodilation and NO free radicals are cytotoxic to microbial and mammalian cells. NOS = nitric oxide synthase. (Courtesy of Dr. Jeffrey Joseph.)

lium, they induce a spectrum of changes—mostly regulated at the level of gene transcription—referred to as *endothelial activation*.[13] In particular, they induce the synthesis of endothelial adhesion molecules, other cytokines, growth factors, eicosanoids, and nitric oxide and increase surface thrombogenicity of the endothelium. TNF also causes aggregation and *priming* of neutrophils, leading to augmented responses of these cells to other mediators, and the release of proteolytic enzymes from mesenchymal cells, thus contributing to tissue damage.

IL-8 is a small (8000 MW) polypeptide secreted by activated macrophages and other cell types (e.g., endothelial cells) that is a powerful chemoattractant and activator of neutrophils, with limited activity on monocytes and eosinophils.[36] Its most important inducers are other cytokines, mainly IL-1 and TNF-α. It belongs to a family of structurally similar small proteins, now called *chemokines*,[36] characterized by four cysteine residues at identical positions. These include, in addition to IL-8, *platelet factor 4 (PF4)*, a cationic protein of platelet alpha granules (see Chapter 4) with chemotactic activity for neutrophils, monocytes, and eosinophils and with histamine-releasing activity for mast cells; *monocyte chemoattractant protein (MCP-1)*, a chemotactic and activating agent that is fairly specific for monocytes, and *RANTES*, which is chemotactic for thymocytes. The chemokines bind to a family of receptors, called *serpentines*, characterized by seven transmembrane domains coupled to G proteins.[37]

Both IL-1 and TNF (as well as IL-6) also induce the systemic *acute-phase responses* (see discussion under section on fever)[38] associated with infection or injury, including fever, the production of slow-wave sleep, the release of neutrophils into the circulation, the release of adrenocorticotropic hormone (ACTH) and corticosteroids, and, particularly with regard to TNF, the hemodynamic effects of septic shock—hypotension, decreased vascular resistance, increased heart rate, and decreased blood pH.

NITRIC OXIDE (NO)

This is a relatively "new" mediator of inflammation, and the history of its discovery deserves brief mention. In 1980, Furchgott showed that vasodilatation produced by acetylcholine requires an intact endothelium.[39] In response to such vasodilatory agents, endothelial cells produced a short-acting factor, endothelium-derived relaxing factor (EDRF), that relaxed vascular smooth muscle. Subsequently, it was shown that vascular endothelium produces NO, and this gas has the physical and biologic properties of EDRF.[40] NO binds to the heme moiety on guanylyl cyclase and activates the enzyme. Through a cascade of kinases, the resultant increase in the concentration of cyclic guanosine monophosphate (cGMP) mediates relaxation and, consequently, produces vasodilatation.

Nitric oxide is a soluble free radical gas that is produced not only by endothelial cells but also by macrophages and specific neurons in the brain. *It is synthesized from L-arginine, molecular oxygen, and NADPH by the enzyme nitric oxide synthase (NOS).* There are two types of NOS (Fig. 3–21). In endothelial cells and neurons, *NOS* is present

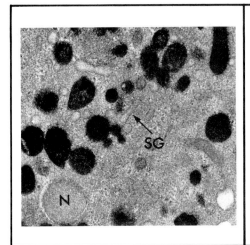

SPECIFIC GRANULES
Lactoferrin
Lysozyme
Alkaline phosphatase
Type IV collagenase
Leukocyte adhesion molecules
Plasminogen activation
Phospholipase A_2

AZUROPHIL GRANULES
Myeloperoxidase
Lysozyme ← Bactericidal factors
Cationic proteins
Acid hydrolases
Elastase
Nonspecific collagenase
BPI
Defensins
Cathepsin G
Phospholipase A_2

Figure 3–22. Ultrastructure of neutrophil granules stained for peroxidase activity and their constituents. The large peroxidase-containing granules are the azurophil granules; the smaller peroxidase-negative ones are the specific granules (SG). N = portion of nucleus; BPI = bactericidal permeability increasing protein.

A   B

constitutively and can be activated rapidly by an increase in cytoplasmic calcium ions in the presence of calmodulin. Influx of calcium into these cells leads to a rapid production of NO. In contrast, *macrophage NOS is induced*, when macrophages are activated by cytokines (e.g., IFN-γ) or other agents; no intracellular increase in calcium is required. Since the *in vivo* half-life of NO is only a matter of seconds, the gas acts only on cells in close proximity to where it is produced. Such a localized activity accounts for the specificity of its actions.

In addition to vascular smooth muscle relaxation, NO plays other important roles in inflammation. It reduces platelet aggregation and adhesion, as described in Chapter 4. The NO produced by macrophages, acting as a free radical, is cytotoxic to certain microbes and tumor cells. It can oxidize sulfhydryl groups on proteins and cause a depletion of cytosolic glutathione, and it can react with superoxide anion to form the strong oxidant nitrogen dioxide and the highly reactive hydroxyl radical ($NO^{\cdot} + O_2^{-} \longrightarrow NO_2^{-} + OH^{\cdot}$).[40] Uncontrolled NO production by activated macrophages in septic shock (see Chapter 4) can lead to massive peripheral vasodilatation and shock, and NO has also been implicated in a variety of inflammatory diseases. Inhibitors of NO production are now being tested clinically and have been shown, for example, to reduce the size of ischemic brain infarcts.

LYSOSOMAL CONSTITUENTS OF LEUKOCYTES

Neutrophils and monocytes contain lysosomal granules, which when released may contribute to the inflammatory response. *Neutrophils* exhibit two main types of granules (Fig. 3–22). The smaller *specific* (or secondary) granules contain lactoferrin,

lysozyme, alkaline phosphatase, the components of NADPH oxidase, the intracytoplasmic pool of integrins, and (in human neutrophils) a collagenase. The large *azurophil* (or primary) granules contain MPO, bactericidal factors (lysozyme, defensins), acid hydrolases, and a variety of neutral proteases (elastase, nonspecific collagenases, proteinase 3). As previously explained, these enzymes are either released after cell death or secreted by a variety of mechanisms. There are, however, differences in the mobilization of specific and azurophil granules. The specific granules are secreted more readily and by lower concentrations of agonists, while the more potentially destructive azurophil granules release their contents primarily within the phagosome and require very high levels of agonists to be released extracellularly.[42]

Acid proteases degrade proteins at an acid pH. Their most likely action is to degrade bacteria and debris *within* the phagolysosomes, where an acid pH is readily reached. *Neutral proteases*, on the other hand, are capable of degrading various extracellular components. These enzymes can attack collagen, basement membrane, fibrin, elastin, and cartilage, resulting in the tissue destruction characteristic of purulent and deforming inflammatory processes. Neutral proteases can also cleave C3 and C5 directly, releasing anaphylatoxins, and release a kinin-like peptide from kininogen. *Monocytes* and *macrophages* also contain acid hydrolases, collagenase, elastase, and plasminogen activator. These may be particularly active in chronic inflammatory reactions.

Lysosomal constituents thus have numerous effects. The initial leukocytic infiltration, if unchecked, can potentiate further increases in vascular permeability, chemotaxis, and tissue damage. These harmful proteases, however, are held in check by a system of *antiproteases* in the serum and tissue fluids. Foremost among these is *alpha₁-antitrypsin*, which is the major inhibitor of neutrophilic elastase. A deficiency of these inhibitors may lead to sustained action of leukocyte proteases, as is the case in patients with alpha$_1$-antitrypsin deficiency (see Chapter 15). *Alpha$_2$-macroglobulin* is another antiprotease found in serum and various secretions.

OXYGEN-DERIVED FREE RADICALS

These metabolites may be released extracellularly from leukocytes after exposure to chemotactic agents, immune complexes, or a phagocytic challenge. Their production is dependent, as we have seen, on the activation of the NADPH oxidative system and generation of superoxide. Superoxide, in turn, is converted to H_2O_2, $OH^{\cdot}$ and, by combining with NO, to toxic NO derivatives.[43] They are implicated in the following responses.

- *Endothelial cell damage, with resultant increased vascular permeability.* Adherent neutrophils, when activated, not only produce their own toxic species but also stimulate xanthine oxidation in endothelial cells themselves, thus elaborating more superoxide.
- *Inactivation of antiproteases,* such as alpha$_1$-antitrypsin, discussed earlier together with *activation of metalloproteinases.* This leads to unopposed protease activity, with increased destruction of ECM.
- *Injury to other cell types* (tumor cells, red cells, parenchymal cells).

Serum, tissue fluids, and target cells possess antioxidant protective mechanisms that detoxify these potentially harmful oxygen-derived radicals. These antioxidants have been discussed in Chapter 1, but to repeat, they include (1) the copper-containing serum protein *ceruloplasmin;* (2) the iron-free fraction of serum, *transferrin;* (3) the enzyme *superoxide dismutase,* which is found or can be activated in a variety of cell types; (4) the enzyme *catalase,* which detoxifies H_2O_2; and (5) *glutathione peroxidase,* another powerful H_2O_2 detoxifier. *Thus, the influence of oxygen-derived free radicals in any given inflammatory reaction depends on the balance between the production and the inactivation of these metabolites by cells and tissues.*

OTHER MEDIATORS

Neuropeptides, such as substance P, cause vasodilatation and increased vascular permeability both directly and by stimulating histamine release and ei-

Table 3–4. SUMMARY OF MEDIATORS OF ACUTE INFLAMMATION

MEDIATOR	SOURCE	ACTION		
		Vascular Leakage	*Chemotaxis*	*Other*
Histamine and serotonin	Mast cells, platelets	+	−	
Bradykinin	Plasma substrate	+	−	Pain
C3a	Plasma protein via	+	−	Opsonic fragment (C3b)
C5a	liver; macrophages	+	+	Leukocyte adhesion, activation
Prostaglandins	Mast cells, from membrane phospholipids	Potentiate other mediators	−	Vasodilation, pain, fever
Leukotriene B$_4$	Leukocytes	−	+	Leukocyte adhesion, activation
Leukotriene C$_4$, D$_4$, E$_4$	Leukocytes, mast cells	+	−	Bronchoconstriction, vasoconstriction
Oxygen metabolites	Leukocytes	+	±	Endothelial damage, tissue damage
PAF	Leukocytes; mast cells	+	+	Bronchoconstriction Leukocyte priming
IL-1 and TNF	Macrophages; other	−	+	Acute phase reactions Endothelial activation
IL-8	Macrophages Endothelium	−	+	Leukocyte activation
Nitric oxide	Macrophages Endothelium			Vasodilation Cytotoxicity

Table 3-5. MOST LIKELY MEDIATORS IN INFLAMMATION

VASODILATION
Prostaglandins
Nitric oxide
INCREASED VASCULAR PERMEABILITY
Vasoactive amines
C3a and C5a (through liberating amines)
Bradykinin
Leukotrienes C_4, D_4, E_4
PAF
CHEMOTAXIS, LEUKOCYTE ACTIVATION
C5a
Leukotriene B_4
Bacterial products
Cytokines (IL-8)
FEVER
IL-1, IL-6, TNF
Prostaglandins
PAIN
Prostaglandins
Bradykinin
TISSUE DAMAGE
Neutrophil and macrophage lysosomal enzymes
Oxygen metabolites
Nitric oxide

cosanoid production by mast cells, and also enhance neutrophil adhesion and chemotaxis.[44]

Growth factors (platelet-derived growth factor [PDGF] and transforming growth factor β [TGF-β]), as we described in Chapter 2, may be chemotactic to leukocytes and mesenchymal cells and have other activities resembling those of cytokines. Indeed, there is so much overlap in the functions of cytokines and growth factors that the terms are now used interchangeably. Additionally, certain *ECM components* or their fragments have chemotactic activity. These will be discussed further under the section on chronic inflammation.

SUMMARY OF CHEMICAL MEDIATORS OF ACUTE INFLAMMATION

Table 3-4 summarizes the major actions of the principal mediators. When Lewis suggested that existence of histamine, one mediator was clearly not enough. Now, we are wallowing in them! Yet, from this menu of substances we can tentatively extract a few mediators that may be relevant *in vivo* (Table 3-5). *For increased vascular permeability, histamine, the anaphylatoxins (C3a and C5a), the kinins, leukotrienes C, D, and E, and PAF are almost certainly involved, at least early in the course of inflammation. For chemotaxis, complement fragment C5a, lipoxygenase products (LTB_4), and other chemotactic lipids are the most likely protagonists. Also, the important role of prostaglandins in vasodilation, pain, and fever and in potentiating edema cannot be denied. IL-1 and TNF are involved with endothelial-leukocyte interactions and with acute-phase reactions. Lysosomal products and oxy-*

gen-derived radicals are the most likely candidates as causes of the ensuing tissue destruction. NO is involved in vasodilatation and cytotoxicity.*

OUTCOMES OF ACUTE INFLAMMATION

The discussion of mediators completed the basic description of the relatively uniform pattern of the inflammatory reaction encountered in most injuries. *Recall that, although hemodynamic, permeability, and white cell changes have been described sequentially and may be initiated in this order, all these phenomena in the fully evolved reaction to injury are concurrent in a seemingly chaotic but remarkably organized multiring circus. As might be expected, many variables may modify this basic process, including the nature and intensity of the injury, the site and tissue affected, and the responsiveness of the host.*

In general, however, acute inflammation may have one of four outcomes (Fig. 3-23):

1. *Complete resolution.* In a perfect world, all inflammatory reactions, once they have succeeded in neutralizing the injurious stimulus, should end with restoration of the site of acute inflammation to normal. This is called *resolution* and is the usual outcome when the injury is limited or short-lived or when there has been little tissue destruction. Resolution involves neutralization of the chemical mediators, with subsequent return of normal vascular permeability, cessation of leukocytic infiltration, and finally removal of edema fluid and protein, leukocytes, foreign agents, and necrotic debris from the battleground (Fig. 3-24). Lymphatics and phagocytes play a role in these events, as we shall see.

2. *Healing by connective tissue replacement (fibrosis)* occurs after substantial tissue destruction, or when the inflammatory injury occurs in tissues that do not regenerate, or when there is abundant fibrin exudation. When the fibrinous exudate in tissue or serous cavities (pleura, peritoneum) cannot be adequately resorbed, connective tissue grows into the area of exudate, converting it into a mass of fibrous tissue—a process also called *organization.*

3. *Abscess formation,* which occurs particularly in infections with pyogenic organisms.

4. Progression of the tissue response to *chronic inflammation,* which will be discussed next, may follow acute inflammation, or the response may be chronic almost from the onset. Acute to chronic transition occurs when the acute inflammatory response cannot be resolved, owing either to the persistence of the injurious agent or to some interference in the normal process of healing. For example, bacterial infection of the lung may begin as a focus of acute inflammation (pneumonia), but

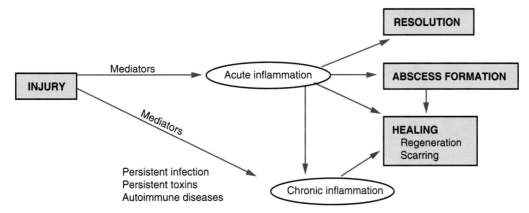

Figure 3-23. Outcome of acute inflammation (see text).

its failure to resolve may lead to extensive tissue destruction and formation of a cavity in which the inflammation continues to smolder, leading eventually to a chronic lung abscess. Another example of chronic inflammation with a persisting stimulus is

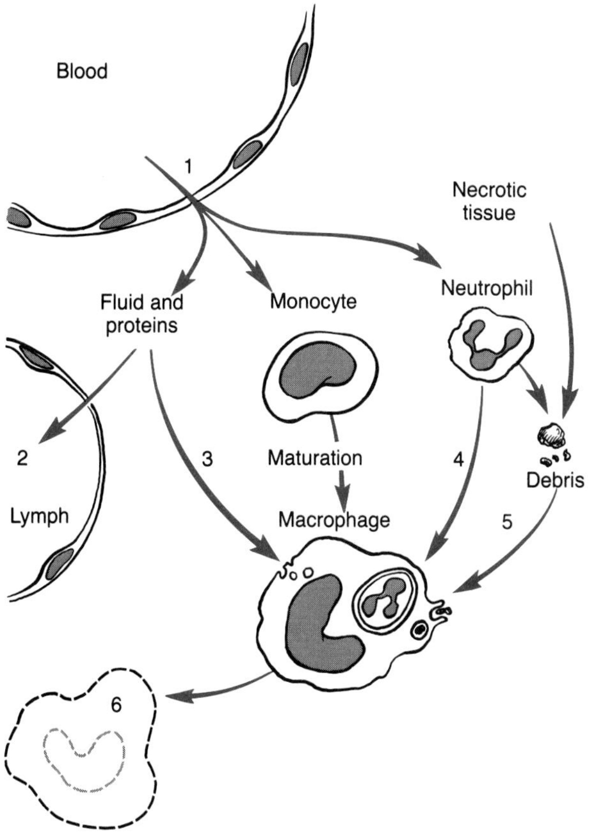

peptic ulcer of the duodenum or stomach. Peptic ulcers may persist for months or years and, as we shall see, are manifested by both acute and chronic inflammatory reactions.

We shall now proceed to a more detailed account of chronic inflammation.

CHRONIC INFLAMMATION

Although difficult to define precisely, chronic inflammation is considered to be *inflammation of prolonged duration* (weeks or months) *in which active inflammation, tissue destruction, and attempts at healing are proceeding simultaneously*. While it may follow acute inflammation, as described earlier, chronic inflammation frequently begins insidiously, as a low-grade, smoldering, often asymptomatic response. Indeed, this latter type of chronic inflammation includes some of the most common and disabling of human diseases, such as rheumatoid arthritis, atherosclerosis, tuberculosis, and the chronic lung diseases. Such inflammation arises under the following settings:

- *Persistent infections* by certain microorganisms, such as tubercle bacilli, *Treponema pallidum* (causative organism of syphilis), and certain fungi. These organisms are of low toxicity and evoke an immune reaction called delayed hypersensitivity (see Chapter 6). The inflammatory response sometimes takes a specific pattern called a *granulomatous reaction*, which is discussed later in this chapter.

- *Prolonged exposure to potentially toxic agents,* either exogenous or endogenous. Examples are nondegradable inanimate material, such as particulate silica inhaled for a prolonged period that results in a lung inflammatory disease called *silicosis* (Chapter 15); and plasma lipid components, which, if chronically elevated, induce *atherosclerosis* (Chapter 11).

- Under certain conditions, immune reactions are set up against the individual's own tissues, lead-

Figure 3-24. Events in the resolution of inflammation: (1) return to normal vascular permeability; (2) drainage of edema fluid and proteins into lymphatics or (3) by pinocytosis into macrophages; (4) phagocytosis of neutrophils; (5) necrotic debris by macrophages; and (6) disposal of macrophages. Note the central role of macrophages in resolution. (Modified from Haslett, C., and Henson, P.M.: *In* Clark, R., and Henson, P.M. (eds.): The Molecular and Cellular Biology of Wound Repair. New York, Plenum Press, 1988.)

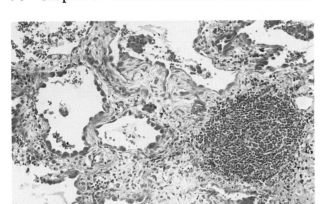

Figure 3-25. Chronic inflammation in the lung, showing all three characteristic histologic features: a collection of chronic inflammatory cells; replacement by connective tissue (fibrosis); and destruction of lung parenchyma— normal alveoli are replaced by spaces lined by cuboidal epithelium.

ing to *autoimmune diseases* (see Chapter 6). In these diseases, autoantigens evoke a self-perpetuating immune reaction that results in several common chronic inflammatory diseases, such as rheumatoid arthritis and lupus erythematosus.

In contrast to acute inflammation, which is manifested by vascular changes, edema, and largely neutrophilic infiltration, *chronic inflammation is characterized by (1) infiltration with mononuclear cells, which include macrophages, lymphocytes, and plasma cells*, a reflection of a persistent *reaction to injury*, (2) *tissue destruction*, largely induced by the inflammatory cells, and (3) attempts at *repair by*

connective tissue replacement, namely proliferation of small blood vessels *(angiogenesis)* and, in particular, *fibrosis* (Fig. 3–25). We shall now review these manifestations of chronic inflammation and discuss the mechanisms underlying them.

MONONUCLEAR INFILTRATION

The *macrophage* is the prima donna of chronic inflammation, and we shall begin our discussion with a brief review of its biology.[46]

Macrophages are but one component of the *mononuclear phagocyte system (MPS)*, previously known as the reticuloendothelial system (RES) (Fig. 3–26). The MPS consists of closely related cells of bone marrow origin, including blood monocytes, and tissue macrophages. The latter are diffusely scattered in the connective tissue or clustered in organs such as the liver (Kupffer's cells), spleen and lymph nodes (sinus histiocytes), and lungs (alveolar macrophages). All arise from a common precursor in the bone marrow, which gives rise to blood monocytes. From the blood, monocytes migrate into various tissue and transform into macrophages. The half-life of blood monocytes is about one day, whereas the life span of tissue macrophages is several months.

As discussed previously, monocytes begin to emigrate relatively early in acute inflammation, and within 48 hours they constitute the predominant cell type. Extravasation of monocytes is governed by the same factors involved in neutrophil emigration, namely adhesion molecules and chemical mediators with chemotactic and activating

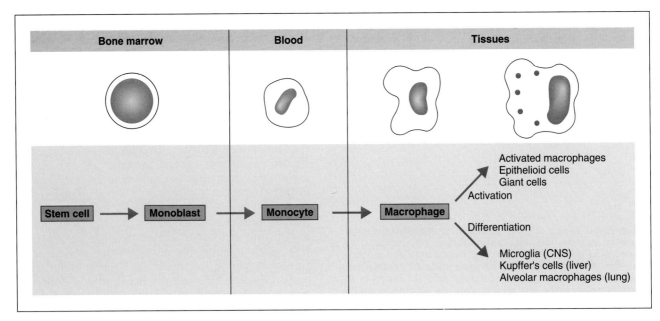

Figure 3-26. Maturation of mononuclear phagocytes. (With permission from Abbas, A. K., et al.: Cellular and Molecular Immunology, 2nd ed. Philadelphia, W.B. Saunders Co., 1994.)

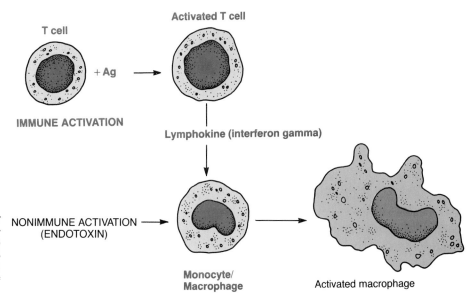

Figure 3–27. Two stimuli for macrophage activation: lymphokines (interferon gamma) from immune-activated T cells and nonimmunologic stimuli such as endotoxin. Ag = antigen.

properties.[45] When the monocyte reaches the extravascular tissue it undergoes transformation into a larger phagocytic cell, *the macrophage.* In addition to performing phagocytosis, macrophages have the potential of being *"activated,"* a process that results in an increase in cell size, increased levels of lysosomal enzymes, more active metabolism, and greater ability to phagocytose and kill ingested microbes. Activation signals include cytokines (e.g., IFN-γ) secreted by sensitized T lymphocytes, bacterial endotoxins, other chemical mediators, and ECM proteins like fibronectin (Fig. 3–27). Following activation, the *macrophages secrete a wide variety of biologically active products* that are important mediators of the tissue destruction, vascular proliferation, and fibrosis characteristic of chronic inflammation (Fig. 3–28 and Table 3–6).

In short-lived acute inflammation, if the irritant is eliminated, macrophages eventually disappear (either dying off or making their way into the lymphatics and lymph nodes). In chronic inflammation macrophage accumulation persists, mediated by different mechanisms, each predominating in different types of reactions (Fig. 3–29):

1. *Continued recruitment of monocytes from the circulation,* which results from the steady expression of adhesion molecules and chemotactic factors. This is numerically the most important source for macrophages. Chemotactic stimuli for monocytes include C5a; cytokines of the IL-8 family (chemokines) produced by activated macrophages and lymphocytes (e.g., MCP-1 for monocytes); certain growth factors, such as PDGF and TGF-β; fragments from the breakdown of collagen and fibronectin, and fibrinopeptides. Each of these may play a role under given circumstances; for example, cytokines are almost certainly involved during delayed-hypersensitivity immune reactions.

2. *Local proliferation of macrophages* after their emigration from the bloodstream. Once thought to be an unusual event, macrophage proliferation is now known to occur prominently in atheromatous plaques (see Chapter 11).

3. *Immobilization of macrophages* within the site of inflammation. Indeed, certain cytokines (macrophage inhibitory factor) and oxidized lipids (see Chapter 11) can cause such immobilization.

The macrophage is a central figure in chronic inflammation because of the great number of biologically active substances it can produce. Some of these are toxic to cells (e.g., oxygen metabolites) or extracellular matrix (proteases), some cause influx of other cell types (e.g., cytokines, chemotac-

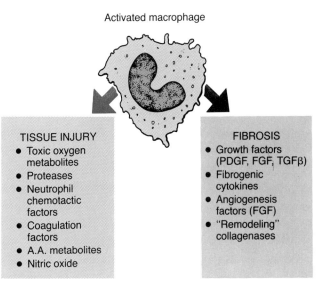

Activated macrophage

TISSUE INJURY
- Toxic oxygen metabolites
- Proteases
- Neutrophil chemotactic factors
- Coagulation factors
- A.A. metabolites
- Nitric oxide

FIBROSIS
- Growth factors (PDGF, FGF, TGFβ)
- Fibrogenic cytokines
- Angiogenesis factors (FGF)
- "Remodeling" collagenases

Figure 3–28. Macrophage products involved in tissue destruction and fibrosis.

Table 3–6. PRODUCTS RELEASED BY MACROPHAGES

Enzymes
    Neutral proteases
        Elastase
        Collagenase
        Plasminogen activator
    Acid hydrolases
        Phosphatases
        Lipases
Plasma proteins
    Complement components (e.g., C1 to C5, properdin)
    Coagulation factors (e.g., factors V, VIII, tissue factor)
Reactive metabolites of oxygen
Eicosanoids
Cytokines (IL-1, TNF, IL-8)
Growth factors (PDGF, EGF, FGF, TGF-β)
Nitric oxide

tic factors), and still others cause fibroblast proliferation and collagen deposition (e.g., growth factors). This impressive arsenal of mediators makes macrophages powerful allies in the body's defense against unwanted invaders, but the very same weaponry can also induce considerable tissue damage when macrophages are inappropriately activated. Thus, *tissue destruction is one of the hallmarks of chronic inflammation.*

Other types of cells present in chronic inflammation are lymphocytes, plasma cells, eosinophils, and mast cells. *Lymphocytes* are mobilized in both antibody- and cell-mediated immune reactions and also, for reasons unknown, in nonimmune-mediated inflammation. Lymphocytes of different types (T, B) or states (naive, activated or memory T cell) use various adhesion molecules (VLA-4/VCAM-1 and ICAM-1/LFA-1 predominantly) and chemical mediators (largely cytokines) to migrate into inflammatory sites. They have a reciprocal relationship to macrophages in chronic inflammation (Fig. 3–30). Lymphocytes can be activated by contact with antigen. Activated lymphocytes produce *lymphokines*, and one of these, IFN-γ is a major stimulator of monocytes and macrophages. Cytokines from activated macrophages *(monokines)*, in turn, activate lymphocytes, which themselves also produce inflammatory mediators—setting the stage for persistence of the inflammatory response (see Chapter 6).

Plasma cells produce antibody directed either against persistent antigen in the inflammatory site or against altered tissue components. *Eosinophils* are characteristic of immune reactions mediated by IgE and of parasitic infections (Fig. 3–31). Like neutrophils, they use adhesion molecules and chemotactic agents (derived from mast cells, lymphocytes, or macrophages) to exit the blood. Eosinophils are phagocytic and undergo activation. Their granules contain major basic protein (MBP), a highly cationic protein that is toxic to parasites but also causes lysis of mammalian epithelial cells.

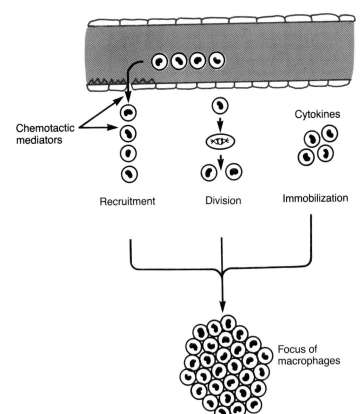

Chemotactic mediators

Cytokines

Recruitment   Division   Immobilization

Focus of macrophages

Figure 3–29. Three mechanisms for macrophage accumulation. The most important is continued recruitment from the microcirculation. (Adapted from Ryan, G., and Majno, G.: Inflammation. Northfield, MN, Scope Publishing Co. Upjohn Co., Kalamazoo, MI.)

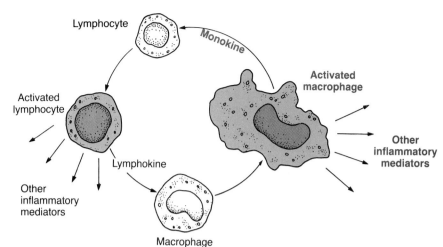

Figure 3-30. Macrophage-lymphocyte interactions in chronic inflammation. Activated lymphocytes and macrophages influence each other and also release inflammatory mediators that affect other cells.

They may thus be of benefit in parasitic infections but contribute to tissue damage in immune reactions.[48]

Although neutrophils are the hallmark of acute inflammation, many forms of chronic inflammation, lasting for months, continue to show large numbers of neutrophils, induced either by the persistent bacteria or by mediators produced by macrophages or necrotic cells. In chronic bacterial inflammation of bone (osteomyelitis), a neutrophilic exudate can persist for many months. Neutrophils are also important in the chronic damage induced in lungs by smoking and other stimuli, as we shall see (see Chapter 15).

REPAIR BY CONNECTIVE TISSUE (FIBROSIS)

As noted, persistent tissue destruction, with damage to both parenchymal cells *and stromal framework,* is a hallmark of chronic inflammation. As a

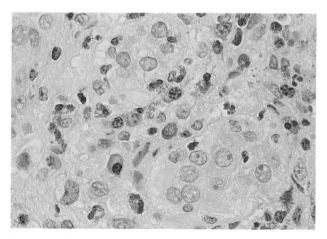

Figure 3-31. A focus of inflammation showing numerous eosinophils.

consequence, repair cannot be accomplished solely by regeneration of parenchymal cells, even in organs whose cells are able to regenerate (see Chapter 2). Attempts at repairing tissue damage then occur by replacement of nonregenerated parenchymal cells by connective tissue, which in time produces *fibrosis* and *scarring.* The process is fundamentally similar to that occurring in the healing of wounds (described later), but because the injury is persistent, and the inflammatory reaction ebbs and flows, the events are less predictable.

There are four components to this process:

- Formation of new blood vessels (angiogenesis)
- Migration and proliferation of fibroblasts
- Deposition of extracellular matrix
- Maturation and organization of the fibrous tissue, also known as *remodeling*

The process of repair begins early in inflammation. Sometimes as early as 24 hours after injury, fibroblasts and vascular endothelial cells being proliferating to form (by 3 to 5 days) the specialized type of tissue (granulation tissue) that is the hallmark of healing. The term *granulation tissue* derives from its pink, soft, granular appearance on the surface of wounds, but it is the histologic features that are characteristic: *the proliferation of new small blood vessels and fibroblasts* (Fig. 3–32). New vessels originate by budding or sprouting of pre-existing vessels, a process called *angiogenesis* or *neovascularization. Angiogenesis* is an important biologic process that, as we shall see (Chapter 7), is also involved in the progressive growth of cancer. Four steps are needed in the development of a new capillary vessel (Fig. 3–33): (1) proteolytic degradation of the basement membrane of the parent vessel to allow formation of a capillary sprout and subsequent cell migration; (2) migration of endothelial cells toward the angiogenic stimulus; (3) proliferation of endothelial cells, just behind the leading front of migrating cells; and (4) matu-

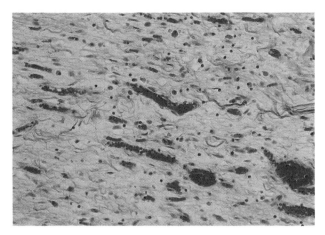

Figure 3–32. Granulation tissue showing abundant new blood vessels filled with red cells, edema, and a few inflammatory cells in the interstitium. Trichrome stain, which stains collagen blue. There is little mature collagen at this time. Compare with Figure 3–41, a more advanced scar, with abundant collagen.

ration of endothelial cells and organization into capillary tubes. These new vessels have leaky interendothelial junctions, allowing the passage of proteins and red cells into the extravascular space. *Thus, new granulation tissue is often edematous.*

Several factors can induce angiogenesis, notably basic fibroblast growth factor (FGF) and vascular endothelial growth factor (VEGF, or vascular permeability factor [VPF]). Basic FGF, as described in Chapter 2, can mediate all the steps in angiogenesis, both *in vitro* and *in vivo,* and is produced by activated macrophages. VEGF/VPF, a 46-kd tumor cell product that causes both angiogenesis and increased vascular permeability,[49] is an excellent candidate for tumor angiogenesis and for blood vessel growth in normal development[50] and may also be involved in chronic inflammation and wound healing.[49]

Migration of fibroblasts to the site of injury and their subsequent *proliferation* are undoubtedly

triggered by growth factors, such as PDGF, EGF, FGF, and TGF-β, and the fibrogenic cytokines, derived in part from inflammatory macrophages. Some of these growth factors also stimulate synthesis of collagen and other connective tissue molecules (see Table 3–9) and modulate the synthesis and activation of *metalloproteinases,* enzymes that serve to degrade these ECM components. The net effect of ECM *synthesis* versus *degradation* results in "remodeling" of the connective tissues framework—an important feature of both chronic inflammation and wound repair. Remodeling and the metalloproteinases will be discussed further in the section on wound healing.

Of the growth factors involved in inflammatory fibrosis TGF-β appears to be most critical, because of the multitude of effects that favor fibrous tissue deposition (Table 3–7). It is produced by platelets, activated macrophages, and other cells, and it is released in an inactive form that needs to be proteolytically cleaved to become functional. TGF-β (predominantly TGF-β1, but also the 2 and 3 isoforms) causes *fibroblast migration and proliferation, increased synthesis of collagen and fibronectin, and decreased degradation of ECM by metalloproteinases.* TGF-β is also chemotactic for monocytes and causes angiogenesis *in vivo,* possibly by inducing macrophage influx. It has been identified in a number of chronic fibrotic diseases in humans and experimental animals.

Having discussed the general features and molecular mechanisms of chronic inflammation, we now turn to a rather specific form of chronic inflammatory response, granulomatous inflammation.

GRANULOMATOUS INFLAMMATION

This is a distinctive pattern of chronic inflammatory reaction in which the predominant cell type is an activated macrophage with a modified epithelial-like (epithelioid) appearance. It is encountered in a rel-

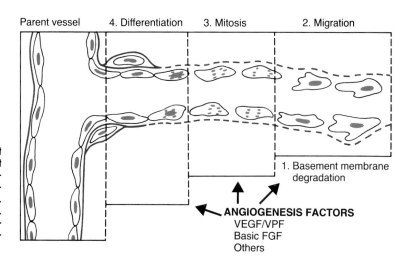

Figure 3–33. Four steps in angiogenesis. Parent mature vessel is on the left. (1) Basement membrane and ECM degradation. (2) Endothelial migration. (3) Endothelial proliferation (mitoses). (4) Organization and maturation. (Adapted from Ausprunk, D. H.: *In* Houck, J. C. (ed.): Chemical Messengers of the Inflammatory Process. Amsterdam, Elsevier North-Holland, 1979.)

Parent vessel   4. Differentiation   3. Mitosis   2. Migration

1. Basement membrane degradation

ANGIOGENESIS FACTORS
VEGF/VPF
Basic FGF
Others

Table 3–7. TRANSFORMING GROWTH
FACTOR-β (TGF-β)

Produced by:
  Platelets, macrophages, other cells
Released in inactive form
Actions
  Monocyte chemotaxis
  Fibroblast migration
  Fibroblast proliferation
  Collagen and ECM
    Increased synthesis
    Decreased degradation

atively few but widespread chronic immune and infectious diseases. Its genesis is firmly linked to immune reactions and thus is described in more detail in Chapter 6. Tuberculosis is the archetype of the granulomatous diseases, but sarcoidosis, cat-scratch disease, lymphogranuloma inguinale, leprosy, brucellosis, syphilis, some of the mycotic infections, berylliosis, and reactions of irritant lipids are also included (Table 3–8). Recognition of the granulomatous pattern in a biopsy specimen is important because of the limited number of possible conditions that cause it.

A granuloma is a focal area of granulomatous inflammation. It consists of a microscopic aggregation of macrophages that are transformed into epi-thelium-like cells surrounded by a collar of mononuclear leukocytes, principally lymphocytes and occasionally plasma cells (see Chapter 6, Fig. 6–15). In the usual hematoxylin and eosin preparations the epithelioid cells have a pale pink granular cytoplasm with indistinct cell boundaries, often appearing to merge into one another. The nucleus is less dense than that of a lymphocyte (vesicular), is oval or elongate, and may show folding of the nuclear membrane. Older granulomas develop an enclosing rim of fibroblasts and connective tissue. Frequently, but not invariably, epithelioid cells fuse to form *giant cells* in the periphery or sometimes in the center of granulomas. These giant cells may attain diameters of 40 to 50 μm. They comprise a large mass of cytoplasm containing 20 or more small nuclei arranged either peripherally (Langhans-type giant cell) or haphazardly (foreign body–type giant cell) (Fig. 3–34).

There are two types of granulomas:

- *Foreign body granulomas*, incited by relatively inert foreign bodies.
- *Immune granulomas.* Two factors determine the formation of immune granulomas: the presence of indigestible particles of organisms (e.g., the tubercle bacillus) and T cell–mediated immunity to the inciting agent. Products of activated T lymphocytes, principally IFN-γ, are important in

Table 3–8. EXAMPLES OF GRANULOMATOUS INFLAMMATIONS

DISEASE	CAUSE	TISSUE REACTION
Bacterial		
Tuberculosis	*Mycobacterium tuberculosis*	Noncaseating tubercle (granuloma prototype): a focus of epithelioid cells, rimmed by fibroblasts, lymphocytes, histiocytes, occasional Langhans' giant cell; caseating tubercle: central amorphous granular debris, loss of all cellular detail; acid-fast bacilli
Leprosy	*Mycobacterium leprae*	Acid-fast bacilli in macrophages; granulomas and epithelioid types
Syphilis	*Treponema pallidum*	Gumma: microscopic to grossly visible lesion, enclosing wall of histiocytes; plasma cell infiltrate; center cells are necrotic without loss of cellular outline
Cat-scratch disease	Gram-negative bacillus	Rounded or stellate granuloma containing central granular debris and recognizable neutrophils; giant cells uncommon
Parasitic		
Schistosomiasis	*Schistosoma mansoni, S. haematobium, S. japonicum*	Egg emboli; eosinophils
Fungal		
	Cryptococcus neoformans	Organism is yeast-like, sometimes budding; 5–10 μm; large, clear capsule
	Coccidioides immitis	Organism appears as spherical (30–80 μm) cyst containing endospores of 3–5 μm each
Inorganic Metals and Dusts		
Silicosis, berylliosis		Lung involvement; fibrosis
Unknown		
Sarcoidosis		Noncaseating granuloma: giant cells (Langhans' and foreign-body types); asteroids in giant cells; occasional Schaumann's body (concentric calcific concretion); no organisms

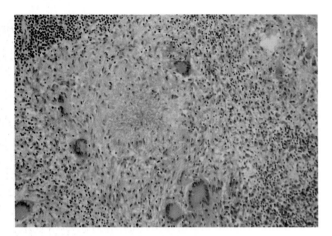

Figure 3–34. Typical tuberculous granuloma showing an area of central necrosis, epithelioid cells, multiple Langhans-type giant cells and lymphocytes.

transforming macrophages into epithelioid cells and multinucleate giant cells (see Chapter 6).[52]

In tuberculosis, the granuloma is referred to as a *tubercle* and is *classically characterized by the presence of central caseous necrosis* (Fig. 3–34). In contrast, caseating necrosis is rare in other granulomatous diseases. The morphologic patterns in the various granulomatous diseases may be sufficiently different to allow reasonably accurate diagnosis by an experienced pathologist (see Table 3–8); however, there are so many atypical presentations that it is always necessary to identify the specific etiologic agent. The agent can be identified histologically (as in the case of a refractile foreign body that can be detected by polarization microscopy), by special stains for organisms (e.g., acid-fast stains for tubercle bacilli), by culture methods (in tuberculosis, fungal disease), and by serologic studies (e.g., in syphilis). In sarcoidosis, the etiologic agent is unknown (see Chapter 15).

To summarize, granulomatous inflammation is a specific type of chronic reaction characterized by accumulations of modified macrophages (epithelioid cells) and initiated by a variety of infectious and noninfectious agents. The presence of *poorly digestible irritants or T cell–mediated immunity to the irritant, or both,* appears to be necessary for granuloma formation.

LYMPHATICS IN INFLAMMATION

The system of lymphatics and lymph nodes filters and "polices" the extravascular fluids. Together with the *mononuclear phagocyte system*, it represents a secondary line of defense that is called into play whenever a local inflammatory reaction fails to contain and neutralize injury.

Lymphatics are extremely delicate channels that are difficult to visualize in ordinary tissue sec-

tions because they readily collapse. They are lined by continuous, thin endothelium with loose, overlapping cell junctions; scant basement membrane; and no muscular support, except in the larger ducts. Lymph flow in inflammation is increased and helps drain the edema fluid from the extravascular space. Because the junctions of lymphatics are loose, lymphatic fluid eventually equilibrates with extravascular fluid. Not only fluid but also leukocytes and cell debris may find their way into lymph. Valves are present in collecting lymphatics, allowing lymph content to flow only proximally. Delicate fibrils, attached at right angles to the walls of the lymphatic vessel, extend into the adjacent tissues and serve to maintain patency of the lymphatic channels.

In severe injuries the drainage may transport the offending agent, be it chemical or bacterial. The lymphatics may become secondarily inflamed (*lymphangitis*), as may the draining lymph nodes (*lymphadenitis*). Therefore, it is not uncommon in infections of the hand, for example, to observe red streaks along the entire arm up to the axilla following the course of the lymphatic channels, accompanied by painful enlargement of the axillary lymph nodes. The nodal enlargement is usually caused by hyperplasia of the lymphoid follicles and also by hyperplasia of the phagocytic cells lining the sinuses of the lymph nodes. This constellation of nodal histologic changes is termed *reactive* or *inflammatory lymphadenitis*.

Fortunately, the secondary barriers sometimes contain the spread of the infection, but in some instances they are overwhelmed, and the organisms drain through progressively larger channels and gain access to the vascular circulation, thus inducing a *bacteremia*. The phagocytic cells of the liver, spleen, and bone marrow constitute the next line of defense, but in massive infections, bacteria seed distant tissues of the body. The heart valves, meninges, kidneys, and joints are favored sites of implantation for blood-borne organisms, and in such a fashion endocarditis, meningitis, renal abscesses, and septic arthritis may develop.

MORPHOLOGIC PATTERNS IN ACUTE AND CHRONIC INFLAMMATION

The severity of the reaction, its specific cause, and the particular tissue and site involved all introduce morphologic variations in the basic patterns of acute and chronic inflammation.

SEROUS INFLAMMATION. Serous inflammation is marked by the outpouring of a thin fluid that, depending on the size of injury, is derived from either the blood serum or the secretions of mesothe-

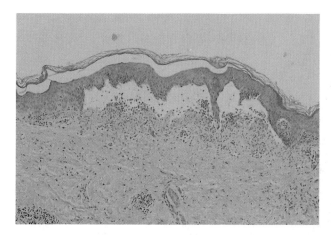

Figure 3–35. A low-power view of a cross-section of a skin blister. The epidermis has been lifted off the dermis by the focal collection of fluid.

lial cells lining the peritoneal, pleural, and pericardial cavities (called *effusion*). The skin blister resulting from a burn or viral infection represents a large accumulation of serous fluid, either within or immediately beneath the epidermis of the skin (Fig.3–35).

FIBRINOUS INFLAMMATION. With more severe injuries and the resulting greater vascular permeability, larger molecules such as fibrin pass the vascular barrier. A fibrinous exudate develops when the vascular leaks are large enough or there is a procoagulant stimulus in the interstitium (e.g., cancer cells). A fibrinous exudate is characteristic of inflammation in body cavities, such as the pericardium and pleura. Histologically, fibrin appears as an eosinophilic meshwork of threads, or sometimes as an amorphous coagulum (Fig. 3–36). Fibrinous exudates may be removed by fibrinolysis, and other debris by macrophages. This process, called *resolution*, may restore normal tissue structure, but when the fibrin is not removed it may stimulate

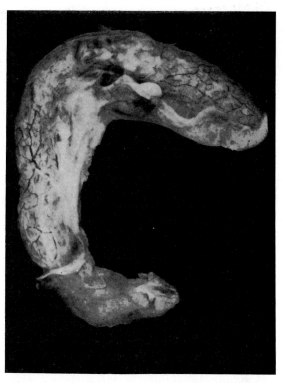

Figure 3–37. A gross view of acute appendicitis. The covering serosa is heavily layered with a pale fibrinosuppurative exudate.

the ingrowth of fibroblasts and blood vessels and thus lead to scarring. Conversion of the fibrinous exudate to scar tissue *(organization)* within the pericardial sac will lead either to opaque fibrous thickening of the pericardium and epicardium in the area of exudation or, more often, to the development of fibrous strands that bridge the pericardial space.

SUPPURATIVE OR PURULENT INFLAMMATION. This form of inflammation is characterized by the production of large amounts of pus or purulent exudate consisting of neutrophils, necrotic cells, and edema fluid. Certain organisms (e.g., staphylococci) produce this localized suppuration and are therefore referred to as pyogenic (pus-producing) bacteria. A common example of an acute suppurative inflammation is acute appendicitis (Fig. 3–37). *Abscesses are focal localized collections of purulent inflammatory tissue* caused by suppuration buried in a tissue, an organ, or a confined space. They are produced by deep seeding of pyogenic bacteria into a tissue. Abscesses have a central region that appears as a mass of necrotic white cells and tissue cells. There is usually a zone of preserved neutrophils about this necrotic focus, and outside this region vascular dilatation and parenchymal and fibroblastic proliferation occur, indicating the beginning of repair. In time, the abscess may become walled off by connective tissue that limits further spread.

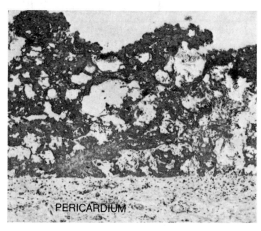

PERICARDIUM

Figure 3–36. The microscopic appearance of the shaggy, amorphous fibrinous exudate on the pericardial surface.

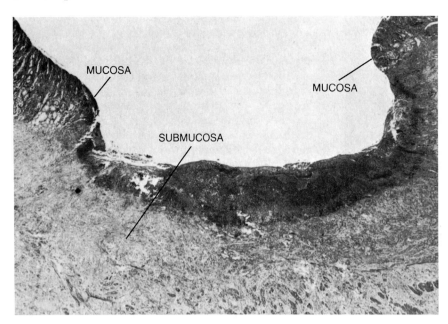

Figure 3–38. A low-power cross-section of duodenal ulcer crater with a dark inflammatory exudate in the base.

ULCERS. *An ulcer is a local defect, or excavation, of the surface of an organ or tissue that is produced by the sloughing (shedding) of inflammatory necrotic tissue* (Fig. 3–38). Ulceration can occur only when an inflammatory necrotic area exists on or near the surface. It is most commonly encountered in (1) inflammatory necrosis of the mucosa of the mouth, stomach, intestines, or genitourinary tract, and (2) subcutaneous inflammations of the lower extremities in older persons who have circulatory disturbances that predispose to extensive necrosis. Ulcerations are best exemplified by the peptic ulcer of the stomach or duodenum. During the acute stage, there is intense polymorphonuclear infiltration and vascular dilatation in the margins of the defect. With chronicity, the margins and base of the ulcer develop fibroblastic proliferation, scarring, and the accumulation of lymphocytes, macrophages, and plasma cells.

SYSTEMIC EFFECTS OF INFLAMMATION

Anyone who has suffered a severe sore throat or a respiratory infection has experienced the systemic manifestations of acute inflammation. Fever is one of the most prominent of such manifestations, especially when an inflammation is associated with infection. Known collectively as *acute-phase reactions,* other systemic manifestations include increase in slow-wave sleep; decreased appetite; increased degradation of proteins; hypotension and other hemodynamic changes; the synthesis of acute-phase proteins by the liver, including C-reactive protein, serum amyloid A, complement, and coagulation proteins; and a variety of changes in peripheral blood leukocytes.

IL-1, IL-6, and TNF are important mediators of these reactions. These cytokines, produced by leukocytes (and other cell types) in response to infectious agents or immunologic and toxic reactions, are released into the circulation. *IL-1 acts directly and also by inducing IL-6, which has essentially similar effects in producing the acute-phase reactions.* Both produce fever by interacting with *vascular* receptors in the thermoregulatory center of the hypothalamus. *Either by the direct action of the cytokines or, more likely, through the induction of local prostaglandin (PGE) production,* information is transmitted from the anterior through the posterior hypothalamus to the vasomotor center, resulting in sympathetic nerve stimulation, vasoconstriction of skin vessels, decrease in heat dissipation, and fever (Fig. 3–39).

Leukocytosis is a common feature of inflammatory reactions, especially those induced by bacterial infection. The leukocyte count usually climbs to 15,000 or 20,000 cells/ml, but sometimes it may reach extraordinarily high levels of 40,000 to 100,000 cells/ml. These extreme elevations are referred to as *leukemoid reactions,* because they are similar to the white cell counts obtained in leukemia. The leukocytosis occurs initially because of *accelerated release* of cells from the bone marrow postmitotic reserve pool (caused by IL-1 and TNF) and is associated with a rise in the number of more immature neutrophils in the blood ("shift to the left"). However, prolonged infection also induces proliferation of precursors in the bone marrow, caused by increased production of *colony-stimulating factors (CSF).* This stimulation of CSF production is also mediated by IL-1 and TNF.

Most bacterial infections induce *neutrophilia,*

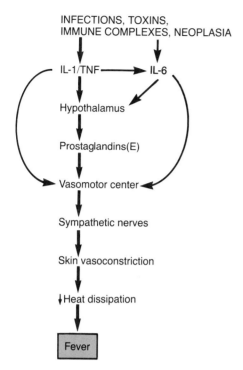

INFECTIONS, TOXINS,
IMMUNE COMPLEXES, NEOPLASIA

IL-1/TNF ——→ IL-6

Hypothalamus

Prostaglandins(E)

Vasomotor center

Sympathetic nerves

Skin vasoconstriction

↓Heat dissipation

Fever

Figure 3–39. Mechanism of fever (see text).

but infectious mononucleosis, mumps, and German measles are exceptions and produce a leukocytosis by virtue of an absolute increase in the number of lymphocytes *(lymphocytosis).* In an additional group of disorders, which includes bronchial asthma, hay fever, and parasitic infestations, there is an absolute increase in the number of eosinophils, creating an *eosinophilia.*

Certain infections (typhoid fever and infections caused by viruses, rickettsiae, and certain protozoa) are associated with a decreased number of circulating white cells *(leukopenia).* Leukopenia is also encountered in infections that overwhelm patients debilitated by disseminated cancer or rampant tuberculosis.

This ends the discussion of the cellular and molecular events in acute and chronic inflammation. We shall conclude this chapter by briefly reviewing the healing of skin wounds, as it represents a finely regulated process that encompasses both inflammation and repair.[52]

WOUND HEALING

The least complicated example of wound repair is the healing of a clean, uninfected surgical incision approximated by surgical sutures (Fig. 3–40). Such healing is referred to as *primary union or healing by first intention.* The incision causes death of a limited number of epithelial cells and connective tissue cells as well as disruption of epithelial basement membrane continuity. The narrow incisional space immediately fills with clotted blood containing fibrin and blood cells; dehydration of the surface clot forms the well-known scab that covers the wound.

Within 24 hours, neutrophils appear at the margins of the incision, moving toward the fibrin clot. The epidermis at its cut edges thickens *as a result of mitotic activity of basal cells,* and within 24 to 48 hours spurs of epithelial cells from the edges both migrate and grow along the cut margins of the dermis, depositing basement membrane components as they move. They fuse in the midline beneath the surface scab, thus producing a continuous but thin epithelial layer.

By day 3, the neutrophils have been largely replaced by macrophages. *Granulation tissue* progressively invades the incision space. Collagen fibers are now present in the margins of the incision, but at first these are vertically oriented and do not bridge the incision. Epithelial cell proliferation continues, thickening the epidermal covering layer.

By day 5, the incisional space is filled with granulation tissue. Neovascularization is maximal. Collagen fibrils become more abundant and begin to bridge the incision. The epidermis recovers its normal thickness, and differentiation of surface cells yields a mature epidermal architecture with surface keratinization.

During the second week, there is continued accumulation of collagen and proliferation of fibroblasts. The leukocytic infiltrate, edema, and increased vascularity have largely disappeared. At this time, the long process of blanching begins, accomplished by the increased accumulation of collagen within the incisional scar, accompanied by regression of vascular channels.

By the end of the first month, the scar comprises a cellular connective tissue devoid of inflammatory infiltrate, covered now by intact epidermis (Fig. 3–41). The dermal appendages that have been destroyed in the line of the incision are permanently lost. Tensile strength of the wound increases thereafter, but it may take months for the wounded area to obtain its maximal strength.

When there is more extensive loss of cells and tissue, as occurs in infarction, inflammatory ulceration, abscess formation, and surface wounds that create large defects, the reparative process is more complicated. *The common denominator in all these situations is a large tissue defect that must be filled.* Regeneration of parenchymal cells cannot completely reconstitute the original architecture. Abundant granulation tissue grows in from the margin to complete the repair. This form of healing is referred to as *secondary union or healing by second intention.*

Secondary healing differs from primary healing in several respects:

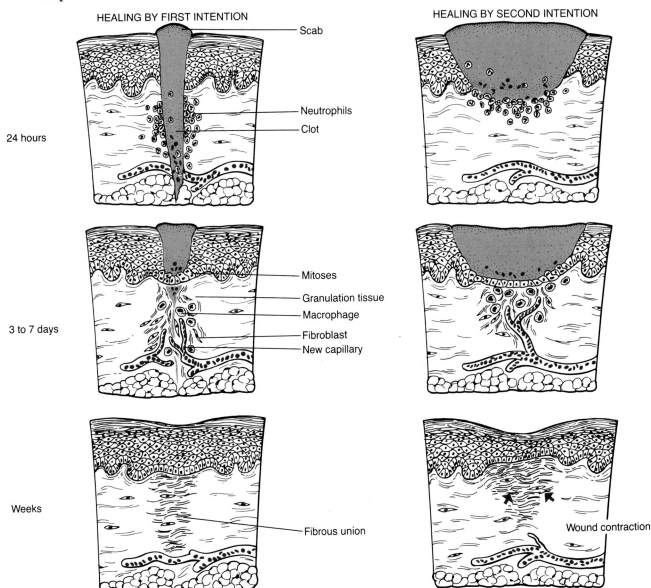

Figure 3–40. Steps in wound healing by first intention (left) and second intention (right). In the latter, the resultant scar is much smaller than the original wound, owing to wound contraction.

1. Inevitably, large tissue defects initially have more fibrin and more necrotic debris and exudate that must be removed. Consequently, the *inflammatory reaction is more intense.*

2. *Much larger amounts of granulation tissue are formed.* When a large defect occurs in deeper tissues, such as in a viscus, granulation tissue with its numerous scavenger white cells bears the full responsibility for its closure, because drainage to the surface cannot occur.

3. Perhaps the feature that most clearly differentiates primary from secondary healing is the phenomenon of *wound contraction*, which occurs in large surface wounds. Large defects in the skin of a rabbit are reduced in approximately 6 weeks to 5 to 10% of their original size, largely by contraction. Contraction has been ascribed, at least in part, to the presence of *myofibroblasts*—altered fibroblasts that have the ultrastructural characteristics of smooth muscle cells.

MECHANISMS OF WOUND HEALING

Wound healing, as we have seen, is a complex (but orderly) phenomenon involving a number of processes, including *induction of an acute inflammatory process by the wounding, regeneration of parenchymal cells, migration and proliferation of both parenchymal and connective tissue cells, synthesis of ECM proteins, remodeling of connective tissue and parenchymal components, and collagenization and acquisition of wound strength.* The mechanisms underlying most of these events have already been discussed: the mediators of acute inflammation earlier in this chapter; the role of growth factors and

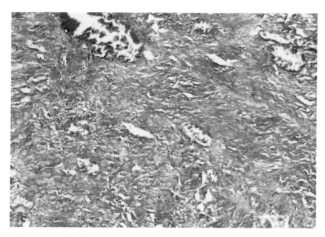

Figure 3–41. Trichrome stain of healed scar, which stains collagen blue, showing dense collagen with only scattered vascular channels. Compare with Figure 3–32, which shows early granulation tissue.

cell-ECM interactions in cell migration, proliferation, and differentiation in Chapter 2; and the mechanisms of angiogenesis and fibrosis in the discussion of chronic inflammation earlier in this chapter.

As noted the deposition of connective tissue matrix, particularly collagen, its remodeling into a scar, and the acquisition of wound strength are the ultimate effects of orderly wound repair. We shall end this discussion of wound healing by considering the determinants of wound collagenization.

Collagen Synthesis and Degradation and Wound Strength

Collagen is the most common protein in the animal world, providing the extracellular framework for all multicellular organisms. Without collagen, a human being would be reduced to a clump of cells, interconnected by a few neurons! The essential product of the fibroblast, collagen, ultimately provides the tensile strength of healing wounds. On the basis of the biochemical composition of the chains that make up the triple helix of the collagen molecule, some 14 types of collagen can be discerned, of which the most well characterized are shown in Table 3–9.[53] Types I, II, and III are the *interstitial* or *fibrillar collagens*. Types IV, V, and VI are amorphous and are present in interstitial tissue and basement membranes.

The main steps in collagen synthesis are shown in Figure 3–42. Following synthesis on ribosomes, the alpha chains are subjected to a number of enzymatic modifications, including hydroxylation of proline in the alpha position, providing collagen with its characteristic high content of hydroxyproline (about 10%). This hydroxylation, which is dependent on the availability of ascorbic acid (vitamin C), is important because it is necessary to hold the three alpha chains together.

At this stage the procollagen molecule is still soluble and contains an extra length of polypeptide and C terminal at the ends of the chain. During or shortly after excretion from the cell, procollagen peptidases clip the terminal peptide chains, promoting formation of fibrils. *True fibrils form in the extracellular space, and these collagen fibrils give strength to connective tissue.* A critical extracellular modification is *lysyl hydroxylysyl oxidation*, because this results in *cross linkages* between alpha chains of adjacent molecules and is *the basis of the structural stability of collagen. Cross linking is a major contributor to the tensile strength of collagen.*

As previously described, collagen synthesis by fibroblasts begins early in wound healing, by day 3 or 5, and continues for several weeks, depending on wound size. Collagen synthesis is stimulated by several factors, including growth factors (PDGF, FGF, TGF-β) and cytokines (IL-1, IL-4), which are secreted by leukocytes and fibroblasts in healing wounds (Table 3–10). *Net collagen accumulation, however, depends not only on synthesis but also on collagen degradation.*

Table 3–9. TYPES OF COLLAGEN

TYPE	CHAINS	CHARACTERISTICS	DISTRIBUTION
I	α 1(I), α 2(I)	Bundles of banded fibers with high tensile strength	Skin (80%), bone (90%), tendons, most other organs
II	α 1(II)	Thin fibrils; structural protein	Cartilage (50%), vitreous humor
III	α 1(III)	Thin fibrils; pliable	Blood vessels, uterus, skin (10%)
IV	α 1, α 2, α 3, α 4, α 5, α 6(IV)	Amorphous	All basement membranes
V	α 1(V, α2(V)), α 3(V)	Amorphous/fine fibrils	2–5% of interstitial tissues, blood vessels
VI	α 1(VI), α 2(VI), α 3(VI)		Interstitial tissues
VII	α 1(VII)	Anchoring filament	Dermal-epidermal junction
VIII	α 1(VIII), α 2(VIII)	Probably amorphous	Endothelium-Descemet's membrane
IX	α 1(IX), α 2(IX), α 3(IX)	Possible role in maturation of cartilage	Cartilage
X	α 1(X)		
XI	α 1(XI), α 2(XI), α 2(XI)		

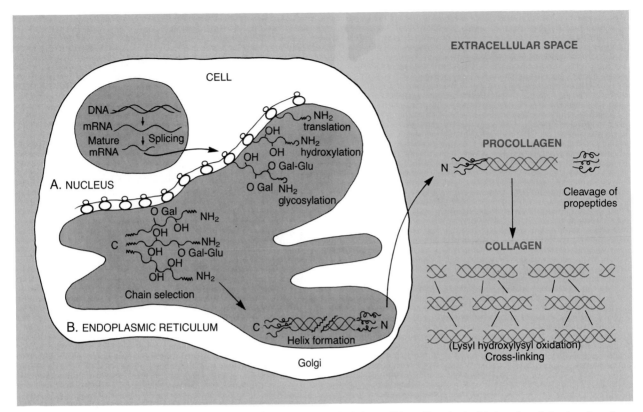

Figure 3–42. Steps in synthesis of collagen (see text). (Adapted from Krieg, T., et al.: Molecular defects of collagen metabolism in the Ehlers-Danlos syndrome. Int. J. Dermatol. 20:415, 1981.)

Degradation of collagen and other ECM proteins is achieved by a family of *metalloproteinases,* which are dependent on zinc ions for their activity.[54] (Neutrophil elastase, cathepsin G, kinins, plasmin, and other important proteolytic enzymes mentioned earlier can also degrade ECM components, but they are *serine proteinases, not metalloenzymes.*) Metalloproteinases consist of *interstitial collagenases,* which cleave the fibrillar collagen types I, II and III; *gelatinases (or type IV collagenases),* which degrade amorphous collagen as well as fibronectin; and *stromelysins,* which act on a variety of ECM components, including proteoglycans, laminin, fibronectin, and amorphous collagens.[55] These enzymes are produced by several cell types (fibroblasts, macrophages, neutrophils, synovial cells, and some epithelial cells), and their secretion is induced by many stimuli, including growth factors (PDGF, FGF), cytokines (IL-1, TNF-α), and phagocytic stimuli (Fig. 3–43). Collagenases cleave collagen under physiologic conditions, cutting the triple helix into two unequal fragments, which are then susceptible to digestion by other proteases. This is potentially harmful to the organism, but the enzyme is elaborated in a latent (procollagenase) form that can be activated by chemicals (HOCl• produced, as you recall, during the oxidative burst of leukocytes) and proteases (plasmin). Once formed, activated collagenases can be rapidly inhibited by a family of specific tissue inhibitors of metalloproteinase (TIMP), which are produced by most mesenchymal cells. There are thus multiple checks against the uncontrolled action of these proteinases, as shown in Fig. 3–43. Nevertheless, it is thought that the collagenases play a role in degrading collagen in inflammation and wound healing. Degradation aids in the débridement of injured sites and also in the remodeling of connective tissue necessary to repair the defect. Indeed, collagenases and their inhibitors have been shown to be spatially and temporally regulated in healing burn wounds.[56]

We now turn to the questions of how long it takes for a skin wound to achieve its maximal strength, and which substances contribute to this strength. When sutures are removed, usually at the end of the first week, wound strength is approximately 10% of the strength of unwounded skin, but it increases rapidly over the next 4 weeks. This rate of increase then slows at approximately the

Table 3–10. GROWTH FACTORS IN WOUND HEALING

Monocyte chemotaxis	PDGF, FGF, TGF-β
Fibroblast migration	PDGF, EGF, FGF, TGF-β, TNF
Fibroblast proliferation	PDGF, EGF, FGF, TNF
Angiogenesis	VEGF, FGF
Collagen synthesis	TGF-β, PDGF, TNF
Collagenase secretion	PDGF, FGF, EGF, TNF, TGF-β inhibits

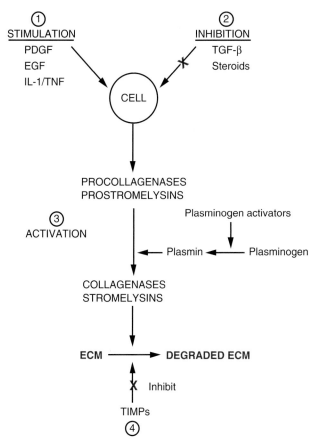

Figure 3–43. Matrix metalloproteinase regulation. The matrix metalloproteinases are regulated in at least four different ways: (1) metalloproteinase synthesis is stimulated by growth factors, cytokines, and tumor promoters; (2) this stimulation can be inhibited by steroids and TGF-*β*; (3) the enzymes are secreted in a latent form and are activated by plasmin; (4) the activity of the enzymes on ECM components can also be blocked by specific tissue inhibitors of metalloproteinases (TIMPs). (Modified from Matrisian, L.M.: Metalloproteinases and their inhibitors in matrix remodeling. Trends Genet *6*:122, 1990.)

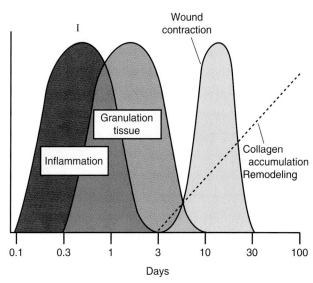

Figure 3–44. The orchestrated phases of orderly wound healing. (Modified from Clark, R.A.: *In* Goldsmith, L.A. (ed.): Physiology, Biochemistry, and Molecular Biology of the Skin, 2nd ed. Vol. I. New York, Oxford University Press, 1991, p. 577; and Clark, R.A.: Cutaneous tissue repair. J. Am. Acad. Dermatol. *13*:702, 1985.)

third month after the original incision and then reaches a plateau at about 70 to 80% of the tensile strength of unwounded skin, which indeed may persist for life. The recovery of tensile strength results from increased collagen synthesis exceeding collagen degradation during the first 2 months, and from structural modifications of collagen fibers (cross-linking, increased fiber size), when collagen synthesis ceases at later times.

We can conclude this discussion of wound healing and collagenization by emphasizing that the healing wound, as a prototype of many other forms of tissue repair, is a dynamic and changing process (Fig. 3–44). The early phase is one of inflammation, followed by a stage of fibroplasia, followed by tissue remodeling and scarring. Different mechanisms occurring at different times trigger the release of chemical signals that modulate the orderly migration, proliferation, and differentiation of cells and the synthesis and degradation of ECM

proteins. These proteins, in turn, directly affect cellular events and modulate cell responsiveness to soluble growth factors.

The magic behind the seemingly precise orchestration of these events under normal conditions remains beyond our grasp, but almost certainly lies in the regulation of specific soluble mediators and their receptors on particular cells, cell-matrix interactions, and a controlling effect of *physical factors*, including forces generated by changes in cell shape and plasticity.[57]

PATHOLOGIC ASPECTS OF INFLAMMATION AND REPAIR

In this chapter we have discussed the usual manifestations of inflammation and repair and we reviewed the orderly healing of wounds in normal persons. But these processes are modified by a number of known influences and some unknown ones, frequently impairing the quality and adequacy of both inflammation and repair.

• *Many systemic and local host factors influence the adequacy of the inflammatory-reparative response. Nutrition* has profound effects on wound healing. Protein deficiency, for example, and particularly vitamin C deficiency, inhibit collagen synthesis and retard healing. *Glucocorticoids* have well-documented anti-inflammatory effects that influence varius components of inflammation and fibroplasia. Of the local factors, *infection* is the single most important cause of delay in healing. *Mechanical factors* such as increased abdom-

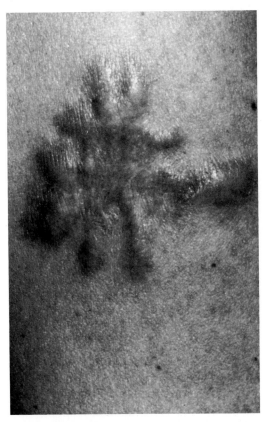

Figure 3–45. Close-up gross photograph of a keloid on the skin of the forearm. The irregular tumor-like lesion is firm and consists of abundant amounts of dense collagen.

inal pressure may cause rupture of abdominal wounds, called *wound dehiscence*. *Inadequate blood supply* usually caused by arteriosclerosis or venous abnormalities that retard venous drainage also impair healing. Finally, *foreign bodies* such as unnecessary sutures or fragments of steel, glass, or even bone constitute impediments to healing.

- Aberrations of growth may occur even in what may begin initially as normal wound healing. The accumulation of excessive amounts of collagen may give rise to a raised tumorous scar known as a *keloid* (Fig. 3–45). Keloid formation appears to be an individual predisposition, and for reasons unknown this aberration is somewhat more common in blacks. We still do not know the mechanisms of keloid formation. Another deviation in wound healing is the formation of excessive amounts of granulation tissue, which protrudes above the level of the surrounding skin and in fact blocks re-epithelialization. This has been called *exuberant granulation* or, with more literary fervor, *proud flesh*. Excessive granulations must be removed by cautery or surgical excision to permit restoration of the continuity of the epithelium. Finally (fortunately rarely), incisional

scars or traumatic injuries may be followed by exuberant proliferations of fibroblasts and other connective tissue elements that may, in fact, recur after excision. Called *desmoids*, or *aggressive fibromatoses*, these lie in the interface between benign proliferations and malignant (though low-grade) tumors. Indeed, the line between the benign hyperplasias characteristic of repair and neoplasia is frequently finely drawn, as we shall see in Chapter 7.

- The mechanisms underlying the fibroplasia of wound repair — cell proliferation, cell-cell interactions, cell-matrix interactions, and ECM deposition — are similar to those that occur in the chronic inflammatory fibrosis of such diseases as rheumatoid arthritis, lung fibrosis, and hepatic cirrhosis. Unlike orderly wound healing, however, the diseases are associated with persistence of initial stimuli for fibroplasia or the development of immune and autoimmune reactions in which lymphocyte-monocyte interactions sustain the synthesis and secretion of growth factors and fibrogenic cytokines, proteolytic enzymes and other biologically active molecules. Collagen degradation by collagenases, for example, which is important in the normal remodeling of healing wounds, causes much of the joint destruction in rheumatoid arthritis (see Chapter 27).

OVERVIEW OF THE INFLAMMATORY-REPARATIVE RESPONSE

At this point, a backward look may help relate the multitude of changes that occur simultaneously or sequentially in the inflammatory-reparative response. Figure 3–46 offers an overview of the possible pathways. This schema re-emphasizes certain important concepts. Not all injuries result in permanent damage; some are resolved with almost perfect repair. More often, the injury and inflammatory response result in residual scarring. Although it is functionally imperfect, the scarring provides a permanent patch that permits the residual parenchyma more or less to continue functioning. Sometimes, however, the scar itself is so large or so situated that it may cause permanent dysfunction, as in a healed myocardial infarct. In this case, the fibrous tissue not only represents a loss of pre-existing contractile muscle but also constitutes a permanent burden to the overworked residual muscle. In chronic inflammation, persistent injury commonly results in tissue destruction and scarring. The processes of inflammation and repair underscore the remarkable capacity of the human

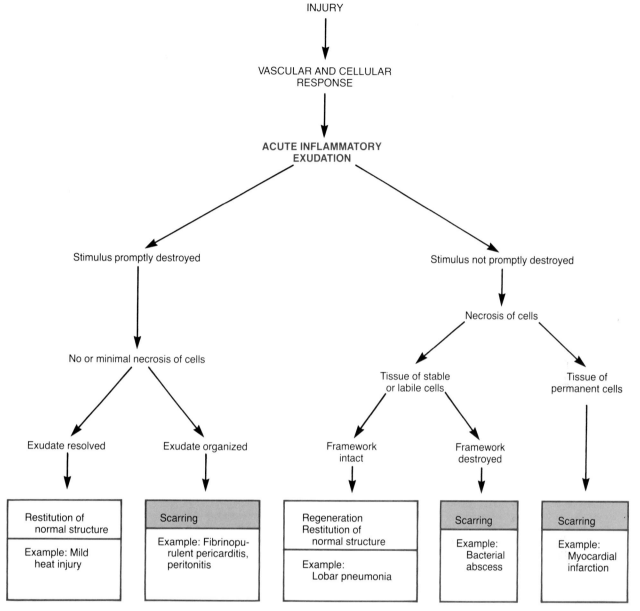

Figure 3-46. Pathways of reparative responses.

body to restore itself, far surpassing any device made by humans.

1. Majno, G.: The Healing Hand: Man and Wound in the Ancient World. Cambridge, Harvard University Press, 1975.
2. Weissman, G.: Inflammation: Historical perspectives. *In* Gallin, J.I., et al. (eds.): Inflammation: Basic Principles and Clinical Correlates, 2nd ed. New York, Raven Press. 1992, pp. 5-13.
3. Hunter, J.: A Treatise of the Blood, Inflammation, and Gunshot Wounds, Vol. 1. London, J. Nicoli, 1794.
4. Cohnheim, J.: Lectures in general Pathology (Translated by McKee, A.D., from the second German edition, Vol. 1). London, New Sydenham Society, 1889.
5. Heifets, L.: Centennial of Metchnikoff's discovery. J. Reticuloendothel. Soc. 31:381, 1982.
6. Cotran, R.S.: Endothelial cells. *In* Kelley, W.N., et al. (eds.): Textbook of Rheumatology, 4th ed. Philadelphia, W.B. Saunders Co., 1993, pp. 327-336.
7. Majno, G.: The capillary then and now: An overview of capillary pathology. Mod. Pathol. 5:9, 1992.
8. Majno, G., and Palade, G.E.: Studies on inflammation. I. The effect of histamine and serotonin on vascular permeability: An electron microscopic study. J. Biophys. Biochem. Cytol. 11:571, 1961; and Majno, G., et al.: Studies on inflammation. II. The site of action of histamine and serotonin along the vascular tree: A topographic study. J. Biophys. Biochem. Cytol. 11:607, 1961.
9. Brett, J., et al.: Tumor necrosis factor/cachectin increases permeability of endothelial cell monolayers by a mechanism involving regulatory G proteins. J. Exp. Med. 169:1977, 1989.
9a. Kohn, S., et al.: Structural basis of hyperpermeability of tumor blood vessels. Lab. Invest. 67:596, 1992.

10. Cochrane, C.G., and Gimbrone, M.A., Jr. (eds.): Leukocyte-endothelial adhesion molecules. *In* Cellular and Molecular Mechanisms of Inflammation, Vol. 3. San Diego, CA, Academic Press, 1992.
11. Springer, T.A.: Traffic signals for lymphocyte circulation and leukocyte migration: The multistep paradigm. Cell 76:301, 1994.
12. Bevilacqua, M.P.: Endothelial-leukocyte adhesion molecules. Annu. Rev. Immunol. 11:767, 1993.
13. Pober, J.S., and Cotran, R.S.: Overview: The role of endothelial cells in inflammation. Transplantation 50:537, 1990.
14. Lorant, D.E., et al.: Inflammatory roles of P-selectin. J. Clin. Invest. 92:559, 1993.
15. Travis, J.T.: Biotech gets a grip on cell adhesion. Science 26:906, 1993.
16. Butcher, E.C.: Leukocyte-endothelial cell recognition: Three or more steps to diversity and sensitivity. Cell 67:1033, 1991.
17. Arnaout, A.M.: Leukocyte adhesion molecule deficiency. Immunol. Rev. 114:145, 1990.
18. Etzioni, A., et al.: Brief Report: Recurrent severe infections caused by a novel leukocyte adhesion deficiency. N. Engl. J. Med. 327:1789, 1992.
19. McEver, R.P.: Leukocyte-endothelial cell interactions. Curr. Opin. Cell Biol. 4:840, 1992.
20. Mayadas, T.N., et al.: Leukocyte rolling and extravasation are severely compromised in P-selectin–deficient mice. Cell 74:541, 1993.
21. Muller, W.A., et al.: PECAM-1 is required for transendothelial migration of leukocytes. J. Exp. Med. 178:449, 1993.
22. Snyderman, R., and Uhuig, R. J.: Chemoattractant stimulus-response coupling. *In* Gallin, J.I., et al. (eds.): Inflammation: Basic Principles and Clinical Correlates, 2nd ed. New York, Raven Press, 1992, pp. 421–441.
23. Stossel, T.P.: On the crawling of animal cells. Science 260:1045, 1993.
24. Wright, I.: Complement receptors and the biology of phagocytosis. *In* Gallin, J.I., et al. (eds.): Inflammation: Basic Principles and Clinical Correlates, 2nd ed. New York, Raven Press, 1992, pp. 730–754.
25. Klebanoff, S.J.: Oxygen metabolites from phagocytes. *In* Gallin, J.I., et al. (eds.): Inflammation: Basic Principles and Clinical Correlates, 2nd ed. New York, Raven Press, 1992, pp. 541–589.
26. Gallin, J.I. (ed.): Disorders of phagocytic cells. *In* Inflammation: Basic Principles and Clinical Correlates, 2nd ed. New York, Raven Press, 1992, pp. 859–875.
27. Lehrer, R.J., et al.: Defensins: Endogenous antibiotic peptides of animal cells. Cell 64:229, 1991.
28. Henson, P.M., et al.: Phagocytosis. *In* Gallin, J.I., et al. (eds.): Inflammation: Basic Principles and Clinical Correlates, 2nd ed. New York, Raven Press, 1992, pp. 511–541.
29. Ross, G.D. (ed.): Immunobiology of the Complement System. San Diego, CA, Academic Press, 1986.
30. Kozik, F., and Cochrane, C.G.: The contact activation system of plasma. *In* Gallin, J.I., et al. (eds.): Inflammation, 2nd ed. New York, Raven Press, 1992, pp. 103–121.
31. Zurier, R.B.: Prostaglandins, leukotrienes, and related compounds. *In* Kelley, W.N., et al. (eds.): Textbook of Rheumatology, 4th ed. Philadelphia, W.B. Saunders Co., 1992, pp. 201–212.
32. Serhan, C.N.: Lipoxin biosynthesis and the impact on inflammatory and vascular events. Biochim. Biophys. Acta 1994 (in press).
33. Leaf, A., and Weber, P.C.: Cardiovascular effects of omega 3 fatty acids. N. Engl. J. Med. 318:549, 1988.
34. Zimmerman, G., et al.: A fluid phase and cell-associated mediator of inflammation. *In* Gallin, J.I., et al. (eds.): Inflammation: Basic Principles and Clinical Correlates, 2nd ed. New York, Raven Press, 1992, pp. 149–176.
35. Tracey, K.J., and Cerami, A.: Tumor necrosis factor, cytokines and disease. Annu. Rev. Cell Biol. 9:317, 1993.
36. Taub, D.D., and Oppenheim, J.J.: Review of the chemokine. The Third International Meeting of Chemotactic Cytokines. Cytokine 5:175, 1993.
37. Kelvin, D.J., et al.: Chemokines and serpentives. J. Leukocyte Biol. 54:605, 1993.
38. Gouldie, J., and Baumann, H.: Cytokines and acute-phase protein expression. *In* Kimball, E.S. (ed.): Cytokines in Inflammation. Boca Raton, FL, CRC Press, 1992, pp. 275–298.
39. Furchgott, R.F., and Zawadzki, J.V.: The obligatory role of endothelial cells in the relaxation of arterial smooth muscle by acetylcholine. Nature 288:373, 1980.
40. Moncada, S., et al.: Nitric oxide. Pharmacol. Rev. 43:109, 1991.
41. Lowenstein, C.J., and Snyder, S.: Nitric oxide, a novel biologic messenger. Cell 70:705, 1992.
42. Venge, P., et al.: Neutrophils and eosinophils. *In* Kelley, W.N., et al. (eds.): Textbook of Rheumatology, 4th ed. Philadelphia, W.B. Saunders Co., 1993, pp. 269–285.
43. Ward, P., and Mulligan, M.S.: Leukocyte oxygen products and tissue damage. *In* Jesaitis, A.J., and Dratz, E. A. (eds.): Molecular Basis of Oxidation Damage by Leukocytes. Boca Raton, FL, CRC Press, 1992, pp. 139–149.
44. Matis, W. L., et al.: Endogenous neuropeptides regulate expression of an endothelial molecule for leukocyte adhesion. Lab. Invest. 62:64, 1990.
45. Beekhuizen, H., and Van Furth, R.: Monocyte adherence to human vascular endothelium. J. Leukocyte Biol. 54:363, 1993.
46. Thomas, R., and Lipsky, P.E.: Monocytes and macrophages. *In* Kelley, W.N., et al. (eds.): Textbook of Rheumatology, 4th ed. Vol. 1. Philadelphia, W.B. Saunders Co., 1993, pp. 286–303.
47. Johnston, R.B., Jr.: Monocytes and macrophages. *In* Lachman, P., et al. (eds.): Critical Aspects of Immunology, 5th ed. London, Blackwell, 1993, pp. 457–480.
48. Gleich, G.J., et al.: The biology of the eosinophilic leukocyte. Annu. Rev. Med. 44:85, 1993.
49. Klagsbrun, M., and Soker, S.: The angiogenesis factor found? Curr. Biol. 3:699, 1993.
50. Senger, D.R., et al.: Vascular permeability factor (VPF/VEGF) in tumor biology. Cancer Metastasis Rev. 12:303, 1993.
51. Roberts, A.B., McCune, B.K., and Sporn, M.B.: TGF-β: Regulation of extracellular matrix. Kidney Int. 41:557, 1992.
52. Cohn, I.K., Diegelman, R.F., and Lindblad, W.J., (eds.): Wound Healing: Biochemical and Clinical Aspects. Philadelphia, W.B. Saunders Co., 1992.
53. Lingenmayer, T.F.: Collagen. *In* Hay, E. (ed.): Cell Biology of the Extracellular Matrix, 2nd ed. New York, Plenum Press, 1992, pp. 7–44.
54. Matrisian, L.M.: The matrix-degrading metalloproteinases. Bioassays 14:455, 1992.
55. Werb, Z., and Alexander, C.M.: Proteinases and matrix degradaton. *In* Kelley, W.N., et al. (eds.): Textbook of Rheumatology, 4th ed. Philadelphia, W.B. Saunders Co., 1993, pp. 248–268.
56. Stricklin, G.P., et al.: Localization of mRNAs representing collagenase and TIMP in healing human burn wounds. Am. J. Pathol. 143:1657, 1993.
57. Wang, N., Butter, J.P., and Tugber, D.E.: Mechanicotransduction across the cell surface and through the cytoskeleton. *Science* 260:1124, 1993.

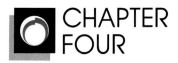

CHAPTER FOUR

Hemodynamic Disorders, Thrombosis, and Shock

Survival of cells and tissues is exquisitely dependent on the oxygen provided in a normal blood supply and, therefore, on delivery of sufficient blood through a patent circulatory system. Cells are also dependent on a normal fluid balance. Approximately 60% of a person's lean body weight is water, with 40% in the intracellular compartment and 20% present extracellularly. Derangements in either blood supply or fluid balance cause some of the most commonly encountered disorders in medical practice: edema, congestion, hemorrhage, shock, and the three interrelated conditions—thrombosis, embolism, and infarction. Not only are these disorders common, but also they are major causes of mortality. Pulmonary edema is often the terminal event in most forms of heart disease. Hemorrhage and shock are virtually daily problems in the emergency rooms of any large hospital. Thrombosis, embolism, and infarction underlie three of the most important disorders in industrialized nations: myocardial infarction, pulmonary embolism, and cerebrovascular accidents (strokes). This chapter, then, deals with predominating causes of morbidity and mortality.

EDEMA

The term *edema* refers to the accumulation of abnormal amounts of fluid in the intercellular tissue spaces or body cavities. There are two main types of edema:

- *Inflammatory edema*, already discussed in detail in Chapter 3, is due to increased vascular permeability.
- *Noninflammatory edema* is caused by alterations in hemodynamic forces across the capillary wall (also called *hemodynamic edema*). This will be the focus of our discussion here.

Edema may occur as a generalized or localized disorder. The term *anasarca* is used when the edema is severe and generalized, producing marked swelling of the subcutaneous tissues. Edematous collections in the various serous cavities of the body are given the special designations *hydrothorax*, *hydropericardium*, and *hydroperitoneum* (more commonly called *ascites*). The fluid of noninflammatory edema is a transudate, low in protein and other colloids, with a specific gravity usually below 1.012. Inflammatory edema, as we have seen, is rich in protein and therefore has a higher specific gravity—usually over 1.020 (an exudate).

Edema is the result of an increase in the forces that tend to move fluids from the intravascular compartment into the interstitial fluid. The normal interchange of fluid, as proposed by Starling, is regulated by the hydrostatic and osmotic pressures within and outside the vascular compartment (Fig.

93

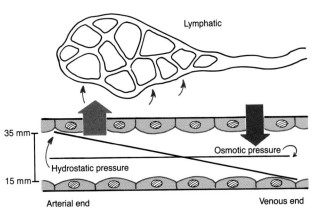

Figure 4-1. Normal formation and drainage of interstitial fluid (see text).

Table 4-1. PATHOPHYSIOLOGIC CATEGORIES OF EDEMA

I. Increased hydrostatic pressure
  A. Impaired venous return
    1. Congestive heart failure
    2. Constrictive pericarditis
    3. Cirrhosis of liver (ascites)
    4. Obstruction or narrowing of veins
      a. Thrombosis
      b. External pressure
      c. Inactivity of the lower extremities with long periods of dependency
  B. Arteriolar dilatation
    1. Heat
    2. Neurohumoral excess or deficit
II. Reduced oncotic pressure of plasma—hypoproteinemia
  A. Protein-losing glomerulopathies—nephrotic syndrome
  B. Cirrhosis of liver (ascites)
  C. Malnutrition
  D. Protein-losing gastroenteropathy
III. Sodium retention
  A. Excessive salt intake with reduced renal function
  B. Increased tubular reabsorption of sodium
    1. Reduced renal perfusion
    2. Increased renin-angiotensin-aldosterone secretion
IV. Lymphatic obstruction
  A. Inflammatory
  B. Neoplastic
  C. Postsurgical
  D. Postirradiation

Modified from Leaf, A., and Cotran, R.S.: Renal Pathophysiology, 3rd ed. New York, Oxford University Press, 1985, p. 146.

4-1). *The opposing effects of intravascular hydrostatic pressure and plasma colloid osmotic pressure are the major factors to be considered in the pathogenesis of edema.* At the arteriolar end of the capillary bed, the hydrostatic pressure is about 35 mm Hg. At the venular end it falls to 12 to 15 mm Hg. The colloid osmotic pressure of the plasma is 20 to 25 mm Hg, rising slightly at the venular end as fluid escapes. Thus, fluid leaves at the arteriolar end of the capillary bed and returns at the venular end. Not all of the fluid in the interstitial spaces returns to the venules; some is drained off through the lymphatics, to be returned to the bloodstream only indirectly.

We can deduce that noninflammatory edema will occur when the following conditions are present:

- *an increase in intravascular hydrostatic pressure*
- *a fall in colloid osmotic pressure of the plasma*
- *an impairment in the flow of lymph.*
- To this list must be added *renal retention of salt and water,* which may be a primary disturbance when there is kidney disease or may be a secondary event contributing to edema of other causes. Table 4-1 lists the primary causes of noninflammatory edema and the associated clinical conditions.

INCREASED HYDROSTATIC PRESSURE

- *Local increases* may result from an impaired venous outflow, most frequently encountered in the lower extremities, secondary to the development of obstructive thromboses. The resulting edema is localized to the legs.
- *Generalized increases* in venous pressure and systemic edema occur most commonly when there is *congestive heart failure* affecting right ventricular function (see Chapter 12). Although increased venous hydrostatic pressure is an important factor, the pathogenesis of cardiac edema is far more complex (Fig. 4-2).[1] Congestive heart failure is associated with reduced cardiac output

and reduced renal blood flow. Through a series of regulatory mechanisms, a reduction in renal perfusion or perfusion pressure triggers the renin-angiotensin-aldosterone axis, resulting in renal retention of sodium and water *(secondary aldosteronism).* Expansion of the intravascular volume resulting from this sequence of events does not improve renal perfusion, since the failing heart is unable to increase cardiac output. With the extra fluid load (which the heart is unable to handle) there is further increase in venous pressure and edema formation. Thus, a vicious circle of fluid retention and worsening edema sets in. Not surprisingly, therefore, restriction of salt intake and administration of diuretics and aldosterone antagonists reduce the edema of congestive heart failure.

REDUCED PLASMA OSMOTIC PRESSURE. This results from excess loss or reduced synthesis of serum albumin. The most important cause of increased *loss of albumin* is the *nephrotic syndrome* (see Chapter 20), a kidney disorder characterized by a leaky glomerular basement membrane and generalized edema. *Reduced synthesis* of serum proteins occurs with diffuse diseases of the liver, such as cirrhosis (Chapter 18), or in association with malnutrition. In all these instances, movement of fluid from the intravascular to the interstitial compartment leads to a contraction of plasma vol-

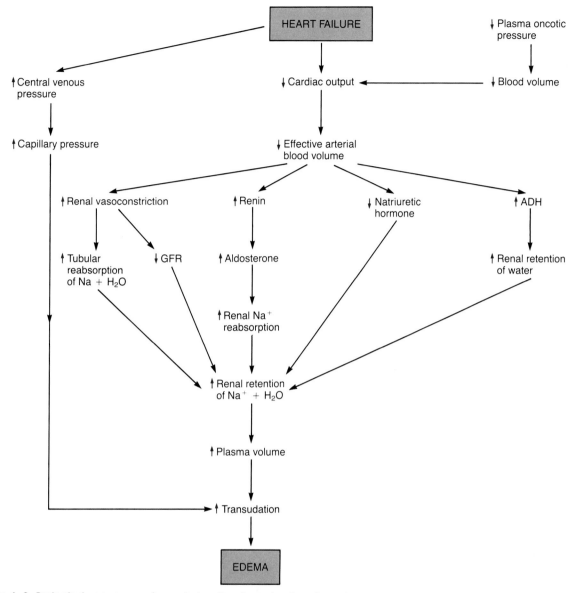

Figure 4–2. Projected sequence of events leading to systemic edema in heart failure and with reduced plasma oncotic pressure, as in the nephrotic syndrome.

ume. Predictably, a reduction in renal perfusion follows, and secondary aldosteronism sets in. However, the retained salt and water cannot correct the deficit in plasma volume, because the primary defect of too little serum proteins persists. Once again, we see that the edema initiated by one mechanism gets complicated by secondary salt and fluid retention.

LYMPHATIC OBSTRUCTION. Impaired lymphatic drainage and consequent lymphedema is usually localized and may result from inflammatory or neoplastic obstruction. Filariasis, a parasitic infection, often causes massive fibrosis of the lymph nodes and lymph channels in the inguinal region. The resulting edema of the external genitalia and the lower limbs is so extreme it is called *elephanti-*

asis (Fig. 4–3). Cancer of the breast is sometimes treated by removal or irradiation of the entire breast along with all or most of the lymph nodes in the axilla. Consequently, postoperative edema of the arm often follows such therapy and can be a troublesome clinical problem.

SODIUM AND WATER RETENTION. This has already been mentioned as a contributing factor in several forms of edema. Salt retention may be a primary cause of edema when there is acute reduction in renal function, as may be encountered in poststreptococcal glomerulonephritis or in acute renal failure (Chapter 20). The retained salt and water cause expansion of intravascular fluid volume and lead secondarily to increased hydrostatic pressure and, consequently, edema.

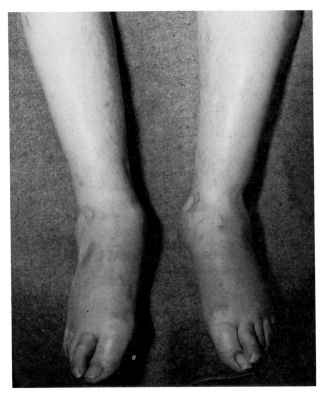

Figure 4–3. Dependent edema of the lower legs illustrating "pitting" about the ankles.

MORPHOLOGY. The morphologic changes of edema are much more evident grossly than microscopically. Although any organ or tissue in the body may be involved, edema is encountered most often in three sites: the subcutaneous tissues, usually in the lower extremities; the lungs; and the brain.

Subcutaneous edema of the lower parts of the body is a prominent manifestation of cardiac failure, particularly failure of the right ventricle. Although right ventricular failure obviously affects the entire systemic venous return to the heart, edema is most prominent in the lower extremities because they are subject to the highest hydrostatic pressures. If the patient is confined to bed, sacral edema may become evident. **Since the distribution of the edema is influenced by gravity, it is termed "dependent."**

Edema produced by **renal dysfunction** and **nephrotic syndrome** tends to be generalized and more severe than cardiac edema, affecting all parts of the body equally. However, it may manifest itself initially in tissues that have a loose connective tissue matrix, such as the eyelids **(periorbital edema).** Such generalized edema merits the designation *anasarca.* Finger pressure over edematous subcutaneous tissue will squeeze out the fluid and produce pitted depressions, hence the common clinical term **pitting edema** (see Fig. 4–3).

Pulmonary edema is a very common clinical problem, discussed in some detail in Chapter 15. The edema is usually confined to, or most marked in, the lower lobes. In far-advanced edema, however, all lobes may be involved and assume a rubbery gelatinous consistency. Sectioning of the lobes permits the free escape of frothy, sanguineous fluid representing a mixture of air and edema fluid (Fig. 4–4). On histologic examination, the edematous fluid first accumulates about the septal capillaries with widening of the septa. As the process evolves, a proteinaceous fluid escapes into the alveolar spaces, marked by a granular, pink coagulate within such spaces.

Edema of the brain is described in Chapter 29. It suffices here that it may be localized to the region about focal lesions (e.g., neoplasms, abscesses) or generalized involving the entire brain, as for example in encephalitis, hypertensive crises, and obstruction to the venous outflow of the brain. Trauma may cause localized or generalized edema, depending on its nature and distribution. When the entire brain is involved it is heavier than

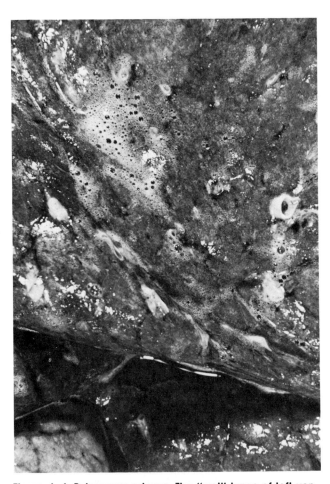

Figure 4–4. Pulmonary edema. The "wet" lungs of left ventricular failure. A frothy fluid oozes out of the transected surface.

normal; the sulci are narrowed, and the swollen gyri are flattened where they press against the skull. On section, the white matter may appear unusually soft and gelatinous, and the peripheral layer of gray matter is widened. Histologically, the edema, whether localized or generalized, is marked by widening of the interfibrillar spaces of the brain substance; this gives a loose appearance to the white and gray matter. Swelling of the neuronal and glial cells may also be present. The perivascular (Virchow-Robin) spaces become unusually widened and form clear halos about the small vessels.

CLINICAL CORRELATIONS. Edema may give rise to minor clinical problems, or it can be lethal. Edema of the subcutaneous tissues in cardiac or renal failure is important chiefly because it indicates underlying disease, but it sometimes impairs healing of wounds or infections. Because edema of the lungs (pulmonary edema) impairs normal ventilatory function, it may be lethal. Edema of the brain can be a serious clinical problem and may cause death if it is sufficiently marked. The increased mass of brain substance may cause herniation of the cerebellar tonsils into the foramen magnum or may cause shearing stresses on the blood supply to the brain stem. Both conditions secondarily impinge on medullary centers to cause death.

HYPEREMIA AND CONGESTION

The terms hyperemia and congestion are elegant medical expressions for an increased volume of blood in an affected tissue or part. *Hyperemia, also called active hyperemia to differentiate it from congestion or passive hyperemia,* occurs when arterial and arteriolar dilatation produces an increased flow of blood into capillary beds, with opening of inactive capillaries. Congestion or passive hyperemia, on the other hand, results from impaired venous drainage.

Active hyperemia causes increased redness in the affected part. The arterial and arteriolar dilatation is brought about by sympathetic neurogenic mechanisms or the release of "vasoactive" substances (as discussed in Chapter 3). Active hyperemia of the skin is encountered whenever excess body heat must be dissipated, such as in muscular exercise and febrile states. Blushing is another example of hyperemia induced by neurogenic mechanisms.

Congestion, or *passive hyperemia,* causes an intensified blue-red coloration in affected parts as venous blood is dammed back. The blue tint is accentuated when the congestion leads to an increase of deoxygenated hemoglobin in the blood

—*cyanosis.* Congestion may occur as a systemic phenomenon in congestive heart failure when both left and right ventricles are decompensated, may affect only the pulmonary circuit in left ventricular failure, or may affect the entire body, sparing the lungs, in right ventricular decompensation. Congestion can, of course, occur as a localized process when, for example, the venous return of blood from an extremity is obstructed, or when it involves only the portal circulation, as occurs in portal hypertension secondary to cirrhosis of the liver. *Congestion of capillary beds is closely related to the development of edema, and so congestion and edema commonly occur together.*

MORPHOLOGY. Cut surfaces of acutely hyperemic and/or congested organs are excessively bloody and wet. With long-standing congestion, called **chronic passive congestion,** the stasis of poorly oxygenated blood causes chronic hypoxia, which may lead to degeneration or even death of parenchymal cells. Minute hemorrhages from capillary rupture may be converted in time to hemosiderin-laden scars. The lungs, liver, and spleen develop the most obvious manifestations of chronic passive congestion.

Acute and chronic passive congestion of the lungs and consequent pulmonary edema are encountered whenever there is elevated left atrial pressure and consequent elevated pulmonary venous pressure. Microscopically, the alveolar capillaries are engorged with blood. Rupture may cause minute intra-alveolar hemorrhages, and the breakdown and phagocytosis of the red cell debris eventually lead to the appearance of hemosiderin-laden macrophages ("heart failure" cells) in the alveolar spaces. Edema fluid collects in alveoli and within the interstitium of the alveolar septa (congestion and edema). In time, the edematous septa become fibrotic and, together with the hemosiderin pigmentation, constitute the basis for the designation **brown induration.** The long-standing congestion and consequent pulmonary hypertension may cause progressive thickening of the walls of the pulmonary arteries and arterioles.

Acute and chronic passive congestion of the liver results from right-sided heart failure or, more rarely, from obstruction of the inferior vena cava or hepatic vein. With chronic congestion, the central regions of the lobule become red-blue, surrounded by a zone of uncongested liver substance, descriptively referred to as **nutmeg liver** (Fig. 4–5). Microscopically, the central vein and the vascular sinusoids of the centrilobular regions are distended with blood. The central hepatocytes frequently become atrophic secondary to chronic hypoxia, whereas the peripheral hepatocytes, suffering from less severe hypoxia, develop fatty change.

With severe cardiac failure the central hepatocytes may become necrotic, and the centrilobular

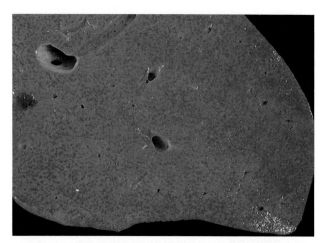

Figure 4-5. Liver: Central congestion and hemorrhagic necrosis. The central areas are red and slightly depressed compared to the pale peripheral portions of the lobules, and thus compose the so-called nutmeg pattern.

zone hemorrhagic, producing so-called **central hemorrhagic necrosis.** This is caused by the hypoxia induced by reduction in the circulating blood volume and hepatic blood flow.[1] Thus, **centrilobular necrosis** may appear in shock from any cause without preceding chronic passive congestion.

Chronic passive congestion of the spleen (congestive splenomegaly) is described in Chapter 14.

HEMORRHAGE

Hemorrhage obviously implies rupture of a blood vessel. Rupture of a large artery or vein is almost always caused by some form of injury, such as trauma, atherosclerosis, and inflammatory or neoplastic erosion of the vessel wall. Rupture of a large artery in the brain is a frequent cause of death in hypertensive patients (Fig. 4-6A). An increased tendency to hemorrhage is encountered in a wide variety of clinical disorders known collectively as the *hemorrhagic diatheses.* These are discussed in Chapter 13.

Hemorrhages may be external and exsanguinating. When the blood is trapped within the tissues of the body, the accumulation is referred to as a *hematoma.* Rupture of the aorta, for example in a dissecting or atherosclerotic aneurysm, may cause a massive retroperitoneal hematoma with sufficient loss of blood to cause death. When the blood accumulates in one of the body cavities it is referred to as *hemothorax, hemopericardium, hemoperitoneum,* or *hemarthrosis.* Minute hemorrhages into the skin, mucous membranes, or serosal surfaces are known as *petechiae.* Slightly larger hemorrhages are designated *purpura* (see Fig. 4-6B). A large (over 1 to 2 cm in diameter) subcutaneous hematoma, an example of which is the common bruise, is called an *ecchymosis.* The released hemoglobin is converted into bilirubin and eventually into hemosiderin. Patients who sustain a large hemorrhage, such as massive gastrointestinal bleeding, a pulmonary hemorrhage or infarct, or a hematoma, sometimes become jaundiced owing to the breakdown of red cells and subsequent release of bilirubin.

The significance of hemorrhage depends on the volume of blood loss, the rate of loss, and the site of hemorrhage. Sudden losses of up to 20% of the blood volume or slow losses of even larger amounts may have little clinical significance. Larger or more acute losses may induce hemorrhagic (hypovolemic) shock, as described later. The site of the hemorrhage is, of course, important; a hemorrhage that would be trivial in the subcutaneous tissues may cause death when located in the brain stem. Repeated external hemorrhages (i.e., those in which the blood is shed—as from the skin, gastrointestinal tract, or female genital tract) represent losses of not only blood volume but also

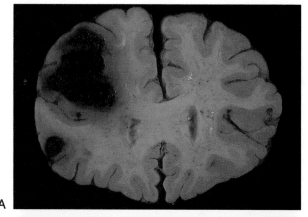

A

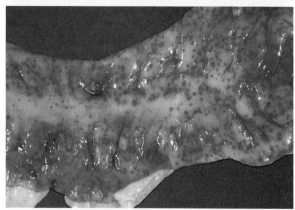

B

Figure 4-6. A, A fatal intracerebral hemorrhage. B, Punctate hemorrhages of the colonic mucosa caused by thrombocytopenia.

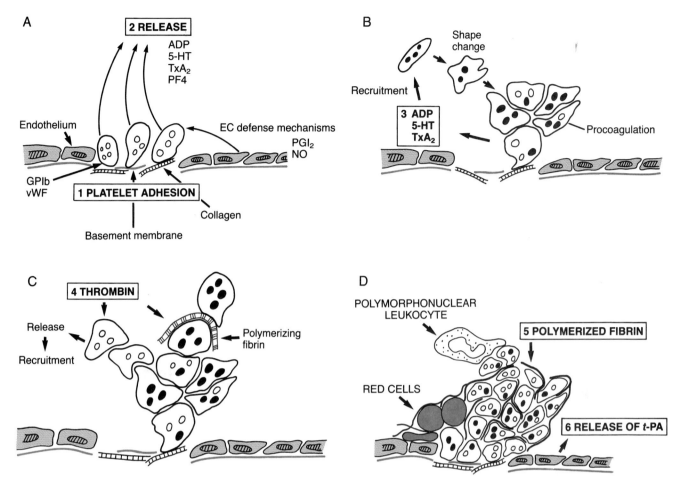

Figure 4–7. Diagrammatic representation of the normal hemostatic process. *A,* Exposure of subendothelium due to vascular damage results in immediate platelet adherence to collagen (1). Collagen induces platelet release of ADP and serotonin (5-HT) and synthesis of thromboxane A₂ (TxA₂) (2). Simultaneously, endothelial cell PGI₂ and NO attempt to limit the size of the thrombus. Concomitant with formation of the releasate, the recruitment phase is initiated. *B,* ADP, 5-HT, and TxA₂ are the most important recruiting components of the platelet releasate (3). They activate additional platelets, which then undergo shape change and aggregate onto the initial layer of activated platelets. Thromboxane and serotonin induce vasoconstriction, which serves to limit the velocity of blood flow. Complex phospholipoproteins are now available on the platelet surface for catalytic activation of proteins of the coagulation system. *C,* Thrombin formation has major consequences that lead to the final stages of platelet thrombus development (4). Platelet activation, release, and recruitment are reinduced, and fibrin formation is initiated. *D,* The consolidated platelet thrombus is now virtually impermeable (5). Neutrophils and erythrocytes are also seen in close contact with platelets. Formation of the platelet thrombus also signals the initiation of fibrinolysis, that is, release of tissue plasminogen activator *t*-PA from endothelial cells (6). (Modified and redrawn from Marcus, A.J., and Safier, L.B.: Thromboregulation: Multicellular modulation of platelet reactivity in hemostasis and thrombosis. FASEB J. 7:516, 1993, from an original by Dr. J.F. Mustard.)

valuable iron. Chronic loss of iron may lead to an iron deficiency anemia.

HEMOSTASIS AND THROMBOSIS

We now come to the core of this chapter, a consideration of how blood remains fluid, how holes in the circulation are plugged, and what happens when these mechanisms go awry. Nature has designed a complex but ingenious system to maintain the blood in the vascular system fluid and free from clots, yet allow the rapid formation of a solid plug of blood to close ruptures or other forms of injury to blood vessels. This process is referred to as *normal hemostasis. Thrombosis,* on the other hand, is a *pathologic process. It denotes the formation of a clotted mass of blood within the noninterrupted vascular system; it represents, to a considerable extent, a pathologic extension of normal hemostasis.* Both are dependent on three important contributors: (1) the *vascular wall,* with its lining endothelium and underlying subendothelial connective tissues; (2) *platelets,* essential for both hemostasis and thrombus formation; and (3) the *coag-*

ulation system. The coagulation proteins, present in the plasma and in certain cells in inactive forms, are poised to be triggered along a cascade that ends in the deposition of the ultimate insoluble product, *fibrin.*

NORMAL HEMOSTASIS

Before we discuss each contributor to hemostasis separately, the sequence of events in the formation of a hemostatic plug, occurring after a vessel is severed or injured, will be summarized[2,3] (Fig. 4–7).

1. *There is first a brief period of vasoconstriction owing to reflex neurogenic mechanisms, possibly augmented by such humoral factors as endothelin, a potent endothelium-derived vasoconstrictor. Such vascular contraction is most evident in vessels that have well-defined muscular walls and serves momentarily to reduce blood loss.*

2. *Much more important, injury to endothelial cells exposes highly thrombogenic subendothelial collagen, to which the platelets adhere and undergo so-called "activation," that is, a shape change and a release reaction. The agonists released—adenosine diphosphate (ADP), thromboxane A$_2$, and serotonin— then recruit additional platelets, which aggregate over the early platelets, to form the hemostatic plug. This platelet reaction occurs within minutes of injury and is called* **primary hemostasis.**

3. *Virtually simultaneously, release of tissue factors at the site of injury, in combination with platelet factors, activates the plasma coagulation sequence, culminating in the formation of thrombin, which converts fibrinogen to fibrin and stimulates further platelet recruitment and release. This requires a longer time for completion and is referred to as* **secondary hemostasis.**

4. *Ultimately, a permanent plug is produced. Polymerized fibrin and platelet aggregates now form a solid mass that prevents hemorrhage from the site of injury.*

We shall now examine the three components involved in the process, endothelium, platelets, and the coagulation system.

Endothelium

Endothelial cells modulate several aspects of the hemostasis-coagulation sequence. On the one hand, they possess antiplatelet, anticoagulant, and fibrinolytic properties; on the other hand, when they are injured or activated they exert procoagulant functions[4,5] (Figs. 4–8 and 4–9). Endothelial activation (see Chapter 3) is induced by infectious products, hemodynamic factors, and plasma constituents (e.g., lipids) but most profoundly by cyto-

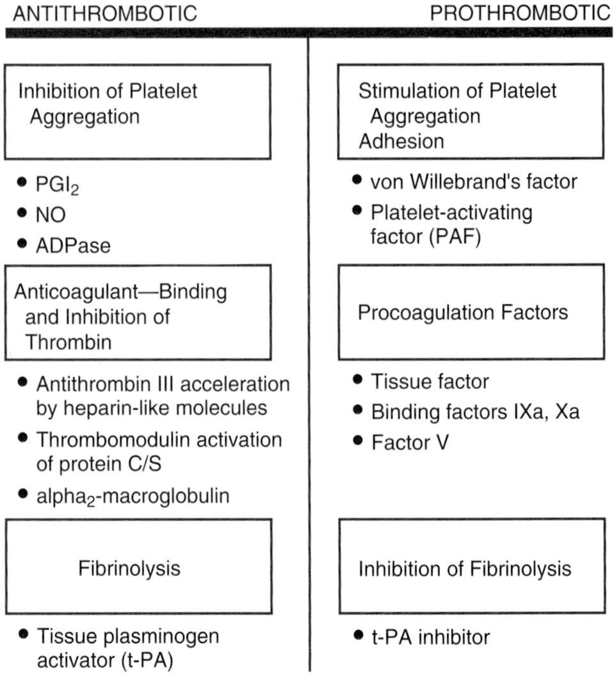

Figure 4–8. The endothelial thrombotic-antithrombotic balance. The major factors favoring and inhibiting thrombosis are shown.

kines. The balance between endothelial antithrombotic and prothrombotic activities often determines whether thrombus formation, propagation, or dissolution occurs.

ANTITHROMBOTIC PROPERTIES. Consider first those aspects of the endothelium that oppose clotting.

• *Antiplatelet effects.* Intact endothelium insulates the blood platelets and coagulation proteins from the highly thrombogenic subendothelial components, principally collagen. Platelets flowing in the bloodstream do not adhere to the endothelium. This antiplatelet function seems intrinsic to the plasma membrane of endothelium. On the other hand, once platelets are "activated" (following focal endothelial injury), they are inhibited from aggregating on the surrounding uninjured endothelial cells by the action of *prostacyclin (PGI$_2$) and nitric oxide, which are powerful inhibitors of platelet aggregation and potent vasodilators.* PGI$_2$, as you recall, is an arachidonic acid derivative, whereas nitric oxide is generated by enzymatic transformation of L-arginine (see Chapter 3). Their synthesis in endothelial cells is stimulated by ADP, thrombin, cytokines, and other factors produced during coagulation.[7]

• *Anticoagulant properties.* These are mediated by membrane-associated heparin-like molecules and thrombomodulin, a specific thrombin receptor (Fig. 4–9). The *heparin-like molecules* act indirectly; they catalyze the actions of naturally occurring anticoagulant protein antithrombin III,

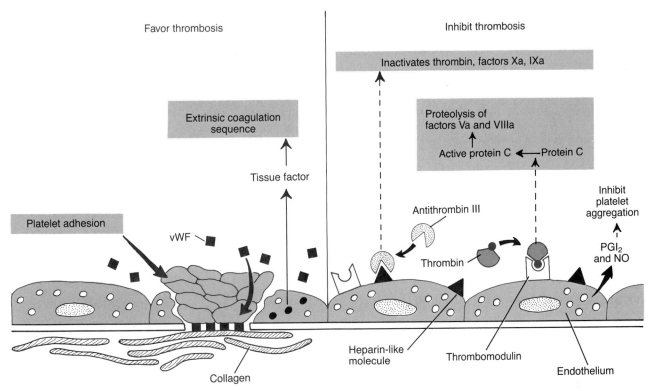

Figure 4–9. Schematic illustration of some of the prothrombotic and antithrombotic activities of endothelial cells. Not shown are the profibrinolytic and antifibrinolytic properties.

which inactivates thrombin and several other coagulation factors, including factor Xa.[8] *Thrombomodulin* also acts indirectly. It binds thrombin and, in so doing, converts thrombin from a procoagulant to an anticoagulant. Thrombin that is bound to thrombomodulin activates protein C, a powerful naturally occurring anticoagulant. Activated protein C inhibits clotting by proteolytic cleavage of factors Va and VIIIa. Protein S, synthesized by endothelial cells, serves as a cofactor for the anticoagulant activity of protein C.[9]

- *Fibrinolytic properties.* Endothelial cells synthesize tissue type plasminogen activators (*t*-PA) that promote fibrinolytic activity and help clear fibrin deposits from endothelial surfaces.[10]

Prothrombotic properties. While on the one hand endothelial cells oppose blood clotting and thrombosis, on the other they have prohemostatic and prothrombotic effects, affecting platelets, coagulation proteins, and the fibrinolytic system. As mentioned earlier, endothelial injury leads to the first step in hemostasis: adhesion of platelets to subendothelial collagen. Endothelial cells synthesize and secrete von Willebrand's factor (vWF), which, as we shall see, is essential for the adhesion of platelets to collagen and other surfaces. Endothelial cells can also be induced by cytokines—interleukin-1 (IL-1)/tumor necrosis factor (TNF)—or bacterial endotoxins to synthesize *tissue factor*, thus activating the extrinsic clotting pathway. Additionally, endothelial cells express binding sites for activated forms of factors IX and X, and cell-bound factors seem to be more active than their counterparts in solution. All these effects are *prothrombotic.* Finally, although endothelial cells produce *t*-PA, thus promoting fibrinolysis, they also secrete an inhibitor of *t*-PA, which depresses fibrinolysis, as we shall see in the discussion of the coagulation system.

In summary, intact endothelial cells, although multifunctional, normally serve to inhibit platelet adherence and initiation of blood clotting. Conversely, injury to endothelial cells represents a loss of anticlotting mechanisms and thus contributes to hemostasis and, as will be seen, to thrombosis. Endothelial activation markedly influences both prothrombotic and antithrombotic properties of endothelial cells, usually favoring thrombosis.

Platelets

It is already evident that *platelets* play a central role in normal hemostasis and therefore also in thrombosis.[7] Despite their lack of a nucleus, head, and heart, these tiny structures (about 2 μm in diameter) are amazingly versatile.

In their circulating form, they appear as relatively smooth discs enclosed within a typical plasma membrane containing a number of receptor glycoproteins of the integrin family. Within the platelets are two specific types of granules. *Alpha granules* contain fibrinogen, fibronectin, factors V and VIII, platelet factor 4 (a heparin-binding chemokine), and growth factors (platelet-derived growth factor [PDGF] and transforming growth factor-beta [TGF-β]). Their membranes also contain the adhesion molecule P-selectin (see Chapter 3). The other form of granules are *electron-dense bodies* that are the storage sites for a nonmetabolic pool of adenine nucleotides (ADP and ATP), ionized calcium, histamine, serotonin, and epinephrine.

With injury to a vessel, platelets are exposed to extracellular matrix in the vascular wall—collagen, proteoglycans, fibronectin, and other adhesive glycoproteins. This initiates the hemostatic cascade, in which platelets undergo three important reactions: *(1) adhesion and shape change, (2) secretion (release reaction), and (3) aggregation, collectively referred to as platelet activation.*

1. Adhesion refers to attachment of platelets to sites of endothelial cell injury, where subendothelial elements, particularly fibrillar collagen, are exposed (Fig. 4–9). The platelets at first attach themselves by long pseudopods but then spread broadly to become tightly adherent. vWF is necessary for such adhesion and serves as a molecular bridge between platelets and collagen, acting through glycoprotein receptors (mostly GpIb) (Fig. 4–10). This reaction is critical in stabilizing platelet adhesion, allowing it to withstand high shear forces generated by flowing blood. Genetic deficiencies of vWF (von Willebrand's disease) or of the glycoprotein receptors result in defects in platelet adhesion.

2. Secretion—the release reaction—of the

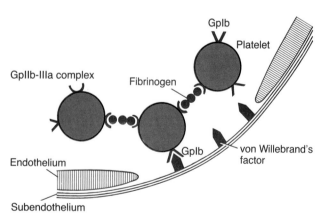

Figure 4–10. Platelet adhesion and aggregation. Von Willebrand's factor serves as a bridge between subendothelial collagen and platelet receptors (GpIb). Aggregation involves fibrinogen, which serves as a link between receptors (GpIIb-IIIa) on adjacent platelets.

contents of both platelet granules follows soon after adhesion. *Alpha granules,* as we have seen, contain coagulation proteins, growth factors, and a variety of enzymes. *Dense bodies* or delta granules are rich in ADP and ionized calcium and also contain vasoactive amines. Calcium is necessary in the coagulation sequence, and *ADP is a potent mediator of platelet aggregation,* as will shortly be discussed. Platelet activation and secretion are initiated by binding of agonists to platelet receptors, phospholipase C activation, and two signal transduction pathways mediated by protein kinase A and C. With platelet activation and the release reaction, *a phospholipid complex* becomes activated or, in some manner, exposed on the platelet surface. This phenomenon is of importance, since it provides a site on the platelet surface where coagulation factors and Ca^{++} bind to activate the intrinsic pathway of blood clotting and the formation of *thrombin,* as will be presently described.

3. *Platelet aggregation (implying platelet-platelet interadherence) closely follows adhesion and secretion.* There are at least three important stimuli for platelet aggregation. One previously described is *ADP.* The second is *thromboxane A$_2$* (TxA$_2$), which is synthesized and released by activated platelets. TxA$_2$ is an eicosanoid that is also a potent vasoconstrictor. These two set into motion an autocatalytic reaction with the build-up of an enlarging platelet aggregation known as the *temporary or primary hemostatic plug.* This primary aggregation is reversible, but with the activation of the coagulation sequence *thrombin* is generated. *Thrombin* is the third powerful platelet agonist, acting by binding to a platelet thrombin receptor. The combination of thrombin, ADP, and TxA$_2$ (and to some extent serotonin) induces further platelet aggregation. This is followed by *platelet contraction* (mediated by intraplatelet actomyosin), creating a fused mass of platelets—*"viscous metamorphosis"*—which constitutes the *definitive or secondary hemostatic plug.* At the same time, *thrombin causes the conversion of fibrinogen to fibrin within and about the platelet aggregate,* producing in essence a mortar for the "platelet bricks," further stabilizing the plug and anchoring it to its site of origin. Thrombin is thus central to the formation of thrombi and, indeed, is a major target in antithrombotic therapy[11] (Fig. 4–11).

Fibrinogen is an important cofactor in platelet aggregation. ADP-activated platelets bind fibrinogen, which then binds to glycoprotein receptors (GPIIb-IIIa) on adjacent platelets, forming a link that enhances platelet aggregation (see Fig. 4–10). Patients with *thrombasthenia* have reduced or absent GPIIb-IIIa, markedly diminished platelet aggregation, and severe bleeding.

Normally, platelet aggregation is inhibited by endothelial derived PGI$_2$ and nitric oxide. PGI$_2$ and TxA$_2$, both arachidonic acid derivatives, have opposing actions: PGI$_2$ inhibits platelet aggregation

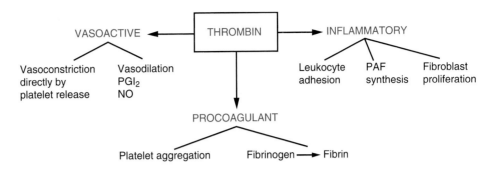

Figure 4–11. The central role of thrombin in hemostasis. Not shown are anticoagulant effects, including inhibition of PAI formation and protein C activation. (Modified and redrawn from Esmon, C.T.: Cell-mediated events that control blood coagulation. Annu. Rev. Cell Biol. 9:1, 1993.)

and is a vasodilator, whereas TxA_2 is a powerful aggregator and vascoconstrictor. *The interplay of PGI_2 and TxA_2 constitutes a finely balanced mechanism for modulation of human platelet function, which, in the normal state, prevents intravascular platelet aggregation and clotting but, following endothelial injury, favors the formation of a hemostatic plug. Nitric oxide, like PGI_2, is also a vasodilator and inhibitor of platelet aggregation* (see Fig. 4–7).

Finally, both erythrocytes and leukocytes can be found in hemostatic plugs. Erythrocytes, by unknown mechanisms, enhance platelet reactivity. Leukocytes adhere to platelets and endothelium through the action of adhesion molecules (P-selectin, ICAM-1) and contribute to the inflammatory response that often accompanies thrombosis. Thrombin again plays an important role in this inflammatory reaction. It stimulates neutrophil and monocyte adhesion and is directly mitogenic for fibroblasts. By causing fibrin formation, it releases fibrin split products, which are chemotactic for leukocytes (see Fig. 4–11).

The complex sequence of platelet events can be summarized as follows (see Fig. 4–7): (1) Platelets recognize sites of endothelial injury and adhere to subendothelial fibrillar collagen, thus becoming activated. (2) With activation they secrete a variety of products stored in granules (among them ADP and fibrinogen) and synthesize thromboxane A_2. (3) Platelet phospholipid complex helps activate several coagulation factors in the intrinsic coagulation sequence. (4) Concomitantly, the release of tissue factor from injured cells and endothelial cells participates in activation of the extrinsic coagulation sequence. (5) The ADP released from platelets initiates the formation of a temporary hemostatic plug of aggregated platelets, soon converted into a larger "secondary plug" under the influence of ADP, thrombin, and thromboxane (platelet agonists). Fibrinogen binding to platelets is critical to platelet aggregation. (6) The deposition of fibrin (derived from platelets and plasma fibrinogen) into and about the platelet aggregation stabilizes and anchors it.

Thus, platelet deficiencies, in either number or function will lead to potentially serious bleeding disorders, as discussed in Chapter 14.

Coagulation System

The *coagulation system* is the third component of the hemostatic process and a major contributor to thrombosis. It is not necessary to describe the details of the coagulation system because it is well presented in Figure 4–12. Only general principles and newer concepts will be highlighted.[13]

- The coagulation sequence comprises, in essence, a series of transformations of proenzymes to activated enzymes culminating in the formation of thrombin, which converts soluble fibrinogen into the insoluble fibrous protein fibrin.

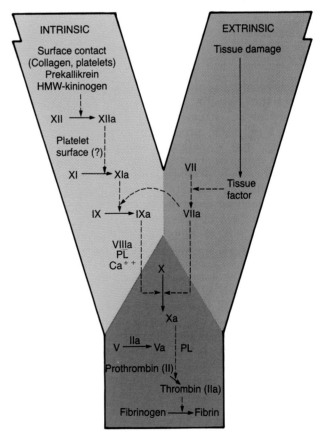

Figure 4–12. The coagulation cascade. Note the common links between the intrinsic and extrinsic coagulation pathways.

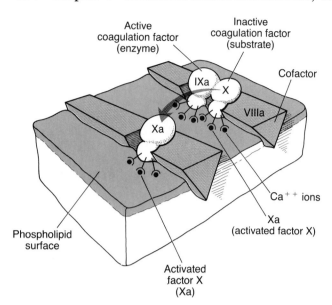

Figure 4–13. Schematic illustration of the conversion of factor X to factor Xa. The reaction complex consisting of an active enzyme (factor IXa), a substrate (factor X), and a reaction accelerator (factor VIIIa) is assembled on phospholipid surfaces. Ca++ ions hold the assembled components together and are essential for reaction. Activated factor Xa then becomes part of a second adjacent complex during the coagulation cascade, and so on. (Modified and redrawn with permission from Mann, K.G., Nesheim, M.E., Hibbard, L.S., et al.: The role of factor V in the assembly of the prothrombinase complex. *In* Walz, D.A., and McCoy, L.E. (eds.): Annals of the New York Academy of Sciences. New York, New York Academy of Sciences, 1981, pp. 378–388.)

- Each reaction in the coagulation pathway results from the assembly of a reaction complex composed of an *enzyme* (activated coagulation factor), a *substrate* (proenzyme form of coagulation factor), and a *cofactor* (reaction accelerator). These components are assembled on a *phospholipid surface* and held together by *calcium ions.* Thus, clotting tends to remain localized to sites where such an assembly can occur, for example, on the surface of activated platelets. One of the key reactions in blood clotting, conversion of factor X to Xa, is illustrated in Figure 4–13.

- It has been customary to divide the blood coagulation scheme into an *extrinsic* and an *intrinsic pathway*, both of which converge at the point where factor X is activated (see Fig. 4–12). The intrinsic pathway is initiated *in vitro* by contact activation of *Hageman factor* (factor XII), which converts factor IX to IXa. The extrinsic pathway is activated by *tissue factor*, a cellular lipoprotein released from damaged tissues or expressed on the surface of activated monocytes, endothelial cells, and other nonvascular cells and which converts factor VII to VIIa. However, there is little evidence that the intrinsic pathway is of primary importance *in vivo*, as patients with factor XII deficiency exhibit no abnormal bleeding. In ad-

dition, it is now clear that tissue factor also plays a role in intrinsic pathway activation, as the factor VIIa–tissue factor complex can also convert factor IX to IXa (see Fig. 4–12).[14]

Once the coagulation cascade has been activated, it must be contained to the local site of vascular injury lest clotting involve the entire vascular tree. The naturally occurring anticoagulants, described earlier in the discussion of endothelium, fall into three basic groups:

1. *Antithrombins*, exemplified by antithrombin III, are characterized by their ability to inhibit the activity of thrombin and other serine proteases — factors IXa, Xa, XIa, and XIIa. Antithrombin is activated by binding to heparin-like molecules on endothelial cells and by the therapeutic administration of heparin.

2. *Proteins C and S* are two vitamin K–dependent proteins characterized by their ability to inactivate cofactors Va and VIIIa. These two, it will be recalled, serve as reaction accelerators in the coagulation cascade. The activation of protein C by endothelium-associated thrombomodulin has already been described.

3. The *plasminogen-plasmin system* serves to break down fibrin and check fibrin polymerization. The proteolytic conversion of plasminogen to its active form, plasmin, is accomplished largely by plasminogen activators (PA). There are two groups of PAs: (1) *urokinase-like PA* (*u*-PA) is present in plasma and various tissues and activates plasminogen in the fluid phase; (2) *t*-PA, synthesized principally by endothelial cells, is active when attached to fibrin. It is noteworthy that plasmin itself converts inactive urokinase (prourokinase) to urokinase, thus amplifying fibrinolysis (Fig. 4–14). Plasminogen is also activated by a bacterial product, streptokinase.

Endothelial cells also elaborate inhibitors of fibrinolysis — plasminogen activation inhibitors (PAI) — which prevent fibrin binding of *t*-PA.[15]

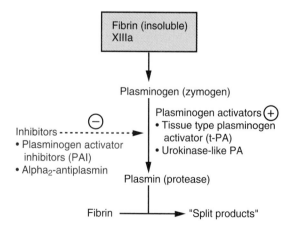

Figure 4–14. The fibrinolytic system illustrating the plasminogen activators and inhibitors.

PAIs also amplify the effect of a circulating factor, alpha$_2$-antiplasmin, which inhibits fibrin binding of plasmin. Thus, the fibrinolytic activity on the surface of thrombi presents a balance between activator and inhibitor properties. This balance can be perturbed by certain stimuli. For example, the cytokines IL-1 and TNF (which, as you recall, augment tissue factor activity) stimulate *t*-PA inhibitor synthesis. Both these activities of the cytokines favor thrombus formation, and indeed these mediators have been implicated in the intravascular thrombosis that sometimes accompanies severe infections. Conversely, certain tumor extracts increase *t*-PA synthesis by endothelium, thus potentiating fibrinolysis.

Against this background of normal hemostasis we can now consider thrombogenesis.

THROMBOSIS

Pathogenesis

Three major influences predispose to thrombosis: (1) injury to endothelium; (2) alterations in normal blood flow, and (3) alterations in the blood (hypercoagulability). Endothelial injury is the major and most frequent influence and the only one that, by and of itself, may lead to thrombosis. However, it is probably not required when the other two influences are operative.

- *Endothelial injury* is particularly important in the formation of thrombi in the heart and arteries. This is amply documented in humans by the frequency with which thrombi develop in the left ventricle at sites of myocardial infarction and on ulcerated plaques in advanced atherosclerosis of the aorta and arteries. Thrombi also develop within the cardiac chambers when there has been injury to the endocardium, as may occur with cardiac surgery, infections of the myocardium, or immunologic myocardial reactions. Valves with inflammatory valve disease and prosthetic valves are favored sites of thrombus formation. In addition to such overt causes, covert damage may be produced by a variety of influences. The hemodynamic stress in hypertension or the turbulent flow in arterial disorders induces a variety of alterations in endothelium, and some of these favor thrombosis. Other potential bases of damage to endothelial cells are radiation injury, chemical agents of exogenous origin (derivatives of cigarette smoke, for example) or of endogenous origin (hypercholesterolemia, homocystine), bacterial toxins or endotoxins, and immunologic injuries (in transplant rejection, immune complex deposition). Whatever the cause of injury to endothelium, it is a potent thrombogenic influence.
- *Alterations in normal blood flow*, as encountered

with turbulence, contribute to the development of arterial and cardiac thrombi, while stasis (sluggish blood flow) contributes to venous thrombosis.[15] In normal laminar flow all the formed blood elements occupy the central "axial" stream. The periphery of the bloodstream adjacent to the endothelial layer moves most slowly and is free from all formed blood elements. Stasis and turbulence (causing countercurrents and local pockets of stasis) provide at least four important dimensions: (1) They disrupt laminar flow and bring platelets into contact with the endothelium; (2) they prevent the dilution by the fresh flow of blood and hepatic clearance of the activated coagulation factors; (3) they retard the inflow of inhibitors of clotting factors and permit the build-up of thrombi; and (4) turbulence may cause dysfunction or damage to the endothelium, favoring platelet and fibrin deposition while at the same time reducing the local release of prostacyclin and *t*-PA.

The roles of turbulence or stasis are clearly documented in many clinical situations involving both the arterial and the venous sides of the circulation. Thrombi often form, as mentioned earlier, overlying ulcerated *atherosclerotic plaques*. Here the ulceration not only exposes subendothelial elements but also causes local turbulence. Thrombi are also prone to occur in the aorta and arteries within abnormal dilatations referred to as *aneurysms*. In the heart, not only do myocardial infarctions provide sites of endothelial injury, but also the necrotic muscle does not contract, and so some element of stasis is added. In healed rheumatic heart disease, for example, mitral stenosis causes the left atrium to expand and fail to empty. When arrhythmias such as atrial fibrillation (common in rheumatic heart disease) supervene, the stage is set for atrial and auricular thrombosis.

Stasis is undoubtedly the prime factor in the more slowly moving venous circulation. Most thrombi that develop in abnormally dilated varicose veins arise within the pockets created by venous valves, where presumably there is increased stasis or turbulence. Certainly there is no discernible evidence of endothelial injury, but hemodynamic alterations have clearly been shown to induce endothelial dysfunction, without evidence of overt injury.[16]

Stasis may have more subtle origins. Hyperviscosity syndromes, such as polycythemia, cryoglobulinemia, and macroglobulinemia, increase resistance to flow and induce stasis in small vessels. In sickle cell anemia the deformed red cells tend to cause a logjam, and the stasis predisposes to thrombosis.[16]

- *Hypercoagulability* can be defined as an alteration of the blood coagulation mechanism that in some way predisposes to thrombosis. This is not a common cause of thrombosis. Hypercoagulable

Table 4–2. HYPERCOAGULABLE STATES

PRIMARY (GENETIC)

Antithrombin III deficiency
Protein C deficiency
Protein S deficiency
Fibrinolysis defects
?Other combined defects

SECONDARY (ACQUIRED)

High Risk

Prolonged bed rest or immobilization	Acute leukemia
Myocardial infarction	Myeloproliferative disorders
Tissue damage (including surgery, fractures, burns)	Prosthetic cardiac valves
Cardiac failure	Disseminated intravascular coagulation
Cancer	Thrombotic thrombocytopenia
	Homocystinuria

Lower Risk

Atrial fibrillation	Hyperlipidemia
Cardiomyopathy	Lupus anticoagulant
Nephrotic syndrome	Sickle cell anemia
Late pregnancy/postdelivery	Smoking
Oral contraceptives	Thrombocytosis

states can be either *primary,* due to a genetic defect in one or several coagulation proteins, or *secondary,* occurring in a variety of clinical conditions associated with recurrent thrombosis (Table 4–2).[17] Often the hypercoagulability has no obvious cause.

The best-understood are those associated with an inherited lack of the anticoagulants antithrombin III, protein C, or protein S. Affected patients present with venous thrombosis and recurrent thromboembolism in adolescence or early adult life. Rarer cases are due to defects in the fibrinolytic system. These hereditary disorders are quite uncommon. However, it has also been suggested that subtle inherited predispositions to thrombosis may result from mutations in two or more of the coagulation protein genes, possibly accounting for patients with recurrent thromboses and no known cause.[18]

It is more difficult to unravel the pathogenesis of the thrombotic diathesis in the secondary hypercoagulable settings such as nephrotic syndrome, severe trauma or burns, late pregnancy, cardiac failure, and disseminated cancer. In some of these conditions, for example with cardiac failure or following trauma, other influences such as stasis or vascular injury may be the most important mechanism. In users of oral contraceptives an increase in concentrations of plasma fibrinogen, prothrombin, and factors VII, VIII, and X can be demonstrated, as can a decrease in fibrinolytic activity; yet it has not been possible to prove a cause-and-effect relationship between the abnormalities in laboratory tests and the increased thromboses. In patients with disseminated cancer, secretion or release of procoagulant tumor products that activate factor X directly, or thromboplastic substances that trigger the extrinsic pathway, have been proposed as the basis for the tendency toward thrombosis. This paraneoplastic syndrome, known as Trousseau's sign, is characterized by migratory thrombosis and is discussed further in Chapter 7.

With *advancing age,* a number of influences, as will be pointed out later, predispose to thrombus formation, but of particular relevance with respect to hypercoagulability is an increased aggregability of platelets, reduced release of PGI_2, and reduced fibrinolytic response. *Smoking* increases the hazard of thrombosis. This is best borne out by data documenting that users of oral contraceptives who are smokers have a substantially greater risk of developing thrombi than those who do not smoke. *Obesity,* in some ill-defined manner, increases the predisposition.

Some patients with high titers of *autoantibodies directed against anionic phospholipids* (cardiolipin) have a high frequency of arterial and venous thrombosis.[19] Some of them have manifestations of a well-defined autoimmune disease such as systemic lupus erythematosus (in whom the antibody is known as *lupus anticoagulant*), but in others thrombosis is the major or only clinical manifestation. The possible mechanisms by which antiphospholipid antibodies promote thrombosis include induction of platelet aggregation, inhibition of prostacyclin or nitric oxide production by endothelial cells, or interference in the generation of protein C.

MORPHOLOGY OF THROMBI. Thrombi may occur anywhere in the cardiovascular system: within the cardiac chambers, arteries, veins, or capillaries. They are of variable size and shape, dictated by their site of origin and the circumstances leading to their development. When thrombi are formed within a cardiac chamber or the aorta, they may have apparent laminations called the **lines of Zahn.** These are produced by alternating layers of paler platelets admixed with some fibrin, separated by darker layers containing more red cells. However, the laminations may not be evident in thrombi formed within smaller arteries or veins. Moreover, thrombi formed in the slower-moving flow in veins sometimes closely resemble coagulated blood, but close inspection will reveal traversing or tangled pale strands of aggregated platelets and fibrin, but well-defined lines of Zahn are rarely evident.

Mural thrombi, that is, thrombi applied to one wall of an underlying structure, occur in the capacious lumina of the heart chambers and aorta. Myocardial infarcts or cardiac arrhythmias are common antecedents to the thrombi that form in

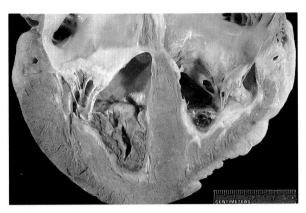

Figure 4-15. Mural thrombus in left ventricle and right ventricle overlying areas of pale white fibrosis.

the heart, while atherosclerosis or aneurysmal dilatations are almost invariable precursors of aortic thrombus formation (Figs. 4-15 and 4-16).

In special circumstances thrombi may be deposited on the heart valves. Blood-borne infections may attack heart valves **(bacterial or infective endocarditis),** creating ideal sites for the development of thrombotic masses. These masses, laden with micro-organisms, are referred to as vegetations. Less commonly, noninfective, **verrucous endocarditis** may appear in patients who have systemic lupus erythematosus. Vegetations may also develop on uninfected valves—**nonbacterial (thrombotic) endocarditis** in older patients with terminal cancers or other chronic ailments, and sometimes in young patients with nonfatal disorders. In these conditions, hypercoagulability of the blood, subtle endothelial injuries, or both are invoked as the causative mechanisms.

Arterial thrombi are usually **occlusive,** although they may be mural in such large vessels as the iliacs and common carotids. Occlusive thrombi

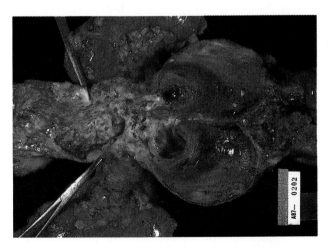

Figure 4-16. Opened abdominal aneurysm showing laminated thrombus totally filling the aneurysm *(right).*

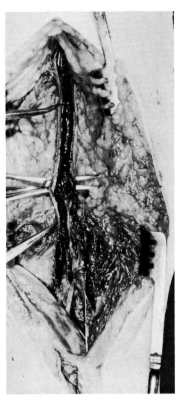

Figure 4-17. Popliteal veins exposed to demonstrate a large thrombus.

are most frequently encountered, in descending order, in the coronary, cerebral, and femoral arteries. Almost always the thrombus is superimposed on an atherosclerotic lesion, but uncommonly, other forms of vascular disease, such as acute vasculitis and traumatic injury, are involved. The thrombi are usually gray-white and friable, made up of tangled strands and layers of fibrin and platelets enmeshed in the clot. Moreover, they are usually firmly attached to the damaged arterial wall. Contraction of the freshly formed thrombus may provide a slit-like lumen, restoring some flow; under this circumstance, the original thrombotic mass may enlarge (propagate) at both the upstream and the downstream ends.

Venous thrombosis, also known as **phlebothrombosis,** is almost invariably occlusive. In fact, the thrombus often creates a long cast of the lumen of the vein (Fig. 4-17). In the slower-moving blood of the veins, the coagulation simulates that in a test tube. Thus, these thrombi have a much richer admixture of erythrocytes and are therefore known as **red, coagulative,** or **stasis thrombi.** On transection, laminations are not well developed, but tangled strands of fibrin can usually be seen. **Phlebothrombosis most commonly affects the veins of the lower extremities (90%) in approximately the following order of frequency: deep calf, femoral, popliteal, and iliac veins.** Less commonly, venous thrombi may develop in the peri-

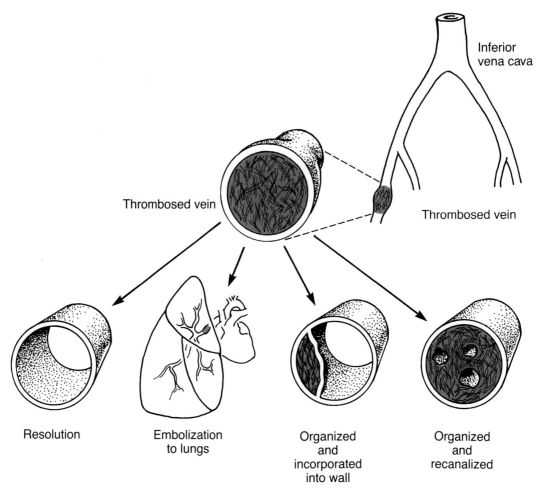

Figure 4–18. The potential outcomes following venous thrombosis.

prostatic plexus, or the ovarian and periuterine veins. Sometimes they occur in the portal vein or its radicles or in the dural sinuses.

Venous thrombi can be readily confused with postmortem clots at autopsy. The postmortem clot forms a cast of the vessel, but it is rubbery and gelatinous. The dependent portions of the clot where the red cells have settled by gravity tend to resemble dark red "currant jelly." The supernatant, free of red cells, has a yellow "chicken fat" appearance. Characteristically, the postmortem clot is not attached to the underlying wall. In contrast, coagulation thrombi are firmer, almost always have a point of attachment, and on transection disclose barely visible tangled strands of pale-gray fibrin.

Arterial and venous thrombi vary enormously in size. They range from small, irregular, roughly spherical masses to enormously elongated, snake-like structures that are formed when a long tail builds up behind the occluding head. In the arterial circulation, the tail builds up retrograde to the direction of flow. On the venous side the tail extends in the direction of the blood flow, that is, toward the heart. Often such propagations extend to the next major vascular branch.

A small or large area of attachment to the underlying vessel or heart wall is characteristic of all thromboses. Frequently, the attachment is firmest at the point of origin, and the propagating tail may or may not be attached. It is this loosely attached tail that, in veins, is most likely to fragment, creating an embolus. On the arterial side of the circulation, embolization usually implies detachment of the entire or almost the entire thrombus.

Fate of the Thrombus

If a patient survives the immediate effects of vascular obstruction, what happens to the thrombus over the course of days and weeks? One of the following sequences evolves (Fig. 4–18):

- *Propagation.* The thrombus may *propagate* and eventually cause obstruction of some critical vessel.

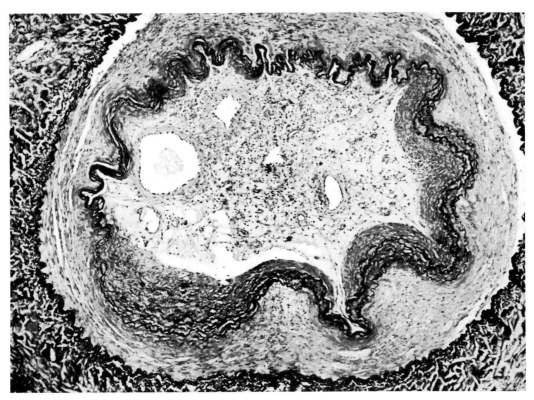

Figure 4–19. Low-power view of a thrombosed artery stained for elastic tissue. The lumen is delineated by the partially degenerated internal elastic membrane and is totally filled with organized clot, now traversed by many newly formed recanalized channels.

- *Embolization.* Thrombi may dislodge to distal sites in the vascular tree.
- *Dissolution.* They may be removed by fibrinolytic activity.
- *Organization and recanalization.* Thrombi may induce inflammation and fibrosis — termed organization — and may eventually become recanalized.

The first two eventualities will be discussed presently under sections on infarction and embolism. There is evidence that fibrinolytic removal may occur. By angiography, pulmonary thromboemboli have been observed to shrink rapidly and even be totally lysed soon after they develop. Such a happy outcome is most likely within the first day or two, presumably because as the thrombus ages and the fibrin undergoes continued polymerization, it is more resistant to proteolysis. It is relevant in this connection to note that infusion of fibrinolytic agents such as recombinant *t*-PA and streptokinase within hours of the acute event is currently employed in the management of massive pulmonary thromboemboli and coronary thrombosis.

When a thrombus persists *in situ* for a few days, it is likely to become *organized* (Fig. 4–19). This term refers to the ingrowth of granulation tissue, subendothelial smooth muscle cells, and mesenchymal cells into the fibrin-rich thrombus. In time the thrombus becomes populated with these spindle cells, and capillary channels are formed. Simultaneously the surface of the thrombus becomes covered with a layer of endothelial cells. The capillary channels may anastomose to create thoroughfares from one end of the thrombus to the other through which blood may flow, re-establishing to some extent the continuity of the lumen of the original vessel. This process is known as *recanalization* of the thrombus (see Fig. 4–19).

In this manner, the thrombus is converted into a vascularized subendothelial mass of connective tissue and eventually incorporated into the wall of the vessel. With the passage of time and the contraction of the mesenchymal cells, only a fibrous lump or thickening may remain to mark the site. Occasionally, instead of becoming organized, the center of the thrombus undergoes enzymic digestion and softens. This action presumably reflects the release of lysosomal enzymes derived from the trapped leukocytes and platelets. This sequence is particularly likely in large thrombi within aneurysmal dilatations or within mural thrombi in the cardiac chambers. If a bacteremia occurs, such softened debris is an ideal culture medium for conversion of the thrombus into a septic mass of pus.

CLINICAL CORRELATIONS. Thrombi are critically important for two reasons: (1) *they cause obstruc-*

tion of arteries and veins and (2) *they provide possible sources of emboli.* Venous thrombi may cause congestion and edema in dependent parts, but a far graver consequence is that thrombi, most frequently those arising in the deep veins of the legs, are responsible for one of the major causes of death in the United States—namely, pulmonary embolization and infarction (see Chapter 15). In contrast, although arterial thrombi may of course embolize, much more important is their obstructive role in myocardial infarction, when the coronary arteries are involved, and in cerebral infarction, when the arteries in the brain are involved.

Venous Thrombosis (Phlebothrombosis).[20,21] As pointed out earlier, most venous thrombi are occlusive. *The great preponderance of these thrombi arise in either the superficial or the deep veins of the leg.* Superficial thrombi usually occur in the saphenous system, particularly when there are varicosities. Such thrombi may cause local congestion and swelling, pain, and tenderness along the course of the involved vein, but only rarely do they embolize. However, the local edema and impaired venous drainage predispose the skin to infections from slight trauma and to the development of *varicose ulcers.* It is the *deep thrombi in the larger outflow veins of the legs (e.g., popliteal, femoral, and iliac veins) that are the most serious because they may embolize.* They may also cause edema of the foot and ankle and produce pain and tenderness on compression of the calf muscles (by either squeezing the calf muscles or forced dorsiflexion of the foot), known as Homans' sign. However, in *approximately half of the patients, such thrombi are entirely asymptomatic* and are recognized only when they have embolized. The venous obstruction is soon compensated for by the opening of collateral bypass channels of drainage. The most serious aspect of venous thrombosis in the deep veins of the leg, as mentioned, is its potential for causing pulmonary embolization and infarction (see also discussion on phlebothrombosis and thrombophlebitis in Chapter 11).

Specific clinical settings in which venous thrombosis is most likely to occur have already been mentioned in the discussion of thrombogenesis but, for emphasis, are repeated here. *They include cardiac failure, severe trauma or burns, postoperative and postpartum states, the nephrotic syndrome, disseminated cancer* (and in fact, all serious illnesses), and the use of oral contraceptives. Regardless of specific clinical setting, advanced age, bed rest, and immobilization increase the hazard. The reduced physical activity in older age lessens the milking action of muscles in the lower leg and so slows venous return. Immobilization and bed rest carry the same implications.

Arterial Thrombosis. *Arterial thrombi are particularly likely to develop in patients with myocardial* infarction, rheumatic heart disease, florid atherosclerosis, and aneurysmal dilatations of the aorta or other major arteries. Myocardial infarction usually is associated with damage to the adjacent endocardium, providing a site for the origin of a mural thrombus, usually within the left ventricle. Stasis and turbulence within the affected cardiac chamber are usually also present because of dyskinetic contraction of the myocardium or the development of cardiac irregularities. Advanced age, bed rest, and impaired circulation compound the problem. Rheumatic heart disease often leads to marked stenosis of the mitral valve and, along with it, stasis within the markedly dilated left atrium and atrial appendage. Concurrently, cardiac arrhythmias may augment the stasis. Florid atherosclerosis is a prime initiator of thromboses for what must now be obvious reasons. But, in addition to all the serious obstructive consequences, thrombi in the aorta and in the cardiac chambers often yield fragments that embolize to such sites as the brain, the kidneys, the legs, and the spleen. Other tissues or organs may also be affected, but the brain, kidneys, and spleen constitute prime targets because of their large blood flow volume.

In closing this discussion of thrombosis, it is important to point out that although many settings are known to significantly increase the risk, thrombogenesis is ultimately a puzzling and unpredictable phenomenon. It may occur at any time, under any conditions, and indeed appears surprisingly often in healthy ambulant individuals without apparent provocation or known predisposition.

DISSEMINATED INTRAVASCULAR COAGULATION (DIC)

A variety of disorders ranging from obstetric difficulties to advanced cancer may be complicated by the sudden or insidious development of myriad fibrin thrombi in the microcirculation—DIC—followed in some cases by active fibrinolysis and a bleeding diathesis.[22] With the development of the multiple thrombi, there is rapid consumption of platelets, prothrombin, fibrinogen, and factors V, VIII, and X (hence the synonyms *consumption coagulopathy* and *defibrination syndrome*); at the same time, the plasminogen-plasmin system is activated, and fibrin(ogen) degradation products are formed, having an anticoagulation effect. In this manner a thrombotic disorder ends up as a bleeding disorder. *It should be emphasized that DIC is not a primary disease; rather it complicates the course of any condition associated with activation of thrombin through either the intrinsic or the extrinsic pathway.* Because it is closely related to thrombotic thrombocytopenic purpura (and several other conditions), it is discussed later along with the bleeding diatheses (see Chapter 13).

EMBOLISM

An embolus is a detached intravascular solid, liquid, or gaseous mass that is carried by the blood to a site distant from its point of origin. Virtually 99% of all emboli arise in thrombi (thromboembolism). Rare forms of emboli include fragments of bone or bone marrow, atheromatous debris from ruptured atherosclerotic plaques, droplets of fat, bits of tumor, foreign bodies such as bullets, and bubbles of air or nitrogen. *Unless otherwise qualified, the term embolus implies thromboembolism.* Inevitably, emboli lodge in vessels too small to permit their further passage, resulting in partial or complete occlusion of the vessel. Depending on their site of origin, emboli may come to rest anywhere within the cardiovascular system and are best discussed from the standpoint of whether they lodge in the pulmonary or systemic circulations, thus producing differing clinical effects.

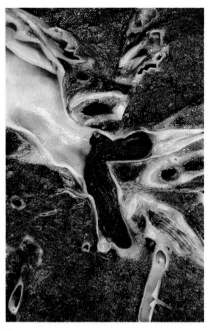

Figure 4–20. Large embolus from the veins of the lower leg in the pulmonary artery.

PULMONARY EMBOLISM

Pulmonary embolism is the most common preventable cause of death in hospitalized patients. This important complication of thrombosis is discussed more fully in Chapter 15; only an overview is presented here.

Occlusion of a large or medium-sized pulmonary artery is embolic in origin until proved otherwise. Thrombotic occlusion of these vessels is very uncommon and is encountered virtually only when pulmonary hypertension has led to atherosclerotic or other hypertensive changes in the pulmonary arterial tree or with chest trauma. Pulmonary embolism is a major clinical problem, especially among hospitalized patients; annually it causes about 50,000 deaths in the United States.

More than 95% of all pulmonary emboli arise in thrombi within the large deep veins of the lower legs—popliteal, femoral, and iliac veins (Figs. 4–20 and 4–21). Thrombi within the superficial veins of the legs (usually associated with varicosities), veins of the calf muscles, or such other sites as the veins in the pelvis—the periprostatic, broad ligament, periovarian, and uterine veins—are uncommon sources of emboli.

Depending on the size and length of the embolic mass, it may occlude the main pulmonary artery (usually when coiled on itself), impact astride the bifurcation (a *saddle embolus*), or pass out into the progressively smaller branching pulmonary arteries. Often, there are multiple emboli, perhaps sequentially, or a large mass fragments to produce a shower of smaller emboli impacting in a number of vessels. Rarely, an embolus may pass through an interatrial or interventricular defect, when the pressure in the right heart exceeds that in the left heart, to gain access to the systemic circulation (*paradoxical embolism*).

The clinical consequences of a pulmonary embolus are discussed in Chapter 15; only some comments will be offered here.

- *Most pulmonary emboli (60 to 80%) are clinically silent* because they are small.
- Sudden death, acute right heart failure (acute cor pulmonale), or cardiovascular collapse may occur when more than 60% of the total pulmonary vasculature is obstructed by a large embolus or multiple, simultaneous, small emboli.
- Obstruction of relatively small pulmonary branches (10 to 15% of cases) that behave as end arteries usually causes pulmonary infarction. Sometimes a more proximal, larger embolus fragments and obstructs smaller vessels and thus produces infarcts hours or even days after the acute embolic event.
- Embolic obstruction of middle-sized arteries (10 to 15% of cases) that are not end-arteries is usually not associated with pulmonary infarction but instead results in more centrally located pulmonary hemorrhage. The bronchial circulation and other anastomoses prevent total ischemia in this setting. However, should there be cardiac failure or underlying pulmonary disease, such proximal emboli may indeed cause large infarcts.
- Uncommonly, multiple emboli lead to pulmonary hypertension, chronic right heart strain (chronic

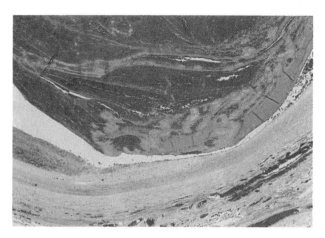

Figure 4–21. Microscopic section of pulmonary embolus. Note platelet-fibrin mass close to the vessel wall and superimposed red clot.

cor pulmonale), and in time pulmonary vascular sclerosis with progressively worsening dyspnea.

What is the fate of an embolus if it does not resolve? As with a thrombus, the thromboembolus may undergo organization and essentially be incorporated within the wall of the pulmonary artery as an endothelium-covered fibrous mass. Such mural projections contribute to the development of pulmonary hypertension and subsequent pulmonary vascular sclerosis, including pulmonary atherosclerosis (see Chapter 15). Occasionally and inexplicably, *organization of a thromboembolus creates delicate, insignificant, bridging fibrous webs.*

SYSTEMIC EMBOLISM

This term refers to emboli that travel through the arterial circulation. *Most arterial emboli (80 to 85%) arise from thrombi within the heart.* About 60 to 65% arise within the left ventricle secondary to myocardial infarction, and only about 5 to 10% from atrial thrombi in rheumatic heart disease. Cardiomyopathy accounts for an additional 5%.[25] Whatever the underlying heart disease, arrhythmias such as atrial fibrillation increase the risk of embolization. Less common sources of arterial emboli include thrombi developing in relation to ulcerated atherosclerotic plaques, aortic aneurysms, infective endocarditis, valvular or aortic prostheses, and paradoxical embolism from venous thrombi that gain access to the left side of the circulation through a right-to-left congenital cardiac anomaly. In about 10 to 15% of patients the source of the embolus is unknown.

In contrast to venous emboli, *arterial emboli follow a much more varied pathway, but they almost always cause infarction.* The major sites of lodgment of all systemic emboli are the *lower ex-*

tremities (70 to 75%), the brain (10%), viscera (10%—includes mesenteric, renal and splenic), and the upper limbs (7 to 8%). The site of lodgment and the size of the embolus within the systemic vessels are obvious critical determinants of its significance. Embolic occlusion of the femoral artery is disastrous inasmuch as it causes infarction (gangrene) of the lower extremity, but it is not necessarily life-threatening. In contrast, a much smaller embolus that occludes the middle cerebral artery may lead to death in days, or even hours. As with pulmonary emboli, prompt diagnosis and effective treatment—general supportive measures, anticoagulation, embolectomy—have greatly improved the prognosis of both life and limb.

AMNIOTIC FLUID EMBOLISM (INFUSION)

This extremely grave complication usually of labor and the immediate postpartum period has become a major cause of maternal mortality as the other fatal complications (e.g., hemorrhage, toxemia, pulmonary embolism) have been better controlled.[25] Fortunately, amniotic fluid embolism, or as some would prefer *amniotic fluid infusion*, is uncommon, with an incidence of about 1 per 50,000 deliveries, but it incurs a mortality rate of 86%. The clinical presentation is striking—suddenly and without warning, profound respiratory difficulty with deep cyanosis and cardiovascular shock appear, followed rapidly in some cases by clonic-tonic convulsions and profound coma. If the patient survives the initial crisis, within a few hours marked pulmonary edema usually becomes evident, and in about half the cases excessive bleeding from the uterus and birth canal. The latter is attributed to the *development of DIC* due to release of thromboplastic substances in amniotic fluid.

The underlying cause is the infusion of amniotic fluid with all of its contents into the maternal circulation following a tear in the placental membranes and rupture of uterine and/or cervical veins. As a consequence, *epithelial squames from fetal skin, lanugo hair, fat from vernix caseosa, mucin from the fetal respiratory or gastrointestinal tract, and occasionally bile from meconium contamination of the amniotic fluid can be found in the victim's pulmonary microcirculation at postmortem examination* (Fig. 4–22). Often there is also marked pulmonary edema and changes typical of acute respiratory distress syndrome (see Chapter 15).

There is a poor correlation at postmortem examination between the amount of amniotic fluid debris found in the vessels and the rapidity of the fatal course. It is suspected that some humoral factor (possibly prostaglandins) in amniotic fluid caus-

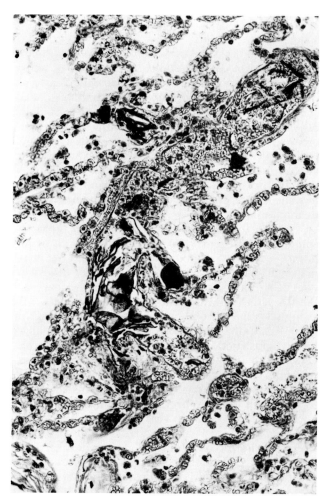

Figure 4-22. Amniotic embolism. Masses of dark mucous debris and desquamated squames are present in the pulmonary vessels and alveolar capillaries.

ing pulmonary vasoconstriction and impaired cardiac contractility is responsible for the respiratory and cardiac decompensation. To date, this cause of maternal death remains unpredictable and largely unpreventable.

AIR EMBOLISM (CAISSON DISEASE)

Bubbles of air or gas within the circulation obstruct vascular flow and damage tissues just as certainly as thrombotic masses.[26] The injury is now referred to as *barotrauma*. Air or gas may gain access to the circulation (1) during delivery or abortion when it is forced into ruptured uterine venous sinuses by the powerful contractions of the uterus, (2) during the performance of a pneumothorax when a large artery or vein is ruptured or entered accidentally, and (3) when injury to the lung or the chest wall opens a large vein and permits the entrance of air during the negative pressure phase of inspiration. These bubbles of air act as physical masses. Many small bubbles may coalesce to produce frothy, gaseous masses, sufficiently large to occlude a major vessel, usually in the lungs or brain. Large quantities of air, probably somewhere in the neighborhood of 100 cc, are required to produce problems.

A specialized form of gas embolism known as *caisson disease* or *decompression sickness* occurs in persons exposed to sudden changes in atmospheric pressure. Those at particular risk are scuba and deep sea divers and workers engaged in underwater tunneling and the construction of foundations for offshore drilling platforms. When the gas is breathed under high pressure, increased amounts dissolve in the blood, tissue fluids, and fat. If the individual decompresses too rapidly, the gases come out of solution as minute bubbles. Oxygen is readily soluble, but nitrogen and helium (which are used at deeper levels) tend to persist to form gaseous emboli within the blood vessels and tissues.

There are two types of decompression sickness, acute and chronic. The *acute form* is commonly known as "the bends" or "the chokes." The acute obstruction of small blood vessels in and around the joints and skeletal muscles causes the patient to double up in pain; a similar process may produce acute respiratory distress, while involvement of the cerebral vessels may lead to obtundation, coma, and sometimes death. *The chronic form of decompression sickness is more properly referred to as caisson disease.* Here, the presumed persistence of gaseous emboli leads to multiple foci of ischemic necrosis throughout the skeletal system, favored sites being the heads of the femurs, tibia, and humeri (see Chapter 9).

When air or gas embolism is suspected, it is necessary at autopsy to open the heart and major pulmonary trunks under water to detect the escaping gas. At times the frothy appearance of the blood calls attention to the presence of the gaseous bubbles.

FAT EMBOLISM

Minute globules of fat can often be demonstrated in the circulation following fractures of the shafts of long bones (which have fatty marrows) and, rarely, with soft tissue trauma and burns. Presumably, the microglobules are released by injury to marrow or adipose tissue and gain access to the circulation by rupture of the marrow vascular sinusoids or venules. It should be emphasized that whereas *traumatic fat embolism can be demonstrated anatomically in approximately 90% of individuals who sustain severe skeletal injuries, only about 1% of these individuals manifest clinical signs or symptoms known as fat embolism syndrome.* It is characterized by pulmonary insufficiency, neurologic symptoms, anemia, and thrombocytopenia. Typically, the symptoms appear after a latent period of 24 to 72 hours after injury. There is the sudden onset of tachypnea, dyspnea, and tachycardia. Neurologic symptoms include irritability and restlessness, which progress to delirium or coma. Petechial skin rash is common. The fat embolism syndrome is fatal in about 10% of cases.

The pathogenesis of this symptom complex is believed to involve both mechanical obstruction and chemical injury.[27] It is proposed that microaggregates of neutral fat cause occlusion of pulmonary or cerebral microvasculature, and the free fatty acids released from fat globules result in toxic injury to the vascular endothelium. The petechial skin rash is related to rapid onset of thrombocytopenia. Presumably, myriad fat globules become coated with platelets, thus depleting circulating platelets.

The microscopic demonstration of fat microglobules in tissues or organs (Fig. 4–23) requires special techniques using frozen sections and fat stains because the emboli are dissolved out of the blood by the usual solvents employed in paraffin embedding of tissues.

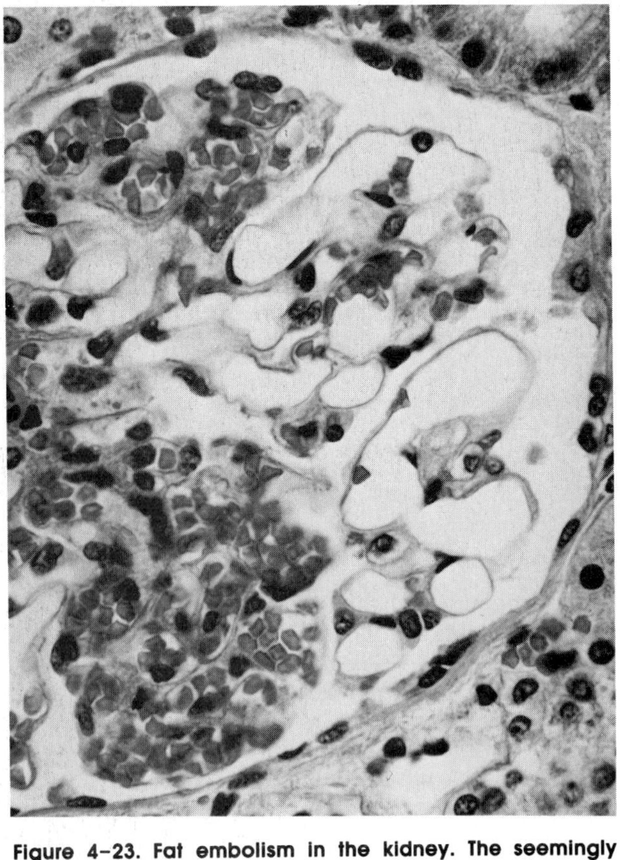

Figure 4–23. Fat embolism in the kidney. The seemingly empty glomerular capillaries are plugged with lipid vacuoles. Contrast with unoccluded congested capillaries on the left.

INFARCTION

An infarct is an area of ischemic necrosis within a tissue or an organ, produced by occlusion of either its arterial supply or its venous drainage. Nearly all infarcts result from thrombotic or embolic occlusion, but sometimes infarction may be caused by other mechanisms, such as ballooning of an atheroma secondary to hemorrhage within a plaque. Other uncommon causes include twisting of the vessels to the ovary or a loop of bowel, compression of the blood supply of a loop of bowel in a hernial sac, or trapping of a viscus under a peritoneal adhesion.

Nearly 99% of infarcts are caused by thromboembolic events, and almost all are the result of arterial occlusions. Emboli arising in the heart or major arteries must impact in arteries. Similarly, venous thromboemboli lodge in the pulmonary arterial system and so cause arterial infarcts. Although venous thrombosis may cause infarction of some tissue or organ, more often it merely induces venous obstruction. Usually, bypass channels develop, providing some outflow from the area, which in turn permits some improvement in the arterial inflow. Infarcts caused by venous thrombosis are more likely in organs having a single venous outflow channel, such as the testis and ovary.

TYPES OF INFARCTS. Infarcts are crudely divided on the basis of their color and the presence or absence of bacterial contamination. Infarcts are either *anemic (white)* or *hemorrhagic (red).*

- *White infarcts are encountered (1) with arterial occlusion and (2) in solid tissues. When a solid tissue is deprived of its arterial circulation, the infarct may be transiently hemorrhagic, but most become pale in a very short time.* At the moment of vascular occlusion, blood from anastomotic peripheral vessels flows into the focus of injury, producing the initial hemorrhagic appearance. If the tissue affected is solid, the seepage of blood is minimal. Soon after the initial extravasation, the red cells are lysed, and the released hemoglobin pigment either diffuses out or is converted to hemosiderin. In solid organs, therefore, the arterial infarct will soon (24 to 48 hours) become pale. *The heart, spleen, and kidneys are representative of solid, compact organs that tend to have pale infarcts* (Fig. 4–24).
- *Red or hemorrhagic infarcts are encountered usually (1) with venous occlusions, (2) in loose tissues, (3) in tissues with a double circulation, and (4) in tissues previously congested.* The loose, honeycombed tissue of the *lung* provides an example of hemorrhagic infarction secondary to arterial obstruction. At the moment of infarction, large amounts of hemorrhage collect in the spongy pulmonary parenchyma, so the arterial

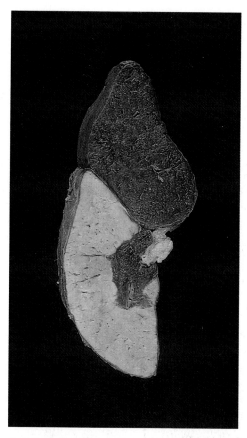

Figure 4–24. Transected surface of a spleen with pale, sharply demarcated infarct.

MORPHOLOGY. Whether hemorrhagic or pale, all infarcts tend to be wedge-shaped, with the apex of the wedge pointing toward the focus of vascular occlusion. Since all the dependent tissue out to the periphery of the organ is affected, the external aspect of the organ forms the base of the wedge.

A few hours after onset, all infarcts are somewhat poorly defined, are slightly darker in color than normal, and have firmer consistency than that of the surrounding normal tissue. During the next 24 hours, the demarcation becomes better defined, and the color change is more intense.

In the course of several days, pale infarcts become yellow-white and sharply demarcated, while the appearance of the pulmonary hemorrhagic infarcts remains relatively unchanged. The margins of both types of infarcts tend to become better defined by a narrow rim of hyperemia due to the marginal inflammatory response. The involved surface of the organ is usually covered by fibrinous exudate.

The characteristic cytologic change of all infarcts, save those in the brain, is ischemic coagulative necrosis of the affected cells (described in Chapter 1). If the vascular occlusion has occurred only a few hours prior to the death of the patient, there may be no demonstrable cellular change,

infarction remains red (Fig. 4–25). Venous occlusion leads to hemorrhagic infarction as occurs, for example, with twisting of the pedicle of the ovary. The thin-walled ovarian veins are occluded first, causing intense congestion and infarction with or without occlusion of the artery. The *small intestine* is another site where hemorrhagic infarcts typically occur. Venous occlusions or even arterial occlusions may cause hemorrhagic infarction of long segments of the intestine. The explanation lies in the rich arterial anastomoses between the many branches of the superior mesenteric artery, which permit arterial flow to the injured segment through anastomosing arcades. Hemorrhagic arterial infarction is sometimes encountered in the *brain* as well. An embolus to a large artery, such as the middle cerebral, may produce a nonhemorrhagic area of cerebral infarction. Soon thereafter, the embolus may shatter, and the fragments may move into smaller, more peripheral branches. Reflow through the major trunk may yield extensive hemorrhage into the primary area of ischemic necrosis.

• Infarcts are also classified as either *septic* or *bland,* depending on the presence or absence of bacterial infection in the area of necrosis.

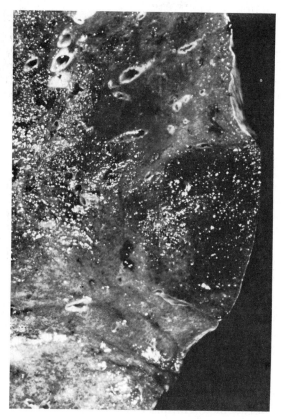

Figure 4–25. Sharply circumscribed hemorrhagic infarct in the lung.

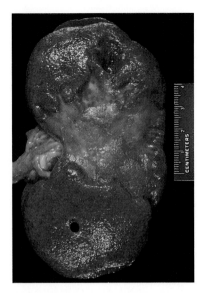

Figure 4-26. Old infarct in the kidney. Note depressed fibrotic scar in the cortex.

since there may have been insufficient time for enzymic alteration of the dead cells. If the patient survives for about 12 to 18 hours, only hemorrhagic suffusion may be present.

Inflammatory exudation begins in the margins in a few hours and becomes better defined in the next few days. The inflammatory reaction is followed by a fibroblastic, reparative response beginning in the preserved margins. Some parenchymal regeneration may occur at the periphery where the underlying framework of the organ has been spared. However, in most cases the necrotic focus is eventually replaced by scar tissue (Fig. 4-26).

The brain is an exception to these generalizations. When it suffers ischemic necrosis the affected area promptly and rapidly undergoes **liquefaction.**

With septic infarction the lesion is converted to an abscess and, if seen at a very late stage, may be unrecognizable as an infarct. The inflammatory reaction is correspondingly greater, but the eventual sequence of organization follows the pattern already described.

FACTORS THAT CONDITION THE DEVELOPMENT OF AN INFARCT. Occlusion of an artery or a vein may have little or no effect on the involved tissue or it may cause death of the tissue and, indeed, of the individual. *The major determinants include (1) the nature of the vascular supply, (2) the rate of development of the occlusion, and (3) the vulnerability of the tissue to hypoxia.*

The availability of an *alternative or newly acquired source of blood supply* is perhaps the most important factor in determining whether occlusion of a vessel will cause damage. As is well known, the lungs have a dual blood supply from pulmonary and bronchial arteries. Hence, blockage of a

radicle of the pulmonary arterial tree may be without effect in a young person who has normal bronchial circulation. The same applies to the liver, with its double blood supply of hepatic artery and portal vein. Infarction or gangrene of the hand or forearm is almost never encountered, because of the double arterial supply through the radial and ulnar arteries, with their numerous interconnections. Conversely, renal and splenic arteries are end-arteries, and thus infarction almost always follows arterial occlusion.

Newly acquired *collateral circulation* may be equally effective in preventing infarction. The coronary arterial supply to the myocardium is an excellent case in point. Small anastomoses normally exist between the three major coronary trunks—that is, the left anterior descending, the left circumflex, and the right coronary arteries. If one of these trunks is slowly narrowed, as by an atheroma, these anastomoses may enlarge sufficiently to prevent infarction, even though the major coronary artery is eventually occluded.

Slowly developing occlusions are less likely to cause infarction, since they provide an opportunity for alternative pathways of flow and anastomotic bypass channels to develop.

The vulnerability of the tissue to hypoxia influences the likelihood of infarction. Neurons of the nervous system undergo irreversible damage when deprived of their blood supply for 3 to 4 minutes. Myocardial cells, although hardier than neurons, are also quite sensitive to anoxia. In contrast, the fibroblasts within the myocardium are unaffected and are quite resistant to hypoxia. The epithelial cells of the proximal renal tubules are much more vulnerable to hypoxia than are the other segments of the nephron.

CLINICAL SIGNIFICANCE OF INFARCTION. In the United States, more than half of all deaths are caused by cardiovascular disease. Most of these cardiovascular deaths result from myocardial and cerebral infarctions. Coronary heart disease alone accounts for about 30% of all the mortality, and myocardial infarction is by far the predominant cause of fatal coronary heart disease. Cerebral infarction (encephalomalacia) is also the most frequent type of central nervous system disease. Pulmonary infarction is an extremely common complication in a variety of clinical settings, as has been indicated in previous considerations. Ischemic necrosis (gangrene) of the lower extremities is a relatively unusual clinical problem in the population at large but is a major concern in diabetics. Infarction of tissues, therefore, is a common cause of clinical illness.

Thrombosis, embolism, and infarction may strike without notice, but even worse, they are proverbial vultures, stalking every ill, bedridden, and aged patient who regrettably is least able to cope with them.

Table 4-3. THE THREE MAJOR TYPES OF SHOCK

TYPE OF SHOCK	CLINICAL EXAMPLES	PRINCIPAL MECHANISMS
Cardiogenic	Myocardial infarction Rupture of heart Arrhythmias Cardiac tamponade Pulmonary embolism	Failure of myocardial pump due to intrinsic myocardial damage or extrinsic pressure or obstruction to outflow
Hypovolemic	Hemorrhage Fluid loss—e.g., vomiting, diarrhea, burns, trauma	Inadequate blood or plasma volume
Septic	Overwhelming bacterial infections: gram-negative septicemia ("endotoxic shock") or gram-positive septicemia	Peripheral vasodilatation and pooling of blood; endothelial activation/injury; leukocyte-induced damage; disseminated intravascular coagulation

SHOCK

Shock, commonly called circulatory collapse, may develop following any serious assault on the body's homeostasis, such as profuse hemorrhage, severe trauma, extensive burns, large myocardial infarction, massive pulmonary embolism, or bacterial sepsis. Whatever the clinical provocation, at the most fundamental level shock constitutes *widespread hypoperfusion of tissues due to reduction in the blood volume or cardiac output, or redistribution of blood, resulting in an inadequate effective circulating volume.* Incident to the perfusion deficit, there is insufficient delivery of oxygen and nutrients to the cells and tissues and inadequate clearance of metabolites. The cellular hypoxia induces a shift from aerobic to anaerobic metabolism, resulting in increased lactate production and sometimes lactic acidosis. While at the outset the hemodynamic and metabolic derangements are correctable and induce reversible injury to cells, persistence or worsening of the shock state leads to irreversible injury and death of cells and sometimes, unhappily, the patient.

Shock is commonly divided into three major types[28] (Table 4-3).

- *Cardiogenic shock,* caused by failure of the myocardial pump due to intrinsic myocardial damage (myocardial infarction), arrhythmias, extrinsic pressure (cardiac tamponade), or outflow obstruction (pulmonary embolism)
- *Hypovolemic* or *hemorrhagic shock,* due to inadequate blood or plasma volume caused by hemorrhage, fluid loss from severe burns, or trauma (*traumatic shock*)
- *Septic shock,* caused by severe bacteremic infections, most commonly by gram-negative bacteria

(endotoxic shock) but also by gram-positive organisms and, occasionally, fungi

Rare types are *neurogenic shock,* due to anesthetic accidents or spinal cord injury and caused by massive peripheral vasodilatation, and *anaphylactic shock* (Chapter 6) initiated by generalized type I hypersensitivity reactions.

A review of the causes and types of shock (see Table 4-3) will indicate that the initiating mechanisms underlying cardiogenic and hypovolemic shock are fairly obvious. As might be expected, they are *associated with low cardiac output, hypotension, impaired tissue perfusion, and cellular hypoxia.* The hemodynamic and metabolic considerations of these types of shock are of great clinical significance but are beyond the scope of this book. Here we shall focus on the pathogenesis of septic shock.

Pathogenesis of Septic Shock

Septic shock is currently the most common cause of death in intensive care units, accounting for some 100,000 deaths annually in the United States.[29] It results from the spread of microbes from severe localized infections (e.g., abscess, peritonitis, pneumonia) into the bloodstream. The majority of cases are caused by endotoxin-producing gram-negative bacilli—*Escherichia coli, Klebsiella pneumoniae, Proteus* species, *Pseudomonas aeruginosa, Serratia,* and *Bacteroides*—hence the term *endotoxic shock.* Endotoxins are bacterial wall lipopolysaccharides (LPS), consisting of a toxic lipid A core component and a complex polysaccharide coat (see Chapter 8). Gram-positive cocci, such as pneumococci and streptococci, and certain fungi, as well as gram-positive bacterial toxins (such as the *toxic shock syndrome toxin 1*) produce a similar syndrome.

All of the hemodynamic and metabolic alterations of septic shock can be mimicked by injections of LPS. LPS forms a complex with an LPS binding protein in the serum, which in turn binds to CD14 receptors on leukocytes, endothelial cells, and other cell types. LPS is then thought to induce its effects in two ways: directly, by causing injury or altering the function of cells, but more importantly *indirectly,* by initiating the synthesis, release, or activation of a cascade of mediators derived from plasma or from cells (monocytes, macrophages, neutrophils, endothelial cells, and others)[30] (Fig. 4-27). These mediators, in turn, affect a number of organ systems, notably the following:

- the *heart,* causing myocardial dysfunction
- the *vascular system,* resulting in vasodilation and hypotension

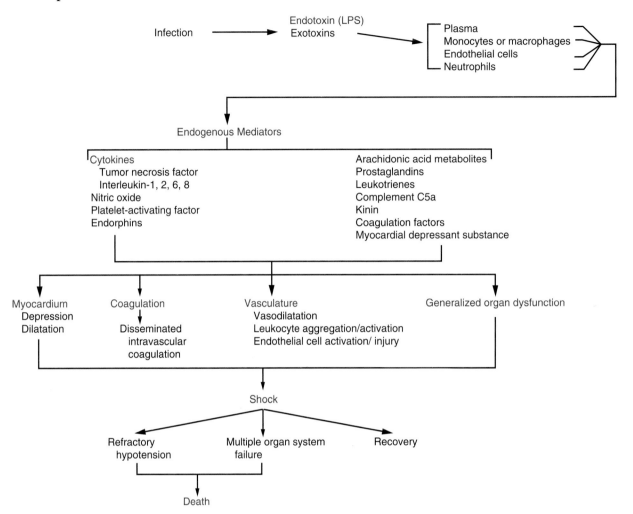

Figure 4–27. Pathogenetic sequence of events in septic shock. Although the mediators are listed in one category, TNF and IL-1 appear central, as they in turn induce other mediators, notably NO, PGs, and PAF. Organ failure occurs from direct effects of mediators or endotoxin and, secondarily, as a result of the anoxia induced by the DIC and vascular changes. (Adapted from Parrillo, J.E.: Pathogenetic mechanisms of septic shock. *The New England Journal of Medicine* 328:1472, 1993.)

- the *microcirculation,* leading to endothelial injury and activation as well as leukocyte aggregation and adhesion
- the *coagulation system,* culminating in disseminated intravascular coagulation
- the *lungs,* leading to the acute respiratory distress syndrome (ARDS)
- the *liver,* resulting in liver failure
- the *kidney,* causing acute renal failure
- the *central nervous system,* culminating in coma

The mediators that have been implicated in causing shock include the following. Most of these have been described in Chapter 3.

- Cytokines (IL-1, TNF, IL-6, IL-8)
- Platelet activating factor
- Nitric oxide
- Complement (C5a and C3a)
- Prostaglandins
- Leukotrienes
- The kinin system
- Oxygen metabolites
- Catecholamines
- Endorphins
- Myocardial depressant factor

The evidence implicating these mediators is more substantial for some than for others and, in many instances, is derived from animal studies whose relevance to humans remains uncertain. However, *it is clear that endotoxin-mediated activation of the mononuclear phagocyte system and the consequent release of IL-1 and TNF-α is a key event in the pathogenesis of septic shock.*[31] These cytokines, as we have seen, *cause endothelial activation and leukocyte adhesion and aggregation, and promote intravascular coagulation and capillary thrombosis. They also signal secondary mediators, including prostaglandins, platelet-activating factor, and*

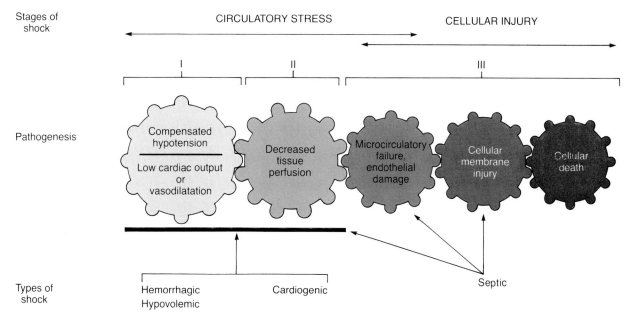

Figure 4–28. Pathogenesis and stages of shock. Stage I is nonprogressive, stage II is progressive, and stage III is irreversible. Note that endotoxic shock is multifactorial; it is associated with vasodilatation, decreased tissue perfusion, endothelial damage, and direct cellular injury. (Modified from Wyngaarden, J.B., and Smith, L.H., Jr.: Cecil Textbook of Medicine, 17th ed. Philadelphia, W.B. Saunders Co., 1985, p. 212.)

nitric oxide.[32] The latter, in turn, cause vasodilatation and other proinflammatory effects. Indeed, most of the metabolic and hemodynamic effects of endotoxins can be mimicked by the infusion of IL-1 or TNF-α or, more profoundly, by combinations of these cytokines in laboratory animals. Conversely, antibodies directed against TNF, or IL-1 receptor antagonists, or deficiency of TNF receptors,[33] protect against septic shock in animals and humans. Similarly, suppression of the mediators induced by these cytokines (i.e., nitric oxide) ameliorates the hemodynamic complications of septic shock in some experimental models.[34]

In addition to causing the release of biologically active mediators, bacterial toxins also cause direct injury to cells and tissues. Thus, even the cells that are well perfused fail to extract adequate oxygen from the blood. This results in the subnormal arteriovenous oxygen difference often noted in septic shock.

Stages of Shock. Shock is a progressive disorder that, if uncorrected, may lead to death. Unless the insult is massive and rapidly lethal (e.g., a massive hemorrhage from a ruptured aortic aneurysm or an extensive infarct affecting the left ventricle), shock tends to evolve through three stages (Fig. 4–28): (1) an initial *nonprogressive phase* during which reflex compensatory mechanisms are activated and perfusion of vital organs is preserved; (2) a *progressive stage* characterized by tissue hypoperfusion and onset of an ever-widening circle of circulatory and metabolic imbalances; and finally (3) an *irreversible stage* that sets in after the body has incurred cellular and tissue injury so severe that

even if therapy corrects the hemodynamic defects survival is not possible. Admittedly, these stages are somewhat arbitrary, but a brief discussion of this sequence will serve to integrate the sequential pathophysiologic and clinical alterations in shock.

During "early shock" (say, following blood loss), a *variety of neurohumoral mechanisms come into play to maintain cardiac output and blood pressure.* These include the baroreceptor reflexes, release of catecholamines, activation of the renin-angiotensin axis, antidiuretic hormone release, and generalized sympathetic stimulation. The effect of all these is to produce *tachycardia, peripheral vasoconstriction, and conservation of fluid by the kidney.* The vasoconstrictor response is responsible for the coolness and pallor of skin seen in cardiac and hypovolemic shock. Since the coronary and cerebral vessels are less affected by the sympathetic response, oxygen continues to be delivered to these vital organs. Obviously, therapeutic maneuvers have the best chance of success at this stage. Uncorrected, shock passes imperceptibly to the progressive phase, during which the vital organs begin to experience significant hypoxia. With persistent oxygen deficit there is impairment of intracellular aerobic respiration, followed by anaerobic glycolysis and excessive production of lactate, which often induces metabolic *lactic acidosis.* The lowering of pH in the tissues obtunds the vasomotor response; arterioles dilate and blood begins to pool in the microcirculation. Peripheral pooling not only worsens the cardiac output but also favors anoxic injury to endothelial cells, thereby setting the stage for DIC. With widespread tissue hypoxia, the function of vital organs begins to deteriorate; often *the patient is confused and the urinary output begins to fall.*

At some point in the downward spiral there is a transition from the reversible to the irreversible stage. Widespread cell injury allows leakage of lysosomal enzymes, which further aggravate the shock state. A *myocardial depressant factor, still currently not well characterized,* worsens the already poor cardiac performance. Endotoxic shock may be superimposed on hypovolemic or cardiogenic shock if the ischemic intestinal mucosa allows intestinal flora to enter the circulation. By this stage *the patient has complete renal shutdown due to acute tubular necrosis.* In closing, one may ask, When does shock become irreversible? Some would argue that if the initiating cause is removed, shock is reversible at any stage. The issue is moot, but one fact is not: death from shock, despite the heroic measures afforded by modern intensive care units, is still an everyday happening.

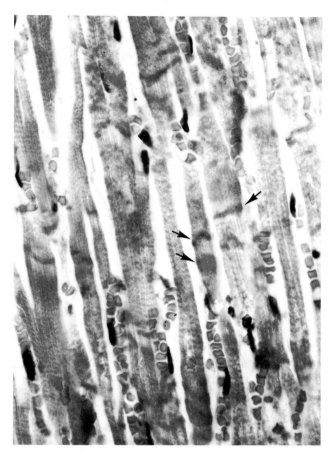

Figure 4–29. Contraction bands *(arrows)* in a heart suffering from hypoperfusion. The heavy bands should not be confused with the more delicate cross striations of cardiac myocytes.

MORPHOLOGY. Shock is characterized by **hypoxic failure of multiple organ systems,** and hence the cellular changes may appear in any tissue. They are particularly evident in the brain, heart, lungs, kidneys, adrenals, and gastrointestinal tract.

The **brain** may develop so-called ischemic encephalopathy, discussed in Chapter 29. The **heart** may undergo a variety of changes. Subendocardial hemorrhages and necrosis, or "zonal lesions," sometimes appear in all forms of shock. The term zonal lesions refers to apparent hypercontraction of a myocyte, inducing shortening and scalloping of the sarcomere, fragmentation of the Z band, distortion of the myofilaments, and displacement of the mitochondria away from the intercalated disc (Fig. 4–29). Subendocardial hemorrhages and zonal lesions are not diagnostic of shock and may be seen following administration of catecholamines or after prolonged use of the heart-lung bypass pump in cardiac surgery. The **kidneys** may be severely affected in shock, and so oliguria, anuria, and electrolyte disturbances constitute major clinical problems. The renal changes are referred to as **acute tubular necrosis,** discussed in Chapter 20. The **lungs** are seldom affected in pure hypovolemic shock because they are resistant to hypoxic injury, but when the vascular collapse is caused by bacterial sepsis or trauma, changes may appear that are referred to as "shock lung." They are referred to as the acute respiratory distress syndrome (see Chapter 15).

The **adrenal** alterations encountered in shock comprise in essence those common to all forms of stress and so might be referred to as **"the stress response."** Early there is focal depletion of lipids in the cortical cells beginning in the zona reticularis and then spreading progressively outward into the zona fasciculata. This loss of corticolipids implies not adrenal exhaustion but rather reversion of the relatively inactive vacuolated cells to metabolically active cells that utilize stored lipids for the synthesis of steroids. The **gastrointestinal tract** may suffer patchy mucosal hemorrhages and necroses, referred to as "hemorrhagic enteropathy." The **liver** may sometimes develop fatty change and, with severe perfusion deficits, central hemorrhagic necrosis (see Chapter 18).

Virtually all of these organ changes may revert to normal if the patient survives. However, loss of neurons from the brain and of myocytes from the heart is, of course, irreversible. However, most patients who suffer shock so severe as to produce irreversible changes succumb before these alterations become well developed.

CLINICAL COURSE. The clinical manifestations depend on the precipitating insult. In hypovolemic and cardiogenic shock, *the patient presents with hypotension; an ashen-gray pallor; cool, clammy skin; weak, thready pulse; and rapid cardiac and respiratory rates. With uncontrolled sepsis, however, the skin may be warm and indeed flushed owing to peripheral vasodilation.* The course of the patient in shock is beset with a sequence of hazards and pitfalls. The initial threat to life stems from the underlying catastrophe that precipitated the shock, such as the myocardial infarct, severe hemorrhage, or uncontrolled bacterial infection. However, the cardiac, cerebral, and pulmonary changes secondary to the shock state materially worsen the problem. Soon electrolyte disturbances and metabolic acidosis make their unwanted contributions. If all of these grave problems are survived, *the patient enters a second phase dominated by renal insufficiency,* as is detailed in Chapter 20. This may appear any time from the second to the sixth day and is marked by a progressive fall in urine output.

It is evident that the postshock course of the patient does not lack for threats to life. The prognosis varies with the origin of shock and its duration. For example, 80% of young, otherwise healthy patients with hypovolemic shock survive with appropriate management, whereas cardiogenic shock associated with extensive myocardial infarction, and gram-negative shock carry a mortality rate of 70 to 80%, even with the best care currently available.

1. Braunwald, E. Pathophysiology of heart failure. *In* Braunwald, E. (ed.): Heart Disease: A Textbook of Cardiovascular Medicine, 4th ed. Philadelphia, W.B. Saunders Co., 1992, pp. 393–418.
2. Marcus, A.J., and Safier, L.B.: Thromboregulation: Multicellular modulation of platelet reactivity in hemostasis and thrombosis. FASEB J. 7:516, 1993.
3. Handin, R.I., and Loscalzo, J.: Hemostasis, thrombosis, fibrinolysis, and cardiovascular disease. *In* Braunwald, E. (ed.): Heart Disease: A Textbook of Cardiovascular Medicine, 4th ed. Philadelphia, W.B. Saunders Co., 1992, pp. 1767–1789.
4. Ware, J.A., and Heistad, D.A.: Platelet-endothelium interactions. N. Engl. J. Med. 328:628, 1993.
5. Gimbrone, M.A., Jr. (ed.): Vascular Endothelium in Hemostasis and Thrombosis. Edinburgh, Churchill Livingstone, 1987.
6. Pober, J.S., and Cotran, R.S.: Cytokines and endothelial cell biology. Physiol. Rev. 70:427, 1990.
7. Hibbs, J.B., et al.: Evidence for cytokine-induced nitric oxide synthesis from L-arginine. J. Clin. Invest. 89:867, 1992.
8. Pratt, C.N., and Church, F.C.: Antithrombin: Structure and function. Semin. Hematol. 28:3, 1991.
9. Esmon, C.T.: The protein C anticoagulant pathway. Arterioscler. Thromb. 12:135, 1992.
10. Benedict, C.R., et al.: Thrombolytic therapy: A state-of-the-art review. Hosp. Pract. 27:6, 1992.
11. Scharfstein, J., and Loscalzo, J.: Molecular approaches to antithrombotic therapy. Hosp. Pract. 27:43, 1992.
12. Esmon, C.T.: Cell-mediated events that control blood coagulation and vascular injury. Annu. Rev. Cell Biol. 9:1, 1993.
13. Furie, B., and Furie, B.C.: The molecular basis of blood coagulation. Cell 53:506, 1988.
14. Furie, B., and Furie, B.C.: Molecular and cellular biology of blood coagulation. N. Engl. J. Med. 326:800, 1992.
15. Collen, D., and Lijuen, H.R.: Basic and clinical aspects of fibrinolysis and thrombolysis. Blood 78:3114, 1991.
16. Davies, P.F., and Tripathi, S.: Mechanical stress mechanisms in cells: An endothelial paradigm. Circ. Res. 72:239, 1993.
17. Schaffer, A.I.: Pathophysiology of thrombosis. *In* Loscalzo, J., et al. (eds.): Vascular Medicine, 1st ed. Boston, Little, Brown & Co., 1992, pp. 307–333.
18. Miletich, J.P.: Inherited predisposition to thrombosis. Cell 72:477, 1993.
19. Eisenberg, G.M.: The antiphospholipid syndrome. Hosp. Pract. 27:119, 1992.
20. Hirsh, J., et al.: Evolution of thrombosis. Ann. NY Acad. Sci. 516:586, 1987.
21. Moser, K.M.: Venous thromboembolism. Am. Rev. Respir. Dis. 141:235, 1990.
22. Moake, J.L. Hypercoagulable states. Adv. Intern. Med. 35:235, 1990.
23. Freiman, D.C., et al.: Frequency of pulmonary embolism in man. N. Engl. J. Med. 27:1278, 1965.
24. England, R., and Magee, H.R.: Peripheral arterial embolism. Aust. N.Z. J. Surg. 57:27, 1987.
25. Price, T.M., et al.: Amniotic fluid embolism: Three case reports with a review of the literature. Obstet. Gynecol. Surv. 40:462, 1985.
26. Gregg, P.J., and Walder, D.N.: Caisson disease of bone. Clin. Orthop. 210:43, 1986.
27. Van Besouw, J.P., and Hinds, C.J.: Fat embolism syndrome. Br. J. Hosp. Med. 42:304, 1989.
28. Weil, M., et al.: Acute circulatory collapse (shock). *In* Braunwald, E. (ed.): Heart Disease: A Textbook of Cardiovascular Medicine, 4th ed. Philadelphia, W.B. Saunders Co., 1992, pp. 569–587.
29. Parrillo, J.E. (moderator): NIH Conference: Septic shock in humans. Ann. Intern. Med. 113:227, 1990.
30. Parrillo, J.E.: Pathogenetic mechanisms of septic shock. N. Engl. J. Med. 328:1471, 1993.
31. Tracey, K.J., and Cerami, A.: Tumor necrosis factor (cachectin) in septic endotoxic shock. *In* Neugebauer, E.A., and Holoday, J.W. (eds.): Handbook of Mediators of Septic Shock. Boca Raton, FL, CRC Press, 1993, pp. 291–308.
32. Dinarello, C.A., and Wolff, S.M.: The role of IL-1 in disease. N. Engl. J. Med. 328:14, 1993.
33. Pfeffer, K., et al.: Mice deficient for the 55-kd TNF receptor are resistant to endotoxic shock. Cell 73:457, 1993.
34. Petros, A., et al.: Effect of nitric oxide synthase inhibitors in hypotension in patients with septic shock. Lancet 338:1557, 1991.
35. Johnston, J.: Molecular science gets its signs on septic shock. J. NIH Res. 3:61, 1991.

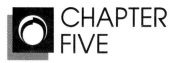

CHAPTER FIVE

Genetic Disorders

NEW GENETICS

Until the recent past, medical genetics was viewed as an obscure subject concerned primarily with the study of rare syndromes and disorders. Since the 1980s, however, progress in molecular genetics has literally revolutionized the study of medicine. The "new genetics" has provided penetrating insights into common diseases, such as cancer, diabetes, and atherosclerosis. Indeed, Victor McKusick, the dean of medical geneticists, has said, "Genetics is to biology what atomic theory is to physical sciences."

Much of the recent progress in medical genetics has resulted from the spectacular advances in molecular biology, involving recombinant DNA technology.[1] The details of these techniques are well known and are not repeated here. Some examples, however, of the impact of recombinant DNA technology on medicine are worthy of attention.

- *Molecular basis of human disease.* Two general strategies have been used to isolate and charac-

terize involved genes (Fig. 5–1). The "classic" approach has been successfully utilized to study a variety of inborn errors of metabolism, such as phenylketonuria and disorders of hemoglobin synthesis. Common to these genetic diseases is a knowledge of the abnormal gene product and the corresponding protein. When the affected protein is known, a variety of methods can be employed to isolate the normal gene, clone it, and ultimately determine the molecular changes that affect the gene in patients with the disorder. Because in many common single-gene disorders, such as cystic fibrosis, there was no clue to the nature of the defective gene product, an alternative strategy called "reverse genetics," or "positional cloning," had to be employed. This approach initially ignores the biochemical clues from the phenotype and relies instead on the chromosomal localization of the mutant gene. The approximate location of the gene is determined by linkage to known "marker genes" that are in close proximity to the disease locus. Once the region in which the mutant gene lies has been localized within reasonably narrow limits,

123

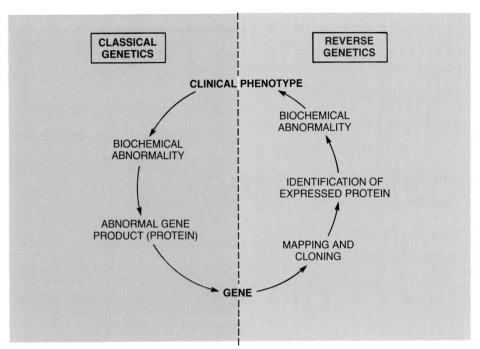

Figure 5–1. Schematic illustration of the strategies employed in classic and reverse genetics. The classic approach begins with relating the clinical phenotype to biochemical-protein abnormalities, followed by isolating the mutant gene. The reverse genetic strategy begins by mapping and cloning the disease gene without any knowledge of the gene product. Identification of the gene product and the mechanism by which it produces the disease follows the isolation of the mutant gene.

the next step is to clone several pieces of DNA from the relevant segment of the genome (positional cloning). Expression of the cloned DNA *in vitro*, followed by identification of the protein products, can then be used to identify the aberrant protein encoded by the mutant genes. This approach has been used successfully in several diseases, such as cystic fibrosis, neurofibromatosis, Duchenne muscular dystrophy (a hereditary disorder characterized by progressive muscle weakness), and most recently Huntington's disease.[2]

Another powerful tool for studying the molecular pathogenesis of human diseases—both genetic and acquired—involves insertion of molecularly cloned human DNA into the germ line of mice. Using appropriate gene constructs, it is possible, in such transgenic mice, to target the expression of the introduced gene in specific tissues such as the beta cells of the pancreatic islets. Transgenic mice are proving to be extremely useful in the study of diseases as diverse as viral hepatitis, diabetes mellitus, and neoplasia.

Refinements in transgenic technology have made it possible to "knock out" the functioning of specific mouse genes. The production of genetic knockouts involves constructing a disrupted gene, which is transfected into embryonic stem (ES) cells *in vitro*. With appropriate breeding, the mutant gene can be transmitted through the germ line, and mice homozygous for the knockout gene are bred. Study of such mutant mice has provided many surprises. In some instances, for example in mice with homozygous loss of the cystic fibrosis gene, the effects are milder than

expected, and in other cases, such as the *src* gene knockouts, the phenotype is different from that expected. The murine models suggest that, on the one hand, evolution may have "padded" animals with several backups to compensate for gene loss, and, on the other hand, researchers may have previously missed some important functions of genes.[3]

- *Production of human biologically active agents.* An array of ultrapure biologically active agents can now be produced in virtually unlimited quantities by inserting the requisite gene into bacteria or other suitable cells in tissue culture. Some examples of genetically engineered products already in clinical use include tissue plasminogen activator (tPA) for the treatment of thrombotic states, growth hormone for the treatment of deficiency states, erythropoietin to reverse the anemia of renal disease, and myeloid growth and differentiation factors (GM-CSF, G-CSF) to enhance production of monocytes and neutrophils in states of poor marrow function.

- *Gene therapy.* The goal of treating genetic diseases by transfer of somatic cells transfected with the normal gene, although not yet attained, is tantalizingly close. Much interest is focused on transplantation of patients' hematopoietic stem cells that have been transfected with the cloned normal gene. The first attempts at human gene therapy have been undertaken in patients with immunodeficiency resulting from a lack of the enzyme adenosine deaminase (ADA). It is expected that the expression of the transferred ADA gene in the marrow cells will restore enzyme levels *in vivo*, thereby reversing the state of immunoincompetence that characterizes ADA-deficient patients. In another strategy, being tested in patients with cystic fibrosis, the normal gene is delivered to the somatic cells by way of a harmless viral vector.

• *Disease diagnosis.* Molecular probes are proving to be extremely useful in the diagnosis of both genetic and nongenetic (e.g., infectious) diseases. The diagnostic applications of recombinant DNA technology are detailed at the end of this chapter.

With this background of "new genetics," we can turn next to the time-honored classification of human diseases into three categories: (1) those environmentally determined, (2) those genetically determined, and (3) those in which both environmental and genetic factors play a role. Microbiologic infections at first sight might appear to be representative of the first category; however, even here, with the expansion of knowledge about the role of immune response genes in the control of immunocompetence, it is evident that microbiologic infections—and all disorders to a greater or lesser degree—are conditioned by the genotype. Into the third category just mentioned fall many of the important diseases of humans, such as peptic ulcer, diabetes mellitus, atherosclerosis, schizophrenia, and probably most cancers, in which clearly both nature and nurture play significant roles.

With recognition of the complexity of this nature-nurture interplay, our interest here is with those diseases in which nature (i.e., the genetic component) plays a major if not determinant role. The genetic diseases encountered in medical practice represent only the tip of the iceberg, that is, those with less extreme genotypic errors permitting full embryonic development and live birth. It is estimated that 50% of spontaneous abortuses during the early months of gestation have a demonstrable chromosomal abnormality; there are in addition numerous smaller detectable errors and many others still beyond our range of identification. About 1% of all newborn infants possess a gross chromosomal abnormality, and approximately 5% of individuals under the age of 25 years develop a serious disease with a significant genetic component.[4] How many more mutations remain hidden?

It is beyond the scope of this book to review normal human genetics. It is necessary, however, to clarify several commonly used terms— *hereditary, familial,* and *congenital.* Hereditary disorders, by definition, are derived from one's parents and are transmitted in the germ line through the generations and therefore are familial. The term *congenital* simply implies "born with." Some congenital diseases are not genetic, as for example congenital syphilis. Not all genetic diseases are congenital; patients with hereditary Huntington's disease, for example, begin to manifest their condition only after the third or fourth decade of life.

MUTATIONS

A mutation may be defined as a permanent change in the DNA. Mutations that affect the germ cells are transmitted to the progeny and may give rise to inherited diseases. Mutations that arise in somatic cells understandably do not cause hereditary diseases but are important in the genesis of cancers and some congenital malformations.

Based on the extent of genetic change, mutations may be classified into three categories.[5] *Ge-*

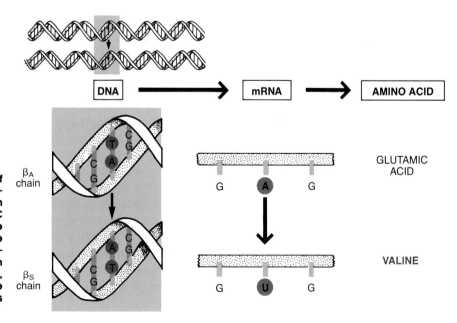

Figure 5-2. Schematic illustration of a point mutation resulting from a single base pair change in the DNA. In the example shown, a CTC to CAC change alters the meaning of the genetic code (GAG to GUG in the opposite strand), leading to replacement of glutamic acid by valine in the polypeptide chain. This change, affecting the sixth amino acid of the normal β-globin ($β_A$) chain, converts it to sickle β-globin ($β_S$).

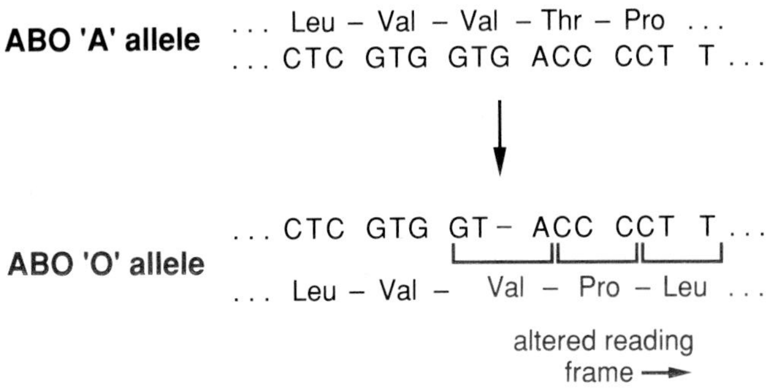

ABO 'A' allele

```
...  Leu – Val – Val – Thr – Pro  ...
...  CTC GTG GTG ACC CCT T ...
```

ABO 'O' allele

```
...  CTC GTG GT– ACC CCT T ...
...  Leu – Val –  Val – Pro – Leu  ...
               altered reading
                   frame →
```

Figure 5–3. Single-base deletion at the ABO (glycosyltransferase) locus, leading to a frameshift mutation responsible for the O allele. (With permission from Thompson, M.W., McInnes, R.R., and Willard, H.F.: Thompson and Thompson Genetics in Medicine, 5th ed. Philadelphia, W.B. Saunders Co., 1991, p. 134.)

nome mutations involve loss or gain of whole chromosomes, giving rise to monosomy or trisomy. *Chromosome mutations* result from rearrangement of genetic material and give rise to visible structural changes in the chromosome. Mutations involving changes in the number or structure of chromosomes are transmitted only infrequently because most are incompatible with survival. The vast majority of mutations associated with hereditary diseases are submicroscopic *gene mutations*. These may result in partial or complete deletion of a gene or more often affect a single base. For example, a single nucleotide base may be *substituted* by a different base, resulting in a *point mutation* (Fig. 5–2). Less commonly, one or two base pairs may be *inserted* into or *deleted* from the DNA, leading to alterations in the reading frame of the DNA strand; hence these are referred to as *frameshift* mutations (Figs. 5–3 and 5–4). The consequences of mutations are varied, depending on several factors, including the type of mutation and the genomic site affected by it. Details of specific mutations and their effects are discussed along with the relevant disorders throughout this text. Here we briefly review some general principles relating to the effects of gene mutations.

• *Point mutations within coding sequences.* A point mutation (single base substitution) may alter the code in a triplet of bases and lead to the replacement of one amino acid by another in the gene product. Because these mutations alter the meaning of the genetic code, they are often termed "missense mutations." An excellent ex-

ample of this type is the sickle mutation affecting the beta-globin chain of hemoglobin (see Chapter 13). Here the nucleotide triplet CTC (or GAG in messenger RNA [mRNA]), which codes for glutamic acid, is changed to CAC (or GUG in mRNA), which codes for valine (see Fig. 5–2). This single amino acid substitution alters the physicochemical properties of hemoglobin, giving rise to sickle cell anemia. Besides producing an amino acid substitution, a point mutation may change an amino acid codon to a chain terminator or *stop codon* ("nonsense mutation"). Taking again the example of β-globin, a point mutation affecting the codon for glutamine (CAG) creates a stop codon (UAG) if U is substituted for C (Fig. 5–5). This change leads to premature termination of β-globin gene translation, and the resulting short peptide is rapidly degraded. The affected individuals lack β-globin chains and develop a severe form of anemia called β^0 thalassemia (see Chapter 13).

• *Mutations within noncoding sequences.* Deleterious effects may also result from mutations that do not involve the exons. As is well known, transcription of DNA is initiated and regulated by promoter and enhancer sequences that are found downstream or upstream of the gene. Point mutations or deletions involving these regulatory sequences may interfere with binding of transcription factors and thus lead to a marked reduction in or total lack of transcription. Such is the case in certain forms of hereditary hemolytic anemias. In addition, point mutations within introns lead to defective splicing of intervening se-

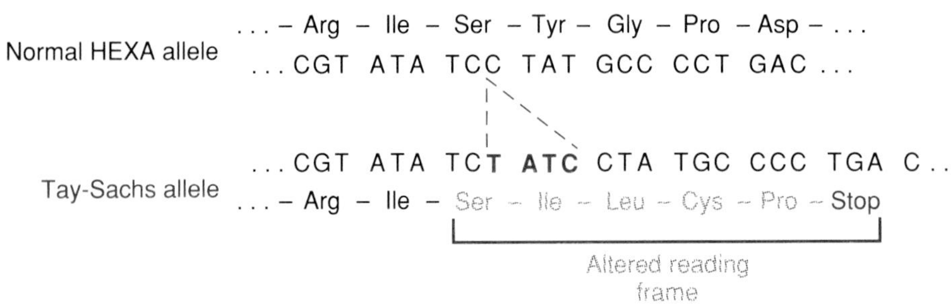

Normal HEXA allele

```
...  – Arg – Ile – Ser – Tyr – Gly – Pro – Asp – ...
...  CGT ATA TCC TAT GCC CCT GAC ...
```

Tay-Sachs allele

```
...  CGT ATA TCT ATC CTA TGC CCC TGA C ...
...  – Arg – Ile – Ser – Ile – Leu – Cys – Pro – Stop
                  Altered reading
                      frame
```

Figure 5–4. Four-base insertion in the hexosaminidase A gene in Tay-Sachs disease, leading to a frameshift mutation. This mutation is the major cause of Tay-Sachs disease in Ashkenazi Jews. (With permission from Thompson, M.W., McInnes, R.R., and Willard, H.F.: Thompson and Thompson Genetics in Medicine, 5th ed. Philadelphia, W.B. Saunders Co., 1991, p. 135.)

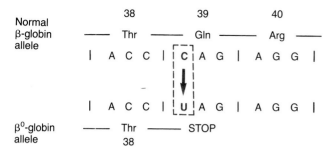

Figure 5–5. Point mutation leading to premature chain termination. Partial mRNA sequence of the β-globin chain of hemoglobin showing codons for amino acids 38 to 40. A point mutation (C → U) in codon 39 changes glutamine (Gln) codon to a stop codon, and hence protein synthesis stops at the 38th amino acid.

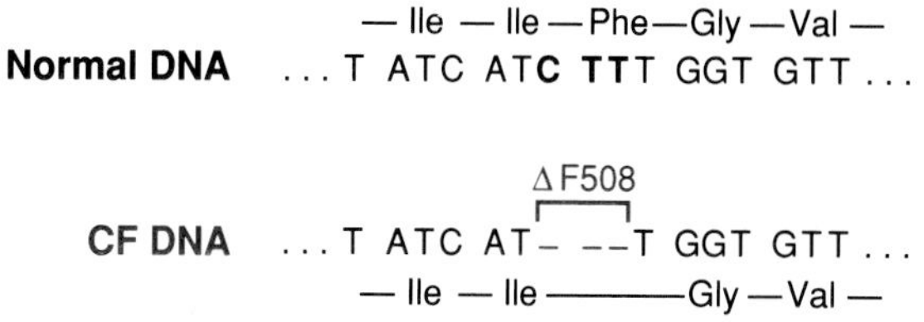

Normal DNA   — Ile — Ile —Phe—Gly —Val —
...T ATC ATC TTT GGT GTT...

ΔF508
CF DNA   ...T ATC AT— ——T GGT GTT...
— Ile — Ile ————Gly —Val —

Figure 5–6. Three-base deletion in the common cystic fibrosis (CF) allele results in synthesis of a protein that is missing amino acid 508 (phenylalanine). Because the deletion is a multiple of three, this is not a frameshift mutation. (With permission from Thompson, M.W., McInnes, R.R., and Willard, H.F.: Thompson and Thompson Genetics in Medicine, 5th ed. Philadelphia, W.B. Saunders Co., 1991, p. 135.)

quences. This, in turn, interferes with normal processing of the initial mRNA transcripts and results in a failure to form mature mRNA transcripts. Therefore, translation cannot take place, and the gene product is not synthesized.

- *Deletions and insertions.* Small deletions or insertions involving the coding sequence lead to alterations in the reading frame of the DNA strand; hence they are referred to as frameshift mutations (see Figs. 5–3 and 5–4). If the number of base pairs involved is three or a multiple of three, frameshift does not occur (Fig. 5–6); instead, an abnormal protein missing one or more amino acids is synthesized.

To summarize, mutations can interfere with protein synthesis at various levels. Transcription may be suppressed with gene deletions and point mutations involving promoter sequences. Abnormal mRNA processing may result from mutations affecting introns or splice junctions, or both. Translation is affected if a stop codon (chain termination mutation) is created within an exon. Finally, some point mutations may lead to the formation of an abnormal protein without impairing any step in protein synthesis.

Mutations occur spontaneously during the process of DNA replication. Certain environmental influences, such as radiation, chemicals, and viruses, increase the rate of so-called spontaneous mutations. Because the mutagenic potential of environmental agents is linked to their role in carcinogenesis, they are discussed later, in Chapter 7.

Against this background, we can now turn our attention to the major categories of genetic disorders. Traditionally, genetic disorders are classified into three categories: (1) those related to mutant genes of large effect, (2) diseases with multifactorial (polygenic) inheritance, and (3) chromosomal disorders. The first category includes many relatively uncommon conditions, such as storage disorders and inborn errors of metabolism, all resulting from single-gene mutations of large effect. Because most of these follow the classic mendelian patterns

of inheritance, they are also referred to as mendelian disorders. The second category includes some of the most common diseases of humans, such as hypertension and diabetes mellitus. They are called multifactorial because they are influenced by both genetic and environmental factors. The genetic component involves the additive result of multiple genes of small effect; the environmental contribution may be small or large, and in some cases, it is required for the expression of disease. The third category includes diseases that result from genomic or chromosomal mutations and are therefore associated with numerical or structural changes in chromosomes. To these three well-known categories must be added a heterogeneous group of *single-gene disorders with nonclassic patterns of inheritance.* This group includes disorders resulting from triplet repeat mutations, those arising from mutations in mitochondrial DNA, and those in which the transmission is influenced by *genomic imprinting.*

MENDELIAN DISORDERS

All mendelian disorders are the result of expressed mutations in single genes of large effect. It is not necessary to detail Mendel's laws here, as every student in biology, and possibly every garden pea, has learned about them at an early age. Only some comments of medical relevance are made.

The number of mendelian disorders known has grown to monumental proportions. In a recent edition of his book, McKusick has listed more than 4500 disorders.[6] It is estimated that every individual is a carrier of five to eight deleterious genes. Fortunately, most of these are recessive and therefore do not have serious phenotypic effects. About 80 to 85% of these mutations are familial. The remainder represent new mutations acquired *de novo* by an affected individual.

Some autosomal mutations produce partial expression in the heterozygote and full expression in the homozygote. Sickle cell anemia is caused by substitution of normal hemoglobin (HbA) by hemoglobin S (HbS). When an individual is homozygous for the mutant gene, all the hemoglobin is of the abnormal HbS type, and even under normal atmospheric pressures of oxygen, the disorder is fully expressed, i.e., sickling deformity of all red cells and hemolytic anemia. In the heterozygote, only a proportion of the hemoglobin is HbS (the remainder being HbA), and therefore red cell sickling and possibly hemolysis occur only when there is exposure to lowered oxygen tension. This is referred to as the sickle cell trait to differentiate it from full-blown sickle cell anemia.

Although gene expression is usually described as dominant or recessive, in some cases, both alleles of a gene pair may be fully expressed in the heterozygote—a condition called *codominance.* Histocompatibility and blood group antigens are good examples of codominant inheritance.

A single mutant gene may lead to many end effects, termed *pleiotropism,* and conversely mutations at several genetic loci may produce the same trait *(genetic heterogeneity).* Sickle cell anemia may serve as an example of pleiotropism. In this hereditary disorder, not only does the point mutation in the gene give rise to HbS, which predisposes the red cells to hemolysis, but also the abnormal red cells tend to cause a logjam in small vessels, inducing, for example, splenic fibrosis, organ infarcts, and bone changes. The numerous differing end-organ derangements all are related to the primary defect in hemoglobin synthesis. On the other hand, profound childhood deafness, an apparently homogeneous clinical entity, results from any of 16 different types of autosomal recessive mutations. Recognition of genetic heterogeneity not only is important in genetic counseling but also is relevant in the understanding of the pathogenesis of some common disorders, such as diabetes mellitus.

TRANSMISSION PATTERNS OF SINGLE-GENE DISORDERS

Mutations involving single genes typically follow one of three patterns of inheritance: autosomal dominant, autosomal recessive, and X-linked. The general rules that govern the transmission of single-gene disorders are well known and will not be repeated here. Only a few salient features are summarized below. Single-gene disorders with non-classic patterns of inheritance are described later.

Autosomal Dominant Disorders

Autosomal dominant disorders are manifested in the heterozygous state, so at least one parent of an index case is usually affected; both males and fe-

males are affected, and both can transmit the condition. When an affected person marries an unaffected one, every child has one chance in two of having the disease. In addition to these basic rules, autosomal dominant conditions are characterized by the following.

- With every autosomal dominant disorder, some patients do not have affected parents. Such patients owe their disorder to new mutations involving either the egg or the sperm from which they were derived. Their siblings are neither affected nor at increased risk for developing the disease. The proportion of patients who develop the disease as a result of a new mutation is related to the effect of the disease on reproductive capability. If a disease markedly reduces reproductive fitness, most cases would be expected to result from new mutations. Many new mutations seem to occur in germ cells of relatively older fathers.

- Clinical features can be modified by reduced penetrance and variable expressivity. Some individuals inherit the mutant gene but are phenotypically normal. This is referred to as *reduced penetrance.* Penetrance is expressed in mathematical terms: Thus 50% penetrance indicates that 50% of those who carry the gene express the trait. The factors that affect penetrance are not clearly understood, but this phenomenon is clearly important for genetic counseling because such phenotypically normal persons can transmit the disease and so belong to a skipped generation. In contrast to penetrance, if a trait is seen in all individuals carrying the mutant gene but is expressed differently among individuals, the phenomenon is called *variable expressivity.* For example, manifestations of neurofibromatosis range from brownish spots on the skin to multiple skin tumors and skeletal deformities.

- In many conditions, the age at onset is delayed: symptoms and signs do not appear until adulthood (as in Huntington's disease).

Two major categories of nonenzyme proteins are usually affected in autosomal dominant disorders: (1) those involved in regulation of complex metabolic pathways, often subject to feedback control (e.g., membrane receptors and transport proteins), and (2) key structural proteins, such as collagen and cytoskeletal components of the red cell membrane (e.g., spectrin). Because up to a 50% loss of enzyme activity can usually be compensated for, mutations of genes that encode enzyme proteins do not usually manifest in an autosomal dominant pattern of inheritance. The mechanisms by which loss of one normal allele gives rise to severe phenotypic effects are not fully understood. In some instances, especially when the gene encodes one subunit of a multimeric protein such as collagen, the product of the mutant allele can interfere

Table 5-1. AUTOSOMAL DOMINANT DISORDERS

SYSTEM	DISORDER
Nervous	Huntington's disease Neurofibromatosis Myotonic dystrophy Tuberous sclerosis
Urinary	Polycystic kidney disease
Gastrointestinal	Familial polyposis coli
Hematopoietic	Hereditary spherocytosis von Willebrand disease
Skeletal	Marfan syndrome* Ehler-Danlos syndrome (some variants)* Osteogenesis imperfecta Achondroplasia
Metabolic	Familial hypercholesterolemia* Acute intermittent porphyria

* Discussed in this chapter. Other disorders listed are discussed in appropriate chapters of this book.

with the function of the normal protein. This is exemplified by the type II variant of osteogenesis imperfecta (see Chapter 27). In this autosomal dominant disorder, there is a missense mutation in the gene that encodes the $\alpha 1$ chain of type I collagen. As expected, 50% of the $\alpha 1$ chains are abnormal in heterozygotes. Because each collagen molecule is a helical trimer composed of two $\alpha 1$ chains and one $\alpha 2$ chain, random association of the normal and mutant $\alpha 1$ chains with normal $\alpha 2$ chains yields three types of type I collagen molecules: (1) normal, i.e., with no mutant $\alpha 1$ chains; (2) with one mutant $\alpha 1$ chain; and (3) with two mutant $\alpha 1$ chains. These three forms occur in the ratio of $1:2:1$. Thus, 75% of all collagen triple helices are abnormal. These trimers assemble poorly and are degraded prematurely ("protein suicide"). The net result is a marked deficiency of collagen and severe skeletal abnormalities. In this instance, the mutant allele is called "dominant negative" because it impairs the function of the normal alleles.

Table 5-1 provides a listing of the more common autosomal dominant disorders. Many are discussed more logically in other chapters. A few conditions not considered elsewhere are discussed later in this chapter as examples of important genetic principles.

Autosomal Recessive Disorders

Autosomal recessive inheritance is the single largest category of mendelian disorders. Because autosomal recessive disorders result only when both alleles at a given gene locus are mutants, such disorders are characterized by the following features: (1) The trait does not usually affect the parents, but siblings may show the disease; (2) siblings have one chance in four of being affected (i.e.,

the recurrence risk is 25% for each birth); (3) if the mutant gene occurs with a low frequency in the population, there is a strong likelihood that the proband is the product of a consanguineous marriage. In contrast to those of autosomal dominant diseases, the following features generally apply to most autosomal recessive disorders.

- The expression of the defect tends to be more uniform than in autosomal dominant disorders.
- Complete penetrance is common.
- Onset is frequently early in life.
- Although new mutations for recessive disorders do occur, they are rarely detected clinically. Since the individual with a new mutation is an asymptomatic heterozygote, several generations may pass before the descendants of such a person mate with heterozygotes and produce affected offspring.
- In many cases, enzyme proteins are affected by the mutation. In heterozygotes, equal amounts of normal and defective enzyme are synthesized. Usually the natural "margin of safety" ensures that cells with half their usual complement of the enzyme function normally.

Autosomal recessive disorders include almost all inborn errors of metabolism. The various consequences of enzyme deficiencies are discussed later. The more common of these conditions are listed in Table 5-2. Most are presented elsewhere; a few prototypes will be discussed later in this chapter.

X-Linked Disorders

All sex-linked disorders are X-linked, almost all X-linked recessive. The only gene assigned with cer-

Table 5-2. AUTOSOMAL RECESSIVE DISORDERS

SYSTEM	DISORDER
Metabolic	Cystic fibrosis Phenylketonuria Galactosemia Homocystinuria Lysosomal storage diseases* α_1-Antitrypsin deficiency Wilson's disease Hemochromatosis Glycogen storage diseases*
Hematopoietic	Sickle cell anemia Thalassemias
Endocrine	Congenital adrenal hyperplasia
Skeletal	Ehlers-Danlos syndrome (some variants)* Alkaptonuria*
Nervous	Neurogenic muscular atrophies Friedreich ataxia Spinal muscular atrophy

* Discussed in this chapter. Many others are discussed throughout the text.

Table 5-3. X-LINKED RECESSIVE DISORDERS

SYSTEM	DISEASE
Musculoskeletal	Duchenne muscular dystrophy
Blood	Hemophilia A and B Chronic granulomatous disease Glucose-6-phosphate dehydrogenase deficiency
Immune	Agammaglobulinemia Wiskott-Aldrich syndrome
Metabolic	Diabetes insipidus Lesch-Nyhan syndrome
Nervous	Fragile X syndrome*

* Discussed in this chapter.

tainty to the Y chromosome is the determinant for testes; although a few additional phenotypic characteristics have tentatively been assigned to the Y chromosome, none has been proved to be Y chromosome–related.

X-linked recessive inheritance accounts for a small number of well-defined clinical conditions. The Y chromosome, for the most part, is not homologous to the X, and so mutant genes on the X are not paired with alleles on the Y. Thus, the male is said to be *hemizygous* for X-linked mutant genes, so these disorders are expressed in the male. An affected male does not transmit the disorder to his sons, but all daughters are carriers. Sons of heterozygous women have, of course, one chance in two of receiving the mutant gene. The heterozygous female usually does not express the full phenotypic change because of the paired normal allele. Because of the random inactivation of one of the X chromosomes in the female, however, females have a variable proportion of cells in which the mutant X chromosome is active. Thus, it is remotely possible for the normal allele to be inactivated in most cells, permitting full expression of heterozygous X-linked conditions in the female. Much more commonly, the normal allele is inactivated in only some of the cells, and thus the heterozygous female expresses the disorder partially. An illustrative condition is *glucose-6-phosphate dehydrogenase (G6PD) deficiency*. Transmitted on the X chromosome, this enzyme deficiency, which predisposes to red cell hemolysis in patients receiving certain types of drugs (see Chapter 13), is expressed principally in males. In the female, a proportion of the red cells may be derived from marrow cells with inactivation of the normal allele. Such red cells are at the same risk for undergoing hemolysis as are the red cells in the hemizygous male. Thus, the female is not simply a carrier of this trait but also is susceptible to drug-induced hemolytic reactions. Because the proportion of defective red cells in heterozygous females depends on the random inactivation of one of the X chromosomes, however, the severity of the hemolytic

reaction is almost always less in heterozygous women than in hemizygous men. Most of the X-linked conditions listed in Table 5–3 are covered elsewhere in the text.

There are only a few *X-linked dominant* conditions. These disorders are transmitted by an affected heterozygous female to half her sons and half her daughters, and by an affected male parent to all his daughters but none of his sons, if the female parent is unaffected.

BIOCHEMICAL AND MOLECULAR BASIS OF SINGLE-GENE (MENDELIAN) DISORDERS

Mendelian disorders result from alterations involving single genes. The genetic defect may lead to the formation of an abnormal protein or a reduction in the output of the gene product. As mentioned earlier, mutations may effect protein synthesis by affecting transcription, mRNA processing, or translation. The phenotypic effects of a mutation may result directly, from abnormalities in the protein encoded by the mutant gene, or indirectly, owing to interactions of the mutant protein with other normal proteins. For example, all forms of Ehlers-Danlos syndrome (described later) are associated with abnormalities of collagen. In some forms (e.g., type IV), there is a mutation in one of the collagen genes, whereas in others (e.g., type VI), the collagen genes are normal, but there is a mutation in the gene that encodes lysyl hydroxylase, an enzyme essential for the cross-linking of collagen. In these patients, collagen weakness is secondary to a deficiency of lysyl hydroxylase.

Virtually any type of protein may be affected in single-gene disorders and by a variety of mechanisms (Table 5–4). To some extent, the pattern of inheritance of the disease is related to the kind of protein affected by the mutation, as will be described later. For the purposes of this discussion, the mechanisms involved in single-gene disorders can be classified into four categories: *(1) enzyme defects and their consequences; (2) defects in membrane receptors and transport systems; (3) alterations in the structure, function, or quantity of nonenzyme proteins; and (4) mutations resulting in unusual reactions to drugs.*

ENZYME DEFECTS AND THEIR CONSEQUENCES. Mutations may result in the synthesis of a defective enzyme with reduced activity or in a reduced amount of a normal enzyme. In either case, the consequence is a metabolic block. Figure 5–7 provides an example of an enzyme reaction in which the substrate S is converted by intracellular enzymes E_1, E_2, and E_3 into an end product P through intermediates I_1 and I_2. In this model, the final product P exerts feedback control on enzyme

Table 5–4. BIOCHEMICAL AND MOLECULAR BASIS OF SOME MENDELIAN DISORDERS

PROTEIN TYPE/FUNCTION	EXAMPLE	MOLECULAR LESION	DISEASE
Enzyme			
	Phenylalanine hydroxylase	Splice site mutation: reduced amount	Phenylketonuria
	Hexosaminidase	Splice site mutation or frame-shift mutation with stop codon: reduced amount	Tay-Sachs disease
	Adenosine deaminase	Point mutations: abnormal protein with reduced activity	Severe combined immunodeficiency
Receptor			
	Low-density lipoprotein receptor	Deletions, point mutations: reduction of synthesis, transport to cell surface, or binding to low-density lipoprotein	Familial hypercholesterolemia
	Vitamin D receptor	Point mutations: failure of normal signaling	Vitamin D–resistant rickets
Transport			
Oxygen	Hemoglobin	Deletions: reduced amount	α Thalassemia
		Defective mRNA processing: reduced amount	β Thalassemia
		Point mutations: abnormal structure	Sickle cell anemia
Ions	Cystic fibrosis transmembrane conductance regulator	Deletions and other mutations	Cystic fibrosis
Structural			
Extracellular	Collagen	Deletions or point mutations cause reduced amount of normal collagen or normal amounts of mutant collagen	Osteogenesis imperfecta; Ehlers-Danlos syndromes
	Fibrillin	Point mutations	Marfan syndrome
Cell membrane	Dystrophin	Deletion with reduced synthesis	Duchenne/Becker muscular dystrophy
	Spectrin, ankyrin, or protein 4.1	Heterogeneous	Hereditary spherocytosis
Enzyme Inhibitor	α_1-Antitrypsin	Missense mutations—impair secretion from liver to serum	Emphysema and liver disease
Hemostasis	Factor VIII	Deletions, insertions, nonsense mutations, and others: reduced synthesis or abnormal factor VIII	Hemophilia A

E_1. A minor pathway producing small quantities of M_1 and M_2 also exists. The biochemical consequences of an enzyme defect in such a reaction may lead to three major consequences:

1. *Accumulation of the substrate,* which, depending on the site of block, may be accompanied by accumulation of one or both intermediates. Moreover, an increased concentration of I_2 may stimulate the minor pathway and thus lead to an excess of M_1 and M_2. Under these conditions, tissue injury may result if the precursor, the intermediates, or the products of alternative minor pathways are toxic in high concentrations. For example, in galactosemia, the deficiency of galactose-1-phosphate uridyltransferase (see Chapter 10) leads to the accumulation of galactose and consequent tissue damage. A deficiency of phenylalanine hydroxylase (see Chapter 10) results in the accu-

mulation of phenylalanine. Excessive accumulation of complex substrates within the lysosomes due to deficiency of degradative enzymes is responsible for a group of diseases generally referred to as *lysosomal storage diseases.*

2. *An enzyme defect can lead to a metabolic block and a decreased amount of end product* that

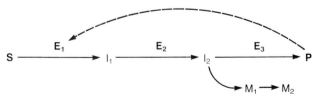

Figure 5–7. Schema illustrating the conversion of a substrate (S) to the end product (P), through several intermediates (I), brought about by enzymes (E). P exerts feedback inhibition of E_1. M denotes products of minor pathways.

may be necessary for normal function. For example, a deficiency of melanin may result from lack of tyrosinase, which is necessary for the biosynthesis of melanin from its precursor, tyrosine. This results in the clinical condition called albinism, to be discussed later. If the end product is a feedback inhibitor of the enzymes involved in the early reactions (in Figure 5–7, it is shown that P inhibits E_1), the deficiency of the end product may permit overproduction of intermediates and their catabolic products, some of which may be injurious at high concentrations. A prime example of a disease with such an underlying mechanism is the Lesch-Nyhan syndrome (see Chapter 27).

3. *Failure to inactivate a tissue-damaging substrate.* This is best exemplified by alpha₁-antitrypsin (α_1-AT) deficiency. Patients who have an inherited deficiency of serum α_1-AT are unable to inactivate neutrophil elastase in their lungs. Unchecked activity of this protease leads to destruction of elastin in the walls of lung alveoli, leading eventually to pulmonary emphysema (see Chapter 15).

DEFECTS IN RECEPTORS AND TRANSPORT SYSTEMS. Many biologically active substances have to be actively transported across the cell membrane. This is generally achieved by one of two mechanisms — by receptor-mediated endocytosis or by a transport protein. A genetic defect in a receptor-mediated transport system is exemplified by familial hypercholesterolemia, in which reduced synthesis or function of low-density lipoprotein (LDL) receptors leads to defective transport of LDL into the cells and secondarily to excessive cholesterol synthesis by complex intermediary mechanisms. In cystic fibrosis, on the other hand, the transport system for Cl⁻ ions across sweat ducts, lungs, and pancreas is defective. By mechanisms not fully understood, impaired Cl⁻ transport leads to serious injury to the lungs and pancreas (see Chapter 10).

ALTERATIONS IN STRUCTURE, FUNCTION, OR QUANTITY OF NONENZYME PROTEINS. Genetic defects resulting in alterations of structural proteins often have widespread secondary effects, as exemplified by sickle cell disease. Indeed, the hemoglobinopathies, sickle cell disease being one, all of which are characterized by defects in the structure of the globin molecule, best exemplify this category. In contrast to the hemoglobinopathies, the group of thalassemias results from mutations in globin genes that affect the amount of globin chains synthesized. Thalassemias are associated with reduced amounts of structurally normal α- or β-globin chains (see Chapter 13). Other examples of genetically defective structural proteins include collagen, spectrin, and dystrophin, giving rise to osteogenesis imperfecta (see Chapter 27), hereditary spherocytosis (see Chapter 13), and muscular dystrophies (see Chapter 29).

GENETICALLY DETERMINED ADVERSE REACTIONS TO DRUGS. Certain genetically determined enzyme deficiencies are unmasked only after exposure of the affected individual to certain drugs. This special area of genetics, called pharmacogenetics, is of considerable clinical importance.[7] The classic example of drug-induced injury in the genetically susceptible individual is associated with a deficiency of the enzyme G6PD. Under normal conditions, G6PD deficiency does not result in disease, but on administration, for example, of the antimalarial drug primaquine, a severe hemolytic anemia results (see Chapter 13).

With this overview of the biochemical basis of single-gene disorders, we now consider selected examples grouped according to the underlying defect.

DISORDERS ASSOCIATED WITH DEFECTS IN STRUCTURAL PROTEINS

Several diseases caused by mutations in genes that encode structural proteins are listed in Table 5–4. Many are discussed elsewhere in the text. Only Marfan syndrome and Ehlers-Danlos syndromes are discussed here, because they affect multiple organ systems.

Marfan Syndrome

Marfan syndrome is a *disorder of the connective tissues of the body, manifested principally by changes in the skeleton, eyes, and cardiovascular system.*[8] Affected individuals have unusually long, slender extremities, particularly elongation of the fingers, termed "spider fingers." Approximately 70 to 85% of the cases are familial and transmitted by autosomal dominant inheritance. The remainder are sporadic and arise from new mutations.

MORPHOLOGY. Skeletal abnormalities are the most striking feature of Marfan syndrome. Typically, the patient is unusually tall with exceptionally long extremities and long, tapering fingers and toes. Because the tall stature is contributed largely by the lower segment of the body, the ratio of the upper segment (top of the head to the pubis) to the lower segment (top of pubic ramus to the floor) is significantly lower than the norm for the age, race, and sex. The joint ligaments in the hands and feet are lax, suggesting that the patient is double-jointed; typically, the thumb can be hyperextended back to the wrist. The head is commonly dolichocephalic (long-headed) with bossing of the frontal eminences and prominent supraorbital ridges. Because President Abraham Lincoln possessed many of these physical characteristics, it is strongly suspected that he had Marfan syndrome. A variety of spinal deformities may appear, including kyphosis, scoliosis, or rotation or slipping of the dorsal or lumbar vertebrae. The chest is classically deformed, presenting either pectus excavatum (deeply depressed sternum) or a pigeon-breast deformity.

The **ocular changes** take many forms. Most characteristic is bilateral subluxation or dislocation (usually outward and upward) of the lens, referred to as ectopia lentis. This abnormality is so uncommon in persons who do not have this genetic disease that the finding of bilateral ectopia lentis should raise the suspicion of Marfan syndrome.

Cardiovascular lesions are the most life-threatening features of this disorder. The two most common lesions are mitral valve prolapse and, of greater importance, dilatation of the ascending aorta owing to cystic medionecrosis. Histologically, the changes in the media are virtually identical to those found in cystic medionecrosis not related to Marfan syndrome (see section on aortic dissection, Chapter 12). **Loss of medial support results in progressive dilatation of the aortic valve ring and the root of the aorta, giving rise to severe aortic incompetence.** Weakening of the media also predisposes to an intimal tear, which may initiate an intramural hematoma that cleaves the layers of the media to produce aortic dissection. After cleaving the aortic layers for considerable distances, sometimes back to the root of the aorta or down to the iliac arteries, the hemorrhage often ruptures through the aortic wall. Such a calamity is the cause of death in 30 to 45% of these individuals.

Although mitral valve lesions are more frequent, they are clinically less important than aortic lesions. Loss of connective tissue support in the mitral valve leaflets makes them soft and billowy, creating the so-called floppy valve (see Chapter 12). Valvular lesions, along with lengthening of the chordae tendineae, frequently give rise to mitral regurgitation. Similar changes may affect the tricuspid and, rarely, the aortic valves. Echocardiography greatly enhances the ability to detect the cardiovascular abnormalities and is therefore extremely valuable in the diagnosis of Marfan syndrome. The great majority of deaths are caused by rupture of aortic dissections, followed in importance by cardiac failure.

Although the lesions just described typify Marfan syndrome, it must be emphasized that there is great variation in the clinical expression of this genetic disorder. Patients with prominent eye or cardiovascular changes may have few skeletal abnormalities, whereas others with striking changes in body habitus have no eye changes. Although variability in clinical expression may be seen within a family, interfamilial variability is much more common and extensive. A possible explanation for the varied expression of Marfan syndrome is genetic heterogeneity, that is, different mutations produce similar phenotypes.

The nature of the Marfan gene and the protein encoded by it remained mysterious for years. The search ended in 1991 with the discovery that Marfan syndrome resulted from mutations in the fibrillin gene.[9] Fibrillin is a glycoprotein secreted by fibroblasts that aggregates either alone or in conjunction with other proteins to form a microfibrillar network in the extracellular matrix. The microfibrillary fibers serve as scaffolding for deposition of elastin and are considered integral components of elastic elements. Although microfibrillar structures are widely distributed, they are particularly abundant in the aorta, in ligaments, and in the ciliary zonules that support the lens.

Molecular studies firmly implicate fibrillin proteins as the primary culprit in Marfan syndrome:

- Immunohistologic studies reveal that fibrillin is either abnormal or deficient in the dermis of patients with Marfan syndrome. In tissue culture, dermal fibroblasts from patients fail to synthesize normal amounts of fibrillin or in some cases secrete it slowly. In other cases, the secreted fibrillin is poorly incorporated into the extracellular matrix.[10]
- In family linkage studies, the locus responsible for Marfan syndrome has been mapped to chromosome 15q21.1, and in independent studies, the gene that encodes one form of fibrillin has been mapped to the same locale.
- Point mutations in the fibrillin gene have been identified in some patients with the sporadic form of Marfan syndrome.

Because of the variable expression of the Marfan defect, it has been hypothesized that Marfan syndrome may be genetically heterogeneous. All studies to date, however, point to mutations in the fibrillin gene on chromosome 15 as the cause of this disease. The variable expressivity may be explained on the basis of allelic mutations within the same locus. Further studies of different families should delineate the number and frequency of such mutations. Until this information is available, direct gene diagnosis of Marfan syndrome is not feasible. Presymptomatic detection, however, is possible by restriction fragment length polymorphism (RFLP) analysis. The principles underlying these two methods of DNA-based diagnosis are described later in this chapter.[11]

Ehlers-Danlos Syndromes

Ehlers-Danlos syndromes (EDS) comprise a clinically and genetically heterogeneous group of disor-

ders that result from some defect in collagen synthesis or structure. As such, they belong to the same category of diseases as osteogenesis imperfecta (see Chapter 27).

The mode of inheritance of EDS encompasses all three mendelian patterns. This should not be surprising because biosynthesis of collagen is a complex process that can be disturbed by genetic errors that may affect any one of the numerous structural collagen genes or by mutations involving the genes encoding enzymes necessary for post-transcriptional modifications of collagen. Because abnormalities of collagen are fundamental in the pathogenesis of EDS, it would be advisable to review collagen structure and synthesis. We should recall that there are at least 12 genetically distinct collagen types, having somewhat characteristic tissue distribution. As we shall see, to some extent the clinical heterogeneity and variable modes of transmission of EDS can be explained based on the specific collagen type involved and the nature of the molecular defects.

On the basis of clinical manifestations and the pattern of inheritance, at least 10 variants of EDS have been recognized. It is beyond the scope of this book to discuss each variant individually, and the interested reader is referred to several excellent reviews for such details.[12] Instead we shall first summarize the important clinical features that are common to most variants and then correlate some of the clinical manifestations with the underlying molecular defects in collagen synthesis or structure.

As might be expected, tissues rich in collagen, such as skin, ligaments, and joints, are frequently involved in most variants of EDS. Because the abnormal collagen fibers lack adequate tensile strength, *skin is hyperextensible and the joints are hypermobile.* These features permit grotesque contortions, such as bending the thumb backward to touch the forearm and bending the knee forward to create almost a right angle. Indeed, it is believed that most contortionists have one of the EDSs. A predisposition to joint dislocation, however, is one of the prices paid for this virtuosity. *The skin is extraordinarily stretchable, extremely fragile, and vulnerable to trauma.* Minor injuries produce gaping defects, and surgical repair or any surgical intervention is accomplished with great difficulty because of the lack of normal tensile strength. *The basic defect in connective tissue may lead to serious internal complications.* These include rupture of the colon and large arteries (EDS type IV), ocular fragility with rupture of cornea and retinal detachment (EDS type VI), and diaphragmatic herniae (EDS type I).

The biochemical and molecular bases of these abnormalities are known in only a few forms of EDS. These will be described briefly because they offer some insights into the perplexing clinical heterogeneity of EDS. Perhaps the best characterized is *type VI, the most common autosomal recessive form of EDS.* It results from reduced activity of lysyl hydroxylase, an enzyme necessary for hydroxylation of lysine residues during collagen synthesis. Because hydroxylysine is essential for the cross-linking of collagen fibers, a deficiency of lysyl hydroxylase results in the synthesis of collagen that lacks normal structural stability. It is interesting to note that only collagen types I and III are affected in this disorder; the hydroxylation of collagen types II, IV, and V is normal. The molecular basis of this difference in hydroxylation is not clear.

Type IV EDS results from abnormalities of type III collagen. This form is genetically heterogeneous because at least three distinct mutations affecting the structural gene for collagen type III can give rise to this variant. At the molecular level, deletions, RNA splice mutations, and point mutations have been detected.[13] Some affect the rate of synthesis of pro α1 (III) chains, others affect the secretion of type III procollagen, and still others lead to the synthesis of structurally abnormal type III collagen. Some mutant alleles behave as dominant negatives (see discussion under autosomal dominant disorders) and thus produce very severe phenotypic effects. These molecular studies provide a rational basis for the pattern of transmission and clinical features that are characteristic of this variant. First, because EDS IV results from mutations involving a structural protein (rather than an enzyme protein), an autosomal dominant pattern of inheritance would be expected. Second, because blood vessels and intestines are known to be rich in collagen type III, an abnormality of this collagen is consistent with severe defects (e.g., spontaneous rupture) in these organs.

In EDS type VII, the fundamental defect is in the conversion of type I procollagen to collagen. This step in collagen synthesis involves cleavage of noncollagen peptides at the N and C terminals of the procollagen molecule. This is accomplished by N-terminal–specific and C-terminal–specific peptidases. *The defect in the conversion of procollagen to collagen in type VII EDS has been traced to mutations that affect one of the two type I collagen genes [i.e., α1 (I) or α2 (I)].* As a result, structurally abnormal pro α1 (I) or pro α2 (I) chains that resist cleavage of N-terminal peptides are formed. In patients with a single mutant allele, only 50% of the type I collagen chains are abnormal, but because these chains interfere with the formation of normal collagen helices, heterozygotes manifest the disease.

Finally, EDS type IX is worthy of brief mention because it illustrates how trace metals can affect connective tissues. The primary defect in this variant involves copper metabolism. These patients have high levels of copper within the cells, but serum copper and ceruloplasmin levels are low.

The molecular basis of abnormal copper distribution is not yet known, but its effect is to reduce the activity of the copper-dependent enzyme lysyl oxidase, which is essential for cross linking of collagen and elastin fibers. Because the genes that regulate copper metabolism map to the X chromosome, this variant of EDS (in contrast to most others) is inherited as an X-linked recessive trait.

The common thread in EDS is some abnormality of collagen. These disorders, however, are extremely heterogeneous. At the molecular level, a variety of defects, varying from mutations involving structural genes for collagen to those involving enzymes that are responsible for post-transcriptional modifications of mRNA, have been detected. Such molecular heterogeneity results in the expression of EDS as a clinically heterogeneous disorder with several patterns of inheritance.

DISORDERS ASSOCIATED WITH DEFECTS IN RECEPTOR PROTEINS

Familial Hypercholesterolemia

This "receptor disease" is the consequence of a *mutation in the gene encoding the receptor for low-density lipoprotein (LDL), which is involved in the transport and metabolism of cholesterol.* As a consequence of receptor abnormalities, there is a loss of feedback control and elevated levels of cholesterol that induce premature atherosclerosis, leading to a greatly increased risk of myocardial infarction.[14]

Familial hypercholesterolemia (FH) is possibly the most frequent mendelian disorder. Heterozygotes with one mutant gene, representing about 1 in 500 individuals, have from birth a twofold to threefold elevation of plasma cholesterol level, leading to tendinous xanthomas and premature atherosclerosis in adult life (see Chapter 11). Homozygotes, having a double dose of the mutant gene, are much more severely affected and may have fivefold to sixfold elevations in plasma cholesterol levels. These individuals develop skin xanthomas and coronary, cerebral, and peripheral vascular atherosclerosis at an early age. Myocardial infarction may develop before the age of 20 years. Large-scale studies have found that familial hypercholesterolemia is present in 3 to 6% of survivors of myocardial infarction.

An understanding of this disorder requires that we briefly review the normal process of cholesterol metabolism and transport. Approximately 7% of the body's cholesterol circulates in the plasma, predominantly in the form of LDL. As might be expected, the level of plasma cholesterol is influenced by its synthesis and catabolism. Figure 5–8 illustrates that liver plays a crucial role in

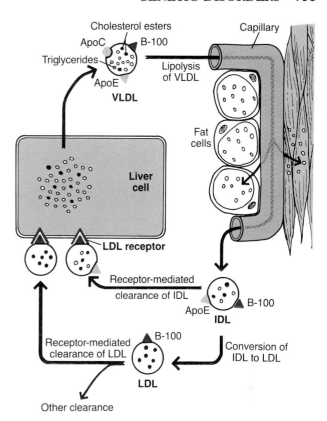

Figure 5–8. Schematic illustration of LDL metabolism and the role of liver in its synthesis and clearance. Lipolysis of VLDL by lipoprotein lipase in the capillaries releases triglycerides, which are then stored in fat cells and used as a source of energy in skeletal muscles.

both these processes.[15] The first step in this complex sequence is the secretion of very low–density lipoproteins (VLDL) by the liver into the bloodstream. VLDL particles are rich in triglycerides, although they do contain lesser amounts of cholesteryl esters. When a VLDL particle reaches the capillaries of adipose tissue or muscle, it is cleaved by lipoprotein lipase, a process that extracts most of the triglycerides. The resulting molecule, called intermediate-density lipoprotein (IDL), is reduced in triglyceride content and enriched in cholesteryl esters, but it retains two of the three apoproteins (B-100 and E) present in the parent VLDL particle (see Fig. 5–8). After release from the capillary endothelium, the IDL particles have one of two fates. Approximately 50% of newly formed IDL is rapidly taken up by the liver through a receptor-mediated transport. The receptor responsible for the binding of IDL to liver cell membrane recognizes both apoprotein B-100 and apoprotein E. It is called the LDL receptor, however, because it is also involved in the hepatic clearance of LDL, as described later. In the liver cells, IDL is recycled to generate VLDL. The IDL particles not taken up by the liver are subjected to further metabolic

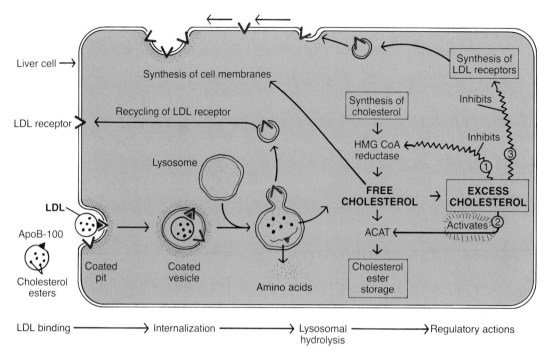

Figure 5-9. Sequential steps in LDL receptor pathway in cultured mammalian cells. LDL = low-density lipoprotein; HMG CoA reductase = 3-hydroxy-3-methyl-glutaryl CoA reductase; ACAT = acyl CoA: cholesterol acyltransferase.

processing that removes most of the remaining triglycerides and apoprotein E, yielding the cholesterol-rich LDL. *It should be emphasized that IDL is the immediate and major source of plasma LDL.* There appear to be two mechanisms for removal of LDL from plasma, one mediated by an LDL receptor–dependent process and the other by an LDL receptor–independent pathway, described later. Although many cell types, including fibroblasts, lymphocytes, smooth muscle cells, hepatocytes, and adrenocortical cells, possess high-affinity LDL receptors, approximately 70% of the plasma LDL appears to be cleared by the liver, utilizing a relatively sophisticated transport process (Fig. 5-9). The first step involves binding of LDL to cell surface receptors, which are clustered in specialized regions of the plasma membrane called *coated pits.* After binding, the coated pits containing the receptor-bound LDL are internalized by invagination to form coated vesicles, after which they migrate within the cell to fuse with the lysosomes. Here the LDL dissociates from the receptor, which is recycled to the surface. In the lysosomes, the LDL molecule is enzymically degraded; the apoprotein part is hydrolyzed to amino acids, whereas the cholesteryl esters are broken down to free cholesterol. This in turn crosses the lysosomal membrane to enter the cytoplasm, where it is used for membrane synthesis and as a regulator of cholesterol homeostasis. Three separate processes are affected by the released intra-cellular cholesterol: (1) Cholesterol *suppresses* cholesterol synthesis within the cell by inhibiting the activity of the enzyme 3-hydroxy-3-methylglutaryl (3HMG) CoA reductase, which is the rate-limiting enzyme in the synthetic pathway; (2) the cholesterol *activates* the enzyme acyl-coenzyme A:cholesterol acyltransferase, favoring esterification and storage of excess cholesterol; and (3) cholesterol *suppresses* the synthesis of LDL receptors, thus protecting the cells from excessive accumulation of cholesterol.

As mentioned earlier, FH results from mutations in the gene specifying the receptor for LDL. Heterozygotes with FH possess only 50% of the normal number of high-affinity LDL receptors, because they have only one normal gene. As a result of this defect in transport, the catabolism of LDL by the receptor-dependent pathways is impaired, and the plasma level of LDL increases approximately twofold. Homozygotes have virtually no normal LDL receptors in their cells and have much higher levels of circulating LDL. In addition to defective LDL clearance, both the homozygotes and heterozygotes have increased synthesis of LDL. The mechanism of increased synthesis that contributes to hypercholesterolemia also results from a lack of LDL receptors (see Fig. 5-8). Recall that IDL, the immediate precursor of plasma LDL, also uses hepatic LDL receptors (apoprotein B-100 and E receptors) for its transport into the liver. In FH, impaired IDL transport into the liver secondarily diverts a greater proportion of plasma IDL into the precursor pool for plasma LDL.

The transport of LDL not involving LDL receptors appears to occur at least in part into the cells of the mononuclear phagocyte system. Mono-

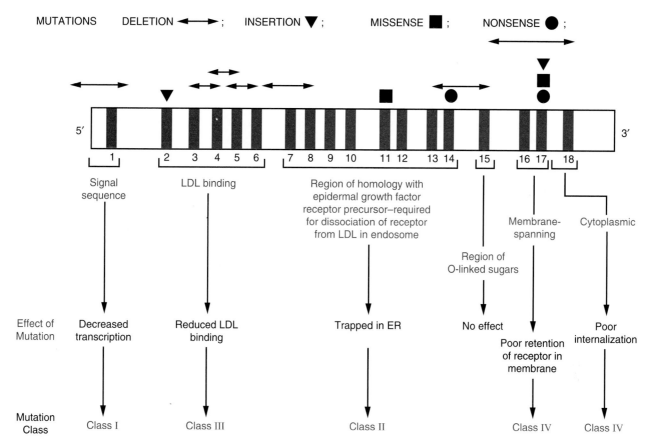

Figure 5-10. The structure of the LDL receptor gene, showing the 18 exons (shaded) and five domains. The effect of some mutations on the synthesis or structure of LDL is indicated. (Modified and reproduced with permission from Goldstein, J.L., and Brown, M.S.: Familial hypercholesterolemia. *In* Scriver, C.R., Beaudet, A.L., Sly, W.S., and Valle, D. (eds.): The Metabolic Basis of Inherited Disease, 6th ed. New York, McGraw-Hill, 1989, p. 1232.)

cytes and macrophages have receptors for chemically altered (e.g., acetylated or oxidized) LDL. Normally, the amount of LDL transported along this "scavenger receptor" pathway is less than that mediated by the receptor-dependent mechanisms. In the face of hypercholesterolemia, however, there is a marked increase in the LDL receptor–independent traffic of LDL cholesterol into the cells of the mononuclear phagocyte system and possibly the vascular walls. This is responsible for the appearance of xanthomas and may also contribute to the pathogenesis of premature atherosclerosis.

The molecular genetics of FH has proved to be extremely complex. The human LDL receptor gene located on chromosome 19 is extremely large, with 18 exons and 5 domains that span a distance of about 45 kb (Fig. 5–10). At least 35 mutations, including insertions, deletions, and missense and nonsense mutations, involving each of the five domains have been identified. These can be classified into four groups: *Class I mutations* are the most common, and they lead to a complete failure of synthesis of the receptor protein (null allele). *Class II mutations* encode receptor proteins that accumulate in the endoplasmic reticulum because they cannot be transported to the Golgi complex (transport-deficiency alleles). *Class III mutations* affect the LDL-binding domain of the receptor; the encoded proteins reach the cell surface but fail to bind LDL or do so poorly (binding-deficient alleles). *Class IV mutations* encode proteins that are synthesized and transported to the cell surface efficiently. They bind LDL normally, but they fail to localize in coated pits and hence the bound LDL is not internalized.[16]

The discovery of the critical role of LDL receptors in cholesterol homeostasis has led to the rational design of drugs that lower plasma cholesterol by increasing the number of LDL receptors.[17] One strategy that has proved to be successful is based on the ability of certain drugs (e.g., lovastatin) to suppress intracellular cholesterol synthesis by inhibiting the enzyme HMG CoA reductase. This in turn allows greater synthesis of LDL receptors (see Fig. 5–9). Such a therapeutic approach lowers plasma cholesterol levels not only in patients with heterozygous FH, but also in patients with the more common nongenetic forms of hypercholesterolemia.[18]

DISORDERS ASSOCIATED WITH DEFECTS IN ENZYMES

Lysosomal Storage Diseases

Lysosomes are key components of the "intracellular digestive tract." They contain a battery of hydrolytic enzymes, which have two special properties. First, they can function in the acid milieu of the lysosomes. Second, these enzymes constitute a special category of secretory proteins that, in contrast to most others, are destined for secretion not into the extracellular fluids but into an intracellular organelle. This latter characteristic requires special processing within the Golgi apparatus, which is reviewed briefly. Similar to all other secretory proteins, lysosomal enzymes (or acid hydrolases, as they are sometimes called) are synthesized in the endoplasmic reticulum and transported to the Golgi apparatus. Within the Golgi complex, they undergo a variety of post-translational modifications, of which one is worthy of special note. This involves the attachment of terminal mannose-6-phosphate groupings to some of the oligosaccharide side chains. The phosphorylated mannose residues may be viewed as an "address label" that is recognized by specific receptors found on the inner surface of the Golgi membrane. Lysosomal enzymes bind to these receptors and are thereby segregated from the numerous other secretory proteins within the Golgi. Subsequently, small transport vesicles containing the receptor-bound enzymes are pinched off from the Golgi and proceed to fuse with the lysosomes. Thus, the enzymes are targeted to their intracellular abode, and, as indicated in Figure 5–11, the vesicles are shuttled back to the Golgi. As will be discussed later, genetically determined errors in this remarkable sorting mechanism may give rise to one form of lysosomal storage disease.

The lysosomal acid hydrolases catalyze the breakdown of a variety of complex macromolecules. These large molecules may be derived from the metabolic turnover of intracellular organelles (autophagy), or they may be acquired from outside the cells by phagocytosis (heterophagy). With an inherited deficiency of a functional lysosomal enzyme, catabolism of its substrate remains incomplete, leading to the accumulation of the partially degraded insoluble metabolite within the lysosomes. Stuffed with incompletely digested macromolecules, these organelles become large and numerous enough to interfere with normal cell functions, giving rise to the so-called *lysosomal storage disorders* (Fig. 5–12). When this category of diseases was first discovered in 1963, it was thought that they resulted exclusively from mutations that lead to reduced synthesis of lysosomal enzymes ("missing enzyme syndromes"). In the last two decades, however, research focusing on

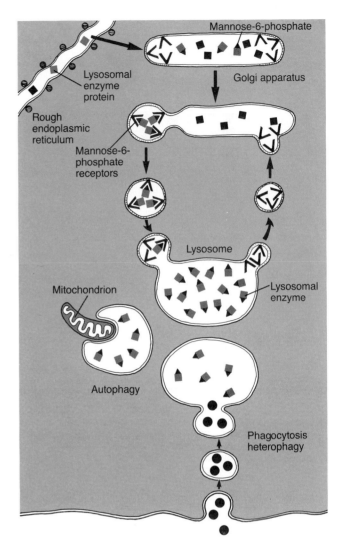

Figure 5–11. Synthesis and intracellular transport of lysosomal enzymes.

the molecular pathology of lysosomal storage diseases has led to the discovery of several other defects.[19] Some of these are as follows:

- Synthesis of a catalytically inactive protein that cross-reacts immunologically with the normal enzyme. Thus, by immunoassays the enzyme levels appear to be normal.
- Defects in post-translational processing of the enzyme protein. Included in this category is a failure to attach the mannose-6-phosphate "marker," the absence of which prevents the enzyme from following its correct path to the lysosome. Instead, the enzyme is secreted outside the cell.
- Lack of an enzyme activator or protector protein.
- Lack of a substrate activator protein. In some instances, proteins that react with the substrate to facilitate its hydrolysis may be missing or defective.

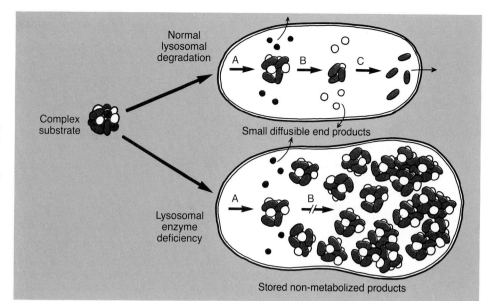

Figure 5–12. A schematic diagram illustrating the pathogenesis of lysosomal storage diseases. In the example illustrated, a complex substrate is normally degraded by a series of lysosomal enzymes (A, B, and C) into soluble end products. If there is a deficiency or malfunction of one of the enzymes (e.g., B), catabolism is incomplete, and insoluble intermediates accumulate in the lysosomes.

Table 5–5. LYSOSOMAL STORAGE DISEASES

DISEASE	ENZYME DEFICIENCY	MAJOR ACCUMULATING METABOLITES
Glycogenosis		
Type 2—Pompe's disease	α-1,4-Glucosidase (lysosomal glucosidase)	Glycogen
Sphingolipidoses		

GM₁ gangliosidosis
  Type 1—infantile, generalized
  Type 2—juvenile
	GM₁ ganglioside β-galactosidase	GM₁ ganglioside, galactose-containing oligosaccharides

GM₂ gangliosidosis
  Tay-Sachs disease
  Sandhoff disease
  GM₂ gangliosidosis, variant AB
	Hexosaminidase—α subunit
	Hexosaminidase—β subunit
	Ganglioside activator protein
		GM₂ ganglioside
		GM₂ ganglioside, globoside
		GM₂ ganglioside

Sulfatidoses		
Metachromatic leukodystrophy	Arylsulfatase A	Sulfatide
Multiple sulfatase deficiency	Arylsulfatases A, B, C; steroid sulfatase; iduronate sulfatase, heparan N-sulfatase	Sulfatide, steroid sulfate, heparan sulfate, dermatan sulfate
Krabbe disease	Galactosylceramidase	Galactocerebroside
Fabry disease	α-Galactosidase A	Ceramide trihexoside
Gaucher disease	Glucocerebrosidase	Glucocerebroside
Niemann-Pick disease: types A and B	Sphingomyelinase	Sphingomyelin
Mucopolysaccharidoses		
MPS I H (Hurler)	α-L-Iduronidase	Dermatan sulfate, heparan sulfate
MPS II (Hunter)	L-Iduronosulfate sulfatase	
Mucolipidoses (ML)		
I-cell disease (ML II) and pseudo–Hurler polydystrophy	Deficiency of phosphorylating enzymes essential for the formation of mannose-6-phosphate recognition marker; acid hydrolases lacking the recognition marker cannot be targeted to the lysosomes but are secreted extracellularly	Mucopolysaccharide, glycolipid
Other diseases of complex carbohydrates		
Fucosidosis	α-Fucosidase	Fucose-containing sphingolipids and glycoprotein fragments
Mannosidosis	α-Mannosidase	Mannose-containing oligosaccharides
Aspartylglycosaminuria	Aspartylglycosamine amide hydrolase	Aspartyl-2-deoxy-2-acetamido-glycosylamine
Other lysosomal storage diseases		
Wolman disease	Acid lipase	Cholesterol esters, triglycerides
Acid phosphate deficiency	Lysosomal acid phosphatase	Phosphate esters

- Lack of a transport protein required for egress of the digested material from the lysosomes.

It should be evident, therefore, that the concept of lysosomal storage disorders has to be expanded to include the lack of any protein essential for the normal function of lysosomes.

Several distinctive and separable conditions are included among the lysosomal storage diseases (Table 5–5). In general, the distribution of the stored material, and hence the organs affected, are determined by two interrelated factors: (1) the site where most of the material to be degraded is found, and (2) the location where most of the degradation normally occurs. *For example, brain is rich in gangliosides, and hence defective hydrolysis of gangliosides as occurs in GM$_1$ and GM$_2$ gangliosidoses results primarily in storage within neurons and neurologic symptoms.* Defects in degradation of mucopolysaccharides affect virtually every organ because mucopolysaccharides are widely distributed in the body. Because cells of the mononuclear phagocyte system are especially rich in lysosomes and are involved in the degradation of a variety of substrates, organs rich in phagocytic cells such as the spleen and liver are frequently enlarged in

several forms of lysosomal storage disorders. The ever-expanding number of lysosomal storage diseases can be divided into rational categories based on the biochemical nature of the accumulated metabolite, thus creating such subgroups as the *glycogenoses, sphingolipidoses (lipidoses), mucopolysaccharidoses,* and *mucolipidoses* (see Table 5–5). Only one among the many glycogenoses results from a lysosomal enzyme deficiency, and so this family of storage diseases is considered later. Only the most common disorders among the remaining groups are considered here; the others must be left to specialized texts and reviews.[20]

TAY-SACHS DISEASE (GM$_2$ GANGLIOSIDOSIS: HEXOSAMINIDASE α-SUBUNIT DEFICIENCY). GM$_2$ gangliosidoses are a group of three lysosomal storage diseases caused by an inability to catabolize GM$_2$ gangliosides. Degradation of GM$_2$ gangliosides requires three polypeptides encoded by three separate loci (Fig. 5–13). The phenotypic effects of mutations affecting these genes are fairly similar because they result from accumulation of GM$_2$ gangliosides. The underlying enzyme defect, however, is different for each. Tay-Sachs disease, the most common form of GM$_2$ gangliosidosis, results

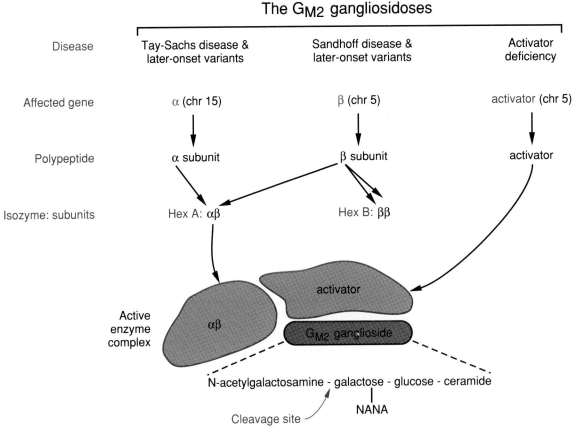

The G$_{M2}$ gangliosidoses

Figure 5–13. The three-gene system required for hexosaminidase A activity, and the diseases that result from defects in each of the genes. The function of the activator protein is to bind the ganglioside substrate and present it to the enzyme. (Modified and reproduced with permission from Sandhoff, K., Conzelmann, E., Neufeld, E.F., et al.: The GM$_2$ gangliosidoses. In Scriver, C.R., Beaudet, A.L., Sly, W.S., and Valle, D. (eds.): The Metabolic Basis of Inherited Disease, 6th ed. New York, McGraw-Hill, 1989, p. 1824.)

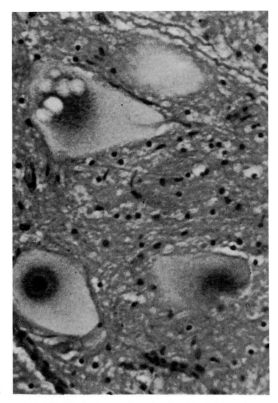 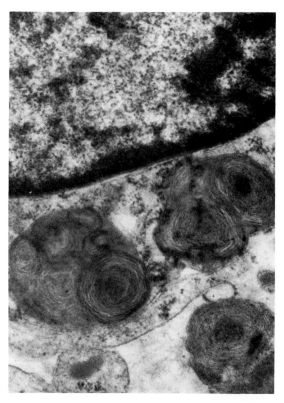

A   B

Figure 5–14. Ganglion cells in Tay-Sachs disease. *A*, Under the light microscope, a large neuron at the top has obvious lipid vacuolation with karyolysis and granularity of nucleus. *B*, A portion of a neuron under the electron microscope shows prominent lysosomes with whorled configurations. Part of the nucleus is shown above. (Electron micrograph courtesy of Dr. Joe Rutledge, University of Texas Southwestern Medical School, Dallas.)

from mutations that affect the α-subunit locus on chromosome 15 and cause a severe deficiency of hexosaminidase A. This disease is especially prevalent among Jews, particularly among those of Eastern European (Ashkenazic) origin, in whom a carrier rate of 1 in 30 has been reported.

MORPHOLOGY. The hexosaminidase A is absent from virtually all the tissues that have been examined, including leukocytes and plasma, and so GM_2 ganglioside accumulates in many tissues (e.g., heart, liver, spleen), but the involvement of neurons in the central and autonomic nervous systems and retina dominates the clinical picture. On histologic examination, the neurons are ballooned with cytoplasmic vacuoles, each of which constitutes a markedly distended lysosome filled with gangliosides (Fig. 5–14). Stains for fat such as oil red O and Sudan black are positive. With the electron microscope, several types of cytoplasmic inclusions can be visualized, the most prominent being whorled configurations within lysosomes composed of onionskin layers of membranes. In time there is progressive destruction of neurons, proliferation of microglia, and accumulation of complex lipids in phagocytes within the brain substance. A similar process occurs in the cerebellum as well as in neurons throughout the basal ganglia, brain stem, spinal cord, and dorsal root ganglia, and in the neurons of the autonomic nervous system. The ganglion cells in the retina are similarly swollen with GM_2-ganglioside, particularly at the margins of the macula. A **cherry-red spot** thus appears in the macula, representing accentuation of the normal color of the macular choroid contrasted with the pallor produced by the swollen ganglion cells in the remainder of the retina. This finding is characteristic of Tay-Sachs disease and other storage disorders affecting the neurons.

Several alleles have been identified at the α-subunit locus, each associated with a variable degree of enzyme deficiency and hence with variable clinical manifestations. With the most profound deficiency of hexosaminidase A, the affected infants appear normal at birth but begin to manifest signs and symptoms at about 6 months of age. There is relentless motor and mental deterioration, beginning with motor incoordination, mental obtundation leading to muscular flaccidity, blindness, and increasing dementia. Sometime during the early course of the disease, the characteristic, but not pathognomonic, cherry-red spot appears in the macula of the eye grounds in almost all patients. Over the span of 1 or 2 years, a complete, pathetic vegetative state is reached, followed by death at two to three years of age.

Antenatal diagnosis and carrier detection are possible by enzyme assays and DNA-based analysis.[21] The clinical features of the two other forms of GM$_2$ gangliosidosis (see Fig. 5–13), Sandhoff disease, resulting from β-subunit defect, and GM$_2$ activator deficiency, are similar to those of Tay-Sachs disease.

NIEMANN-PICK DISEASE. This designation refers to a group of disorders that are clinically, biochemically, and genetically heterogeneous.[22] The unifying feature of the Niemann-Pick group of diseases is the lysosomal accumulation of sphingomyelin and cholesterol. Biochemically, *two major groups of patients can be distinguished:* those with a deficiency of the sphingomyelin-cleaving enzyme sphingomyelinase (types A and B), and others in whom this enzyme activity is normal or nearly so (types C and D). In the latter types, there is a primary defect in intracellular cholesterol esterification and transport, but the defective gene product has yet to be identified. All types are rare, so our remarks will be confined largely to sphingomyelinase-deficient, type A variant, representing 75 to 80% of all cases. *This is the severe infantile form with extensive neurologic involvement, marked visceral accumulations of sphingomyelin, and progressive wasting and early death within the first 3 years of life.* To provide a perspective on the differences between the variants of Niemann-Pick disease, we need only point out that in type B, for example, patients have organomegaly but generally no central nervous system involvement. They usually survive into adulthood.

MORPHOLOGY. In the classic infantile type A variant, the deficiency of sphingomyelinase is almost complete. Sphingomyelin is a ubiquitous component of cellular (including organellar) membranes, and so the enzyme deficiency blocks degradation of the lipid, resulting in its progressive accumulation within lysosomes, particularly within cells of the mononuclear phagocyte system (Fig. 5–15). Affected cells become enlarged, sometimes to 90 μm in diameter, secondary to the distention of lysosomes with sphingomyelin and cholesterol. Innumerable small vacuoles of relatively uniform size are created, imparting a foaminess to the cytoplasm. In frozen sections of fresh tissue, the vacuoles stain for fat with Sudan black B and oil red O. Electron microscopy confirms that the vacuoles are engorged secondary lysosomes that often contain membranous cytoplasmic bodies (MCB) resembling concentric lamellated myelin figures. Sometimes the lysosomal configurations take the form of parallel palisaded lamellae, creating so-called zebra bodies.

The lipid-laden phagocytic foam cells are widely distributed in the spleen, liver, lymph nodes,

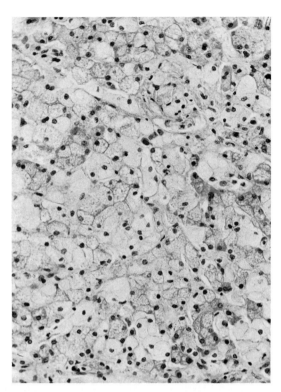

Figure 5–15. Niemann-Pick disease in bone marrow. The marrow space is virtually filled with fairly regular lipid-filled macrophages.

bone marrow, tonsils, gastrointestinal tract, and lungs. The involvement of the spleen generally produces massive enlargement, sometimes to 10 times its normal weight, but the hepatomegaly is usually not quite so striking. The lymph nodes are generally moderately to markedly enlarged throughout the body. Often the color of these organs is paler than usual owing to the massive accumulations of sphingomyelin.

Involvement of the brain and eye deserves special mention. In brain, the gyri are shrunken and the sulci widened. The neuronal involvement is diffuse, affecting all parts of the nervous system. Vacuolation and ballooning of neurons constitute the dominant histologic change, which in time leads to cell death and loss of brain substance. A retinal cherry-red spot similar to that seen in Tay-Sachs disease is present in about one-third to one-half of affected individuals. Its origin is similar to that described in Tay-Sachs disease except that the accumulated metabolite is sphingomyelin.

Clinical manifestations may be present even at birth, but almost certainly become evident by six months of age. Infants typically have a protuberant abdomen because of the hepatosplenomegaly. Accumulation of sphingomyelin and cholesterol in subcutaneous phagocytic cells may produce small skin xanthomas. Once the manifestations appear, they are followed by progressive failure to thrive, vomiting, fever, and generalized lymphadenopathy as well as progressive deterioration of psychomotor function. Death comes as a release, usually within the first or second year of life.

The diagnosis is established by biochemical assays for sphingomyelinase activity in liver or bone marrow biopsy. The sphingomyelinase gene has been cloned, and hence individuals affected with types A and B, as well as carriers, can be detected by DNA-probe analysis.

GAUCHER DISEASE. This eponym refers to a cluster of autosomal recessive disorders resulting from mutations at the glucocerebrosidase locus on chromosome 1q21. The affected gene encodes glucocerebrosidase, an enzyme that normally cleaves the glucose residue from ceramide. As a result, glucocerebroside accumulates principally in the phagocytic cells of the body but in some forms also in the central nervous system. Glucocerebrosides are continually formed from the catabolism of glycolipids derived mainly from the cell membranes of senescent leukocytes and erythrocytes. Three clinical subtypes of Gaucher disease have been distinguished. The most common, accounting for 99% of cases, is called type I, or the chronic non-neuronopathic form. In this type, *storage of glucocerebrosides is limited to the mononuclear phagocytes throughout the body without involving the brain. Splenic and skeletal involvements dominate this pattern of the disease.* It is found principally in Jews of European stock. Patients with this disorder have reduced but detectable levels of glucocerebrosidase activity. Longevity is shortened but not markedly. Type II, or acute neuronopathic, Gaucher disease is the *infantile acute cerebral pattern. This infantile form has no predilection for Jews. In these patients, there is virtually no detectable glucocerebrosidase activity in the tissues.* Hepatosplenomegaly is also seen in this form of Gaucher disease, but the clinical picture is dominated by progressive central nervous system involvement, leading to death at an early age. A third pattern, type III, is sometimes distinguished, intermediate between types I and II. These patients are usually juveniles and have the systemic involvement characteristic of type I but have progressive central nervous system disease that usually begins in the second or third decade of life. These specific patterns run within families, resulting from different allelic mutations in the structural gene for the enzyme.[23]

MORPHOLOGY. The glucocerebrosides accumulate in massive amounts within phagocytic cells throughout the body in all forms of Gaucher disease. The distended phagocytic cells, known as **Gaucher cells,** are found in the spleen, liver, bone marrow, lymph nodes, tonsils, thymus, and Peyer patches. Similar cells may be found in both the alveolar septa and the air spaces in the lung. In contrast to the lipid storage diseases already discussed, Gaucher cells rarely appear vacuolated but instead have a fibrillary type of cytoplasm likened to crumpled tissue paper (Fig. 5–16). Gaucher cells are often enlarged, sometimes up to 100 μm in diameter, and have one or more dark, eccentrically placed nuclei. Periodic acid–Schiff (PAS) staining is usually intensely positive. With the electron microscope, the fibrillary cytoplasm can be resolved as elongated, distended lysosomes, containing the stored lipid in stacks of bilayers.[24]

The accumulation of Gaucher cells produces a variety of gross anatomic changes. The spleen is enlarged in the type I variant, sometimes up to 10 kg. It too may appear uniformly pale or have a mottled surface owing to focal accumulations of Gaucher cells. The lymphadenopathy is mild to moderate and is body-wide. The accumulations of Gaucher cells in the bone marrow may produce small focal areas of bone erosion or large, soft, gray tumorous masses that cause skeletal deformities or destroy sufficient bone to give rise to fractures. In patients with cerebral involvement, Gaucher cells are seen in the Virchow-Robin spaces, and arterioles are surrounded by swollen adventitial cells. There is no convincing evidence for the storage of lipids in the neurons, yet neurons appear shriveled and are progressively destroyed. It is suspected that the lipids that accumulate in the phagocytic cells around blood vessels are in some manner toxic to neural tissue.

The clinical course of Gaucher disease depends on the clinical subtype. In the type I pattern, symptoms and signs first appear in adult life and are related to splenomegaly or bone involvement. Most commonly, there is pancytopenia or thrombocytopenia secondary to hypersplenism. Pathologic fractures and bone pain occur if there has been extensive expansion of the marrow space. Although the disease is progressive in the adult, it is compatible with long life. In types II and III, central nervous system dysfunction, convulsions, and progressive mental deterioration dominate, although organs such as the liver, spleen, and lymph nodes are also affected.

The diagnosis of homozygotes and the detection of heterozygous carriers can be made through measurement of glucocerebrosidase activity in peripheral blood leukocytes or in extracts of cultured skin fibroblasts. Because there is substantial overlap between the enzyme levels in normals and heterozygotes, the detection of specific mutations is a more precise tool.[25]

As with all lysosomal storage diseases, the prospects for treatment are not encouraging. Replacement therapy with recombinant enzymes is

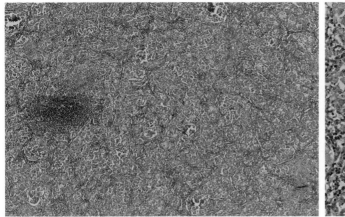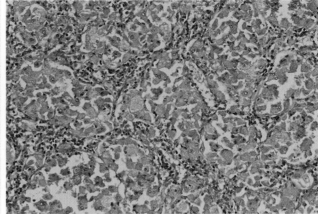

Figure 5–16. Gaucher disease involving the spleen. The left frame (at low magnification) shows expansion of red pulp in between and around the lymphoid white pulp. The right frame (at higher magnification) shows Gaucher cells with abundant lipid-laden granular cytoplasm and eccentric nuclei. (Courtesy of Dr. Trace Worrell, Department of Pathology, University of Texas Southwestern Medical School, Dallas.)

effective but extremely expensive. Because the fundamental defect resides in mononuclear phagocytic cells originating from marrow stem cells, bone marrow transplantation has been attempted. More recent attempts are directed toward correction of the enzyme defect by transfer of the normal glucocerebrosidase gene into the patient's cells. A mouse model of Gaucher disease has been produced by targeted disruption ("gene knockout") of the murine glucocerebrosidase gene.[26] This animal model is likely to prove useful in designing gene therapy for Gaucher disease.

MUCOPOLYSACCHARIDOSES. The mucopolysaccharidoses (MPS) are another form of lysosomal storage disease. They constitute a group of closely related syndromes that result from genetically determined deficiencies of specific lysosomal enzymes involved in the degradation of mucopolysaccharides (glycosaminoglycans). The glycosaminoglycans that accumulate in the MPS are dermatan sulfate, heparan sulfate, keratan sulfate, and chondroitin sulfate.[27] The enzymes involved in the degradation of these molecules cleave terminal sugars from the polysaccharide chains disposed along a polypeptide or "core protein." When there is a block in the removal of a terminal sugar, the remainder of the polysaccharide chain is not further degraded, and thus these chains accumulate within lysosomes in various tissues and organs of the body. Severe somatic and neurologic changes result.

Several clinical variants of MPS, classified numerically from MPS I to MPS VII, have been described, each resulting from the deficiency of one specific enzyme. All the MPS except one are inherited as autosomal recessive traits; the one variant, called Hunter syndrome, is an X-linked recessive. Within a given group (e.g., MPS I, characterized by a deficiency of α-L-iduronidase)

subgroups exist that result from different mutant alleles at the same genetic locus. Thus, the severity of enzyme deficiency and the clinical picture even within subgroups are often different.

In general, the MPS are progressive disorders, characterized by involvement of multiple organs, including liver, spleen, heart, and blood vessels. Most are associated with *coarse facial features, clouding of the cornea, joint stiffness, and mental retardation.* Urinary excretion of the accumulated mucopolysaccharides is often increased.

MORPHOLOGY. The accumulated mucopolysaccharides are generally found in mononuclear phagocytic cells, endothelial cells, intimal smooth muscle cells, and fibroblasts throughout the body. Common sites of involvement are thus the spleen, liver, bone marrow, lymph nodes, blood vessels, and also the heart.

Microscopically, affected cells are distended and have apparent clearing of the cytoplasm to create so-called balloon cells. The cleared cytoplasm can be resolved as numerous minute vacuoles, which, with the electron microscope, can be visualized as swollen lysosomes filled with a finely granular PAS-positive material that can be identified biochemically as mucopolysaccharide. Similar lysosomal changes are found in the neurons of those syndromes characterized by central nervous system involvement. In addition, however, some of the lysosomes in neurons are replaced by lamellated zebra bodies similar to those seen in Niemann-Pick disease. **Hepatosplenomegaly, skeletal deformities, valvular lesions, and subendothelial arterial deposits, particularly in the coronary arteries and lesions in the brain, are common threads that run through all the MPS.** In many of the more protracted syndromes, coronary subendothelial lesions lead to myocardial ischemia. Thus, myocardial infarction and cardiac decompensation are important causes of death.

Of the seven recognized variants, only two well-characterized syndromes are described briefly here. *Hurler syndrome,* also called MPS I H, results from a deficiency of α-L-iduronidase. It is one of the most severe forms of MPS. The affected children appear normal at birth but develop hepatosplenomegaly by 6 to 24 months. Their growth is retarded and, as in other forms of MPS, they develop coarse facial features and skeletal deformities. Death occurs by 6 to 10 years of age and is often due to cardiovascular complications. *Hunter syndrome,* also called MPS II, differs from Hurler syndrome in its mode of inheritance (X-linked), the absence of corneal clouding, and its milder clinical course.

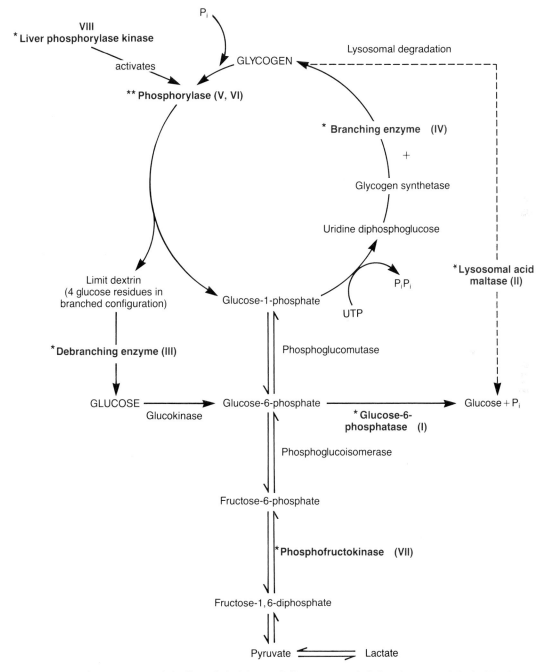

Figure 5–17. Pathways of glycogen metabolism. Asterisks mark the enzyme deficiencies associated with glycogen storage diseases. Roman numerals indicate the type of glycogen storage disease associated with the given enzyme deficiency. Types V and VI result from deficiencies of muscle and liver phosphorylases, respectively. (Modified and reproduced with permission from Hers, H., Van Hoof, F., and Barsy, T.: Glycogen storage diseases. *In* Scriver, C.R., Beaudet, A.L., Sly, W.S., and Valle, D. (eds.): The Metabolic Basis of Inherited Disease, 6th ed. New York, McGraw-Hill, 1989, p. 425.)

Glycogen Storage Diseases (Glycogenoses)

A number of genetic syndromes have been identified that result from some metabolic defect in the synthesis or catabolism of glycogen. The best understood and most important category includes the *glycogen storage diseases*, resulting from a hereditary deficiency of one of the enzymes involved in the synthesis or sequential degradation of glycogen. Depending on the tissue or organ distribution of the specific enzyme in the normal state, *glycogen storage in these disorders may be limited to a few tissues, may be more widespread while not affecting all tissues, or may be systemic in distribution.*

The significance of a specific enzyme deficiency is best understood from the perspective of the normal metabolism of glycogen (Fig. 5–17). As is well known, glycogen is a storage form of glucose. Glycogen synthesis begins with the conversion of glucose to glucose-6-phosphate by the action of a hexokinase (glucokinase). A phosphoglucomutase then transforms the glucose-6-phosphate to glucose-1-phosphate, which in turn is converted to uridine diphosphoglucose. A highly branched, very large polymer is then built up (molecular weight up to 100,000,000), containing up to 10,000 glucose molecules linked together by α-1,4-glucoside bonds. The glycogen chain and branches continue to be elongated by the addition of glucose molecules mediated by glycogen synthetases. During degradation, distinct phosphorylases in the liver and muscle split glucose-1-phosphate from the glycogen until about four glucose residues remain on each branch, leaving a branched oligosaccharide called limit dextrin. This can be further degraded only by the debranching enzyme. In addition to these major pathways, glycogen is also degraded in the lysosomes by acid maltase. If the lysosomes are deficient in this enzyme, the glycogen contained within them is not accessible to degradation by cytoplasmic enzymes such as phosphorylases.

On the basis of specific enzyme deficiencies and the resultant clinical pictures, glycogenoses have traditionally been divided into a dozen or so syndromes designated by roman numerals, and the list continues to grow. Rather than describing each syndrome, we offer a more manageable classification that is based on the pathophysiology of these disorders.[28] According to this approach, glycogenoses can be divided into three major subgroups.

• *Hepatic forms.* As is well known, liver is a key player in glycogen metabolism. It contains enzymes that synthesize glycogen for storage and ultimately break it down into free glucose, which is then released into the blood. An inherited deficiency of hepatic enzymes that are involved in

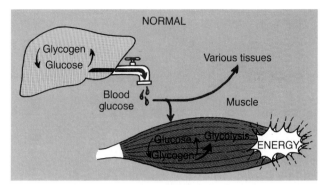

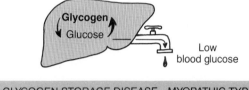

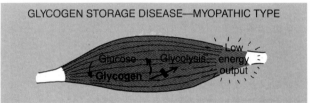

Figure 5–18. Simplified schema of normal glycogen metabolism in the liver and skeletal muscles *(top)*. The middle panel illustrates the effects of an inherited deficiency of hepatic enzymes involved in glycogen metabolism. The lower panel shows the consequences of a genetic deficiency in the enzymes that metabolize glycogen in skeletal muscles.

glycogen metabolism therefore leads not only to the storage of glycogen in the liver but also to a reduction in blood glucose level (hypoglycemia) (Fig. 5–18). Deficiency of the enzyme glucose-6-phosphatase (von Gierke disease, or type I glycogenosis) is a prime example of the hepatic-hypoglycemic form of glycogen storage disease (Table 5–6). Other examples include lack of liver phosphorylase and debranching enzyme, both involved in the breakdown of glycogen (see Fig. 5–17). In all these cases, glycogen is stored in many organs, but the *hepatic enlargement and hypoglycemia dominate the clinical picture.*

• *Myopathic forms.* In the striated muscles, as opposed to the liver, glycogen is used predominantly as a source of energy. This is derived by glycolysis, which leads ultimately to the formation of lactate (see Fig. 5–18). If the enzymes that fuel the glycolytic pathway are deficient, glycogen storage occurs in the muscles and is associated with muscular weakness owing to impaired energy production. Examples in this category include deficiencies of muscle phosphory-

Table 5-6. PRINCIPAL SUBGROUPS OF GLYCOGENOSES

CLINICOPATHOLOGIC CATEGORY	SPECIFIC TYPE	ENZYME DEFICIENCY	MORPHOLOGIC CHANGES	CLINICAL FEATURES
Hepatic type	Hepatorenal—von Gierke disease (type I)	Glucose-6-phosphatase	Hepatomegaly—intracytoplasmic accumulations of glycogen and small amounts of lipid; intranuclear glycogen Renomegaly—intracytoplasmic accumulations of glycogen in cortical tubular epithelial cells	Failure to thrive, stunted growth, hepatomegaly, and renomegaly. Hypoglycemia due to failure of glucose mobilization, often leading to convulsions. Hyperlipidemia and hyperuricemia resulting from deranged glucose metabolism; many patients develop gout and skin xanthomas. Bleeding tendency due to platelet dysfunction. Mortality approximately 50%
Myopathic type	McArdle syndrome (type V)	Muscle phosphorylase	Skeletal muscle only—accumulations of glycogen predominant in subsarcolemmal location	Painful cramps associated with strenuous exercise. Myoglobinuria occurs in 50% of cases. Onset in adulthood (>20 years of age). Muscular exercise fails to raise lactate level in venous blood. Compatible with normal longevity
Miscellaneous types	Generalized glycogenosis—Pompe disease (type II)	Lysosomal glucosidase (acid maltase)	Mild hepatomegaly—ballooning of lysosomes with glycogen creating lacy cytoplasmic pattern Cardiomegaly—glycogen within sarcoplasm as well as membrane-bound Skeletal muscle—similar to heart (see Cardiomegaly)	Massive cardiomegaly, muscle hypotonia, and cardiorespiratory failure within 2 years. A milder adult form with only skeletal muscle involvement presenting with chronic myopathy

lase (McArdle disease, or type V glycogenosis), muscle phosphofructokinase (type VII glycogen storage disease), and several others.[29] *Typically, patients with the myopathic forms present with muscle cramps following exercise and a failure of exercise-induced rise in blood lactate levels owing to a block in glycolysis.*

- Glycogen storage diseases associated with (1) deficiency of α-glucosidase (acid maltase) and (2) lack of branching enzyme do not fit into the hepatic or myopathic categories just described. They are associated with glycogen storage in many organs and death early in life. Acid maltase is a lysosomal enzyme, and hence its deficiency leads to lysosomal storage of glycogen (type II glycogenosis, or Pompe disease) in all organs, but cardiomegaly is most prominent (Fig. 5-19). Brancher glycogenosis (type IV) is associated with widespread deposition of an abnormal form

of glycogen with detrimental effects on the brain, heart, skeletal muscles, and liver.

The principal features of some important examples from each of the aforementioned three categories are summarized in Table 5-6. Details of other forms may be found in specialized texts.[30]

Alkaptonuria (Ochronosis)

In this autosomal recessive disorder, *the lack of homogentisic oxidase blocks the metabolism of phenylalanine-tyrosine at the level of homogentisic acid.* Thus, homogentisic acid accumulates in the body. A large amount is excreted, imparting a black color to the urine if allowed to stand and undergo oxidation.[31]

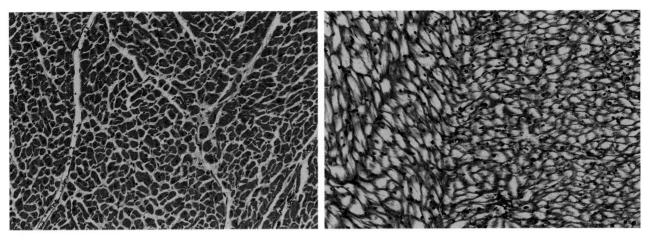

Figure 5-19. Pompe disease (glycogen storage disease type II). The left frame shows normal myocardium with abundant eosinophilic cytoplasm. The right frame (at the same magnification) from a patient with Pompe disease shows the myocardial fibers full of glycogen seen as clear spaces. (Courtesy of Dr. Trace Worrell, Department of Pathology, University of Texas Southwestern Medical School, Dallas.)

MORPHOLOGY. The retained homogentisic acid selectively binds to collagen in connective tissues, tendons, and cartilage, imparting to these tissues a blue-black pigmentation **(ochronosis)** most evident in the ears, nose, and cheeks. **The most serious consequences of ochronosis, however, stem from deposits of the pigment in the articular cartilages of the joints.** In some obscure manner, the pigmentation causes the cartilage to lose its normal resiliency and become brittle and fibrillated.[32] Wear-and-tear erosion of this abnormal cartilage leads to denudation of the subchondral bone, and often tiny fragments of the fibrillated cartilage are driven into the underlying bone, worsening the damage. The vertebral column, particularly the intervertebral disc, is the prime site of attack, but later the knees, shoulders, and hips may be affected. The small joints of the hands and feet are usually spared.

Although the metabolic defect is present from birth, the degenerative arthropathy develops slowly and usually does not become clinically evident until the fourth decade of life. Although it is not life-threatening, it may be severely crippling. The disability may be as extreme as that encountered in the severe forms of osteoarthritis (see Chapter 27) of the elderly, but, unfortunately, in alkaptonuria the arthropathy occurs at a much earlier age.

DISORDERS ASSOCIATED WITH DEFECTS IN PROTEINS THAT REGULATE CELL GROWTH

Normal growth and differentiation of cells is regulated by two classes of genes: proto-oncogenes and tumor-suppressor genes, whose products promote or restrain cell growth (see Chapters 2 and 7). It is now well established that mutations in these two classes of genes are important in the pathogenesis of tumors. In the vast majority of cases, cancer-causing mutations affect somatic cells and hence are not passed in the germ line. In approximately 5% of all cancers, however, mutations transmitted through the germ line contribute to the development of cancer. Most familial cancers are inherited in an autosomal dominant fashion, but a few recessive disorders have also been described. This subject is discussed in greater detail in Chapter 7. Here we provide an example of two common familial neoplasms.

Neurofibromatosis: Types 1 and 2

Neurofibromatoses comprise at least two autosomal dominant disorders, affecting approximately 100,000 people in the United States. They are referred to as neurofibromatosis type 1 (also called von Recklinghausen disease) and neurofibromatosis type 2 (also called acoustic neurofibromatosis). Although there is some overlap in clinical features, these two entities are genetically distinct.[33] Neurofibromatosis-1 is a relatively common disorder with a frequency of almost 1 in 3000. Although approximately 50% of the patients have a definite family history consistent with autosomal dominant transmission, the remainder appear to represent new mutations. In familial cases, the expressivity of the disorder is extremely variable, but the penetrance is 100%. Neurofibromatosis-1 has three major features: (1) *multiple neural tumors dispersed anywhere on or in the body;* (2) *numerous pigmented skin lesions, some of which are "café au lait" spots;* and (3) *pigmented iris hamartomas, also called*

Lisch nodules. A bewildering assortment of other abnormalities (cited later) may accompany these cardinal manifestations.

MORPHOLOGY. The neurofibromas arise within or are attached to nerve trunks anywhere in the skin, including the palms and soles, as well as in every conceivable internal site, including the cranial nerves (particularly the acoustic nerve). Acoustic neuromas when they occur in classic neurofibromatosis-1 are unilateral, in contrast to the bilateral tumors in neurofibromatosis-2, to be described later. On the surface of the body, neurofibromas generally occur in profusion and range from discrete, soft, yielding, subcutaneous nodules less than 1 cm in diameter; to moderate-sized pedunculated lesions; to huge, multilobar pendulous masses, 20 cm or more in greatest diameter. The last, referred to as plexiform neurofibromas, diffusely involve subcutaneous tissue and contain numerous tortuous, thickened nerves; the overlying skin is frequently hyperpigmented. These may grow to massive proportions, causing striking enlargement of a limb or some other body part. Similar tumors may occur internally, and in general the deeply situated lesions tend to be large. Microscopically neurofibromas are composed of a proliferation of all the elements in the peripheral nerve, including neurites, Schwann cells, and fibroblasts. Typically, these components are dispersed in a loose, disorderly pattern, often in a loose, myxoid stroma. Elongated, serpentine Schwann cells predominate, with their slender, spindle-shaped nuclei. The loose disorderliness of the microscopic architecture helps differentiate these neural tumors from related neurilemmomas (schwannomas). Neurilemmomas composed entirely of Schwann cells virtually never undergo malignant transformation, whereas the neurofibromas of von Recklinghausen disease become malignant in about 3% of patients.[34] Malignant transformation is most common in the very large plexiform tumors attached to large nerve trunks of the neck or extremities. The superficial lesions, despite their size, rarely become malignant.

The cutaneous pigmentations, the second major component of this syndrome, are present in more than 90% of patients. Most commonly they appear as light brown **café au lait** macules, with generally smooth borders, often located over nerve trunks. They are usually round to ovoid, with their long axes parallel to the underlying cutaneous nerve. Although normal individuals may have a few café au lait spots, it is a clinical maxim that when six or more spots over 1.5 cm in diameter are present, the patient is likely to have neurofibromatosis.

Lisch nodules (pigmented hamartomas in the iris) are present in more than 94% of patients who are six years old or older. They do not produce any symptoms but are helpful in establishing the diagnosis.

A wide range of associated abnormalities has been reported in these patients. Perhaps most common (seen in 30 to 50% of patients) are skeletal lesions, which take a variety of forms, including (1) erosive defects due to contiguity of neurofibromas to bone, (2) scoliosis, (3) intraosseous cystic lesions, (4) subperiosteal bone cysts, and (5) pseudarthrosis of the tibia. Patients with von Recklinghausen disease have a twofold to fourfold greater risk of developing other tumors, especially meningiomas, optic gliomas, and pheochromocytomas.

Although some patients with this condition have normal mentality, there is an unmistakable tendency for reduced intelligence. When neurofibromas arise within the gastrointestinal tract, intestinal obstruction or gastrointestinal bleeding may occur. Narrowing of a renal artery by a tumor may induce hypertension. Owing to variable expression of the gene, the range of clinical presentations is almost limitless, but ultimately the diagnosis rests on the concurrence of multiple café au lait spots and multiple skin tumors. The neurofibromatosis-1 (NF-1) gene has been mapped to chromosome 17q11.2. It encodes a protein called neurofibromin, which down-regulates the function of the p21 *ras* oncoprotein (see section on oncogenes, Chapter 7). NF-1 therefore belongs to the family of tumor suppressor genes.[35]

Type 2 neurofibromatosis is much less frequent than type 1. In these patients, bilateral acoustic nerve tumors are invariably present with or without skin tumors. Café au lait spots are present, but Lisch nodules in the iris are not found. The gene for type 2 neurofibromatosis is also a tumor suppressor gene, which has been mapped to chromosome 22.[36] It encodes a protein that links integral membrane proteins with the cytoskeleton. How such a protein is involved in tumorigenesis is not known.

DISORDERS WITH MULTIFACTORIAL INHERITANCE

As pointed out earlier, the multifactorial disorders are believed to result from the combined actions of environmental influences and two or more mutant genes having additive effects. The genetic component, then, exerts a dosage effect—the greater the number of inherited deleterious genes, the more severe the expression of the disease. Because environmental factors significantly influence the expression of these genetic disorders, the term polygenic inheritance should not be used.

A number of normal phenotypic characteristics are governed by multifactorial inheritance, such as hair color, eye color, skin color, height, and intelligence. These characteristics exhibit a continuous variation in population groups, producing the standard bell-shaped curve of distribution. Environmental influences, however, significantly modify the phenotypic expression of multifactorial traits. For example, certain subsets of diabetes mellitus have many of the features of a multifactorial disorder. It is well recognized clinically that individuals often first manifest this disease following weight gain. Thus, obesity as well as other environmental influences unmasks the diabetic genetic trait. Nutritional influences may cause even monozygous twins to achieve different heights. The culturally deprived child cannot achieve his or her full intellectual capacity.

The following features characterize multifactorial inheritance. These have been established for the multifactorial inheritance of congenital malformations and, in all likelihood, obtain for other multifactorial diseases.[37]

- *The risk of expressing a multifactorial disorder is conditioned by the number of mutant genes inherited. Thus, the risk is greater in sibs of patients having severe expressions of the disorder.*
- *Environmental influences significantly modify the risk of expressing the disease.*
- *The rate of recurrence of the disorder (in the range of 2 to 7%) is the same for all first-degree relatives, i.e., parents, sibs, and offspring, of the affected individual. Thus, if parents have had one affected child, the risk that the next child will be affected is between 2 and 7%. Similarly, there is the same chance that one of the parents will be affected.*
- *The likelihood that both identical twins will be affected is significantly less than 100% but is much greater than the chance that both nonidentical twins will be affected. Experience has proved, for example, that the frequency of concordance for identical twins is in the range of 20 to 40%.*
- *The risk of recurrence of the phenotypic abnormality in subsequent pregnancies depends on the outcome in previous pregnancies. When one child is affected, there is up to a 7% chance that the next child will be affected, but after two affected sibs, the risk rises to about 9%.*
- *Severity of expression of the disease may range along a bell-shaped curve or may be discontinuous. Despite the polygenic mode of inheritance, a threshold may exist beyond which individuals are at risk. Thus, for some multifactorial disorders, it appears that inheritance of a certain number of mutant genes is required before the disorder is expressed. As stated before, however, environmental influences still play a role.*

Table 5–7. MULTIFACTORIAL DISORDERS

DISORDER	CHAPTER
Cleft lip or cleft palate (or both)	Chapter 16
Congenital heart disease	Chapter 12
Coronary heart disease	Chapter 12
Hypertension	Chapter 11
Gout	Chapter 27
Diabetes mellitus	Chapter 19
Pyloric stenosis	Chapter 17

Assigning a disease to this mode of inheritance must be done with caution. It depends on many factors but first of all on familial clustering and the exclusion of mendelian and chromosomal modes of transmission. A range of levels of severity of a disease is suggestive of multifactorial inheritance, but, as pointed out earlier, variable expressivity and reduced penetrance of mendelian mutant genes may also account for this phenomenon. Because of these difficulties, there is often disagreement as to whether the pedigree conforms to a mendelian or multifactorial pattern, as is the case, for example, with diabetes mellitus and epilepsy. The problem is well put in the statement: "Multifactorial inheritance is a geneticist's nightmare."

In contrast to the mendelian disorders, which must be considered uncommon, the multifactorial group includes some of the most common ailments to which humans are heir (Table 5–7). Most of these disorders are described in appropriate chapters elsewhere in this book.

THE NORMAL KARYOTYPE

As is well known, human somatic cells contain 46 chromosomes; these comprise 22 homologous pairs of autosomes and two sex chromosomes, XX in the female and XY in the male. The study of chromosomes—karyotyping—is the basic tool of the cytogeneticist. The usual procedure of producing a chromosome spread is to arrest mitosis in cultured cells in metaphase by the use of colchicine and then to stain the chromosomes. In a metaphase spread, the individual chromosomes take the form of two chromatids connected at the centromere. Before 1970, the techniques utilized in karyotyping resulted in solid, dark staining of the chromosomes, and hence only limited distinction of chromosomes was possible; they were classified into seven groups (A through G) based on their size and the position of the centromere.

In 1970, Caspersson and colleagues described the identification of each individual chromosome on the basis of a distinctive and reliable pattern of alternating light and dark bands along the length of the chromosome. Although a number of *banding techniques* have since been developed, G (Giemsa)

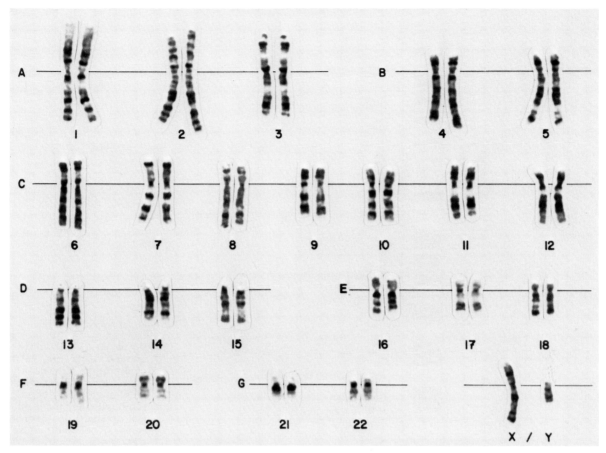

Figure 5-20. A normal male karyotype with G banding. (Courtesy of Dr. Nancy R. Schneider, Department of Pathology, University of Texas Southwestern Medical Center, Dallas.)

banding is the most widely used. A normal male karyotype with G banding is illustrated in Figure 5-20. With G banding, approximately 300 to 500 bands per haploid set can be detected. Because genes vary greatly in size, each band may harbor anywhere from a few to many individual genes. In recent years, the resolution obtained by banding techniques has been dramatically improved by obtaining the cells in prophase. The individual chromosomes appear markedly elongated, and up to 1500 bands per karyotype may be recognized.[38] The use of these banding techniques permits certain identification of each chromosome as well as delineation of precise breakpoints and other subtle alterations, to be described later.

Before this discussion of the normal karyotype is concluded, reference must be made to commonly used cytogenetic terminology. Karyotypes are usually described using a shorthand system of notations. In general, the following order is used: Total number of chromosomes is given first, followed by the sex chromosome complement, and finally the description of any abnormality. For example, a male with trisomy 21 is designated 47,XY,+21. The notations denoting structural alterations of chromosomes are described along with

the abnormalities in a later section. Here we should mention that the short arm of a chromosome is designated "p" (for petit) and the long arm is referred to as "q" (the next letter of alphabet). In a banded karyotype, each arm of the chromosome is divided into two or more regions by prominent bands. The regions are numbered (e.g., 1, 2, 3) from the centromere outward. Each region is further subdivided into bands and sub-bands, and these are ordered numerically as well (Fig. 5-21). Thus, the notation Xp21.2 refers to a chromosomal segment located on the short arm of the X chromosome, in region 2, band 1 and sub-band 2.

INTERPHASE CYTOGENETICS. Until recently, karyotyping was the only method available for the study of chromosomes. A major limitation of karyotyping is that it is applicable only to cells that are dividing or can be induced to divide in culture. With DNA probes, this problem can be overcome, at least partly. For example, it is possible to construct DNA probes that recognize chromosome-specific repetitive sequences. Such DNA probes can be labeled with fluorescent dyes and applied to interphase nuclei. The probe binds to its target site in the DNA and thus labels the specific chromosome.

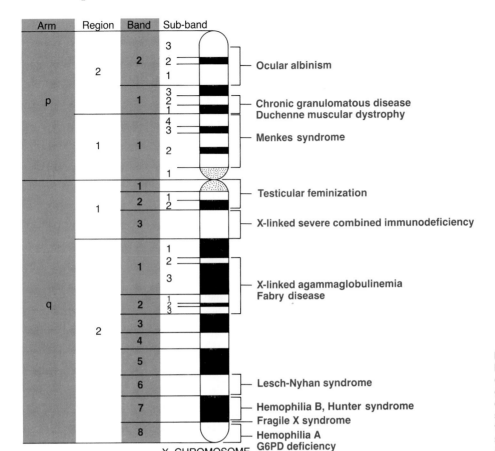

Arm	Region	Band	Sub-band

Ocular albinism

Chronic granulomatous disease
Duchenne muscular dystrophy

Menkes syndrome

Testicular feminization

X-linked severe combined immunodeficiency

X-linked agammaglobulinemia
Fabry disease

Lesch-Nyhan syndrome

Hemophilia B, Hunter syndrome
Fragile X syndrome
Hemophilia A
G6PD deficiency

X–CHROMOSOME

Figure 5–21. Details of a banded karyotype of the X chromosome (also called idiogram). Note the nomenclature of arms, regions, bands, and sub-bands. On the right side, the approximate locations of some genes that cause disease are indicated.

This technique is called fluorescent *in situ* hybridization (FISH). An example of its application is to enumerate chromosomes in interphase nuclei. In a normal diploid cell, a chromosome-specific fluorescent probe is seen as two bright dots when examined under ultraviolet light (Fig. 5–22). "Chromosome painting" is an emerging extension of this technique that uses a collection of probes that recognize unique DNA sequences along the entire length of a given chromosome. This then causes the entire chromosome to fluoresce after *in situ* hybridization with the collection of sequences.

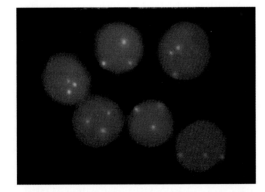

Figure 5–22. Fluorescent *in situ* hybridization (FISH). Interphase nuclei of a childhood hepatic cancer (hepatoblastoma) stained with a fluorescent DNA probe that hybridizes to chromosome 20. Under ultraviolet light each nucleus reveals three bright yellow fluorescent dots representing three copies of chromosome 20. Normal diploid cells (not shown) have two fluorescent dots. (Courtesy of Dr. Vijay Tonk, Department of Pathology, University of Texas Southwestern Medical School, Dallas.)

CYTOGENETIC DISORDERS

The aberrations underlying cytogenetic disorders (chromosome mutations) may take the form of an abnormal number of chromosomes or alterations in the structure of one or more chromosomes. The normal chromosome count is expressed as 46,XX for the female and 46,XY for the male. Any exact multiple of the haploid number is called *euploid*. If an error occurs in meiosis or mitosis, however, and a cell acquires a chromosome complement that is not an exact multiple of 23, it is referred to as *aneuploidy*. The usual causes for aneuploidy are *nondisjunction* and *anaphase lag*. The former occurs when a homologous pair of chromosomes fails to disjoin at the first meiotic division, or the two chromatids fail to separate either at the second meiotic division or in somatic cell divisions, resulting in two aneuploid cells. When nondisjunction occurs during gametogenesis, the gametes formed have either an extra chromosome (n + 1) or one less chromosome (n − 1). Fertilization of such gametes by normal gametes would result in two types of zygotes—trisomic (2n + 1) or monosomic (2n − 1). In anaphase lag, one homologous chromosome in meiosis or one chromatid in mitosis lags behind and is left out of the cell nucleus. The result is one normal cell and one cell with monosomy. As will be seen, monosomy or trisomy involving the sex chromosomes, or even more bizarre aberrations, is compatible with life and is usually associated with variable degrees of phenotypic abnormalities. *Monosomy involving an autosome generally represents loss of too much genetic information to permit live birth or even embryogenesis, but a number of autosomal trisomies do permit survival.* With the exception of trisomy 21, all yield severely handicapped infants who almost invariably die at an early age.

Occasionally, *mitotic errors in early development give rise to two or more populations of cells in the same individual, a condition referred to as mosaicism.* This can result from mitotic errors during the cleavage of the fertilized ovum or in somatic cells. Mosaicism affecting the sex chromosomes is relatively common. In the division of the fertilized ovum, an error may lead to one of the daughter cells receiving three sex chromosomes, whereas the other receives only one, yielding, for example, a 45,X/47,XXX mosaic. All descendent cells derived from each of these precursors thus have either a 47,XXX count or a 45,X count. Such a patient would be a mosaic variant of Turner syndrome, with the extent of phenotypic expression dependent on the number and distribution of the 45,X cells. If the error occurs at a later cleavage, the mosaic will have three populations of cells, with some possessing the normal 46,XX complement, i.e., 45,X/46,XX/47,XXX. Repeated mitotic errors may lead to many populations of cells.

Autosomal mosaicism appears to be much less common than that involving the sex chromosomes. An error in an early mitotic division affecting the autosomes usually leads to a nonviable mosaic with autosomal monosomy. Rarely, the loss of a nonviable cell in embryogenesis is tolerated, yielding a mosaic, e.g., 46,XY/47,XY,+21. Such a patient would be a trisomy 21 mosaic with partial expression of the Down syndrome, depending on the proportion of cells expressing the trisomy.

A second category of chromosomal aberrations is associated with changes in the structure of chromosomes. To be visible by currently available banding techniques, a fairly large amount of DNA (approximately 4 million base pairs), containing several genes, must be involved. Structural changes in chromosomes usually result from chromosome breakage followed by loss or rearrangement of material. Such alterations occur spontaneously at a low rate that is increased by exposure to environmental mutagens, such as chemicals and ionizing radiations. In addition, several rare autosomal recessive genetic disorders—Fanconi anemia, Bloom syndrome, and ataxia-telangiectasia—are associated with such a high level of chromosomal instability that they are known as "chromosome-breakage syndromes." As discussed later, in Chapter 7, there is a significantly increased risk of cancers in all these conditions. In the following section, we briefly review the more common forms of alterations in chromosome structure and the notations used to signify them.

Deletion refers to loss of a portion of chromosome. It may be terminal or interstitial. Terminal deletions result from a single break in the arm of a chromosome, producing a fragment with no centromere, which is then lost at the next cell division. This might be designated as 46,XY,16p− to indicate loss of some part of the short arm of chromosome 16 (see Fig. 5–23). One can specify in which region and at what band the break and deletion has occurred, as, for example, 46,XY,del(16)(p14), meaning a break point in region 1 band 4 of the short arm of chromosome 16. Interstitial deletions occur when there are two breaks in the chromosome followed by loss of the region between the breaks.

In *translocation*, a segment of one chromosome is transferred to another (Fig. 5–23). In one form, called *balanced reciprocal translocation*, there are single breaks in each of two chromosomes, with exchange of material. Such a translocation might not be disclosed without banding techniques. A balanced reciprocal translocation between the long arm of chromosome 2 and the short arm of chromosome 5 would be written 46,XX,t(2;5)(q31;p14). This individual has 46 chromosomes with altered morphology of one of the chromosomes 2 and one of the chromosomes 5. Because there has been no loss of genetic material, the individual will be phenotypically normal. A balanced translocation carrier, however, is at increased risk for producing abnormal gametes. For example, in the case previously cited, a gamete containing one normal chromosome 2 and a translocated chromosome 5 may be formed. Such a gamete would be unbalanced, since it would not contain the normal complement of genetic material. Subsequent fertilization by a normal gamete would lead to the formation of an abnormal (unbalanced) zygote, resulting in spontaneous abortion or birth of a malformed child. The other important pattern of translocation is called a *Robertsonian translocation* (or centric fusion), a reciprocal translocation between two acrocentric chromosomes. Typically the breaks occur close to the centromeres of each chromosome, affecting the long arm in one and the short arm in the other. Transfer of the segments then leads to one very large chromosome and one extremely small one. Often, the small product is lost (see Fig. 5–23); however, it carries so little genetic information that this loss is compatible

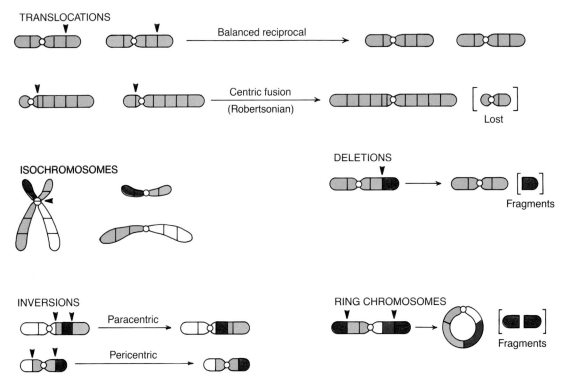

Figure 5–23. Types of chromosomal rearrangements.

with a normal phenotype, and Robertsonian translocation between two chromosomes is encountered in apparently normal individuals. The significance of this form of translocation also lies in the production of abnormal progeny, as discussed later with Down syndrome.

Isochromosome formation results when one arm of a chromosome is lost and the remaining arm is duplicated, resulting in a chromosome consisting of two short arms only or of two long arms (see Fig. 5–23). An isochromosome has genetic information that is morphologically identical in both arms. The most common isochromosome present in live births involves the long arm of the X and is designated i(Xq). The i(Xq) isochromosome is associated with monosomy for genes on the short arm of X and with trisomy for genes on the long arm of X.

A *ring chromosome* is a special form of deletion. It is produced when a deletion occurs at both ends of a chromosome with fusion of the damaged ends (see Fig. 5–23). If significant genetic material is lost, phenotypic abnormalities result. This might be expressed as 46,XY,r(14). Ring chromosomes do not behave normally in meiosis or mitosis and usually result in serious consequences.

Inversion refers to a rearrangement that involves two breaks within a single chromosome with reincorporation of the inverted segment (see Fig. 5–23). Such an inversion involving only one arm of the chromosome is known as paracentric. If the breaks are on opposite sides of the centromere, it

is known as pericentric. Inversions are perfectly compatible with normal development.

Many more numerical and structural aberrations are described in specialized texts, and the number of abnormal karyotypes encountered in genetic diseases increases with each passing month. As pointed out earlier, the clinically important chromosome disorders represent only the "tip of the iceberg." It is estimated that approximately 7.5% of all conceptions have a chromosomal abnormality, most of which are not compatible with survival or live birth. Thus, chromosome abnormalities are identified in 50% of early spontaneous abortuses and in 5% of stillbirths and infants who die in the immediate postnatal period. Even in live-born infants, the frequency is approximately 0.5 to 1.0%. It is beyond the scope of this book to discuss most of the clinically recognizable chromosomal disorders. Hence we focus our attention on those few that are most common.

CYTOGENETIC DISORDERS INVOLVING AUTOSOMES

Trisomy 21 (Down Syndrome)

Down syndrome is the most common of the chromosomal disorders and a major cause of mental retardation. In the United States, the incidence in newborns is about 1 in 800.[39] Approximately 95%

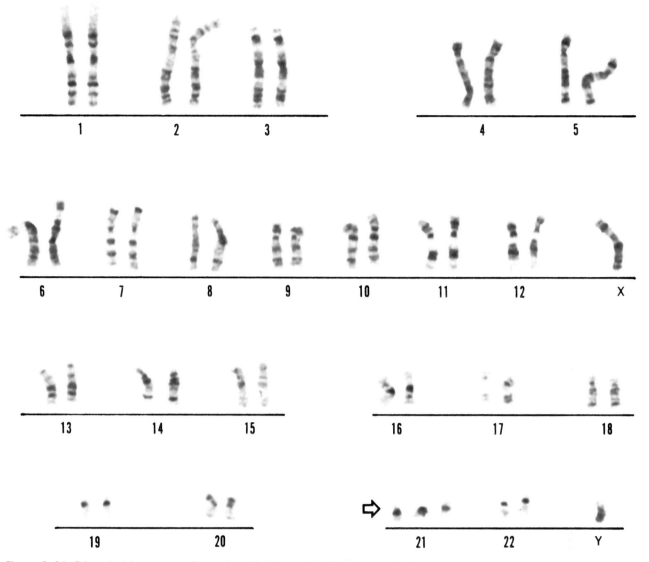

Figure 5-24. G-banded karyotype of a male with trisomy 21. (Courtesy of Dr. Patricia Howard-Peebles, University of Texas, Southwestern Medical School, Dallas.)

of affected individuals have trisomy 21, so their chromosome count is 47 (Fig. 5-24); most others have normal chromosome numbers, but the extra chromosomal material is present as a translocation. As mentioned earlier, the most common cause of trisomy and therefore of Down syndrome is meiotic nondisjunction. The parents of such children have a normal karyotype and are normal in all respects.

Maternal age has a strong influence on the incidence of Down syndrome. It occurs once in 1550 live births in women under the age of 20 years, in contrast to 1 in 25 live births for mothers over 45 years of age.[5] The correlation with maternal age suggests that in most cases the meiotic nondisjunction of chromosome 21 occurs in the ovum. Indeed, studies in which DNA polymorphisms were used to trace the parental origin of chromosome 21

have revealed that in 95% of the cases with trisomy 21, the extra chromosome is of maternal origin.[40] Although many hypotheses have been advanced, the reason for the increased susceptibility of the ovum to nondisjunction remains unknown.

In about 4% of all cases of Down syndrome, the extra chromosomal material derives from the presence of a Robertsonian translocation of the long arm of chromosome 21 to another acrocentric chromosome, e.g., 22 or 14. Because the fertilized ovum already possesses two normal autosomes 21, the translocated material provides the same triple gene dosage as in trisomy 21. Such cases are frequently (but not always) familial, and the translocated chromosome is inherited from one of the parents, who is a carrier of a Robertsonian translocation, for example, mother with karyotype 45,XX,−14,−21,+t(14q 21q). In those cases where neither parent is a carrier of the transloca-tion, the rearrangement occurs during gametogen-esis. Theoretically the carrier parent has a one in three chance of bearing a live child with Down syndrome; however, the observed frequency of af-fected children in such cases is much lower. The reasons for this discrepancy are not well under-stood.

Approximately 1% of Down syndrome patients are mosaics, usually having a mixture of cells with 46 and 47 chromosomes. This results from mitotic nondisjunction of chromosome 21 during an early stage of embryogenesis. Symptoms in such cases are variable and milder, depending on the propor-tion of abnormal cells. Clearly, in cases of translo-cation or mosaic Down syndrome, maternal age is of no importance.

The diagnostic clinical features of this condi-tion, illustrated in Figure 5-25, are usually readily evident, even at birth. The flat facial profile, oblique palpebral fissures, and epicanthic folds ac-count for the older, unfortunate designations "mongolism" and "mongolian idiocy." Down syn-drome is a leading cause of mental retardation. The mental retardation is severe; approximately 80% of those afflicted have an intelligence quotient (IQ) of 25 to 50. Ironically, these severely disadvantaged children usually have a gentle, shy manner and are far more easily directed than their more fortunate siblings, less burdened with chromosomes. It should be pointed out that some mosaics with Down syndrome have very mild phenotypic changes and may even have normal or near-normal intelligence.

In addition to the phenotypic abnormalities and the mental retardation already noted, some other clinical features are worthy of note.

- Approximately 40% of the patients have congen-ital heart disease, most commonly defects of the endocardial cushion, including ostium primum, atrial septal defect, atrioventricular valve malfor-mations, and ventricular septal defects. Cardiac problems are responsible for the majority of the deaths in infancy and early childhood.
- Children with trisomy 21 have a 10-fold to 20-fold increased risk of developing acute leukemia. Both acute lymphoblastic leukemias and acute nonlymphoblastic leukemias occur. The relative distribution of these two types of leukemia is similar for children with and without Down syn-drome.
- Virtually all patients with trisomy 21 older than 40 years of age develop neuropathologic changes characteristic of Alzheimer disease, a form of se-nile dementia.[41]
- Patients with Down syndrome have abnormal im-mune responses that predispose them to serious infections, particularly of the lungs, and to thy-roid autoimmunity. Although several abnormali-ties, affecting mainly T cell subsets, have been

reported, the cellular basis of immunologic dis-turbances is not clear.[42]

Despite all these problems, improved medical care has increased the longevity of patients with trisomy 21. Currently more than 80% survive to age 30 or beyond.

Although the karyotype and clinical features of trisomy 21 have been known for well over three decades, little is known about the molecular basis of Down syndrome. Advances in gene mapping, however, have begun to penetrate the mystery.[43] By a careful study of patients with the transloca-tion variant of Down syndrome who exhibit partial trisomy 21, it has been determined that the region of chromosome 21 that is required for the expres-sion of the facial, neurologic, and cardiovascular changes is limited to the 21q22.2 and 21q22.3 re-gion. Genes located within this "obligate Down syndrome region" must be critical to the patho-genesis of the Down syndrome phenotype (Fig. 5-26). Although this region of chromosome 21 is large enough to accommodate several hundred genes, only a handful have been assigned to this area. Mapping of additional genes and relating their molecular effects to the phenotypic changes is progressing rapidly.

Other Trisomies

A variety of other trisomies, involving chromo-somes 8, 9, 22, 18, and 13, have been described. Only trisomy 18 (Edwards syndrome) and trisomy 13 (Patau syndrome) are common enough to merit brief mention here. As noted in Figure 5-25, they share several karyotypic and clinical features with trisomy 21. Thus, most cases result from meiotic nondisjunction and therefore carry a complete extra copy of chromosome 18 or 13. As in Down syndrome, an association with increased maternal age is also noted. In contrast to trisomy 21, how-ever, the malformations are much more severe and wide-ranging. As a result, only rarely do these in-fants survive beyond the first year of life. Most succumb within a few weeks to months.

Cri du Chat Syndrome (5p−)

Deletion of the short arm of chromosome 5 (5p−) was so named because affected infants up to the age of one year have the characteristic cry of a cat. The major clinical features include severe mental retardation, microcephaly, and round facies. In general, these children thrive better than those with the trisomies, and some survive into adult life. As the infant grows older, the kitten cry and high

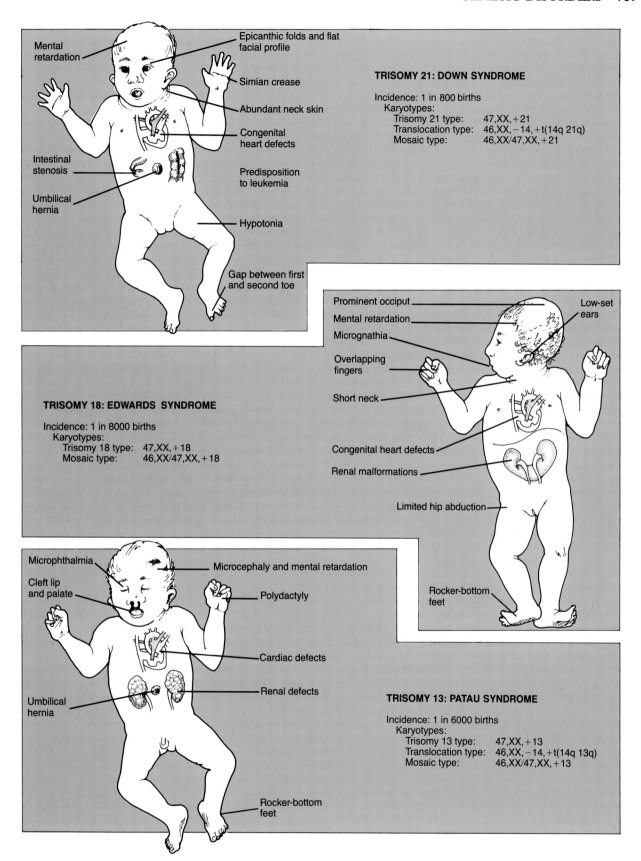

TRISOMY 21: DOWN SYNDROME

Incidence: 1 in 800 births
Karyotypes:
Trisomy 21 type: 47,XX,+21
Translocation type: 46,XX,−14,+t(14q 21q)
Mosaic type: 46,XX/47,XX,+21

TRISOMY 18: EDWARDS SYNDROME

Incidence: 1 in 8000 births
Karyotypes:
Trisomy 18 type: 47,XX,+18
Mosaic type: 46,XX/47,XX,+18

TRISOMY 13: PATAU SYNDROME

Incidence: 1 in 6000 births
Karyotypes:
Trisomy 13 type: 47,XX,+13
Translocation type: 46,XX,−14,+t(14q 13q)
Mosaic type: 46,XX/47,XX,+13

Figure 5–25. Clinical features of karyotypes of selected autosomal trisomies.

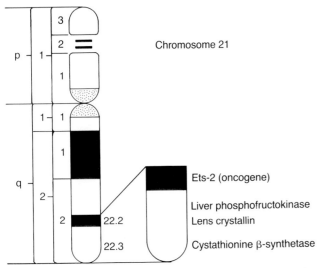

Figure 5–26. Idiogram of chromosome 21. The obligate Down syndrome region of 21q22.2 and 21q22.3 is enlarged, and genes mapped to this region are indicated. The orientation of these genes with respect to each other is not certain.

vocal register improve, rendering clinical diagnosis more difficult.

CYTOGENETIC DISORDERS INVOLVING SEX CHROMOSOMES

The genetic diseases associated with karyotypic changes involving the sex chromosomes are far more common than those related to autosomal aberrations. Furthermore, imbalances (excess or loss) of sex chromosomes are much better tolerated than similar imbalances of autosomes. In large part, this latitude relates to two factors that are peculiar to the sex chromosomes: (1) lyonization or inactivation of all but one X chromosome, and (2) the small amount of genetic material carried by the Y chromosome. We discuss these features briefly to aid our understanding of sex-chromosomal disorders.

In 1961, Mary Lyon outlined the X-inactivation, or what is commonly known as the Lyon, hypothesis. It states that *(1) only one of the X chromosomes is genetically active, (2) the other X of either maternal or paternal origin undergoes heteropyknosis and is rendered inactive, (3) inactivation of either the maternal or paternal X occurs at random among all the cells of the blastocyst on or about the 16th day of embryonic life, and (4) inactivation of the same X chromosome persists in all the cells derived from each precursor cell.* Thus, the great preponderance of normal females are in reality mosaics and have two populations of cells, one with an inactivated maternal X and the other with an inactivated paternal X. Herein lies the explanation of why females have the same dosage of X-linked active genes as in the male. The inactive X can be seen in the interphase nucleus as a darkly staining small mass in contact with the nuclear membrane known as the Barr body or X chromatin. Barr bodies are present in all somatic cells of normal females, but they are most readily demonstrated in smears of buccal squamous epithelial cells.

Although the basic tenets of the Lyon hypothesis have stood the test of time, several modifications have been made. For example, at first it was thought that all the genes on the inactive X are "shut off." More recent molecular studies have revealed that many genes escape X-inactivation (Fig. 5–27). It is believed that at least some of the genes that are expressed from both X chromosomes are important for normal growth and development. This notion is supported by the fact that patients with monosomy of the X chromosome (Turner syndrome: 45,X) have severe somatic and gonadal abnormalities. If a single dose of X-linked genes were sufficient, no detrimental effect would be expected in such cases. Furthermore, although one X chromosome is inactivated in all cells during embryogenesis, it is selectively reactivated in germ cells before the first meiotic division. Thus, it seems that both X chromosomes are required for normal oogenesis.

The molecular basis of X-inactivation has remained mysterious, but breakthroughs are on the horizon. It is now certain that a gene that maps to Xq13 serves as a master switch that is critical for silencing the vast majority of genes on the inactive X chromosome. Quite surprisingly, this gene, called X-inactive–specific transcript gene (XIST), does not code for a protein. Apparently, the RNA transcript of the XIST gene never leaves the nucleus and, in some unexplained manner, prevents transcription of other genes on the X chromosome.[44] Abnormalities of the XIST gene that prevent normal X-inactivation may explain why in certain families female-to-female transmission of X-linked traits such as hemophilia occurs.

With respect to the Y chromosome, it is well known that this chromosome is both necessary and sufficient for male development. Indeed, *regardless of the number of X chromosomes, the presence of a single Y determines the male sex.* The gene that dictates testicular development (*Sry*: sex-determining region Y gene) has been located on its distal short arm.[45]

With this background, we can review some features that are common to all sex chromosome disorders.

- *In general, they induce subtle, chronic problems relating to sexual development and fertility.*
- *They are often difficult to diagnose at birth, and many are first recognized at the time of puberty.*
- *In general, the higher the number of X chromo-*

Genes known to be subject to X inactivation / Genes known to escape X inactivation

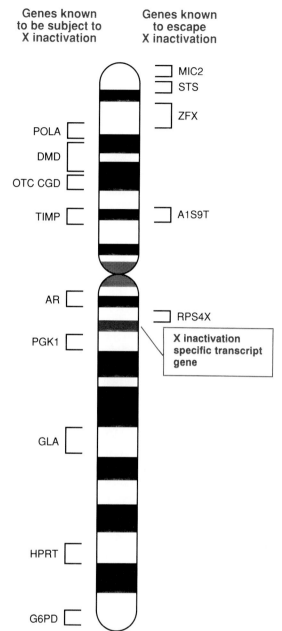

Figure 5–27. Schematic of X chromosome. Only a few important gene loci are indicated. Selected genes that are known to be subject to X-inactivation are shown at the left. Genes that escape inactivation and are expressed from both active and inactive Xs are shown on the right. The position of the X-inactivation specific transcript gene in Xq13 is shown in red. (Gene acronyms include *POLA*, DNA polymerase-alpha; *DMD*, Duchenne muscular dystrophy; *OTC*, ornithine transcarbamylase; *CGD*, chronic granulomatous disease; *TIMP*, tissue inhibitor of metalloproteinases; *AR*, androgen receptor; *PGK1*, phosphoglycerate kinase 1; *GLA*, alpha-galactosidase; *HPRT*, hypoxanthine phosphoribosyl-transferase; *G6PD*, glucose-6-phosphate dehydrogenase; *MIC2*, cell surface protein MIC2; *STS*, steroid sulfatase; *ZFX*, zinc-finger protein; *AIS9T*, ubiquitin-activating enzyme E1; *RPS4X*, ribosomal protein S4. (Modified with permission from Thompson, M.W., McInnes, R.R., and Willard, H.F.: Thompson and Thompson Genetics in Medicine, 5th ed. Philadelphia, W.B. Saunders Co., 1991, p. 237.)

somes, in both male and female, the greater the likelihood of mental retardation.

The most important disorders arising in aberrations of sex chromosomes are described briefly here.

Klinefelter Syndrome

Klinefelter syndrome is best defined as male hypogonadism that occurs when there are two or more X chromosomes and one or more Y chromosomes. It is one of the most frequent forms of genetic disease involving the sex chromosomes as well as one of the most common causes of hypogonadism in the male. The incidence of this condition is approximately 1 in 850 live male births. It can rarely be diagnosed before puberty, particularly because the testicular abnormality does not develop before early puberty. Most patients have a distinctive body habitus with an increase in length between the soles and the pubic bone, which creates the appearance of an elongated body. Also characteristic are the eunuchoid body habitus with abnormally long legs, the small atrophic testes often associated with a small penis, and the lack of such secondary male characteristics as deep voice, beard, and male distribution of pubic hair. The mean IQ is somewhat lower than normal, but mental retardation is uncommon. It should be noted, however, that this typical pattern is not seen in all cases, the only consistent finding being hypogonadism. Plasma gonadotropin levels, particularly follicle-stimulating hormone (FSH), are consistently elevated, whereas testosterone levels are variably reduced. Mean plasma estradiol levels are elevated by an as yet unknown mechanism. The ratio of estrogens and testosterone determines the degree of feminization in individual cases.

Klinefelter syndrome is the principal cause of male infertility. The reduced spermatogenesis is related to several patterns of morphologic change in the testis. In some patients, the testicular tubules are totally atrophied and replaced by pink, hyaline, collagenous ghosts. In others, the dysgenesis is manifested by apparently normal tubules interspersed with atrophic tubules. In some patients, all tubules are primitive and appear embryonic, consisting of cords of cells that never developed a lumen or progressed to mature spermatogenesis. Leydig cells appear prominent, owing to the atrophy and crowding of tubules.

The classic pattern of Klinefelter syndrome is associated with a 47,XXY karyotype (82% of cases). This complement results from nondisjunction during the meiotic divisions in one of the parents. Paternal nondisjunction at the first meiotic division accounts for a little more than half of the cases. Most of the remaining result from nondisjunction during the first maternal meiotic division. There is no phenotypic difference between those who receive the extra X chromosome from their father and those who receive it from their mother. Maternal age is increased in the cases associated with errors in oogenesis. In addition to this classic karyotype, approximately 15% of the patients with Klinefelter syndrome have been found to have a variety of mosaic patterns, most of them being 46,XY/47,XXY. Other patterns are 47,XXY/48,XXXY and variations on this theme. Rare individuals have also been found to possess 48,XXXY or 49,XXXXY karyotypes. Such polysomic X individuals have further physical abnormalities, including cryptorchidism, hypospadias, more severe hypoplasia of the testes, and skeletal changes, such as prognathism and radioulnar synostosis.

XYY Syndrome

Supernumerary Y chromosomes may be found in the male, giving rise to 47,XYY, or even greater Y polysomy. Approximately 1 in 1000 live-born males has one of these karyotypes. Nearly all are phenotypically normal, but the individuals frequently are excessively tall and may be susceptible to severe acne. From present data, it appears that the intelligence of these individuals is in the normal range.

The impact of extra Y chromosomes on behavior is uncertain and controversial. These karyotypes have been identified with increased frequency among inmates of penal institutions. The behavioral difficulties take the form of antisocial (not violent), delinquent, impulsive acting-out disorders.[46] From more recent studies, it appears that only about 1 to 2% of individuals with XYY phenotypes exhibit such deviant behavior; the overwhelming preponderance are no more antisocial than their peers who have fewer Y chromosomes.

Turner Syndrome

This syndrome results from complete or partial monosomy of the X chromosome and is characterized primarily by hypogonadism in phenotypic females.[47] In approximately 57% of the patients, an entire X chromosome is missing, resulting in the 45,X karyotype. The remaining 43% have other abnormalities as described subsequently. It should be emphasized that only about 1% of fetuses with the 45,X karyotype survive to birth. The surviving infants are severely affected, and in contrast to several other sex-chromosomal aneuploidies, the diagnosis of the 45,X variant of Turner syndrome can often be made at birth or in early childhood.

More than half of those who do not have the 45,X karyotype have structural abnormalities of the X chromosome. These include, in the order of their frequency, the following: (1) deletion of the small arm, resulting in the formation of an isochromosome of the long arm, 46,X,i(Xq); (2) deletions of portions of the short or long arm, 46,XXq− or 46,XXp−; and (3) deletion of portions of both the short and the long arm, resulting in the formation of ring chromosome 46,X,r(X). The remaining patients are mosaics, with karyotypes such as 45,X/46,XY or 45,X/47,XXX. It is important to appreciate the karyotypic heterogeneity associated with Turner syndrome because it is responsible for significant variations in phenotype. In contrast to the patients with monosomy X, those who are mosaics or who have deletions (e.g., 46,XXq−) may have an almost normal appearance and may present only with primary amenorrhea.

The most severely affected infants generally present during infancy with edema (owing to lymph stasis) of the dorsum of the hand and foot and sometimes swelling of the nape of the neck. The latter is related to markedly distended lymphatic channels, producing a so-called cystic hygroma (see Chapter 11). As these infants develop, the swellings subside but often leave bilateral neck webbing and persistent looseness of skin on the back of the neck. Congenital heart disease is also common, particularly preductal coarctation of the aorta and aortic stenosis with endocardial fibroelastosis, anomalies that may account for some of the early deaths.

The principal clinical features in the adolescent and adult are illustrated in Figure 5–28. At puberty, there is failure to develop normal secondary sex characteristics. The genitalia remain infantile, breast development is inadequate, and there is little pubic hair. The mental status of these patients is usually normal, but a few may exhibit some retardation. Of particular importance in establishing the diagnosis in the adult is the shortness of stature (rarely exceeding 150 cm in height) and the amenorrhea. To be noted, *Turner syndrome is the single most important cause of primary amenorrhea*, accounting for approximately one-third of the cases.

As mentioned earlier, both X chromosomes are active during oogenesis and are essential for normal development of the ovaries. To understand the pathogenesis of Turner syndrome, it is essential to review normal ovarian development. It has been said that the ovary is "the most precisely doomed structure in the human body: it carries in its makeup the destruction of its own seeds."[48] During fetal development, ovaries contain as many as 7 million oocytes. The oocytes begin to disappear *in utero*, however, so that by birth there are about 3 million left, and by menarche their numbers have already dwindled to a mere 400,000. Further loss continues after puberty, and when menopause occurs fewer than 10,000 remain. In Turner syndrome, fetal ovaries develop normally early in embryogenesis, but the absence of the second X chromosome leads to an accelerated loss of oocytes, which is complete by the age of 2 years. In a sense, therefore, "menopause occurs before menarche,"[48] and the ovaries are reduced to atrophic

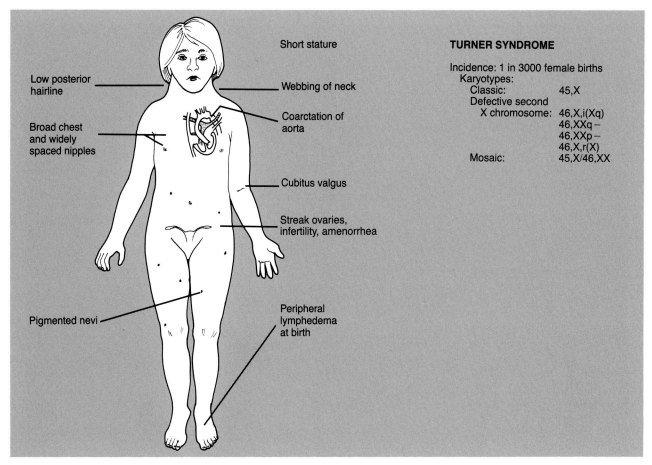

Figure 5-28. Clinical features and karyotypes of Turner syndrome.

fibrous strands, devoid of ova and follicles ("*streak ovaries*"). The reduced estrogen output by the ovaries leads to elevated pituitary gonadotropin secretion.

Multi-X Females

Karyotypes with one to three extra X chromosomes have been described and are not uncommon, being found in about 1 in 1200 newborn females. Most of these women, according to current thought, are entirely normal. A variety of random findings, however, may be present. As mentioned, there is an increased tendency to mental retardation in proportion to the number of extra X chromosomes. Thus, mental retardation is seen in all with the 49,XXXXX karyotype, whereas most with 47,XXX are unaffected. Some women have amenorrhea or occasionally other menstrual irregularities.

Hermaphroditism and Pseudohermaphroditism

The problem of sexual ambiguity is exceedingly complex, and only limited observations are possible here. For more details, reference should be made to specialized texts.[49] It will be no surprise to medical students that the sex of an individual can be defined on several levels. *Genetic sex* is determined by the presence or absence of a Y chromosome. No matter how many X chromosomes are present, a single Y chromosome dictates testicular development and the genetic male gender. The initially indifferent gonads of both the male and the female embryos have an inherent tendency to feminize, unless influenced by Y chromosome-dependent masculinizing factors. *Gonadal sex* is based on the histologic characteristics of the gonads. *Ductal sex* depends on the presence of derivatives of the müllerian or wolffian ducts. *Phenotypic* or *genital sex* is based on the appearance of the external genitalia. Sexual ambiguity is present whenever there is disagreement among these various criteria for determining sex.

The term "true hermaphrodite" implies the presence of both ovarian and testicular tissue. In contrast, a pseudohermaphrodite represents a disagreement between the phenotypic and gonadal sex: i.e., a female pseudohermaphrodite has ovaries but male external genitalia; a male pseudohermaphrodite has testicular tissue but female-type genitalia.

True hermaphroditism, implying the presence of both ovarian and testicular tissue, is an extremely rare condition. In some cases, there is a testis on one side and an ovary on the other, whereas in other cases, there may be combined ovarian and testicular tissue, referred to as ovotestes. The karyotype is 46,XX in two-thirds of patients; most of the remaining are mosaics (e.g., XX/XXY) in which a Y-bearing cell line is present. In those with the 46,XX karyotype, there seems to be a translocation of the Y chromosome to the X chromosome or an autosome. Mosaics, obviously, have both X and Y chromosomes. Thus, true hermaphrodites are a heterogeneous group, having in common the presence of two X chromosomes as well as a complete or partial Y chromosome, in at least some of the cells.

Female pseudohermaphroditism is much less complex. The genetic sex in all cases is XX, and the development of the gonads (ovaries) and internal genitalia is normal. Only the external genitalia are ambiguous or virilized. The basis of female pseudohermaphroditism is excessive and inappropriate exposure to androgenic steroids during the early part of gestation. Such steroids are most commonly derived from the fetal adrenal affected by congenital adrenal hyperplasia, which is transmitted as an autosomal recessive trait. Biosynthetic defects in the pathway of cortisol synthesis are present in these cases that lead secondarily to excessive synthesis of androgenic steroids by the fetal adrenal cortex (see Chapter 25).

Male pseudohermaphroditism represents the most complex of all disorders of sexual differentiation. These individuals possess a Y chromosome, and thus their gonads are exclusively testes, but the genital ducts or the external genitalia are incompletely differentiated along the male phenotype. Their external genitalia are either ambiguous or completely female. Male pseudohermaphroditism is extremely heterogeneous, with a multiplicity of causes. Common to all is defective virilization of the male embryo, which usually results from genetically determined defects in androgen synthesis or action or both. The most common form, called *complete androgen insensitivity syndrome (testicular feminization)*, results from mutations in the gene for the androgen receptor. This gene is located at Xq11-Xq12, and hence this disorder is inherited as an X-linked recessive.

SINGLE-GENE DISORDERS WITH NONCLASSIC INHERITANCE

It has become increasingly evident that transmission of certain single-gene disorders does not follow classic mendelian principles. This group of disorders can be classified into three categories:

- Diseases caused by triplet-repeat mutations
- Disorders caused by mutations in mitochondrial genes
- Disorders associated with genomic imprinting

Clinical and molecular features of some single-gene diseases that exemplify nonclassic patterns of inheritance are described next.

TRIPLET REPEAT MUTATIONS — FRAGILE X SYNDROME

Fragile X syndrome is the prototype of diseases in which the mutation is characterized by a long repeating sequence of three nucleotides. Although the specific nucleotide sequence that undergoes amplification differs in the four disorders included in this group, all affected sequences share the nucleotides guanine (G) and cytosine (C). In the ensuing discussion, we shall consider the clinical features and inheritance pattern of the fragile X syndrome, to be followed by the causative molecular lesion. Two of the remaining disorders in this group—Huntington disease, a neurodegenerative disorder,[2] and myotonic dystrophy, a common inherited disease of muscles—are discussed later, in Chapter 28. The fourth, spinal and bulbar muscular atrophy, is quite rare.

Fragile X syndrome is one of the most common causes of familial mental retardation. It is an X-linked disorder characterized by an inducible cytogenetic abnormality in the X chromosome. The cytogenetic alteration is seen as a discontinuity of staining or as a constriction in the long arm of the X chromosome (Fig. 5–29). This abnormality is referred to as a fragile site because it is particularly liable to chromatid breaks when cells are cultured

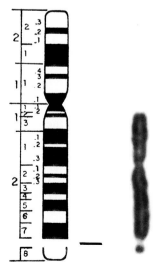

Figure 5–29. Fragile X, seen as discontinuity of staining. (Courtesy of Dr. Patricia Howard-Peebles, University of Texas Southwestern Medical School, Dallas.)

in folate-deficient media. The affected males are *mentally retarded,* with an IQ in the range of 40 to 70. They express a characteristic physical phenotype that includes a *long face with a large mandible, large everted ears, and large testicles (macroorchidism).* It should be noted, however, that these and other physical abnormalities described in this condition are not always present and, in some cases, are quite subtle. *The only distinctive feature that can be detected in at least 80% of postpubertal males is macro-orchidism.*[50]

As with all X-linked diseases, fragile X syndrome affects males. Analysis of several pedigrees, however, reveals some patterns of transmission not typically associated with other X-linked recessive disorders. These include:

- *Carrier males.* Approximately 20% of males who by pedigree analysis are known to carry the fragile X mutation are clinically and cytogenetically normal. Because carrier males transmit the trait through all their daughters (phenotypically normal) to affected grandchildren, they are called "transmitting males."
- *Affected females.* Approximately 30% of carrier females are affected (i.e., mentally retarded), a number much higher than that in other X-linked recessive disorders.
- *Risk of phenotypic effects.* This depends on the position of the individual in the pedigree. For example, brothers of transmitting males are at a 9% risk of having mental retardation, whereas grandsons of transmitting males incur a 40% risk. This positional risk is sometimes referred to as Sherman's paradox.
- *Anticipation.* This refers to the observation that clinical features of fragile X worsen with each successive generation, as if the mutation becomes more and more deleterious as it is transmitted from a man to his grandsons and great-grandsons.

These unusual patterns perplexed geneticists for years, but molecular studies have finally begun to unravel some of these complexities.[51,52] The first breakthrough came when linkage studies localized the mutation responsible for this disease to Xq27.3, within the cytogenetically abnormal region. Cloning and sequencing of the DNA revealed a section within this region that is characterized by multiple tandem repeats of the nucleotide sequence CGG. In the normal population, the number of CGG repeats is small, ranging from 6 to 54 (average 29). The presence of clinical symptoms and a cytogenetically detectable fragile site seem related to the extent of amplification of the CGG repeats. Thus, normal transmitting males and carrier females carry 52 to 200 CGG repeats. Expansions of this size are called *"premutations."* In contrast, affected individuals have an extremely large expansion of the repeat region (250 to 4000 repeats or *"full mutations"*). Full mutations are believed to arise by further amplification of the CGG

repeats seen in premutations. How this process takes place is quite peculiar. Carrier males transmit the repeats to their progeny with small changes in repeat number. When the premutation is passed on by a carrier female, however, there is a dramatic amplification of the CGG repeats, leading to mental retardation in most of the males and 30% of female offspring. Thus, *it appears that during the process of oogenesis, but not in spermatogenesis, premutations can be converted to mutations by triplet repeat amplification.* This explains Sherman's paradox, that is, the likelihood of mental retardation is much higher in grandsons than in brothers of transmitting males, because grandsons incur the risk of inheriting a premutation from their grandfather that is amplified to a "full mutation" in their mother's ova. By comparison, brothers of transmitting males, being "higher up" in the pedigree, are less likely to have a full mutation. These molecular details also provide a satisfactory explanation of anticipation—a phenomenon observed by clinical geneticists but not believed by molecular geneticists until triplet repeat mutations were identified.

Although the triplet repeat mutations appear to be causally related to the fragile X syndrome, it is still not clear how these mutations give rise to mental retardation and other phenotypic abnormalities. The CGG repeats occur within the transcriptional open reading frame of the newly discovered FMR-1 gene. The protein product of this gene has not yet been identified but is likely to be discovered soon. It is assumed that disruption of the FMR-1 gene and the consequent loss of the gene product is responsible for the clinical features of fragile X syndrome.

Until recently, cytogenetic demonstration of the fragile X (see Fig. 5–29) was the only method of laboratory diagnosis. Direct DNA-based molecular diagnosis, however, is now the method of choice. With Southern blot analysis, distinction between premutations and mutations can be made prenatally as well as postnatally. Hence this technique is valuable not only for establishing the diagnosis but also for genetic counseling.

MUTATIONS IN MITOCHONDRIAL GENES—LEBER HEREDITARY OPTIC NEUROPATHY

As is well known, the vast majority of genes are located on chromosomes in the cell nucleus. Mendelian inheritance applies to such genes. There exist several mitochondrial genes, however, which are inherited in quite a different manner. *A feature unique to mitochondrial DNA (mtDNA) is maternal inheritance.* This peculiarity results from the fact that ova contain mitochondria within their abundant cytoplasm, whereas spermatozoa contain few, if any, mitochondria. Hence, the mtDNA complement of the zygote is derived entirely from the ovum. Thus, mothers transmit mtDNA to all their offspring—male and female; however, daughters but not sons transmit the DNA further to their progeny. Several other features apply to mitochondrial inheritance.[53]

- Because mtDNA encodes enzymes involved in oxidative phosphorylation, mutations affecting these genes exert their deleterious effects primarily on the organs most dependent on oxidative phosphorylation. These include the central nervous system, skeletal muscle, cardiac muscle, liver, and kidneys.
- During cell division, mitochondria and their contained DNA are randomly distributed to the daughter cells. Thus, when a cell containing normal and mutant mtDNA divides, the proportion of the normal and mutant mtDNA in daughter cells is extremely variable. Therefore the expression of disorders resulting from mutations in mtDNA is quite variable.

As mentioned above, many diseases associated with mitochondrial inheritance affect the neuromuscular system. All are rare, and hence only one —Leber hereditary optic neuropathy—is described briefly. This is a neurodegenerative disease that manifests itself as progressive bilateral loss of central vision. Visual impairment is first noted between 15 and 35 years of age and it leads, in due course, to blindness. Cardiac conduction defects and minor neurologic manifestations have also been observed in some families.[54]

GENOMIC IMPRINTING—PRADER-WILLI AND ANGELMAN SYNDROMES

As is well known, we all inherit two copies of each gene, carried on homologous maternal and paternal chromosomes. Until recently it was assumed that there is no difference between the genes derived from the mother or the father: All that was needed for normal development was inheritance of two normal copies of each gene. Recent studies have challenged this notion, and there is accumulating evidence that, at least with respect to some genes, there are functional differences between the paternal and the maternal gene. In other words, there are "parent of origin" effects on the function of certain genes.[55,56] Differences in the function of the two parental chromosomes appear to result from an epigenetic process called *genomic imprinting* whereby paternal and maternal chromosomes are marked differentially. As is often the case in medicine, genomic imprinting is best illustrated by considering two uncommon genetic disorders: Prader-Willi syndrome and Angelman syndrome.

The *Prader-Willi syndrome* is characterized by mental retardation, short stature, hypotonia, obesity, small hands and feet, and hypogonadism. In 50 to 60% of cases, an interstitial deletion of band q12 in the long arm of chromosome 15, i.e., del(15)(q11q13) can be detected. In many patients without a detectable cytogenetic abnormality, DNA probe analysis reveals smaller deletions within the same region. *It is striking that in all cases the deletion affects the paternally derived chromosome 15.* In contrast with the Prader-Willi syndrome, patients with the phenotypically distinct Angelman syndrome are *born with a deletion of the same chromosomal region derived from their mothers.* Patients with Angelman syndrome are also mentally retarded, but in addition they present with ataxic gait, seizures, and inappropriate laughter. Because of their laughter and ataxia, they are also called "happy puppets." A comparison of these two syndromes clearly demonstrates the "parent of origin" effects on gene function. If all the paternal and maternal genes contained within chromosome 15 were expressed in an identical fashion, clinical features resulting from these deletions would be expected to be identical regardless of the parental origin of chromosome 15. Molecular studies of the cytogenetically normal patients with the Prader-Willi syndrome have revealed that in some cases both of the structurally normal chromosome 15's are derived from the mother. This situation, that is, inheritance of both chromosomes of a pair from one parent, is called *uniparental disomy.* Angelman syndrome, as might be expected, can also result from uniparental disomy of paternal chromosome 15. These examples further illustrate the concept that for normal development certain homologous genes must be inherited from each parent.

The molecular basis of imprinting is still not clear. There is little doubt that changes associated with imprinting are epigenetic. There is no alteration of the genetic code, but perhaps some biochemical alteration of the DNA influences the expression of the imprinted genes. Because methylation of DNA is known to affect gene expression, it is strongly suspected that imprinting is associated with differential patterns of DNA methylation. Regardless of the mechanism, it is believed that the marking of paternal and maternal chromosomes occurs during gametogenesis, and thus it seems that from the very moment of conception some chromosomes remember where they came from.

It should be pointed out that the importance of imprinting is not restricted to rare chromosomal disorders. Parent-of-origin effects have been identified in a variety of inherited diseases, such as Huntington disease, myotonic dystrophy, and neurofibromatosis.[57]

MOLECULAR DIAGNOSIS

Medical applications of recombinant DNA technology have come of age. With the rapid transfer of technology from "the bench to the bedside," it is now clear that DNA probes can be powerful tools for the diagnosis of human disease, both genetic and acquired.[58,59] Molecular diagnostic techniques have found application in virtually all areas of medicine. These include the following:

- Detection of inherited mutations that underlie the development of genetic diseases either prenatally or after birth
- Detection of acquired mutations that underlie the development of neoplasms
- Accurate diagnosis and classification of neoplasms, especially those that originate in the hematopoietic system
- Diagnosis of infectious diseases, including human immunodeficiency virus (HIV) disease
- Determination of relatedness and identity in transplantation, paternity testing, and forensic medicine

In the next section, we briefly review the diagnostic applications of molecular techniques as they relate to genetic disorders.

GENETIC DISEASES

Historically, the diagnosis of mendelian or "simple" genetic diseases has depended on the identification of abnormal gene products (e.g., mutant hemoglobin or enzymes) or their clinical effects such as anemia or mental retardation (e.g., phenylketonuria). It is now possible, however, to identify gene mutations and offer gene diagnosis for several mendelian disorders, and the list continues to grow. Molecular diagnosis of inherited diseases has several distinct advantages over other techniques.

- First, it is remarkably sensitive. The amount of DNA required for diagnosis can be readily obtained from approximately 10^5 cells. Furthermore, with the polymerase chain reaction (PCR), target DNA can be amplified up to a million fold, and hence as few as one cell may suffice.[60]
- Second, all cells of the body contain the same DNA, and therefore all are affected in inherited genetic disorders. In other words, the test is not dependent on a gene product that may be produced only in certain cells (e.g., erythroid cells) or expression of a gene that may occur late in life. These two features have profound implications for in utero (prenatal) diagnosis because enough cells can be obtained either by removing amniotic fluid or from biopsy of chorionic villus.

The latter can be performed as early as the first trimester.

There are two fundamentally different approaches to the identification of genetic diseases related to an aberrant gene: *(1) direct gene diagnosis involving detection of the mutation and (2) gene tracking, an indirect method based on detecting linkage of the disease gene with a harmless "marker gene." Each of these is discussed briefly.*

Direct Gene Diagnosis

This may well be considered the "diagnostic biopsy of the human genome."[61] The principle of detecting the mutant gene is the same as for a traditional diagnostic test, i.e., to detect some important qualitative difference from normal in the DNA sequence of the gene in question. There are two variations of direct gene diagnosis that depend on the nature of the mutation.

- One technique relies on the fact that some mutations alter or destroy certain restriction sites on the normal DNA. For example, in the normal beta-globin gene (HbA), there are three sites that are specifically recognized by the restriction enzyme Mst II (Fig. 5–30). The sickle mutation responsible for sickle cell anemia (see Chapter 13) involves a single base pair change from *CCTGAGG* to *CCTGTGG*, in the sixth codon of the β-globin chain. The enzyme Mst II recognizes and cleaves the normal *CTGAGG* sequence but not the altered sequence; hence the mutant (hemoglobin S) gene loses one of the three Mst II cutting sites. When DNA from a normal individual is digested with Mst II and hybridized with the radioactive cDNA probe specific for the 5′ end of β-globin gene, a single 1.15 kb band that reacts with the probe is detected on Southern blot analysis (such a band results from the formation of identical 1.15 kb fragments from each of the two normal chromosomes). A similar analysis of DNA from the cells of a patient homozygous for the HbS gene leads to the formation of a single 1.35 kb band, owing to the loss of the Mst II sites from both chromosomes. In individuals heterozygous for the sickle mutation, the normal chromosome yields a 1.15 kb band, whereas the chromosome carrying the mutation gives rise to the 1.35 kb band. Thus, Southern blot analysis reveals two different-sized bands, allowing the detection of a heterozygote carrier. Other diseases in which point mutations alter restriction sites include hemophilia A and X-linked ornithine transcarbamylase deficiency.
- If the mutation that causes disease does not alter the cutting sites of any known restriction enzyme, an alternative technique based on the use of allele-specific oligonucleotides can be applied.

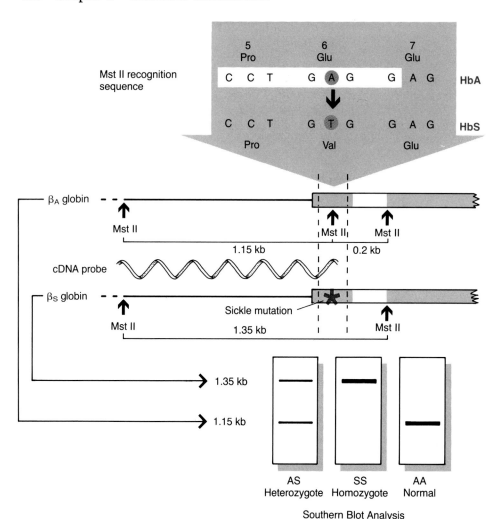

Figure 5–30. Direct gene diagnosis: detection of the sickle mutation by Southern blot analysis. An A → T substitution in the sixth codon of the β_A globin gene yields the β_S allele. This substitution eliminates an Mst II recognition site in the β globin DNA. Thus, when digested with Mst II and probed with an appropriate cDNA, the β_S allele generates a 1.35-kb fragment rather than the normal 1.15-kb fragment.

An illustrative example is that of α_1-antitrypsin (α_1-AT) deficiency, which in many cases is associated with single G → A change in the α_1-AT gene, producing the so-called Z allele (see emphysema, Chapter 15). Two short (18 to 20 bases long) oligonucleotides that have at their center the single base by which the normal and mutant genes differ are synthesized. Such allele-specific oligonucleotides can be radiolabeled and used in a Southern blot analysis (Fig. 5–31). The oligonucleotide containing the sequence of the normal gene hybridizes with both the normal and the mutant DNA, but hybridization to the mutant DNA is unstable owing to the single base pair mismatch. Thus, under stringent conditions of hybridization, the labeled normal probe produces a strong autoradiographic signal with DNA from a normal individual, no signal in the DNA extracted from a patient homozygous for the mutant gene, and a faint signal with DNA from a heterozygote. With the probe containing the mutant sequence, the pattern of hybridization is reversed. Of course, heterozygotes react with both probes because they carry one normal and one mutant gene.

Indirect DNA Diagnosis: Gene Tracking

It must be evident from the preceding discussion that direct gene diagnosis is possible only if the structure of the mutant gene and that of its normal counterpart are known. In a large number of genetic diseases, information about the gene sequence or sometimes even the chromosomal location of the gene is lacking. Obviously, direct gene diagnosis is not possible in these situations. Therefore, alternative strategies, such as "gene tracking," have to be used. *Stated simply, gene tracking asks the question "Has this family member or fetus inherited the same relevant chromosome region(s) as a previously affected family member?"*[62] This principle can be illustrated by considering an autosomal recessive disease. A child who has the disease must have received two chromosomes carrying the mutant gene, one from each of the two unaffected heterozygous parents. In a subsequent pregnancy, such a couple could be expected to give birth to an affected, carrier, or normal child. In a situation like this, an antenatal determination of the fetal genotype can be made by detecting

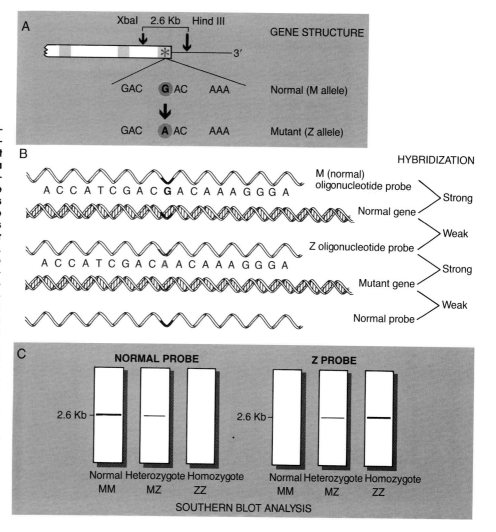

Figure 5–31. Direct gene diagnosis by using an oligonucleotide probe, and Southern blot analysis. Panel A shows that a G → A change converts a normal α_1-antitrypsin allele (allele M) to a mutant Z allele. This change involves exon V of the α_1-antitrypsin gene, which lies between restriction sites for the enzymes Xba I and Hind III. Panel B illustrates the principle of oligonucleotide probe analysis. Two synthetic oligonucleotide probes, one corresponding in sequence to the normal allele (M allele probe) and the other corresponding to the mutant allele (Z allele probe), are lined up against normal and mutant genes, and the expected pattern of hybridization with different combinations is indicated on the right. Panel C diagrams the results of Southern blot analysis when DNA from normal individuals or those heterozygous or homozygous for the mutant Z allele is digested (with Xba I and Hind III) and probed with the normal (M) or Z oligonucleotide probe.

whether the conceptus had inherited both, one, or neither of the parental chromosomes that carry the mutant gene. It follows, therefore, that the success of such a strategy depends on the ability to distinguish the chromosome that carries the mutation from its normal homologous counterpart. This is accomplished by exploiting naturally occurring variations in DNA sequences that can be used to "track" individual chromosomes. Two types of DNA polymorphism are useful in this regard: (1) RFLPs and (2) variable number of tandem repeats (VNTR). Because RFLPs form the backbone of indirect DNA diagnosis, these are discussed first.

Examination of DNA from any two persons reveals variations in the DNA sequences involving approximately one nucleotide in every 200 to 500 base pair stretch. Most of these variations occur in noncoding regions of the DNA and are hence phenotypically silent. These single base pair changes, however, may abolish or create recognition sites for restriction enzymes, thereby altering the length of DNA fragments produced after digestion with certain restriction enzymes. Using appropriate cDNA probes that hybridize with sequences in the vicinity of the polymorphic sites, it is possible to detect the DNA fragments of different lengths by Southern blot analysis. *The term "restriction fragment length polymorphism" refers to variation in fragment length between individuals that results from DNA sequence polymorphisms.*

VNTRs represent a different kind of polymorphism. They are generated by the presence of short sequences of DNA that are arranged in a head-to-tail fashion and repeated several times in a tandem array. Because the number of repeats varies from one chromosome to another, VNTRs can be used to distinguish different chromosomes (Fig. 5–32). VNTR polymorphism is so great that VNTRs are useful for not only linkage analysis but also identification of individuals.

With this background, we can discuss how RFLPs can be used in gene tracking. As illustrated in Figure 5–33, if an individual is heterozygous for an RFLP, it is often possible to distinguish the bands produced by each of the two chromosomes in a Southern blot analysis. In the illustrated example, chromosome A has two restriction sites (7.6 kb apart), whereas chromosome B has a DNA se-

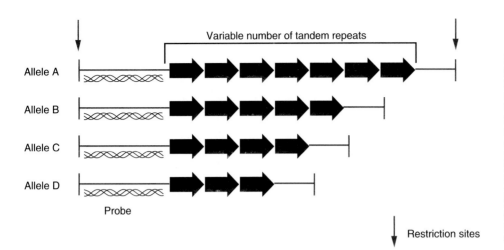

Figure 5–32. Schematic illustration of DNA polymorphisms resulting from a variable number of tandem repeats. When DNA is digested with a restriction enzyme that cuts outside the tandem repeats, different-sized fragments are produced. These can be detected by using a probe that lies outside the tandem repeats (as shown) or a probe that detects the DNA sequence within the tandem repeats. ↓ indicates restriction sites.

quence polymorphism that results in the creation of an additional (third) restriction site for the same enzyme. When DNA from such an individual is digested with the appropriate restriction enzyme and probed with a cloned DNA fragment that hybridizes with a stretch of sequences between the restriction sites, chromosome A yields a 7.6 kb band, whereas chromosome B produces a smaller

6.8 kb band. Thus, on Southern blot analysis, two bands are noted. We can now discuss how this technique was used to perform indirect gene diagnosis of the autosomal recessive disease cystic fibrosis (CF). (Because the CF gene has been cloned, direct DNA diagnosis can be used for most patients with this disease.) Let us assume that chromosomes A and B represent two number 7

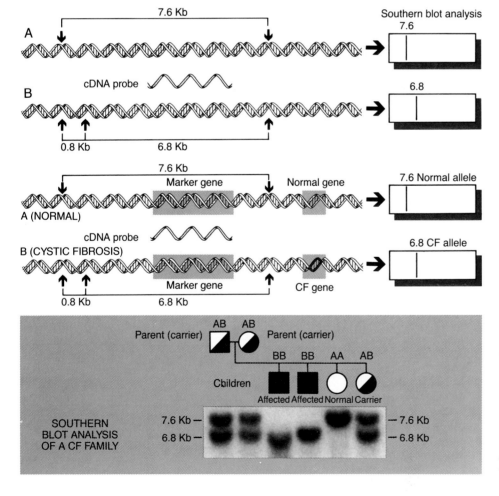

Figure 5–33. Schematic illustration of the principles underlying RFLP analysis in the diagnosis of genetic diseases. Details are described in the text. Note that the distance between the marker gene (p met D) and the CF gene is approximately 600 Kb. They are shown closer for simplicity and to emphasize linkage. The Southern blot analysis shown in the lower panel was performed on Bam 1 digest of DNA probed with the p met D probe. (Southern blot courtesy of Dr. Arthur L. Beaudet, Howard Hughes Medical Institute and Baylor College of Medicine, Houston, Texas.)

chromosomes of an individual who is heterozygous for the CF gene, and that the CF gene and its normal counterpart are in close proximity to the polymorphic DNA site. Also present in this region is a "marker" gene that is distinct from the CF gene but whose presence can be detected by available cDNA probes. Under these conditions, Southern blot analysis of DNA extracted from the parents and siblings of a patient with cystic fibrosis could be expected to produce an RFLP pattern like that indicated in Figure 5–33. Such an analysis makes it possible to track the transmission of a single chromosome region through a family and to see if a particular single-gene disease is coinherited with a polymorphic site. It is therefore possible to use this method for antenatal diagnosis by examining fetal DNA. Because the probe does not identify the disease gene itself, however, certain limitations become apparent:

- First, for prenatal diagnosis, several relevant family members must be available for testing. With an autosomal recessive disease, for example, a DNA sample from a previously affected child is necessary to determine the RFLP pattern that is associated with the homozygous genotype.
- Second, key family members must be heterozygous for an RFLP; i.e., the two homologous chromosomes must be distinguishable. This may require the use of multiple restriction enzymes and several different probes for closely linked genes.
- Third, normal exchange of chromosomal material between homologous chromosomes (recombination) during gametogenesis may lead to "separation" of the mutant gene from the polymorphism pattern with which it had been previously coinherited. This may lead to an erroneous genetic prediction in a subsequent pregnancy. Obviously, the closer the linkage, the lower the degree of recombination and thus a false test. The likelihood of such an error is also minimized by probing for two closely linked marker genes that flank the disease gene.

The probes utilized in RFLP studies may be complementary to functional genes that are linked to the disease gene or to DNA sequences of no known function ("anonymous probes"). An additional advantage of this technique is that if the chromosomal location of the marker gene is known, the chromosomal location of the polymorphic site (and thus the linked mutant gene) can be determined. It is in this manner that the location of the CF gene was mapped to chromosome 7, leading ultimately to the cloning of the gene. The list of single-gene disorders in which linkage analysis has been useful continues to grow and includes Duchenne muscular dystrophy, fragile X syndrome, polycystic kidney disease, and neurofibromatosis.

OTHER DIAGNOSTIC APPLICATIONS OF RECOMBINANT DNA TECHNIQUES

Three other areas in which DNA probe analysis is proving to be of value are (1) the diagnosis of cancer, (2) forensic pathology, and (3) the diagnosis of infectious diseases. As alluded to earlier in this chapter, there is little doubt that neoplastic transformation is associated with somatic mutations. The nature of the genetic alterations that are related to carcinogenesis is discussed in Chapter 7. Suffice it to say here that recombinant DNA techniques can be readily applied to detect the subtlest of alterations in gene structure or expressions that may accompany malignant transformation.

DNA probe analysis has obvious implications for forensic pathology because each human has a unique set of expressed genes and silent DNA polymorphisms. Thus, definite identification of individuals or their tissues can be accomplished by utilizing appropriate, usually multiple, gene probes. Specimens of hair, semen, and blood are being used to provide "molecular fingerprints" of considerable value in cases of rape, violent crime, and disputed paternity.

Because every organism has a DNA sequence that is unique to that microbe, DNA probes can be used not only to detect infectious agents but also to distinguish closely related organisms. This technique can be applied to virtually all classes of pathogens, that is, bacteria, viruses, and parasites. It is particularly advantageous if the organisms are impossible or difficult to grow or are present in extremely small numbers. PCR allows detection of vanishingly small amounts of DNA, as, for example in HIV infection.

So we come to the end of this chapter, but by no means the end of the role of genetics in the diseases of humans. Additional instances appear throughout this book.

1. Craig, R.K.: Methods in molecular medicine. Br. Med. J. 295:646, 1987.
2. The Huntington's Disease Collaborative Research Group: A novel gene containing a trinucleotide repeat that is expanded and unstable on Huntington's disease chromosomes. Cell 72:971, 1993.
3. News. Genetic knockouts: Surprises, lessons, and dreams. J. N.I.H. Res. 4:34, 1992.
4. Baird, P.A., et al.: Genetic disorders in children and young adults: A population study. Am. J. Hum. Genet. 42:677, 1988.
5. Thompson, M.W., et al: Thompson and Thompson Genetics in Medicine, 5th ed. Philadelphia, W.B. Saunders Co., 1991, p. 116.
6. McKusick, V.A.: Mendelian Inheritance in Man, 10th ed. Baltimore, Johns Hopkins University Press, 1992.
7. Agarwal, D.P., and Goedde, H.W.: Pharmacogenetics and ecogenetics. Experientia 42:1148, 1986.
8. Pyeritz, R.E.: The Marfan syndrome. Am. Fam. Physician 34:83, 1986.

9. McKusick, V.A.: The defect in Marfan's syndrome. Nature 352:279, 1991.
10. Milewicz, D.M., et al.: Marfan syndrome: Defective synthesis, secretion, and extracellular matrix formation of fibrillin by cultured dermal fibroblasts. J. Clin. Invest. 89:79, 1992.
11. Pyeritz, R.E.: Marfan's syndrome. In Emery, A.E., and Rimoin, D.L. (eds.): Principles and Practice of Medical Genetics, 2nd ed. New York, Churchill Livingstone, 1990, p. 1047.
12. Byers, P.H., and Holbrook, K.A.: Ehlers-Danlos syndrome. In Emery, A.E., and Rimoin, D.L. (eds.): Principles and Practice of Medical Genetics, 2nd ed. New York, Churchill Livingstone, 1990, p. 1065.
13. Kuivaniemi, H., et al.: Mutations in collagen genes: Causes of rare and some common disorders in humans. FASEB J. 5:2052, 1991.
14. Goldstein, J.L., and Brown, M.S.: Familial hypercholesterolemia. In Scriver, C.R., et al. (eds.): The Metabolic Basis of Inherited Disease, 6th ed. New York, McGraw-Hill, 1989, p. 1215.
15. Vega, G.L., and Grundy, S.M.: Mechanisms of primary hypercholesterolemia in humans. Am. Heart J. 113:493, 1987.
16. Hobbs, H.H., et al.: The LDL receptor locus in familial hypercholesterolemia. Annu. Rev. Genet. 24:133, 1990.
17. Illingworth, D.R., and Sexton, G.J.: Hypocholesterolemic effects of mevinolin in patients with heterozygous familial hypercholesterolemia. J. Clin. Invest. 74:1972, 1984.
18. Hunninghake, D.B., et al.: The efficacy of intensive dietary therapy alone or combined with lovastatin in outpatients with hypercholesterolemia. N. Engl. J. Med. 328:1213, 1993.
19. Tager, J.M.: Inborn errors of cellular organelles: An overview. J. Inherit. Metab. Dis. 10(Suppl. 1):3, 1987.
20. Glew, R.H., et al.: Lysosomal storage diseases. Lab. Invest. 53:250, 1985.
21. Triggs-Raine, B.L., et al.: Screening for carriers of Tay-Sachs disease among Ashkenazi Jews: A comparison of DNA-based and enzyme-based tests. N. Engl. J. Med. 323:6, 1990.
22. Elleder, M.: Niemann-Pick disease. Pathol. Res. Pract. 185:293, 1989.
23. Beutler, E.: Gaucher's disease. N. Engl. J. Med. 325:1354, 1991.
24. Lee, R.E., et al.: Gaucher's disease: Clinical, morphologic, and pathogenetic considerations. Pathol. Annu. 12:309, 1977.
25. Mistry, P.K., et al.: Genetic diagnosis of Gaucher's disease. Lancet 339:889, 1992.
26. Tybulewicz, V.L.J., et al.: Animal model of Gaucher's disease from targeted disruption of mouse glucocerebrosidase gene. Nature 357:407, 1992.
27. Muenzer, J.: Mucopolysaccharidoses. Adv. Pediatr. 33:269, 1986.
28. Beaudet, A.L.: The glycogen storage diseases. In Wilson, J.D., et al. (eds.): Harrison's Principles of Internal Medicine, 12th ed. New York, McGraw-Hill, 1991, p.1854.
29. DiManro, S., et al.: Metabolic myopathies. Am. J. Med. Genet. 25:635, 1986.
30. Hers, H., et al.: Glycogen storage diseases. In Scriver, C.L., et al. (eds.): The Metabolic Basis of Inherited Diseases, 6th ed. New York, McGraw-Hill, 1989, p. 425.
31. La Du, B.N.: Alcaptonuria. In Scriver C.R., et al. (eds.): The Metabolic Basis of Inherited Disease, 6th ed. New York, McGraw-Hill, 1989, p. 775.
32. Gaines, J.J., Jr.: The pathology of alkaptonuric ochronosis. Hum. Pathol. 20:40, 1989.
33. Mulvihill, J.J. (moderator): NIH conference. Neurofibromatosis 1 (Recklinghausen's disease) and neurofibromatosis 2 (bilateral acoustic neurofibromatosis): An update. Ann. Intern. Med. 113:39, 1990.
34. Bader, J.L.: Neurofibromatosis and cancer. Ann. N.Y. Acad. Sci. 486:57, 1986.
35. Gutmann, D.H., and Collins, F.S.: The neurofibromatosis type 1 gene and its protein product, neurofibromin. Neuron 10:335, 1993.
36. Rouleau, G.A., et al.: Alteration in a new gene encoding a putative membrane-organizing protein causes neurofibromatosis type 2. Nature 363:515, 1993.
37. Nelson, K., and Holmes, L.B.: Malformations due to presumed spontaneous mutations in newborn infants. N. Engl. J. Med. 320:19, 1989.
38. Francke, U., and Oliver, N.: Quantitative analysis of high-resolution trypsin-Giemsa bands of human prometaphase chromosomes. Hum. Genet. 45:137, 1978.
39. Cooley, W.C., and Graham, J.M.: Down syndrome—an update and review for the primary pediatrician. Clin. Pediatr. 30:233, 1991.
40. Antonarakis, S.E., et al.: Parental origin of the extra chromosome in trisomy 21 as indicated by analysis of DNA polymorphisms. N. Engl. J. Med. 324:872, 1991.
41. Cork, L.C.: Neuropathology of Down syndrome and Alzheimer disease. Am. J. Med. Genet. Suppl. 7:282, 1990.
42. Ugazio, A.G., et al.: Immunology of Down syndrome: A review. Am. J. Med. Genet. Suppl. 7:204, 1990.
43. Korenberg, J.R., et al.: Down syndrome: Toward a molecular definition of the phenotype. Am. J. Med. Genet. Suppl. 7:91, 1990.
44. Brown, C.J., et al.: The human XIST gene: Analysis of a 17-kb inactive X-specific RNA that contains conserved repeats and is highly localized within the nucleus. Cell 71:527, 1992.
45. McLaren, A.: News and Views: What makes a man a man. Nature 346:216, 1990.
46. Money, J., et al.: Cytogenetics, hormones, and behavior disability: Comparison of XXY and XYY syndromes. Clin. Genet. 6:370, 1974.
47. Lippe, B.: Turner syndrome. Endocrinol. Metab. Clin. North Am. 20:121, 1991.
48. Federman, D.D.: Mapping the X-chromosome: Minding its p's and q's. N. Engl. J. Med. 317:161, 1987.
49. Grumbach, M.M., and Conte, F.A.: Disorders of sex differentiation. In Wilson, J.D., and Foster, D.W. (eds.): Williams Textbook of Endocrinology, 8th ed. Philadelphia, W.B. Saunders Co., 1992, p. 853.
50. Howard-Peebles, P.N., et al.: Fragile X syndrome. In Rosenberg, R.N., et al. (eds.): The Molecular and Genetic Basis of Neurologic Disease. Stoneham, MA, Butterworth-Heinemann, 1993, p. 79.
51. Mandel, J.-L., and Heitz, D.: Molecular genetics of the fragile X syndrome: A novel type of unstable mutation. Curr. Opin. Genet. Dev. 2:422, 1992.
52. Caskey, C.T., et al.: Triplet repeat mutations in human disease. Science 256:754, 1992.
53. Wallace, D.C.: Diseases of mitochondrial DNA. Annu. Rev. Biochem. 61:1175, 1992.
54. Brown, M.D., et al.: Leber's hereditary optic neuropathy: A model for mitochondrial neurodegenerative diseases. FASEB J. 6:2791, 1992.
55. Hall, J.G.: Genomic imprinting and its clinical implications. N. Engl. J. Med. 326:827, 1992.
56. Reik, W.: Genomic imprinting and genetic disorders in man. Trends Genet. 5:331, 1989.
57. Hall, J.G.: Genetic imprinting: Review and relevance to human diseases. Am. J. Hum. Genet. 46:857, 1990.
58. Cooper, D.N., and Schmidtke, J.: Molecular genetic approaches to the analysis and diagnosis of human inherited disease: An overview. Ann. Med. 24:29, 1992.
59. Fenoglio-Preiser, C.M., and William, C.L. (eds.): Molecular Diagnostic Pathology. Baltimore, Williams & Wilkins, 1991.
60. Markham, A.F.: The polymerase chain reaction: A tool for molecular medicine. Br. Med. J. 306:441, 1993.
61. McKusick, V.A.: The morbid anatomy of the human genome: A review of gene mapping in clinical medicine. Medicine 67:1, 1988.
62. Pembrey, M.: Impact of molecular biology on clinical genetics. Br. Med. J. 295:711, 1987.

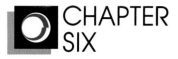 CHAPTER SIX

DISEASES OF IMMUNITY

GENERAL FEATURES OF THE IMMUNE SYSTEM

Although vital to survival, the immune system is like the proverbial two-edged sword. On the one hand, immunodeficiency states render humans easy prey to infections and possibly tumors; on the other hand, a hyperactive immune system may cause fatal disease, as in the case of an overwhelming allergic reaction to the sting of a bee. In yet another series of derangements, the immune system may lose its normal capacity to distinguish self from nonself, resulting in the emergence of immunity against one's own tissues and cells (autoimmunity). In this chapter, we consider diseases caused by too little immunity as well as those re-

sulting from too much immunologic reactivity. We also consider amyloidosis, a disease in which an abnormal protein, derived in some cases from fragments of immunoglobulins, is deposited in tissues.

First, we review some advances in the understanding of lymphocyte biology, and then a brief description of the histocompatibility genes is given because their products are relevant to several immunologically mediated diseases and to the rejection of transplants.

CELLS OF THE IMMUNE SYSTEM

T LYMPHOCYTES

As is well known, cellular immunity is mediated by thymus-derived (T) lymphocytes. In the blood, T

171

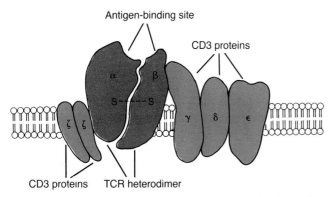

Figure 6-1. The T-cell receptor (TCR) complex. A schematic illustration of TCRα and TCRβ polypeptide chains linked to the CD3 molecular complex.

cells constitute 60 to 70% of peripheral lymphocytes. *T lymphocytes are also found in the paracortical areas of lymph nodes and periarteriolar sheaths of the spleen.* Each T cell is genetically programmed to recognize a specific cell-bound antigen by means of an antigen-specific T-cell receptor (TCR).[1] In approximately 95% of T cells, the TCR consists of a disulfide-linked heterodimer made up of an alpha (α) and a beta (β) polypeptide chain (Fig. 6-1), each having a variable (antigen-binding) and a constant region. In a minority of peripheral blood T cells, another type of TCR, composed of gamma (γ) and delta (δ) polypeptide chains, is found. The TCRγ/δ cells tend to aggregate at epithelial interfaces, such as the mucosa of the respiratory and gastrointestinal tracts. Both the α/β and γ/δ TCRs are noncovalently linked to a cluster of five polypeptide chains, referred to as the CD3 molecular complex. The CD3 proteins are nonvariable. They do not bind antigen but are involved in the transduction of signals into the T cell after it has bound the antigen. TCR diversity is generated by somatic rearrangement of the genes that encode the α, β, γ, and δ TCR chains. As might be expected, every somatic cell has TCR genes from the germ line. During ontogeny, somatic rearrangements of these genes occur only in T cells; hence the *demonstration of TCR gene rearrangements by Southern blot analysis is a molecular marker of T-lineage cells.* Such analyses are used in classification of lymphoid malignancies (see Chapter 14). Furthermore, because each T cell has a unique DNA rearrangement (and hence a unique TCR), it is possible to distinguish polyclonal (nonneoplastic) T-cell proliferations from monoclonal (neoplastic) T-cell proliferations.

In addition to CD3 proteins, T cells express a variety of other nonpolymorphic functions–associated molecules, including CD4, CD8, and many so-called accessory molecules, such as CD2, CD11a, CD28, and CD43. Of these, CD4 and CD8 are particularly important.[2] They are expressed on two mutually exclusive subsets of T cells. CD4 is expressed on approximately 60% of

mature CD3+ T cells, whereas CD8 is expressed on about 30% of T cells. Thus in normal healthy persons, the CD4-CD8 ratio is about 2 : 1. These T-cell membrane–associated glycoproteins serve as coreceptors in T-cell activation. During antigen presentation, CD4 molecules bind to the nonpolymorphic portions of class II major histocompatibility complex (MHC) molecules expressed on antigen-presenting cells. In contrast, CD8 molecules bind to class I MHC molecules. Because of these properties, CD4+ helper/inducer T cells can recognize antigen only in the context of class II MHC antigens, whereas the CD8+ cytotoxic/suppressor T cells recognize cell-bound antigens only in association with class I MHC antigens.

The CD4+ and CD8+ T cells perform distinct but somewhat overlapping functions. The CD4+ T cell can be viewed as a master regulator—the conductor of a symphony orchestra, so to speak. By secreting soluble factors (cytokines), CD4+ T cells influence the function of virtually all other cells of the immune system, including other T cells, B cells, macrophages, and natural killer (NK) cells. The central role of CD4+ T cells is tragically illustrated when the human immunodeficiency virus (HIV) cripples the immune system by selective destruction of this T-cell subset. In recent years, two functionally different populations of CD4+ helper cells have been recognized. The T-helper-1 (T$_H$1) subset synthesizes and secretes interleukin-2 (IL-2) and interferon-gamma (IFN-γ) but not IL-4 or IL-5, whereas T$_H$2 cells produce IL-4 and IL-5 but not IL-2 or IFN-γ.[3] This distinction is significant because the cytokines secreted by these subsets have different effects on other immune cells. In general, the T$_H$1 subset is involved in facilitating the macrophage-dependent immune responses, including induction of delayed hypersensitivity and production of opsonizing antibodies. The T$_H$2 subset aids in the synthesis of other classes of antibodies. The CD8+ T cells, in contrast to CD4+ T cells, mediate their functions primarily by acting as cytotoxic cells.

B LYMPHOCYTES

B lymphocytes constitute 10 to 20% of the circulating peripheral lymphocyte population. They are also present in bone marrow; peripheral lymphoid tissues such as lymph nodes, spleen, or tonsils; and extralymphatic organs, such as the gastrointestinal tract. In lymph nodes, they are found in the superficial cortex. In the spleen, they are found in the white pulp. At both sites, they are aggregated in the form of lymphoid follicles, which on activation develop pale-staining germinal centers (Fig. 6-2).

On antigenic stimulation, B cells form plasma cells that secrete immunoglobulins, which in turn are the mediators of humoral immunity. B cells

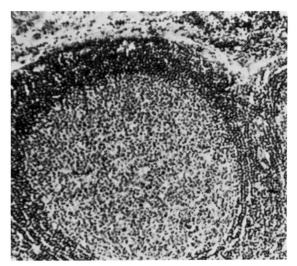

Figure 6-2. Lymph node cortex, showing lymphoid follicles, the B cell-containing area.

recognize antigen via the B-cell antigen receptor complex. Immunoglobulin M (IgM), present on the surface of all B cells, constitutes the antigen-binding component of the B cell receptor. As with T cells, each B-cell receptor has a unique antigen specificity, derived in part from somatic rearrangements of immunoglobulin genes. *Thus the presence of rearranged immunoglobulin genes in a lymphoid cell is used as a molecular marker of B-lineage cells.* It has recently been recognized that, in addition to membrane IgM, the B-cell antigen receptor complex contains a heterodimer of nonpolymorphic transmembrane proteins: Igα and Igβ. Like the CD3 proteins of the TCR, Igα and Igβ do not bind antigen but are essential for signal transduction through the receptor. B cells also express several other nonpolymorphic molecules that are essential for B cell function.[4] These include complement receptors, Fc receptors, and CD19. It is worthy of note that complement receptor-2 (CD21) is also the receptor for the Epstein-Barr virus (EBV), and hence B cells are readily infected by EBV. CD19, a signal transducing molecule, is B-cell restricted and appears early in B-cell differentiation. It is therefore useful in identification of B-cell tumors.

MACROPHAGES

Macrophages are a part of the mononuclear phagocyte system, and, as such, their origin, differentiation, and role in inflammation are discussed in Chapter 3. Here we need only to emphasize that macrophages play several roles in the immune response.

• First, they are required to process and present antigen to immunocompetent T cells. Because T cells (in contrast to B cells) cannot be activated

by soluble antigens, presentation of processed, membrane-bound antigens by macrophages or other antigen-presenting cells (e.g., Langerhans' cells, discussed later) is obligatory for induction of cell-mediated immunity.
• They produce a variety of cytokines. Some, such as IL-1 and TNF-α, are pro-inflammatory as well as fibrogenic (see Chapter 3).
• Macrophages lyse tumor cells by secreting toxic metabolites and proteolytic enzymes and, as such, may play a role in immunosurveillance.
• Macrophages are important effector cells in certain forms of cell-mediated immunity, such as the delayed hypersensitivity reaction. As mentioned earlier, macrophage functions are facilitated by cytokines produced by the T_H1 subset of CD4+ cells.

DENDRITIC AND LANGERHANS' CELLS

Dendritic cells and Langerhans' cells comprise two populations that are characterized by dendritic cytoplasmic processes and the presence of large amounts of cell-surface class II molecules. Dendritic cells are widely distributed. They are found in lymphoid tissue and in the interstitium of many nonlymphoid organs, such as the heart and lungs. Similar cells within the epidermis have been called Langerhans' cells. By virtue of cell-surface class II molecules, dendritic cells and Langerhans' cells are extremely efficient in antigen presentation, and some investigators believe that they are the most important antigen-presenting cells in the body. It should be noted that although they share antigen-presenting capacity with macrophages, in contrast to the latter cell type, they are weakly or not at all phagocytic.

NATURAL KILLER (NK) CELLS

Approximately 10 to 15% of the peripheral blood lymphocytes do not bear TCR or cell-surface immunoglobulins.[5] In the past, these non-T, non-B cells were called "null cells." It is now recognized that these lymphocytes are endowed with an innate ability to lyse a variety of tumor cells, virally infected cells, and some normal cells, *without prior sensitization.* Hence they are called NK cells (Fig. 6-3). NK cells are believed to be a part of the "natural" (as opposed to adaptive) immune system that may be the first line of defense against neoplastic or virus-infected cells. Selective deficiency of NK cells, although rare, is associated with recurrent viral infections.[6]

Although they share some surface markers with T cells (e.g., CD2), NK cells do not rearrange TCR genes and are CD3-. Two cell-surface molecules, CD16 and CD56, are widely used to iden-

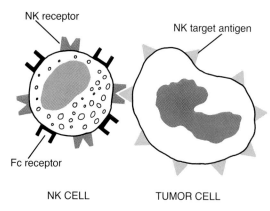

NK receptor

NK target antigen

Fc receptor

NK CELL   TUMOR CELL

Figure 6–3. Schematic representation of direct tumor cell killing by NK cells. Note that the Fc receptor of NK cells is not involved.

tify NK cells. Of these, CD16 is of functional significance. It represents the Fc receptor for IgG and hence endows NK cells with another function—the ability to lyse IgG-coated target cells. This phenomenon, known as antibody-dependent cytotoxicity (ADCC), is described in greater detail later in this chapter under hypersensitivity disorders.

In addition to cytolytic ability, NK cells are also endowed with immunoregulatory functions. These are mediated by the secretion of cytokines, such as IFN-γ. In the early phase of microbial infections, NK cells are believed to be the most important source of IFN-γ.

Morphologically, NK cells are somewhat larger than T and B lymphocytes and, in contrast to these two cell types, contain azurophilic cytoplasmic granules. Hence NK cells are sometimes referred to as large granular lymphocytes.

CYTOKINES: MESSENGER MOLECULES OF THE IMMUNE SYSTEM

The induction and regulation of the immune responses involve multiple interactions among lymphocytes, monocytes, inflammatory cells (e.g., neutrophils), and endothelial cells. Many such interactions are cognitive and so depend on cell-to-cell contact; however, many interactions and effector functions are mediated by short-acting soluble mediators, called *cytokines*. This term includes the previously designated lymphokines (lymphocyte-derived); monokines (monocyte-derived); and several other polypeptides that regulate the immunologic, inflammatory, and reparative host responses. Most cytokines have a wide spectrum of effects, and some are produced by several different cell types.

We shall not attempt to list the currently well-characterized and molecularly cloned cytokines because any such list would soon be dwarfed by the torrent of new cytokines being isolated and reported every day. Instead we shall classify the currently known cytokines into four categories and list some of their general properties.

- Cytokines that mediate natural immunity. Included in this group are IL-1, tumor necrosis factor-alpha (TNF-α), type 1 interferons, and the IL-8 family. Certain of these cytokines (e.g., interferons) protect against viral infections, whereas others (e.g., IL-1, TNF-α, IL-8) initiate nonspecific inflammatory responses.
- Cytokines that regulate lymphocyte growth, activation, and differentiation. Within this category are IL-2, IL-4, IL-5, IL-12, and transforming growth factor-beta (TGF-β). Although some, such as IL-2 and IL-4, favor lymphocyte growth and differentiation, others such as IL-10 and TGF-β, down-regulate immune responses.
- Cytokines that activate inflammatory cells. In this category are IFN-γ, TNF-α, lymphotoxin (TNF-β), migration inhibitory factor, and IL-8. Most of these cytokines serve to activate the functions of nonspecific effector cells.
- Cytokines that stimulate hematopoiesis. Many cytokines derived from lymphocytes or stromal cells stimulate the growth and production of new blood cells by acting on hematopoietic progenitor cells. Several members of this family are called colony-stimulating factors (CSFs) because they were initially detected by their ability to promote the *in vitro* growth of hematopoietic cell colonies from the bone marrow. In this category, granulocyte-macrophage (GM) CSF and granulocyte (G) CSF act on committed progenitor cells, whereas stem cell factor (c-kit ligand) acts on pluripotent stem cells.

It should be noted that this subdivision of cytokines into functional groups, although convenient, is somewhat arbitrary because, as will be noted subsequently, many cytokines, such as IL-1, TNF-α, and IFN-γ, are pleiotropic in their effects.

General Properties of Cytokines

- Many individual cytokines are produced by several different cell types. For example, IL-1 and TNF-α can be produced by virtually any cell.
- The effects of cytokines are pleiotropic: They act on many cell types. For example, IL-2, initially discovered as a T-cell growth factor, is known to affect the growth and differentiation of B cells and NK cells as well.
- Cytokines induce their effects in three ways: (1) they act on the same cell that produces them (*autocrine* effect), such as occurs when IL-2 produced by activated T cells promotes T-cell growth; (2) they affect other cells in their vicin-

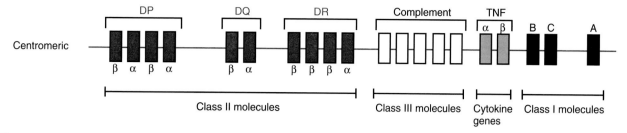

Figure 6-4. Schematic representation of the HLA complex and its subregions. The relative distances between various genes and regions are not drawn to scale.

ity (*paracrine* effect), as occurs when IL-7 produced by marrow stromal cells promotes the differentiation of B-cell progenitors in the marrow; and (3) they affect many cells systemically (*endocrine* effect), the best examples in this category being IL-1 and TNF-α, which produce the acute-phase response during inflammation.

- Cytokines mediate their effects by binding to specific high-affinity receptors on their target cells. For example, IL-2 activates T cells by binding to high-affinity IL-2 receptors (IL-2R). Blockade of the IL-2R by specific anti-receptor monoclonal antibodies prevents T-cell activation. This observation provides a means by which T-cell activation, when undesirable (as in transplant rejection), may be controlled.

The knowledge gained about cytokines has practical therapeutic ramifications. First, by regulating cytokine production or action, it may be possible to control the harmful effects of inflammation or tissue-damaging immune reactions. Second, recombinant cytokines can be administered to enhance immunity against cancer or microbial infections (immunotherapy). Both these avenues are currently being pursued on an experimental basis in humans.

STRUCTURE AND FUNCTION OF HISTOCOMPATIBILITY ANTIGENS

Although originally identified as antigens that evoke rejection of transplanted organs, histocompatibility molecules are now known to be extremely important for the induction and regulation of the immune response and for certain nonimmunologic functions. *The principal physiologic function of the cell surface histocompatibility molecules is to bind peptide fragments of foreign proteins for presentation to appropriate antigen-specific T cells.* Recall that T cells (in contrast to B cells) can recognize only membrane-bound antigens, and hence histocompatibility antigens are critical to the induction of T-cell immunity. The histocompatibility

molecules and the corresponding genes are complex in structure and are still incompletely understood. Here we summarize only the salient features of human histocompatibility antigens, primarily to facilitate understanding of their role in rejection of organ transplants and in disease susceptibility. Several genes code for histocompatibility antigens, but those that code for the most important transplantation antigens are clustered on a small segment of chromosome 6. This cluster constitutes the human major histocompatibility complex (MHC) and is also known as the human leukocyte antigen (HLA) complex (Fig. 6-4) because MHC-encoded antigens were initially detected on the white cells. The HLA system is highly polymorphic. This, as we shall see, constitutes a barrier in organ transplantation.

Based on their chemical structure, tissue distribution, and function, the MHC gene products are classified into three categories. Class I and class II genes encode cell surface glycoproteins, and class III genes encode components of the complement system. The latter, as is well known, are soluble proteins; they are not discussed in this section.

Class I antigens are expressed on all nucleated cells and platelets. They are encoded by three closely linked loci, designated HLA-A, HLA-B, and HLA-C (see Fig. 6-4). Each of these molecules is a heterodimer, consisting of a polymorphic alpha (α), or heavy, chain (44-kd) linked noncovalently to a smaller (12-kd) nonpolymorphic peptide called beta$_2$-microglobulin. The latter is not encoded within the MHC. The extracellular region of the heavy chain is divided into three domains: α_1, α_2, and α_3 (Fig. 6-5). Crystal structure of class I molecules has revealed that the α_1 and α_2 domains contain a cleft, or groove, where peptides bind to the MHC molecule. Biochemical analyses of several different class I alleles have revealed that almost all polymorphic residues line the sides or the base of the peptide-binding groove. As a result, different class I alleles bind to different peptide fragments. In general, class I MHC molecules bind to those peptides that are derived from proteins, such as viral antigens, synthesized within the cell. The generation of peptide fragments within the cells, and their association with MHC molecules

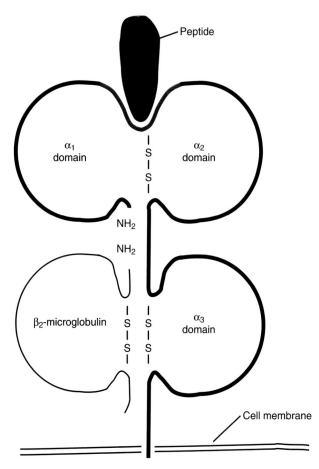

Figure 6-5. Schematic diagram of HLA class I molecule.

called HLA-D, which has three subregions: HLA-DP, HLA-DQ, and HLA-DR. Each class II molecule is a heterodimer consisting of a noncovalently associated α chain and β chain. Both chains are polymorphic, and each of three HLA-D subregions encodes one or more α chains and β chains (see Fig. 6-4). The extracellular portions of the α and β chains have two domains: α_1, α_2 and β_1, β_2. Crystal structure of class II molecules has revealed that, like class I molecules, they have an antigen-binding cleft facing outwards.[8] In contrast to class I molecules, however, the antigen-binding groove is formed by an interaction of the α_1 and β_1 domains of both the chains, and it is in this portion that most class II alleles differ. Thus, it seems that, as with class I molecules, polymorphism of class II molecules is associated with differential binding of antigenic peptides. The nature of peptides that bind to class II molecules is different from that of peptides that bind to class I molecules. In general, class II molecules present exogenous antigens (e.g., extracellular microbes, soluble proteins) that are first internalized and processed in the endosomes or lysosomes. Peptides resulting from proteolytic cleavage then associate with class II heterodimers assembled in the ER. Finally, the peptide-MHC complex is transported to the cell surface,[9] where it can be recognized by CD4+ helper T cells. In

and transport to the cell surface, is a complex process.[7] Involved in this sequence are proteolytic complexes (proteosomes), which digest antigenic proteins into short peptides, and transport proteins, which ferry peptide fragments from the cytoplasm to the endoplasmic reticulum (ER). Within the ER, peptides bind to the antigen-binding cleft of newly synthesized class I heavy chains, which then associate with beta$_2$-microglobulin to form a stable trimer that is transported to the cell surface for presentation to the CD8+ cytotoxic T lymphocytes (Fig. 6-6). In this interaction, the TCR recognizes the MHC-peptide complex; the CD8 molecule, acting as a coreceptor, then binds to the nonpolymorphic, alpha$_3$, domain of the class I heavy chain. It is important to note that CD8+ cytotoxic T cells can recognize viral (or other) peptides only if presented as a complex with self class I antigens. In the eyes of T cells, self MHC molecules are those that they "grew up" with during maturation within the thymus. Because one of the important functions of CD8+ T cells is to eliminate virus-infected T cells, it makes "good sense" to have widespread expression of class I HLA antigens.

Class II antigens are coded for in a region

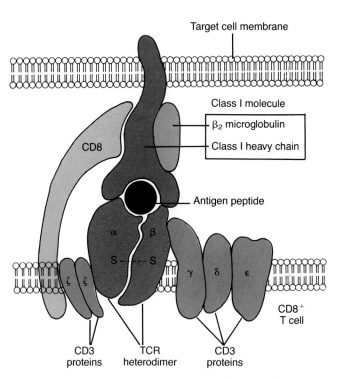

Figure 6-6. Schematic illustration of antigen recognition by CD8+ T cells. Note that the T cell receptor (TCR heterodimer) recognizes a complex formed by the peptide fragment of the antigen and class I MHC molecule. The CD8 molecule binds to the nonpolymorphic portion of the class I molecule and thus acts as an accessory structure during antigen recognition.

this interaction, the CD4 molecule acts as the co-receptor. Because CD4+ T cells can recognize antigens only in the context of self class II molecules, they are referred to as "class II restricted."

The role of class II antigens in the induction of helper T cells has an important bearing on the genetic regulation of the immune response.

- How class II molecules regulate immune responses is not entirely clear, but there are two plausible mechanisms. One possibility rests on the fact that different antigenic peptides bind to different class II gene products. It follows that an individual will mount a vigorous immune response against an antigen only if he or she inherits the gene(s) for those class II molecule(s) that can bind the nominal antigen and present it to helper T cells. The consequences of inheriting a given class II gene depend on the nature of the antigen bound by the class II molecule. For example, if the antigen was ragweed pollen, the individual would be genetically prone to type I hypersensitivity disease. An inherited capacity to bind a bacterial peptide may provide resistance to disease by evoking an antibody response.
- The other possibility is related to the role of MHC molecules in shaping the T-cell repertoire. During intrathymic differentiation, only T cells that can recognize self-MHC molecules are selected for export to the periphery (see later discussion of immunologic tolerance). Thus, the type of MHC molecules that T cells encounter during their differentiation influences the functional capacity of mature peripheral T cells.

HLA and Disease Association

A variety of diseases have been found to be associated with certain HLA types (Table 6–1). The best known is the association between ankylosing spondylitis and HLA-B27; individuals who possess this antigen have a 90-fold greater chance (relative risk) of developing the disease than those who are negative for HLA-B27. The diseases that show association with HLA can be broadly grouped into the following categories: (1) *inflammatory diseases*, including ankylosing spondylitis and several postinfectious arthropathies, all associated with HLA-B27; (2) *inherited errors of metabolism*, such as hemochromatosis (HLA-A3) and 21-hydroxylase deficiency (HLA-BW47); and (3) *autoimmune diseases*, including autoimmune endocrinopathies, associated with alleles at the DR locus. The mechanisms underlying these associations are not understood at present. In view of the physiologic role of the HLA complex in regulation of the immune response, it is somewhat easier to speculate on the possible mechanisms that may underlie the associations with immunologically mediated diseases. As has already been discussed, HLA class II genes can regulate immune responsiveness. Accordingly, an association between certain autoimmune diseases and HLA-DR antigens may result from an exaggerated immune response to autoantigens.

DISORDERS OF THE IMMUNE SYSTEM

Having reviewed some fundamentals of basic immunology, we can now turn to general disorders of the immune system and some specific immunologic diseases. These are discussed under four broad headings: (1) *hypersensitivity reactions*, which form the mechanisms of immunologic injury in a variety of diseases discussed throughout this book; (2) *autoimmune diseases*, which are caused by immune reactions against self; (3) *immunologic deficiency syndromes*, which result from relatively distinct, genetically determined or acquired defects in some components of the normal immune response; and (4) *amyloidosis*, a poorly understood disorder having immunologic association.

MECHANISMS OF IMMUNOLOGIC TISSUE INJURY (HYPERSENSITIVITY REACTIONS)

Humans live in an environment teeming with substances capable of producing immunologic responses. Contact with antigen leads not only to induction of a protective immune response, but also to reactions that can be damaging to tissues. Exogenous antigens occur in dust, pollens, foods, drugs, microbiologic agents, chemicals, and many blood products used in clinical practice. The im-

Table 6–1. ASSOCIATION OF HLA WITH DISEASE

DISEASE	HLA ALLELE	RELATIVE RISK
Ankylosing spondylitis	B27	87.4
Postgonococcal arthritis	B27	14.0
Acute anterior uveitis	B27	14.6
Rheumatoid arthritis	DR4	5.8
Chronic active hepatitis	DR3	13.9
Primary Sjögren's syndrome	DR3	9.7
Insulin-dependent diabetes	DR3	5.0
	DR4	6.8
	DR3/DR4	14.3
Hemochromatosis	A3	8.2
21-Hydroxylase deficiency	BW47	15.0

Table 6-2. MECHANISMS OF IMMUNOLOGICALLY MEDIATED DISORDERS

TYPE	PROTOTYPE DISORDER	IMMUNE MECHANISM
I Anaphylactic type	Anaphylaxis, some forms of bronchial asthma	Formation of IgE (cytotropic) antibody → immediate release of vasoactive amines and other mediators from basophils and mast cells followed by recruitment of other inflammatory cells
II Cytotoxic type	Autoimmune hemolytic anemia, erythroblastosis fetalis, Goodpasture's syndrome	Formation of IgG, IgM → binds to antigen on target cell surface → phagocytosis of target cell or lysis of target cell by C8,9 fraction of activated complement or antibody-dependent cellular cytotoxicity (ADCC)
III Immune complex disease	Arthus reaction, serum sickness, systemic lupus erythematosus, certain forms of acute glomerulonephritis	Antigen-antibody complexes → activated complement → attracted neutrophils → release of lysosomal enzymes and other toxic moieties
IV Cell-mediated (delayed) hypersensitivity	Tuberculosis, contact dermatitis, transplant rejection	Sensitized T lymphocytes → release of lymphokines and T cell–mediated cytotoxicity

mune responses that may result from such exogenous antigens take a variety of forms, ranging from annoying but trivial discomforts such as itching of the skin to potentially fatal disease such as bronchial asthma. The various reactions produced are called *hypersensitivity reactions,* and these can be initiated either by the interaction of antigen with humoral antibody or by cell-mediated immune mechanisms.

Tissue-damaging immune reactions may be evoked not only by exogenous antigens, but also by those that are intrinsic to the body (endogenous). This distinction is of value because it indicates that some disorders—those due to exogenous antigens—are essentially environmental and as such are theoretically preventable. Poison ivy contact dermatitis could be eradicated as a disease by mere avoidance of contact with the plant, as could hay fever resulting from inhalation of plant pollens. However, many of the most important immune diseases are caused by antigens intrinsic to humans. Some anti-self immune reactions are triggered by homologous antigens that differ among humans with different genetic backgrounds. Transfusion reactions and graft rejection are examples of immunologic disorders evoked by homologous antigens. Another category of disorders, those incited by autologous antigens, constitutes the important group of autoimmune diseases, to be discussed later in this chapter. These diseases appear to arise because of the emergence of immune responses against self-antigens.

Hypersensitivity diseases can be classified on the basis of the immunologic mechanism that mediates the disease (Table 6–2). This approach is of value in clarifying the manner in which the immune response ultimately causes tissue injury and disease.

- In *type I disease,* the immune response releases vasoactive and spasmogenic substances that act on vessels and smooth muscle, thus altering their function.
- In *type II disorders,* humoral antibodies participate directly in injuring cells by predisposing them to phagocytosis or lysis.
- *Type III disorders* are best remembered as "immune complex diseases," in which humoral antibodies bind antigens and activate complement. The fractions of complement then attract neutrophils, which, partly through the release of neutrophilic lysosomal enzymes, produce tissue damage.
- *Type IV disorders* involve tissue injury in which cell-mediated immune responses with sensitized lymphocytes are the cause of the cellular and tissue injury.

Prototypes of each of these immune mechanisms are presented in the following sections.

TYPE I HYPERSENSITIVITY (ANAPHYLACTIC TYPE)

Type I hypersensitivity may be defined as a rapidly developing immunologic reaction occurring within minutes after the combination of an antigen with antibody bound to mast cells or basophils in individuals previously sensitized to the antigen. It may occur as a systemic disorder or as a local reaction. The systemic reaction usually follows an intravenous injection of an antigen to which the host has already become sensitized. Often within minutes a state of shock is produced, which is sometimes fatal. Local reactions depend on the portal of entry of the allergen and take the form of localized cuta-

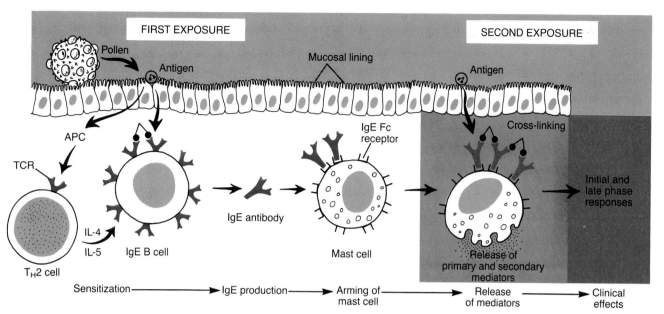

Figure 6–7. Sequence of events leading to type I hypersensitivity. TCR = T cell receptor; APC = antigen-presenting cell; T$_H$2 = T-helper 2 CD4+ cells.

neous swellings (skin allergy, hives), nasal and conjunctival discharge (allergic rhinitis and conjunctivitis), hay fever, bronchial asthma, or allergic gastroenteritis (food allergy). It is now recognized that many local type I hypersensitivity reactions have two well-defined phases: the initial response, characterized by vasodilatation, vascular leakage, and, depending on the location, smooth muscle spasm or glandular secretions. These changes usually become evident within 5 to 30 minutes after exposure to an allergen and tend to subside in 60 minutes. In many instances (e.g., allergic rhinitis and bronchial asthma), a second, "late phase," reaction sets in 2 to 8 hours later without additional exposure to antigen and lasts for several days. This late phase reaction is characterized by more intense infiltration of tissues with eosinophils, neutrophils, basophils, and monocytes as well as tissue destruction in the form of mucosal epithelial cell damage.

Because mast cells and basophils are central to the development of type I hypersensitivity, we shall first review some of their salient characteristics and then discuss the immune mechanisms that underlie this form of hypersensitivity. Mast cells are bone marrow–derived cells that are widely distributed in the tissues. They are found predominantly near blood vessels and nerves and in subepithelial sites, where local type I reactions tend to occur.[10] As is well known, mast cell cytoplasm contains membrane-bound granules that possess a variety of biologically active mediators. In addition, mast cell granules contain acidic proteoglycans that bind basic dyes such as toluidine blue. Because the stained granules often acquire a color

that is different from that of the native dye, they are referred to as "metachromatic" granules. As is detailed next, mast cells and basophils are activated by the cross-linking of high-affinity IgE Fc receptors; in addition, mast cells may also be triggered by several other stimuli, such as complement components C5a and C3a (anaphylatoxins), both of which act by binding to their receptors on the mast cell membrane. Other mast cell secretagogues include macrophage-derived cytokines (e.g., IL-8), some drugs such as codeine and morphine, mellitin (present in bee venom), and physical stimuli (e.g., heat, cold, sunlight). Reactions resulting from non-IgE–mediated release of mast cell contents are sometimes called "anaphylactoid" to indicate the similarity of the resultant clinical manifestations with those seen in anaphylaxis. Basophils are similar to mast cells in many respects, including the presence of cell-surface IgE Fc receptors as well as cytoplasmic granules. In contrast to mast cells, however, basophils are not normally present in tissues but rather circulate in the blood in extremely small numbers. Like other granulocytes, they can be recruited to inflammatory sites.

In humans, type I reactions are mediated by IgE antibodies. An allergen stimulates B lymphocyte production of IgE, principally at the mucosal site of entry of the antigen and in the draining lymph nodes. This process requires the assistance of the T$_H$2 subset of CD4+ helper T cells. IgE antibodies formed in response to an allergen have a strong tendency to attach to mast cells and basophils, which possess high-affinity receptors for the Fc portion of IgE (Fig. 6–7). *When a mast cell or basophil, armed with cytophilic IgE antibodies, is*

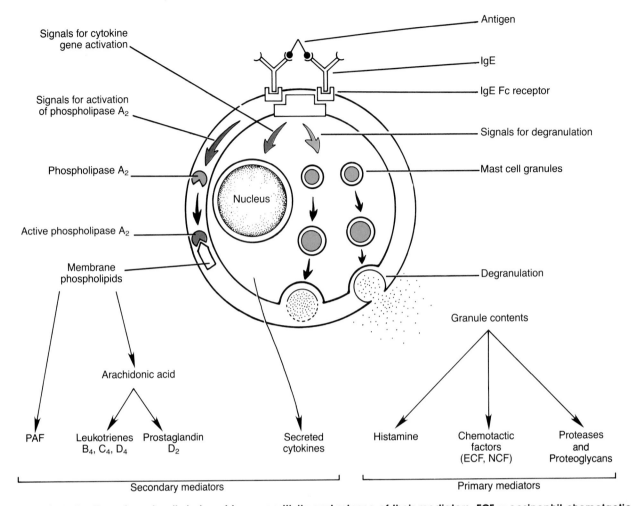

Figure 6-8. Activation of mast cells in type I hypersensitivity and release of their mediators. ECF = eosinophil chemotactic factor; NCF = neutrophil chemotactic factor.

re-exposed to the specific allergen, a series of reactions takes place, leading eventually to the release of a variety of powerful mediators responsible for the clinical expression of type I hypersensitivity reactions. In the first step in this sequence, antigen (allergen) is bound to the IgE antibodies previously attached to the mast cells. In this process, multivalent antigens bind to more than one IgE molecule and cause cross-linkage of adjacent IgE antibodies. The bridging of IgE molecules leads to perturbations of the IgE Fc receptors and initiates two parallel and interdependent processes (Fig. 6–8)— one leading to *mast cell degranulation with discharge of preformed (primary) mediators* and the other involving *de novo synthesis and release of secondary mediators, such as arachidonic metabolites.* These mediators are directly responsible for the initial, sometimes explosive, symptoms of type I hypersensitivity, and they also set into motion the events that lead to the late phase response.

PRIMARY MEDIATORS. Primary mediators contained within mast cell granules can be divided into four categories.[11]

- *Biogenic amines.* These include histamine and adenosine. Histamine causes intense bronchial smooth muscle contraction; increased vascular permeability; and increased secretion by nasal, bronchial, and gastric glands. Adenosine enhances mast cell mediator release, causes bronchoconstriction, and inhibits platelet aggregation.
- *Chemotactic mediators.* These include eosinophil chemotactic factor and neutrophil chemotactic factor.
- *Enzymes.* These are contained in the granule matrix and include proteases (chymase, tryptase) and several acid hydrolases. The enzymes lead to the generation of kinins and activated components of complement (e.g., C3a) by acting on their precursor proteins.
- *Proteoglycans.* These include heparin, a well-known anticoagulant.

SECONDARY MEDIATORS. These include two classes of compounds: (1) lipid mediators and (2) cytokines. The lipid mediators are generated by sequential reactions in the mast cell membranes that lead to activation of phospholipase A_2, an enzyme that acts on membrane phospholipids to yield *arachidonic acid.* This, you may recall, is the parent compound from which leukotrienes and prostaglandins are derived by the 5-lipoxygenase and cyclooxygenase pathways (see Chapter 3).

- *Leukotrienes* are extremely important in the pathogenesis of type I hypersensitivity. *Leukotrienes C_4 and D_4* are the most potent vasoactive and spasmogenic agents known. On a molar basis, they are several thousand times more active than histamine in increasing vascular permeability and causing bronchial smooth muscle contraction. *Leukotriene B_4* is highly chemotactic for neutrophils, eosinophils, and monocytes.
- *Prostaglandin D_2* is the most abundant mediator derived by the cyclooxygenase pathway in mast cells. It causes intense bronchospasm as well as increased mucus secretion.
- *Platelet-activating factor* (PAF) (see Chapter 3) is a secondary mediator that causes platelet aggregation, release of histamine, bronchospasm, increased vascular permeability, and vasodilatation. In addition, it has important proinflammatory actions. PAF is chemotactic for neutrophils and eosinophils. At higher concentrations, it activates the newly elicited inflammatory cells, causing them to aggregate and degranulate. Because of its ability to recruit and activate inflammatory cells, it is considered important in the initiation of the late phase response. Although its production is also triggered by the activation of phospholipase A_2, it is not a product of arachidonic acid metabolism.
- *Cytokines.* These polypeptides play an important role in the pathogenesis of type I hypersensitivity reactions because of their ability to recruit and activate inflammatory cells. Mast cells are believed to produce a variety of cytokines, including TNF-α, IL-1, IL-3, IL-4, IL-5, IL-6, and GM-CSF.[12] In experimental models, TNF-α has been shown to be an important mediator of IgE-dependent cutaneous reactions. TNF-α, it may be recalled, is a potent proinflammatory cytokine that can attract neutrophils and eosinophils, favor their transmigration through the vasculature, and activate them in the tissues (see Chapter 3). In addition, IL-4 is important for the recruitment of eosinophils. Inflammatory cells that accumulate at the sites of type I hypersensitivity reactions are additional sources of cytokines and of histamine-releasing factors that cause further mast cell degranulation.

A variety of chemotactic, vasoactive, and spasmogenic compounds, listed in Table 6–3, mediate type I hypersensitivity reactions. Some, such as histamine and leukotrienes, are released rapidly from sensitized mast cells and are believed to be responsible for the intense immediate reactions characterized by edema, mucus secretion, and smooth

Table 6–3. SUMMARY OF THE ACTION OF MAST CELL MEDIATORS IN TYPE I HYPERSENSITIVITY

ACTION	MEDIATOR
Cellular infiltration	Leukotriene B_4 Eosinophil chemotactic factor of anaphylaxis Neutrophil chemotactic factor of anaphylaxis PAF* Cytokines, e.g., TNF-α*
Vasoactive (vasodilatation, increased vascular permeability)	Histamine PAF Leukotrienes C_4, D_4, E_4 Neutral proteases that activate complement and kinins Prostaglandin D_2
Smooth muscle spasm	Leukotrienes C_4, D_4, E_4 Histamine Prostaglandins PAF

* Important for late-phase reactions.
PAF = Platelet-activating factor.

muscle spasm; many others, exemplified by leukotrienes, PAF, and TNF-α, set the stage for the late phase response by recruiting additional leukocytes—basophils, neutrophils, and eosinophils. Not only do these inflammatory cells release additional waves of mediators (including cytokines), but they also cause epithelial cell damage.

Among the cells that are recruited in the late phase reaction, *eosinophils* are particularly important. Their armamentarium of mediators is as extensive as that of mast cells, and in addition they produce major basic protein (MBP) and eosinophil cationic protein (ECP), which are toxic to epithelial cells. Activated eosinophils and other leukocytes also produce leukotriene C4 and PAF and directly activate mast cells to release mediators. Thus the recruited cells amplify and sustain the inflammatory response without additional exposure to the triggering antigen.

CYTOKINE-MEDIATED REGULATION OF TYPE I HYPERSENSITIVITY. Cytokines are important not only in the inflammatory phase of type I hypersensitivity but also in the regulation of reactions at several other levels.

- *IgE synthesis.* It is evident that synthesis of IgE by B cells is critical to the development of type I hypersensitivity. This response depends on the presence of IL-4, IL-5, and IL-6, all secreted by the T_H2 subset of CD4+ cells. Of these, IL-4 is absolutely essential for the turning on of IgE-producing B cells. It is postulated that the proclivity of certain antigens to cause allergic reactions is related in part to their ability to activate the T_H2 cells. In contrast, some cytokines produced by T_H1 cells, e.g., IFN-γ, down-regulate IgE synthesis.[13]

- *Mast cell growth.* Increased tissue concentration of mast cells is a feature of type I hypersensitivity. Growth and differentiation of mast cells are favored by several cytokines, including IL-3, IL-4, and the c-kit ligand (stem cell factor).
- *Eosinophil growth and activation.* The T_H2 cell–derived cytokine IL-5 is extremely important for the production of eosinophils from its progenitors. It also activates mature eosinophils.

With this consideration of the basic mechanisms of type I hypersensitivity, we turn to some conditions that are important examples of IgE-mediated disease.

Systemic Anaphylaxis

In humans, systemic anaphylaxis may occur after administration of heterologous proteins (e.g., antisera), hormones, enzymes, polysaccharides, and drugs (such as the antibiotic penicillin).[14] The severity of the disorder varies with the level of sensitization. The shock dose of antigen, however, may be exceedingly small, as, for example, the tiny amounts used in ordinary skin testing for various forms of allergies. Within minutes after exposure, itching, hives, and skin erythema appear, followed shortly thereafter by a striking contraction of respiratory bronchioles and the appearance of respiratory distress. Laryngeal edema results in hoarseness. Vomiting, abdominal cramps, diarrhea, and laryngeal obstruction follow, and the patient may go into shock and even die within the hour. At autopsy, some patients may be found to have pulmonary edema and hemorrhage, whereas others show hyperdistention of the lungs along with right-sided cardiac dilatation, a reflection of the constricted pulmonary vasculature. It is obvious that the effects of anaphylaxis must always be borne in mind when a therapeutic agent is administered. Although patients at risk can generally be identified by a previous history of some form of allergy, the absence of such a history does not preclude the possibility of an anaphylactic reaction.

Local Anaphylaxis

These reactions are exemplified by so-called atopic allergy. The term "atopy" implies a genetically de-termined predisposition to develop localized anaphylactic reactions to inhaled or ingested allergens. About 10% of the population suffers from allergies involving localized anaphylactic reactions to extrinsic allergens, such as pollen, animal dander, house dust, fish, and the like. Specific diseases include urticaria, angioedema, allergic rhinitis (hay fever), and some forms of asthma, all discussed elsewhere in this book. Of interest is the familial predisposition to the development of this type of allergy. A positive family history of allergy is found in 50% of atopic individuals. The basis of familial predisposition is not clear. Although there are no significant associations between specific HLA antigens and atopic diseases as a group, the occurrence of atopic allergy has been correlated with specific HLA haplotypes in certain families. Atopic individuals also tend to have higher serum IgE levels, as compared with the general population. Perhaps in those genetically prone to develop allergies, environmental antigens preferentially activate the T_H2 pathway. Such genetic predisposition can be clearly demonstrated in experimental animals exposed to helminth infections.

TYPE II HYPERSENSITIVITY

Type II hypersensitivity is mediated by antibodies directed toward antigens present on the surface of cells or other tissue components. The antigenic determinants may be intrinsic to the cell membrane, or they may take the form of an exogenous antigen adsorbed on the cell surface. In either case, the hypersensitivity reaction results from the binding of antibodies to normal or altered cell-surface antigens. Three different antibody-dependent mechanisms involved in this type of reaction are depicted in Figure 6–9 and described next.

Complement-Dependent Reactions

There are two mechanisms by which antibody and complement may mediate type II hypersensitivity: direct lysis and opsonization. In the first pattern, antibody (IgM or IgG) reacts with an antigen present on the surface of the cell, causing activation of the complement system and resulting in the assembly of the membrane attack complex that disrupts membrane integrity by "drilling holes" through the lipid bilayer. In the second pattern, the cells become susceptible to phagocytosis by fixation of antibody or C3b fragment to the cell surface (opsonization). This form of type II hypersensitivity most commonly involves blood cells—red blood cells, white blood cells, and platelets—

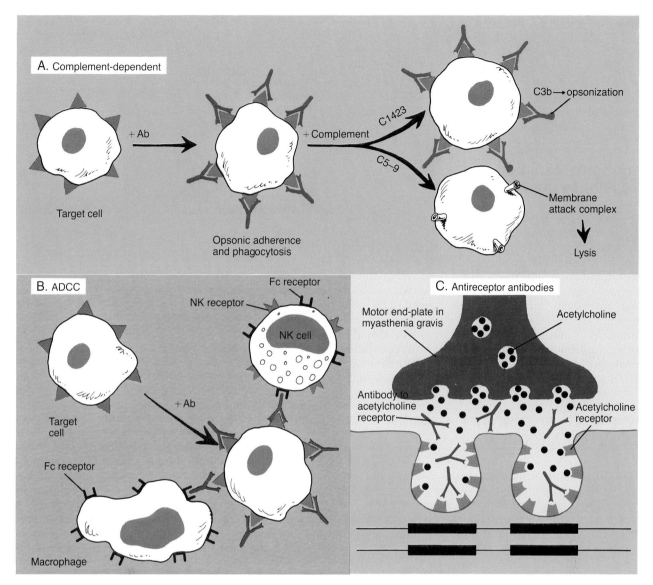

Figure 6-9. Schematic illustration of three different mechanisms of antibody-mediated injury in type II hypersensitivity. *A,* Complement-dependent reactions that lead to lysis of cells or render them susceptible to phagocytosis. *B,* Antibody-dependent cellular cytotoxicity. IgG-coated target cells are killed by cells that bear Fc receptors for IgG (e.g., NK cells, macrophages). *C,* Antireceptor antibodies disturb the normal function of receptors. In this example, acetylcholine receptor antibodies impair neuromuscular transmission in myasthenia gravis.

but the antibodies can also be directed against extracellular tissue (e.g., glomerular basement membrane in anti–glomerular basement membrane nephritis (see Chapter 20). Clinically such reactions occur in the following situations: (1) *transfusion reactions,* in which cells from an incompatible donor react with autochthonous antibody of the host; (2) *erythroblastosis fetalis,* in which there is an antigenic difference between the mother and the fetus, and antibodies (of the IgG class) from the mother cross the placenta and cause destruction of fetal red cells; (3) *autoimmune hemolytic anemia, agranulocytosis, or thrombocytopenia,* in which individuals produce antibodies to their own blood cells, which are then destroyed; (4) *certain drug reactions,* in which antibodies are produced that react with the drug, which may be complexed to red cell antigen.

Antibody-Dependent Cell-Mediated Cytotoxicity (ADCC)

This form of antibody-mediated cell injury does not involve fixation of complement but instead requires the cooperation of leukocytes. The target cells, coated with low concentrations of IgG antibody, are killed by a variety of *nonsensitized* cells that have Fc receptors. The latter bind to the target by their receptors for the Fc fragment of IgG, and *cell lysis proceeds without phagocytosis.* ADCC may be mediated by monocytes, neutrophils, eosinophils, and NK cells. Although in most instances IgG antibodies are involved in ADCC, in certain cases (e.g., eosinophil-mediated cytotoxicity against parasites) IgE antibodies are utilized. ADCC may be relevant to the destruction of targets too large to be phagocytosed, such as parasites or tumor cells, and it may also play some role in graft rejection.

Antibody-Mediated Cellular Dysfunction

In some cases, antibodies directed against cell surface receptors impair or dysregulate function without causing cell injury or inflammation. For example, in myasthenia gravis, antibodies reactive with acetylcholine receptors in the motor end plates of skeletal muscles impair neuromuscular transmission and therefore cause muscle weakness. The converse, i.e., antibody-mediated stimulation of cell function, is noted in Graves' disease. In this disorder, antibodies against the thyroid-stimulating hormone (TSH) receptor on thyroid epithelial cells stimulate the cells, resulting in hyperthyroidism.

TYPE III HYPERSENSITIVITY (IMMUNE COMPLEX–MEDIATED)

Type III hypersensitivity reaction is induced by antigen-antibody complexes that produce tissue damage as a result of their capacity to activate a variety of serum mediators, principally the complement system. The toxic reaction is initiated when antigen combines with antibody, whether within the circulation (circulating immune complexes) or at extravascular sites where antigen may have been deposited (*in situ* immune complexes). Some forms of glomerulonephritis in which immune complexes are formed *in situ* following initial implantation of the antigen on the glomerular basement membrane are discussed later. Complexes formed in the circulation produce damage, particularly as they localize within blood vessel walls or when they are trapped in filtering structures, such as the renal glomerulus. *It should be pointed out at the outset that the mere formation of antigen-antibody complexes in the circulation does not imply the presence of disease;* indeed, immune complexes are formed during many immune responses and may perhaps represent a normal mechanism of antigen removal. The factors that determine whether the immune complexes formed in circulation will be pathogenic are not fully understood, but some possible influences are discussed later.

Two general types of antigens cause immune complex–mediated injury: (1) The antigen may be *exogenous*, such as a foreign protein, a bacterium, or a virus, but (2) under some circumstances, the

Table 6–4. SOME ANTIGENS ASSOCIATED WITH IMMUNE COMPLEX DISORDERS

ANTIGENS		CLINICAL MANIFESTATIONS
Exogenous		
Infectious agents		
Bacteria:	Streptococci	Glomerulonephritis, infective endo-carditis
	Yersinia enterocolitica	Arthritis
	Treponema pallidum	Glomerulonephritis
Viruses:	Hepatitis B	Polyarteritis nodosa
	Cytomegalovirus	
Parasites:	Plasmodium sp.	Glomerulonephritis
	Schistosoma sp.	
Fungi:	Actinomycetes	Farmer's lung
Drugs or chemicals		
Foreign serum (antithymocyte globulin)		Serum sickness
Quinidine		Hemolytic anemia
Heroin		Glomerulonephritis
Endogenous		
Nuclear antigens		Systemic lupus erythematosus
Immunoglobulins		Rheumatoid arthritis
Tumor antigens		Glomerulonephritis

individual can produce antibody against self components—*endogenous antigens* (Table 6–4). The latter can be trace components present in the blood or, more commonly, antigenic components in cells and tissues. Immune complex–mediated diseases can be *generalized*, if immune complexes are formed in the circulation and are deposited in many organs, or *localized* to particular organs, such as the kidney (glomerulonephritis), joints (arthritis), or the small blood vessels of the skin if the complexes are formed and deposited locally (the local Arthus reaction). These two patterns are considered separately.

Systemic Immune Complex Disease

Acute serum sickness is the prototype of a systemic immune complex disease; it was at one time a frequent sequel to the administration of large amounts of foreign serum (e.g., horse antitetanus serum) used for passive immunization. It is now seen infrequently and in different clinical settings. For example, in one report, 11 of 12 patients who were injected with horse antithymocyte globulin for treatment of aplastic anemia developed serum sickness.[15]

For the sake of simplicity, the pathogenesis of systemic immune complex disease can be resolved into three phases: *(1) formation of antigen-antibody complexes in the circulation and (2) deposition of the immune complexes in various tissues, thus initiating (3) an inflammatory reaction in dispersed sites throughout the body* (Fig. 6–10). The *first*

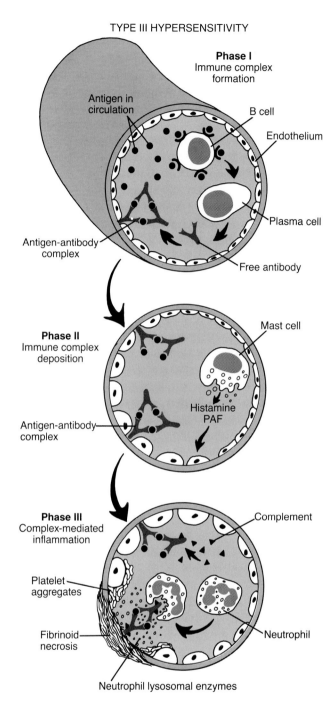

TYPE III HYPERSENSITIVITY

Phase I
Immune complex formation

Antigen in circulation

B cell

Endothelium

Plasma cell

Free antibody

Antigen-antibody complex

Phase II
Immune complex deposition

Mast cell

Histamine PAF

Antigen-antibody complex

Phase III
Complex-mediated inflammation

Complement

Platelet aggregates

Neutrophil

Fibrinoid necrosis

Neutrophil lysosomal enzymes

Figure 6-10. Schematic illustration of the three sequential phases in the induction of systemic type III (immune complex) hypersensitivity.

determine whether immune complex formation will lead to tissue deposition and disease are not fully understood, but two possible influences are the size of the immune complexes and the functional status of the mononuclear phagocyte system (MPS):

- Very large complexes formed in great antibody excess are rapidly removed from the circulation by the MPS cells and are therefore relatively harmless. The most pathogenic complexes are of small or intermediate size (formed in slight antigen excess), circulate longer, and bind less avidly to phagocytic cells.
- Because the mononuclear phagocyte system normally filters out the circulating immune complexes, its overload or intrinsic dysfunction increases the probability of persistence of immune complexes in circulation and tissue deposition.

In addition, several other factors, such as charge of the immune complexes (anionic versus cationic), valency of the antigen, avidity of the antibody, the affinity of the antigen to various tissue components, the three-dimensional (lattice) structure of the complexes, and hemodynamic factors, influence their tissue deposition. Because most of these influences have been investigated with reference to deposition of immune complexes in the glomeruli, they are discussed further in Chapter 20. In addition to the renal glomeruli, the favored sites of immune complex deposition are joints, skin, heart, serosal surfaces, and small blood vessels.

For complexes to leave the microcirculation and deposit within or outside the vessel wall, an increase in vascular permeability must occur. One possibility is that IgE antibody induced by the antigen shortly after injection binds to circulating basophils and releases histamine and PAF. These mediators then separate the endothelial cells and allow the complexes to enter the vessel wall. Alternatively (or additionally), immune complexes bind to inflammatory cells through their Fc or C3b receptors and trigger release of vasoactive mediators as well as permeability-enhancing cytokines. Once complexes are deposited in the tissues, they initiate an acute inflammatory reaction *(phase three)*. It is during this phase (approximately 10 days after antigen administration) that clinical features such as fever, urticaria, arthralgias, lymph node enlargement, and proteinuria appear.

Wherever complexes deposit, the tissue damage is similar (Fig. 6-11). *Central to this mechanism is activation of the complement cascade and the elaboration of biologically active fragments.* As will be recalled from the discussion in Chapter 3, complement activation has several proinflammatory effects:

- Release of C3b, the opsonin that promotes phagocytosis of particles and organisms.
- Production of chemotactic factors, which direct

phase is initiated by the introduction of antigen into the circulation and its interaction with immunocompetent cells, resulting in the formation of antibodies. Approximately 5 days after serum injection, antibodies directed against the serum components are produced; these react with the antigen still present in the circulation to form antigen-antibody complexes. In the *second phase,* antigen-antibody complexes formed in the circulation are deposited in various tissues. The factors that

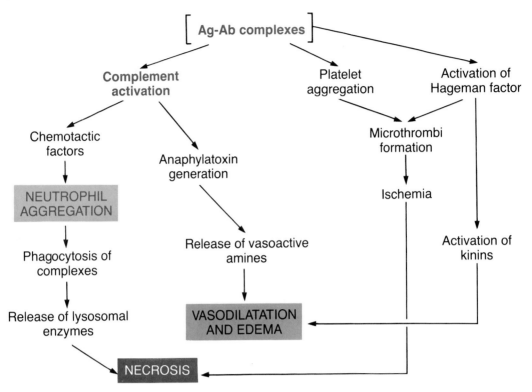

Figure 6–11. Schematic representation of the pathogenesis of immune complex–mediated tissue injury. The morphologic consequences are depicted as boxed areas.

the migration of polymorphonuclear leukocytes and monocytes (C5 fragments, C5b67).

- Release of anaphylatoxins (C3a and C5a), which increase vascular permeability and cause contraction of smooth muscle.
- Formation of membrane attack complex (C5–9), causing cell membrane damage or even cytolysis.

Phagocytosis of antigen-antibody complexes by leukocytes drawn in by the chemotactic factors results in the release or generation of a variety of additional proinflammatory substances, including prostaglandins, vasodilator peptides, and chemotactic substances, as well as several lysosomal enzymes, including proteases capable of digesting basement membrane, collagen, elastin, and cartilage. Tissue damage is also mediated by free oxygen radicals produced by activated neutrophils. Immune complexes have several other effects: They cause aggregation of platelets and activate Hageman factor; both of these reactions augment the inflammatory process and initiate the formation of microthrombi (see Fig. 6–11). The resultant pathologic lesion is termed vasculitis if it occurs in blood vessels, glomerulonephritis if it occurs in renal glomeruli, arthritis if it occurs in the joints, and so on.

It is clear from the foregoing that complement-fixing antibodies (i.e., IgG and IgM) induce these lesions. Because IgA can activate complement by the alternate pathway, IgA-containing complexes may also induce tissue injury. The important role of complement in the pathogenesis of the tissue injury is supported by the observation that experimental depletion of serum complement levels greatly reduces the severity of the lesions, as does depletion of neutrophils. *During the active phase of the disease, consumption of complement decreases the serum levels.*

The morphologic consequences of immune complex injury are dominated by acute necrotizing vasculitis, with deposits of fibrinoid and intense neutrophilic exudation permeating the entire arterial wall, much like the changes that we shall describe for polyarteritis nodosa (Fig. 6–12). Affected glomeruli are hypercellular because of swelling and proliferation of endothelial and mesangial cells, accompanied by neutrophilic and monocytic infiltration. *The complexes can be seen on immunofluorescence microscopy as granular lumpy deposits of immunoglobulin and complement* and on electron microscopy as electron dense deposits along the glomerular basement membrane (see Figs. 6–26 and 6–27). If the disease results from a single large exposure to antigen (e.g., acute poststreptococcal glomerulonephritis and acute serum sickness), all lesions tend to resolve, owing to catabolism of the immune complexes.

A chronic form of serum sickness results from repeated or prolonged exposure to an antigen. Continuous antigenemia is necessary for the development of chronic immune complex disease be-

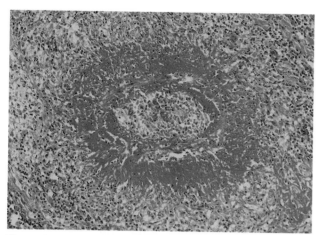

Figure 6–12. Immune complex vasculitis. The necrotic vessel wall is replaced by smudgy, pink "fibrinoid" material. (Courtesy of Dr. Trace Worrell, Department of Pathology, University of Texas Southwestern Medical School, Dallas.)

cause, as stated earlier, complexes in antigen excess are the ones most likely to be deposited in vascular beds. This occurs in several human diseases, such as systemic lupus erythematosus (SLE), which is associated with persistent exposure to autoantigens. Often, however, despite the fact that the morphologic changes and other findings suggest immune complex disease, the inciting antigens are unknown. Included in this category are rheumatoid arthritis, polyarteritis nodosa, membranous glomerulonephritis, and several other vasculitides.

Local Immune Complex Disease (Arthus Reaction)

The Arthus reaction may be defined as a localized area of tissue necrosis resulting from acute immune complex vasculitis, usually elicited in the skin. The reaction can be produced experimentally by intracutaneous injection of antigen in *an immune animal having circulating antibodies against the antigen.* Because of the excess of antibodies, as the antigen diffuses into the vascular wall, large immune complexes are formed, which precipitate locally and trigger the inflammatory reaction already discussed. In contrast to IgE-mediated type I reactions, which appear immediately, the Arthus lesion develops over a few hours and reaches a peak 4 to 10 hours after injection, when it can be seen as an area of visible edema with severe hemorrhage followed occasionally by ulceration. Immunofluorescent stains will disclose complement, immunoglobulins, and fibrinogen precipitated within the vessel walls, usually the venules. On light microscopy, these produce a smudgy eosinophilic deposit that obscures the underlying cellular detail, an appearance termed *"fibrinoid" necrosis* of the vessels (see Fig. 6–12). Rupture of these vessels may produce local hemorrhages, but more often the vascular lu-

mina undergo thrombosis, adding an element of local ischemic injury.

TYPE IV HYPERSENSITIVITY (CELL-MEDIATED)

The cell-mediated type of hypersensitivity is initiated by specifically sensitized T lymphocytes. It includes the classic *delayed-type hypersensitivity reactions initiated by CD4+ T cells and direct cell cytotoxicity mediated by CD8+ T cells.* It is the principal pattern of immunologic response to a variety of intracellular microbiologic agents, particularly *Mycobacterium tuberculosis,* but also to many viruses, fungi, protozoa, and parasites. So-called contact skin sensitivity to chemical agents and graft rejection are other instances of cell-mediated reactions. The two forms of type IV hypersensitivity are described next.

Delayed-Type Hypersensitivity

The best-known example of delayed hypersensitivity is the *tuberculin reaction,* which is produced by the intracutaneous injection of tuberculin, a protein-lipopolysaccharide component of the tubercle bacillus. In a previously sensitized individual, reddening and induration of the site appear in 8 to 12 hours, reach a peak in 24 to 72 hours, and thereafter slowly subside. An extremely sensitive patient may develop necrosis at the site of injection. Morphologically, delayed-type hypersensitivity is characterized by the accumulation of mononuclear cells in the subcutaneous tissue and deep and superficial dermis (Fig. 6–13). There is predominant accumulation around small veins and venules, producing a characteristic perivascular "cuffing." There is an associated increased microvascular permeability resulting from the formation of interendothelial gaps. Not unexpectedly, there is an escape of plasma proteins, giving rise to dermal edema and deposition of fibrin in the interstitium. The latter appears to be the main cause of induration, which is characteristic of delayed hypersensitivity skin lesions. In fully developed lesions, the lymphocyte-cuffed venules show marked endothelial hypertrophy and, in some cases, hyperplasia. Immunoperoxidase staining of the lesions not unexpectedly reveals a preponderance of CD4+ (helper) T lymphocytes (Fig. 6–14).[16]

With certain persistent or nondegradable antigens, the initial perivascular lymphocytic infiltrate is replaced by macrophages over a period of 2 or 3 weeks. The accumulated macrophages often undergo a morphologic transformation into epithelium-like cells and are then referred to as epithelioid cells. *A microscopic aggregation of epithelioid cells, usually surrounded by a collar of lympho-*

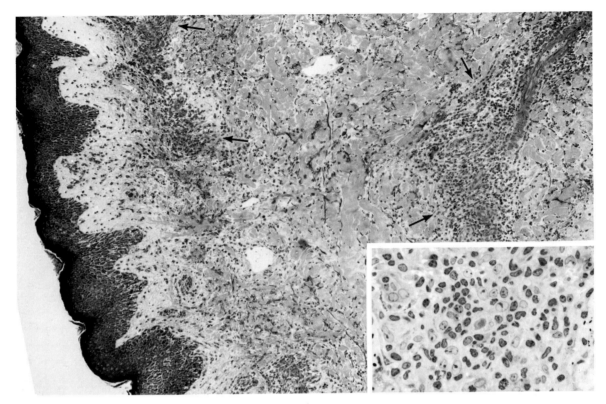

Figure 6–13. A 48-hour delayed hypersensitivity skin reaction in a man elicited with tuberculin. There are superficial and deep perivascular infiltrates of mononuclear cells *(arrows)*. Note edema *(pale areas)* of superficial dermis. *Inset:* Higher-power view of mononuclear perivascular infiltrate. (With permission from Dvorak, H.: Delayed hypersensitivity. *In* Zweifach, B.W., et al. (eds.): The Inflammatory Process, Vol III. New York, Academic Press, 1974.)

cytes, is referred to as a granuloma (Fig. 6–15). This pattern of inflammation that is characteristic of type IV hypersensitivity is called granulomatous inflammation.

The sequence of cellular events in delayed hy-persensitivity can be exemplified by the tuberculin reaction, which begins with the first exposure of the individual to tubercle bacilli. Naive CD4+ T cells recognize peptides derived from tubercle ba-cilli in association with class II molecules on the

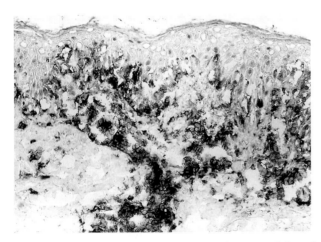

Figure 6–14. Experimentally induced cutaneous delayed hypersensitivity against the chemical dinitrochloroben-zene. Immunoperoxidase staining reveals a cellular infil-trate *(dark outlines)* that marks positively with anti-CD4 an-tibodies. (Courtesy of Dr. George Murphy, Department of Pathology, University of Pennsylvania, Philadelphia.)

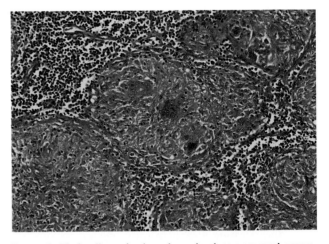

Figure 6–15. Section of a lymph node shows several granu-lomas, each made up of an aggregate of epithelioid cells and surrounded by lymphocytes. The granuloma in the center shows several multinucleate giant cells. (Courtesy of Dr. Trace Worrell, Department of Pathology, University of Texas Southwestern Medical School, Dallas.)

surface of monocytes or other antigen-presenting cells. This initial encounter drives the differentiation of naive CD4+ T cells to T_H1 cells. The induction of T_H1 cells is of signal importance because the expression of delayed hypersensitivity depends in large part on the cytokines secreted by T_H1 cells. Why certain antigens preferentially induce the T_H1 response is not entirely clear, but the cytokine milieu in which naive CD4+ T cells are activated seems to be relevant.[17] In the unimmunized host, microbes are first attacked by macrophages, albeit inefficiently. Nevertheless, this interaction leads, in some cases, to the production of IL-12 by the macrophages; this cytokine drives the differentiation of naive CD4+ T cells toward the T_H1 type. Thus it seems that induction of delayed-type hypersensitivity may be linked to IL-12 production. The sensitized T_H1 cells so formed enter the circulation and remain there for long periods, sometimes years. On intracutaneous injection of tuberculin in an individual previously exposed to tubercle bacilli, the memory T_H1 cells interact with the antigen on the surface of antigen-presenting cells and are activated (i.e., they undergo blast transformation and proliferation). These changes are accompanied by the secretion of the T_H1 type cluster of cytokines, which are responsible for the expression of delayed-type hypersensitivity (Fig. 6-16). Cytokines most relevant to this reaction and their actions are as follows.

- IFN-γ is an extremely important mediator of delayed-type hypersensitivity. It is a powerful activator of macrophages. Activated macrophages are altered in several ways: Their ability to phagocytose and kill microorganisms is markedly augmented; they express more class II molecules on the surface, thus facilitating further antigen presentation; their capacity to kill tumor cells is enhanced; and they secrete several polypeptide growth factors, such as platelet-derived growth factor and TGF-β, that stimulate fibroblast proliferation and augment collagen synthesis. Thus activated, macrophages serve to eliminate the offending antigen, and if the activation is sustained, fibrosis results.
- IL-2 causes autocrine and paracrine proliferation of T cells, which accumulate at sites of delayed hypersensitivity; included in this infiltrate are some antigen-specific CD4+ T cells and many more bystander T cells activated by IL-2.
- TNF-α and lymphotoxin are two cytokines that exert important effects on endothelial cells: (1) increased secretion of prostacyclin, which in turn favors increased blood flow by causing local vasodilatation; (2) increased expression of ELAM-1 (see Chapter 3), an adhesion molecule that promotes attachment of the passing lymphocytes and monocytes; and (3) induction and secretion of low–molecular weight chemotactic

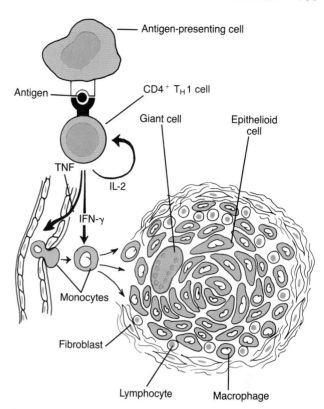

Figure 6-16. Schematic illustration of the events that give rise to the formation of granuloma in type IV hypersensitivity reactions. Note the role played by T_H1 cell–derived cytokines.

factors such as IL-8. Together all these changes in the endothelium facilitate the extravasation of lymphocytes and monocytes at the site of the delayed hypersensitivity reaction. TNF-α is also considered to be important in the formation of granulomas.[18]

This type of hypersensitivity is a major mechanism of defense against a variety of intracellular pathogens, including mycobacteria, fungi, and certain parasites, and may also be involved in transplant rejection and tumor immunity.

T Cell–Mediated Cytotoxicity

In this variant of type IV hypersensitivity, sensitized CD8+ T cells kill antigen-bearing target cells. Such effector cells are called cytotoxic T lymphocytes (CTLs). CTLs, directed against cell surface histocompatibility antigens, play an important role in graft rejection, to be discussed next. They also play a role in resistance to virus infections. In a virus-infected cell, viral peptides associate with the class I molecules within the cell, and the two are transported to the cell surface in the form of a complex. It is this complex that is recognized by cytotoxic CD8+ T lymphocytes. The lysis of infected cells before viral replication is completed leads in due course to the elimination of the infection. It is believed that many tumor-associated antigens (see tumor immunity, Chapter 7) may also be similarly presented on the cell surface. CTLs therefore may also be involved in tumor immunity.

TRANSPLANT REJECTION

Transplant rejection is discussed here because it appears to involve several of the hypersensitivity reactions discussed earlier. One of the goals of present-day immunologic research is successful transplantation of tissues in humans without immunologic rejection. Although the surgical expertise for the transplantation of skin, kidneys, heart, lungs, livers, spleen, bone marrow, and endocrine organs is now well in hand, it regrettably outpaces thus far our ability to confer on the recipient permanent acceptance of foreign grafts.

Mechanisms Involved in Rejection

Graft rejection depends on recognition by the host of the grafted tissue as foreign. The antigens responsible for such rejection in humans are those of the major histocompatibility antigen (HLA) system. *Rejection is a complex process in which both cell-mediated immunity and circulating antibodies play a role;* moreover, the relative contributions of these two mechanisms to rejection vary among grafts and are often reflected in the histologic features of the rejected organs.

T CELL–MEDIATED REACTIONS. The critical role of T cells in transplant rejection has been documented both in humans and in experimental animals. But how do T lymphocytes cause graft destruction? Both activation of CD8+ CTLs and delayed hypersensitivity reactions triggered by activated CD4+ helper cells seem to be involved. The generation of CTLs and antibodies in response to allogeneic HLA antigens is depicted schematically in Figure 6–17. The T cell–mediated reaction is initiated when the recipient's lymphocytes encounter the donor's HLA antigens. It is believed that interstitial dendritic cells carried in the donor organs are the most important immunogens. The host T cells encounter the dendritic cells within the grafted organ or after these cells migrate to the draining lymph nodes. The CD4+ helper T-cell subset is triggered into proliferation by recognition of the class II specificities. At the same time, precursors of CD8+ CTL (prekiller T cells), which bear receptors for class I HLA antigens, differentiate into mature CTLs. This process of differentiation is complex and incompletely understood. Involved are interactions of antigen-presenting cells;

T-cell subsets; and release of cytokines, such as IL-2, IL-4, and IL-5 (see Fig. 6–17). Once mature CTLs are generated, they lyse the grafted tissue. In addition to the specific cytotoxic T cells, lymphokine-secreting CD4+ T cells are also generated by sensitization, and they are believed to play an extremely important role in graft rejection. As in delayed hypersensitivity reactions, cytokines derived from the activated CD4+ T cells cause increased vascular permeability and local accumulation of mononuclear cells (lymphocytes and macrophages). According to some investigators, the delayed hypersensitivity with its attendant microvascular injury, tissue ischemia, and destruction mediated by accumulated macrophages is the most important mechanism of graft destruction.[19] It is more likely, however, that the relative importance of CD8+ T cell–mediated cytotoxicity versus CD4+ T cell–mediated reactions depends on the nature of HLA disparities between the donor and the host.

The molecular basis of allorecognition by T cells is incompletely understood.[20-22] It is unlikely that host T cells recognize allogeneic class I or class II MHC molecules directly; as with other forms of T-cell recognition, T-cell receptors of the recipient can react only with peptides that are within the antigen-binding groove of MHC molecules. Within this framework, there are two possibilities: Foreign MHC molecules shed from the surface of donor cells are processed by host antigen-presenting cells, and the derived peptides are presented in the groove of self-MHC molecules; alternatively, the host T cells recognize donor cell–derived peptides presented in the groove of allo-MHC molecules. The relative importance of these two possibilities is under investigation.[23]

ANTIBODY-MEDIATED REACTIONS. Although there is little doubt that T cells are pivotal in the rejection of organ transplants, antibodies evoked against alloantigens can also mediate rejection. This process can take two forms. *Hyperacute rejection occurs when preformed antidonor antibodies are present in the circulation of the recipient.* Such antibodies may be present in a recipient who has already rejected a kidney transplant. Multiparous women who develop anti-HLA antibodies against paternal antigens shed from the fetus may also have preformed antibodies to grafts taken from their husbands or children. Prior blood transfusions from HLA-nonidentical donors can also lead to presensitization because platelets and white cells are particularly rich in HLA antigens. In such circumstances, rejection occurs immediately after transplantation because the circulating antibodies react with and deposit rapidly on the vascular endothelium of the grafted organ. Complement fixation occurs, and an Arthus-type reaction follows. Fortunately, with the current practice of cross-

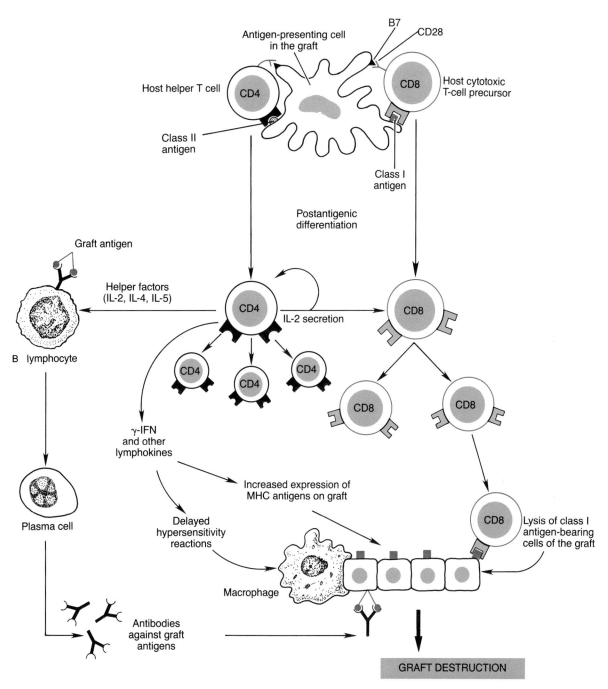

Figure 6–17. Schematic representation of the events that lead to the destruction of histoincompatible grafts. Donor class I and class II antigens along with B7 molecules are recognized by CD8+ cytotoxic T cells and CD4+ helper T cells, respectively, of the host. The interaction of the CD4+ cells with peptides presented by class II antigens leads to proliferation of CD4+ cells and the release of interleukin 2 (IL-2) from the cells. IL-2 further augments the proliferation of CD4+ cells and also provides helper signals for the differentiation of class I–specific CD8+ cytotoxic cells. In addition to IL-2, a variety of other soluble mediators (lymphokines) that promote B-cell differentiation and participate in the induction of a local delayed hypersensitivity reaction are produced by CD4+ helper cells. Eventually, several mechanisms converge to destroy the graft: (1) lysis of cells that bear class I antigens by CD8+ cytotoxic T cells, (2) antigraft antibodies produced by sensitized B cells, and (3) nonspecific damage inflicted by macrophages and other cells that accumulate as a result of the delayed hypersensitivity reaction.

matching, that is, testing recipient's serum for antibodies against donor's lymphocytes, hyperacute rejection is no longer a significant clinical problem.

In recipients not previously sensitized to transplantation antigens, exposure to the class I and class II HLA antigens of the donor may evoke antibodies, as depicted in Figure 6–17. The antibodies formed by the recipient may cause injury by several mechanisms, including complement-dependent cytotoxicity, antibody-dependent cell-mediated cytolysis, and the deposition of antigen-antibody complexes. *The initial target of these antibodies in rejection appears to be the graft vasculature.* Thus, antibody-dependent rejection phenomena in the kidney are reflected histologically by a vasculitis, sometimes referred to as "rejection vasculitis."

MORPHOLOGY OF REJECTION REACTIONS. On the basis of the morphology and the underlying mechanism, **rejection reactions are classified as hyperacute, acute, and chronic. The morphologic changes in these patterns are described as they relate to renal transplants.**[24] Similar changes are encountered in any other vascularized organ transplant.

Hyperacute Rejection. This form of rejection occurs within minutes or hours after transplantation and can sometimes be recognized by the surgeon just after the graft vasculature is anastomosed to the recipient's. In contrast to the nonrejecting kidney graft, which rapidly regains a normal pink coloration and normal tissue turgor and promptly excretes urine, a hyperacutely rejecting kidney rapidly becomes cyanotic, mottled, and flaccid and may excrete a mere few drops of bloody urine. The histologic lesions are characteristic of the classic Arthus reaction. There is a rapid accumulation of neutrophils within arterioles, glomeruli, and peritubular capillaries. Immunoglobulin and complement are deposited in the vessel wall, and electron microscopy discloses early endothelial injury together with fibrin-platelet thrombi. **These early lesions point to an antigen-antibody reaction at the level of vascular endothelium.** Subsequently these changes become diffuse and intense, the glomeruli undergo thrombotic occlusion of the capillaries, and fibrinoid necrosis occurs in arterial walls. The kidney cortex then undergoes outright infarction (necrosis), and such nonfunctioning kidneys are removed.

Acute Rejection. This may occur within days of transplantation in the untreated recipient or may appear suddenly months or even years later, when immunosuppression has been employed and terminated. As suggested earlier, acute graft rejection is a combined process in which both cellular and humoral tissue injuries play parts. In any one pa-

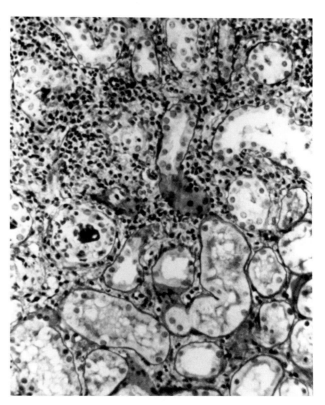

Figure 6–18. Acute cellular rejection of renal allograft manifested by a diffuse mononuclear cell infiltrate and interstitial edema. (Courtesy of Dr. Helmut Rennke, Department of Pathology, Brigham and Women's Hospital, Boston.)

tient, one or the other mechanism may predominate. Histologically, humoral rejection is associated with vasculitis, whereas cellular rejection is marked by an interstitial mononuclear cell infiltrate.

Acute cellular rejection is most commonly seen within the initial months after transplantation and is heralded by an elevation of serum creatinine level followed by clinical signs of renal failure. Histologically, there may be extensive interstitial mononuclear cell infiltration and edema as well as mild interstitial hemorrhage (Fig. 6–18). In humans, the mononuclear cell infiltrate consists primarily of medium-sized and small lymphocytes, along with some large "transformed" lymphocytes, which have abundant basophilic cytoplasm and a vesicular nucleus. As might be expected, immunoperoxidase staining reveals both CD4+ and CD8+ lymphocytes. In many cases, IL-2 receptors, which appear on activated T cells, can be demonstrated. Glomerular and peritubular capillaries contain large numbers of mononuclear cells that may also invade the tubules, causing focal tubular necrosis. The recognition of cellular rejection is important because, in the absence of an accompanying arteritis, patients promptly respond to immunosuppressive therapy. Cyclosporine, a widely used immunosuppressive drug, is also nephrotoxic, and hence the histologic changes resulting from cyclosporine may be superimposed.

Acute rejection vasculitis (humoral rejection) is seen most commonly in the first few months after transplantation or when immunosuppressive therapy is discontinued. Such patients show immediate, persistent poor function of the graft and do not respond to high-dose immunosuppressive therapy. The histologic lesions consist of necrotizing vasculitis with endothelial necrosis; neutrophilic infiltration; deposition of immunoglobulins, complement, and fibrin; and thrombosis. The process may evolve to extensive glomerular necrosis and cortical arteriolar thrombosis, with resulting cortical infarction. Almost all these patients also have evidence of acute cellular rejection. More common than this acute type of vasculitis is so-called **subacute vasculitis,** which is also seen in greatest intensity during the first few months after transplantation. Clinically, patients with subacute vasculitis have a course punctuated by repeated episodes of clinical rejection with altered renal function. The arterial lesions are rather characteristic. **The major alterations are in the intima,** which is markedly thickened by a cushion of proliferating fibroblasts, myocytes, and foamy macrophages, often leading to luminal narrowing or obliteration. The thickened intima may be infiltrated by scattered neutrophils and mononuclear cells, and the walls of most of these arteries show deposits of immunoglobulin and complement (Fig. 6–19).

Chronic Rejection. Because most instances of acute graft rejection are more or less controlled by immunosuppressive therapy, chronic changes are commonly seen in the renal allograft. Patients with chronic rejection present clinically with a progressive rise in serum creatinine level over a period of 4 to 6 months. The **vascular changes** consist of dense intimal fibrosis, principally in the cortical arteries, the lesion probably being the end stage of the proliferative arteritis described in acute and subacute stages. These vascular lesions result in renal ischemia manifested by glomerular ischemic simplification and obsolescence, interstitial fibrosis and tubular atrophy, and shrinkage of the renal parenchyma. Together with the vascular lesions, chronically rejecting kidneys usually have interstitial mononuclear cell infiltrates containing large numbers of plasma cells and numerous eosinophils. This is taken as an indication of chronic cell-mediated rejection, but in truth it must be said that delineation of the pathogenetic mechanisms in chronic graft rejection is much more difficult than it is in the acute forms.

The glomeruli in chronic graft rejection show no consistent pattern of injury. They may be entirely normal in appearance or may show ischemic changes that may be difficult to distinguish from recurrent glomerular disease.[25]

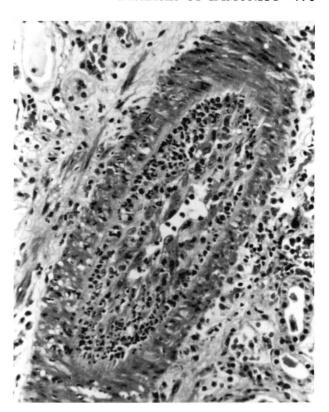

Figure 6–19. Acute humoral rejection of a renal allograft manifested by subacute vasculitis. The vascular intima is markedly thickened and inflamed. (Courtesy of Dr. Helmut Rennke, Department of Pathology, Brigham and Women's Hospital, Boston.)

Methods of Increasing Graft Survival

Because HLA antigens are the major targets in transplant rejection, minimization of the HLA disparity between the donor and the recipient would be expected to influence graft survival.[26] Indeed, in the case of intrafamilial (related donor) kidney transplants, a markedly beneficial effect of matching for class I antigens has been observed. In cadaver renal transplants, matching for HLA class I antigens (HLA-A and HLA-B) has at best a modest effect on graft acceptance. Additional matching for class II antigens (HLA-DR) results in a definite improvement in graft survival. In all likelihood, this benefit is derived because class II antigen-reactive CD4+ helper cells, which play an important role in the induction of both cellular and humoral immunity, are not triggered. It should be noted, however, that effective immunosuppression, particularly with cyclosporine, may mask the beneficial effects of HLA matching.

Except in the case of identical twins, who are obviously matched for all possible histocompatibility antigens, *immunosuppressive therapy* is a practical necessity in all other donor-recipient combinations.[27] Even HLA-identical siblings may differ at several minor histocompatibility loci, which can evoke slow rejection. At present, drugs such as azathioprine, steroids, cyclosporine, antilymphocyte globulins, and monoclonal anti–T cell antibodies (e.g., monoclonal anti-CD3) are employed.

As mentioned earlier, introduction of cyclosporine as an immunosuppressive agent has had a major impact on clinical organ transplantation. Cyclosporine suppresses T cell–mediated immunity by inhibiting activation of cytokine genes, in particular the gene for IL-2. FK506, another drug under clinical trial, like cyclosporine, suppresses T-cell activation. Although immunosuppression has produced significant gains in terms of graft survival, it should be remembered that immunosuppressive therapy is like the proverbial double-edged sword. The price paid in the form of increased susceptibility to opportunistic fungal, viral, and other infections is not small. These patients are also at increased risk for developing EBV-induced lymphomas (see Chapter 14). To make the anti–T cell therapy more selective, current attempts are directed toward eliminating only those T cells that are activated and therefore express the IL-2 receptor. Administration of anti–IL-2 receptor antibodies provides one such approach. Because adhesion molecules such as ICAM-1 play an extremely important role in immune cell interactions and extravasation of inflammatory cells, antibodies directed against such molecules are also being tested in experimental models.[28]

Transplantation of Other Solid Organs

The success of kidney transplantation has spurred the efforts to transplant a variety of organs, such as the liver (see Chapter 18), heart (see Chapter 12), lungs, and pancreas. Transplantations of the liver and the heart are now performed at most major medical centers in the United States. In contrast to the case with kidney transplantation, no effort is made to match HLA antigens of the donor and host. Because the transplanted liver or heart has to fit snugly into the space previously occupied by the host organ, the size and availability of the donor organ is of major importance, and it takes precedence over HLA match. With effective immunosuppression, the detrimental effects of an HLA mismatch can be greatly reduced.

Transplantation of Hematopoietic Cells

Use of this form of therapy for hematologic malignancies, aplastic anemias, and certain immunodeficiency states is increasing. Transplantation of ge-

netically engineered hematopoietic stem cells is also likely to be useful for somatic cell gene therapy. Several features distinguish bone marrow transplants from solid organ transplants. In most of the conditions in which bone marrow transplantation is indicated, the recipient is irradiated with lethal doses either to destroy the malignant cells (e.g., leukemias) or to create a graft bed (aplastic anemias). Two major problems arise in bone marrow transplantation: graft-versus-host (GVH) disease and transplant rejection.

GVH disease occurs in any situation in which immunologically competent cells or their precursors are transplanted into immunologically crippled recipients. GVH disease occurs most commonly in the setting of allogeneic bone marrow transplantation but may also follow transplantation of solid organs rich in lymphoid cells (e.g., the liver) or following transfusion of unirradiated blood.[29]

Recipients of bone marrow transplants are immunodeficient because of either primary disease or prior treatment of the disease with drugs or irradiation. When such recipients receive normal bone marrow cells from allogeneic donors, the immunocompetent T cells derived from the donor marrow recognize the recipient's HLA antigens as "foreign" and react against them. With sensitization, antirecipient CD4+ and CD8+ T cells are generated.

Acute GVH disease occurs within days to weeks after allogeneic bone marrow transplantation. Although any organ may be affected, predominant manifestations result from the involvement of the *immune system and epithelia of skin, liver, and intestines.* Affected individuals are profoundly immunosuppressed and are easy prey to infections. Cutaneous involvement is manifested by a generalized rash leading to desquamation in severe cases. Destruction of small bile ducts gives rise to jaundice, and mucosal ulceration of the gut results in bloody diarrhea.

Chronic GVH disease may follow the acute syndrome or may occur insidiously. These patients have extensive cutaneous injury, with destruction of skin appendages and fibrosis of the dermis. The changes may resemble systemic sclerosis, discussed later in this chapter. Chronic liver disease manifested by cholestatic jaundice is also frequent. Damage to the gastrointestinal mucosa may cause esophageal strictures. The immune system is devastated, with involution of the thymus and depletion of lymphocytes in the lymph nodes. Not surprisingly, the patients experience recurrent and life-threatening infections.

Because GVH disease is mediated by T lymphocytes contained in the donor bone marrow, depletion of donor T cells before transfusion virtually eliminates GVH disease. This protocol, however, has proved to be the proverbial double-edged sword: GVH disease is ameliorated, but the incidence of graft failures and the recurrence of disease in leukemic patients increases. It seems that the schizophrenic T cells not only mediate GVH but also are required for engraftment of the transplanted marrow stem cells and control of leukemic cells.

The mechanisms reponsible for rejection of allogeneic bone marrow transplants are poorly understood. It seems to be mediated by natural killer cells and T cells that survive in the irradiated host.

AUTOIMMUNE DISEASES

The evidence is now compelling that an immune reaction against "self-antigens"—autoimmunity—is the cause of certain diseases in humans. A growing number of diseases have been attributed to autoimmunity (Table 6–5), but it must be confessed that in many the evidence is not firm. This is because autoantibodies can be found in the serum or tissues of a remarkably large number of apparently normal individuals, particularly in older age groups. Apparently innocuous autoantibodies are also formed following damage to tissue and may serve a physiologic role in the removal of tissue breakdown products. Furthermore, cellular interactions involved in the normal immune response require recognition of self histocompatibility antigens. These observations indicate that some forms of autorecognition are normal and physiologic. How, then, does one define "pathologic" autoimmunity?[30]

Ideally, at least three requirements should be

Table 6–5. AUTOIMMUNE DISEASES

SINGLE ORGAN OR CELL TYPE	SYSTEMIC
Probable	*Probable*
Hashimoto's thyroiditis	Systemic lupus erythematosus
Autoimmune hemolytic anemia	Rheumatoid arthritis
Autoimmune atrophic gastritis of pernicious anemia	Sjögren's syndrome
Autoimmune encephalomyelitis	Reiter's syndrome
Autoimmune orchitis	*Possible*
Goodpasture's syndrome*	Inflammatory myopathies
Autoimmune thrombocytopenia	Systemic sclerosis (scleroderma)
Insulin-dependent diabetes mellitus	Polyarteritis nodosa
Myasthenia gravis	
Graves' disease	
Possible	
Primary biliary cirrhosis	
Chronic active hepatitis	
Ulcerative colitis	
Membranous glomerulonephritis	

* Target is basement membrane of glomeruli and alveolar walls.

met before a disorder can be categorized as truly due to autoimmunity: (1) the presence of an autoimmune reaction, (2) clinical or experimental evidence that such a reaction is *not secondary* to tissue damage but is of primary pathogenetic significance, and (3) the absence of another well-defined cause of the disease. Unfortunately, these requirements are met in only a few diseases, such as systemic lupus erythematosus and autoimmune blood dyscrasias.

The autoimmune disorders form a spectrum on one end of which are conditions in which autoantibodies are directed against a single organ or tissue, therefore resulting in localized tissue damage. A classic example is Hashimoto's thyroiditis, in which the antibodies have absolute specificity for thyroid constituents. At the other end of the spectrum is SLE, in which a diversity of antibodies results in widespread lesions throughout the body. In SLE, autoantibodies react with nuclear constituents of virtually every cell within the organism. In the middle of the spectrum falls Goodpasture's syndrome, in which antibodies to basement membranes of lung and kidney induce lesions and symptoms in these organs. It is obvious that autoimmunity implies loss of self-tolerance, and the question arises as to how this happens. Before we look for answers to this question, we should review the mechanisms of immunologic tolerance and self-tolerance.

IMMUNOLOGIC TOLERANCE

Immunologic tolerance is a state in which the individual is incapable of developing an immune response to a specific antigen. Self-tolerance refers to lack of responsiveness to an individual's antigens, and obviously it underlies our ability to live in harmony with our own cells and tissues. Several mechanisms, albeit not well understood, have been postulated to explain the tolerant state.[31,32] Three of these are worthy of consideration: clonal deletion, clonal anergy, and peripheral suppression. They are illustrated in Figure 6–20 and briefly described here.

• *Clonal deletion.* This refers to loss of self-reactive T and B lymphocytes during their maturation. Experiments with transgenic mice provide abundant evidence that T lymphocytes that bear receptors for self-antigens are deleted within the thymus during the process of T-cell maturation.[33] It is proposed that many autologous protein antigens are expressed in the thymus in association with self-MHC molecules. The developing T cells that express high-affinity receptors for such self-antigens are "negatively selected," or deleted, and therefore the peripheral T-cell pool is lacking or deficient in self-reactive cells. An issue not yet settled is whether there is extrathymic dele-

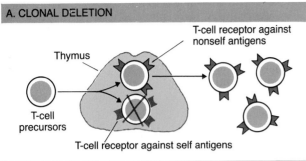

A. CLONAL DELETION

Thymus

T-cell receptor against nonself antigens

T-cell precursors

T-cell receptor against self antigens

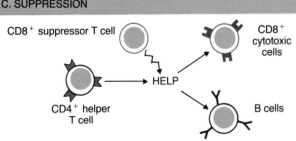

B. CLONAL ANERGY

B7

APC

Antigen

Co-stimulation

CD28

ON signal

Clonal activation

T cell

OFF signal

Clonal anergy

APC

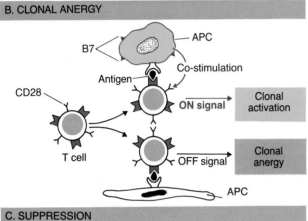

C. SUPPRESSION

CD8+ suppressor T cell

CD8+ cytotoxic cells

HELP

CD4+ helper T cell

B cells

Figure 6–20. Schematic illustration of the three possible mechanisms of self-tolerance.

tion of potentially self-reactive T cells that have not encountered autologous antigens within the thymus.[34] As with T cells, clonal deletion is also operative in B cells. Again by using transgenic mice, it has been documented that when developing B cells encounter a membrane-bound antigen within the bone marrow, they undergo deletion.[35] It should be pointed out, however, that clonal deletion of self-reactive lymphocytes is far from perfect. That there is "slippage" in this system is evidenced by the presence of B cells that bear receptors for a variety of self-antigens, including thyroglobulin, collagen, DNA, and myelin in the normal human peripheral blood.

• *Clonal anergy.* This refers to prolonged or irreversible functional inactivation of lymphocytes, induced by encounter with antigens under certain conditions. For example, it is well established that activation of antigen-specific CD4+ cells requires two signals: recognition of peptide antigen in association with class II MHC molecules on the surface of antigen-presenting cells (APCs) and a set of second co-stimulatory signals provided by APCs. To initiate second signals, certain T cell–associated molecules, such as CD28, must bind to its ligand (called B7) on APCs. If the antigen is presented by cells that do not bear the CD28 ligand, a negative signal is delivered, and the cell becomes anergic. Such a cell then fails to be activated even if the relevant antigen is presented by competent APCs (e.g., macrophages, dendritic cells) that can deliver co-stimulation. Clonal anergy of T cells may occur during development in the thymus, if the thymic APCs fail to deliver the second signal, or it may occur in peripheral tissues.[36] A special form of peripheral unresponsiveness may occur if a T cell that bears receptors for self-antigen encounters the antigen on a cell that does not express MHC class II molecules. For example, T cells reactive to an organ-specific antigen expressed on thyroid cells (but not within the thymus) may not be clonally deleted in the thymus. Such cells fail to be activated in the thyroid because normal thyroid acini do not express MHC class II molecules. As mentioned earlier, interactions between the CD4 coreceptor and MHC class II molecules are essential for the triggering of CD4+ T cells. Clonal anergy affects B cells as well and is probably the major mechanism for B-cell tolerance to self-antigens. It is believed that if B cells encounter antigen before they are fully mature, the antigen-receptor complex is endocytosed but, in contrast to mature B cells, such cells never reexpress their immunoglobulin receptors. Understandably, such cells are unable to respond to subsequent antigenic stimulation. In addition to antigen-induced loss of surface immunoglobulin receptors, other mechanisms of B-cell anergy are also postulated to exist.

• *Peripheral suppression by T cells.* Although clonal deletion and anergy are the primary mechanisms of self-tolerance, it is believed that additional fail-safe mechanisms must also exist. Many factors, both cellular and humoral, that can actively suppress autoreactive lymphocytes have been described. Most interest, however, has focused on suppressor T cells. These cells, like cytotoxic T cells, are CD8+ but are believed to comprise a distinct subset. A subset of CD4+ cells that can regulate T-cell autoreactivity against pancreatic beta cells has also been demonstrated.[37] The molecular mechanisms by which suppressor T cells recognize antigens and exert their suppressive effects have remained elusive. There is some evidence that peripheral suppression of autoreactivity may be mediated in part by the regulated secretion of cytokines. Suppressor cells may inhibit autoreactivity by secreting cytokines, such as TGF-β_1, known to down-regulate many immune responses. As evidence, targeted disruption of the TGF-β_1 gene in mice gives rise to inflammatory lesions that are similar to those seen in many autoimmune diseases.[38]

Prevention of autoimmunity is so vital to survival that several mechanisms have evolved to protect us from our "protectors." There is firm evidence for clonal deletion as well as clonal anergy; their relative importance in maintaining self-tolerance is not established and may well vary with the nature of the autoantigen (e.g., cell-bound versus soluble). Because helper T cells are critical control elements for both cellular and humoral immunity, *tolerance of self-reactive T cells is extremely important for prevention of autoimmune diseases.* Most self-antigens are T dependent; therefore, autoantibody formation may be prevented by tolerance of either hapten-specific B cells or the relevant helper T cells or both. Lymphocytes (both T and B cells) that "leak" through the barriers of clonal deletion or anergy are restrained by suppressor mechanisms.

MECHANISMS OF AUTOIMMUNE DISEASES

Although it would be attractive to explain all autoimmune diseases by a single mechanism, it is now clear that there are a number of ways by which tolerance can be bypassed, thus terminating a previously unresponsive state to autoantigens. More than one defect might be present in each disease, and the defects vary from one disorder to the other. Furthermore, the pathogenesis of autoimmunity appears to involve immunologic, genetic, and viral factors interacting through complicated mechanisms that are poorly understood. Here we can only scratch the surface of the rapidly evolving area of investigation into the mechanisms of autoimmunity. First we discuss the initiating immunologic mechanisms, and then the role of genetic and viral factors is reviewed briefly.

The initiating mechanisms in autoimmunity can best be understood in terms of those discussed for tolerance. Four general mechanisms for loss of self-tolerance have been postulated.

BYPASS OF HELPER T CELL TOLERANCE. It can be deduced from our earlier discussion that tolerance of CD4+ helper T cells is critical to the prevention of autoimmunity. Tolerance to a self-antigen is often associated with clonal deletion or anergy of carrier-specific helper T cells in the presence of fully competent hapten-specific B cells. Therefore, tolerance may be broken if the need for tolerant helper T cells is bypassed or substituted. This can be accomplished experimentally in several ways, some of which may have relevance to human autoimmunity.

Modification of the Molecule. If a potentially autoantigenic determinant (hapten) is complexed to a new carrier, the carrier part of the complex may be recognized by nontolerant T cells as foreign. The latter would then cooperate with the hapten-specific B cells, leading to the production of autoantibodies. This modification of the molecule could arise in several ways:

- *Complexing of self-antigens with drugs or microorganisms.* Autoimmune hemolytic anemia associated with drugs (e.g., antihypertensive agent alpha-methyldopa) may be due to an alteration of the red cell surface, thus providing a new carrier for an Rh antigen-hapten that stimulates B cells.
- *Partial degradation of autoantigen.* This could expose new antigenic determinants. Thus, partially degraded collagen and enzymically altered thyroglobulin or gamma globulin are more immunogenic than the native species. The autoantibodies to gamma globulin (rheumatoid factor) induced during some bacterial, viral, and parasitic infections may well be due to alterations of gamma globulin by either the microorganisms or lysosomal hydrolases.

Molecular Mimicry. Several infectious agents cross-react with human tissues through their haptenic determinants (B-cell epitopes).[39] The infecting microorganisms may trigger an antibody response by presenting the cross-reacting haptenic determinant in association with their own carrier, to which the helper T cells are not tolerant. The antibody so formed may then damage the tissue that shares the cross-reacting determinants. There is evidence that rheumatic heart disease sometimes follows streptococcal infection because an antibody to streptococcal M protein cross-reacts with the M protein in the sarcolemma of cardiac muscle. Molecular mimicry or cross-reactions may also apply to T-cell epitopes. Once the infectious agents provoke tissue damage, their continued presence is not necessary because tissue injury releases more self-antigens.

POLYCLONAL LYMPHOCYTE ACTIVATION. As mentioned earlier, tolerance in some cases is maintained by clonal anergy. Autoimmunity may occur if such self-reactive but anergic clones are stimulated by antigen-independent mechanisms. Several microorganisms and their products are capable of causing polyclonal (i.e., antigen nonspecific) activation of B cells. The best investigated among these is bacterial lipopolysaccharide (endotoxin), which can induce mouse lymphocytes to form anti-DNA, antithymocyte, and anti–red cell antibodies in vitro. Infection of B cells with EBV could also achieve the same effect because human B cells bear receptors for EBV.

IMBALANCE OF SUPPRESSOR-HELPER T-CELL FUNCTION. It may be expected from our discussion of suppressor T cells that any loss of suppressor T-cell function will contribute to autoimmunity, and, conversely, excessive T-cell help may drive B cells to extremely high levels of autoantibody production. Some experimental evidence supports this concept. There is an age-associated loss of suppressor T cells in the NZB × NZW (F1) mice, which develop an autoimmune disease similar to SLE as they age. Defects in suppressor T cell function or numbers (or both) have also been reported in human SLE, but this subject remains controversial. Enhanced helper T cell function manifested in the form of chronic hypersecretion of cytokines is seen in the lupus erythematosus–prone MRL-1pr/1pr mice, and a somewhat similar increase in helper T cell activity is also noted in certain patients with SLE.

EMERGENCE OF A SEQUESTERED ANTIGEN. Regardless of the exact mechanism by which self-tolerance is achieved (clonal deletion or suppressive influences), it is clear that induction of tolerance requires interaction between the antigen and the immune system. Thus, any self-antigen that is completely sequestered during development is likely to be viewed as foreign if introduced into the circulation, and an immune response will develop. Spermatozoa, myelin basic protein, and lens crystallin may fall into this category of antigens. Indeed, trauma to the testes involving the release of sperm into the tissues is followed by the appearance of antibodies to spermatozoa. This mechanism of autoimmune reactions is applicable only to the special situations cited.

GENETIC FACTORS IN AUTOIMMUNITY. There is little doubt that, both in laboratory animals and in humans, genetic factors determine the frequency and the nature of autoimmune diseases.[40] This conclusion is based on several lines of evidence: (1) familial clustering of several human autoimmune diseases, such as SLE, autoimmune hemolytic anemia, and autoimmune thyroiditis; (2) linkage of several autoimmune diseases with HLA, especially class II, antigens;[41] and (3) induction of autoimmune disease in transgenic rats.[42] In humans, HLA-B27 is strongly associated with certain autoimmune diseases, such as ankylosing spondylitis (see Chapter 27). Rats carrying the human HLA-B27 transgene develop ankylosing spondylitis and several other autoimmune disorders. This provides direct evidence for regulation of autoimmunity by a human MHC gene.

The precise mechanism by which certain genes predispose to autoimmunity is not clear, but attention is focused on the relationship of autoimmunity to class II MHC molecules.[43] At least two mechanisms can explain this association.

• It may be recalled that CD4+ helper cells are triggered by peptide antigens bound to class II MHC molecules. A class II allele that can bind to a given self-antigen may facilitate an autoimmune response. Molecular analyses of class II antigens have provided support for this hypothesis. The majority of patients with rheumatoid arthritis (an autoimmune disease of joints; see Chapter 27) carry the HLA-DR4 or HLA-DR1, or both alleles. These two alleles share a common stretch of four amino acids located in the antigen-binding cleft of the DR molecule. Thus the association between rheumatoid arthritis and certain DR molecules may be explained by the capacity of these DR molecules to bind an arthritogenic antigen, which in turn activates CD4+ T cells.

• Another possibility involves the effect of MHC class II molecules on the T-cell repertoire of the individual. It is postulated that MHC antigens influence the clonal deletion of potentially autoreactive T cells within the thymus. Because clonal deletion in the thymus is based on high-affinity binding of the T-cell receptors with self-antigens presented by class II molecules, it follows that if a given MHC allele presents an autoantigen poorly, the relevant autoreactive T-cell clone may not be deleted. Individuals who inherit such class II molecules may therefore be at increased risk for developing autoimmunity.

MICROBIAL AGENTS IN AUTOIMMUNITY. A variety of microbes, including bacteria, mycoplasmas, and viruses, have been implicated in triggering autoimmunity at one time or another.

Microbes may trigger autoimmune reactions in several ways. First, viral antigens and autoantigens may become associated to form immunogenic units and bypass T-cell tolerance, as described earlier. Second, some viruses (e.g., EBV) are nonspecific, polyclonal B-cell mitogens and may thus induce formation of autoantibodies. Third, viral infection may result in loss of suppressor T-cell function by mechanisms that at present are not entirely clear. Viruses and other microbes, particularly certain bacteria such as streptococci and Klebsiella, may share cross-reacting epitopes with self-antigens. Certain infectious agents cause powerful activation and proliferation of CD4+ T cells. The lymphokines produced under these conditions can break tolerance in anergic T cells.[44] In a transgenic mouse, production of IL-2 in the pancreatic islets led to autoimmune diabetes. Apparently IL-2 was able to activate beta cell–specific T cells that were otherwise anergic.[45] It must be obvious that there is no dearth of possible and some plausible mechanisms by which infectious agents may participate in the pathogenesis of autoimmunity. At present, however, there is no clear evidence to implicate any microbe in the causation of human autoimmune diseases.

Against this background, we can proceed to discuss the consequences of the loss of self-tolerance, that is, autoimmune diseases. As stated earlier, the autoimmune diseases of humans range from those in which the target is a single tissue,

Table 6-6. THE 1982 REVISED CRITERIA FOR CLASSIFICATION OF SYSTEMIC LUPUS ERYTHEMATOSUS*

CRITERION	DEFINITION
1. Malar rash	Fixed erythema, flat or raised, over the malar eminences, tending to spare the nasolabial folds
2. Discoid rash	Erythematous raised patches with adherent keratotic scaling and follicular plugging; atrophic scarring may occur in older lesions
3. Photosensitivity	Skin rash as a result of unusual reaction to sunlight, by patient history or physician observation
4. Oral ulcers	Oral or nasopharyngeal ulceration, usually painless, observed by a physician
5. Arthritis	Nonerosive arthritis involving two or more peripheral joints, characterized by tenderness, swelling, or effusion
6. Serositis	(a) Pleuritis—convincing history of pleuritic pain or rub heard by a physician or evidence of pleural effusion, or (b) Pericarditis—documented by electrocardiogram or rub or evidence of pericardial effusion
7. Renal disorder	(a) Persistent proteinuria greater than 0.5 g/dl or greater than 3+ if quantitation not performed, or (b) Cellular casts—may be red blood cell, hemoglobin, granular, tubular, or mixed
8. Neurologic disorder	(a) Seizures—in the absence of offending drugs or known metabolic derangements, e.g., uremia, ketoacidosis, or electrolyte imbalance, or (b) Psychosis—in the absence of offending drugs or known metabolic derangements, e.g., uremia, ketoacidosis, or electrolyte imbalance
9. Hematologic disorder	(a) Hemolytic anemia—with reticulocytosis, or (b) Leukopenia—less than 4.0×10^9/L (4000/mm^3) total on two or more occasions, or (c) Lymphopenia—less than 1.5×10^9/L (1500/mm^3) on two or more occasions, or (d) Thrombocytopenia—less than 100×10^9/L (100×10^3/mm^3) in the absence of offending drugs
10. Immunologic disorder	(a) Positive lupus erythematosus cell preparation, or (b) Anti-DNA antibody to native DNA in abnormal titer, or (c) Anti-Sm—presence of antibody to Sm nuclear antigen, or (d) False-positive serologic test for syphilis known to be positive for at least 6 months and confirmed by negative *Treponema pallidum* immobilization or fluorescent treponemal antibody absorption test
11. Antinuclear antibody	An abnormal titer of antinuclear antibody by immunofluorescence or an equivalent assay at any point in time and in the absence of drugs known to be associated with drug-induced lupus syndrome

* The proposed classification is based on 11 criteria. For the purpose of identifying patients in clinical studies, a person shall be said to have systemic lupus erythematosus if any 4 or more of the 11 criteria are present, serially or simultaneously, during any interval of observation.

With permission from Tan, E.M., et al: The revised criteria for the classification of systemic lupus erythematosus. Arthritis Rheum. 25:1271, 1982.

such as the autoimmune hemolytic anemias and thyroiditis, to those in which a host of self-antigens evoke a constellation of reactions against many organs and systems. In this chapter, we deal principally with those presumed autoimmune diseases that are primarily of a systemic nature, and we leave most single-tissue diseases to specific chapters throughout the book. For reference, however, Table 6-5 lists both systemic and organ-specific autoimmune disorders.

SYSTEMIC LUPUS ERYTHEMATOSUS (SLE)

Systemic lupus erythematosus is the classic prototype of the multisystem disease of autoimmune origin, characterized by a bewildering array of autoantibodies, particularly antinuclear antibodies (ANAs). *Acute or insidious in its onset, it is a chronic, remitting and relapsing, often febrile illness characterized principally by injury to the skin, joints, kidney, and serosal membranes.* Virtually every other organ in the body, however, may also be affected. Indeed, the clinical presentation of SLE is so variable that the American Rheumatism

Association has developed criteria for diagnosis of this disorder (Table 6-6). SLE is a fairly common disease, with a prevalence that may be as high as 1 in 2500 in certain populations.[46] Like most autoimmune diseases, SLE is predominantly a disease of women, with a frequency of 1 in 700 among women between the ages of 20 and 64 and a female-to-male ratio of 9:1. The disease is more common and severe in American black women (1 in 245). Although lupus erythematosus usually arises in the second and third decades, it may become manifest at any age, even in early childhood.

ETIOLOGY AND PATHOGENESIS. The cause of SLE remains unknown, but the existence of a seemingly limitless number of antibodies in these patients against self-constituents indicates that the *fundamental defect in SLE is a failure of the regulatory mechanisms that sustain self-tolerance.* Antibodies have been identified against an array of nuclear and cytoplasmic components of the cell that are neither organ nor species specific. Apart from their value in the diagnosis and management of patients with SLE, these antibodies are of major pathogenetic significance, as, for example, in the immune complex–mediated glomerulonephritis so typical of this disease.

ANAs are directed against several nuclear antigens and can be grouped into four categories[47]: *(1) antibodies to DNA, (2) antibodies to histones, (3) antibodies to nonhistone proteins bound to RNA, and (4) antibodies to nucleolar antigens.* Table 6–7 lists several ANAs and their association with SLE as well as with other autoimmune diseases to be discussed later. Several techniques are used to detect ANAs. Clinically, the most commonly utilized method is indirect immunofluorescence, which detects a variety of nuclear antigens, including DNA, RNA, and proteins (collectively called generic ANAs). The pattern of nuclear fluorescence suggests the type of antibody present in the patient's serum. Four basic patterns are recognized.

- *Homogeneous or diffuse nuclear staining* usually reflects antibodies to chromatin, histones, and, occasionally, double-stranded DNA.
- *Rim or peripheral staining* patterns are most commonly indicative of antibodies to double-stranded DNA.
- *Speckled pattern* refers to the presence of uniform or variable-sized speckles. This is one of the most commonly observed patterns of fluorescence and therefore the least specific. It reflects the presence of antibodies to non-DNA nuclear constituents. These components of the nucleus are easily extractable with buffered salt solutions, and hence they are also called *extractable nuclear antigens* (ENAs). Examples of ENAs include Sm antigen, ribonucleoprotein (RNP), and SS-A and SS-B reactive antigens (see Table 6–7).
- *Nucleolar pattern* refers to the presence of a few discrete spots of fluorescence within the nucleus and represents antibodies to nucleolar RNA. This pattern is reported most often in patients with systemic sclerosis.

It must be emphasized, however, that the patterns are not absolutely specific for the type of antibody, and because many autoantibodies may be present, combinations of patterns are frequent. *The immunofluorescence test for ANA is positive in virtually every patient with SLE; hence this test is very sensitive, but it is not specific because patients with other autoimmune diseases also frequently score positive* (see Table 6–7). *Furthermore, approximately 5 to 15% of normal individuals have low titers of these antibodies.* The incidence increases with age.

Detection of antibodies to specific nuclear antigens requires specialized techniques. Of the approximately 30 nuclear antigen-antibody systems,[48] some that are clinically useful are listed in Table 6–7. It should be noted that *antibodies to double-stranded DNA (dsDNA) and the so-called Smith (Sm) antigen are virtually diagnostic of SLE.*

There is some, albeit imperfect, correlation between the presence or absence of certain antinuclear antibodies and clinical manifestations. For example, high titers of dsDNA antibodies are usually associated with active renal disease. Conversely, the risk of nephritis is low if anti–SS-B antibodies are present.[49]

In addition to ANAs, lupus patients have a host of other autoantibodies. Some are directed against elements of the blood, such as red cells, platelets, and lymphocytes; others are directed against phospholipids. In recent years, there has been much interest in antiphospholipid antibodies. They are present in 20 to 40% of lupus patients and react with a wide variety of anionic phospholipids. Some bind to cardiolipin antigen, used in syphilis serology, and therefore lupus patients may have a false-positive test result for syphilis. Because phospholipids are required for blood clotting, patients with antiphospholipid antibodies may display abnormalities of *in vitro* clotting tests, such as partial thromboplastin time. Therefore these antibodies are sometimes referred to as "lupus anticoagulant." Despite having a circulating anticoagulant that delays clotting *in vitro*, these patients have complications associated with a *procoagulant* state.[50] They have venous and arterial thromboses, which may be associated with recurrent spontaneous miscarriages and focal cerebral or ocular ischemia. The pathogenesis of thrombosis in patients with antiphospholipid antibodies is unknown. Proposed mechanisms include direct endothelial cell injury, antibody-mediated platelet activation, and inhibition of endogenous anticoagulants such as protein C.

Given the presence of all these autoantibodies, we still know little about the mechanism of their emergence. Three converging lines of investigation hold center stage today: genetic predisposition, some nongenetic (environmental) factors and a fundamental abnormality in the immune system.

GENETIC FACTORS. The evidence that supports a genetic predisposition takes many forms.

- Family members have an increased risk of developing SLE.
- Up to 20% of clinically unaffected first-degree relatives reveal autoantibodies and other immunoregulatory abnormalities.
- There is a higher rate of concordance (24%) in monozygotic twins when compared with dizygotic twins (1 to 3%).[51] Quite interestingly, monozygotic twins who are discordant for SLE have similar patterns and titers of autoantibodies. These data suggest that the genetic makeup regulates the formation of autoantibodies, but the expression of the disease (i.e., tissue injury) is influenced by nongenetic (possibly environmental) factors.
- Studies of HLA associations further support the concept that MHC genes regulate production of specific autoantibodies, rather than conferring a generalized predisposition to SLE. Specific polymorphisms of the HLA-DQ locus have been

Table 6–7. ANTINUCLEAR ANTIBODIES IN VARIOUS AUTOIMMUNE DISEASES

NATURE OF ANTIGEN	ANTIBODY SYSTEM	DISEASE, % POSITIVE					
		SLE	Drug-Induced LE	Systemic Sclerosis—Diffuse	Limited Scleroderma—CREST	Sjögren's Syndrome	Inflammatory Myopathies
Many nuclear antigens (DNA, RNA, proteins)	Generic ANA (indirect IF)	>95	>95	70–90	70–90	50–80	40–60
Native DNA	Anti–double-stranded DNA	40–60	<5	<5	<5	<5	<5
Histones	Antihistone	50–70	>95	<5	<5	<5	<5
Core proteins of small nuclear ribonucleoprotein particles (Smith antigen)	Anti-Sm	20–30	<5	<5	<5	<5	<5
Ribonucleoprotein (U1RNP)	Nuclear RNP	30–40	<5	15	10	<5	<5
RNP	SS-A(Ro)	30–50	<5	<5	<5	70–95	10
RNP	SS-B(La)	10–15	<5	<5	<5	60–90	<5
DNA topoisomerase I	Scl-70	<5	<5	28–70	10–18	<5	<5
Centromeric proteins	Anticentromere	<5	<5	22–36	90	<5	<5
Histidyl–t-RNA synthetase	Jo-1	<5	<5	<5	<5	<5	25

Boxed entries indicate high correlation.

SLE = Systemic lupus erythematosus; LE = lupus erythematosus; ANA = antinuclear antibodies; RNP = ribonucleoprotein.

Data from Tan, E.M., et al.: Antinuclear antibodies (ANAs): Diagnostically specific immune markers and clues towards understanding systemic autoimmunity. Clin. Immunol. Immunopathol. 47:121, 1988; McCarty, G.A.: Autoantibodies and their relation to rheumatic diseases. Med. Clin. North Am. 70:237, 1986; and Bernstein, R.M., and Matthews, M.B.: Autoantibodies to intracellular antigens, with particular reference to t-RNA and related proteins in myositis. J. Rheumatol. 14(Suppl. 13):83, 1987.

linked to the production of anti-dsDNA, anti-Sm, and antiphospholipid antibodies.[52] In addition, linkage to certain non-MHC genes, especially TCRβ chain genes, has also been noted.

- Some lupus patients (approximately 6%) have inherited deficiencies of early complement components, such as C2 or C4. Lack of complement presumably impairs removal of circulating immune complexes by the mononuclear phagocyte system, and favors tissue deposition.

NONGENETIC FACTORS. There are many indications that, in addition to genetic factors, several *environmental* or nongenetic factors must be involved in the pathogenesis of SLE. The clearest example comes from the observation that *drugs* such as hydralazine, procainamide, and D-penicillamine can induce an SLE-like response in humans.[53] Exposure to *ultraviolet light* is another environmental factor that exacerbates the disease in many individuals. How ultraviolet light acts is not entirely clear, but it is strongly suspected of modulating the immune response. For example, it induces keratinocytes to produce IL-1, a factor known to influence the immune response. *Viruses* have also been suspected of causing SLE. Although viruses could well initiate autoimmune reactions by a variety of mechanisms that were discussed earlier, there is no hard evidence to support any role for viruses or other infectious agents in human SLE. *Sex hormones* seem to exert an important influence on the occurrence and manifestations of SLE. During the reproductive years, the frequency of SLE is 10 times greater in women than in men, and exacerbation has been noted during normal menses and pregnancy.

IMMUNOLOGIC FACTORS. With all the immunologic findings in SLE patients, there can be little doubt that some fundamental derangement of the immune system is involved in the pathogenesis of SLE. Although a variety of immunologic abnormalities affecting both T cells and B cells have been detected in patients with SLE,[54] it has been difficult to relate any one of them to the causation of this disease. For years it had been thought that an intrinsic B-cell hyperactivity is fundamental to the pathogenesis of SLE. Indeed, polyclonal B-cell activation can be readily demonstrated in patients with SLE and in murine models of this disease. Recent molecular analyses of anti-dsDNA antibodies, however, strongly suggest that pathogenic autoantibodies are not derived from polyclonally activated B cells. Instead it appears that the production of tissue-damaging antibodies is driven by self-antigens and results from an oligoclonal B-cell response not dissimilar to the response to foreign antigens. Furthermore, helper T cells cloned from the peripheral blood of lupus patients can induce autologous B cells to secrete anti-dsDNA antibodies *in vitro*. These anti-DNA antibodies are cationic—a feature associated with deposition in

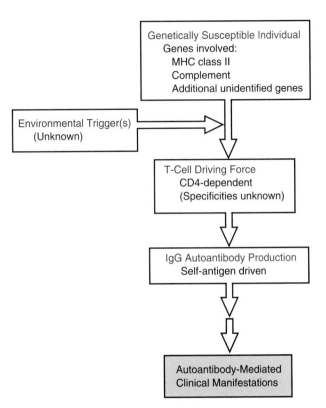

Figure 6–21. A model for the pathogenesis of systemic lupus erythematosus. (With permission from Drake, C.G., and Kotzin, B.L.: Genetic and immunological mechanisms in the pathogenesis of systemic lupus erythematosus. Curr. Opin. Immunol. 4:733, 1992.)

renal glomeruli—whereas the anti-DNA antibodies produced by polyclonally activated B cells are anionic and nonpathogenic. These observations have shifted the onus of driving the autoimmune response squarely on helper T cells. Expanded populations of helper T cells, some with an unusual phenotype (CD4–, CD8–), have been detected in patients with active SLE.[55] Based on these findings, a model for the pathogenesis of SLE, illustrated in Figure 6–21, has been proposed. It must be remembered, however, that SLE is a heterogeneous disease, and as mentioned earlier, the production of different autoantibodies is regulated by distinct genetic factors. Hence, there may well be distinct immunoregulatory disturbances in patients with different genetic backgrounds and autoantibody profiles.[56]

Regardless of the exact sequence by which autoantibodies are formed, they are clearly the mediators of tissue injury. *Most of the visceral lesions are mediated by immune complexes (type III hypersensitivity).* DNA–anti-DNA complexes can be detected in the glomeruli and small blood vessels. Low levels of serum complement and granular deposits of complement and immunoglobulins in the glomeruli further support the immune complex nature of the disease. *Autoantibodies against red cells, white cells, and platelets mediate their effects via*

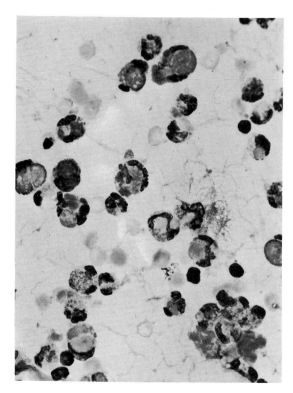

Figure 6–22. A cluster of LE cells (in vitro reaction) demonstrating homogeneous inclusions that have distorted the enclosing polymorphonuclear leukocytes.

Table 6–8. CLINICAL MANIFESTATIONS OF SYSTEMIC LUPUS ERYTHEMATOSUS

CLINICAL MANIFESTATION	PREVALENCE IN PATIENTS, %
Hematologic	100
Arthritis	90
Skin	85
Fever	83
Fatigue	81
Weight loss	63
Renal	50
Pleurisy	46
Myalgia	33
Pericarditis	25
Gastrointestinal	21
Raynaud's phenomenon	20
Central nervous system	20
Ocular	15
Peripheral neuropathy	14
Pneumonitis	11
Parotid gland enlargement	8
Liver disease	2

With permission from Condemi, J.J.: The autoimmune diseases. J.A.M.A. *258*:2920–2929, 1987. Copyright 1987, American Medical Association.

type II hypersensitivity. There is no evidence that ANAs, which are involved in immune complex formation, can penetrate intact cells. If cell nuclei are exposed, however, the ANAs can bind to them. In tissues, nuclei of damaged cells react with ANAs, lose their chromatin pattern, and become homogeneous, to produce so-called *LE bodies or hematoxylin bodies. Related to this phenomenon is the LE cell, which is readily seen in vitro. Basically, the LE cell is any phagocytic leukocyte (neutrophil or macrophage) that has engulfed the denatured nucleus of an injured cell* (Fig. 6–22). Sometimes LE cells are found in pericardial or pleural effusions in patients. The demonstration of LE cells *in vitro* involves the microscopic examination of white cells. If the withdrawn blood is agitated, a sufficient number of leukocytes can be damaged, thus exposing their nuclei to ANAs. The binding of ANAs to nuclei denatures them, and subsequent fixation of complement renders antibody-coated nuclei strongly chemotactic for phagocytic cells. The LE cell test is positive in up to 70% of the patients with SLE. With new techniques for detection of ANAs, however, this test is now largely of historical interest.

To summarize, *SLE appears to be a complex disorder of multifactorial origin resulting from interactions among genetic, hormonal, and environmental factors acting in concert to cause activation of helper T cells and B cells that results in the secretion of several species of autoantibodies. In this complex web, each factor may be necessary but not enough for the clinical expression of the disease; the relative importance of various factors may vary from individual to individual.*

MORPHOLOGY. The morphologic changes in SLE are extremely variable, reflecting the variability of the clinical manifestations and the course of the disease in individual patients. It can also be said that none of these morphologic changes is pathognomonic. The constellation of clinical, serologic, and morphologic changes is essential for diagnosis (see Table 6–6). The frequency of individual organ involvement is shown in Table 6–8. The most characteristic lesions result from the deposition of immune complexes and are found in the blood vessels, kidneys, connective tissue, and skin.

An acute necrotizing vasculitis involving small arteries and arterioles may be present in any tissue although skin and muscles are most commonly affected. The arteritis is characterized by fibrinoid deposits in the vessel walls. In chronic stages, vessels undergo fibrous thickening with luminal narrowing. In the spleen, these vascular lesions involve the central penicilliary arteries and are characterized by marked perivascular fibrosis, producing so-called **onionskin** lesions (Fig. 6–23).

Kidney. On light microscopic examination, the kidney appears to be involved in 60 to 70% of cases, but if immunofluorescence and electron microscopy are included in the examination of biopsy material, almost all cases of SLE show some renal abnormality.[57] According to the World Health Organization (WHO) morphologic classification of

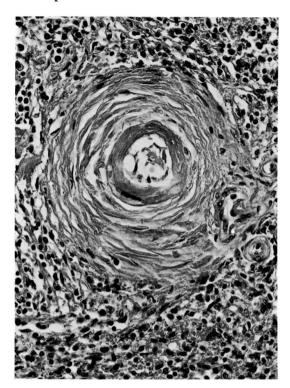

Figure 6–23. Lupus erythematosus—concentric periarterial fibrosis in the spleen.

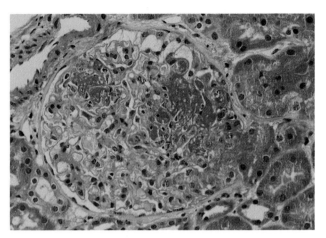

Figure 6–24. Lupus nephritis. There are two focal necrotizing lesions at 11 and 2 o'clock. Hematoxylin and eosin stain. (Courtesy of Dr. Helmut Rennke, Department of Pathology, Brigham and Women's Hospital, Boston.)

lupus nephritis, five patterns are recognized: (1) normal by light, electron, and immunofluorescent microscopy (class I), which is quite rare; (2) mesangial lupus glomerulonephritis (class II); (3) focal proliferative glomerulonephritis (class III); (4) diffuse proliferative glomerulonephritis (class IV); and (5) membranous glomerulonephritis (class V). It should be noted, however, that none of these patterns is specific for lupus.

Mesangial lupus glomerulonephritis is the mildest of the lesions and is seen in those patients who have minimal clinical manifestations, such as mild hematuria or transient proteinuria. It occurs in approximately 25% of patients. There is a slight-to-moderate increase in the intercapillary mesangial matrix as well as in the number of mesangial cells. Despite the very mild histologic changes, **granular mesangial deposits of immunoglobulin and complement are always present.** Such deposits presumably reflect the earliest change because filtered immune complexes accumulate primarily in the mesangium. The other changes to be described are usually superimposed on the mesangial changes.

Focal proliferative glomerulonephritis is seen in about 20% of initial biopsies of these patients. As the name implies, this is a focal lesion, affecting usually fewer than 50% of the glomeruli and generally only portions of each glomerulus. Typically one or two tufts in an otherwise normal glomerulus exhibit swelling and proliferation of endothelial and mesangial cells, infiltration with neutrophils, and

sometimes fibrinoid deposits and intracapillary thrombi (Fig. 6–24). Focal lesions are associated with proteinuria, sometimes in the nephrotic range (see Chapter 20). Hematuria is more pronounced than in the mesangial form. Renal insufficiency is present in one-third of the patients. Others may progress to renal failure.

Diffuse proliferative glomerulonephritis is the most serious of the renal lesions in SLE, occurring in 35 to 40% of patients who are biopsied. Anatomic changes are dominated by proliferation of endothelial, mesangial, and sometimes epithelial cells (Fig. 6–25), producing in some cases epithelial crescents that fill the Bowman's space (see Chapter 20). The presence of fibrinoid necrosis and hyaline thrombi indicates active disease. Most or all glomeruli are involved in both kidneys, and the entire glomerulus is almost always affected. Patients

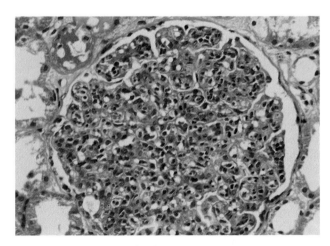

Figure 6–25. Lupus nephritis, diffuse proliferative type. Note the marked increase in cellularity throughout the glomerulus. Hematoxylin and eosin stain. (Courtesy of Dr. Helmut Rennke, Department of Pathology, Brigham and Women's Hospital, Boston.)

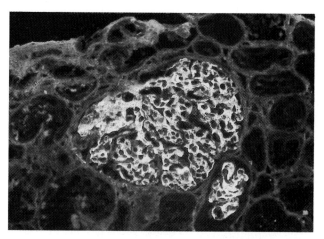

Figure 6–26. Immunofluorescence micrograph stained with fluorescent anti-IgG from a patient with diffuse proliferative lupus nephritis. One complete glomerulus and part of another one are seen. Note the mesangial and capillary wall deposits of IgG. (Courtesy of Dr. Helmut Rennke, Department of Pathology, Brigham and Women's Hospital, Boston.)

with diffuse lesions are usually overtly symptomatic, showing microscopic or gross hematuria as well as proteinuria that is severe enough to cause the nephrotic syndrome in more than 50% of patients. Hypertension and mild-to-severe renal insufficiency are also common.

Membranous glomerulonephritis occurs in 15% of patients and is a designation given to glomerular disease in which the principal histologic change consists of widespread thickening of the capillary walls. The lesions are similar to those encountered in idiopathic membranous glomerulonephritis, described more fully in Chapter 20. Patients with this histologic change almost always have severe proteinuria with the nephrotic syndrome.

All four types are thought to have the same general pathogenetic mechanism, that is, the deposition of DNA–anti-DNA complexes within the glomeruli. As mentioned earlier, cationic anti-DNA antibodies are most pathogenic because they bind to anionic sites in the glomeruli. Granular deposits of immunoglobulin and complement are regularly present in the mesangium alone, or along the entire basement membrane and sometimes massively throughout the entire glomerulus (Fig. 6–26). Why this same pathogenetic mechanism produces such different histologic lesions (and clinical manifestations) in different patients is not entirely clear.

Electron microscopy demonstrates electron-dense immune complexes that may be mesangial, intramembranous, subepithelial, or subendothelial in location: (1) All histologic types show large amounts of deposits in the mesangium; (2) in membranous glomerulonephritis (class V), the deposits are predominantly between the basement membrane and the visceral epithelial cell (subepithelial), a location similar to that of deposits in other types of membranous nephropathy; (3) subendothelial deposits (between the endothelium and the basement membrane) are most commonly seen in the diffuse proliferative variety (Fig. 6–27). When extensive, subendothelial deposits create a peculiar thickening of the capillary wall, which can be seen by means of light microscopy as a "wire loop" lesion (Fig. 6–28). Such "wire loops" are often found in the diffuse proliferative type of glomerulonephritis (class IV) but can also be present in the focal (class III) and membranous types (class V). They usually reflect active disease and generally indicate a poor prognosis.

The natural history of lupus nephritis is not fully understood. It is generally believed that mesangial lupus nephritis represents mild disease that progresses to other, more serious forms in approximately 5% of cases. In contrast, focal (class III) disease is usually considered to be an earlier stage of diffuse (class IV) disease. Transformation from class III or IV to membranous (class V) disease can also occur.[57] Changes in the **interstitium and tubules are also frequently present in patients with SLE,** especially in association with diffuse proliferative glomerulonephritis. In a few cases, tubulointerstitial lesions may be the dominant abnormality. As we shall see in Chapter 20, granular deposits composed of immunoglobulin and complement similar to those seen in glomeruli are present in the tubular basement membranes in about 50% of patients with SLE, a pattern indicative of so-called tubular immune complex disease.

Skin. The skin is involved in the majority of patients. Characteristic erythema affects the facial "butterfly" area (bridge of the nose and cheeks) in approximately 50% of patients, but a similar rash may also be seen on the extremities and trunk. Urticaria, bullae, maculopapular lesions, and ulcerations also occur. **Exposure to sunlight incites or accentuates the erythema.** Histologically, the involved areas show liquefactive degeneration of the basal layer of the epidermis together with edema at the dermal junction (Fig. 6–29). In the dermis, there is variable edema and perivascular mononuclear infiltrates. Vasculitis with fibrinoid necrosis of the vessels may be prominent. Immunofluorescence microscopy shows deposition of immunoglobulin and complement along the dermoepidermal junction (see Fig. 6–29). Similar deposits may be present in uninvolved skin. The presence of immunoglobulin and complement at the dermoepidermal junction is not diagnostic of SLE because similar deposits are sometimes seen in the skin of patients with scleroderma or dermatomyositis.

Joints. Joint involvement is frequent, the typical lesion being a nonerosive synovitis with little deformity. The latter fact distinguishes this arthritis from that seen in rheumatoid disease. In the acute phases of arthritis in SLE, there is exudation of neutrophils and fibrin into the synovium and a perivas-

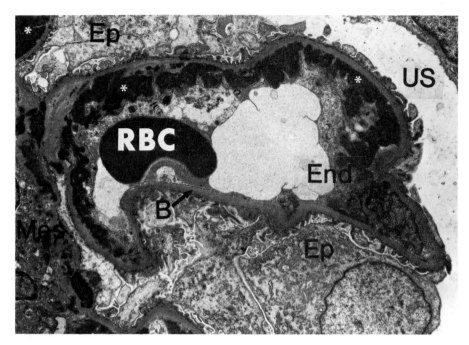

Figure 6-27. Electron micrograph of renal glomerular capillary loop from patient with systemic lupus erythematosus nephritis. Subendothelial dense deposits correspond to "wire loops" seen by light microscopy. End = endothelium; Mes = mesangium; Ep = epithelial cell with foot processes; RBC = red blood cell in capillary lumen; B = basement membrane; US = urinary space; * = electron-dense deposits in subendothelial location. (Courtesy of Dr. Edwin Eigenbrodt, Department of Pathology, University of Texas Southwestern Medical School, Dallas.)

cular mononuclear cell infiltrate in the subsynovial tissue.

Central Nervous System. The pathologic basis of central nervous system (CNS) symptoms is not entirely clear. It has often been ascribed to acute vasculitis with resultant focal neurologic symptoms. Histologic studies, however, of the nervous system in patients with neuropsychiatric manifestations of SLE fail to reveal significant vasculitis. Instead noninflammatory occlusion of small vessels by intimal proliferation is sometimes noticed. These changes are believed to result from damage to the endothelium by antiphospholipid antibodies. In addition, recent studies suggest that antibodies against a

synaptic membrane protein may play a role in the pathogenesis of CNS symptoms.[58]

Pericarditis and Other Serosal Cavity Involvement. Inflammation of the serosal lining membranes may be acute, subacute, or chronic. During the acute phases, the mesothelial surfaces are sometimes covered with fibrinous exudate. Later they become thickened, opaque, and coated with a shaggy fibrous tissue that may lead to partial or total obliteration of the serosal cavity.

Cardiovascular system involvement is manifested primarily in the form of pericarditis. Symptomatic or asymptomatic pericardial involvement is present in the vast majority of patients. Myocarditis, manifested as nonspecific mononuclear cell infiltration, may also be present but is less common. It may cause resting tachycardia and electrocardiographic abnormalities. Valvular endocarditis may occur, but it is clinically insignificant. In the era before the widespread use of steroids, the so-called Libman-Sacks endocarditis was more common. This **nonbacterial verrucous endocarditis** takes the form of single or multiple irregular 1- to 3-mm warty deposits on any valve in the heart, distinctively on **either surface of the leaflets** (i.e., on the surface exposed to the forward flow of the blood or on the underside of the leaflet) (Fig. 6-30). By comparison, the vegetations in infective endocarditis are considerably larger, and those in rheumatic heart disease (see Chapter 12) are smaller and confined to the lines of closure of the valve leaflets.

An increasing number of patients have clinical evidence of coronary artery disease (angina, myocardial infarction) owing to coronary atherosclerosis. This complication is noted particularly in young

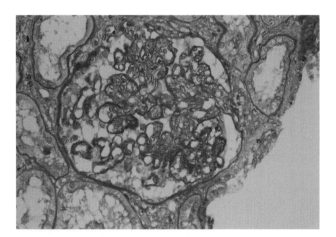

Figure 6-28. Lupus nephritis. A glomerulus with several "wire loop" lesions representing extensive subendothelial deposits of immune complexes. PAS stain. (Courtesy of Dr. Helmut Rennke, Department of Pathology, Brigham and Women's Hospital, Boston.)

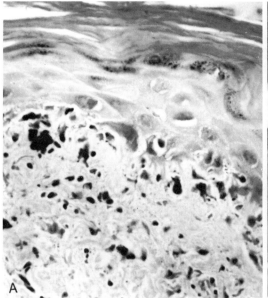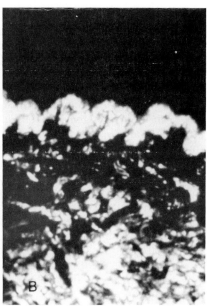

Figure 6-29. Systemic lupus erythematosus involving the skin. *A,* Hematoxylin and eosin-stained section shows liquefactive degeneration of the basal layer of epidermis and edema at the dermoepidermal junction. *B,* Immunofluorescence micrograph stained for IgG reveals deposits of immunoglobulin along the dermoepidermal junction. (Courtesy of Dr. Candace Kasper, Department of Pathology, University of Texas Southwestern Medical School, Dallas.)

patients with long-standing disease and especially in those who have been treated with corticosteroids. The pathogenesis of accelerated coronary atherosclerosis is unclear. Coronary endothelium may be damaged by antiphospholipid antibodies and/or immune complex and thus become predisposed to atherosclerosis.[59]

Spleen. The spleen may be moderately enlarged. Capsular thickening is common, as is follicular hyperplasia. Plasma cells are usually numerous in the pulp and can be shown to contain immunoglobulins of the IgG and IgM variety by fluorescence microscopy. As mentioned earlier, the central penicilliary arteries show thickening and perivascular fibrosis, producing the so-called onionskin lesions.

Lungs. Pleuritis and pleural effusions are the most common pulmonary manifestations, affecting almost 50% of patients. Less commonly there is evidence of alveolar injury in the form of edema and hemorrhage. In some cases, there is chronic interstitial fibrosis. None of these changes is specific for SLE.

Other Organs and Tissues. Acute vasculitis may be seen in the portal tracts of the liver accompanied by lymphocytic infiltrates, creating nonspecific portal triaditis. LE cells in the bone marrow may be strongly indicative of lupus erythematosus. Lymph nodes may be enlarged and contain hyperactive follicles as well as plasma cells, changes that are indicative of B-cell activation.

CLINICAL COURSE. It should be evident from Tables 6-6 and 6-8 that SLE is a multisystem disease, and as such it is highly variable in its clinical presentation. Typically the patient is a young woman with a butterfly rash over the face, fever, pain but no deformity in one or more peripheral joints (feet, ankles, knees, hips, fingers, wrists, elbows, shoulders), pleuritic chest pain, and photosensitivity. In many patients, however, the presentation of SLE is subtle and puzzling, taking forms

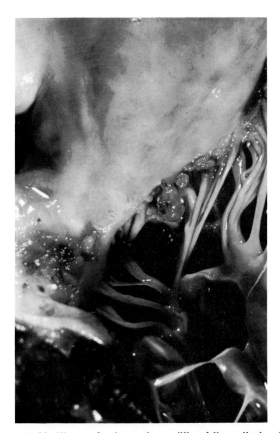

Figure 6-30. Libman-Sacks endocarditis of the mitral valve in lupus erythematosus. The small vegetations attached to the margin of the valve leaflet are easily seen.

such as a febrile illness of unknown origin, abnormal urinary findings, or joint disease masquerading as rheumatoid arthritis or rheumatic fever. ANAs can be found in virtually 100% of patients. ANAs, however, can also be found in patients with other autoimmune disorders (see Table 6–7). *As mentioned earlier, antibodies against double-stranded DNA and Sm antigen are virtually diagnostic of SLE.* A variety of clinical findings may point toward renal involvement, including hematuria, red cell casts, proteinuria, and, in some cases, the classic nephrotic syndrome (see Chapter 20). Laboratory evidence of some hematologic derangement is seen in virtually every case, but in some patients, they may be the presenting manifestation as well as the dominant clinical problem. In still others, mental aberrations, including psychosis or convulsions, may constitute prominent clinical problems.

The course of the disease is variable and almost unpredictable. Rare acute cases result in death within weeks to months. More often, with appropriate therapy, the disease is characterized by flareups and remissions spanning a period of years or even decades. During acute flareups, increased formation of immune complexes and the accompanying complement activation often results in hypocomplementemia. Disease exacerbations are usually treated by corticosteroids or other immunosuppressant drugs. Even without therapy, in some patients the disease may run a benign course with skin manifestations and mild hematuria for years. The outcome has improved significantly in the recent past, and an approximately 70% 10-year survival can be expected. *The most common causes of death are renal failure and intercurrent infections, followed by diffuse CNS disease.* Patients treated with steroids and immunosuppressive drugs incur the usual risks associated with such therapy.

As mentioned earlier, involvement of skin along with multisystem disease is fairly common in SLE. In addition, two syndromes have been recognized in which the cutaneous involvement is the most prominent or exclusive feature.

CHRONIC DISCOID LUPUS ERYTHEMATOSUS. Chronic discoid lupus erythematosus is a disease in which the skin manifestations may mimic SLE, but systemic manifestations are rare. It is characterized by the presence of skin plaques showing varying degrees of edema, erythema, scaliness, follicular plugging, and skin atrophy surrounded by an elevated erythematous border. The face and scalp are usually affected, but widely disseminated lesions occasionally occur. The disease is usually confined to the skin, but 5 to 10% of patients with discoid lupus erythematosus develop multisystem manifestations after many years. Conversely, some patients with SLE may have prominent discoid lesions in the skin. Approximately 35% of patients show a positive ANA test but antibodies to double-stranded DNA are rarely present. Immunofluores-

cence studies of skin biopsies show the same deposition of immunoglobulin and C3 at the dermo-epidermal junction that is seen in SLE.

SUBACUTE CUTANEOUS LUPUS ERYTHEMATOSUS. This condition also presents with predominant skin involvement and can be distinguished from chronic discoid lupus erythematosus by several criteria. It is characterized by widespread but superficial and nonscarring lesions and mild systemic disease. Furthermore, there is a strong association with antibodies to the SS-A antigen and with the HLA-DR3 genotype. Thus, the term subacute lupus erythematosus seems to define a group intermediate between SLE and lupus erythematosus localized only to skin.[60]

DRUG-INDUCED LUPUS ERYTHEMATOSUS. An interesting lupus erythematosus–like syndrome develops in patients receiving a variety of drugs, including hydralazine (given for hypertension), procainamide, isoniazid, and D-penicillamine, to name only a few of the many therapeutic agents that have been implicated.[61] Many are associated with the development of ANAs, but most do not have symptoms of lupus erythematosus. For example, 80% of the patients receiving procainamide are positive for ANAs, but only one-third of these manifest clinical symptoms, such as arthralgias, fever, and serositis. *Although multiple organs are affected, renal and CNS involvement is distinctly uncommon.* As compared with idiopathic SLE, there are serologic and genetic differences as well. Anti–double-stranded DNA antibodies are rare, but there is an extremely high frequency of anti-histone antibodies. Persons with the HLA-DR4 antigen are at a greater risk of developing lupus erythematosus after administration of hydralazine. Fortunately, the disease remits after withdrawal of the offending drug.

SJÖGREN'S SYNDROME

Sjögren's syndrome is a clinicopathologic entity characterized by dry eyes (keratoconjunctivitis sicca) and dry mouth (xerostomia) resulting from immunologically mediated destruction of the lacrimal and salivary glands. It occurs as an isolated disorder (primary form), also known as the *sicca syndrome,* or more often in association with another autoimmune disease (secondary form). Among the associated disorders, rheumatoid arthritis is the most common, but some patients have SLE, polymyositis, scleroderma, vasculitis, mixed connective tissue disease, or thyroiditis.

ETIOLOGY AND PATHOGENESIS. As we shall see in the description of morphology, the decrease in tears and saliva (sicca syndrome) is the result of *lymphocytic infiltration* and fibrosis of the lacrimal and salivary glands. The infiltrate contains predominantly activated CD4+ helper T cells and some B cells, including plasma cells that secrete antibody locally.[62] It is not clear, however, whether the tissue damage is mediated by the few cytotoxic T cells that infiltrate the gland or by autoantibodies, several of which can be found in the serum. About 75% of patients have rheumatoid factor regardless of whether coexisting rheumatoid arthritis is present or not. ANAs are detected in 50 to 80% of patients, and a positive LE test result is present in 25%. A whole host of other organ-specific and non–organ-specific antibodies have also been identified. Most important, however, are antibodies directed against two RNP antigens, SS-A (Ro) and SS-B (La) (see Table 6–7), which can be detected in up to 90% of patients. Those with high titers of antibodies to SS-A are more likely to have extraglandular manifestations, such as cutaneous vasculitis and CNS disease.

It should be recalled that these autoantibodies are also present in a smaller percentage of patients with SLE and hence are not diagnostic of Sjögren's syndrome. As with other autoimmune diseases, Sjögren's syndrome shows association with HLA class II alleles. Recent studies suggest linkage of the primary form with HLA-DR3 as well as HLA-DQA1 and HLA-DQB1 loci; the secondary form, like rheumatoid arthritis, is associated with HLA-DR4.[63] *To summarize, Sjögren's syndrome is associated with several autoantibodies, although the spectrum is not as broad as in SLE. Anti–SS-A and anti–SS-B are the two most common antibodies; hence they are considered to be important serologic markers of this disorder.*

How autoimmune reactions are initiated remains mysterious. EBV infection has been cited as a culprit, and circumstantial evidence supporting a role for EBV has been gathered.[64] As might be expected from the presence of autoantibodies, a variety of functional abnormalities has been detected in the T cells, B cells, and macrophages. The significance of these in the pathogenesis of Sjögren's syndrome is not clear. Of interest are studies that indicate the presence of a monoclonal B-cell population within the salivary glands that gives rise to monoclonal immunoglobulins or light chains in the serum. Whether or not these are the precursor of lymphomas, known to occur in these patients, is under investigation.[65]

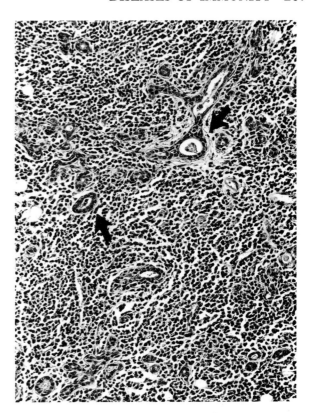

Figure 6–31. Sjögren's syndrome—submandibular gland. The intense lymphocytic and plasma cell infiltration virtually obscures the native architecture. Only a few residual ducts (arrows) can be identified.

MORPHOLOGY. As mentioned earlier, lacrimal and salivary glands are the major targets of the disease, although other exocrine glands, including those lining the respiratory and gastrointestinal tracts and the vagina, may also be involved.

The earliest histologic finding in both the major and the minor salivary glands is **periductal and perivascular lymphocytic infiltration.**[62] Eventually, the lymphocytic infiltrate becomes extensive, and in the larger salivary glands lymphoid follicles with germinal centers may be seen (Fig. 6–31). The ductal lining epithelial cells may show hyperplasia, thus obstructing the ducts. Later there is atrophy of the acini, fibrosis, and hyalinization and, still later in the course, atrophy and replacement of parenchyma with fat. In some cases, the lymphoid infiltrate may be so intense as to give the appearance of a lymphoma; however, the benign appearance of the lymphocytes, the heterogeneous population of cells, and the preservation of lobular architecture of the gland differentiate the lesions from those of lymphoma.

The lack of tears leads to drying of the corneal epithelium, which becomes inflamed, eroded, and ulcerated; the oral mucosa may atrophy, with inflammatory fissuring and ulceration; and dryness and crusting of the nose may lead to ulcerations and even perforation of the nasal septum. In approximately 25% of cases, extraglandular tissues, such as kidneys, lungs, skin, CNS, and muscles, are also involved. As mentioned earlier, these are more common in patients with high titers of anti–SS-A antibodies. **In contrast to SLE, glomerular lesions are extremely rare in Sjögren's syndrome.** Defects of tubular function, however, including renal tubular acidosis, uricosuria, and phosphaturia, are often seen and are associated histologically with a **tubulointerstitial nephritis** (see Chapter 20).

CLINICAL MANIFESTATIONS. Approximately 90% of patients with Sjögren's syndrome are women between the ages of 40 and 60 years. As might be expected, symptoms result from inflammatory destruction of the exocrine glands. The keratoconjunctivitis produces blurring of vision, burning, and itching, and thick secretions accumulate in the conjunctival sac. The xerostomia results in difficulty in swallowing solid foods, a decrease in the ability to taste, cracks and fissures in the mouth, and dryness of the buccal mucosa. Parotid gland enlargement is present in half the patients; dryness of the nasal mucosa, epistaxis, recurrent bronchitis, and pneumonitis are other symptoms. The 60% of patients who have an accompanying autoimmune disorder, such as rheumatoid arthritis, also have the symptoms and signs of that disorder.

The combination of lacrimal and salivary gland inflammatory involvement was once called *Mikulicz's disease.* The name has now been replaced, however, by *Mikulicz's syndrome,* broadened to include lacrimal and salivary gland enlargement of whatever cause. Sarcoidosis, leukemia, lymphoma, and other tumors likewise produce Mikulicz's syndrome. Thus, *biopsy of the lip (to examine minor salivary glands) is essential for the diagnosis of Sjögren's syndrome.*

The lymph nodes of patients with Sjögren's syndrome show not only enlargement, but also a pleomorphic infiltrate of cells with frequent mitoses. The appearance has been described as "pseudolymphoma" because not all the criteria of malignant lymphoma are satisfied. Clear-cut non-Hodgkin's lymphomas, however, mostly of the B-cell type, have developed in the salivary glands and lymph nodes in some patients, and it is believed that patients with Sjögren's syndrome have an approximately 40-fold higher risk of developing lymphoid malignancies. This has led to the statement that the disorder lies "somewhere between hyperplasia and neoplasia."

SYSTEMIC SCLEROSIS (SCLERODERMA)

Although the term "scleroderma" is ingrained in the literature through common usage, this disease is better named systemic sclerosis because it is characterized by excessive fibrosis *throughout the body.* The skin is most commonly affected, but the gastrointestinal tract, kidneys, heart, muscles, and lungs also are frequently involved. In some patients, the disease appears to remain confined to the skin for many years, but in the majority, it progresses to visceral involvement with death from renal failure, cardiac failure, pulmonary insufficiency, or intestinal malabsorption. In recent years, the clinical heterogeneity of systemic sclerosis has been recognized by classifying the disease into two major categories[66]: (1) *diffuse scleroderma,* characterized by widespread skin involvement at onset, with rapid progression and early visceral involvement, and (2) *localized scleroderma,* associated with relatively limited skin involvement often confined to fingers, forearms, and face. Visceral involvement occurs late; hence, the clinical course is relatively benign. Because of the somewhat higher incidence of *c*alcinosis, *R*aynaud's phenomenon, *e*sophageal dysmotility, *s*clerodactyly, and *t*elangiectasia, these patients are sometimes said to have the CREST syndrome.

Several other variants and related conditions, such as eosinophilic fasciitis, are far less frequent and are not described here.

ETIOLOGY AND PATHOGENESIS. Systemic sclerosis is a disease of unknown cause. Excessive deposition of collagen, the hallmark of systemic sclerosis, results from multiple interacting factors that ultimately lead to the production of a variety of fibroblast growth factors. Both immunologic derangements and vascular abnormalities play a role in fibrogenesis.[67,68]

According to the *immunologic hypothesis,* fibrosis is secondary to abnormal activation of the immune system. It is proposed that T cells responding to an as yet unidentified antigen accumulate in the skin and release cytokines that recruit inflammatory cells, including mast cells and macrophages. Several mast cell–derived and monocyte-derived mediators, such as histamine, heparin, IL-1, TNF-α, PDGF, and TGF-β, can enhance fibroblast growth or up-regulate collagen synthesis. In support of this hypothesis, activated CD4+ helper T cells can be found in the skin of many patients with systemic sclerosis. Accumulation of mast cells and activation of monocytes have also been documented.[69] The possibility that the immune system may be playing a role in the pathogenesis of systemic sclerosis is further supported by the finding that several features of this disease (including the cutaneous sclerosis) are found in chronic graft-versus-host disease, a disorder that results from activation of T cells.

The *vascular hypothesis* rests on the consistent presence of microvascular disease early in the course of systemic sclerosis. Intimal fibrosis is evident in 100% of digital arteries of patients with systemic sclerosis. Capillary dilatation as well as destruction are also common. Nailfold capillary loops are distorted early in the course of disease, and later they disappear. Thus there is unmistakable morphologic evidence of microvascular injury. Telltale signs of endothelial injury (increased levels of factor VIII–von Willebrand factor) and increased platelet activation (increased percentage of circulating platelet aggregates) have also been noted. It is proposed that repeated cycles of endothelial injury followed by platelet aggregation lead to release of platelet factors (e.g., PDGF, TGF-β)

that trigger periadventitial fibrosis. Activated or injured endothelial cells themselves may release PDGF and factors chemotactic for fibroblasts. Eventually, widespread narrowing of the microvasculature leads to ischemic injury as well.

What triggers injury to the endothelium is not clear. Both immunologic and nonimmunologic factors have been blamed. A protease released from activated T cells or mast cells has been implicated,[68] but this issue is not settled yet.

Although in the schema outlined here disturbances in the T-cell immunity have been emphasized and may well be important in the pathogenesis of systemic sclerosis, there is abundant evidence for disordered humoral immunity. Virtually all patients have ANAs that react with a variety of intranuclear targets.[70] Two ANAs more or less unique to systemic sclerosis have been described. One of these, directed against DNA topoisomerase I (anti–Scl 70), is highly specific. Depending on the assay, it is present in 28 to 70% of patients with diffuse systemic sclerosis. Patients who have this antibody are more likely to have pulmonary fibrosis and peripheral vascular disease. The other, an anticentromere antibody, is found in 22 to 36% of patients with this disease.[71] More important, 96% of those with the anticentromere antibody have the CREST syndrome. Hence this antibody, in contrast to the anti–DNA topoisomerase antibody, is restricted largely to patients with limited systemic sclerosis. It is rare to have both antibodies in the same patient.

To summarize, systemic sclerosis is associated with excessive fibrosis, changes in the microvasculature, and a variety of immunologic abnormalities. Although the antigens that trigger the (auto-)immune response have not been identified, it has been postulated that immunologic mechanisms lead to fibrosis either by elaboration of cytokines that activate fibroblasts or by inflicting damage on the small blood vessels, or by both (Fig. 6–32).

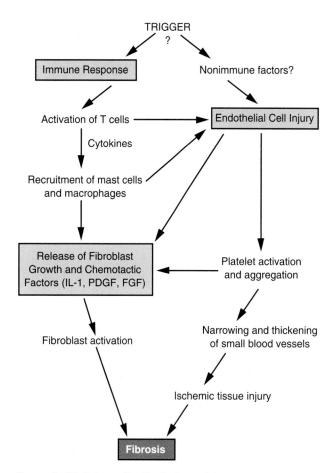

Figure 6–32. Schematic illustration of the possible mechanisms leading to systemic sclerosis.

MORPHOLOGY. Virtually all organs may be involved in systemic sclerosis. The prominent changes occur in the skin, alimentary tract, musculoskeletal system, and kidney, but lesions also are often present in the blood vessels, heart, lungs, and peripheral nerves.

Skin. A great majority of patients have diffuse, sclerotic atrophy of the skin, which usually begins in the fingers and distal regions of the upper extremities and extends proximally to involve the upper arms, shoulders, neck, and face. In the early stages, affected skin areas are somewhat edematous and have a doughy consistency. Histologically, there are edema and perivascular infiltrates containing CD4+ T cells, together with swelling and degeneration of collagen fibers, which become eosinophilic. Capillaries and small arteries (150 to 500 μm in diameter) may show thickening of the basal lamina, endothelial cell damage, and partial occlusion. With progression, the edematous phase is replaced by progressive fibrosis of the dermis, which becomes tightly bound to the subcutaneous structures. There is marked increase of compact collagen in the dermis along with thinning of the epidermis, loss of rete pegs, atrophy of the dermal appendages, and hyaline thickening of the walls of dermal arterioles and capillaries (Fig. 6–33). Focal and sometimes diffuse subcutaneous calcifications may develop, especially in patients with the CREST syndrome. In advanced stages, the fingers take on a tapered, claw-like appearance with limitation of motion in the joints (Fig. 6–34), and the face becomes a drawn mask. Loss of blood supply may lead to cutaneous ulcerations and to atrophic changes in the terminal phalanges. Sometimes the tips of the fingers undergo autoamputation.

Alimentary Tract. The alimentary tract is affected in more than half the patients. Progressive atrophy and collagenous fibrous replacement of the muscularis may develop at any level of the gut but is most severe in the esophagus. The lower two-thirds of the esophagus often develops a rubber-hose in-

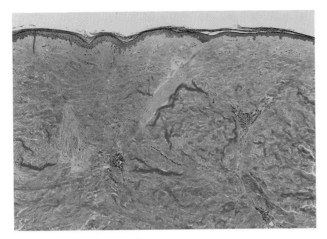

Figure 6-33. Systemic sclerosis. Note the extensive deposition of dense collagen in the dermis with virtual absence of appendages and thinning of epidermis. (Courtesy of Dr. Trace Worrell, Department of Pathology, University of Texas Southwestern Medical School, Dallas.)

flexibility. The mucosa is thinned and may be ulcerated, and there is excessive collagenization of the lamina propria and submucosa. Loss of villi and microvilli in the small bowel is the anatomic basis for the malabsorption syndrome sometimes encountered.

Musculoskeletal System. Inflammation of the synovium, associated with hypertrophy and hyperplasia of the synovial soft tissues, is common in the early stages; fibrosis later ensues. It is evident that these changes are closely reminiscent of rheumatoid arthritis, but joint destruction is not common in systemic sclerosis. In a small subset of patients (approximately 10%), inflammatory myositis indistinguishable from polymyositis may develop.

Kidneys. Renal abnormalities occur in two-thirds of patients with systemic sclerosis. The most prominent are those in the vessel walls. Interlobular arteries (150 to 500 μm in diameter) show intimal thickening as a result of deposition of mucinous or finely collagenous material, which stains histochemically for glycoprotein and acid mucopolysaccharides. There is also concentric proliferation of intimal cells. These changes may resemble those seen in malignant hypertension, but it has been stressed that in scleroderma the alterations are restricted to vessels 150 to 500 μm in diameter and are not always associated with hypertension. Hypertension, however, occurs in 30% of patients with scleroderma, and in 20% it takes an ominously malignant course (malignant hypertension). In hypertensive patients, vascular alterations are more pronounced and are often associated with fibrinoid necrosis involving the arterioles together with thrombosis and infarction. When this occurs, it becomes difficult to differentiate the lesions of scleroderma from those of other types of malignant hypertension (see Chapter 20). Such patients often die of renal failure,

which accounts for about 50% of deaths in patients with this disease. There are no specific glomerular changes.

Lungs. The lungs are involved in more than 50% of patients with systemic sclerosis. A diffuse interstitial and alveolar fibrosis may appear with variable fibrous thickening of small pulmonary vessels. In some instances, the alveolar walls thicken, and in others, there is an apparent distention of alveolar spaces and rupture of septa, leading to cyst-like cavities. Thus, patients with systemic sclerosis have a pulmonary picture similar to that of idiopathic pulmonary fibrosis, and systemic sclerosis must be considered in the differential diagnosis of diffuse pulmonary interstitial disease.

Heart. Pericarditis with effusion and myocardial fibrosis, along with thickening of intramyocardial arterioles, occurs in one-third of the patients. Clinical myocardial involvement, however, is less common.

CLINICAL COURSE. Systemic sclerosis is primarily a disease of women (female-to-male ratio, 3 : 1) with a peak incidence in the 50- to 60-year age group.[72] It must be apparent from the described anatomic changes that systemic sclerosis shares many features with SLE, with rheumatoid arthritis (de-

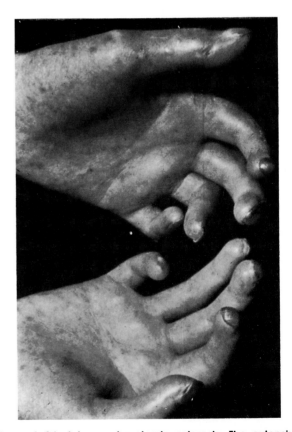

Figure 6-34. Advanced systemic sclerosis. The extensive subcutaneous fibrosis has virtually immobilized the fingers, creating a claw-like flexion deformity.

scribed in Chapter 27), and with polymyositis (see below under "Inflammatory Myopathies"). Its distinctive features are the striking cutaneous changes. Often Raynaud's phenomenon, manifested as episodic vasoconstriction of the arteries and arterioles of the extremities, precedes all other symptoms. Dysphagia attributable to esophageal fibrosis and its resultant hypomotility is present in more than 50% of patients. Eventually, destruction of the esophageal wall leads to atony and dilatation, especially at its lower end. Abdominal pain, intestinal obstruction, or malabsorption syndrome with weight loss and anemia reflect involvement of the small intestine. Respiratory difficulties due to the pulmonary fibrosis may result in right-sided cardiac dysfunction, and myocardial fibrosis may cause either arrhythmias or cardiac failure. Mild proteinuria occurs in up to 70% of patients, but rarely is the proteinuria so severe as to cause a nephrotic syndrome. The most ominous manifestation is malignant hypertension, with the subsequent development of fatal renal failure, but in its absence progression of the disease may be slow. The disease tends to be more severe in blacks, especially black women.

As mentioned earlier, the CREST syndrome is seen in some patients with limited systemic sclerosis. It is characterized by calcinosis, Raynaud's phenomenon, esophageal dysfunction, sclerodactyly, telangiectasia, and the presence of anticentromere antibodies. Patients with the CREST syndrome have relatively limited involvement of skin, often confined to fingers, forearms, and face, and calcification of the subcutaneous tissues. Raynaud's phenomenon and involvement of skin are the initial manifestations and often the only manifestations for several years. Involvement of the viscera, including esophageal lesions, pulmonary hypertension, and biliary cirrhosis, occurs late, and in general the patients live longer than those with systemic sclerosis with its diffuse visceral involvement at the outset.

INFLAMMATORY MYOPATHIES

Inflammatory myopathies comprise an uncommon, heterogeneous group of disorders characterized by possible immunologically mediated injury and inflammation of skeletal muscles. Three relatively distinct disorders, *dermatomyositis, polymyositis,* and *inclusion-body myositis,* are included in this category.[73] These may occur alone or with other immune-mediated diseases, particularly systemic sclerosis. The distinctive clinical features of each disorder will be presented first to facilitate discussion of pathogenesis and morphologic changes.

DERMATOMYOSITIS. As the name indicates, patients with dermatomyositis have involvement of the skin as well as the skeletal muscles. Dermato-myositis may occur in children or adults and is characterized by a distinctive skin rash that may accompany or precede the onset of muscle disease. The *classic rash takes the form of a lilac or heliotrope discoloration of the upper eyelids with periorbital edema.* It is often accompanied by a scaling erythematous eruption or dusky red patches over the knuckles, elbows, and knees (Grotton's lesions). *Muscle weakness* is slow in onset, is bilaterally symmetric, and *typically affects the proximal muscles first.* Thus tasks such as getting up from a chair and climbing steps become increasingly difficult. Fine movements controlled by distal muscles are affected late in the disease. Sometimes, especially in children, there are extramuscular manifestations, such as ulcerations of the gastrointestinal tract and soft-tissue calcification. As compared with the normal population, adult women with dermatomyositis have a slightly higher risk of developing visceral cancers (lung, ovary, stomach).[74]

POLYMYOSITIS. In this inflammatory myopathy, the pattern of symmetric proximal muscle involvement is similar to that seen in dermatomyositis. It differs from dermatomyositis by the lack of cutaneous involvement and its occurrence mainly in adults. There is a slight but statistically insignificant increase in the risk of developing visceral cancers.

INCLUSION-BODY MYOSITIS. This is the most recently identified inflammatory myopathy. In contrast with the other two entities, inclusion-body myositis begins with the *involvement of distal muscles,* especially extensors of the foot and flexors of fingers. Furthermore, muscle weakness may be *asymmetric.* This is an insidiously developing disorder that typically affects individuals over the age of 50 years.

ETIOLOGY AND PATHOGENESIS. The etiology of inflammatory myopathies is unknown, but the tissue injury seems to be mediated by immunologic mechanisms. In dermatomyositis, capillaries seem to be the principal targets. The microvasculature is attacked by antibodies and complement, giving rise to foci of myocyte necrosis. This hypothesis is supported by the presence of a higher-than-normal percentage of B cells within the muscles, and a relative absence of lymphocytes within the areas of myofiber injury. CD4+ T cells that presumably provide helper function for B cells are seen in the muscles. Polymyositis and inclusion-body myositis, in contrast, seem to be caused by cell-mediated injury. CD8+ cytotoxic T cells and macrophages are seen near damaged muscle fibers, and the expression of HLA class I molecules is increased on the sarcolemma of normal fibers. It may be recalled from the earlier discussion in this chapter that cytotoxic CD8+ T cells recognize antigens only when presented by class I MHC molecules.

How and why autoreactive B cells and T cells develop is as mysterious in the inflammatory my-

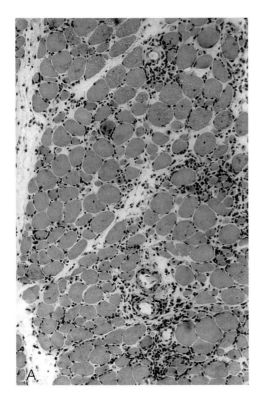

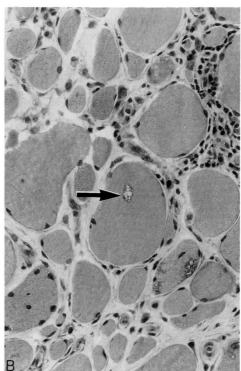

Figure 6–35. (A) Polymyositis with inflammatory infiltrate of muscle and endomysial fibrosis, features characteristic of an inflammatory myopathy. (Courtesy of Dr. U. De-Girolami, Brigham and Women's Hospital, Boston, MA). (B) Inclusion body myositis with rimmed vacuole (*arrow*) within a myocyte. (Courtesy of Dr. R. Heffner, Buffalo, NY.)

opathies as it is in other presumed autoimmune diseases. Similar to other diseases in this category, ANAs are present in a variable number of cases (see Table 6–7). The specificities of the autoantibodies are quite varied,[75] but those directed against tRNA synthetases seem to be more or less specific for inflammatory myopathies. One such antibody, referred to as anti–Jo-1, is noted in 15 to 25% of all patients within this group. Although the pathogenetic significance of this antibody is unknown, its presence is a marker of coexisting interstitial pulmonary fibrosis. This antibody may be present with any of the three histologic patterns of inflammatory myopathy.

MORPHOLOGY. The histologic features of the individual forms of myositis are quite distinctive and will be described separately.

Dermatomyositis. The inflammatory infiltrates in dermatomyositis are located predominantly around small blood vessels and in the perimysial connective tissue. Typically, a few layers of atrophic fibers are present at the periphery of fascicles. Perifascicular atrophy is sufficient for diagnosis even if the inflammation is mild or absent. Quantitative analyses reveal a dramatic reduction in the intramuscular capillaries, believed to result from vascular endothelial injury and fibrosis. In addition, there are several nonspecific changes indicative of muscle fiber necrosis and regeneration.

Polymyositis. In this condition, caused by direct injury to the myofibers by CD8+ T cells, the inflam-

matory cells are found in the endomysium. Lymphoid cells can be seen to surround and invade healthy muscle fibers. Both necrotic and regenerating fibers are present. There is no evidence of vascular injury (Fig. 6–35A).

Inclusion-Body Myositis. The diagnostic finding in this form of myositis is the presence of rimmed vacuoles, seen only in frozen section (Fig. 6–35B). The vacuoles are present within myocytes, and they are marked by basophilic granules at their periphery. Under the electron microscope, the granules consist of lamellated membranous structures. In the vicinity of the rimmed vacuoles, tubular filamentous inclusions are seen. The pattern of the inflammatory cell infiltrate is similar to that seen in polymyositis.

The diagnosis of myositis is based on clinical symptoms, electromyography, levels of muscle-related enzymes in serum, and biopsy. In a patient with muscle weakness, electromyography allows distinction between inflammatory muscle disease and diseases of neurons and receptors. As might be expected, muscle injury is associated with elevated serum levels of creatine kinase. Biopsy is required for definitive diagnosis.

MIXED CONNECTIVE TISSUE DISEASE (MCTD)

This term was coined in 1972 to describe the disease seen in a group of patients who were identi-

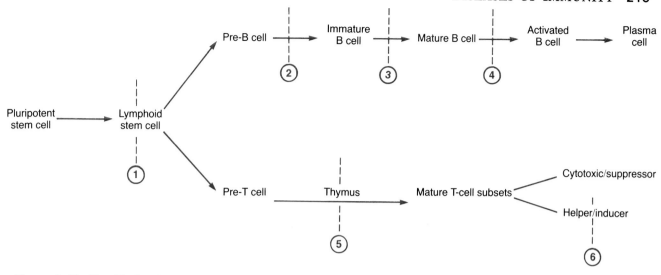

Figure 6-36. Simplified schema of lymphocyte development. Numbers indicate cells or steps affected in various immunodeficiency states: 1, severe combined immunodeficiency: defects in lymphoid stem cells, as depicted, are rare; most cases result from T cell defects; 2, Bruton's agammaglobulinemia; 3, isolated IgA deficiency, affects only immature IgA-positive B cells; 4, one form of common variable immunodeficiency; 5, DiGeorge's syndrome; and 6, AIDS.

fied clinically by the coexistence of features suggestive of SLE, polymyositis, and systemic sclerosis and *serologically by high titers of antibodies to RNP particle–containing U1RNP.*[76] Two other factors have been considered important in lending distinctiveness to mixed connective tissue disease (MCTD)—the paucity of renal disease and an extremely good response to corticosteroids, both of which could be considered as indicative of a good long-term prognosis.

MCTD may present with arthritis, swelling of the hands, Raynaud's phenomenon, abnormal esophageal motility, myositis, leukopenia and anemia, fever, lymphadenopathy, and hypergammaglobulinemia. These manifestations suggest SLE, polymyositis, and systemic sclerosis. Over the last 20 years, as more patients with clinical and serologic features consistent with the diagnosis of MCTD have been identified, a controversy has developed over whether MCTD constitutes a distinct disease or is a heterogeneous mixture of subsets of SLE, systemic sclerosis, and polymyositis. According to this view, because overlapping of clinical features is common among autoimmune diseases and antibodies to U1RNP are not restricted to any specific disease entity (see Table 6–7), MCTD cannot be considered a distinct clinicopathologic entity; furthermore, many patients with an initial diagnosis of MCTD develop features most consistent with systemic sclerosis.[70,77] We can leave the resolution of this semantic issue to experts, but take note that although in general the various "rheumatic diseases" present with distinctive clinical and serologic features, several patients manifest overlapping features that defy simple categorization.

POLYARTERITIS NODOSA AND OTHER VASCULITIDES

Polyarteritis nodosa belongs to a group of diseases characterized by necrotizing inflammation of the walls of blood vessels and showing strong evidence of an immunologic pathogenetic mechanism. The general term *noninfectious necrotizing vasculitis* differentiates these conditions from those due to direct infection of the blood vessel wall (such as occurs in the wall of an abscess) and serves to emphasize that any type of vessel may be involved —arteries, arterioles, veins, or capillaries.

Noninfectious necrotizing vasculitis is encountered in many clinical settings. A detailed classification and description of vasculitides is presented in Chapter 11 on the diseases of blood vessels, where the immunologic mechanisms are also discussed.

IMMUNOLOGIC DEFICIENCY SYNDROMES

The immunologic deficiency syndromes are experiments of nature that allow insights into the complexities of the human immune system. Nowhere has the relevance of the individual components of immunologic function been more distinctly shown than when deficiencies of single components have given rise to distinctive disorders. Indeed, many of the important concepts of immunology either arose from or were confirmed by the study of clinical examples of specific immunodeficiencies. Traditionally, immunodeficiency disorders are considered according to the primary component or components involved (i.e., the B cell, the T cell, the undifferentiated stem cell, or complement); however, in view of the extensive cell interactions between T and B lymphocytes and macrophages, these distinctions are not always clear-cut (Fig. 6–36).

Immunodeficiencies can also be divided into the primary immunodeficiency disorders, which are almost always genetically determined, and secondary immunodeficiency states, arising as complications of infections; malnutrition; aging; or side effects of immunosuppression, irradiation, or chemotherapy for cancer and other autoimmune diseases. Here we briefly discuss some of the more important primary immunodeficiencies, to be followed by a more detailed description of the acquired immunodeficiency syndrome (AIDS), the most devastating example of secondary immunodeficiency.

PRIMARY IMMUNODEFICIENCIES

Most primary immunodeficiency diseases are genetically determined and affect specific immunity (i.e., humoral and cellular) or nonspecific host defense mechanisms mediated by complement proteins and cells such as phagocytes or NK cells. Although originally thought to be quite rare, some forms, such as IgA deficiency, are common, and collectively they are a significant health problem, especially in children. Most primary immunodeficiencies manifest themselves in infancy, between six months and two years of life, and they are noted because of the susceptibility of infants to recurrent infections. Detailed classification of the primary immunodeficiencies according to the suggested cellular defect may be found in the WHO report on immunodeficiency and in other specialized sources.[78] Only a few examples are presented here.

X-Linked Agammaglobulinemia of Bruton

This is one of the most common forms of primary immunodeficiency and is characterized by the virtual absence of serum immunoglobulins, although small amounts of IgG may sometimes be present. It is an X-linked disease restricted to males. Severe recurrent infections usually begin at eight to nine months of age, when the infant becomes depleted of maternal immunoglobulins. The most common offending organisms are pyogenic (e.g., staphylococcus, *Haemophilus influenzae*), and patients have recurrent conjunctivitis, pharyngitis, otitis media, bronchitis, pneumonia, and skin infections. Most viral and fungal infections are handled normally

because cell-mediated immunity, the predominant mode of defense against these pathogens, is normal. There are, however, some curious and important exceptions to this generalization; affected individuals are at particular risk for development of vaccine-associated paralytic poliomyelitis as well as fatal echovirus encephalitis. They are also at increased risk for development of *Pneumocystis carinii* pneumonia. Persistent intestinal infections with *Giardia lamblia* may also occur and give rise to malabsorption.

Autoimmune diseases occur with increased frequency in patients with Bruton's disease. Nearly half of these children develop a condition similar to rheumatoid arthritis that clears remarkably with restitutive immunoglobulin therapy. Similarly, lupus erythematosus, dermatomyositis, and other autoimmune disorders are more common in these patients. The basis of these peculiar associations is not known.

The classic characteristics, first described by Bruton, are those that would be expected from a primary B-cell deficiency. B cells are virtually absent in the blood except in rare cases. Pre-B cells, which are large lymphoid cells with intracytoplasmic IgM but no surface immunoglobulins, are found in normal numbers in the bone marrow. The lymph nodes and spleen lack germinal centers, and plasma cells are absent from the lymph nodes, spleen, bone marrow, and connective tissue. Tonsils in particular are poorly developed or rudimentary. There are, however, normal numbers of circulating and tissue T cells, and T-cell function as measured by delayed hypersensitivity tests and allograft rejection is normal. The gene responsible for X-linked agammaglobulinemia has been cloned by positional cloning. It encodes a protein-tyrosine kinase, dubbed *Atk* (to denote *a*gammaglobulinemia *t*yrosine *k*inase), expressed in B cells but not in T cells.[79] Protein tyrosine kinases are known to be involved in signal transduction pathways, and it is suspected that *Atk* is critical for transducing signals that drive pre-B cells to become B cells.

Common Variable Immunodeficiency (CVI)

This relatively common but poorly defined derangement represents a heterogeneous group of disorders. It may be congenital or acquired, sporadic or familial (with an inconstant mode of inheritance). *The feature common to all patients is hypogammaglobulinemia, generally affecting all the antibody classes but sometimes only IgG.*[80] The basis of immunoglobulin deficiency is varied, but it is distinct from that in X-linked agammaglobulinemia. In contrast to the latter, most patients with common variable immunodeficiency (CVI) have normal numbers of B cells in the blood and lymphoid tissues. These B cells, however, are not able to differentiate into plasma cells. In the vast majority of cases, the defect in terminal differentiation of B cells is intrinsic to B lymphocytes, that is, they fail to secrete normal levels of immunoglobulins even when helper T cells are provided and any potential suppressor T cells are removed.

The molecular basis of abnormal B-cell differentiation is varied. Some patients have mutations that regulate expression of immunoglobulin genes[81]; others have defective B cells as well as functional abnormalities of CD4+ (helper) or CD8+ (suppressor) T cells. In one subgroup, the number of CD4+ T cells is normal, but they produce subnormal amounts of IL-2 and IFN-γ on activation.[82] Because cytokines are essential for immunoglobulin secretion, these T-cell defects contribute to hypogammaglobulinemia. In other patients, the problem is not a lack of T-cell help but, rather, an absolute increase in the numbers of CD8+ T cells that can suppress antibody secretion by normal B cells *in vitro*. Even in these patients, however, culture of purified B cells *in vitro* does not fully restore normal immunoglobulin production, pointing to a coexistent primary B-cell defect. Recent studies point to the existence of genetic factors that predispose to CVI.[83] Several genes within the HLA complex have been implicated, but curiously the association seems strongest with the complement genes. Many patients have deletions of the C4A gene or possess rare alleles of the C2 gene. These studies have revealed that genetic susceptibility to selective IgA deficiency (see later) is also regulated by the same gene complex. Furthermore, both CVI and selective IgA deficiency can affect different members of the same family, leading some to suggest that these two disorders are related and may represent different expression of a common genetic defect.

The clinical manifestations of CVI are those of antibody deficiency—that is, recurrent bacterial infections. In contrast to X-linked agammaglobulinemia, CVI affects both sexes equally, and the onset of symptoms is later—in childhood or adolescence. Histologically, the B-cell areas of the lymphoid tissues (i.e., lymphoid follicles in nodes, spleen, and gut) are hyperplastic. The enlargement of B-cell areas probably reflects defective immunoregulation, that is, B cells can proliferate in response to antigen, but because antibody production is impaired, the normal feedback inhibition by IgG is absent. In addition to bacterial infections, patients with CVI are also prone to severe enteroviral infections, recurrent herpes zoster, and persistent diarrhea caused by *Giardia lamblia*.

These patients have a high frequency of autoimmune diseases (approximately 20%), including rheumatoid arthritis, pernicious anemia, and hemolytic anemia. The risk of lymphoid malignancy is also increased. All these features suggest widespread defects in immunoregulation.

Isolated IgA Deficiency

Isolated IgA deficiency is a very common immunodeficiency. In the United States, it occurs in about 1 in 600 individuals of European descent. It is far less common in blacks and Asians. Affected individuals have extremely low levels of *both serum and secretory IgA*. It may be familial or acquired in association with toxoplasmosis, measles, or some other virus infection. The association of IgA deficiency with common variable immunodeficiency, and their linkage to HLA genes, was mentioned earlier. It is generally believed that most individuals with this disease are completely asymptomatic, but according to some authorities, IgA deficiency is commonly associated with some form of illness.[84] Because IgA is the major immunoglobulin in external secretions, mucosal defenses are weakened, and infections occur in the respiratory, gastrointestinal, and urogenital tracts. Symptomatic patients commonly present with recurrent sinopulmonary infections and diarrhea. It is now apparent that some individuals previously classified as having selective IgA deficiency are also deficient in IgG_2 and IgG_4 subclasses of immunoglobulin G. This group of patients is particularly prone to developing infections.[85] In addition, IgA-deficient patients have a high frequency of respiratory tract allergy and a variety of autoimmune diseases, particularly SLE and rheumatoid arthritis. The basis of the increased frequency of autoimmune and allergic diseases is not known. Because secretory IgA normally acts as a mucosal barrier against foreign proteins and antigens, it could be speculated that unregulated absorption of foreign protein antigens triggers abnormal immune responses *in vivo*.

The basic defect is in the differentiation of IgA B lymphocytes. In most patients with selective IgA deficiency, the number of IgA-positive B cells is normal, but most of them express the immature phenotype characterized by co-expression of surface IgD and IgM. Only a very few of these cells can be induced to transform into IgA plasma cells *in vitro*. Serum antibodies to IgA are found in approximately 40% of the patients. Whether this finding is of any etiologic significance is unknown, but it has important clinical implications. When transfused with blood containing normal IgA, some of these patients develop severe, even fatal anaphylactic reactions.

DiGeorge's Syndrome (Thymic Hypoplasia)

This is an example of selective T-cell deficiency that derives from failure of development of the third and fourth pharyngeal pouches. The latter give rise to the thymus, the parathyroids, some of the clear cells of the thyroid, and the ultimobranchial body.

Thus, these patients have total absence of cell-mediated immune responses (owing to hypoplasia or lack of the thymus), tetany (owing to lack of the parathyroids), and congenital defects of the heart and great vessels. In addition, the appearance of the mouth, ears, and facies may be abnormal. Absence of cell-mediated immunity is reflected in low levels of circulating T lymphocytes and a poor defense against certain fungal and viral infections. Plasma cells are present in normal numbers in lymphoid tissues, but the thymic-dependent paracortical areas of the lymph nodes and the periarteriolar sheaths of the spleen are depleted. Immunoglobulin levels tend to be normal.

DiGeorge's syndrome is not genetically determined but appears to be the result of intrauterine fetal damage around the eighth week of gestation. Patients with "partial" DiGeorge's syndrome, who have an extremely small but histologically normal thymus, have also been recorded. T-cell function improves with age in these children, so by 5 years of age, many have no T-cell deficit. In those with a complete absence of thymus, transplantation of fetal thymus may be of benefit.

Severe Combined Immunodeficiency Diseases (SCID)

This group of immunodeficiency diseases is characterized by combined T-cell and B-cell defects. Affected infants are susceptible to recurrent, severe infections by a wide range of pathogens, including *Candida albicans, Pneumocystis carinii, Pseudomonas,* cytomegalovirus, varicella, and a whole host of bacteria. Some patients develop graft-versus-host disease mediated by transplacental transfer of maternal T cells. Without bone marrow transplantation, death occurs within the first year of life. Despite the common clinical manifestations, the underlying defects are quite different and in many cases unknown. The so-called classic form, initially described in Swiss infants and believed to result from a defect in the common lymphoid stem cell, is extremely uncommon (see Fig. 6–36). More commonly, the severe combined immunodeficiency disease (SCID) defect resides in the T-cell compartment, with a secondary impairment of humoral immunity. The T-cell defects may occur at any stage of the T-cell differentiation and activation pathway. If the differentiation of mature T cells is impaired, the patients are lymphopenic, with reduced T-cell counts and normal B-cell numbers.

Depending on the location of the mutant gene and the nature of the genetic defect, two patterns of inheritance are seen: autosomal recessive and X-linked recessive. Among the autosomal recessive forms of SCID, approximately 40% lack the enzyme adenosine deaminase (ADA). Deficiency of ADA leads to accumulation of deoxyadenosine and its derivatives (e.g., deoxy-ATP), which are particularly toxic to immature lymphocytes, especially

those of T lineage. Hence T-lymphocyte numbers may be markedly reduced in severe cases. Patients with ADA deficiency have been treated with bone marrow transplantation and, more recently, with gene therapy. The ADA gene may be introduced into the patient's bone marrow cells before reinfusion. Alternatively, T cells harvested from the patient's peripheral blood are expanded *in vitro*, transfected with the ADA gene, and then returned to the patient.[83] Both forms of therapy are under investigation.

Defects in T-cell activation are less common causes of autosomal recessive SCID. They are extremely interesting, however, because they aid in the understanding of T-cell biology. In these patients, T cells are normal in number but deficient in one of several molecules that lie within the T-cell activation pathway. It may be recalled that T-cell activation depends on the recognition of antigenic peptides bound to class I or class II MHC molecules by the TCR complex. The latter includes CD3 proteins that are essential for transmitting signals into the cells. Intracellular signaling involves several proteins, some of which activate the transcription of cytokines (e.g., IL-2) and their receptor genes. Not surprisingly, the SCID phenotype is known to result from genetic defects in the expression of MHC molecules, mutations in the CD3 polypeptides, and deficiencies of nuclear transcription factor responsible for activation of the IL-2 gene.[86]

Approximately 50% of patients with SCID have an X-linked recessive pattern of inheritance. These patients have a mutation that affects a protein shared by the receptors for IL-2, IL-4, and IL-7, thus pointing to the importance of these cytokines in the development of lymphocytes.[87,88]

The histologic findings in SCID depend on the underlying defect. In the two most common forms (ADA deficiency and receptor mutation), the thymus is small and devoid of lymphoid cells. In the ADA-negative SCID, remnants of Hassall's corpuscles can be found, whereas in the X-linked recessive SCID, the thymus contains lobules of undifferentiated epithelial cells resembling fetal thymus.[89] In either case, other lymphoid tissues are hypoplastic as well, with marked depletion of T-cell areas and in some cases both T-cell and B-cell zones.

Currently, bone marrow transplantation is the mainstay of treatment, but with the elucidation of genetic defects, specific gene therapy is on the horizon.

Immunodeficiency with Thrombocytopenia and Eczema (Wiskott-Aldrich Syndrome)

This remarkable syndrome has been deemed "curious," "enigmatic," or "confusing" because its immunologic defects are so difficult to explain. *It is an X-linked recessive disease characterized by thrombocytopenia, eczema, and a marked vulnerability to recurrent infection, ending in early death.* The thymus is morphologically normal, at least early in the course of the disease, but there is progressive secondary depletion of T lymphocytes in the peripheral blood and in the paracortical (thymus-dependent) areas of the lymph nodes, with variable loss of cellular immunity. Patients may exhibit normal responses to such protein antigens as tetanus and diphtheria toxoid, but classically they show a poor antibody response to polysaccharide antigens. IgM levels in the serum are low, but levels of IgG are usually normal. Paradoxically, the levels of IgA and IgE are often elevated. Patients are also prone to developing malignant lymphomas. Recent studies have revealed a defect common to lymphocytes and platelets: an instability of cell surface sialoglycoproteins.[83] One such sialoglycoprotein, CD43, is partially depleted from the surface of lymphocytes. Loss of platelet-associated sialoglycoproteins reduces their life span. The CD43 gene maps to chromosome 16, and hence a mutation at this locus cannot be the primary cause of the disease. More likely, an unidentified gene on the X chromosome affects the stability of CD43 and related proteins.

Genetic Deficiencies of the Complement System

The various components of the complement system play a critical role in inflammatory and immunologic responses. Hereditary deficiencies have been described for virtually all components of the complement system and two of the inhibitors.[90] As might be expected, deficiency of complement components, especially C3, which is critical for both the classic and the alternative pathways, results in an increased susceptibility to infection with pyogenic bacteria. Inherited deficiencies of C1q, C2, and C4 increase the risk of immune complex–mediated disease (e.g., SLE), possibly by impairing the clearance of immune complexes from circulation. The absence of C1 esterase inhibitor allows uncontrolled C1 esterase activation with the generation of vasoactive C2 kinin. These patients develop *hereditary angioedema*, characterized by recurrent episodes of localized edema affecting skin and mucous membranes. The deficiencies of the later-acting components of the classic pathway (C5 to 8) result in recurrent neisserial (gonococcal, meningococcal) infections.

ACQUIRED IMMUNODEFICIENCY SYNDROME (AIDS)

In June 1981, the Centers for Disease Control of the United States reported that five young homosexual men in the Los Angeles area had contracted *Pneumocystis carinii* pneumonia. Two of the patients had died. This report signaled the beginning of an epidemic of a *retroviral disease characterized by profound immunosuppression associated with opportunistic infections, secondary neoplasms, and neurologic manifestations, which has come to be known as AIDS.* It is projected that by late 1993 approximately 300,000 patients with AIDS will have been diagnosed in the United States, and, based on serologic data, it is estimated that 1.5 to 2 million individuals have been infected with HIV, the agent that causes AIDS. Worldwide, an estimated 10 million people are infected, with Africa bearing the largest burden of some 6 million HIV-infected individuals. AIDS extracts a heavy toll. In the United States, it is currently the fourth leading cause of mortality for men between the ages of 15 and 54 years.[91] In the past decade, there has been an explosion of new knowledge relating to HIV and its remarkable ability to cause this modern plague. So rapid is the pace of research on the molecular biology of HIV and its effects that any review of this rapidly changing field is destined to be "out of date" by the time it is published. It is with this humbling realization that an attempt is made here to summarize the currently available data on the epidemiology, cause, pathogenesis, and clinical features of HIV infection.

EPIDEMIOLOGY. Although AIDS was first described in the United States and this country has the majority of the reported cases, AIDS has now been reported from more than 163 countries around the world, and the pool of HIV-infected persons in Africa and Asia is large and expanding. Epidemiologic studies in the United States have identified five groups of adults at risk for developing AIDS. The case distribution in these groups is as follows.

- *Homosexual or bisexual males* constitute by far the largest group, accounting for 60% of the reported cases. This includes 5% who were intravenous drug abusers as well.
- *Intravenous drug abusers* with no previous history of homosexuality compose the next largest group, representing about 23% of all patients. They represent the majority of all cases among heterosexuals.
- *Hemophiliacs*, especially those who received large amounts of factor VIII concentrates before 1985, make up 1% of all cases.
- *Recipients of blood and blood components* who are not hemophiliacs but who received transfusions of HIV-infected whole blood or components (e.g., platelets, plasma) account for 2% of patients. (Organs obtained from HIV-infected donors can also transmit AIDS.)
- *Heterosexual contacts* of members of other high-risk groups (chiefly intravenous drug abusers) constitute 6% of the patient population.

In approximately 6% of cases, the risk factors cannot be determined.

Close to 2% of all AIDS cases occur in the pediatric population. In this group, more than 80% have resulted from transmission of the virus from mother to child (discussed later). The remaining 20% are hemophiliacs and others who received blood or blood products before 1985.

Although the risk factors listed here apply to the U.S. population at large, two additional facts must be emphasized. First, the distribution of risk factors is influenced by social and demographic factors, and hence the proportion of transmission categories varies considerably within different regions. For example, in the San Francisco area, the great majority of patients with AIDS (>90%) are homosexual or bisexual men without a history of intravenous drug abuse, but in New York City, drug abuse is an extremely important risk factor.

Second, there has been a major demographic shift in the AIDS epidemic in the last few years. Although white homosexual and bisexual men are currently the largest group affected by AIDS in the United States, the largest increase in the rate of AIDS is now occurring in heterosexuals, women, and among the minorities (blacks, Hispanics). The basis for these changes will become apparent in the ensuing discussion.

It should be apparent from the preceding discussion that transmission of HIV occurs under conditions that facilitate exchange of blood or body fluids containing the virus or virus-infected cells. Hence the three major routes of transmission are *sexual contact, parenteral inoculation,* and *passage of the virus from infected mothers to their newborns.*

Bidirectional venereal transmission is clearly the predominant mode of infection worldwide. Because the majority of patients in the United States are homosexual or bisexual men, most sexual transmission has occurred among homosexual men. It is believed that the virus is carried in the lymphocytes present in the semen and enters the recipient's body through abrasions in rectal mucosa. Hence receptive anal intercourse increases the probability of infection. Heterosexual transmission, although initially of less quantitative importance in the United States, is globally the most common mode by which HIV is spread. Since 1985, however, even in the United States, *the rate of increase of heterosexual transmission is beginning to outpace transmission by other means.* Such spread is occurring most rapidly in female sex partners of male intravenous drug abusers. Not surprisingly therefore, the incidence of AIDS acquired by this route is highest in those areas with a high prevalence of intravenous drug abuse (e.g., metropolitan New York and Florida). In contrast to the U.S. experience, heterosexual transmission is the dominant mode of HIV infection in Asia and Africa.

In addition to male-to-male and male-to-female transmission, there is evidence supporting female-to-male transmission, presumably via HIV present in vaginal secretions and cervical cells of infected women. This form of heterosexual spread, however, is approximately two-fold less efficient than male-to-female transmission[92] and is probably far more important in Africa than in the United States. All forms of sexual transmission of HIV are aided and abetted by coexisting sexually transmitted diseases, especially those associated with genital ulceration (e.g., herpes-simplex and syphilis).[93]

Parenteral transmission of HIV has occurred in three groups of individuals: intravenous drug abusers, hemophiliacs who received factor VIII concentrates, and random recipients of blood transfusion. Of these three, intravenous drug abusers constitute by far the largest group. Transmission occurs by sharing of needles, syringes, and other paraphernalia contaminated with HIV-containing blood. This group occupies a pivotal position in the AIDS epidemic because it represents the principal link in the transmission of HIV to other adult populations through heterosexual activity.

Transmission of HIV by transfusion of blood or blood products such as lyophilized factor VIII concentrates has been virtually eliminated. This happy outcome resulted from three public health measures: screening of donated blood and plasma for antibody to HIV, heat treatment of clotting factor concentrates, and screening of donors on the basis of history. There persists, however, an extremely small but definite risk of acquiring AIDS through transfusion of seronegative blood because a recently infected individual may be antibody-negative. Currently, this risk is estimated to range from 1 in 40,000 to 1 in 250,000 per unit of blood transfused. Although it is possible to detect HIV-associated p24 antigens in the blood before the development of humoral antibodies, this test is not routinely performed because in large studies (involving 1.5 million units of donated blood), no p24 antigen–positive, antibody-negative donors were detected.[94] This may change, however, with the development of the next generation of tests based, for example, on polymerase chain reaction (PCR) technology.

As alluded to earlier, *mother-to-infant transmission* is the major cause of pediatric AIDS. Infected mothers can transmit the infection to their offspring by three routes: *in utero* by transplacental spread, during delivery through an infected birth canal, and after birth by ingestion of breast milk. In one large European study, the rate of vertical transmission was approximately 14%, but in other studies, it has varied from 7 to 39%.[95]

Because of the uniformly fatal outcome of AIDS, there has been much concern in the lay public and among health care workers regarding spread of HIV infection outside the high-risk groups. Extensive studies indicate that *HIV infection cannot be transmitted by casual personal con-*

tact in the household, workplace, or school. No convincing evidence for spread by insect bites has been obtained. Regarding transmission of HIV infection to health care workers, there seems to be an extremely small but definite risk. Seroconversion has been documented after accidental needlestick injury or exposure of nonintact skin to infected blood in laboratory accidents. Following such accidents, the risk of seroconversion is believed to be about 0.3%.[96] By comparison, approximately 30% of those accidently exposed to hepatitis B–infected blood become seropositive.[97] Although much publicized, and a cause of justifiable concern, the transmission of AIDS from an infected health care provider to a patient is extremely rare.

ETIOLOGY. There is little doubt that AIDS is caused by HIV, a human retrovirus belonging to the lentivirus family. Included in this group are feline immunodeficiency virus, simian immunodeficiency virus, visna virus of sheep, and the equine infectious anemia virus. These nontransforming retroviruses have several features in common:

- A long incubation period, followed by a slowly progressive fatal outcome
- Tropism for hematopoietic and nervous systems
- An ability to cause immunosuppression
- Cytopathic effects *in vitro*

Two genetically different but related forms of HIV, called HIV-1 and HIV-2, have been isolated from patients with AIDS. HIV-1 is the most common type associated with AIDS in the United States, Europe, and Central Africa, whereas HIV-2 causes a similar disease principally in West Africa. Although distinct, HIV-1 and HIV-2 share some antigens; because of the serologic cross-reactivity, most (but not all) cases of HIV-2 infection can be detected by the enzyme-linked immunosorbent assay (ELISA) test for HIV-1 used by blood banks.

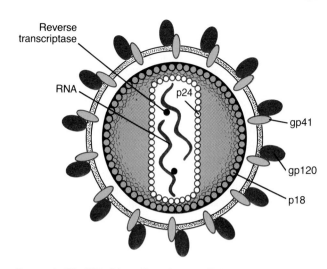

Figure 6–37. HIV virion. The virus particle is covered by a membrane that is derived from the host cell. Studding the membrane are viral glycoproteins gp41 and gp120. Inside there is a core made up of proteins designated p18 and p24. The viral RNA and the enzyme reverse transcriptase are carried in the core.

Specific tests for HIV-2, however, are now available, and blood collected for transfusion is routinely screened for HIV-2 seropositivity. The ensuing discussion relates primarily to HIV-1 and diseases caused by it, but it is generally applicable to HIV-2 as well.

Like most C-type retroviruses, the HIV-1 virion is spherical and contains an electron-dense core surrounded by a lipid envelope derived from the host cell membrane.[98] The virus core contains four core proteins, including p24 and p18, two strands of genomic RNA, and the enzyme reverse transcriptase (Fig. 6–37). Studding the viral envelope are two viral glycoproteins, gp 120 and gp 41, that are critical for HIV infection of cells. The HIV-1 proviral genome contains the *gag, pol,* and

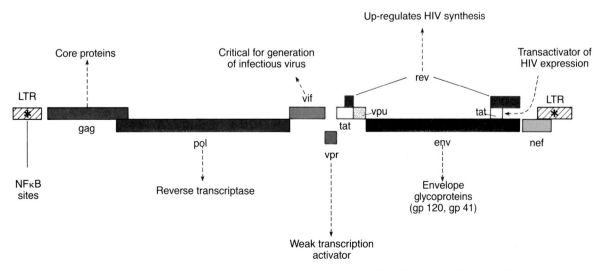

Figure 6–38. HIV proviral genome. Several viral genes and their recognized functions are illustrated. The genes outlined in red are unique to HIV; others are shared by all retroviruses. Like *vif, vpu* favors generation of infectious virus.

env genes that code for the core proteins, reverse transcriptase, and envelope proteins (Fig. 6–38). *In addition to these three standard retroviral genes, HIV contains several other genes,* including *tat, rev, vif, nef, vpr,* and *vpu,* which regulate the synthesis and assembly of infectious viral particles.[99] The product of the *tat* (transactivator) gene, for example, is critical for virus gene expression. The *tat* protein functions by causing a 7-fold to 40-fold increase in the transcription of viral genes. Like *tat, rev* is also essential for HIV-1 replication, but it exerts its effects at a post-transcriptional level by regulating the transport of viral mRNAs from the nucleus to the cytoplasm. The products of the *vpu* and *vif* genes act late in the viral life cycle and seem to be essential for the budding of virions from infected cells *(vpu)* and for endowing the cell-free virus with the ability to infect other cells *(vif)*. From this brief review of the functions of HIV-1 genes, it should be apparent that the products of regulatory genes are important for the pathogenicity of HIV, and hence there is considerable interest in developing therapeutic agents that can block the action of these genes.

PATHOGENESIS. There are two major targets of HIV: the immune system and the CNS. The effects of HIV infection on each of these two will be discussed separately.

Immunopathogenesis of HIV Disease. Profound immunosuppression, primarily affecting cell-mediated immunity, is the hallmark of AIDS. This results chiefly from a severe loss of CD4+ T cells as well as an impairment in the function of surviving helper T cells. Because depletion of CD4+ T cells is critical to the pathogenesis of AIDS, we shall focus our attention first on the events that lead to the infection and destruction of T cells, after which HIV infection of monocytes and its consequences will be discussed.

There is abundant evidence that *the CD4 molecule is in fact a high-affinity receptor* for HIV. This explains the selective tropism of the virus for CD4+ T cells and its ability to infect other CD4+ cells, particularly macrophages (Fig. 6–39). The initial step in infection is the binding of gp120 envelope glycoprotein to CD4 molecules. This is followed by fusion of the virus to the cell membrane and internalization. It is believed that fusion requires a postbinding step in which viral gp 41 makes contact with a yet to be identified component of the cell membrane. The binding of gp120 with the CD4 molecule has been scrutinized in great detail because this step provides a potential target for therapy designed to limit or even prevent HIV from infecting cells. For example, genetically engineered soluble CD4 molecules, or their fragments containing the gp120-binding domains, can bind free virus and thereby prevent infection of CD4+ T cells *in vitro*.

Whether CD4− cells can be infected by HIV remains uncertain. According to some investigators, cells such as astrocytes, skin fibroblasts, and bowel epithelial cells (all lacking detectable CD4) are infected through an entirely different receptor. The identity of an alternative receptor, if it exists, remains uncertain.

Once internalized, the viral genome undergoes reverse transcription, leading to formation of cDNA (proviral DNA). In quiescent T cells, HIV cDNA may remain in the cytoplasm in a linear episomal form.[100] In dividing T cells, the cDNA circularizes, enters the nucleus, and is then integrated into host genome. Following this, the provirus may remain locked into the chromosome for months or years, and hence the infection may become latent. Alternatively, proviral DNA may be transcribed, with the formation of complete viral particles that bud from the cell membrane. Such productive infection, when associated with extensive viral budding, leads to cell death (see Fig. 6–39). It is important to note that although HIV-1 can infect resting T cells, the initiation of proviral DNA transcription (and hence productive infection) occurs only when the infected cell is activated by an exposure to antigens or cytokines. It is obvious therefore that physiologic stimuli that promote activation and growth of normal T cells lead to the death of HIV-infected T cells.

It might be surmised from the preceding discussion that productive infection of T cells is the mechanism by which HIV causes lysis of CD4+ T cells. Despite the relentless, and eventually profound, loss of CD4+ cells from the peripheral blood, however, there is a relative paucity of productively infected T cells (0.01 to 0.1%) in circulation, especially early in the course of the disease. Even with the most sensitive *in situ* PCR techniques, only 0.1 to 13% of the peripheral blood cells score positive for HIV.[101] This paradox has spawned many hypotheses that attempt to explain the loss of CD4+ T cells by mechanisms other than direct cytolysis.[102] Although some of the proposed alternative mechanisms, to be described later, may indeed be important, a plausible solution to this puzzle has emerged from the discovery of large numbers of infected CD4+ cells in lymphoid organs, such as lymph nodes, tonsils, and spleen.[103,104] Even during the early stages of HIV infection, approximately 20 to 30% of the CD4+ T cells in the lymph nodes contain HIV DNA. Although most cells within the lymphoid organs harbor latent infection, the frequency of productively infected T cells in lymph nodes is significantly greater than in the peripheral blood. Based on these studies, *it has been proposed that early in the course of the disease, there is heavy infection of CD4+ T cells in the lymphoid tissues.* With antigenic exposure, productive infection is continually activated in a fraction of latently infected cells,

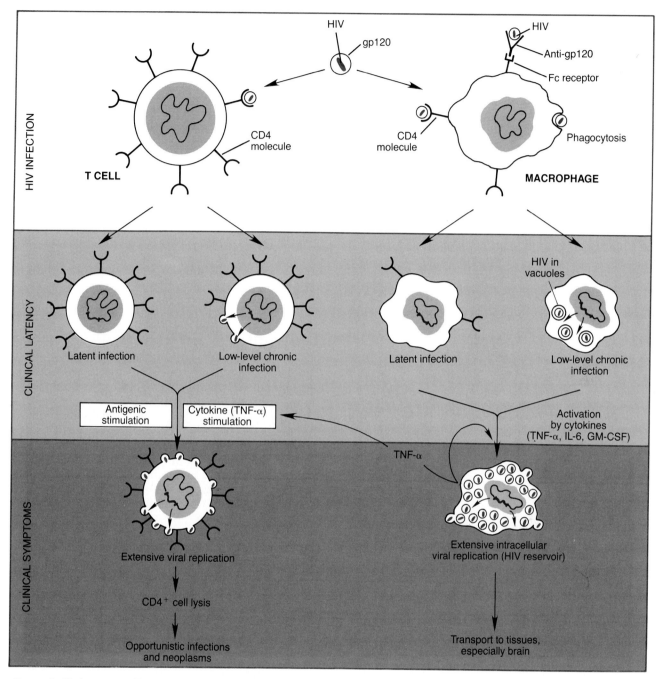

Figure 6-39. Immunopathogenesis of HIV infection. CD4+ T cells and macrophages are the major targets of HIV. Infection of these two cell types leads to somewhat distinctive events that eventually lead to a marked loss of CD4+ T cells and dissemination of HIV into various tissues, especially the CNS.

which are then destroyed. Thus there is a steady, gradual attrition of the CD4+ population systemically.

In addition to cell death resulting from productive infection of CD4+ T cells, several other indirect mechanisms could contribute to the loss of helper T lymphocytes.[105] These include the following.

- Loss of immature precursors of CD4+ T cells, either by direct infection of thymic progenitor cells or by infection of accessory cells that secrete cytokines essential for CD4+ T-cell differentiation.

- Fusion of infected and uninfected cells, with formation of syncytia (giant cells) (Fig. 6-40). In tissue culture, the gp120 expressed on productively infected cells binds to CD4 molecules on uninfected T cells, followed by cell fusion. Fused cells develop "ballooning" and usually die within a few hours.

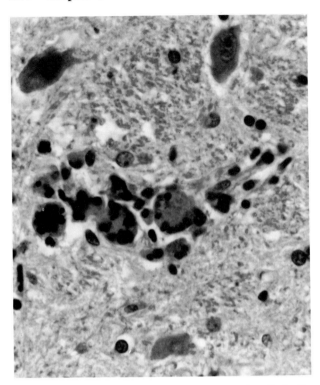

Figure 6–40. HIV infection. Formation of giant cells in the brain. (Courtesy of Dr. Dennis Burns, Department of Pathology, University of Texas Southwestern Medical School, Dallas.)

- Autoimmune destruction of both infected and uninfected CD4+ T cells. Soluble gp120 released from infected cells can bind to CD4 molecules on uninfected cells. Because many patients have circulating anti-gp120 antibodies, these gp120-coated cells could be destroyed by ADCC.

Loss of CD4+ cells by direct and indirect mechanisms leads to an inversion of the CD4-CD8 ratio in the peripheral blood. It may be recalled that the normal CD4-CD8 ratio is close to 2, whereas in patients with AIDS, a ratio close to 0.5 is not uncommon. Such an inversion, although a consistent finding in AIDS, should not be considered diagnostic because it may also occur with certain other viral infections.

Although marked reduction in CD4+ T cells, a hallmark of AIDS, can account for most of the immunodeficiency late in the course of HIV infection, there is compelling evidence for *qualitative defects in T cells that can be detected even in asymptomatic HIV-infected persons.* Such defects include a reduction in antigen-induced T-cell proliferation, impaired production of cytokines such as IL-2 and IFN-γ, defects in intracellular signaling, and many more. There is also a selective loss of the memory subset of CD4+ helper T cells early in the course of disease. This observation explains the inability of peripheral blood T cells to be activated when challenged with common recall antigens. The

basis of T-cell dysfunction is multifactorial. Included in the list of possible mechanisms are anergy resulting from the binding of gp120 antigen-antibody complexes to CD4 molecules, impairment of antigen presentation by anti-gp120 antibodies that cross-react with and bind to class II HLA molecules on antigen-presenting cells, and anergy of large numbers of T cells resulting from binding of HIV-derived superantigens to beta chains of TCRs.

In addition to infection and loss of CD4+ T cells, *infection of monocytes and macrophages is also extremely important in the pathogenesis of HIV infection.* Like T cells, the majority of the *macrophages that are infected by HIV are found in the tissues and not in peripheral blood.* A relatively high frequency (10 to 50%) of productively infected macrophages is detected in certain tissues, such as brain and lungs. Several important differences between HIV infection of T cells and macrophages, however, need to be emphasized.

- Because many macrophages express low levels of CD4, HIV may infect these cells by the gp120-CD4 pathway; in addition, HIV may enter macrophages by phagocytosis or by Fc receptor–mediated endocytosis of antibody-coated HIV particles (see Fig. 6–39).
- Infected macrophages bud relatively small amounts of virus from the cell surface, but these cells contain large numbers of virus particles located exclusively in intracellular vacuoles. Despite the fact that macrophages allow viral replication, in contrast to CD4+ T cells, they are quite resistant to the cytopathic effects of HIV.

HIV infection of macrophages has two important implications. First, monocytes and macrophages represent a veritable virus factory and reservoir, whose output remains largely protected from host defenses. Second, macrophages provide a safe vehicle for HIV to be transported to various parts of the body, particularly the nervous system.

In contrast to tissue macrophages, the number of monocytes in circulation infected by HIV is low; yet there are unexplained functional defects that have important bearing in host defense. These defects include impaired microbicidal activity, decreased chemotaxis, decreased secretion of IL-1, inappropriate secretion of TNF-α, and, most important, poor capacity to present antigens to T cells.

Recent studies have documented that, in addition to macrophages, *follicular dendritic cells (FDCs) in the germinal centers of lymph nodes are also important reservoirs* of HIV. Although some FDCs are infected by HIV, most virus particles are found on the surface of their dendritic processes. FDCs have receptors for the Fc portion of immunoglobulins, and hence they trap HIV virions coated with anti-HIV antibodies.[104] FDC-associated viral particles readily infect CD4+ T cells as they traverse the intricate meshwork formed by the dendritic processes of the FDC.

These studies provide clear evidence that CD4+ T cells, macrophages, and FDC contained in the lymphoid tissues, and not the cells in the blood, are the major sites of HIV infection and persistence.

Low-level chronic or latent infection of T cells and macrophages is an important feature of HIV infection. Early in the course of this infection, only rare CD4+ T cells in the blood or lymph nodes express infectious virus, whereas in the lymph nodes, up to 30% can be demonstrated by PCR to harbor the HIV genome. It is widely believed that integrated provirus, without virus expression (latent infection), can remain in the cells from months to years. Completion of the viral life cycle in latently infected cells occurs only after cell activation, which in the case of CD4+ T cells results in cell lysis. To understand the molecular basis of release from latency, we must briefly consider the events that are associated with activation of CD4+ helper T cells. It is well known that antigen-induced or mitogen-induced activation of T cells is associated with transcription of genes encoding the cytokine IL-2 and its receptor (IL-2R). At the molecular level, this is accomplished in part by the induction of a nuclear binding factor called NF kB (nuclear factor kB), which binds to enhancer sequences (kB sites) within the promoter regions of IL-2 and IL-2R genes. Quite remarkably, the LTR sequences that flank the HIV genome also contain similar kB sites that can be triggered by the same nuclear regulatory factors. Imagine now a latently infected CD4+ cell that encounters an environmental antigen. Induction of NF kB in such a cell (a physiologic response) activates the transcription of HIV proviral DNA (a pathologic outcome) and leads ultimately to the production of virions and to cell lysis. Furthermore, TNF-α, a cytokine produced by activated macrophages, also leads to transcriptional activation of HIV-mRNA by production of nuclear factors that bind to kB-enhancer elements of HIV. The production of HIV-1 by macrophages is also up-regulated by cytokines, such as TNF-α, TNF-β, IFN-γ, IL-6, and GM-CSF. Many of these cytokines are produced during a normal immune response. Of these, TNF-α, produced by macrophages, is particularly important because it can act in both an autocrine and a paracrine manner.[106] Thus it seems that HIV thrives when the host macrophages and T cells are physiologically activated, an act that can be best described as "subversion from within." Such activation *in vivo* may result from antigenic stimulation, especially by other infecting microorganisms, such as cytomegalovirus, EBV, hepatitis B virus, and herpes simplex virus. The lifestyle of most HIV-infected patients in the United States places them at increased risk for recurrent exposure to other sexually transmitted diseases, and in Africa, socioeconomic conditions probably impose a higher

burden of chronic microbial infections. It is easy to visualize how in patients with AIDS a vicious cycle of cell destruction may be set up. Multiple infections to which these patients are prone because of diminished helper T-cell function lead to increased TNF-α production, which in turn stimulates more HIV production, followed by infection and loss of additional CD4+ T cells.

Although much attention has been focused on T cells and macrophages because they can be infected by HIV, patients with AIDS also display profound abnormalities of B cell function. Paradoxically, these patients have hypergammaglobulinemia and circulating immune complexes owing to polyclonal B-cell activation. This may result from multiple interacting factors, such as infection with cytomegalovirus and EBV, both of which are polyclonal B-cell activators; gp120 itself can promote B-cell growth and differentiation, and HIV-infected macrophages produce increased amounts of IL-6, which favors activation of B cells. *Despite the presence of spontaneously activated B cells, patients with AIDS are unable to mount an antibody response to a new antigen.* This could in part be due to lack of T-cell help, but antibody responses against T-independent antigens are also suppressed, and hence there may be other defects in B cells as well. Impaired humoral immunity renders these patients prey to disseminated infections caused by encapsulated bacteria, such as *Streptococcus pneumoniae* and *Haemophilus influenzae*, both of which require antibodies for effective opsonization.

In closing this discussion of immunopathogenesis, it must be recalled the CD4+ T cells play a pivotal role in regulating the immune response: They produce a plethora of cytokines, such as IL-2, IL-4, IL-5, IFN-γ, macrophage chemotactic factors, and hematopoietic growth factors, such as GM-CSF. Therefore loss of this "master cell" has ripple effects on virtually every other cell of the immune system, as illustrated in Figure 6–41 and summarized in Table 6–9.

Pathogenesis of Central Nervous System Involvement. The pathogenesis of neurologic manifestations deserves special mention because, in addition to the lymphoid system, the nervous system is a major target of HIV infection.[107] Macrophages and cells belonging to the monocyte and macrophage lineage (microglia) are the predominant cell types in the brain that are infected with HIV. Hence it is widely believed that HIV is carried into the brain by infected monocytes. The mechanism of HIV-induced damage of the brain, however, remains obscure. According to some workers, HIV-infected macrophages produce soluble factors that may be cytotoxic for neuronal cells or impair their function without direct cytotoxicity.[108] Included among the soluble factors are cytokines, such as IL-1. Direct damage of neurons by soluble HIV

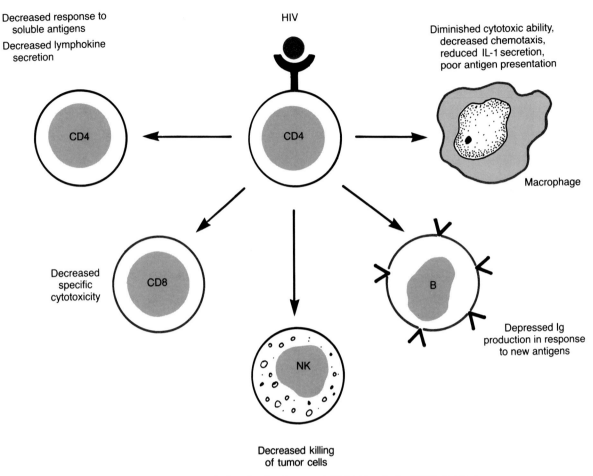

Figure 6–41. The multiple effects of loss of CD4+ T cells by HIV infection.

Table 6–9. MAJOR ABNORMALITIES OF IMMUNE FUNCTION IN AIDS

LYMPHOPENIA
Predominantly due to selective loss of the CD4+ helper-inducer T-cell subset; inversion of CD4-CD8 ratio
DECREASED T-CELL FUNCTION *IN VIVO*
Preferential loss of memory T cells
Susceptibility to opportunistic infections
Susceptibility to neoplasms
Decreased delayed-type hypersensitivity
ALTERED T-CELL FUNCTION *IN VITRO*
Decreased proliferative response to mitogens, alloantigens, and soluble antigens
Decreased specific cytotoxicity
Decreased helper function for pokeweed mitogen-induced B-cell immunoglobulin production
Decreased IL-2 and IFN-γ production
POLYCLONAL B-CELL ACTIVATION
Hypergammaglobulinemia and circulating immune complexes
Inability to mount *de novo* antibody response to a new antigen
Refractoriness to the normal signals for B-cell activation *in vitro*
ALTERED MONOCYTE OR MACROPHAGE FUNCTIONS
Decreased chemotaxis and phagocytosis
Decreased HLA class II antigen expression
Diminished capacity to present antigen to T cells
Increased spontaneous secretion of IL-1, TNF-α, IL-6

gp120 has also been postulated. Support for most of the proposed mechanisms comes in large part from studies *in vitro*, and hence their relevance to neuronal injury and dysfunction *in vivo* remains speculative.

Comparison of HIV isolated from the brain with virus recovered from the lymphocytes indicates that HIV isolates from the brain constitute a special subgroup of the AIDS virus. These strains seem to grow equally well in macrophages and T cells, whereas those recovered from CD4+ lymphocytes seem to grow preferentially in T cells. This difference in tropism can be localized to a specific domain of the gp120 molecule.[109] Therefore it may well be that the risk of CNS damage is related to the strain of HIV. According to this view, those HIV strains that grow preferentially in T cells may be less prone to cause CNS disease. Some workers have reported that HIV is present in the brain in cell types other than macrophages, including astrocytes, oligodendrocytes, and endothelial cells. These reports suggest a much wider tissue tropism for HIV as well as additional, possibly more direct, mechanisms for brain parenchymal injury. At present, however, pathways of HIV-induced brain damage that do not depend on

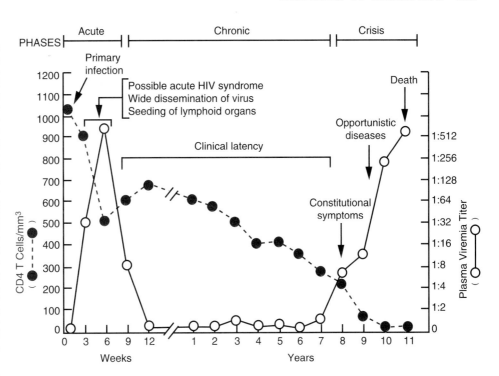

Figure 6-42. Typical course of HIV infection. During the early period after primary infection there is widespread dissemination of virus and a sharp decrease in the number of CD4+ T cells in peripheral blood. An immune response to HIV ensues, with a decrease in detectable viremia followed by a prolonged period of clinical latency. The CD4+ T-cell count continues to decrease during the following years, until it reaches a critical level below which there is a substantial risk of opportunistic diseases. (Redrawn and reproduced with permission from Pantaleo, G., Graziosi, C., and Fauci, A.S.: The immunopathogenesis of human immunodeficiency virus infection. *The New England Journal of Medicine* 328:327, 1993.)

macrophage transport must be considered "suggestoid" rather than proven.

NATURAL HISTORY OF HIV INFECTION. The course of HIV infection can be best understood in terms of an interplay between HIV and the immune system. *Three phases reflecting the dynamics of virus-host interaction can be recognized: an early, acute phase; a middle, chronic phase; and a final, crisis phase* (Fig. 6-42).[102] We first present the cardinal features of the three phases of HIV infection and their associated clinical syndromes and then recount the sequential virologic and immunologic findings during the course of HIV infection.

The early, acute phase represents the initial response of an immunocompetent adult to HIV infection. It is characterized initially by a high level of virus production, viremia, and widespread seeding of the lymphoid tissues. The initial infection, however, is readily controlled by the development of an antiviral immune response. Clinically, this phase is associated with self-limited acute illness that develops in 50 to 70% of adults infected with HIV. Nonspecific symptoms such as sore throat, myalgias, fever, rash, and sometimes aseptic meningitis develop 3 to 6 weeks after infection and resolve spontaneously 2 to 3 weeks later.

The middle, chronic phase represents a stage of relative containment of the virus, associated with a period of clinical latency. The immune system is largely intact, but *there is smoldering, low-level HIV replication, predominantly in the lymphoid tissues, which may last for several years.* Patients are either asymptomatic or develop persistent generalized lymphadenopathy. Constitutional symptoms are usually absent or mild. Persistent lymphadenopathy with significant constitutional symptoms (fever, rash, fatigue) reflects the onset of immune system decompensation, escalation of viral replication, and the onset of the "crisis" phase.

The final or crisis phase is characterized by a breakdown of host defense, resultant recrudescence of viral replication, and clinical disease. Typically the patients present with long-lasting fever (longer than a month), fatigue, loss of weight, and diarrhea; the CD4+ cell count is reduced. After a variable period, serious opportunistic infections, secondary neoplasms, or clinical neurologic disease supervenes, and the patient is said to have developed AIDS. In addition, according to current guidelines of the Centers for Disease Control, any HIV-infected person with fewer than 200 CD4+ T cells/μl is considered to have AIDS.[110]

In the absence of treatment, most if not all patients with HIV infection progress to AIDS after a chronic phase lasting from 7 to 10 years. This *clinical latent phase* is shorter in those who receive a large parenteral inoculum of HIV, as occurs with blood transfusions, or may be especially long in those who receive prophylactic antiretroviral therapy.

With this overview of the three phases of HIV infection, we can consider some details of host-parasite relationships during the course of HIV infection. As mentioned earlier, when a normal immunocompetent adult is first exposed to HIV, there is a transient period of active viral replication associated with an abrupt, sometimes severe, reduction in CD4+ T cells. During this period, HIV can be readily isolated from the blood, and there are high levels of HIV p24 antigen in serum. Soon, however, a virus-specific immune response develops, evidenced by seroconversion (usually within 3 to 7 weeks of presumed exposure) and, more important, by development of virus-specific CD8+ cytotoxic T cells. *HIV-specific cytotoxic T cells are detected in blood at about the time viral titers begin to fall and are most likely responsible for the containment of HIV infection.* As viral replication in the peripheral blood mononuclear cells abates, CD4+ T cells return to nearly normal numbers, signaling the end of the early acute phase.[111] It should be remembered, however, that although plasma viremia declines, there is widespread dissemination and seeding of the virus, especially in the lymphoid organs. With the formation of anti-HIV antibodies, immune complexes containing virions are trapped by follicular dendritic cells (FDCs) in the germinal centers. As discussed earlier, proviral DNA can be found in a large number of CD4+ T cells and macrophages within the lymph nodes, and viral particles are readily detected on the surface of FDCs. During the middle or chronic phase, there is a continuing battle between HIV and the host immune system. The CD8+ cytotoxic T-cell response remains activated, *viral replication is restrained but not absent,* and the patients have few or mild symptoms. There is, however, a gradual erosion of the CD4+ T cells, and their numbers decline by 50 to 100 cells/μl per year. With disease progression, the rate of loss of CD4+ T cells becomes more brisk. Concomitant with the loss of CD4+ T cells, host defenses begin to wane, and the proportion of the surviving CD4+ cells infected with HIV increases, as does the viral burden per CD4+ cell. Not unexpectedly, HIV spillover into the plasma increases. *From a practical standpoint, CD4+ T-cell counts in the blood are reasonably accurate prognosticators of disease progression.*[112] Hence current classification recognizes CD4+ cell counts as an important barometer of the severity of HIV disease. Accordingly, HIV infection is stratified into three categories: CD4+ cells greater than or equal to 500 cells/μl; 200 to 499 cells/μl; and fewer than 200 cells/μl. An absolute CD4+ T-cell count below 200 cells/μl or a rapidly falling cell count correlates with disease progression, whereas CD4+ cell counts above 500 cells/μl have a much lower probability of rapid progression.

It should be evident from our discussion that in each of the three phases of HIV infection, variable degrees of viral replication continue to occur. Even in the clinical latent phase, when the majority of infected cells have the provirus locked into the genome, productive infection of T cells, chiefly in the lymphoid organs, is maintained. In other words, *HIV infection lacks a phase of true microbiologic latency,* that is, a phase during which *all* the HIV is in the form of proviral DNA, and no cell is productively infected. It is for this reason

that a strong case has been made for commencing antiretroviral therapy during the asymptomatic period. According to some, such therapeutic intervention slows the progression to AIDS as well as improves survival,[113] but this issue is far from being settled.

CLINICAL FEATURES. The clinical manifestations of HIV infection can be readily surmised from the foregoing discussion. They range from a mild acute illness to severe disease. Because the salient clinical features of the acute early and chronic middle phases of HIV infection were described earlier, here we shall summarize the clinical manifestations of the terminal phase, commonly known as AIDS.

In the United States, the typical adult patient with AIDS is a young homosexual man or an intravenous drug abuser who presents with fever, weight loss, diarrhea, generalized lymphadenopathy, multiple opportunistic infections, neurologic disease, and, in many cases, secondary neoplasms. The infections and neoplasms listed in Table 6–10 are included in the surveillance definition of AIDS.[114]

Pneumonia caused by the opportunistic fungus *P. carinii* (representing reactivation of a prior latent infection) is the presenting feature in about

Table 6–10. AIDS-DEFINING OPPORTUNISTIC INFECTIONS AND NEOPLASMS FOUND IN PATIENTS WITH HIV INFECTION

INFECTIONS

Protozoal and Helminthic Infections

   Cryptosporidiosis or isosporidiosis (enteritis)
   Pneumocytosis (pneumonia or disseminated infection)
   Toxoplasmosis (pneumonia or CNS infection)

Fungal Infections

   Candidiasis (esophageal, tracheal, or pulmonary)
   Cryptococcosis (CNS infection)
   Coccidioidomycosis (disseminated)
   Histoplasmosis (disseminated)

Bacterial Infections

   Mycobacteriosis ("atypical," e.g., *M. avium-intracellulare,* disseminated or extrapulmonary; *M. tuberculosis,* pulmonary or extrapulmonary)
   Nocardiosis (pneumonia, meningitis, disseminated)
   Salmonella infections, disseminated

Viral Infections

   Cytomegalovirus (pulmonary, intestinal, retinitis, or CNS infections)
   Herpes simplex virus (localized or disseminated)
   Varicella-zoster virus (localized or disseminated)
   Progressive multifocal leukoencephalopathy

NEOPLASMS

   Kaposi's sarcoma
   Non-Hodgkin's lymphomas (Burkitt's, immunoblastic)
   Primary lymphoma of the brain
   Invasive cancer of uterine cervix

   CNS = Central nervous system.

50% of cases, and approximately 70 to 80% of AIDS patients develop this infection at some time during the course of their illness. The risk of developing this infection is extremely high in individuals with fewer than 200 CD4+ cells/μl. Approximately 12% of patients present with an opportunistic infection other than *P. carinii* pneumonia. Among the most common pathogens are Candida species, cytomegalovirus, atypical and typical mycobacteria, *Cryptococcus neoformans*, *Toxoplasma gondii*, Cryptosporidium species, herpes simplex virus, papovaviruses, and *Histoplasma capsulatum*.[115]

Candidiasis of the oral cavity (thrush) and esophagus is extremely common in patients with AIDS. In asymptomatic HIV-infected individuals, oral candidiasis is a sign of immunologic decompensation, and it often heralds the transition to AIDS. *Cytomegalovirus* may cause disseminated disease or, more commonly, affects the eye and gastrointestinal tract. Chorioretinitis occurs in approximately 20% of patients, whereas gastrointestinal disease, seen in about 10% of cases, manifests as esophagitis, hepatitis, and colitis. Disseminated bacterial infection with *atypical mycobacteria (M. avium-intracellulare)* occurs late, in the setting of severe immunosuppression. Approximately 18 to 29% of the patients with AIDS have clinical evidence of disseminated infection, but the incidence at autopsy approaches 70%. Coincident with the AIDS epidemic, the incidence of tuberculosis has risen dramatically. Patients with AIDS have reactivation of latent pulmonary disease as well as outbreaks of primary infection.[116] As with tuberculosis in other settings, the infection may be confined to lungs or may involve other organs as well. In the setting of HIV infection, tuberculosis is more common among intravenous drug abusers, blacks, Hispanics, and Haitians. Most worrisome are recent reports indicating that a growing number of isolates are resistant to multiple drugs. *Cryptococcosis* occurs in about 10% of AIDS patients. Among fungal infections that prey on HIV-infected individuals, it is second only to candidiasis. As with other causes of immunosuppression, meningitis is the major clinical manifestation. In contrast to Cryptococcus, *Toxoplasma gondii*, another frequent invader of the CNS in AIDS, causes encephalitis. *Herpes simplex virus infection* is manifested by mucocutaneous ulcerations involving the mouth, esophagus, external genitalia, and perianal region. *Persistent diarrhea*, so common in patients with AIDS, is often caused by Cryptosporidium or *Isospora belli* infections. These patients have chronic profuse watery diarrhea with massive fluid loss. Diarrhea may also result from infection with enteric bacteria, such as Salmonella and Shigella. Depressed humoral immunity renders AIDS patients susceptible to severe, recurrent bacterial pneumonias.

Patients with AIDS have a high incidence of certain tumors.[117] The basis of the increased risk of malignancy is multifactorial: profound defects in T-cell immunity, dysregulated B-cell and monocyte functions, and multiple infections with known (e.g., EBV, HPV) and unknown viruses.

Kaposi's sarcoma, a tumor that is otherwise rare in the United States, is the most common neoplasm in patients with AIDS. At the onset of the AIDS epidemic, up to 40% of the reported cases had Kaposi's sarcoma, but in recent years there has been a definite and unexplained decline in its incidence. There are several peculiar features of this tumor in patients with AIDS. It is far more common in homosexual or bisexual men than in intravenous drug abusers or patients belonging to other risk categories. Its relationship to immune suppression is also unclear. The current incidence of about 15% in AIDS patients contrasts with 0.05% incidence in immunosuppressed transplant recipients.[118] By comparison, the 3% incidence of malignant lymphomas in patients with AIDS is roughly equivalent to that in immunosuppressed transplant patients. Furthermore, Kaposi's sarcoma sometimes arises early in the course of HIV infection, before the onset of severe immunodeficiency. Thus it appears that in patients with AIDS, Kaposi's sarcoma is not induced by immunosuppression alone. To complicate matters further, the cell of origin of this tumor has not been identified with certainty. Endothelial cells, smooth muscle cells, and pericytes all have been implicated. According to current hypotheses, Kaposi's sarcoma results from abnormal growth of primitive mesenchymal cells under the influence of autocrine and paracrine growth factors, including cytokines such as TNF-α, IL-1β, fibroblast growth factor, and IL-6; oncostatin (a novel cytokine); and HIV-1–derived *tat* protein. What pulls the trigger remains unknown. Clinically, the AIDS-associated Kaposi's sarcoma is quite different from the sporadic form (see Chapter 11). In HIV-infected individuals, the tumor is generally widespread, affecting the skin, mucous membranes, gastrointestinal tract, lymph nodes, and lungs. These tumors also tend to be more aggressive than the classic Kaposi's sarcoma.

With prolonged survival, the number of AIDS patients who develop non-Hodgkin's lymphoma has increased steadily. In a review of approximately 100,000 patients with AIDS, 3% were found to have non-Hodgkin's lymphoma.[119] As mentioned earlier, the risk of developing these lymphomas (approximately 60-fold higher than the general population) in patients with AIDS is comparable to that seen in other states of immunosuppression. Thus, in contrast to Kaposi's sarcoma, immunodeficiency is firmly implicated as the central predisposing factor. Indeed, it appears that patients with CD4+ cell counts below 50/μl incur an extremely high risk.[120] There are several features that characterize AIDS-associated non-Hodgkin's lymphomas: They are almost exclusively of B-cell origin, are highly aggressive, and have a penchant for extra-nodal involvement. The brain is the most common extranodal site affected, and hence primary lymphoma of the brain is considered an AIDS-defining condition. In keeping with their aggressive clinical course, approximately two-thirds of the tumors are of high-grade histology (see Chapter 14). The pathogenesis of AIDS-associated B-cell lymphomas probably involves sustained polyclonal B-cell activation followed by the emergence of monoclonal or oligoclonal B-cell populations. It is believed that during the frenzy of proliferation, some clones undergo somatic mutations and neoplastic transformation (see discussion Chapter 14). There is morphologic evidence of B-cell activation in lymph nodes, and it is believed that at least in some cases B-cell proliferation is triggered by activation of EBV infection. Patients with **AIDS** have an increase in anti-EBV immunoglobulins and in the number of EBV-infected B cells. Other evidence of EBV infection includes oral hairy leukoplakia (white fibrillar projections on the tongue), believed to result from EBV-driven squamous cell proliferation of the oral mucosa (see Chapter 16). Molecular analyses of AIDS-associated lymphomas reveal the presence of EBV genome in approximately 30 to 50% of the tumors, lending support to the postulated role of EBV in the genesis of these tumors. In cases in which molecular footprints of EBV infection cannot be detected, other viruses and microbes may initiate polyclonal B-cell proliferation. There is no evidence that HIV by itself is capable of causing neoplastic transformation.

In 1993, the U.S. Centers for Disease Control added invasive cancer of the uterine cervix to the list of AIDS-defining conditions. This change reflects the greatly increased prevalence of HPV infection in patients with **AIDS**. This virus is believed to be intimately associated with squamous cell carcinoma of the cervix and its precursor lesions—cervical dysplasia and carcinoma in situ (see Chapter 23). HPV-associated cervical dysplasia is ten times more common in HIV-infected women, as compared with uninfected women attending family planning clinics. Hence it is recommended that gynecologic examination be part of a routine work-up of HIV-infected women.

A large variety of other neoplasms, including Hodgkin's disease and T-cell lymphomas, have been reported in patients with **AIDS**. It is not clear, however, whether the incidence of these tumors is increased with HIV infection.

Involvement of the CNS is a common and important manifestation of AIDS. *Seventy to ninety per cent of patients demonstrate some form of neurologic involvement at autopsy, and 30 to 50% have clinically manifest neurologic dysfunction.* Quite important, in some patients neurologic manifestations may be the sole or earliest presenting feature of HIV infection. In addition to opportunistic infections and neoplasms, several virally determined

neuropathologic changes occur. These include a self-limited meningoencephalitis occurring at the time of seroconversion, aseptic meningitis, vacuolar myelopathy, peripheral neuropathies, and, most commonly, a progressive encephalopathy designated clinically as the AIDS-dementia complex (see Chapter 29).

MORPHOLOGY. The anatomic changes in the tissues (with the exception of lesions in the brain) are neither specific nor diagnostic. In general, the pathologic features of AIDS are those characteristic of widespread opportunistic infections, Kaposi's sarcoma, and lymphoid tumors. Most of these lesions are discussed elsewhere because they also occur in patients who do not have HIV infection. To appreciate the distinctive nature of lesions in the CNS, they are discussed in the context of other disorders affecting the brain. Here we concentrate on changes in the lymphoid organs.

Biopsy specimens from enlarged lymph nodes in the early stages of HIV infection reveal a **marked follicular hyperplasia.**[121] The enlarged follicles have irregular, sometimes serrated borders, and they are present not only in the cortex but also in the medulla and may even extend outside the capsule. The mantle zones that surround the follicles are markedly attenuated, and hence the germinal centers seem to merge with the interfollicular area. These changes, affecting primarily the B-cell areas of the node, are the morphologic reflections of the polyclonal B-cell activation and hypergammaglobulinemia seen in patients with AIDS. In addition to B-cell expansion within germinal centers, activated monocytoid B cells are present within and around the sinusoids and trabecular blood vessels. Under the electron microscope and by *in situ* hybridization, HIV particles can be detected within the germinal centers. Here they seem to be concentrated on the villous processes of follicular dendritic cells, presumably trapped in the form of immune complexes. During the early phase of HIV infection, viral DNA can be found within the nuclei of CD4+ T cells located predominantly in the follicular mantle zone. With disease progression, the frenzy of B-cell proliferation subsides and gives way to a pattern of severe follicular involution. The follicles are depleted of cells, and the **organized network of follicular dendritic cells is disrupted.** The germinal centers may even become hyalinized. During this advanced stage, viral burden in the nodes is reduced, in part because of the disruption of the follicular dendritic cells. These "burnt-out" lymph nodes are atrophic and small and may harbor numerous opportunistic pathogens. Because of profound immunosuppression, the inflammatory response to infections both in the lymph nodes and at extranodal sites may be sparse or atypical. For example, mycobacteria do not evoke granuloma formation because CD4+

cells are deficient. In the empty-looking lymph nodes and in other organs, the presence of infectious agents may not be readily apparent without the application of special stains. As might be expected, lymphoid depletion is not confined to the nodes; in later stages of AIDS, spleen and thymus also appear to be "wastelands."

Non-Hodgkin's lymphomas, involving the nodes as well as extranodal sites, such as the liver, gastrointestinal tract, and bone marrow, are primarily high-grade diffuse B-cell neoplasms (see Chapter 14).

Since the emergence of AIDS in 1981, the concerted efforts of epidemiologists, immunologists, and molecular biologists have resulted in spectacular advances in our understanding of this disorder. Despite all this progress, however, the prognosis of patients with AIDS remains dismal. Of the initial 200,000 patients reported, more than 100,000 are dead. With time, true mortality figures are likely to be much higher, perhaps approaching 100%. Although a causative virus has been identified, many hurdles remain to be crossed before a vaccine can be developed. Molecular analyses have revealed an alarming degree of polymorphism in viral isolates from different patients; this renders the task of producing a vaccine remarkably difficult.

AMYLOIDOSIS

Immunologic mechanisms are suspected of contributing to a large number of diseases in addition to those already described in this chapter. Some of the entities are discussed in the chapters dealing with individual organs and systems. One disease—amyloidosis—requires description at this point. There is strong evidence that in most patients some derangement in the immune apparatus underlies this disease, and as a systemic disease it cannot be assigned to any single organ or system.

Amyloid is a pathologic proteinaceous substance, deposited between cells in various tissues and organs of the body in a wide variety of clinical settings. Because amyloid deposition appears so insidiously and sometimes mysteriously, its clinical recognition ultimately depends on morphologic identification of this distinctive substance in appropriate biopsy specimens. *With the light microscope and standard tissue stains, amyloid appears as an amorphous, eosinophilic, hyaline, extracellular substance that, with progressive accumulation, encroaches on and produces pressure atrophy of adjacent cells.* To differentiate amyloid from other hyaline deposits (e.g., collagen, fibrin), a variety of histochemical techniques, described later, are used. Perhaps most widely used is the Congo red

stain, which under ordinary light imparts a pink or red color to tissue deposits, but far more dramatic and specific is the green birefringence of the stained amyloid when observed by polarizing microscopy (Fig. 6–43).

Despite the fact that all deposits have a uniform appearance and tinctorial characteristics, *it is quite clear that amyloid is not a chemically distinct entity.* There are two major and several minor biochemical forms. These are deposited by several different pathogenetic mechanisms, and therefore *amyloidosis should not be considered a single disease; rather it is a group of diseases having in common the deposition of similar-appearing proteins.*[122] At the heart of the morphologic uniformity is the remarkably uniform physical organization of amyloid protein, which we consider first. This is followed by a discussion of the chemical nature of amyloid.

PHYSICAL NATURE OF AMYLOID. *By electron microscopy, amyloid is seen to be made up largely of nonbranching fibrils of indefinite length and a diameter of approximately 7.5 to 10 nm.* This electron microscopic structure is identical in all types of amyloidosis. X-ray crystallography and infrared spectroscopy demonstrate a characteristic cross beta-pleated sheet conformation (Fig. 6–44). This conformation is seen regardless of the clinical setting or chemical composition and is responsible for the distinctive staining and birefringence of Congo red–stained amyloid. In addition to amyloid fibrils, a minor second component is always present in amyloid, known as the P component. With the electron microscope, it appears as a pentagonal, doughnut-shaped structure.

CHEMICAL NATURE OF AMYLOID. Approximately 95% of the amyloid material consists of fibril proteins, the remaining 5% being the P component, which is a glycoprotein. *Of the 15 biochemically distinct forms of amyloid proteins that have been identified, two are most common: One, called AL (amyloid light chain) is derived from plasma cells (immunocytes) and contains immunoglobulin light chains; the other, designated AA (amyloid-associated), is a unique nonimmunoglobulin protein synthesized by the liver.*

These two amyloid proteins are deposited in distinct clinicopathologic settings. The AL protein is made up of complete immunoglobulin light chains, the NH_2-terminal fragments of light chains, or both. Most of the AL proteins analyzed are composed of lambda light chains (particularly lambda VI type) or their fragments, but in some cases kappa chains have been identified. As might be expected, the amyloid fibril protein of the AL type is produced by immunoglobulin-secreting cells, and their deposition is associated with some form of monoclonal B cell proliferation.

The second major class of amyloid fibril protein (AA) does not have structural homology to

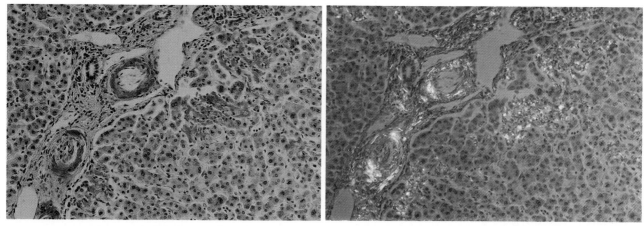

Figure 6–43. Amyloidosis. *A,* Section of the liver stained with Congo red reveals pink-red deposits of amyloid in the walls of blood vessels and along sinusoids. *B,* Note the yellow-green birefringence of the deposits when observed by polarizing microscope. (Courtesy of Dr. Trace Worrell and Sandy Hinton, Department of Pathology, University of Texas Southwestern Medical School, Dallas.)

immunoglobulins. It has a molecular weight of 8500 and consists of 76 amino acid residues. The AA protein is found in those clinical settings described clinically as "secondary amyloidosis." AA fibrils are derived from a larger (12,000 daltons) precursor in the serum called SAA (serum amyloid–associated) protein that is synthesized in the liver and circulates in association with the HDL3 subclass of lipoproteins.

Several other biochemically distinct proteins have been found in amyloid deposits in a variety of clinical settings.

• *Transthyretin* (TTR) is a normal serum protein that binds and transports thyroxine and retinol, hence the name *trans-thy-retin.* It was previously

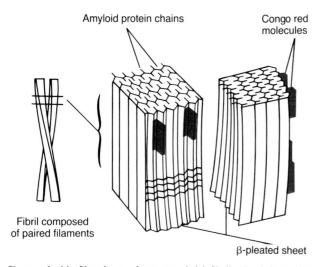

Amyloid protein chains

Congo red molecules

Fibril composed of paired filaments

β-pleated sheet

Figure 6–44. Structure of an amyloid fibril, depicting the beta-pleated sheet structure and binding sites for the Congo red dye, which is used for diagnosis of amyloidosis. (Modified from Glenner, G.G.: Amyloid deposit and amyloidosis. The *β*-fibrilloses. N. Engl. J. Med. 52:148, 1980, by permission of The New England Journal of Medicine.)

called prealbumin because it precedes serum albumin on serum electrophoresis. *A mutant form of transthyretin (and its fragments) is deposited in a group of genetically determined disorders referred to as familial amyloid polyneuropathies.*[123] Amyloid transthyretin (ATTR) deposited in the tissues differs from its normal counterpart by a single amino acid. Transthyretin is also deposited in the heart of aged individuals (senile cardiac amyloidosis), but in such cases the transthyretin molecule is structurally normal.

• *Beta$_2$-microglobulin,* a component of the MHC class I molecules and a normal serum protein, has been identified as the amyloid fibril subunit (Aβ_2m) in amyloidosis that complicates the course of patients on *long-term hemodialysis.* Aβ_2m fibers are structurally similar to normal β_2m protein.

• *Beta$_2$-amyloid protein* (Aβ), not to be confused with beta$_2$-microglobulin, is a 4000-dalton peptide that constitutes the core of cerebral plaques found in Alzheimer's disease as well as the amyloid deposited in walls of cerebral blood vessels in patients with Alzheimer's disease. The Aβ protein is derived from a much larger transmembrane glycoprotein, called amyloid precursor protein (APP).

• In addition to the foregoing, amyloid deposits derived from diverse precursors such as hormones (procalcitonin) and keratin have also been reported.

The P component, a glycoprotein, is distinct from the amyloid fibrils but is closely associated with them in all forms of amyloidosis. It has a striking structural homology to C-reactive protein, a well-known acute phase reactant. The serum P component has an affinity for amyloid fibrils, and it may be necessary for tissue deposition. Its pres-

Table 6-11. CLASSIFICATION OF AMYLOIDOSIS

CLINICOPATHOLOGIC CATEGORY	ASSOCIATED DISEASES	MAJOR FIBRIL PROTEIN	CHEMICALLY RELATED PRECURSOR PROTEIN
Systemic (Generalized) Amyloidosis			
Immunocyte dyscrasias with amyloidosis (primary amyloidosis)	Multiple myeloma and other monoclonal B-cell proliferations	AL	Immunoglobulin light chains, chiefly λ type
Reactive systemic amyloidosis (secondary amyloidosis)	Chronic inflammatory conditions	AA	SAA
Hemodialysis-associated amyloidosis	Chronic renal failure	$A\beta_2m$	β_2-microglobulin
Hereditary amyloidosis			
Familial Mediterranean fever	—	AA	SAA
Familial amyloidotic neuropathies (several types)	—	ATTR	Transthyretin*
Localized Amyloidosis			
Senile cardiac	—	ATTR	Transthyretin*
Senile cerebral	Alzheimer's disease	$A\beta_2$	APP
Endocrine			
Medullary carcinoma of thyroid	—	A Cal	Calcitonin
Islet of Langerhans	Type II diabetes	AIAPP	Islet amyloid peptide
Isolated atrial amyloidosis	—	AANF	Atrial natriuretic factor

* Transthyretin is also known as prealbumin.

ence in amyloid is responsible for staining with periodic acid–Schiff (PAS), which led early observers to believe that amyloid was a saccharide.

CLASSIFICATION OF AMYLOIDOSIS. According to the most recent recommendation of "amyloidologists," who congregate every few years to discuss their favorite protein, amyloid should be classified based on its constituent chemical fibrils into categories such as AL, AA, and ATTR and not based on clinical syndromes.[124] Because a given biochemical form of amyloid (e.g., AA) may be associated with amyloid deposition in diverse clinical settings, we shall follow a combined biochemical-clinical classification for our discussion (Table 6–11). Amyloid may be _systemic_ (generalized), involving several organ systems, or it may be _localized_, when deposits are limited to a single organ, such as the heart. As should become evident, several different biochemical forms of amyloid are encompassed by such a segregation.

On clinical grounds, the systemic, or generalized, pattern is subclassified into _primary amyloidosis_, when associated with some immunocyte dyscrasia, or _secondary amyloidosis_, when it occurs as a complication of an underlying chronic inflammatory or tissue destructive process. _Hereditary_ or familial amyloidosis constitutes a separate, albeit heterogeneous group, with several distinctive patterns of organ involvement.

Immunocyte Dyscrasias with Amyloidosis ("Primary Amyloidosis"). Amyloid in this category is usually systemic in distribution and is of the AL type. In the United States, this is the most common form of amyloidosis (75% of cases).[125] In many of these cases, the patients have some form of plasma

cell dyscrasia. Best defined is the occurrence of systemic amyloidosis in 5 to 15% of patients with multiple myeloma, a form of plasma cell neoplasia characterized by multiple osteolytic lesions throughout the skeletal system (see Chapter 14). The malignant B cells characteristically synthesize abnormal amounts of a single specific immunoglobulin (monoclonal gammopathy), producing an M (myeloma) protein spike on serum electrophoresis. In addition to the synthesis of whole immunoglobulin molecules, only the light chains (referred to as Bence Jones protein) of either the kappa or the lambda variety may be elaborated and found in the serum. By virtue of the small molecular size of the Bence Jones protein, it is frequently excreted in the urine. Almost all the patients with myeloma who develop amyloidosis have Bence Jones proteins in the serum or urine, or both, but it should be remembered that a great majority of myeloma patients who have free light chains do not develop amyloidosis. Clearly, therefore, _the presence of Bence Jones proteins, although necessary, is by itself not enough to produce amyloidosis._ We discuss later the other factors, such as the type of light chain produced ("amyloidogenic potential") and the subsequent handling (possibly degradation) that may have a bearing on whether Bence Jones proteins are deposited as amyloid.

The great majority of patients with AL amyloid do not have classic multiple myeloma or any other overt B-cell neoplasm; such cases have been traditionally classified as primary amyloidosis because their clinical features derive from the effects of amyloid deposition without any other associated disease. In virtually all such cases, however, monoclonal immunoglobulins or free light chains, or both, can be found in the serum or urine. Most of these patients also have a modest increase in the number of plasma cells in the bone marrow, which presumably secrete the precursors of AL protein. Clearly these patients have an underlying B-cell dyscrasia ("covert myeloma") in which production of an abnormal protein, rather than production of tumor masses, is the predominant manifestation. Whether the condition of most of these patients would evolve into multiple myeloma if they lived long enough can only be a matter for speculation.

Reactive Systemic Amyloidosis. The amyloid deposits in this pattern are systemic in distribution and are composed of AA protein. This category is commonly referred to as *secondary amyloidosis* because it is secondary to the associated inflammatory condition. The feature common to most of the conditions associated with reactive systemic amyloidosis is protracted breakdown of cells resulting from a wide variety of infectious and noninfectious chronic inflammatory conditions. At one time, tuberculosis, bronchiectasis, and chronic osteomyelitis were the most important underlying conditions, but with the advent of effective antimicrobial chemotherapy, the importance of these conditions has diminished. More commonly now, reactive systemic amyloidosis complicates rheumatoid arthritis, other connective tissue disorders such as ankylosing spondylitis, and inflammatory bowel disease, particularly regional enteritis and ulcerative colitis. Among these, the most frequent associated condition is rheumatoid arthritis. Amyloidosis is reported to occur in approximately 3% of patients with rheumatoid arthritis. Recent studies indicate that heroine abusers who inject the drug subcutaneously have a high occurrence rate of generalized AA amyloidosis. The chronic skin infections associated with "skin-popping" of narcotics seem to be responsible for amyloidosis in this group of patients.

Reactive systemic amyloidosis may also occur in association with nonimmunocyte-derived tumors, the two most common being renal cell carcinoma and Hodgkin's disease.

Hemodialysis-Associated Amyloidosis. Patients on long-term hemodialysis for renal failure develop amyloidosis owing to deposition of beta$_2$-microglobulin. This protein is present in high concentrations in the serum of patients with renal disease and is retained in circulation because it cannot be filtered through the cuprophane dialysis membranes. In some series, as many as 70% of the patients on long-term dialysis developed amyloid deposits in the synovium, joints, and tendon sheaths.

Heredofamilial Amyloidosis. A variety of familial forms of amyloidosis have been described. Most of them are rare and occur in limited geographic areas. The most common and best studied is an autosomal recessive condition called *familial Medi-*

terranean fever. This is a febrile disorder of unknown cause characterized by attacks of fever accompanied by inflammation of serosal surfaces, including peritoneum, pleura, and synovial membrane. This disorder is encountered largely in individuals of Armenian, Sephardic Jewish, and Arabic origins. It is associated with widespread tissue involvement indistinguishable from reactive systemic amyloidosis. The amyloid fibril proteins are made up of AA proteins, suggesting that this form of amyloidosis is related to the recurrent bouts of inflammation that characterize this disease.

In contrast to familial Mediterranean fever, a group of autosomal dominant familial disorders is characterized by deposition of amyloid predominantly in the nerves—peripheral and autonomic.[123] These familial amyloidotic polyneuropathies have been described in different parts of the world. For example, neuropathic amyloidosis has been identified in individuals in Portugal, Japan, Sweden, and the United States. As mentioned previously, in all of these genetic disorders, the fibrils are made up of mutant transthyretins (ATTR).

Localized Amyloidosis. Sometimes amyloid deposits are limited to a single organ or tissue without involvement of any other site in the body. The deposits may produce grossly detectable nodular masses or be evident only on microscopic examination. Nodular (tumor-forming) deposits of amyloid are most often encountered in the lung, larynx, skin, urinary bladder, tongue, and the region about the eye. Frequently there are infiltrates of lymphocytes and plasma cells in the periphery of these amyloid masses, raising the question of whether the mononuclear infiltrate is a response to the deposition of amyloid or instead is responsible for it. At least in some cases, the amyloid consists of AL protein and may therefore represent a localized form of immunocyte-derived amyloid.

Endocrine Amyloid. Microscopic deposits of localized amyloid may be found in certain endocrine tumors, such as medullary carcinoma of the thyroid gland, islet tumors of the pancreas, pheochromocytomas, and undifferentiated carcinomas of the stomach, and in the islets of Langerhans in patients with type II diabetes mellitus. In these settings, the amyloidogenic proteins seem to be derived either from polypeptide hormones (medullary carcinoma) or from unique proteins (e.g., islet amyloid polypeptide, IAPP).

Amyloid of Aging. Two well-documented forms of amyloid deposition occur with aging.

Senile cardiac amyloidosis refers to the deposition of amyloid in the heart of elderly patients (usually in the eighth and ninth decades of life). It may occur in two forms: deposition of transthyretin, involving the ventricles, or deposition of atrial natriuretic peptide, involving the atria. Such deposition is usually asymptomatic but can cause serious

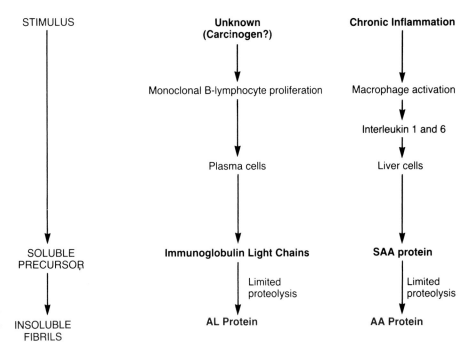

Figure 6-45. Proposed schema of the pathogenesis of two major forms of amyloid fibrils

cardiac dysfunction. In addition to cardiac involvement, there may also be deposition of amyloid in the lungs, pancreas, or spleen, suggesting that senile cardiac amyloidosis may well be a systemic disorder.

Senile cerebral amyloidosis refers to the deposition of Aβ_2 protein in the cerebral blood vessels and plaques of patients with Alzheimer's disease (see Chapter 29).

PATHOGENESIS. Although the precursors of the two major amyloid proteins have been identified, several aspects of their origins still are not clear. In reactive systemic amyloidosis, it appears that long-standing tissue destruction and inflammation lead to elevated SAA levels (Fig. 6-45). SAA is synthesized by the liver cells under the influence of cytokines such as IL-6 and IL-1; however, increased production of SAA by itself is not sufficient for the deposition of amyloid. Elevation of serum SAA levels is common to inflammatory states but in most instances does not lead to amyloidosis. There are two possible explanations for this. According to one view, SAA is normally degraded to soluble end products by the action of monocyte-derived enzymes. Conceivably, individuals who develop amyloidosis have an enzyme defect that results in incomplete breakdown of SAA, thus generating insoluble AA molecules. Alternatively, a genetically determined structural abnormality in the SAA molecule itself renders it resistant to degradation by monocytes. In the case of immunocyte dyscrasias, there is an excess of immunoglobulin light chains, and amyloid can be derived by proteolysis of Ig light chains *in vitro*. Again, defective degradation has been invoked,

and perhaps particular light chains are resistant to complete proteolysis.

In contrast to the two examples already cited, in familial amyloidosis the deposition of transthyretins as amyloid fibrils does not result from overproduction of transthyretins. It has been proposed that genetically determined alterations of structure render the transthyretins prone to abnormal aggregation and proteolysis.

The cells involved in the conversion of the precursor proteins into the fibrils are not fully characterized, but macrophages seem to be the most likely candidates.

MORPHOLOGY. There are no consistent or distinctive patterns of organ or tissue distribution of amyloid deposits in any of the categories cited. Nonetheless, a few generalizations can be made. Amyloidosis secondary to chronic inflammatory disorders tends to yield the most severe systemic involvements. Kidneys, liver, spleen, lymph nodes, adrenals, and thyroid as well as many other tissues are classically involved. Although immunocyte-associated amyloidosis cannot reliably be distinguished from the secondary form by its organ distribution, more often it involves the heart, gastrointestinal tract, peripheral nerves, skin, and tongue. In addition, bizarre distributions, such as amyloidosis of the eye and respiratory tract, are encountered more often in patients with immunocyte-associated amyloidosis.

Macroscopically, the affected organs are often enlarged and firm and have a waxy appearance. If the deposits are sufficiently large, painting the cut surface with iodine imparts a yellow color that is transformed to blue violet after application of sulfuric acid.

As noted earlier, the histologic diagnosis of amyloid is based almost entirely on its staining characteristics. The most commonly used staining technique utilizes the dye Congo red, which under ordinary light imparts a pink or red color to amyloid deposits. Under polarized light, the Congo red–stained amyloid shows a green birefringence (Fig. 6–43). This reaction is shared by all forms of amyloid and is due to the cross-beta-pleated configuration of amyloid fibrils. Other methods of differentiating amyloid from hyaline deposits include somewhat less specific histochemical techniques. For example, amyloid stains metachromatically (violet to pink) with crystal violet or methyl violet. It yields secondary fluorescence in ultraviolet light with the dyes thioflavine T and S. For routine diagnosis, birefringence after Congo red staining is the most widely practiced and reliable tool. Confirmation can be obtained by electron microscopy. AA, AL, and transthyretin amyloid can be distinguished in histologic sections. AA protein loses affinity for Congo red after pretreatment with potassium permanganate, whereas other forms of amyloid do not. Immunoperoxidase staining with specific antibodies reactive with various chemical forms of amyloid is also useful in the identification of amyloid fibril proteins.

Because the pattern of organ involvement in different clinical forms of amyloidosis is variable, each of the major organ involvements is described separately.

Kidney. Amyloidosis of the kidney is the most common and potentially the most serious form of organ involvement. In most reported series of patients with amyloidosis, renal amyloidosis is the major cause of death. On gross inspection, the kidney may appear normal in size and color, or it may be enlarged. In advanced cases, it may be shrunken and contracted owing to vascular narrowing induced by the deposition of amyloid within arterial and arteriolar walls.

Histologically, the amyloid is deposited primarily in the glomeruli, but the interstitial peritubular tissue, arteries, and arterioles are also affected. The glomerular deposits first appear as subtle thickenings of the mesangial matrix, accompanied usually by uneven widening of the basement membranes of the glomerular capillaries. In time, the mesangial depositions and the deposits along the basement membranes cause capillary narrowing and distortion of the glomerular vascular tuft. With progression of the glomerular amyloidosis, the capillary lumina are obliterated, and the obsolescent glomerulus is flooded by confluent masses or interlacing broad ribbons of amyloid (Fig. 6–46).

Spleen. Amyloidosis of the spleen may be inapparent grossly or may cause moderate to marked

splenomegaly (up to 800 gm). For completely mysterious reasons, one of two patterns of deposition is seen. In one, the deposit is largely limited to the splenic follicles, producing tapioca-like granules on gross inspection, designated "sago spleen." Histologically the entire follicle may be replaced in advanced cases. In the other pattern, the amyloid appears to spare the follicles and instead involves the walls of the splenic sinuses and connective tissue framework in the red pulp. Fusion of the early deposits gives rise to large, map-like areas of amyloidosis, creating what has been designated the "lardaceous" spleen.

Liver. Here again the deposits may be grossly inapparent or may cause moderate to marked hepatomegaly. The amyloid appears first in the space of Disse and then progressively encroaches on adjacent hepatic parenchymal cells and sinusoids. In time, deformity, pressure atrophy, and disappearance of hepatocytes occur, causing total replacement of large areas of liver parenchyma. Vascular involvement and Kupffer cell depositions are frequent. Normal liver function is usually preserved despite sometimes quite severe involvement of the liver.

Heart. Amyloidosis of the heart may occur in any form of systemic amyloidosis, much more commonly in persons with immunocyte-derived disease. In some patients, it represents an isolated organ involvement, and almost invariably the patient is over 70 years of age **(amyloid of aging).** The heart may be enlarged and firm, but more often it shows no significant changes on cross section of the myocardium. Histologically, the deposits begin in focal subendocardial accumulations and within the myocardium between the muscle fibers. Expansion of these myocardial deposits eventually causes pressure atrophy of myocardial fibers (Fig. 6–47). In most cases, the deposits are separated and widely

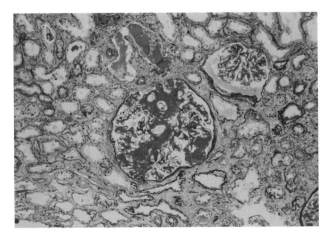

Figure 6–46. Amyloidosis of the kidney. The glomerular architecture is almost totally obliterated by the massive accumulation of amyloid.

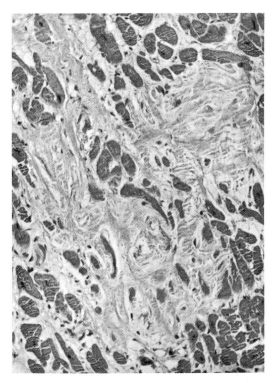

Figure 6-47. Amyloidosis of aging in the heart. The amyloid surrounds isolated myocardial fibers and has caused atrophy of others.

distributed, but when they are subendocardial, the conduction system may be damaged, accounting for the electrocardiographic abnormalities noted in some patients.

Other Organs. Amyloidosis of other organs is generally encountered in systemic disease. The adrenals, thyroid, and pituitary are common sites of involvement. In the adrenals, the intercellular deposits begin adjacent to the basement membranes of the cortical cells, usually first in the zona glomerulosa. With progression, large sheets of amyloid may replace considerable amounts of the cortical parenchyma. Similar patterns are seen in the thyroid and pituitary. The gastrointestinal tract may be involved at any level, from the oral cavity (gingiva, tongue) to the anus. The early lesions mainly affect blood vessels, but eventually extend to involve the adjacent areas of the submucosa, muscularis, and subserosa.

Nodular depositions in the tongue may cause macroglossia, giving rise to the designation **tumor-forming amyloid of the tongue.** The respiratory tract may be involved focally or diffusely from the larynx down to the smallest bronchioles. As mentioned earlier, a distinct chemical form of amyloid has been found in the brain of patients with Alzheimer's disease. It involves so-called plaques as well as blood vessels (see Chapter 29). Amyloidosis of peripheral and autonomic nerves is a feature of several familial amyloidotic neuropathies. Curiously,

depositions of amyloid in patients on long-term hemodialysis are most prominent in the carpal ligament of the wrist, resulting in compression of the median nerve (carpal tunnel syndrome). These patients may also have extensive amyloid deposition in the joints.

CLINICAL CORRELATION. Amyloidosis may be found as an unsuspected anatomic change, having produced no clinical manifestations, or it may cause death. The symptoms depend, as you might expect, on the magnitude of the deposits and on the particular sites or organs affected. Clinical manifestations at first are often entirely nonspecific, such as weakness, weight loss, lightheadedness, or syncope. Somewhat more specific findings appear later and most often relate to renal, cardiac, and gastrointestinal involvement, but hepatomegaly and splenomegaly and alterations in serum protein levels may also be present.

Renal involvement is the dominating and most life-threatening feature of most cases of systemic amyloidosis, including those patients with familial Mediterranean fever. It gives rise to proteinuria, and is an important cause of the nephrotic syndrome (see Chapter 20). Progressive obliteration of glomeruli in advanced cases ultimately leads to renal failure and uremia.

Cardiac amyloidosis is extremely common in patients with immunocyte-derived amyloidosis, but it is less frequently present in those with reactive systemic amyloidosis. It is also encountered as an isolated involvement in patients of advanced age. When symptomatic, the typical presentation is the insidious onset of congestive heart failure. The most serious aspects of cardiac amyloidosis are the conduction disturbances and arrhythmias that may prove fatal. Occasionally cardiac amyloidosis produces a restrictive pattern of cardiomyopathy and masquerades as chronic constrictive pericarditis (see Chapter 12).

Gastrointestinal amyloidosis may be entirely asymptomatic, or it may present in a variety of ways. Amyloidosis of the tongue may cause sufficient enlargement and inelasticity to hamper speech and swallowing. Depositions in the stomach and intestine may lead to malabsorption, diarrhea, and disturbances in digestion.

The diagnosis of amyloidosis depends upon demonstration of amyloid deposits in tissues. The most common sites biopsied are the kidney, when renal manifestations are present, or rectal or gingival tissues in patients suspected of having systemic amyloidosis. Examination of abdominal fat aspirates stained with Congo red is an extremely useful technique for the diagnosis of systemic amyloidosis. Binding of radiolabeled P component to amyloid deposits has been used in the diagnosis of systemic amyloidosis.[126]

In suspected cases of immunocyte-associated

amyloidosis, serum and urine protein electrophoresis and immunoelectrophoresis should be performed. Bone marrow aspirates in such cases often show plasmacytosis even in the absence of overt multiple myeloma.

The prognosis for patients with generalized amyloidosis is poor. Those with immunocyte-derived amyloidosis (not including multiple myeloma) have a median survival of 2 years after diagnosis. Patients with myeloma-associated amyloidosis have a poorer prognosis.[125] The outlook for patients with reactive systemic amyloidosis is somewhat better and depends to some extent on the control of the underlying condition. Resorption of amyloid after treatment of the associated condition has been reported, but this is a rare occurrence.

1. Weiss, A.: Structure and function of the T cell antigen receptor. J. Clin. Invest. 86:1015, 1990.
2. Springer, T.A.: Adhesion receptors of the immune system. Nature 346:425, 1990.
3. Romagnani, S.: Human T_H-1 and T_H-2 subsets: Doubt no more. Immunol. Today 12:256, 1991.
4. van Noesel, C.J.M., et al.: Dual recognition by B cells. Immunol. Today 14:9, 1993.
5. Kumar, V., and Bennett, M.: Natural killer cells. In Frank, M.M. et al. (eds.): Samters Immunologic Diseases. 5th ed. Boston, Little, Brown and Co., 1994 (in press).
6. Biron, C.A., et al.: Severe herpesvirus infections in an adolescent without natural killer cells. N. Engl. J. Med. 320(26):1731, 1989.
7. Monaco, J.J.: A molecular model of MHC class-I–restricted antigen processing. Immunol. Today 13:173, 1992.
8. Brown, J.H.: Three-dimensional structure of the human class II histocompatibility antigen HLA-DR1. Nature 364:33, 1993.
9. Neefjes, J.J., and Ploegh, H.L.: Intracellular transport of MHC class II molecules. Immunol. Today 13:179, 1992.
10. Galli, S.: New concepts about the mast cell. N. Engl. J. Med. 328:257, 1993.
11. Borish, L., and Joseph, B.: Inflammation and allergic response. Med. Clin. North Am. 76:765, 1992.
12. Galli, S.J., et al.: Cytokine production by mast cells and basophils. Curr. Opin. Immunol. 3:865, 1991.
13. Tan, H.P., et al.: Regulatory role of cytokines in IgE-mediated allergy. J. Leukoc. Biol. 52:115, 1992.
14. Bochner, B.S., and Lichtenstein, L.M.: Anaphylaxis. N. Engl. J. Med. 324:1785, 1991.
15. Lawley, J.J., et al.: A prospective clinical and immunologic analysis of patients with serum sickness. N. Engl. J. Med. 311:1407, 1984.
16. Waldorf, H.A., et al.: Early cellular events in evolving cutaneous delayed hypersensitivity in humans. Am. J. Pathol. 138:477, 1991.
17. Scott, P.: IL-12: Initiation cytokine for cell-mediated immunity. Science 260:496, 1993.
18. Amiri, P., et al.: Tumor necrosis factor α restores granulomas and induces parasite egg-laying in schistosome-infected SCID mice. Nature 356:604, 1992.
19. Rosenberg, A., and Singer, A.: Cellular basis of skin allograft rejection: An in vivo model of immune-mediated destruction. Annu. Rev. Immunol. 10:333, 1992.
20. Lechler, R., and Lombardi, G.: Structural aspects of allorecognition. Curr. Opin. Immunol. 3:715, 1991.
21. Bradley, J.A., et al.: Processed MHC class I alloantigen as the stimulus for CD4+ T-cell–dependent antibody-mediated graft rejection. Immunol. Today 13:434, 1992.
22. Sherman, L.A., and Chattopadhyay, S.: The molecular basis of allorecognition. Annu. Rev. Immunol. 11:385, 1993.
23. Wecker, H., and Auchincloss, H.: Cellular mechanisms of rejection. Curr. Opin. Immunol. 4:561, 1992.
24. Pardo-Mindan, F.J., et al.: Pathology of renal transplantation. Semin. Diagn. Pathol. 9(3):185, 1992.
25. Paul, L.C., and Fellström, B.: Chronic vascular rejection of the heart and kidney—have rational treatment options emerged? Transplantation 53:1169, 1992.
26. Takemoto, S., et al.: Survival of nationally shared, HLA-matched kidney transplants from cadaveric donors. N. Engl. J. Med. 327:834, 1992.
27. Lu, C.Y., et al.: Prevention and treatment of renal allograft rejection: New therapeutic approaches and new insights into established therapies. J. Am. Soc. Nephrol. 4:1239, 1993.
28. Isobe, M., et al.: Specific acceptance of cardiac allografts after treatment with antibodies to ICAM-1 and LFA-1. Science 255:1125, 1992.
29. Ferrara, J.L., and Deeg, H.J.: Graft-versus-host disease. N. Engl. J. Med. 324:667, 1991.
30. Naparstek, Y., and Plotz, P.H.: The role of autoantibodies in autoimmune disease. Annu. Rev. Immunol. 11:79, 1993.
31. Lo, D.: T-cell tolerance. Curr. Opin. Immunol. 4:711, 1992.
32. Goodnow, C.: B-cell tolerance. Curr. Opin. Immunol. 4:703, 1992.
33. Speiser, D.E., et al.: Clonal deletion induced by either radioresistant thymic host cells or lymphohemopoietic donor cells at different stages of class I–restricted T cell ontogeny. J. Exp. Med. 175:1277, 1992.
34. Jones, L.A., et al.: Peripheral clonal elimination of functional T cells. Science 250:1726, 1990.
35. Okamoto, M., et al.: A transgenic model of autoimmune hemolytic anemia. J. Exp. Med. 175:71, 1992.
36. Tan, P., et al.: Induction of alloantigen-specific hyporesponsiveness in human T lymphocytes by blocking interaction of CD28 with its natural ligand B7/BB1. J. Exp. Med. 177:165, 1993.
37. Fowell, D., and Mason, D.: Evidence that the T cell repertoire of normal rats contains cells with the potential to cause diabetes: Characterization of the CD4+ T cell subset that inhibits autoimmune potential. J. Exp. Med. 177:627, 1993.
38. Shull, M., et al.: Targeted disruption of the mouse transforming growth factor-β1 gene results in multifocal inflammatory disease. Nature 359:693, 1992.
39. Barnett, L.A., and Fujinami, R.S.: Molecular mimicry: A mechanism for autoimmune injury. FASEB J. 6:840, 1992.
40. Shoenfeld, Y., and Schwartz, R.S.: Immunologic and genetic factors in autoimmune disease. N. Engl. J. Med. 311:1019, 1984.
41. Dalton, T.A., and Bennett, J.C.: Autoimmune diseases and the major histocompatibility complex: Therapeutic implications. Am. J. Med. 92:183, 1992.
42. Hammer, R.E., et al.: Spontaneous inflammatory disease in transgenic rats expressing HLA-B27 and human beta 2m: An animal model of HLA-B27–associated human disorders. Cell. 63(5):1099, 1990.
43. Nepom, G.T., and Erlich, H.: MHC class II molecules and autoimmunity. Annu. Rev. Immunol. 9:493, 1991.
44. Röcken, M., et al.: Infection breaks T-cell tolerance. Nature 359:79, 1992.
45. Heath, W.R., et al.: Autoimmune diabetes as a consequence of locally produced interleukin-2. Nature 359:547, 1992.
46. Michet, C.J., Jr., et al.: Epidemiology of systemic lupus erythematosus and other connective tissue diseases in Rochester, Minnesota, 1950 through 1979. Mayo Clin. Proc. 60:105, 1985.
47. Reichlin, M., and Harley, J.B.: Antinuclear antibodies: An overview. In Wallace, D.J., and Hahn, B.H. (eds.):

Dubois' Lupus Erythematosus, 4th ed. Philadelphia, Lea & Febiger, 1993, p. 188.

48. Tan, E.M.: Antinuclear antibodies: Diagnostic markers for autoimmune diseases and probes for cell biology. Adv. Immunol. 44:93, 1989.

49. Harley, J., and Scofield, R.H.: Systemic lupus erythematosus: RNA-protein autoantigens, models of disease heterogeneity, and theories of etiology. J. Clin. Immunol. 11:297, 1991.

50. Eisenberg, G.M.: Antiphospholipid syndrome: The reality and implications. Hosp. Pract. 27:119, 1992.

51. Deapen, D., et al.: A revised estimate of twin concordance in systemic lupus erythematosus. Arthritis Rheum. 35:311, 1992.

52. Arnett, F.C.: Genetic aspects of human lupus. Clin. Immunol. Immunopathol. 63:4, 1992.

53. Hess, E.V., and Mongey, A.B.: Drug-related lupus. Bull. Rheum. Dis. 40:1, 1991.

54. Tsokos, G.C.: Lymphocyte abnormalities in human lupus. Clin. Immunol. Immunopathol. 63:7, 1992.

55. Shivakumar, S., et al.: T cell receptor α/β expressing double negative (CD4−/CD8−) and CD4+ T helper cells in humans augment the production of pathogenic anti-DNA autoantibodies associated with lupus nephritis. J. Immunol. 143:103, 1989.

56. Steinberg, A.D.: Concepts of pathogenesis of systemic lupus erythematosus. Clin. Immunol. Immunopathol. 63:19, 1992.

57. Pollak, V.E., and Pirani, C.L.: Lupus nephritis. In Wallace, D.J., and Hahn, B.H. (eds.): Dubois' Lupus Erythematosus, 4th ed. Philadelphia, Lea & Febiger, 1993, p. 525.

58. Hanson, V., et al.: Systemic lupus erythematosus patients with central nervous system involvement show autoantibodies to a 50-kD neuronal membrane protein. J. Exp. Med. 176:565, 1992.

59. Godeau, P., et al.: The multiple clinical aspects of lupus. Clin. Exp. Rheumatol. 8(Suppl. 5):27, 1990.

60. Sontheimer, R.: Subacute cutaneous lupus erythematosus. Clin. Dermatol. 3:58, 1985.

61. Stevens, M.B.: Drug-induced lupus. Hosp. Pract. 27(3A):27, 1992.

62. Fox, R.I., and Kang, H.I.: Pathogenesis of Sjögren's syndrome. Rheum. Dis. Clin. North Am. 18:517, 1992.

63. Reveille, J.D., and Arnett, F.C.: The immunogenetics of Sjögren's syndrome. Rheum. Dis. Clin. North Am. 18:539, 1992.

64. Fox, R.I., et al.: Reactivation of Epstein-Barr virus in Sjögren's syndrome. Springer Semin. Immunopathol. 13:217, 1991.

65. Tzioufas, A.G., et al.: Sjögren's syndrome: An oligo-monoclonal B cell process. Clin. Exp. Rheumatol. 8(Suppl. 5):17, 1990.

66. Geppert, T.: Southwestern Internal Medicine Conference: Clinical features, pathogenic mechanisms, and new developments in the treatment of systemic sclerosis. Am. J. Med. Sci. 299:193, 1990.

67. Kahaleh, M.B.: The role of vascular endothelium in fibroblast activation and tissue fibrosis, particularly in scleroderma (systemic sclerosis) and pachydermoperiostosis (primary hypertrophic osteoarthropathy). Clin. Exp. Rheumatol. 10(Suppl. 7):51, 1992.

68. LeRoy, E.C.: A brief overview of the pathogenesis of scleroderma (systemic sclerosis). Ann. Rheum. Dis. 51:286, 1992.

69. Frieri, M.: Systemic sclerosis: The role of mast cells and cytokines. Ann. Allergy 69:385, 1992.

70. Sontheimer, R.D., et al.: Antinuclear antibodies: Clinical correlations and biologic significance. Adv. Dermatol. 7:3, 1991.

71. Rothfield, N.: Autoantibodies in scleroderma. Rheum. Dis. Clin. North Am. 18:483, 1992.

72. Silman, A.J.: Epidemiology of scleroderma. Ann. Rheum. Dis. 50:846, 1991.

73. Dalakas, M.C.: Polymyositis, dermatomyositis, and inclusion-body myositis. N. Engl. J. Med. 325:1487, 1991.

74. Sigurgeirsson, B., et al.: Risk of cancer in patients with dermatomyositis or polymyositis: A population-based study. N. Engl. J. Med. 326:363, 1992.

75. Targoff, I.N.: Autoantibodies in polymyositis. Rheum. Dis. Clin. North Am. 18:455, 1992.

76. Lundberg, I., and Hedfors, E.: Clinical course of patients with anti-RNP antibodies: A prospective study of 32 patients. J. Rheumatol. 18:1511, 1991.

77. Maddison, P.J.: Mixed connective tissue disease, overlap syndromes, and eosinophilic fasciitis. Ann. Rheum. Dis. 50:887, 1991.

78. Amman, A.J.: Mechanisms of immunodeficiency. In Stites, D.P., and Terr, A.T. (eds.): Basic and Clinical Immunology, 7th ed. East Norwalk, CT, Appleton & Lange, 1991, p. 320.

79. Vetrie, D., et al.: The gene involved in X-linked agammaglobulinemia is a member of the src family of protein-tyrosine kinases. Nature 361:226, 1993.

80. Sneller, M.C. (moderator): New insights into common variable immunodeficiency. Ann. Intern. Med. 118:720, 1993.

81. Kaneko, H., et al.: Expression of immunoglobulin genes in common variable immunodeficiency. J. Clin. Immunol. 11:262, 1991.

82. Sneller, M.C., and Strober, W.: Abnormalities of lymphokine gene expression in patients with common variable immunodeficiency. J. Immunol. 144:3762, 1990.

83. Matsumoto, S., et al.: Progress in primary immunodeficiency. Immunol. Today 13:4, 1992.

84. Buckley, R.H.: Immunodeficiency diseases. J.A.M.A. 258:2841, 1987.

85. Hanson, L.A., et al.: The heterogeneity of IgA deficiency. J. Clin. Immunol. 8:159, 1988.

86. Arnaiz-Villera, A., et al.: Human T cell activation deficiencies. Immunol. Today 13:260, 1992.

87. Noguchi, M., et al.: Interleukin-2 receptor γ chain mutation results in X-linked severe combined immunodeficiency in humans. Cell 73:147, 1993.

88. Russell, S.M., et al.: Interleukin-2 receptor γ chain: A functional component of the interleukin-4 receptor. Science 262:1880, 1993.

89. Huber, J., et al.: Pathology of congenital immunodeficiencies. Semin. Diagn. Pathol. 9:31, 1992.

90. Morgan, B.P., and Walport, M.J.: Complement deficiency and disease. Immunol. Today 12:301, 1991.

91. Boring, C.C., et al.: Cancer statistics. CA Cancer J Clin 44:7, 1994.

92. European Study Group on Heterosexual Transmission of HIV: Comparison of female-to-male and male-to-female transmission of HIV in 563 stable couples. Br. Med. J. 304:809, 1992.

93. Kwan, D.J., and Lowe, F.C.: Acquired immunodeficiency syndrome: A venereal disease. Urol. Clin. North Am. 19:13, 1992.

94. Alter, H.J., et al.: Prevalence of human immunodeficiency virus type 1 p24 antigen in U.S. blood donors— an assessment of the efficacy of testing in donor screening. N. Engl. J. Med. 323:1312, 1990.

95. European Collaborative Study: Risk factors for mother-to-child transmission of HIV-1. Lancet 339:1007, 1992.

96. Jefferies, D.J.: Doctors, patients, and HIV. Br. Med. J. 304:1258, 1992.

97. Geberding, J.L., et al.: Risk of transmitting the human immunodeficiency virus to health care workers exposed to patients with AIDS and AIDS-related conditions. J. Infect. Dis. 156:1, 1987.

98. Green, W.C.: The molecular biology of human immunodeficiency virus type I infection. N. Engl. J. Med. 324:308, 1991.

99. Karn, J.: Control of human immunodeficiency virus replication by the tat, rev, nef, and protease genes. Curr. Opin. Immunol. 3:526, 1991.

100. Bukrinsky, M.I., et al.: Quiescent T lymphocytes as an inducible virus reservoir in HIV-1 infection. Science 254:423, 1991.

101. Bagasra, O., et al.: Detection of human immunodeficiency virus type I provirus in mononuclear cells by in situ polymerase chain reaction. N. Engl. J. Med. 326:1385, 1992.

102. Pantaleo, G., et al.: The immunopathogenesis of human immunodeficiency virus infection. N. Engl. J. Med. 328:327, 1993.

103. Pantaleo, G., et al.: HIV infection is active and progressive in lymphoid tissue during the clinically latent stage of disease. Nature 362:355, 1993.

104. Embretson, J., et al.: Massive covert infection of helper T lymphocytes and macrophages by HIV during the incubation period of AIDS. Nature 362:359, 1993.

105. Greenberg, P.: Immunopathogenesis of HIV infection. Hosp. Pract. 27(2):109, 1992.

106. Poli, G., and Fauci, A.S.: The effect of cytokines and pharmacologic agents on chronic HIV infection. AIDS Res. Hum. Retroviruses 8:191, 1992.

107. Berger, J.R., and Levy, J.A.: The human immunodeficiency virus type I: The virus and its role in neurologic disease. Semin. Neurol. 12:1, 1992.

108. Pulliam, L., et al.: Human immunodeficiency virus–infected macrophages produce soluble factors that cause histological and neurochemical alterations in cultured human brains. J. Clin. Invest. 87:503, 1991.

109. Hwang, S.S., et al.: Identification of the envelope V3 loop as the primary determinant of cell tropism in HIV-1. Science 253:71, 1991.

110. Buehler, J.W., and Ward, J.W.: A new definition for AIDS surveillance. Ann. Intern. Med. 118:390, 1993.

111. Tindall, B., and Cooper, D.A.: Primary HIV infection: Host responses and intervention strategies. AIDS 5:1, 1991.

112. Phillips, A.N., et al.: Serial CD4+ lymphocyte counts and development of AIDS. Lancet 337:389, 1991.

113. Graham, N.M.H., et al.: The effects on survival of early treatment of human immunodeficiency virus infection. N. Engl. J. Med. 326:1037, 1992.

114. Centers for Disease Control and Prevention 1993 revised classification system and expanded surveillance definition for AIDS among adolescents and adults. MMWR 41(RR-17):1, 1992.

115. Kessler, H.A., et al.: AIDS: Part II. Dis. Mon. 38:695, 1992.

116. Daley, C.L., et al.: An outbreak of tuberculosis with accelerated progression among persons infected with the human immunodeficiency virus: An analysis using restriction fragment length polymorphisms. N. Engl. J. Med. 326:231, 1992.

117. Safai, B., et al.: Malignant neoplasms associated with human immunodeficiency virus infection. CA Cancer J. Clin. 42:74, 1992.

118. Roth, W.K., et al.: Cellular and molecular features of HIV-associated Kaposi's sarcoma. AIDS 6:895, 1992.

119. Beral, V., et al.: AIDS-associated non-Hodgkin's lymphoma. Lancet 337:805, 1991.

120. Yarchoan, R., et al.: CD4 count and the risk of death in patients infected with HIV receiving antiretroviral therapy. Ann. Intern. Med. 115:184, 1991.

121. Knowles, D.M., and Chadburn, A.: Lymphadenopathy and the lymphoid neoplasms associated with the acquired immune deficiency syndrome. In Knowles, D.M. (ed.): Neoplastic Hematopathology. Baltimore, Williams & Wilkins, 1992, p. 773.

122. Sipe, J.D.: Amyloidosis. Annu. Rev. Biochem. 61:947, 1992.

123. Benson, M.D.: Inherited amyloidosis. J. Med. Genet. 28:73, 1991.

124. Jacobson, D.R., and Buxbaum, J.N.: Genetic aspects of amyloidosis. Adv. Hum. Genet. 20:69, 1991.

125. Kyle, R.A., and Gertz, M.A.: Systemic amyloidosis. Crit. Rev. Oncol. Hematol. 10:49, 1990.

126. Hawkins, P.N., et al.: Evaluation of systemic amyloidosis by scintigraphy with ^{123}I-labeled serum amyloid P component. N. Engl. J. Med. 323:508, 1990.

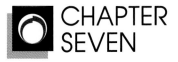

CHAPTER SEVEN

Neoplasia

In the United States each year, well over 1 million individuals learn for the first time that they have some type of cancer. Fortunately, many of these tumors can be cured. Nonetheless, according to American Cancer Society estimates, cancer caused approximately 538,000 deaths in 1994, accounting for about 23% of all deaths.[1] Only cardiovascular diseases cause more deaths. The discussion that follows deals with both benign tumors and cancers; understandably the latter receive more attention. The focus is on the basic morphologic and behavioral characteristics and our present understanding of the molecular basis of carcinogenesis. We also discuss the interactions of the tumor with the host and the host response to tumor. Although the discussion of therapy is beyond our scope, with many forms of malignancy, notably the leukemias and lymphomas, there are now dramatic improvements in 5-year survival rates. A greater proportion of cancers are being cured or arrested today than ever before.

DEFINITIONS

Neoplasia literally means "new growth," and the new growth is a "neoplasm." The term "tumor" was originally applied to the swelling caused by inflammation. Neoplasms also may induce swellings, but by long precedent, the non-neoplastic usage of "tumor" has passed into limbo; thus, the term is now equated with neoplasm. Oncology (Greek "oncos" = tumor) is the study of tumors or neoplasms. *Cancer is the common term for all malignant tumors.* Although the ancient origins of this term are somewhat uncertain, it probably derives from the Latin for crab, "cancer" — presumably because a cancer "adheres to any part that it seizes upon in an obstinate manner like the crab."

Although all physicians know what they mean when they use the term "neoplasm," it has been surprisingly difficult to develop an accurate definition. The eminent British oncologist Sir Rupert Willis has come closest: "A neoplasm is an abnormal mass of tissue, the growth of which exceeds and is uncoordinated with that of the normal tissues and persists in the same excessive manner after cessation of the stimuli which evoked the change."[2] To this characterization we might add that the abnormal mass is purposeless, preys on the host, and is virtually autonomous. It preys on the host insofar as the growth of the neoplastic tissue competes with normal cells and tissues for energy supplies and nutritional substrate. Inasmuch as these masses may flourish in a patient who is wasting away, they are to a degree autonomous. Later it becomes evident that such autonomy is not complete. All neoplasms ultimately depend on the host for their nutrition and vascular supply; many forms of neoplasia require endocrine support.

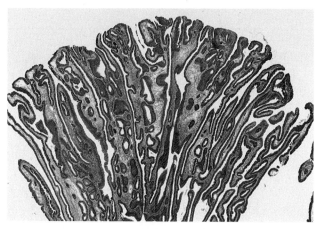

Figure 7–1. Papilloma of the colon with finger-like projections into the lumen. (Courtesy of Dr. Trace Worrell, Department of Pathology, University of Texas Southwestern Medical School, Dallas.)

NOMENCLATURE

All tumors, benign and malignant, have two basic components: (1) proliferating neoplastic cells that constitute their *parenchyma* and (2) *supportive stroma* made up of connective tissue and blood vessels. Although parenchymal cells represent the proliferating "cutting edge" of neoplasms and so determine their nature, the growth and evolution of neoplasms are critically dependent on their stroma. An adequate stromal blood supply is requisite, and the stromal connective tissue provides the framework for the parenchyma. In some tumors, the stromal support is scant, and so the neoplasm is soft and fleshy. Sometimes the parenchymal cells stimulate the formation of an abundant collagenous stroma—referred to as *desmoplasia.* Some tumors, for example some cancers of the female breast, are stony hard or scirrhous. The nomenclature of tumors is, however, based on the parenchymal component.

BENIGN TUMORS. In general, these are designated by attaching the suffix "-oma" to the cell of origin. Tumors of mesenchymal cells generally follow this rule. For example, a benign tumor arising from fibroblastic cells is called a *fibroma.* A cartilaginous tumor is a *chondroma,* and a tumor of osteoblasts is an *osteoma.* In contrast, nomenclature of benign epithelial tumors is more complex. They are variously classified, some based on their cells of origin, others on microscopic architecture, and still others on their macroscopic patterns.

Adenoma is the term applied to the benign epithelial neoplasm that forms glandular patterns as well as to the tumors derived from glands but not necessarily reproducing glandular patterns. On this basis, a benign epithelial neoplasm that arises from renal tubular cells growing in the form of numerous tightly clustered small glands would be termed an adenoma, as would a heterogeneous

mass of adrenal cortical cells growing in no distinctive pattern. Benign epithelial neoplasms producing microscopically or macroscopically visible finger-like or warty projections from epithelial surfaces are referred to as *papillomas* (Fig. 7–1). Those that form large cystic masses, as in the ovary, are referred to as *cystadenomas.* Some tumors produce papillary patterns that protrude into cystic spaces and are called *papillary cystadenomas.* When a neoplasm, benign or malignant, produces a macroscopically visible projection above a *mucosal* surface and projects, for example, into the gastric or colonic lumen, it is termed a *polyp.* The term polyp preferably is restricted to benign tumors. Malignant polyps are better designated polypoid cancers.

MALIGNANT TUMORS. The nomenclature of malignant tumors essentially follows the same schema used for benign neoplasms, with certain additions. *Malignant tumors arising in mesenchymal tissue are usually called sarcomas* (Greek "sar" = fleshy) because they have little connective tissue stroma and so are fleshy, e.g., fibrosarcoma, liposarcoma, and leiomyosarcoma for smooth muscle cancer and rhabdomyosarcoma for a cancer that differentiates toward striated muscle. *Malignant neoplasms of epithelial cell origin, derived from any of the three germ layers, are called carcinomas.* Thus cancer arising in the epidermis of ectodermal origin is a carcinoma, as is a cancer arising in the mesodermally derived cells of the renal tubules and the endodermally derived cells of the lining of the gastrointestinal tract. Carcinomas may be further qualified. One with a glandular growth pattern microscopically is termed an *adenocarcinoma,* and one producing recognizable squamous cells arising in any epithelium of the body would be termed a

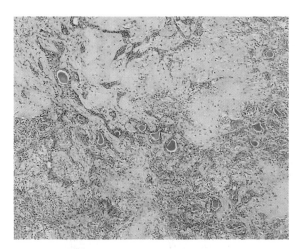

Figure 7-2. Mixed tumor of the parotid gland contains epithelial cells forming ducts and myxoid stroma that resembles cartilage. (Courtesy of Dr. Trace Worrell, Department of Pathology, University of Texas Southwestern Medical School, Dallas.)

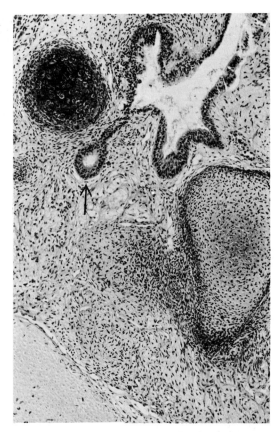

Figure 7-3. Teratoma. Three distinct types of adult tissues are seen: a circular island of darkly stained cartilage (mesodermal) in the upper left, a large nest of stratified squamous epithelial cells (ectodermal) on the right, and in the center a gland space lined by columnar cells resembling intestinal tract mucosa (endodermal) (arrow).

squamous cell carcinoma. It is further common practice to specify, when possible, the organ of origin, e.g., a renal cell adenocarcinoma or bronchogenic squamous cell carcinoma. Not infrequently, however, a cancer is composed of undifferentiated cells and must be designated merely as a poorly differentiated or undifferentiated malignant tumor.

In most neoplasms, benign and malignant, the parenchymal cells bear a close resemblance to each other, as though all were derived from a single cell, as indeed we know to be the case with most cancers. Infrequently divergent differentiation of a single line of parenchymal cells creates what are called *mixed tumors.* The best example is the *mixed tumor of salivary gland origin.* These tumors contain epithelial components scattered within a myxoid stroma that sometimes contains islands of apparent cartilage or even bone (Fig. 7–2). All these elements, it is believed, arise from epithelial and myoepithelial cells of salivary gland origin; thus the preferred designation of these neoplasms is *pleomorphic adenoma.* This schizophrenic morphology presumably reflects variable expression of several programs of differentiation that are repressed in the genome of all cells. The great majority of neoplasms, even mixed tumors, are composed of cells representative of a single germ layer. The *teratoma,* in contrast, is made up of a variety of parenchymal cell types representative of more than one germ layer, usually all three. They arise from totipotential cells and so are principally encountered in the gonads but rarely in sequestered primitive cell rests elsewhere. These totipotential cells differentiate along various germ lines, producing, for example, tissues that can be identified as skin, muscle, fat, gut epithelium, tooth structures, and, indeed, any tissue of the body (Fig. 7–3). A particularly common pattern is seen in the ovarian *cystic teratoma* (dermoid cyst), which differentiates principally along ectodermal lines to create a cystic tumor lined by skin replete with hair, sebaceous glands, and tooth structures.

The nomenclature of the more common forms of neoplasia is presented in Table 7–1. It is evident from this compilation that there are some inappropriate but deeply entrenched usages. For generations, carcinomas of melanocytes have been called "melanomas," although correctly they should be referred to as melanocarcinomas. Analogously carcinomas of testicular origin are stubbornly called "seminomas." Other instances will be encountered in which innocent designations belie ugly behavior. Irrational as such usage may be, it is probably more irrational to expect humans to be rational. The converse is also true when ominous terms are applied to usually trivial lesions. An ectopic rest of normal tissue is sometimes called a *choristoma*—as, for example, a rest of adrenal cells

Table 7-1. NOMENCLATURE OF TUMORS

TISSUE OF ORIGIN	BENIGN	MALIGNANT
I. Composed of One Parenchymal Cell Type		
A. Mesenchymal tumors		
1. Connective tissue and derivatives	Fibroma	Fibrosarcoma
	Lipoma	Liposarcoma
	Chondroma	Chondrosarcoma
	Osteoma	Osteogenic sarcoma
2. Endothelial and related tissues		
Blood vessels	Hemangioma	Angiosarcoma
Lymph vessels	Lymphangioma	Lymphangiosarcoma
Synovium		Synovial sarcoma
Mesothelium		Mesothelioma
Brain coverings	Meningioma	Invasive meningioma
3. Blood cells and related cells		
Hematopoietic cells		Leukemias
Lymphoid tissue		Malignant lymphomas
4. Muscle		
Smooth	Leiomyoma	Leiomyosarcoma
Striated	Rhabdomyoma	Rhabdomyosarcoma
B. Epithelial tumors		
1. Stratified squamous	Squamous cell papilloma	Squamous cell or epidermoid carcinoma
2. Basal cells of skin or adnexa		Basal cell carcinoma
3. Epithelial lining		
Glands or ducts	Adenoma	Adenocarcinoma
	Papilloma	Papillary carcinoma
	Cystadenoma	Cystadenocarcinoma
4. Respiratory passages		Bronchogenic carcinoma
		Bronchial "adenoma" (carcinoid)
5. Neuroectoderm	Nevus	Malignant melanoma
6. Renal epithelium	Renal tubular adenoma	Renal cell carcinoma
7. Liver cells	Liver cell adenoma	Hepatocellular carcinoma
8. Urinary tract epithelium (transitional)	Transitional cell papilloma	Transitional cell carcinoma
9. Placental epithelium (trophoblast)	Hydatidiform mole	Choriocarcinoma
10. Testicular epithelium (germ cells)		Seminoma
		Embryonal carcinoma
II. More Than One Neoplastic Cell Type— Mixed Tumors		
1. Salivary glands	Pleomorphic adenoma (mixed tumor of salivary origin)	Malignant mixed tumor of salivary gland origin
2. Breast	Fibroadenoma	Malignant cystosarcoma phyllodes
3. Renal anlage		Wilms' tumor
III. More Than One Neoplastic Cell Type Derived From More Than One Germ Layer —Teratogenous		
1. Totipotential cells in gonads or in embryonic rests	Mature teratoma, dermoid cyst	Immature teratoma, teratocarcinoma

under the kidney capsule. Occasionally a pancreatic nodular rest in the mucosa of the small intestine may mimic a neoplasm, providing some partial justification for the use of a term that implies a tumor. Analogously, aberrant differentiation may produce a mass of disorganized but mature specialized cells or tissue indigenous to the particular site, referred to as a *hamartoma*. Thus a hamartoma in the lung may contain islands of cartilage, blood vessels, bronchial-type structures, and lymphoid tissue. Sometimes the lesion is purely cartilaginous or purely angiomatous. Although these might be construed as benign neoplasms, the complete resemblance of the tissue to normal cartilage or blood vessels and the occasional admixture of other elements favor a hamartomatous origin. In any event, the hamartoma is totally benign.

The nomenclature of tumors is important because specific designations have specific clinical implications. The historically sanctified term "seminoma" connotes a form of carcinoma that tends to spread to lymph nodes along the iliac arteries and aorta. Further, these tumors are extremely radiosensitive and can be eradicated by radiotherapy; thus, very few patients with seminomas die of the neoplasm. By contrast, the embryonal carcinoma of the testis is not radiosensitive and tends to invade locally beyond the confines of the testis and spread

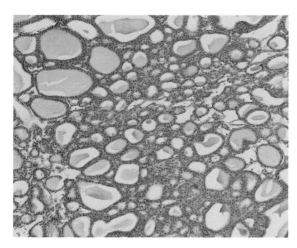

Figure 7-4. Benign tumor (adenoma) of thyroid. Note the normal-looking (well-differentiated) colloid-filled thyroid follicles. (Courtesy of Dr. Trace Worrell, Department of Pathology, University of Texas Southwestern Medical School, Dallas.)

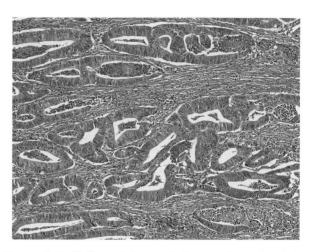

Figure 7-5. Malignant tumor (adenocarcinoma) of the colon. Note that as compared to the well-formed and normal-looking glands characteristic of a benign tumor (see Fig. 7-4), the cancerous glands are irregular in shape and size and do not resemble the normal colonic glands. This tumor is considered differentiated because gland formation can be seen. The malignant glands have invaded the muscular layer of the colon. (Courtesy of Dr. Trace Worrell, Department of Pathology, University of Texas Southwestern Medical School, Dallas.)

throughout the body. There also are other varieties of testicular neoplasms, and so the designation "cancer of the testis" tells little of its clinical significance.

CHARACTERISTICS OF BENIGN AND MALIGNANT NEOPLASMS

In the great majority of instances, the differentiation of a benign from a malignant tumor can be made morphologically with considerable certainty; sometimes, however, a neoplasm defies categorization. It has been said, "All tumors need not of necessity be either benign or malignant." Certain anatomic features may suggest innocence, whereas others point toward cancerous potential. Ultimately all morphologic diagnosis is subjective and constitutes prediction of the future course of a neoplasm. Occasionally this prediction is confounded by a marked discrepancy between the morphologic appearance of a tumor and its biologic behavior: An innocent face may mask an ugly nature. Such deception or ambiguity, however, is not the rule; in general, there are criteria by which benign and malignant tumors can be differentiated, and they behave accordingly. These differences can conveniently be discussed under the following headings: (1) differentiation and anaplasia, (2) rate of growth, (3) local invasion, and (4) metastasis.

DIFFERENTIATION AND ANAPLASIA

The terms *differentiation* and *anaplasia* apply to the parenchymal cells of neoplasms. *Differentiation* refers to the extent to which parenchymal cells resemble comparable normal cells, both morphologically and functionally. Well-differentiated tumors are thus composed of cells resembling the mature normal cells of the tissue of origin of the neoplasm. Poorly differentiated or undifferentiated tumors have primitive-appearing, unspecialized cells. *In general, benign tumors are well differentiated* (Fig. 7-4). The neoplastic cell in a benign smooth muscle tumor—a leiomyoma—so closely resembles the normal cell as to make it impossible to recognize it as a tumor cell on high-power examination. Only the massing of these cells into a nodule discloses the tumorous nature of the lesion. One may get so close to the tree that one loses sight of the forest.

Malignant neoplasms, in contrast, range from well differentiated to undifferentiated. Malignant neoplasms composed of undifferentiated cells are said to be anaplastic. Indeed, lack of differentiation, or anaplasia, is considered a hallmark of malignant transformation. Literally anaplasia means "to form backward," implying a reversion from a high level of differentiation to a lower level. There is substantial evidence, however, that cancers arise from stem cells present in all specialized tissues. The well-differentiated cancer (Fig. 7-5) evolves from maturation or specialization of undifferentiated cells as they proliferate, whereas the undifferentiated malignant tumor derives from proliferation without maturation of the transformed cells. Lack of differentiation then is not the consequence of dedifferentiation.

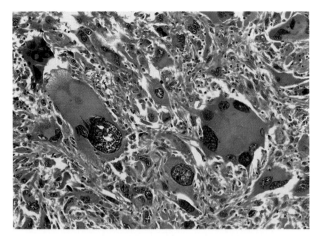

Figure 7–6. Anaplastic tumor of the skeletal muscle (rhabdomyosarcoma). Note the marked cellular and nuclear pleomorphism, hyperchromatic nuclei, and tumor giant cells. (Courtesy of Dr. Trace Worrell, Department of Pathology, University of Texas Southwestern Medical School, Dallas.)

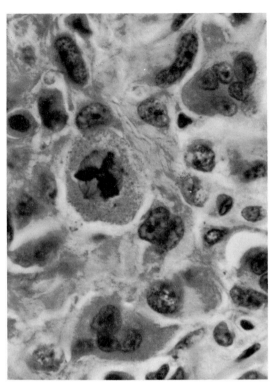

Figure 7–7. High-power detail of anaplastic tumor cells showing cellular and nuclear variation in size and shape. The prominent cell in the center of the field has an abnormal tripolar spindle.

Lack of differentiation, or *anaplasia,* is marked by a number of morphologic and functional changes. Both the cells and the nuclei characteristically display *pleomorphism*—variation in size and shape (Fig. 7–6). Cells may be found that are many times larger than their neighbors, and other cells may be extremely small and primitive appearing. Characteristically the nuclei contain an abundance of DNA and are extremely dark staining *(hyperchromatic).* The nuclei are disproportionately large for the cell, and the nuclear-cytoplasmic ratio may approach 1:1 instead of the normal 1:4 or 1:6. The nuclear shape is usually extremely variable, and the chromatin is often coarsely clumped and distributed along the nuclear membrane. Large nucleoli are usually present in these nuclei.

As compared with benign tumors and some well-differentiated malignant neoplasms, undifferentiated tumors usually possess large numbers of mitoses, reflecting the higher proliferative activity of the parenchymal cells. It should be noted, however, that *the presence of mitoses does not necessarily indicate that a tumor is malignant or that the tissue is neoplastic.* Many normal tissues exhibiting rapid turnover, such as bone marrow, have numerous mitoses, and non-neoplastic proliferations such as hyperplasias contain many cells in mitosis. More important as a morphologic feature of malignant neoplasia are atypical, bizarre mitotic figures sometimes producing tripolar, quadripolar, or multipolar spindles (Fig. 7–7).

Another feature of anaplasia is the formation of *tumor giant cells,* some possessing only a single huge polymorphic nucleus, whereas others have two or more nuclei. These giant cells are not to be confused with inflammatory Langhans or foreign body giant cells, which possess many small, normal-appearing nuclei. In the cancer giant cell, the nucleus is hyperchromatic and is very large in relation to the cell. In addition to the cytologic abnormalities described here, the *orientation of anaplastic cells is markedly disturbed.* Sheets or large masses of tumor cells grow in an anarchic, disorganized fashion. Although these growing cells obviously require a blood supply, often the connective tissue–vascular stroma is scant, and indeed in many anaplastic tumors, large central areas undergo ischemic necrosis. As mentioned at the outset, malignant tumors differ widely in the extent to which their morphologic appearance deviates from the norm. On one end of the spectrum are the extremely undifferentiated, anaplastic tumors, and at the other end are cancers that bear striking resemblance to their tissues of origin. Certain well-differentiated adenocarcinomas of the thyroid, for example, may form normal-appearing follicles, and some squamous cell carcinomas contain cells that do not differ cytologically from normal squamous epithelial cells (Fig. 7–8). Thus the morphologic diagnosis of malignancy in well-differentiated tumors may sometimes be quite difficult. In between the two extremes lie tumors that are loosely referred to as "moderately well differentiated."

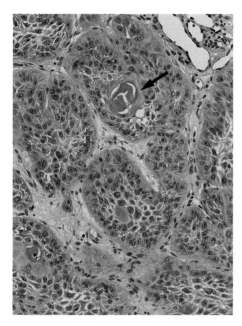

Figure 7–8. Well-differentiated squamous cell carcinoma of the skin. The tumor cells are strikingly similar to normal squamous epithelial cells, with intercellular bridges and nests of keratin pearls (arrow). (Courtesy of Dr. Trace Worrell, Department of Pathology, University of Texas Southwestern Medical School, Dallas.)

changes that do not involve the entire thickness of epithelium may be reversible, and with removal of the putative inciting causes, the epithelium may revert to normal.

Turning to the functional differentiation of neoplastic cells, as you might presume, the better the differentiation of the cell, the more completely it retains the functional capabilities found in its normal counterparts. Thus, benign neoplasms and well-differentiated carcinomas of endocrine glands frequently elaborate the hormones characteristic of their origin. Well-differentiated squamous cell carcinomas of the epidermis elaborate keratin, just as well-differentiated hepatocellular carcinomas elaborate bile. There are few differences in the enzyme profiles of well-differentiated tumor cells from those of their normal counterparts. As one descends the scale of differentiation, enzymes and specialized pathways of metabolism are lost and the cells undergo functional simplification. Highly anaplastic undifferentiated cells then, whatever their tissue of origin, come to resemble each other more than the normal cells from which they have arisen. In some instances, however, unanticipated functions emerge. Some tumors may elaborate fe-

Before we leave the subject of differentiation and anaplasia, we should discuss *dysplasia*, a term used to describe disorderly but non-neoplastic proliferation. Dysplasia is encountered principally in the epithelia. *It is a loss in the uniformity of the individual cells as well as a loss in their architectural orientation.* Dysplastic cells exhibit considerable pleomorphism (variation in size and shape) and often possess deeply stained (hyperchromatic) nuclei, which are abnormally large for the size of the cell. Mitotic figures are more abundant than usual, although almost invariably they conform to normal patterns. Frequently the mitoses appear in abnormal locations within the epithelium. Thus, in dysplastic stratified squamous epithelium, mitoses are not confined to the basal layers and may appear at all levels and even in surface cells. There is considerable architectural anarchy. For example, the usual progressive maturation of tall cells in the basal layer to flattened squames on the surface may be lost and replaced by a disordered scrambling of dark basal-appearing cells. When dysplastic changes are marked and involve the entire thickness of the epithelium, the lesion is considered a preinvasive neoplasm and is referred to as *carcinoma in situ* (Fig. 7–9). Although dysplastic changes are often found adjacent to foci of invasive carcinoma and, in long-term studies of cigarette smokers, epithelial dysplasia almost invariably antedates the appearance of cancer, *dysplasia does not necessarily progress to cancer*. Mild to moderate

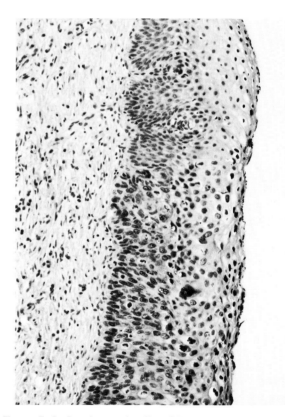

Figure 7–9. Carcinoma in situ of the uterine cervix. In the lower part the entire thickness of the epithelium is replaced by atypical, dysplastic cells, with loss of orderly differentiation. The basement membrane is intact, and there are no tumor cells in the subepithelial stroma. Compare with normal mucosa above.

tal proteins (antigens) not produced by the comparable cells in the adult. Analogously carcinomas of nonendocrine origin may assume hormone synthesis to produce so-called ectopic hormones. For example, bronchogenic carcinomas may produce adrenocorticotropic hormone, parathyroid-like hormone, insulin, and glucagon as well as others. More is said about these phenomena later. *Despite exceptions, the more rapidly growing and the more anaplastic a tumor, the less likely there will be specialized functional activity.*

The cells in benign tumors are almost always well differentiated and resemble their normal cells of origin; the cells in cancer are more or less differentiated, but some loss of differentiation is always present.

RATE OF GROWTH

The generalization can be made that *most benign tumors grow slowly over a period of years, whereas most cancers grow rapidly, sometimes at an erratic pace,* and eventually spread and kill their hosts. Such an oversimplification, however, must be extensively qualified. Some benign tumors have a higher growth rate than malignant tumors. Moreover, the rate of growth of benign as well as malignant neoplasms may not be constant over time. Factors such as hormone dependence, adequacy of blood supply, and likely unknown influences may affect their growth. For example, leiomyomas (benign smooth muscle tumors) of the uterus are common. Not infrequently, repeated clinical examination of women bearing such neoplasms over the span of decades discloses no significant increase in size. After the menopause, the neoplasms may atrophy and later be found to be replaced largely by collagenous, sometimes calcified, tissue. Leiomyomas frequently enter a growth spurt during pregnancy. These neoplasms to some extent depend on the circulating levels of steroid hormones, particularly estrogens.

In general, *the growth rate of tumors correlates with their level of differentiation, and thus most malignant tumors grow more rapidly than do benign lesions.* There is, however, a wide range of behavior. Some malignant tumors grow slowly for years and then suddenly increase in size virtually under observation, explosively disseminating to cause death within a few months of discovery. It is believed that such behavior results from the emergence of an aggressive subclone of transformed cells. At the other extreme are those that grow more slowly than benign tumors and may even enter periods of dormancy lasting for years. On occasion, cancers have been observed to decrease in size and even spontaneously disappear, but the handful of "miracles" fills only a small volume. To examine this variable behavior more closely, we consider what is known about the life history of cancer, including the cell kinetics of cancer growth and the influences that modify the growth of malignant tumors, in a later section.

LOCAL INVASION

Nearly all benign tumors grow as cohesive expansile masses that remain localized to their site of origin and do not have the capacity to infiltrate, invade, or metastasize to distant sites, as do malignant tumors. Because they grow and expand slowly, they usually develop a rim of compressed connective tissue, sometimes called a fibrous *capsule*, that separates them from the host tissue. This capsule is derived largely from the stroma of the native tissue as the parenchymal cells atrophy under the pressure of expanding tumor. Such encapsulation tends to contain the benign neoplasm as a discrete, readily palpable, and easily movable mass that can be surgically enucleated (Figs. 7–10 and 7–11). Although a well-defined cleavage plane exists around most benign tumors, in some it is lacking. Thus hemangiomas (neoplasms composed of tangled blood vessels) are often "unencapsulated" and may appear to permeate the site in which they arise (commonly the dermis of the skin).

The growth of cancers is accompanied by progressive infiltration, invasion, and destruction of the surrounding tissue. In general, they are poorly demarcated from the surrounding normal tissue, and a well-defined cleavage plane is lacking (Figs. 7–12 and 7–13). Slowly expanding malignant tumors, however, may develop an apparently enclosing fibrous capsule and may push along a broad front into adjacent normal structures (Fig. 7–14). Histologic examination of such apparently encapsulated masses almost always discloses tiny crab-like feet penetrating the margin and infiltrating the adjacent structures.

Most malignant tumors are obviously invasive and can be expected to penetrate the wall of the colon or uterus, for example, or fungate through the surface of the skin. They recognize no normal anatomic boundaries. Such invasiveness makes their surgical resection difficult, and even if the tumor appears well circumscribed, it is necessary to remove a considerable margin of apparently normal tissues about the infiltrative neoplasm; this is referred to as "radical surgery." *Next to the development of metastases, invasiveness is the most reliable feature that differentiates malignant from benign tumors.* We noted earlier that some cancers seem to evolve from a preinvasive stage referred to as *carcinoma in situ.* This is best illustrated by carcinoma of the uterine cervix (see Chapter 23). *In situ cancers display the cytologic features of malignancy without invasion of the basement membrane.* They may be considered one step removed from

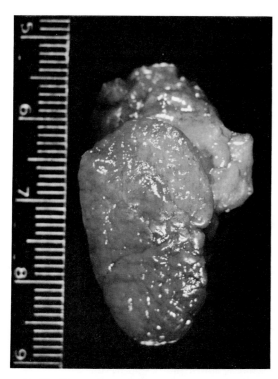

Figure 7-10. Gross view of fibroadenoma of breast. The discrete tumor bulges above the level of the surrounding breast substance as it extrudes from its tight encapsulation.

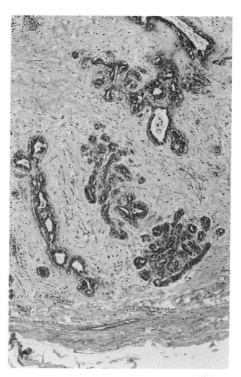

Figure 7-11. Microscopic view of fibroadenoma of breast seen in Figure 7-10. The fibrous capsule *(below)* sharply delimits the tumor from the surrounding tissue. (Courtesy of Dr. Trace Worrell, Department of Pathology, University of Texas Southwestern Medical School, Dallas.)

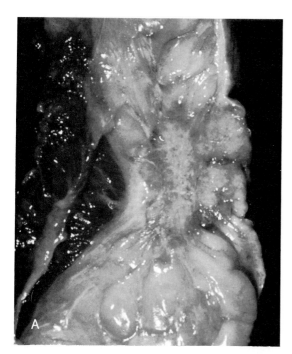

Figure 7-12. Close-up view of the cut surface of a cancer of the female breast. The tumor has infiltrated and eroded through the skin *(right)*, and its crab-like extensions pull on the adjacent fat and dark pectoral muscles.

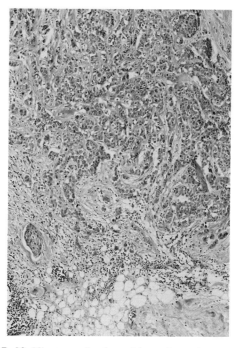

Figure 7-13. Microscopic view of breast carcinoma seen in Figure 7-12 illustrates the invasion of breast stroma and fat by nests and cords of tumor cells (compare with Fig. 7-11). The absence of a well-defined capsule should be noted. (Courtesy of Dr. Trace Worrell, Department of Pathology, University of Texas Southwestern Medical School, Dallas.)

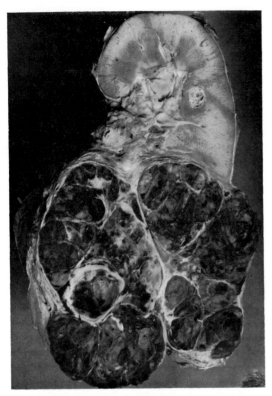

Figure 7-14. Renal cell carcinoma. The malignancy deceptively appears to be well encapsulated.

invasive cancer, and indeed with time most penetrate the basement membrane and invade the subepithelial stroma.

METASTASIS

Metastases are tumor implants discontinuous with the primary tumor. *Metastasis unequivocally marks a tumor as malignant because benign neoplasms do not metastasize.* The invasiveness of cancers permits them to penetrate into blood vessels, lymphatics, and body cavities, providing the opportunity for spread. *With few exceptions, all cancers can metastasize.* The major exceptions are most malignant neoplasms of the glial cells in the central nervous system, called gliomas, and basal cell carcinomas of the skin. Both are highly invasive forms of neoplasia (the latter being known in the older literature as rodent ulcers because of their invasive destructiveness), but they rarely metastasize. It is evident then that the properties of invasion and metastasis are separable.

In general, the more aggressive, the more rapidly growing, and the larger the primary neoplasm, the greater the likelihood that it will metastasize or already has metastasized. However, there are innumerable exceptions. Small, well-differentiated, slowly growing lesions sometimes metastasize widely, and conversely, some rapidly growing

lesions remain localized for years. No judgment can be made then about the probability of metastasis from pathologic examination of the primary tumor. Many factors relating to both invader and host are involved, as is pointed out later.

Approximately 30% of newly diagnosed patients with solid tumors (excluding skin cancers other than melanomas) present with metastases. Metastatic spread strongly reduces the possibility of cure; hence short of prevention of cancer, no achievement would confer greater benefit on patients than methods to prevent distant spread.

Pathways of Spread

Dissemination of cancers may occur through one of three pathways: (1) direct seeding of body cavities or surfaces, (2) lymphatic spread, and (3) hematogenous spread. Although direct transplantation of tumor cells, as for example on surgical instruments, may theoretically occur, it is rare and, in any event, an artificial mode of dissemination that is not discussed further. Each of the three major pathways is described separately.

SEEDING OF BODY CAVITIES AND SURFACES. This may occur whenever a malignant neoplasm penetrates into a natural "open field." Most often involved is the peritoneal cavity, but any other cavity—pleural, pericardial, subarachnoid, and joint spaces—may be affected. Such seeding is particularly characteristic of carcinomas arising in the ovaries, when, not infrequently, all peritoneal surfaces become coated with a heavy layer of cancerous glaze. Remarkably the tumor cells may remain confined to the surface of the coated abdominal viscera without penetrating into the substance. Sometimes mucus-secreting ovarian and appendiceal carcinomas fill the peritoneal cavity with a gelatinous neoplastic mass referred to as *pseudomyxoma peritonei*.

LYMPHATIC SPREAD. Transport through lymphatics is the most common pathway for the initial dissemination of carcinomas (Fig. 7–15), but it should be remembered that sarcomas may also use this route. The emphasis on lymphatic spread for carcinomas and hematogenous spread for sarcomas is misleading because ultimately there are numerous interconnections between the vascular and lymphatic systems. *The pattern of lymph node involvement follows the natural routes of drainage.* Because carcinomas of the breast usually arise in the upper outer quadrants, they generally disseminate first to the axillary lymph nodes. Cancers of the inner quadrant may drain through lymphatics to the nodes within the chest along the internal mammary arteries. Thereafter the infraclavicular and supraclavicular nodes may become involved. Carcinomas of the lung arising in the major respiratory passages metastasize first to the perihilar tracheobron-

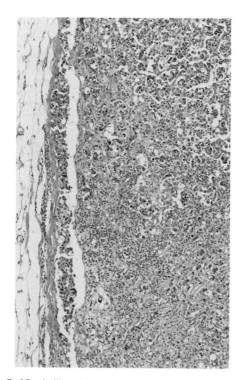

Figure 7-15. Axillary lymph node with metastatic breast carcinoma. The subcapsular sinus (left) is distended with tumor cells. Nests of tumor cells have also invaded the subcapsular cortex. (Courtesy of Dr. Trace Worrell, Department of Pathology, University of Texas Southwestern Medical School, Dallas.)

chial and mediastinal nodes. Local lymph nodes, however, may be bypassed—"skip metastasis"—because of venous-lymphatic anastomoses or because inflammation or radiation has obliterated channels.

In many cases, the regional nodes serve as effective barriers to further dissemination of the tumor, at least for a time. Conceivably the cells, after arrest within the node, may be destroyed. A tumor-specific immune response may participate in this cell destruction. Drainage of tumor cell debris or tumor antigens, or both, also induces reactive changes within nodes. Thus, enlargement of nodes may be caused by (1) the spread and growth of cancer cells or (2) reactive hyperplasia (see Chapter 14). It should be noted therefore that *nodal enlargement in proximity to a cancer does not necessarily mean dissemination of the primary lesion*.

HEMATOGENOUS SPREAD. This pathway is typical of sarcomas but is also used by carcinomas. Arteries, with their thicker walls, are less readily penetrated than are veins. Arterial spread, however, may occur when tumor cells pass through the pulmonary capillary beds or pulmonary arteriovenous shunts or when pulmonary metastases themselves give rise to additional tumor emboli. In such arterial spread, a number of factors (to be discussed) condition the patterns of distribution of the metastases. With venous invasion, the blood-borne cells follow the venous flow, draining the site of the neoplasm. Understandably the liver and lungs are most frequently involved secondarily in such

Figure 7-16. Carcinoma metastatic to liver. Note umbilication (arrow) of large implant caused by central necrosis of tumor. (Courtesy of Dr. Lawrence Weiss, Brigham and Women's Hospital, Boston.)

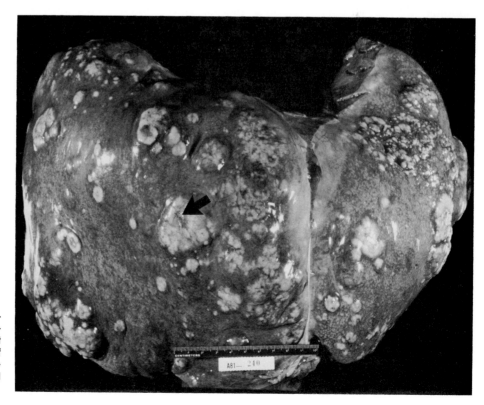

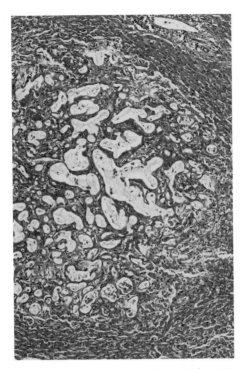

Figure 7–17. Microscopic view of liver metastasis. A pancreatic adenocarcinoma has formed a metastatic nodule in the liver. (Courtesy of Dr. Trace Worrell, Department of Pathology, University of Texas Southwestern Medical School, Dallas.)

hematogenous dissemination (Figs. 7–16 and 7–17). All portal area drainage flows to the liver, and all caval blood flows to the lungs. Cancers arising in close proximity to the vertebral column often embolize through the paravertebral plexus, and this pathway is probably involved in the frequent vertebral metastases of carcinomas of the thyroid and prostate.

Certain cancers have a propensity for invasion of veins. Renal cell carcinoma often invades the branches of the renal vein and then the renal vein itself to grow in a snake-like fashion up the inferior vena cava, sometimes reaching the right side of the heart. Hepatocarcinomas often penetrate portal and hepatic radicles to grow within them into the main venous channels. Remarkably such intravenous growth may not be accompanied by widespread dissemination. Histologic evidence of penetration of small vessels at the site of the primary neoplasm is obviously an ominous feature. Such changes, however, must be viewed guardedly because, for reasons discussed later, they do not indicate the inevitable development of metastases.

The differential features discussed in this overview of the specific characteristics of benign and malignant tumors are summarized in Table 7–2.

With this background on the structure and behavior of neoplasms, we now discuss the origin of tumors, starting with insights gained from the epidemiology of cancer and followed by the molecular basis of transformation.

EPIDEMIOLOGY

Because cancer is a disorder of cell growth and behavior, its ultimate cause has to be defined at the cellular and subcellular levels. Study of cancer patterns in populations, however, can contribute substantially to knowledge about the origins of cancer. For example, the concept that chemicals can cause cancer arose from the astute observations of Sir Percival Pott, who related the increased incidence of scrotal cancer in chimney sweeps to chronic exposure to soot. Thus major insights into the etiology of cancer can be obtained by epidemiologic studies that relate particular environmental, racial (hereditary?), and cultural influences to the occurrence of malignant neoplasms. In addition, certain diseases associated with an increased risk of developing cancer can provide insights into the pathogenesis of malignancy. Therefore, in the following discussion, we shall first summarize the overall incidence of cancer to provide an insight into the magnitude of the cancer problem and then review a number of factors relating to both the patient and the environment that influence predisposition to cancer.

Table 7–2. COMPARISONS BETWEEN BENIGN AND MALIGNANT TUMORS

CHARACTERISTICS	BENIGN	MALIGNANT
Differentiation/anaplasia	Well-differentiated; structure may be typical of tissue of origin	Some lack of differentiation with anaplasia; structure is often atypical
Rate of growth	Usually progressive and slow; may come to a standstill or regress; mitotic figures are rare and normal	Erratic and may be slow to rapid; mitotic figures may be numerous and abnormal
Local invasion	Usually cohesive and expansile well-demarcated masses that do not invade or infiltrate surrounding normal tissues	Locally invasive, infiltrating the surrounding normal tissues; sometimes may be seemingly cohesive and expansile
Metastasis	Absent	Frequently present; the larger and more undifferentiated the primary, the more likely are metastases

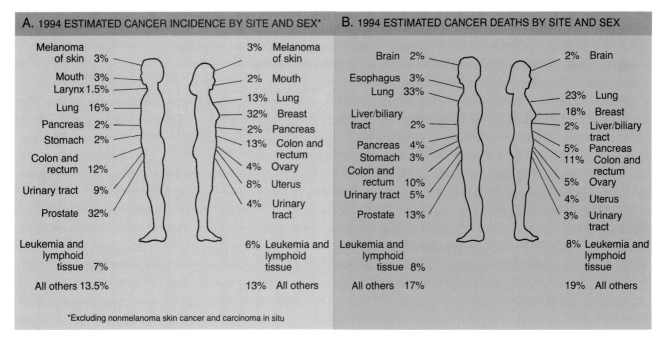

A. 1994 ESTIMATED CANCER INCIDENCE BY SITE AND SEX*

Melanoma of skin 3%
Mouth 3%
Larynx 1.5%
Lung 16%
Pancreas 2%
Stomach 2%
Colon and rectum 12%
Urinary tract 9%
Prostate 32%
Leukemia and lymphoid tissue 7%
All others 13.5%

3% Melanoma of skin
2% Mouth
13% Lung
32% Breast
2% Pancreas
13% Colon and rectum
4% Ovary
8% Uterus
4% Urinary tract
6% Leukemia and lymphoid tissue
13% All others

*Excluding nonmelanoma skin cancer and carcinoma in situ

B. 1994 ESTIMATED CANCER DEATHS BY SITE AND SEX

Brain 2%
Esophagus 3%
Lung 33%
Liver/biliary tract 2%
Pancreas 4%
Stomach 3%
Colon and rectum 10%
Urinary tract 5%
Prostate 13%
Leukemia and lymphoid tissue 8%
All others 17%

2% Brain
23% Lung
18% Breast
2% Liver/biliary tract
5% Pancreas
11% Colon and rectum
5% Ovary
4% Uterus
3% Urinary tract
8% Leukemia and lymphoid tissue
19% All others

Figure 7–18. Cancer incidence and mortality by site and sex. (Adapted from Boring, C.C., Squires, T.S., Tong, T., and Montgomery, S.: Cancer statistics. CA 44:9, 1994.)

CANCER INCIDENCE

In some measure, an individual's likelihood of developing a cancer is expressed by national incidence and mortality rates. For example, it is sobering to realize that residents of the United States have about a one in five chance of dying of cancer. There were, it is estimated, about 538,000 deaths from cancer in 1994, representing 23% of all mortality.[1] These data do not include an additional 700,000, for the most part readily curable, nonmelanoma cancers of the skin and 100,000 cases of carcinoma in situ, largely of the uterine cervix but also of the breast. The major organ sites affected and overall frequency are cited in Figure 7–18.

The age-adjusted death rates (number of deaths per 100,000 population) for many forms of cancer have significantly changed over the years (Fig. 7–19). Many of the temporal comparisons are noteworthy. In males, the overall cancer death rate has significantly increased, whereas in females, it has fallen slightly. The increase in males can be laid largely at the doorstep of lung cancer. The improvement in females is mainly attributable to a significant decline in death rates from cancers of the uterus, stomach, and liver, notably carcinoma of the cervix, one of the frequent forms of malignant neoplasia in females. Striking is the alarming increase in deaths from carcinoma of the lung in both sexes. Although the deaths from lung cancer seem to have plateaued in males, the curve in females continues to point upward—an unfortunate consequence of the increasing use of cigarettes by women. In females, carcinomas of the breast are about three times more frequent than those of the lung. Because of a striking difference in the cure rates of these two cancers, however, bronchogenic carcinoma has become the leading cause of cancer deaths in women. The decline in the number of deaths caused by uterine, including cervical, cancer probably relates to earlier diagnosis and more cures made possible by the Papanicolaou smear. Much more mysterious is the downward trend in deaths from stomach and liver carcinomas. Could this be due to a decrease in some dietary carcinogens?

GEOGRAPHIC AND ENVIRONMENTAL FACTORS

Remarkable differences can be found in the incidence and death rates of specific forms of cancer around the world. For example, the death rate for stomach carcinoma in both males and females is seven to eight times higher in Japan than in the United States. In contrast, the death rate from carcinoma of the lung is slightly more than twice as great in the United States as in Japan, and in Belgium it is even higher than in the United States. Skin cancer deaths, largely caused by melanocarcinomas, are six times more frequent in New Zealand than in Iceland, which is probably attributable to differences in sun exposure. Although racial predispositions cannot be ruled out, it is generally believed that most of these geographic differences are the consequence of environmental influences. This is best brought out by comparing mortality

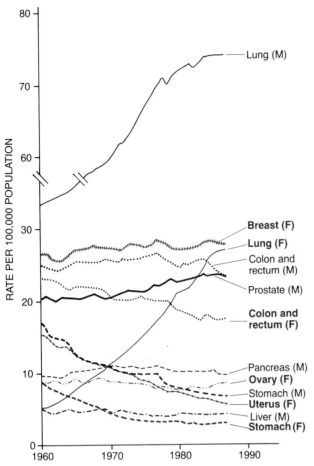

Figure 7–19. Age-adjusted cancer death rates for selected sites in the United States. M = male; F = female. (Adapted from Boring, C.C., Squires, T.S., and Tong, T.: Cancer statistics. CA 43:9, 1993.)

creases the risk of carcinomas of the oropharynx (excluding lip), larynx, and esophagus and, through the intermediation of alcoholic cirrhosis, carcinoma of the liver. Smoking, particularly of cigarettes, has been implicated in cancer of the mouth, pharynx, larynx, esophagus, pancreas, and bladder but most significantly is responsible for about 77% of lung cancer among males and 43% among females (see also Chapter 9). Indeed, cigarette smoking has been called the single most important environmental factor contributing to premature death in the United States. Alcohol and tobacco together multiply the danger of incurring cancers in the upper aerodigestive tract. The risk of cervical cancer is linked to age at first intercourse and the number of sex partners. These associations point to a possible causal role for venereal transmission of cervical viral infections. It begins to appear that everything one does to gain a livelihood or for pleasure is fattening, immoral, illegal, or, even worse, oncogenic.

AGE

Age is an important influence on the likelihood of being afflicted with cancer. As everyone knows, most carcinomas occur in the later years of life (55 years and over). Each age group has its own predilection to certain forms of cancer, as is evident in Tables 7–3 and 7–4. Here the striking increase in mortality from cancer in the age group 55 to 74 years should be noted. The decline in deaths in the 75-year-and-over group merely reflects the dwindling population reaching this age. Also to be noted is that children under the age of 15 are not spared. Indeed, cancer accounts for slightly more than 10% of all deaths in this group in the United States and is second only to accidents. Acute leukemia and neoplasms of the central nervous system are responsible for approximately 60 to 75% of these deaths. The common neoplasms of infancy and childhood include neuroblastoma, Wilms' tumor, retinoblastoma, acute leukemias, and rhabdomyosarcomas. These are discussed in Chapter 10 and elsewhere in the text.

HEREDITY

One frequently asked question is: "My mother and father both died of cancer. Does that mean I am doomed to get it?" Based on current knowledge, the answer must be carefully qualified.[3] The evidence now indicates that for a large number of types of cancer, including the most common forms, there exist not only environmental influences but also hereditary predispositions. For example, lung cancer is in most instances clearly related to cigarette smoking, yet mortality from lung cancer has

rates for Japanese immigrants to the United States and Japanese born in the United States of immigrant parents (Nisei) with those of long-term residents of both countries. Figure 7–20 indicates that cancer mortality rates for first-generation Japanese immigrants are intermediate between those of natives of Japan and of California, and the two rates come closer with each passing generation. This points strongly to environmental and cultural rather than genetic predisposition. There is no paucity of environmental factors: They lurk behind virtually every door. They are found in the ambient environment, in the workplace, in food, and in personal practices.

The carcinogenicity of ultraviolet rays and many drugs will be discussed in a later section. Asbestos, vinyl chloride, and 2-naphthylamine can serve as examples of occupational hazards, and many others are discussed in Chapter 9; the risks may be incurred in lifestyle and personal exposures (for example, dietary influences). Overall, mortality data indicate that persons more than 25% overweight have a higher death rate from cancer than do their "trim" neighbors. Alcohol abuse alone in-

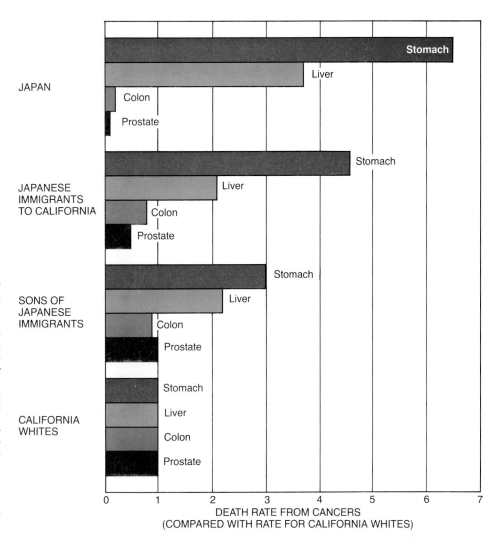

Figure 7–20. Change in incidence of various cancers with migration from Japan to the United States provides evidence that the cancers are caused by components of the environment that differ in the two countries. The incidence of each kind of cancer is expressed as the ratio of the death rate in the population being considered to that in a hypothetical population of California whites with the same age distribution; the death rates for whites are thus defined as 1. The death rates among immigrants and immigrants' sons tend consistently toward California norms. (With permission from Cairns, J.: The cancer problem. *In* Readings from Scientific American— Cancer Biology. New York, W.H. Freeman and Co., 1986, p. 13. © 1975 by Scientific American, Inc. All rights reserved.)

been shown to be four times greater among nonsmoking relatives (parents and siblings) of lung cancer patients than among nonsmoking relatives of controls.

Hereditary forms of cancers can be divided into three categories (Table 7–5).[4]

INHERITED CANCER SYNDROMES. These include several well-defined cancers in which inheritance of a single mutant gene greatly increases the risk of developing a tumor. The predisposition to these tumors shows an autosomal dominant pattern of inheritance. Childhood retinoblastoma offers the most striking example in this category. Approximately 40% of retinoblastomas are familial. Carriers of this gene have a 10,000-fold increased risk of developing retinoblastoma, usually bilateral. They also have a greatly increased risk of developing a second cancer, particularly osteogenic sarcoma. As is discussed later, a "cancer suppressor" gene has been implicated in the pathogenesis of this tumor. Familial adenomatous polyposis is another hereditary disorder marked by an extraordinarily high risk of cancer. Individuals who inherit

the autosomal dominant mutation have at birth, or soon thereafter, innumerable polypoid adenomas of the colon and in virtually 100% of cases are fated to develop a carcinoma of the colon by age 50.

There are several features that characterize inherited cancer syndromes:

- In each syndrome, tumors involve specific sites and tissues. For example, in the multiple endocrine neoplasia syndrome type 2, thyroid, parathyroid, and adrenals are involved. There is no increase in predisposition to cancers in general.
- Tumors within this group are often associated with a specific marker phenotype. For example, there may be multiple benign tumors in the affected tissue, as occurs in familial polyposis of the colon and in multiple endocrine neoplasia. Sometimes there are abnormalities in tissue that are not the target of transformation (e.g., Lisch nodules and café au lait spots in neurofibromatosis type 1; see Chapter 5).
- As in other autosomal dominant conditions, both incomplete penetrance and variable expressivity are noted.

Table 7–3. MORTALITY FOR THE FIVE LEADING CANCER SITES FOR MALES BY AGE GROUP, UNITED STATES, 1990

ALL AGES	UNDER 15	15–34	35–54	55–74	75+
All cancer 268,283	All cancer 949	All cancer 3,788	All cancer 27,005	All cancer 141,787	All cancer 94,739
Lung 91,091	Leukemia 344	Leukemia 719	Lung 8,882	Lung 56,225	Lung 25,770
Prostate 32,378	Brain & CNS 248	Non-Hodgkin's lymphomas 485	Colon & rectum 2,412	Colon & rectum 14,190	Prostate 19,622
Colon & rectum 28,635	Endocrine 113	Brain & CNS 441	Non-Hodgkin's lymphomas 1,542	Prostate 12,423	Colon & rectum 11,842
Pancreas 12,199	Non-Hodgkin's lymphomas 66	Skin 289	Brain & CNS 1,454	Pancreas 6,771	Pancreas 4,128
Leukemia 10,192	Connective tissue 41	Hodgkin's disease 279	Skin 1,252	Esophagus 4,516	Bladder 3,694

With permission from Boring, C.C., Squires, T.S., Tong, T., and Montgomery, S.: Cancer statistics. CA 44:13, 1994.

FAMILIAL CANCERS. Virtually all the common types of cancers that occur sporadically have also been reported to occur in familial forms. Examples include carcinomas of colon, breast, ovary, and brain. Features that characterize familial cancers include early age at onset, tumors arising in two or more close relatives of the index case, and sometimes multiple or bilateral tumors. Familial cancers are not associated with specific marker phenotypes. For example, in contrast to the familial adenomatous polyp syndrome, familial colonic cancers do not arise in pre-existing benign polyps. The transmission pattern of familial cancers is not clear. In general, sibs have a relative risk between 2 and 3. Segregation analyses of large families usually reveals that predisposition to the tumors is dominant, but multifactorial inheritance cannot be easily ruled out.

AUTOSOMAL RECESSIVE SYNDROMES OF DEFECTIVE DNA REPAIR. Besides the dominantly inherited precancerous conditions, a small group of autosomal recessive disorders is collectively characterized by chromosomal or DNA instability.[5] One of the best studied examples is xeroderma pigmentosum, in which DNA repair is defective. This and other familial disorders of DNA instability are described in a later section.

It is impossible to estimate the contribution of heredity to the fatal burden of human cancer. The

Table 7–4. MORTALITY FOR THE FIVE LEADING CANCER SITES FOR FEMALES BY AGE GROUP, UNITED STATES, 1990

ALL AGES	UNDER 15	15–34	35–54	55–74	75+
All cancer 237,039	All cancer 748	All cancer 3,458	All cancer 29,041	All cancer 110,545	All cancer 93,235
Lung 50,194	Leukemia 232	Breast 643	Breast 9,192	Lung 29,729	Colon & rectum 15,524
Breast 43,391	Brain & CNS 212	Leukemia 484	Lung 5,417	Breast 20,096	Lung 14,924
Colon & rectum 28,895	Endocrine 89	Uterus 358	Uterus 2,071	Colon & rectum 11,205	Breast 13,458
Pancreas 12,883	Connective tissue 49	Brain & CNS 301	Colon & rectum 1,998	Ovary 6,575	Pancreas 6,376
Ovary 12,762	Bone 39	Skin 197	Ovary 1,728	Pancreas 5,674	Non-Hodgkin's lymphomas 4,310

With permission from Boring, C.C., Squires, T.S., Tong, T., and Montgomery, S.: Cancer statistics. CA 44:13, 1994.

Table 7–5. INHERITED PREDISPOSITION TO CANCER

Inherited Cancer Syndromes (Autosomal Dominant)
Inherited predisposition indicated by strong family
  history of uncommon cancer and/or associated
  marker phenotype
    Familial retinoblastoma
    Familial adenomatous polyps of the colon
    Multiple endocrine neoplasia syndromes
    Neurofibromatosis types 1 and 2
    Von Hippel–Lindau syndrome

Familial Cancers
Evident familial clustering of cancer but role of
  inherited predisposition may not be clear in an
  individual case
    Breast cancer
    Ovarian cancer
    Colon cancers other than familial adenomatous polyps

Autosomal Recessive Syndromes of Defective DNA Repair
    Xeroderma pigmentosum
    Ataxia-telangiectasia
    Bloom's syndrome
    Fanconi's anemia

Modified from Ponder, B.A.J.: Inherited predisposition to cancer.
Trends Genet. 6:213, 1990.

best "guesstimates," however, suggest that no
more than 5 to 10% of all human cancers are included in the three categories just listed. What can
be said about the influence of heredity on the
large preponderance of malignant neoplasms? It
could be argued that they are entirely or largely of
environmental origin. There is increasing realization, however, that lack of family history does not
preclude a genetic hereditary component. For example, if a dominant cancer-susceptibility gene has
low penetrance, familial cases will be very uncommon. Furthermore, the genotype can significantly
influence the likelihood of developing environmentally induced cancers. It is likely that inherited
variations (polymorphisms) of enzymes that metabolize procarcinogens to their active carcinogenic
forms (see Initiation of Carcinogenesis) may well
influence the susceptibility to cancer. Of interest
in this regard are genes that encode the cytochrome P-450 enzymes. It has been suggested
that polymorphism at one of the P-450 loci confers
inherited susceptibility to lung cancers in cigarette
smokers.[6] More such correlations are likely to be
found, and it is suspected that genetic predisposition contributes to many, if not most, "spontaneous" tumors of humans.

ACQUIRED PRENEOPLASTIC DISORDERS

The only certain way of avoiding cancer is not to
be born; to live is to incur the risk. The risk is
greater than average, however, under many circumstances, as is evident from the predisposing influences discussed earlier. Certain clinical condi-

tions are also of importance. Because cell replication is involved in cancerous transformation, regenerative, hyperplastic, and dysplastic proliferations are fertile soil for the origin of a malignant
neoplasm. There is a well-defined association between certain forms of endometrial hyperplasia and
endometrial carcinoma and between cervical dysplasia and cervical carcinoma (see Chapter 23).
The bronchial mucosal metaplasia and dysplasia of
habitual cigarette smokers are ominous antecedents
of bronchogenic carcinoma. About 80% of hepatocellular carcinomas arise in cirrhotic livers, which
are characterized by active parenchymal regeneration (see Chapter 18). Other examples could be
offered, but although these settings constitute important predispositions, it must be appreciated that
in the great majority of instances they are not
complicated by neoplasia.

Certain non-neoplastic disorders—*the chronic
atrophic gastritis of pernicious anemia; solar keratosis of the skin; chronic ulcerative colitis; and leukoplakia of the oral cavity, vulva, and penis*—have
such a well-defined association with cancer that
they have been termed "precancerous conditions."
This designation is somewhat unfortunate because
in the great majority of instances no malignant
neoplasm emerges. Nonetheless, the term persists
because it calls attention to the increased risk.
Analogously certain forms of benign neoplasia also
constitute "precancerous conditions." The villous
adenoma of the colon, as it increases in size, develops cancerous change in up to 50% of cases. It
might be asked: Is there not a risk with all benign
neoplasms? Although some risk may be inherent, a
large cumulative experience indicates that *most benign neoplasms do not become cancerous.* Nonetheless, numerous examples could be offered of
cancers arising, albeit rarely, in benign tumors: for
example, a leiomyosarcoma beginning in a leiomyoma, and carcinoma appearing in long-standing
pleomorphic adenomas. Generalization is impossible because each type of benign neoplasm is associated with a particular level of risk ranging from
virtually never to frequently. Only follow-up studies of large series of each neoplasm can establish
the level of risk, and always the question remains:
Was the tumor an indolent form of cancer from the
outset, or was there a malignant focus in the benign tumor?

MOLECULAR BASIS OF CANCER

Despite wide variations in the gross and microscopic features of individual malignant tumors,
they share certain fundamental characteristics that
typify their growth and behavior. In this section,
we discuss the molecular changes that form the
basis of such alterations. Before delving into the

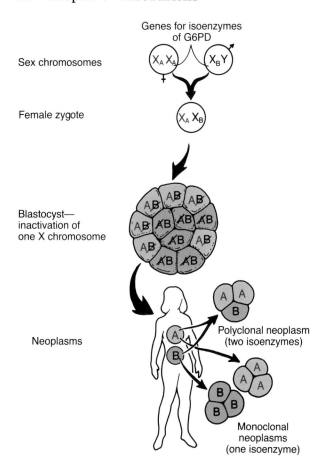

Figure 7-21. Diagram depicting the use of isoenzyme cell markers as evidence of the monoclonality of neoplasms.

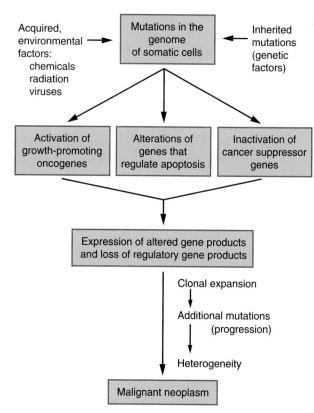

Figure 7-22. Flow chart depicts a simplified scheme of cancer pathogenesis.

details of the genetic basis of cancer, however, it would be profitable to list some of the basic principles:

- *Nonlethal genetic damage lies at the heart of carcinogenesis.* Such genetic damage (or mutation) may be acquired (in somatic cells) by the action of environmental agents, such as chemicals, radiation, or viruses, or it may be inherited in the germ line. The genetic hypothesis of cancer implies that a tumor mass results from the clonal expansion of a single progenitor cell that has incurred the genetic damage; i.e., tumors are monoclonal. This expectation has been realized in the vast majority of tumors that have been analyzed. Clonality of tumors is assessed quite readily in women who are heterozygous for polymorphic X-linked markers, such as the enzyme glucose-6-phosphate dehydrogenase (G6PD) or X-linked restriction fragment length polymorphisms (RFLPs). The principle underlying such an analysis is illustrated in Figure 7–21.

- *It is established that two classes of normal regulatory genes—the growth-promoting proto-oncogenes and the growth-inhibiting cancer suppressor genes (anti-oncogenes)—are the principal targets of genetic damage.* Mutant alleles of proto-oncogenes are considered dominant because they transform cells despite the presence of their normal counterpart. In contrast, both normal alleles of the tumor suppressor genes must be damaged for transformation to occur, so this family of genes is sometimes referred to as recessive oncogenes.

- There is emerging evidence that *a third category of genes—those that control programmed cell death, or apoptosis—*are also important in carcinogenesis. Some of the apoptosis-regulating genes are unique, whereas others function as proto-oncogenes or anti-oncogenes as well.

- *Carcinogenesis is a multistep process at both the phenotypic and genetic level.* A malignant neoplasm has several phenotypic attributes, such as excessive growth, local invasiveness, and the ability to form distant mestastases. These characteristics are acquired in a stepwise fashion—a phenomenon called *tumor progression.* At the molecular level, progression results from accumulation of genetic lesions.

With this overview (Fig. 7–22) we can address in some detail the molecular pathogenesis of cancer and then discuss the carcinogenic agents that inflict genetic damage.

ONCOGENES AND CANCER

Oncogenes, or cancer-causing genes, are derived from proto-oncogenes, cellular genes that promote normal growth and differentiation. As often happens in science, the discovery of proto-oncogenes was not straightforward. These cellular genes were first discovered as "passengers" within the genome of *acute transforming retroviruses*, which cause rapid induction of tumors in animals and can also transform animal cells *in vitro*. Molecular dissection of their genomes revealed the presence of unique transforming sequences (viral oncogenes or v-*oncs*) not found in the genomes of nontransforming retroviruses. Most surprisingly, molecular hybridization revealed that the v-*onc* sequences were almost identical to sequences found in the normal cellular DNA. From this evolved the concept that during evolution, retroviral oncogenes were *transduced* (captured) by the virus through a chance recombination with the DNA of a (normal) host cell that had been infected by the virus. Because they were discovered initially as "viral genes," proto-oncogenes are named after their viral homologs. Each v-*onc* is designated by a three-letter word that relates the oncogene to the virus from which it was isolated. Thus the v-*onc* contained in *feline* sarcoma virus is referred to as v-*fes*, whereas the oncogene in *simian* sarcoma virus is called v-*sis*. The corresponding proto-oncogenes are referred to as *fes* and *cis* by dropping the prefix.

It is important to note that v-*oncs* are not present in several cancer-causing RNA viruses. One such example is a group of so-called slow transforming viruses that cause leukemias in rodents after a long latent period. The mechanism by which they cause neoplastic transformation implicates, once again, proto-oncogenes. Molecular dissection of the cells transformed by these leukemia viruses has revealed that the proviral DNA is always found to be integrated (inserted) near a proto-oncogene. One consequence of proviral insertion near a proto-oncogene is to induce a structural change in the cellular gene, thus converting it into a c-*onc*. Alternatively, strong retroviral promoters inserted in the vicinity of the proto-oncogenes lead to dysregulated expression of the cellular gene. This mode of proto-oncogene activation is called *insertional mutagenesis*.

Although the study of transforming animal retroviruses provided the first glimpse of proto-oncogenes, these investigations did not explain the origin of human tumors, which (with rare exceptions) are not caused by infection with retroviruses. Hence the question was raised: Do nonviral tumors contain oncogenic DNA sequences? The answer was provided by experiments involving DNA-mediated gene transfer (DNA transfection). When DNA extracted from several different human tumors was transfected into mouse fibroblast cell lines *in vitro*, the recipient cells underwent malignant transformation. The conclusion from such experiments was inescapable: DNA of spontaneously arising cancers contains oncogenic sequences, or oncogenes. Many of these transforming sequences have turned out to be homologous to the *ras* proto-oncogenes that are the forbears of v-*oncs* contained in Harvey (H) and Kirsten (K) sarcoma viruses. Others, such as the c-*erb* B2 oncogene, represent novel transforming sequences that have never been detected in retroviruses. *To summarize, proto-oncogenes may become oncogenic by retroviral transduction (v-oncs) or by influences that alter their behavior in situ, thereby converting them into cellular oncogenes (c-oncs).* Two questions follow: (1) What are the functions of oncogene products? (2) How do the normally "civilized" proto-oncogenes turn into "enemies within"? These issues are discussed next.

Protein Products of Oncogenes

Oncogenes encode proteins called *oncoproteins*, which resemble the normal products of proto-oncogenes, with the exception that oncoproteins are devoid of important regulatory elements and their production in the transformed cells does not depend on growth factors or other external signals. To aid in the understanding of the nature and functions of oncoproteins, it is necessary to review briefly the sequence of events that characterize normal cell proliferation. (These are discussed in more detail in Chapter 2.) Under physiologic conditions, cell proliferation can be readily resolved into the following steps:

- The binding of a growth factor to its specific receptor on the cell membrane
- Transient and limited activation of the growth factor receptor, which in turn activates several signal-transducing proteins on the inner leaflet of the plasma membrane
- Transmission of the transduced signal across the cytosol to the nucleus via second messengers
- Induction and activation of nuclear regulatory factors that initiate DNA transcription and ultimately cell division

With this background, we can readily identify oncogenes and oncoproteins as altered versions of their normal counterparts and group them on the basis of their role in the signal transduction cascade[7,8] (Table 7–6).

GROWTH FACTORS. A number of polypeptide growth factors that stimulate proliferation of normal cells have been described (Chapter 2), and many are suspected to play a role in tumorigenesis.[9] Mutations of genes that encode growth factors can render them oncogenic. Such is the case with

Table 7–6. SELECTED ONCOGENES, THEIR MODE OF ACTIVATION, AND ASSOCIATED HUMAN TUMORS

CATEGORY	PROTO-ONCOGENE	MECHANISM	ASSOCIATED HUMAN TUMOR
Growth Factors			
PDGF-β chain	sis	Overexpression	Astrocytoma
			Osteosarcoma
Fibroblast growth	hst-1	Overexpression	Stomach cancer
factors	int-2		Bladder cancer
			Breast cancer
			Melanoma
Growth Factor Receptors			
EGF-receptor family	erb-B1	Overexpression	Squamous cell carcinomas of lung
	erb-B2	Amplification	Breast, ovarian, lung, and stomach cancers
	erb-B3	Overexpression	Breast cancers
CSF-1 receptor	fms	Point mutation	Leukemia
Proteins Involved in Signal Transduction			
GTP-binding	ras	Point mutations	A variety of human cancers, including lung, colon, pancreas; many leukemias
Non-receptor tyrosine kinase	abl	Translocation	Chronic myeloid leukemia
			Acute lymphoblastic leukemia
Nuclear Regulatory Proteins			
Transcriptional	myc	Translocation	Burkitt's lymphoma
activators	N-myc	Amplification	Neuroblastoma
			Small cell carcinoma of lung
	L-myc	Amplification	Small cell carcinoma of lung

the proto-oncogene c-sis, which encodes the beta chain of PDGF. This oncogene was first discovered in the guise of the viral oncogene contained in the v-sis. Subsequently, several human tumors, especially astrocytomas and osteosarcomas, have been found to produce PDGF. Furthermore, it appears that the same tumors also express receptors for PDGF and are hence subject to autocrine stimulation. Although an autocrine loop is considered to be an important element in the pathogenesis of several tumors, in most instances the growth factor gene itself is not altered or mutated. More commonly, products of other oncogenes such as ras (that lie along the signal transduction pathway) cause overexpression of growth factor genes, thus forcing the cells to secrete large amounts of growth factors, such as transforming growth factor-alpha (TGF-α). This growth factor, you may recall, is related to epidermal growth factor (EGF) and induces proliferation by binding to the EGF receptor. TGF-α is often detected in carcinomas that express high levels of EGF receptors.

In addition to c-sis, a group of related oncogenes that encode homologs of fibroblast growth factors (FGFs) (e.g., hst-1 and int-2) is activated in several gastrointestinal and breast tumors[10]; bFGF, a member of the fibroblast growth factor family, is expressed in human melanomas but not in normal melanocytes. Small cell lung carcinomas produce bombesin-like peptides that stimulate their proliferation.

Despite extensive documentation of growth factor–mediated autocrine stimulation of transformed cells, it must be noted that increased growth factor production is not sufficient for neoplastic transformation. Extensive cell proliferation,

in all likelihood, contributes to the malignant phenotype by increasing the risk of spontaneous or induced mutations in the cell population.

GROWTH FACTOR RECEPTORS. The next group in the sequence of signal transduction involves growth factor receptors, and, not surprisingly, several oncogenes that encode growth factor receptors have been found. Both structural alterations and pathologic overexpression of growth factor receptors have been found in tumors. To understand how mutations affect the function of these receptors, it should be recalled that several growth factor receptors are transmembrane proteins with an external ligand-binding and a cytoplasmic tyrosine kinase domain. In the normal forms of these receptors, the kinase activity is *transiently* activated by binding of their specific growth factors, followed rapidly by tyrosine phosphorylation of several substrates that are a part of the mitotic cascade. The oncogenic versions of these receptors are associated with persistent activation of the tyrosine kinase activity of the cytoplasmic domain without binding to the growth factor. Hence the mutant receptors deliver continuous mitogenic signals to the cell. The mutations that affect growth factor receptors may take one of two forms: truncation of the receptor and point mutations. v-erb B, the transforming oncogene of avian erythroblastosis virus, encodes a mutant EGF receptor that is missing most of its external EGF-binding domain; such truncation leads to constitutive activation of its intracellular tyrosine kinase. A similar truncation of the EGF receptor has been found in some human astrocytomas. In myeloid leukemias, point mutations that activate c-fms, the gene encoding the colony-stimulating factor 1 (CSF-1) receptor, have been detected.[11] Far more common than mutations that derail the regulatory function of these proto-oncogenes is overexpression of the normal forms of growth factor receptors. The three known members of the EGF receptor family are the ones most commonly involved.[12] The normal form of c-erb B1, the EGF receptor gene, is overexpressed in up to 80% of squamous cell carcinomas of the lung and, less commonly, in carcinomas of the urinary bladder, gastrointestinal tract, and astrocytomas. In some cases, increased receptor expression results from gene amplification. In most others, the molecular basis of increased receptor expression is not known. In contrast, the c-erb B2 gene (also called c-neu), the second member of the EGF receptor family, is amplified in a high percentage of human adenocarcinomas arising within the breast, ovary, lung, stomach, and salivary glands.[13] The ligand for the c-erb B2 gene has been identified,[14] and transcripts of this novel growth factor have been detected in the same tissues that express the receptor.

A third member of the EGF receptor family, c-erb B3, has recently been isolated, and this gene is also overexpressed in breast cancers. It might be suspected that tumors that overexpress the growth factor receptors, such as c-erb B2, would be exquisitely sensitive to the growth-promoting effects of a very small amount of growth factors and hence likely to be more aggressive. This hypothesis is supported by the observation that high levels of c-erb B2 protein on breast cancer cells is a harbinger of poor prognosis.

SIGNAL-TRANSDUCING PROTEINS. Several examples of oncoproteins that mimic the function of normal cytoplasmic signal-transducing proteins have been found. Most such proteins are strategically located on the inner leaflet of the plasma membrane, where they receive signals from outside the cell (e.g., by activation of growth factor receptors) and transmit them to the cell's nucleus. Biochemically, the signal-transducing proteins are heterogeneous, but they can be grouped into two major categories: *guanosine triphosphate (GTP)–binding proteins (e.g., c-ras) and non–receptor-associated tyrosine kinases (e.g., c-abl)*. Each of these two classes is discussed separately.

GTP-Binding Proteins. These include the *ras* family of proteins and the well-known G proteins. Approximately 30% of all human tumors contain mutated versions of *ras* proteins. In some tumors (e.g., carcinomas of the colon, pancreas, and thyroid), the incidence of *ras* mutation is even higher.[15] *Indeed mutation of the* ras *gene is the single most common abnormality of dominant oncogenes in human tumors*. Several studies indicate that *ras* plays an important role in mitogenesis induced by growth factors. For example, blockade of *ras* function by microinjection of specific antibodies blocks

the proliferative response to EGF, PDGF, and CSF-1. Normal *ras* proteins flip back and forth between an activated, signal-transmitting form and an inactive, quiescent state. In the inactive state, *ras* proteins bind guanosine diphosphate (GDP); when cells are stimulated by growth factors or other receptor-ligand interactions, *ras* becomes activated by exchanging GDP for GTP (Fig. 7–23). The activated *ras* in turn excites downstream regulators of proliferation, such as MAP kinases and protein kinase C. In normal cells, the activated signal-transmitting stage of *ras* protein is transient because its intrinsic GTPase activity hydrolyzes GTP to GDP, thereby returning *ras* to its quiescent ground state. This orderly cycling of the *ras* protein depends on two reactions: (1) nucleotide exchange (GDP by GTP), which activates *ras* protein, and (2) GTP hydrolysis, which converts the GTP-bound, active *ras* to the GDP-bound, inactive form.[16,17] Both these processes are enzymatically regulated. The release of bound GDP from inactive *ras* is catalyzed by a family of guanine-releasing factors (GRF). Much more importantly, the GTPase activity intrinsic to normal *ras* proteins is dramatically accelerated by GTPase-activating proteins (GAPs). These widely distributed proteins bind to the active *ras* and augment its GTPase activity by more than 1000-fold, leading to rapid hydrolysis of GTP to GDP and termination of signal transduction.[18] Thus GAPs function as "brakes" that prevent uncontrolled *ras* activity. It is the response to this braking action of GAPs that seems to falter when mutations affect the *ras* gene. *Mutant* ras *proteins bind GAP, but their GTPase activity fails to be augmented*. Hence the mutant proteins are "trapped" in their excited GTP-bound form, causing in turn a pathologic activation of the mitogenic signaling pathway. The importance of GTPase activation in normal growth control is underscored by the fact that a disabling mutation of neurofibromin (NF-1), a GTPase-activating protein, is also associated with neoplasia (see Cancer Suppressor Genes).

In contrast to *ras*, the signal-transducing function of G proteins is much better understood. Only one G protein, however, the stimulatory subunit that controls the activity of adenyl cyclase, GαS, has been implicated as an oncoprotein. Mutant GαS is detected in subsets of hormone-secreting tumors of the pituitary, adrenal, and thyroid.

Non–Receptor-Associated Tyrosine Kinases. These proteins, like the GTP-binding proteins, lie on the inner leaflet of the plasma membrane and serve to phosphorylate intracellular targets in response to external growth-promoting stimuli. As with the proto-oncogenes that encode growth factor receptors, mutations of the non–receptor-associated tyrosine kinases that increase their kinase activity turn them into oncogenes. Mutant forms of non–receptor-associated tyrosine kinases that have acquired transforming potential are com-

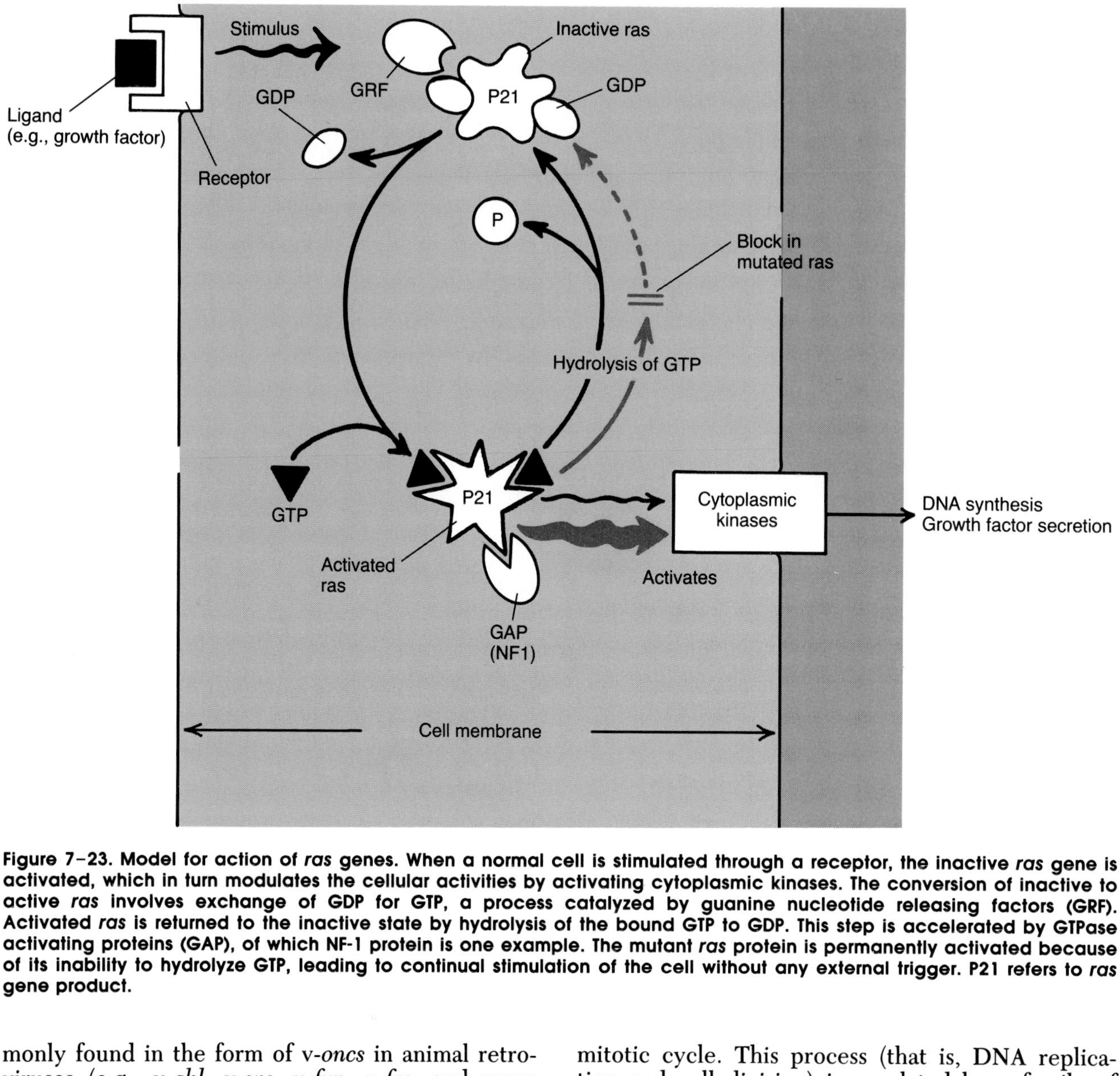

Figure 7-23. Model for action of *ras* genes. When a normal cell is stimulated through a receptor, the inactive *ras* gene is activated, which in turn modulates the cellular activities by activating cytoplasmic kinases. The conversion of inactive to active *ras* involves exchange of GDP for GTP, a process catalyzed by guanine nucleotide releasing factors (GRF). Activated *ras* is returned to the inactive state by hydrolysis of the bound GTP to GDP. This step is accelerated by GTPase activating proteins (GAP), of which NF-1 protein is one example. The mutant *ras* protein is permanently activated because of its inability to hydrolyze GTP, leading to continual stimulation of the cell without any external trigger. P21 refers to *ras* gene product.

monly found in the form of v-*oncs* in animal retroviruses (e.g., v-*abl*, v-*src*, v-*fyn*, v-*fes*, and many others). However, with the exception of c-*abl*, they are rarely activated in human tumors. The *abl* proto-oncogene has tyrosine kinase activity, which is dampened by negative regulatory domains. In chronic myeloid leukemia and some acute lymphoblastic leukemias, however, this activity is unleashed because the c-*abl* gene is translocated from its normal abode on chromosome 9 to chromosome 22; here it fuses with part of the *bcr* (break-point cluster region) gene on chromosome 22, and the hybrid gene has potent tyrosine kinase activity. Although the substrates phosphorylated by the *abl-bcr* chimera are not known, it is suspected that they regulate cellular proliferation.

NUCLEAR REGULATORY PROTEINS. Ultimately, all signal transduction pathways enter the nucleus and impact on a large bank of responder genes that orchestrate the cells' orderly advance through the

mitotic cycle. This process (that is, DNA replication and cell division) is regulated by a family of genes whose products are localized to the nucleus, where they control the transcription of growth-related genes. Not surprisingly, therefore, mutations affecting genes that encode nuclear transcription factors are associated with malignant transformation. A whole host of oncoproteins, including products of the *myc*, *myb*, *jun*, and *fos* oncogenes, have been localized to the nucleus. Of these, the *myc* gene is most commonly involved in human tumors, and hence a brief overview of its function is warranted.[19] The c-*myc* proto-oncogene is expressed in virtually all eukaryotic cells and belongs to the immediate early growth response genes (see Chapter 2), which are rapidly induced when quiescent cells receive a signal to divide. Following a transient increase of c-*myc* mRNA, the expression declines to a basal level. The importance of c-*myc* in cell proliferation is underscored by experiments in which specific inhibition of c-*myc* expression by

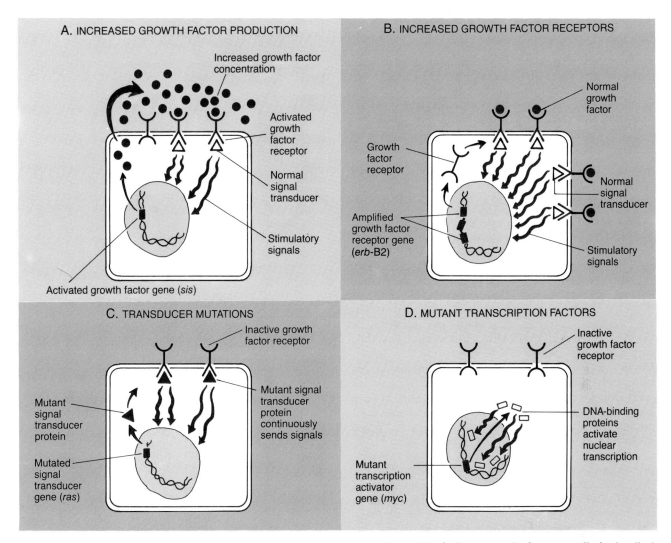

Figure 7-24. Mechanisms by which an oncogene may promote cell growth. *A,* It may code for a growth factor that stimulates the tumor cell by autocrine mechanisms. *B,* It may encode a growth factor receptor and be amplified, thus increasing the number of receptors on tumor cells. *C,* It may encode for defective signal transducers that transmit growth-promoting signals without an external trigger. *D,* It may encode a transcription factor that binds to DNA and stimulates cell growth.

antisense oligonucleotides prevents the entry of cells into the S-phase.

The molecular basis of c-*myc* function in cell replication is not entirely clear, but some general principles have emerged. Following translation, the c-*myc* protein is rapidly translocated to the nucleus. Either before or after transport to the nucleus, it forms a heterodimer with another protein, called *max.* Next the c-*myc*/*max* complex binds to specific DNA sequences, presumably in the vicinity of genes that are essential for cell proliferation. From this strategic location, *myc* activates the transcription of the nearby growth-related genes.[20] The identity of the growth-promoting genes that are the targets of transcriptional activation by *myc* is yet to be determined, but several candidates, including c-*sis*, which encodes the beta chain of PDGF, have been identified. In contrast to the regulated expression of c-*myc* during normal cell

proliferation, oncogenic versions are associated with persistent expression, and in some cases overexpression, of the *myc* protein. This may lead to sustained transcription of critical target genes and possibly neoplastic transformation. Dysregulation of c-*myc* expression occurs in Burkitt's lymphoma, a B-cell tumor; the related N-*myc* and L-*myc* genes are amplified in neuroblastomas and small cell cancers of lung.

Some mechanisms by which oncogenes promote cell growth are summarized in Figure 7-24.

Activation of Oncogenes

In the preceding section we discussed how mutant forms of proto-oncogenes may provide gratuitous growth-stimulating signals. Next we focus on mechanisms by which proto-oncogenes are transformed into oncogenes. This is brought about by two broad categories of changes:

- Changes in the *structure* of the gene, resulting in the synthesis of an abnormal gene product (oncoprotein) having an aberrant function
- Changes in *regulation* of gene expression, resulting in enhanced or inappropriate production of the structurally normal growth-promoting protein

We can now discuss the specific lesions that lead to structural and regulatory changes that affect proto-oncogenes.

POINT MUTATIONS. The *ras* oncogene represents the best example of activation by point mutations. Several distinct mutations have been identified, all of which dramatically reduce the GTPase activity of the *ras* proteins. As mentioned in an earlier section, the intrinsic GTPase activity of normal *ras* proteins is augmented greatly by GAPs; in contrast, the GTPase activity of mutant *ras* proteins is poorly stimulated by GAPs. The mutant *ras* thus remains in the active GTP bound form.

A large number of human tumors carry *ras* mutations. The frequency of such mutations varies with different tumors, but in some types it is very high. For example, 90% of pancreatic adenocarcinomas and cholangiocarcinomas contain a *ras* point mutation, as do about 50% of colon, endometrial, and thyroid cancers and 30% of lung adenocarcinomas and myeloid leukemias. Interestingly, *ras* mutations are infrequent or even nonexistent in certain other cancers, particularly those arising in the uterine cervix or breast. It should be obvious, therefore, that *although ras mutations are extremely common, their presence is not essential for carcinogenesis*. As discussed later, there are many pathways to cancer and *ras* mutations happen to lie on one of the well-traveled roads. In addition to *ras*, activating point mutations have been found in the c-*fms* gene in some cases of acute myeloid leukemia.

CHROMOSOMAL TRANSLOCATIONS. Rearrangement of genetic material brought about by *chromosomal translocation usually results in overexpression of proto-oncogenes, but in some cases the gene may incur structural changes as well*. Translocation-induced overexpression of a proto-oncogene is best exemplified by Burkitt's lymphoma. All such tumors carry one of three translocations, each involving chromosome 8q24, where the c-*myc* gene has been mapped, as well as one of the three immunoglobulin gene-carrying chromosomes. At its normal locus, the expression of the *myc* gene is tightly controlled and is expressed only during certain stages of the cell cycle (see Chapter 2). In Burkitt's lymphoma, the most common form of translocation results in the movement of the c-*myc*–containing segment of chromosome 8 to

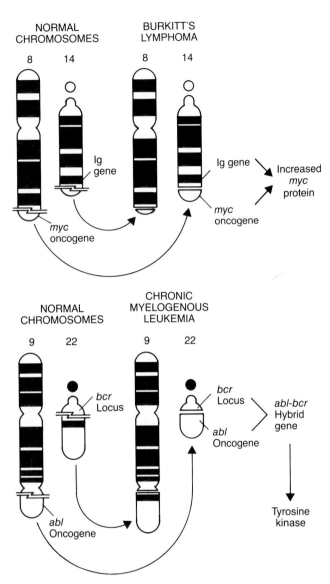

Figure 7–25. Chromosomal translocations and associated oncogenes in Burkitt's lymphoma and chronic myelogenous leukemia.

chromosome 14q band 32 (Fig. 7–25). This places c-*myc* close to the immunoglobulin heavy-chain (Cμ) gene. The molecular mechanisms of the translocation-associated activation of c-*myc* are variable, as are the precise breakpoints within the gene. In some cases, the translocation renders the c-*myc* gene subject to relentless stimulation by the adjacent enhancer element of the immunoglobulin gene. In others, the translocation causes mutations in the regulatory sequences of the *myc* gene. In all instances, the coding sequences of the gene remain intact, and the c-*myc* gene is constitutively expressed at high levels. The invariable presence of the translocated c-*myc* gene in Burkitt's lymphomas attests to the importance of c-*myc* overexpression in the pathogenesis of this tumor. This notion has been verified by the occurrence of B-cell lymphomas in transgenic mice that carry the *myc* gene under the control of an immunoglobulin enhancer.[21]

Overexpression of the *bcl-2* gene (to be described later) occurs by a mechanism similar to that of the *myc* gene. In virtually all follicular B-cell lymphomas, the *bcl-2* gene, mapped to 18q21, is shifted to chromosome 14q32, near the immunoglobulin heavy-chain locus.

The Philadelphia chromosome, characteristic of chronic myeloid leukemia and a subset of acute lymphoblastic leukemias, provides an example of genetic damage wrought by translocation. In these cases, a reciprocal translocation between chromosomes 9 and 22 relocates a truncated portion of the proto-oncogene c-*abl* (from chromosome 9) to the *breakpoint cluster region (bcr)* on chromosome 22. The hybrid c-*abl-bcr* gene encodes a chimeric protein that has tyrosine kinase activity (see Fig. 7–25). Although the translocations are cytogenetically identical in chronic myeloid leukemia and acute lymphoblastic leukemias, they differ at the molecular level. In chronic myeloid leukemia, the chimeric protein has a molecular weight of 210 kd, whereas in the more aggressive acute leukemias, a slightly different, 180-kd, *abl-bcr* fusion protein is formed. The latter has much greater tyrosine kinase activity than does the 210-kd protein.[22] In addition to these examples, a whole array of translocations, many of which give rise to oncogenic fusion proteins, is being uncovered with increasing regularity.[23]

GENE AMPLIFICATION. Activation of proto-oncogenes associated with overexpression of their products may result from reduplication and manifold amplification of their DNA sequences. Such amplification may produce several hundred copies of the proto-oncogene in the tumor cell. The amplified genes can be readily detected by molecular hybridization with the appropriate DNA probe. In some cases, the amplified genes produce cytogenetic changes that can be identified microscopically. Two mutually exclusive patterns are seen: multiple small, chromosome-like structures called *double minutes* (dms) or *homogeneous staining regions* (HSRs). The latter derive from the assembly of amplified genes into new chromosomes; because these regions containing amplified genes lack a normal banding pattern, they appear homogeneous in a G-banded karyotype (Fig. 7–26). The most interesting cases of amplification involve N-*myc* in neuroblastoma and c-*erb B2* in breast cancers. These genes are amplified in 30 to 40% of these two tumors, and in both settings this amplification is associated with poor prognosis.[24] Similarly amplification of L-*myc* and N-*myc* correlates strongly with disease progression in small cell cancer of the lung.

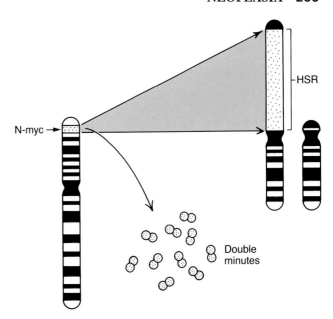

Figure 7–26. Amplification of the N-*myc* gene in human neuroblastomas. The N-*myc* gene, present normally on chromosome 2p, becomes amplified and is seen either as extra chromosomal double minutes or as a chromosomally integrated homogeneous staining region. The integration involves other autosomes, such as 4, 9, or 13. (Modified from Brodeur, G.M.: Molecular correlates of cytogenetic abnormalities in human cancer cells: Implications for oncogene activation. *In* Brown, E.B. (ed.): Progress in Hematology, Vol. 14. Orlando, FL, Grune & Stratton, 1986, pp. 229–256.)

CANCER SUPPRESSOR GENES

Although proto-oncogenes encode proteins that promote cell growth, the products of tumor suppressor genes apply brakes to cell proliferation. In a sense, the term "tumor suppressor genes" is a misnomer because the physiologic function of these genes is to regulate cell growth, not to prevent tumor formation. Because the loss of these genes is a key event in many, possibly all, human tumors, and because their discovery resulted from the study of tumors, the name tumor suppressor or anti-oncogene persists.

Like many discoveries in medicine, the cancer suppressor genes were excavated by digging among rare diseases, in this case retinoblastoma, a tumor that affects about 1 in 20,000 infants and children. Approximately 60% of retinoblastomas are sporadic, and the remaining 40% are familial, with the predisposition to develop the tumor being transmitted as an autosomal dominant trait. To explain the familial and sporadic occurrence of an apparently identical tumor, Knudson proposed his now famous "two hit" hypothesis of oncogenesis. He suggested that in hereditary cases, one genetic change ("first hit") is inherited from an affected parent and is therefore present in all somatic cells of the body, whereas the second mutation ("second hit") occurs in one of the many retinal cells (which already carry the first mutation). In sporadic cases, however, both mutations (hits) occur somatically within a single retinal cell, whose progeny then form the tumor. Knudson's hypothesis has been amply substantiated by cytogenetic and molecular studies and can now be formulated in more precise terms:

- The mutations required to produce retinoblastoma involve the *Rb* gene, located on chromosome 13q14. In some cases, the genetic damage is large enough to be visible in the form of a deletion of 13q14.
- Both normal alleles of the *Rb* locus must be inactivated ("two hits") for the development of retinoblastoma (Fig. 7–27). In familial cases, children are born with one normal and one defective copy of the *Rb* gene. They lose the intact copy in the retinoblasts through some form of somatic mutation (point mutation, interstitial deletion of 13q14, or even complete loss of the normal chromosome 13). In sporadic cases, both normal *Rb* alleles are lost by somatic mutation in one of the retinoblasts. The end result is the same—a retinal cell that has lost both normal copies of the *Rb* gene gives rise to cancer.
- Patients with familial retinoblastoma are also at greatly increased risk of developing osteosarcoma and some other soft tissue sarcomas. Furthermore, inactivation of the *Rb* locus has been noted in several other tumors, including adenocarcinoma of the breast, small cell carcinoma of the lung, and bladder carcinoma.[25] Thus the loss of *Rb* genes has implications beyond the development of retinoblastoma.

At this point, we should clarify some terminology. A child carrying an inherited mutant *Rb* allele in all somatic cells is perfectly normal (save for the increased risk of developing cancer). Because such a child is heterozygous at the *Rb* locus, it implies that heterozygosity for the *Rb* gene does not affect cell behavior. *Cancer develops when the cell becomes homozygous for the mutant allele or, put another way, loses heterozygosity for the normal Rb gene. Because the Rb gene is associated with cancer when both normal copies are lost, it is sometimes referred to as a "recessive cancer gene."*

The *Rb* gene stands as a paradigm for several other genes that act similarly. For example, one or more genes on the short arm of chromosome 11 play a role in the formation of Wilms' tumor, hepatoblastoma, and rhabdomyosarcoma. Among the more common tumors, loss of heterozygosity for certain loci on chromosomes 13, 3, 5, 17, and 18 has been associated with cancers of the breast (13), lung (3), and colon (5, 17, 18).[26] Consistent and nonrandom loss of heterozygosity has provided important clues to the location of several cancer suppressor genes.[26] A list of some tumor suppressor genes and brief comments relating to them follow:

- *p53:* Located on chromosome 17p13.1, the *p53* gene is the single most common target for genetic alterations in human cancer.[27,28] Homozygous loss of the *p53* gene is found in 70% of colon cancers, 30 to 50% of breast cancers, and 50% of lung cancers—the three "biggies" in the cancer parade. Mutations of *p53* are not restricted to epithelial tumors—they have been found in a diverse array of neoplasms, including leukemias, lymphomas, sarcomas, and neurogenic tumors. Although in most instances *p53* mutations are acquired in somatic cells, inherited forms of *p53* alterations have also been described. As with the *Rb* gene, inheritance of a mutant *p53* allele in the Li-Fraumeni syndrome predisposes individuals to the development of cancers. In contrast to those who inherit a defective *Rb* gene, however, patients with the Li-Fraumeni syndrome are at a high risk of developing a wide range of tumors, including breast carcinomas, sarcomas, and brain tumors.[29] The central role played by the *p53* tumor suppressor gene in the origin of human tumors has been confirmed by studies in *p53* knockout mice. With homozygous loss of both *p53* alleles, these mice develop a variety of tumors in young adulthood.[30]
- *APC and NF-1.* These genes, similar to the *Rb* gene, are involved in the pathogenesis of hereditary tumors but with a slight twist to their action. Germ line mutations at these loci are associated with the development of benign tumors that are precursors of carcinomas that develop later. In the case of the APC (*a*denomatous *p*olyposis *c*oli) gene, inherited loss of one allele predisposes to the formation of multiple colonic polyps by the end of the second or third decade of life (familial adenomatous polyposis and Gardner's syndrome; see Chapter 17). A proportion of these adenomas then become malignant. This sequence raises the question: Is inherited mutation affecting one copy of the APC gene sufficient to create tumors, albeit benign adenomas, and is the inactivation of a second allele by somatic mutations required for malignant transformation? If this were the case, as seems likely, the APC gene (in contrast to many other tumor suppressor genes) may not be "recessive" at the cellular level.

In addition to cancers arising in the setting of familial colonic polyposis, the majority of nonfamilial colorectal carcinomas and benign adenomas also contain a mutated APC gene.[31] Interestingly only 30% of the sporadic tumors (adenomas and carcinomas) have homozygous loss of the APC gene, suggesting that inactivation of both alleles may not be essential for tumorigenesis. The molecular mechanisms whereby mutations affecting a single allele of a tumor suppressor

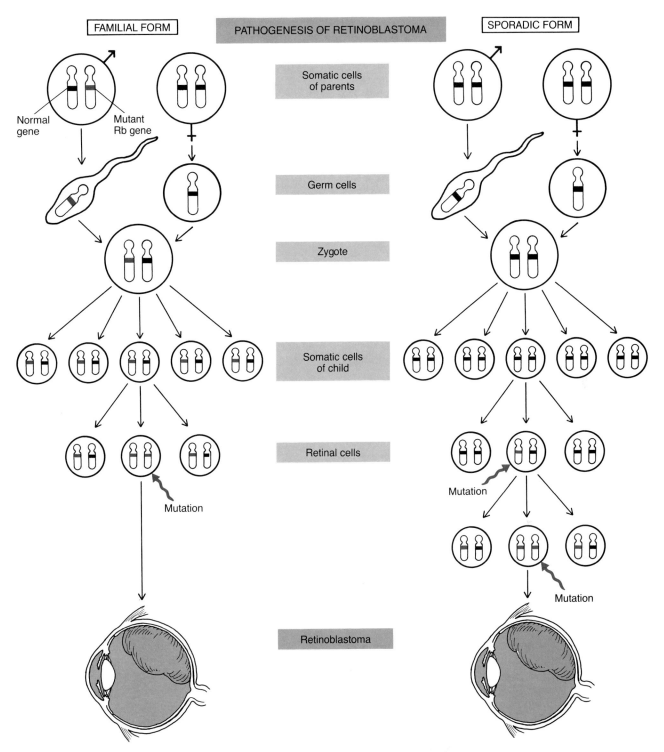

Figure 7–27. Pathogenesis of retinoblastoma. Two mutations at the Rb locus on chromosome 13q14 lead to neoplastic proliferation of the retinal cells. In the familial form, all somatic cells inherit one mutant Rb gene from a carrier parent. The second mutation affects the Rb locus in one of the retinal cells after birth. In the sporadic form, on the other hand, both mutations at the Rb locus are acquired by the retinal cells after birth.

gene may affect cell growth are discussed later (see section on biochemical functions of *p53* gene). The loss of the APC gene is not restricted to colonic neoplasms; it is also mutated in several gastric and pancreatic cancers.[32]

The neurofibromatosis type 1 (NF-1) gene behaves much like the APC gene. Individuals who inherit a mutant allele develop numerous benign neurofibromas, some of which progress to neurofibrosarcomas.

Table 7–7. TUMOR SUPPRESSOR GENES INVOLVED IN HUMAN NEOPLASMS

GENE	CHROMOSOMAL LOCATION	NEOPLASMS ASSOCIATED WITH SOMATIC MUTATIONS	NEOPLASMS ASSOCIATED WITH INHERITED (GERM-LINE) MUTATIONS
Rb	13q14	Retinoblastoma; osteosarcoma; carcinomas of breast, prostate, bladder, and lung	Retinoblastoma; osteosarcoma
p53	17p13.1	Most human cancers	Li-Fraumeni syndrome: carcinomas of breast and adrenal cortex; sarcomas; leukemias; brain tumors
APC	5q21	Carcinomas of colon, stomach, and pancreas	Familial adenomatous polyposis coli; carcinomas of colon
WT-1	11p13	Wilms' tumor	Wilms' tumor
DCC	18q21	Carcinomas of colon and stomach	Unknown
NF-1	17q11	Schwannomas	Neurofibromatosis type 1: neural tumors
NF-2	22q12	Schwannomas and meningiomas	Neurofibromatosis type 2: central (acoustic) schwannomas; meningiomas
VHL	3p25	Unknown	von Hippel-Lindau disease: retinal and cerebellar hemangioblastomas; renal cell carcinomas; angiomas and cysts of many visceral organs

Data from Harris, C.C., and Hollstein, M.: Clinical implication of the *p53* tumor suppressor gene. N. Engl. J. Med. *329*:1318, 1993.

- *Deleted in Colon Carcinoma (DCC):* This rather uninteresting designation refers to a gene mapped to 18q21. This locus, like many other sites that harbor putative cancer suppressor genes, was identified because of the frequent loss of heterozygosity in colorectal cancers. Deletions of the DCC gene have more recently been noted in carcinomas of the stomach as well.[33] As is discussed later, the biochemical nature of the DCC gene sets it apart from other tumor suppressor genes.

- *WT-1:* This cancer suppressor gene, located on chromosome 11p13, is believed to predispose to another childhood neoplasm, Wilms' tumor, which, like retinoblastoma, occurs in both inherited and sporadic forms. In contrast to retinoblastoma, however, it seems that Wilms' tumor is pathogenetically heterogeneous: Not all cases are related to the loss of WT-1. Two other putative tumor suppressor genes, located at 11p15 and 16q13, are implicated in some of the cases.[34]

A listing of several tumor suppressor genes is provided in Table 7–7.

Biochemical Functions of Tumor Suppressor Genes

The signals and signal-transducing pathways for growth inhibition are much less well understood than those for growth promotion. Nevertheless, it is reasonable to assume that, like mitogenic signals, growth inhibitory signals originate outside the cell and use receptors, signal transducers, and nuclear transcription regulators to accomplish their effects. The tumor suppressor genes seem to encode various components of this growth inhibitory pathway.

CELL SURFACE MOLECULES. The DCC gene encodes a transmembrane protein that has structural similarity with cell adhesion molecules—proteins involved in cell-cell or cell–extracellular matrix interactions. It is likely therefore that the DCC gene product is involved in transmission of negative signals responsible for phenomena such as contact inhibition, a property that is lost on malignant transformation. Homozygous loss of the DCC gene is seen in more than 70% of colorectal cancers and in large (precancerous) colonic adenomas.[35]

MOLECULES THAT REGULATE SIGNAL TRANSDUCTION. Down-regulation of growth factor–derived signals is another potential site at which products of tumor suppressor genes may be operative. The product of the NF-1 gene falls in this category. Recall that the *ras* protein, involved in transmission of growth-promoting signals, flips back and forth between active and inactive states. *The normal NF-1 gene encodes a GTPase-activating protein (GAP) that binds to active ras and greatly augments its GTPase activity.*[18] This interaction leads to rapid hydrolysis of GTP to GDP, thus terminating signal transduction. With loss of normal NF-1, *ras* is trapped in its active signal-emitting state. The molecular structure of the recently cloned von Hippel-Lindau disease tumor suppressor gene also suggests that the encoded protein regulates signal transduction.[36]

MOLECULES THAT REGULATE NUCLEAR TRANSCRIPTION. Ultimately, all positive and negative signals converge on the nucleus, where decisions to divide or not to divide are made. Not surprisingly therefore products of several tumor suppressor genes (*Rb*, WT-1, and p53) are localized to the nucleus.

Much is known about the *Rb* gene because this was the first tumor suppressor gene discovered. pRb, the product of the *Rb* gene, is a nuclear

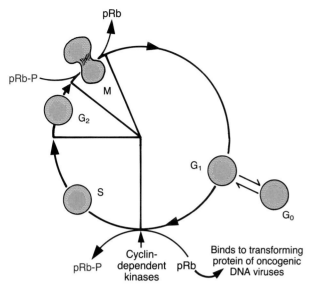

pRb

pRb-P

M

G_2

G_1

S

G_0

pRb-P

Cyclin-
dependent
kinases

pRb

Binds to transforming
protein of oncogenic
DNA viruses

Figure 7–28. Proposed mechanism of action of the *Rb* protein (pRb) in regulation of cell cycle. Oncoproteins of some DNA viruses (e.g., SV40, human papillomavirus) bind to unphosphorylated *pRb* and neutralize its action.

phosphoprotein that regulates the cell cycle. It is expressed in every cell type examined, where it exists in an active underphosphorylated and an inactive hyperphosphorylated state. It is proposed that in its active state *Rb* protein serves as a brake on the advancement of cells from the G_0/G_1 to the S phase of the cell cycle (Fig. 7–28). When the cells are stimulated to divide, the *Rb* protein is inactivated by phosphorylation (pRb-P), the brake is released, and the cell undergoes mitosis. During mitosis, the dephosphorylated form of *Rb* is regenerated and the daughter cells enter G_1.

Recent studies have begun to reveal the molecular basis of this braking action. *Quiescent cells (in G_0 or early G_1) contain the active hypophosphorylated form of pRb. In this state, pRb prevents cell replication by binding, and thereby sequestering, transcription factors. Such factors include the product of the c-myc oncogene and the so-called E2F protein.*[19,37,38] *When nondividing cells are stimulated by growth factors or other mitogenic signals, cyclin-dependent kinases phosphorylate pRb (in the late G_1 phase), causing the pRb to release nuclear factors essential for cell proliferation. During or immediately after mitosis, a phosphatase returns pRb to its active hypophosphorylated state, allowing cells to return to G_0 or G_1. As might be predicted, factors that inhibit cell growth (e.g., TGF-β) have an opposite effect; they favor maintenance of the active form of pRb by preventing its phosphorylation.*

Mutations of the *Rb* gene typically involve the transcription factor binding domain, the so-called *Rb* pocket, of the pRb. With deletions or mutations of the *Rb* gene, uncontrolled cycling of cells occurs because the activity of transcription factors cannot

be regulated. Rather striking evidence pointing to the critical role of the *Rb* gene in neoplastic transformation emerged quite unexpectedly from the study of oncogenic DNA viruses. It has been revealed that the transforming proteins of several animal and human DNA viruses (e.g., SV40, human papillomaviruses) bind to the hypophosphorylated form of pRb. Even more remarkably, the binding occurs within the same pRb pocket that serves to sequester the transcription factors. With its binding sites occupied by virus-encoded proteins, pRb is functionally deleted. Thus it seems that the oncogenicity of such tumor viruses may be based in part on their ability to inhibit the function of Rb and certain other tumor suppressor genes.[39]

The *p53* gene, like the *Rb* gene, is a nuclear phosphoprotein that regulates DNA replication, cell proliferation, and cell death.[39a] Although the precise mechanisms by which *p53* acts as a tumor suppressor gene are not known, accumulating evidence suggests that normal (wild-type) *p53* acts as a "molecular policeman" that prevents propagation of genetically damaged cells.[40,41] Under physiologic conditions, *p53* has a very short half-life, measured in minutes, and there is no evidence that this protein is required for normal cell division. Once cells are exposed to mutagenic agents such as chemicals or irradiation, however, there are dramatic changes in *p53*. Through post-translational modifications, *p53* is stabilized, and it accumulates within the nucleus. The accumulated wild-type *p53* binds to DNA and causes cells to arrest in the G_1 phase of the cell cycle.[27] This reversible pause in cell cycling is welcome because it allows the cells time to repair the DNA damage inflicted by the mutagenic agent. If for some reason the repair mechanisms fail, *p53* seems to "sense" the risk of allowing mutated cells to divide and hence as a last ditch measure triggers cell death by apoptosis (Fig. 7–29). In view of its protective functions, *p53* has rightly been called "guardian of the genome."[40] With loss of normal *p53* (common in many tumors), cells exposed to mutagenic agents replicate the damaged DNA, and thus mutations become fixed in the genome. Although no single mutation is sufficient to transform cells, the loss of the *p53* pathway predisposes cells to additional mutations and, ultimately, malignant transformation (see Fig. 7–29). Inactivation of the *p53* gene occurs most commonly by missense mutations. These abnormal proteins fail to bind to DNA but have a remarkably long half-life, and hence they can be readily detected in tumor cells by immunocytochemical staining. Indeed *p53* proteins detected in this manner are almost always associated with mutation.[42]

In addition to mutations, there are two other mechanisms by which normal *p53* function may be subverted. As with pRb, the transforming proteins of several DNA viruses (SV40, adenoviruses, human papillomaviruses) can bind and sequester nor-

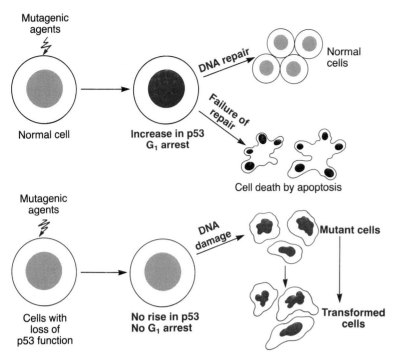

Figure 7–29. Proposed model for the action of normal and mutant *p53*.

mal *p53*. Products of certain nuclear oncogenes also seem to inactivate the tumor suppressor activity of *p53* by binding to it.

Thus far we have discussed *p53* as a negative regulator of cell growth. Amazingly, however, it appears that *p53* is quite versatile and can function as an oncogene as well as a cancer suppressor gene. Indeed, for many years after its discovery, *p53* was considered solely to be an oncogene because some mutant forms of *p53* can transform cells *in vitro*, as several oncogenes do. The molecular basis of the "yin and yang" behavior can be related at least in part to its tumor suppressor activity. It seems that certain mutant forms of *p53* not only lose their normal function but also gain the ability to bind and inactivate normal *p53* protein. Thus a cell with one mutant and one normal allele behaves as if it has no functional *p53* at all. Mutations of this type are called "dominant negative" because the mutant allele acts dominantly to nullify or cripple the normal allele. As alluded to earlier, the APC gene may also behave as a dominant negative.

GENES THAT REGULATE APOPTOSIS

For many years, oncogenes and cancer suppressor genes held center stage in understanding the molecular basis of tumorigenesis. Although they act quite differently, ultimately genes belonging to both of these classes regulate cell proliferation. Only recently has it become apparent that genes that prevent or induce programmed cell death are also important variables in the cancer equation.[43]

The discovery of *bcl-2*, the prototypic gene in this category, began with the observation that approximately 85% of B-cell lymphomas of the follicular type (see Chapter 14) carry a characteristic t(14;18)(q32;q21) translocation. Recall that 14q32, the site where Ig heavy-chain genes are found, is also involved in Burkitt's lymphoma. Juxtaposition of this transcriptionally active locus with *bcl-2* (located at 18q21) causes overexpression of the *bcl-2* protein. *By mechanisms not yet clear, bcl-2 prevents programmed cell death. Presumably by extending cell survival, overexpression of bcl-2 allows other mutations that affect proto-oncogenes and cancer suppressor genes to supervene.* This notion is supported by the observation that transgenic mice in which human *bcl-2* is overexpressed initially develop a polyclonal B-cell proliferation that after a long latent period transforms into an aggressive monoclonal malignant lymphoma. Not only is the function of *bcl-2* unusual, but also its location is atypical: the inner mitochondrial membrane, the nuclear envelope, and endoplasmic reticulum. The biochemical basis of *bcl-2* action is not fully elucidated. Recent studies suggest that, in many cases, apoptosis results from lethal injury caused by reactive oxygen species and that *bcl-2* inhibits apoptosis by regulating an antioxidant pathway.[44] Because *bcl-2* prevents apoptosis, one might ask: Are there any genes that have the opposite effect, that is, do they trigger programmed cell death? In other words, are there any "cell death genes?" Such genes (e.g., *ced-8*) have been found in nematodes and in mammalian cells. A partial answer to this question has been revealed by the study of the c-*myc* oncogene and *p53* anti-oncogene. Although c-*myc* has been traditionally viewed as a transcriptional activator that promotes cell growth, recent evidence indicates that if cells driven by overactive c-*myc* do not have sufficient growth factors in their environment, they undergo apoptosis. If *bcl-2* is overexpressed in such cells, however, apoptosis is prevented. Thus it seems that unless the *bcl-2* gene "cooperates," c-*myc* activation, brought about for example by translocation, is lethal. Whether or not *p53*, also known to cause apoptosis, collaborates with *bcl-2* in a similar fashion is currently unknown.

MOLECULAR BASIS OF MULTISTEP CARCINOGENESIS

The notion that malignant tumors arise from a protracted sequence of events is supported by epidemiologic, experimental, and molecular studies. Many eons ago, before oncogenes and antioncogenes had infiltrated the scientific literature, cancer epidemiologists had suggested that the age-associated increase in cancers could best be explained by postulating that five or six independent steps were required for tumorigenesis. This idea received initial support from experimental models of chemical carcinogenesis in which the process of tumor formation could be divided into distinct steps, such as initiation and promotion. The study of oncogenes and tumor suppressor genes has provided a firm molecular footing for the concept of multistep carcinogenesis:[45,46]

- DNA transfection experiments reveal that no single oncogene (e.g., *myc*, *ras*) can fully transform cells *in vitro* but that together *ras* and *myc* can transform fibroblasts. Such cooperation is required because each oncogene is specialized to induce part of the phenotype necessary for full transformation. In this example, *ras* oncogene induces cells to secrete growth factors and enables them to grow without anchorage to a normal substrate (anchorage independence), whereas *myc* oncogene renders cells more sensitive to growth factors and immortalizes cells. As mentioned earlier, *myc* and *bcl-2* also cooperate in neoplastic transformation.
- *Every human cancer that has been analyzed reveals multiple genetic alterations involving activation of several oncogenes and loss of two or more cancer suppressor genes.* Each of these alterations represents a crucial step in the progression from a normal cell to a malignant tumor. A dramatic example of incremental acquisition of the malignant phenotype is documented by the study of colon carcinoma.[35] These lesions are believed to evolve through a series of morphologically identifiable stages: colon epithelial hyperplasia followed by formation of adenomas that progressively enlarge and ultimately undergo malignant transformation (see Chapter 17). The proposed

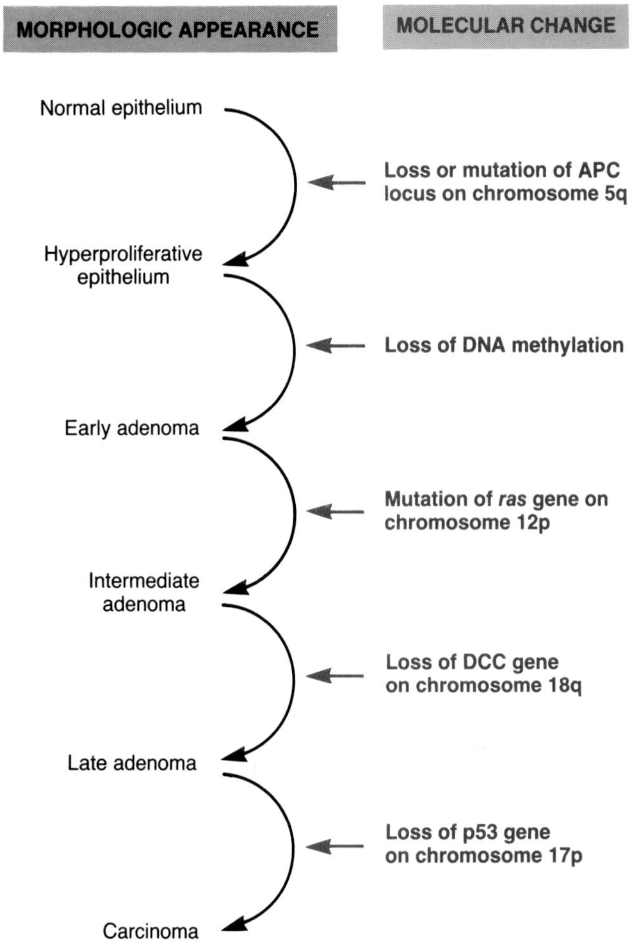

Figure 7–30. Molecular model for the evolution of colorectal cancers through the adenoma-carcinoma sequence. (Based on studies of Fearon, E.R., and Vogelstein, B.: A genetic model of colorectal carcinogenesis. Cell 61:759, 1990. Copyright 1990, Cell Press.)

molecular correlates of this adenoma-carcinoma sequence are illustrated in Figure 7–30. According to this scheme, inactivation of the APC tumor suppressor gene occurs first, followed by activation of *ras* and ultimately loss of DCC and *p53* genes. Although Figure 7–30 suggests a temporal sequence of mutations in specific genes, it should be noted that the order of mutations is considered less important than their total accumulation. Thus in some cases, loss of APC genes precedes *ras* mutation; in others, the sequence is reversed.

- Given the fact that multiple mutations underlie carcinogenesis, one might ask whether the numerous mutations in cancer cells arise independently, or do they result from genetic damage to one or more master "mutator genes"? Although this question is yet to be answered in its entirety, evidence points to the existence of a gene on chromosome 2p15-16 that in some way regulates or influences mutations at hundreds or possibly thousands of other loci. Because this gene was discovered in hereditary nonpolyposis colonic cancer (not associated with colonic polyposis), it has been called *familial colon carcinoma* (FCC) gene.[47] Approximately 13% of sporadic colonic cancers also have mutations in the FCC gene. The product of the FCC gene is involved in DNA repair. When a strand of DNA is being copied, the FCC protein seems to act as a "spell checker." If there is an error that leads to mispairing of bases (e.g., pairing of G with T, rather than the normal A with T), the FCC gene product "directs" the DNA repair machinery to correct it. Without this "spell checker," errors slowly accumulate in several genes, including those that regulate cell growth[47a].

KARYOTYPIC CHANGES IN TUMORS

The genetic damage that activates oncogenes or inactivates tumor suppressor genes may be subtle (e.g., point mutations) or be large enough to be detected in a karyotype. In certain neoplasms, karyotypic abnormalities are nonrandom and common. Specific abnormalities have been identified in most leukemias and lymphomas and in an increasing number of nonhematopoietic tumors. The common types of nonrandom structural abnormalities in tumor cells are (1) balanced translocations, (2) deletions, and (3) cytogenetic manifestations of gene amplification. In addition, whole chromosomes may be gained or lost.[48,49]

The study of chromosomal changes in tumor cells is important on two accounts. First, molecular cloning of genes in the vicinity of chromosomal breakpoints or deletions has been extremely useful in identification of oncogenes (e.g., *bcl*-2, c-*abl*) and tumor suppressor genes (e.g., APC, *Rb*). Second, certain karyotypic abnormalities are specific enough to be of diagnostic value, and in some cases they are predictive of clinical course. Several examples of karyotypic changes were provided in the discussion of carcinogenesis. Many others are described with later considerations of specific forms of neoplasia. Only a few additional examples are presented here.

BALANCED TRANSLOCATIONS. Balanced translocations are extremely common, especially in hematopoietic neoplasms. Most notable is the Philadelphia (Ph[1]) chromosome in chronic myelogenous leukemia (CML), comprising a reciprocal and balanced translocation between chromosomes 22 and, usually, 9. As a consequence, chromosome 22 appears somewhat abbreviated. *This cytogenetic change, seen in more than 95% of cases of CML, is a reliable marker of the disease. The few "Ph[1]-negative" cases*

of CML have molecular evidence of bcr-c-abl *rearrangement. Patients lacking either cytogenetic or molecular evidence of* bcr-c-abl *fusion cannot be classified as having CML and tend to have a worse prognosis (see Chapter 14).* As another example, in more than 90% of cases of Burkitt's lymphoma, the cells have a translocation, usually between chromosomes 8 and 14. In follicular B-cell lymphomas, a reciprocal translocation between chromosomes 14 and 18 is extremely common.

DELETIONS. Chromosome deletions are the second most prevalent structural abnormality in tumor cells. *As compared with translocations, deletions are more common in nonhematopoietic solid tumors.* As discussed, deletions of chromosome 13q band 14 are associated with retinoblastoma. Deletions of 17p, 5q, and 18q, all noted in colorectal cancers, inactivate three tumor suppressor genes. Deletion of 3p is extremely common in small cell lung carcinomas and renal cell carcinomas, raising the suspicion that one or more cancer suppressor genes will be found at this locale. Deletions of 1p band 11-12 are observed in many different tumor types, most notably malignant melanoma, breast adenocarcinomas, and pleural mesotheliomas, making this region a hot area of pursuit by molecular oncologists.

GENE AMPLIFICATIONS. There are two karyotypic manifestations of gene amplification: homogeneously staining regions (HSRs) on single chromosomes and double minutes (see Fig. 7–26), which are seen as small paired fragments of chromatin. As discussed in an earlier section, neuroblastomas and breast cancers are the best-studied examples of gene amplification, involving the N-*myc* and c-*erb B2* genes, respectively.

BIOLOGY OF TUMOR GROWTH

The natural history of most malignant tumors can be divided into four phases: (1) malignant change in the target cell, referred to as *transformation*, (2) *growth* of the transformed cells, (3) local *invasion*, and (4) distant *metastases*. In this sequence, the molecular basis of transformation has already been considered. Next we discuss the factors that affect the growth of transformed cells and, last, the biochemical and molecular basis of invasion and metastasis.

The formation of a tumor mass by the clonal descendants of a transformed cell is a complex process that is influenced by many factors. Some, such as doubling time of tumor cells, are intrinsic

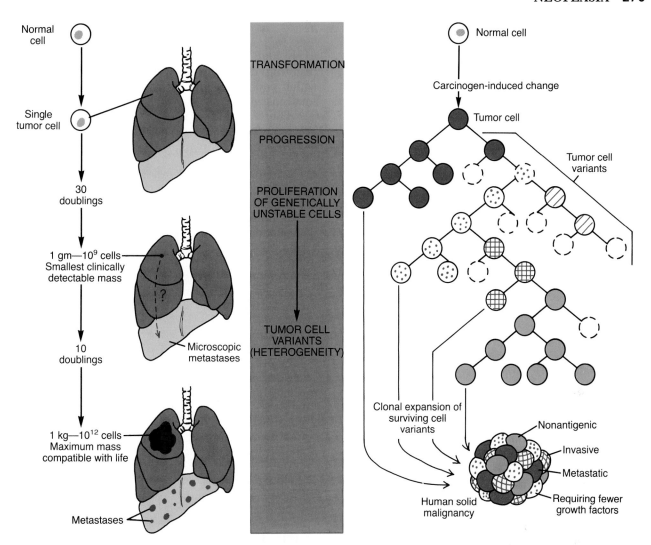

Figure 7–31. Biology of tumor growth. The left panel depicts minimal estimates of tumor cell doublings that precede the formation of a clinically detectable tumor mass. It is evident that by the time a solid tumor is detected, it has already completed a major portion of its life cycle as measured by cell doublings. The right panel illustrates clonal evolution of tumors and generation of tumor cell heterogeneity. New subclones arise from the descendants of the original transformed cell, and with progressive growth the tumor mass becomes enriched for those variants that are more adept at evading host defenses and are likely to be more aggressive. (Adapted from Tannock, I.F.: Biology of tumor growth. Hosp. Pract. 18:81, 1983.)

to the tumor cells, whereas others, such as angiogenesis, represent host responses elicited by tumor cells or their products. The multiple factors that influence tumor growth are considered under three headings: (1) kinetics of tumor cell growth, (2) tumor angiogenesis, and (3) tumor progression and heterogeneity.

KINETICS OF TUMOR CELL GROWTH

One can begin the consideration of tumor cell kinetics by asking the question: How long does it take to produce a clinically overt tumor mass? It can be readily calculated that the original transformed cell (approximately 10 μm in diameter)

must undergo at least 30 population doublings to produce 10^9 cells (weighing approximately 1 gm), which is the smallest clinically detectable mass. In contrast, only 10 further doubling cycles are required to produce a tumor containing 10^{12} cells (weighing approximately 1 kg), which is usually the maximum size compatible with life (Fig. 7–31). These are minimal estimates, based on the assumption that all descendants of the transformed cell retain the ability to divide and that there is no loss of cells from the replicative pool. This concept of tumor as a "pathologic dynamo" is not entirely correct, as we shall discuss.[50] Nevertheless, this calculation highlights an extremely important concept about tumor growth, i.e., *by the time a solid tumor is clinically detected, it has already completed a major portion of its life cycle.* This, as we

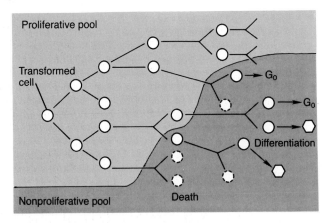

Figure 7-32. Schematic representation of tumor growth. As the cell population expands, a progressively higher percentage of tumor cells leaves the replicative pool by reversion to G_0, differentiation, and death.

see subsequently, is a major impediment in the treatment of cancer. But first let us examine the veracity of the assumption that a malignant tumor is a pathologic dynamo—a mass of rapidly and relentlessly dividing cells! To resolve this issue, it is necessary to address the following questions that relate to tumor cell kinetics:

• What is the doubling time of tumor cells?
• What is the fraction of tumor cells that are in the replicative pool?
• What is the rate at which cells are shed and lost in the growing lesion?

The cell cycle of tumors, like that of all other cells, has the same five phases observed in normal cells (G_0, G_1, S, G_2, and M). Although intuitively one may think that tumor cells divide more rapidly than do normal cells, actual measurements speak to the contrary. In reality, total cell cycle time for many tumors is equal to or longer than that of corresponding normal cells. *Thus it can be safely concluded that growth of tumors is not commonly associated with a shortening of cell cycle time.*

The proportion of cells within the tumor population that are in the proliferative pool is referred to as the *growth fraction*. Clinical and experimental studies suggest that during the early, submicroscopic phase of tumor growth, the vast majority of transformed cells are in the proliferative pool (Fig. 7–32). As tumors continue to grow, cells leave the replicative pool in ever-increasing numbers owing to shedding or lack of nutrients, by differentiating and by reversion to G_0. Indeed, most cells within cancers remain in the G_0 or G_1 phase. Thus by the time a tumor is clinically detectable, most cells are not in the replicative pool. Even in some rapidly growing tumors, the growth fraction is approximately 20%.

Ultimately then the progressive growth of tumors and the rate at which they grow are determined by the *excess of cell production over cell loss.* In some tumors, especially those with a relatively high growth fraction, the imbalance is large, resulting in more rapid growth than in those in which cell production exceeds cell loss by only a small margin.

There are several important conceptual and practical lessons to be learned from these studies of tumor cell kinetics:

• The rate of tumor growth depends on the growth fraction and the degree of imbalance between cell production and cell loss. Some leukemias and lymphomas and certain lung cancers (small cell carcinoma) have a relatively high growth fraction, and their clinical course is rapid. By comparison, many common tumors such as cancer of the colon and breast have low growth fractions, and cell production exceeds cell loss by only about 10%; they tend to grow at a much slower pace.
• The growth fraction of tumor cells has a profound effect on their susceptibility to cancer chemotherapy. Because most anticancer agents act on cells that are actively synthesizing DNA, it is not difficult to imagine that a tumor that contains 5% of all cells in the replicating pool will be slowly growing but relatively refractory to treatment with drugs that kill dividing cells. Paradoxically otherwise aggressive tumors (such as certain lymphomas) that contain a large pool of dividing cells literally melt away with chemotherapy, and even cures may be effected.
• Frequency of mitoses in a neoplasm is at best a crude reflection of rate of growth. If the cell cycle time is prolonged, as occurs in some tumors, many more mitoses are visible at any given time, but whether the tumor grows rapidly or not depends on other factors, such as growth fraction and rate of cell loss.

We can now return to the question posed earlier: How long does it take for one transformed cell to produce a clinically detectable tumor containing 10^9 cells? If every one of the daughter cells remained in cell cycle and no cells were shed or lost, we could anticipate the answer to be 90 days (30 population doublings, with a cell cycle time of 3 days; see Fig. 7–31). In reality, *the latent period before which a tumor becomes clinically detectable is quite unpredictably long, probably years, emphasizing once again that human cancers are diagnosed only after they are fairly advanced in their life cycle.* After they become clinically detectable, the average volume-doubling time for such common killers as cancer of the lung and colon is about 2 to 3 months. As might be anticipated from the discussion of the variables that affect growth rate, however, the range of doubling time values is extremely broad, varying from less than 1 month for some childhood cancers to more than 1 year for certain salivary gland tumors. Cancer is indeed an unpredictable disorder.

TUMOR ANGIOGENESIS

Factors other than cell kinetics modify the rate of growth. Most important among these is blood supply. Folkman has demonstrated that tumor cells in culture can grow in the absence of vascularization only up to nodules in the range of 1 to 2 mm in diameter.[51] When these nodules are implanted in tissue, however, and develop a blood supply from the surrounding host tissues, further growth ensues. Support for the idea that tumor growth is absolutely dependent on vascularization also comes from observations of human tumors *in vivo*. Necrosis commonly occurs in solid tumors. A careful examination often reveals that the necrotic region is parallel to a tumor blood vessel and separated from it by a 1- to 2-mm zone of viable tumor cells. Presumably, the 1- to 2-mm zone around blood vessels represents the maximal distance across which oxygen and other nutrients in blood can readily diffuse. In addition to providing nutrition to growing tumor cells, angiogenesis is also critical for distant spread of tumors; without access to vessels or lymphatics, the tumor would fail to metastasize. Several studies suggest that there is a correlation between the extent of angiogenesis and the probability of metastases in several human tumors, including melanoma, invasive breast cancer, and lung cancer.[52,53]

How do growing tumors develop a blood supply? Several studies indicate that tumors contain factors that are capable of effecting the entire series of events involved in the formation of new capillaries (see Chapter 3). Tumor-associated angiogenic factors may be produced by tumor cells or may be derived from inflammatory cells (e.g., macrophages) that infiltrate tumors. A very large number of tumor-associated angiogenic factors have been isolated. Among the best characterized is a family of heparin-binding fibroblast growth factors (FGFs). These molecules possess a triad of functions: They are chemotactic and mitogenic for endothelial cells, and they induce production of proteolytic enzymes that allow penetration of the stroma by endothelial sprouts. Other tumor-derived angiogenic factors include TGF-α, TGF-β, EGF, PDGF, and vascular endothelial growth factor (VEGF). Not all tumor-derived angiogenic factors act directly on endothelial cells. For example, TFG-β inhibits growth of endothelial cells *in vitro* but is angiogenic *in vivo*. It seems likely that TGF-β attracts macrophages, which then release a variety of angiogenic factors, such as FGFs and TNF-α.

Because angiogenesis is critical for the growth and spread of tumors, much attention is focused on how angiogenesis is switched on and what can be done to retard it. In answer to the first, it should be recalled that several angiogenic molecules, such as FGFs, are products of proto-oncogenes that are activated by mutations. FGFs, however, lack a signal sequence for their secretion from cells, and so they may be released only after tumor cell death. Other angiogenic factors, such as VEGF, are secretory glycoproteins that can induce vascularization around actively growing tumor cells.[54] Tumor angiogenesis may also involve loss of an angiogenesis-inhibiting factor encoded by a putative cancer suppressor gene.[55] Thus it seems that growth autonomy and angiogenesis may well be the consequences of similar genetic events. Can the basic knowledge about angiogenic factors be exploited for tumor therapy? In principle, inhibition of factor production could starve the tumor cells, and hence much effort is directed toward this novel approach of tumor therapy.

TUMOR PROGRESSION AND HETEROGENEITY

It is well established that over a period of time many tumors become more aggressive and acquire greater malignant potential. Indeed, in some instances (e.g., colon cancer; see Chapter 17), there is an orderly progression from preneoplastic lesions to benign tumors and, ultimately, invasive cancers. This phenomenon is referred to as tumor *progression*. Careful clinical and experimental studies reveal that increasing malignancy (e.g., accelerated growth, invasiveness, and ability to form distant metastases) is often acquired in an incremental fashion. *This biologic phenomenon is related to the sequential appearance of subpopulations of cells that differ with respect to several phenotypic attributes, such as invasiveness, rate of growth, metastatic ability, karyotype, hormonal responsiveness, and susceptibility to antineoplastic drugs. Thus, despite the fact that most malignant tumors are monoclonal in origin, by the time they become clinically evident, their constituent cells are extremely heterogeneous.* At the molecular level, tumor progression and associated heterogeneity most likely result from multiple mutations that accumulate independently in different cells, thus generating subclones with different characteristics.

What predisposes the original transformed cell to additional genetic damage is not entirely clear. Many investigators believe that transformed cells are genetically unstable.[56] This renders them susceptible to a high rate of random, spontaneous mutations during clonal expansion (Fig. 7–31). Additionally, mutations in certain master "mutator genes," such as the familial colon cancer (FCC) gene, discussed earlier, may predispose to widespread genetic instability. Some of these mutations may be lethal; others may spur cell growth by affecting proto-oncogenes or cancer suppressor genes. As discussed earlier, mutations in the *p53* tumor suppressor genes allow cells with damaged DNA to divide and thus potentiate accumulation of additional mutations. All of these mechanisms lead to the generation of subclones that are subjected to immune and nonimmune selection pressures. For example, cells that are highly antigenic are destroyed by host defenses, whereas those with reduced growth factor requirements are positively selected. *A growing tumor therefore tends to be enriched for those subclones that "beat the odds" and are adept at survival, growth, invasion, and metastases.* Although progression is most obvious after a tumor is diagnosed, it should be recalled (see Fig. 7–31) that during the latent period many cell doublings occur, and hence *generation of heterogeneity begins well before the tumor is clinically evident.*

The rate at which mutant subclones are generated is quite variable. In some tumors, such as osteosarcomas, metastatic subclones are already present when the patient walks into the doctor's office. In others, typified by certain salivary gland tumors, aggressive subclones develop late and infrequently. Knowledge of such biologic differences is of obvious importance to the clinical potential of cancers and to the management of cancer patients.

MECHANISMS OF INVASION AND METASTASIS

Invasion and metastasis are biologic hallmarks of malignant tumors. They are the major cause of cancer-related morbidity and mortality and hence the subjects of intense scrutiny. For tumor cells to break loose from a primary mass, enter blood vessels or lymphatics, and produce a secondary growth at a distant site, they must go through a series of steps[57] that are summarized in Figure 7–33. Each step in this sequence is subject to a multitude of influences, and hence at any point in the sequence the breakaway cell may not survive. Studies in mice reveal that although millions of cells are released into the circulation each day from a primary tumor, only a few metastases are produced. What then is the basis of the apparent inefficiency of this process? To understand this, it must be recalled that cells within a tumor are heterogeneous with respect to metastatic potential; only certain subclones possess the right combination of gene products to complete all the steps outlined in Figure 7–33. For the purpose of discussion, the metastatic cascade can be divided into two phases: invasion of the extracellular matrix, and vascular dissemination and homing of tumor cells.

Invasion of Extracellular Matrix

As is well known, our tissues are organized into a series of compartments separated from each other by two types of extracellular matrix (ECM): basement membranes and interstitial connective tissue. Although organized differently, each of these components of ECM is made up of collagens, glycoproteins, and proteoglycans. A review of Figure 7–33 reveals that tumor cells must interact with the ECM at several stages in the metastatic cascade. A carcinoma must first breach the underlying basement membrane, then traverse the interstitial connective tissue, and ultimately gain access to the circulation by penetrating the vascular basement membrane. This cycle is repeated when tumor cell emboli extravasate at a distant site. Invasion of the ECM is an active process that can be resolved into several steps:

- Detachment ("loosening up") of the tumor cells from each other
- Attachment to matrix components
- Degradation of ECM
- Migration of tumor cells

Normal cells are neatly glued to each other and their surroundings by a variety of adhesion molecules. Of these, the cadherin family of transmembrane glycoproteins is of particular importance.[58] Epithelial (E) cadherins mediate homotypic adhesions in epithelial tissue, thus serving to keep the epithelial cells together. In several epithelial tumors, including adenocarcinomas of the colon and breast, there is a down-regulation of E-cadherin expression.[59] Presumably, this reduces the ability of cells to adhere to each other and facilitates their detachment from the primary tumor and their advance into the surrounding tissues.

To penetrate the surrounding ECM, the tumor cells must first adhere to the matrix components (Fig. 7–34). There is substantial evidence that receptor-mediated attachment of tumor cells to laminin and fibronectin is important for invasion and metastasis.[60] Normal epithelial cells express high-affinity receptors for basement membrane laminin that are polarized to their basal surface. In contrast, carcinoma cells have many more receptors, and they are distributed all around the cell membrane. Much more important, there seems to be a correlation between the invasiveness and the density of laminin receptors in carcinomas of the breast and colon.[61] In addition to laminin-specific receptors, tumor cells also express integrins that can serve as receptors for many components of the ECM, including fibronectin, laminin, collagen, and vitronectin.[62] As with laminin receptors, there seems to be a correlation between the expression of $\alpha_4\beta_1$ integrin (VLA-4) on melanoma cells and their ability to metastasize. Such a relationship, however, is not universal, and hence it is likely

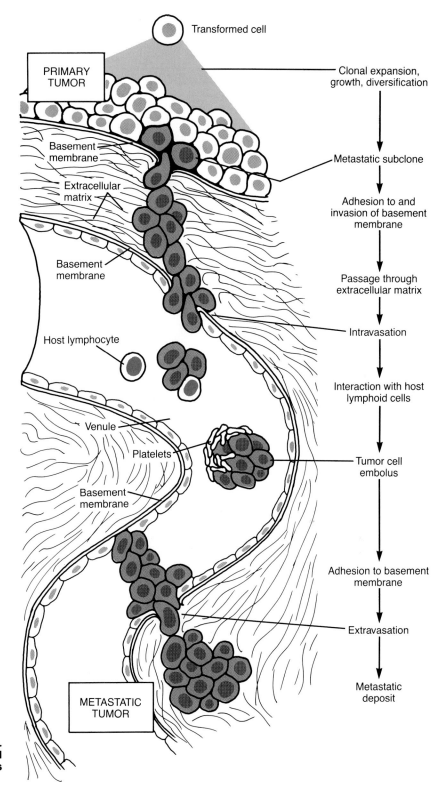

Figure 7–33. The metastatic cascade. Schematic illustration of the sequential steps involved in the hematogenous spread of a tumor.

that tumor cells use several different mechanisms to adhere to ECM.

After attachment to the components of the basement membrane or interstitial ECM, tumor cells must create passageways for migration. Invasion of the matrix is not due merely to passive growth pressure but requires active enzymatic degradation of the ECM components.[63] Tumor cells secrete proteolytic enzymes themselves or induce host cells (e.g., stromal fibroblasts and infiltrating macrophages) to elaborate proteases. Three classes of proteases have been identified: the ser-

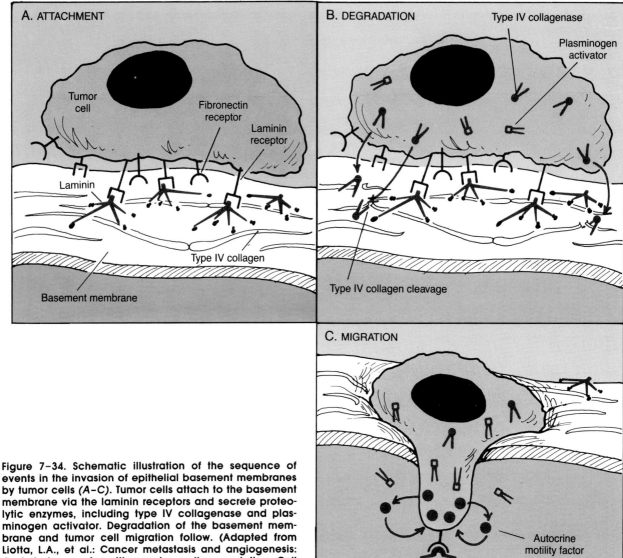

Figure 7–34. Schematic illustration of the sequence of events in the invasion of epithelial basement membranes by tumor cells (A–C). Tumor cells attach to the basement membrane via the laminin receptors and secrete proteolytic enzymes, including type IV collagenase and plasminogen activator. Degradation of the basement membrane and tumor cell migration follow. (Adapted from Liotta, L.A., et al.: Cancer metastasis and angiogenesis: An imbalance of positive and negative regulation. Cell 64:327, 1991. Copyright 1991, Cell Press.)

ine, cysteine, and metalloproteinases. Type IV collagenase is a metalloproteinase that cleaves type IV collagen of epithelial and vascular basement membranes. Liotta and colleagues have provided compelling evidence supporting the role of type IV collagenase in tumor cell invasion:[60]

- Several invasive carcinomas, melanomas, and sarcomas contain high levels of type IV collagenase.
- In situ lesions and adenomas of breast and colon have much lower levels of type IV collagenase content than do invasive lesions.
- In experimental animals, chemical inhibitors of type IV collagenases greatly reduced metastases. Thus it seems that metalloproteinase inhibitors may be of value in the treatment of cancer. Two natural tissue inhibitors of metalloproteinase (TIMPs) have been isolated, and their genes have been cloned. In a preliminary study, injection of

recombinant human **TIMP** greatly reduced experimentally induced metastases in mice.[64]

Cathepsin D (a cysteine proteinase) and urokinase-type plasminogen activator (a serine proteinase) are also important in the degradation of ECM. These enzymes act on a large variety of substrates, including fibronectin, laminin, and protein cores of proteoglycans. Levels of these enzymes are elevated in several animal and human tumors. Levels of cathepsin D in the serum seem to be prognostic in patients with breast cancer. Patients with elevated levels, presumably harboring more invasive tumors, fare less well than those without elevations.[65]

Locomotion is the next step of invasion, propelling tumor cells through the degraded basement membranes and zones of matrix proteolysis. Migration seems to be mediated by tumor cell–derived cytokines, such as *autocrine motility factor*. This 55-kd protein is secreted by a variety of tumor cells and seems to induce motility by binding to a specific receptor.[66] In addition, cleavage products of matrix components (e.g., collagen, laminin) and some growth factors (e.g., insulin-like growth factors I and II) have chemotactic activity for tumor cells. The latter could play a role in organ-selective homing of tumor cells.

The most obvious effect of matrix destruction is to create a passage for invasion by tumor cells. In addition, *cleavage products of matrix components, derived from collagen and proteoglycans, have growth-promoting, angiogenic, and chemotactic activities*. The latter may promote the migration of tumor cells into the loosened ECM.

Vascular Dissemination and Homing of Tumor Cells

Once in circulation, tumor cells are particularly vulnerable to destruction by natural and adaptive immune defenses. The details of tumor immunity are considered later. Suffice it to say that natural killer (NK) cells seem to be particularly important in controlling hematogenous spread of tumors.

Within the circulation, tumor cells tend to aggregate in clumps. This is favored by homotypic adhesions among tumor cells as well as heterotypic adhesion between tumor cells and blood cells, particularly platelets (see Fig. 7–33). Formation of platelet-tumor aggregates seems to enhance tumor cell survival and implantability. Arrest and extravasation of tumor emboli at distant sites involves adhesion to the endothelium, followed by egress through the basement membrane. Involved in these processes are adhesion molecules (integrins, laminin receptors) and proteolytic enzymes, discussed earlier. Of particular interest is an adhesion molecule called CD44, which is expressed on normal T lymphocytes and is used by these cells to migrate to selective sites in the lymphoid tissue. Such migration is accomplished by the binding of CD44 to high endothelial venules. Recent studies reveal that some tumors express variant forms of CD44 and possibly use these molecules to implant themselves in the lymph nodes.[67] Thus, it appears that tumor cells with high levels of CD44 are likely to be adept at extravascular dissemination. This notion is borne out by studies of some human and animal tumors.[62]

The site at which circulating tumor cells leave the capillaries to form secondary deposits is related in part to the anatomic localization of the primary tumor. Many observations, however, suggest that natural pathways of drainage do not wholly explain the distributions of metastases. For example, prostatic carcinoma preferentially spreads to bone, bronchogenic carcinomas tend to involve the adrenals and the brain, and neuroblastomas spread to the liver and bones. Such organ tropism may be related to the following three mechanisms:[68]

- Because the first step in extravasation is adhesion to the endothelium, tumor cells may express adhesion molecules whose ligands are expressed preferentially on the endothelial cells of the target organ.
- Some target organs may liberate chemoattractants that tend to recruit tumor cells to the site. Examples include insulin-like growth factors I and II.
- In some cases, the target tissue may be an unpermissive environment, unfavorable soil, so to speak, for the growth of tumor seedlings. For example, inhibitors of proteases could prevent the establishment of a tumor colony.

Despite the foregoing considerations, however, the precise localization of metastases cannot be predicted with any form of cancer. Evidently many tumors have not read textbooks of pathology!

Molecular Genetics of Metastases

It can be asked: Are there oncogenes or tumor suppressor genes that elicit metastases as their principal or sole contribution to tumorigenesis? This question is of more than academic interest because if altered forms of certain genes promote or suppress the metastatic phenotype, their detection in a primary tumor may have prognostic as well as therapeutic implications. At present, no single "metastasis gene" has been found. Indeed, some have argued that because metastatic cells must acquire multiple properties (e.g., expression of adhesion receptors, production of collagenases, motility factors), no single genetic alteration is likely to render a cell metastasis-prone. Nevertheless, some interesting correlations have emerged. Transfection of cells with mutant *ras* genes not only confers growth autonomy but also induces other changes that render cells metastatic. For example, there is induction of degradative enzymes such as metalloproteinases as well as decreased expression of their inhibitors (TIMPs).[69] The molecular basis of these pleiotropic effects is under investigation. Even more intriguing is the possibility that there exist some metastasis-specific tumor suppressor genes. When normal cells are fused with metastatic tumor cells, some of the hybrids remain tumorigenic but fail to metastasize.[60] These experiments suggest that some normal genes specifically suppress one or more properties essential for metastasis. Several candidate metastasis suppressor genes have been isolated by subtractive hybridization of cDNA libraries obtained from metastatic tumor cell lines and their nonmetastatic but transformed counterparts.[70] One such gene, called *nm23*, has attracted considerable attention. In murine models, the expression of *nm23* is high in lines with low metastatic potential and is reduced tenfold in lines with high metastatic ability. In a series of human breast cancers, the *nm23* levels were highest in the tumors that had three or fewer involved nodes and were uniformly low in tumors that had extensive nodal metastases. The applicability of these findings to other tumors, however, remains to be established. Studies of *nm23* expression in human colon cancer failed to implicate this gene in metastasis suppression.[71] To muddy the waters further, the *nm23* gene has been found to be amplified and overexpressed in aggressive childhood neuroblastomas.[72] There is no satisfactory explanation for these confusing observations. It may be that *nm23* acts as a metastasis suppressor in a tissue-specific manner, serving this role in breast but not colonic epithelium.

CARCINOGENIC AGENTS AND THEIR CELLULAR INTERACTIONS

A large number of agents cause genetic damage and induce neoplastic transformation of cells. They fall into the following categories: (1) chemical carcinogens, (2) radiant energy, and (3) oncogenic viruses. Radiant energy and certain chemical carcinogens are documented causes of cancer in humans, and the evidence linking certain viruses to human cancers grows ever stronger. In the following discussion, each group of agents is considered separately, but it is important to note that several may act in concert or synergize the effects of others.

CHEMICAL CARCINOGENESIS

Although John Hill earlier called attention to the association of "immoderate use of snuff" and the development of "polypusses" (polyps), we owe largely to Sir Percival Pott our awareness of the potential carcinogenicity of chemical agents. Pott astutely related the increased incidence of scrotal skin cancer in chimney sweeps to chronic exposure to soot. A few years later, based on this observation, the Danish Chimney Sweeps Guild ruled that its members must bathe daily. No public health measure since that time has so successfully controlled a form of cancer! Over the succeeding two centuries, hundreds of chemicals have been shown to transform cells *in vitro* and to be carcinogenic in animals. Some of the most potent (e.g., the polycyclic aromatic hydrocarbons) have been extracted from fossil fuels or are products of incomplete combustions. Some are synthetic products created by industry or for the study of chemical carcinogenesis. Some are naturally occurring components

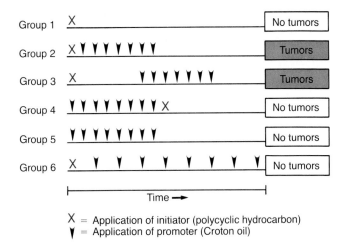

X = Application of initiator (polycyclic hydrocarbon)
Y = Application of promoter (Croton oil)

Figure 7–35. Experiments demonstrating the initiation and promotion phases of carcinogenesis in mice. Group 2—application of promoter repeated at twice-weekly intervals for several months; group 3—application of promoter delayed for several months and then applied twice weekly; group 6—promoter applied at monthly intervals.

of plants and microbial organisms. Most important, a significant number (including, ironically, some medical drugs) have been strongly implicated in the causation of cancers in humans.

Steps Involved in Chemical Carcinogenesis

It was discussed earlier that carcinogenesis is a multistep process. This is most readily demonstrated in experimental models of chemical carcinogenesis, in which cancer induction can be broadly divided into two stages: initiation and promotion.[73] The classic experiments that allowed the distinction between initiation and promotion were performed on mouse skin and are outlined in Figure 7–35. The following concepts relating to the initiation-promotion sequence have emerged from these experiments:

- Initiation results from exposure of cells to an appropriate dose of a carcinogenic agent (initiator); an initiated cell is in some manner altered, rendering it likely to give rise to a tumor (groups 2 and 3). Initiation alone, however, is not sufficient for tumor formation (group 1).
- Initiation causes permanent DNA damage (mutations). It is therefore rapid and irreversible and has "memory." This is illustrated by group 3, in which tumors were produced even if the application of the promoting agent was delayed for several months after a single application of the initiator.
- *Promoters can induce tumors in initiated cells, but they are nontumorigenic by themselves* (group 5). Furthermore, tumors do not result when the promoting agent is applied before, rather than

after, the initiating agent (group 4). This indicates that, *in contrast to the effects of initiators, the cellular changes resulting from the application of promoters do not affect DNA directly and are reversible.*

• That the effects of promoters are reversible is further documented in group 6, in which tumors failed to develop in initiated cells if the time between multiple applications of the promoter was sufficiently extended.

• Because the effects of initiators are irreversible, multiple divided doses achieve the same result as a comparable dose administered at one time. In contrast, there is a threshold level for promoters; thus subthreshold or widely spaced doses are without effect.

Although the concepts of initiation and promotion have been derived largely from experiments involving induction of skin cancer in mice, more recent studies indicate that these stages are also discernible in the development of cancers of the liver, urinary bladder, breast, colon, and respiratory tract.[74,75]

It should be noted that some chemicals possess the capability of both initiation and promotion, as evidenced by their ability to induce tumors without any added factors. They are called "complete carcinogens" to distinguish them from "incomplete carcinogens," which are defined as agents capable only of initiation. With this brief overview of the two major steps in carcinogenesis, we can examine initiation and promotion in more detail, following the outline in Figure 7–36.[76]

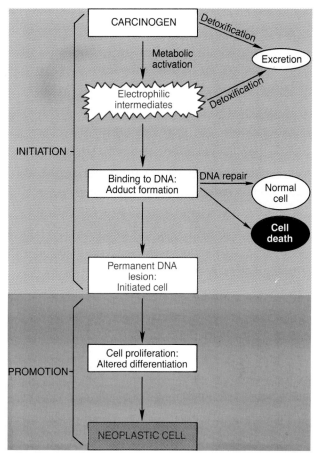

Figure 7–36. General schema of events in chemical carcinogenesis. (Modified from Tannock, I.F., and Hill, R.P. (eds.): The Basic Science of Oncology. New York, Pergamon Press, 1987, p. 92.)

Initiation of Carcinogenesis

Chemicals that initiate carcinogenesis are extremely diverse in structure and include both natural and synthetic products (Table 7–8). They fall into one of two categories: (1) *direct-acting* compounds, which do not require chemical transformation for their carcinogenicity, or (2) *indirect-acting* or *procarcinogens*, which require metabolic conversion *in vivo* to produce *ultimate carcinogens* capable of transforming cells. All direct-acting and ultimate carcinogens have one property in common: They *are highly reactive electrophiles* (have electron-deficient atoms) *that can react with nucleophilic (electron-rich) sites in the cell.* These reactions are nonenzymatic and result in the formation of covalent adducts (addition products). The electrophilic reactions may attack several electron-rich sites in the target cells, including DNA, RNA, and proteins, thus sometimes producing lethal damage. In initiated cells, the interaction is obviously nonlethal, and, as should be evident, DNA is the primary target.

METABOLIC ACTIVATION OF CARCINOGENS. Save for the few direct-acting alkylating and acylating agents that are intrinsically electrophilic, most chemical carcinogens require metabolic activation for conversion into ultimate carcinogens. Other metabolic pathways may lead to the inactivation (detoxification) of the procarcinogen or its derivatives. Thus the carcinogenic potency of a chemical is determined not only by the inherent reactivity of its electrophilic derivative but also by the balance between metabolic activation and inactivation reactions.

Most of the known carcinogens are metabolized by cytochrome P-450–dependent mono-oxygenases. Several factors, both environmental and genetic, are known to affect the activity of these oxidative enzymes, and hence the potency of the procarcinogen. In mice, for example, it has been possible to correlate the carcinogenic potency of polycyclic hydrocarbons with genetically determined levels of the enzyme (aryl hydrocarbon hydroxylase) involved in the formation of reactive metabolites. In humans, a similar correlation be-

Table 7–8. MAJOR CHEMICAL CARCINOGENS

DIRECT-ACTING CARCINOGENS

Alkylating Agents
  Beta-propiolactone
  Dimethyl sulfate
  Diepoxybutane
  Anticancer drugs (cyclophosphamide, chlorambucil, nitro-
    soureas, and others)

Acylating Agents
  1-Acetyl-imidazole
  Dimethylcarbamyl chloride

PROCARCINOGENS THAT REQUIRE METABOLIC ACTIVATION

Polycyclic and Heterocyclic Aromatic Hydrocarbons
  Benz(a)anthracene
  Benzo(a)pyrene
  Dibenz(a,h)anthracene
  3-Methylcholanthrene
  7,12-Dimethylbenz(a)anthracene

Aromatic Amines, Amides, Azo Dyes
  2-Naphthylamine (beta-naphthylamine)
  Benzidine
  2-Acetylaminofluorene
  Dimethylaminoazobenzene (butter yellow)

Natural Plant and Microbial Products
  Aflatoxin B$_1$
  Griseofulvin
  Cycasin
  Safrole
  Betel nuts

Others
  Nitrosamine and amides
  Vinyl chloride, nickel, chromium
  Insecticides, fungicides
  Polychlorinated biphenyls

tween genetically determined levels of aryl hydro-carbon hydroxylase and occurrence of lung cancer in smokers has been noted in some (but not all) studies. Drugs, such as phenobarbital, that are known to induce microsomal enzymes may enhance tumorigenesis in experimental animals by increasing the levels of the cytochrome P-450 oxygenase system. Suffice it to say that numerous factors, including age, sex, species, and hormonal and nutritional status of the individual, may modify the carcinogenic effect of a chemical by affecting its metabolism.

MOLECULAR TARGETS OF CHEMICAL CARCINOGENS. Because malignant transformation results from mutations that affect oncogenes, cancer suppressor genes, and genes that regulate apoptosis, it will come as no surprise that the vast majority of initiating chemicals are mutagenic. Their mutagenic potential has been investigated, most commonly using the *Ames test.* This test uses the ability of a chemical to induce mutations in the bacterium *Salmonella typhimurium.* The vast majority (70 to 90%) of known chemical carcinogens score positive in the Ames test. Conversely, most but not all chemicals that are mutagenic *in vitro* are carcinogenic *in vivo.* Because of the high

correlation between mutagenicity and carcinogenicity, the Ames test is frequently used to screen chemicals for their carcinogenic potential.

That DNA is the primary target for chemical carcinogens seems fairly well established, but there is no single or unique alteration that can be associated with initiation of chemical carcinogenesis. Furthermore, carcinogen-induced changes in DNA do not necessarily lead to initiation because several forms of DNA damage can be repaired by cellular enzymes. Indeed, it is very likely that environmentally induced insults to DNA are far more common than is the occurrence of cancer. This is best exemplified by the rare hereditary disorder xeroderma pigmentosum, which is associated with a defect in DNA repair and a greatly increased vulnerability to skin cancers caused by ultraviolet light and some chemicals (see Radiation Carcinogenesis).

Although virtually any gene may be targeted by chemical carcinogens, *ras* mutations are particularly common in several chemically induced tumors in rodents. Molecular analyses of mutant *ras* genes isolated from such tumors reveals that the change in nucleotide sequence is precisely that predicted from the known sites of reaction of the carcinogen with specific bases in DNA. Thus, it seems that each carcinogen produces a molecular "fingerprint" that can link specific chemicals with their mutational effects.[77] These observations raise the possibility that molecular analysis of the mutations found in human tumors may provide clues to the identity of the initiating agent. For example, in certain geographic areas, hepatocellular carcinoma has been linked to the ingestion of the fungal metabolite aflatoxin B1, whereas in other regions of the world, it follows chronic hepatitis B virus infection. In all cases, there is mutation of the *p53* gene. The mutation site and base change for hepatic cancers in aflatoxin B1–contaminated areas is quite distinct, however, and different from the *p53* mutations seen in areas where hepatitis B is endemic.[78]

THE INITIATED CELL. In the preceding sections, we noted that unrepaired alterations in the DNA are essential first steps in the process of initiation. Changes in DNA, however, are not enough to produce an initiated cell. *For the change to be heritable, the damaged DNA template must be replicated. Thus, for initiation to occur, carcinogen-altered cells must undergo at least one cycle of proliferation, so that the change in DNA becomes "fixed" or permanent.* In the liver, many chemicals are activated to reactive electrophiles, yet most of them do not produce cancers unless the liver cells proliferate within 72 to 96 hours of the formation of DNA adducts. In tissues that are normally quiescent, the mitogenic stimulus may be provided by the carcinogen itself because many cells die owing to toxic effects of the carcinogenic chemical, thereby stimulating regeneration in the surviving cells. Alternatively, cell proliferation may be induced by concurrent exposure to biologic agents such as viruses and parasites, dietary factors, or hormonal influences.[79]

Promotion of Carcinogenesis

It was mentioned earlier that carcinogenicity of some chemicals is augmented by subsequent administration of "promoters" (such as phorbol esters, hormones, phenols, and drugs) that by themselves are nontumorigenic. The initiation-promotion sequence of chemical carcinogenesis raises an important question: *Since promoters are not mutagenic, how do they contribute to tumorigenesis?* Although the effects of tumor promoters are pleiotropic, induction of cell proliferation is a *sine qua non* of tumor promotion. TPA, a phorbol ester and the best-studied tumor promoter, is a powerful activator of protein kinase C, an enzyme that phosphorylates several substrates involved in signal transduction pathways, including those activated by growth factors. TPA also causes growth factor secretion by some cells. The ability of TPA to activate protein kinase C rests on its structural similarity to diacylglycerol, the physiologic activator of protein kinase C. Okadoic acid, another tumor promoter, affects signal transduction by a related but distinct mechanism. It is a powerful inhibitor of protein phosphatases and hence prevents dephosphorylation of substrates that promote signal transduction in their phosphorylated form.

It seems most likely therefore that although the application of an initiator may cause the mutational activation of an oncogene such as *ras,* subsequent application of promoters leads to proliferation and clonal expansion of initiated (mutated) cells. Such cells (especially after *ras* activation) have reduced growth factor requirements and may also be less responsive to growth inhibitory signals in their extracellular milieu. Forced to proliferate, the initiated clone of cells suffers additional mutations, developing eventually into a malignant tumor. Although tumor promoters are not mutagenic, recent evidence indicates that they can affect DNA in other ways. TPA can cause singlestranded DNA breaks in some cells by generation of oxygen-derived free radicals. It is suspected that this effect of phorbol esters leads to cell death, which in turn induces a regenerative response.

The concept that sustained cell proliferation increases the risk of mutagenesis, and hence neoplastic transformation, is also applicable to human carcinogenesis. For example, pathologic hyperplasia of the endometrium (see Chapter 23) and increased regenerative activity that accompanies chronic liver cell injury are associated with the development of cancer in these organs.

Carcinogenic Chemicals

Before closing this discussion of chemical carcinogenesis, we briefly describe some initiators (see Table 7–8) and promoters of chemical carcinogenesis, with special emphasis on those that have been linked to cancer development in humans.

DIRECT-ACTING ALKYLATING AGENTS. These agents are activation independent, and in general they are weak carcinogens. Nonetheless, they have importance because many therapeutic agents (e.g., cyclophosphamide, chlorambucil, busulfan, melphalan, and others) fall into this category. These are used as anticancer drugs but regrettably have been documented to induce lymphoid neoplasms, leukemia, and other forms of cancer. Some alkylating agents, such as cyclophosphamide, are also powerful immunosuppressive agents and are therefore used in treatment of immunologic disorders, including rheumatoid arthritis and Wegener's granulomatosis. Although the risk of induced cancer with these agents is low, judicious use of them is indicated. Alkylating agents appear to exert their therapeutic effects by interacting with and damaging DNA, but it is precisely these actions that render them also carcinogenic.

POLYCYCLIC AROMATIC HYDROCARBONS. These agents represent some of the most potent carcinogens known. They require metabolic activation and can induce tumors in a wide variety of tissues and species. Painted on the skin, they cause skin cancers; injected subcutaneously, they evoke sarcomas; introduced into a specific organ, they cause cancers locally. The polycyclic hydrocarbons are of particular interest as carcinogens because they are produced in the combustion of tobacco, particularly with cigarette smoking, and may well contribute to the causation of lung cancer. They are also produced from animal fats in the process of broiling meats and are present in smoked meats and fish.

AROMATIC AMINES AND AZO DYES. The carcinogenicity of most aromatic amines and azo dyes is exerted mainly in the liver, where the "ultimate carcinogen" is formed by the intermediation of the cytochrome P-450 oxygenase systems. Thus, fed to rats, acetylaminofluorene and the azo dyes induce hepatocellular carcinomas but not cancers of the gastrointestinal tract. An agent implicated in human cancers, beta-naphthylamine, is an exception. In the past, it has been responsible for a 50-fold increased incidence of bladder cancer in heavily exposed workers in aniline dye and rubber industries.[80] After absorption, it is hydroxylated into an active form and then detoxified by conjugation with glucuronic acid. When excreted in the urine, the nontoxic conjugate is split by the urinary enzyme glucuronidase to release the electrophilic reactant again, thus inducing bladder cancer.

Regrettably humans are one of the few species to possess the urinary glucuronidase. Some of the azo dyes were developed to color food, e.g., butter yellow to give margarine the appearance of butter and scarlet red to impart the seductive coloration of certain foods such as maraschino cherries. These dyes are now federally regulated in the United States because of the fear that they may be dangerous to humans.

NATURALLY OCCURRING CARCINOGENS. Among the approximately 30 known chemical carcinogens produced by plants and microorganisms, the potent hepatic carcinogen aflatoxin B1 is most important. It is produced by some strains of *Aspergillus flavus* that thrive on improperly stored grains and peanuts. A strong correlation has been found between the dietary level of this hepatocarcinogen and the incidence of hepatocellular carcinoma in some parts of Africa and the Far East. It may be noted that infection with hepatitis B virus has also been strongly correlated with these cancers, raising the possibility that the aflatoxin and the virus collaborate in the production of this form of neoplasia.

NITROSAMINES AND AMIDES. These carcinogens are of interest because of the possibility that they are formed in the gastrointestinal tract of humans and so may contribute to the induction of some forms of cancer, particularly gastric carcinoma. Similar to most other carcinogens, the nitroso-compounds require activation, which again involves the microsomal P-450 system.

MISCELLANEOUS AGENTS. *Scores of other chemicals* have been indicted as carcinogens. Only a few that represent important industrial hazards are mentioned.[81] Occupational exposure to *asbestos* has been associated with an increased incidence of bronchogenic carcinomas, mesotheliomas, and gastrointestinal cancers, as discussed in Chapter 15. Concomitant cigarette smoking heightens the risk of bronchogenic carcinoma manyfold. *Vinyl chloride* is the monomer from which the polymer polyvinyl chloride is fabricated. It was first identified as a carcinogen in animals, but investigations soon disclosed a scattered incidence of the extremely rare hemangiosarcoma of the liver among workers exposed to this chemical. *Chromium, nickel,* and other metals, when volatilized and inhaled in industrial environments, have caused cancer of the lung. Skin cancer associated with arsenic is also well established. Similarly, there is reasonable evidence that many insecticides, such as aldrin, dieldrin, and chlordane and the polychlorinated biphenyls, are carcinogenic in animals, and the unpleasant citations could be continued.

PROMOTERS OF CHEMICAL CARCINOGENESIS. Certain promoters may contribute to cancers in humans. It has been argued that promoters are at least as important as initiating chemicals because cells initiated by exposure to environmental carcinogens are innocuous unless subjected to repeated assault by promoters. Saccharin and cyclamates have been shown to promote the induction of bladder cancer in rats previously given marginal doses of carcinogens. Whether these artificial sweeteners are also initiators or promoters in humans in a hotly debated issue.[82] Epidemiologic studies, although yielding conflicting results, disclose no solid evidence of carcinogenicity in the dosages customarily used by humans. Hormones such as estrogens serve in animals as promoters of liver tumors. The prolonged use of diethylstilbestrol is implicated in the production of postmenopausal endometrial carcinoma and in the causation of vaginal cancer in offspring exposed in utero, as discussed in Chapter 23. Intake of high levels of dietary fat has been associated with increased risk of colon cancer. This may be related to an increase in synthesis of bile acids, which have been shown to act as promoters in experimental models of colon cancer.

RADIATION CARCINOGENESIS

Radiant energy, whether in the form of the ultraviolet rays of sunlight or as ionizing electromagnetic and particulate radiation, can transform virtually all cell types *in vitro* and induce neoplasms *in vivo* in both humans and experimental animals. Ultraviolet light is clearly implicated in the causation of skin cancers, and ionizing radiations of medical, occupational, and, lamentably, atomic bomb origins have produced a variety of forms of malignant neoplasia. Although the contribution of radiation to the total human burden of cancer is probably small, the well-known latency of radiant energy and its cumulative effect require extremely long periods of observation and make it difficult to ascertain its total significance. Only now, four decades later, an increased incidence of breast cancer has become apparent among females exposed during childhood to the A-bomb.[83] Moreover, its possible additive or synergistic effects on other potential carcinogenic influences add yet another dimension. The effects of ultraviolet light on DNA differ somewhat from those of ionizing radiations. Because the cellular and molecular effects of ionizing radiation are discussed in Chapter 9, the following discussion focuses in large part on the carcinogenic effects of ultraviolet rays.

Ultraviolet Rays

There is ample evidence from epidemiologic studies that *ultraviolet rays* derived from the sun induce an increased incidence of squamous cell carcinoma, basal cell carcinoma, and melanocarcinoma of the skin.[84] The degree of risk depends on the type of ultraviolet rays, the intensity of exposure, and the quantity of light-absorbing "protective mantle" of melanin in the skin. Persons of European origin who have fair skin that repeatedly gets sunburned but stalwartly refuses to tan and who live in locales receiving a great deal of sunlight (for example, Queensland, Australia, close to the equator) have the highest incidence of melanoma. The ultraviolet portion of the solar spectrum can be divided into three wavelength ranges: UVA (320 to 400 nm), UVB (280 to 320 nm), and UVC (200 to 280 nm). Of these, UVB is believed to be responsible for the induction of cutaneous cancers. UVC, although a potent mutagen, is not considered significant because it is filtered out by the ozone shield around the earth (hence the concern about ozone depletion). UVA, until recently considered harmless, has now been determined to cause cancer in animals, and therefore there is renewed interest in its role in human cancer.

Ultraviolet rays have a number of effects on cells, including inhibition of cell division, inactivation of enzymes, induction of mutations, and in sufficient dosage, killing of cells. *The carcinogenicity of UVB light is attributed to its formation of pyrimidine dimers in DNA. When unrepaired, these dimers lead to larger transcriptional errors and, in some instances, cancer.* Studies in mice suggest that more is involved than ultraviolet-induced mutations alone. The ultraviolet light simultaneously impairs cell-mediated immunity.[85] Whether these findings apply to humans is not documented, but it is likely that ultraviolet-induced mutations serve as the initiating mechanism and the immune changes as either potentiators or promoters.

As with other carcinogens, UVB also causes mutations in oncogenes and tumor suppressor genes.[86] In particular, mutant forms of the *ras* and *p53* genes have been detected both in human skin cancers and in UVB-induced cancers in mice. These mutations occur mainly at dipyridimine sequences within the DNA, thus implicating UVB-induced genetic damage in the causation of skin cancers.

Ionizing Radiation

Electromagnetic (x-rays, gamma rays) and particulate (alpha particles, beta particles, protons, neutrons) radiations are all carcinogenic.[83] The evidence is so voluminous that only a few examples will suffice. Many of the pioneers in the development of roentgen rays developed skin cancers. Miners of radioactive elements in central Europe and the Rocky Mountain region of the United States have suffered a tenfold increased incidence of lung cancers. Most telling is the follow-up of survivors of the atomic bombs dropped on Hiroshima and Nagasaki. Initially, there was a marked increase in the incidence of leukemias—

principally acute and chronic myelocytic leukemia —after an average latent period of about 7 years. Subsequently, the incidence of many solid tumors with longer latent periods (e.g., breast, colon, thyroid, and lung) has increased.

Even therapeutic irradiation has been documented to be carcinogenic. Thyroid cancers have developed in approximately 9% of those exposed during infancy and childhood to head and neck radiation. The previous practice of treating a form of arthritis of the spine known as ankylosing spondylitis with therapeutic irradiation has yielded a 10- to 12-fold increase in the incidence of leukemia years later.

To conclude this doleful litany, mention should be made of the residents of the Marshall Islands, who were exposed on one occasion to accidental fallout from a hydrogen bomb test that contained thyroid-seeking radioactive iodines. As many as 90% of the children under the age of ten years on Rongelap Island developed thyroid nodules within 15 years, and it is significant that about 5% of these nodules proved to be thyroid carcinomas. It is evident that radiant energy—whether absorbed in the pleasant form of sunlight, through the best intentions of a physician, or by tragic exposure to an atomic bomb blast—has awesome carcinogenic potential.

In humans, there is a hierarchy of vulnerability to radiation-induced cancers. Most frequent are the leukemias, save for chronic lymphocytic leukemia, which, for unknown reasons, almost never follows radiation injury. Cancer of the thyroid follows closely but only in the young. In the intermediate category are cancers of the breast, lungs, and salivary glands. In contrast, skin, bone, and the gastrointestinal tract are relatively resistant to radiation-induced neoplasia, even though the gastrointestinal mucosal cells are vulnerable to the cell-killing effects of radiation and the skin is in the pathway of all external radiation. Nonetheless, the physician dare not forget: *Any* cell can be transformed into a cancer cell by sufficient exposure to radiant energy.

DNA Repair Defects

Important insights into the molecular processes that affect the response of cells to radiations have been provided by the study of rare inherited diseases characterized by defects in DNA repair.[87] These autosomal recessive disorders include xeroderma pigmentosum, Bloom's syndrome, ataxia-telangiectasia, and Fanconi's anemia. Together they are characterized by hypersensitivity to one or more DNA-damaging agents and by a predisposition to cancer. Patients with *xeroderma pigmentosum* have extreme photosensitivity, a very high incidence of cancers in sun-exposed skin, and, in some cases, neurologic abnormalities. The molecular basis of degenerative changes in sun-exposed skin and occurrence of cutaneous tumors rests on an inherited inability to repair ultraviolet light–induced DNA damage. As mentioned earlier, ultraviolet light causes formation of pyrimidine dimers; cells from patients with xeroderma pigmentosum are markedly deficient in the excision repair of pyrimidine dimers. Xeroderma pigmentosum is genetically heterogeneous—with at least seven different variants. Each of these forms is caused by a mutation in one of several genes involved in nucleotide excision repair.[88] *Ataxia-telangiectasia*, in contrast to xeroderma pigmentosum, is associated with defective response to damage induced by ionizing radiation and a greatly increased risk of developing lymphoid malignancies. In addition, as the name indicates, these patients have progressive cerebellar ataxia and oculocutaneous telangiectasia. They are also immunodeficient and susceptible to recurrent sinopulmonary infection. Like xeroderma pigmentosum, ataxia-telangiectasia is also genetically heterogeneous, with at least six molecular variants. Patients with *Fanconi's anemia* have a predisposition to leukemias, progressive aplastic anemia (see Chapter 13), and congenital malformations. Their cells are extremely sensitive to DNA cross-linking agents, presumably as a result of a deficiency of enzymes that eliminate interstrand cross-links that form after exposure to genotoxic agents. *Bloom's syndrome* differs from all other disorders in this group because patients with this disease seem to be hypersensitive to a variety of different DNA-damaging agents (e.g., ultraviolet light, irradiation). Thus, it appears that they have a more generalized DNA repair defect. Cytologically, cells from these patients are characterized by a greatly increased frequency of apparently spontaneous sister-chromatid exchange, resulting presumably from some defect in DNA ligation. Clinically, patients with Bloom's syndrome have severe immunodeficiency, growth retardation, and predisposition to several types of cancers. Because these syndromes are inherited as autosomal recessives, it can be concluded that both copies of the relevant DNA repair genes are mutated or inactivated in these cancer-prone patients. In this respect, genes involved in DNA repair may be considered tumor suppressor genes.

VIRAL CARCINOGENESIS

A large number of DNA and RNA viruses have proved to be oncogenic in a wide variety of animals, ranging from amphibia to our first cousins, the primates, and the evidence grows ever stronger that certain forms of human cancer are of viral origin. In the following discussion, the better characterized and most intensively studied human oncogenic viruses are presented.

DNA Oncogenic Viruses

Several DNA viruses have been associated with the causation of cancer in animals. Some, such as adenoviruses, cause tumors only in laboratory animals, whereas others, such as the bovine papillomaviruses, cause benign as well as malignant neoplasms in their natural hosts. Of the various human DNA viruses, three (papillomaviruses, Epstein-Barr virus [EBV], and hepatitis B virus [HBV]) are of particular interest because they have been implicated in the causation of human cancer. Before we discuss the role of these viruses in carcinogenesis, a few general comments relating to transformation by DNA viruses are offered:

- Transforming DNA viruses form stable associations with the host cell genome. The integrated virus is unable to complete its replicative cycle because the viral genes essential for completion of replication are interrupted during integration of viral DNA.
- Those viral genes that are transcribed early (early genes) in the viral life cycle are important for transformation. They are expressed in transformed cells.

HUMAN PAPILLOMAVIRUS. Approximately 65 genetically distinct types of human papillomavirus (HPV) have been identified. Some types (e.g., 1, 2, 4, and 7) definitely cause benign squamous papillomas (warts) in humans. HPVs have also been implicated in the genesis of several cancers, particularly squamous cell carcinoma of the cervix and anogenital region.[89] Epidemiologic studies suggest that carcinoma of the cervix is caused by a sexually transmitted agent, and HPV is a prime suspect. DNA sequences of HPV types 16 and 18 and, less commonly, types 31, 33, 35, and 51 are found in approximately 85% of invasive squamous cell cancers and their presumed precursors (severe dysplasias and carcinoma in situ). In contrast to cervical cancers, genital warts with low malignant potential are associated with distinct HPV types, predominantly HPV-6 and HPV-11 ("low-risk" types).

Molecular analyses of HPV-associated carcinomas and benign genital warts reveals differences that may be pertinent to the transforming activity of these viruses. In benign warts and in preneoplastic lesions, the HPV genome is maintained in an episomal (nonintegrated) form, whereas in cancers, the viral DNA is usually integrated into the host cell genome. This suggests that integration of viral DNA is important in malignant transformation. Although the site of viral integration in host chromosomes is random (the viral DNA is found at different locations in different cancers), the pattern of integration is clonal, that is, the site of integration is identical within all cells of a given cancer. This would not be expected if HPV were merely a passenger that infects cells after transformation. Molecular analysis of several HPV-associated cancers has revealed that the site at which the viral DNA is interrupted in the process of integration is fairly constant: It is almost always within the E1/E2 open reading frame of the viral genome. Because the E2 region of the viral DNA normally represses the transcription of the E6 and E7 early viral genes, its interruption causes overexpression of the E6 and E7 proteins of HPV-16 and HPV-18.[90] The oncogenic potential of HPV-16 and HPV-18 can be related to these two early viral gene products. The E7 protein binds to and presumably sequesters the underphosphorylated form of the tumor suppressor protein pRb, whereas the E6 protein binds to and facilitates the degradation of the *p53* gene product. The affinity of these viral proteins for the products of tumor suppressor genes differs depending on the oncogenic potential of HPV. E6 and E7 proteins derived from high-risk HPVs (types 16, 18, and 31) bind to *Rb* and *p53* with high affinity, whereas the E6 and E7 gene products of low-risk HPVs (types 6 and 11) bind with low affinity. That the oncogenic potential of HPV-16 is related to E6 and E7 proteins is further documented by the occurrence of neuroepithelial tumors in mice transgenic for these early viral genes.[91]

Although these observations implicate certain HPV types in the pathogenesis of human cancer, it should be noted that when human keratinocytes are transfected with DNA from HPV 16, 18, or 31 *in vitro* they are immortalized, but they do not form tumors in experimental animals. Cotransfection with a mutated *ras* gene results in full malignant transformation. These data strongly suggest that although HPV very likely plays a role in human carcinogenesis, the virus does not act alone. In all likelihood, other genetic events that occur in cells released from growth restraint by HPV infection are superimposed, or possibly other environmental factors collaborate with the virus.

EPSTEIN-BARR VIRUS. This virus, a member of the herpes family, has been implicated in the pathogenesis of four types of human tumors: the African form of Burkitt's lymphoma; B-cell lymphomas in immunosuppressed individuals, particularly after human immunodeficiency virus (HIV) infection and organ transplantation; some cases of Hodgkin's disease; and nasopharyngeal carcinomas.[92,93] These neoplasms are reviewed elsewhere in this book, and therefore only their association with EBV is discussed here.

EBV infects epithelial cells of the oropharynx and B lymphocytes. It gains entry into cells via the CD21 molecule, which is expressed on B cells and oropharyngeal mucosa. Within B lymphocytes, the linear genome of EBV circularizes to form an episome in the cell nucleus. The infection of B cells is latent, that is, there is no replication of the virus,

and the cells are not killed. The latently infected B cells are immortalized and acquire the ability to propagate indefinitely *in vitro*. The molecular basis of B-cell immortalization by EBV is complex. Involved in this process is the latent membrane protein-1 (LMP-1), which prevents apoptosis by interacting with the *bcl-2* gene; the *EBNA-1* gene, which maintains the virus in latent stage; and the *EBNA-2* gene, which transactivates several viral and host cell genes important for B-cell growth.[94] With this brief review of EBV infection, we can turn to its role in the causation of B-cell tumors.

Burkitt's lymphoma is a neoplasm of B lymphocytes that is the most common childhood tumor in Central Africa and New Guinea. A morphologically identical lymphoma occurs sporadically throughout the world. The association between African Burkitt's lymphoma and EBV is quite strong:

- More than 90% of African tumors carry the EBV genome.
- One hundred per cent of the patients have elevated antibody titers against viral capsid antigens.
- Serum antibody titers against viral capsid antigens are correlated with the risk of developing the tumor.

Although these data strongly support the idea that EBV is intimately involved in the causation of Burkitt's lymphoma, several other observations suggest that additional factors must be involved. *First*, EBV infection is not limited to the geographic locales where Burkitt's lymphoma is found. EBV is a ubiquitous virus that asymptomatically infects almost all adults worldwide. *Second*, EBV is known to cause infectious mononucleosis, a self-limited disorder (see Chapter 8) in which B cells are infected. *Third*, the EBV genome can be found in only 15 to 20% of cases of Burkitt's lymphoma outside Africa, but both the endemic (African) and the sporadic cases of Burkitt's lymphoma have a t(8;14) or, less commonly, variant translocations that lead to dysregulated expression of the c-*myc* oncogene. *Finally*, although EBV infection immortalizes B cells *in vitro*, these cells do not form tumors when injected into appropriately conditioned mice *in vivo*. Indeed, there are significant differences in the patterns of viral gene expression in EBV-transformed (but not tumorigenic) B-cell lines and Burkitt's lymphoma cells. For instance, the tumor cells do not express several viral-encoded membrane proteins that are known to be targeted by host cytotoxic T cells.

It appears, therefore, that EBV serves as one factor in the multistep development of Burkitt's lymphoma (Fig. 7–37). In normal individuals, EBV infection is readily controlled by effective immune responses directed against viral antigens expressed on the cell membranes, and hence the vast majority of infected individuals remain asymptomatic or

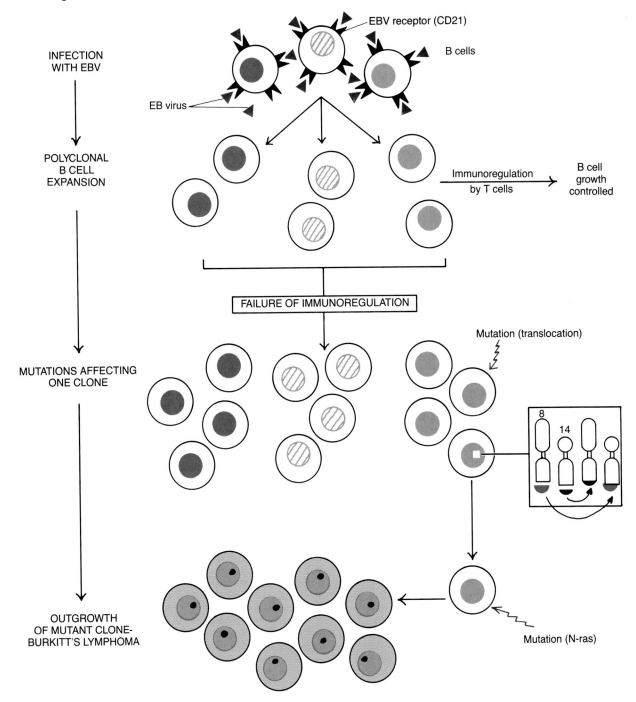

INFECTION
WITH EBV

POLYCLONAL
B CELL
EXPANSION

MUTATIONS AFFECTING
ONE CLONE

OUTGROWTH
OF MUTANT CLONE-
BURKITT'S LYMPHOMA

EBV receptor (CD21)

B cells

EB virus

Immunoregulation
by T cells

B cell
growth
controlled

FAILURE OF IMMUNOREGULATION

Mutation (translocation)

Mutation (N-ras)

Figure 7-37. Schema depicting the possible evolution of EBV-induced Burkitt's lymphoma.

develop self-limited infectious mononucleosis. In regions of Africa where Burkitt's lymphoma is endemic, poorly understood cofactors (e.g., chronic malaria) favor sustained proliferation of B cells immortalized by EBV. The actively dividing B-cell population is at increased risk for developing mutations, such as the t(8;14) translocation, that juxtapose c-*myc* with one of the immunoglobulin gene loci. This provides growth advantage to the affected cell owing to activation of c-*myc*. Overexpression of the c-*myc* oncogene by itself is not

sufficient for malignant transformation. In all likelihood, it represents one of multiple steps in lymphomagenesis. Additional mutations, possibly affecting the N-*ras* oncogene, occur in the B cells immortalized by the EBV. Together these changes lead to the emergence of a monoclonal B-cell neoplasm (see Fig. 7-37). According to this view then, EBV itself is not directly oncogenic, but by acting as a polyclonal B-cell mitogen, it sets the stage for the acquisition of the t(8;14) translocation and other mutations, which ultimately release the cells from normal growth regulation. Concurrent with these changes, there is alteration in viral gene expression as well, such that the display of antigens that could be recognized by cytotoxic T cells is reduced.

The role played by host immune response in controlling EBV-transformed B cells is illustrated dramatically by the occurrence of B-cell lymphomas in immunosuppressed patients. Some patients with acquired immunodeficiency syndrome (AIDS) and those who receive long-term immunosuppressive therapy for preventing allograft rejection present with multifocal B-cell tumors within lymphoid tissue or in the central nervous system. These tumors are polyclonal at the outset but can develop into monoclonal proliferations. The expression of viral antigen such as LMP-1 remains high on these cells, and hence these tumors seem to represent the *in vivo* counterparts of the B-cell lines immortalized by EBV infection *in vitro*. That the growth of these EBV-driven cells is sensitive to immunologic regulation is evident from the observation that in some cases the tumors regress after relaxation of immunosuppressive therapy.

Nasopharyngeal carcinoma is the other tumor associated with EBV infection. This tumor is endemic in Southern China, in some parts of Africa, and in Arctic Eskimos. In contrast to Burkitt's lymphoma, 100% of nasopharyngeal carcinomas obtained from all parts of the world contain EBV DNA. In addition, antibody titers to viral capsid antigens are greatly elevated, and in endemic areas patients develop IgA antibodies before the appearance of the tumor. The 100% correlation between EBV and nasopharyngeal carcinoma suggests that EBV plays a role in the genesis of this tumor, but (as with Burkitt's tumor) the restricted geographic distribution indicates that genetic or environmental cofactors, or both, also contribute to its etiology.[95]

The relationship of EBV with the pathogenesis of Hodgkin's disease is less well established and is discussed in Chapter 14.

HEPATITIS B VIRUS. Epidemiologic studies, discussed in greater detail in Chapter 18, strongly suggest a close association between HBV infection and the occurrence of liver cancer (hepatocellular carcinoma). HBV is endemic in countries of the Far East and Africa, and correspondingly these areas have the highest incidence of hepatocellular carcinoma. For example, in Taiwan, those who are infected with HBV have a greater than 200-fold increased risk of developing liver cancer as compared with uninfected individuals in the same area. Studies in experimental animals also support a role for HBV in the development of liver cancer. Although HBV infection is restricted to humans and chimpanzees, related hepadnaviruses cause hepatocellular cancers in woodchucks.[96] Despite compelling epidemiologic and experimental evidence, the precise role of HBV in the causation of

human liver cancer is not clear. In virtually all cases of HBV-related liver cell cancer, the viral DNA is integrated into the host cell genome and, as with HPV, the tumors are clonal with respect to these insertions. The HBV genome, however, does not encode any oncoproteins, and there is no consistent pattern of integration in the vicinity of any known proto-oncogene. It is likely therefore that the effect of HBV is indirect and possibly multifactorial.[97] *First*, by causing chronic liver cell injury and accompanying regenerative hyperplasia, HBV expands the pool of cells at risk for subsequent genetic changes. In the mitotically active liver cells, mutations may arise spontaneously or be inflicted by environmental agents, such as dietary aflatoxins. Mutational inactivation of *p53* is noted in areas of the world where exposure to HBV as well as aflatoxins is endemic. *Second*, HBV encodes a regulatory element called HBx protein that disrupts normal growth control of infected liver cells by transcriptional activation of several host cell proto-oncogenes. *Third*, the HBx protein activates protein kinase C, a critical component of several signal transduction pathways, and thus mimics the action of the tumor promoter TPA.[98] The important role played by HBx in the pathogenesis of liver cell cancers is buttressed by the observation that mice transgenic for the HBx gene develop hepatic cancers.

RNA Oncogenic Viruses

Although the study of animal retroviruses has provided spectacular insights into the molecular basis of cancer, only one human retrovirus, human T-cell leukemia virus type 1 (HTLV-1), is firmly implicated in the causation of cancer.

HUMAN T-CELL LEUKEMIA VIRUS TYPE 1. HTLV-1 is associated with a form of T-cell leukemia/lymphoma that is endemic in certain parts of Japan and the Caribbean basin but is found sporadically elsewhere, including the United States. Similar to the AIDS virus, HTLV-1 has tropism for CD4$^+$ T cells, and hence this subset of T cells is the major target for neoplastic transformation. Human infection requires transmission of infected T cells via sexual intercourse, blood products, or breastfeeding. Leukemia develops in only about 1% of the infected individuals after a long latent period of 20 to 30 years. In addition to leukemia, HTLV-1 is also associated with a demyelinating neurologic disorder called tropical spastic paraparesis (see Chapter 29).

There is little doubt that HTLV-1 infection of T lymphocytes is necessary for leukemogenesis, but the molecular mechanisms of transformation are not entirely clear. In contrast to several murine retroviruses, HTLV-1 does not contain a v-*onc*, and no consistent integration next to a proto-oncogene

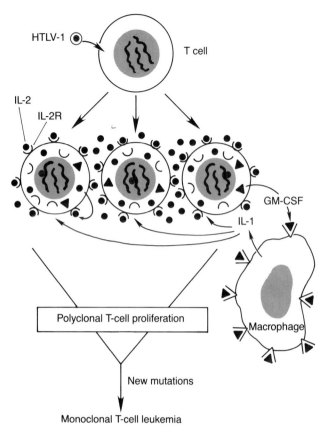

Figure 7–38. Pathogenesis of HTLV-1–induced T-cell leukemia/lymphoma. HTLV-1 infects many T cells and initially causes polyclonal proliferation by autocrine and paracrine pathways. Ultimately, a monoclonal T-cell leukemia/lymphoma results when one proliferating T cell suffers additional mutations.

has been discovered. In leukemic cells, however, viral integration shows a clonal pattern. The genomic structure of HTLV-1 reveals the *gag, pol, env,* and long terminal repeat (LTR) regions typical of other retroviruses, but, in contrast to other leukemia viruses, it contains another region, referred to as *tax.* It seems that the secrets of its transforming activity are locked in the *tax* gene. The product of this gene is essential for viral replication because it stimulates transcription of viral mRNA by acting on the 5' LTR. Recent findings indicate that the *tax* protein can also activate the transcription of several host cell genes, including c-*fos*, c-*sis*, genes encoding the cytokine IL-2 and its receptor, and the gene for myeloid growth factor GM-CSF.[99] From these and other observations, the following scenario is emerging (Fig. 7–38): HTLV-1 infection stimulates proliferation of T cells. This is brought about by the *tax* gene, which turns on genes that encode a T-cell growth factor, interleukin-2 (IL-2), and its receptor, setting up an autocrine system for proliferation. At the same time, a paracrine pathway is activated by the increased production of GM-CSF. This myeloid growth factor, by acting on neighboring macro-

phages, induces increased secretion of other T-cell mitogens, such as IL-1. Initially the T-cell proliferation is polyclonal because the virus infects many cells. The proliferating T cells are at increased risk of secondary transforming events (mutations), which lead ultimately to the outgrowth of a monoclonal neoplastic T-cell population.

HOST DEFENSE AGAINST TUMORS — TUMOR IMMUNITY

Neoplastic transformation, as we have discussed, results from a series of genetic alterations, some of which may result in the expression of cell surface antigens that are seen as nonself by the immune system. The idea that tumors are not entirely self was conceived by Ehrlich, who proposed that immune-mediated recognition of autologous tumor cells may be a "positive mechanism" capable of eliminating transformed cells. Subsequently Lewis Thomas and McFarlane Burnet formalized this concept by coining the term "immune surveillance" to refer to recognition and destruction of nonself tumor cells on their appearance. The fact that cancers occur suggests that immune surveillance is imperfect; however, because some tumors escape such policing does not preclude the possibility that others may have been aborted. It is necessary therefore to explore certain questions about tumor immunity: What is the nature of tumor antigens? What host effector systems may recognize tumor cells? Is antitumor immunity effective against spontaneous neoplasms? Can immune reactions against tumors be exploited for immunotherapy?

TUMOR ANTIGENS

Antigens that elicit an immune response have been demonstrated in many experimentally induced tumors and in some human cancers. They can be broadly classified into two categories: *tumor-specific antigens* (TSAs), which are present only on tumor cells and not on any normal cells, and *tumor-associated antigens* (TAAs), which are present on tumor cells and also on some normal cells.

TUMOR-SPECIFIC ANTIGENS. TSAs are most clearly demonstrated in chemically induced tumors of rodents. In experimental model systems, tumor antigenicity is usually assessed by (1) the ability of an animal to resist a live tumor implant following previous immunization with live or killed tumor cells, (2) the ability of tumor-free host animals to resist challenge when infused with sensitized T cells from a tumor-immunized syngeneic donor, and (3) the demonstration *in vitro* of tumor cell destruction by cytotoxic T cells derived from a tumor-immunized animal. By these methods, it has been found that many chemically induced tumors express "private" or "unique" antigens not shared by other (histologically identical) tumors induced by the same chemical, even in the same animal.

The nature of TSAs in experimentally induced tumors and their existence on human tumors remained elusive until the molecular basis of T-cell recognition was understood. With the realization that T-cell receptors recognize peptides bound to the antigen-binding cleft of major histocompatibility complex (MHC) molecules (see Chapter 6), it became evident that TSAs that evoke a cytotoxic T cell response must be derived from peptides that are uniquely present within tumor cells and presented on the cell surface by class I MHC molecules. What is the nature of proteins that give rise to tumor-specific antigens? The answer to this question came from a series of elegent experiments performed by Boon and colleagues.[100] In a genetic analysis of mouse tumor cell lines, they found three mechanisms by which TSAs are derived:

- According to the first scenario, illustrated in Figure 7–39, TSAs are derived from mutant forms of normal cellular proteins. In normal cells, a diverse array of cellular proteins gives rise to peptides that are transported to the cell surface after binding to class I MHC molecules within the endoplasmic reticulum. They do not induce an immune response because T cells that recognize normal self peptide–class I complexes were clonally deleted or rendered anergic during development (see Self-Tolerance, Chapter 6). During transformation, several mutations occur; some affect oncogenes and tumor-suppressor genes, but many others affect genes that encode other normal cellular proteins, and hence altered forms of these proteins are generated. The peptide–class I complex assembled from such mutant proteins is seen as nonself, just as a complex derived from a noncellular (e.g., viral) protein would be viewed as foreign. This accounts for the antigenicity of tumor cells. The uniqueness of TSAs results from the fact that in each tumor a different array of normal cellular genes is randomly affected by mutations. Thus in different neoplasms, altered forms of distinct normal proteins are generated, each giving rise to a distinctive complex when bound by normal MHC antigens.
- Another mechanism for the formation of TSAs became evident when it was found that normal cells contain several peptides that do not possess the structural motifs required for binding to the class I MHC molecules of the host; such peptides are never displayed on the cell surface. A mutation in the gene encoding such proteins can convert the peptide into a form that can bind to

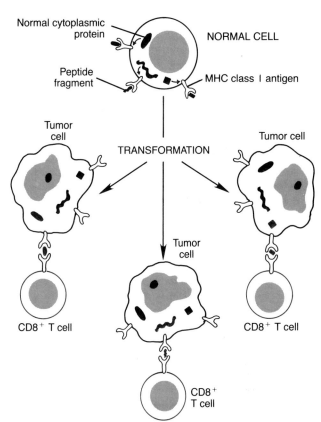

Figure 7–39. The molecular nature of tumor specific antigens (TSAs). During transformation several normal cellular proteins may be altered owing to mutations. A different protein is altered in each of the three transformed cells shown. Each mutant protein forms a distinct tumor antigen in association with MHC class I protein. The unique TSAs so formed are recognized by different CD8+ cytotoxic T lymphocytes.

MHC molecules and thus be displayed as a tumor-specific antigen on the cell surface.
- TSAs may also be generated by gene activation. During transformation, a mutation may lead to the transcription of a gene that is normally silent. Peptides derived from the protein product of the activated genes may fit into the groove of an MHC molecule and be recognized by T cells.

On the heels of these observations in mice came the discovery that approximately 40% of human melanomas, 20% of breast carcinomas, and 30% of small cell carcinomas of lung express a TSA referred to as *melanoma antigen-1* (MAGE-1). Molecular analysis has revealed that the gene encoding MAGE-1 is present in normal cells as well as in tumor cells, and there is no evidence that it is mutated in cancer cells. However, as in some animal tumors referred to earlier, *the gene is silent in normal adult cells;* whether or not it is expressed during development remains to be determined.[101] CD8+ cytotoxic T cells specific for MAGE-1 can be obtained by culturing tumor cells with patients' lymphocytes *in vitro*. There is every reason to believe that there are other human TSAs waiting to be discovered and that a given tumor may express more than one TSA.

Thus far we have considered TSAs derived from normal cellular proteins of unknown functions. Another category of tumor antigens are the products of oncogenes and anti-oncogenes. Altered versions of these genes not only may lead to growth advantage but also may generate novel antigens. In principle, these antigens would be uniquely tumor specific. Preliminary studies suggest that mutant forms of *ras* and *p53* proteins give rise to peptides that are immunogenic. The product of the *bcr-abl* fusion gene is also capable of evoking an immune response in mice. Whether or not lymphocytes from tumor-bearing patients can be sensitized to these mutant oncoproteins is currently being investigated.[102]

TUMOR-ASSOCIATED ANTIGENS. The majority of the currently recognized human tumor antigens are not unique to tumors; rather they are shared by certain normal cells. Such TAAs fall into three general categories: *tumor-associated carbohydrate antigens (TACAs), oncofetal antigens,* and *differentiation-specific antigens.* Because TAAs are normal self proteins, they do not evoke an immune response in humans and are of little functional significance in tumor rejection. Detection of these antigens is nevertheless of value in the diagnosis of certain tumors, and antibodies raised against them can be useful for immunotherapy.

TACAs have been extensively investigated as targets for antibody-based therapy.[103] They represent abnormal forms of widely expressed glycoproteins and glycolipids, such as blood group antigens and epithelial mucins. One example is a mucin-associated antigen detected in pancreatic and breast cancers. Because of incomplete glycosylation, an epitope that is concealed on fully glycosylated normal mucins becomes exposed in tumor mucins. Many other examples are discussed in a recent review.[103]

Oncofetal antigens, or embryonic antigens, are normally expressed in developing (embryonic) tissues but not in normal adult tissues. Their expression in some types of cancer cells is presumably due to derepression of genetic programs. The two best examples of oncofetal antigens—alpha-fetoprotein and carcinoembryonic antigen—are described later in this chapter.

Differentiation antigens are peculiar to the differentiation state at which cancer cells are arrested. For example, CD10 (CALLA antigen), an antigen expressed in early B lymphocytes, is expressed in B-cell leukemias and lymphomas. Similarly, prostate-specific antigen is expressed on normal as well as cancerous prostatic epithelium. Both serve as useful differentiation markers in the diagnosis of lymphoid and prostatic cancers.

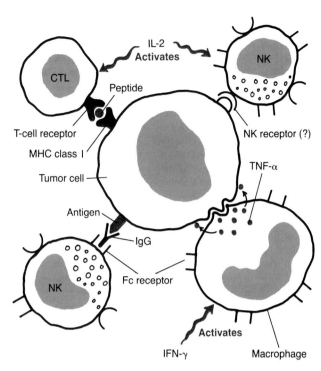

Figure 7–40. Cellular effectors of antitumor immunity and some cytokines that modulate antitumor activities. The nature of antigen recognized by T cells is depicted in Figure 7–39.

ANTITUMOR EFFECTOR MECHANISMS

Both cell-mediated and humoral immunity can have antitumor activity. The cellular effectors that mediate immunity were described in Chapter 6, so it is necessary here only to characterize them briefly (Fig. 7–40):

- *Cytotoxic T lymphocytes.* The role of specifically sensitized cytotoxic T cells in experimentally induced tumors is well established. In humans, they seem to play a protective role, chiefly against virus-associated neoplasms (e.g., EBV-induced Burkitt's lymphoma and HPV-induced tumors). The presence of HLA-restricted cytotoxic T cells within several human tumors suggests a wider role for protective T-cell immunity.
- *NK cells.* NK cells are lymphocytes that are capable of destroying tumor cells without prior sensitization. After activation with IL-2, NK cells can lyse a wide range of human tumors, including many that appear to be nonimmunogenic for T cells. So NK cells may provide the first line of defense against many tumors. Neither the target antigens recognized by NK cells nor the relevant NK-cell receptors have been identified. Because a wide variety of unrelated tumors can be lysed by NK cells without apparent specificity, it appears that the target antigens might be highly conserved tissue antigens whose expression is enhanced or altered on transformed cells. In ad-

dition to direct lysis of tumor cells, NK cells can also participate in antibody-dependent cellular cytotoxicity (ADCC), as described in Chapter 6.

- *Macrophages.* Activated macrophages exhibit somewhat selective cytotoxicity against tumor cells *in vitro*. T cells and macrophages may collaborate in antitumor reactivity because interferon gamma (IFN-γ), a T cell–derived cytokine, is a potent activator of macrophages. These cells may kill tumors by mechanisms similar to those used to kill microbes (e.g., production of reactive oxygen metabolites) or by secretion of tumor necrosis factor-alpha (TNF-α). In addition to its many other effects, this cytokine is lytic for several tumor cells.

- *Humoral* mechanisms may also participate in tumor cell destruction by two mechanisms: activation of complement and induction of ADCC by NK cells.

IMMUNOSURVEILLANCE

Given the host of possible and potential antitumor mechanisms, is there any evidence that they operate *in vivo* to prevent emergence of neoplasms? The strongest argument for the existence of immunosurveillance is the increased frequency of cancers in immunodeficient hosts. About 5% of persons with congenital immunodeficiencies develop cancers, about 200 times the expected prevalence. Analogously, immunosuppressed transplant recipients and patients with AIDS have more malignancies. It should be noted that most (but not all) of these neoplasms are lymphomas, often immunoblastic B-cell lymphomas. Particularly illustrative is the rare X-linked recessive immunodeficiency disorder termed XLP.[92] When affected boys develop an EBV infection, it does not take the usual self-limited form of infectious mononucleosis but in the vast majority of cases evolves into a fatal form of infectious mononucleosis. Approximately 25% of XLP patients develop malignant lymphoma.

Most cancers occur in persons who do not suffer from any overt immunodeficiency. It is evident then that *tumor cells must develop mechanisms to escape* or evade the immune system in immunocompetent hosts. Several such mechanisms may be operative. During tumor progression, strongly immunogenic subclones are likely to be eliminated by host effector cells, thus favoring selective outgrowth of *antigen-negative variants.* In some instances, tumor cells express *reduced levels of HLA class I molecules;* this impairs presentation of antigenic peptides to cytotoxic T cells. In addition to class I molecules, several accessory molecules, such as integrins (CD11a), are also essential for the interaction of T cells with their tumor targets. Some tumors, e.g., renal cell carcinomas, tend to escape attack by down-regulating expression of ICAM-1,

the ligand of CD11a. Many oncogenic agents (e.g., chemicals, ionizing radiation) suppress host immune responses. Tumors or tumor products may also be immunosuppressive. For example, transforming growth factor-β (TGF-β), secreted in large quantities by many tumors, is a potent immunosuppressant. In some cases, the immune response induced by the tumor (e.g., activation of suppressor T cells) may itself inhibit tumor immunity.

Although the increased occurrence of tumors in immunodeficient hosts supports the existence of immunosurveillance, the strongest argument against the concept of immunosurveillance also derives from the study of immunosuppressed patients. The most common forms of cancers in immunosuppressed and immunodeficient patients are lymphomas, notably immunoblastic B-cell lymphomas, which could be the consequence of abnormal immunoproliferative responses to microbes such as EBV or to the various therapeutic agents administered to these patients. Significantly an increased incidence of the most common forms of cancer — lung, breast, gastrointestinal tract — and multiple neoplasms might be anticipated in immunologic cripples but does not occur.

IMMUNOTHERAPY AND GENE THERAPY OF TUMORS

Even if immune surveillance exists, for the patient who develops cancer this protective mechanism has clearly failed. Can something be done to shore up defenses? The premise of immunotherapy and gene therapy is either to replace the suppressed components of the immune system or to stimulate endogenous responses.[104] Three general approaches are being tested in humans.

ADOPTIVE CELLULAR THERAPY. Because incubation of peripheral blood lymphocytes with IL-2 generates lymphokine-activated killer (LAK) cells with potent antitumor activity *in vitro*, such cells have been used for adoptive immunotherapy. The patients' blood lymphocytes are cultured with IL-2 *in vitro*, and the LAK cells (generated principally from expansion of blood NK cells) are reinfused along with additional IL-2. Human LAK trials have met with limited success in the treatment of advanced metastatic tumors.

Based on the assumption that tumor-specific cytotoxic T cells are likely to be enriched among tumor-infiltrating lymphocytes (TILs), several investigators are using expanded and activated populations of TILs for immunotherapy. Lymphocytes harvested from surgically resected tumor masses are cultured in IL-2 and then reinfused into the patient. To increase the potency of TILs, they may be transfected with the gene for TNF-α, a potent antitumor cytokine. It is hoped that cytotoxic TILs will seek and kill tumor cells and also deliver lethal concentrations of TNF-α to the tumor site. The efficacy of these modalities is being evaluated.

CYTOKINE THERAPY. Because cytokines can activate specific and nonspecific (inflammatory) host defenses, several cytokines, alone or in combination with other forms of treatment, are being evaluated for antitumor therapy. The use of IL-2 has already been mentioned. In addition, interferon-α (IFN-α) and IFN-γ, TNF-α, and hematopoietic growth factors GM-CSF and G-CSF are also being tested in cancer patients. IFN-α has already shown considerable promise. It activates NK cells, increases expression of MHC molecules on tumor cells, and is also directly cytostatic. The most impressive results with IFN-α have been obtained in the treatment of hairy cell leukemia (see Chapter 14). In addition to their proinflammatory effects, cytokines can also enhance immune recognition of tumor cells. When cytokine genes are inserted into poorly immunogenic tumor cells before infusion into experimental animals, potent antitumor responses are generated. A similar approach is now being attempted for the treatment of advanced human cancers.

ANTIBODY-BASED THERAPY. Although antibodies against TAA by themselves have not proved to be efficacious, current interest lies in using antibodies as targeting agents for delivery of cell toxins. In one approach, monoclonal antibodies against certain B-cell lymphomas are conjugated with ricin (a potent toxin), and the resulting "immunotoxin" is infused into patients. The efficacy of such "magic bullets" in the treatment of leukemias and lymphomas is under investigation.

CLINICAL FEATURES OF TUMORS

Neoplasms are essentially parasites. Some cause only trivial mischief, but others are catastrophic. All tumors, even benign ones, may cause morbidity and mortality. Moreover, every new growth requires careful appraisal lest it be cancerous. This differential comes into sharpest focus with "lumps" in the female breast. Both cancers and many benign disorders of the female breast present as palpable masses. In fact, benign lesions are more common than cancers. Although clinical evaluation may suggest one or the other, "the only unequivocally benign breast mass is the excised and anatomically diagnosed one." This is equally true of all neoplasms. There are, however, instances when adherence to this dictum must be tempered by clinical judgment. Subcutaneous lipomas, for example, are quite common and readily recognized by their soft, yielding consistency. Unless they are uncomfortable, subject to trauma, or aesthetically

disturbing, small lesions are often merely observed for significant increase in size. A few other examples might be cited, but it suffices that *with a few exceptions, all masses require anatomic evaluation.* Besides the concern malignant neoplasms arouse, even benign ones may have many adverse effects. The sections that follow consider (1) the effects of a tumor on the host, (2) the grading and clinical staging of cancer, and (3) the laboratory diagnosis of neoplasms.

EFFECTS OF TUMOR ON HOST

Obviously, cancers are far more threatening to the host than benign tumors are. Nonetheless, both types of neoplasia may cause problems because of (1) location and impingement on adjacent structures, (2) functional activity such as hormone synthesis, (3) bleeding and secondary infections when they ulcerate through adjacent natural surfaces, and (4) initiation of acute symptoms caused by either rupture or infarction. Any metastasis has the potential to produce these same consequences. Cancers may also be responsible for cachexia (wasting) or paraneoplastic syndromes.

Local and Hormonal Effects

An example of disease related to critical location is the pituitary adenoma. Although benign and possibly not productive of hormone, expansile growth of the tumor can destroy the remaining pituitary and thus lead to serious endocrinopathy. Analogously cancers arising within or metastatic to an endocrine gland may cause an endocrine insufficiency by destroying the gland. Neoplasms in the gut, both benign and malignant, may cause obstruction as they enlarge. Infrequently the peristaltic pull telescopes the neoplasm and its affected segment into the downstream segment, producing an obstructing intussusception (see Chapter 17).

Neoplasms arising in endocrine glands may produce manifestations by elaboration of hormones. Such functional activity is more typical of benign tumors than of cancers, which may be sufficiently undifferentiated to have lost such capability. A benign beta-cell adenoma of the pancreatic islets less than 1 cm in diameter may produce sufficient insulin to cause fatal hypoglycemia. In addition, nonendocrine tumors may elaborate hormones or hormone-like products. The erosive destructive growth of cancers or the expansile pressure of a benign tumor on any natural surface, such as the skin or mucosa of the gut, may cause ulcerations, secondary infections, and bleeding. Indeed, melena (blood in the stool) and hematuria, for example, are characteristic of neoplasms of the gut and urinary tract. Neoplasms may cause disease in unusual ways. A mobile organ bearing a large tumor may, in some unknown manner, undergo torsion, thereby cutting off the venous drainage and sometimes also the arterial supply. This complication most often occurs with benign ovarian neoplasms that become infarcted and so cause acute lower abdominal pain and sometimes bleeding into the peritoneal cavity. Neoplasms, benign as well as malignant, may then cause problems in varied ways, but all are far less common than the cachexia of malignancy.

Cancer Cachexia

Patients with cancer commonly suffer progressive loss of body fat and lean body mass accompanied by profound weakness, anorexia, and anemia. This wasting syndrome is referred to as cachexia.

The origins of cancer cachexia are obscure. There is little doubt, however, that cachexia is not caused by the nutritional demands of the tumor. Cancers rarely grow as rapidly as the fetus, yet many a postpartum mother when getting on the scale laments that she did not suffer just a little bit of "cachexia"! Current evidence indicates that cachexia results from the action of soluble factors such as cytokines produced either by the tumor or by the host in response to the tumor.

Clinically, anorexia is a common problem in patients with cancer, even in those who do not have mechanical obstruction caused by gastrointestinal tumors. Reduced food intake has been related to abnormalities in taste and central control of appetite, but reduced intake alone is not sufficient to explain the cachexia of malignancy. There are ill-understood metabolic changes that lead to reduced synthesis and storage of fat and increased mobilization of fatty acids from adipocytes. Many of the changes associated with cancer cachexia, including loss of appetite and alterations in fat metabolism, are mimicked by the administration of TNF-α in experimental animals. It is suspected therefore that TNF-α, produced by macrophages or possibly some tumor cells, is a mediator of the wasting syndrome that accompanies cancer.[105] TNF-α, however, is not likely to be the sole mediator of cachexia. Elevations of plasma TNF-α levels are not detected in cancer patients. Other cytokines, such as IL-1 and IFN-γ, synergize with TNF-α, and the possibility exists that several soluble factors collaborate in contributing to malnutrition in cancer patients.

Paraneoplastic Syndromes

Symptom complexes in cancer-bearing patients that cannot readily be explained, either by the local or distant spread of the tumor or by the elaboration of hormones indigenous to the tissue from which the tumor arose, are known as *paraneoplastic syndromes*.[106] These occur in about 10% of patients with advanced malignant disease. Despite their relative infrequency, paraneoplastic syndromes are important to recognize:

- First, they may represent the earliest manifestation of an occult neoplasm.
- Second, in affected patients, they may represent significant clinical problems and may even be lethal.
- Third, they may mimic metastatic disease and therefore confound treatment.

A classification of paraneoplastic syndromes and their presumed origins is presented in Table 7–9. A few comments on some of the more common and interesting syndromes follow.

The *endocrinopathies* are frequently encountered paraneoplastic syndromes. Because the native cells giving rise to the cancer are not of endocrine origin, the functional activity is referred to as *ectopic hormone production*.[107] Among the endocrinopathies, Cushing's syndrome is the most common. Approximately 50% of the patients with this endocrinopathy have carcinoma of the lung, chiefly the small cell type. It is caused by excessive production of ACTH or ACTH-like peptides. The precursor of ACTH is a large molecule known as proopiomelanocortin (POMC). Lung cancer patients with Cushing's syndrome have elevated serum levels of POMC as well as ACTH. The former is not found in serum of patients with a pituitary source of excess ACTH.

Hypercalcemia is probably the most common paraneoplastic syndrome, and conversely, overtly symptomatic hypercalcemia is most often related to some form of cancer rather than to hyperparathyroidism. Two general processes are involved in cancer-associated hypercalcemia: (1) osteolysis induced by cancer, whether primary in bone, such as multiple myeloma, or metastatic to bone from any primary lesion, and (2) the production of calcemic humoral substances by extraosseous neoplasms. Several humoral factors have been associated with hypercalcemia of malignancy.[108] Perhaps the most important is a molecule related to, but distinct from, parathyroid hormone (PTH). The so-called parathyroid hormone–related protein (PTHrP) resembles the native hormone only in its amino terminus. It shares several biologic actions with PTH and acts by binding to the PTH receptor. In contrast to PTH, PTHrP is produced by many normal tissues, including keratinocytes, muscles, bone, and ovary. The amounts produced by normal cells, however, are small. At present, the physiologic significance or normal functions of PTHrP are not clear. In addition to PTHrP, several other factors, such as IL-1, TGF-α, TNF-α, and dihydroxyvitamin D, have also been implicated in causing the hypercalcemia of malignancy. The most common neo-

Table 7-9. PARANEOPLASTIC SYNDROMES

CLINICAL SYNDROMES	MAJOR FORMS OF UNDERLYING CANCER	CAUSAL MECHANISM
Endocrinopathies		
Cushing's syndrome	Small cell carcinoma of lung Pancreatic carcinoma Neural tumors	ACTH or ACTH-like substance
Syndrome of inappropriate antidiuretic hormone secretion	Small cell carcinoma of lung Intracranial neoplasms	Antidiuretic hormone or atrial natriuretic hormones
Hypercalcemia	Squamous cell carcinoma of lung Breast carcinoma Renal carcinoma Adult T-cell leukemia/lymphoma Ovarian carcinoma	Parathyroid hormone related peptide TGF-α, TNF-α, IL-1
Hypoglycemia	Fibrosarcoma Other mesenchymal sarcomas Hepatocellular carcinoma	Insulin or insulin-like substance
Carcinoid syndrome	Bronchial adenoma (carcinoid) Pancreatic carcinoma Gastric carcinoma	Serotonin, bradykinin, ?histamine
Polycythemia	Renal carcinoma Cerebellar hemangioma Hepatocellular carcinoma	Erythropoietin
Nerve and Muscle Syndromes		
Myasthenia Disorders of the central and peripheral nervous systems	Bronchogenic carcinoma Breast carcinoma	?Immunologic, ?toxic
Dermatologic Disorders		
Acanthosis nigricans	Gastric carcinoma Lung carcinoma Uterine carcinoma	?Immunologic, ?secretion of epidermal growth factor
Dermatomyositis	Bronchogenic, breast carcinoma	?Immunologic, ?toxic
Osseous, Articular, and Soft Tissue Changes		
Hypertrophic osteoarthropathy and clubbing of the fingers	Bronchogenic carcinoma	Unknown
Vascular and Hematologic Changes		
Venous thrombosis (Trousseau's phenomenon)	Pancreatic carcinoma Bronchogenic carcinoma Other cancers	Tumor products (mucins) that activate clotting
Nonbacterial thrombotic endocarditis	Advanced cancers	Hypercoagulability
Anemia	Thymic neoplasms	Unknown
Others		
Nephrotic syndrome	Various cancers	Tumor antigens, immune complexes

plasm associated with hypercalcemia is the squamous cell bronchogenic carcinoma, rather than small cell cancer of the lung (more often associated with endocrinopathies).

The *neuromyopathic paraneoplastic syndromes* take diverse forms, such as peripheral neuropathies, cortical cerebellar degeneration, a polymyopathy resembling polymyositis, and a myasthenic syndrome similar to *myasthenia gravis.* The etiology of these syndromes is poorly understood. In some cases, antibodies, presumably induced against tumor cells that cross-react with neuronal cells, have been detected.[109]

Acanthosis nigricans is characterized by gray-black patches of verrucous hyperkeratosis on the skin. This disorder occurs rarely as a genetically determined disease in juveniles or adults. In addition, particularly in those over the age of 40, the appearance of such lesions is associated in about 50% of cases with some form of cancer. Sometimes the skin changes appear before discovery of the cancer.[110]

Clubbing of fingers and hypertrophic osteoarthropathy, described more fully in Chapter 27, are encountered in 1 to 10% of patients with bronchogenic carcinomas. Rarely, other forms of cancer are involved. Although the osteoarthropathy is seldom seen in noncancer patients, clubbing of the fingertips may be encountered in liver diseases, diffuse lung disease, congenital cyanotic heart disease, ulcerative colitis, and other disorders.

Several *vascular and hematologic manifestations* may appear in association with a variety of forms of cancer. As mentioned in the earlier discussion of thrombosis (see Chapter 4), *migratory thrombophlebitis* (Trousseau's syndrome) may be encountered in association with deep-seated cancers, most often with carcinomas of the pancreas or lung. Disseminated intravascular coagulation (DIC) may complicate a diversity of clinical disorders, as pointed out in Chapter 13. Acute DIC is most commonly associated with acute promyelocytic leukemia and prostatic adenocarcinoma. Bland, small, nonbacterial fibrinous vegetations sometimes form on the cardiac valve leaflets (more often on left-sided valves), particularly in patients with advanced mucin-secreting adenocarcinomas. These lesions, called *nonbacterial thrombotic endocarditis*, are described further in Chapter 12. The vegetations are potential sources of emboli that can further complicate the course of cancer.

GRADING AND STAGING OF TUMORS

Comparison of end results of various forms of cancer treatment, particularly between clinics, requires some degree of comparability of the neoplasms being assayed. To this end, systems have been derived to express, at least in semiquantitative terms, the level of differentiation, or *grade*, and extent of spread of a cancer within the patient, or *stage*, as parameters of the clinical gravity of the disease.

Grading of a cancer is based on the degree of differentiation of the tumor cells and the number of mitoses within the tumor as presumed correlates of the neoplasm's aggressiveness. Thus cancers are classified as grades I to IV with increasing anaplasia. Criteria for the individual grades vary with each form of neoplasia and so are not detailed here, but all attempt, in essence, to judge the extent to which the tumor cells resemble or fail to resemble their normal counterparts. It should be noted that although histologic grading is useful, the correlation between histologic appearance and biologic behavior is less than perfect. In recognition of this problem and to avoid spurious quantification, it is common practice to characterize a particular neoplasm in descriptive terms, for example, well-differentiated, mucin-secreting adenocarcinoma of the stomach, or highly undifferentiated, retroperitoneal malignant tumor—probably sarcoma. In general, with a few exceptions, such as soft tissue sarcomas, grading of cancers has proved of less clinical value than has staging.

The staging of cancers is based on the size of the primary lesion, its extent of spread to regional lymph nodes, and the presence or absence of blood-borne metastases. Two major staging systems are currently in use, one developed by the Union Internationale Contre Cancer (UICC) and the other by the American Joint Committee (AJC) on Cancer Staging. The UICC employs a so-called *TNM system—T* for primary tumor, *N* for regional lymph node involvement, and *M* for metastases. The TNM staging varies for each specific form of cancer, but there are general principles. With increasing size, the primary lesion is characterized as T1 to T4. T0 is added to indicate an in situ lesion, N0 would mean no nodal involvement, whereas N1–N3 would denote involvement of an increasing number and range of nodes. M0 signifies no distant metastases, whereas M1 or sometimes M2 indicates the presence of blood-borne metastases and some judgment as to their number.

The AJC employs a somewhat different nomenclature and divides all cancers into stages 0 to IV, incorporating within each of these stages the size of the primary lesion as well as the presence of nodal spread and distant metastases. The use of these systems of staging and more details are described later in the consideration of specific tumors. It merits emphasis here, however, that staging of neoplastic disease has assumed great importance in the selection of the best form of therapy for the patient. Indeed, staging has proved to be of greater clinical value than grading.

LABORATORY DIAGNOSIS OF CANCER

Every year the approach to laboratory diagnosis of cancer becomes more complex, more sophisticated, and more specialized. It may come as a rude surprise that for virtually every neoplasm mentioned in this text, a number of subcategories have been characterized by the experts; but we must walk before we can run. Each of the following sections attempts to present the "state of the art," avoiding details of method.

HISTOLOGIC AND CYTOLOGIC METHODS. The laboratory diagnosis of cancer is, in most instances, not difficult. The two ends of the benign-malignant spectrum pose no problems; however, in the middle lies a "no man's land" where wise men tread cautiously. This issue was sufficiently emphasized earlier; here the focus is on the roles of the clinician (often a surgeon) and the pathologist in facilitating the correct diagnosis.

Clinicians tend to underestimate the important contributions they make to the diagnosis of a neoplasm. Clinical data are invaluable for optimal pathologic diagnosis. Radiation changes in the skin or mucosa can be similar to cancer. Sections taken from a healing fracture can mimic remarkably an

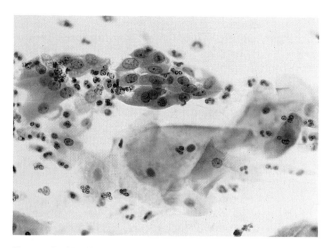

Figure 7–41. Normal cervicovaginal smear shows large flattened squamous cells and groups of metaplastic cells; interspersed are some neutrophils. There are no malignant cells. (Courtesy of Dr. P.K. Gupta, Department of Pathology and Laboratory Medicine, University of Pennsylvania Medical Center, Philadelphia.)

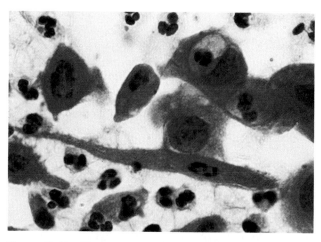

Figure 7–42. Abnormal cervicovaginal smear shows numerous malignant cells, which have pleomorphic, hyperchromatic nuclei; interspersed are some normal polymorphonuclear leukocytes. (Courtesy of Dr. P.K. Gupta, Department of Pathology and Laboratory Medicine, University of Pennsylvania Medical Center, Philadelphia.)

osteosarcoma. Moreover, the laboratory evaluation of a lesion can be only as good as the specimen made available for examination. It must be adequate, representative, and properly preserved. Several sampling approaches are available: (1) excision or biopsy, (2) needle aspiration, and (3) cytologic smears. When excision of a small lesion is not possible, selection of an appropriate site for biopsy of a large mass requires awareness that the margins may not be representative and the center largely necrotic. Analogously with disseminated lymphoma (involving many nodes), those in the inguinal region draining large areas of the body often have reactive changes that may mask neoplastic involvement. Appropriate preservation of the specimen is obvious, yet it involves such actions as prompt immersion in a usual fixative (for example, formalin solution) or instead preservation of a portion in a special fixative (e.g., glutaraldehyde) for electron microscopy or prompt refrigeration to permit optimal hormone or receptor analysis. Requesting "quick-frozen section" diagnosis is sometimes desirable, for example, in determining the nature of a breast lesion or in evaluating the margins of an excised cancer to ascertain that the entire neoplasm has been removed. This method allows sectioning of a "quick-frozen" sample and permits histologic evaluation within minutes. In experienced, competent hands, frozen-section diagnosis is highly accurate, but there are particular instances in which the better histologic detail provided by the more time-consuming routine methods is needed—for example, when extremely radical surgery, such as the amputation of an extremity, may be indicated. Better to wait a day or two despite the drawbacks than to perform inadequate or unnecessary surgery.

Fine needle aspiration of tumors provides another approach that is widely used. The procedure involves aspirating cells and attendant fluid with a small-bore needle, followed by cytologic examination of the stained smear. This method is used most commonly for the assessment of readily palpable lesions in sites such as the breast, thyroid, lymph nodes, and, with the aid of a special needle, the prostate. Modern imaging techniques enable the method to be extended to lesions in deep-seated structures, such as pelvic lymph nodes. Fine needle aspiration is less invasive and more rapidly performed than are needle biopsies. In experienced hands, it is an extremely reliable, rapid, and useful technique.

Cytologic (Papanicolaou or "Pap") smears provide yet another method for the detection of cancer. This approach is widely used for the discovery of carcinoma of the cervix, often at an in situ stage, but it is also used with many other forms of suspected malignancy, such as endometrial carcinoma, bronchogenic carcinoma, bladder and prostatic tumors, and gastric carcinomas; for the identification of tumor cells in abdominal, pleural, joint, and cerebrospinal fluids; and, less commonly, with other forms of neoplasia.

As pointed out earlier, cancer cells have lowered cohesiveness and exhibit a range of morphologic changes encompassed by the term anaplasia. Thus, shed cells can be evaluated for the features of anaplasia indicative of their origin in a cancer (Figs. 7–41 and 7–42). In contrast to the histologist's task, judgment here must be rendered based on individual cell cytology or (at most, perhaps) on that of a clump of a few cells without the supporting evidence of architectural disarray, loss of orientation of one cell to another, and (perhaps most

Table 7–10. INTERMEDIATE FILAMENTS AND THEIR DISTRIBUTION

Keratins	Carcinomas
	Mesothelioma
Desmin	Muscle tumors: smooth, striated
Vimentin	Mesenchymal tumors, some carcinomas
Glial filaments	Gliomatous tumors
Neurofilaments	Neuronal tumors

important) evidence of invasion. This method permits differentiation among normal, dysplastic, and cancerous cells and in addition permits the recognition of cellular changes characteristic of carcinoma in situ. The gratifying control of cervical cancer is the best testament to the value of the cytologic method.

Although histology and exfoliative cytology remain the most commonly used methods in the diagnosis of cancer, new techniques are being constantly added to the tools of the surgical pathologist. Some, such as immunocytochemistry, are already well established and widely used; others, including molecular methods, are rapidly finding their way into the "routine" category. Only some highlights of these diagnostic modalities are presented.

IMMUNOCYTOCHEMISTRY. The availability of specific monoclonal antibodies has greatly facilitated the identification of cell products or surface markers. For example, antibodies directed against intermediate filaments have proved to be of value in the classification of otherwise poorly differentiated tumors.[111] Table 7–10 lists the five major types of intermediate filaments and the types of tumors in which they are found. The presence of cytokeratin (detected by immunoperoxidase staining), for example, allows distinction between a poorly differentiated carcinoma and a large cell lymphoma. Both may look similar by routine staining, but only carcinomas contain keratin (Fig. 7–43). Vimentin, the predominant intermediate filament of mesenchymal cells, is less specific because certain epithelial tumors (e.g., renal cell carcinomas) may coexpress keratin and vimentin. Desmin is specific for neoplasms showing muscle differentiation.

Immunocytochemistry (in conjunction with immunofluorescence) has also proved useful in the identification and classification of tumors arising from T and B lymphocytes and from mononuclear-phagocytic cells. Monoclonal antibodies directed against various lymphohemopoietic cells are listed in Chapter 14. Immunocytochemistry can also be applied for detection of molecular changes within tumor. For example, mutations of the p53 gene lead to accumulation of the mutant protein within tumor cells, which can be readily detected in paraffin-embedded tissues.[112] Immunocytochemical de-

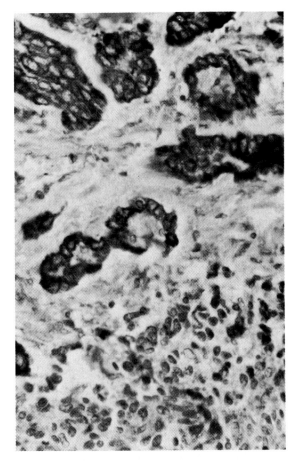

Figure 7–43. Antikeratin immunoperoxidase stain of a carcinoma of the lung. The atypical gland patterns above are stained dark, indicating a positive antikeratin reaction.

tection of the p53 protein is virtually restricted to neoplastic cells. Immunostaining of oncogene products (e.g., c-erb B2) allows detection of gene amplification.

MOLECULAR DIAGNOSIS. Molecular biology has moved from the research laboratory to the bedside. There are several examples of molecular techniques—some established, others emerging—that have been applied for diagnosis or in some cases predicting behavior of tumors. It is possible to identify T-cell and B-cell neoplasms based on clonal rearrangement of their receptor genes by using Southern blot analysis. Amplification of the N-myc oncogene (neuroblastomas) and the c-erb B2 gene (breast carcinomas) has proved to be of prognostic value. The extent of amplification can be detected by Southern blot analysis of tumor DNA or by Northern blot analysis of tumor RNA. Precise molecular diagnosis of chronic myeloid leukemia is established by the detection of bcr-abl fusion gene. Following treatment of this leukemia, the presence of minimal disease or the onset of a relapse can also be monitored by polymerase chain reaction—

Table 7–11. SELECTED TUMOR MARKERS

MARKERS	ASSOCIATED CANCERS
Hormones	
Human chorionic gonadotropin	Trophoblastic tumors, nonseminomatous testicular tumors
Calcitonin	Medullary carcinoma of thyroid
Catecholamine and metabolites	Pheochromocytoma and related tumors
Ectopic hormones	See Paraneoplastic Syndromes in Table 7–9
Oncofetal Antigens	
Alpha-fetoprotein	Liver cell cancer, nonseminomatous germ cell tumors of testis
Carcinoembryonic antigen	Carcinomas of the colon, pancreas, lung, stomach, and breast
Isoenzymes	
Prostatic acid phosphatase	Prostate cancer
Neuron-specific enolase	Small cell cancer of lung, neuroblastoma
Specific Proteins	
Immunoglobulins	Multiple myeloma and other gammopathies
Prostate-specific antigen	Prostate cancer
Mucins and Other Glycoproteins	
CA-125	Ovarian cancer
CA-19-9	Colon cancer, pancreatic cancer
CA-15-3	Breast cancer

based amplification of *bcr-abl* transcripts. The expression of the MyoD1 gene is restricted to cells of muscle lineage; hence the presence of MyoD1 transcripts allows the diagnosis of rhabdomyosarcomas in difficult cases. Mutations of the K-*ras* gene detected in stool samples have been proposed as a noninvasive method for the diagnosis of colonic tumors.[113] Several other diagnostic applications of recombinant DNA technology are cited with the discussion of specific tumors.

FLOW CYTOMETRY. Flow cytometry can rapidly and quantitatively measure several individual cell characteristics, such as membrane antigens and the DNA content of tumor cells. Identification of cell surface antigens by flow cytometry is widely utilized in the classification of leukemias, and lymphomas (see Chapter 14). Flow cytometric detection of ploidy is applied to specimens from a variety of sources, such as fresh-frozen surgical biopsy specimens (from which nuclei can be extracted), pleural or peritoneal effusions associated with cancer, bone marrow aspirations, and cells obtained by irrigation of the urinary bladder. A relationship between abnormal DNA content and prognosis is becoming apparent for a variety of malignancies. In general, aneuploidy seems to be associated with poorer prognosis in early-stage breast cancer, carcinoma of the urinary bladder, lung cancer, colorectal cancer, and prostate cancer.

TUMOR MARKERS. Tumor markers are biochemical indicators of the presence of a tumor. They include cell surface antigens, cytoplasmic proteins, enzymes, and hormones. In clinical practice, however, the term usually refers to a molecule that can be detected in plasma or other body fluids.[114] *Tumor markers cannot be construed as primary modalities for the diagnosis of cancer.* Their main utility in clinical medicine has been as a laboratory test to support the diagnosis. Some tumor markers are also of value in determining the response to therapy and in indicating relapse during the follow-up period.

A host of tumor markers have been described, and new ones appear every year.[115,116] Only a few have stood the test of time and proved to have clinical usefulness. The application of several markers, listed in Table 7–11, is considered with specific forms of neoplasia discussed in other chapters, so only two widely used examples will suffice here.

Carcinoembryonic antigen (CEA), normally produced in embryonic tissue of the gut, pancreas, and liver, is a complex glycoprotein that is elaborated by many different neoplasms. Depending on the serum level adopted as a significant elevation, it is variously reported to be positive in 60 to 90% of colorectal, 50 to 80% of pancreatic, and 25 to 50% of gastric and breast carcinomas. Much less consistently, elevated CEA has been described in other forms of cancer. CEA elevations have also been reported in many benign disorders, such as alcoholic cirrhosis, hepatitis, ulcerative colitis, Crohn's disease, and others. Occasionally levels of this antigen are elevated in apparently healthy smokers. Thus *CEA assays lack both specificity and the sensitivity required for the detection of early cancers.* Preoperative CEA levels have some bearing on prognosis because the level of elevation is correlated with body burden of tumor. In colon cancer, the levels correlate with the widely used Dukes grading system (see Chapter 17). In patients with CEA-positive colon cancers, the presence of elevated CEA levels 6 weeks after therapy indicates residual disease. Recurrence is indicated by a rising CEA level, with an increase in tumor marker level often preceding clinically detectable disease. Serum CEA is also useful in monitoring the treatment of metastatic breast cancer.

Alpha-fetoprotein (AFP) is another well-established tumor marker, discussed in some detail in Chapter 22. This glycoprotein is synthesized normally early in fetal life by the yolk sac, fetal liver, and fetal gastrointestinal tract. Abnormal plasma elevations are encountered in adults with cancer arising principally in the liver and germ cells of the testis. Elevated plasma AFP is also found less regularly in carcinomas of the colon, lung, and pancreas. Similar to CEA, non-neoplastic conditions, including cirrhosis, toxic liver injury, hepatitis, and pregnancy (especially with fetal distress or death), also may cause minimal to moderate plasma elevations of AFP. Although there is then some problem with specificity, marked elevations of the plasma AFP level have proved to be a useful indicator of hepatocellular carcinomas and germ cell tumors of the testis. AFP levels decline rapidly after surgical resection of liver cell cancer or treatment of germ cell tumors. Serial post-therapy measurements of AFP (and human chorionic gonadotropin) levels in patients with germ cell tumors of the testis provide a sensitive index of response to therapy and recurrence.

This cursory overview suffices to indicate the many laboratory approaches in use for detection and diagnosis of tumors.

1. Boring, C.C., et al.: Cancer statistics, 1994. CA *44*:7, 1994.
2. Willis, R.A.: The Spread of Tumors in the Human Body. London, Butterworth & Co., 1952.
3. Ponder B.A.J.: Genetic predisposition to cancer. *In* Holland, J.F., et al. (eds.): Cancer Medicine, 3rd ed. Philadelphia, Lea & Febiger, 1993, p. 198.
4. Ponder, B.A.J.: Inherited predisposition to cancer. Trends Genet. *6*:213, 1990.
5. Digweed, M.: Human genetic instability syndromes: Single gene defects with increased risk of cancer. Toxicol. Lett. *67*:259, 1993.
6. Gough, A.C., et al.: Identification of the primary gene defect at the cytochrome P450 CYP2D locus. Nature *347*:773, 1990.
7. Klein, G.: Oncogenes. *In* Holland, J.F., et al. (eds.): Cancer Medicine, 3rd ed. Philadelphia, Lea & Febiger, 1993, p. 65.
8. Weinberg, R.A.: The integration of molecular genetics into cancer management. Cancer *70*:1653, 1992.
9. Pusztal, L., et al.: Growth factors: Regulation of normal and neoplastic growth. J. Pathol. *169*:191, 1993.
10. Goldfarb, M.: The fibroblast growth factor family. Cell Growth Diff. *1*:439, 1990.
11. Aaronson, S.A., and Tronick, S.R.: Growth factors. *In* Holland, J.F., et al. (eds.): Cancer Medicine, 3rd ed. Philadelphia, Lea & Febiger, p. 33.
12. Gullick, W.J.: Prevalence of aberrant expression of the epidermal growth factor receptors in human cancers. Br. Med. Bull. *47*:87, 1991.
13. Hynes, N.E.: Amplification and overexpression of the *erb B*-2 gene in human tumors: Its involvement in tumor development, significance as a prognostic factor, and potential as a target for cancer therapy. Semin. Cancer Biol. *4*:19, 1993.
14. Holmes, W.E., et al.: Identification of heregulin, a specific activator of p185erbB2. Science *249*:1552, 1992.
15. Anderson, M.W., et al.: Role of proto-oncogene activation in carcinogenesis. Environ. Health Perspect. *98*:13, 1992.
16. Feig, L.: The many roads that lead to *Ras*. Science *260*:767, 1993.
17. McCormick, F.: How receptors turn *Ras* on. Nature *363*:15, 1993.
18. Polakis, P., and McCormick, F.: Interactions between p21ras proteins and their GTPase activating proteins. Cancer Surv. *12*:25, 1992.
19. Koskinen, P.J., and Alitalo, K.: Role of *myc* amplification and overexpression in cell growth, differentiation, and death. Semin. Cancer Biol. *4*:3, 1993.
20. Kato, G.J., and Dang, C.V.: Function of the c-*myc* oncoprotein. FASEB J. *6*:3065, 1992.
21. Sheer, D.: Chromosomes and cancer. *In* Franks, L.M., and Teich, N.M. (eds.): Introduction to the Cellular and Molecular Biology of Cancer, 2nd ed. Oxford, Oxford University Press, 1991, p. 289.
22. Sawyers, C.L., et al.: Leukemia and disruption of normal hematopoiesis. Cell *64*:337, 1991.
23. Nichols, J., and Nimer, S.D.: Transcription factors, translocation, and leukemia. Blood *80*:2953, 1992.
24. Schwab, M.: Amplification of N-*myc* as a prognostic marker for patients with neuroblastoma. Semin. Cancer Biol. *4*:13, 1993.
25. Benedict, W.F., et al.: Role of retinoblastoma gene in the initiation and progression of human cancer. J. Clin. Invest. *85*:988, 1990.
26. Fearon, E.R., and Vogelstein, B.: Tumor suppressor genes and cancer. *In* Holland, J.F., et al. (eds.): Cancer Medicine, 3rd ed. Philadelphia, Lea & Febiger, 1993, p. 77.
27. Zambetti, G.P., and Levine, A.J.: A comparison of the biologic activities of wild type and mutant p53. FASEB J. *7*:855, 1993.
28. Chang, F., et al.: The p53 tumor suppressor gene as a common cellular target in human carcinogenesis. Am. J. Gastroenterol. *88*:174, 1993.
29. Frebourg, T., and Friend, S.H.: Cancer risks from germline p53 mutations. J. Clin. Invest. *90*:1637, 1992.
30. Donehower, L.A., et al.: Mice deficient for p53 are developmentally normal but susceptible to spontaneous tumors. Nature *356*:215, 1992.
31. Powell, S.M., et al.: APC mutations occur early during colorectal tumorigenesis. Nature *359*:235, 1992.
32. Horii, A., et al.: Frequent somatic mutations of the APC gene in human pancreatic cancer. Cancer Res. *52*:6696, 1992.
33. Uchino, S., et al.: Frequent loss of heterozygosity at the DCC locus in gastric cancer. Cancer Res. *52*:3099, 1992.
34. Maw, M.A., et al.: A third Wilms' tumor locus on chromosome 16q. Cancer Res. *52*:3094, 1992.
35. Fearon, E.R.: Genetic alterations underlying colorectal tumorigenesis. Cancer Surv. *12*:119, 1992.
36. Latif, F., et al.: Identification of the von Hippel–Lindau disease tumor suppressor gene. Science *260*:1317, 1993.
37. Goodrich, D.W., and Lee, W.: Abrogation by c-*myc* of G₁ phase arrest induced by Rb protein but not by p53. Nature *360*:177, 1992.
38. Wiman, K.: The retinoblastoma gene: Role in cell cycle control and cell differentiation. FASEB J. *7*:841, 1993.
39. Weinberg, R.A.: The retinoblastoma gene and gene product. Cancer Surv. *12*:43, 1992.
39a. Harris C.C., and Hollstein, M.: Clinical implications of the p53 tumor suppressor gene. N. Engl. J. Med. *329*:1318, 1993.
40. Lane, D.P.: p53, guardian of the genome. Nature *358*:15, 1992.
41. Lane, D.P.: A death in the life of p53. Nature *362*:786, 1993.
42. Kaklamanis, L., et al.: p53 expression in colorectal adenomas. Am. J. Pathol. *142*:87, 1993.
43. Korsmeyer, S.J.: Bcl-2: An antidote to programmed cell death. Cancer Surv. *12*:105, 1992.
44. Hockenberry, D.M., et al.: Bcl-2 functions in an antioxidant pathway to prevent apoptosis. Cell *75*:241, 1993.
45. Adams, J.M., and Cory, S.: Oncogene cooperation in leukemogenesis. Cancer Surv. *15*:119, 1992.

46. Sugimura, T., et al.: Multiple genetic alterations in human carcinogenesis. Environ. Health Perspect. 98:5, 1992.
47. Marx, J.: Research news: New colon cancer gene discovered. Science 260:751, 1993.
47a. Bodmer, W., et al.: Genetic steps in colorectal cancer. Nature Genetics 6:217, 1994.
48. Solomon, E., et al.: Chromosome aberrations and cancer. Science 254:1153, 1991.
49. Nowell, P.C.: Cancer, chromosomes, and genes. Lab. Invest. 66:407, 1992.
50. Tannock, I.F.: Cell proliferation. In Tannock, I.F., and Hill, R.P. (eds.): The Basic Science of Oncology, 2nd ed. New York, McGraw-Hill, 1992, p. 154.
51. Folkman, J.: Tumor angiogenesis. In Holland, J.F., et al. (eds.): Cancer Medicine. 3rd ed. Philadelphia, Lea & Febiger, 1993, p. 153.
52. Macchiarini, P., et al.: Relation of neovascularization to metastasis of non–small cell lung cancer. Lancet 340:145, 1992.
53. Horak, E.R., et al.: Angiogenesis, assessed by platelet/endothelial adhesion molecule antibodies, as indicator of node metastases and survival in breast cancer. Lancet 340:1120, 1992.
54. Berkman, R.A., et al.: Expression of vascular permeability factor/vascular endothelial growth factor gene in central nervous system neoplasms. J. Clin. Invest. 91:153, 1993.
55. Bouck, N.: Tumor angiogenesis: The role of oncogenes and tumor suppressor genes. Cancer Cells. 2:179, 1990.
56. Hill, R.P.: Tumor progression: Potential role of unstable genomic changes. Cancer Metastasis Rev. 9:137, 1990.
57. Hart, I.R., and Saini, A.: Biology of tumor metastasis. Lancet 339:1453, 1992.
58. Takeichi, M.: Cadherin cell adhesion receptors as a morphogenetic regulator. Science 251:1451, 1991.
59. Dorudi, S., et al.: E-Cadherin expression in colorectal cancer. Am. J. Pathol. 142:981, 1993.
60. Liotta, L.A., et al.: Invasion and metastasis. In Holland, JF., et al. (eds.): Cancer Medicine, 3rd ed. Philadelphia, Lea & Febiger, 1993, p. 138.
61. Cioce, V., et al.: Increased expression of laminin receptor in human colon cancer. J. Natl. Cancer Inst. 83:29, 1991.
62. Albelda, S.M.: Role of integrins and other cell-adhesion molecules in tumor progression and metastasis. Lab. Invest. 68:4, 1993.
63. Steeg, P.S.: Invasion and metastasis. Curr. Opin. Oncol. 4:134, 1992.
64. Alvarez, O.A., et al.: Inhibition of collagenolytic activity and metastasis of tumor cells by recombinant human tissue inhibitor of metalloproteinases. J. Natl. Cancer Inst. 82:589, 1990.
65. Tandon, A.K., et al.: Cathepsin D and prognosis in breast cancer. N. Engl. J. Med. 322:297, 1990.
66. Nabi, I.R., et al.: Autocrine motility factor and its receptor: Role in cell locomotion and metastasis. Cancer Metastasis Rev. 11:5, 1992.
67. Kahn, P.: Cancer research: Adhesion protein studies provide new clue to metastases. Science 257:614, 1992.
68. Rusciano, D., and Burger, M.: Why do cancer cells metastasize into particular organs. Bioessays 14:185, 1992.
69. Chambers, A.F., and Tuck, A.B.: Ras-responsive genes and tumor metastasis. Crit. Rev. Oncog. 4:95, 1993.
70. Hart, I.R., and Easty, D.: Identification of genes controlling metastatic behavior. Br. J. Cancer 63:9, 1991.
71. Myeroff, L.L., and Markowitz, S.D.: Increased nm23-H1 and nm23-H2 mRNA expression and absence of mutations in colon carcinomas of low and high metastatic potential. J. Natl. Cancer Inst. 85:147, 1993.
72. Leone, A., et al.: Evidence for nm23 overexpression, DNA amplification and mutation in aggressive childhood neuroblastomas. Oncogene 8:855, 1993.
73. Harris, C.C.: Chemical and physical carcinogenesis: Advances and perspectives for the 1990s. Cancer Res. (Suppl.) 51:5023s, 1991.
74. Farber, E., and Sarma, D.S.R.: Hepatocarcinogenesis: A dynamic cellular perspective. Lab. Invest. 56:4, 1987.
75. Slaga, T.J. (ed.): Mechanisms of Tumor-Promotion: Tumor Promotion in Internal Organs. Boca Raton, FL, CRC Press, 1983.
76. Wigley, C., and Balmain, A.: Chemical carcinogenesis and precancer. In Franks, L.M., and Teich, N.M. (eds.): Introduction to the Cellular and Molecular Biology of Cancer, 2nd ed. Oxford, Oxford University Press, 1991, p. 148.
77. Vogelstein, B., and Kinzler, K.W.: Carcinogens leave fingerprints. Nature 355:209, 1992.
78. Hsu, I., et al.: Mutational hot spot in the p53 gene in human hepatocellular carcinomas. Nature 350:427, 1991.
79. Cohen, S.M., and Ellwein, L.B.: Genetic errors, cell proliferation, and carcinogenesis. Cancer Res. 51:6493, 1991.
80. Kleinfeld, M., et al.: Bladder tumors in a coal tar dye plant. Ind. Med. Surg. 35:570, 1966.
81. Pitot, H.C.: Fundamentals of Oncology, 3rd. ed. New York, Marcel Dekker, 1986, p. 228.
82. Ellwein, L.B., and Cohen, S.M.: The health risks of saccharin revisited. Toxicology 20:311, 1990.
83. Rauth, A.M.: Radiation carcinogenesis. In Tannock, I.F., and Hill, R.P. (eds.): The Basic Science of Oncology, 2nd ed. New York, McGraw-Hill, 1992, p. 119.
84. Cleaver, J.E., and Mitchell, D.L.: Ultraviolet radiation carcinogenesis. In Holland, J.F., et al. (eds.): Cancer Medicine, 3rd ed. Philadelphia, Lea & Febiger, 1993, p. 245.
85. Kripke, M.L.: Effects of UV radiation on tumor immunity. J. Natl. Cancer Inst. 82:1392, 1990.
86. Kanjilal, S., et al.: Ultraviolet radiation in the pathogenesis of skin cancers: Involvement of ras and p53 genes. Cancer Bull. 45:205, 1993.
87. Smith, P.J.: Carcinogenesis: Molecular defenses against carcinogens. Br. Med. Bull. 47:3, 1991.
88. Hoeijmakers, J.H.J., and Bootsma, D.: DNA repair: Two pieces of the puzzle. Nature Genet. 1:313, 1992.
89. Lancaster, W.D.: Viral role in cervical and liver cancer. Cancer 70:1794, 1993.
90. Vousden, K.: Interaction of human papillomavirus transforming proteins with products of tumor suppressor genes. FASEB J. 7:872, 1993.
91. Arbeit, J.M., et al.: Neuroepithelial carcinomas in mice transgenic with human papilloma virus type 16 E6/E7 ORFs. Am. J. Pathol. 142:1187, 1993.
92. Purtillo, D.T., et al.: Epstein-Barr virus–associated lymphoproliferative disorders. Lab. Invest. 67:5, 1992.
93. Straus, S.E., et al.: Epstein-Barr virus infections: Biology, pathogenesis, and management. Ann. Intern. Med. 118:45, 1993.
94. Young, L.S., and Renee, M.: Epstein-Barr virus, lymphomas, and Hodgkin's disease. Semin. Cancer Biol. 3:273, 1992.
95. Raab-Traub, N.: Epstein-Barr virus and nasopharyngeal carcinoma. Semin. Cancer Biol. 3:297, 1992.
96. Buendia, M.A.: Mammalian hepatitis B viruses and primary liver cancer. Semin. Cancer Biol. 3:309, 1992.
97. Ganem, D.: Oncogenic viruses: Of marmosets and men. Nature 347:230, 1990.
98. Kekule, A.S., et al.: Hepatitis B virus transactivator HBx uses a tumor promoter signalling pathway. Nature 361:742, 1993.
99. Sherman, M.P., et al.: Human T-cell lymphoma/leukemia retroviruses and malignancy. Cancer Treat. Res. 64:79, 1993.
100. Boon, T.: Teaching the immune system to fight cancer. Sci. Am. 268:82, 1993.
101. Carrel, S., and Johnson, J.P.: Immunologic recognition of malignant melanoma by autologous lymphocytes. Curr. Opin. Oncol. 5:383, 1993.

102. Lynch, S.A., and Houghton, A.N.: Cancer immunology. Curr. Opin. Oncol. 5:145, 1993.

103. Hakamori, S.: Possible function of tumor-associated carbohydrate antigens. Curr. Opin. Immunol. 3:646, 1991.

104. Rosenberg, S.A.: Gene therapy for cancer. J.A.M.A. 268:2416, 1992.

105. Beutler, B.: Cytokines and cancer cachexia. Hosp. Pract. 28:45, 1993.

106. Richardson, G.E., and Johnson, B.E.: Paraneoplastic syndromes in thoracic malignancies. Curr. Opin. Oncol. 3:320, 1991.

107. Odell, W.D.: Paraendocrine syndromes of cancer. Adv. Intern. Med. 34:325, 1989.

108. Rosol, T.J., and Capen, C.C.: Mechanisms of cancer induced hypercalcemia. Lab. Invest. 67:680, 1992.

109. Anderson, N.E.: Anti-neuronal antibodies and neurologic paraneoplastic syndromes. Aust. N.Z. J. Med. Sci. 19:379, 1989.

110. Poole, S., and Fenske, N.A.: Cutaneous markers of internal malignancy. II. Paraneoplastic dermatoses and environmental carcinogens. J. Am. Acad. Dermatol. 28:147, 1993.

111. Ordonez, N.G.: Immunocytochemistry in the diagnosis of soft tissue sarcomas. Cancer Bull. 45:13, 1993.

112. Porter, P.L., et al.: Widespread p53 overexpression in human malignant tumors. Am. J. Pathol. 140:145, 1992.

113. Sidransky, D., et al.: Identification of ras oncogene mutations in the stool of patients with curable colorectal tumors. Science 256:102, 1992.

114. Liu, F.J.: Serum tumor marker assays in cancer patient care. Cancer Bull. 45:55, 1993.

115. Virji, M.A., et al.: Tumor markers in cancer diagnosis and prognosis. CA 38:104, 1988.

116. Carney, W.: Human tumor antigens and specific tumor therapy. Immunol. Today 9:363, 1988.

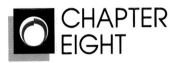

CHAPTER EIGHT

Infectious Diseases

JOHN SAMUELSON, M.D., Ph.D., and FRANZ VON LICHTENBERG, M.D.

GENERAL PRINCIPLES OF MICROBIAL PATHOGENESIS

Despite improved living conditions, widespread vaccination, and availability of effective antibiotics, infectious diseases continue to take a heavy toll in the United States among persons with acquired immune deficiency syndrome (AIDS), debilitated with chronic disease, or treated with immunosuppressive drugs. In developing countries, unsanitary living conditions and malnutrition contribute to a massive burden of infectious disease that kills more than 10 million persons each year.[1] Most of these deaths are among children, who suffer respiratory and diarrheal infections caused by viruses and bacteria.

Our understanding of infectious disease is based on Koch's postulates, which establish criteria for linking a specific microorganism to a specific disease: (1) The organism is regularly found in the lesions of the disease, (2) the organism can be isolated as single colonies on solid medium, (3) inoculation of this culture causes lesions in an experimental animal, and (4) the organism can be recovered from lesions in the animals. In the past 10 years, the revolution in molecular biology has led to a molecular form of Koch's postulates, which links a particular trait of an organism to a particular disease process:[2] (1) The phenotype or trait should be associated with virulent strains of the organism and not with avirulent strains; (2) specific inactivation of the gene associated with virulence—for example, by replacing the normal (called the wild-type) gene with a changed or mutant gene—should lead to a measurable decrease in pathogenicity; (3) replacement of the mutant gene with the wild-type gene should restore full pathogenicity to the organism.

In discussing the mechanisms of infectious disease, two separate but inter-related aspects must be considered: (1) the specific properties of the organisms causing the infection, and (2) the host response to the infectious agents. This chapter begins with a review of the categories of infectious agents and a discussion of the mechanisms by which these organisms cause disease. These general principles are then illustrated with a selection of major human infectious diseases, organized by the organ system involved or the groups of patients frequently infected and including descriptions of the lesions caused by each organism.[3,4] Detailed discussions of many other infectious diseases are presented elsewhere in this book (e.g., viral hepatitis in Chapter 18; pneumococcal pneumonia in Chapter 15; and human immunodeficiency virus (HIV) infection and AIDS in Chapter 6).

CATEGORIES OF INFECTIOUS AGENTS

Infectious organisms, which can enter the human host (endoparasites), belong to a wide range of classes and vary in size from the 2-nm poliovirus to 10-m tapeworms (Table 8–1). In addition, several classes of arthropods are ectoparasites, that is, cause damage only via the skin.

Viruses

All viruses depend on host cell metabolism for their replication, that is, are obligate intracellular parasites. They are classified by the nucleic acid content of their core (DNA or RNA) and by the shape of their protein coat or capsid, which can be spherical if capsid proteins form an icosahedron or cylindrical if they form a helix. Many of the more than 400 viral species known to inhabit humans do not cause any disease, but some are frequent causes of acute illness (e.g., colds, influenza). Others are capable of lifelong latency and of long-term reactivation (herpesviruses) or may give rise to chronic disease (e.g., hepatitis B, [HBV]). Together, viral pathogens account for a major share of all human

infections (Table 8–2). Different viral species can give rise to the same clinical picture (e.g., upper respiratory infection; see section on viral respiratory infections[16]); conversely, a single virus can cause different lesions depending on host age or immune status (e.g., cytomegalovirus [CMV]).

Bacteriophages, Plasmids, Transposons

These are mobile genetic elements that encode bacterial virulence factors (e.g., adhesins, toxins, or enzymes that confer antibiotic resistance). They can infect bacteria and incorporate themselves into their genome, thus converting an otherwise harmless bacterium into a virulent one or an antibiotic-sensitive organism into a resistant one. Exchange of these elements between bacterial strains and species therefore endows the recipients with a survival advantage, or with the capacity to cause disease, or both.

Bacteria

Bacterial cells are prokaryotes, which lack nuclei and endoplasmic reticulum. Their cell walls are relatively rigid, composed either of two phospholipid bilayers with a peptidoglycan layer sandwiched in between (gram-negative species) or of a single bilayer covered by peptidoglycan (gram-positive bacteria). Bacteria synthesize their own DNA, RNA, and proteins but depend on the host for favorable growth conditions. Some thrive mainly on the body's surface layers; normal persons carry 10^{12} bacteria on the skin, including *Staphylococcus epidermidis* and *Propionibacterium acnes*, the agent responsible for adolescent pimples. Normally, 10^{14} bacteria reside inside the gastrointestinal tract, 99.9% of which are anaerobic, including Bacteroides species. Many bacterial pathogens invade host tissue and are capable of extracellular division (e.g., Pneumococcus) or of both extracellular and intracellular division (e.g., *Mycobacterium tuberculosis*). Next to viruses, bacteria are the most frequent and diverse class of human pathogens and include many of the major pathogens discussed in this chapter. A microbiologic categorization of the bacterial pathogens and the diseases they induce are shown in Table 8–3. Only some of these will be discussed later in the chapter.

Chlamydiae, Rickettsiae, Mycoplasmas

These infectious agents are grouped together because they are similar to bacteria in that they di-

Table 8–1. CLASSES OF HUMAN ENDOPARASITES AND THEIR HABITATS

TAXONOMIC CLASS	SIZE	SITE OF PROPAGATION	SAMPLE SPECIES AND ITS DISEASE	
Viruses	20–30 nm	Obligate intracellular	Poliovirus	Poliomyelitis
Chlamydiae	200–1000 nm	Obligate intracellular	*C. trachomatis*	Trachoma
Rickettsiae	300–1200 nm	Obligate intracellular	*R. prowazekii*	Typhus fever
Mycoplasmas	125–350 nm	Extracellular	*M. pneumoniae*	Atypical pneumonia
Bacteria, spirochetes, mycobacteria	0.8–15 μm	Cutaneous Mucosal Extracellular Facultative intracellular	*Staphylococcus epidermidis* *Vibrio cholerae* *Streptococcus pneumoniae* *M. tuberculosis*	Wound infection Cholera Pneumonia Tuberculosis
Fungi imperfecti	2–200 μm	Cutaneous Mucosal Extracellular Facultative intracellular	*Trichophyton* sp. *Candida albicans* *Sporothrix schenkii* *Histoplasma capsulatum*	Tinea pedis (athlete's foot) Thrush Sporotrichosis Histoplasmosis
Protozoa	1–50 mm	Mucosal Extracellular Facultative intracellular Obligate intracellular	*G. lamblia* *Trypanosoma gambiense* *Trypanosoma cruzi* *L. donovani*	Giardiasis Sleeping sickness Chagas' disease Kala-azar
Helminths	3 mm–10 m	Mucosal Extracellular Intracellular	*Enterobius vermicularis* *Wuchereria bancrofti* *Trichinella spiralis*	Oxyuriasis Filariasis Trichinosis

vide by binary fission and are susceptible to antibiotics but lack certain structures (e.g., Mycoplasma lacks a cell wall), or metabolic capabilities (e.g., Chlamydiae lack adenosine triphosphate [ATP] synthesis). Chlamydiae, which are frequent causes of genitourinary infections, conjunctivitis, and respiratory infections of newborn infants, are discussed with the sexually transmitted diseases.

Most rickettsiae are transmitted by insect vectors, including lice (epidemic typhus), ticks (Rocky Mountain spotted fever [RMSF], Q fever), and mites (scrub typhus).[5] Rickettsiae are obligate intracellular agents that replicate in the cytoplasm of endothelial cells (see section on vector-borne infections). By injuring the endothelial cells, rickettsiae cause a hemorrhagic vasculitis often visible as a skin rash but may also cause a transient pneumonia or hepatitis (Q fever) or injure the central nervous system and cause death (RMSF and epidemic typhus).

Mycoplasmas and the closely related genus Ureaplasma are the tiniest free-living organisms known (125 to 300 nm). *Mycoplasma pneumoniae* spreads from person to person by aerosols; binds to the surface of epithelial cells in the airways via an adhesin called P1; and causes an atypical pneumonia, characterized by peribronchiolar infiltrates of lymphocytes and plasma cells[6] (see Chapter 15). Ureaplasmas are transmitted venereally and may cause nongonococcal urethritis.

Fungi

Fungi posess thick, ergosterol-containing cell walls and grow as perfect, sexually reproducing forms in nature and as imperfect forms *in vivo*, which include budding yeast cells and slender tubes (hyphae) (Fig. 8–1). Some produce spores, which are resistant to extreme environmental conditions, whereas hyphae may produce fruiting bodies called *conidia*. Some fungal species, for example, those of the Tinea group causing "athletes foot," are confined to the superficial layers of the human skin; other "dermatophytes" preferentially damage the hair shafts or nails. Certain fungal species invade the subcutaneous tissue, causing abscesses or granulomas, as happens in sporotrichosis and in tropical mycoses. Deep fungal infections can spread systemically, destroying vital organs in immunocompromised hosts, whereas these fungal lesions heal spontaneously or remain latent in otherwise normal hosts. Some deep fungal species are limited to a particular geographic region (e.g., Coccidioides, Histoplasma, and Blastomyces). Opportunistic fungi (Candida, Aspergillus, Mucor), by contrast, are ubiquitous contaminants colonizing the normal human skin or gut without causing illness. Only in immunosuppressed individuals do opportunistic fungi give rise to life-threatening infections. In addition, AIDS patients, late in their course, are frequent victims of the opportunistic fungus-like organism *Pneumocystis carinii*.

Protozoa

Parasitic protozoa are single-celled organisms endowed with motility, pliable plasma membranes, and complex cytoplasmic organelles (Table 8–4). The flagellate *Trichomonas vaginalis* is transmitted

Table 8–2. HUMAN VIRAL DISEASES AND THEIR PATHOGENS

VIRAL PATHOGEN	VIRAL FAMILY	GENOMIC TYPE	DISEASE EXPRESSION
Respiratory			
Adenovirus	Adeno	DS DNA	Upper and lower respiratory tract infections (URI, LRI); conjunctivitis, diarrhea
Echovirus	Picorna	SS RNA*	URI, pharyngitis, skin rash
Rhinovirus	Picorna	SS RNA*	URI
Coxsackie virus	Picorna	SS RNA*	Pleurodynia, herpangina, hand-foot-and-mouth disease
Coronavirus	Corona	SS RNA*	URI
Influenza A, B	Orthomyxo	SS RNA†,‡	Influenza
Parainfluenza virus 1–4	Paramyxo	SS RNA†	URI, LRI, croup
Respiratory syncytial virus	Paramyxo	SS RNA†	Bronchiolitis, pneumonia
Digestive			
Mumps virus	Paramyxo	SS RNA†	Mumps, pancreatitis, orchitis
Rotavirus	Reo	DS RNA‡	Childhood diarrhea
Norwalk agent	Calici ?	SS RNA	Gastroenteritis
Hepatitis A virus	Picorna	SS RNA*	Acute viral hepatitis
Hepatitis B virus	Hepadna	DS DNA	Acute or chronic hepatitis
Hepatitis D		SS RNA	With HBV, acute or chronic hepatitis
Hepatitis C virus	Flavi	SS RNA	Acute or chronic hepatitis
Hepatitis E virus	Norwalk-like	SS RNA	Enterically transmitted hepatitis
Systemic with Skin Eruptions			
Measles virus	Paramyxo	SS RNA†	Measles (rubeola)
Rubella virus	Toga	SS RNA*	German measles (rubella)
Parvovirus	Parvo	SS DNA	Erythema infectiosum
			Asplastic anemia
Vacciniavirus	Pox	DS DNA	Smallpox vaccine
Varicella-zoster	Herpes	DS DNA	Chickenpox, shingles
Herpes simplex virus I	Herpes	DS DNA	"Cold sore"
Herpes simplex virus II	Herpes	DS DNA	Genital herpes
Systemic with Hematopoietic Disorders			
Cytomegalovirus (CMV)	Herpes	DS DNA	Cytomegalic inclusion disease
Epstein-Barr (EBV) virus	Herpes	DS DNA	Infectious mononucleosis
HTLV I virus	Retro	SS RNA§	Adult T-cell leukemia; tropical spastic paraparesis
HTLV II virus	Retro	SS RNA§	Role still uncertain
HIV I and II virus	Retro	SS RNA§	AIDS
Arboviral and Hemorrhagic Fevers			
Denguevirus 1–4	Toga	SS RNA*	Dengue, hemorrhagic fever
Yellow fever	Toga	SS RNA*	Yellow fever
Colorado tick	Reo (Orbi)	SS RNA‡	Colorado tick fever
Regional hemorrhagic fever viruses	Arena	SS RNA†,‡	Bolivian, Argentinian, Lassa
	Bunya	SS RNA†,‡	Crimean-Congo, Hantaan, sandfly fever
	Filo?	SS RNA	Ebola, Marburg disease
	Hanta	SS RNA	Korean, USA pneumonia
Warty Growths			
Papillomavirus (HPV)	Papova	DS DNA	Condyloma; cervical carcinoma
Molluscum virus	Pox	DS DNA	Molluscum contagiosum
Central Nervous System			
Poliovirus	Picorna	SS RNA*	Poliomyelitis
Rabiesvirus	Rhabdo	SS RNA†	Rabies
JC virus	Papova	DS DNA	Progressive multifocal leukoencephalopathy (opportunistic)
Arboviral Encephalitis viruses	Toga	SS RNA*	Eastern, Western, Venezuelan, St. Louis, California
	Bunya	SS RNA†,‡	group

HTLV, human T-cell leukemia virus; HIV, human immunodeficiency virus.
* Positive-sense genome (nucleotide sequences directly translated).
† Negative-sense genome (complementary to positive-sense strand).
‡ Segmented genome.
§ DNA step required in retroviral replication.

Table 8-3. BACTERIAL, SPIROCHETAL, AND MYCOBACTERIAL DISEASES

CLINICAL OR MICROBIOLOGIC CATEGORY	SPECIES	FREQUENT DISEASE PRESENTATIONS
Infections by Pyogenic Cocci	Staphylococcus aureus, epidermidis	Abscess, cellulitis, pneumonia, septicemia
	Streptococcus pyogenes, beta hemolytic	URI, erysipelas, scarlet fever, septicemia
	Streptococcus pneumoniae (pneumococcus)	Lobar pneumonia, meningitis
	Neisseria meningitidis (meningococcus)	Cerebrospinal meningitis
	Neisseria gonorrhoeae (gonococcus)	Gonorrhea
Gram-Negative Infections, Common	* Escherichia coli	
	* Klebsiella pneumoniae	
	* Enterobacter (Aerobacter) aerogenes	
	* Proteus spp. (mirabilis, morgagni, etc.)	Urinary tract infection, wound infection, abscess, pneumonia, septicemia, endotoxemia, endocarditis, etc.
	* Serratia marcescens	
	* Pseudomonas spp. (aeruginosa, etc.)	Anaerobic infections
	Bacteroides sp. (fragilis, etc.)	
	* Legionella spp. (pneumophilia, etc.)	Legionnaires' disease
Gram-Negative Infections, Rare	Klebsiella rhinoscleromatis, ozenae	Rhinoscleroma, ozena
	Haemophilus ducreyi	Chancroid (soft chancre)
	Calymmatobacterium donovani	Granuloma inguinale
	Bartonella bacilliformis	Carrión's disease (Oroya fever)
Contagious Childhood Bacterial Diseases	Hemophilus influenzae	Meningitis, URI, LRI
	Hemophilus pertussis	Whooping cough
	Corynebacterium diphtheriae	Diphtheria
Enteropathic Infections	Enteropathogenic E. coli	
	Shigella sp.	
	Vibrio cholerae, etc.	Invasive or noninvasive gastroentero-colitis, some with septicemia
	Campylobacter fetus, jejuni	
	Yersinia enterocolitica	
	Salmonella spp. (1000 strains)	
	Salmonella typhi	Typhoid fever
Clostridial Infections	Clostridium tetani	Tetanus (lockjaw)
	Clostridium botulinum	Botulism (paralytic food poisoning)
	Clostridium perfringens, septicum, etc.	Gas gangrene, necrotizing cellulitis
	* Clostridium difficile	Pseudomembranous colitis
Zoonotic Bacterial Infections	Bacillus anthracis	Anthrax (malignant pustule)
	* Listeria monocytogenes	Listeria meningitis, listeriosis
	Yersinia pestis	Bubonic plague
	Francisella tularensis	Tularemia
	Brucella melitensis, suis, abortus	Brucellosis (undulant fever)
	Pseudomonas mallei, pseudomallei	Glanders, melioidosis
	Leptospira spp. (many groups)	Leptospirosis, Weil's disease
	Borrelia recurrentis	Relapsing fever
	Borrelia burgdorferi	Lyme borreliosis
	Rochalimaea henseli	Cat-scratch disease; bacillary angiomatosis
	Spirillum minus, Streptobacillus moniliformis	Rat-bite fever
Human Treponemal Infections	Treponema pallidum	Venereal, endemic syphilis (bejel)
	Treponema pertenue	Yaws (frambesia)
	Treponema carateum (herrejoni)	Pinta (carate, mal del pinto)
Mycobacterial Infections	* Mycobacterium tuberculosis bovis (Koch's bacillus)	Tuberculosis
	M. leprae (Hansen's bacillus)	Leprosy
	* M. kansasii, avium, intracellulare, etc.	Atypical mycobacterial infections
	M. ulcerans	Buruli ulcer
Actinomycetaceae	* Nocardia asteroides	Nocardiosis
	Actinomyces israelii	Actinomycosis

* Important opportunistic infections.

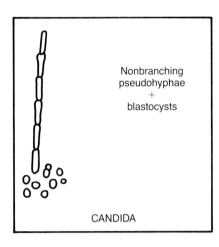

Nonbranching
pseudohyphae
+
blastocysts

CANDIDA

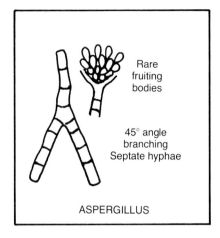

Rare
fruiting
bodies

45° angle
branching
Septate hyphae

ASPERGILLUS

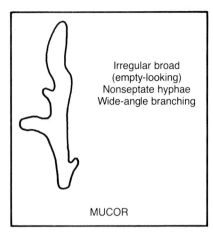

Irregular broad
(empty-looking)
Nonseptate hyphae
Wide-angle branching

MUCOR

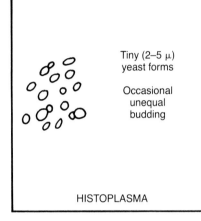

Tiny (2–5 μ)
yeast forms

Occasional
unequal
budding

HISTOPLASMA

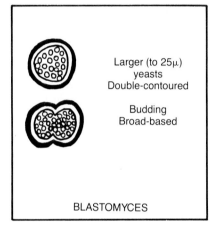

Larger (to 25μ)
yeasts
Double-contoured

Budding
Broad-based

BLASTOMYCES

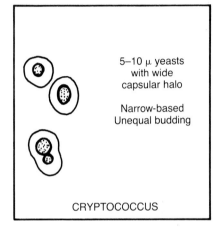

5–10 μ yeasts
with wide
capsular halo

Narrow-based
Unequal budding

CRYPTOCOCCUS

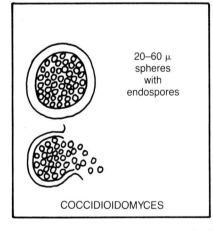

20–60 μ
spheres
with
endospores

COCCIDIOIDOMYCES

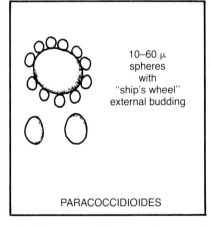

10–60 μ
spheres
with
"ship's wheel"
external budding

PARACOCCIDIOIDES

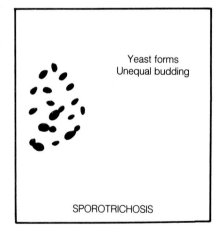

Yeast forms
Unequal budding

SPOROTRICHOSIS

Figure 8–1. Characteristic tissue forms of fungi.

sexually from person to person. The intestinal protozoa (e.g., *Entamoeba histolytica* and *Giardia lamblia*) are spread by the fecal-oral route. Blood-borne protozoa (e.g., plasmodium species and Leishmania species) are transmitted by blood-sucking insects, in which they undergo a complex succession of life stages before being passed to new human hosts. *Toxoplasma gondii* is acquired either

by contact with oocyst-shedding kittens or by eating cyst-ridden, undercooked meat.

Helminths

Parasitic worms are highly differentiated multicellular organisms. Their life cycles are complex; most

Table 8–4. PROTOZOA PATHOGENIC FOR HUMANS

SPECIES	ORDER	FORM, SIZE*	DISEASE
Luminal or Epithelial			
Entamoeba histolytica	Amebae	Trophozoite 15–50 μm	Amebic dysentery
			Liver abscess
Balantidium coli	Ciliates	Trophozoite 50–100 μm	Colitis
Naegleria fowleri	Ameboflagellates	Trophozoite 10–20 μm	Meningoencephalitis
Acanthamoeba sp.	Ameboflagellates	Trophozoite 15–30 μm	Same or ophthalmitis
Giardia lamblia	Mastigophora	Trophozoite 11–18 μm	Diarrheal disease
			Malabsorption
Isospora belli	Coccidia	Oocyst 10–20 μm	⎱ Chronic enterocolitis or malab-
Cryptosporidium sp.	Coccidia	Oocyst 5–6 μm	⎰ sorption, or both
Enterocytozoon bieneusi	Microsporidia	Spore	Diarrhea in AIDS patients
Trichomonas vaginalis	Mastigophora	Trophozoite 10–30 μm	Urethritis, vaginitis
Bloodstream			
Plasmodium vivax	Hemosporidia	⎫ Trophozoites, schizonts, ga-	Benign tertian malaria
P. ovale	Hemosporidia	⎬ metes (all small and inside	Benign tertian malaria
P. malariae	Hemosporidia	⎪ red cells)	Quartan malaria
P. falciparum	Hemosporidia	⎭	Malignant tertian malaria
Babesia microti, bovis	Hemosporidia	Trophozoites inside red cells	Babesiosis
Trypanosoma brucei, rhode-siense, gambiense	Hemoflagellates	Trypomastigote 14–33 μm	African sleeping sickness
Intracellular			
Trypanosoma cruzi	Hemoflagellates	Trypomastigote 20 μm	Chagas' disease
Leishmania donovani	Hemoflagellates	Amastigote 2 μm	Kala-azar
Leishmania tropica; mexicana, brasiliensis	Hemoflagellates	Amastigote 2 μm	Cutaneous and mucocu-taneous leishmaniasis
Toxoplasma gondii	Coccidia (Eimeriae)	Tachyzoite 4–6 μm (cyst larger)	Toxoplasmosis

alternate between sexual reproduction in the definitive host and asexual multiplication in an intermediary host or vector. Thus, depending on parasite species, humans may harbor either adult worms (e.g., Ascaris) or immature stages (e.g., *Toxocara canis*), or asexual larval forms (e.g., Echinococcus). Adult worms, once resident in humans, do not multiply in number but generate eggs or larvae destined for the next phase of the cycle. An exception is Strongyloides, the larvae of which can become infective inside the gut, and cause overwhelming autoinfection in immunosuppressed persons. There are two important consequences of the lack of replication of adult worms: (1) Disease is often caused by inflammatory responses to the eggs or larvae rather than adults (e.g., schistosomiasis), and (2) disease is in proportion to the number of organisms that have infected the individual (e.g., 10 hookworms cause little pathology, whereas 1000 hookworms cause severe anemia by consuming 100 ml of blood per day). Fortunately, most persons in endemic areas harbor few worms and are free from disease, and only a minority are heavily infected and ill.

Parasitic worms are of three classes. The first class, *Roundworms* (nematodes), is characterized by a collagenous tegument and a nonsegmented structure. These include Ascaris, hookworms, and strongyloides among the intestinal worms and the filariae and Trichinella among the tissue invaders. The second class, *Flatworms* (cestodes), comprises gutless worms, whose head (scolex) sprouts a ribbon of flat segments (proglottids) covered by an absorptive tegument. This class includes the pork, beef, and fish tapeworms and the cystic tapeworm larvae (cysticerci and hydatid cysts). The third class, *Flukes* (trematodes), which are primitive leaf-like worms with syncytial integument, includes the oriental liver and lung flukes and the blood-dwelling schistosomes, discussed later.

Ectoparasites

Ectoparasites are arthropods (lice, ticks, bedbugs, fleas) that attach to and live on the skin. In addition, skin lesions can be caused by the stings of mosquitoes and bees. Scabies is an example of severe dermatitis elicited by mites burrowing into the stratum corneum (see Chapter 26). Skin nodules caused by burrowing botfly larvae are intensely inflamed and eosinophil-enriched. In addition, attached arthropods can be vectors for other pathogens that make characteristic skin lesions (e.g., the expanding erythematous plaque caused by the Lyme disease spirochete *Borrelia Burgdorferi*, which is transmitted by ticks).

HOST BARRIERS TO INFECTION AND HOW MICROORGANISMS ESCAPE THEM

The first and most formidable barriers to infection are the intact host skin and mucosal surfaces and their secretory-excretory products.[7] For example, lysozyme secreted by the tear glands degrades the peptidoglycans of bacterial cell walls and protects the eyes from infection. Acid gastric juice is lethal for some enteric pathogens; for example, normal volunteers do not become infected by *Vibrio cholerae* unless fed 10^{11} organisms. In contrast, Shigella and Giardia are relatively resistant to acid, and fewer than 100 organisms of each species are infective. In general, skin infections in normal persons tend to arise in damaged sites, that is, wounds, cuts, or burns, and can be caused by resident bacteria of relatively low virulence. In contrast, infections transmitted by the respiratory, gastrointestinal, or genitourinary route generally require virulent organisms capable of damaging or penetrating normal mucosal barriers.

Respiratory Tract

City inhabitants inhale some 10,000 microorganisms per day, including viruses, bacteria, and fungi. Most of the larger inhaled microbes are trapped in the mucociliary blanket of the upper air passages. Those that manage to reach the trachea are either coughed up or pushed backward toward the throat by ciliary action, then swallowed and cleared. Only particles 5 μm or smaller in size reach the alveoli, where they are attacked and interiorized by alveolar macrophages or by neutrophils attracted to the site by cytokines. This normal clearing system (see Chapter 15) is quite efficient, but mucociliary action can be impaired by smoking, by viscous secretions in cystic fibrosis, by aspiration of acid stomach contents, or by the trauma of intubation. It is also weakened by viral infection, which favors superinfection by bacteria. Some respiratory viruses (e.g., influenza viruses) possess hemagglutinins, which attach to epithelial surface carbohydrates and thus prevent mucociliary clearance. Others also have neuraminidases, which degrade respiratory mucus and thereby prevent viral entrapment. Some respiratory bacterial pathogens (e.g., Haemophilus and Bordetella) elaborate toxins that paralyze mucosal cilia. *Mycobacterium tuberculosis*, in contrast gains its foothold in normal alveoli because of its resistance to killing by nonactivated macrophages.

Gastrointestinal Tract

Most gastrointestinal pathogens are transmitted by food or drink contaminated with fecal material. Exposure can therefore be reduced by sanitary disposal of waste and vermin, clean drinking water, hand washing, and thorough cooking of food. Where hygiene fails, diarrheal disease becomes rampant.

Normal defenses against ingested pathogens include (1) acid gastric juice, (2) the viscous mucous layer covering the gut, (3) lytic pancreatic enzymes and bile detergents, and (4) secreted IgA antibodies. In addition, pathogenic organisms must compete for nutrients with abundant commensal bacteria resident in the lower gut, and all gut microbes are intermittently expelled by defecation. Host defenses are weakened by low gastric acidity, by antibiotics that unbalance the normal bacterial flora (e.g., pseudomembranous colitis; see Chapter 17), or when there is stalled peristalsis or mechanical obstruction (e.g., blind loop syndrome). Most enveloped viruses are killed by the digestive juices, but nonenveloped ones may be resistant (e.g., the hepatitis A virus, rotaviruses, reoviruses, and Norwalk agents). Rotaviruses directly damage the intestinal epithelial cells they infect, whereas reoviruses pass through mucosal M cells into the bloodstream without any detectable local cell injury.

Enteropathogenic bacteria elicit gastrointestinal disease by a variety of mechanisms: (1) While growing on contaminated food, certain staphylococcal strains release powerful enterotoxins that, on ingestion, cause food-poisoning symptoms without any bacterial multiplication in the gut. (2) *Vibrio cholerae* and toxigenic *Escherichia coli* multiply inside the mucous layer overlying the gut epithelium and release exotoxins that cause the gut epithelium to secrete excessive volumes of watery diarrhea. (3) By contrast, Shigella, Salmonella, and Campylobacter invade and damage the intestinal mucosa and lamina propria and so cause ulceration, inflammation, and hemorrhage, clinically manifested as dysentery. (4) *Salmonella typhi* passes from the damaged mucosa through Peyer's patches and mesenteric lymph nodes and into the bloodstream, resulting in a systemic infection.

Fungal infection of the gastrointestinal tract occurs mainly in immunologically compromised patients. Candida shows a predilection for stratified squamous epithelium, causing oral thrush or membranous esophagitis but may also disseminate to the stomach, lower gastrointestinal tract, and systemic organs.

The cyst forms of intestinal protozoa are essential for their transmission because cysts resist stomach acid. In the gut, cysts convert to motile trophozoites and attach to sugars on the intestinal epithelia via surface lectins. Thereafter, there is wide species variation: *Giardia lamblia* attaches to the epithelial brush border, whereas cryptosporidia are taken up by enterocytes, in which they form gametes and spores. *Entamoeba histolytica* causes contact-mediated cytolysis analogous to that of cytotoxic T lymphocytes by releasing a channel-forming pore protein that depolarizes and kills its cellular prey. In this manner, the colonic mucosa is ulcerated and invaded. Intestinal helminths, as a rule, cause disease only when present in large numbers or in ectopic sites, for example, by obstructing the gut or invading and damaging the bile ducts (Ascaris). Hookworms may cause iron deficiency anemia by chronic loss of blood, sucked from intestinal villi; the fish tapeworm, Diphyllobothrium, competes with and can deplete its host of vitamin B_{12}, giving rise to an illness resembling pernicious anemia. Finally, the larvae of several helminth parasites pass through the gut briefly on their way toward another organ habitat, for example, Trichinella larvae preferentially encyst in muscle, Echinococcus larvae in the liver or lung.

Urogenital Tract

Even though urine can support the growth of many bacteria, the urinary tract is normally sterile. The mechanisms by which urinary infection is initiated are critical to the pathogenesis of renal infection (pyelonephritis) and are discussed in detail in Chapter 20.

Skin

The human skin is normally inhabited by a variety of bacterial and fungal species, including some potential opportunists such as *Staphylococcus epidermidis* and *Candida albicans*. This rich cutaneous flora maintains itself in metabolic equilibrium and thus inhibits overgrowth of any single resident species or virulent newcomer pathogen. In addition, the dense, keratinized outer skin layer bearing resident microbes is constantly shed and renewed. The low pH and fatty acid content of normal skin favor commensal bacteria over bacterial pathogens; however, heat and moisture can weaken resistance to dermatophytic and opportunistic fungi. In addition, when moist skin is chafed or traumatized, as occurs during sexual intercourse, it can be breached by a variety of venereal pathogens, including *Treponema pallidum*, the agent of syphilis. Skin that is soiled and moist invites infections of its superficial layers by gram-positive cocci (e.g., staphylococcal impetigo). Most other pathogens enter via skin lesions, including surgical incisions, burn sites (e.g., Staphylococcus and Pseudomonas), pressure sores, and ischemic or diabetic sores of the extremities. When the skin is pierced by needles, catheters, or prostheses, microbes may be introduced directly into the bloodstream as well as into the local site. In intravenous drug addicts, this is a frequent route for HIV-1 and HBV infection as well as for bacteria and fungi capable of implanting on heart valves (see Chapter 12). In hospitalized patients with indwelling catheters, opportunistic infections by *Staphylococcus epidermidis* or by Candida species are not infrequent.

Many important pathogens bypass the human skin via an insect bite. These range from viruses (e.g., dengue fever) through rickettsiae (spotted fevers) and bacteria (Lyme disease) to protozoa (malaria, leishmaniasis) and even helminths (filariasis). Animal or human bites can transmit microbial agents (e.g., rabies virus). In some cases (e.g., sandfly bites), parasite infectivity is enhanced by spreading factors or enzymes secreted by insect saliva.[8] Helminth larvae (e.g., hookworm, Schistosoma) actively enter unbroken human skin from soil or water by vigorous burrowing and secretion of lytic proteases.

Spread and Dissemination of Microbes

Once implanted, the spread of microbes on the surface of moist and warm mucosae is faster than on cool and dry skin. Some of the superficial pathogens stay confined to the lumen of hollow viscera (e.g., cholera); others adhere to or proliferate exclusively in or on epithelial cells (e.g., papillomaviruses, dermatophytes). A variety of pathogenic bacteria, fungi, and helminths are invasive pathogens, that is, have the ability to invade the interstitium by virtue of their motility or lytic enzyme production (e.g., streptococcal hyaluronidase, schistosome proteases). Microbial spread initially follows tissue planes of least resistance, for example, along aponeurotic compartments. Spread through serosal cavities (pleura, peritoneum, meninges) is particularly fast and dangerous. Microbes may also ascend the lymphatics from their entry site to the regional nodes and hence into the bloodstream (Fig. 8–2). Thus, untreated staphylococcal infections may progress from a localized abscess or furuncle to regional lymphadenitis followed by bacteremia, endocarditis, or formation of multiple pyemic abscesses in distant metastatic sites (brain, kidney, bone). Depending on microbial species, secondary foci of infection, established via the bloodstream, take the form of abscesses or granulomas. They can be single and large (a solitary abscess or tuberculoma) or multiple and tiny, the size of millet seeds (e.g., miliary tuberculosis or Candida microabscesses). Viruses may propagate from cell to cell by fusion or axonal transport (e.g., poliovirus), but like other intracellular pathogens (e.g., tubercle bacilli), they can enter the bloodstream and be carried to distant sites by migratory macrophages (HIV-1), or by circulating red cells (Colorado tick fever virus).

Sometimes, therefore *the major manifestations of infectious disease arise at sites distant from those of parasite entry.* For example, chickenpox and measles viruses enter via the airways but manifest themselves first as skin rashes; poliovirus is ingested and multiplies inside the gut wall before proceeding to viremic invasion and killing of motor

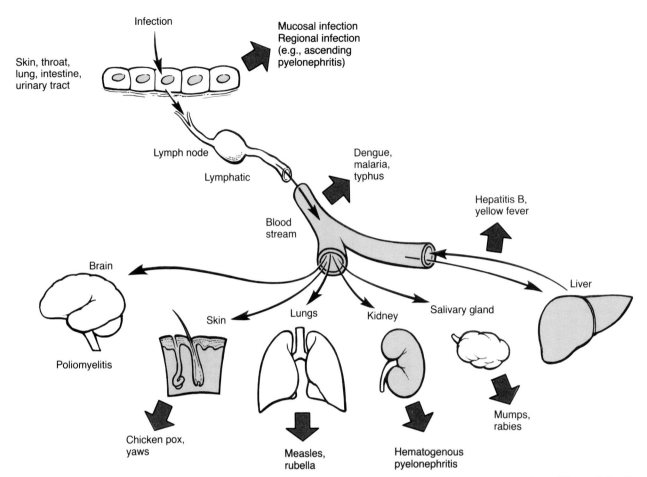

Figure 8-2. Routes of entry, dissemination, and release of microbes from the body. (Adapted from Mims, C.A.: The Pathogenesis of Infectious Disease, 3rd ed. San Diego, CA, Academic Press, 1987.)

neurons. Several helminth parasites (e.g., hookworm) enter the skin as penetrating larvae but complete their migratory cycle and maturation inside the gut.

Bloodstream invasion by sporadic low-virulence or nonvirulent microbes is a common event but is quickly suppressed by the normal host defenses. By contrast, sustained bloodstream invasion and dissemination of pathogens, that is, viremia, bacteremia, fungemia, or parasitemia is a serious insult and manifests itself by fever, low arterial pressure, and multiple other systemic "septic" signs and symptoms. These alarming events are triggered by a cascade of cytokines and other mediators that are activated by bacterial endotoxin or by lytic products of damaged host cells (see Chapter 3). Massive bloodstream invasion by bacteria or their endotoxins can rapidly become fatal, even for previously healthy individuals.

When infectious organisms reach the pregnant uterus via the cervical orifice or the bloodstream and are able to traverse the placenta, severe damage to the fetus may result. Bacterial or mycoplasmal placentitis may cause premature delivery or stillbirth. *Treponema pallidum* infecting the mother, unless treated, breaches the placenta by the end of the second trimester and causes manifestations of congenital syphilis in the infant, ranging from dental deformities to stillbirth. By contrast, vertical transmission of maternal viruses or of Toxoplasma infections is most dangerous during early pregnancy and can result in flagrant systemic disease of the fetus (e.g., cytomegalovirus), fetal maldevelopment, deafness, and congenital heart disease (e.g., rubella). Central nervous system damage is particularly common in the so-called TORCH infections (*T*oxoplasma, *r*ubella, *C*MV, *h*erpesviruses, and *o*ther) (see Chapter 10). The same agents can also cause more subtle mental retardation or learning disabilities during childhood. Fetuses infected late during pregnancy or during passage through the birth canal and infants receiving virus via maternal milk usually fare better than those infected during early embryonal life; their lesions may resemble those of adult patients. Stillbirth and maldevelopment of infants occurs increasingly in HIV-1–infected mothers. Although fewer than half of affected children develop the typical childhood manifestations of AIDS, they are currently the fastest growing group of AIDS victims. Maternal transmission of Hepatitis B virus (HBV) is common in Third World countries and among the drug-addicted. Such children are at high risk for liver cancer later during adult life.

Release and Transmission of Microbes

For transmission to occur, microbial pathogens must be able to leave the host organism. Depending on the location of infection, release may be accomplished by skin shedding, mucosal contact, coughing, sneezing, shouting, or voiding of urine or feces. Microbes directly transmissible from person to person via contact or aerosol (e.g., measles or chickenpox) are termed *contagious.* Viruses infecting the salivary glands (e.g., herpesviruses, mumps viruses) are released principally by kissing or spitting. Other pathogens are infective mainly by prolonged, intimate or mucosal contact, as occurs during sexual transmission (e.g., HIV-1, herpes simplex virus (HSV-2), papillomaviruses, chlamydiae, syphilis). Bacteria and fungi transmitted by the respiratory route are infective only when lesions are open to the airways and not via "closed lesions" (e.g., pulmonary tuberculosis). Many pathogens, from viruses to helminths, are transmitted by the fecal-to-oral route, that is, by ingestion of stool-contaminated food or water. To ensure transmission, such organisms may form bacterial spores, protozoan cysts, or thick-shelled helminth eggs, which can survive in a cool and dry environment. Alternatively, some enteric pathogens are shed for long periods by asymptomatic carrier hosts (e.g., salmonellae). For transmission of microbes from skin to insect to occur during feeding, the pathogen must circulate in the blood or reside in the skin, even if the lesion is elsewhere (e.g., onchocerciasis and river blindness). Some parasitic helminths shedding eggs via the excreta gain access to new hosts via larval skin penetration rather than by oral intake (e.g., hookworms, schistosomes). Higher parasite phyla, that is, protozoa and helminths, have evolved complex transmission cycles involving a chain of intermediary and vector hosts bearing successive developmental parasite stages (e.g., the liver flukes). Transmission of pathogens by the various routes listed occurs not only from human to human but also from animal to human (e.g., field mice are the "reservoir hosts" for Lyme disease) and vice versa. Diseases of this type are termed *zoonotic infections.* By contrast, transmission of HBV and HIV infections via blood and blood products is frequently caused by human agency, that is, needle sharing by addicts, viral-contaminated blood transfusions, cuts, needlesticks, and other accidents.

HOW MICROORGANISMS CAUSE DISEASE

Infectious agents establish infection and damage tissues in three ways:

1. They can contact or enter host cells and directly cause cell death.

2. They may release endotoxins or exotoxins that kill cells at a distance, release enzymes that degrade tissue components, or damage blood vessels and cause ischemic necrosis.

3. They induce host-cellular responses that, although directed against the invader, may cause additional tissue damage, including suppuration, scarring, and hypersensitivity reactions. Thus, the defensive responses of the host are a two-edged sword: they are necessary to overcome the infection but at the same time directly contribute to tissue damage. Here we describe some of the particular mechanisms whereby viruses and bacteria damage host tissues.

Viral Damage to Host Cells

Viruses damage host cells by entering the cell and replicating at the host's expense.[9] Viruses have on their surface specific viral proteins that bind to specific host surface receptor proteins, many of which have known functions. For example, HIV binds to the protein involved with antigen presentation on helper lymphocytes (CD4), Epstein-Barr virus (EBV) binds to the complement receptor on macrophages (CD2), rabies virus binds to the acetylcholine receptor on neurons, and rhinoviruses bind to the adhesion protein ICAM-1 on mucosal cells. One reason for viral tropism (the tendency to infect some cells but not others) is the presence or absence of host cell receptors that allow the virus to attach. A second major cause of viral tropism is the ability of the virus to replicate inside some cells but not in others. For example, JC papovavirus, which causes leukoencephalopathy, is restricted to oligodendroglia in the central nervous system because JC virus promoter and enhancer DNA sequences upstream from the viral genes are active in glial cells but not in neurons or endothelial cells.

Once attached, the entire virion or a portion containing the genome and essential polymerases *penetrates* into the cell cytoplasm by one of three ways: (1) Translocation of the entire virus across the plasma membrane, (2) fusion of the viral envelope with the cell membrane, or (3) receptor-mediated endocytosis of the virus and fusion with endosomal membranes.[10] Within the cell, the virus uncoats, separating its genome from its structural components and losing its infectivity. Viruses then replicate using enzymes, which are distinct for each virus family. For example, RNA polymerase is

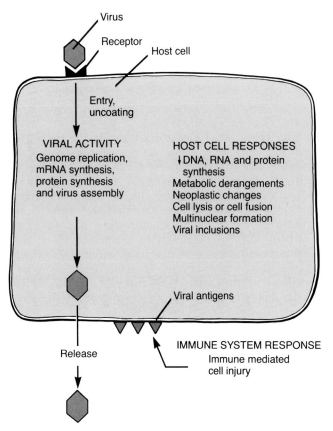

Figure 8-3. Mechanisms by which viruses cause injuries to cells.

used by negative-stranded RNA viruses to generate positive-stranded mRNA, whereas reverse transcriptase is used by retroviruses to generate DNA from their RNA template and to integrate that DNA into the host genome. Viruses also use host enzymes for viral synthesis, which may be present in some differentiated tissues and not in others. Newly synthesized viral genomes and capsid proteins are then assembled into progeny virions in the nucleus or cytoplasm and are released directly (unencapsulated viruses) or bud through the plasma membrane (encapsulated viruses).

Viral infection can be *abortive* (with incomplete viral replicative cycle), *latent* (e.g., herpes zoster virus persists in a cryptic state within the dorsal root ganglia and then presents as painful shingles), or *persistent* (virions are synthesized continuously, with or without altered cell function [e.g., hepatitis B]).

Viruses kill host cells in a number of ways (Fig. 8-3):

• Viruses inhibit host cell DNA, RNA, or protein synthesis. For example, poliovirus inactivates cap-binding protein, which is essential for protein synthesis directed by capped host cell mRNAs, while allowing protein synthesis from uncapped poliovirus mRNAs.

• Viral proteins insert into the host cell's plasma membrane and directly damage its integrity or promote cell fusion (HIV, measles virus, and herpesviruses).

• Viruses replicate efficiently and lyse host cells (e.g., liver cells by yellow fever virus, and neurons by poliovirus).

• *Slow virus infections* (e.g., subacute sclerosing panencephalitis [SSPE] caused by measles virus) culminate in severe progressive disease after a long latency period.

• Viral proteins on the surface of the host cells are recognized by the immune system, and the host lymphocytes attack the virus-infected cells (e.g., liver cells infected with HBV).

• Viruses damage cells involved in host antimicrobial defense, leading to secondary infections. For example, viral damage to respiratory epithelium allows subsequent pneumonias caused by Pneumococcus or Haemophilus, and HIV depletes CD4+ helper lymphocytes, which normally suppress opportunistic infections that kill other host cells.

• Viral killing of one cell type causes the death of other cells that depend on them (e.g., degeneration of muscle cells denervated by the attack of poliovirus on motor neurons).

• Finally, viruses cause *cell transformation* (e.g., human T-cell lymphotropic virus [HTLV-1], HBV, human papillomavirus, or EBV), which results in neoplastic growth (see Chapter 7).

Bacterial Adhesins and Toxins

Bacterial damage to host tissues depends on their ability to adhere to and enter host cells or to deliver bacterial toxins. The coordination of bacterial adherence and toxin delivery is so important to bacterial virulence that the genes encoding adherence proteins and toxins are frequently regulated together by specific environmental signals.[11] For example, the virulence of enterotoxic *E. coli* depends on the coordinate expression of adherence proteins that allow the bacteria to bind to the intestinal epithelial cells and the synthesis and release of heat-labile or heat-stable toxins by the bacteria that cause intestinal cells to secrete isotonic fluids.

BACTERIAL ADHESINS. Bacterial adhesins that bind bacteria to host cells are limited in type but have a broad range of host cell specificity.[12] The *fibrillae* covering the surface of gram-positive cocci such as Streptococcus are composed of M protein and lipoteichoic acids (Fig. 8-4).[13] *Lipoteichoic acids* are hydrophobic and bind to the surface of all eukaryotic cells, although with a higher affinity to particular receptors on blood cells and oral epithelial cells. *Fimbriae* or *pili* on the surface of gram-negative rods and cocci are nonflagellar filamentous

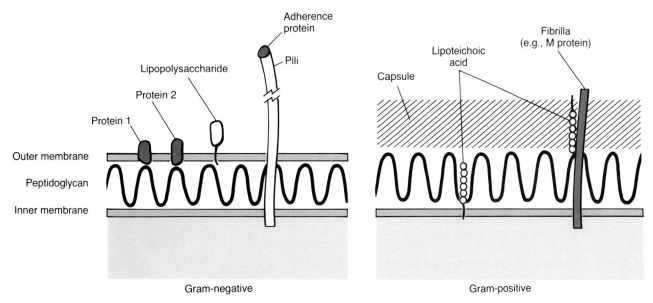

Figure 8–4. Molecules on the surface of gram-negative and gram-positive bacteria involved in pathogenesis (see text).

structures composed of repeating subunits (Fig. 8–5). Sex pili are used to exchange genes carried on plasmids or transposons from one bacterium to another; other pili mediate adherence of bacteria to host cells. The base of the subunit that anchors the

pili to the bacterial cell wall is similar for widely divergent bacteria. At the tips of the pili are minor protein components that determine to which host cells the microbes will attach (bacterial tropism). In *E. coli*, these minor proteins are antigenically

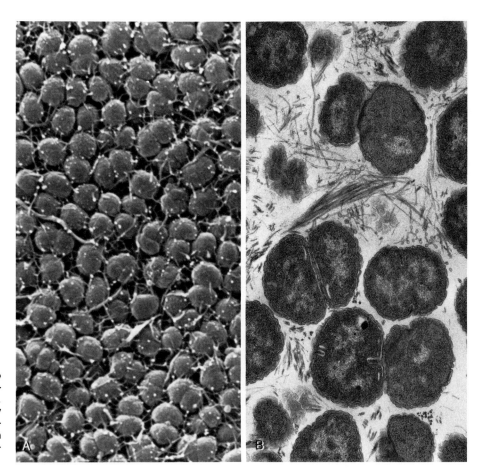

Figure 8–5. Gonococcal culture showing pili as seen by scanning electron microscopy *(A)*, and in clusters, as seen by transmission electron microscopy *(B)*. (Courtesy of Dr. John Swanson, Rocky Mountain Laboratories, Hamilton, Montana.)

distinct and are associated with particular infections (e.g., type I proteins bind mannose and cause urinary tract infections, type P proteins bind galactose and cause pyelonephritis, and type S proteins bind sialic acid and cause meningitis). A single bacterium can express more than one type of pili as well as nonpilar adhesins.

In contrast to viruses, which can infect a broad range of host cells, facultative intracellular bacteria infect mainly epithelial cells (Shigella and enteroinvasive E. coli), macrophages (Mycobacterium tuberculosis and M. leprae, Legionella pneumophila, and Yersinia) or both cell types (Salmonella typhi). Many bacteria attach to host cell integrins, the plasma membrane proteins that bind complement or extracellular matrix proteins (see Chapters 2 and 3). For example, Legionella, M. tuberculosis, and the protozoan Leishmania all bind to CR3, the cell receptor for complement C3bi. Some intracellular bacteria are unable to penetrate the host cells directly but are interiorized by endocytosis in epithelial cells and in macrophages. Subsequently they may use a hemolysin to escape from the endocytic vacuole into the cytoplasm.[14] Once in the cytoplasm, certain bacteria (Shigella and E. coli) inhibit host protein synthesis, rapidly replicate, and lyse the host cells. In contrast, others, such as Salmonella, Mycobacteria, and Yersinia replicate within the phagolysosome of the macrophage; whereas Legionella and the protozoan Toxoplasma inhibit the acidification that normally occurs when the endosome fuses with the lysosome. Many bacteria can replicate within macrophages in the absence of a host immune response (e.g., lepromatous leprosy, M. avium infection in AIDS patients), but activated macrophages kill these bacteria and slow or suppress the infection.

BACTERIAL ENDOTOXIN. Bacterial endotoxin is a lipopolysaccharide (LPS) that is a structural component in the outer cell wall of gram-negative bacteria. LPS is composed of a long-chain fatty acid anchor (lipid A) connected to a core sugar chain, both of which are the same in all gram-negative bacteria. Attached to the core sugar is a variable carbohydrate chain (O antigen), which is used to serotype and discriminate different bacteria. All biologic activities of LPS, including the induction of fever, macrophage activation, and B-cell mitogenicity, come from lipid A and the core sugars and are mediated by induction of host cytokines, including tumor necrosis factor (TNF) and interleukin-1 (IL-1) (see p. 70).

BACTERIAL EXOTOXINS. Bacteria secrete a variety of enzymes (leukocidins, hemolysins, hyaluronidases, coagulases, fibrinolysins). These act on their respective substrates in vitro, but their role in human disease remains presumptive. In contrast, the role of bacterial exotoxins is well established, and the molecular mechanisms of most of their actions are known. The mechanism of action of diph-

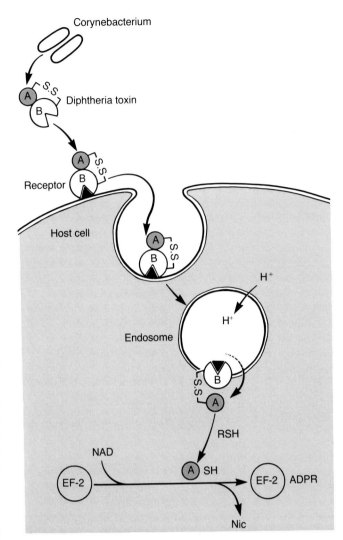

Figure 8–6. Inhibition of cellular protein synthesis by diphtheria toxin. (Adapted from Collier, R.J.: Corynebacteria. In Davis, B.D., Dulbecco, R., Eisen, H.N., and Ginsberg, H.S. (eds.): Microbiology, 3rd ed. New York, Harper & Row, 1990.)

theria toxin, for example, is well understood.[15] The toxin is composed of fragment B, which is at the carboxyl end of the molecule and is essential for attachment to host cells, and fragment A, which is at the amino end and linked to fragment B by a disulfide bridge (Fig. 8–6). Bound diphtheria toxin enters the acidic endosome of cells, where it fuses with the endosomal membrane and enters the cell cytoplasm. There the disulfide bond of the toxin is broken, releasing the enzymatically active fragment A that catalyzes the covalent transfer of adenosine diphosphate ribose (ADPR) from nicotinamide-adenine dinucleotide (NAD) to EF-2; the latter, a ribosomal elongation factor involved in protein synthesis, is thus inactivated. One molecule of diphtheria toxin can kill a cell by ADP-ribosylating more than a million EF-2 molecules. Diphtheria toxin creates a layer of dead cells in the throat, on which Corynebacterium diphtheria outgrows competing bacteria. Subsequently, wide dissemination of diphtheria toxin causes the characteristic neural and myocardial dysfunction of diphtheria.

The heat-labile enterotoxins of *Vibrio cholerae* and of *E. coli* also have an A-B structure and are ADP-ribosyl transferases, but these enzymes catalyze transfer from NAD to the guanyl-nucleotide–dependent regulatory component of adenylate cyclase. This generates excess cyclic adenosine monophosphate (cAMP), which causes intestinal epithelial cells to secrete isosmotic fluid, resulting in voluminous diarrhea and loss of water and electrolytes.

Another well-understood toxin is the alpha toxin produced by the gram-positive anaerobic *Clostridium perfringens,* the agent of gas gangrene. Alpha toxin is a lecithinase that disrupts plasma membranes of erythrocytes, leukocytes, and endothelial cells, resulting in tissue injury.

IMMUNE EVASION BY MICROBES

The humoral and cellular immune responses that protect the host from most infections and the mechanisms of immune-mediated damage to host tissues induced by microbes (e.g., anaphylactic reactions, immune complex reactions) were discussed in Chapter 6. Conversely microorganisms can escape the immune system by several mechanisms, including (1) inaccessibility to immune response, (2) resistance to complement-mediated lysis and phagocytosis, (3) varying or shedding antigens, and (4) causing specific or nonspecific immunosuppression. Here we cite some examples of these phenomena.

Microbes that propagate in the lumen of the intestine (e.g., toxin-producing *Clostridium difficile*) or gallbladder (e.g., *Salmonella typhi*) are inaccessible to the host immune defenses, including secretory IgA. Viruses that are shed from the luminal surface of epithelial cells (e.g., CMV in urine or milk and poliovirus in stool) or those that infect the keratinized epithelium (poxviruses, which cause molluscum contagiosum) are also inaccessible to the host humoral immune system. Some organisms establish infections by rapidly invading host cells before the host humoral response becomes effective (e.g., malaria sporozoites entering liver cells; Trichinella and *Trypanosoma cruzi* entering skeletal or cardiac muscles). Some larger parasites (e.g., the larvae of tapeworms) form cysts in host tissues that are covered by a dense fibrous capsule that walls them off from host immune responses.

The carbohydrate capsule on the surface of all the major pathogens that cause pneumonia or meningitis (pneumococcus, meningococcus, Haemophilus) makes them more virulent by shielding bacterial antigens and preventing phagocytosis of the organisms by neutrophils. Pseudomonas bacteria secrete a leukotoxin that kills neutrophils. Some *E. coli* have K antigens that prevent activation of complement by the alternative pathway and lysis of the cells. Conversely, some gram-negative bacteria have very long polysaccharide O antigens, which bind host antibody and activate complement at such distance from the bacterial cells that the organisms fail to lyse. Staphylococci are covered by protein A molecules that bind the Fc portion of the antibody and so inhibit phagocytosis. Neisseria, Haemophilus, and Streptococcus all secrete proteases that degrade antibodies.

Viral infection evokes neutralizing *antibodies* that prevent viral attachment, penetration, or uncoating. This highly specific immunity is the basis of antiviral vaccination, but it cannot protect against viruses with many antigenic variants (e.g., rhinoviruses or influenza viruses). Pneumococci are capable of more than 80 permutations of their capsular polysaccharides, so in repeated infection the host is unlikely to recognize the new serotype. *Neisseria gonorrheae* have pilar (attachment) proteins composed of a constant region and a hypervariable region.[16] The latter allows Neisseria to change its antigens during infection and prevent immune clearance. Similarly, the spirochete *Borrelia recurrentis* causes a relapsing fever by repeatedly switching its surface antigens before each successive clone is eliminated by the host. Successive clones of African trypanosomes also vary their major surface antigen to escape host antibody responses.[17] Cercariae of *Schistosoma mansoni* shed parasite antigens that are recognized by host antibodies or activate complement by the alternative pathway, within minutes of penetrating the skin. Finally, viruses that infect lymphocytes (HIV and EBV) directly damage the host immune system and cause opportunistic infections (AIDS).

SPECIAL TECHNIQUES FOR DIAGNOSING INFECTIOUS AGENTS

Some infectious agents or their products can be directly observed in hematoxylin and eosin–stained sections (e.g., the inclusion bodies formed by CMV and herpesvirus; bacterial clumps, which usually stain blue; Candida and Mucor, among the fungi; most protozoans; and all helminths). Many infectious agents, however, are best visualized by special stains that identify organisms based on particular characteristics of their cell walls or coat—Gram, acid-fast, silver, mucicarmine, and Giemsa stains—or after labeling with specific antibody probes (Table 8–5). Regardless of the staining technique, organisms are usually best visualized at the advancing edge of a lesion rather than at its center, particularly if there is necrosis. Because these morphologic techniques cannot define species of organisms, determine drug sensitivity, or

Table 8–5. SPECIAL TECHNIQUES FOR DIAGNOSING INFECTIOUS AGENTS

Gram stain	Most bacteria
Acid-fast stain	Mycobacteria, Nocardia (modified)
Silver stains	Fungi, Legionella, Pneumocystis
Periodic acid–Schiff	Fungi, amebae
Mucicarmine	Cryptococci
Giemsa	Campylobacteria, Leishmania, malaria
Antibody probes	Viruses, rickettsiae
Culture	All classes
DNA probes	Viruses, bacteria, protozoa

identify virulence characteristics, cultures of lesional tissue are performed. DNA probes identify microbes that grow slowly in culture (mycobacteria or CMV) or do not culture at all (hepatitis B and C viruses). In addition, DNA sequence analysis has been used to classify bacteria that have never been cultured, including those that cause Whipple's disease (a gram-positive actinobacterium related to actinomyces and streptomyces[18]) and bacillary angiomatosis (genus Rochalimaea).

Regardless of the method of microbial identification, the final step in diagnosis of infectious pathogens is correlation of the suspect organism with the lesion caused and the signs and symptoms produced.

SPECTRUM OF INFLAMMATORY RESPONSES TO INFECTION

In contrast to the vast molecular diversity of microbes, the patterns of tissue responses to these agents are limited. At the microscopic level, therefore, many pathogens produce identical reaction patterns, and few features are unique or pathognomonic of each agent. Moreover, it is the interaction between the microorganism and the host that determines the histologic features of the inflammatory response. Thus, in a profoundly neutropenic host, pyogenic bacteria, which normally evoke vigorous leukocyte responses, may cause rapid tissue necrosis with little leukocyte exudation. Similarly, in a normal patient, *M. tuberculosis* causes well-formed granulomas with few mycobacteria present whereas in an AIDS patient, the same mycobacteria multiply profusely in macrophages, which fail to coalesce into granulomas.

Organisms induce five major patterns of tissue reaction.

SUPPURATIVE (POLYMORPHONUCLEAR) INFLAMMATION. Suppurative inflammation is characterized by increased vascular permeability and leukocytic infiltration, predominantly of neutrophils. The neutrophils are attracted to the site of infection by release of chemoattractants from the rapidly dividing, "pyogenic" bacteria that evoke this response, mostly extracellular gram-positive cocci and gram-negative rods. The bacterial chemoattractants include secreted bacterial peptides, which contain *N*-formyl methionine residues at their amino termini that are recognized by specific receptors on neutrophils. Alternatively, bacteria attract neutrophils indirectly by releasing endotoxin that stimulates macrophages to secrete IL-1 or TNF, or by cleaving complement into chemoattractant peptides. Massing of neutrophils results in the formation of pus. The sizes of exudative lesions vary from tiny microabscesses formed in multiple organs in bacterial septicemia to diffuse involvement of entire lobes of the lung in pneumococcal infections. How destructive the lesions are depends on their location and the organism involved. For example, pneumococci spare alveolar walls, whereas staphylococci and Klebsiella species destroy them and form abscesses. Bacterial pharyngitis heals without sequelae, whereas untreated acute bacterial inflammation of a joint can destroy it in a few days.

Mononuclear and Granulomatous Inflammation

Diffuse, predominantly mononuclear interstitial infiltrates occur in response to viruses, intracellular bacteria, spirochetes, intracellular parasites, or helminths. Which mononuclear cell predominates within the inflammatory lesion depends on the host immune response to the organism. For example, mostly plasma cells are seen in the chancres of primary syphilis and mostly lymphocytes, with active HBV infection or Lyme disease, or in viral infections of the brain (Fig. 8–7). These lymphocytes reflect cell-mediated immunity against the pathogen or the pathogen-infected cells. *Granulomatous inflammation* occurs when aggregates of altered macrophages form, sometimes around a central necrotic focus or fuse together to form giant cells (see Chapter 3). These very distinctive lesions are usually evoked by relatively slowly dividing infectious agents (e.g., *M. tuberculosis* or Histoplasma) or by those of relatively large size (e.g., schistosome eggs) in the presence of T cell–mediated immunity. At the other extreme, macrophages may become filled with organisms, as occurs in *M. avium* infections in AIDS patients, who can mount no immune response to the organisms. For *Mycobacterium leprae* and for cutaneous *leishmaniasis*, some individuals mount a strong immune response so their lesions contain few organisms, few macrophages, and many lymphocytes, whereas other individuals with a weak immune response have lesions with many organisms, many macrophages, and few lymphocytes.

Cytopathic-Cytoproliferative Inflammation

These reactions are characteristic of viral-mediated damage to individual host cells in the absence of host inflammatory response. Some viruses replicate within cells and make viral aggregates that are visible as inclusion bodies (e.g., CMV or adenovirus) or induce cells to fuse and form polykaryons (e.g., measles or herpesviruses). Focal cell damage may cause epithelial cells to become discohesive and form blisters (e.g., herpes; Fig. 8–8). Viruses can also cause epithelial cells to proliferate and form unusual individual and aggregate morphologies (e.g., venereal warts caused by human papillomavirus or the umbilicated papules of molluscum contagiosum caused by poxviruses). Finally, viruses can cause dysplastic changes and cancers in epithelial cells and lymphocytes as discussed in Chapter 7.

Necrotizing Inflammation

Clostridium perfringens and other organisms that secrete very strong toxins cause such rapid and severe tissue damage that cell death is the dominant feature. Because so few inflammatory cells are involved, these lesions resemble ischemic necrosis with disruption or loss of basophilic nuclear staining and preservation of cellular outlines. Similarly, the parasite *Entamoeba histolytica* causes colonic ulcers and liver abscesses characterized by extensive tissue destruction with liquefactive necrosis, in the absence of a prominent inflammatory infiltrate. By entirely different mechanisms, viruses can cause necrotizing inflammation when host cell damage is particularly widespread and severe, as exemplified

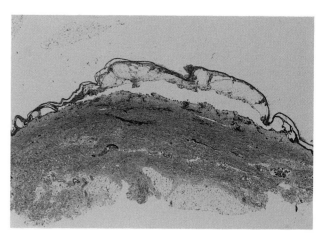

Figure 8–8. Herpes virus blister in mucosa. See Figure 8–25 for viral inclusions.

by total destruction of the temporal lobes of the brain by herpesvirus or the liver by HBV.

Chronic Inflammation and Scarring

The final common pathway of many infections is chronic inflammation, which may lead either to complete healing or to extensive scarring. For some organisms that are relatively inert, the exuberant scarring response is a major cause of dysfunction (e.g., the "pipe-stem" fibrosis of the liver caused by schistosome eggs or the constrictive fibrous pericarditis in tuberculosis).

These patterns of tissue reaction are useful as working tools in analyzing microscopic features of infective processes, but they rarely appear in pure form because they frequently overlap. For example, a cutaneous lesion of leishmaniasis may contain two separate histopathologic regions: a central ulcerated area filled with neutrophils and a peripheral region containing a mixed infiltrate of lymphocytes and mononuclear cells, where the leishmanial parasites are located. The lung of an AIDS patient may be infected with CMV that causes cytolytic changes and Pneumocystis that causes interstitial inflammation. Similar patterns of inflammation can also be seen in tissue responses to physical or chemical agents and in inflammatory diseases of unknown cause.

This concludes our discussion of the general principles in the pathogenesis and pathology of infectious disease. We now turn to brief descriptions of specific infections as they affect different organ systems and distinct patient populations. In each of these categories, we begin with viral infections, followed by bacterial, fungal, or parasitic diseases. In this discussion, we emphasize *pathogenetic mechanisms* and *pathologic changes*, rather than details of clinical features, which are available in clinical textbooks.

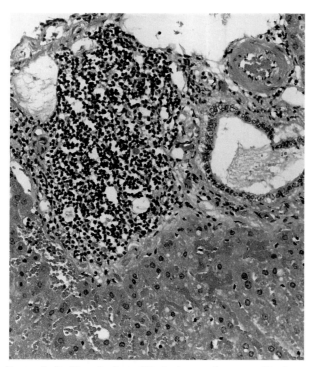

Figure 8–7. Chronic hepatitis in Lyme disease with dense infiltrate of lymphocytes. (Courtesy of Dr. Paul Duray, Brigham and Women's Hospital, Boston.)

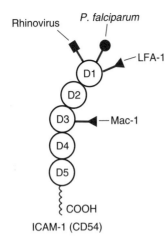

Figure 8-9. ICAM-1, a multifunctional receptor, binds to rhinovirus, *P. falciparum*, and integrins LFA-1 and Mac-1. D1 and D5 are Ig domains of the molecule.

SELECTED HUMAN INFECTIOUS DISEASES

RESPIRATORY INFECTIONS

Viral Respiratory Infections

Viral respiratory disorders are the most frequent and least preventable of all infectious diseases and range in severity from the discomforting but self-limited common cold to life-threatening pneumonias, occurring most often in debilitated or immunosuppressed individuals. Moreover, viral infections damage bronchial epithelium and obstruct airways and so may lead to superinfection with bacteria, including Pneumococcus, Staphylococcus, and Haemophilus. Of the many viruses capable of causing upper respiratory infections (rhinitis, sinusitis, otitis media, pharyngitis, and tonsillitis) and lower respiratory infections (laryngotracheobronchitis, bronchiolitis, interstitial pneumonia, and pleuritis), *rhinovirus* and *influenza virus* are the most important and the best studied.

RHINOVIRUSES. Rhinoviruses, which cause more than 50% of common colds, are members of the picornavirus family (small RNA viruses), which includes poliovirus, hepatitis A virus, and coxsackievirus. Rhinoviruses have a single-stranded RNA genome, surrounded by an unencapsulated, icosahedral capsid composed of four proteins that vary in their antigenicity and account for more than 100 serotypes.[19] There is a cleft, or "canyon," in the rhinovirus surface, inaccessible to antibody, that does not vary among immunotypes and is the presumed site of attachment of the virus to host cells. *The human rhinovirus receptor is intercellular adhesion molecule 1 (ICAM-1 or CD 54)*,[20] a member of the immunoglobulin gene superfamily (Fig. 8-9). The site of binding of rhinovirus on the

ICAM-1 molecule is the same as that used by the leukocyte adhesion molecule LFA-1, the integrin on the surface of lymphocytes that mediates T lymphocyte–specific, antigen-specific responses and leukocyte emigration into inflammatory sites (see Chapter 3).

Rhinoviruses infect humans and higher primates, who have ICAM-1 on their epithelial cells. The infection confined to the upper respiratory tract because the viruses grow best at 33 to 35°C. The injury to epithelial cells is relatively slight, but inflammatory mediators such as bradykinins cause the excessive mucous secretions characteristic of the common cold. Rhinoviruses induce serotype-specific IgG and IgA antibodies, which prevent reinfection with the same rhinovirus but not with other serotypes.

INFLUENZA VIRUSES. Influenza viruses are larger and more complex than rhinoviruses. The genome of influenza is composed of eight helices of single-stranded RNA, each encoding a single gene and each bound by a nucleoprotein that determines the type of influenza virus (A, B, or C). The spherical surface of influenza virus is a lipid bilayer (envelope) containing the viral hemagglutinin and neuraminidase, which determine the subtype of the virus (H1-H3; N1 or N2). The rod-shaped hemagglutinin binds to sialic acid–containing proteins and lipids on host cells and mediates the entry of the virus into the endosome.[21] When the endosome fuses with the lysosome and becomes acidified, the viral hemagglutinin undergoes pH-dependent conformational changes, which mediates fusion with the host cell membrane and injection of the virus into the cytosol. This process is reminiscent of diphtheria toxin entry into the cytosol, described earlier. The neuraminidase forms a mushroom-like projection on the viral surface and, by removing sialic acids, may be important in the release of viruses from host cells. Host antibodies to the hemagglutinin and neuraminidase prevent and ameliorate, respectively, future infection with the flu virus. Two mechanisms account for the clearance of primary influenza virus infection: cytotoxic T cells kill virus-infected cells, and an intracellular anti-influenza protein (called Mx1) is induced in macrophages by the cytokines interferon-alpha and beta.[22]

Influenza viruses of type A infect humans, pigs, horses, and birds and are the major cause of pandemic and epidemic flu infections. Remarkably, a single subtype of influenza virus A predominates throughout the world at a given time. The pandemic of influenza in 1918 that killed 20 million people occurred when both the hemagglutinin and the neuraminidase were replaced through recombination of RNA segments with those of animal viruses, making all individuals susceptible to the new influenza virus (*antigenic shift*).[23] Epidemics of influenza, which are less severe and more local than pandemics, occur through mutations of the hemagglutinin and neuraminidase that allow the virus to escape most host antibodies *(antigenic drift)*. Influenza virus types B and C, which do not show antigenic drift or shift, infect mostly children, who develop antibodies against reinfection in a manner similar to chickenpox, mumps, and other childhood viral illnesses. Rarely, influenza virus may cause interstitial myocarditis or, following aspirin therapy, Reye's syndrome (see Chapter 18).

> **MORPHOLOGY.** Viral upper respiratory infections are marked by mucosal hyperemia and swelling with a predominantly lymphomonocytic and plasmacytic infiltration of the submucosa accompanied by overproduction of mucous secretions. The swollen mucosa and viscid exudate may plug the nasal channels, sinuses, or Eustachian tubes and lead to suppurative secondary bacterial infection. Virus-induced tonsillitis with enlargement of the lymphoid tissue within Waldeyer's ring is frequent in children, although lymphoid hyperplasia is not usually associated with suppuration or abscess formation, such as is encountered with streptococci or staphylococci.
>
> In **laryngotracheobronchitis** and **bronchiolitis,** there is vocal cord swelling and abundant mucous exudation. Impairment of bronchociliary function invites bacterial superinfection with more marked suppuration. Plugging of small airways may give rise to focal lung atelectasis. In the more severe bronchiolar involvement, widespread plugging of secondary and terminal airways by cell debris, fibrin, and inflammatory exudate may, when prolonged, cause organization and fibrosis, resulting in obliterative bronchiolitis and permanent lung damage. Viral pneumonias, like bacterial pneumonias, take a variety of anatomic forms, which are described in Chapter 15.

Bacterial Respiratory Infections

Bacterial pneumonias are some of the most common bacterial infections in humans and are particularly important because they are most frequently cited as the *immediate cause* of death in hospitalized patients. Almost any type of virulent bacterial species can cause pneumonia, and the pathogenesis and pathology of the most common pneumonias are described in detail in Chapter 15. Here we cover only infections caused by *Haemophilus influenzae* and *Mycobacterium tuberculosis*.

HAEMOPHILUS INFLUENZAE INFECTION. *H. influenzae* is a pleomorphic, gram-negative organism that is a major cause of life-threatening acute lower respiratory tract infections and meningitis in young children. *H. influenzae* is a ubiquitous colonizer of the pharynx, where it exists in two forms—encapsulated (5%) and unencapsulated (95%). The encapsulated *H. influenzae* dominates the unencapsulated forms by secreting an antibiotic called haemocin that kills the unencapsulated *H. influenzae*.[24] Although there are six serotypes of the encapsulated form (a–f), type b, which has a polyribosephosphate capsule, is the most frequent cause of severe invasive disease. Nonencapsulated forms, however, may also spread along the surface of the upper respiratory tract and produce otitis media (infection of the middle ear), sinusitis, and bronchopneumonia.

Fimbriae and other adhesins on the surface of *H. influenzae* mediate adherence of the organisms to the respiratory epithelium. In addition, *H. influenzae* secrete a factor that disorganizes ciliary beating, and a protease that degrades IgA, the major class of antibody secreted into the airways. Survival of *H. influenzae* in the bloodstream correlates with the presence of the capsule, which, like that of *Pneumococcus*, prevents opsonization by complement and phagocytosis by host cells. Antibodies against the capsule protect the host from *H. influenzae* infection, so the capsular polysaccharide b is incorporated in a vaccine for children against *H. influenzae*. In *H. influenzae* meningitis, a lipopolysaccharide endotoxin induces leukocyte chemotaxis and leukocytosis, and a cell wall peptidoglycan damages the vascular endothelium and disrupts the blood-brain barrier.[25]

> **MORPHOLOGY.** *H. influenzae* respiratory infections range from trivial involvement of the pharynx, middle ear, sinuses, or tonsils, which resemble viral upper respiratory infections, to severe febrile bacteremic illnesses that may be resistant to routine antibiotics. Acute epiglottitis and related involvement are more frequently caused by *H. influenzae* than by any other pathogen. The uvula, epiglottic folds, and vocal cords swell rapidly and may suffocate the child within less than 24 hours if an open airway is not promptly established.
>
> **H. influenzae pneumonia,** which may follow a viral respiratory infection, is a pediatric emergency and has a high mortality rate. Descending laryngotracheobronchitis results in airway obstruction as the smaller bronchi are plugged by dense, fibrin-rich exudate of polymorphonuclear cells, similar to that seen in pneumococcal pneumonias. Pulmonary consolidation is usually lobular and patchy but may be confluent and involve the entire lung lobe.
>
> *H. influenzae* is one of the most common causes of suppurative meningitis in children up to five years of age, the pathology of which is described in Chapter 29. *H. influenzae* also causes an acute, purulent conjunctivitis (pink eye) in children and, in predisposed older patients, may cause septicemia, endocarditis, pyelonephritis, cholecystitis, and suppurative arthritis.

TUBERCULOSIS (MYCOBACTERIUM TUBERCULOSIS).

M. tuberculosis infects about one-third of the world's population and kills about 3 million patients each year and so is the single most important infectious cause of death on earth.[26] With alleviation of overcrowding, which causes the spread of *M. tuberculosis,* and with the introduction of effective antibiotics in the 1950s, the United States and Western countries enjoyed a long decline in the rates of *M. tuberculosis* infections and deaths until the mid-1980s. Since that time, tuberculosis has been increasing here and in Europe and especially in Africa, in part because *M. tuberculosis* frequently and dramatically infects persons with AIDS.[27] These individuals, who have a diminished T cell–mediated resistance to *M. tuberculosis* (see later), develop disease at much higher rates than do healthy persons, have more abundant pulmonary disease, and are more likely to transmit *M. tuberculosis* to others. In addition, multidrug-resistant *M. tuberculosis* has appeared among AIDS patients, threatening close contacts and health care workers. This multidrug-resistant *M. tuberculosis* causes an 80% fatality rate in patients with AIDS and a 50% mortality rate in nonimmunosuppressed individuals, similar to the 50% mortality rate of untreated *M. tuberculosis* in nonimmunosuppressed individuals.[28] Tuberculosis is discussed further in Chapter 15. Here, we shall review general aspects of etiology and pathogenesis and review the morphology of only selected features of the disease.

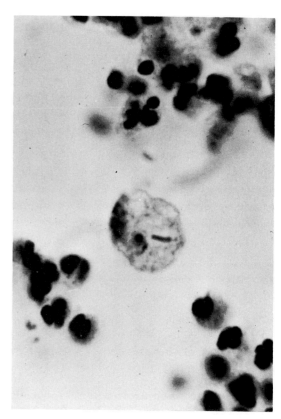

Figure 8–10. A macrophage with an engulfed tubercle bacillus (acid-fast stain).

Etiology and Pathogenesis. Two species of Mycobacterium cause tuberculosis: *M. tuberculosis* and *M. bovis*. *M. tuberculosis* is transmitted by inhalation of infective droplets coughed or sneezed into the air by a patient with tuberculosis. *M. bovis* is transmitted by milk from diseased cows and first produces intestinal or tonsillar lesions. In developed countries, control of *M. bovis* in dairy herds and pasteurization of milk have virtually eradicated this organism. *M. avium* and *M. intracellulare,* two closely related mycobacteria, have no virulence in normal hosts but cause disseminated infections in 15 to 24% of patients with AIDS.[29] *M. leprae* is the cause of leprosy, discussed later in this chapter.

Mycobacteria are aerobic, non–spore-forming, nonmotile bacilli with a waxy coat that causes them to retain the red dye when treated with acid ("red snappers") in the acid-fast stains. The growth of these mycobacteria in culture is very slow (20 to 100 times slower than that of other bacteria), so it takes 4 to 6 weeks to obtain a colony of *M. tuberculosis* for identification or drug-sensitivity studies. In lieu of culture results, a positive tuberculin test, a demonstration of delayed-type hypersensitivity to a purified protein derivative of *M. tuberculosis* (PPD) injected beneath the skin, confirms previous exposure to the mycobacteria but does not prove

active mycobacterial infection. Currently, molecular techniques are being developed to identify mycobacterial species more rapidly.

There are three important considerations in the pathogenesis of tuberculosis: (1) the basis of the virulence of the organism, (2) the relationship of hypersensitivity to immunity against infection, and (3) the pathogenesis of tissue destruction and caseous necrosis.

As to virulence, *M. tuberculosis* has no known exotoxins, endotoxins, or histolytic enzymes. Instead, its pathogenicity is related to its ability to escape killing by macrophages and induce delayed-type hypersensitivity (Fig. 8–11). This has been attributed to several components of the *M. tuberculosis* cell wall. First is *cord factor,* a surface glycolipid that causes *M. tuberculosis* to grow in serpentine cords *in vitro.* Virulent strains of *M. tuberculosis* have cord factor on their surface, whereas avirulent strains do not, and injection of purified cord factor into mice induces characteristic granulomas. Second are *sulfatides,* which are surface glycolipids containing sulfur that are present on virulent but not avirulent *M. tuberculosis.* They prevent fusion of phagosomes of macrophages containing *M. tuberculosis* with the lysosomes. Third, *LAM,* a major heteropolysaccharide similar in structure to the endotoxin of gram-negative bacteria, inhibits macrophage activation by interferon-gamma. LAM also induces macrophages to secrete TNF-α, which causes fever, weight loss, and tissue damage, and IL-10, which suppresses mycobacteria-induced T-cell proliferation (see Chapter 6).[30] Fourth, a highly immunogenic 65-kd *M. tuberculosis heat-shock protein* is similar to human heat-shock proteins (see Chapter 1) and may have a role in autoimmune reactions induced by *M. tuberculosis*.[31] Finally, *complement* activated on the surface of mycobacteria may opsonize the organism and facilitate its uptake via the macrophage complement receptor CR3 (MAC-1 integrin) without triggering the respiratory burst necessary to kill the organisms.

The development of cell-mediated, or type IV, hypersensitivity to the tubercle bacillus probably explains the organism's destructiveness in tissues and also the emergence of resistance to the organisms. On the initial exposure to the organism, the inflammatory response is nonspecific, resembling the reaction to any form of bacterial invasion. Within 2 or 3 weeks, coincident with the appearance of a positive skin reaction, the reaction becomes granulomatous and the centers of granulomas become caseous, forming typical "soft tubercles." The sequence of events following an initial lung infection is outlined in Figure 8–11. The pattern of host response depends on whether the infection represents a *primary* first exposure to the organism or *secondary* reaction in an already sensitized host.

Primary *M. Tuberculosis*. The primary phase of *M. tuberculosis* infection begins with inhalation of the mycobacteria and ends with a T cell–mediated immune response that induces hypersensitivity to the organisms and controls 95% of infections. Most often in the periphery of one lung, inhaled *M. tuberculosis* is first phagocytosed by alveolar macrophages and transported by these cells to hilar lymph nodes. Naive macrophages are unable to kill the mycobacteria, which multiply, lyse the host cell, infect other macrophages, and sometimes disseminate through the blood to other parts of the lung and elsewhere in the body. After a few weeks, T cell–mediated immunity develops that is demonstrable by a positive PPD test and involves mycobacteria-activated T cells interacting with macrophages in two ways.[32] First, CD4+ helper T cells secrete interferon-gamma, which activates macrophages to kill intracellular mycobacteria via reactive nitrogen intermediates, including NO, NO_2, and HNO_3. This is associated with the formation of epithelioid cell granulomas (see Chapter 3) and clearance of the mycobacteria. Second, CD8+ suppresser T cells kill macrophages that are infected with mycobacteria, resulting in the formation of caseating granulomas (delayed-type hypersensitivity reactions; Fig. 8–12). Direct toxicity of the mycobacteria to the macrophages may also contribute to the necrotic centers. Regardless of

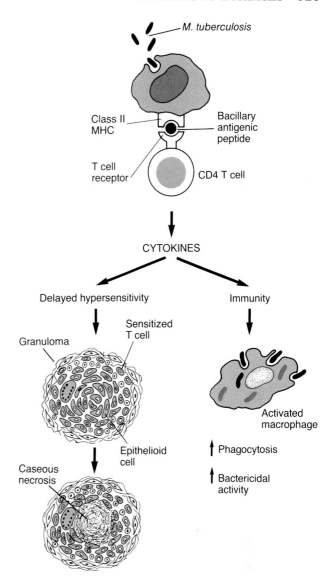

Figure 8–11. Tuberculosis: The dual consequences of macrophage activation and sensitization.

the cause of caseation, mycobacteria cannot grow in this acidic, extracellular environment lacking in oxygen, and so the mycobacterial infection is controlled. The ultimate residuum of the primary infection is a calcified scar in the lung parenchyma and in the hilar lymph node, together referred to as the *Ghon complex* (see Chapter 15).

Secondary and Disseminated Tuberculosis. Some individuals become reinfected with mycobacteria, reactivate dormant disease, or progress directly from the primary mycobacterial lesions into disseminated disease. This may be because the strain of mycobacterium is particularly virulent or the host is particularly susceptible. In mice, susceptibility to mycobacterial (as well as Salmonella and Leishmania) infection is determined by an autosomal dominant gene called *Bcg*, which encodes a membrane transport protein.[33] Whether the effect

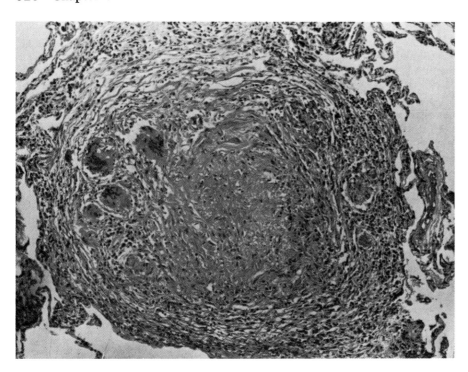

Figure 8–12. Granuloma caused by *M. tuberculosis* with central caseation and giant cells.

of this protein is at the level of the plasma membrane or interferes with bacterial killing in the phagolysosome is unclear. Granulomas of secondary tuberculosis most often occur in the apex of the lungs but may be widely disseminated in the lungs, kidneys, meninges, marrow, and other organs. These granulomas, which fail to contain the spread of the mycobacterial infection, are the major cause of tissue damage in tuberculosis and are a reflection of delayed-type hypersensitivity. Two special features of secondary tuberculosis are the presence of caseous necrosis and of cavities, which rupture into blood vessels, spreading mycobacteria throughout the body, and break into airways, releasing infectious mycobacteria in aerosols.

MORPHOLOGY. The histopathology of primary and secondary pulmonary tuberculosis is described in Chapter 15. **Miliary tuberculosis** refers to hematogenous dissemination of tuberculous lesions throughout the body. The term miliary is descriptive of the small, yellow-white lesions, which resemble millet seeds fed to birds, and are present in the lungs and systemic organs (see Chapter 15, Fig. 15–26). Certain tissues are relatively resistant to tuberculous infection, so it is rare to find tubercles in the heart, striated muscle, thyroid, and pancreas. In certain instances, hematogenously spread organisms are destroyed in all tissues but persist in only one organ (isolated end-organ disease). This occurrence is most frequent in the lungs, cervical lymph nodes (scrofula), meninges (tuberculous

meningitis), kidneys, adrenals, bones (tuberculous osteomyelitis), Fallopian tubes, and epididymis. In vertebral tuberculosis (Pott's disease), long fistulas may form along the psoas muscle to open and drain into the groin region.

***M. tuberculosis* and *M. avium-intracellulare* Lesions in AIDS.** Mycobacterial infection in patients with AIDS can take three forms, depending on the degree of immunosuppression: (1) In developing countries, where *M. tuberculosis* infection is frequent, HIV-infected individuals often have primary and secondary *M. tuberculosis* infection with the usual, well-formed granulomas composed of epithelioid cells, Langhans' giant cells, and lymphocytes. In these lesions, acid-fast mycobacteria are few and often difficult to find. (2) When HIV-positive patients develop AIDS and are moderately immunosuppressed (less than 200 CD4+ helper T cells per mm^3), *M. tuberculosis* infection is frequently caused by reactivation or by exposure to new mycobacteria. Because HIV infects both T cells and macrophages, defects in the host immune response to *M. tuberculosis* may be secondary to the failure of helper T cells to secrete lymphokines that activate macrophages to kill mycobacteria or the failure of HIV-infected and mycobacteria-infected macrophages to respond to lymphokines. The relative increase in the number of CD8+ cytotoxic T cells may also cause macrophage destruction in the *M. tuberculosis* lesions. Histologically, granulomas are less well formed, are more frequently necrotic, and contain more abundant

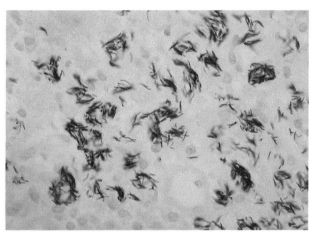

Figure 8-13. *M. avium* infection in a patient with AIDS, showing massive infection with acid-fast organisms. (Courtesy of Dr. Arlene Sharpe.)

acid-fast organisms. Neutrophils may be present where tuberculous cavities have eroded into the airways. Although the sputum is positive for acid-fast organisms in 31 to 82% of patients with AIDS, only 33% of patients are reactive to PPD. Extrapulmonary tuberculosis occurs in 70% of such patients, involving lymph nodes, blood, central nervous system, and bowel. Despite the severity of *M. tuberculosis* infection in AIDS patients, treatment with multiple drugs clears all but the multidrug-resistant organisms. (3) Opportunistic infections with *M. avium-intracellulare* occurs in severely immunosuppressed patients (less than 60 CD4+ cells per mm^3). Most infections with these organisms originate in the gastrointestinal tract, although some begin in the lung. *M. avium-intracellulare* infections are usually widely disseminated throughout the reticuloendothelial systems, causing enlargement of involved lymph nodes, liver, and spleen. There may be a yellowish pigmentation to these organs secondary to the large number of *M. avium-intracellulare* present in swollen macrophages (as many as 10^{10} organisms per gram of tissue) (Fig. 8-13). Granulomas, lymphocytes, and tissue destruction are rare.

Respiratory Infections by Dimorphic and Geographic Fungi

Histoplasmosis and *coccidioidomycosis* are discussed together because (1) both are granulomatous diseases of the lungs that may resemble tuberculosis, (2) both are caused by fungi that are thermally dimorphic in that they grow as hyphae that produce spores at environmental temperatures but grow as yeasts (spherules or ellipses) at body temperature within the lungs and (3) each fungus is geographic in that it causes disease primarily among persons living along the Ohio and Mississippi Rivers and in the Caribbean (Histoplasma) and in the Southwest and Far West of the United States and in Mexico (Coccidioidomyces).

HISTOPLASMOSIS. *Histoplasma capsulatum* infection is acquired by inhalation of dust particles from soil contaminated with bird or bat droppings that contain small spores (microconidia), the infectious form of the fungus. Like *M. tuberculosis*, *H. capsulatum* are intracellular parasites of macrophages. The clinical presentations and morphologic lesions of histoplasmosis also strikingly resemble those of tuberculosis, including (1) a self-limited and often latent primary pulmonary involvement, which may result in coin lesions on chest x-ray; (2) chronic, progressive, secondary lung disease, which is localized to the lung apices and causes cough, fever, and night sweats; (3) localized lesions in extrapulmonary sites, including mediastinum, adrenals, liver, or meninges; and (4) a widely disseminated involvement, particularly in immunosuppressed patients. Differentiation of histoplasmosis from tuberculosis is made by eliciting a delayed-type hypersensitivity response to skin injection of a fungal lysate (histoplasmin test, similar to the tuberculin test) or by identification of the fungus in lung, lymph node, or bone marrow biopsy specimens in patients with disseminated histoplasmosis.

Unopsonized Histoplasma conidia (infectious form) and yeasts (tissue form) bind to the beta-chain of the integrins receptors LFA-1 (CD11a/CD18) and MAC-1 (CD11b/CD18). Histoplasma yeasts are phagocytosed by the unstimulated macrophages, multiply within the phagolysosome, and lyse the host cells. Histoplasma infections are controlled by helper T cells that recognize fungal cell wall antigens and heat-shock proteins and subsequently secrete interferon-gamma that activates macrophages to kill intracellular yeasts. In addition, Histoplasma induces macrophages to secrete TNF-α, which stimulates other macrophages to kill Histoplasma.[35] Lacking cellular immunity, patients with AIDS are susceptible to disseminated infection with Histoplasma, which is a major opportunistic pathogen in this disease.

MORPHOLOGY. In the lungs of otherwise healthy adults, Histoplasma infections produce epithelioid cell granulomas, which usually undergo coagulative necrosis and coalesce to produce large areas of consolidation but may also liquefy to form cavities. With spontaneous or drug control of the infection, these lesions undergo fibrosis and calcification (Fig. 8-14). Histologic differentiation from tuberculosis, sarcoidosis, and coccidioidomycosis requires identification of the 2 to 5 μm, thin-walled yeast forms (stained with methenamine silver) that may persist in tissues for years.

In **chronic histoplasmosis,** gray-white granulomas are usually present in the apices of the lungs,

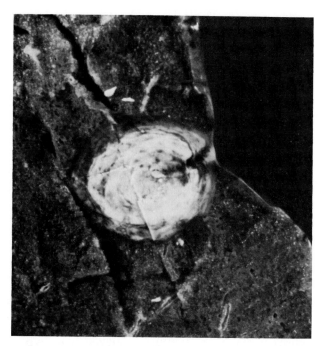

Figure 8-14. Laminated Histoplasma granuloma of the lung.

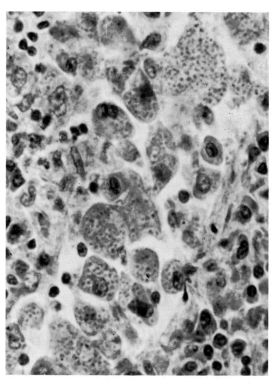

Figure 8-15. *Histoplasma capsulatum* yeast forms fill phagocytes in a lymph node of a patient with disseminated histoplasmosis.

with retraction and thickening of the pleura, and in the hilar nodes. Further progression involves more and more of the lung parenchyma, with cavity formation less frequent than in tuberculosis.

In **fulminant disseminated histoplasmosis,** which occurs in immunosuppressed individuals, epithelioid cell granulomas are not formed, but instead there are focal accumulations of mononuclear phagocytes filled with fungal yeasts throughout the tissues and organs of the body. The overloading of the reticuloendothelial system with macrophages stuffed with organisms resembles that found in severe cases of visceral leishmaniasis (Fig. 8–15), described later.

COCCIDIOIDOMYCOSIS. Almost everyone who inhales the spores of *Coccidioides immitis* becomes infected and develops a delayed-type hypersensitivity to the fungus, so that more than 80% of persons in endemic areas of the Southwest and Western United States have a positive skin test. One reason for the high rate of infectivity by *C. immitis* is the fact that infective arthroconidia, when ingested by alveolar macrophages, block fusion of the phagosome and lysosome and so resist intracellular killing.[36] As is the case with Histoplasma, most primary infections with *C. immitis* are asymptomatic, but 10% of persons have lung lesions, fever, cough, and pleuritic pains, accompanied by erythema nodosum or erythema multiforme (the San Joaquin Valley fever complex). Fewer than 1% of persons develop disseminated *C. immitis* infection, which frequently involves the skin and meninges.

MORPHOLOGY. The primary and secondary lung lesions of *C. immitis* are similar to the granulomatous lesions of Histoplasma. Within macrophages or giant cells, *C. immitis* is present as thick-walled, nonbudding spherules 20 to 60 μm in diameter, often filled with small endospores (Fig. 8–16). A pyogenic reaction is superimposed when the spherules rupture to release the endospores, which are not infectious. In contrast, infectious *C. immitis* boxcar-like arthrospores produced in culture are easily detached and disseminated by air, so extreme caution is needed in handling this fungus in the laboratory. Rare progressive *C. immitis* disease involves the lungs, meninges, skin, bones, adrenals, lymph nodes, spleen, or liver. At all these sites, the inflammatory response may be purely granulomatous, pyogenic, or mixed. Purulent lesions dominate in patients with diminished resistance and with widespread dissemination.

GASTROINTESTINAL (GI) INFECTIONS

The clinicopathologic features of GI infections are discussed in Chapter 17, and in this chapter attention is directed largely to pathogenetic mechanisms. Table 8–6 lists the major causes of GI infection.

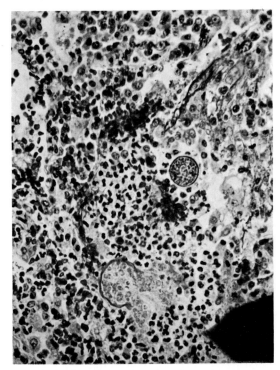

Figure 8–16. Coccidioidomycosis with an intact spherule and a ruptured spherule releasing endospores.

Viral Enteritis and Diarrhea

Acute, self-limited infectious diarrhea, which is a major cause of morbidity among children, is most frequently caused by enteric viruses, including rotaviruses, Norwalk-like viruses, coronaviruses, adenoviruses, and astroviruses. In infants, infectious diarrhea may cause severe dehydration and metabolic acidosis, which may result in hospitalization in Developed Countries and death in developing countries.

Rotavirus, which is an encapsulated virus with a segmented double-stranded RNA genome, is the major cause of diarrhea in infants.[37] Like other enteric viruses, rotavirus is spread by the fecal-oral route. Rotaviruses invade and destroy mature host epithelial cells in the middle and upper villus. Viral diarrhea is caused by a decreased absorption of sodium and water from the bowel lumen, in contrast to toxin-mediated bacterial diarrheas, which are caused by increased secretion from host epithelial cells. Because secretory immunity to rotavirus surface antigens develops, older children and adults are resistant to infection. These antirotavirus antibodies are present in mother's milk, so rotavirus infection is most frequent at the time of weaning. Although rotaviruses were initially diagnosed in the stool by electron microscopy, these viruses are now identified by enzyme-linked immunoabsorbent assays (ELISAs).[38]

Norwalk-like viruses, which are small icosahedral viruses containing a single-stranded RNA genome, cause epidemic gastroenteritis with diarrhea, nausea, and vomiting among children. *Coronaviruses* are pleomorphic enveloped viruses, which have large club-shaped projections (crowns). Coronaviruses cause diarrhea and upper respiratory tract infections and are usually endemic rather

Table 8–6. MAJOR INFECTIOUS CAUSES OF DIARRHEA

ORGANISM	COMMENT
Viruses	
Rotaviruses	Principally in children under age six. Sporadic—from contaminated water, may become epidemic; also direct fecal-oral transmission
Enteric adenoviruses	Common in infants and children, mostly sporadic
Norwalk virus	Young and old, mainly epidemic; fecal-oral
Bacteria	
Enterotoxigenic *E. coli*	Major cause of traveler's diarrhea, food- and water-borne, previously unencountered strains
Campylobacter jejuni	Major global cause, any age, mainly children, transmission by contaminated water and food
Yersinia enterocolitica	Similar to above
Shigella	Major global offender, children and adults, fecal-oral direct transmission and contaminated water and food, endemic and epidemic
Enteropathogenic *E. coli*	Children and nursery outbreaks
Salmonella spp.	Large number serotypes with range of clinical syndromes, children and adults, food- and water-borne, human and animal reservoirs
Clostridium difficile	Antibiotic-associated, hospital-acquired, mainly in predisposed adults
Vibrio cholerae	Major cause of pandemic and epidemic diarrhea in developing infections
Parasites	
Giardia lamblia	Carrier state common, major cause of traveler's diarrhea, contaminated drinking water, high infection rate in Russia, northwestern United States, other locales; may become epidemic
Entamoeba histolytica	Large reservoir of asymptomatic carriers in developed countries and endemic in developing areas, fecal-oral, sexual transmission particularly among homosexuals, and from contaminated water and food

than epidemic. *Enteric adenoviruses,* distinguished from adenoviruses that cause respiratory disease by their failure to grow easily in culture, are the second leading cause of diarrhea among infants.

MORPHOLOGY. Although the enteric viruses are genetically and morphologically very different from each other, the lesions they cause in the intestinal tract are similar.[39] There is a blunting and destruction of the villus epithelial cells, which contain viruses visible by electron microscopy or immunofluorescence staining. There is secondary hyperplasia of the mucosal crypts and a mixed inflammatory infiltrate of the lamina propria.

Bacterial Enteritis

SHIGELLA BACILLARY DYSENTERY. Dysentery refers to diarrhea with abdominal cramping and tenesmus in which loose stools contain blood, pus, and mucus. Bacillary dysentery, which results in as many as 500,000 deaths among children in developing countries each year, is caused by *Shigella dysenteriae, S. flexneri, S. boydii,* and *S. sonnei* as well as certain O-type enterotoxic *E. coli.* Amebic dysentery is caused by the protozoan parasite *Entamoeba histolytica,* discussed later in this chapter. Shigella species are gram-negative facultative anaerobes, which in contrast to Salmonella infect only humans.[14] Transmission is fecal-oral and is remarkable for the small number of organisms that may cause disease (10 ingested organisms cause illness in 10% of volunteers, and 500 organisms cause disease in 50% of volunteers). *S. flexneri* is the major cause of bacillary dysentery in endemic locations of poor hygiene, including large regions of the developing world and institutions in the developed world. Epidemic shigellosis occurs when individuals consume uncooked foods at picnics or other events.

Shigella bacteria invade the intestinal mucosal cells but do not usually go beyond the lamina propria. They cause diarrhea by unclear mechanisms. Dysentery is caused when the bacteria escape the epithelial cell phagolysosome, multiply within the cytoplasm, and destroy host cells. Shigella genes, some of which are plasmid-encoded, associated with bacterial virulence include those that encode (1) a master regulatory protein; (2) a lipopolysaccharide capsule; (3) bacterial proteins that bind to host cells; (4) a hemolysin associated with breakdown of the phagolysosome; (5) proteins involved with intercellular spread; (6) superoxide dismutase, which protects bacteria from killing by macrophages; and (7) Shiga toxin, which, like the *E. coli* Shiga-like toxin blocks host cell protein synthesis

by cleaving the 28S ribosomal RNA. This toxin is also involved in the genesis of the hemolytic-uremic syndrome associated with both Shigella and *E. coli* infections (see Chapter 20). In addition, chronic arthritis secondary to *S. flexneri* infection in HLA-B27 individuals, called Reiter's syndrome, may be caused by a bacterial antigen that crossreacts with the HLA-B27 host protein.

MORPHOLOGY. In severe bacillary dysentery, the colonic mucosa becomes hyperemic and edematous; enlargement of the lymphoid follicles creates small, projecting nodules. Within the course of 24 hours, a fibrinosuppurative exudate first patchily, then diffusely covers the mucosa and produces a dirty gray-to-yellow pseudomembrane (Fig. 8-17). The inflammatory reaction within the intestinal mucosa builds up, the mucosa becomes soft and friable, and irregular superficial ulcerations appear. If the infection is severe, large tracts may be denuded, leaving only islands of preserved mucosa.

Histologically, there is a predominantly mononuclear leukocytic infiltrate within the lamina propria, but the surfaces of the ulcers are covered with an acute, suppurative, neutrophilic reaction accompanied by congestion, marked edema, fibrin deposition, and thromboses of small vessels. As the disease progresses, the ulcer margins are transformed into active granulation tissue. When the disease remits, this granulation tissue fills the defect, and the ulcers heal by regeneration of the mucosal epithelium.

CAMPYLOBACTER ENTERITIS. This comma-shaped, flagellated, gram-negative organism was once classified with the vibrios. Only when special culture conditions permitted its isolation did it become ap-

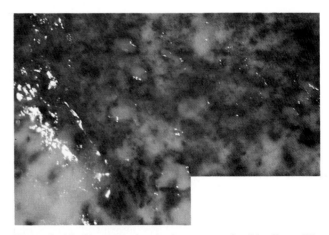

Figure 8–17. Closeup of colonic mucosa in shigella colitis with erythema, ulceration, and pseudomembrane formation (white plaques).

parent that Campylobacter was an important cause of chronic gastritis, enterocolitis, and septicemia in humans that had frequently been missed by routine cultures for enterobacteria. The role of *Helicobacter pylori*, previously called *Campylobacter*, in gastritis and peptic ulceration is discussed in detail in Chapter 17; here our attention is directed to the enteritis. Currently, *Campylobacter jejuni* is responsible for 5 to 11% of all cases of diarrhea and dysentery in United States hospitals, equaling or surpassing the salmonellae as an enteric pathogen.[40] Infection with Campylobacter species occurs by ingestion, most often of contaminated liquid or solid food, such as milk, poultry, or water. Epidemics are usually modest in size, affecting both children and adults. Sporadic infections may be derived from human or zoonotic sources; domestic dogs are frequent carriers.

Campylobacter species induce disease by three mechanisms, shared with other enteric pathogens. One is toxin-induced disease with watery diarrhea similar to cholera. Another type involves invasion and proliferation within the intestinal epithelium, leading to cell death. This is manifested clinically by bloody diarrhea and inflammatory cells in the stool. A third mechanism is termed translocation, whereby the organisms penetrate the intestinal mucosa and proliferate within the lamina propria and mesenteric lymph nodes. This may produce an enteric fever without frank dysentery.[41]

> **MORPHOLOGY.** Inflammation may involve the entire gut from the jejunum to the anus. In invasive infection, the colonic mucosa appears friable or superficially eroded on proctoscopy. By light microscopy, hyperemia; edema; and inflammatory infiltrates of neutrophils, lymphocytes, and plasma cells are seen. There may be colonic crypt abscesses and ulcerations resembling those of chronic ulcerative colitis. In the small bowel, there is some decrease in the crypt-villus ratio.[42]

YERSINIA ENTERITIS. *Y. enterocolitica* and *Y. pseudotuberculosis* are gram-negative facultative intracellular bacteria related to *Y. pestis*, which causes epidemic plague. *Y. enterocolitica* and *Y. pseudotuberculosis* cause fecal-oral–transmitted ileitis and mesenteric lymphadenitis, which is most frequent among children but may affect adults as well.[43] Although Yersinia infections respond to appropriate antibiotics, patients with Yersinia bacteria in the appendix or with chronic ileocolitis are often surgically explored for appendicitis. Extraintestinal manifestations of Yersinia infection include arthritis, erythema nodosum, and glomerulonephritis.

Y. pseudotuberculosis has a variety of molecules on its surface involved in attachment to and phagocytosis by host epithelial cells, including a protein called invasin, which binds to host cell $\beta 1$-integrins that also bind fibronectin and collagen.[44] Within host cells, *Y. pseudotuberculosis* secretes a serine/threonine kinase and a protein tyrosine phosphatase, which damage host cells, presumably by disrupting the normal signal transduction pathways.[45]

> **MORPHOLOGY.** *Y. enterocolitica* and *Y. pseudotuberculosis* most frequently involve the distal ileum and colon, although they can cause pharyngitis and tonsillitis. The ulcerative intestinal lesions resemble those of typhoid fever, although there may also be a diffuse enteritis with villus shortening, crypt hyperplasia, and mucosal microabscesses. Within submucosal tissues, yersiniae produce microabscesses rimmed by activated macrophages, which resemble the stellate granulomas of lymphogranuloma venereum and cat-scratch disease.

Salmonellosis and Typhoid Fever

Salmonellae are flagellated, gram-negative bacteria that cause a self-limited food-borne and water-borne gastroenteritis (*S. enteritidis*, *S. typhimurium*, and others), or a life-threatening systemic illness marked by fever (*S. typhi*). In the United States, Salmonella species cause approximately 500,000 reported cases of food poisoning, and many cases go unreported. Because Salmonella species (other than *S. typhi*) infect most commercially raised chickens and many cows, the major sources of Salmonella in the United States are feces-contaminated meat and chicken that are insufficiently washed and cooked. In contrast, humans are the only host of *S. typhi*, which is shed in the feces, urine, vomitus, and oral secretions by acutely ill persons and in the feces by chronic carriers without overt disease. Therefore typhoid fever is a disease largely of developing countries where sanitary conditions are insufficient to stop its spread. Typhoid fever is a protracted disease that includes bacteremia with fever and chills during the first week; widespread reticuloendothelial involvement with rash, abdominal pain, and prostration in the second week; and ulceration of Peyer's patches with intestinal bleeding and shock during the third week.

Salmonellae invade nonphagocytotic intestinal epithelial cells as well as tissue macrophages. Invasion of intestinal epithelial cells is controlled by different invasion genes that are induced by the low oxygen tension found in the gut. These genes encode proteins involved in adhesion and in recruitment of host cytoskeletal proteins that internalize the bacterium.[11] Mutant bacteria unable to penetrate epithelial cells *in vitro* are not in-

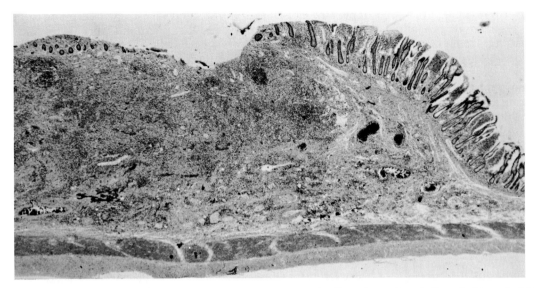

Figure 8-18. Typhoid fever. Low-power view of cross-section of a markedly enlarged and disrupted lymphoid follicle in ileum, with necrosis of overlying mucosa.

fectious when given orally but are infectious when injected into the peritoneum. In contrast, Salmonella mutants, which are unable to grow within macrophages *in vitro*, are not infectious *in vivo*. Some 20 different genes, which are also coregulated by starvation of bacteria *in vitro*, are induced by the acid pH within the macrophage phagolysosome.[46] Other bacterial genes, which are turned on by the growth of Salmonella *in vivo*, may be virulence factors.[47]

MORPHOLOGY. Lesions induced by *S. enteritides* or *typhimurium* are limited to the ileum and colon and include erosion of the epithelium and mixed inflammation in the lamina propria. Variable numbers of polymorphonuclear neutrophils are found in the stools, depending on the severity of the infections. *S. typhi* causes proliferation of phagocytes with enlargement of reticuloendothelial and lymphoid tissues throughout the body. Peyer's patches in the terminal ileum become sharply delineated, plateau-like elevations up to 8 cm in diameter, with enlargement of draining mesenteric lymph nodes. In the second week, the mucosa over the swollen lymphoid tissue is shed, resulting in oval ulcers with their long axes in the direction of bowel flow (Fig. 8-18), a pattern also seen with Yersinia infections. In contrast, intestinal tuberculosis produces circular or transverse ulcers. Microscopically, macrophages containing bacteria, red blood cells (erythrophagocytosis), and nuclear debris form small nodular aggregates in Peyer's patches. Intermingled with the phagocytes are lymphocytes and plasma cells, whereas neutrophils are present near the ulcerated surface. The *spleen* is enlarged, soft, and bulging, with uniformly pale red pulp, obliterated follicular markings, and prominent sinus histiocytosis and reticuloendothelial proliferation. The *liver* shows small, randomly scattered foci of parenchymal necrosis in which the hepatocytes are replaced by a phagocytic mononuclear cell aggregate, called a "typhoid nodule." These distinctive nodules also occur in the bone marrow and lymph nodes. *Gallbladder* colonization, which may be associated with gallstones, causes a chronic carrier state that may require cholecystectomy to eliminate bacterial shedding.

Cholera

Vibrio cholerae are comma-shaped, gram-negative bacteria that have been the cause of seven great long-lasting epidemics (pandemics) of diarrheal disease, the latest one during the years 1961 to 1974. Many of these pandemics begin in the Ganges Valley of India and Bangladesh, which is never free from cholera, and then move east. Smaller cholera epidemics have appeared in Peru and elsewhere in Latin America. The severe, watery diarrhea of cholera is caused by an enterotoxin secreted by 01-serotype *V. cholerae*. In addition, a non-01 serotype causes diarrhea associated with eating contaminated shellfish from the Gulf of Mexico and elsewhere.

The vibrios never invade the enteric epithelium but instead remain within the lumen and secrete their enterotoxin. Therefore, the most important of the some 17 known virulence-associated genes are those necessary for colonization and toxin secretion. Flagellar proteins involved in motility and attachment are necessary for efficient

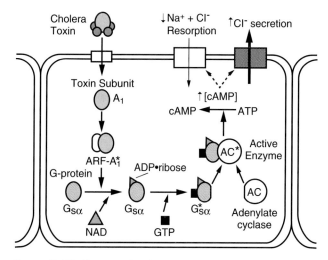

Figure 8–19. The mechanism of action of cholera toxin. (Courtesy of Dr. Jeffrey Joseph.)

bacterial colonization. This is in contrast to Shigella species and certain *E. coli* strains, which are nonmotile and yet invasive. The Vibrio hemagglutinin, which is a metalloprotease, is important for detachment of Vibrio from epithelial cells, analogous to the neuraminidase of influenza virus.

Secretory diarrhea is caused by release of an enterotoxin, called cholera toxin, which is nearly identical to *E. coli* enterotoxin.[49] It is composed of five binding peptides B and a catalytic peptide A. The peptides B bind to carbohydrates on GM_1 ganglioside on the surface of epithelial cells. Within the cell, the disulfide bond linking the two fragments of peptide A (A1 and A2) is cleaved, and catalytic peptide A1 interacts with 20-kd cytosolic G-proteins called ADP-ribosylation factors (ARFs). ARFs and GTP increase the activity of cholera toxin, which ADP-ribosylates a 49-kd *G*-protein (called $G_{s\alpha}$), which in turn stimulates adenyl cyclase. ADP-ribosylated $G_{s\alpha}$ is permanently in an active GTP-bound state (similar to activated *ras* mutants described in Chapter 7), resulting in persistent activation of adenylate cyclase; high levels of intracellular cAMP; and massive secretion of chloride, sodium, and water. The reabsorptive function of the colon is overwhelmed, and liters of dilute "ricewater" diarrhea containing flecks of mucus but few leukocytes are produced. Because overall absorption in the gut remains intact, massive sodium, chloride, and bicarbonate and fluid losses can be replaced by oral formulas and reduce the mortality rate from 50% to less than 1%. A second cholera toxin, identified in mutants lacking the primary cholera toxin, causes a milder diarrhea by disrupting intercellular tight junctions.

MORPHOLOGY. *V. cholerae* bacteria do not invade the gut mucosa and consequently cause minor histopathologic changes that underestimate the

physiologic damage caused by the secreted toxin. There is usually congestion of the mucosal lamina propria, moderate infiltration of mononuclear inflammatory cells, and hyperplasia of Peyer's patches. In contrast, non-01 *V. cholerae* invade the intestinal mucosa and cause necrosis of the luminal epithelium.

Amebiasis

The protozoan parasite *Entamoeba histolytica* infects approximately 500 million persons in developing countries, such as India, Mexico, and Colombia, resulting in approximately 40 million cases of dysentery and liver abscess.[50] *E. histolytica* cysts, which have a chitin wall and four nuclei, are the infectious form of the parasite because they are resistant to gastric acid. In the colonic lumen, cysts release trophozoites, the ameboid form, that reproduce under anaerobic conditions without harming the host. Because the parasites lack mitochondria or Krebs cycle enzymes, amebae are obligate fermenters of glucose to ethanol. Metronidazole, the best drug to treat invasive infections with entamoebae (as well as infections with Giardia, trichomonads, and anaerobic bacteria), targets ferredoxin-dependent pyruvate-oxidoreductase, an enzyme critical in such fermentation, which is present in these organisms but is absent in humans.[51]

Amebae cause dysentery—bloody diarrhea, intestinal pain, fever—when they attach to the colonic epithelium, lyse colonic epithelial cells, and invade the bowel well. Ameba proteins that may be involved in tissue invasion include (1) a lectin on the parasite surface that binds to carbohydrates on the surface of colonic epithelial cells; (2) a channel-forming protein that contains an amphipathic helix that induces pores in the plasma membrane of colonic epithelial cells and lyses them; and (3) cysteine proteinases, which are able to break down proteins of the extracellular matrix.[52]

A major unresolved question in the pathogenesis of amebiasis is why only 10% of persons infected develop dysentery. One explanation supported by immunologic and molecular studies is the existence of two genetically distinct forms of *E. histolytica*. The cysts of virulent and nonvirulent amebae have a similar structure in stool, but the presence of trophozoites containing ingested red blood cells is indicative of tissue invasion by virulent *E. histolytica* parasites.

MORPHOLOGY. Amebiasis most frequently involves the cecum and ascending colon, followed in order by the sigmoid, rectum, and appendix. In severe,

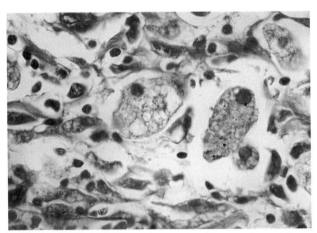

Figure 8-20. Amebiasis of the colon with a portion of three *E. histolytica* trophozoites.

full-blown cases, however, the entire colon is involved. Amebae can mimic the appearance of macrophages because of their comparable size and large number of vacuoles; the parasites, however, have a smaller nucleus, which contains a large karyosome (Fig. 8-20). Amebae invade the crypts of the colonic glands, burrow through the tunica propria, and are halted by the muscularis mucosae. There the amebae fan out laterally to create a flask-shaped ulcer with a narrow neck and broad base. As the lesion progresses, the overlying surface mucosa is deprived of its blood supply and sloughs. The earliest amebic lesions show neutrophilic infiltrates in the mucosa, which later develop into ulcers that contain few host inflammatory cells and areas of extensive liquefactive necrosis. The mucosa between ulcers is often normal or mildly inflamed. An uncommon lesion is the *ameboma*, a napkin-like constrictive lesion, which represents a focus of profuse granulation tissue response to the parasites and is sometimes mistaken for a colonic tumor.

In about 40% of patients with amebic dysentery, parasites penetrate portal vessels and embolize to the liver to produce solitary, or less often multiple, discrete abscesses, some exceeding 10 cm in diameter. **Amebic liver abscesses** have a scant inflammatory reaction at their margins and a shaggy fibrin lining. Because of hemorrhage into the cavities, the abscesses are sometimes filled with a chocolate-colored, odorless, pasty material likened to anchovy paste. Secondary bacterial infection may make these abscesses purulent. As the amebic abscesses enlarge, they produce pain by pressing on the liver capsule and can be visualized with ultrasound. Amebic liver abscesses are treated with drainage and drugs or with drugs alone. Rarely, amebic abscesses reach the lung and the heart by direct extension or spread through the blood into the kidneys and brain.

Giardiasis

Giardia lamblia is the most prevalent pathogenic intestinal protozoan worldwide. Infection may be subclinical or may cause acute or chronic diarrhea, steatorrhea, or constipation. Because Giardia cysts are not killed by chlorine, Giardia is endemic in public water supplies that are not filtered through sand and in streams accessed by campers. In the United States, Giardia infections are especially frequent in institutions for the retarded and in day care centers. Giardia, like Entamoeba, ferments glucose, lacks mitochondria and exists in two forms: (1) a dormant but infectious cyst spread by the fecal-oral route from person to person (as well as from cats, bears, and beavers to persons) and (2) trophozoites that multiply in the intestinal lumen and cause disease. In contrast to Entamoeba, Giardia trophozoites have two nuclei rather than one, are flagellated, reside in the duodenum rather than the colon, adhere to but do not invade intestinal epithelial cells, and so cause diarrhea rather than dysentery.[53]

Giardia trophozoites adhere to sugars on intestinal epithelial cells via a parasite lectin that is activated when cleaved by proteases, which are plentiful in the lumen of the duodenum.[54] Tight contact between the parasite and the epithelial cell is made via a sucker-like disc, composed of cytoplasmic tubulin and a unique intermediate filament called *giardin*. No enterotoxins have been isolated from Giardia, and so the diarrhea caused by the parasites appears to be secondary to nutrient malabsorption rather than excess electrolyte secretion.[55] Giardia may block nutrient absorption by covering the surface of the epithelial cells, or by mechanically damaging the microvilli thus reducing the absorptive area. Antibody-mediated immunity, including secretory IgA, is important in resistance to Giardia because agammaglobulinemic individuals are severely affected by the parasite. Immunity to Giardia, however, is limited by the fact that the parasite is able to vary its major surface proteins into antigenically distinct forms.

MORPHOLOGY. In stool smears, *Giardia lamblia* trophozoites are pear-shaped and binucleate, resembling a cartoonist's drawing of a ghost. Duodenal biopsy specimens are often teeming with sickle-shaped trophozoites, which are tightly bound via the concave attachment disc to the villous surface of the epithelial cells (Fig. 8-21). Although the intestinal morphology may range from virtually normal to markedly abnormal, most commonly Giardia causes clubbing of villi, a decreased villus-to-crypt ratio, and a mixed inflammatory infiltrate of the lamina propria. The brush borders of the absorptive cells are irregular, and sometimes there is virtual absence of villi, resembling the atrophic stage of

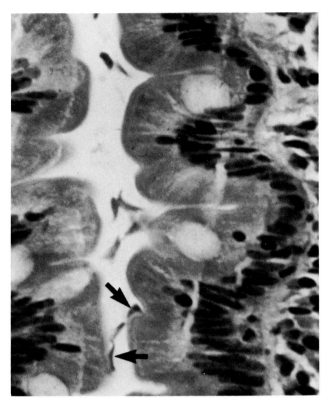

Figure 8–21. *Giardia lamblia* trophozoite adhering to the duodenal epithelium *(arrows).*

gluten-induced enteropathy (see Chapter 17). Giardia in individuals with immunoglobulin deficiencies causes follicular hypertrophy of the mucosal lymphoid tissue.

GRAM-POSITIVE PYOGENIC BACTERIAL INFECTIONS

Staphylococcal Infections

Staphylococcus aureus organisms are pyogenic, nonmotile, gram-positive cocci that tend to form grape-like clusters. Staphylococci cause a myriad of skin lesions (boils, carbuncles, impetigo, and scalded skin) and also cause pharyngitis, pneumonia, endocarditis, food poisoning, and toxic shock syndrome (Fig. 8–22). Here we review the general characteristics of *S. aureus* infection. Specific organ infections are described in other chapters. *S. aureus* is the major cause of infection of patients with severe burns and surgical wounds and is second only to *E. coli* as a cause of hospital-acquired infections. *Staphylococcus epidermidis*, a species

that is related to *S. aureus*, causes opportunistic infections in catheterized patients, patients with prosthetic cardiac valves, and drug addicts. Most staphylococci lack a capsule, and so these cocci are typed by their ability to be infected by bacteriophages. In addition, staphylococci are distinguished by their large number of plasmids, which encode enzymes involved in antibiotic resistance and other virulence factors.

S. aureus and other virulent staphylococci possess a multitude of virulence factors, which include surface proteins involved in adherence to host cells, secreted enzymes that degrade host proteins, and secreted toxins that damage host cells:

- *S. aureus* has, on its surface, receptors for fibrinogen, fibronectin, and vitronectin and uses these molecules as a bridge to bind to host endothelial cells.[56]
- *S. aureus* has a laminin receptor which is similar to metastatic tumor cells and allows bacteria to bind to host extracellular matrix proteins and invade host tissues.[57]
- Staphylococci infecting prosthetic valves and catheters have an exopolysaccharide capsule that allows them to attach to the artificial materials and to resist host cell phagocytosis.
- The lipase of *S. aureus* degrades lipids on the skin surface, and its expression is correlated with the ability of the bacteria to produce skin abscesses.
- *S. aureus* produces multiple hemolytic toxins, including alpha toxin, which is a pore-forming protein that intercalates into the plasma membrane of host cells and depolarizes them;[58,59] beta-toxin, a sphingomyelinase; and delta-toxin, which is an amphipathic (detergent-like) peptide.
- *S. aureus* enterotoxins are associated with food poisoning and appear to act by stimulating emetic receptors in the abdominal viscera and so cause vomiting and diarrhea. In addition, *S. aureus* enterotoxins are superantigens. They bind to macrophage major histocompatibility complex (MHC) class II molecules at a conserved site away from the hypervariable groove and then to the site of the T-cell receptor beta chain, rather than to its variable face that recognizes conventionally processed antigens bound to the MHC.[60] This leads to massive stimulation of host T cells and release of cytokines, which mediate the systemic effects of *S. aureus* enterotoxin.
- Exfoliative toxins of *S. aureus* are associated with the staphylococcal *scalded-skin syndrome,* in which cells in the granular layer of the epidermis detach from each other and form skin blisters.
- Toxic shock syndrome toxin (TSST-1) is secreted by *S. aureus* colonizing the vagina of women using tampons and causes shock by mechanisms similar to those of *S. aureus* enterotoxins, which it resembles in structure.[61]

STAPHYLOCOCCAL INFECTIONS

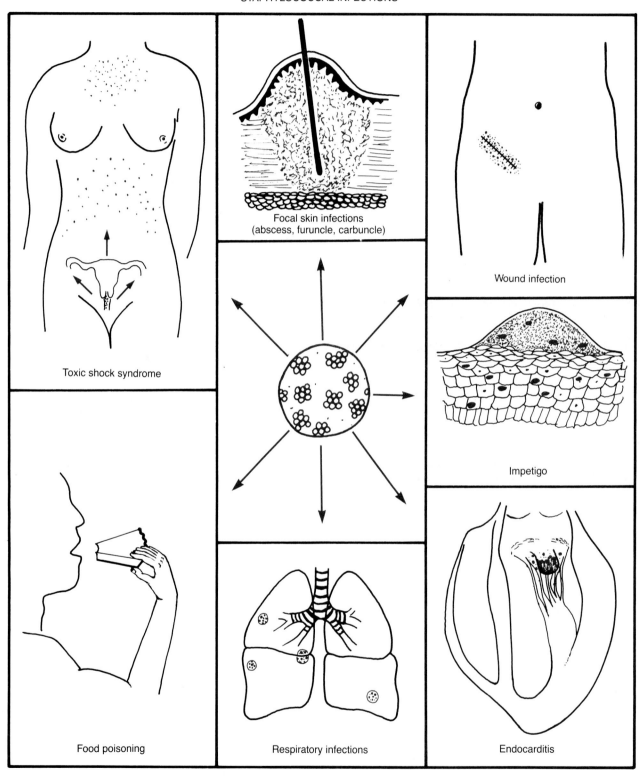

Figure 8-22. The many consequences of staphylococcal infection.

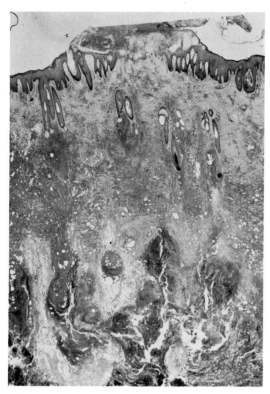

Figure 8–23. Low-power view of staphylococcal carbuncle showing deep-seated suppuration.

Whether the lesion is located in the skin, lungs, bones, or heart valves, *S. aureus* causes pyogenic inflammation that is distinctive for its local destructiveness. Excluding impetigo, which is a staphylococcal or streptococcal infection restricted to the superficial epidermis, staphylococcal skin infections are centered around the hair follicles.

A *furuncle,* or *boil,* is a focal suppurative inflammation of the skin and subcutaneous tissue, either solitary or multiple, or recurrent in successive crops. Furuncles are most frequent in moist, hairy areas, such as the face, axillae, groin, legs, and submammary folds. Beginning in a single hair follicle, a boil develops into a growing and deepening abscess that eventually "comes to a head" by thinning and rupturing the overlying skin. A *carbuncle* is associated with deeper suppuration that spreads laterally beneath the deep subcutaneous fascia and then burrows superficially to erupt in multiple adjacent skin sinuses (Fig. 8–23). Carbuncles typically appear beneath the skin of the upper back and posterior neck, where fascial planes favor their spread. Persistent abscess formation of apocrine gland regions, most frequently of the axilla, is known as *hidradenitis suppurativa.* Those of the nailbed *(paronychia)* or on the palmar side of the fingertips *(felons)* are exquisitely painful. They may follow trauma or embedded splinters and, if

deep enough, destroy the bone of the terminal phalanx or detach the fingernail.

Staphylococcus scalded skin syndrome (SSSS), also called Ritter's disease, is a toxin-mediated, exfoliative dermatitis that most frequently occurs in children with staphylococcal infections of the nasopharynx or skin. In SSSS, there is a sunburn-like rash that spreads over the entire body and forms fragile bullae that lead to partial or total skin loss. The intraepithelial split in SSSS is in the granulosa layer, distinguishing it from toxic epidermal necrolysis (TEN), or Lyell's disease, which is secondary to drug hypersensitivity and causes splitting at the epidermal-dermal junction (see Chapter 26).

Streptococcal Infections

Streptococci are facultative anaerobic, gram-positive cocci that grow in pairs or chains and cause a myriad of suppurative infections of the skin, oropharynx, lungs, and heart valves and also cause poststreptococcal syndromes, including rheumatic fever (see Chapter 12), immune complex glomerulonephritis (see Chapter 20), and erythema nodosum (see Chapter 26). Most streptococci are beta-hemolytic and are typed according to their surface (Lancefield) antigens and include *S. pyogenes* (group A), which causes pharyngitis, scarlet fever, erysipelas, impetigo, rheumatic fever, and glomerulonephritis; *S. agalactiae* (group B), which causes neonatal sepsis and urinary tract infections; and *Enterococcus faecalis* (group D), which causes endocarditis and urinary tract infections. *S. viridans,* which is alpha-hemolytic and thus green on blood agar plates, comprises a group of untypable variants that can cause endocarditis (see Chapter 12). *Streptococcus pneumoniae* (pneumococcus) is typed by its capsular antigens and is the major cause of community-acquired pneumonia in the United States and a major cause of bacterial meningitis among adults. Finally, *Streptococcus mutans* is the major cause of dental caries.

As is the case with many other microbial pathogens, multiple virulence-associated genes of Streptococcus are coregulated in response to environmental stimuli. These include M-protein, a rod-like surface protein that prevents bacteria from being phagocytosed;[13] a surface protein that binds the Fc receptor of host immunoglobulins; and a complement C5a peptidase, which degrades this chemotactic peptide. Streptococci also have surface molecules, including lipoteichoic acid, that bind to the host extracellular matrix protein laminin, and pneumococci have a polysaccharide capsule that prevents phagocytosis.[62] Streptococci secrete a phage-encoded pyrogenic exotoxin that causes fever and rash in scarlet fever. *S. mutans* produces caries by metabolizing sucrose to lactic

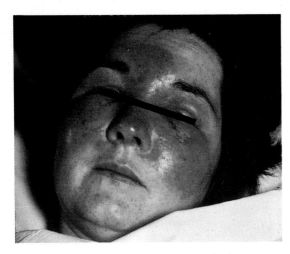

Figure 8–24. Streptococcal erysipelas.

acid (which causes demineralization of tooth enamel) and by secreting high-molecular-weight glucans that promote aggregation of bacteria and plaque formation.[63] Streptococci secrete other enzymes that may be involved in virulence, including hemolysins, neuraminidase, proteases that cleave immunoglobulins, and streptokinase that cleaves thrombin. Poststreptococcal autoimmune diseases of the heart (rheumatic fever) may result from antistreptococcal M-protein antibodies that cross-react with cardiac myosin.[64]

MORPHOLOGY. Streptococcal infections are characterized by diffuse interstitial neutrophilic infiltrates with minimal destruction of host tissues. The skin lesions caused by streptococci (furuncles, carbuncles, and impetigo) resemble those of staphylococci, although there is less tendency to form discrete abscesses.

Erysipelas is most common among middle-aged persons in warm climates and is caused by exotoxins released chiefly from group A and occasionally group C streptococci. It is characterized by rapidly spreading, erythematous cutaneous swelling that may begin on the face or, less frequently, on the body or an extremity. The rash has a sharp, well-demarcated, serpiginous border and may form a "butterfly" distribution on the face (Fig. 8–24). Histologically, there is a diffuse, acute edematous, neutrophilic, interstitial reaction in the dermis and epidermis extending into the subcutaneous tissues. The leukocytic infiltration is more intense about vessels and the skin adnexa. Microabscesses may be formed, but tissue necrosis is usually minor.

Streptococcal pharyngitis, which is the major antecedent of poststreptococcal glomerulonephritis (see Chapter 20), is marked by edema, epiglottic swelling, and punctate abscesses of the tonsillar crypts, sometimes accompanied by cervical lymphadenopathy. With extension of the pharyngeal infection, there may be encroachment on the

airways, especially if there is peritonsillar or retropharyngeal abscess formation **(quinsy sore throat).** Microscopically, these lesions show vasodilation, spreading edema, and intense diffuse neutrophilic exudation, often with a liberal admixture of mononuclear phagocytes.

Pneumococci are important causes of lobar pneumonia (described in Chapter 15).

Scarlet fever, associated with streptococcal group A pharyngitis and tonsillitis, is most frequent between the ages of 3 and 15 years. It is manifested by a punctate erythematous rash that is most abundant over the trunk and inner aspects of the arms and legs. The face is also involved, but usually a small area about the mouth remains relatively unaffected, to produce a circumoral pallor. Microscopically, there is a characteristic acute, edematous, neutrophilic inflammatory reaction within the affected tissues (i.e., the oropharynx, skin, and lymph nodes). The inflammatory involvement of the epidermis is usually followed by hyperkeratosis of the skin, which accounts for the scaling during defervescence.

ANAEROBIC BACTERIAL INFECTIONS

Clostridial Infections

Clostridium species are gram-positive bacilli that grow under anaerobic conditions and produce spores which are frequently present in the soil. There are four types of Clostridium that cause human disease:

1. *C. perfringens (welchii)*, *C. septicum,* and other species invade traumatic and surgical wounds and cause an anaerobic cellulitis or myonecrosis *(gas gangrene)*, contaminate illegal abortions and cause uterine myonecrosis, cause mild food poisoning, and infect the small bowel of ischemic or neutropenic patients to produce severe sepsis.

2. *C. tetani* proliferates in puncture wounds and in the umbilical stump of newborn infants in developing countries and releases a potent neurotoxin, called tetanospasmin, that causes convulsive contractions of skeletal muscles (lockjaw).

3. *C. botulinum* grows in inadequately sterilized canned foods and releases a potent neurotoxin that blocks synaptic release of acetylcholine and causes a severe paralysis of respiratory and skeletal muscles (botulism).

4. *C. difficile* overgrows other intestinal flora in antibiotic-treated patients, releases multiple toxins, and causes pseudomembranous colitis (see Chapter 17).

Severe trauma, gross contamination, and delayed surgical débridement all contribute to high rates of gas gangrene during wars. In peacetime, 50% of the severe *C. perfringens* infections follow accidents, whereas the other 50% follow intestinal and gallbladder surgery. Tetanus toxoid (formalin-fixed neurotoxin) is part of the DPT (diphtheria, pertussis, and tetanus) immunizations given to children that has greatly decreased the incidence of tetanus in the United States and in developing countries.

Clostridia release collagenase and hyaluronidase that degrade extracellular matrix proteins and contribute to bacterial invasiveness, but their most powerful virulence factors are the great variety of toxins they produce. *C. perfringens* secrete 12 toxins, the most important of which is *alpha toxin*.[65] Alpha toxin is a phospholipase C that degrades lecithin, a major component of cell membranes, and so destroys red blood cells, platelets, and muscle cells, *causing myonecrosis*. Alpha toxin also has a sphingomyelinase activity that contributes to nerve-sheath damage. *Theta toxin* binds cholesterol and forms a membrane-destabilizing pore that causes leukocyte lysis, explaining the paucity of polymorphonuclear leukocytes in the lesions of gas gangrene. *Beta toxin* is a major cause of enteritis in sheep, calves, and pigs and causes food poisoning in malnourished persons who eat the meat of infected animals. *Enterotoxin* forms pores in the target epithelial cell membranes and lyses the cells and is the major cause of *C. perfringens* food poisoning.

C. tetani tetanospasmin, the sole toxin that causes tetanus, is composed of an A domain, which is catalytic, and a B domain, which binds gangliosides and the receptor for thyroid-stimulating hormone.[66] Tetanus toxin is bound by peripheral nerves, transported to the nucleus within the axon, released, and taken up by inhibitory neurons, which are blocked from secreting inhibitory neurotransmitters that normally control muscle spasms.

Botulinum neurotoxin is the most potent toxin known; 1 μg of toxin can kill 200,000 mice. In contrast to other exotoxins, botulinum toxin is not secreted but is released when the organisms die and autolyse. Toxin-infected neurons are unable to release acetylcholine at the neuromuscular junction and at the synaptic ganglia and parasympathetic motor end plates of the autonomic nervous system, leading to descending paralysis from the cranial nerves down to the extremities. Another botulinum toxin, exoenzyme C3, ADP-ribosylates a 21-kd G-protein called *rho*, which is related to the oncogene *ras* and is important for actin stress-fiber formation.[67]

C. difficile produces *toxin A*, which is an enterotoxin and a potent chemoattractant for granulocytes, and *toxin B*, a cytotoxin, which causes distinctive cytopathic effects in cultured cells and is used in the diagnosis of *C. difficile* infections.[68]

MORPHOLOGY. Clostridial cellulitis, which originates in wounds, can be differentiated from infection caused by pyogenic cocci by its foul odor; its thin, discolored exudate; and the relatively prompt and wide tissue destruction. Microscopically, the amount of tissue necrosis is disproportionate to the number of neutrophils and gram-positive bacteria present. Clostridial cellulitis, which often has granulation tissue at its borders, is treatable by débridement and antibiotics.

In contrast, **clostridial gas gangrene** is life-threatening and is characterized by marked edema and enzymatic necrosis of involved muscle cells 1 to 3 days after injury. An extensive fluid exudate, which is lacking in inflammatory cells, causes swelling of the affected region and the overlying skin, forming large, bullous vesicles that rupture. Gas bubbles caused by bacterial fermentations appear within the gangrenous tissues. As the infection progresses, the inflamed muscles become soft, blue-black, friable, and semifluid as a result of the massive proteolytic action of the released bacterial enzymes. Microscopically, there is severe **myonecrosis,** extensive hemolysis, and marked vascular injury, with thrombosis. *C. perfringens* is also associated with dusk-colored, wedge-shaped infarcts in the small bowel, particularly of neutropenic patients. Regardless of the location of the source, when *C. perfringens* disseminates hematogenously, there is widespread formation of gas bubbles. Despite the severe neurologic damage caused by botulinum and tetanus toxins, the neuropathologic changes are subtle and nonspecific.

Non–Spore-Forming Anaerobic Infections

Anaerobic non–spore-forming bacteria are the most frequent commensal organisms in the gastrointestinal tract (99.9%), female genitals, mouth, and skin.[69] These organisms include gram-negative bacilli (Bacteroides, Prevotella, and Fusobacterium), gram-positive bacilli (Actinomyces and *Propionibacterium acnes*), and gram-positive cocci (Peptostreptococcus). In contrast to the spore-forming anaerobes — *Clostridium species* — the non–spore-forming anaerobes do not secrete toxins. Instead these organisms are for the most part opportunistic pathogens, causing acne in the oil-laden pores of adolescents (Propionibacterium), intra-abdominal abscesses secondary to surgery or perforation (*Bacteroides fragilis* and others), septic abortion and salpingitis (Prevotella), and periodontal abscesses (*Bacteroides melaninogenicus*).

MORPHOLOGY. *Bacteroides melaninogenicus,* alone or in association with aerobic organisms, is found in abscesses and phlegmons mostly above the diaphragm (e.g., in the floor of the mouth, the retropharynx, and even the lung and brain). *Bac-*

teroides fragilis is typically a cause of, or a participant in, intra-abdominal and retroperitoneal sepsis and in pelvic peritonitis of women beyond their twenties; sometimes it infects surgical abdominal wounds. It may also be present in lung abscesses. In all these lesions, the pus is often discolored and foul smelling, especially in lung abscesses, and the suppuration is often poorly walled off. Otherwise, these lesions pathologically resemble those of the common pyogenic infections.

SEXUALLY TRANSMITTED INFECTIONS (STI)

Although the classic sexually transmitted diseases —gonorrhea, syphilis, and chlamydia—have been greatly reduced in some segments of Western societies, these diseases are increasing at epidemic rates among certain urban populations in the United States.[70] Worldwide epidemics of HIV (see Chapter 6) and HBV (see Chapter 18) remain uncontrolled and involve adults of both sexes and children of infected mothers. In addition, viruses spread by intimate contact include those that cause oral and genital sores (HSV-1 and HSV-2), infectious mononucleosis (EBV), and opportunistic congenital infections in infants with AIDS (CMV) (Table 8–7). Here we shall review selected important STIs that are not covered elsewhere in the book.

Herpesvirus Infections

Herpesviruses are large encapsulated viruses that have a double-stranded DNA genome that encodes approximately 70 proteins. Eight types of herpesviruses, belonging to three groups, have been isolated from humans: neurotropic alpha-group viruses, including HSV-1, HSV-2, and varicella-zoster (VZV); lymphotropic beta-group viruses, including CMV, human herpesvirus 6 (which causes exanthum subitum, a benign rash of infants), and human herpesvirus 7 (which is not yet associated with a specific disease); and gamma-group virus, EBV. In addition, herpesvirus simiae (HVS) is an Old World monkey virus that resembles HSV-1 and may cause fatal neurologic disease in animal handlers. Here we discuss the lesions induced by HSV-1 and HSV-2.

NATURAL HISTORY OF HSV-1 AND HSV-2 INFECTIONS. HSV-1 and HSV-2 are genetically similar and cause a similar set of primary and recurrent infections.[71] Both viruses replicate in the skin and the mucous membranes at the site of entrance of the virus (oropharynx or genitals), where they cause vesicular lesions of the epidermis and infect the neurons that innervate these locations. Within the nucleus of host epithelial cells, HSV-encoded

Table 8–7. SEXUALLY TRANSMITTED INFECTIOUS DISEASES

A. Exclusively or regularly transmitted by sexual contact

CAUSAL AGENT	DISEASE MANIFESTATIONS
Viral	
HIV-I, HIV-II	Acquired immunodeficiency syndrome
Herpesvirus 1, 2 (HSV-1, 2)	Herpes lesions
Papillomaviruses	Condyloma acuminatum, cervical dysplasia, neoplasia
Chlamydial, Mycoplasmal	
Chlamydia trachomatis (L type)	Lymphogranuloma venereum
C. trachomatis	Nongonorrheal urethritis, cervicitis
Ureaplasma urealyticum	Nongonorrheal urethritis, cervicitis
Bacterial	
Neisseria gonorrhoeae	Gonorrhea
Treponema pallidum	Syphilis (lues venerea)
Haemophilus ducreyi	Chancroid
Calymmatobacterium donovani	Granuloma inguinale
Protozoal	
Trichomonas vaginalis	Trichomoniasis
By Arthropod	
Phthirus pubis	Pediculosis pubis (crabs)

B. Transmissible sexually or by other means

Viral
Cytomegalovirus, hepatitis B virus, Epstein-Barr virus, molluscum contagiosum virus

Bacterial
Group B streptococci; gram-negative bacilli

Fungal
Candida

Protozoal
Entamoeba histolytica

proteins form a replication compartment where viral DNA is made and capsid proteins are attached. The viral envelope is attached to the nucleocapsid in the cytoplasm. In immunocompetent hosts, primary HSV infection resolves in a few weeks, although herpesviruses remain latent in the nerve cells. Latency is operationally defined as the inability to recover infectious particles from disrupted cells that harbor the virus, although viral DNA and a few viral mRNAs may be identified by molecular methods.[72] Reactivation of HSV-1 and HSV-2 may occur repeatedly with or without symptoms and results in the spread of virus from the neurons to the skin or to mucous membranes.

HSV-1 is the major infectious cause of corneal blindness in the United States, secondary to stromal conjunctivitis; such inflammation appears to be immune-mediated because it responds to corticosteroids, and the lesions show numerous mononuclear cells surrounding keratinocytes.[73] HSV-1 is

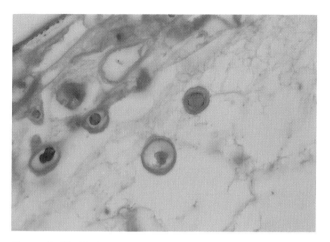

Figure 8-25. High-power view of cells from blister in Figure 8-8 showing glassy intranuclear herpes simplex inclusion bodies.

also the major cause of fatal sporadic encephalitis in the United States, when viruses spread to the brain, particularly the temporal lobes. In addition, neonates and individuals with decreased cellular immunity secondary to **AIDS** or to antitransplant rejection chemotherapy may suffer disseminated herpesvirus infections.

MORPHOLOGY. All HSV lesions are marked by formation of large, pink-to-purple (Cowdry type A) intranuclear inclusions that contain intact and disrupted virions and push darkly stained host cell chromatin to the edges of the nucleus (Fig. 8-25). Although cell and nuclear size increase only slightly, herpesvirus produces inclusion-bearing multinucleated syncytia, which are diagnostic in smears of blister fluid.

HSV-1 and HSV-2 cause lesions ranging from self-limited cold sores and gingivostomatitis to life-threatening disseminated visceral infections and encephalitis. **Fever blisters or cold sores** favor the facial skin around mucosal orifices (lips, nose), where their distribution is frequently bilateral and independent of skin dermatomes. Intraepithelial vesicles (blisters), which are formed by intracellular edema and ballooning degeneration of epidermal cells, frequently burst and crust over, but some may result in superficial ulcerations.

Gingivostomatitis, which is usually encountered in children, is caused by HSV-1. It is a vesicular eruption extending from tongue to retropharynx and causing cervical lymphadenopathy. Coxsackievirus also causes oral vesicular eruptions in children, although the lesions are milder and limited to the pharynx and tonsils.

Two forms of **corneal lesions** are caused by HSV. **Herpes epithelial keratitis** shows typical viral-induced cytolysis of the superficial epithelium and is sensitive to antiviral drugs. In contrast, **herpes**

stromal keratitis shows infiltrates of mononuclear cells around keratinocytes and endothelial cells, leading to neovascularization, scarring, opacification of the cornea, and eventual blindness. This is an immunologic reaction to the HSV infection and responds to corticosteroid therapy.

Herpes simplex encephalitis is described in Chapter 29.

Disseminated skin and visceral herpes infections are usually encountered in hospitalized patients with some form of underlying cancer or under immunosuppressive treatment. **Kaposi's varicelliform eruption** is a generalized vesiculating involvement of the skin, whereas **eczema herpeticum** is characterized by confluent, pustular, or hemorrhagic blisters, often with bacterial superinfection and viral dissemination to internal viscera. **Herpes esophagitis** is frequently complicated by superinfection with bacteria or fungi. **Herpes bronchopneumonia,** which may be introduced with an airway inserted through oral herpes lesions, is often necrotizing, and **herpes hepatitis** may cause liver failure.

Genital herpes is characterized by vesicles on the genital mucous membranes as well as external genitalia, which are rapidly converted into superficial ulcerations, rimmed by an inflammatory infiltrate. HSV-2 is transmitted to neonates during passage through the birth canal of infected mothers. Although HSV-2 disease in the neonate may be mild, it is more often fulminating with generalized lymphadenopathy, splenomegaly, and necrotic foci throughout the lungs, liver, adrenals, and central nervous systems (see also Chapter 23).

Chlamydial Infections

Chlamydia trachomatis is an obligate intracellular pathogen of columnar epithelial cells that causes venereal urethritis, lymphogranuloma venereum, and trachoma (Table 8-8). Closely related, *C. pneumoniae* and *C. psittaci* cause mild and severe pneumonias, respectively. *C. trachomatis* causes more than a half million reported cases of nongonorrheal urethritis in the United States each year, which are more frequently symptomatic in men than in women. In some men, *C. trachomatis* infection causes *Reiter's syndrome*, a triad of conjunctivitis, polyarthritis, and genital infection. Lymphogranuloma venereum is caused by a specific strain of *C. trachomatis* and results in granulomatous inflammation of the inguinal and rectal lymph nodes. Infants born to mothers with *C. trachomatis* cervicitis may develop inclusion conjunctivitis or neonatal pneumonia. Trachoma or chronic keratoconjunctivitis, a leading global cause of blindness, is a disease of poverty and overcrowding, transmitted from eye to eye by aerosols or by hand contact.

Chlamydiae exist in two forms: elementary

Table 8–8. HUMAN CHLAMYDIAL DISEASES AND SPECIES

SPECIES AND SEROTYPE	DISEASES	TRANSMISSION
Chlamydia psittaci	Ornithosis (psittacosis)	Aspiration of bird-contaminated particles
Chlamydia pneumoniae	Mild pneumonia	Aerosols (person-to-person)
Chlamydia trachomatis		
A, B, Ba, C	Trachoma	Repeated contact, fomites, insects
D, E, F, G, H, I, J, K	Inclusion conjunctivitis	Birth canal infection (infants)
		Sexual contact, swimming (adults)
"	Nongonorrheal urethritis	Sexual contact
"	Postgonorrheal urethritis	Sexual contact
"	Proctitis, pharyngitis, cervicitis, arthritis	Sexual contact
L_1, L_2, L_3	Lymphogranuloma venereum	Sexual contact

bodies, which never divide but are infectious, and reticulate bodies, which multiply within vacuoles of host cells but are not infectious.[74,75] Elementary bodies have a cell wall that is made rigid by disulfide bonds rather than cross-linked peptidoglycans found in most bacteria, and thus *chlamydiae are not susceptible to penicillin.* Elementary bodies have adhesins on their surface, which bind to microvilli on host columnar epithelial cells. Depending on the chlamydia species and type of host cell, organisms enter host cells via endosomes or phagosomes. Within endosome-bound inclusion bodies that fail to fuse with host lysosomes, elementary bodies transform to reticulate bodies and multiply to as many as 500 organisms per host cell. Because chlamydiae are unable to synthesize ATP, the organisms induce host cell mitochondria (which make ATP) to closely appose the inclusion body. Reticulate bodies then transform back to elementary bodies, which cause bursting of host cells, infecting neighboring cells.

MORPHOLOGY. Inclusions of chlamydial forms in epithelial cells are best seen with fluorescent anti-Chlamydia antibodies. Chlamydial urethritis or cervicitis may also be diagnosed by culture on McCoy cells and by detecting anti-Chlamydia antibodies in patients' sera.

Lymphogranuloma venereum causes a small epidermal vesicle at the site of infection on the genitalia. The vesicle ulcerates and oozes a neutrophilic exudate. At the base of this ulcer, there is a zone of chronic, often granulomatous inflammation. In addition, lymphogranuloma venereum causes rapid swelling of the inguinal, pelvic, and rectal lymph nodes, caused by a mixture of suppurative and granulomatous inflammation (Fig. 8–26). Irregular, stellate abscesses form when granulomas with suppurative centers fuse. These abscesses are rimmed by a layer of epithelioid macrophages and resemble lesions seen in cat-scratch disease. Later lesions in lymphogranuloma venereum show fewer granulomas, plasma cell infiltrates, and increasing fibrosis.

Inclusion conjunctivitis is a self-limited disease of infants born to mothers with cervical infections with *C. trachomatis.* The conjunctivae are hyperemic and edematous and show a monocytic infiltrate.

Chlamydia psittaci is excreted from infected

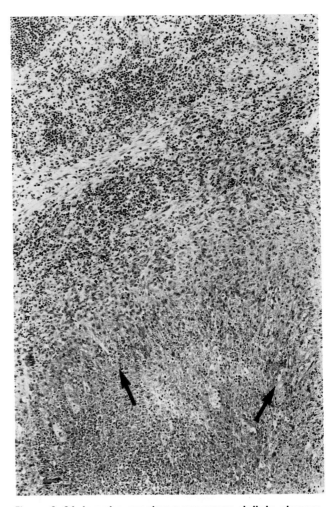

Figure 8–26. Lymphogranuloma venereum stellate abscess in a lymph node. The area of necrosis *(below)* is rimmed by a granulomatous reaction *(arrows).*

birds and inhaled with dust particles. Although human infection may be asymptomatic or mild, *C. psittaci* also causes a severe pneumonia, also known as **ornithosis.** Lethal generalized disease, most frequent during epidemics, is marked by focal areas of necrosis in the liver and spleen and diffuse mononuclear infiltrates in the kidneys, heart, and (sometimes) brain.

Gonorrhea

Neisseria gonorrhoeae is a pyogenic, encapsulated, gram-negative diplococcus. There are nearly 700,000 reported cases of gonorrheal urethritis in the United States each year, but *N. gonorrhoeae* can also cause pharyngitis or proctitis, depending upon sexual practices. In men, the gonococcus may cause urethral strictures and chronic infections of the epididymis, prostate, and seminal vesicles. Infection of the fallopian tubes in women (salpingitis) may result in scars, which increase rates of sterility and ectopic pregnancy or lead to chronic infections with anaerobic bacteria. Gonococcal bacteremia leads to an arthritis-dermatitis syndrome, whereas conjunctivitis may appear in adults from autoinoculation.

N. gonorrhoeae is genetically very similar to *N. meningitidis*. *N. meningitidis* frequently resides as a commensal in the upper respiratory mucosa but may invade host tissues and cause meningitis (see Chapter 29), bacteremia, and in fatal cases diffuse intravascular coagulation (DIC) with the Waterhouse-Friderichsen syndrome (see Chapter 25).

N. gonorrhoeae is a facultative intracellular pathogen that binds to and invades host epithelial cells. Binding is mediated by adhesins or pili, which show antigenic variation based on intragenomic recombination and on recombination following incorporation of exogenous DNA from lysed gonococci.[17] Internalization is based on a second set of adhesins (called the opacity outer membrane proteins, or P.II), which show antigenic variation via genetic mechanisms different from those of pili.[77] Capsular polysaccharides contribute to virulence by inhibiting phagocytosis in the absence of antigonococcal antibodies. Pathogenic Neisseria secrete a protease that cleaves IgA. In addition, Neisseria release peptidoglycans and endotoxins, which induce host cell secretion of TNF-α that may cause shock and multisystem failure. Damage to the epithelial cells of the fallopian tubes by *N. gonorrhoeae* may also be mediated by TNF-α, which induces the same lesions when instilled into fallopian tubes as those caused by gonococci.[78]

All gonococcal lesions show exudative and purulent reactions followed by granulation tissue formation, plasma cell infiltration, and fibrosis. Gonococci in men cause a mucopurulent discharge from an edematous and inflamed urethral meatus 2 to 7 days after exposure. If untreated, suppurative inflammation with focal abscesses spread to the posterior urethra, epididymis, prostate, and seminal vesicles. Chronic inflammation may lead to urethral strictures and sterility.

In women, urethral inflammation is less prominent, whereas abscesses frequently cause bulging of Bartholin's and Skene's glands. Gonococcal cervicitis results in few sequelae, whereas salpingitis may seal the fallopian tubes, which become massively distended with pus and may be left severely scarred. Tubo-ovarian abscesses and pelvic peritonitis (pelvic inflammatory disease) result from further extension and may create multiple adhesions and points of blockage of the oviducts (see also Chapter 23).

Syphilis

Treponema pallidum is the microaerophilic spirochete that causes syphilis, a systemic venereal disease with multiple clinical presentations (the great impostor). Other closely related treponemas cause yaws *(T. pertenue)*, pinta *(T. carateum)*, and periodontal disease *(T. denticola)*. Like the Borrelia spirochetes of Lyme disease and relapsing fever, described later, *T. pallidum* organisms have an axial periplasmic flagella wound around a slender, helical protoplasm, all of which are covered by a unit membrane called the outer sheath. *T. pallidum* spirochetes have not been cultured but are detectable by silver stains, dark-field examination, and immunofluorescence techniques. Sexual intercourse is the usual mode of transmission, although bacteria-laden secretions can transfer the disease by other intimate contact. Transplacental transmission of *T. pallidum* occurs readily, and active disease during pregnancy results in congenital syphilis.

CLINICAL FEATURES OF SYPHILIS (Fig. 8–27). The *primary stage* of syphilis, occurring approximately 3 weeks after contact with an infected individual, features a single firm, nontender, raised, red lesion (chancre) located at the site of treponemal invasion on the penis, cervix, vaginal wall, or anus. Although spirochetes seed the body via hematogenous spread, the chancre heals in a few weeks with or without therapy. The *secondary stage* of syphilis, which occurs 2 to 10 weeks after the primary chancre, is characterized by a diffuse rash, particularly of the palms and soles, that may be accompanied by white oral lesions, fever, lymphadenopa-

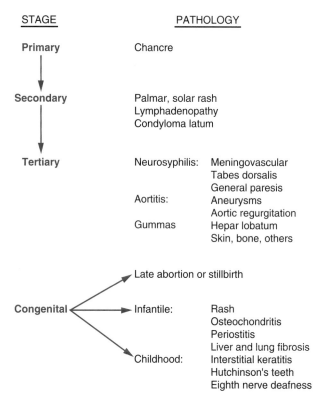

STAGE	PATHOLOGY	
Primary	Chancre	
Secondary	Palmar, solar rash	
	Lymphadenopathy	
	Condyloma latum	
Tertiary	Neurosyphilis:	Meningovascular
		Tabes dorsalis
		General paresis
	Aortitis:	Aneurysms
		Aortic regurgitation
	Gummas	Hepar lobatum
		Skin, bone, others
Congenital	Late abortion or stillbirth	
	Infantile:	Rash
		Osteochondritis
		Periostitis
		Liver and lung fibrosis
	Childhood:	Interstitial keratitis
		Hutchinson's teeth
		Eighth nerve deafness

Figure 8–27. The protean manifestations of syphilis.

thy, headache and arthritis. These lesions as well resolve spontaneously. The *tertiary stage*, which occurs years after the primary lesion, is characterized either by active inflammatory lesions of the aorta, heart (see Chapter 12), and central nervous system (see Chapter 29) or by quiescent lesions (gummas) involving the liver, bones, and skin. Congenital syphilis is described subsequently.

PATHOGENESIS. Whatever the stage of the disease and location of the lesions, the histologic hallmarks of syphilis are obliterative endarteritis and plasma cell–rich mononuclear infiltrates. The endarteritis is secondary to the binding of spirochetes to endothelial cells, mediated by host fibronectin molecules bound to the surface of the spirochetes.[79] The mononuclear infiltrates reflect an immunologic response. In animal models, a delayed-type hypersensitivity response is more important than antibodies in limiting the initial localized infection.[80] The antibodies may be against spirochete-specific antigens (the basis of treponemal serologic tests) or against antigens that cross-react with host molecules (the basis of nontreponemal tests, including the Wasserman and Venereal Disease Research Laboratory [VDRL] tests). Host humoral and cellular immune responses may prevent the formation of a chancre on subsequent infections with *T. pallidum* but are insufficient to clear the spirochetes. This may be because the outer sheath is lacking in immunogenic molecules[81] or may be secondary to down-regulation of helper T cells of the T_H1 class.

MORPHOLOGY. In primary syphilis, a chancre occurs on the penis or scrotum of 70% of men and on the vulva or cervix of 50% of women. The chancre is a slightly elevated, firm, reddened papule, up to several centimeters in diameter, that erodes to create a clean-based, shallow ulcer. The contiguous induration creates a button-like mass directly subjacent to the eroded skin, providing the basis of the designation hard chancre (Fig. 8–28A). Histologically, the chancre contains an intense infiltrate of plasma cells, with scattered macrophages and lymphocytes and an obliterative endarteritis (see Fig. 8–28B). Treponemes are visible with silver stains or immunofluorescence techniques at the surface of the ulcer. The regional nodes are usually enlarged and may show nonspecific acute or chronic lymphadenitis, plasma cell–rich infiltrates, or focal epithelioid granulomas.

In **secondary syphilis,** widespread mucocutaneous lesions involve the oral cavity, palms of the hands, and soles of the feet. The rash is frequently macular, with discrete red-brown spots less than 5 mm in diameter, but may be follicular, pustular, annular, or scaling. Reddened mucous patches in the mouth or vagina contain the most organisms and are the most infectious. Papular lesions in the region of the penis or vulva form 2 to 3-cm elevated, red-brown plaques, which are called **condylomata lata** (not to be confused with venereal warts, which are called condylomata acuminata; (see Chapter 22). Histologically, the lesions of secondary syphilis show the same plasma cell infiltrate and obliterative endarteritis as the primary chancre, although the inflammation is often less intense.

Tertiary syphilis occurs years after the initial infection and most frequently involves the aorta (80 to 85%); the central nervous system (5 to 10%); and the liver, bones and testes (gummas). **Aortitis** is manifested by aortic aneurysms in which there is inflammatory scarring of the tunica media, widening and incompetence of the aortic valve ring, and narrowing of the mouths of the coronary ostia (see Chapter 11). **Neurosyphilis** takes one of several forms, designated meningovascular syphilis, tabes dorsalis, and general paresis (see Chapter 29). **Syphilitic gummas** are white-gray and rubbery, occur singly or multiply, and vary in size from microscopic defects resembling tubercles to large tumor-like masses. They occur in most organs, but particularly in skin, subcutaneous tissue, bone, and joints. In the liver, scarring as a result of gummas may cause a distinctive hepatic lesion known as hepar lobatum (Fig. 8–31). Histologically, the gummas contain a center of coagulated, necrotic material and margins composed of plump or palisaded macrophages and fibroblasts surrounded by large numbers of mononuclear leukocytes, chiefly plasma cells. Treponemes are scant in these gummas and are difficult to demonstrate.

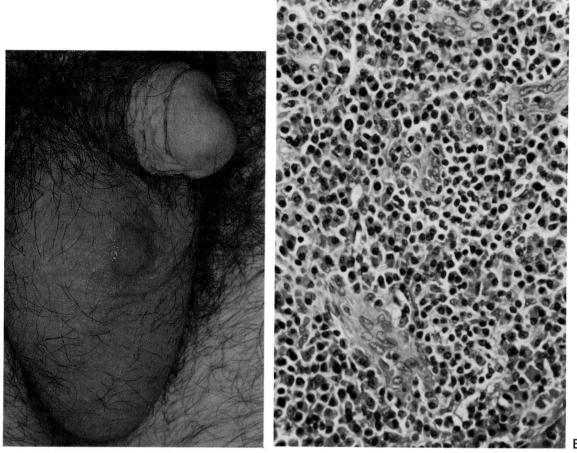

Figure 8–28. *A,* Syphilitic chancre in the scrotum. *B,* Histology of chancre with diffuse plasmacytic infiltrate and endothelial proliferation. (Courtesy of Dr. Richard Johnson, New England Deaconess Hospital.)

Congenital syphilis is most severe when the mother's infection is recent. Because treponemes do not invade the placental tissue or the fetus until the fifth month of gestation, syphilis causes late abortion, stillbirth, or death soon after delivery, or it may persist in latent form to become apparent only during childhood or adult life. In **perinatal and infantile syphilis,** a diffuse rash develops, which differs from that of the acquired secondary stage in that there is extensive sloughing of the epithelium, particularly on the palms, soles, and skin about the mouth and anus. These lesions teem with spirochetes. **Syphilitic osteochondritis and periostitis** affect all bones, although lesions of the nose and lower legs are most distinctive. Destruction of the vomer causes collapse of the bridge of the nose and, later on, the characteristic saddle nose deformity. Periostitis of the tibia leads to excessive new bone growth on the anterior surfaces and anterior bowing, or saber shin. There is also widespread disturbance in endochondral bone formation. The epiphyses become widened as the cartilage overgrows, and cartilage is found as displaced islands within the metaphysis.

The **liver** is often severely affected in congenital syphilis. Diffuse fibrosis permeates lobules to isolate hepatic cells into small nests, accompanied by the characteristic white cell infiltrate and vascular changes. Gummas are occasionally found in the liver, even in early cases. The **lungs** may be affected by a diffuse interstitial fibrosis. In the syphilitic stillborn, the lungs appear as pale, airless organs (pneumonia alba). The generalized spirochetemia may lead to diffuse interstitial inflammatory reactions in virtually any other organ of the body (e.g., the pancreas, kidneys, heart, spleen, thymus, endocrine organs, and central nervous system).

The late-occurring form of congenital syphilis is distinctive for the **triad of interstitial keratitis, Hutchinson's teeth, and eigth nerve deafness.** Eye changes consist of interstitial keratitis and choroiditis with abnormal pigment production causing a spotted retina. The dental changes involve the incisor teeth, which are small and shaped like a screwdriver or a peg, often with notches in the enamel (Hutchinson's teeth). Eighth nerve deafness and optic nerve atrophy develop secondary to meningovascular syphilis.

Trichomoniasis

Trichomonas vaginalis, a sexually transmitted anaerobic, flagellated protozoan parasite, infects some 3 million new persons each year. *T. vaginalis* is the simplest of all protozoan parasites: There is only a trophozoite form, which adheres to and causes superficial lesions of the mucosal surfaces of the male and female genital tracts but fails to invade host tissues. *T. vaginalis* infection in women is often associated with loss of acid-producing Doderlein bacilli, may be asymptomatic, but frequently causes itching and a profuse watery vaginal discharge. It is exacerbated by menstruation and by pregnancy. Urethral colonization by *T. vaginalis* causes urinary frequency and dysuria. *T. vaginalis* infection of men is mostly asymptomatic but may result in nongonococcal urethritis and rarely prostatitis. Infants infected with *T. vaginalis* during the birth process spontaneously clear the parasites in a few weeks.

MORPHOLOGY. Trichomonads cause a spotty reddening and edema of the affected mucosa, sometimes with small blisters or papules, referred to as "strawberry mucosa." Histologically, the mucosa and superficial submucosa are infiltrated by lymphocytes, plasma cells, and polymorphonuclear leukocytes. The discharge is rarely purulent, as in gonorrheal or chlamydial infection. The turnip-shaped trichomonads are best seen in fresh preparations diluted with warm saline, where they are rapidly motile, or in Giemsa-stained smears.

INFECTIONS OF CHILDHOOD AND ADOLESCENCE

Measles

Measles (rubeola) virus is the cause of more than 2 million deaths per year among Third World children, who by reasons of poor nutrition are 10 to 1000 times more likely to die of measles pneumonia than are Western children.[82] In the United States, the incidence of measles has decreased by 95% since 1963, when a measels vaccine was licensed, but miniepidemics of measles still occur among unvaccinated individuals and among vaccinated individuals who did not develop protective immunity (primary vaccine failure).

Measles virus is an RNA virus of the paramyxovirus family that includes mumps, respiratory syncytial virus (the major cause of lower respiratory infections in infants), and parainfluenza virus (the cause of croup). There is only one strain of measles virus. It has an envelope that contains a hemagglutinin that binds to host cells, and a small glycoprotein that has hemolytic activity and mediates penetration of the virus into the cytosol. Measles virus are spread by respiratory droplets and multiply within upper respiratory epithelial cells and mononuclear cells, including B and T lymphocytes and macrophages. A transient viremia spreads the measles virus throughout the body and may cause croup, pneumonia, diarrhea with protein-losing enteropathy, keratitis with scarring and blindness, encephalitis, and hemorrhages ("black measles"). Most children, however, develop T cell–mediated immunity to measles virus that controls the viral infection and produces the measles rash, a hypersensitivity reaction to viral antigens in the skin. The rash does not occur in patients with deficiencies in cell-mediated immunity but does occur in agammaglobulinemic patients. Antibody-mediated immunity to measles virus protects against reinfection. Subacute sclerosing panencephalitis (SSPE; described in Chapter 29) and measles inclusion body encephalitis (in immunocompromised individuals) are rare late complications of measles, caused by hypermutated, "defective" viruses that cannot produce matrix or envelope proteins.[83]

MORPHOLOGY. The blotchy, reddish-brown rash of measles virus infection on the face, trunk, and proximal extremities is produced by dilated skin vessels, edema, and a moderate, nonspecific, mononuclear perivascular infiltrate. Ulcerated mucosal lesions in the oral cavity near the opening of Stensen's ducts (the pathognomonic Koplik spots) are marked by necrosis, neutrophil exudate, and neovascularization. The lymphoid organs typically have marked follicular hyperplasia, large germinal centers, and randomly distributed multinucleate giant cells, called Warthin-Finkeldey cells, which have eosinophilic nuclear and cytoplasmic inclusion bodies. These are pathognomonic of measles and are also found in the lung and sputum (Fig. 8–29). The milder forms of measles pneumonia show the same peribronchial and interstitial mononuclear infiltration seen in other nonlethal viral infections. In severe or neglected cases, bacterial superinfection may be a cause of death.

Mumps

Mumps virus causes a transient inflammation of the parotid glands and, less often, of the testes, pancreas, and central nervous system. Mumps virus is

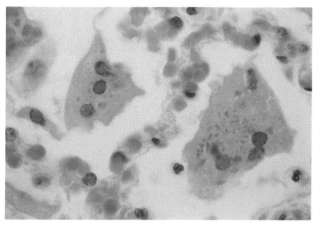

Figure 8-29. Measles giant cells in the lung. Note glassy eosinophilic intranuclear inclusions.

similar in structure to measles virus except for the fact that the large glycoprotein on its surface has both hemagglutinin and neuraminidase activities. Mumps viruses are spread by respiratory droplets and multiply within upper respiratory epithelial cells, salivary glands, and T cells in lymph nodes. A transient viremia spreads the mumps virus to other glands and the central nervous system via the choroid plexus. Mumps virus is a rare cause of aseptic meningitis and encephalitis.

MORPHOLOGY. In mumps parotitis, which is bilateral in 70% of cases, affected glands are enlarged, have a doughy consistency, and are moist, glistening, and reddish brown on cross-section. Microscopically, the gland interstitium is edematous and diffusely infiltrated by histiocytes, lymphocytes, and plasma cells that compress acini and ducts. Neutrophils and necrotic debris may fill the ductal lumen and cause focal damage to the ductal epithelium.

In **mumps orchitis,** testicular swelling may be marked, caused by edema, mononuclear cell infiltration, and focal hemorrhages. Because the testis is tightly contained within the tunica albuginea, parenchymal swelling may compromise the blood supply and cause areas of infarction. Sterility, when it occurs, is caused by scars and atrophy of the testis after resolution of viral infection.

In the enzyme-rich pancreas, lesions may be very destructive, causing parenchymal and fat necrosis and polymorphonuclear cell infiltration. Mumps encephalitis causes perivenous demyelinization and perivascular mononuclear cuffing.

Infectious Mononucleosis (Epstein-Barr virus)

Infectious mononucleosis (IM) is a benign, self-limited lymphoproliferative disease caused by EBV, a gamma-group herpesvirus. IM is characterized by fever, generalized lymphadenopathy, splenomegaly, sore throat, and the appearance in the blood of atypical activated T lymphocytes (mononucleosis cells). Some patients develop hepatitis, meningoencephalitis, and pneumonitis. IM occurs principally in late adolescents or young adults (it delights in college students) among upper socioeconomic classes in developed nations. In the rest of the world, primary infection with EBV occurs in childhood, is usually asymptomatic, and confers immunity to subsequent reinfection.

PATHOGENESIS. EBV is transmitted by close human contact, frequently with the saliva during kissing. An EBV envelope glycoprotein binds to CD21 protein, the complement receptor CR2[84] (see Chapter 3) present on epithelial cells and B cells. The virus enters the cytoplasm of epithelial cells by directly fusing with the plasma membrane, and of B cells by fusing with endosomal membranes. The virus initially penetrates nasopharyngeal, oropharyngeal, and salivary epithelial cells (Fig. 8-30). Simultaneously, it spreads to underlying lymphoid tissue and, more specifically, to B lymphocytes. Infection of B cells may take one of two forms. In a minority of B cells there is productive infection with lysis of infected cells and release of virions which reinfect oropharyngeal epithelium, and persist as a subclinical productive infection. Thus, the agent is shed in the saliva. In the vast majority of B cells, however, the virus associates with the host cell genome, giving rise to latent infection. B cells that harbor the EBV genome undergo polyclonal activation and proliferation. Two EBV proteins, EBNA2 and LMP-1, are associated with such B cell immortalization.[85] B cells then disseminate in the circulation and secrete antibodies with several specificities, including the well-known heterophil anti-sheep red blood cell antibodies used for the diagnosis of IM.

A normal immune response is important in controlling the proliferation of EBV-infected B cells and suppressing cell-free virus. Early in the course of the infection IgM, and, later, IgG, antibodies are formed against viral capsid antigens. The latter persist for life. IgA antibodies prevent infection of B cells but increase infectivity of EBV for epithelial cells.[86] More important in the control of polyclonal B-cell proliferation are cytotoxic CD8+ T cells and natural killer (NK) cells. Curiously, however, a large number of activated T cells with the phenotypic attributes of suppressor cells are also generated. They are not specific for EBV-infected B cells, so their role in recovery from EBV infection is not clear. Together with the virus-specific cytotoxic T cells, these suppressor T cells appear in the circulation as atypical lymphocytes, so characteristic of this disease. It is significant to note that in otherwise healthy persons the fully developed humoral and cellular responses to

EBV INFECTION

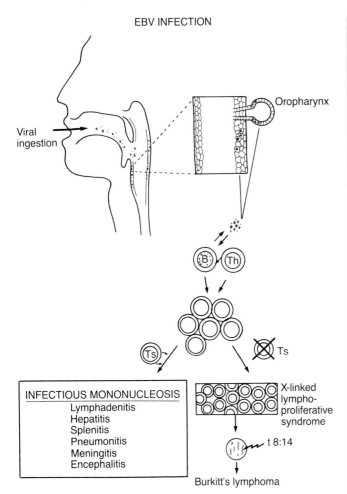

INFECTIOUS MONONUCLEOSIS
Lymphadenitis
Hepatitis
Splenitis
Pneumonitis
Meningitis
Encephalitis

X-linked lympho-proliferative syndrome

t 8:14

Burkitt's lymphoma

Figure 8–30. The pathways of transmission of the Epstein-Barr virus leading in a normal individual to infectious mononucleosis or in those with a cell-mediated deficit to the X-linked lymphoproliferative syndrome and possibly to Burkitt's lymphoma when combined with an 8:14 autosomal translocation. Th = T helper cells. EBV can also cause nasopharyngeal carcinoma (see Chapter 7).

EBV act as brakes on viral shedding, limiting the number of infected B cells rather than eliminating them. Latent EBV remains in a few B cells as well as in oropharyngeal epithelial cells and, as described in Chapter 7, is associated with the development of Burkitt's lymphoma and nasopharyngeal carcinoma, respectively. In addition, as will be seen, impaired immunity in the host can have disastrous consequences.

MORPHOLOGY. The major alterations involve the blood, lymph nodes, spleen, liver, central nervous system, and, occasionally, other organs. The **peripheral blood** shows absolute lymphocytosis with a total white cell count between 12,000 and 18,000 per microliter, more than 60% of which are lymphocytes. Many of these are large, **atypical lymphocytes,** 12 to 16 μm in diameter, character-

ized by an abundant cytoplasm containing multiple clear vacuolations and an oval, indented, or folded nucleus (Fig. 8–31). These atypical lymphocytes, most of which bear T-cell markers, are usually sufficiently distinctive to permit the diagnosis from examination of a peripheral blood smear.

The **lymph nodes** are typically discrete and enlarged throughout the body, principally in the posterior cervical, axillary, and groin regions. Histologically, the lymphoid tissue is flooded by atypical lymphocytes, which occupy the paracortical (T-cell) areas. There is, in addition, some B-cell reaction, with enlargement of follicles. Although the underlying architecture is usually preserved, it may be blurred by intense lymphoproliferation. Occasionally, cells resembling Reed-Sternberg (RS) cells may also be found in the nodes. Together these features sometimes make it difficult to distinguish the nodal morphology from that seen in malignant lymphomas, particularly Hodgkin's disease. Differentiation then depends on recognition of the atypical lymphocytes. Similar changes commonly occur in the tonsils and lymphoid tissue of the oropharynx.

The **spleen** is enlarged in most cases, weighing between 300 and 500 gm. It is usually soft and fleshy, with a hyperemic cut surface. The histologic changes are analogous to those of the lymph nodes, showing a heavy infiltration of atypical lymphocytes, which may result either in prominence of the splenic follicles or in some blurring of the architecture. These spleens are especially vulnerable to rupture, possibly resulting in part from infiltration of the trabeculae and capsule by the lymphocytes.

Liver function is almost always transiently impaired to some degree, although hepatomegaly is at most moderate. Histologically, atypical lymphocytes are seen in the portal areas and sinusoids, and scattered, isolated cells or foci of parenchymal necrosis filled with lymphocytes may be present. This histologic picture may be difficult to distinguish from that of viral hepatitis.

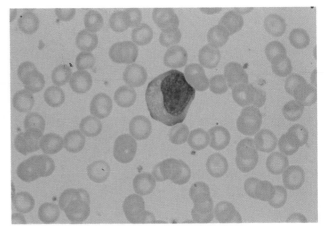

Figure 8–31. Atypical lymphocyte in infectious mononucleosis. (Courtesy of Dr. David Weinberg.)

The **central nervous system** may show congestion, edema, and perivascular mononuclear infiltrates in the leptomeninges. Myelin degeneration and destruction of axis cylinders have been described in the peripheral nerves.

Although classically IM presents with fever, sore throat, lymphadenitis, and the other features mentioned earlier, quite often it is more aberrant in behavior. It may present with little or no fever and only malaise, fatigue, and lymphadenopathy, raising the specter of leukemia-lymphoma; as a fever of unknown origin without significant lymphadenopathy or other localized findings; as hepatitis that is difficult to differentiate from one of the hepatotropic viral syndromes; or as a febrile rash resembling rubella. *Ultimately, the diagnosis depends on the following findings (in increasing order of specificity): (1) lymphocytosis with the characteristic atypical lymphocytes in the peripheral blood, (2) a positive heterophil reaction (Monospot test), and (3) specific antibodies for EBV antigens (viral capsid antigens, early antigens, or Epstein-Barr nuclear antigen).* In the great majority of patients, IM resolves within 4 to 6 weeks, but sometimes the fatigue lasts longer. Occasionally, one or more complications supervene. They may involve virtually any organ or system in the body. Perhaps most common is marked hepatic dysfunction with jaundice, elevated hepatic enzyme levels, disturbed appetite, and rarely, even liver failure. Other complications involve the nervous system, kidneys, bone marrow, lungs, eyes, heart, and spleen (splenic rupture has been fatal). A more serious complication in those suffering from some form of immunodeficiency, such as acquired immunodeficiency syndrome (AIDS), or receiving immunosuppressive therapy (perhaps post-transplant) is that the polyclonal B-cell proliferation may run amok, leading to death. True monoclonal B-cell lymphomas have also appeared, sometimes preceded by polyclonal lymphoproliferation. These unfortunate consequences were described in a family suffering from an X-linked recessive T-cell defect, and so the condition has been designated Duncan's disease or X-linked lymphoproliferation (XLP) syndrome.

Poliovirus Infection

Poliovirus is a spherical, unencapsulated RNA virus of the enterovirus family. Other members of the family cause childhood diarrhea as well as rashes (coxsackievirus A), conjunctivitis (enterovirus 70), viral meningitis (coxsackieviruses and echovirus), myopericarditis (coxsackievirus B), and jaundice (hepatitis A virus). It is also similar in structure to the rhinoviruses that cause the common cold. The 7500-bp genome encodes four structural proteins, two proteases, and an RNA-dependent RNA polymerase. There are three major strains of poliovirus, each of which is included in the Salk formalin-fixed (killed) vaccine and the Sabin oral, attenuated (live) vaccine.[87] These vaccines have nearly eliminated poliovirus from the United States and other Western countries, although poliomyelitis is still a major crippling disease in developing countries.

Poliovirus, like other enteroviruses, first infects tissues in the oropharynx, is secreted into the saliva and swallowed, and then multiplies in the intestinal mucosa and lymph nodes, causing a transient viremia and fever. In 1 of 100 infected persons, poliovirus invades the central nervous system and replicates in motor neurons of the spinal cord (spinal poliomyelitis) or brain stem (bulbar poliomyelitis). Although it is clear that antivirus antibodies control the disease in most cases and that poliovirus binds to ICAM-1 receptors on neurons, it is not known why most individuals clear the virus, while others do not. Virus spread to the nervous system may be secondary to viremia or by retrograde transport of the virus along axons of motor neurons.[88] Rare cases of poliomyelitis that occur after vaccination are caused by mutations of the attenuated viruses to wild-type forms. The neuropathology of poliovirus infection is described in Chapter 29.

Varicella Zoster Infection (Chickenpox and Shingles)

Like HSV, varicella zoster virus (VZV) infects mucous membranes, skin, and neurons and causes a self-limited primary infection in immunocompetent individuals. In contrast to HSV, VZV is transmitted in epidemic fashion by aerosols, disseminates hematogenously, and causes widespread vascular skin lesions (chickenpox). VZV infects primarily satellite cells around neurons in the dorsal root ganglia and may recur many years after the primary infection, causing shingles. Localized recurrences of VZV, are most frequent and painful in dermatomes innervated by the trigeminal ganglia, where VZV is most likely to exist in a state of latency. One reason why VZV recurs less frequently than HSV is that the genes involved in reactivation in HSV are missing in VSV.[72] In addition, immune surveillance may prevent VSV recurrences because shingles occurs most frequently in immunosuppressed or elderly persons.

MORPHOLOGY. The **chickenpox** rash occurs approximately 2 weeks after respiratory infection and travels in multiple waves centrifugally from the torso to the head and extremities. Each lesion progresses rapidly from a macule to a vesicle, which resembles "a dewdrop on a rose petal." Histologi-

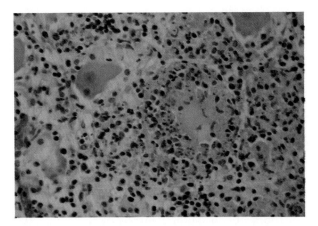

Figure 8–32. Dorsal root ganglion with varicella-zoster virus infection. Note ganglion cell necrosis and associated inflammation. (Courtesy of Dr. James Morris, Radcliffe Infirmary, Oxford, England.)

cally, chickenpox vesicles contain intranuclear inclusions of the epithelial cells identical to those of HSV-1 (see Fig. 8–10). After a few days, most chickenpox vesicles rupture, crust over, and heal by regeneration, leaving no scars, whereas traumatic rupture of some vesicles with bacterial superinfection may lead to destruction of the basal epidermal layer and residual scarring.

Shingles occurs when VZVs, which have long remained latent in the dorsal root ganglia after a previous chickenpox infection, are activated and infect sensory nerves that carry viruses to one or more dermatomes. There VZVs cause vesicular lesions, differentiated from chickenpox by the often intense itching, burning, or sharp pain, because of the simultaneous radiculoneuritis. This pain is especially strong when the trigeminal nerves are involved, rarely involving the geniculate nucleus and causing facial paralysis (Ramsay Hunt syndrome). In the sensory ganglia, there is a dense, predominantly mononuclear infiltrate, with herpetic intranuclear inclusions within neurons and their supporting cells (Fig. 8–32). VZV also causes interstitial pneumonia, encephalitis, transverse myelitis, and necrotizing visceral lesions, particularly in immunosuppressed patients.

Whooping Cough

Whooping cough, caused by the gram-negative coccobacillus *Bordetella pertussis*, is an acute, highly communicable illness characterized by violent coughing paroxysms followed by a loud inspiratory "whoop." Although the DPT vaccine, which contains heat-killed *B. pertussis* bacteria, has reduced greatly the prevalence of whooping cough in the United States, *B. pertussis* infects tens of millions of children and causes hundreds of thousands of deaths annually in the developing world.

The pathogenesis of *B. pertussis* infection is linked largely to its toxins. *B. pertussis* colonizes the brush border of the bronchial epithelium and also invades respiratory macrophages. Conditions in the upper respiratory tract induce *B. pertussis* to coordinately produce numerous virulence factors, including a filamentous hemagglutinin, fimbriae, pertussis toxin, and an adenylate cyclase–hemolysin toxin. The filamentous hemagglutinin binds to carbohydrates on the surface of respiratory epithelial cells as well as to CR3 (MAC-1) integrins on macrophages.[89] Pertussis toxin is an exotoxin composed of five distinct peptides, including a catalytic peptide S1 that shows homology with the catalytic peptides of cholera toxin and *E. coli* heat-labile toxin.[90] Like cholera toxin, pertussis toxin ADP-ribosylates and inactivates guanine-nucleotide–binding proteins, so that these G-proteins no longer transduce signals from host plasma membrane receptors. Other *B. pertussis* toxins include a hemolysin important in early colonization, a bacterial lipopolysaccharide that has endotoxin activity, and a small peptidoglycan toxin that competes for 5-hydroxytryptamine sites on respiratory epithelial cells. Together these toxins reduce the number of ciliated respiratory epithelial cells and decrease the quantity of cilia per cell.[91]

MORPHOLOGY. Bordetella bacteria cause a laryngotracheobronchitis that in severe cases features bronchial mucosal erosion, hyperemia, and copious mucopurulent exudate (Fig. 8–33). Unless superinfected, the lung alveoli remain open and intact. In parallel with a striking peripheral lymphocytosis (up to 90%), there is hypercellularity and enlargement of the mucosal lymph follicles and peribronchial lymph nodes.

Diphtheria

Diphtheria is caused by a slender, gram-positive rod *Corynebacterium diphtheriae*, which is passed from person to person via aerosols or skin shedding. *C. diphtheriae* causes a range of illnesses from asymptomatic carriage, to skin lesions in neglected wounds of combat troops in the tropics, to a life-threatening syndrome that includes formation of a tough pharyngeal membrane and toxin-mediated damage to the heart, nerves, and other organs. In contrast to Bordetella and other bacteria, *C. diphtheriae* has only one toxin, which is encoded by a lysogenic phage and described in detail previously. Inclusion of diphtheria toxoid (formalin-fixed toxin) in the childhood vaccines does not prevent colonization with *C. diphtheriae* but protects immunized individuals from the lethal effects of released toxin.

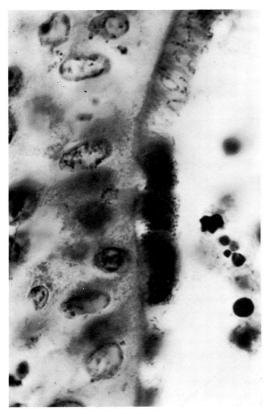

Figure 8-33. Whooping cough showing bacilli covering the cilia of bronchial columnar epithelial cells.

MORPHOLOGY. Inhaled *C. diphtheriae* proliferate at the site of attachment on the mucosa of the nasopharynx, oropharynx, larynx, or trachea but also form satellite lesions in the esophagus or lower airways. Release of exotoxin causes necrosis of the epithelium, accompanied by an outpouring of a dense fibrinosuppurative exudate. The coagulation of this exudate on the ulcerated necrotic surface creates a tough, dirty gray-to-black, superficial membrane (Fig. 8-34). Neutrophilic infiltration in the underlying tissues is intense and is accompanied by marked vascular congestion, interstitial edema, and fibrin exudation. When the membrane sloughs off its inflamed and vascularized bed, bleeding and asphyxiation may occur. With control of the infection, the membrane is coughed up or removed by enzymatic digestion, and the inflammatory reaction subsides.

Although the bacterial invasion remains localized, generalized reticuloendothelial hyperplasia of the spleen and lymph nodes ensues, owing to the absorption of soluble exotoxin into the blood. The exotoxin may cause fatty myocardial change with isolated myofiber necrosis, polyneuritis with degeneration of the myelin sheaths and axis cylinders, and (less commonly) fatty change and focal necroses of parenchymal cells in the liver, kidneys, and adrenals.

OPPORTUNISTIC AND AIDS-ASSOCIATED INFECTIONS

Infections that are usually innocuous or dormant in normal individuals appear with increased frequency in "altered" hosts with genetic or acquired immunodeficiencies. Such opportunistic infections occur in particular in patients receiving cytotoxic and immunosuppressive therapy for tumors, tissue transplants, or autoimmune disease and most dramatically in patients with AIDS (see Chapter 6). Viral, bacterial, fungal, and parasitic infections all

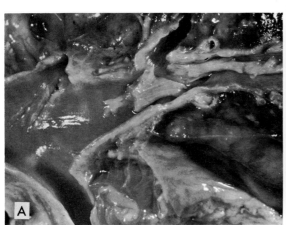
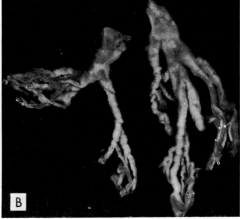

Figure 8-34. Membrane of diphtheria lying within a transverse bronchus (*A*) and forming a perfect cast (removed from the lung) of the branching respiratory tree (*B*).

fall into this category, and we shall discuss some of the more important examples.

Cytomegalic Inclusion Disease

CMV is a beta-group herpesvirus that causes an asymptomatic or mononucleosis-like infection in healthy individuals. CMV, however, can also cause devastating systemic infections in neonates and in immunosuppressed patients. CMV is spread by (1) intrauterine transmission, (2) perinatal transmission at childbirth, (3) mother's milk, (4) respiratory droplets, (5) semen and vaginal fluid, (6) blood transfusions (in about 5% of blood donors, the circulating leukocytes contain latent CMV), and (7) transplantation of virus-infected grafts from a donor with a latent infection. In immunocompetent individuals, CMV infects and remains latent in white blood cells. In immunocompromised patients, CMV causes esophagitis, colitis, hepatitis, pneumonitis, renal tubulitis, chorioretinitis, and meningoencephalitis. In patients with AIDS, CMV pneumonitis is almost always accompanied by *Pneumocystis carinii*, which determines the outcome of infection. In contrast, CMV causes an interstitial pneumonitis in recipients of autologous marrow transplants, which is usually not complicated by *P. carinii* infection and appears to be facilitated by graft-versus-host reactions.[92]

Although 90% of CMV-infected neonates have no sequelae, full-blown congenital CMV infection resembles erythroblastosis fetalis. Affected infants manifest a hemolytic form of anemia, jaundice, thrombocytopenia, purpura, hepatosplenomegaly (due to extramedullary hematopoiesis), pneumonitis, deafness, chorioretinitis, and extensive brain damage. At least half the infants with such severe disease die; some of the survivors are mentally retarded.

MORPHOLOGY. The lesions caused by disseminated CMV infection in the newborn and in immunosuppressed patients are similar and so will be described together. Cells infected with CMV are markedly enlarged, with large purple intranuclear inclusions surrounded by a clear halo, and smaller basophilic cytoplasmic inclusions (Fig. 8–35). Disseminated CMV causes focal necrosis with minimal inflammation in virtually any organ but most often in the salivary glands, kidneys, liver, lungs, gut, pancreas, thyroid, adrenals, and brain. Cytomegalic inclusions are present in both endothelial and epithelial cells and are most abundant in the renal tubular epithelium, hepatocytes, and lining cells of portal bile ducts. In the lung, CMV also infects alveolar epithelial cells, macrophages, and endothelial cells and causes an interstitial pneumonitis with intra-alveolar edema, proteinaceous exudate, and focal hyaline membranes. CMV causes sharply

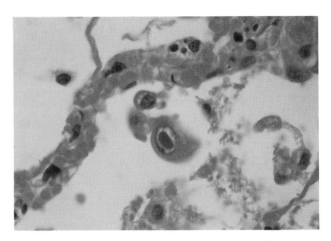

Figure 8–35. CMV distinct nuclear and ill-defined cytoplasmic inclusions in lung. (Courtesy of Dr. Arlene Sharpe.)

punched-out ulcerations in the small and large intestines.

CMV encephalitis is most frequent in congenital infections, in which there are focal acute inflammatory changes with inclusion-bearing giant cells distributed in a narrow band in the subependymal and subpial tissue as well as necrotic lesions irregularly scattered in the cerebrum. CMV lesions are often located about the lateral ventricles, aqueduct, and fourth ventricle and may become calcified. CMV chorioretinitis can occur alone or together with other organ involvements, and is a frequent cause of blindness in patients with AIDS.

Pseudomonas Infection

Pseudomonas aeruginosa is an opportunistic gram-negative bacterium that is a frequent, deadly pathogen of patients with cystic fibrosis, severe burns, or neutropenia.[93] Most patients with cystic fibrosis die of pulmonary failure secondary to chronic infection with *P. aeruginosa*. Although gram-positive cocci are most frequently present soon after thermal injury, *P. aeruginosa* eventually predominate, spread locally, and cause sepsis. *P. aeruginosa* is the third leading cause of hospital-acquired infections (after *S. aureus* and *E. coli*); it has been cultured from wash basins, respirator tubing, nursery cribs, and even antiseptic-containing bottles.

P. aeruginosa also causes corneal keratitis in wearers of contact lenses, endocarditis and osteomyelitis in intravenous drug abusers, external otitis (swimmer's ear) in normal individuals, and severe external otitis in diabetics.

Like other gram-negative bacteria, *P. aeruginosa* has coregulated pili and adherence proteins that mediate adherence to epithelial cells and lung mucin, as well as an endotoxin that causes the symptoms and signs of gram-negative sepsis. Pseudomonas also has a number of virulence factors

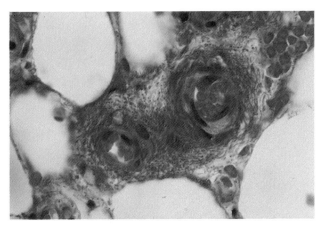

Figure 8–36. Pseudomonas vasculitis in which masses of organisms form a perivascular blue haze.

that are distinctive: (1) Pseudomonas bacteria in the lungs of patients with cystic fibrosis form mucoid colonies that are resistant to antibacterial antibodies, complement, and phagocytes. (2) The organisms secrete exotoxin A, which is similar in structure to diphtheria toxin and, like diphtheria toxin, inhibits protein synthesis by ADP-ribosylating elongation factor 2, a ribosomal G-protein.[94] (3) *P. aeruginosa* secretes exoenzyme S, which ADP-ribosylates small G-proteins, including p21^{ras}, and so may interfere with host cell growth.[95] (4) They secrete a phospholipase C that lyses red blood cells and degrades pulmonary surfactant, and an elastase that degrades IgGs and extracellular matrix proteins and so may be important in tissue invasion and destruction of the cornea in keratitis. (5) Finally, *P. aeruginosa* secretes iron-containing compounds that are extremely toxic to endothelial cells and so may cause the vascular lesions characteristic of this infection.[96]

MORPHOLOGY. Pseudomonas pneumonia, particularly in the altered host, is the prototype of **necrotizing inflammation,** distributing through the terminal airways in a "fleur-de-lis" pattern, with striking whitish necrotic centers and red hemorrhagic peripheral areas. Microscopically, masses of organisms cloud the host tissue with a bluish haze, concentrating in the wall of blood vessels, where host cells undergo coagulation necrosis and nuclei fade away (Fig. 8–36). This picture of gram-negative vasculitis accompanied by thrombosis and hemorrhage, although not pathognomonic, is highly suggestive of *P. aeruginosa*.

Bronchial obstruction caused by mucous plugging and *P. aeruginosa* infection are characteristic of cystic fibrosis. Despite antibiotic treatment and the host immune response against the bacteria, chronic *P. aeruginosa* infection results in bronchiectasis and pulmonary fibrosis (see Chapter 15).

In skin burns. *P. aeruginosa* proliferate widely, penetrating deeply into the veins to induce massive bacteremias. Well-demarcated necrotic and hemorrhagic skin lesions of oval shape often arise during these bacteremias, called *ecthyma gangrenosum*. DIC is a frequent complication of bacteremia.

Legionnaires' Disease

When a lethal pneumonia struck a group of participants at the 1976 convention of the American Legion in Philadelphia, the microbe hunt that ensued led to a hitherto unknown gram-negative bacterial pathogen, *Legionella pneumophila*. Although *L. pneumophila* was not a new pathogen and had caused at least one outbreak of fever in Pontiac, Michigan, in 1968, the bacterium had been missed because the organisms demand culture on special media and are visible in tissue sections only after silver staining. *L. pneumophila* is resistant to chlorine, and epidemic foci have been associated with aerosols from cooling systems of buildings. The same *L. pneumophila* bacterium causes a mild, self-limited fever (Pontiac fever) in otherwise healthy individuals or a severe pneumonia (legionnaire's disease) in smokers, the elderly, individuals with chronic lung disease, and immunosuppressed patients. *L. pneumophila* is unique among bacteria because it is a facultative intracellular parasite of macrophages and of the aquatic amebae *Hartmannella vermiformis* and *Tetrahymena pyriformis*. *L. pneumophila* bacteria enter the macrophage in two ways: (1) In nonimmune serum, complement-coated bacteria bind to macrophage CR1 and CR3 complement receptors and are engulfed by pseudopods, and (2) when coated with anti–*L. pneumophila* antibodies, bacteria bind the macrophage Fc receptors and enter via conventional "zipper" phagocytosis.[97] Within the macrophage, *L. pneumophila* fails to induce a respiratory burst; they block phagosome fusion with the lysosome, multiply, and eventually lyse the host cell. A 24-kd protein on the surface of the bacteria (called macrophage infectivity potentiator) is necessary for growth in the macrophages and amebae and for infectivity in animal models.[98]

MORPHOLOGY. Legionella species produce a multifocal pneumonia of fibrinopurulent type that is initially nodular but may become confluent or lobar. The lesions are focused on the alveoli and distal bronchioles, with sparing of the proximal bronchioles and bronchi. A high ratio of mononuclear phagocytes to neutrophils is characteristic, with many destroyed phagocytes at the center of the lesions (leukocytoclasis), surrounded by intact macrophages. Silver-stained bacteria are copious in the leukocytoclastic areas and are also present locally inside large, bubbly-appearing macrophages and in hilar lymph nodes. Secondary inflammation of the walls of small pulmonary arteries and veins is often intense and accompanied by thrombosis. Abscesses are frequent but tend to be small and rarely confluent. These destructive lesions explain the tendency toward organization and scarring.

Candidiasis

Candida species, which are part of the normal flora of the skin, mouth, and GI tract, are the most frequent cause of human fungal infections. (The most common is *C. albicans.*) These infections vary from superficial lesions in healthy persons to disseminated infections in neutropenic patients. Candida grow as yeast forms, tandem arrays of elongated forms without hyphae (pseudohyphae), and true hyphae with septae. All may be mixed together in the same tissue, and all are stained with Gram, periodic acid–Schiff, or methenamine silver. Candida grows best on warm, moist surfaces and so frequently causes vaginitis (particularly during pregnancy), diaper rash, and oral thrush. Dishwashers, diabetics, and burn patients are also particularly susceptible to superficial candidiasis. Chronic mucocutaneous candidiasis occurs in persons with AIDS, in individuals with inherited or iatrogenic defects in T cell–mediated immunity, and in persons with polyendocrine deficiencies (hypoparathyroidism, hypoadrenalism, and hypothyroidism). Severe disseminated candidiasis is associated with neutropenia secondary to chronic granulomatous disease, leukemia, anticancer therapy, or immunosuppression after transplantation. Candida is directly introduced into the blood by intravenous lines, catheters, peritoneal dialysis, cardiac surgery, or intravenous drug abuse. Although the course of candidal sepsis is less rampant than that of bacterial sepsis, disseminated Candida eventually causes shock and DIC.

Candida has numerous molecules on its surface that mediate its adherence to host tissues, including (1) a receptor homologous to the human CR3 integrin, which binds RGD groups on C3bi, fibrinogen, fibronectin, and laminin; (2) a lectin that binds sugars on epithelial cells; and (3) mannose-containing proteins that bind to lectin-like molecules on epithelial cells.[99] Other virulence-associated factors include a secreted aspartyl proteinase, which may be involved in tissue invasion by degrading extracellular matrix proteins, and secreted adenosine, which blocks neutrophil oxygen radical production and degranulation.[100]

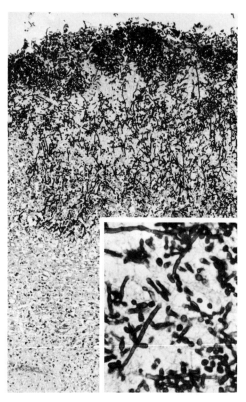

Figure 8–37. Silver stain of a candidal ulcer of the esophagus with slender filamentous and yeast forms.

MORPHOLOGY. Candida infections of the oral cavity (thrush) and vagina produce superficial, white patches or large, almost fluffy membranes that are easily detached, leaving a reddened, irritated underlying surface. Spread of oral candidasis, as by a nasogastric tube, may lead to similar lesions in the esophagus (Fig. 8–37). Candida also causes cutaneous eczematoid lesions in moist areas of the skin (i.e., between the fingers and toes and in inguinal creases, inframammary folds, and the anogenital region). Microscopically, these lesions contain acute and chronic inflammation with microabscesses, but in their chronic states granulomatous reactions may develop. Sometimes hypersensitivity dermal reactions develop in sites remote from the infections, and these lesions are known as **candidids** or **id reactions**.

Severe, invasive candidiasis associated with immunosuppression or with phagocyte depletion involves the **kidney** in 90% of cases, causing multiple microabscesses in both the cortex and the medulla. Microscopically, the yeast or pseudohyphal forms of the fungus occupy the center of the lesion, with a surrounding area of necrosis and polymorphonuclear infiltrate. Some fungal cells may be found inside glomerular capillary loops. Candida right-sided **endocarditis**, resulting from direct inoculation of the fungi into the bloodstream, most often in drug addicts, gives rise to large, friable vegetations that frequently break off into emboli. In the lungs, lesions are extensive and polymorphous and often are hemorrhagic and infarct-like owing to fungal invasion of vascular walls. Meningitis, intracerebral abscesses, hepatic abscesses, enteritis, endophthalmitis, multiple subcutaneous abscesses, arthritis, and osteomyelitis are some of the other presentations of disseminated candidiasis. In any of these locations, the fungus may evoke little or no inflammatory reaction, cause the usual suppurative response, or occasionally produce granulomas.

Cryptococcosis

Cryptococcus neoformans is an encapsulated yeast that can cause meningoencephalitis in normal individuals but more frequently in patients with AIDS, leukemia, lymphoma, systemic lupus erythematosus, Hodgkin's disease, sarcoidosis, or transplant recipients. Many of these patients receive high-dose corticosteroids, a major risk factor for cryptococcus infection.

C. neoformans is present in the soil and in bird (particularly pigeon) droppings and infects patients when it is inhaled. Three properties of C. neoformans are associated with virulence. These include (1) the capsular polysaccharide, a surface molecule that stains bright red with mucicarmine in tissues, stains negative in India ink preparations in cerebrospinal fluid (CSF), and can be detected with antibody-coated beads in the CSF; (2) resistance to killing by alveolar macrophages; and (3) production of phenoloxidase. This enzyme consumes host epinephrine in the synthesis of fungal melanin, thus protecting the fungi from the epinephrine oxidative system present in the host nervous system.[101] One reason why C. neoformans preferentially infects the brain may be that the CSF lacks alternative pathway complement components (present in serum) that bind to the carbohydrate capsule and facilitate phagocytosis and killing by polymorphonuclear cells.

MORPHOLOGY. Although the lung is the primary site of localization, pulmonary infection with C. neoformans is usually mild and asymptomatic, even while the fungus is spreading to the central nervous system. C. neoformans, however, may form a solitary pulmonary granuloma similar to the coin lesions caused by Histoplasma. The major pathology of C. neoformans is in the central nervous system, including the meninges, cortical gray matter, and basal nuclei. The tissue response to cryptococci is extremely variable. In immunosuppressed patients, organisms may evoke virtually no inflammatory reaction, so gelatinous masses of fungi grow in the

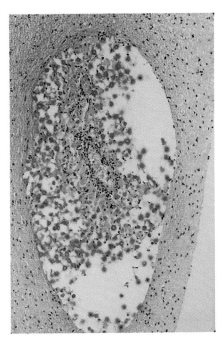

Figure 8–38. Mucicarmine stain of cryptococci (staining red) in a Virchow-Robin perivascular space of the brain (soap-bubble lesion).

meninges or in small cysts within the gray matter (soap-bubble lesions; Fig. 8–38) as though in a culture medium. In nonimmunosuppressed patients or in those with protracted disease, the fungi induce a chronic granulomatous reaction composed of macrophages, lymphocytes, and foreign body-type giant cells. Neutrophils and suppuration may also occur, as well as a rare granulomatous arteritis of the circle of Willis. In severely immunosuppressed persons, C. neoformans may disseminate widely to the skin, liver, spleen, adrenals, and bones.

Aspergillosis

Aspergillus is an ubiquitous mold that causes allergies (brewer's lung) in otherwise healthy persons and serious *sinusitis*, *pneumonia*, and *fungemia* in neutropenic persons. Aspergillus species secrete three toxins that may be important in human disease. The carcinogen *aflatoxin* is made by Aspergillus species growing on the surface of peanuts and may be a major cause of liver cancer in Africa (see Chapter 18). *Restrictocin* and *mitogillin* are ribotoxins that inhibit host cell protein synthesis by degrading mRNAs. In addition, mitogillin is a potent inducer of IgE and so may be involved in host allergic responses to Aspergillus.[102] Sensitization to the Aspergillus spores produces an allergic alveolitis by inducing type III and type IV hypersensitivity reactions (see Chapter 15). *Allergic bronchopulmonary aspergillosis*, which is associated with hypersensitivity arising from superficial coloniza-

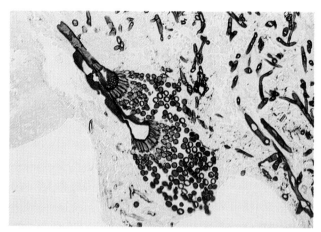

Figure 8–39. Aspergillus colony showing fruiting body and septate hyphae in nasal septum. Silver stain.

tion of the bronchial mucosa and often occurs in asthmatic patients, may eventually result in chronic obstructive lung disease.

MORPHOLOGY. Colonizing aspergillosis (aspergilloma) implies growth of the fungus in pulmonary cavities with minimal or no invasion of the tissues. The cavities usually result from pre-existing tuberculosis, bronchiectasis, old infarcts, or abscesses. Proliferating masses of fungal hyphae called "fungus balls" form brownish masses lying free within the cavities. The surrounding inflammatory reaction may be sparse, or there may be chronic inflammation and fibrosis. Patients with aspergillomas usually have recurrent hemoptysis.

Invasive aspergillosis is an opportunistic infection confined to immunosuppressed and debilitated hosts. The primary lesions are usually in the lung, but widespread hematogenous dissemination with involvement of the heart valves, brain, and kidneys is common. The pulmonary lesions take the form of necrotizing penumonia with sharply delineated, rounded, gray foci with hemorrhagic borders, often referred to as **target lesions.** Aspergillus forms fruiting bodies (particularly in cavities) and septate filaments, 5 to 10 μm thick, branching at acute angles (40 degrees) (Fig. 8–39). Aspergillus has a tendency to invade blood vessels, and thus areas of hemorrhage and infarction are usually superimposed on the necrotizing, inflammatory tissue reactions. Rhinocerebral Aspergillus infection in immunosuppressed individuals resembles that caused by phycomycetes (e.g., mucormycosis).

Mucormycosis

Mucormycosis is an opportunistic infection of neutropenic persons and ketoacidotic diabetics, caused by "breadmold fungi," including Mucor, Absidia,

Rhizopus, and Cunninghamella, which are collectively referred to as the Phycomycetes. These fungi, which are widely distributed in nature and cause no harm to immunocompetent individuals, infect immunosuppressed patients somewhat less frequently than do Candida or Aspergillus.

MORPHOLOGY. The three primary sites of Mucor invasion are the nasal sinuses, lungs, and gastrointestinal tract, depending on whether the spores (widespread in dust and air) are inhaled or ingested. In diabetics, the fungus may spread from nasal sinuses to the orbit, and brain, giving rise to **rhinocerebral mucormycosis.** The phycomycetes cause local tissue necrosis, invade arterial walls, and penetrate the periorbital tissues and cranial vault. Meningoencephalitis follows, sometimes complicated by cerebral infarctions when fungi invade arteries and induce thrombosis. Phycomycetes form nonseptate, irregularly wide (6 to 50 μm) fungal hyphae with frequent right-angle branching, which are readily demonstrated in the necrotic tissues by hematoxylin and eosin or special fungal stains (Fig. 8–40).

Lung involvement with Mucor may be second-

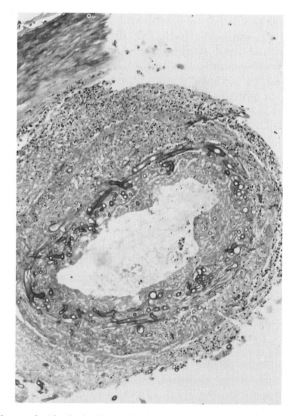

Figure 8–40. Periodic acid–Schiff stain of mucormycosis showing hyphae, which have an irregular width and right-angle branching, invading an artery wall.

ary to rhinocerebral disease, or it may be primary in patients with hematologic neoplasms. The lung lesions combine areas of hemorrhagic pneumonia with vascular thrombi and distal infarctions.

Pneumocystis Pneumonia

Pneumocystis carinii is a ubiquitous organism that produces no disease in normal individuals but causes a severe pneumonia in most patients with AIDS and in children with protein-calorie malnutrition.[103] Pneumocystis pneumonia is frequently the first diagnosed opportunistic infection in HIV-1–infected persons and is the leading cause of death in AIDS. Pneumocystis is diagnosed by the demonstration of 4 to 6 μm cup-shaped or boat-shaped cysts in bronchoalveolar lavage fluid, sputum, or transbronchial biopsy stained by silver, Giemsa, or toluidine blue stain. Aggressive treatment with pentamidine and with folic acid inhibitors greatly reduces the morbidity caused by Pneumocystis in AIDS but often fails to clear the infection and is complicated by adverse drug reactions.

P. carinii was long considered a protozoan parasite because of its multiple forms, including one that is trophozoite-like. Studies, however, have strongly suggested that *P. carinii* is a fungus, based on properties of its cell wall, the paucity of its intracellular organelles, and phylogenetic analysis of its small-subunit ribosomal RNA sequence.[104] Inhaled *P. carinii* attach to type 1 alveolar epithelial cells and multiply within the alveolar space. In mice with severe combined immunodeficiency, which lack B and T cells but have normal macrophages, resistance to *P. carinii* infection is transferred by either CD4+ helper T cells or by hyperimmune serum.[105] In HIV-1–infected persons, *P. carinii* infection occurs when the CD4+ helper T cells fall below 200 per mm³, and anti–*P. carinii* antibodies appear to have no effect on host resistance to the organisms.

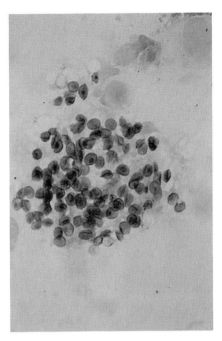

Figure 8–41. Silver stain of cup-shaped *Pneumocystis carinii* organisms within a sputum sample of an AIDS patient.

Cryptosporidiosis

Cryptosporidium parvum is a protozoan parasite that has long been known to cause diarrhea in cattle but has only recently been shown to cause a transient watery diarrhea in normal children, and a chronic, debilitating diarrhea in patients with AIDS. This is in contrast to Entamoeba and Giardia, which have an increased incidence among homosexual men but do not cause increased pathology in patients with AIDS.[106] C. parvum oocytes are not killed by chlorine but instead must be removed by filtration through sand, so that epidemics of cryptosporidiosis, in which tens of thousands of persons have diarrhea, occur when municipal water filtration systems break down.[107]

C. parvum has a complicated life cycle that includes infectious, environmentally resistant oocysts resembling those of Entamoeba and Giardia as well as asexual sporozoites and merozoites and sexual gametes that resemble malaria parasites.[108] Sporozoites have a lectin on their surface that mediates adherence to intestinal and colonic epithelial cells. Malabsorption and a secretory diarrhea occur when sporozoites disrupt the microvilli and enter the cytoplasm of epithelial cells. *Cryptosporidia* also enter M cells and macrophages in underlying Peyer's patches. Although both normal persons and patients with AIDS produce antiparasite IgAs, intact T cell–mediated immunity (lacking in AIDS) appears to be necessary for clearing the parasites. Similarly, mice with severe combined immunodeficiency, which are chronically infected with *C. parvum*, clear the parasite when they receive transplants of T_H1 CD4+ T cells.[109]

MORPHOLOGY. *P. carinii* causes a diffuse or patchy pneumonia. Affected lungs are airless, red, and beefy. Histologically, the alveolar spaces are filled by an amphophilic, foamy, amorphous material resembling proteinaceous edema fluid, composed of proliferating parasites and cell debris (Fig. 8–41). Usually there is an accompanying mild interstitial inflammatory reaction, with widening of the septa, protein and fibrin exudation, pneumocyte proliferation, escape of red cells, and formation of hyaline membranes. Frequently, there is concurrent infection by opportunistic bacteria, fungi, or viruses, especially CMV, which may overshadow the pathology caused by *P. carinii*.

Cryptosporidia adhere to the apical brush border of absorptive gut epithelia, enveloped by a host cell membrane. There is mixed inflammation of the lamina propria. Cryptosporidia shed in the stool are best visualized after staining with a modified acid-fast stain.

Toxoplasmosis

Toxoplasma gondii is an obligate intracellular protozoan that commonly causes subclinical infection or mild lymphadenopathy in normal persons yet produces severe opportunistic infections in infants *in utero*, patients with AIDS, and patients receiving bone marrow and organ transplants.

PATHOGENESIS. Like Giardia, Toxoplasma infects a wide range of animals. Sexual reproduction occurs only in the intestinal epithelium of the cat, but humans can be infected with Toxoplasma either by ingesting oocysts from cat feces or by ingesting incompletely cooked lamb or pork; the latter contain Toxoplasma cysts filled with intracystic organisms, called bradyzoites. Entering through the gut, *T. gondii* spreads systemically and penetrates into any type of host cell, a unique property of this parasite. Bow-shaped *T. gondii* tachyzoites spread from cell to cell until T cell–mediated immunity develops and macrophages are activated by TNF and other lymphokines to kill the intracellular parasites. Some *T. gondii* cysts containing bradyzoites may remain dormant for years in muscle and visceral cells.

After primary *T. gondii* infection of the mother during the first trimester of pregnancy, disseminated and often fatal parasitemias occur in 25% of fetuses. *T. gondii* tachyzoites travel through the placenta into the fetus and destroy the developing heart, brain, and lung tissues. Congenital infection with *T. gondii* is also the most common cause of chorioretinitis in the United States, which may result in blindness in one or both eyes. In patients with AIDS, Toxoplasma reactivated from dormant cysts causes encephalitis, which frequently produces mass lesions. Iatrogenic immunosuppression in organ transplant patients results in toxoplasmosis from (1) reactivation of the cysts within the grafted kidney, heart, liver, or lungs or (2) the recipient's own tissues after bone marrow graft.[110]

T. gondii is able to infect all types of cells because the parasites bind the extracellular matrix protein laminin to their surface, in turn attaching to laminin receptors on the surface of host cells. During host cell penetration, Toxoplasma releases numerous proteins from special secretory organelles called *rhoptries* and enters vacuoles that fail to fuse to lysosomes and so do not become acidified. This route of entry of the *T. gondii* parasites appears to be important in preventing acidification, as organisms covered with antiparasite antibodies and entering host cells via Fc receptors enter acidified vacuoles.

MORPHOLOGY. In otherwise normal adults, Toxoplasma causes lymphadenitis characterized by follicular hyperplasia; focal proliferation of transformed, histiocytoid B cells; and scattered accumulations of enlarged, epithelioid-type macrophages, which do not form well-defined granulomas. Lesions are more frequent in young women than in men, posterior cervical lymph nodes are most often affected, and the diagnosis can be confirmed by serologic titers to Toxoplasma antigens or by staining for parasite antigens by immunohistochemical techniques.

In **neonatal toxoplasmosis,** destructive lesions of the central nervous system are composed of microglial nodules containing many tachyzoites, located about the ventricles and aqueduct, which may be obstructed and so cause hydrocephalus. These lesions are often accompanied by extensive central nervous system necrosis, vascular thrombosis, and intense inflammation. In addition, the liver, heart, lungs, and adrenals all may become necrotic.

In **Toxoplasma chorioretinitis,** destruction of the retina by tachyzoites is accompanied by a granulomatous reaction in the choroid and sclera. Central nervous system involvement with Toxoplasma is discussed and illustrated in Chapter 29 (see Fig. 29–25).

ZOONOTIC AND VECTOR-BORNE INFECTIONS

Rickettsial Infections

Rickettsiae are vector-borne obligate intracellular bacteria that cause epidemic typhus (*R. prowazekii*), scrub typhus (*R. tsutsugamushi*), and spotted fevers (*R. rickettsii* and others) (Table 8–9).[5]

In contrast, Q fever, which is caused by the related organism *Coxiella burnetii* and produces pneumonia and fever, is transmitted by aerosols. *Ehrlichia chaffeensis*, a newly discovered intracellular organism related to the rickettsiae, causes an acute febrile illness similar to the spotted fevers, but without a rash. It is tick transmitted. Epidemic typhus, which is transmitted from person to person via body lice, is particularly associated with wars and human suffering, when persons are forced to live in close contact without changing clothes. Scrub typhus, transmitted by chiggers, was a major problem for U.S. soldiers in the Pacific in World War II and in Vietnam. *Rocky Mountain spotted fever*, transmitted to humans by rodent and dog ticks, is most frequent in the southeastern and

Table 8-9. RICKETTSIAL DISEASES AND PATHOGENS

DISEASE	GEOGRAPHY	AGENT	TRANSMISSION	DISTINCTIVE FEATURES
Typhus Group (No eschar)				
Epidemic typhus	Worldwide (war, famine)	R. prowazekii	Louse feces	Endothelial infection; centrifugal-type rash
Brill-Zinsser disease	That of epidemic typhus	R. prowazekii	Late reactivation	Those of epidemic typhus, but generally milder
Flying squirrel typhus	Southeastern United States	R. prowazekii	Fleas, lice of flying squirrel	Similar to epidemic typhus, but mortality is lower
Murine typhus	Worldwide (rat-related)	R. typhi (mooseri)	Rat flea feces	Similar to epidemic typhus, but mortality is lower
Spotted Fever Group				
Rocky Mountain spotted fever	North and South America	R. rickettsii	Tick bite	Endothelia and vascular smooth muscle infected; rash is centripetal; eschar rarely seen
Boutonneuse fever	Mediterranean, India	R. conorii	Tick bite	Prominent eschar, "tache noire"
North Asian and Queensland tick typhus	USSR, China, etc. Australia	R. sibirica R. australia	Tick bite	Both diseases are typical spotted fevers commonly with eschar
Rickettsial pox	United States, USSR, Korea, Africa	R. akari	Mite bite	Prominent eschar; papulovesicular rash (milder than RMSF)
Scrub Typhus	East Asia, Pacific	R. tsutsugamushi	Chigger bite	Frequent eschar and lymphadenopathy
Q Fever	Worldwide	Coxiella burnetii	Droplet inhalation	No eschar or rash; fever, pneumonia, ring granuloma
Ehrlichiosis	Not yet fully known	Ehrlichia sennetsu, E. canis	Tick bite	Fever, lymphadenopathy, no eschar or rash

southwestern United States. Rickettsiae enter the skin with the bite or with scratching of the skin covered with insect feces.

Regardless of the route of infection, rickettsiae predominantly infect host endothelial and vascular smooth muscle cells, causing a widespread vasculitis that may be complicated by thrombi and hemorrhages. Rickettsiae bind to cholesterol-containing receptors, are endocytosed into phagolysosomes, escape into the cytosol, and multiply until they burst the cells. Rickettsiae have an endotoxin but lack secreted toxins. In addition, R. rickettsii activate host kallikrein and kinins and so cause local clotting. Coxiella and Ehrlichia predominantly infect leukocytes.[111] Antibody-dependent and cell-dependent immunity may prevent reinfection with rickettsiae but may not prevent reactivation of typhus after many years, which is referred to as Brill-Zinsser disease. Diagnosis of rickettsial infections may be made by immunostaining of organisms or by detection of antibodies in the serum. Against this background we can turn to the morphology of rickettsial infections with particular emphasis on typhus fever and Rocky Mountain spotted fever.

Typhus Fever

In milder cases, the gross changes are limited to a skin rash and small hemorrhages incident to the vascular lesions, described below. In more severe cases there may be areas of necrosis of the skin with gangrene of the tips of the fingers, nose, ear lobes, scrotum, penis, and vulva. In such cases, irregular ecchymotic hemorrhages may be found internally, principally in the brain, heart muscle, testes, serosal membrane, lungs, and kidneys.

The most prominent microscopic changes are the small vessel lesions that underlie the rash, and the focal areas of hemorrhage and inflammation in the various organs and tissues affected. Endothelial proliferation and swelling in the capillaries, arterioles, and venules may narrow the lumina of these vessels. Surrounding the involved vessels, a cuff of inflammatory mixed leukocytes is usually present. The vascular lumina are sometimes thrombosed, but necrosis of the vessel wall is unusual in typhus, as compared with Rocky Mountain spotted fever. It is the vascular thromboses that lead to the gangrenous necroses of the skin and other structures. In the brain characteristic typhus nodules are composed of focal microglial proliferations mixed with leukocytes (Fig. 8-42).

Rocky Mountain Spotted Fever (RMSF)

An eschar at the site of the tick bite followed by a hemorrhagic rash that extends over the entire body, including the palms of the hands and soles of the feet, is the hallmark of RMSF. The vascular lesions that underlie the rash often lead to acute necrosis, fibrin extravasation, and thrombosis of the small blood vessels, including arterioles (Fig. 8-43). In severe RMSF, foci of necrotic skin are thus induced, particularly on the fingers, toes, elbows,

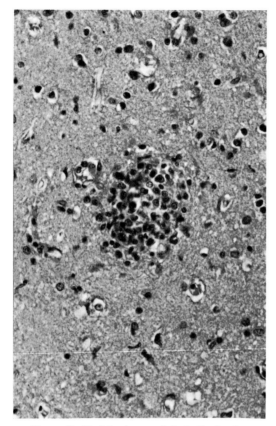

Figure 8-42. A typhus nodule in the brain.

Plague

Yersinia pestis is a gram-negative facultative intracellular bacterium that is transmitted by flea bites or by aerosols and causes a highly invasive, frequently fatal systemic infection called *plague*. Plague, also named Black Death, caused three great pandemics that killed an estimated 100 million persons in Egypt and Byzantium in the 6th century; one quarter of Europe's population in the 14th and 15th centuries; and tens of millions in India, Burma, and China at the beginning of the 20th century.[112] Currently, wild rodents in the western United States are infected with *Y. pestis*, which are rarely transmitted to humans. Most cases of plague occur in urban foci in Southeast Asia, where rats are the reservoir of infection. *Y. enterocolitis* and *Y. pseudotuberculosis* are genetically similar to *Y. pestis*; these bacteria cause fecal-orally transmitted ileitis and mesenteric lymphadenitis, as described earlier.

Y. pestis makes a plasmid-encoded secreted protease that activates plasminogen and cleaves complement C3 at a specific site.[113] This secreted protease is essential for spread of the bacteria from the local site of inoculation and inflammation into the bloodstream, so mutant bacteria lacking this protease are 1 million times less virulent to mice when inoculated into the skin.

ears, and scrotum. Vascular necrosis and thrombosis are far more frequent with RMSF than with typhus and may mimic the necrotizing vasculitis of the collagen-vascular diseases. Despite frequent local thrombi, systemic DIC is rare, even in the most severe cases. The perivascular inflammatory response is similar to that of typhus, particularly in the brain, skeletal muscle, lungs, kidneys, testes, and heart muscle. The vascular necroses in the brain may involve larger vessels and produce focal areas of ischemic demyelinization or microinfarcts. A pneumonitis of primary rickettsial origin is present in severely affected patients and often predisposes to a secondary bacterial infection.

Other Rickettsial Infections

Coxiella infections (Q fever) mainly involve the lungs, producing an interstitial pneumonitis that resembles viral pneumonia. In severe cases, small granulomas may appear in the spleen, liver, and bone marrow along with focal perivascular inflammatory infiltrates.

Scrub typhus, or mite-borne infection, is usually a milder version of typhus fever. The rash is usually transitory or may not appear. Vascular necrosis or thrombosis is rare, but there may be a prominent inflammatory lymphadenopathy.

MORPHOLOGY. Plague causes lymph node enlargement (bubo), pneumonia, or sepsis, all with a striking neutrophilia. The distinctive histological features include (1) massive proliferation of the organisms, (2) early appearance of protein-rich and polysaccharide-rich effusions with few inflammatory cells but with marked tissue swelling, (3) necrosis of tissues and blood vessels with hemorrhage and thrombosis, and (4) neutrophilic infiltrates that accumulate adjacent to necrotic areas as healing begins.

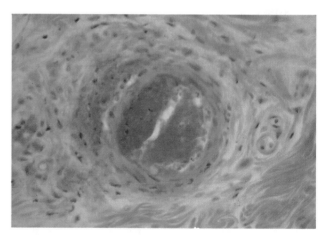

Figure 8-43. Rocky Mountain spotted fever with thrombosed vessel and vasculitis.

In **bubonic plague,** the site of entry is usually on the legs and is marked by a small pustule or ulceration. The nodes of drainage enlarge dramatically within a few days and become soft, pulpy, and plum-colored and may infarct or rupture through the skin. In **pneumonic plague,** there is a severe, confluent, hemorrhagic, and necrotizing bronchopneumonia, often with fibrinous pleuritis. In **septicemic plague,** lymph nodes throughout the body as well as reticuloendothelial organs develop foci of necrosis. Fulminating bacteremias also induce DIC with widespread hemorrhages and thrombi.

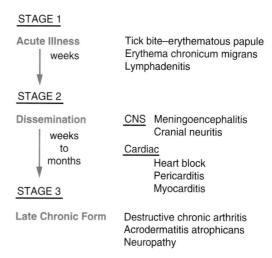

Figure 8–44. The clinical stages of Lyme disease.

Relapsing Fever

Relapsing fever is caused by helical *Borrelia spirochetes (B. recurrentis)*, which are transmitted from person to person by body lice or from animals to humans by soft ticks. Louse-transmitted Borrelia, associated with overcrowding owing to poverty or war, caused multiple large epidemics in Africa, Eastern Europe, and Russia in the first half of the 20th century, infecting 15 million persons and killing 5 million, and is still a problem in some developing countries.[114]

PATHOGENESIS. In both lice- and tick-transmitted borreliosis there is a 1- to 2-week latent period after the bite as the spirochetes multiply in the serum. Clinical infection is heralded by shaking chills, fever, headache, and fatigue, followed by DIC and multiorgan failure. Spirochetes are cleared from the blood by anti-Borrelia antibodies that target a single major surface protein, called the variable major protein.[115] After a few days, bacteria bearing a different surface antigen reach high densities in the blood, and symptoms return until a second set of host antibodies clears these organisms. This process of changing surface molecules in response to antibodies, which is called *antigenic variation*, also occurs in African trypanosomiasis, discussed later. The lessening severity of successive attacks of relapsing fever and its spontaneous cure in many untreated patients have been attributed to the limited genetic repertoire of Borrelia, enabling the host to build up cross-reactive as well as clone-specific antibodies. Antibiotic treatment of Borrelia infections may cause a massive release of endotoxin, resulting in a dangerous rise in temperature with rigors, fall in blood pressure, and leukopenia (the Jarish-Herxheimer reaction).

MORPHOLOGY. In fatal louse-borne disease, the spleen is moderately enlarged (300 to 400 gm) and contains focal necroses and miliary collections of leukocytes, including neutrophils, and numerous

borreliae. There is congestion and hypercellularity of the red pulp with erythrophagocytosis. The liver may also be enlarged and congested with prominent Kupffer's cells and septic foci. Scattered hemorrhages resulting from DIC may be found in serosal and mucosal surfaces, skin, and viscera. Pulmonary bacterial superinfection is a frequent complication.

Lyme Disease

Lyme disease, named for the Connecticut town where in the mid-1970s there was an epidemic of arthritis associated with skin erythema, is caused by the spirochete *Borrelia burgdorferi*. Lyme disease, spread by rodents to people by tiny deer ticks (*Ixodes scapularis [dammini], I. ricinus,* and others), is the major arthropod-borne disease currently in the United States and is also frequent in Europe and Japan.[116] In the northeastern United States, the incidence of Lyme disease is now increasing because as many as 50% of ticks are infected with Borrelia, and the tick population is growing in parallel to the increasing numbers of white-tailed deer.

As in another major spirochetal disease, syphilis, clinical disease caused by Lyme spirochetes involves multiple organ systems and is usually divided into three stages.[117] In *stage 1* (Fig. 8–44) at the site of the tick bite, Borrelia spirochetes multiply and spread locally within the dermis, causing an expanding area of redness, often with an indurated or pale center. This skin lesion, called *erythema chronicum migrans*, may be accompanied by fever and lymphadenopathy but usually disappears in a few weeks' time. In *stage 2, the early disseminated stage,* spirochetes spread hematogenously throughout the entire body and cause secondary annular skin lesions, lymphadenopathy, migratory joint and muscle pain, cardiac arrhythmias, and meningitis often with cranial nerve involvement. In untreated patients, antibodies develop to spirochete flagellar proteins and to two major outer membrane proteins; these antibodies are useful for serodiagnosis of Borrelia infection. Antibody-covered Borrelia are phagocytosed by macrophages by means of the same coiling process used in the uptake of Legionella, Trypanosoma, and Leishmania. Some spirochetes, however, escape host antibody and T-cell responses by sequestering themselves in the central nervous system or (as intracellular forms) within endothelial cells.[118] In *stage 3, the late disseminated stage,* 2 or 3 years after the initial bite, Lyme Borrelia cause a chronic arthritis sometimes with severe damage to large joints, and an encephalitis that varies from mild to debilitating. The host immune response is out of proportion to the scant number of organisms detectable, and may be caused by antibodies to spirochete heat-shock proteins that cross-react with host tissues.[119]

MORPHOLOGY. Skin lesions caused by *B. burgdorferi* are characterized by edema and a lymphocytic–plasma cell infiltrate. In early Lyme arthritis, the synovium resembles that of early rheumatoid arthritis, with villous hypertrophy, lining cell hyperplasia, and abundant lymphocytes and plasma cells in the subsynovium. A distinctive feature of Lyme arthritis is an arteritis, with onionskin-like lesions resembling those seen in hypertension (see Chapter 20).[120] In late Lyme disease, there may be extensive erosion of the cartilage in large joints. In Lyme meningitis, the CSF is hypercellular, shows a marked lymphoplasmacytic, and contains antispirochete IgGs.

Malaria

Malaria caused by the intracellular protozoan parasite *Plasmodium falciparum* is a worldwide infection that affects 100 million and kills 1 to 1.5 million persons per year and so is the major parasitic cause of death. *P. falciparum* and the three other malaria parasites that infect humans (*P. vivax, P. ovale, P. malariae*) are transmitted by more than a dozen species of Anopheles mosquitoes widely distributed throughout Africa, Asia, and Latin America.[121] The wide geographic distribution of malaria is due to the failure of a massive campaign from the 1950s to 1980s to eradicate malaria. This campaign produced mosquitoes that are resistant to DDT and malathion and *P. falciparum* parasites resistant to chloroquine and pyrimethamine.

P. vivax and *P. malariae* cause mild anemia and, in rare instances, splenic rupture and nephrotic syndrome. Acute *P. falciparum* infections produce high parasitemias, severe anemia, cerebral symptoms, renal failure, pulmonary edema, and death. Therefore, the focus of the discussion that follows will be on the pathology caused by *P. falciparum.*

LIFE CYCLE AND PATHOGENESIS. Malaria sporozoites are released into the blood with the bite of an infected mosquito and within minutes attach to and invade liver cells by binding to the hepatocyte receptor for the serum proteins thrombospondin and properdin, located on the basolateral surface of hepatocytes (Fig. 8–45).[122] The binding is accomplished because of the presence of sporozoite surface proteins that contain a domain homologous to the binding domain of thrombospondin. Within liver cells, malaria parasites multiply rapidly, so as many as 30,000 merozoites (asexual, haploid blood forms) are released when the hepatocyte ruptures. The HLA-B53–associated resistance to *P. falciparum* infections exhibited by many Africans appears to be caused by the ability of HLA-B53 to present liver stage–specific malaria antigens to cytotoxic T cells, which then kill malaria-infected hepatocytes.[123]

Once released, *P. falciparum* merozoites bind via a parasite lectin-like molecule to sialic residues on glycophorin molecules on the surface of red blood cells. (*P. vivax* merozoites bind via a homologous lectin to the Duffy antigens on red blood cells, so many Africans who are Duffy-negative are resistant to this parasite.) The merozoites release multiple proteases from a special organelle called the *rhoptry,* also found, as we have seen, in Toxoplasma, Cryptosporidium and Babesia parasites. Within the red blood cells, the parasites multiply in a membrane-bound digestive vacuole, hydrolyzing hemoglobin via secreted enzymes that include a heme polymerase. The latter neutralizes the potentially toxic heme by forming a paracrystalline precipitate called *hemozoin or malaria pigment.* This heme polymerase is inhibited by chloroquine, which accumulates in the digestive vacuole.[124] Individuals with the sickle cell trait are resistant to malaria because their red blood cells sickle when parasitized and so are removed by the spleen. Although most malaria parasites within the red blood cells develop into merozoites, rupture the cell, and then infect new red blood cells, some parasites develop into sexual forms called *gametocytes* that infect the mosquito when it takes its blood meal.

As the malaria parasites mature within red blood cells, they change morphology from ring to schizont form and secrete proteins that form 100-nm bumps on the red blood cell surface, called *knobs.* Malaria proteins on the surface of the knobs, called *sequestrins,*[125] bind to endothelial cells via ICAM-1 (Fig. 8–9), the thrombospondin-receptor, and the glycophorin CD46 and so cause malaria-infected red blood cells to be removed from circulation.[126] In this way, red blood cells

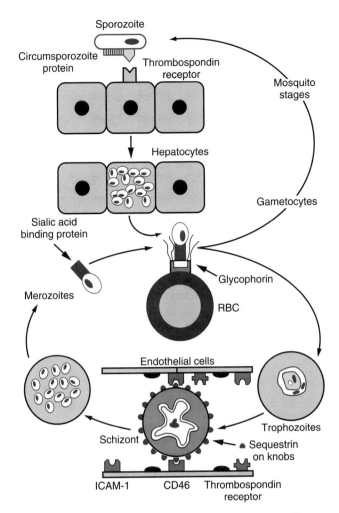

Figure 8–45. Life cycle of *Plasmodium falciparum*. (Drawn by Dr. Jeffrey Joseph, Brigham and Women's Hospital, Boston.)

antigenically distinct sequestrins at rates similar to those of the variant surface glycoproteins produced by trypanosomes.[127]

MORPHOLOGY. P. falciparum infection initially causes congestion and enlargement of the **spleen,** which may eventually exceed 1000 gm in weight. Parasites are present within red blood cells, and there is increased phagocytic activity of the reticuloendothelial cells. In chronic malaria infection, the spleen becomes increasingly fibrotic and brittle, with a thick capsule and fibrous trabeculae. The parenchyma is gray or black because of phagocytotic cells containing granular, brown-black, faintly birefringent hemozoin pigment. In addition, macrophages with engulfed parasites, red blood cells, and debris are numerous.

The **liver** becomes progressively enlarged and pigmented with progression of malaria. Kupffer's cells are heavily laden with malarial pigment, parasites, and cellular debris, while some pigment is also present in the parenchymal cells. Pigmented phagocytic cells may be found dispersed throughout the bone marrow, lymph nodes, subcutaneous tissues, and lungs. The kidneys are often enlarged and congested with a dusting of pigment in the glomeruli and hemoglobin casts in the tubules.

In **malignant cerebral malaria** caused by *P. falciparum*, brain vessels are plugged with parasitized red cells, each cell containing dots of hemozoin pigment (Fig. 8–46). About the vessels, there are ring hemorrhages that are probably related to local hypoxia incident to the vascular stasis and small focal inflammatory reactions (called malarial or Dürck's granulomas). With more severe hypoxia, there is degeneration of neurons, focal ischemic softening, and occasionally scant inflammatory infiltrates in the meninges.

Nonspecific focal hypoxic lesions in the **heart** may be induced by the progressive anemia and circulatory stasis in chronically infected patients. In some, the myocardium shows focal interstitial infiltrates. Finally, in the nonimmune patient, pulmonary edema or shock with DIC may cause death, sometimes in the absence of other characteristic lesions.

containing immature ring forms of the parasite, which are flexible and can pass through the spleen, circulate in the blood, whereas red blood cells containing mature schizonts, which are more rigid, avoid sequestration in the spleen. In addition, sequestrin causes red blood cells to bind to and form rosettes with thrombospondin uninfected red blood cells.

Cerebral involvement by *P. falciparum*, which causes as many as 80% of deaths in children, is due to adhesion of the *P. falciparum* parasites to endothelial cells within the brain. Patients with cerebral malaria have increased amounts of ICAM-1, thrombospondin receptor, and CD46 on their cerebral endothelial cells (perhaps activated by cytokines such as TNF) to which the malaria-infected red blood cells bind. Adults, who are resistant to cerebral malaria, have antibodies to the parasite-encoded sequestrins on the red cell knobs, so malaria-infected red blood cells are cleared. This immunity, however, may be incomplete because *P. falciparum* parasites are able to produce a family of

Babesiosis

Babesia microti are malaria-like protozoans transmitted by the same deer ticks that carry Lyme disease. Babesiae parasitize red blood cells and cause fever and hemolytic anemia. The symptoms are mild except in debilitated or splenectomized individuals, who develop severe and fatal parasitemias. Splenectomized persons may also be infected by *Babesia bovis*, which causes an economically important disease in cattle (Texas cattle fever).

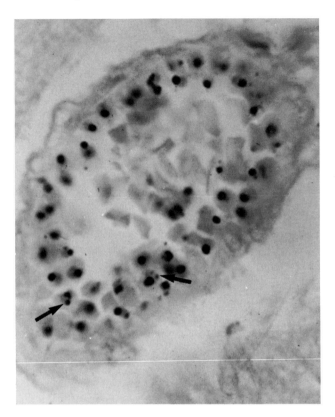

Figure 8–46. _P. falciparum_-infected red cells marginating within a vein in cerebral malaria.

MORPHOLOGY. In blood smears, Babesia resemble _P. falciparum_ ring stages, although they lack hemozoin pigment. They form characteristic tetrads, which are diagnostic. The level of _B. microti_ parasitemia is a good indication of the severity of infection: 1% in mild cases and up to 30% in splenectomized persons, who also show marked erythrophagocytosis associated with the red cell destruction. In fatal cases, the anatomic findings are related to shock and hypoxia and include jaundice, hepatic necrosis, acute renal tubular necrosis, hemolysis, and visceral hemorrhages.

Trichinellosis

Trichinella spiralis is a nematode parasite that is acquired by ingestion of improperly cooked meat from pigs, which have themselves been infected by eating _T. spiralis_-infected rats or pork. In the United States, the number of _T. spiralis_-infected pigs was reduced from 11 to 0.5% from 1950 to 1968, with a consequent decrease in _T. spiralis_ infection at autopsy from 16 to 4%. Still trichinosis is widespread where undercooked pork is eaten.

In the human gut, _T. spiralis_ parasites develop into adults that mate and release larvae, which penetrate into the tissues. Larvae disseminate hematogenously and penetrate muscle cells, causing fever, myalgias, marked eosinophilia, and periorbital edema. Much less commonly patients develop dyspnea (because of invasion of the diaphragm), encephalitis, and cardiac failure. In striated skeletal muscle, _T. spiralis_ larvae become intracellular parasites, increase dramatically in size, and modify the host muscle cell (referred to as the nurse cell), so that it loses its striations, gains a collagenous capsule, and develops a plexus of new blood vessels around itself.[128] The nurse cell–parasite complex is largely asymptomatic and may exist for years before it calcifies. Antibodies to larvae may reduce reinfection and are useful for serodiagnosis of infections. Although eosinophils are numerous, their precise role is uncertain, since mice depleted of eosinophils with antibodies to IL-5, the lymphokine that stimulates eosinophils, are not more susceptible to primary infection or reinfection with _T. spiralis_.[129]

MORPHOLOGY. During the invasive phase of trichinosis, cell destruction can be widespred but is rarely lethal. In the **heart,** there is a patchy interstitial myocarditis characterized by many eosinophils and giant cells. The myocarditis may lead to scarring. Larvae do not encyst and are difficult to identify, as they die and disappear. In the **lungs,** trapped larvae cause focal edema and hemorrhages, sometimes with an allergic eosinophilic infiltrate. In the **central nervous system,** larvae cause a diffuse lymphocytic and eosinophilic infiltrate, with focal gliosis in and about small capillaries of the brain.

T. spiralis preferentially encysts in striated skeletal muscles with the richest blood supply, including the diaphragm, extraocular eye, laryngeal, deltoid, gastrocnemius, and intercostal muscles (Fig. 8–47). Coiled larvae are approximately 1 mm long and are surrounded by membrane-bound vacuoles within nurse cells, which in turn are surrounded by new blood vessels and a lymphocytic and plasmacytic infiltrate. This infiltrate is greatest around dying parasites, which eventually calcify and leave behind characteristic scars useful for retrospective diagnosis of trichinosis.

Cysticercosis

Taenia solium is a cestode parasite. Depending on the route of infection, it produces either mild abdominal symptoms, caused by a solitary adult tapeworm in the gut lumen, or convulsions, increased intracranial pressure, and mental disturbances caused by _T. solium_ cysts in brain tissue. Adult tapeworms are derived from the ingestion of undercooked pork that contains *T. solium* cysticerci. *T. solium* tapeworms, which may be many inches long, attach to the intestinal wall via hook-like scolices and release proglottid segments with thousands of eggs in the feces each day. When eggs are ingested, the larvae hatch, penetrate the gut wall, disseminate hematogenously, and encyst in the central nervous system, causing cerebral cysticercosis. *T. solium* cysts secrete a protein called antigen B, which binds collagen and the first component of complement, thus inhibiting initiation of the classic complement pathway.[130]

MORPHOLOGY. Cysticerci may be found in any organ, but preferred locations include the brain, muscles, skin, and heart. Cerebral symptoms depend on the precise location of the cysts, which includes the meninges, gray and white matter, Sylvian aqueduct, and ventricular foramina. The cysts are ovoid, white to opalescent, rarely exceeding 1.5 cm, and contain an invaginated scolex with hooklets, which are bathed in clear cyst fluid (Fig. 8–48). The cyst wall is more than 100 μm thick, is rich in glycoproteins, and evokes little host reaction when intact. When cysts degenerate, however, there is inflammation, followed by focal scarring, and calcifications, which may be visible by x-ray.

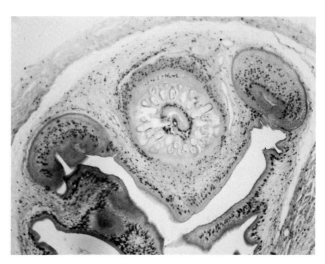

Figure 8–48. Cysticercus in subcutaneous tissue with an inverted scolex and sectioned hooklets (center) and suction cups (both sides).

TROPICAL INFECTIONS

Trachoma

Trachoma is a chronic suppurative eye disease, manifested by follicular keratoconjunctivitis and caused by subtypes of *Chlamydia trachomatis* (see Table 8–3).[75] It is one of the leading global causes of blindness. *Progressive trachoma is seen mostly in dry and sandy regions and among poor people and nomads*, where the infection is acquired during childhood. Trachoma is transmitted by direct human contact, by contaminated particles (fomites), and possibly by flies.

Infections can be either self-limiting or progressive; the latter type begins with a suppurative stage to deeper tissue involvement, with lymphoplasmacytic infiltration and the formation of lymphoid follicles. The upper limbus of the cornea and the upper tarsal plate tend to be most severely involved by epithelial hyperplasia and follicular hypertrophy.[131,132] Soon, the conjunctiva ulcerates, and penetration into the cornea leads to pannus formation, fibroblast ingrowth, scarring, and eventual blindness. The scarring also hampers closure of the eyelids, in turn promoting bacterial superinfection. Furrowing of the mucosa overlying the tarsal plate and pitting of the upper rim of the limbus are characteristic late deformities of trachoma.

Leprosy

Leprosy, or Hansen's disease, is a slowly progressive infection caused by *Mycobacterium leprae*, af-

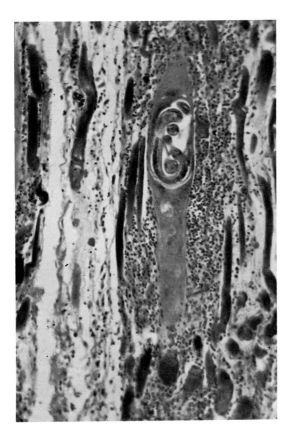

Figure 8–47. Coiled *Trichinella spiralis* larva within a skeletal muscle cell.

fecting the skin and peripheral nerves and resulting in disabling deformities. *M. leprae* is for the most part contained within the skin, but leprosy is believed to be transmitted from person to person via aerosols from lesions in the upper respiratory tract. Inhaled *M. leprae*, like *M. tuberculosis*, is taken up by alveolar macrophages, disseminates through the blood, but grows only in relatively cool tissues of the skin and extremities. Despite its low communicability, leprosy remains endemic among an estimated 10 to 15 million people living in poor tropical countries.[133] Transmission has ceased in the United States, although patients continue to reside in a single specialized facility located in Carville, Louisiana.

PATHOGENESIS AND TYPES OF LEPROSY. *M. leprae* is an acid-fast obligate intracellular organism, which has not been grown in culture but can be grown in the nine-banded armadillo. It grows more slowly than other mycobacteria and grows best at 32 to 34°C, the temperature of the human skin and the core temperature of armadillos. Like *M. tuberculosis*, *M. leprae* secretes no toxins, but its virulence is based on properties of its cell wall. The cell wall is similar enough to that of *M. tuberculosis* that immunization to BCG alone confers 50% protection against *M. leprae* infection.[134] Cell-mediated immunity is reflected by delayed-type hypersensitivity reactions to dermal injections of a bacterial extract called *lepromin*. Antibodies to *M. leprae* antigens, many of which are heat-shock proteins, have no ability to control *M. leprae* infection. *Leprosy is a bipolar disease, determined by the host cellular immune response* (Fig. 8–49). Two forms of the disease occur, depending on whether the host mounts a T cell–mediated immune response (*tuberculoid leprosy*) or is anergic (*lepromatous leprosy*).

Patients with *tuberculoid leprosy* form granulomas similar to those seen in tuberculosis, containing epithelioid macrophages, giant cells, and few surviving mycobacteria. The 48-hour lepromin skin test is strongly positive. At the circumference of the granulomas are CD4+ type 1 helper T cells, that like mouse T_H1 cells secrete IL-2 and interferon-gamma.[135] There are also a few CD8+ lymphocytes in the center of the tuberculoid leprosy lesions. Damage to the nervous system occurs and granulomas form in the nerve sheaths.

In contrast, patients with *lepromatous leprosy* lack T cell–mediated immunity, are anergic to lepromin, and have diffuse lesions containing foamy macrophages stuffed with large numbers of mycobacteria. Lepromatous leprosy lesions lack CD4+ type 1 T cells at their margins but instead contain many CD8+ suppressor T cells in a diffuse pattern. The CD8+ suppressor T cells secrete IL-10, which inhibits helper T cells and may mediate the anergy seen in lepromatous leprosy. These CD8+ suppressor T cells also secrete IL-4, which induces antibody production by B cells. The antibody is not protective, and indeed the formation of antigen-antibody complexes in lepromatous leprosy leads to erythema nodosum leprosum, a life-threatening vasculitis and glomerulonephritis. In lepromatous leprosy, damage to the nervous system comes from widespread invasion of the mycobacteria into Schwann cells and into endoneural and perineural macrophages. Because of the diffuse, parasite-filled lesions, patients with lepromatous leprosy are more infectious than those with tuberculoid leprosy.

MORPHOLOGY. Tuberculoid leprosy begins with localized skin lesions that are at first flat and red but enlarge and develop irregular shapes with indurated, elevated, hyperpigmented margins and depressed pale centers (central healing). Neuronal involvement dominates tuberculoid leprosy, as nerves become enclosed within granulomatous inflammatory reactions and, if small enough (e.g., the peripheral twigs), are destroyed (Fig. 8–50). Nerve degeneration causes skin anesthesias and skin and muscle atrophy that render the patient liable to trauma of the affected parts, with the development of indolent skin ulcers. Contractures, paralyses, and autoamputation of fingers or toes may ensue. Facial nerve involvement can lead to paralysis of the lids, with keratitis and corneal ulcerations. Microscopically, all sites of involvement disclose granulomatous lesions closely resembling hard tubercles, and bacilli are almost never found. Because leprosy pursues an extremely slow course, spanning decades, most patients die with leprosy rather than of it.

Lepromatous (anergic) leprosy involves the skin, peripheral nerves, anterior eye, upper airways (down to the larynx), testes, hands, and feet. The vital organs and central nervous system are rarely affected, presumably because the core temperature is too high for growth of *M. leprae*. Lepromatous lesions contain large aggregates of lipid-laden macrophages (lepra cells), often filled with masses of acid-fast bacilli (globi; Fig. 8–51). Macular, papular, or nodular lesions form on the face, ears, wrists, elbows, and knees. With progression, the nodular lesions coalesce to yield a distinctive leonine facies. Most skin lesions are hypoesthetic or anesthetic. Lesions in the nose may cause persistent inflammation and bacilli-laden discharge. The peripheral nerves, particularly the ulnar and peroneal nerves where they approach the skin surface, are symmetrically invaded with mycobacteria, with minimal inflammation. Loss of sensation and trophic changes in the hands and feet follow the nerve lesions. Lymph nodes show aggregation of foamy histiocytes in the paracortical (T cell) areas, with enlargement of germinal centers. In advanced disease, aggregates of macrophages are also present in the splenic red pulp and the liver. The

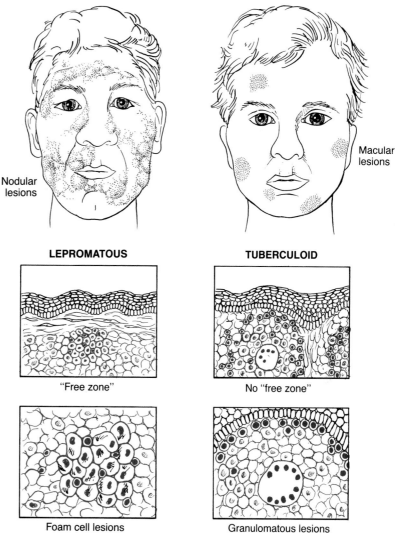

Nodular lesions

Macular lesions

LEPROMATOUS

TUBERCULOID

"Free zone"

No "free zone"

Foam cell lesions

Granulomatous lesions

Figure 8-49. A comparison of the polar extremes of leprosy. The nodular lepromatous form on the left demonstrates aggregates of lipid and bacilli-laden "lepra" cells deep to the epidermis (free zone). In contrast is the tubercular pattern on the right with macular skin lesions produced by a granulomatous reaction directly in contact with the epidermis (no free zone). Bacilli are extremely rare.

testes are usually extensively involved, with destruction of the seminiferous tubules and consequent sterility.

Leishmaniasis

Leishmaniasis is a chronic inflammatory disease of the skin, mucous membranes, or viscera caused by obligate intracellular, kinetoplastid protozoan parasites, transmitted through the bite of infected sandflies. Leishmaniasis is endemic throughout the Middle East, South Asia, Africa, and Latin America. Leishmaniasis may also be epidemic, as is tragically the case in southern Sudan, where tens of thousands of persons have died of visceral leishmaniasis. The infective stage of Leishmania is a slender, flagellated parasite, released into the host dermis along with the sandfly saliva, which potentiates parasite infectivity.[8] Leishmaniae are phago-

cytosed by macrophages and transform into round amastigotes, which lack flagellae but contain a single large mitochondrium-like structure called the kinetoplast. Amastigotes divide only within the phagolysosomes of macrophages, rupture the cells, and infect other macrophages.

ETIOLOGY AND PATHOGENESIS. How far the amastigotes spread throughout the body is determined by the Leishmania species: Cutaneous disease is caused by *L. major* and *L. aethiopica* in the Old World and *L. mexicana* and *L. braziliensis* in the New World, mucocutaneous disease (also called espundia) is caused by *L. braziliensis*, and visceral pathology involving the liver and spleen is caused by *L. donovani* in the Old World and *L. chagasi* in the New World. One explanation for the tropism of Leishmania appears to be temperature, as parasites that cause visceral disease grow at 37°C *in vitro*, whereas parasites that cause mucocutaneous disease grow only at 34°C. As is the case with *M. leprae* infection, the severity of dis-

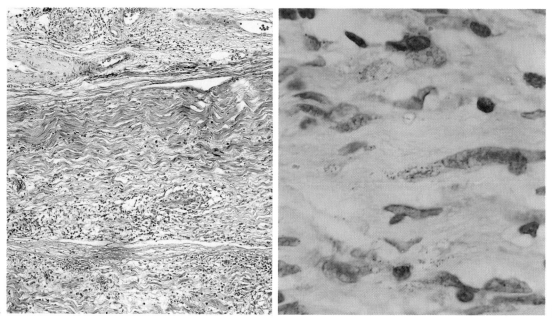

Figure 8–50. Leprosy. *A,* Peripheral nerve. Note inflammatory cell infiltrates in the endoneural and epineural compartments. *B,* Cell within endoneurium contains acid-fast positive lepra bacilli. (Courtesy of E.P. Richardson, Jr., and U. De Girolami, Harvard Medical School).

ease caused by Leishmania is determined by the host immune response. Hosts with parasite-specific, cell-mediated immunity control the infection or make granulomas with few parasites present, whereas anergic hosts have diffuse lesions composed of macrophages stuffed with parasites.

Leishmania amastigotes are the only protozoan parasites that survive and reproduce in macrophage phagolysosomes, which have a pH of 4.5. Amastigotes are protected from the intravacuolar acid by a proton-transporting ATPase, which maintains the intracellular parasite pH at 6.5.[136] Leishmania parasites also have on their surface two abundant glycoconjugates anchored to lipid anchors, which appear to be important for their virulence.[137] The first, *lypophosphoglycans,* are glycoli-

pids that form a dense glycocalyx and bind C3b or C3bi. Organisms, however, resist lysis by complement C5-C9 and are phagocytosed by macrophages via complement receptors CR1 (LFA-1) and CR3 (MAC-1 integrin). Lypophosphoglycans may also protect the parasites within the phagolysosomes by scavenging oxygen radicals and by inhibiting lysosomal enzymes. The second glycoconjugate, *gp63,* is a zinc-dependent proteinase that cleaves complement and some lysosomal antimicrobial enzymes. Its expression correlates with infectivity.

Leishmania parasites are cleared from the body by cell-mediated immune mechanisms, which is reflected by a positive, delayed-type hypersensitivity reaction to extracts of Leishmania injected into the skin *(leishmanin test).*[138] Parasite-specific CD4+ helper T lymphocytes of the T_H1 class secrete interferon-gamma, which, along with TNF-α, secreted by other macrophages activate phagocytes to kill the parasites via toxic metabolites of oxygen or nitric acid (or both). In contrast, down-regulation of the immune response that leads to anergy, and progressive disease may be caused by parasite-specific, CD4+ helper T cells of the T_H2 class that secrete IL-4, which inhibits macrophage activation by interferon-gamma and inhibits secretion of TNF-α.

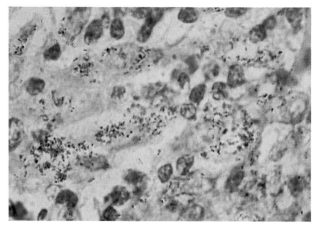

Figure 8–51. Lepromatous leprosy with acid-fast bacilli (red snappers) proliferating in macrophages.

MORPHOLOGY. Leishmania species produce four different lesions in humans: visceral, cutaneous, mucocutaneous, and diffuse cutaneous. In **visceral leishmaniasis,** *L. donovani* or *L. chagasi* parasites

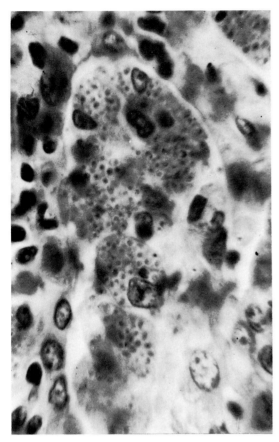

Figure 8–52. *L. donovani* parasites within macrophages of a lymph node in visceral leishmaniasis (kala-azar).

invade macrophages throughout the reticuloendothelial system and cause severe systemic disease marked by hepatosplenomegaly, lymphadenopathy, pancytopenia, fever, and weight loss. The spleen may weigh as much as 3 kg, and the lymph nodes may measure 5 cm in diameter. Phagocytic cells are enlarged and filled with Leishmania, many plasma cells are present, and the normal architecture of the spleen is obscured (Fig. 8–52). In the late stages, the liver becomes increasingly fibrotic. Phagocytic cells crowd the bone marrow and may also be found in the lungs, gastrointestinal tract, kidneys, pancreas, and testes. Often there is hyperpigmentation of the skin in the extremities, which is why the disease is called kala-azar or "black fever" in Hindi. In the kidneys, there may be an immune complex–mediated mesangioproliferative GN (see Chapter 20), and in advanced cases amyloid deposition. The overloading of the reticuloendothelial system with parasites predisposes the patients to bacterial infections, the usual cause of death. Hemorrhages related to thrombocytopenia may also be fatal.

Cutaneous leishmaniasis, caused by *L. major*, *L. mexicana*, and *L. braziliensis*, is a relatively mild, localized disease consisting of a single ulcer on exposed skin. The lesion (often called "*tropical sore*") begins as an itching papule surrounded by induration; changes into a shallow, slowly expanding ulcer with irregular borders; and usually heals by involution within 6 months without treatment. Microscopically, the lesion is granulomatous, usually with many giant cells and few parasites.

Mucocutaneous leishmaniasis, caused by *L. braziliensis,* is found only in the New World. Moist, ulcerating, or nonulcerating lesions, which may be disfiguring, develop in the larynx and at the mucocutaneous junctions of the nasal septum, anus, or vulva. Microscopically, there is a mixed inflammatory infiltrate with parasite-containing histiocytes in association with lymphocytes and plasma cells. Later the tissue reaction becomes granulomatous, and the number of parasites declines. Eventually, the lesions remit and scar, although reactivation may occur after long intervals by mechanisms not currently understood.

Diffuse cutaneous leishmaniasis is a rare form of dermal infection, thus far found only in Ethiopia and adjacent East Africa and in Venezuela, Brazil, and Mexico. Diffuse cutaneous leishmaniasis begins as a single skin nodule, which continues spreading until the entire body is covered by bizarre nodular lesions. These lesions, which resemble keloids or large verrucae, are frequently confused with the nodules of lepromatous leprosy, so patients may be incorrectly sent to leprosaria. The lesions do not ulcerate but contain vast aggregates of foamy macrophages stuffed with leishmania. Patients are usually anergic not only to leishmanin but also to other skin antigens, and the lesions often respond poorly to treatment.

African Trypanosomiasis

African trypanosomes are kinetoplastid parasites that proliferate as extracellullar forms in the blood and cause sustained or intermittent fevers, lymphadenopathy, splenomegaly, progressive brain dysfunction (sleeping sickness), cachexia, and death. *Trypanosoma rhodesiense* infection is often acute and virulent. Its tsetse fly vector prefers the savannah plains of East Africa. *T. gambiense* infection tends to be chronic and occurs most frequently in the West African bush. *T. brucei brucei,* to which humans have become refractory, ravages cattle and sheep over millions of square miles of East Africa.

PATHOGENESIS. African trypanosomes are covered by a single, very abundant, glycolipid-anchored protein called the variable surface glycoprotein (VSG). As parasites increase in numbers in the bloodstream, the host produces antibodies to the VSG, which, in association with phagocytes, kill most of the organisms, causing a spike of fever. A small number of parasites, however, undergo a genetic rearrangement and produce a different VSG on their surface and so escape for a while the host immune response.[17] These successor clones multiply until the host recognizes their VSG and kills them, allowing another clone with a new VSG to take over. In this way, African trypanosomes cause waves of fever before they finally break down the host defenses and invade the central nervous system. A second important way in which the parasites trick the host immune system is by secreting a lymphocyte-triggering factor that binds to CD8 molecules on suppressor T cells and causes these cells to secrete interferon-gamma, which is a strong stimulator of growth of the parasites.[139] The precise mechanisms of tissue injury are unknown, although antigen-antibody complexes and release of lysosomal enzymes from degenerating phagocytes may be involved.

MORPHOLOGY. A large, red, rubbery chancre forms at the site of the insect bite, where large numbers of parasites are surrounded by a dense, largely mononuclear, inflammatory infiltrate. With chronicity, the lymph nodes and spleen enlarge owing to hyperplasia and infiltration by lymphocytes, plasma cells, and macrophages, which are filled with killed parasites. Trypanosomes, which are small and difficult to visualize, concentrate in capillary loops, such as the choroid plexus and glomeruli. When parasites breach the blood-brain barrier and invade the central nervous system, a leptomeningitis extends into the perivascular Virchow-Robin spaces, and eventually a demyelinating panencephalitis occurs. Plasma cells containing glycoprotein globules are frequent and are referred to as **flame cells** or **Mott cells.** Chronic disease leads to progressive cachexia, and patients, devoid of energy and normal mentation, waste away.

Chagas' Disease

Trypanosoma cruzi is a kinetoplastid, intracellular protozoan parasite that causes American trypanosomiasis or Chagas' disease, the most frequent cause of heart failure in Brazil and neighboring Latin American countries. *T. cruzi* parasites are transmitted from person to person via "kissing bugs" (triatomids), which hide in the cracks of rickety houses, feed on the sleeping inhabitants, and pass infectious parasites in the feces; the latter enter the host via damaged skin or through mucous membranes. At the site of skin entry, there may be a transient, erythematous nodule called a *chagoma.*

PATHOGENESIS. *Trypanosoma cruzi* has on its surface a homologue of the human complement regulatory protein, decay-accelerating factor (DAF).[140] Like human DAF, the parasite homologue is an-

chored by means of a glycosyl phosphatidylinositol linkage, binds C3b, and inhibits C3 convertase formation and alternative pathway complement activation.

At least two different proteins on the surface of *T. cruzi* are involved in parasite entry into macrophages and other cells. The first, a parasite *transialidase*, removes host cell sialic residues and transfers them to a parasite surface protein (Ssp-3), which binds to host cells. The second, a protein called *penetrin*, on the surface of *T. cruzi* binds extracellular matrix proteins, heparin, heparan sulfate, and collagen and mediates invasion of the parasites into host cells.[141] *T. cruzi* avoids killing by macrophages by rapidly moving from the lysosome into the host cell cytosol. Again two parasite proteins are involved: (1) A parasite *neuraminidase* removes sialic acids from host proteins lining the lysosomes and so destabilizes this organelle. (2) Stimulated by acid pH within the lysosome, parasites release *hemolysins* that form pores in and disrupt the lysosomal membranes.[142] Parasites reproduce as rounded amastigotes in the cytoplasm of host cells and then develop flagella, burst host cells, enter the bloodstream, and penetrate smooth, skeletal, and heart muscles or infect kissing bugs when the insects take a blood meal.

In acute Chagas' disease, which is mild in most individuals, cardiac damage results from direct invasion of myocardial cells by the organisms and from the consequent inflammatory changes. Rarely, acute Chagas' patients present with high parasitemia, fever, or progressive cardiac dilatation and failure, often with generalized lymphadenopathy or splenomegaly. In *chronic Chagas' disease*, which occurs in 20% of infected patients 5 to 15 years after initial infection, cardiac and digestive tract damage appears to result from an autoimmune response induced by *T. cruzi* parasites. At this time, there may be no detectable parasitemia, but there is a striking inflammatory infiltration of the myocardium, out of proportion to the scant number of organisms present. Patients have antibodies and T cells that react with parasite proteins and cross-react with host myocardial and nerve cells, lymphocytes, and extracellular proteins such as laminin.[143] Damage to myocardial cells and to conductance pathways causes a dilated cardiomyopathy and cardiac arrhythmias, whereas damage to the myenteric plexus causes dilated colon and esophagus. Autoimmune damage in an experimental mouse model is mediated by CD4+ helper T cells.[144]

MORPHOLOGY. In lethal acute myocarditis, the changes are diffusely distributed throughout the heart. Clusters of leishmanial forms cause swelling of individual myocardial fibers and create intracellular pseudocysts. There is focal myocardial cell necrosis accompanied by extensive, dense, acute in-

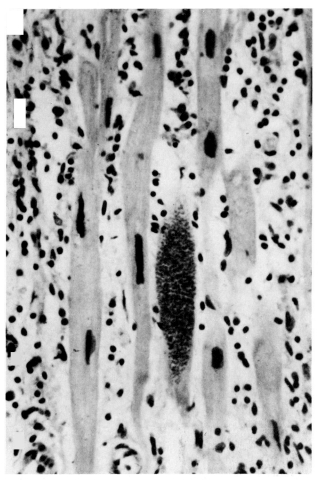

Figure 8-53. Chagasic myocarditis with *T. cruzi*-filled pseudocyst, interstitial edema, and mononuclear infiltrate.

terstitial inflammatory infiltration throughout the myocardium (Fig. 8-53), and there is often four-chamber cardiac dilatation.

In **chronic Chagas' disease,** the heart is typically dilated, rounded, and increased in size and weight. Often there are mural thrombi that, in about one-half of autopsy cases, have given rise to pulmonary or systemic emboli or infarctions. Histologically, interstitial and perivascular inflammatory infiltration is composed of lymphocytes, plasma cells, and monocytes and is heaviest in the right bundle branch of the cardiac conduction system.[145] There are scattered foci of myocardial cell necrosis and interstitial fibrosis, especially toward the apex of the left ventricle, which may undergo aneurysmal dilation and thinning. In the Brazilian endemic foci, as many as one-half of the patients with lethal carditis also have dilatation of the esophagus or colon, apparently related to damage to the intrinsic innervation of these organs. At the late stages, however, when such changes appear, parasites cannot be found within these ganglia.

Schistosomiasis

Schistosomiasis is the most important helminth disease, infecting approximately 200 million persons and killing approximately 250,000 annually. Most of the mortality comes from hepatic granulomas and fibrosis, caused by *Schistosoma mansoni* in Latin America, Africa, and the Middle East and *S. japonicum* and *S. mekongi* in East Asia. In addition, *S. haematobium,* found in Africa, causes hematuria and granulomatous disease of the bladder, resulting in chronic obstructive uropathy.

LIFE CYCLE. Schistosomiasis is transmitted via freshwater snails that live in the slow-moving water of tropical rivers, lakes, and irrigation ditches, which ironically link agricultural development with spread of schistosomiasis (Fig. 8-54). Infectious schistosome larvae swim through fresh water and penetrate human skin with the aid of powerful proteolytic enzymes that degrade the keratinized layer. Within the skin, schistosome larvae shed a surface glycocalyx that protects the organisms from osmotic shock; this glycocalyx, however, activates complement by the alternative pathway and is recognized by many human antischistosome antibodies. *Schistosomes* migrate into the peripheral vasculature, traverse to the lung, and settle in the portal or pelvic venous system, where they develop into adult male and female schistosomes. Attachment in the portal system is mediated by carbohydrates on the parasite surface that bind to receptors on vascular endothelial cells.[146] Females produce hundreds of eggs per day, around which granulomas and fibrosis form, the major pathologic manifestation in schistosomiasis. Some schistosome eggs are passed from the portal veins through the intestinal wall into the colonic lumen, are shed with the feces, and release into freshwater miracidia that infect the snails to complete the life cycle.

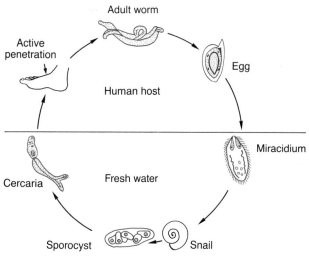

Figure 8-54. Schistosomal life cycle.

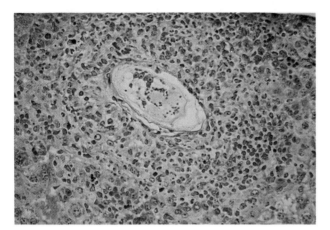

Figure 8-55. *Schistosoma mansoni* granuloma with a miracidium-containing egg *(center)* and numerous scattered eosinophils.

PATHOGENESIS. *Schistosoma mansoni* eggs cause liver pathology in multiple ways. First, substances released from schistosome eggs are directly hepatotoxic, since lesions do occur in mice with severe combined immunodeficiency lacking both B and T cells.[147] Second, eggs induce macrophage accumulation and granuloma formation, mediated by TNF and T_H1 and T_H2 helper cells. T_H2 helper T cells are responsible for the eosinophilia, mastocytosis, and high levels of serum IgE in human schistosomiasis, as these cells secrete IL-4, which induces IgE synthesis by B cells; IL-3 and IL-4, which stimulate mastocytosis; and IL-5, which is a growth factor for eosinophils. Resistance to reinfection by schistosomes after treatment correlates with IgE levels, whereas eosinophil major basic protein may destroy larval schistosomula.[148] Third, eggs release factors that stimulate lymphocytes to secrete a fibrogenic lymphokine that stimulates fibroblast proliferation and portal fibrosis.[149] This exuberant fibrosis, which is out of proportion to the injury caused by the eggs and granulomas, occurs in 5% of persons infected with schistosomes and causes severe portal hypertension, esophageal varices, and ascites, the hallmarks of severe schistosomiasis.

MORPHOLOGY. In mild S. mansoni or S. japonicum infections, white, pinhead-sized granulomas are scattered throughout the gut and liver. The center of the granuloma is the schistosome egg, which contains a miracidium; this degenerates over time and calcifies. The granulomas are composed of macrophages, lymphocytes, neutrophils, and eosinophils; the last-mentioned are distinctive for helminth infections (Fig. 8-55). The liver is darkened by regurgitated heme-derived pigments from the schistosome gut, which like malaria pigments are iron-negative and accumulate in Kupffer's cells and splenic macrophages.

In severe S. mansoni or S. japonicum infections, inflammatory patches or pseudopolyps may form in the colon. The surface of the liver is bumpy, whereas cut surfaces reveal granulomas and a widespread fibrous portal enlargement without distortion of the intervening parenchyma by regenerative nodules. Because these fibrous triads resemble the stem of a clay pipe, the lesion is named "*pipe-stem*" *fibrosis* (see Fig. 8-56). Many of these portal triads lack a vein lumen, causing presinusoidal portal hypertension and severe congestive splenomegaly, esophageal varices, and ascites. Schistosome eggs, diverted to the lung via portal collaterals, may produce granulomatous pulmonary arteritis with intimal hyperplasia, progressive arterial obstruction, and ultimately heart failure (cor pulmonale). Histologically, arteries in the lungs show disruption of the elastica layer by granulomas and scars, luminal organizing thrombi, and angiomatoid lesions similar to those of idiopathic pulmonary hypertension (see Chapter 15). Patients with hepatosplenic schistosomiasis also have an increased frequency of mesangioproliferative or membranous glomerulopathy (see Chapter 20), in which glomeruli contain deposits of immunoglobulin and complement but rarely schistosome antigen.

In S. haematobium infection, bladder inflammatory patches owing to massive egg deposition and granulomas appear early and, when they erode, cause hematuria. Later the granulomas calcify and develop a "sandy" appearance, which if severe may line the wall of the bladder and cause a dense concentric rim (calcified bladder) on x-ray

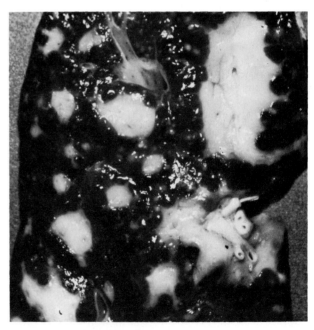

Figure 8-56. Pipe-stem fibrosis of the liver due to chronic *Schistosoma japonicum* infection.

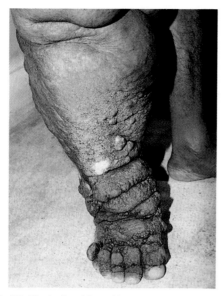

Figure 8–57. Filariasis of leg. (Courtesy of Dr. Willy Piessens, Harvard School of Public Health.)

films. The most frequent complication of S. haematobium infection is inflammation and fibrosis of the ureteral walls, leading to obstruction, hydronephrosis, and chronic pyelonephritis. There is also an association between urinary schistosomiasis and squamous carcinoma of the bladder (see Chapter 21).

Lymphatic Filariasis

Lymphatic filariasis is transmitted by mosquitoes and is caused by two closely related nematodes, *Wuchereria bancrofti* and *Brugia malayi*, which are responsible for 90% and 10%, respectively, of the 90 million infections worldwide. In endemic areas, which include parts of Latin America, sub-Saharan Africa, and Southeast Asia, filariasis causes a spectrum of diseases, including (1) asymptomatic microfilaremia, (2) chronic lymphadenitis with swelling of the dependent limb or scrotum (elephantiasis), and (3) tropical pulmonary eosinophilia. As is the case with leprosy and leishmanial infections, some of the different disease manifestations caused by lymphatic filariae may be understood in the context of varying patterns of host T-cell responses to the parasites.[150]

PATHOGENESIS. Infective larvae released by mosquitoes into the tissues during the blood meal develop within lymphatic channels into adult males and females, which mate and release microfilariae that enter into the bloodstream. Experiments in nude mice suggest that adult filariae secrete factors that, by themselves, are capable of causing lymphatic dilatation, lymphedema, and elephantia-

sis.[151] In contrast, microfilariae, even in massive numbers in microfilaremic hosts, are not directly toxic to the host.

In chronic lymphatic filariasis, damage to the lymphatics is caused directly by the adult parasites and by a T_H1 helper T cell–mediated immune response, which forms granulomas around the adult parasites. Microfilariae are absent from the bloodstream, secondary to immune damage to the adults and to microfilariae.

In contrast, there is a *hypoimmune response* to circulating parasites in microfilaremic individuals, associated with filaria-specific T_H2 helper cells that down-regulate T_H1 cells and inhibit granuloma formation. Because most microfilaremic individuals come from areas endemic with filariasis, there is speculation that the hypoimmune response is caused by prenatal exposure to parasite antigens that may tolerize the host.

Finally, there is an *IgE-mediated hypersensitivity* to microfilariae in *tropical pulmonary eosinophilia*. Both IgE and eosinophils may be secondary to secretion of IL-4 and IL-5, respectively, by filaria-specific T_H2 helper T cells. Tropical pulmonary eosinophilia results in restrictive lung disease, discussed in Chapter 15.

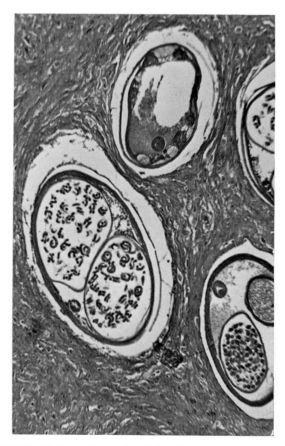

Figure 8–58. Gravid female of *Onchocerca volvulus* in a subcutaneous fibrous nodule.

MORPHOLOGY. Chronic filariasis is characterized by persistent lymphedema of the scrotum, penis, vulva, leg, or arm (Fig. 8–57). Frequently, there is hydrocele and lymph node enlargement. In severe and long-lasting infections, chylous weeping of the enlarged scrotum may ensue, or a chronically swollen leg may develop tough subcutaneous fibrosis and epithelial hyperkeratosis, termed *elephantiasis*. Elephantoid skin shows dilatation of the dermal lymphatics with widespread lymphocytic infiltrates and focal cholesterol deposits; the epidermis is thickened and hyperkeratotic. Adult filarial worms—live, dead, or calcified—are present in the scrotal draining lymphatics or nodes, surrounded by (1) mild or no inflammation, (2) an intense eosinophilia with hemorrhage and fibrin (recurrent filarial funiculoepididymitis), or (3) granulomas not dissimilar to those found in mycobacterial infections.[152] Organization of the endolymphatic exudate results in polypoid infoldings of the vessels with persisting eosinophilic and lymphocytic infiltrates. In time, hydrocele fluid, which often contains cholesterol crystals, red cells, and hemosiderin, induces thickening and calcification of the tunica vaginalis.

Lung involvement by microfilariae is marked by eosinophilia caused by circulating antimicrofilarial IgEs that trigger mast cell degranulation (tropical eosinophilia) or by dead microfilariae surrounded by stellate, hyaline, eosinophilic precipitates embedded in small epithelioid granulomas (Meyers-Kouvenaar bodies). Typically, these patients lack any other manifestations of filarial disease.

Onchocerciasis

Onchocerca volvulus, a filarial nematode transmitted by blackflies, is a major cause of blindness in equatorial Africa, where the parasite infects 20 million persons. Adult *O. volvulus* parasites mate in the dermis, where they are surrounded by a mixed infiltrate of host cells that produces a characteristic subcutaneous nodule (*onchocercoma*). The major pathology, however, which includes blindness and chronic pruritic dermatitis, is caused by large numbers of microfilariae, released by females, that accumulate in the skin and in the eye chambers. *Punctate keratitis* is caused by inflammation around a degenerating microfilaria. It is sometimes accentuated by treatment with antifilarial drugs ("Mazzotti reaction"[153]), resulting in blindness. Damage to the retina is disproportionate to the number of parasites in the posterior eye chamber; it is probably caused by antibodies to a 44-kd parasite antigen that cross-reacts with retinal pigment epithelial cells.[154]

MORPHOLOGY. Severe infection with *O. volvulus* causes chronic, itchy dermatitis with focal darkening or loss of pigment and scaling referred to as "leopard," "lizard," or "elephant" skin. Foci of epidermal atrophy and elastic fiber breakdown may alternate with areas of hyperkeratosis, hyperpigmentation with pigment incontinence, dermal atrophy, and fibrosis. The subcutaneous onchocercoma is composed of a fibrous capsule surrounding adult worms and a mixed chronic inflammatory infiltrate that includes fibrin, neutrophils, eosinophils, lymphocytes, and giant cells (Fig. 8–58). The progressive eye lesions begin with punctate keratitis along with small, fluffy opacities of the cornea caused by degenerating microfilariae, which evoke an eosinophilic infiltrate. This is followed by a sclerosing keratitis that opacifies the cornea, beginning at the scleral limbus. Microfilariae in the anterior chamber cause iridocyclitis and glaucoma, whereas involvement of the choroid and retina results in atrophy and loss of vision.

1. Walsh, J.: Estimating the burden of illness in the tropics. *In* Warren, K.S., and Mahmoud, A.A.F. (eds.): Tropical and Geographical Medicine, 2nd ed. New York, McGraw-Hill, 1990.
2. Falkow, S.: Molecular Koch's postulates applied to microbial pathogenicity. Rev. Infect. Dis. *10*:S274, 1988.
3. von Lichtenberg, F.: Pathology of Infectious Disease. New York, Raven Press, 1991.
4. Binford, C.H., and O'Connor, D.H.: Pathology of Tropical and Extraordinary Diseases, Vols. 1 and 2. Washington, DC, Armed Forces Institute of Pathology, 1976.
5. Walker, D.H.: Pathology and pathogenesis of the vasculotropic rickettsiosis. *In* Walker, D.H. (ed.): Biology of Rickettsial Diseases. Boca Raton, FL, CRC Press, 1988.
6. Woods, G.L., and Guttierrez, Y.: Diagnostic Pathology of Infectious Diseases. Philadelphia, Lea & Febiger, 1993.
7. Mims, C.A.: The Pathogenesis of Infectious Disease, 3rd ed. San Diego, CA, Academic Press, 1987.
8. Titus, R.G., and Ribeiro, J.M.C.: Salivary gland lysates from the sandfly *Lutzomyia longipalpis* enhance Leishmania infectivity. Science *239*:1306, 1988.
9. Sharpe, A.H., and Fields, B.N.: Pathogenesis of viral infections: Basic concepts derived from the reovirus model. N. Engl. J. Med. *312*:486, 1985.
10. Marsh, M., and Helenius, A.: Virus entry into animal cells. Adv. Virus Res. *36*:107, 1989.
11. Falkow, S., et al.: The interaction of bacteria with mammalian cells. Annu. Rev. Cell Biol. *8*:333, 1992.
12. Baddour, L.M., et al.: Microbial adherence. *In* Mandell, G.L., Douglas, R.G., and Bennet, J.E. (eds.): Principles and Practice of Infectious Disease. New York, Churchill Livingstone, 1990.
13. Fischetti, V.A.: Streptococcal M protein. Sci. Am. *264*:58, 1991.
14. Hale, T.L.: Genetic basis of virulence in *Shigella* species. Microbiol. Rev. *55*:206, 1991.
15. Choe, S., et al.: The crystal structure of diphtheria toxin. Nature *357*:216, 1992.
16. Seifert, H.S., and So, M.: Genetic mechanisms of bacterial antigenic variation. Microbiol. Rev. *52*:327, 1988.
17. Borst, P.: Discontinuous transcription and antigenic variation in trypanosomes. Annu. Rev. Biochem. *55*:701, 1986.

18. Relman, D.A., et al.: Identification of the uncultured bacillus of Whipple's disease. N. Engl. J. Med. 327:293, 1992.

19. Rossman, M.G., and Johnson, J.E.: Icosahedral virus structure. Annu. Rev. Biochem. 58:533, 1989.

20. Staunton, D.E., et al.: The arrangement of the immunoglobulin-like domains of ICAM-1 and the binding sites for LFA-1 and rhinovirus. Cell 61:243, 1990.

21. Wiley, D.C., and Skehel, J.J.: The structure and function of the hemagglutinin membrane glycoprotein of influenza virus. Annu. Rev. Biochem. 56:365, 1987.

22. Arnheiter, H., et al.: Transgenic mice with intracellular immunity to influenza virus. Cell 62:51, 1990.

23. Gorman, O.T., et al.: Evolutionary processes in influenza viruses: Divergence, rapid evolution, and stasis. Curr. Top. Microbiol. Immunol. 176:75, 1992.

24. LiPuma, J.J., et al.: Haemocin, the bacteriocin produced by Haemophilus influenzae: Species distribution and role in colonization. Infect. Immun. 58:1600, 1990.

25. Burroughs, M., et al.: Bacterial components and pathophysiology of injury to the blood-brain barrier: Does cell wall add to the effects of endotoxin in gram-negative meningitis? J. Infect. Dis. 165:S82, 1992.

26. Bloom, B.R., and Murray, C.J.L.: Tuberculosis: Commentary on a reemergent killer. Science 257:1055, 1992.

27. Daley, C.L., et al.: An outbreak of tuberculosis with accelerated progression among persons infected with the human immunodeficiency virus. N. Engl. J. Med. 326:231, 1992.

28. Goble, M., et al.: Treatment of 171 patients with pulmonary tuberculosis resistant to isoniazid and rifampin. N. Engl. J. Med. 328:527, 1993.

29. Horsburgh, C.R., Jr.: Mycobacterium avium complex infection in the acquired immunodeficiency syndrome. N. Engl. J. Med. 324:1332, 1991.

30. Barnes, P.F., et al.: Cytokine production induced by Mycobacterium tuberculosis lipoarabinomannan. J. Immunol. 149:541, 1992.

31. Young, D.B., et al.: Stress proteins are immune targets in leprosy and tuberculosis. Proc. Natl. Acad. Sci. 81:848, 1988.

32. Dannenberg, A.M., Jr.: Delayed-type hypersensitivity and cell-mediated immunity in the pathogenesis of tuberculosis. Immunol. Today 12:228, 1991.

33. Vidal, S.M., et al.: Natural resistance to infection with intracellular parasites: Isolation of a candidate for Bcg. Cell 73:469, 1993.

34. Newman, S.L., et al.: Phagocytosis of Histoplasma capsulatum yeast and microconidia by human cultured macrophages and alveolar macrophages. J. Clin. Invest. 85:223, 1990.

35. Wu-Hsieh, B.A., et al.: Early activation of splenic macrophages by tumor necrosis factor alpha is important in determining the outcome of experimental histoplasmosis in mice. Infect. Immun. 60:4230, 1992.

36. Murphy, J.W.: Mechanisms of natural resistance to human pathogenic fungi. Annu. Rev. Microbiol. 45:509, 1991.

37. Estes, M.K., and Cohen, J.: Rotavirus structure and function. Microbiol. Rev. 53:410, 1989.

38. Zentner, B.S., et al.: Detection of rotavirus-specific antibodies by immunoperoxidase assay and enzyme-linked immunosorbent assay. J. Virol. Methods 11:199, 1985.

39. Hall, G.A.: Comparative pathology of infection by novel diarrhea viruses. Ciba Found. Symp. 128:192, 1987.

40. Blaser, M.J., and Reller, L.B.: Campylobacter enteritis. N. Engl. J. Med. 305:1444, 1983.

41. Walker, R.I., et al.: Pathophysiology of Campylobacter enteritis. Microbiol. Rev. 50:81, 1986.

42. Colgan, T., et al.: Campylobacter jejuni enterocolitis: A clinicopathologic study. Arch. Pathol. Lab. Med. 104:571, 1980.

43. O'Loughlin, E.V., et al.: Clinical, morphological, and biochemical alterations in acute intestinal yersiniosis. Pediatr. Res. 20:602, 1986.

44. Isberg, R.R., and Leong, J.M.: Multiple chain integrins are receptors for invasin, a protein that promotes bacterial penetration into mammalian cells. Cell 60:861, 1990.

45. Galyov, E.E., et al.: A secreted protein kinase of Y. pseudotuberculosis is an indispensible virulence determinant. Nature 361:730, 1993.

46. Alpuche Aranda, C.M., et al.: Salmonella typhimurium activates gene transcription within acidified macrophage phagosomes. Proc. Natl. Acad. Sci. U.S.A. 89:10079, 1992.

47. Mahan, M.J., et al.: Selection of bacterial virulence genes that are specifically induced in host tissues. Science 259:686, 1993.

48. DiRita, V.J., et al.: Regulatory cascade controls virulence in Vibrio cholerae. Proc. Natl. Acad. Sci. U.S.A. 88:5403, 1991.

49. Spangler, B.D.: Structure and function of cholera toxin and the related Escherichia coli heat-labile enterotoxin. Microbiol. Rev. 56:622, 1992.

50. Walsh, J.A.: Problems in recognition and diagnosis of amebiasis: Estimation of the global magnitude of morbidity and mortality. Rev. Infect. Dis. 8:228, 1986.

51. Muller, M.: Energy metabolism of protozoa without mitochondria. Annu. Rev. Microbiol. 42:465, 1988.

52. Horstmann, R., et al.: Recent progress in the molecular biology of Entamoeba histolytica. Trop. Med. Parasitol. 43:213, 1992.

53. Nash, T.: Surface antigen variability and variation in giardia. Parasitol. Today 8:229, 1992.

54. Lev, B., et al.: Lectin activation in Giardia lamblia by host protease: A novel host-parasite interaction. Science 232:71, 1986.

55. Adam, R.D.: The biology of Giardia spp. Microbiol. Rev. 55:706, 1991.

56. Cheung, A.L., et al.: Fibrinogen acts as a bridging molecule in the adherence of Staphylococcus aureus to cultured human endothelial cells. J. Clin. Invest. 87:2236, 1991.

57. Lopes, J.D., et al.: Presence of laminin receptors in Staphylococcus aureus. Science 229:275, 1985.

58. Bhakdi, S., and Tranum-Jensen, J.: Alpha-toxin of Staphylococcus aureus. Microbiol. Rev. 55:733, 1991.

59. Iandolo, J.J.: Genetic analysis of extracellular toxins of Staphylococcus aureus. Annu. Rev. Microbiol. 43:375, 1989.

60. Swaminathan, S., et al.: Crystal structure of staphylococcal enterotoxin B, a superantigen. Nature 359:801, 1992.

61. See, R.H., and Chow, A.W.: Microbiology of toxic shock syndrome. Rev. Infect. Dis. 11:S55, 1989.

62. Johnston, R.B.: Pathogenesis of pneumococcal pneumonia. Rev. Infect. Dis. 13:S509, 1991.

63. Loeche, W.J.: Role of Streptococcus mutans in human dental decay. Microbiol. Rev. 50:353, 1986.

64. Cunningham, M.W., et al.: Cytotoxic and viral neutralizing antibodies cross-react with streptococcal M protein, enteroviruses, and human cardiac myosin. Proc. Natl. Acad. Sci. U.S.A. 89:1320, 1992.

65. Rood, J.I., and Cole, S.T.: Molecular genetics and pathogenesis of Clostridium perfringens. Microbiol. Rev. 55:621, 1991.

66. Simpson, L.L.: Molecular pharmacology of botulinum toxin and tetanus toxin. Annu. Rev. Pharmacol. 26:247, 1986.

67. Chardin, P., et al.: The mammalian G protein rhoC is ADP-ribosylated by Clostridium botulinum exoenzyme C3 and affects actin microfilament in Vero cells. EMBO J. 8:1087, 1989.

68. Triadofilopoulos, G., et al.: Differential effects of Clostridium difficile toxins A and B on rabbit ileum. Gastroenterology 93:273, 1987.

69. Brook, I.: Encapsulated anaerobic bacteria in synergistic infections. Microbiol. Rev. 50:452, 1986.

70. Aral, S.O., and Holmes, K.K.: Sexually transmitted diseases in the AIDS era. Sci. Am. 264:62, 1991.

71. Stanbury, L.R.: Pathogenesis of herpes simplex virus infection and animal models for its study. Curr. Top. Microbiol. Immunol. *179*:15, 1992.

72. Croen, K.D., and Straus, S.E.: Varicella-zoster virus latency. Annu. Rev. Microbiol. *45*:265, 1991.

73. Doymaz, M.Z., and Rouse, B.T.: Immunopathology of herpes simplex virus infections. Curr. Top. Microbiol. Immunol. *179*:121, 1992.

74. Patton, D.L., and Taylor, H.R.: The histopathology of experimental trachoma: Ultrastructural changes in the conjunctival epithelium. J. Infect. Dis. *153*:870, 1986.

75. Moulder, J.W.: Interaction of chlamydiae and host cells in vitro. Microbiol. Rev. *55*:143, 1991.

76. Olyhoek, T., Crowe, B.A., and Achtman, M.: Clonal population structure of *Neisseria meningitidis* serogroup A isolated from epidemics and pandemics between 1915 and 1983. Rev. Infect. Dis. *9*:665, 1987.

77. Makino, S., van Putten, J.P., and Meyer, T.F.: Phase variation of the opacity outer membrane protein controls invasion by *Neisseria gonorrhoeae* into human epithelial cells. EMBO J. *10*:1307, 1991.

78. McGee, Z.A., et al.: Local induction of tumor necrosis factor as a molecular mechanism of mucosal damage by gonococci. Microb. Pathog. *12*:333, 1992.

79. Thomas D.D., et al.: Enhanced levels of attachment of fibronectin-primed *Treponema pallidum* to extracellular matrix. Infect. Immun. *52*:736, 1986.

80. Fitzgerald, T.J.: The Th$_1$/Th$_2$-like switch in syphilitic infection: Is it detrimental? Infect. Immun. *60*:3475, 1992.

81. Cox, D.L., et al.: The outer membrane, not a coat of host proteins, limits antigenicity of virulent *Treponema pallidum*. Infect. Immun. *60*:1076, 1992.

82. Halsey, N.A., and Job, J.S.: Measles. *In* Warren, K.S., and Mahmoud, A.A.F. (eds.): Tropical and Geographic Medicine, 2nd ed. New York, McGraw-Hill, 1990.

83. Cattaneo, R., and Billeter, M.A.: Mutations and A/I hypermutations in measles virus persistent infections. Curr. Top. Microbiol. Immunol. *176*:63, 1992.

84. Birkenbach, M., et al.: Characterization of an Epstein-Barr virus receptor on human epithelial cells. J. Exp. Med. *176*:1405, 1992.

85. Sample, C., and Kleff, E.: Molecular basis for Epstein-Barr virus–induced pathogenesis and disease. Springer Semin. Immunopathol. *13*:133, 1991.

86. Sixbey, J.W., and Yao, Q.-Y.: Immunoglobulin A–induced shift of Epstein-Barr virus tissue tropism. Science *255*:1578, 1992.

87. Minor, P.D.: The molecular biology of polioviruses vaccines. J. Gen. Virol. *73*:3065, 1992.

88. Ren, R., and Racaniello, V.R.: Poliovirus spreads from muscle to the central nervous system by neural pathways. J. Infect. Dis. *166*:747, 1992.

89. Relman, D., et al.: Recognition of a bacterial adhesion by an integrin: macrophage CR3 (alpha M beta 2, CD11b/CD18) binds filamentous hemagglutinin of *Bordetella pertussis*. Cell *61*:1375, 1990.

90. Gierschik, P.: ADP-ribosylation of signal-transducing guanine nucleotide-binding proteins by Pertussis toxin. Curr. Top. Microbiol. Immunol. *175*:69, 1992.

91. Wilson, R., et al.: Effects of *Bordetella pertussis* infection on human respiratory epithelium in vivo and in vitro. Infect. Immun. *59*:337, 1991.

92. Grundy, J.E.: Virologic and pathogenetic aspects of cytomegalovirus infections. Rev. Infect. Dis. *12*:S711, 1990.

93. Pier, G.B.: Pulmonary disease associated with *Pseudomonas aeruginosa* in cystic fibrosis: Current status of the host-bacterium interaction. J. Infect. Dis. *151*:575, 1985.

94. Pastan, I., et al.: Recombinant toxins as novel therapeutic agents. Annu. Rev. Biochem. *61*:331, 1992.

95. Coburn, J.: *Pseudomonas aeruginosa* exoenzyme S. Curr. Top. Microbiol. Immunol. *175*:133, 1992.

96. Britigan, B.E., et al.: Interaction of the *Pseudomonas aeruginosa* secretory products pyocyanin and pyochelin generates hydroxyl radical and causes synergistic damage to endothelial cells. J. Clin. Invest. *90*:2187, 1992.

97. Horowitz, M.A.: Phagocytosis of legionnaires' disease bacterium (*Legionella pneumophila*) occurs by a novel mechanism: Engulfment within a pseudopod coil. Cell *36*:27, 1984.

98. Cianciotto, N.P., and Fields, B.S.: *Legionella pneumophila mip* gene potentiates intracellular infection of protozoa and human macrophages. Proc. Natl. Acad. Sci. U.S.A. *89*:5188, 1992.

99. Calderone, R.A., and Braun, P.C.: Adherence and receptor relationships of *Candida albicans*. Microbiol. Rev. *55*:1, 1991.

100. Cutler, J.E.: Putative virulence factors of *Candida albicans*. Annu. Rev. Microbiol. *45*:187, 1991.

101. Polacheck, I., et al.: Catecholamines and virulence of *Cryptococcus neoformans*. Infect. Immun. *58*:2919, 1990.

102. Arruda, L.K., et al.: *Aspergillus fumigatus* allergen I, a major IgE-binding protein, is a member of the mitogillin family of cytotoxins. J. Exp. Med. *172*:1529, 1990.

103. Phair, J., et al.: The risk of *Pneumocystis carinii* pneumonia among men infected with human immunodeficiency virus type 1. N. Engl. J. Med. *322*:161, 1990.

104. Edman, J.C., et al.: Ribosomal RNA sequence shows *Pneumocystis carinii* to be a member of the fungi. Nature *334*:519, 1988.

105. Roths, J.B., and Sidman, C.L.: Both immunity and hyperresponsiveness to *Pneumocystis carinii* result from transfer of CD4+ but not CD8+ T cells into severe combined immunodeficiency mice. J. Clin. Invest. *90*:673, 1992.

106. Lockwood, D.N.J., and Weber, J.N.: Parasite infections in AIDS. Parasitol. Today *5*:310, 1989.

107. Hayes, E.B., et al.: Large community outbreak of cryptosporidiosis due to contamination of a filtered water supply. N. Engl. J. Med. *320*:1372, 1989.

108. Peterson, C.: Cellular biology of *Cryptosporidium parvum*. Parasitol. Today *9*:87, 1993.

109. McDonald, V., et al.: Immune responses to *Cryptosporidium muris* and *Cryptosporidium parvum* in adult immunocompetent or immunocompromised (nude and SCID) mice. Infect. Immun. *60*:3325, 1992.

110. Ambrose-Thomas, P., and Pelloux, H.: Toxoplasmosis—congenital and in immunocompromised patients: A parallel. Parasitol. Today *9*:61, 1993.

111. Maeda, K., et al.: Human infection with *Ehrlichia canis*, a leukocytic rickettsia. N. Engl. J. Med. *316*:853, 1987.

112. Cravens, G., and Marr, J.S.: The Black Death. New York, Ballantine Books, 1977.

113. Sodeinde, O.A., et al.: A surface protease and the invasive character of plague. Science *258*:1004, 1992.

114. Ahmed, M.A.M., et al.: Louse-borne relapsing fever in the Sudan: A historical review and a clinicopathological study. Trop. Geogr. Med. *32*:106, 1980.

115. Barbour, A.G., et al.: Variable antigen genes of the relapsing fever agent *Borrelia hermsii* are activated by promoter addition. Mol. Microbiol. *5*:489, 1991.

116. Jaenson, T.G.T.: The epidemiology of Lyme borreliosis. Parasitol. Today *7*:39, 1991.

117. Steere, A.C.: Lyme arthritis. N. Engl. J. Med. *321*:586, 1989.

118. Ma, Y., et al.: Intracellular localization of *Borrelia burgdorferi* within human cells. Infect. Immun. *59*:671, 1991.

119. Szczepanski, A., and Benach, J.L.: Lyme borreliosis: Host responses to *Borrelia burgdorferi*. Microbiol. Rev. *55*:21, 1991.

120. Lyme Disease and Related Disorders—2nd International Symposium, Vienna, Austria, September 17–19, 1985. Vienna Hygiene Institute, University of Vienna, p. 75.

121. Miller, L.H., and Warrell, D.A.: Malaria. *In* Warren, K.S., and Mahmoud, A.A.F. (eds.): Tropical and Geographical Medicine, 2nd ed. New York, McGraw-Hill, 1990.

122. Cerami, C.: The basolateral domain of the hepatocyte plasma membrane bears receptors for the circumsporozoite protein of *Plasmodium falciparum* sporozoites. Cell *70*:1021, 1992.

123. Hill, A.V.S., et al.: Molecular analysis of the association of HLA-B53 and resistance to severe malaria. Nature 360:434, 1992.

124. Slater, A.F., and Cerami, A.: Inhibition by chloroquine of a novel haem polymerase enzyme activity in malaria trophozoites. Nature 355:167, 1992.

125. Biggs, B.A., et al.: Antigenic variation in *Plasmodium falciparum*. Proc. Natl. Acad. Sci. U.S.A. 88:9171, 1991.

126. Nakamura, K.I., et al.: *Plasmodium falciparum*–infected erythrocyte receptor(s) for CD36 and thrombospondin are restricted to knobs on the erythrocyte surface. J. Histochem. Cytochem. 40:1419, 1992.

127. Roberts, D.J., et al.: Rapid switching to multiple antigenic and adhesive phenotypes in malaria. Nature 357:689, 1992.

128. Despommier, D.D.: *Trichinella spiralis*: The worm that would be a virus. Parasitol. Today 6:193, 1990.

129. Herndon, F.J., and Kayes, S.G.: Depletion of eosinophils by anti–IL-5-monoclonal antibody treatment of mice infected with *Trichinella spiralis* does not alter parasite burden or immunological resistance to reinfection. J. Immunol. 149:3642, 1992.

130. LaClette, J.P., et al.: Paramyosin inhibits complement C1. J. Immunol. 148:124, 1992.

131. Gordon, F.B., and Quan, A.L.: Isolation of the trachoma agent in cell culture. Proc. Soc. Exp. Biol. Med. 118:354, 1965.

132. Patton, D.L., and Taylor, H.R.: The histopathology of experimental trachoma: Ultrastructural changes in the conjunctival epithelium. J. Infect. Dis. 153:870, 1986.

133. Bloom, B.R., and Godal, T.: Selective primary health care: Strategies for control of disease in the developing world. V. Leprosy Rev. Infect. Dis. 5:765, 1983.

134. Convit, J., et al.: Immunoprophylactic trial with combined *Mycobacterium leprae*/BCG vaccine against leprosy: Preliminary results. Lancet 339:446, 1992.

135. Yamamura, M., et al.: Defining protective response to pathogens: Cytokine profiles in leprosy lesions. Science 254:277, 1991.

136. Chang, K.P., and Chauduri, G.: Molecular determinants of Leishmania virulence. Annu. Rev. Microbiol. 44:499, 1990.

137. Moser, D.M., et al.: Leishmania promastigotes require opsonic complement to bind to the human leucocyte integrin Mac-1 (CD11b/CD18). J. Cell Biol. 116:511, 1992.

138. Alexander, J., and Russell, D.G.: The interaction of Leishmania species with macrophages. Adv. Parasitol. 31:175, 1992.

139. Ollson, T., et al.: CD8 is critically involved in lymphocyte activation by a *T. brucei brucei*–released molecule. Cell 72:715, 1993.

140. Norris, K.A., et al.: Characterization of a *Trypanosoma cruzi* C3 binding protein with functional and genetic similarities to the human complement regulatory protein, decay-accelerating factor. J. Immunol. 147:2240, 1993.

141. Ortega-Barria, E., and Pereira, M.E.A.: A novel *T. cruzi* heparin-binding protein promotes fibroblast adhesion and penetration of engineered bacteria and trypanosomes into mammalian cells. Cell 67:411, 1991.

142. Andrews, N.W., et al.: *T. cruzi*–secreted protein immunologically related to the complement component C9: Evidence for membrane pore-forming activity at low pH. Cell 61:1227, 1990.

143. Van Voorhis, W.C., Schlekewy L., and Trong, H.L.: Molecular mimicry by *Trypanosoma cruzi*: The F1-160 epitope that mimics mammalian nerve can be mapped to a 12-amino acid peptide. Proc. Natl. Acad. Sci. U.S.A. 88:5993, 1991.

144. Ribiero dos Santos, R., et al.: Anti-CD4 abrogates rejection and reestablishes long-term tolerance to syngeneic newborn hearts grafted in mice chronically infected with *Trypanosoma cruzi*. J. Exp. Med. 175:29, 1992.

145. Andrade, Z.A., et al.: Histopathology of the conducting tissue of the heart in Chagas' myocarditis. Am. Heart J. 95:316, 1978.

146. Ko, A.I., et al.: A *Schistosoma mansoni* epitope recognized by a protective monoclonal antibody is identical to the stage-specific embryonic antigen 1. Proc. Natl. Acad. Sci. U.S.A. 87:4159, 1990.

147. Amiri, P., et al.: Tumour necrosis factor alpha restores granulomas and induces parasite egg-laying in schistosome-infected SCID mice. Nature 356:604, 1992.

148. Dessein, A.J., et al.: Environmental, genetic, and immunological factors in human resistance to *Schistosoma mansoni*. Immunol. Invest. 21:423, 1992.

149. Prakash, S., and Wyler, D.J.: Fibroblast stimulation in schistosomiasis. J. Immunol. 148:3583, 1992.

150. Ottesen, E.A.: Wellcome Trust Lecture: Infection and disease in lymphatic filariasis: An immunological perspective. Parasitology 104:S71, 1992.

151. Vincent, A.L., et al.: The lymphatic pathology of *Brugia pahangi* in nude (athymic) and thymic mice C3H/HeN. J. Parasitol. 70:48, 1984.

152. von Lichtenberg, F.: Wellcome Trust Lecture: Inflammatory responses to filarial connective tissue parasites. Parasitology 94:S100, 1987.

153. Greene, B.M.: Onchocerciasis. *In* Warren, K.S., and Mahmoud, A.A.F. (eds.): Tropical and Geographical Medicine, 2nd ed. New York, McGraw-Hill, 1990.

154. Braun, G., et al.: Immunological crossreactivity between a cloned antigen of *Onchocerca volvulus* and a component of the retinal pigment epithelium. J. Exp. Med. 174:169, 1991.

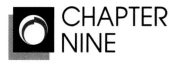

Environmental and Nutritional Diseases

ENVIRONMENTAL DISEASE

All diseases not purely genetic in nature must, of necessity, be of environmental origin. But even genetic diseases are influenced by environmental factors—witness the effect of diet on the expression of phenylketonuria, and, conversely, even though obesity results basically from an excess of calories, in some instances genetic background may be a contributing factor (see Chapter 5). Despite these difficulties in segregating genetic diseases from environmental ones, it is still possible to identify a number of conditions imposed on humans by humankind, many related to our progressively deteriorating environment. Only an overview can be presented because the scope of the problem boggles the mind. The consideration that follows will be divided into (1) the magnitude of the environmental problem; (2) the adverse effects of air pollution, with particular attention to smoking; (3) injuries induced by chemicals, including drugs; (4) the hazards engendered by physical agents, with emphasis on radiation injury; and (5) the health consequences of under- and overnutrition.

MAGNITUDE OF THE ENVIRONMENTAL PROBLEM

It is no exaggeration to say that present trends in population expansion and global environmental deterioration threaten the survival of the human race on this planet. The expansion of the population has now reached the point where grain consumption exceeds production. It is estimated that over a half billion persons consume insufficient calories to maintain normal growth and health.[1] The growing numbers and activities of humans have resulted in serious pollution of air and water supplies; loss of large amounts of arable land; depletion of vital for-

379

ests; extinction of many biologic species; accumulation of wastes, some radioactive, for which no satisfactory method of disposal has yet been developed; and destruction of atmospheric ozone, exposing us to potentially dangerous levels of ultraviolet (UV) radiation, opening the threat of global warming, and contaminating outer space.

The inter-related problems of ozone loss and global warming are paradigms of environmental problems that constitute clear and present threats.[2] Ozone (O_3) is produced by the combination of molecular and atomic oxygen, the latter produced by the action of solar radiation on the scant molecules of oxygen and nitrogen dioxide (NO_2) present in outer space. A layer of ozone in outer space is critically important to our survival because it prevents the sun's UV light, particularly the UVC and UVB regions of UV light, from penetrating into our environment. Regrettably, a large number of chemicals used by humans destroy ozone. All of these essentially provide active free radicals that convert ozone to oxygen. The major offenders are the chlorofluorocarbons (CFCs), used as aerosols and refrigerants, and NO_2 produced by internal combustion engines, many industrial processes, and microbial activity. The CFCs are now banned in the United States, but global production of these chemicals continues to increase. Just as destructive is the bromine radical, notably present within halons used in fire extinguishers. Consider the large reservoir of halons impounded in fire extinguishers around the world. Depletion of the ozone layer first came to the world's attention during the present decade, when an area centered over the Antarctic was discovered to have sustained ozone losses of 40 to 50%. The "hole" in the ozone layer has expanded over the past few years and currently is continental in size. A similar depletion of ozone has now been recorded over the North Pole.

The consequences of the depletion of the ozone layer are diverse. There has been a remarkable rise in the incidence of nonmelanomatous skin carcinomas and of melanomas among whites (see Chapter 26). An almost 100% increase in the incidence of skin melanomas has already appeared in the United States, with greater increases recorded in other countries (e.g., Australia and New Zealand). The Environmental Protection Agency estimates a 0.3 to 2% increase in melanoma incidence among United States whites for each 1% loss of ozone. Increased UVB exposure may have other health consequences, among them increased predisposition to cataracts. There are also suggestions that the increased exposure to UV radiation also impairs the skin's immune response and systemic immunity as well.

Beyond these forms of direct injury to humans, the loss of stratospheric ozone and increased UVB radiation may have grave indirect effects. Ultraviolet B radiation penetrates several meters below the surface of the ocean. Phytoplankton, which require sunlight, are extremely vulnerable to UVB radiation. These lowly life forms constitute the beginning of the food chain for all aquatic animals, on which humans depend for a considerable portion of their food supply. The ripples expand in ever-widening circles.

A closely related problem is global warming, referred to as the "greenhouse effect." The accumulation of carbon dioxide (CO_2) and other gases (CFCs, methane, NO_2) in the atmosphere traps the earth's infrared radiation while permitting free penetration of visible light and warming solar radiation. The net effect is the accumulation of heat at the earth's surface, that is, the "greenhouse phenomenon." The level of CO_2 in the earth's atmosphere will double by 2030 to 2080 if present trends continue. Factors contributing to this increase include loss of vegetation and forests that utilize CO_2 and increased emissions by the expanded number of "human machines." The global temperature has risen about 1°F over the past century and is projected to reach 4 to 9°F in the next 50 to 100 years. The consequences of this warming are far-reaching: evaporation of surface water will transform large land masses into deserts, and the melting of the polar icecaps may raise the sea level a meter or more, threatening coastal cities, contaminating freshwater supplies with refluxed saltwater, destroying tidal ecosystems with dire consequences to edible fishlife, and, in general, causing serious disruption of life as we now know it. More directly, it is suggested that even a slight change in the ambient temperature will increase heat-related mortality, raise the potential for microbiologic epidemics, and predispose to respiratory disease.[3] The litany could be continued, but it suffices that the deterioration of our environment has become life threatening, demanding immediate and effective action.

AIR POLLUTION

Daily, we inhale 10,000 to 20,000 liters of air, bearing myriad pollutants in the forms of bacteria, gases, fibers, and particles. Some of these are only annoying, others injurious; some are dangerous. The particular consequences of air pollution for the respiratory tract depend on the specific pollutant or combination of pollutants inhaled, their levels in the environment, and the duration of exposure. The changes range from simple irritation of the airways to the induction of pulmonary emphysema (Fig. 9–1), fibrosing, debilitating chronic lung disease, and cancer. The various patterns of injury are listed in Table 9–1 and will be described more completely in Chapter 15.

Some pollutants are restricted to particular industries (e.g., silica and coal dust) and are carefully monitored by regulatory agencies; in general, these

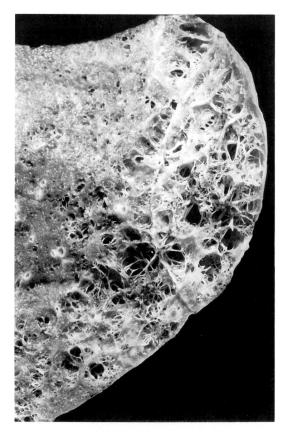

Figure 9-1. The apex of a lung *(to the right)* in a heavy cigarette smoker with severe emphysema (enlargement and distortion of the airspaces).

no longer present public health hazards. Other pollutants are widespread in the ambient atmosphere (e.g., sulfur dioxide, nitrogen dioxide, carbon monoxide, ozone, lead, and a smorgasbord of particulates). Regulatory agencies in most industrialized countries have established air quality standards for some of these pollutants, but many have proved difficult to regulate. Ozone is a case in point. Trace amounts of ozone are found in the air

Table 9-1. PATTERNS OF LUNG INJURY RELATED TO AIR POLLUTION

LUNG RESPONSE	PATHOGENIC MECHANISM
Acute or chronic inflammation (e.g., chronic bronchitis)	Direct cell injury
Emphysema	Enhanced proteolysis
Asthma	Allergic or irritant effect
Hypersensitivity pneumonitis	Immunologic injury
Pneumoconiosis	Fibrotic reactions caused by cytokines released from macrophages and other recruited leukocytes
Neoplasia	Mutagenic and promoting effects

we breathe because of some mixing of stratospheric ozone with air at ground level. In some heavily polluted areas, ozone contributes to the atmospheric "soup" called "smog." Both ozone and nitrogen dioxide are highly oxidant gases that may injure the mucosa of the respiratory passages and alveolar walls. A survey of the 90 largest urban centers in the United States revealed that in 65 the level of ozone exceeded the National Ambient Air Quality Standard.[4] Nitrogen dioxide, the other major oxidant pollutant, has proved equally difficult to control. Fortunately, in most cities, unhealthful levels of these gases occur only transiently (for days), but there is growing concern about their possible long-term effects.

The quality of indoor air is fast becoming a greater concern than the pollution of the outdoor air, which at least can be monitored and, in some measure, regulated. The impressive roster of indoor air pollutants and their health effects are summarized in Table 9-2. Only a few words follow about radon. Asbestos is discussed in detail in Chapter 15, and tobacco smoke in the next section.

Radon, a radioactive gas, is a decay product of uranium widely distributed in the soil. Unexpectedly, radon gas emanating from the earth is quite prevalent in homes and other indoor environments, sometimes in concentrations exceeding those found in underground mines. Even at the very low levels most often present in polluted homes, there is still a risk of lung cancer because the effects of radiation are cumulative and there is no safe threshold level below which there is no risk. Indeed, in Great Britain radon in homes is thought to be second only to cigarette smoking as a cause of lung cancer. Moreover, there is a synergism between the carcinogenic effects of cigarette smoking and radon inhalation.[5]

TOBACCO SMOKING

The adverse consequences of cigarette smoke totally dwarf those of all the other pollutants combined. In the United States, almost 400,000 persons died in 1985 of various diseases directly attributable to cigarette smoking, representing 21% of all mortality. It has repeatedly been referred to as "the single most important preventable cause of premature death in the United States." Happily, the percentage of Americans who smoke has fallen from about 45% in 1958 to about 30% in 1987, but there are still more than 50 million cigarette smokers who damage not only themselves but also, unfortunately, bystanders (passive smokers), a subject that will be addressed later. It should be noted at the outset that although cigarette smoking is the prime culprit, pipe and cigar smoking, although less hazardous, are not without risk, and smokeless tobacco (e.g., chewing tobacco,

Table 9-2. THE PRINCIPAL INDOOR AIR POLLUTANTS AND THEIR SOURCES*

POLLUTANT	TYPICAL SOURCES	PRINCIPAL EFFECTS
SO_2, respirable particles	Tobacco smoke, wood and coal stoves, fireplaces, outside air	Irritant to respiratory epithelium
NO, NO_2	Gas ranges and pilot lights	Irritant to respiratory epithelium
CO	Gas ranges and pilot lights, outside air	Forms carboxyhemoglobin
Infectious or allergenic biologic materials	Dust mites and cockroaches, pollens, animal dander, bacteria, fungi, viruses	Allergic reactions, infections
Formaldehyde	Urea formaldehyde foam insulation, glues, fiberboard, plywood, particle board	Allergic reactions
Radon and radon daughters	Ground beneath buildings	Lung cancer
Volatile organic compounds: benzene, styrene	Outgassing from water, solvents, paints, cleaning compounds; combustion	Respiratory toxin, cancer
Semivolatile organics: chlorinated hydrocarbons and polycyclic compounds, such as benzopyrene, polychlorinated biphenyls (PCBs)	Pesticides, herbicides, combustion of wood, tobacco, and charcoal	See Table 9-8
Asbestos	Building insulation	Pneumoconiosis, cancer

* Exclusive of unique industrial pollutants that result in pneumoconioses.

tobacco pouches, snuff dipping) has emerged as a major influence in the causation of cancers of the oral cavity and upper aerodigestive tract.

ACTIVE SMOKING AND DISEASE. Mainstream smoke that enters the mouth with each cigarette puff is a veritable "satanic brew." The precise composition varies with a number of factors, such as type of tobacco, length of the cigarette, and presence and effectiveness of filter tips, but nonetheless usually present are (1) well-recognized carcinogens in lower animals (e.g., polycyclic hydrocarbons, beta-naphthylamine, nitrosamines), (2) cell irritants and toxins (e.g., ammonia, formaldehyde, oxides of nitrogen), (3) carbon monoxide, and (4) nicotine, having a variety of effects on the sympathetic system, blood pressure, and heart rate and many other actions. The average one-pack-a-day smoker draws in this potent mix of products about 70,000

Table 9-3. SUMMARY OF ESTIMATED RELATIVE RISKS FOR CURRENT CIGARETTE SMOKERS IN THE UNITED STATES, 1982 to 1986, MEN AND WOMEN AGED 35 YEARS AND OLDER

UNDERLYING CAUSE OF DEATH	MEN	WOMEN
Cancer		
Lung	22.36	11.94
Lip, oral cavity, pharynx	27.48	5.59
Larynx	10.48	17.78
Esophagus	7.60	10.25
Pancreas	2.14	2.23
Coronary artery disease		
Age < 35	1.94	1.78
Age 35–64	2.81	1.78
Cerebrovascular lesions		
Age < 35	2.24	1.84
Age 35–64	3.67	4.80
Chronic obstructive pulmonary disease	9.65	10.47

Data from Sherman, C.B.: Health effects of cigarette smoking. Clin. Chest Med. *12*:643, 1991. Originally from U.S. Department of Health and Human Services: Reducing the Health Consequences of Smoking: 25 Years of Progress: A Report of the Surgeon General. Atlanta, GA, Centers for Disease Control, 1989.

times a year; no small wonder that it has adverse consequences, summarized in Table 9–3.

Coronary heart disease, particularly myocardial infarction (MI), is the number one cause of death related to cigarette smoking; MI is responsible for more than 20% of all deaths from heart disease.[6] Cancer of the lung closely follows. Cigarette smoking is also a major risk factor for chronic obstructive pulmonary disease (chronic bronchitis and emphysema) and for other forms of cancer as well, as is evident in Table 9–3. Collectively, these cancer-related deaths approximate 300,000 annually in the United States. Indeed, smoking is the single most significant cause of cancer mortality in the United States, thought to contribute to about one-third of all cancer deaths and almost all of the more than 140,000 lung cancer deaths. The risk of mortality is dose related—the more pack-years of smoking (number of packs per day times number of years), the higher the risk of mortality. Males bear the brunt of this toll, but, unhappily, females are catching up. Similarly, smoking is largely responsible for the 57,000 deaths related to chronic obstructive pulmonary disease (see Chapter 15). These major causes of mortality are diagrammed in Figure 9–2.

The unborn child and the infant are also adversely influenced by maternal smoking. Numerous studies have shown a well-defined association between cigarette smoking and an increased incidence of low birth weight, prematurity, spontaneous abortions, stillbirths, and infant mortality. Furthermore, there are strong suggestions that smoking increases the likelihood of some complications of pregnancy, such as abruptio placentae, placenta previa, and premature rupture of the

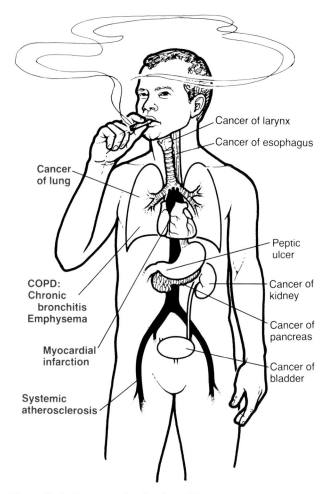

Cancer of larynx

Cancer of esophagus

Cancer of lung

Peptic ulcer

Cancer of kidney

COPD: Chronic bronchitis Emphysema

Cancer of pancreas

Myocardial infarction

Cancer of bladder

Systemic atherosclerosis

Figure 9–2. Adverse effects of smoking. The more common *(on the left)* **and somewhat less common** *(on the right).*

membranes. Even more invidious is the strong suspicion that smoking impairs physical and intellectual development of the fetus and neonate.[7]

INVOLUNTARY SMOKE EXPOSURE (PASSIVE SMOKING). It has become increasingly clear that inhalation of smoke-contaminated air is detrimental to health. Ambient cigarette smoke derives from sidestream smoke that escapes between puffs and from exhaled mainstream smoke. Obviously, the intensity of exposure depends on many factors, such as the volume of air in the room, number of active smokers, rate of air exchange, and duration of exposure. The infant or small child of a smoking mother is likely to have the most intense exposure. Although the data from various studies differ somewhat, there is substantial evidence that involuntary smoke exposure (passive smoking) incurs an increased risk of lung cancer (relative risk 1.5). There is also some increased risk of cardiovascular disease, particularly MI, and a higher incidence of lower respiratory tract illnesses in the infants and children of smoking parents.[8] The evidence is less ironclad but suggests possible retardation of physi-

cal and intellectual maturation during infancy and childhood in the smoke-exposed child. These hazards of involuntary smoking have been recognized only within the past decade, and so the story is not yet complete.

BENEFITS OF CESSATION OR REDUCING EXPOSURE TO CIGARETTE SMOKE. Cessation of smoking is slowly followed by a reduction in excess mortality. The level does not reach baseline until 20 or more smoke-free years. The increased risks of lung cancer and laryngeal cancer begin to decline within 1 to 2 years of smoking cessation, but the rate of decline and its magnitude vary with the amount smoked and its duration. However, even with abstinence for 20 to 30 years, former smokers have a slightly increased risk of lung cancer, which is, nevertheless, a substantial improvement over the 10 to 20× relative risk for current cigarette smokers. Much more prompt is the reduction in the risk of MI, which begins to appear within a year but does not approach that of those who have never smoked until 5 to 20 years. Although lung function appears to improve relatively soon after avoidance of cigarettes, perhaps related to decreased irritation, inflammation, and hyper-responsiveness of the airways, once chronic obstructive pulmonary disease has developed, smoking cessation does not appear to offer any significant benefits.

The question is often asked, will smoking filter-tip or other forms of low-yield cigarettes protect against the adverse consequences of unmodified cigarettes? Various techniques, most commonly the use of filter-tips, have been employed to reduce the yield of tar, nicotine, and other "delectables," and epidemiologic studies indicate that long-term smokers of only such modified cigarettes have a 30 to 50% lower risk of lung cancer than that of smokers of the "good old-fashioned" cigarettes.[9] Presumably, the other adverse consequences of cigarette smoking will also be attenuated, but despite all the ingenious attempts to remove tobacco smoke from smoking, the safest cigarette clearly is the unsmoked one.

CHEMICAL AND DRUG INJURY

All chemicals and drugs are capable of causing injury or death; even such innocuous substances as table salt in sufficient amounts can be damaging. Some agents have been implicated in catastrophic, sometimes industrial, exposures (recall Bhopal, India, where more than 2000 were killed, and another 2000 injured, by an explosion that released gaseous cyanide). In other instances, the injury is the consequence of "accidental exposure" (e.g., the child who swallows a toxic household cleaning product). But in still other instances the injury is the consequence of self-administered agents (sometimes suicidal overdosage). The "street drugs"—for example, heroin and cocaine—fall into this category. Finally, the physiologic response to a therapeutic agent is sometimes unpredictable and, occasionally, harmful; this is known as an adverse drug reaction (ADR).

Some concept of the scope of the chemical and drug problem can be gained from the 1990 Annual Report of the American Association of Poison Control Centers.[10] In that year, more than 1.7 million human exposures to injurious chemicals and drugs were reported. Children younger than six years of age were involved in more than half of the instances. Overall, 80% of exposures were accidental, and almost 7% were suicides; ADRs represented fewer than 1% of total exposures. Only 612 of the almost two million exposures proved fatal, and more than 50% of these were suicides; ADRs were judged to be responsible for only ten of these deaths.

ADVERSE DRUG REACTIONS (ADRs)

An ADR is defined as "any response to a drug that is noxious and unintended and that occurs at doses used in humans for prophylaxis, diagnosis, or therapy, excluding failure to accomplish the intended purpose." More than 15,000 ADRs were reported to the national network of Poison Control Centers in the United States in 1990, but as noted above, they were responsible for only ten fatalities. Only rarely are the ADRs the consequence of physician failures, for example, inadequately monitored use or overuse of an agent, failure to recognize drug interactions, and ill-considered administration of potentially dangerous drugs. These have been aptly called "ADRs that count."[11]

The overwhelming majority of ADRs can be segregated into two categories: (1) exaggeration of the intended pharmacologic effect—largely predictable reactions, or (2) an unpredictable response unrelated to the drug's primary activity. In the first category fall the known adverse consequences of a large variety of powerful drugs now available to treat potentially fatal diseases, such as cancer and leukemia. For example, secondary acute myeloid leukemia may appear in children treated with intensive chemotherapy for acute lymphoid leukemia, and, analogously, the use of large cumulative total doses of daunorubicin or doxorubicin in the attempt to treat a form of cancer may lead to cardiotoxicity (a well-known side effect of these agents; see Cardiomyopathy, Chapter 12). In the second category, unpredictable ADRs are, fortunately, much less common than those that are predictable. These largely idiosyncratic reactions appear when the drug evokes an immunologic

reaction or has totally unanticipated cytotoxicity. Some examples include the development of anaphylaxis following an otherwise innocuous dose of penicillin and the extensive hepatic necrosis that may develop after the use of therapeutic levels of acetaminophen or halothane. Equally unanticipated is the development of hemolytic anemia in individuals not known to have a genetic deficiency of glucose-6-phosphate dehydrogenase when administered an antimalarial drug, such as primaquine.

Table 9–4. SOME COMMON ADVERSE DRUG REACTIONS AND THEIR AGENTS

REACTION	MAJOR OFFENDERS
Blood Dyscrasias (feature of almost half of all drug-related deaths)	
Granulocytopenia, aplastic anemia, pancytopenia	Antineoplastic agents, immunosuppressives, and chloramphenicol
Hemolytic anemia, thrombocytopenia	Penicillin, methyldopa, quinidine
Cutaneous	
Urticaria, macules, papules, vesicles, petechiae, exfoliative dermatitis, fixed drug eruptions	Antineoplastic agents, sulfonamides, hydantoins, many others
Cardiac	
Arrhythmias	Theophylline, hydantoins
Cardiomyopathy	Doxorubicin, daunorubicin
Renal	
Glomerulonephritis	Penicillamine
Acute tubular necrosis	Aminoglycoside antibiotics, cyclosporine, amphotericin B
Tubulointerstitial disease with papillary necrosis	Phenacetin, salicylates
Pulmonary	
Asthma	Salicylates
Acute pneumonitis	Nitrofurantoin
Interstitial fibrosis	Busulfan, nitrofurantoin, bleomycin
Hepatic	
Fatty change	Tetracycline
Diffuse hepatocellular damage	Halothane, isoniazid, acetaminophen
Cholestasis	Chlorpromazine, estrogens, contraceptive agents
Systemic	
Anaphylaxis	Penicillin
Lupus erythematosus syndrome (drug-induced lupus)	Hydralazine, procainamide
Central Nervous System	
Tinnitus and dizziness	Salicylates
Acute dystonic reactions and parkinsonian syndrome	Phenothiazine antipsychotics
Respiratory depression	Sedatives

Table 9–5. A FEW OF THE COMMON AGENTS IMPLICATED IN FATAL REACTIONS

AGENT	ADVERSE REACTION	BASIS OF REACTION	MECHANISM OF INJURY
Tricyclic antidepressants, e.g., ipramine, desipramine, nortriptyline, alprazolam	Few morphologic changes —central nervous system depression, seizures, respiratory arrest, cardiac arrhythmias and arrest	Varies with specific agent —most are potentiated by concurrent alcohol or barbiturates	Poorly understood, may increase synaptic concentrations of neurotransmitters, e.g., dopamine, serotonin? inhilbition of postsynaptic receptors
Acetaminophen—the active metabolite of phenacetin (Tylenol, paracetamol)	*Hepatic necrosis* preceded by nausea, vomiting, diarrhea, and shock	Overdose accidental or suicidal. Usual dose 0.5 mg —toxic dose above 15 mg	Converted in liver to a toxic metabolite that binds to glutathione. With depletion of glutathione toxic metabolite binds to liver macromolecules Aggregation of polymorphonuclear neutrophils in hepatic microcirculation may cause ischemia
Aspirin Acute	*Fluid and electrolyte imbalances*—respiratory alkalosis followed by metabolic acidosis	Overdose: 2–4 gm in children, 10–30 gm in adults Accidental or suicidal	Direct stimulant effect on respiratory center, with hyperventilation followed by respiratory depression and CO_2 retention
Chronic	*Central nervous system syndrome*—from vertigo and tinnitus to convulsions and coma	Prolonged ingestion 2–4 gm	
	Gastritis—gastric ulcer with bleeding	Prolonged ingestion 2–4 gm	Damages gastric mucosal barrier to H^+ permeation
	Bleeding tendency	Prolonged ingestion 2–4 gm	Inhibition of cyclooxygenase and formation of thromboxane
	Renal papillary necrosis	Prolonged use of proprietary mixtures of aspirin and phenacetin	See Chapter 20
Halothane	*Hepatic necrosis*—mild to massive Prodrome fever and jaundice	Anesthetic—toxicity most often follows previous exposure but rarely after first	?Hypersensitivity reaction— ?genetic predisposition to deranged metabolism, with formation of toxic metabolites

Some of the more common ADRs and implicated agents are presented in Table 9–4. A few details about the therapeutic agents most often implicated in fatal drug reactions (usually suicides) are offered in Table 9–5.

Exogenous Estrogens and Oral Contraceptives (OCs)

Because of the well-known contribution of endogenous hyperestrinism to the development of endometrial carcinoma (see Chapter 23.) and possibly breast carcinoma, there has long been reluctance to recommend exogenous estrogens for the prevention or alleviation of postmenopausal changes, most important, postmenopausal osteoporosis. It has been argued that there is insufficient evidence that exogenous estrogens do indeed prevent the development of postmenopausal osteoporosis and that, moreover, a number of studies in the past pointed to an increased risk of endometrial carcinoma and a modest increased risk of breast carcinoma with long-term use. Continuing studies with modified schedules of estrogen administration have shown (as will be pointed out) that estrogens are of clear value in the prevention and possible alleviation of osteoporosis, and so there are strong reasons for their administration. A consensus on the following points has thus been developing with regard to natural (as opposed to synthetic) estrogens, although, admittedly, contrary findings still appear in the literature.

• *Endometrial carcinoma.* Endometrial carcinoma was thought to develop much more frequently (relative risk 1.7 to 2.0) with the long-term postmenopausal use of unopposed estrogens. However, with the monthly interpolation of progestins for 10 to 14 days, the increased risk is totally neutralized, albeit at the price of withdrawal, "pseudomenstrual" bleeding.[12]
• *Breast carcinoma.* Although some studies continue to point to an increased risk of this form of

cancer with the use of unopposed estrogens and, indeed, with synthetic estrogen (commonly estradiol)–progestin therapy,[13] the weight of evidence favors the view that postmenopausal low-dose natural estrogens do not enhance the likelihood of breast carcinoma. The addition of cyclic progestin may reduce the risk even more.[14]

* *Cardiovascular disease.* Cardiovascular disease is definitely reduced in frequency among postmenopausal women with the use of low doses of natural estrogens. Prior to the menopause, women are remarkably shielded from MI (see Chapter 12), but following the menopause, the risk progressively rises with time to approach that of men. With replacement therapy, the relative risk was lowered to 0.5, compared with postmenopausal women who had never used estrogens, and was reduced even more when the therapy was continued after the time of the study.[15] Natural estrogens in low doses raise the level of high-density lipoprotein (HDL) and lower the levels of low-density lipoprotein (LDL) and very low-density lipoprotein (VLDL), all of which tend to protect against coronary atherosclerosis and MI. The addition of sequential progestins did not alter the benefits of estrogen regimens.[15a]

* *Venous thrombosis and pulmonary embolism.* There is a dose-dependent, increased predisposition to venous thrombosis and pulmonary embolism with the postmenopausal use of synthetic estrogens (e.g., diethylstilbestrol). This effect is not entirely understood but may be related to elevated blood levels of a number of clotting factors, possibly accompanied by decreases in antithrombin III and fibrinolytic activity. With the use of low doses of natural estrogens (in contrast with synthetic estrogens), the increased tendency to venous thrombosis virtually disappears.

* *Osteoporosis.* An important indication for the use of postmenopausal estrogens was an attempt to treat, or at least prevent, the development of postmenopausal osteoporosis. Evidence is accumulating that, indeed, the development of this bone disease can be largely or completely prevented with hormone replacement, in combination with calcium supplementation when initiated just prior to or soon after the menopause.[16] The addition of progestins does not diminish the benefits of estrogens. To be noted—hormonal replacement therapy is maximally effective when it is begun immediately or soon after the onset of the menopause. Much less well established is the efficacy of such regimens begun some time later, when osteoporosis has already developed. There are, however, strong suggestions that even established osteoporosis may be improved.

For completeness' sake, the postmenopausal use of estrogens increases the risk of reversible cholestasis (bile stasis) and gallbladder disease but does not predispose to hypertension or cerebrovas-

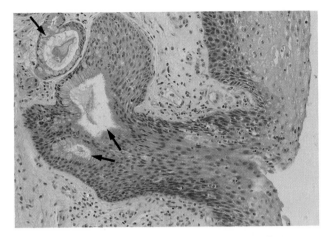

Figure 9–3. Vaginal adenosis. The normal stratified squamous vaginal mucosa is seen on the right and at the bottom of the tongue-like invagination are seen several inclusions of regular columnar clear cells *(arrows)*. (Courtesy of Dr. William Welch, Brigham and Women's Hospital, Boston.)

cular stroke. Substitute estrogens (diethylstilbestrol, but not steroid hormones), once used during pregnancy for threatened abortion, produced in some female offspring in their second to third decades of life vaginal adenosis and, very rarely, superimposed clear cell adenocarcinoma (Fig. 9–3); a topic discussed more completely in Chapter 23.

Oral Contraceptives (OCs)

Before considering the possible adverse consequences of the use of OCs, three important factors must be kept in mind.

1. Almost all the market preparations of OCs employ combinations of synthetic steroids, for example, ethinyl estradiol as the estrogen and some derivative of 19-nortestosterone as the progestogen. The effects of these synthetic steroids may differ from those of natural compounds.

2. The amounts of estrogenic and progestogenic steroids in OCs have been steadily reduced over the past years, and the amounts relative to each other have been altered so that the effects of the current "minipills" are likely to be different from those of the preparations used in the past.

3. Any adverse consequences of the OCs must be balanced against the morbidity and mortality associated with the unwanted pregnancies resulting from their unavailability or nonuse.

The changing formulary and varying dosage schedules ("minipills" have been in use for only about 10 to 15 years) have often led to contradictory conclusions about the consequences of OCs, producing "more heat than light." The following statements, therefore, are offered with the recognition that future studies may require their revision.

- *Venous thrombosis.* The OCs, as used in the past, are associated with a five- to tenfold increased risk of pulmonary thromboembolism, mostly in older women who are cigarette smokers. The data on the use of the "minipills," with their combinations of estrogen and progestogen, do not indicate any increased risk, particularly in nonsmokers younger than 35 years of age, in the absence of other predisposing influences (e.g., hypertension, diabetes, and hyperlipoproteinemia).
- *Myocardial infarction (MI).* Despite the protective effect of natural estrogens, there is controversy about an increased incidence of MI with OC use.[17] Although many studies point to a significantly increased risk, particularly in smokers older than 35, two recent large-scale surveys failed to reveal any association between OC use and MI. These contradictory results may reflect the difference between the OCs of the past and the present.[17]
- *Breast cancer.* Few topics have aroused more disagreement than the relationship of OC use to the development of breast cancer. Despite the disagreements, the prevailing opinion is that, for women younger than 60 years of age, OC use as currently formulated does not increase the risk of breast cancer.[18] However, in the cohort of women younger than 46 who have taken the combined OCs for at least ten years, there is a modest increased relative risk (1.2 to 1.4).
- *Endometrial cancer.* There is no increased risk— there is very likely a protective effect.
- *Cervical cancer.* There is some increased risk, correlated with duration of use and level of sexual activity.
- *Ovarian cancer.* OCs protect against ovarian cancer; the longer the use, the greater the protection, which persists for some time after OC use has been stopped.
- *Benign breast disease.* OCs reduce the incidence of malignant transformation of fibrocystic change.
- *Hepatic adenoma.* There is a well-defined association between the use of OCs and this rare benign tumor, correlated with years of use. There is further an increased predisposition to spontaneous rupture of these neoplasms and hemorrhage, both probably a consequence of rapid tumor growth.
- *Other correlations.* These include an increased predisposition to liver cancer, hypertension, cholestasis (Fig. 9–4), and gallbladder disease, correlated with years of use, but there is no increased incidence of thrombotic or hemorrhagic stroke with the newer formulations.

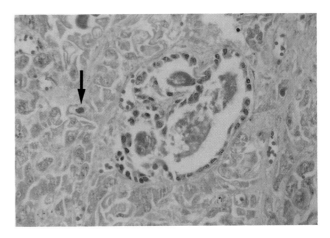

Figure 9–4. Cholestasis. A cluster of small hepatic ductules contains inspissated aggregations of bile. Smaller bile plugs *(arrow)* are seen in hepatocytes.

When viewed in the context of the benefits of OC use, the risks may well be acceptable.

Other Therapeutic Agents

Of the numberless other drugs having possible undesirable side effects, the few mentioned here were selected because of the frequency or significance of their adverse reactions.

Antineoplastic agents have both saved and ended lives. Most act on dividing cells at some specific point in the cell cycle, for example, deoxyribonucleic acid (DNA) synthesis, transcription, and formation of the mitotic spindle. Unfortunately, they therefore may injure normal actively dividing cells, such as those in the bone marrow, intestinal epithelium, and hair follicles. Moreover, these agents have the potential to induce nonlethal mutations in cells. Thus, the adverse consequences of antineoplastic drugs include (1) bone marrow suppression, leading to severe anemia, leukopenia, and thrombocytopenia; (2) immunosuppression, rendering the patient vulnerable to all manner of infection (discussed below); and (3) the initiation of some form of cancer, most often acute myeloid leukemia.[19] So it is that sometimes the successful control of a cancer with a drug ends up a Pyrrhic victory.

Immunosuppressive agents have made possible the present era of organ transplantation and control of some immunologically mediated diseases, but they also have their "dark side." The agents in most common use are corticosteroids, cyclosporine, and the antimetabolite azathioprine. Although each of the agents has specific actions, all suppress humoral or cell-mediated immunity, and sometimes both. These patients are thus rendered vulnerable to microbial infections, particularly with always waiting opportunists such as cytomegalovirus, *Pneumocystis carinii, Candida,* and *Aspergillus.* Recall the plight of the patient with acquired immunodeficiency syndrome (AIDS). In addition, the immunosuppressed patient is at risk for developing graft-versus-host disease following marrow transplantation (see Chapter 6). Other adverse consequences include an increased risk of developing lymphomas, principally immunoblastic. Were these unpleasant consequences not enough, the various long-term immunosuppressive agents have specific cytotoxicities. Cyclosporine is a well-recognized cause of renal injury, and azathioprine may produce interstitial pneumonitis. It is evident that these extremely useful agents may provoke adverse reactions.

Antimicrobial agents have dramatically altered the frequency, severity, and mortality of infectious diseases, but they are also capable of causing mischief.

- Hypersensitivity reactions may result, ranging from trivial, self-limited skin rashes, to life-threatening anaphylaxis, to exfoliative dermatitis.
- In the Darwinian struggle for survival, drug-resistant organisms have emerged, giving rise to drug-resistant, sometimes nosocomial infections and to difficult to control epidemics in the community and hospitals.
- Eradication of the normal microflora of the body may permit opportunists to proliferate, with the emergence of a disease more serious than the initial infection (e.g., a disseminated fungal infection).

All these potentials make understandable the basis for the judicious use of anti-infective drugs.

NONTHERAPEUTIC AGENTS

Only a few of the many potentially injurious, nontherapeutic agents will be discussed, because of their social, public health, or clinical importance.

Ethyl Alcohol

It has been variously estimated that about one-third of the adult population of the United States are abstainers, another third are light to moderate "social" drinkers, and the remaining third are heavy drinkers, many of them alcohol dependent or addicted. Alcohol, as is well known, has major acute effects; less well known are the consequences of protracted use on the organs and tissues of the body but clearly it alters mitochondrial and microsomal function. Still uncertain is whether ethanol itself or its metabolites, notably acetaldehyde, are responsible for these effects. Concomitant malnutrition, such as avitaminoses (the "empty calories" of ethanol substituting for proper food), has largely been ruled out as the basis for most of

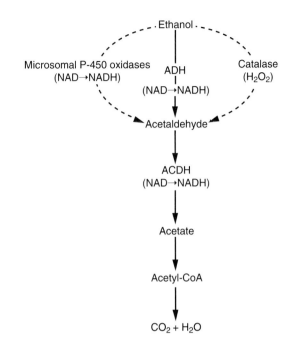

ADH = Hepatic alcohol dehydrogenase
ACDH = Hepatic acetaldehyde dehydrogenase
NAD = Nicotinamide-adenine dinucleotide
NADH = Reduced nicotinamide-adenine dinucleotide

Figure 9–5. Metabolism of alcohol. The major (rate-limiting) pathway is via ADH.

the ill effects of chronic alcohol consumption, save in the case of some of the nervous system changes (as will be detailed). There are approximately 10 gm of ethanol in 12 ounces of beer, 4 ounces of unfortified wine, and 1.5 ounces of 80 proof liquor; the effects of these various drinks depend solely on their ethanol content. Only about 2 to 10% of the ethanol consumed is excreted directly through the lungs, urine, or sweat. The amount exhaled is in direct proportion to the blood level and forms the basis of the breath test employed by law enforcement agencies.

With ingestion, a small amount of ethanol is directly metabolized in the stomach by gastric mucosal alcohol dehydrogenase. The remainder is rapidly absorbed in the stomach and small intestine and can be detected in the blood within minutes. Once in the blood, alcohol is metabolized in the liver through three pathways (Fig. 9–5). The major one involves hepatic alcohol dehydrogenase, yielding acetaldehyde, which is then rapidly converted to acetate by aldehyde dehydrogenase. In these conversions, nicotinamide-adenine dinucleotide (NAD) is converted to reduced NAD (NADH). The increased NADH:NAD ratio may be responsible for some of the metabolic consequences of chronic alcoholism. A second, clearly inducible pathway utilizes the hepatic microsomal P-450 system, also mobilized in the detoxification of a variety of drugs. It too yields acetaldehyde, oxidizable to acetate. In the adult of average size, both of these pathways are capable of metabolizing approximately one drink of beverage ethanol, 10 gm, per hour. A third, less frequently utilized metabolic pathway utilizes peroxisomal catalase. With this background, we can now examine the effects of acute and chronic alcoholism.

Acute alcoholism exerts its effects mainly on the central nervous system (CNS), but it may also, remarkably quickly, induce hepatic and gastric changes that are reversible. (The hepatic changes are described in Chapter 18, and the gastric changes in Chapter 17.) In the CNS, alcohol itself is a powerful depressant, having effects similar to those of ether. Inhibitory control centers are depressed, thereby releasing excitatory pathways that account for the widespread belief that it is a stimulant. The extent of CNS depression depends on blood alcohol levels. The cortex is affected first. As the levels climb, however, other systems also become depressed: first the limbic system, then the cerebellum, and finally the lower brain stem. Consequently, a "party syndrome" develops, with euphoria and some disordered cognitive and motor function. These changes can be seen at blood alcohol levels as low as 20 to 30 mg/dl, possibly resulting from only one or two drinks within a relatively brief time. The legal level of intoxication is generally set at 100 mg/dl; narcosis in the nonhabituated often occurs at blood levels of 200 to 250 mg/dl. Coma and fatal respiratory arrest become likely at 300 to 400 mg/dl. Fortunately, fatal levels are rarely encountered because "blessed stupor" intervenes to protect against continued imbibing. In passing, brief mention should be made of "blackouts" (episodes of forgetting much of what transpired during drinking), which sometimes appear with acute alcoholism. The mechanisms underlying these episodes are not well understood, but ethanol, through its action on membrane receptors for the inhibitory neurotransmitter gamma-aminobutyric acid (GABA), may potentiate GABA-activated inhibition of cerebral neurons.[20]

Chronic alcoholism induces morphologic alterations in virtually all organs and tissues in the body. Some concept of the range of these changes is offered in Table 9–6. Some limited explanatory comments follow.

- *Hepatic changes* are the most common consequence of chronic alcoholism. These are discussed in adequate detail in Chapter 18, and so it suffices to note here that fatty change typically appears within a few days of even modest alcohol consumption. Although the liver cells may be distended with fat vacuoles, the fat can be mobilized when the exposure to alcohol is discontinued. Alcoholic hepatitis is seen with bouts of heavy drinking. It may cause acute liver insufficiency, may or may not be preceded by steatosis, and may or may not be followed by cirrhosis,

Table 9–6. MAJOR CONSEQUENCES OF CHRONIC ALCOHOLISM

	LESION	MECHANISM
Liver	Fatty change	Direct toxicity
	Acute hepatitis	Direct toxicity
	Alcoholic cirrhosis (see Chapter 18)	Direct toxicity
Central nervous system	Wernicke's syndrome	Thiamine deficiency
	Korsakoff's syndrome	Combined thiamine deficiency and direct toxicity
	Cerebral atrophy (questionable)	Direct toxicity
	Cerebellar degeneration	Nutritional deficiency
Nerves	Peripheral neuropathy	Thiamine deficiency
Heart	Congestive cardiomyopathy	Direct toxicity
Skeletal muscle	Acute and chronic fiber rhabdomyolysis	Direct toxicity
Testes	Atrophy	Unclear
Pancreas	Chronic pancreatitis	Unclear
Fetal alcohol syndrome	Retardation of physical and mental development, malformations	?Direct toxicity

which is the end stage of liver disease in the chronic abuser of alcohol.

- *Central nervous system changes* take many forms. Perhaps the most common is *Wernicke's encephalopathy*. It may appear in nonalcoholics who become thiamine deficient but is most commonly encountered in the United States in chronic alcoholics and responds promptly to thiamine administration. The chronic alcoholic subsists on a grossly inadequate diet, and the alcohol itself impairs intestinal absorption of thiamine (discussed later). Why only a subset of chronic alcoholics develop this condition remains unclear, but it is speculated that they have an inherited or acquired abnormality of a thiamine-dependent transketolase (involved in cerebral glucose and energy metabolism), reducing its affinity for thiamine. Clinically, this syndrome is characterized by ataxia, global confusion, ophthalmoplegia, and often nystagmus.

The underlying morphology is quite characteristic and includes foci of symmetric discoloration, and sometimes softening with congestion, and punctate hemorrhages in the paraventricular regions of the thalamus and hypothalamus, in the mammillary bodies, about the aqueduct in the midbrain, in the floor of the fourth ventricle, and in the anterior cerebellum. Microscopically, the focal lesions reveal vascular dilatations and endothelial proliferation ringed by hemorrhages, accompanied by some demyelinization, and loss of neuropil. The neurons may be relatively spared in early disease but eventually reveal degenerative changes and cell death.

Following treatment of Wernicke's encephalopathy with thiamine, a minority of patients reveal a profound memory deficit, both remote and recent, referred to as *Korsakoff's syndrome.* There are no specific morphologic lesions with Korsakoff's syndrome, other than those related to the pre-existing encephalopathy, yet the memory impairment only infrequently responds to continued thiamine treatment. It is believed, therefore, that Korsakoff's syndrome is caused by the direct neurotoxicity of ethanol, perhaps compounded by a lack of thiamine.

Whether *cortical atrophy* is a potential consequence of chronic alcoholism is controversial, because various anatomic studies do not reveal consistent reduction of brain weight in long-term abusers of alcohol. By contrast, *cerebellar degeneration,* related to loss of Purkinje's cells in the cerebellar cortex, is a well-documented change found in a minority of chronic alcoholics. Most studies suggest that this lesion relates to thiamine deficiency rather than to direct ethanol toxicity.

• *Peripheral nerves* suffer a demyelinative polyneuropathy, occasionally mononeuropathy (when accompanied by prolonged compression of a nerve), which is fairly common in chronic alcoholics who are malnourished. The basis is thought to be thiamine deficiency rather than ethanol toxicity.

• *Cardiovascular consequences* of alcohol abuse are wide-ranging. On the one hand, direct injury to the myocardium may produce a dilated congestive cardiomyopathy (see Cardiomyopathy, Chapter 12). On the other hand, moderate consumption of alcohol increases the levels of HDL and decreases the incidence of coronary heart disease. However, heavy consumption leading to liver injury results in lower levels of the HDL fraction of lipoproteins, accompanied by an increased likelihood of coronary heart disease.

• *Miscellaneous changes* take many forms. In low doses, ethanol tends to reduce the blood pressure, but with three or more drinks a day there is a distinct tendency to hypertension. Alcoholics suffer higher incidences of acute and chronic pancreatitis and regressive changes in skeletal muscle, referred to as alcoholic myopathy. Even more unhappily, the use of ethanol during pregnancy can cause microcephaly and mental retardation in the child, sometimes accompanied by facial malformations and cardiac defects. This fetal-alcohol syndrome has appeared in infants of mothers whose alcohol intake was only two or three drinks per day. An increased risk of cancer of the mouth or of the pharynx, larynx, esophagus, stomach, and, possibly, rectum and lung is encountered with chronic alcohol abuse. The increased risk is not trivial; the cumulative rate of these cancers is tenfold greater in alcoholics than in the general population. We can conclude that it is bad enough that acute alcoholism often unhinges the rudder of the ship; chronic abuse may sink it.

Lead

Lead is a furtive villain; it creeps in "on little cat's feet" as small increments silently accumulate to reach toxic levels. Sometimes in adults the poisoning announces itself relatively early, with abdominal pain, fatigue, and arthralgia, but in infants and children "low-level" lead exposure may produce serious impairment of mental development even before there is any awareness of the intoxication.[21] Even worse, in the child, the poisoning may first become apparent by a catastrophic encephalopathic crisis.

There are innumerable sources of lead in our environment. For children, flaking lead paint is the major threat, but there are many other sources, such as lead-contaminated dust, soil, root vegetables, and newsprint. For adults the main threats are occupational—lead mining and smelting and battery fabrication and salvage. However, exposure to lead in the United States is nearly universal, in some part a legacy of the past use of leaded gasoline, with a deposit from lead-contaminated exhaust in the environment. Lead water pipes or soldered joints, mineral deposits in the earth, hair dyes, soldered tin cans, pottery glazes, and home distilled whiskey are additional hazards.

Environmental lead is absorbed either through the gastrointestinal tract or via the lungs into the blood. Urban adults have a daily intake of 100 to 150 μg of lead in water and food, only about 10% of which is absorbed. A deficiency of iron, calcium, or zinc enhances absorption. By contrast, most volatilized lead is absorbed in the lungs. Children have, on average, a lower intake but absorb about 50%. Lead poisoning may, in fact, begin *in utero.* It has been difficult to establish "safe" upper limits of lead in the body. At one time it was thought that a blood lead level of 25 μg/dl was "safe." However, recent surveys have shown a risk of abnormally low IQ scores in children with blood lead levels as low as 10 to 15 μg/dl, with an inverse correlation between the exact level and the IQ score.[22] Thus, in October 1991, the theoretically "safe" blood lead level was lowered to 10 μg/dl in the United States.

Absorbed lead is mainly (80 to 85%) taken up by bone and developing teeth in children; the blood accumulates about 5 to 10%; and the remainder is distributed throughout the soft tissues.

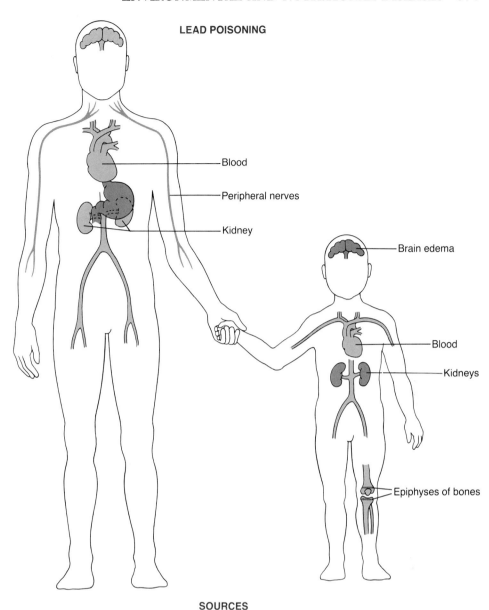

LEAD POISONING

Blood

Peripheral nerves

Kidney

Brain edema

Blood

Kidneys

Epiphyses of bones

SOURCES

OCCUPATIONAL
Spray painting
Foundry work
Mining and extracting lead
Battery burning
Automotive exhaust

NONOCCUPATIONAL
Water supply
Paint dust and flakes
House dust
Urban soil
Newsprint

Figure 9–6. Lead poisoning. The major sites of lead-induced morphologic changes.

Although the soft tissue deposits have a half-life measured in hours to days, the skeletal deposits persist until the contaminated bone salts are recycled. In children, the bony deposits are located particularly in the epiphyses. In a sense, this skeletal sequestration protects the other tissues, but the slow turnover of bone mineral maintains elevated levels of lead in the blood for months to years. Excretion occurs via the kidneys, thereby exposing these organs to potential damage.

Lead poisons enzymes by binding to sulfhydryl groups and denaturing proteins. Recently, binding and cleavage of transfer ribonucleic acid (tRNA) and derangement of phosphokinase C function (a part of a second messenger system in the brain) have also been proposed as additional biologic effects of lead. The major anatomic targets of lead are the blood, nervous system, gastrointestinal tract, and kidneys (Fig. 9–6).

MORPHOLOGY. Blood changes are fairly early and characteristic. Lead interferes with aminolevulinic acid dehydratase (ALA-D) and ferroketolase, in-

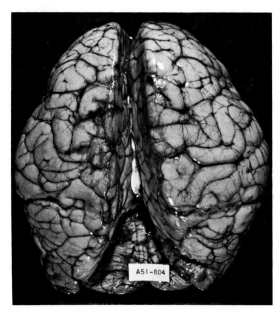

Figure 9-7. Cerebral edema in lead poisoning. The gyri are flattened and widened, and the sulci are narrowed and relatively inapparent.

volved in the incorporation of iron into the heme molecule. As a consequence, the iron is displaced, and zinc protoporphyrin is formed. Thus, the level of zinc protoporphyrin or its product, free erythrocyte protoporphyrin, constitutes blood parameters of lead poisoning. **Typically, there appear a microcytic, hypochromic, mild hemolytic anemia and even more distinctive punctate basophilic stippling of the erythrocytes.**

Children are particularly vulnerable to brain damage; as noted before, it may be very subtle and only functional, or massive and lethal.[23] The anatomic changes underlying the more subtle functional deficits are ill defined and poorly understood (possibly related to phosphokinase-C function, mentioned before), but there is concern that some of the cognitive defects may be permanent. At the more severe end of the spectrum there is marked edema of the brain, with flattening of the gyri and narrowing of the sulci (Fig. 9-7). Microscopically there may be demyelinization of the cerebral and cerebellar white matter and death of cortical neurons, with diffuse astrocytic proliferation. Often there is proliferation of the endothelium of small capillaries in the areas of damage. In the adult, the central nervous system is less often affected, but **frequently a peripheral demyelinating neuropathy appears,** typically involving the motor innervation of the extensor muscles of the wrist and fingers, producing **wrist and foot drop.**

The gastrointestinal tract is a major source of clinical manifestations in adults. Lead "colic," characterized by extremely severe, poorly localized abdominal pain, is often associated with suf-

ficient spasm and rigidity of the abdominal wall to create the impression of an acute "surgical abdomen." No intestinal morphologic changes have been identified, but often there is a "lead line" of precipitated lead sulfide along the gingival margins. It is rare in children and not seen in edentulous individuals. Moreover, although this line is typical of lead poisoning, it may be encountered in other circumstances, such as mercury poisoning.

The **kidneys** are affected less often than the blood or nervous system, but nonetheless they may develop a chronic tubulointerstitial nephritis (see Chapter 20), or so-called Fanconi's syndrome, marked by glycosuria, aminoaciduria, and phosphaturia secondary to altered tubular cell transport mechanisms. Often there is proteinuria, and reabsorption of the urinary proteins leads to **large eosinophilic droplets in the tubular epithelial cells.** As the poisoning progresses, the glomerular filtration rate falls, and some patients develop renal failure.[24] The renal damage impedes normal excretion of uric acid and leads to hyperuricemia and so-called **saturnine gout.**

The clinical diagnosis of lead poisoning is too frequently delayed. Sometimes, the first clues are anemia and basophilic stippling of the red blood cells. Almost always, the diagnosis requires the confirmatory findings of elevated blood lead and free erythrocyte protoporphyrin (above 50 μg/dl) or, alternatively, elevated zinc protoporphyrin levels. Other supportive findings are increased excretion of aminolevulinic acid in the urine and reduced erythrocyte ALA-D activity. If further exposure can be controlled and the blood lead levels reduced with chelators, the hematologic, peripheral nerve, and renal changes can be reversed, but neurologic defects may persist.

Environmental and Occupational Carcinogens

As was pointed out in Chapter 7, we virtually "swim in a sea of carcinogens," a few of which are discussed in some detail in other sections (cigarette smoke, asbestos). According to the Environmental Protection Agency, about 20% of the tens of thousands of substances in current commercial use are putative carcinogens. The term "carcinogenic," however, is open to challenge, since it is often based on epidemiologic and animal studies of arguable relevance. Without getting mired in this scientific and political controversy, we can say that there is no doubt that a large number of environmental and industrial substances are carcinogenic and, indeed, if cigarette smoking is included, are directly responsible, in whole or in part, for more

Table 9-7. SOME MAJOR ENVIRONMENTAL AND OCCUPATIONAL CARCINOGENS

AGENT	TYPE OF CANCER
Arsenic (miners, insecticide manufacturers and users, chemical workers)	Skin, lung, liver carcinomas
Asbestos (see Chapter 15)	Bronchogenic carcinoma, mesothelioma, others
Benzene (rubber cement workers, distillers, dye users)	Myelogenous leukemia
Beta-naphthylamine (rubber, dye industries)	Bladder carcinoma
Cadmium (miners, processors)	Prostate, kidney carcinoma
Chromium (producers and processors)	Nasal cavity, sinus, lung, and laryngeal carcinomas
Cigarette smoke	Bronchogenic carcinoma, others
Nickel (miners and processors)	Nasal sinus, lung cancers
Nitrites (Chapter 17)	Stomach carcinoma
Uranium (miners and processors)	Lung carcinoma
Vinyl chloride (plastic industries)	Liver angiosarcoma

than half of all clinical cancers.[25] Some of the major implicated agents are listed in Table 9-7.

For further details, reference should be made to an authoritative review.[26]

Street Drugs

Drug abuse—the "recreational" use of psychoactive drugs, such as marijuana, cocaine, and heroin—has become almost as widespread in the United States and other privileged societies as cigarette smoking and alcohol abuse. In 1991, more than half of the high school seniors in the United States had used marijuana, and the numbers become more staggering every year. According to the National Institute of Drug Abuse, there were just over 5 million cocaine users in 1974 in the United States, almost 22 million in 1982, and more than 25 million in 1986. Because most addicts have used more than one drug, it has been difficult to sort out the adverse effects of one from those of another. Recognizing this problem, we follow this brief overview with a discussion of marijuana, cocaine, and heroin, the latter in more detail because it is the most common and most dangerous abused substance.

MARIJUANA. At one time, the use of marijuana ("pot") was thought to be a relatively benign ac-

tivity, limited mainly to the years of adolescence and young adulthood. Continuing studies have made clear, however, that marijuana use is far from benign and is not limited to the young or immature. The active substance in marijuana is delta-9-tetrahydrocannabinol (THC), found in the resin of the *Cannabis sativa* plant. Preparations of leaves and flowering tops of cannabis are most often smoked in cigarettes, called "joints," but they can be eaten with foodstuffs or, less commonly, can be drunk as extracts or even injected intravenously. When the active resin is volatilized in smoking, about 50% is absorbed through the lungs; by contrast, only 10% is absorbed when ingested. Hashish, the dried resin, contains about 10% of THC.

Heavy use of marijuana has been associated with adverse behavioral and psychologic reactions and with detrimental pulmonary, reproductive, and possibly immunologic consequences. However, it is necessary to emphasize that these adverse effects are encountered mainly with heavy use, and, moreover, some of the studies on which these opinions are based were poorly controlled. Thus, the data require further investigation.

- *Behavioral and psychologic changes* are almost universally experienced with the smoking of even a single "joint." The smoker's intention is to achieve euphoria, relaxation, and various alterations of sensory perceptions. With continued use, these changes may progress to cognitive and psychomotor impairment, such as the inability to judge time, speed, and distance, delayed reaction time, and other deficits that have the potential to lead to injury and accidental death. Indeed, marijuana use is thought to contribute to a significant fraction of all fatal automobile accidents among adolescents.[27] A number of other cognitive aberrations have been recorded, including psychotic breaks, but it is uncertain whether these symptoms of psychosis are induced by marijuana or merely unmasked by it.
- In the *respiratory tract*, the smoking of three or four marijuana cigarettes a day is associated with the same frequency of acute and chronic bronchitis as the smoking of 20 cigarettes of tobacco. Concern grows that protracted smoking of marijuana may also eventually predispose to cancer of the lungs.
- *Reproductive changes*, such as reduced fertility, diminished sperm motility, and decreased circulating testosterone levels, have been reported in laboratory animals, and there are a few reports of similar effects in humans after intensive marijuana exposure. All these changes require further confirmation.
- *Fetal abnormalities* have been attributed to the heavy use of marijuana during pregnancy. Retarded development of the fetus, low birth weight, and an increased frequency of leukemia

COCAINE INTOXICATION

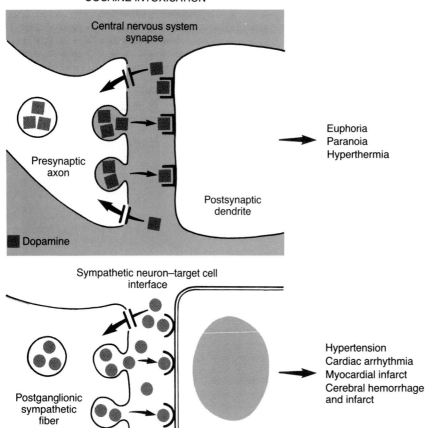

Figure 9-8. The effect of cocaine on neurotransmission. The drug inhibits reuptake of the neurotransmitters dopamine and norepinephrine by presynaptic neurons, leading to excess stimulation of postsynaptic fibers or effector cells.

in the offspring are among the more serious consequences.[28] Similar consequences have been found in a large number of animals, ranging from rodents to monkeys, lending credence to the reliability of these findings in humans.

• Depressed cell-mediated and humoral immune responses are well documented in chronic users of this agent, predisposing to infectious illnesses.

There is, however, a brighter side to the equation. Marijuana has been shown to reduce the nausea of cancer chemotherapy and to be effective in the treatment of glaucoma, convulsive seizures, and asthma when other drugs have failed. Prohibiting the use of marijuana for such medicinal purposes is akin to throwing out the baby with the bath water.

COCAINE AND CRACK. The magnitude of the "cocaine problem" was alluded to earlier, but it is startling to learn that according to a 1986 survey in the United States by the National Institute on Drug Abuse, there were 5000 new cocaine users daily and 6 million regular users, among whom 2 million could be called addicts.[29] Cocaine, an alka-

loid extracted from the leaves of the coca plant, is usually sold as a water-soluble powder (cocaine hydrochloride), liberally diluted with talcum powder or some other similar-appearing white look-alike. Extraction of the pure alkaloid from the cocaine hydrochloride yields a solid form of "freebase" called "crack" because of the sound it produces when heated. Although the pharmacologic actions of cocaine and crack are identical, the latter is much more potent. Both forms of cocaine are absorbed from all sites, that is, the nasal mucosa when snorted (vapors of the heated crack), the lungs when smoked with tobacco, and the gastrointestinal tract when ingested, as well as when taken subcutaneously and intravenously.

The pharmacologic actions of cocaine are varied. As is well known, it is widely used as a local anesthetic, usually in procedures in the oral cavity. In sufficient amounts, it is a potent CNS stimulant, blocking the reuptake of norepinephrine, dopamine, and serotonin at presynaptic nerve terminals, thus increasing the amount of these neurotransmitters at postsynaptic receptor sites[30] (Fig. 9-8). In addition, it also increases the synthesis of norepinephrine and dopamine. The increased levels of dopamine induce a sense of euphoria, and at the same time the norepinephrine causes adrenergic potentiation, with hypertension, tachycardia, and vasoconstriction. Thus, as will be seen, cocaine may cause severe coronary artery narrowing and fatal myocardial ischemic events. In addition, it may also produce calcium-dependent vasoconstriction of vascular smooth muscle, independent of its actions on the sympathetic nervous system. Less well understood is an increased thrombotic tendency, which may lead to thromboses at points of arterial vasospastic narrowing.

With such widespread physiologic effects, cocaine users may experience any or all of the following symptoms:

- Intense euphoria—a "high"—may appear within a few minutes and disappear after 15 to 40 minutes, often followed by depression. To maintain the "high," doses must be repeated frequently; this brings about an intense craving for the substance, rather than a true addiction. However, repeated exposure leads to some level of physiologic tolerance. Thus, the euphoria gradually grows briefer and less intense unless the dose of the drug is increased, an action that, in turn, raises concomitantly the risks of seizures, respiratory depression, and death.
- Cocaine is associated with serious *cardiovascular disease*.[31] Besides hypertension and tachycardia, discussed above, its effects include the following:

  - Arrhythmias and sudden death
  - Myocardial infarction, with or without coronary atherosclerosis
  - Myocarditis and dilated cardiomyopathy; it is not clear whether the myocardial disease results from an intercurrent infection, from a hypersensitivity reaction to the drug, from widespread ischemic injury due to small vessel vasospasm, or from catecholamine-induced injury
  - Rupture of the ascending aorta, presumably related to the hypertension

The hazards of cocaine abuse extend to *pregnancy and the developing fetus*. These hazards include abruptio placentae, premature labor, retarded fetal development, stillbirth, and newborn hyperirritability. It is evident that cocaine is a dangerous way to "escape."

HEROIN. Although not as widely used as cocaine, heroin is the most hazardous street drug. It is an opiate closely related to morphine, methadone, and codeine, all derived from the poppy plant. Heroin is sinister because it produces a true addiction and intense fear of withdrawal ("I'll die without it"). It is sold on the street "cut" with some similar-appearing white powder, often talc or quinine. Dissolved in water (which is sometimes

grossly contaminated), it is self-administered intravenously or subcutaneously along with an abundant "fauna and flora." The resultant feelings of well-being, tranquility, and sedation last only a few hours and can be maintained only by repeated injections. However, opiates produce a progressive tolerance and the need for increasing doses to achieve the desired effects. Thus comes about the dependence and the addiction that often drive victims to violent crime to finance "their habit."

All opiates act on the same specific receptors as the normal endogenous opioid peptides, for example, the enkephalins, endorphins, and dynorphins. These receptors are widely distributed in the body but are mainly found in the CNS and the endocrine, gastrointestinal, and cardiovascular systems. Heroin has a particular affinity for the CNS. Although relatively nontoxic in small doses, it has a large number of adverse effects.

- *Sudden death*, usually related to overdosage, is an everpresent threat to the heroin addict. The actual dose being used is a total unknown because street samples range from 2 to 90% heroin. Understandably, most heroin sold by pushers is very dilute, but an easy way of disposing of "a nuisance" is to provide an uncut preparation. Tolerance to the drug may be lost (as during a period of incarceration), potentiating a severe reaction. Three overdose syndromes have been identified: (1) profound respiratory depression, (2) arrhythmias and cardiac arrest, and (3) severe pulmonary edema (Fig. 9–9).[32]
- *Pulmonary complications* include moderate to severe edema, septic embolism, lung abscess, opportunistic infections, and foreign body granulomas from talc and other adulterants (Fig. 9–10).[33]
- *Granulomas* may occur in the lungs and are sometimes found in the mononuclear-phagocyte system, particularly in the lymph nodes draining the upper extremities, spleen, and liver. A polarized light often highlights the trapped talc crystals (from the diluent), sometimes enclosed within foreign body giant cells.
- *Infectious complications* are extremely frequent. The four sites most commonly affected are the skin and subcutaneous tissue, heart valves, liver, and lungs. *Cutaneous lesions* are probably the most frequent telltale signs of heroin addiction —scarring at injection sites, hyperpigmentation over commonly used veins, thrombosed veins, and skin abscesses, cellulitis, and ulcerations usually secondary to subcutaneous injections ("skin-popping"). The chronicity of these infections sometimes leads to systemic amyloidosis. Endocarditis is a frequent complication. It takes a distinctive form often involving right-sided heart valves, particularly the tricuspid. Most cases are caused by *Staphylococcus aureus*, but fungi and every other organism in the "toilet" have been

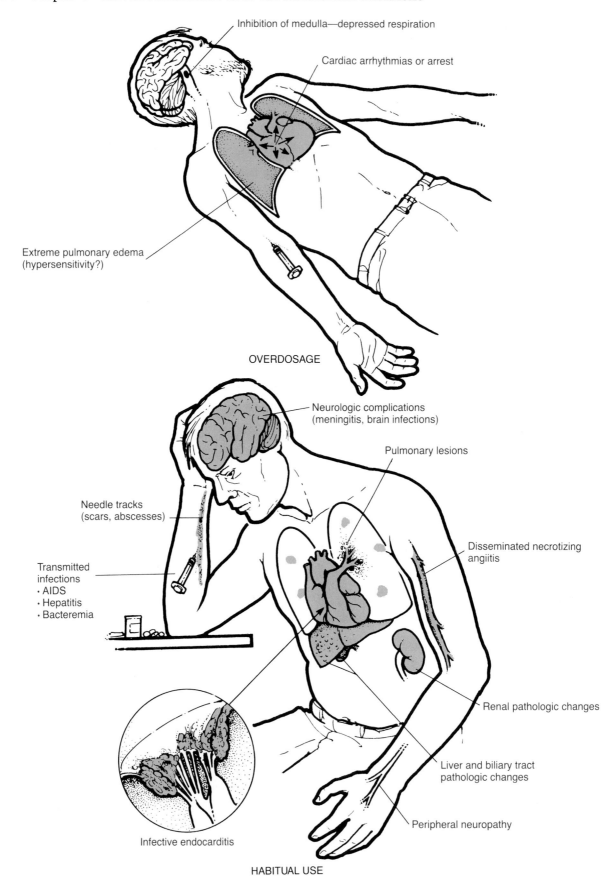

Figure 9–9. The major consequences of heroin addiction—overdosage *(above)* and less catastrophic consequences *(below)*.

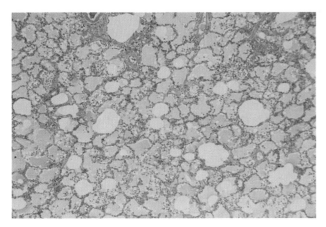

Figure 9-10. Severe pulmonary edema resulting from a hypersensitivity reaction in a heroin addict.

implicated. *Viral hepatitis* is the most common infection among addicts and is acquired by the casual interchange of needles. As is well known, addicts constitute a high-risk group for AIDS. Finally, as mentioned, pulmonary infections also exact their toll and, in many instances, are caused by organisms of low virulence (e.g., *Pneumocystis carinii*).

- *Kidney disease* is a relatively common hazard. The two forms most frequently encountered are amyloidosis (see Chapter 6) and focal glomerulosclerosis (see Chapter 20). Both induce heavy proteinuria and the nephrotic syndrome.

Were all these complications not sufficient, a miscellany of additional hazards faces the heroin addict, including the risk of tetanus, peripheral neuropathy, acute and chronic myopathy, osteomyelitis, and acute disseminated vasculitis. The price of heroin addiction is clearly more than the cost of the drug. Some of the major consequences of heroin use are presented in Figure 9-9.

Table 9-8. UNCOMMON, POTENTIALLY FATAL NONTHERAPEUTIC AGENTS

AGENT	SOURCE	EFFECT	MECHANISM OF INJURY
Methanol	Solvents, sterno, antifreezes	Inebriation, toxic necrosis of retinal ganglion cells with blindness	Metabolized to formaldehyde and formic acid
Carbon monoxide			
Acute poisoning	Fossil fuel exhaust, cigarette smoke	Cherry-red skin, mucous membranes Variable hypoxic injury to brain, liver, renal tubules	Carboxy-Hb (replaces Hb) unable to transport O_2
Chronic poisoning		Diffuse neuronal loss, particularly basal ganglia Occasionally, focal cerebral demyelination	Protracted low-level hypoxia. Once formed, carboxy-Hb is slowly replaced by mass action of O_2
Mercury			
Some organic compounds	Industrial contamination of ocean: from bacteria to fish to humans; interior latex paint	With chronic ingestion—central nervous system disturbances, hearing loss, blindness, spasticity, paralysis (Minamata disease); acrodynia	Neuronal toxicity with focal softenings; cerebral and cerebellar atrophy
Inorganic compounds	Industrial exposure and ingestion	Membranous glomerulopathy with proteinuria, hyaline droplets to necrosis of proximal tubular epithelium	Inactivates wide variety of enzymes
Cyanide	Released by combustion of wool, silk, plastic upholstery —most likely in smoke inhalation in burning dwellings	Hypoxic injury to brain, liver, kidneys, other organs	Binds to cytochrome oxidase and inhibits cellular respiration
Mushroom poisoning	*Amanita phalloides* (potentially lethal) *A. muscaria* (rarely lethal)	Vomiting, abdominal cramps—central nervous system changes, centrilobular hepatic necrosis to massive necrosis, renal tubular necrosis	*A. phalloides* toxin inhibits RNA polymerase
Insecticides			
Chlorinated hydrocarbons	Agricultural and home use: DDT, chlordane, dieldrin	Hyperexcitability, delirium, convulsions, coma	Toxic neuronal injury
Organophosphates	Tri-orthocresylphosphate (TOCP)	Muscle twitching to paralysis, cardiac arrhythmias	Inhibits cholinesterase with synaptic build-up of acetylcholine

OTHER NONTHERAPEUTIC AGENTS

The number of other nontherapeutic agents capable of causing injury or even death is almost limitless. All are quite uncommon, and so only a few have been singled out for capsule characterization in Table 9–8.

PHYSICAL INJURIES

The many forms of physical energy that may give rise to injury can be classified into four groups: mechanical forces, changes in temperature, changes in atmospheric pressure, and electromagnetic energy. Mechanical force exemplified by the everyday occurrence of automobile accidents is, by far, the most frequent cause of physical injury. Changes in atmospheric pressure and hypothermia are uncommon causes of injury, but all too common is hyperthermia producing most often burns. Radiation is a well-known potential cause of injury and, in the past, assumed tragic proportions at Hiroshima and Nagasaki and the Marshall Islands.

INJURIES INDUCED BY MECHANICAL FORCE

Mechanical force may inflict (1) soft tissue injuries, (2) bone injuries, and (3) head injuries. Injuries of the bones and of the head are considered elsewhere. Soft tissue injuries can be subdivided into (1) superficial, involving mainly the skin, and (2) deep, associated with visceral damage. The skin injuries can be further subclassified as follows:

ABRASION. This type of skin injury represents basically a scrape, in which superficial epidermal cells are torn off by friction or a glancing blow. There is no perforation of the skin, and so regeneration without scarring occurs promptly unless infection complicates the process.

LACERATION VERSUS INCISION. A laceration is essentially an irregular tear in the skin produced by overstretching. It may be linear or stellate, depending on the tearing force. Typical of a laceration are the bridging strands of fibrous tissue or blood vessels across the wound, not seen in an incision. The immediate margins of the laceration are frequently hemorrhagic and traumatized. In contrast, an incision is made by a sharp cutting object, such as a knife (scalpel) and a piece of glass. The margins of the incision are usually relatively clean, and there are no bridging strands of tissue. The incision, in contrast with the laceration, can usually be neatly approximated by sutures, leaving little or no scar. Deep tissues and organs may sustain lacerations from an external blow with or without apparent superficial injury. For example, when the unrestrained body impacts on the steering wheel in a head-on collision, the liver may well sustain fatal lacerations. Analogously, improperly worn lap safety belts may violently compress and rupture hollow viscera, such as the intestine, in effect causing a through-and-through laceration of the visceral wall.

CONTUSION. This is an injury caused by a blunt force that injures small blood vessels and causes interstitial bleeding usually without disruption of the continuity of the tissue. With superficial contusions, the bleeding is usually evident almost at once, but with deeper contusions, of skeletal muscle for example, the bleeding may not be evident for many hours or, in fact, may never be seen, leaving only swelling and tenderness at the site. Older individuals, with small vessel fragility, may sustain extensive hematomas at contused sites.

GUNSHOT WOUNDS. Injuries of this nature fall largely into the domain of forensic pathology, a specialty unto itself, dealing with trauma and medicolegal issues. We can no more than scratch the surface of this highly specialized area with some limited observations about the wounds themselves, which may assume great importance, as was the case in the death of President John F. Kennedy.

The character of a gunshot wound at entry and exit and the extent of injury depend on the type of gun used (handgun or rifle) and on a large number of variables, including the caliber of the bullet, the type of ammunition, the distance of the firearm from the body, the locus of the injury, the trajectory of the missile (at right angles to the skin or oblique), and the gyroscopic stability of the bullet (the presence or absence of wobbling or tumbling).

With handguns held at close range (within a foot of the skin surface), there is a gray-black discoloration about the wound of entrance (fouling) produced by the heat, smoke, and burned powder deposits exiting with the bullet from the muzzle. In addition, there may be discrete, larger particles of unburned powder producing a halo of stippling about the entrance wound, the diameter of which depends on the distance of the gun from the body (Fig. 9–11). When firearms are held more than a foot away, but within 3 feet, there may be only stippling without fouling. At greater distances, neither is present. Generally, the perforating cutaneous wound is slightly smaller than the diameter of the bullet and has a narrow enclosing rim of abrasion. When the trajectory of the bullet is angled into the skin, the abrasion is asymmetric, having its greatest width at the margin closest to the origin of the bullet. Depending on the size and velocity of the bullet and the distance between the target and the muzzle of the firearm, when the skin is closely applied to underlying bone, as in the scalp, entering gas may elevate the overlying skin and, in some instances, produce stellate lacerations about the

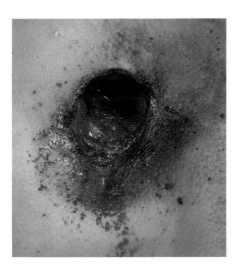

Figure 9–11. An entry gunshot wound at close range revealing the prominent black discoloration *(bottom right)* produced by unburned powder, heat, and smoke as well as the more peripheral stippling resulting from larger particles of unburned powder. (Courtesy of George Katsas, M.D., Forensic Pathologist, Boston.)

perforating wound. Similarly, large-caliber, high-velocity missiles, after penetrating the skin and subcutaneous tissues, may traverse internal organs and, by their mass and velocity, cause extending massive lacerations through the liver or other viscera. In contrast, smaller, low-velocity bullets, even though they penetrate the organ, may produce only fairly restricted burrowing or through-and-through tracts with limited surrounding injury.

Cutaneous exit wounds are generally more irregular than wounds of entrance, because in passing through the tissues the bullet almost inevitably develops a wobbling or yawing trajectory. In fact, with high-velocity rifle bullets, the exit wound may be considerably larger than the entrance wound. The margins of the wound may be everted, and there is no fouling or stippling and, often, little surrounding abrasion. To the experienced eye, it is evident that gunshot wounds tell a story.

INJURIES RELATED TO CHANGES IN TEMPERATURE

Homeothermic humans must maintain their internal temperature within the relatively narrow range of 30°C and 42°C, and even these limits can be tolerated only briefly. Abnormally high and low temperatures produce different patterns of tissue damage and, so, must be discussed separately. Because hyperthermic injuries are so much more common than hypothermic ones, the brunt of attention will be directed to them.

Hyperthermic Injuries

Localized hyperthermia, causing mostly cutaneous burns, is responsible for about 5000 deaths annually in the United States, a large proportion being particularly tragic because they involve children and young adults. Systemic hyperthermia is largely a functional disorder and will be treated briefly.

Cutaneous Burns

The clinical significance of a burn depends on many factors:

- Percentage of total body surface involved
- Depth of the burn
- Possible presence of internal injuries from inhalation of hot gases and fumes
- Promptness and efficacy of the postburn therapy, in particular, fluid and electrolyte management, prevention of shock, and prevention or control of wound infection

Continuous improvement in such therapy has almost invalidated the notion that there is an upper limit of burn area compatible with survival. Nonetheless, any burn exceeding 50% of the total body surface, whether superficial or deep, is grave and potentially fatal. Obviously, depth modifies the outlook. Currently, this is expressed by the terms *"partial-thickness"* and *"full-thickness"* burns. In *partial-thickness burns,* the dermis with its skin appendages is spared, and often the epidermis, even though devitalized, continues to provide a cover to the burned area. Such burns are characterized by blistering and, more important, by the regeneration of the epidermis from preserved islands or dermal appendages. Endothelial injury leads to vascular dilatation, proteinaceous fluid exudation, and a mild inflammatory reaction. Depending on the severity of the burn injury, the epidermal cells may reveal evidence of deranged membrane permeability, with nuclear and cellular swelling, or may disclose nuclear pyknosis and granular coagulation of the cytoplasm.

By contrast, *full-thickness burn* implies total destruction of the entire epidermis, extending into the dermis and sometimes even more deeply. Epithelial regeneration can occur only from the margins, and hence resort must often be made to skin grafting. With incineration of the epidermis, the dermal collagen may take on the appearance of a homogeneous gel, and the cytologic changes described for the partial-thickness burn may be seen in the deeper fibroblasts, endothelial cells, and subcutaneous deeper structures. The inflammatory reaction in the underlying vital tissues is commensurately greater than that in partial-thickness burns.

The *systemic consequences* of a burn are far more important than the local injury. In large burns neurogenic shock may appear almost immediately. This may be followed by hypovolemic shock, owing to the copious loss of exudate from the burn surface. The water loss has been calculated to be 0.3 to 0.4 ml/cm² of burn surface per day. Recognition of this problem and the prompt institution of fluid replacement have substantially reduced the postburn mortality. The loss of plasma protein in the exudate may induce sufficient hypoproteinemia to produce generalized edema and, particularly, pulmonary edema.

Yet another hazard the burn victim faces in the early postburn period is colonization of the devitalized tissue and exudate by microbes that proliferate as in a culture flask. The dominant invaders are *Pseudomonas aeruginosa* and antibiotic-resistant strains common in the hospital, such as *Staphylococcus aureus*, and fungi, in particular, Candida species. These wound infections sometimes lead to regional thrombophlebitis, infective endocarditis, pneumonia, cellulitis, and contamination of every square inch of body surface, in particular, the sites of intravascular lines (e.g., heparin locks). Depressed lymphocyte and phagocyte function with impaired humoral and cellular immunity contribute to the microbial growth, which may progress to direct bacteremic spread or the release of bacterial toxins and endotoxins into the circulation. Septic shock with renal failure and/or the acute respiratory distress syndrome may now rear their ugly heads. Thus, in the clinical management of extensive burns, a great effort is extended to prevent secondary infection, for example, débridement of devitalized tissue, the application of topical antibiotics, and provision of temporary or definitive burn covers or grafts.

There are many other problems that bedevil the postburn period. With excess heat loss from the burn wound, there develops a hypermetabolic state that, together with the loss of plasma proteins, may induce serious fluid, electrolyte, and nutritional imbalances. Tissue proteins are mobilized to compensate for the loss of essential proteins; the imbalance may lead to a clinical picture not unlike starvation. Internal injuries in individuals trapped in burning buildings may further complicate the situation. The temperatures within burning rooms may reach 2000°C, and at this level even so-called nonflammable materials ignite or volatilize, with the possible release of inorganic and organic cyanides (from plastics), hydrogen chloride, and acrolein. Sometimes, the oxygen within the closed space is so rapidly consumed that the victim dies of anoxia within minutes. Oral cavity and upper airway injuries may be sustained, ranging from the equivalent of partial-thickness burns to charring of the mucosal surface. If the victim survives, lower airway obstruction may occur as a result of sloughing of necrotic debris, inhalation of inflammatory exudate, mucosal and submucosal edema, and bronchospasm. No small wonder that specialized institutions — "burn hospitals" — have been created to better cope with these very complex clinical problems.

Systemic Hyperthermia — Heat Stroke

Abnormal elevation of the core body temperature above 40°C occurs in two clinical settings:

- *Exertional heat stroke*, seen mostly in marathon runners, football players, laborers, military recruits, and workers in foundries and boiler rooms
- *Classic heat stroke*, seen in the very young and the elderly, the chronically ill, alcoholics, and the morbidly obese, associated usually with febrile illnesses and hot humid weather

Exertional heat stroke is typically associated with hot, dry skin and cessation of sweating (but sometimes occurs with sweating) and, almost always, a lactic acidosis. Rhabdomyolysis, myoglobinemia, myoglobinuria, and acute tubular necrosis (ATN; see Chapter 20) appear in about one-third of these individuals, sometimes complicated by disseminated intravascular coagulation (DIC) and its attendant organ injuries (see Chapter 11).

Classic heat stroke, by contrast, is rarely accompanied by sweating but rather by hot, dry skin and so is sometimes precipitated by drugs that depress sweating (e.g., anticholinergics and phenothiazines). Instead of a lactic acidosis, there is usually a respiratory alkalosis, as carbon dioxide is blown off owing to an increased respiratory rate. Rhabdomyolysis is uncommon, as is ATN. Only infrequently is the course complicated by DIC. However, redistribution of blood to the skin often produces marked hypotension, with central nervous system hypoperfusion causing fainting and sometimes coma.

Abnormally Low Temperatures

The effects of hypothermia depend on whether there is whole body exposure or exposure only of parts. Death may result when the whole body is exposed, without inducing apparent necrosis of cells or tissues, because with slowing of metabolic processes, particularly in the brain and medullary centers, death may appear before apparent changes in cells or tissues. Fortunately, the reduction in metabolic rate that accompanies the hypothermia sometimes permits successful resuscitation of those in coma without significant damage to the brain and viscera — recall the children who have recovered totally after hours of submersion in icy waters.

LOCAL REACTIONS. Chilling or freezing of cells and tissues causes injury in two ways:

1. Direct effects are probably mediated by physical dislocations within cells and the high salt concentrations incident to the crystallization of the intra- and extracellular water.
2. Indirect effects are exerted by circulatory changes. Depending on the rate at which the tem-

perature drops and the duration of the drop, slowly developing chilling may induce vasoconstriction and increased permeability, leading to edematous changes. Such changes are typical of *"trench foot."* Atrophy and fibrosis may follow. Alternatively, with sudden sharp drops in temperature that are persistent, the vasoconstriction and increased viscosity of the blood in the local area may cause ischemic injury and degenerative changes in peripheral nerves. In this situation, only after the temperature begins to return toward normal do the vascular injury and increased permeability with exudation become evident. However, during the period of ischemia, hypoxic changes and infarction necrosis of the affected tissues may develop (e.g., gangrene of toes or feet).

INJURIES RELATED TO CHANGES IN ATMOSPHERIC PRESSURE

Depending on the direction of change (increase or decrease), its rate of development, and the magnitude of change, four separable syndromes are produced:

- High-altitude illness
- Blast injury
- Air or gas embolism
- Decompression disease—also known as caisson disease—which is sometimes referred to as barotrauma

HIGH-ALTITUDE ILLNESS. As is well known, this is encountered in mountain climbers in the rarefied atmosphere encountered at altitudes above 4000 m. The lowered oxygen tension produces progressive mental obtundation and may be accompanied by poorly understood increased capillary permeability with systemic and, in particular, pulmonary edema.

BLAST INJURY. This form of injury obviously implies a violent increase in pressure either in the atmosphere (air blast) or in water (immersion blast). With *air blast*, the compression wave impinges on the side toward the explosion and so may collapse the thorax or violently compress the abdomen, with rupture of internal organs. The pressure wave may enter the airways and damage the alveoli. The following wave of decreased pressure, with its sudden expansion of the abdomen and thorax, may rupture the intestines or lungs. In *immersion blast*, the pressure is supplied to the body from all sides, inducing injuries similar to those of air blast.

AIR OR GAS EMBOLISM. This may occur as a complication of scuba diving, mechanical positive-pressure ventilatory support, and hyperbaric oxygen therapy and only rarely as a manifestation of decompression disease (see below). Common to all these settings is an abnormal increase in intra-al-veolar air or gas pressure, leading to tearing of tissue with entrance of air into the interstitium and small blood vessels. Pulmonary, mediastinal, and subcutaneous emphysema may result, and in some instances, the coalescence of numerous small air or gas emboli that gain access to the arterial circulation may lead acutely to stroke-like syndromes or a myocardial ischemic episode. Either the neurologic or the myocardial embolism may cause sudden death.[34]

DECOMPRESSION (CAISSON) DISEASE. As the name implies, this disorder is encountered in deep-sea divers and underwater workers who spend long periods of time in caissons or tunnels, under increased atmospheric pressure. The injury, encountered with too rapid decompression, is a function of Henry's law, which in essence states that the solubility of a gas in a liquid (e.g., blood) is proportional to the partial pressure of that gas in the environment. As the underwater depth and consequent atmospheric pressure increase, larger and larger amounts of oxygen and accompanying gases (nitrogen or helium) dissolve in the blood and tissue fluids. Once the ascent begins (decompression), the dissolved gases come out of solution and form minute bubbles in the bloodstream and tissues. Coalescence of these bubbles produces ever larger masses capable of becoming significant emboli in the bloodstream. The oxygen bubbles are soluble in blood and tissues and so redissolve. The nitrogen and helium dissolve only slowly. Periarticular bubbles produce *"the bends."* Bubbles formed within the lung or gaseous emboli give rise to respiratory difficulties, with severe substernal pain referred to as the *"chokes."* Various CNS manifestations may appear, ranging from headache and visual disturbances to behavioral disorientation. Involvement of the inner ear may produce vertigo and the *"staggers."* All these manifestations may appear within hours of the too rapid ascent, but sometimes days later skeletal manifestations—*caisson disease of bone*—may appear. It takes the form of foci of aseptic necrosis typically of femoral and humeral heads, and medullary foci particularly in the lower femur and upper tibia, attributed to embolic occlusion of the vascular supply.[35]

ELECTRICAL INJURIES

The passage of an electric current through the body may be without effect; may cause sudden death by disruption of neural regulatory impulses, producing, for example, cardiac arrest; or may cause thermal injury to organs interposed in the pathway of the current. Many variables are involved, but principally the resistance of the tissues to the conductance of the electric current and the intensity of the current. The greater the resistance of tissues, the greater the heat generated. Although all tissues of the body are conductors of electricity, their resistance to flow varies inversely to their water content. Dry skin is particularly resistant, but when skin is wet or immersed in water its resistance is greatly decreased. Thus, an electric current may cause only a surface burn of dry skin but, when transmitted through wet skin, may cause death by disruption of regulatory pathways, producing, for example, ventricular fibrillation or respiratory paralysis without injury to the skin.

The thermal effects of the passage of an electric current depend on its intensity. High-intensity current, such as lightning coursing along the skin, produces linear arborizing burns known as *lightning marks*. Sometimes the intense current is conducted around the victim (so-called flashover), blasting and disrupting the clothing but doing little injury.[36] When lightning is transmitted internally, it may produce sufficient heat and steam to explode solid organs, fracture bones, or char areas of organs. Focal hemorrhages from rupture of small vessels may be seen in the brain. Sometimes, death is preceded by violent convulsions related to brain damage. Less intense voltage may heat, coagulate, or rupture vessels and cause hemorrhages or, in solid organs such as the spleen and kidneys, cause infarctions or ruptures. The vagaries of electric shocks are almost limitless but, in essence, are permutations of interruption of neural pathways or burn injuries.

RADIATION INJURY

Ionizing radiation has proved to be most valuable, for example, in clinical diagnosis and radiotherapy. However, inadvertent exposure to relatively high doses of ionizing radiation is capable of injuring and killing cells, inducing mutations, producing developmental abnormalities in fetuses exposed *in utero*, or even producing latent cancers. On earth it is impossible to escape exposure to radiation. Cosmic rays bathe the earth continuously, as do terrestrial concentrations of radionuclides, such as radon gas. The two constitute natural "background" radiation. Few humans in developed countries escape diagnostic x-rays, and many require radiotherapy as a potential cure for various types of neoplasia. The "early" injurious effects of radiation appear only when certain cumulative levels of exposure to radiation—thresholds—have been exceeded. However, the later appearing consequences may have no thresholds; hence, the public's concern about the possible carcinogenicity of even low-level exposures.[37] Even the nonionizing UV spectrum of sunlight is conceded to be a major factor in the causation of basal and squamous cell carcinomas and melanomas of the skin among whites (see Chapter 26).

Radiation comprises the physical transfer of energy from its site of origin to the biologic target, *inducing ionization of its atoms.* With sufficient transfer of energy, radiation can eject electrons orbiting about the nucleus of atoms to produce ion pairs consisting of the ejected electron and the positive residual nucleus—hence the term "ionizing radiation." The two forms of ionizing radiation are (1) electromagnetic waves, including x-rays and gamma rays (comprising bundles of energy called photons), and (2) particulate radiation, consisting of neutrons and charged particles (e.g., alpha particles, beta particles, protons, deuterons, and mesons).

Mechanisms of Action

In general, the molecular events involved in the ionization of matter are described by two mechanisms: (1) the *"direct" or "target" effect* and (2) the *"indirect" effect.*

The *direct effect* theory proposes that ionizing radiation acts by direct hits on target atoms. All atoms or molecules within the cell, such as enzymatic and structural proteins and RNA, are vulnerable to radiation injury. However, the principal target is DNA, in which radiation produces single- or double-stranded chromosomal breaks. If such breaks are not repaired before mitosis, they may lead to mutations, such as the formation of intramolecular or intermolecular cross-linkages that have the potential to impair the ability of DNA to act as a template.

The *indirect effect* theory proposes that ionizing radiation exerts its effect by radiolysis of cellular water, with the formation of free "hot" radicals. Water represents about 80% of the weight of living organisms. These free radicals (unpaired electrons) then interact with critical atoms and molecules, particularly DNA, to produce chemical modifications and deleterious effects (see Chapter 1).

If the radiation dose is sufficient, the potential effects of these molecular events on the cell are as follows:

1. Reversible injury occurs, with temporary cell swelling and clumping of nuclear chromatin.

2. Cell death, with nuclear pyknosis or karyorrhexis, is accompanied by pronounced cell swelling and disruption.

3. Inhibition of mitotic division in rapidly dividing cells is followed by cell death—*"reproductive death."* Sometimes, irradiated cells undergo nuclear division without the formation of daughter cells, thus producing multinucleate giant cells.

4. Derangements of the mitotic process yield cells with abnormal nuclear morphology and mitotic figures destined to die.

5. More subtle genetic injuries, such as DNA strand breaks, ultimately are responsible for translocations and deletions, accounting for the muta-

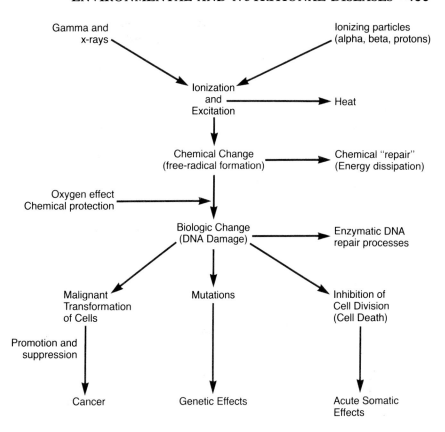

Figure 9–12. Development of radiation injury. (Reproduced with the kind permission of Dr. John B. Little, Harvard School of Public Health. From Little, J.B.: Biologic effects of low-level radiation exposure. In Taveras, J.M., and Ferrucci, J.T. (eds.): Radiology, Diagnosis — Imaging — Intervention, Vol. 1. Philadelphia, J.B. Lippincott Co., 1985.)

genic, teratogenic, and carcinogenic potentials of ionizing radiation that become evident years later. During this long time interval, it is assumed that sequential mitotic divisions are occurring that ultimately "come to the surface." Thus it is said that radiation effects have *"latency"* (Fig. 9–12).

Factors Governing the Biologic Response

Two sets of factors govern the biologic effects of ionizing radiation: (1) those related to the radiation itself and (2) those related to the particular cell and tissue targets affected by the radiation.

Factors related to the radiation comprise the type of radiation, the cumulative dose administered, and the rate of delivery (i.e., time over which the dose is given) because, as will be seen, some repair may take place between divided doses.

The various types of radiation differ in penetrability, energy per unit of radiation, and pattern of deposition of the energy.

When radiation is administered in divided doses, as is usual in the radiotherapy of tumors to spare the normal tissue located over the cancer, its effects are, to an extent, cumulative. The radiation dose administered is usually expressed in rads or centigrays (cGy). One *rad* or 1 *centigray* (1 gray [Gy] corresponds to 100 rad) is the dose of radiation that results in absorption of 100 erg of energy per gram of tissue. In the Systeme Internationale (SI) 1 *sievert* = 100 rem, where a rem equals a rad times a radiation potency factor called a "quality factor." When radionuclides are used as the source of ionizing radiation, it is usually quantitated in terms of *becquerels* (replacing curies). One becquerel denotes 1 decay per second. The half-life of a radionuclide defines the time during which one-half of its unstable atoms will have decayed. It should be noted that the becquerel does not characterize the type of emitted radiation (e.g., gamma rays or beta particles).

None of these quantitations expresses the ability of a given dose of radiation to induce a desired biologic effect. To this end, the following terms are employed.

* *Linear energy transfer* (LET) of the various types of radiation expresses the energy loss or transfer per unit of distance traveled. *The LET thus indicates the likelihood of the radiation's* having an effect within a specific target area and depends on mass, charge, and velocity of the particle or bundle of energy. For example, an alpha particle of large mass but low velocity will deliver its energy within a relatively short distance and have a high LET value. Conversely, gamma rays of high velocity penetrate deeply but generate few interactions along their paths and have a low LET value.

* *Relative biologic effectiveness* (RBE), as the term

implies, compares the effectiveness of different forms of radiation in inducing the same biologic effect.

Whatever the characteristics of a particular form of radiation, the quantity of the radiation is a major factor in determining its potential consequences.

The last consideration relative to the radiation itself is the *time over which a given dose is administered.* Repair of radiation injury, such as repair of a strand break, may occur between divided doses, and so radiant energy is cumulative only to the extent that repair does not nullify some of its effects.

Factors related to the target cells and tissues significantly modify the potential biologic effects of radiation. Of particular importance are (1) the radiosensitivity of different types of normal cells and their tumors, (2) the cells' capacity to repair radiation damage, (3) the phase of the cell cycle during which cells are exposed to the radiation, and (4) the degree of oxygenation of the cells and tissues.

The *cells and tissues of the body and hence their tumors vary in their capacity to sustain radiation injury and survive.* Some are radiosensitive, and others radioresistant.

In general, cells and their tumors are sensitive in the short term to ionizing radiation in direct proportion to their reproductive or mitotic activity, and in inverse proportion to their level of specialization.[38] (Table 9–9). However, the terms "radiosensitive" and "radiocurable," with respect to tumors, are not synonymous. Curability depends on many factors, such as the depth of a neoplasm within the body, the ability to deliver a killing dose of ionizing radiation to it without producing unacceptable damage to surrounding structures, the shielding of the tumor by surrounding structures, and the extent of radiation-induced vascular injury to the blood supply of the tumor. Based on these considerations, a theoretically radiosensitive type of tumor may in fact not be radiocurable, or *vice versa.*

The *phase of the cell cycle* in a population of proliferating cells significantly affects the extent of injury sustained by the cells. Peak sensitivity occurs during G_2 and mitosis, with reduced sensitivity in G_1 and the least sensitivity in the late S phase. Thus, *cells with a high turnover rate, such as those of the bone marrow and mucosa of the small intestine, are particularly vulnerable to radiation injury.* By contrast, such nondividing cells as neurons and muscle cells are less radiosensitive. However, it should be emphasized that all types of cells in the body, whether proliferating or not, can be affected by sufficient quantities of ionizing radiation.

In the normal individual, *cells are capable of repair of sublethal radiation injury.* For example, radiation-induced breaks of a single strand of DNA can be fairly rapidly repaired using the intact

Table 9–9. RADIOSENSITIVITY OF NORMAL TISSUES AND TUMORS

RADIOSENSITIVITY	NORMAL CELLS	TUMORS
High	Lymphoid, hematopoietic, spermatogonia, ovarian follicles	Leukemia-lymphoma, seminoma, dysgerminoma
Fairly high	Acute reactions for gastrointestinal and mucosal epithelium, hair follicles, endothelium Late reactions for lung, kidney	Squamous cell carcinoma of skin, head and neck, and cervix Adenocarcinoma of breast Neuroblastoma
Medium	Late reactions for gastrointestinal tract, endothelium, glandular epithelium of breast, glandular epithelium of pancreas, epithelium of bladder, growing cartilage, bone, and normal brain	Carcinoma of lung, esophagus, pancreas, bladder, medulloblastoma, ovarian cancer
Low	Bone, mature cartilage, muscle, peripheral nerves	Gliomas, large sarcomas, melanoma, renal cell cancer, osteosarcoma

With the gracious help of Dr. Norman Coleman, Harvard Medical School.

strand as a template. However, double-stranded breaks are likely to be irreparable. Analogously, when ionizing radiation causes dimerization or point mutations, the defect can be excised and replaced in most instances. However, in rapidly dividing populations, these small genetic defects, which are compatible with cell survival, may lead to ever larger DNA changes with repeated cell divisions, leading ultimately to a measurable effect. The importance of postirradiation cell repair is amply documented by the small group of autosomal recessive hereditary diseases characterized by some anomaly in DNA metabolism. These diseases are currently thought to involve a cell replication regulator tumor suppressor gene,[39] rendering the cells vulnerable to dysregulation of cell growth and tumorigenesis. These disorders are described in Chapter 7, and so it suffices to recall xeroderma pigmentosum, with its marked predisposition to the development of skin cancers in areas of the body exposed to UV light.

The *oxygenation of tissues* modifies the extent of injury induced by a given quantity of radiation, called the "oxygen enhancement ratio." Oxygenation amplifies low LET radiation damage to a greater extent than high LET radiation. Thus, poorly vascularized regions of tumors having lowered oxygen tensions are less vulnerable to radiotherapy. It is speculated that the "oxygen effect" involves the fixation of radiolesions that would otherwise be reparable.

Morphologic Changes in Cells and Organs Induced by Acute Radiation Injury

Acute changes in this context are those that appear within 60 days of exposure. All cells in the body are vulnerable to radiation injury at some level of exposure. However, even in a uniform population, the amount of injury sustained by individual cells varies. First, the observable general effects on cells will be considered, and then those in specific organs and tissues that are frequent targets of radiation injury.

GENERAL EFFECTS. Although the manifestations of radiation injury may appear in the cytoplasm, the nucleus is the prime target. With sufficient exposure, the nucleus appears swollen, and the chromatin clumped. At higher levels, there is pyknosis and even fragmentation of the nucleus. Abnormal mitotic figures and bizarre nuclear morphology may appear, along with aneuploidy and polyploidy. The cytoplasmic changes include cell swelling, mitochondrial distortion, and degeneration of the endoplasmic reticulum. Plasma membrane focal defects and breaks may appear, and indeed the cell may be disrupted. It should be noted that none of these cellular changes are diagnostic of radiation exposure and that they can be mimicked by the action of various chemotherapeutic agents.

Vascular changes (dose–rate dependent) are prominent in all irradiated tissues. Although endothelial cells are not highly radiosensitive, with sufficient exposure, radiational changes may appear, particularly with antineoplastic radiotherapy. During the immediate postirradiation period, vessels in the skin may show only dilatation, producing some erythema. Later or with higher dosages, there is endothelial swelling and vacuolation or even destruction of endothelial cells, particularly in the microvasculature, with secondary thromboses or hemorrhages. At a later stage, intimal hyperplasia and collagenous hyalinization with thickening of the media develop. Such changes in arterioles and small arteries result in marked narrowing or even obliteration of the vascular lumina.

The *skin* is in the pathway of externally delivered radiation. The area of skin exposed appears to be as critical as dose and type of radiation–the skin being more resistant to necrosis when only small areas are exposed. A range of changes may appear, from mild postirradiation erythema (2 to 3 days), sometimes followed by edema (2 to 3 weeks), to epithelial blistering and desquamation (4 to 6 weeks), to a chronic radiodermatitis (months to years) or even the development of skin cancer. The radiodermatitis takes many forms, including

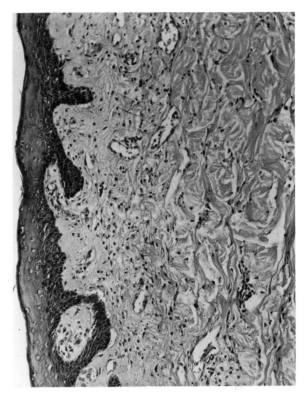

Figure 9–13. Chronic radiodermatitis. There is collagenous hyalinization of dermis, atrophy of skin appendages, and numerous dilated vascular telangiectases.

blotchy increased pigmentation or depigmentation, hyperkeratosis, epilation, skin atrophy, dermal and subcutaneous fibrosis, and, in some instances, telangiectasia and ulcerations (Fig. 9–13). The epidermal cells may show any of the general cytologic alterations described, while the underlying dermis exhibits the characteristic radiation-induced vascular changes accompanied by hyaline collagenization of connective tissue and basophilic degeneration of elastic fibers. The atrophy, depigmentation, and telangiectasia commonly persist for decades. The development of chronic, resistant ulcers is ominous, since they are often forerunners of skin cancer, as experienced by the early x-ray workers.

The *hematopoietic and lymphoid systems* are extremely susceptible to radiant injury. With high dose levels and large exposure fields, severe lymphopenia may appear within hours, along with shrinkage of the lymph nodes and spleen. With sublethal doses of irradiation, regeneration is prompt from viable precursors, leading to restoration of the lymphocytes in the blood within weeks to months. The circulating granulocyte count begins to fall toward the end of the first week, with possibly disappearance of these cells in the circulating blood during the second week. If the patient survives, the normal neutrophil count returns within 2 to 3 months. Platelets are similarly affected, with the nadir of the count occurring

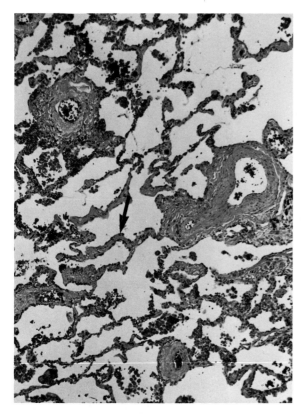

Figure 9–14. Chronic radiation damage to lungs. Note collagenous hyaline thickening of blood vessel walls and fibrosis of septal walls *(arrow)*.

somewhat later than that of the granulocytes; the recovery is similarly delayed. Erythrocytes themselves are radioresistant, but their precursors may be destroyed by heavy exposure, leading in time to severe anemias. Obviously, the severity of the blood and marrow depletion depends on the dose-rate of exposure. Whole body irradiation may be lethal, whereas localized exposure may have no effect on the circulating blood counts. The neutropenia and thrombocytopenia are responsible for increased susceptibility to infections and bleeding diatheses during the postirradiation period. However, if the patient survives, normal marrow function may be restored.

Studies of the survivors of the atomic bomb blasts and radiation accidents have unmistakably demonstrated the leukemogenic effect of radiation.

The *gonads* in both the male and the female, particularly the germinal epithelium, are highly vulnerable to radiation. Sclerosis of the germinal tubules may be evident, but Sertoli's cells and interstitial cells may persist and, in the ovaries, only sclerosed follicles remain. Hence, sterility is a hazard of sufficient gonadal radiation. In passing, it might be noted that the uterus and cervix are relatively radioresistant, and so radionuclides can be inserted into the uterine cavity for the treatment of cervical and endometrial carcinomas.

The *lungs*, because of their rich vascularization, are vulnerable to radiation injury. During the immediate postirradiation period, the endothelial cell changes described in the blood vessels are seen in the alveolar capillaries. The increased vascular permeability may lead to marked pulmonary congestion and edema and the other changes encountered in adult respiratory distress syndrome (ARDS; see Chapter 15). Later, there is fibrosis of the alveolar walls, with the described vascular wall thickening and luminal narrowing (Fig. 9–14). The respiratory dysfunction can be crippling or fatal, since the radiation "pneumonitis" creates a profound alveolocapillary block.

The *gastrointestinal tract* is very radiosensitive and is frequently affected in all forms of deep radiation. The esophagus and rectum are relatively radioresistant, but the midportions of the tract, particularly the colon and small intestine, are quite sensitive. It is the intestinal epithelium (crypt cells) with its high turnover rate that bears the brunt of the damage, with all forms of nuclear and cellular

Table 9–10. RADIATION CHANGES IN VARIOUS ORGANS

ORGAN	EARLY AND LATE CHANGES	DELAYED CONSEQUENCES
Heart	Fibrinous pericarditis, myocardial edema, "radiation cardiomyopathy"	Pericardial fibrosis, myocardial interstitial fibrosis
Kidney	Acute tubular injury, vascular sclerosis	Cortical atrophy with tubular sclerosis and glomerular hyalinization, "chronic radiation nephritis"
Bladder	Acute damage to lining epithelium —"radiation cystitis"—with ulceration	Persistent mucosal atrophy, fibrosis of bladder wall
Cartilage and bone	In fetus and child, growing bone and cartilage are radiosensitive with the potential for later skeletal distortion; in the adult they are radioresistant, save for the possible development of areas of aseptic necrosis where the vascular supply is obliterated	Late appearing osteogenic sarcoma
Central nervous system	In developing fetus, the embryonic brain is radiosensitive; mature nervous tissue is radioresistant	Areas of demyelination and ganglion cell degenerative changes secondary to radiation-induced ischemia
Breast		Late appearing cancers

Table 9–11. ACUTE RADIATION SYNDROME CLASSIFICATION

CATEGORY	WHOLE-BODY DOSE, rem	SIGNS AND SYMPTOMS Early	SIGNS AND SYMPTOMS Definitive	PROGNOSIS
Subclinical	≤ 200	Mild nausea and vomiting lasting 24 hr or less; lymphocytes < 1500/mm³	Usually asymptomatic to minimal prodromal symptoms; depression of neutrophils and platelets by week 4–5 at higher dose range	Essentially 100% survival in healthy adults; evidence of some damage at higher dose range
Hematopoietic (mild form)	200–400	Intermittent nausea and vomiting in nearly all patients for 2–4+ days; lymphocytes < 1000/mm³	Maximum hematopoietic depression at 3 weeks	Recovery in 5–6 weeks; complete recovery in 4–6 months
Hematopoietic (severe form)	400–600*	Severe hematopoietic complications; mild evidence of gastrointestinal damage on upper dose range	Severe neutrophil and platelet depression in 3–5 weeks; evidence of infection and hemorrhage may appear	Zero to 100% mortality in untreated cases; requires bone marrow transplants and other supportive measures; rarely fatal with adequate replacement therapy
Gastrointestinal	600–1000	Severe prodromal symptoms of nausea, vomiting, and diarrhea; difficult management of patient; lymphocytes < 500/mm³	Some recovery, then return of severe diarrhea with blood and electrolyte loss; severe neutrophil and platelet depression by day 10 or earlier; hemorrhage and infection within 1–3 weeks	High mortality even among those given functional replacement therapy; progression to shock and death in 10–14 days; effectiveness of bone marrow therapy not yet evaluated
Central nervous system	≥ 1000	Severe, intractable nausea and vomiting; central nervous system symptoms; burning sensation at exposure and confusion; lymphocytes essentially lacking	Partial recovery, then progressive confusion and shock; central nervous system damage	100% mortality likely independent of therapy given; death in 14–36 hr; marrow therapy trial indicated

* The human whole-body LD$_{50}$ at 60 days is approximately 400–500 rem.

From Castronovo F.P.: Radiation accidents. In Wilkins, E.W., Jr. (ed.): Emergency Medicine: Scientific Foundations and Current Practice, 3rd ed. Baltimore, Williams & Wilkins, 1989. With permission of Dr. Castronovo, Dept. of Radiology, Brigham & Women's Hospital, Boston, MA, and Williams & Wilkins Publishing.

pleomorphism, mitotic abnormality, and cell necrosis. Later, ulcerations may appear, accompanied by vascular and connective tissue changes such as are encountered elsewhere. The late effects of intestinal injury comprise mucosal and submucosal atrophy and fibrosis, occasionally producing esophageal and intestinal strictures. Cancers may appear later if the individual survives.

The changes in *other organs* are briefly characterized in Table 9–10.

Whole Body Radiation

Exposure of large areas of the body to even 100 rad, especially when it is whole body irradiation, may have devastating effects and may induce an "acute radiation syndrome." To place this in context, 4000 rad or more is often used in divided doses in carefully shielded patients in the radiotherapy of tumors. The consequences of whole body exposure can be segregated into hematopoi-etic, gastrointestinal, and CNS syndromes, as shown in Table 9–11.

Late Effects of Radiation

As mentioned earlier, the late effects take the forms of mutations, anomalies in fetuses exposed *in utero*, and cancer induction.

Radiation is a mutagen when delivered in sufficient quantities. The various molecular forms of injury to DNA have already been mentioned. A variety of karyotypic alterations have been observed in lymphocytes (known to be very radiosensitive) of individuals who have received significant doses of ionizing radiation. Any of these mutations may provide the subsoil for the later development of a cancer.

The *in utero effects* of radiation are of obvious concern to pregnant women who have received significant exposures to ionizing radiation. Regrettably, the numerous studies of this problem have failed to yield definitive answers. On the one hand, studies of those exposed to radiation *in utero* point to an increased rate of stillbirths, mental retardation, and congenital malformation and an increased frequency of various forms of cancer before age 20 years (principally leukemias and lymphomas).[40] On the other hand, a very careful comparison of a large cohort of individuals whose parents had been exposed to radiation during the bombing of Hiroshima and Nagasaki comparing them with an equally large age- and sex-matched cohort of individuals born of parents living in these two cities but who were not exposed to radiation revealed no significant differences between the two groups with respect to a large number of variables, including congenital defects, stillbirths, and cancer at an early age.[41] So the issue is still controversial and requires continued study.

The *carcinogenic potential of radiant energy* has been amply documented in lower animals and humans. Much of the documentation was cited in Chapter 7. Here it will suffice to point out the increased frequency of various forms of cancer among survivors of the atomic bomb blasts at Hiroshima and Nagasaki. A 20-fold increased incidence of acute leukemia has occurred in those who were younger than 10 years or older than 50 years of age at the time of the blasts. All forms of leukemia have appeared save, for mysterious reasons, chronic lymphocytic leukemia. In children younger than 10 years of age at the time of exposure, there has been an increased incidence of breast cancer (in females) and thyroid cancer as well as, possibly, lymphoma, multiple myeloma, and cancers of the stomach, esophagus, urinary tract, and salivary glands. Individuals 50 years of age or older at the time of exposure have suffered a notable increase in the incidence of lung cancer. In addition, atomic bomb survivors have developed lenticular opacities.

Although the atomic blasts will never again be repeated, we trust, postirradiation cancers have appeared in patients receiving radiation for ankylosing spondylitis, and second cancers have appeared following successful treatment of a primary tumor by radiotherapy sometimes coupled with chemotherapy. Because of these examples of the potential nonthreshold carcinogenicity of ionizing radiation, there is, understandably, great concern about low-level radiation, as may be emitted from nuclear reactors and nuclear waste sites. But these fears must not be permitted to undermine the great value of radiation in clinical diagnosis and tumor therapy.

NUTRITIONAL DISEASE

Malnutrition, and more particularly undernutrition, constitute globally the most important category of environmental disease. Although there are

Table 9–12. MAJOR CAUSES OF SECONDARY MALNUTRITION

DECREASED INTAKE

Poor teeth
Dysphagia
Systemic disease inducing anorexia
Bizarre or restricted food habits
Anorexia nervosa

MALABSORPTION

Biliary and pancreatic diseases
Enteric malabsorption syndromes
Vitamin B_{12} malabsorption (pernicious anemia)

INCREASED REQUIREMENTS

Rapid growth in infancy, in childhood, and at puberty
Pregnancy, particularly repeated
Trauma
Burns
Excessive losses, as in protein-losing enteropathies and nephropathies

SPECIAL CATEGORIES

Total parenteral nutrition
Drug-induced interference with absorption
Genetic disorders interfering with conversion or utilization of nutrients

many forms of malnutrition—for example, obesity from consumption of excessive calories and avitaminoses from inadequate diet or malabsorption—the dominant problem confronting the world is protein-calorie undernutrition, indeed starvation, as is rampant in many parts of Africa. In the following sections, we shall address this dominating problem first, followed by a consideration of deficiencies of specific vitamins and minerals and concluding with a discussion of some examples of nutritional excesses and imbalances.

Malnutrition and undernutrition are not restricted to the Third World; they are also common even in affluent societies. A lack of all kinds of food and, in particular, protein (so-called primary malnutrition) may be encountered in industrialized nations in pockets of poverty. More common in the industrialized nations is secondary, or "conditioned malnutrition," having many possible origins (Table 9–12).

Whether the nutritional disorder is primary or secondary, overt morphologic lesions are relatively late manifestations and may be preceded for long periods of time by functional deficits. For example, the first manifestation of chronic starvation may be merely listlessness or apathy. Iron deficiency may induce reduced physical and mental capacity, impaired learning ability, and deranged white blood cell function long before the appearance of anemia. Thus, most deficiency states require clinical and biochemical tests for their early discovery, because by the time morphologic changes, if any, appear the malnutrition must be present for a long time.

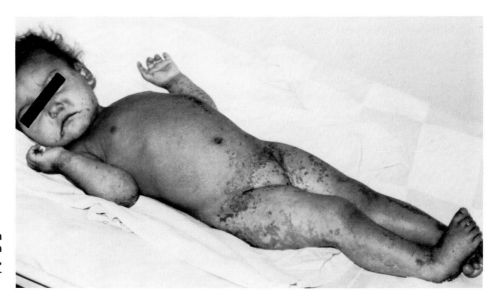

Figure 9-15. An infant with kwashiorkor revealing moon face, generalized edema, and skin rash over the extremities and lower trunk.

PROTEIN-CALORIE UNDERNUTRITION

Protein-calorie undernutrition, also called protein-energy malnutrition (PEM), is rampant in Third World countries, particularly among infants and children. Multiple pregnancies and malnutrition of the mother favor prematurity and low birth weights, predisposing these infants to protein-calorie malnutrition from the day of their birth. Although precise data are not available, the World Health Organization (WHO) estimates that there are more than half a billion individuals suffering from mild to severe undernutrition, and even more staggering, 10 million people, mostly children, die of starvation annually.[43] Grossly oversimplified, crop failures due to loss of arable land and inadequate rain, coupled with global maldistribution of food and uncontrolled parasitic and microbial infections, underlie this massive tragedy. However, PEM is not confined to less developed countries. Mild disease, and sometimes severe PEM, are encountered in industrialized nations, such as the United States, in individuals who have been severely ill or who live in extreme poverty and, particularly, among the very young and the elderly, pregnant women, drug addicts, and the homeless and in both medical and surgical patients, particularly those in chronic care hospitals. Prolonged protein-calorie undernutrition produces a spectrum of syndromes from kwashiorkor at one end, caused by a critical lack of protein despite a sufficient caloric intake, to marasmus at the other end, caused by an overall lack of calories, or more bluntly starvation. The term "kwashiorkor" in the Ga language means "the disease of the displaced child," when a newborn assumes breastfeeding and the older child is weaned to a diet almost entirely of carbohydrates. Between these two extremes are many intermediate syndromes that, in fact, are more common than the well-defined ends of the spectrum. Contributing significantly to the problem, particularly in infants and children, are the virtually universal contagious diseases, microbial-induced diarrhea, and infestations with worms (e.g., ascariasis, trichuriasis, strongyloidiasis, and amebiasis). The protein-calorie malnutrition impairs the immune response, giving rise to a vicious cycle: the infections worsen the protein-calorie imbalance, and *vice versa*. In addition, there is, understandably, almost always a concomitant deficiency of one or more of the vitamins. By examining the classic syndromes of kwashiorkor and marasmus, we can understand the intermediate stages of malnutrition.

Kwashiorkor is characterized by apathy, peripheral edema, subcutaneous fat, moon face, enlarged fatty liver, and low serum albumin (Fig. 9-15). The edema is usually generalized, and often, but not invariably, there are dermatoses presenting as "flaky paint" areas of depigmentation or hyperpigmentation. The hair often develops a fine texture, is loosely rooted, and has a pale reddish hue, with alternating bands of depigmentation and pigmentation, the former reflecting periods of poor nutrition, and the latter more adequate nutrition (Fig. 9-16). Typically there is a moderate to severe anemia. The basis for these morphologic changes is not clear. The edema could be attributed to hypoalbuminemia, along with sodium retention. The fatty liver has been thought to be related to impaired hepatic synthesis of the acceptor proteins necessary for the formation of the lipoproteins that are involved in the mobilization of lipids from liver cells. Recently, however, it has been suggested that the hepatic damage is due to aflatoxin toxicity and chronic free radical exposure,

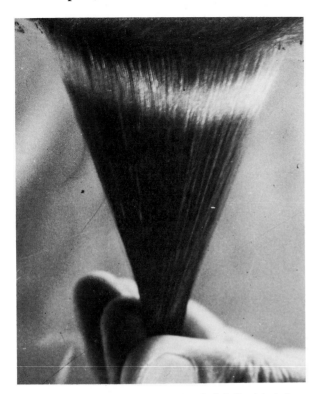

Figure 9–16. Kwashiorkor "flag sign." A tuft of hair in an infant showing a striking band of depigmentation, marking a period of severe malnutrition. (Courtesy of Dr. N. Scrimshaw, Massachusetts Institute of Technology; and the Institute of Nutrition of Central America and Panama.)

marasmus than in kwashiorkor, (2) peripheral edema in kwashiorkor but not in marasmus, and (3) loss of body fat and atrophy of the muscle mass in marasmus. The many hybrid forms obviously share the features of both syndromes.

The **liver** fatty change in kwashiorkor is not different from that encountered under other circumstances. With restoration of an adequate diet, fat is mobilized and no residuals are left. Rarely, if ever, does cirrhosis supervene.

The **small bowel** in kwashiorkor (rarely in marasmus) may reveal mucosal atrophy, with loss of villi and microvilli, and disappearance of mitoses in the epithelium of the crypts. Almost invariably there are secondary changes induced by the masses of worms (previously cited) found in these victims.

The **bone marrow** in both kwashiorkor and marasmus is often hypoplastic, owing mainly to depressed numbers of red blood cell precursors. The resultant anemia is usually related to an iron deficiency worsened by the ever-present intestinal worms. However, a dietary deficiency of folates may lead to a mixed microcytic-macrocytic anemia. Adequate diet and control of infections promptly correct the hematologic abnormalities.

The **brain** in infants of malnourished mothers

secondary to a lack of antioxidant nutrients in the diet, for example, vitamin E. These new theories are considered speculative at this time.

Marasmus can be succinctly characterized as "wasting." These tragic infants and children have stunted growth and a total loss of subcutaneous fat with atrophy of muscles, producing broomstick arms and legs from which the skin hangs pathetically loose. The facies are pinched and wizened, imparting a prematurely aged appearance. In contrast with those with kwashiorkor, these children are alert and hungry and will eat ravenously if given food. There is no edema or hepatic enlargement in the pure marasmic syndrome. However, in the hybrid forms, such as edematous marasmus, features of both ends of the spectrum are present.

The basis for marasmus is all too evident — inadequate food consumption — but the contribution of infection is extremely material. Numerous studies have documented that infants and children on marginal diets can be prevented from developing protein-calorie undernutrition by control of intercurrent infections and by oral rehydration therapy when persistent diarrhea has been a problem.[44]

MORPHOLOGY. The central anatomic changes in PEM are (1) growth failure, more marked in

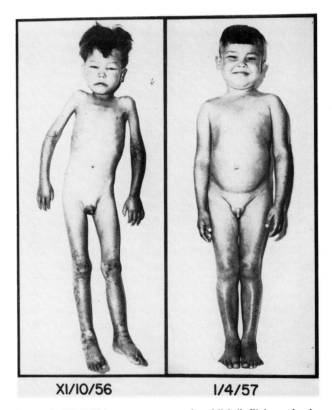

XI/10/56   I/4/57

Figure 9–17. Within every marasmic child *(left)* is a sturdy, smiling youngster, seen *(right)* after 2 months of adequate nutrition. (Courtesy of Dr. N. Scrimshaw, Massachusetts Institute of Technology; and the Institute of Nutrition of Central America and Panama.)

suffering from PEM is reported by some observers to show cerebral atrophy during the first 1 to 2 years of life, a reduced number of neurons, and impaired myelinization of the white matter. However, there is no universal agreement on these findings.

Many **other changes** may be present, including thymic and peripheral lymph node atrophy and other alterations incident to deficiencies of other essential elements, such as iodine.

With restoration of an adequate diet and control of infections, most of the changes in PEM are reversible, including "catch-up growth" and restoration of physical health in all but the terminally ill (Fig. 9–17). Some uncertainty persists as to whether "intellectual health" can be completely restored, but it is not certain whether such cognitive deficits as may be present are of nutritional origin rather than social or cultural.

VITAMINS

Vitamins are organic micronutrients found in a large variety of foods, which are essential for health because they serve as critical catalytic cofactors or prosthetic groups on enzymes involved in vital metabolic reactions. Four vitamins—A, D, E, and K—are fat soluble, and nine—C and the vitamin B complex—are water soluble. Small amounts of vitamins D and K, niacin, and biotin (the last two part of the vitamin B complex) can be synthesized endogenously; however, exogenous sources of all are required to maintain health. As with other nutrients, a deficiency of vitamins may be primarily dietary in origin or may be secondary to some derangement in absorption, transport, storage, or metabolic conversion. Primary deficiencies almost always involve multiple vitamins and, frequently, protein-calorie undernutrition as well. Secondary, conditioned deficiency states, however, may be quite specific, as is the case, for example, with vitamin B_{12} in pernicious anemia. Under certain circumstances, conditioned deficiencies involve multiple vitamins, as is the case in fat malabsorption states (e.g., biliary tract and pancreatic disease). The fat-soluble vitamins can be stored in the body and mobilized as needed during long periods of deprivation. The amounts stored vary with the particular vitamins, as will become evident. The water-soluble vitamins are not stored in comparable amounts, permitting deficiency states to occur after relatively short periods of deprivation.

Although vitamin deficiencies are much more common in Third World countries, they are surprisingly prevalent in industrialized countries as well, and most are dietary in origin, related to socioeconomic factors. Of particular importance are poverty and ignorance of the nutritional composition of foods. But deficiency states are also often encountered in alcoholics and in the very elderly with their restricted diets even in the midst of plenty. A survey of the various vitamins is offered in Table 9–13.

FAT-SOLUBLE VITAMINS

Hypovitaminoses of the fat-soluble vitamins, A and D, on the basis of primary malnutrition are very common in the underprivileged of tropical areas of the world but are also surprisingly common among the poor in industrialized countries, who for economic reasons subsist on restricted diets. Primary deficiencies of vitamins E and K are much less common, for reasons that will become apparent later. However, conditioned deficiencies of any one of the fat-soluble vitamins occur sporadically throughout the world, even in individuals in affluent societies in the presence of biliary tract or pancreatic dysfunction or the intestinal malabsorption syndromes.

Vitamin A

The well-established consequences of vitamin A deficiency are xerophthalmia (conjunctival keratinization), keratomalacia (corneal softening and ulceration), corneal scarring and blindness, impaired maintenance of special epithelia with squamous metaplasia of transitional epithelium and columnar mucus-secreting surfaces, and impaired immune responses with increased mortality from infections (in children) (Fig. 9–18).

Possible consequences of vitamin A deficiency are impaired reproduction (in laboratory animals), impaired skeletal growth (in laboratory animals), and increased predisposition to cancers of the skin, lungs, and other sites (in laboratory animals and possibly in humans).

Next to protein-calorie undernutrition, vitamin A deficiency is the most prevalent nutritional disorder in the world. It is rampant in Southeast Asia, parts of China and Africa, and many other Third World countries. It is estimated that, in these regions, there are about five to ten million new cases of xerophthalmia annually, resulting in blindness in about a quarter million people. It is less widely appreciated that marginal deficiencies of vitamin A are sometimes found among the poor in industrialized countries.

A number of compounds have vitamin A activity; the most important and most active is retinol, but its derivatives retinal (the aldehyde) and retinoic acid also have some vitamin A activity. The important dietary sources of these retinoids are such animal-derived foods as eggs, butter, meat, whole milk, and fish livers. There also are well

Table 9-13. VITAMINS: MAJOR ROLES AND DEFICIENCY SYNDROMES

VITAMIN	ROLES	DEFICIENCY SYNDROMES
Fat-Soluble		
Vitamin A	A component of visual pigment Maintenance of specialized epithelia Maintenance of resistance to infection	Night blindness, xerophthalmia, and blindness Squamous metaplasia Vulnerability to infections, particularly measles
Vitamin D	Facilitates intestinal absorption of Ca and PO_4, and mineralization of bone	Rickets in children Osteomalacia in adults
Vitamin E	Major antioxidant; scavenges free radicals	Spinocerebellar degeneration
Vitamin K	Cofactor in hepatic carboxylation of procoagulants—factors II (prothrombin), VII, IX, and X	Bleeding diathesis
Water-Soluble		
Vitamin B_1 (thiamine)	As pyrophosphate, is coenzyme in decarboxylation reactions Facilitates conduction of impulses in peripheral nerves	Dry and wet beriberi, Wernicke's syndrome, ?Korsakoff's syndrome
Vitamin B_2 (riboflavin)	Converted to coenzymes flavin mononucleotide (FMN) and flavin-adenine dinucleotide (FAD), cofactors for many enzymes in intermediary metabolism	Ariboflavinosis, cheilosis, stomatitis, glossitis, dermatitis, corneal vascularization
Niacin	Incorporated into nicotinamide-adenine dinucleotide (NAD) and NAD phosphate (NADP) involved in a variety of redox reactions	Pellagra—three "D's": dementia, dermatitis, diarrhea
Vitamin B_6 (pyridoxine)	Derivatives serve as coenzymes in many intermediary reactions	Cheilosis, glossitis, dermatitis, peripheral neuropathy
Vitamin B_{12} (cyanocobalamin)	Requisite for normal folate metabolism and DNA synthesis Maintenance of myelinization of spinal cord tracts	Combined system disease (megaloblastic pernicious anemia and degeneration of posterolateral spinal cord tracts)
Vitamin C	Serves in many oxidation-reduction (redox) reactions and hydroxylation of collagen	Scurvy
Folate	Essential for transfer and utilization of 1-carbon units in DNA synthesis	Megaloblastic anemia
Pantothenic acid	Incorporated in coenzyme A	No nonexperimental syndrome recognized
Biotin	Cofactor in carboxylation reactions Widely abundant in foods	No clearly defined clinical syndrome

over 2000 synthetic analogs of vitamin A that have some, but not necessarily all, of its biologic activities. The term "retinoid" encompasses both naturally occurring and synthetic forms of vitamin A. There are, in addition, the *carotenoids,* which are vitamin A precursors, the most important of these being beta-carotene, consisting essentially of two linked molecules of retinol. The carotenoids are richly abundant in leafy green and yellow vegetables, such as spinach, carrots, sweet potatoes, and squash.

Only a few comments will be made about the normal metabolism of vitamin A; further details are available in the review by Tee.[45] As with all fats, the digestion and absorption of carotenes and reti-noids requires bile salts, pancreatic enzymes, and some level of concomitant fat absorption. Storage occurs in the liver; the reserves are sufficient for many months of deprivation. As needed, the esters are hydrolyzed, and the retinol is bound to a specific retinol-binding protein (RBP) called transthyretin for transport in the blood, to the cells of the body. All cells appear to have specific membrane receptors for RBP, and cytosolic retinol-binding proteins (CRBPs) for transport to the nucleus. However, the precise intracellular function of vitamin A is, for the most part, not understood, as will become clear, but it is suspected that in some way it is involved in genomic expression and cell growth and replication.

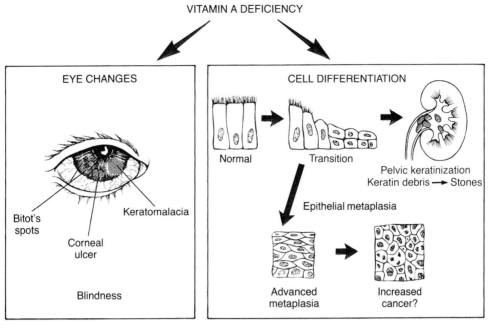

Figure 9-18. Vitamin A deficiency: its major consequences in the eye, in the production of keratinizing metaplasia of specialized epithelial surfaces, and its possible role in potentiating neoplasia.

CONSEQUENCES OF A DEFICIENCY. In humans, the major defined functions of vitamin A can be categorized as the following:

- Maintenance of specialized, mainly mucus-secreting, epithelia
- Provision of a critical prosthetic group in the visual pigments in the retina
- Enhancement of immunity to infections, particularly in children
- Antioxidant function, particularly the carotenoids
- Putative anticarcinogenic action resulting from an apparent regulatory effect on cell growth

In animals, vitamin A appears to be involved in growth and reproduction, but no comparable effects have been found in humans. *Squamous metaplasia of specialized epithelium* occurs with vitamin A deficiency. Curiously, some epithelia are less severely affected than others. For example, in the intestines, there is some loss of mucus-secreting cells but no squamous replacement, whereas in the cornea and conjunctivae, upper respiratory tract, urinary tract, and pancreatic and salivary glands the squamous metaplasia is pronounced. The consequences of such changes in the eyes are extremely serious, as will be detailed. In the respiratory tract, the loss of the "antimicrobial" mucociliary escalator predisposes to respiratory infections. Desquamated squames in the urinary tract provide a nidus for stone formation. Shedding of epithelial cells in the small lumina of the salivary glands and pancreas promotes secretory obstruction and infections. Squamous metaplasia of the se-

baceous and sweat glands of the skin may cause *follicular hyperkeratosis* and predispose to acne.

Vision, particularly in reduced light, is critically dependent on vitamin A. The four kinds of visual pigment in the retina comprise retinal rhodopsin in the rods, the most light-sensitive pigment and, therefore, important in reduced light, and three iodopsins in cone cells, each responsive to specific colors in bright light. Retinol from the blood is oxidized to all-*trans*-retinal and, then, isomerized to 11-*cis*-retinal, which interacts with opsin (a protein) to form rhodopsin. When light impinges on the dark-adapted retina, rhodopsin undergoes a sequence of configurational changes, ultimately yielding all-*trans*-retinal and opsin. In the process, a signal is generated (by changes in membrane potential) that is transmitted over neural pathways to the brain. During dark adaptation, some of the all-*trans*-retinal is reconverted to 11-*cis*-retinal, but most is reduced to retinol and lost to the retina, dictating the need for a continuous supply of retinal. We owe to George Wald and his collaborators this elegant delineation of the function of Vitamin A, which is indeed the only clearly understood function of retinol in the body.[46] Hence, impaired vision in reduced light—*"night blindness"* (nyctalopia)—is an early manifestation of vitamin A deficiency.

In addition to visual changes, vitamin A deficiency may lead to total blindness. Replacement of the normal, moist corneal and conjunctival surfaces by nonsecretory squamous, keratinizing epithelium (xerosis) leads to a "dry eye," or *xerophthalmia*. This is followed by the appearance of small, gray-

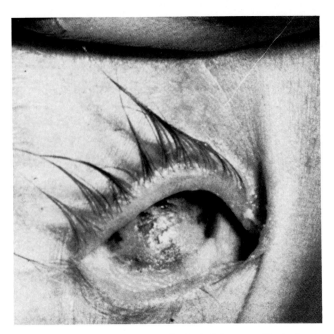

Figure 9–19. Advanced vitamin A deficiency with destruction of the eye. (Reproduced with the kind permission of Dr. Donald S. McLaren, Department of Medicine, Royal Infirmary, Edinburgh. From McLaren, D.: A Colour Atlas of Nutritional Disorders. London, Wolfe Medical Publications, Ltd., 1981, p. 26.)

white plaques of piled-up squamous cells, producing *Bitot's spots*. With more severe vitamin A deficiency, the dry conjunctival and corneal surfaces are prone to ulceration and infection with corneal softening, termed *keratomalacia*. Subsequent scarring or extrusion of the lens may then occur, producing irreversible *blindness*. Vitamin A deficiency is a leading cause of blindness in the world (Fig. 9–19).

Impaired immunity and increased vulnerability to childhood infections appear to be other consequences of vitamin A deficiency. The supporting evidence is somewhat contradictory and still accumulating. But in several studies, the mortality rate from childhood infections (e.g., measles, among children in Indonesia with mild xerophthalmia) was reported to be about four times higher than that of control subjects. Analogously, vitamin A supplementation in the same area reduced the mortality by about 50%.[47] However, attempts to document depressed immune functions in vitamin A–depleted patients have failed to detect any significant impairment in either humoral or cell-mediated immunity.

Mention was made earlier of the possibility that a deficiency of vitamin A may increase the predisposition to certain forms of cancer, is still under study. Here it will suffice that derivatives of vitamin A have proved to be successful in the treatment of several types of skin disease characterized by keratinizing epithelial hyperplasia, such as acne, actinic keratosis, and psoriasis, and have

remarkably controlled acute promyelocytic leukemia by inducing transient maturation of the leukemic myeloid forms (see Chapter 14).

HYPERVITAMINOSIS A TOXICITY. The long-term use of large doses of vitamin A derivatives as an antiproliferative (and particularly retinol) must take into consideration possible adverse consequences. These include headaches, nausea and vomiting, diarrhea, irritability, drowsiness, immunologic abnormalities, and loss of hair. With chronic toxicity, lymphadenopathy and painful, bony hyperostoses may appear. In the infant, there may be premature closure of the fontanelles. Recovery usually promptly follows discontinuance of the vitamin excess, but in pregnant women, long-term treatment with the synthetic retinoids has induced an increased incidence of congenital malformations in the embryo.

An excess of carotenoids is without toxicity. However—rabbits and carrot freaks here take note—hypercarotenemia can induce yellowing of the skin but, unlike the jaundice of hyperbilirubinemia, not of the sclerae.

Vitamin D

The well-established deficiency states are rickets in children, osteomalacia in adults, and hypocalcemic tetany.

The function of vitamin D, or more properly of its metabolites, is the maintenance of adequate serum levels of calcium and phosphate for normal mineralization of bone. *A deficiency of vitamin D function in adults impairs or blocks the normal mineralization of osteoid laid down in the remodeling of bone, producing osteomalacia. In growing children, not only is there inadequate mineralization of osteoid, but also there is inadequate provisional mineralization of epiphyseal cartilage, inducing rickets.* Although both conditions may be caused by a dietary lack of vitamin D, there are many other causes as well.

Humans have two possible sources of vitamin D—endogenous synthesis in the skin from the precursor 7-dehydrocholesterol converted to vitamin D_3 by UV light, and exogenous dietary sources such as deep-sea fish, dairy products fortified with vitamin D, and grains. These foods contain ergosterol, which is converted to vitamin D_2 in the body. Since vitamins D_3 and D_2 have virtually identical functional activities, they hereafter will be referred to as vitamin D.

Before vitamin D can subserve its function in maintaining the serum calcium and phosphate levels, it must first undergo metabolic conversion to its active metabolite involving the following steps, which have been schematized in Figure 9–20:

NORMAL VITAMIN D METABOLISM

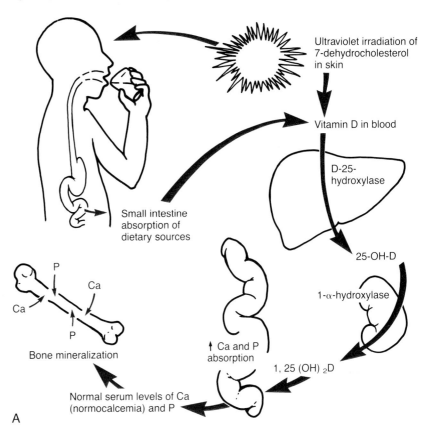

A

VITAMIN D DEFICIENCY

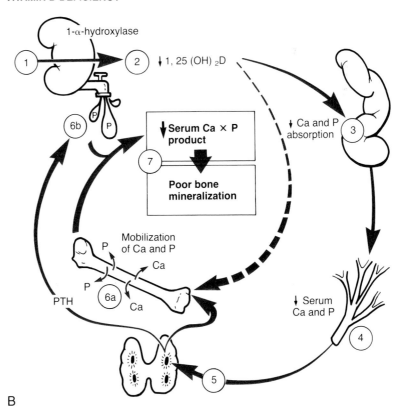

B

Figure 9–20. *A*, Schema of normal vitamin D metabolism. *B*, Hypovitaminosis D. There is inadequate substrate for the renal hydroxylase (1) yielding a deficiency of 1,25-(OH)₂ (2) and deficient absorption of calcium and phosphorus from the gut (3), with consequent depressed serum levels of both (4). The hypocalcemia activates the parathyroid glands (5), causing, along with the vitamin D deficiency, mobilization of calcium and phosphorus from bone (6a). Simultaneously, the parathormone (PTH) induces wasting of phosphate in the urine (6b). Consequently, the serum levels of calcium are normal or nearly normal, but the phosphate is low; hence, mineralization is impaired.

- Whether of endogenous or exogenous origin, vitamin D (and its metabolites) are transported in the blood, bound chiefly to an alpha globulin-vitamin D-binding protein (DBP).
- This complex is transported to the liver, where a P-450 mixed-function oxidase, vitamin D-25-hydroxylase converts it to 25-OH-D, which in physiologic amounts is largely biologically inert.
- The 25-OH-D bound to DBP is then transported to the kidneys, where it is converted into its active metabolite 1,25-dihydroxyvitamin D (1,25-$(OH)_2$D) — calcitriol — by a renal tubular mitochondrial hydroxylase.

The active metabolite acts directly on organs that play principal roles in calcium homeostasis — the intestines, bones, and kidneys.

At the molecular level, the active metabolite interacts with a specific receptor protein in cells, and the complex is taken up by the nucleus in a manner analogous to the steroid hormones.[48]

In the intestinal mucosal cells, through genomic and possibly nongenomic mechanisms, the incorporated 1,25-$(OH)_2$D stimulates increased transcriptional activity of RNA with increased synthesis of calcium-binding protein (CaBP). In addition, 1,25-$(OH)_2$D directly increases the permeability of the brush border membrane of the mucosal cell to calcium and the CaBP facilitates the transfer across the cell into the blood.

The precise roles of 1,25-$(OH)_2$D and CaBP in the normal mineralization of bone and in the mobilization of calcium to support the plasma level are not well understood. In the kidney, calcitriol may participate with parathyroid hormone in increasing tubular reabsorption of calcium, but this role is also not clearly established.

PREVALENCE AND CONSEQUENCES OF A DEFICIENCY. Rickets and osteomalacia are worldwide skeletal diseases, but in developed countries, they are rarely the result of dietary deficiency. However, these conditions may appear whenever there is some derangement in vitamin D absorption or metabolism or, alternatively, in calcium or phosphorus homeostasis. Thus, a wide variety of clinical conditions may be associated with rickets or osteomalacia, as indicated in Table 9–14.

MORPHOLOGY. The anatomic changes in both rickets and osteomalacia are basically the consequences of delayed and/or inadequate mineralization leading to an excess of unmineralized matrix. The changes in rickets, however, are complicated by inadequate provisional calcification of epiphyseal cartilage, deranging endochondral bone growth. All of the changes are most easily understood after a review of normal bone development and maintenance (see Chapter 27). The sequence of events in rickets comprises the following:

Table 9–14. PATHOPHYSIOLOGIC MECHANISMS ASSOCIATED WITH RICKETS OR OSTEOMALACIA

INADEQUATE ENDOGENOUS SYNTHESIS AND DIETARY LACK*

In *developing countries,* occurs because of varying combinations of dark skin, inadequate exposure to sunlight, and primary malnutrition. Infants predisposed by poor maternal nutrition and deficient postnatal reserves, and children because of increased demands of growth.

In *industrialized countries,* occurs mainly in infancy and childhood. Contributory factors are nonuse of fortified foods, e.g., vitamin D–supplemented milk; Northern hemisphere with little sunlight; poverty with general malnutrition; poor maternal nutrition. Osteomalacia apt to occur in *the elderly* because of such factors as avoidance of sunlight and restricted or bizarre diets.†

MALABSORPTION

Occurs with any disease that impairs intestinal absorption of fats (e.g., cholestatic liver disease or extrahepatic biliary tract obstruction), pancreatic insufficiency, celiac sprue, extensive small bowel disease (e.g., regional enteritis). Also occurs with abnormally rapid small intestinal transit following gastrectomy.

DERANGEMENTS IN METABOLISM OF VITAMIN D

Diffuse liver disease—interference with synthesis of the vitamin D transport protein DBP.

Chronic renal failure—due to decreased conversion of 25-OH-D to 1,25-$(OH)_2$D. Azotemia and acidosis also impair intestinal absorption of calcium. The osteomalacia in renal failure may be complicated by osteitis fibrosa related to secondary hyperparathyroidism producing so-called renal osteodystrophy.

Nephrotic syndrome—excessive excretion of vitamin D binding protein.

Drugs such as phenytoin, phenobarbital, and rifampin induce P-450 enzymes accelerating the rate of degradation of sterols, among them vitamin D and its metabolites.

Vitamin D–dependent rickets type I (autosomal recessive) —genetic lack of or defect in 1-alpha-hydroxylase with an inability to convert 25-OH-D into 1,25-$(OH)_2$D.

END-ORGAN RESISTANCE TO VITAMIN D

Vitamin D–dependent rickets type II—attributed to defective receptors with inadequate calcium absorption in the intestine accompanied perhaps by deranged vitamin D function in other organs (e.g., bone).

OTHER RARE CAUSES

X-linked hypophosphatemic rickets, marked by hypophosphatemia, normocalcemia, and low to normal plasma levels of calcitriol. Basic defects: renal phosphate wasting and possibly impaired intestinal absorption of calcium. Most cases X-linked dominant.

Tumor-induced osteomalacia, rickets (oncogenic osteomalacia-rickets), attributed to some tumor-produced product, causing phosphate wasting.

Chronic use of antacids (e.g., Maalox, Mylanta)—aluminum hydroxide binds to phosphate and interferes with absorption.

* Belton, N.R.: Rickets—not only the "English disease." Acta Paediatr. (Suppl.) Scand. *323:*68, 1986.
† Bouillon, R.A., et al.: Vitamin D status in the elderly: Seasonal substrate deficiency causes 1,25-dihydroxycholecalciferol deficiency. Am. J. Clin. Nutr. *45:*755, 1987.

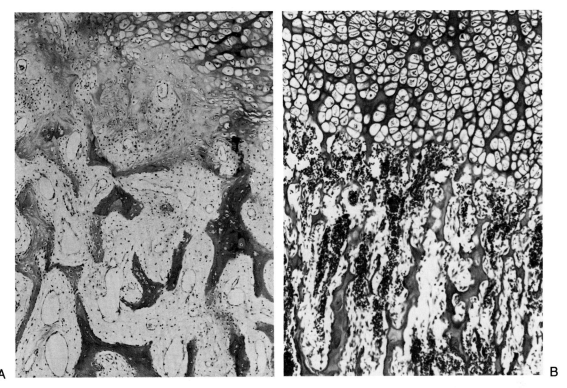

A   B

Figure 9–21. *A,* A detail of a rachitic costochondral junction. The palisade of cartilage is lost. Some of the trabeculae are old, well-formed bone, but the paler ones consist of unmineralized osteoid tissue. *B,* For comparison, normal costochondral junction from a young child demonstrates the orderly transition from cartilage to newly formed bone.

- Overgrowth of inadequately mineralized epiphyseal cartilage due to failure of the cartilage cells to mature and disintegrate
- Persistence of distorted, irregular masses of cartilage, many of which project into the marrow cavity
- Deposition of osteoid matrix on inadequately mineralized cartilaginous remnants; increased numbers and activity of osteoblasts and osteoclasts
- Disruption of the orderly replacement of cartilage by osteoid matrix, with enlargement and lateral expansion of the osteochondral junction (Fig. 9–21A and B)
- Abnormal overgrowth of capillaries in the disorganized zone, with marrow fibrosis
- Deformation of the skeleton due to the loss of structural rigidity of the developing bones

The conformation of the gross skeletal changes depends on the severity of the rachitic process, its duration, and in particular the age of the patient and the stresses to which individual bones are subjected. During the nonambulatory stage of infancy the head and chest sustain the greatest stresses. The softened occipital bones may become flattened, and the parietal bones can be buckled inward by pressure, but with the release of the pressure, elastic recoil snaps the bones back into their original positions—**craniotabes.** An excess of

osteoid produces **frontal bossing** and a **squared appearance to the head.** Deformation of the chest results from overgrowth of cartilage and osteoid tissue at the costochondral junction, producing the **"rachitic rosary."** The weakened metaphyseal areas of the ribs are subject to the pull of the respiratory muscles and thus bend inward, creating anterior protrusion of the sternum—**pigeon-breast deformity.** The inward pull at the margin of the diaphragm creates **Harrison's groove,** girdling the thoracic cavity at the lower margin of the rib cage. The pelvis may become deformed. When the ambulating child develops rickets, deformities are likely to affect the spine, pelvis, and long bones (e.g., tibia), causing most notably **lumbar lordosis** and **bowing of the legs.**

Osteomalacia in the adult is much more subtle and is characterized by loss of skeletal mass or "too little" bone, referred to as **osteopenia.** It must therefore be differentiated, often with difficulty, from other osteopenias such as osteoporosis, osteitis fibrosa, and certain stages of Paget's disease of the bone (see Chapter 27). In these conditions there is no defect in mineralization and, in fact, an increased rate. In contrast, osteomalacia is marked by inadequate mineralization and hence an excess of unmineralized osteoid.[49] Looser's zones or Milkman's fractures (described below) are sometimes present. These may be appreciated only radiologically. Skeletal deformities do not appear in osteomalacia—only apparent loss of bone density and cortical thickness, as visualized by radiography or other techniques. Not surprisingly, with marked osteomalacia the "too-little bone" is subject to fractures, most often of the vertebrae, hips, wrists, and ribs, and to kyphoscoliotic deformity of the vertebral column.

CLINICAL COURSE. In the growing child, full-blown rickets presents no clinical diagnostic challenge. In addition to the skeletal changes cited, circulating levels of 25-OH-D and $1,25\text{-}(OH)_2D$ may be low when the condition is related to a dietary lack of the nutrient or malabsorption of it. However, there are forms of rickets in which the circulating levels of these vitamin metabolites are normal, for example, vitamin D–dependent rickets, type II, and oncogenic rickets.

In adults, the biochemical and radiologic evidence of osteomalacia is often deceptively subtle, and therefore the clinical diagnosis is often difficult. Sometimes, however, the condition can be suspected on the basis of the background of malnutrition, renal failure, or some malabsorption state. The differentiation of osteomalacia from other forms of osteopenia may be exceedingly difficult (see Chapter 27). An early pathognomonic feature of rickets and osteomalacia, but uncommonly present, comprises radiographic changes of Looser's zones or Milkman's fractures. These are radiolucent narrow lines that lie either at right angles or obliquely to the cortical outlines of bones and often transect them. They commonly are bilateral and symmetric and most often are found at the axillary margins of the scapula, lower ribs, neck of the proximal femurs, and posterior margins of the proximal ulnas. Looser's zones or Milkman's fractures are related either to stress fractures that are inadequately healed and calcified or to mechanical erosion by penetrating nutrient arteries. They are obvious sites for future serious fractures. Only rarely is bone biopsy resorted to for diagnostic purposes. In most instances, a trial of vitamin D and calcium therapy is implemented.[50]

VITAMIN D TOXICITY. Large excesses of vitamin D are well tolerated. Extreme acute overdosage is very uncommon but may cause hypercalcemia, which is transient unless the vitamin D excess is continued. Chronic toxicity, with its increased levels of blood calcium, may give rise to metastatic calcifications and renal stones (see Chapter 1).

Vitamin E

The deficiency states are spinocerebellar degeneration; skeletal muscle changes; hemolytic anemia in infants.

Four closely related tocopherols and tocotrienols have *vitamin E* activity, among which

Table 9–15. DISORDERS INDUCING VITAMIN E DEFICIENCY

Abetalipoproteinemia	Autosomal recessive disorder characterized by inability to synthesize apoprotein B, an essential component of chylomicrons, low density and very low density lipoproteins leading to defective transport of vitamin E in the plasma
Intrahepatic and extrahepatic cholestasis	Deficient delivery of bile to the small intestine with fat malabsorption
Cystic fibrosis of the pancreas	Inadequate pancreatic enzymes and bile flow with fat malabsorption
Small intestinal disorders	Celiac disease, extensive regional enteritis, radiation injury, and small bowel resection, for example, all may lead to steatorrhea and fat malabsorption
Isolated vitamin E deficiency (rare)	No generalized fat malabsorption, but specific obscure defects of vitamin E absorption, autosomal recessive
Low birth weight neonates	Physiologic immaturity of the liver and gastrointestinal tract, aggravated by formulas high in polyunsaturated fatty acid (PUFA) and low in alpha-tocopherol

Modified with permission from Harding, A.E.: Vitamin E and the nervous system. C.R.C. Crit. Rev. Neurobiol. 3:89, 1987.

alpha-tocopherol is the most potent. All serve principally as antioxidants and so have the important functions of scavenging free radicals formed in redox reactions throughout the body and protecting the polyunsaturated fatty acids in cellular and subcellular membranes from free radical peroxidation. Thus diets rich in polyunsaturated fatty acids increase the need for vitamin E, and, conversely, other antioxidants (e.g., selenium) can reduce the need. The tocopherols are widely distributed in vegetables, grains and their oils, and fish. After absorption, they are transported in chylomicrons in the blood, which rapidly equilibrate with the plasma lipoproteins, mainly LDLs. They are stored throughout the body, but mostly in adipose tissue, liver, and muscle. Vitamin E does not appear to need a specific carrier protein for its transport in the blood, nor is metabolic conversion necessary. Because of its wide distribution in virtually all foods, a dietary deficiency is rare, even in less developed countries. Much more commonly, deficiency is encountered with some underlying disorder (Table 9–15).

CONSEQUENCES OF A DEFICIENCY STATE. There is now good evidence that vitamin E deficiency produces in humans spinocerebellar, particularly posterior column, abnormalities, skeletal muscle disease, and pigmented retinopathy. Why these particular tissues are affected is unclear, as well as the precise mechanism by which the vitamin is transferred to the brain, spinal cord, and muscle. All that is known with any degree of certainty is that the neurologic sites affected normally tend to have lower vitamin E content than other brain regions, and this may reflect higher rates of utilization and greater vulnerability to deprivation.[51]

MORPHOLOGY. Some of the earliest neuropathologic changes are swollen dystrophic axons (spheroids) in the posterior columns of the spinal cord and peripheral sensory nerves. The gracile and cuneate nuclei of the brain stem undergo secondary demyelinization. With more severe or prolonged vitamin E deficiency, there is degeneration of the dorsal and ventral spinocerebellar tracts and atrophy of the cerebellum overall, as well as disappearance (dying-back) of neurons in the dorsal root nuclei and of the third and fourth cranial nerves. Accompanying these neuropathologic changes is the accumulation of lipopigment in dorsal root sensory neurons and the Schwann cells of peripheral nerves. The accumulation of lipofuscin may well reflect the peroxidation of membrane lipids of damaged organelles.

Two types of skeletal muscle lesions are encountered in vitamin E deficiency. One is the consequence of denervation-renervation, leading to so-called fiber-type grouping (see Chapter 28). The other lesion constitutes the accumulation of fine, grain-like, autofluorescent, basophilic deposits within the muscle fibers. Electron microscopy suggests that they are cigar-shaped secondary lysosomes containing lipopigment.

A pigment retinopathy is encountered in older patients with abetalipoproteinemia. Significantly, the rods of the retina are rich in unsaturated fatty acids.

CLINICAL COURSE. The clinical manifestations of vitamin E deficiency are virtually only recognizable in association with one of the well-defined conditions mentioned above that impair the absorption of the tocopherols. Most characteristic are depressed (or, more often, absent) tendon reflexes, ataxia, dysarthria, loss of position and vibration sense, and loss of pain sensation. In addition, there may be impaired vision and disorders of eye movement, sometimes progressing to total ophthalmoplegia. Muscle weakness may be present, more likely related to the neurologic changes. Anemia caused by a shortened red blood cell half-life is sometimes present in premature infants suffering from vitamin E deficiency, but its origin may well be multifactorial.

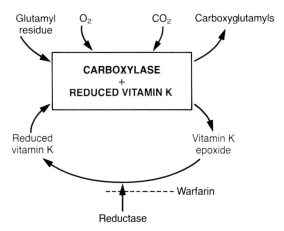

Figure 9–22. The biochemical events in the carboxylation of vitamin K–dependent proteins.

TOXICITY. Modest excesses of vitamin E are of little significance, but massive overdosage has been reported to induce gastrointestinal disturbances, interference with absorption of vitamins A and K, and predisposition to enteritis in infants.

Vitamin K

The deficiency state is hypoprothrombinemia and a bleeding diathesis.

Vitamin K is a fat-soluble cofactor for a liver microsomal carboxylase required for conversion of glutamyl residues in certain proteins into gamma-carboxyglutamates. In the course of this carboxylation reaction, the vitamin is oxidized to its inactive epoxide, which is then restored to its active form by a reductase (Fig. 9–22). Four clotting factors require such carboxylation: factors II (prothrombin), VII, IX, and X. The carboxylation provides the calcium binding sites necessary for the calcium-dependent interaction of these clotting factors with a phospholipid surface involved in the generation of thrombin. In addition, plasma proteins C and S require carboxylation for their function. Protein C is a circulating zymogen of a natural anticoagulant that is activated by thrombin in the presence of thrombomodulin. Activated protein C inhibits coagulation by inactivating factors VIIIa and Va. This activity of protein C is enhanced by protein S. Another glutamate-containing protein is osteocalcin in bone, possibly involved in the calcification of osteoid matrix (see Chapter 27).

Vitamin K is widely available in the diet in green vegetables, dairy products, liver, and bacon. Absorption, as with all fats, requires normal biliary and pancreatic function. There is, in addition, some endogenous synthesis of vitamin K by the normal intestinal flora, but only small amounts are absorbed. However, the relatively efficient recycling of vitamin K after its involvement in carboxylation reactions obviates the need for all but small amounts of dietary vitamin K. Only relatively small amounts are stored in the liver and other parenchymal organs, and so a negative balance may soon lead to a deficiency state. In the adult, conditioned deficiencies may appear with (1) any fat malabsorption syndrome, particularly with biliary tract disease; (2) the systemic administration of broad-spectrum antibiotics, which appear to inhibit the hepatic epoxide reductase involved in recycling vitamin K; (3) diffuse liver disease, impairing the hepatic synthesis of the vitamin K–dependent coagulation precursors (this form of vitamin K deficiency can be differentiated from that caused by malabsorption because of the absence in the circulation of the uncarboxylated precursor proteins); and (4) the intentional administration of the anticoagulant vitamin K antagonists (e.g., warfarin and dicumarol), which interfere with the action of the hepatic reductase.

The neonate is much more vulnerable to vitamin K deficiency, for several reasons. Very small amounts of the vitamin are transported across the placenta from the mother, and so the fetal reserves are low. After birth, the fetal gut is sterile, and therefore there is little neonatal synthesis until the normal intestinal flora becomes established, usually toward the end of the first week of postnatal life. Furthermore, breast milk is a relatively poor source of vitamin K, as compared with commercial formulas.

CONSEQUENCES OF A DEFICIENCY STATE. Whatever its origin, hypoprothrombinemia secondary to deficient vitamin K function induces hemorrhagic disease. In adults, this bleeding diathesis is of major concern in those requiring surgery, particularly on the biliary tract (for correction of obstructive jaundice, the major predisposition to malabsorption of the vitamin). More often, the bleeding diathesis develops in the neonate and has the potential to produce intracranial hemorrhage and also bleeding from any other site, including skin, umbilicus, and viscera. It is estimated that 1 to 3% of neonates have some degree of vitamin K deficiency, warranting, according to some experts, prophylactic therapy.

Excessive consumption of foodstuffs rich in vitamin K is without toxicity, but rare instances of hemolytic anemia have been reported following the parenteral administration of large doses of synthetic water-soluble derivatives.

WATER-SOLUBLE VITAMINS

This category encompasses a complex of B vitamins, including thiamine, riboflavin, niacin, vitamin B_6, folic acid, and vitamin B_{12}, and vitamin C (ascorbic acid). In addition, biotin and pantothenic acid are sometimes referred to as B vitamins, but they have not been associated with well-defined clinical deficiency states. Most of the water-soluble vitamins are widely available and, by and large, are readily absorbed, chiefly in the small intestine. A variety of foods are rich sources of the B vitamins, principally cereals, leafy green vegetables, yeast, liver, and milk. Analogously, vitamin C, as is well known, is widely available in citrus fruits, vegetables, and some meats. Thus, deficiency states of the water-soluble vitamins are not global problems, in comparison with that of vitamin A, for example. However, primary and conditioned deficiencies are encountered sporadically throughout the world. Further comments will be restricted to vitamin B_1 (thiamine) and vitamin C. The remaining vitamins are briefly characterized in Table 9–13 and vitamin B_{12} and folic acid are discussed with their related anemias.

Thiamine

The deficiency states are "dry" beriberi, "wet" beriberi, and Wernicke-Korsakoff syndrome.

Thiamine is widely available in natural foods, but refined foods such as polished rice, white flour, and white sugar contain very little. Although the normal diet contains more than is required, items such as raw, freshwater fish, strong tea and coffee, and factors in myoglobin and hemoglobin act as antithiamines and reduce the dietary content of this vitamin. Reserves are relatively limited and are found mainly in skeletal muscle but also in heart, liver, kidney, and brain. Two mechanisms are involved in absorption: passive diffusion at high dietary concentrations, and active, energy-dependent transport at low concentrations. During absorption, thiamine undergoes phosphorylation to produce thiamine pyrophosphate (TPP), the functionally active coenzyme form of the vitamin. Thiamine pyrophosphate has three major functions: (1) oxidative decarboxylation of alpha-ketoacids, leading to the synthesis of ATP; (2) as a cofactor for transketolase in the pentose phosphate pathway; and (3) in maintaining neural membranes and normal nerve conduction, chiefly of peripheral nerves, although the mechanism is poorly understood.

CONSEQUENCES OF A DEFICIENCY. In addition to many nonspecific manifestations, to be detailed later, a deficiency of thiamine damages peripheral nerves ("dry" beriberi), the heart ("wet" beriberi), and the CNS (Wernicke-Korsakoff syndrome). In less developed countries, when a large part of the scant diet constitutes polished rice, as occurs in many areas of Southeast Asia, thiamine deficiency sometimes develops. Beriberi has also been observed among maltreated prisoners of war. In developed countries clinically evident thiamine deficiency is uncommon on a strictly dietary basis, but surveys point to subclinical deficiencies among populations not having fortified foods available.[52]

In virtually all countries, overt thiamine deficiency is commonly encountered in chronic alcoholics, affecting as many as one-quarter of those admitted to general hospitals in the United States. Contributing to the impact of the hypovitaminosis B in this population is an apparent transketolase abnormality transmitted, in some instances as an autosomal recessive trait, which seems to be common in chronic alcoholics. A deficiency state may also be seen as a result of pernicious vomiting of pregnancy, long-term unsupplemented parenteral nutrition, or debilitating illnesses that impair the appetite, predispose to vomiting, or cause protracted diarrhea. Because thiamine is required for carbohydrate metabolism, a subclinical deficiency state may be converted into overt disease by extended intravenous glucose therapy or refeeding of chronically malnourished individuals (e.g., alcoholics) unless adequate amounts of thiamine are administered concurrently.

MORPHOLOGY. The major targets of thiamine deficiency are (1) the heart, (2) the peripheral nerves, and (3) the brain.

The heart may be normal, have subtle changes, or be markedly enlarged and globular (owing to four-chamber dilatation) with pale, flabby myocardium. The dilatation thins the ventricular walls. Mural thrombi are often present, particularly in the dilated atria. The histologic changes are inconstant and unimpressive; they include interstitial myocardial edema, myofiber swelling and sometimes fatty change, and individual myofiber necrosis. Similar changes may occur in alcoholic cardiomyopathy (see Chapter 12.). The cardiac lesions in beriberi then are not pathognomonic (Fig. 9–23A).

In the peripheral nerves, the earliest changes are a symmetric, nonspecific polyneuropathy involving motor, sensory, and reflex arcs beginning particularly in the nerves of the feet and lower legs. With progression, the changes extend proximally while at the same time nerves of the upper extremities and trunk and even the vagus and phrenic nerves become involved. At the outset there is myelin degeneration, but depending on duration and severity of the deficiency, it may progress to disruption of axons. Sometimes the changes extend proximally to involve the associated anterior horn neurons and posterior columns of the spinal cord (see Fig. 9–23B).

The CNS lesions of the Wernicke-Korsakoff syndrome were discussed earlier, but in essence they comprise foci of hemorrhage and necrosis in the mammillary bodies and about the ventricular regions of the thalamus and hypothalamus, about the aqueduct in the midbrain, and in the floor of the fourth ventricle and anterior region of the cerebellum (see Fig. 9–23C).

The reasons that the nervous system and the heart are the two major targets of thiamine deficiency are still poorly understood. With respect to the heart, it is theorized that deficient TPP impairs the function of key enzymes (e.g., transketolase involved in glucose metabolism) and so impairs ATP synthesis, on which myocardial cell function is dependent. The impaired glucose metabolism affects brain function; but how then to explain the focal nature of the lesions? In alcoholics the basis of the changes in the heart and nervous system is even more uncertain. Alcohol itself is known to damage the heart, peripheral nerves, and brain. Moreover, Korsakoff's psychosis (a feature of the deficiency state) responds poorly to the administration of thiamine. It is evident there is much yet to be learned about the pathophysiology of vitamin B_1.

CLINICAL COURSE. The clinical manifestations of thiamine deficiency at the outset are very nonspecific (e.g., anorexia, weakness, weight loss), but as the condition progresses three distinctive syndromes can be recognized: (1) a polyneuropathy (dry beriberi), (2) a cardiovascular syndrome (wet beriberi), and (3) the Wernicke-Korsakoff syndrome. Typically, the three syndromes appear in the sequence given, but on occasion the deficiency state is manifested by only one of them. The polyneuropathy is manifested first by numbness and tingling of the feet and lower legs. Then the upper extremities may become involved. There is progressive sensory loss in affected parts accompanied by muscle weakness and hypo- or areflexia. Beriberi heart disease (wet beriberi) is associated with peripheral vasodilatation leading to more rapid arteriovenous shunting of blood, rapid circulation, and "high-output failure." With the onset of failure, decreased renal blood flow leads to vasoconstriction in the vascular bed of the kidney and retention of salt and water with the development of peripheral edema. When the deficiency state occurs particularly acutely, a fulminant form of heart failure may arise, referred to as *shoshin beriberi.*[53]

In protracted, severe deficiency states, most often encountered in chronic alcoholics in the Western world, Wernicke-Korsakoff syndrome may appear. In most instances, it develops against a background of peripheral neuropathy and cardiac insufficiency, but in some instances it is the presenting and only manifestation of thiamine deficiency. The clinical features of this neurologic condition are discussed with ethyl alcohol toxicity, but here we should note that Wernicke's encephalopathy and Korsakoff's psychosis are not distinct syndromes but rather successive stages of a single CNS disease having the same pathologic substrate.[54]

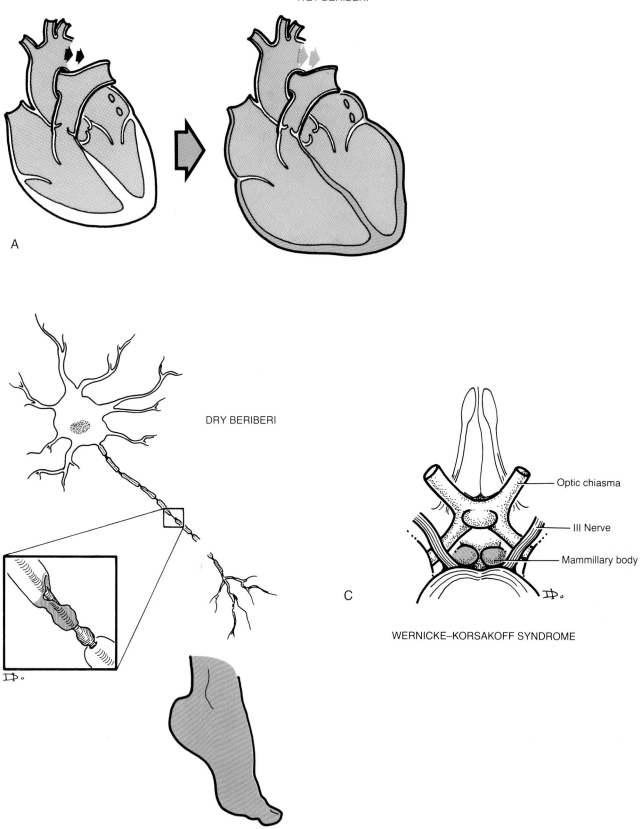

Figure 9-23. *A,* The flabby, four-chambered, dilated heart of "wet" beriberi. *B,* The peripheral neuropathy with myelin degeneration leading to foot drop, wrist drop, and sensory changes in "dry" beriberi. *C,* Hemorrhages into the mammillary bodies in the Wernicke-Korsakoff syndrome.

TOXICITY. Although the administration of thiamine sometimes produces dizziness and flushing, these manifestations are mild and transient. No serious untoward effects from massive doses have been recorded.

Vitamin C (Ascorbic Acid)

The deficiency state is scurvy.

Humans, unlike most mammals and even lower life forms, cannot synthesize ascorbic acid and so are dependent on a dietary source. This vitamin is widely available in the human diet, but the richest sources are citrus fruits, leafy green vegetables, peppers, and tomatoes. Absorptive capacity in the small intestine is relatively limited, and so the larger the daily intake, the smaller the proportion absorbed. For this reason, the ingestion of mega-dose pills of vitamin C have little effect on the levels of ascorbic acid in the plasma. Reserves are limited, and 2 to 3% of the total body pool is catabolized daily; so a deficiency could appear after 30 to 40 days if none were available in the diet. Moreover, emotional and physical stresses, such as trauma, surgery, and febrile illnesses, increase the daily requirement, as does lactation. Smokers, too, appear to have an increased need for, or reduced capacity to absorb, vitamin C.

Ascorbic acid, like vitamin E, is a powerful antioxidant and reducing agent. It is thus involved, like vitamin E, in scavenging free radicals and in maintaining the prosthetic metals Fe^{++} and Cu^+ on various oxygenases in a reduced state. It therefore functions to protect lipids against peroxidation. In addition, it participates in collagen metabolism, in the biosynthesis of neurotransmitters, in carnitine biosynthesis, as a component of the P-450 mixed-function oxidases, and, in some poorly understood manner, in immune functions. It also enhances the intestinal absorption of nonheme iron and, by virtue of its reducing potential, prevents the oxidation of tetrahydrofolate.

Perhaps best understood is the role of ascorbic acid in collagen synthesis. The collagen molecule contains a large number of proline and lysine amino acid residues that are post-translationally hydroxylated. The requisite proline and lysine hydroxylases involved in the hydroxylation require ferrous iron for their maximal function, and it is the role of ascorbic acid to maintain the iron in its reduced state. The other functions of ascorbic acid presumably also involve the maintenance of enzymatic prosthetic groups in reduced states, accounting for the wide-ranging biochemical functions of ascorbic acid.[55]

CONSEQUENCES OF A DEFICIENCY STATE. With the disappearance of seamen who went on long sea voyages without fresh food, scurvy has become uncommon. However, it is sometimes encountered in the economically deprived, the elderly—with their restricted diets—and food faddists, such as strict devotees of macrobiotic diets. It is also worth noting that vitamin C–containing foods can be seriously depleted by prolonged storage and excessive cooking, especially boiling, since ascorbic acid is readily dissolved out and is heat sensitive.

MORPHOLOGY. Scurvy in the growing child is far more dramatic than in the adult. **Hemorrhages** constitute one of the most striking features related to the defect in collagen synthesis and inadequate support of vascular walls. Purpura and ecchymoses often appear in the skin, most prominently along the backs of the lower legs and in the gingival mucosa, particularly at the margins. Loose attachments of the periosteum and the hemorrhagic diathesis lead to extensive **subperiosteal hematomas** and bleeding into the joints. More threatening are retrobulbar, subarachnoid, and **intracerebral hemorrhages,** which may prove fatal.

Skeletal changes may appear in the growing child. The primary disturbance is in the formation of the collagen-rich osteoid matrix, not in mineralization or calcification, such as is typical of rickets. Both membranous and endochondral bone formation may be disrupted. The lack of sufficient production of osteoid matrix leads to disruption of epiphyseal bone growth, with long spicules and plates of cartilage projecting into the metaphyseal region of the marrow cavity, and sometimes lateral overgrowth of the epiphyses (Fig. 9–24A and B). Further disrupting the epiphyseal area are hemorrhages occasioned by poorly supported microvessels, and the defective osteoid. The poorly formed bone yields to the stresses of weight bearing and muscle tension, with bowing of the long bones of the lower legs and abnormal depression of the sternum, with outward projection of the ends of the ribs, creating the so-called **scorbutic rosary.** Further distorting the skeletal system are hematomas beneath the periosteum. The deranged bone formation also involves the jaws and alveolar bone. Thus, the teeth are abnormally mobile and may be displaced or fall out. Gingival swelling, hemorrhages, and secondary bacterial periodontal infection are common in severely scorbutic patients.

A distinctive **perifollicular, hyperkeratotic papular rash,** sometimes ringed by hemorrhages, often appears. **Wound healing and localization of focal infections** are both impaired. Anemia is also a common finding. Most often it is normochromic and normocytic, related to the bleeding into the various tissues and to the impaired absorption of iron, but sometimes the anemia is macrocytic or megaloblastic, owing to a lack of folate. The major features of scurvy in the child are summarized in Figure 9–25.

The changes in the adult are similar to those in the child, but skeletal deformation does not occur.

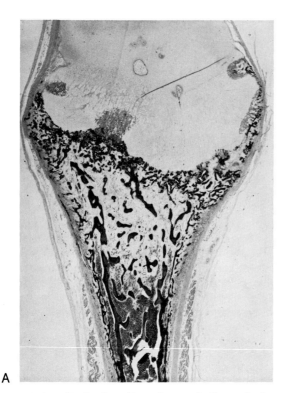
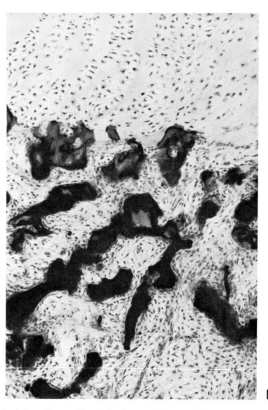

A   B

Figure 9-24. *A*, Longitudinal section of a scorbutic costochondral junction with widening of the epiphyseal cartilage and projection of masses of cartilage into the adjacent bone. *B*, Detail of a scorbutic costochondral junction. The orderly palisade is totally destroyed. There is dense mineralization of the spicules present but no evidence of newly formed osteoid.

Thus the major anatomic changes relate to the bleeding tendency, skin rash, anemia, and, often prominently, hemorrhagic gingival enlargement accompanied by periodontal infection.

CLINICAL COURSE. Because of its rarity, the diagnosis of scurvy requires an awareness of the clinical settings in which it is most likely to appear. The earliest manifestations at all ages are nonspecific, including lethargy, malaise, and weakness. More specific findings in the adult have already been detailed, but particularly characteristic are skin purpura over the lower leg, easy bruisability, friable bleeding gums, and hematoma formation in virtually any site exposed to trauma. The friability of the microvessels may lead to the appearance of a shower of petechiae over the arm after the application of a blood pressure cuff. Unrecognized bleeding into the tissues, together with iron or folate deficiency, may lead to a severe anemia.

Childhood scurvy is characterized by essentially the same findings, but they tend to occur in the context of skeletal system changes. Subperiosteal hemorrhages, with pain and swelling along the involved bones, and joint hemorrhages, with pain and limitation of motion, are particularly characteristic. Severe scurvy may retard growth and pro-

duce skeletal deformities, as described above. At all ages, the course may suddenly take a downturn because of intracranial bleeding, which may prove fatal.

Confirmation of the diagnosis requires documentation of abnormally low levels of ascorbic acid in serum or plasma.

THE MEGADOSE CONTROVERSY. Claims have been made that megadoses of ascorbic acid (more than 1 gm/day), in comparison to the average daily requirement of 100 mg or more, would increase resistance to the common cold, alleviate its symptoms, and also be effective in the treatment of advanced cancer. These claims would have aroused little notice, save that their chief advocate was a respected Nobel laureate. Numerous studies have followed that almost uniformly discredit any benefit in the treatment of advanced cancer. However, with the common cold the results have been somewhat contradictory; on balance, they do not point to any decrease in the incidence of the common cold, but perhaps some decrease in the duration and severity of the symptoms (possibly as a result of the mild antihistaminic action of ascorbic acid).[56]

The slender and somewhat doubtful benefits of megadoses of vitamin C must be placed in the perspective of possible untoward effects. Multigram

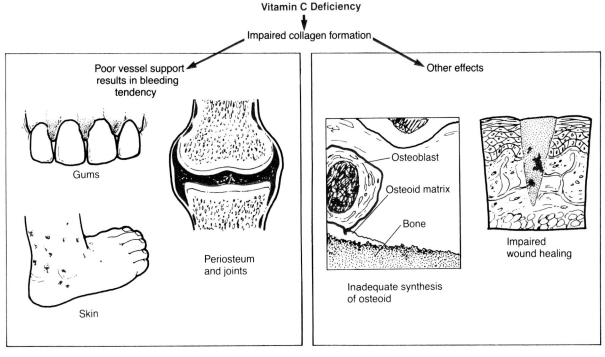

Figure 9-25. The major consequences of vitamin C deficiency.

daily amounts of ascorbic acid have induced urico-suria, increased absorption of nonheme iron, with the potential of iron overload (in predisposed individuals), systemic acidosis in those individuals with chronic renal disease, and hemolysis in infants with diminished glucose-6-phosphate dehydrogenase activity, whose mothers had consumed multigram doses of ascorbic acid during pregnancy.

NUTRITIONAL EXCESSES AND IMBALANCES

The well-defined nutritional diseases discussed thus far all stem from deficiencies of essential dietary components. However, other nutritional and dietary imbalances may also be important, causing or contributing to such conditions as obesity and systemic diseases (e.g., non–insulin-dependent diabetes). Whether the diet may also predispose to cancer continues to be debated. These topics are considered in the following discussions.

OBESITY

Few problems are more talked about, are less often resolved, and have supported more authors (of diet books) than obesity. It is an extremely common problem in the United States. About one-quarter of adult Americans are overweight, almost half of

whom are markedly overweight. This frequency must be viewed in the context of the millions of starving "have-nots" in Third World countries, many of whom will die for lack of nutrition.

It has proved surprisingly difficult to objectively characterize the degree of obesity in individuals. Perhaps most widely used are the following approaches:

• Weight for height, corrected for gender and age, referred to as the body-mass index (BMI)
• Skin fold measurements, taken in specified locations—biceps, triceps, subcapsular, and suprailiac
• Waist-hip circumference ratio
• A wide variety of other more elaborate systems[57]

All approaches have flaws. For example, elderly people lose muscle mass and balance the loss with deposits of fat without change in the BMI. Even more important, the BMI does not give any indication of the distribution of the body fat. When obesity develops, both men and women accumulate abdominal fat. In addition, women are likely to develop deposits of fat in the gluteal regions and the upper part of the legs. This distribution has been referred to as "gynoid," in contrast with the abdominal obesity of males, which is referred to as "android"; more colorfully, we become "pears" and "apples." Many studies suggest that it is abdominal obesity which is particularly linked to increased disease risk.

For years, it has been conventional wisdom that *obesity is the result of "too much food and too*

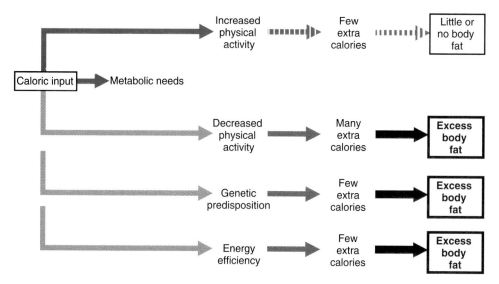

Figure 9-26. Obesity. The varying pathways to the accumulation of excess fat.

little exercise." While this maxim is largely correct, the etiology of obesity can be much more complex. There is a well-documented familial tendency, but whether this is of environmental or genetic origin is unclear. Studies of twins separated at birth and living apart provide strong evidence for a substantial genetic influence. Children of overweight parents, when adopted by "lean" families, have a greater tendency to become obese than do adoptees from nonobese natural parents. "Energy efficiency" may contribute to obesity; with reserves of fat deposits readily available to metabolize in the obese, a given amount of activity requires a smaller expenditure of energy. This theory has been invoked by those who complain that they "gain weight whether they eat or not," and indeed there is evidence of differences in energy efficiency among individuals. Similarly, obesity has been attributed to abnormally low basal metabolic rates (BMRs), since obese individuals do show lower BMRs. However, this fact is due to an artifact of BMR measurement; a larger proportion of the total fat mass of an obese person is inert, low-metabolizing fat, a fact that skews BMR calculations lower. When BMRs are recalculated on the basis of lean body mass, obese individuals do not, in general, have low rates. Obesity itself imposes an increased burden when physical activity is undertaken, since energy is expended to move the expanded body mass. Lack of exercise is probably as important in the development of obesity as the number of calories consumed; regrettably, as fat accumulates, activity tends to dwindle. Other speculations might be offered, but ultimately, and until proved otherwise, *obesity is the consequence of storing excess calories in fat depots,* and without excess calories from too little energy expenditure, obesity would not exist (Fig. 9-26).

CONSEQUENCES OF OBESITY. In addition to the psychologic and social implications of obesity, it is a health hazard. There is a clear association between average length of life and BMI; the greater the BMI, the greater the risk of death, irrespective of age. The various disorders that account for this increased mortality follow (Fig. 9-27).

Insulin resistance appears with increasing obesity. Studies indicate that the enlarged fat cells have a decreased number of insulin receptors per unit of cell surface, but they also apparently develop a postreceptor abnormality manifested as impaired glucose utilization.

Diabetes mellitus, the non–insulin-dependent, so-called adult onset diabetes, is strongly associated with obesity. More than 80% of patients with this disorder are more than 20% overweight. Indeed, the diabetic state is often unmasked by the accumulation of fat and often reverts to a subclinical state with weight loss (see Chapter 19).

Hypertension is unmistakenly correlated with obesity. A risk of developing hypertension among previously normotensive individuals was proportional to the degree of excess weight gain. It is variously said to be from three to eight times greater among obese individuals who are more than 20% over their optimal weight than among the nonobese.

Hyperlipidemia is only weakly associated with obesity. The correlation is much greater for hypertriglyceridemia than for hypercholesterolemia.

Heart disease is found more often among the obese than among the nonobese. With the accumulation of fat depots, blood and stroke volume and left ventricular filling pressure all increase, predisposing eventually to left ventricular hypertrophy and heart failure. Hypertension is a strong ancillary contributor.

OBESITY

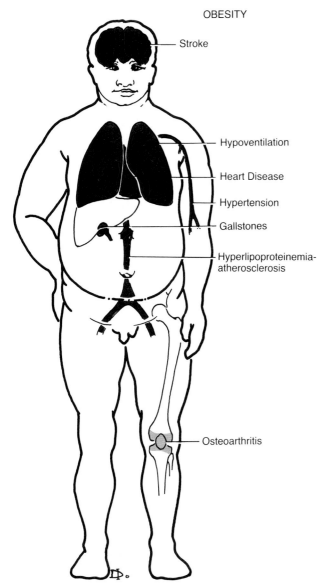

Stroke

Hypoventilation

Heart Disease

Hypertension

Gallstones

Hyperlipoproteinemia-atherosclerosis

Osteoarthritis

Figure 9–27. The major adverse consequences of obesity.

Coronary heart disease was the major contributor to the higher mortality among obese individuals in a population study of 750,000 men and women. Mortality from coronary heart disease was nearly 50% greater among men and women 30 to 40% above ideal weight as compared with control subjects. Clearly, hypertension, diabetes, and hyperlipidemia contribute to this predisposition to coronary atherosclerosis and coronary heart disease.

Other conditions are also associated with obesity. There is an increased incidence of cholesterol gallstones among those who are significantly overweight. Respiratory problems are much more prone to appear in individuals who are significantly overweight, attributed to an increased breathing workload and decreased functional reserve capac-

ity. Such problems have been called "Pickwickian syndrome," after the fat lad who was constantly falling asleep in Dickens' *Pickwick Papers.* Hypersomnolence, both at night and during the day, is characteristic and is often associated with apneic pauses during sleep. Osteoarthritis, particularly in the knee joints, is more likely to become symptomatic as total body weight increases.

The relationship between obesity and cancer will be taken up in a following section.

DIET AND SYSTEMIC DISEASES

Throughout the book, there are repeated references to the contribution of the diet to the development of various diseases. Holding center stage is the role of diet in the genesis of atherosclerosis and associated heart disease. As pointed out in Chapter 11, there is a large body of evidence that diets high in cholesterol and saturated fats raise the plasma cholesterol level, and, conversely, diets low in cholesterol and low in the ratio of saturated to polyunsaturated fats lower plasma cholesterol levels. Although some disbelievers persist, the evidence linking the level of cholesterol consumption to the predisposition to atherosclerosis and coronary artery disease is nearly irrefutable. Most of this evidence has been cited in the earlier discussion of atherosclerosis, but a few considerations merit emphasis.

The average adult in the United States consumes about 140 gm of fat per day and about 500 mg of cholesterol. The ratio of saturated to polyunsaturated fatty acids in this fat is about 3:1. Lowering the saturates to the level of the polyunsaturates effects a reduction in the dietary cholesterol to about 200 to 300 mg, with a 10 to 15% reduction in serum cholesterol level within a few weeks. Vegetable oils, such as corn and safflower oils, and fish oils contain highly polyunsaturated fatty acids. Fish oil fatty acids belonging to the "omega-3" or "N-3" family have more double bonds than the "omega-6" or "N-6" fatty acids found in vegetable oils. Substitution of a portion of the saturated fat with a fish oil for a 4-week period induced a substantial reduction in serum lipid levels, particularly in triglycerides and VLDLs, which was greater than that induced by vegetable oils.[58] Significantly, a recent study of Dutch men whose usual daily diet contained 30 gm of fish revealed a substantially lower frequency of death from coronary heart disease than that among comparable control subjects.[59] The conclusion seems inescapable — animal fat, with its cholesterol content, is no "friend of the heart."

To turn to other examples of the effect of diet on health and life, calorie restriction in experimental animals clearly prolongs life, and repeated studies have pointed to small indigenous populations with strikingly extended life spans, whose calorie intake is substantially lower than that of the average American. Hypertension is beneficially affected by restricting sodium intake. A deficiency in dietary fiber or roughage resulting in decreased fecal bulk is thought to be responsible for, or predispose to, diverticulosis of the colon (see Chapter 17). The effect of calories and obesity on diabetes was pointed out in a previous discussion. Other examples could be cited, but it is clear that disease and diet have many important interactions.

Diet and Cancer

There is great concern today in governmental, scientific, and lay circles about the possibility that what we eat or fail to eat contributes to the causation of cancer.[60,61] Cancer of the stomach is about five times more frequent in Japan than in the United States, whereas the reverse holds true for cancer of the colon. Successive generations of Japanese families who migrated to the United States progressively have acquired an incidence rate for both forms of cancer ever closer to that of their new home, attributed to change in diet (see Chapter 7).[62]

Even more convincing is the laboratory evidence. Restriction of dietary intake lowers the spontaneous incidence of cancers in a variety of animals and also reduces the incidence and progression of experimentally induced neoplasms. But what underlies this association of diet with cancer?[63]

Three aspects of the diet are of concern: (1) its possible content of exogenous carcinogens, (2) the potential that carcinogens might be endogenously synthesized from dietary components, and (3) a possible lack of protective factors.[64] *Relative to exogenous carcinogens*, it was pointed out in Chapter 7 that some naturally occurring carcinogens may be present in the diet (e.g., aflatoxins). The high incidence of hepatocarcinoma in Africa may be attributable in part to contamination of grains and nuts by aflatoxin B, resulting from the growth of *Aspergillus flavus*. Aromatic polycylic hydrocarbons could be produced in the broiling and smoking of meats and fish. Of great current interest is the controversy about the dangers of the artificial sweeteners saccharin and cyclamates (hence the search for natural, potentially safer agents). However, many analyses have failed to reveal any significant increase in the frequency of bladder cancer among users of saccharin and cyclamates. Thus, although saccharin and cyclamates are probably not initiators of cancer, the possibility that they might enhance the action of concurrent carcinogenic influences has not been ruled out.

Concern about the *endogenous synthesis of carcinogens* or *promoters* from components of the diet relates principally to gastric, mammary, and endometrial carcinomas. With gastric carcinoma, nitrosamines and nitrosamides are in the spotlight. These compounds could be formed in the body from nitrites and amines or amides derived from proteins or be found in foods to which nitrite is added as a preservative, as in processed meats that are not heated sufficiently to destroy botulinal spores. Furthermore, nitrates are abundant in the soil and water and can be reduced to nitrites by bacterial action in the gut. There is, then, the potential for the endogenous production of carcinogenic agents from dietary components, which might well have an effect on the stomach exposed to the highest concentrations.

With carcinoma of the breast in postmenopausal women, several epidemiologic studies implicate diets high in animal meats and fats and overnutrition (obesity). There is no shortage of theories to explain these associations, but all are highly speculative. The association of breast carcinoma with the level of dietary fat is further buttressed by animal studies showing an increased incidence of carcinogen-induced breast cancers when the fat level in the diet is raised. Seductive as these observations may be, a large number of epidemiologic studies refute an association between breast cancer and dietary animal fats or obesity. For the present, we must conclude that there is no solid evidence that diet plays a significant role in this form of cancer.

Low fiber and a high animal fat intake has been implicated in the causation of colon cancer. The most convincing attempt to explain these associations is the following. A high animal fat diet might have two effects. The high fat intake would increase the level of bile acids in the gut, which in turn would modify the intestinal flora, favoring the growth of microaerophilic bacteroides. It is then proposed that either the bile acids themselves, or metabolites of the bile acids produced by the bacteroides, might serve as carcinogens or promoters. Furthermore, a low fiber content in the diet would decrease stool bulk and slow transit time, thereby exposing the mucosa to the putative offenders longer. Alternatively, certain types of fiber might bind carcinogens and thereby protect the mucosa. Reduction in stool bulk would also lessen the dilution of offending products. Unfortunately, attempts to document these theories in patients and experimental animals have, on the whole, led to contradictory results.

There are many other ramifications to the story, for example, the possible protective roles of vitamins A, C, and E; the contribution of a lack of selenium to a predisposition to cancer; and the growing anxiety (sometimes hysteria) about the use of food additives and agricultural pesticides and fungicides. Nevertheless, at present, while there are reasons for being cautious about the role of the diet in the development of certain forms of cancer, definitive proof or even persuasive evidence is still lacking.

1. The World Commission on Environment and Development: Our Common Future. Oxford, England, Oxford University Press, 1987.
2. McCally, M., and Cassil, C.K.: Medical responsibility and global environmental change. Ann. Intern. Med. *113:*467, 1990.
3. Leaf, A.: Potential health effects of global climatic and environmental changes. N. Engl. J. Med. *321:*1577, 1989.
4. Beckett, W.S.: Ozone, air pollution, and respiratory health. Yale J. Biol. Med. *64:*167, 1991.
5. Pershagen, G., et al.: Residential radon exposure and lung cancer in Sweden. N. Engl. J. Med. *330:*159, 1994.
6. Manson, J.E., et al.: The primary prevention of myocardial infarction. N. Engl. J. Med. *326:*1406, 1992.
7. U.S. Department of Health and Human Services: The Health Consequences of Smoking for Women: A Report of the Surgeon General. Bethesda, MD, United States Department of Health and Human Services, Office of the Assistant Secretary for Health, Office on Smoking and Health, 1980.
8. Sherman, C.B.: Health effects of cigarette smoking. Clin. Chest Med. *12:*643, 1991.
9. Hoffman, D., et al.: Lung cancer and the changing cigarette. International Agency for Research on Cancer (IARC) Sci. Publ. *105:*449, 1991.
10. Litovitz, T.L., et al.: 1990 Annual Report. American Association of Poison Control Centers, National Data Collection System, p. 461.
11. Ingelfinger, F.J.: Adverse drug reactions that count. N. Engl. J. Med. *294:*1003, 1976.
12. Voigt, L.F., et al.: Progestogen supplementation of exogenous oestrogens and risk of endometrial cancer. Lancet *338:*274, 1991.
13. Bergkvistel, L.: The risk of breast cancer after estrogen and estrogen-progestin replacement. N. Engl. J. Med. *321:*293, 1989.
14. Gambrell, R.D.: Estrogen-progestogen replacement and cancer risk. Hosp. Pract. *25:*81, 1990.
15. Stampfer, M.J., et al.: Postmenopausal estrogen therapy and cardiovascular disease: Ten-year follow-up from the Nurses' Health Study. N. Engl. J. Med. *325:*756, 1991.
15a. Martin, K.A., and Freeman, M.W.: Postmenopausal hormone replacement therapy. N. Engl. J. Med. *328:*1115, 1993.
16. Riggs, B.L., and Melton, L.J., III: Drug therapy: The prevention and treatment of osteoporosis. N. Engl. J. Med. *327:*614, 1992.
17. Wynn, V.: Oral contraceptives and coronary heart disease. J. Reprod. Med. *36:*219, 1991.
18. Baird, D.T., and Glasier, A.F.: Hormonal contraception. N. Engl. J. Med. *328:*1543, 1993.
19. Kaldor, J.M., et al.: Leukemia following Hodgkin's disease. N. Engl. J. Med. *322:*7, 1990.
20. Charness, M.E.: Ethanol and the nervous system. N. Engl. J. Med. *321:*442, 1989.
21. Baghurst, P.A., et al.: Environmental exposure to lead and children's intelligence at the age of seven years. N. Engl. J. Med. *327:*1279, 1992.
22. Needleman, H.L., and Bellinger, D.: The health effects of low level exposure to lead. Annu. Rev. Public Health *12:*111, 1991.
23. Chisolm, J.J.: The continuing hazard of lead exposure and its effects in children. Neurotoxicology *5:*23, 1984.
24. Bennett, W.M.: Lead nephropathy. Kidney Int. *28:*212, 1985.
25. Ernst, P., and Theriault, G.: Known occupational carcinogens and their significance. Can. Med. Assoc. J. *130:*863, 1984.
26. Haley, T.J.: Occupational cancer and chemical structure: Past, present, and future. Drug Metab. Rev. *15:*919, 1984.
27. Committee on Adolescence; Committee on Substance Abuse: Marijuana: A continuing concern for pediatricians. Pediatrics *88:*1070, 1991.
28. Nahas, G., and Latour, C.: The human toxicity of marijuana. Med. J. Aust. *156:*495, 1992.
29. Kozel, N.J., and Adams, E.H.: Epidemiology of drug abuse: An overview. Science *234:*970, 1986.
30. Volpe, J.J.: Effects of cocaine use on the fetus. N. Engl. J. Med. *327:*399, 1992.
31. Virmani, R.: Cocaine-associated cardiovascular disease: Clinical and pathological aspects. NIDA Res. Monogr. *108:*220, 1991.
32. Ostor, A.G.: The medical complications of narcotic addiction. Med. J. Aust. *1:*410, 448, 497, 1977.
33. Stern, W.Z., and Subarrao, K.: Pulmonary complications of drug addiction. Semin. Roentgenol. *18:*183, 1983.
34. Melamed, Y., et al.: Medical problems associated with underwater diving. N. Engl. J. Med. *326:*30, 1992.
35. Gregg, P.J., and Walder, D.N.: Caisson disease of bone. Clin. Orthop. *210:*43, 1986.
36. Tribble, C.G., et al.: Lightning injuries. Compr. Ther. *11:*32, 1985.
37. Upton, A.C.: Radiation diagnosis and management. Cancer Detect. Prev. *15:*241, 1991.
38. Withers, H.R.: Biological basis of radiation therapy for cancer. Lancet *339:*156, 1992.
39. Lane, D.P.: Guardian of the genome. Nature *358:*15, 1992.
40. Yoshimoto, Y., et al.: Risk of cancer among children exposed in utero to A bomb radiations, 1950–1984. Lancet *2:*665, 1988.
41. Neel, J.V.: Update on the genetic effects of ionizing radiation. J.A.M.A. *698:*266, 1991.
42. Michaelson, S.M., et al.: Fundamental and Applied Aspects of Nonionizing Radiation. New York, Plenum Press, 1975.
43. Latham, M.C.: Protein energy malnutrition (PEM)—its epidemiology and control. J. Environ. Pathol. Toxicol. Oncol. *10:*168, 1990.
44. Stephenson, L.S., et al.: Treatment with a single dose of albendazole improves growth of Kenyan schoolchildren with hookworm, *Trichuris trichiura,* and *Ascaris lumbricoides* infections. Am. J. Trop. Med. Hyg. *41:*78, 1989.
45. Tee, E.-S.: Carotenoids and retinoids in human nutrition. Crit. Rev. Food Sci. Nutr. *31:*103, 1992.
46. Wald, G.: Molecular basis of visual excitation. Science *162:*230, 1968.
47. West, C.E., et al.: Vitamin A and immune function. Proc. Nutr. Soc. *50:*251, 1991.
48. Kumar, R.: Vitamin D and calcium transport. Kidney Int. *40:*1177, 1991.
49. Bordier, P., et al.: Vitamin D metabolites and bone mineralization in man. J. Clin. Endocrinol. Metab. *46:*284, 1978.
50. Hutchinson, F.N., and Bell, N.H.: Osteomalacia and rickets. Semin. Nephrol. *12:*127, 1992.
51. Sokol, R.J.: Vitamin E and neurologic function in man. Free Radic. Biol. Med. *6:*189, 1989.
52. Anderson, S.H., et al.: Adult thiamine requirements and the continuing need to fortify processed cereals. Lancet *2:*85, 1986.
53. Pang, J.A., et al.: Shoshin beriberi: An underdiagnosed condition. Intensive Care Med. *12:*380, 1986.
54. Harper, C.G., et al.: Clinical sign in the Wernicke-Korsakoff complex: A retrospective analysis of 131 cases discovered at necropsy. J. Neurol. Neurosurg. Psychiatry *49:*341, 1986.
55. Padh, H.: Vitamin C: Newer insights into its biochemical function. Nutr. Rev. *49:*65, 1991.

56. Hemila, H.: Vitamin C and the common cold. Br. J. Nutr. *67*:3, 1992.

57. Flynn, M.A.T., and Gibney, M.J.: Obesity and health: Why slim? Proc. Nutr. Soc. *50*:413, 1991.

58. Phillipson, B.E., et al.: Reduction of plasma lipids, lipoproteins, and apoproteins by dietary fish oils in patients with hypertriglyceridemia. N. Engl. J. Med. *312*:1210, 1985.

59. Kromhout, D.: The inverse relation between fish consumption and twenty-year mortality from coronary heart disease. N. Engl. J. Med. *312*:1205, 1985.

60. Editorial: Obesity: The cancer connection. Lancet *1*:1223, 1982.

61. Gori, G.B.: Dietary and nutritional implications in the multifactorial etiology of certain prevalent human cancers. Cancer *43*:2151, 1979.

62. Haenszel, W., and Kurihara, M.: Studies of Japanese migrants. I. Mortality from cancer and other diseases among Japanese in the United States. J. Natl. Cancer Inst. *40*:43, 1968.

63. Habs, M., and Schmahl, D.: Diet and cancer. J. Cancer Res. Clin. Oncol. *96*:1, 1980.

64. Manousos, O.N.: Diverticular disease of the colon. Dig. Dis. *7*:86, 1989.

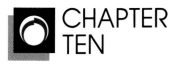

CHAPTER
TEN

Diseases of Infancy and Childhood

DEBORAH SCHOFIELD, M.D., and RAMZI S. COTRAN, M.D.

Children are not merely "little people," nor are their disorders merely variants of the diseases of adult life. Most childhood conditions are unique to, or at least take distinctive forms in, this stage of life and so merit the designation pediatric diseases. Collectively, they exact a heavy toll. Considering all ages from birth to senility, "certain conditions originating in the perinatal period" are currently the twelfth leading cause of death in the United States. As would be expected, the chances for survival of live-born infants improve with each passing week. The mortality rate in the first week of life is more than ten times greater than in the second week. Ironically, this striking differential represents, at least in part, a triumph of improved medical care. Better prenatal care, more effective methods of monitoring the condition of the fetus, and more frequent resort to cesarean section before term when there is evidence of fetal distress all contribute to bringing onto this "mortal coil" liveborn infants who in past years might have been stillborn. These represent, then, an increased number of "high-risk" infants. Nonetheless, the infant mortality rate in the United States has shown a decline from a level of 20.0 deaths per 1000 population in 1970 to about 11 currently. Sadly, the United States still ranks 19th in infant mortality

among industrialized nations, and American blacks have twice (18 per 1000) the infant mortality rate of American whites.

Each stage of development of the infant and child is prey to a somewhat different group of disorders. The data available permit a survey of four time spans: (1) the neonatal period (the first 4 weeks of life), (2) infancy (the first year of life), (3) 1 to 4 years of age, and (4) 5 to 14 years of age. The single most hazardous period of life is unquestionably the neonatal period. Never again is the individual confronted with more dramatic challenges than in the transition from dependent, intrauterine existence to independent, postnatal life. From the moment the umbilical cord is severed, the circulation to the heart is radically rerouted. Respiratory function must take over the role of oxygenation of the blood. Maintenance of body temperature and other homeostatic constants must now be borne alone by the fledgling organism. All these adaptations render the neonate particularly vulnerable.

The major causes of death in infancy and childhood are cited in Table 10–1. Congenital anomalies, respiratory distress syndrome, immaturity, birth trauma, birth asphyxia, complications of pregnancy, pneumonia, meningitis, and diseases of

431

Table 10–1. CAUSES OF DEATH AND AGE

CAUSES*	RATE
Under 1 Yr: All Causes†	692† (992.9§)
1Perinatal conditions	
Intrauterine growth retardation/low birth weight	
Respiratory distress syndrome	
Intrauterine hypoxia/birth asphyxia	
Birth trauma	
Others	
Congenital anomalies	
Sudden infant death syndrome	
Pneumonia	
Gastrointestinal disorders	
1–4 Yr: All Causes‡	43.3‡
Injuries	
Congenital anomalies	
Malignant neoplasms	
Homicide	
Diseases of the heart**	
5–9 Yr: All Causes¶	18.5‖
Injuries	
Malignant neoplasms	
Congenital anomalies	
Homicide	
Diseases of the heart**	
10–14 Yr: All Causes¶	18.5‖
Injuries	
Malignant neoplasms	
Suicide	
Homicide	
Congenital anomalies	
15–24 Yr†† : All Causes§	52.0‡
Injuries	
Suicide	
Homicide	
Malignant neoplasms	
Diseases of the heart**	

    * Listed in decreasing order of frequency.
    † Adapted from Monthly Vital Statistics Report 37(13):16, 26, 1989. Ranking is for 1988.
    ‡ 1988 (Prov.) rate per 100,000 population.
    § 1988 (Prov.) rate per 100,000 live births.
    ¶ Leading causes of death by age, 1985. National Center for Health Statistics.
    ‖ Mortality rate per 100,000 population ages 5–14 yr for 1988 (Prov.).
    ** Excludes congenital heart anomalies.
    †† Ranking is for ages 15–19 in 1985.
    Modified from Behrman, R.E., et al. (eds.): Nelson Textbook of Pediatrics, 14th ed. Philadelphia, W.B. Saunders Co., 1992, p. 2.

the gastrointestinal system represent the leading causes of death in the first 12 months of life.

Once the infant survives the first year of life, the outlook brightens measurably. However, it is sobering to realize that in the next two age groups —1 to 4 and 5 to 14—injuries resulting from accidents have become the leading cause of death (see Table 10–1). Among the natural diseases, in order of importance, congenital anomalies and malignant neoplasms assume major significance. It would appear then that, in a sense, life is an obsta-

cle course. Fortunately for the great majority of us, the obstacles are surmounted, or even better, bypassed. We can now take a closer look at the specific conditions encountered during the various stages of infant and child development.

BIRTH WEIGHT AND GESTATIONAL AGE

It has been known for many years that infants born before completion of the normal gestation period have higher morbidity and mortality rates than full-term infants. Understandably, the vital organs of preterm infants are immature and therefore unable to adapt readily to early extrauterine existence. Infants who have failed to complete normal intrauterine growth weigh less than full-term infants, and in the past, premature infants were defined as those having a birth weight of less than 2500 gm. However, it is inaccurate to define prematurity by birth weight alone, because weight is but one of several measures of intrauterine growth. For example, an infant weighing 2300 gm and born at 34 weeks of gestation is likely to be physiologically immature and therefore at greater risk for suffering the consequences of organ system immaturity (e.g., respiratory distress syndrome or transient hyperbilirubinemia) than a full-term infant also weighing 2300 gm, but with corresponding functional maturity of most organ systems. Therefore, a system of classification that takes into account both gestational age and birth weight has been adopted. Infants are classified as being (1) *appropriate for gestational age (AGA)*, (2) *small for gestational age (SGA)*, and (3) *large for gestational age (LGA)*. Those whose birth weight falls between the 10th and the 90th percentiles for a given gestational age are considered AGA, whereas those who fall above or below these norms are classified as LGA or SGA, respectively. With respect to gestational age, infants born before 37 or 38 weeks are considered *preterm*, whereas those delivered after the 42nd week are considered *post-term*. The usefulness of this classification system is illustrated in Figure 10–1,[1] which graphically depicts the correlation among gestational age, birth weight, and risk of perinatal mortality. For example, an AGA 1500-gm infant born at 32 weeks of gestation has a mortality risk up to 20%, whereas an SGA, 700-gm infant born at a similar gestational age has a mortality risk approaching 65%. The variation in mortality (and morbidity) rates seen in these different birth weight–gestational age groups is a reflection of the different and distinctive diseases with which these infants are afflicted. We shall briefly discuss the group of infants that are small for gestational age, as prematurity and low

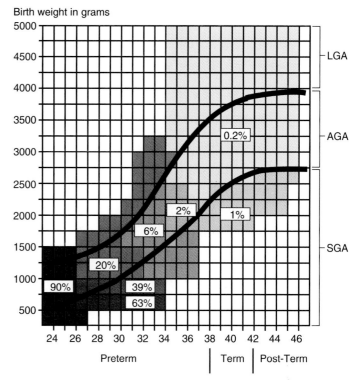

Birth weight in grams

WEEKS OF GESTATION

Figure 10–1. Neonatal mortality risk based on actual data from 14,413 live births at the University of Colorado Health Sciences Center from 1974 to 1980. Differentially shaded areas correspond to different mortality risks. For example, an infant born at 36 weeks of gestation and weighing 1250 gm has a mortality risk of 6%. If the same infant weighs 3000 gm, the risk of mortality falls to 0.2%. (Redrawn with permission from Koops, B., Morgan, L., Battaglia, F.: Neonatal mortality risk in relation to birth weight and gestational age: Update. J. Pediatr. *101:*969, 1982.)

birth weight are factors accounting for a significant proportion of perinatal mortality (see Table 10–1).

INTRAUTERINE GROWTH RETARDATION

It is generally accepted that at least one-third of infants who weigh less than 2500 gm are born at term and that they are therefore undergrown rather than immature. Hence, intrauterine growth retardation (IUGR) commonly underlies SGA. IUGR can be detected prior to delivery by ultrasonographic measurement of various fetal parameters, such as biparietal diameter, head circumference, abdominal circumference, head-to-abdomen circumference ratio, and total intrauterine volume. Although in a significant percentage of infants with IUGR the etiology is unknown, those factors known to result in IUGR can be divided into three main groups: fetal, placental, and maternal.

FETAL. Fetal factors are those that intrinsically reduce its growth potential despite an adequate supply of nutrients from the mother. Prominent among such fetal conditions are *chromosomal disorders* (in particular trisomies 13, 18 and 21, liveborn monosomy X and triploidy), *congenital anomalies*, and *congenital infections*.[2] Infants who are SGA due to "fetal" factors are characterized by symmetric growth retardation (also referred to as

proportionate, or type I, IUGR), meaning that all organ systems are similarly affected.[3]

PLACENTAL. In the third trimester of pregnancy, vigorous fetal growth places heavy demands on the uteroplacental supply line. *Uteroplacental insufficiency, therefore, is an important cause of growth retardation.* This may result from *placental abruption, placenta previa, placental thrombosis and infarction, placental infections,* or *multiple gestations* (see Chapter 23). In some cases, the placenta may be small without any detectable underlying cause.

Confined placental mosaicism is an additional, recently discovered, possible cause of IUGR.[4] Chromosomal mosaicism, in general, results from viable genetic mutations occurring after zygote formation. Depending on the developmental timing and cell of origin of the mutation, variable forms of chromosomal mosaicism result. For example, genetic mutations occurring at the time of the first or second postzygotic division result in generalized constitutional mosaicism of the fetus and placenta. On the other hand, should the mutation occur later and within dividing trophoblast or extraembryonic progenitor cells of the inner cell mass, a genetic abnormality limited ("confined") to the placenta results (Fig. 10–2).

Placental (and maternal) causes of IUGR result in disproportionate (or type II) growth retardation of the fetus — considered disproportionate because of relative sparing of the brain. Uteroplacental insufficiency is suspected as the cause of IUGR when

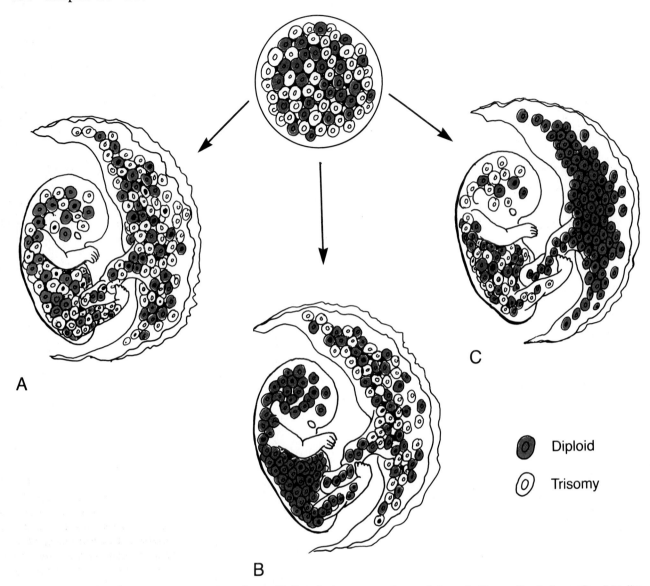

Figure 10–2. Diagrammatic representation of constitutional chromosomal mosaicism. *A*, Generalized; *B*, confined to the placenta; and *C*, confined to the embryo. (Modified and redrawn from Kalousek, D.K.: Confined placental mosaicism and intrauterine development. Pediatr. Pathol. *10*:69, 1990.)

in utero measurements of fetal growth reveal body size decreased out of proportion to head size.

MATERNAL. By far the most common factors associated with SGA infants are maternal, as many maternal conditions result in decreased placental blood flow. Vascular diseases, such as *toxemia* and *chronic hypertension*, are often the underlying cause. *Maternal malnutrition* may also affect fetal growth, but the association between SGA infants and the nutritional status of the mother is complex. The list of other maternal conditions associated with SGA infants is long,[5] but some of the avoidable factors worth mentioning are maternal *narcotic abuse, alcohol intake,* and *heavy cigarette smoking.* Drugs causing IUGR include both classic teratogens, such as antimetabolites, and some commonly administered therapeutic agents, such as Dilantin (diphenylhydantoin).

The SGA infant faces a difficult course, not only in the perinatal period, while struggle for survival is the main objective, but also in childhood and adult life. Depending on the underlying etiology of IUGR and, to a lesser extent, the degree of prematurity, there is a significant risk of morbidity in the form of a major handicap, cerebral dysfunction, learning disability, or hearing and visual impairment.

IMMATURITY OF ORGAN SYSTEMS

A major problem confronting the preterm infant regardless of birth weight is the functional and sometimes structural immaturity of various organs.

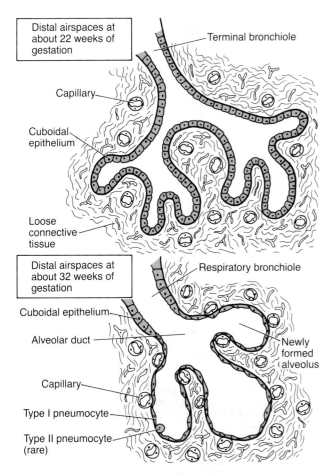

Distal airspaces at about 22 weeks of gestation

Terminal bronchiole

Capillary

Cuboidal epithelium

Loose connective tissue

Distal airspaces at about 32 weeks of gestation

Respiratory bronchiole

Cuboidal epithelium

Alveolar duct

Newly formed alveolus

Capillary

Type I pneumocyte

Type II pneumocyte (rare)

Figure 10-3. Schematic diagrams of fetal lung maturation.

Those who are also SGA are, understandably, the most seriously handicapped. Because immaturity may be the direct cause of death in very early preterm infants and significantly biases the probable outcome in others, it is appropriate to consider the features of immaturity of the more vital organs.

LUNGS. During the first half of fetal life, the development of the lungs consists essentially of the formation of a system of branching tubes from the foregut that eventually give rise to the trachea, bronchi, and bronchioles. The alveoli only begin to differentiate at approximately the seventh month of gestation. They are at first imperfectly formed, with thick walls and large amounts of inter- and intralobular connective tissue. The vascularization is buried within this connective tissue and is not in immediate contact with the alveolar spaces (Fig. 10-3). The epithelium lining the airspaces at this time is cuboidal and not anatomically suited to effecting the rapid transfer of oxygen to the blood. Between the 26th and 32nd weeks of gestation, the cuboidal epithelium shows transition to the flat, type I alveolar epithelial cells as well as type II cells that contain lamellar bodies (see Chapter 15). Further maturation of the lungs leads to reduction in

the interstitial tissues and increasing numbers of capillaries. However, even at full term the alveoli are small and the septa are considerably thicker than in the adult. Most of the cells lining the alveoli are type I cells. The type II cells appear in small clusters, mainly at the branching points of alveolar ducts. Development of alveoli continues after birth, and the full adult complement of alveoli is reached at about 8 years of age.

The immature lungs, then, are grossly unexpanded, red, and meaty. The alveolar spaces are incompletely expanded and usually contain pink proteinaceous precipitate and occasional squamous epithelial cells. The presence of large amounts of amniotic debris, such as squames, lanugo hair, and mucus, usually indicates prenatal respiratory distress.

KIDNEYS. In the preterm infant the formation of glomeruli is incomplete. Primitive glomeruli can be seen in the subcapsular zone. These structures have an organoid, glandular appearance imparted by the presence of cuboidal cells in the parietal and visceral layers of Bowman's capsule. However, the deeper glomeruli are well formed, and renal function is adequate to permit survival.

BRAIN. The brain is also incompletely developed in the preterm infant. The surface is relatively smooth and devoid of the typical convolutions found in the cerebral hemispheres of the adult. The brain substance is soft, gelatinous, and easily torn, and the definition between white and gray matter is somewhat ill defined. This lack of separation is, in large part, attributable to poorly developed myelination of the nerve fibers. To the best of our present knowledge, despite this underdevelopment, the vital brain centers are sufficiently developed, even in the very immature infant, to sustain normal central nervous system function. However, homeostasis is not perfect, and the preterm infant has difficulty in maintaining a constant normal level of temperature and has poor vasomotor control, irregular respirations, muscular inertia, and feeble sweating.

LIVER. The liver, although large relative to the size of the preterm infant, suffers from lack of physiologic maturity. Some of this increase in size is due to persistence of extramedullary hematopoiesis in this organ. Many or most of the functions of the liver are marginally adequate to carry out the demands placed on them. Almost all newborns and particularly those of low birth weight have a transient period of **physiologic jaundice** within the first postnatal week. This jaundice stems from both breakdown of fetal red cells and inadequacy of the biliary excretory function of liver cells. Deficiencies of bilirubin glucuronyl transferase, hydroxylating enzymes, and protein synthetic capacity, to name only a few hepatic systems, all characterize the immature liver.

Table 10-2. EVALUATION OF THE NEWBORN INFANT

SIGN	0	1	2
Heart rate	Absent	Below 100	Over 100
Respiratory effort	Absent	Slow, irregular	Good, crying
Muscle tone	Limp	Some flexion of extremities	Active motion
Response to catheter in nostril (tested after oropharynx is clear)	No response	Grimace	Cough or sneeze
Color	Blue, pale	Body pink, extremities blue	Completely pink

Sixty seconds after the complete birth of the infant (disregarding removal of the cord and placenta) the five objective signs are evaluated and each is given a score of 0, 1, or 2. A total score of 10 indicates an infant in the best possible condition.
Modified from Apgar, V.: A proposal for a new method of evaluation of the newborn infant. Anesth. Analg. 32:260, 1953.

APGAR SCORE

The Apgar score, devised by Dr. Virginia Apgar, represents a clinically useful method of evaluating the physiologic condition and responsiveness of the newborn infant, and hence its chances of survival.[6] Table 10-2 indicates the five parameters to be scored and how they are quantitated. The newborn infant may be evaluated at 1 minute or at 5 minutes. A total score of 10 indicates an infant in the best possible condition. The correlation between the Apgar score and the mortality during the first 28 days of life is very impressive. Infants with a 5-minute Apgar score of 0 to 1 have a 50% mortality within the first month of life. This drops to 20% with a score of 4, and to almost 0% when the score is 7 or better.[7] Despite the established value of the Apgar score in predicting perinatal morbidity, particularly in normal-birth-weight infants, it is not a reliable indicator of long-term neurologic morbidity.[8]

BIRTH INJURIES

Birth injuries constitute important causes of illness or death in infants as well as in children during the first years of life. No infant is immune to birth injury, although the risk and type of injury vary from the LGA infant to the preterm AGA or SGA infant. These injuries most commonly involve the head, skeletal system, liver, adrenals, and peripheral nerves. Considering the violent expulsive forces to which the fragile fetus is exposed, it is quite surprising that birth injuries are so relatively uncommon.

Morbidity associated with birth injury may be acute (e.g., that due to fractures) or the result of later-appearing sequelae (e.g., following damage to nerves or the brain). The distribution of injuries in a large municipal hospital, in descending order of frequency, is as follows:[9] clavicular fracture, facial nerve injury, brachial plexus injury, intracra-

nial injury, humeral fracture, and lacerations. Not surprisingly, LGA infants are at greater risk for birth injury, in particular those involving the skeletal system and peripheral nerves. We shall briefly discuss only injuries involving the head, as they are the most ominous.[10]

Intracranial hemorrhage is the most common important birth injury. These hemorrhages are generally thought to be related to excessive molding of the head or sudden pressure changes in its shape as it is subjected to the pressure of forceps or sudden precipitate expulsion. Prolonged labor, hypoxia, hemorrhagic disorders, or intracranial vascular anomalies are important predispositions. The hemorrhage may arise from tears in the dura, particularly in the falx cerebri and tentorium cerebelli; the dural sinuses may be stretched beyond their elastic limit and may rupture; the substance of the brain may be torn or bruised, leading to intraventricular hemorrhages or bleeding into the brain substance; or vessels that traverse the subdural space may be ruptured. Whatever their origin, intracranial hemorrhages are of great importance, as they cause sudden increases in intracranial pressure; damage to the brain substance; herniation of the medulla or base of the brain into the foramen magnum; and serious, frequently fatal depression of function of the vital medullary centers.

Caput succedaneum and *cephalhematoma* are so common, even in normal uncomplicated births, that they hardly merit the designation "birth injury." The first refers to progressive accumulation of interstitial fluid in the soft tissues of the scalp, giving rise to a usually circular area of edema, congestion, and swelling at the site where the head begins to enter the lower uterine canal. Because the fluid accumulates in the subcutaneous tissue, it may extend across the suture lines. Hemorrhage may occur into the scalp, producing a cephalhematoma. Usually the blood accumulates subperiosteally, and therefore the overlying swelling does not cross the cranial sutures. Both forms of injury are of little clinical significance and are of importance only insofar as *they must be differentiated from skull fractures with attendant hemorrhage and edema. In approximately 25% of cephalhematomas there is an underlying skull fracture.*

The skull bones may be fractured or may override each other, particularly when there is some disturbance in the ordinary mechanism of labor. Precipitate or sudden delivery with incomplete molding of the head, inappropriate use of forceps, and prolonged intense labor with disproportion between the size of the fetal head and birth canal are some of the clinical circumstances that surround the occurrence of these skull injuries.

CONGENITAL MALFORMATIONS

Congenital malformations are morphologic defects that are present at birth, although they may not become clinically apparent until later in life. The term *congenital* does not imply or exclude a genetic basis for malformations. It is estimated that about 3% of newborns have a *major malformation,* defined as a malformation having either cosmetic or functional significance.[11] As indicated in Table 10–1, they are a major cause of infant mortality.[12] Moreover, they continue to be a significant cause of illness, disability, and death throughout the early years of life. In a real sense, malformations found in live-born infants represent the less serious developmental failures in embryogenesis that are compatible with live birth. Perhaps 20% of fertilized ova are so anomalous that they are blighted from the outset. Less severe anomalies may be compatible with early fetal survival, only to lead to spontaneous abortion. As they become progressively less severe, a level is reached that permits more prolonged intrauterine survival, with some disorders terminating in stillbirth, and those still less significant permitting live birth despite the handicaps imposed.

DEFINITIONS. Before proceeding, it is important to define some of the terms used for various kinds of errors in morphogenesis—*malformations, deformations, disruptions, sequences,* and *syndromes.*

- *Malformations* represent intrinsic abnormalities occurring during the developmental process. Malformations may present in several patterns. Some, such as congenital heart defects and anencephaly (absence of brain), involve single body systems, whereas in other cases multiple malformations involving many organs may coexist. Malformations will be further discussed shortly.
- In contrast to malformations, *deformations* arise later in fetal life and represent an alteration in form or structure resulting from mechanical factors. They usually manifest as abnormalities in shape, form, or position of the body and, in gen-

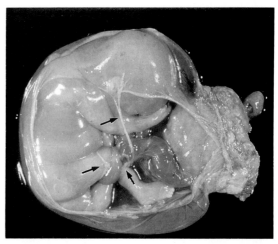

Figure 10–4. Amniotic band syndrome. Note placenta at right of diagram and band of amnion extending from the top portion of the amniotic sac to encircle the leg of the fetus. *(arrows).* (Courtesy of Dr. Theonia Boyd, Children's Hospital of Boston.)

eral, are associated with much less risk of recurrence in subsequent siblings. Uterine constraint is the most common underlying factor in infants born with deformations. This is partially due to the fact that between the 35th and the 38th weeks of gestation, the rapidly increasing growth of the fetus outpaces the growth of the uterus, while at the same time, there is a relative decrease in the amount of amniotic fluid (which normally acts as a cushion). Thus, even the normal fetus is subjected to some form of uterine constraint. Several factors increase the likelihood of excessive compression of the fetus resulting in deformations. *Maternal factors* include first pregnancy, small uterus, malformed (bicornuate) uterus, and leiomyomas. *Fetal* or *placental factors* include oligohydramnios, multiple fetuses, and abnormal fetal presentation. Examples of deformations include clubfeet, often a component of Potter's sequence, described below.

- *Disruptions,* the third main error in morphogenesis, result from secondary destruction of or interference with an organ or body region that was previously normal in development. Disruptions may be caused by either extrinsic factors or internal interferences, such as vascular insults, and are not heritable. *Amniotic bands,* denoting rupture of the amnion resulting in formation of "bands" that may compress, attach to, or encircle parts of the developing fetus, are the classic example of a disruption (Fig. 10–4).
- *Multiple congenital anomalies* may have their origin in a single localized aberration in organogenesis (malformation, disruption, or deformation) leading to secondary effects in other organs. Such a pattern of cascade anomalies is called a *sequence.* A good example is the *oligohydramnios (or Potter's) sequence* (Fig. 10–5). Oligohydramnios (decreased amniotic fluid) may be caused by

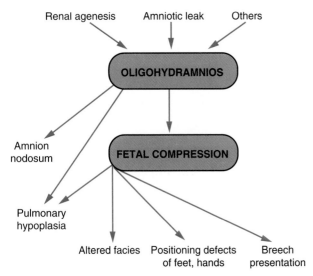

Figure 10-5. Schematic diagram of the pathogenesis of the oligohydramnios (Potter's) sequence.

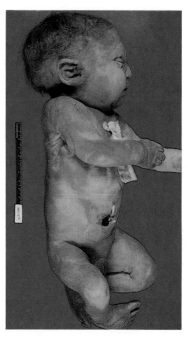

Figure 10-6. Infant with oligohydramnios/Potter's sequence. Note flattened facial features and deformed right foot. (talipes equinovarus).

a variety of unrelated maternal, placental, or fetal abnormalities. Chronic leakage of amniotic fluid due to rupture of the amnion, uteroplacental insufficiency resulting from maternal hypertension or severe toxemia, and renal agenesis in the fetus (as fetal urine is a major constituent of amniotic fluid) all are causes of oligohydramnios. The fetal compression associated with significant oligohydramnios in turn results in a classic phenotype in the newborn infant, including flattened facies and positional abnormalities of the hands and feet (Fig. 10–6). The hips may be dislocated. Growth of the chest wall and the contained lungs is also compromised so that the lungs are frequently hypoplastic, occasionally to the degree that they are the cause of fetal demise. Nodules in the amnion *(amnion nodosum)* are frequently present.

- The corollary of a sequence is a *syndrome*. In a syndrome, a patient may have several defects, felt to be pathogenetically related, that cannot be explained on the basis of a single, localized initiating anomaly. Syndromes are most often caused by a single etiologic agent, such as a viral infection or specific chromosomal abnormality, that simultaneously affects several tissues. When the underlying cause of the condition becomes known, for example the diagnosis of neurofibromatosis is made in a child with café-au-lait spots and numerous soft tissue masses, the syndrome is referred to as a *disease*.

- In addition to the above global definitions, a few organ-specific terms should be defined. *Agenesis* refers to the complete absence of an organ and its associated primordium. A closely related term, *aplasia*, refers also to the absence of an organ, but due to failure of the developmental anlage to develop. *Atresia* describes the absence

of an opening, usually of a hollow visceral organ, such as the trachea and intestine. *Hypoplasia*, or incomplete development or underdevelopment of an organ with decreased numbers of cells, is a less severe form of aplasia, whereas *hyperplasia* refers to the converse, that is, overdevelopment of an organ associated with increased numbers of cells. An abnormality in an organ or a tissue due to an increase or a decrease in the size (rather than the number) of individual cells defines *hypertrophy* or *hypotrophy*, respectively. Finally, *dysplasia*, in the context of malformations (vs. neoplasia) describes an abnormal organization of cells.

CAUSES OF MALFORMATIONS. At one time, it was believed that the presence of visible, external malformation was divine punishment for wickedness, occasionally jeopardizing the mother's life. Although we have a different understanding of malformations today, the exact cause remains unknown in at least half of the cases. Malformations can be grouped into two major categories—genetic and environmental (Table 10–3).

Genetic. Malformations that are known to be genetic in origin can be divided into three groups: (1) those associated with karyotypic aberrations, (2) those arising in single gene mutations, and (3) those suspected of resulting from multifactorial inheritance, a term that implies the interaction of two or more genes of small effect with environmental factors.

Virtually all the *chromosomal syndromes* (Chapter 5) are characterized by congenital anomalies.

Table 10–3. CAUSES OF CONGENITAL MALFORMATIONS IN HUMANS

CAUSE	MALFORMED LIVE BIRTHS (%)
Genetic	
Chromosomal aberrations	10–15
Mendelian inheritance	2–10
Multifactorial	20–25
Environmental	
Maternal/placental infections	2–3
Rubella	
Toxoplasmosis	
Syphilis	
Cytomegalovirus	
Human immuno- deficiency virus (HIV)	
Maternal disease states	6–8
Diabetes	
Phenylketonuria	
Endocrinopathies	
Drugs and chemicals	~1
Alcohol	
Folic acid antagonists	
Androgens	
Phenytoin	
Thalidomide	
Warfarin	
13-cis-Retinoic acid	
Others	
Irradiation	~1
Unknown	40–60

Adapted from Stevenson, R.E., et al. (eds.): Human Malformations and Related Anomalies. New York, Oxford University Press, 1993, p. 115.

Karyotypic abnormalities (see Chapter 5) are present in approximately 10 to 15% of live-born infants with congenital malformations. Only one reaches the birth frequency of 1 in 1000 total births, namely, trisomy 21 (Down syndrome). Next in order of frequency are Klinefelter's syndrome, Turner's syndrome, and trisomy 13 (Patau's syndrome). The remaining chromosomal syndromes associated with malformations are far rarer. *The great preponderance of these cytogenetic aberrations arise as defects in gametogenesis and so are not familial.* There are, however, transmissible chromosomal abnormalities, as for example the translocation form of Down syndrome passed from one generation to the next, thus constituting a familial pattern of structural abnormalities.

Single gene mutations of large effect may underlie major malformations, which, as expected, follow Mendelian patterns of inheritance. On the whole these are relatively uncommon and do not have a birth frequency of 1 in 1000 births. Among these rare entities are the relatively less serious limb malformations: polydactyly, syndactyly, and brachydactyly. However, there is still some question about the mode of transmission of some of these, and multifactorial inheritance cannot be totally excluded. In addition, there are a number of malformation syndromes in which multiple anomalies occur in disorders having Mendelian modes of transmission, for example Marfan's syndrome and the mucopolysaccharidoses (see Chapter 5).

Environmental. Environmental influences, such as viral infections, drugs, and irradiation, to which the mother was exposed during pregnancy may induce malformations in the fetus and infant.[15] As will be discussed later, many agents known to be carcinogenic postnatally are teratogenic to the fetus. Many viruses have been implicated, including the agents responsible for rubella, cytomegalic inclusion disease, herpes simplex, varicella-zoster infection, influenza, mumps, and other infections. Among these, the rubella virus and the cytomegalovirus are the most extensively investigated. With all viruses, the gestational age at which the infection occurs in the mother is critically important. *The at-risk period for rubella infection extends from shortly before conception to the 16th week of gestation,* the hazard being greater in the first 8 weeks than in the second 8 weeks. The incidence of malformations is reduced from 50% to 20% or 7%, respectively, if infection occurs in the first, second, or third month of gestation. The fetal defects are extremely varied, but the major triad comprises cataracts, heart defects (persistent ductus arteriosus, pulmonary artery hypoplasia or stenosis, ventricular septal defect, tetralogy of Fallot), and deafness, referred to as *rubella syndrome.*

Intrauterine infection with the cytomegalovirus, mostly asymptomatic, is the most common fetal viral infection. Its prevalence is estimated to be 0.4 to 7.4%.[16] This viral disease is considered in detail in Chapter 8, and it suffices here to indicate that the highest at-risk period is the second trimester of pregnancy. Because organogenesis is largely completed by the end of the first trimester, congenital malformations occur less frequently than in rubella; nevertheless, the effects of virus-induced injury on the formed organs are often severe. Involvement of the central nervous system is a major feature, and the most prominent clinical changes are mental retardation, microcephaly, deafness, and hepatosplenomegaly.

A variety of drugs and chemicals have been suspected to be teratogenic, but perhaps fewer than 1% of congenital malformations are caused by these agents. The list includes thalidomide, folate antagonists, androgenic hormones, alcohol, anticonvulsants, warfarin (oral anticoagulant), and 13-cis-retinoic acid used in the treatment of severe acne. For example, *thalidomide,* once used as a tranquilizer in Europe, caused an extremely high frequency (50 to 80%) of malformations. Limb abnormalities range from severe, such as amelia (absence of limbs) and phocomelia ("seal limbs," absence of limb with hands or feet attached directly to the trunk), to minor, such as hypoplasia of the thumb. *Alcohol,* perhaps the most widely used agent today, has only recently been recognized as

Table 10–4. APPROXIMATE FREQUENCY OF THE MORE COMMON CONGENITAL MALFORMATIONS IN THE UNITED STATES

MALFORMATION	FREQUENCY PER 10,000 TOTAL BIRTHS
Hypospadias	28.23
Clubfoot without neural defects	25.61
Ventricular septal defect	15.23
Cleft lip with or without cleft palate	9.05
Congenital dislocation of hip without neural defects	8.92
Patent ductus arteriosus	7.50
Spina bifida without anencephaly	4.78
Anencephaly	3.14
Atrial septal defect	1.70
Cystic disease of kidney	1.30

Adapted from Edmonds, L.D., and James, L.M.: Temporal trends in the incidence of malformations in the United States: Selected years, 1970–71, 1982–83. MMWR (CDC Surveillance Summaries), 34(No. 255):155, 355, 1985.

a teratogen.[16] Affected infants show growth retardation, microcephaly, atrial septal defect, short palpebral fissures, maxillary hypoplasia, and several other minor anomalies. These together are labeled the *fetal alcohol syndrome.*[17]

Radiation, in addition to being mutagenic and carcinogenic, is teratogenic. Exposure to heavy doses of radiation during the period of organogenesis leads to malformations, such as microcephaly, blindness, skull defects, spina bifida, and other deformities. Such exposure occurred in the past when radiation was used to treat cervical cancer.

The genetic and environmental factors just discussed can account for no more than one-half of human congenital malformations. The causes of the vast majority of birth defects, including some relatively common disorders such as cleft lip and cleft palate, remain unknown. In these malformations, it would appear that inheritance of a certain number of mutant genes and their interaction with the environment is required before the disorder is expressed. In the case of congenital dislocation of the hip, for example, depth of the acetabular socket and laxity of the ligaments are believed to be genetically determined, whereas a significant environmental factor is believed to be frank breech position *in utero,* with hips flexed and knees extended. In most instances, unfortunately, the nature of genetic and environmental factors and their interplay are unknown. The approximate frequency of some common malformations in the United States is presented in Table 10–4.

MECHANISMS OF MALFORMATIONS. The pathogenesis of congenital malformations is complex and still poorly understood. Certain general principles of developmental pathology that are relevant regardless of the etiologic agent will be discussed first.

- *The timing of the prenatal teratogenic insult has an important impact on the occurrence and the type of malformation produced*[11] (Fig. 10–7).

  The intrauterine development of humans can be divided into two phases: the embryonic period occupying the first 9 weeks of pregnancy, and the fetal period terminating at birth. In the *early embryonic period* (first 3 weeks after fertilization), an injurious agent damages either enough cells to cause death and abortion, or only a few cells, presumably allowing the embryo to recover without developing defects. Between the third and the ninth weeks the embryo is extremely susceptible to teratogenesis, and the peak sensitivity during this period is between the fourth and the fifth weeks. It is during this period that organs are being created out of the germ cell layers. The *fetal period* that follows organogenesis is marked chiefly by the further growth and maturation of the organs, with greatly reduced susceptibility to teratogenic agents. Instead the fetus is susceptible to growth retardation or injury to already formed organs. It is therefore possible for a given agent to produce different malformations if exposure occurs at different times of gestation.

- *Teratogens and genetic defects may act at several levels. These include cell proliferation, cell migration, differentiation, and damage to formed differentiated organs.* These events are influenced, during development, by the same growth regulatory molecules (e.g., growth factors, apoptosis-associated genes) and cell-matrix interactions that we have discussed in Chapter 2 and that are also involved in wound healing and neoplasia. For example, the TGF-β family includes, in addition to TGF-β-1, 2 and 3 described earlier, molecules that induce mesoderm (activin), influence bone morphogenesis (bone morphogenetic protein), and cause inhibition of Müllerian duct development.[18] There are an increasing number of examples in which spontaneous or experimentally induced aberrations in growth factors are associated with congenital malformations. There is an association, for example, between rare mutations of TGF-α and cleft palate,[19] and mutations in some of the TGF-β family genes cause malformations in mice.[18] Another dramatic example is the role of the Wilms' tumor gene (WT-1), which as you recall (see Chapter 7 and later in this chapter) is a tumor suppressor gene that acts as a transcriptional repressor after growth factor stimulation. The WT-1 gene is expressed at critical times of urogenital development. Mutations in WT-1 are associated with urogenital malformations, and deletion of the gene in transgenic mice causes renal agenesis (absent kidneys).[20]

  Orderly migrations take place in extracellular matrices and involve adhesive glycoproteins. Genetically engineered mice with aberrations or deficiencies in fibronectin or some of the inte-

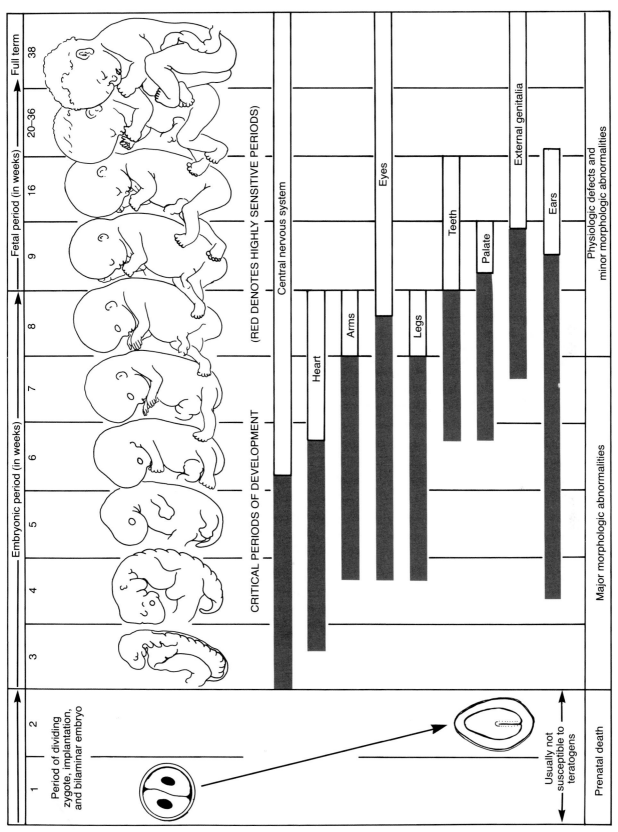

Figure 10–7. Critical periods of development for various organ systems and the resultant malformations. (Modified and redrawn from Moore, K.L.: The Developing Human, 5th ed. Philadelphia, W.B. Saunders Co., 1993, p. 156.)

441

grins either die as embryos or are born with congenital defects.[20a] Teratogens may disrupt cell migrations. For example, in experimental animals, disturbance in collagen-matrix formation by cadmium produces major craniofacial anomalies because the migration of neural crest cells is inhibited. Anticonvulsant drugs, on the other hand, impair the appropriate differentiation of the mesenchyme and give rise to cleft palate in rodents.

• *Morphogenesis genes.* Since many congenital malformations reflect failure of normal morphogenesis during development, it is reasonable to expect that alterations of genes that control these events might cause birth defects.[21] Classes of genes known to be important in embryonic patterning include those that contain conserved regions thought to be important in transcriptional regulation. One such class, the Hox genes, were first identified from study of the Drosophila mutant, *antennapedia*, in which legs appear in the position normally occupied by the antennae. Hox genes have a 180 nucleotide motif, dubbed the "homeobox," which has DNA binding properties and is conserved between species as divergent as insects and humans. Introduction of altered Hox genes in transgenic mice, embryonic exposure to chemical agents known to increase or decrease expression of Hox genes, and deletion of those genes ("knock outs") frequently produce malformations concordant with their presumed role in embryonic patterning.[22]

While it is presumed that the Hox gene products influence development by interacting with other genes, their downstream targets have not yet been identified. However, *retinoic acid* has been shown to be an upstream regulator of some Hox genes in normal morphogenesis.[23] Inasmuch as *retinoic acid is a known human teratogen*, mechanisms of action are of considerable interest. Currently, it is thought that retinoic acid can "turn on" Hox genes via another class of genes important in patterning (e.g., Hedgehog.[23a] The mechanism by which these genes interact to generate a normal embryo is unclear but is probably related to differential temporal and spatial expression of receptors (e.g., retinoic acid receptors) and cellular-cytoplasmic binding proteins (e.g., cellular retinoic acid–binding protein [CRABP], which bind retinoic acid or its metabolites) (Fig. 10–8, *left*).[24] In animals, retinoic acid exposure produces reproducible changes in Hox gene expression and causes a wide range of structural congenital malformations, the nature of which are determined by the dosage and timing of exposure.[24a] Correspondingly, infants born to mothers treated with retinoic acid for severe acne have a predictable phenotype (*retinoic acid embryopathy*), including central nervous system, cardiac, and craniofacial

defects[25] (Fig. 10–8). It remains to be seen whether other known teratogens have similarly specific effects on such genes.

Another family of developmental genes, the "paired-box," or *PAX genes*, constitute a group encoding DNA-binding proteins that, when mutated, cause human malformations. PAX-3 is mutated in Waardenburg's syndrome, characterized by congenital pigment abnormalities and deafness, and PAX-6 mutations may cause congenital absence of the iris—aniridia. Their mechanism of action is still unknown, but PAX genes may also induce neoplastic transformation or spontaneously occurring tumors, such as alveolar rhabdomyosarcoma.[25a] Much is currently being learned about the molecular mechanisms in morphogenesis and progress in our understanding of related congenital malformations is bound to be rapid.

PERINATAL INFECTIONS

Infections of the embryo, fetus, and neonate are manifested in a variety of ways and are mentioned as etiologic factors in Chapter 8 (Infectious Diseases) and numerous other sections within this chapter. Here we shall discuss only the general routes of infections. In general, fetal and perinatal infections are acquired via one of two primary routes—transcervically (also referred to as ascending) or transplacentally (hematologic). Occasionally, infections occur by a combination of the two routes in that an ascending microorganism infects the endometrium and then the fetal bloodstream via the chorionic villi.

TRANSCERVICAL, OR ASCENDING, INFECTIONS. Most bacterial and a few viral (e.g. herpes simplex II) infections are acquired by way of the cervicovaginal route. Infections that occur via this route may be acquired *in utero* or around the time of birth. In general, the fetus acquires the infection either by "inhaling" infected amniotic fluid into the lungs shortly before birth or by passing through an infected birth canal during delivery. Preterm birth of these infants is not uncommon and may be related to either damage and rupture of the amniotic sac as a direct consequence of the inflammation or to the induction of labor associated with a release of prostaglandins by the infiltrating neutrophils or microorganisms. Chorioamnionitis of the placental membranes and funisitis (inflammation of the umbilical cord) are usually demonstrable, although the presence or absence and severity of chorioamnionitis does not necessarily correlate with the severity of the fetal infection.

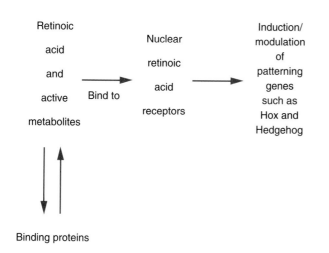

POSTULATED ROLE OF RETINOIC ACID IN NORMAL DEVELOPMENT

Retinoic acid and active metabolites → Bind to → Nuclear retinoic acid receptors → Induction/modulation of patterning genes such as Hox and Hedgehog

Binding proteins

RETINOIC ACID EMBRYOPATHY

Craniofacial malformations, including
    microtia/anotia (small/absent ears)
    facial bone and calvarial abnormalities
    micrognathia
    cleft palate

Congenital heart disease, including
    conotruncal malformations
    aortic arch abnormalities

Thymic ectopia, hypoplasia, or aplasia

Central nervous system malformations,
    including
    hydrocephalus
    cerebellar hypoplasia or vermis agenesis
    microcephaly

Limb abnormalities

Figure 10–8. Schematic representation of postulated role of retinoic acid in normal development and the features associated with retinoic acid embryopathy. Free retinoic acid (or its active metabolites) enters the cytoplasm of the cell, where it may be bound to cytoplasmic (or cellular) binding proteins. The unbound retinoic acid remains available for binding to nuclear retinoic acid receptors. Some of these retinoic acid–receptor complexes may then act as transcriptional regulators of various patterning genes, such as Hox and Hedgehog. Expression of the binding proteins and receptors in various tissues and at various times during embryogenesis may be a mechanism of selectively modulating the action of retinoic acid. This differential expression may also relate to the pattern of abnormalities seen in retinoic acid embryopathy.

TRANSPLACENTAL, OR HEMATOLOGIC, INFECTIONS. Most parasitic and viral infections, and a few bacterial (i.e., Listeria, treponema) infections gain access to the fetal bloodstream transplacentally via the chorionic villi. This hematogenous transmission may occur at any time during gestation or occasionally, as may be the case with hepatitis B and human immunodeficiency virus (HIV), at the time of delivery via maternal-to-fetal transfusion. In contrast to the fetus infected via inhalation of amniotic fluid, in which pneumonia, sepsis, and frequently meningitis are the most common sequelae, the effects of transplacental infection are more widespread. The clinical manifestations of these infections are highly variable, depending largely on the gestational timing and microorganism involved. Infections occurring early in gestation may result in more chronic sequelae, such as growth retardation, congenital malformations, and disruptions. Some infections, such as those with parvovirus B19 (which causes fifth disease in the mother), have been associated with spontaneous abortion and hydrops fetalis.[26] While the virus can bind to different cell types, replication occurs only in erythroid cells, and diagnostic viral cytopathic effect can be recognized in late erythroid progenitor cells of infected infants (Fig. 10–9). Examination of the placenta in these infants tends to reveal a villitis, corresponding directly with the transplacental mode of infection.

TORCH infections are caused by Toxoplasma (T), rubella (R), cytomegalovirus (C), herpes virus (H), and a number of other (O) bacterial and viral agents. They are grouped together because they may evoke similar clinical and pathologic manifestations. The latter include fever, encephalitis, chorioretinitis, hepatosplenomegaly, pneumonitis, myocarditis, hemolytic anemia, and vesicular/hemorrhagic skin lesions. Such infections, occurring early in gestation may also cause chronic sequelae in the child, including growth and mental retardation, cataracts, congenital cardiac anomalies, and bone defects.

Perinatal infections can also be grouped clinically by whether they tend to result in "early" versus "late" onset sepsis. For example, group B streptococci and *Escherichia coli* infections acquired at, or shortly prior to birth, tend to result in clinical signs and symptoms of pneumonia, sepsis, and occasionally meningitis within 4 or 5 days of

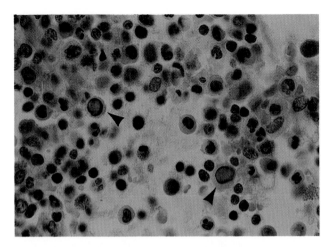

Figure 10–9. Bone marrow from an infant infected with parvovirus B19. The arrowheads point to two erythroid precursors with large homogeneous intranuclear inclusions and a surrounding peripheral rim of residual chromatin.

life — "early" sepsis. Infections with Listeria and Candida, on the other hand, require a latent period between the time of microorganism inoculation and the appearance of clinical symptomatology — "late" sepsis.

RESPIRATORY DISTRESS SYNDROME IN NEWBORN

Respiratory distress is one of the most common and life-threatening complications to confront the newborn infant, affecting 60,000 to 70,000 infants each year in the United States. It can have many origins, including (1) excessive sedation of the mother with consequent depression of respiration in the infant; (2) brain injury with failure of the central respiratory centers; (3) feeble respiratory efforts secondary to immaturity of the lungs and skeletal muscles (primary atelectasis); (4) aspiration during birth of blood clot and amniotic fluid when the amniotic debris (i.e., desquamated keratotic squames, mucus, lanugo hairs, proteinaceous precipitate, and blood) blocks ventilatory function; and (5) asphyxiating coils of umbilical cord about the neck of the infant. *But more important than all these by an order of magnitude is the idiopathic respiratory distress syndrome (RDS).* Despite the striking improvement in neonatal intensive care in the last 2 decades, RDS or its complications still take the lives of about 25,000 infants every year in the United States.

RDS is also known as hyaline membrane disease (HMD), highlighting one of the major pulmonary anatomic findings in this disease. In most cases this disorder presents in stereotyped fashion, which is best characterized by the following typical clinical setting. The infant is almost always preterm and appropriate for gestational age, and there are strong, but not invariable, associations with diabetes in the mother and with delivery by cesarean section. Resuscitation may be necessary at birth, but usually within a few minutes rhythmic breathing and normal color are reestablished. However, soon afterward, often within 30 minutes, breathing becomes more difficult, there is retraction of the lower ribs and sternum on inspiration, and an expiratory grunt becomes audible. Over the span of the next few hours the respiratory distress becomes worse, and cyanosis becomes evident. Fine rales can now be heard over both lung fields. A chest x-ray film at this time usually reveals uniform minute reticulogranular densities, producing a so-called "ground-glass" picture. At first the administration of oxygen to the infant lessens the cyanosis; indeed, during the next 12 to 24 hours recovery may ensue, but in the full-blown condition the respiratory distress persists, cyanosis increases, and even the administration of 80% oxygen by a variety of ventilatory methods fails to improve the situation. Flaccidity, unresponsiveness, and periods of apnea may now appear and may presage death. However, if therapy staves off death for the first 3 or 4 days, the baby has an excellent chance of recovery.[27]

ETIOLOGY AND PATHOGENESIS. Immaturity of the lungs is the most important subsoil on which this condition develops. It may be encountered in full-term infants but is much less frequent than in those "born before their time into this breathing world."[28] The incidence of RDS is inversely proportional to gestational age. It is estimated to occur in about 60% of infants born at less than 28 weeks of gestation, 15 to 20% of those born between 32 and 36 weeks, and less than 5% of those born after 37 weeks of gestation.[29]

The *fundamental defect in RDS is a deficiency of pulmonary surfactant.* As described in Chapter 15, surfactant consists predominantly of dipalmitoyl phosphatidylcholine, smaller amounts of phosphatidylglycerol, and at least two proteins that are thought to be important for normal surfactant function *in vivo*.[30] Surfactant reduces surface tension within the alveoli so that less pressure is required to hold alveoli open, and it maintains alveolar expansion by varying surface tension with alveolar size. It is synthesized by type II alveolar cells most abundantly after the 35th week of gestation in the fetus. At birth, the first breath of life requires high inspiratory pressures to expand the lungs. With normal levels of surfactant the lungs retain up to 40% of the residual air volume after the first breath; thus, subsequent breaths require far lower inspiratory pressures. With a deficiency of surfactant the lungs collapse with each successive breath, and so the infant must work as hard with each successive breath as it did with the first. The problem of "stiff" atelectatic lungs is com-

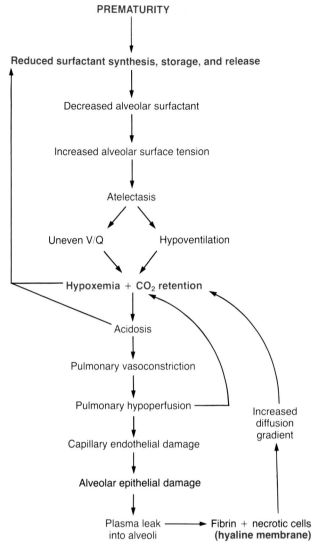

PREMATURITY

↓

Reduced surfactant synthesis, storage, and release

↓

Decreased alveolar surfactant

↓

Increased alveolar surface tension

↓

Atelectasis

Uneven V/Q ← → Hypoventilation

↓

Hypoxemia + CO_2 retention

↓

Acidosis

↓

Pulmonary vasoconstriction

↓

Pulmonary hypoperfusion

Increased diffusion gradient

↓

Capillary endothelial damage

↓

Alveolar epithelial damage

↓

Plasma leak ──→ Fibrin + necrotic cells
into alveoli   (hyaline membrane)

Figure 10–10. Schematic outline of pathophysiology of respiratory distress syndrome. V/Q = ventilation-perfusion ratio. (From Oh, W., and Stern, L.: Respiratory diseases of the newborn. *In* Stern, L., and Vert, P. (eds.): Neonatal Medicine. New York, Masson Publishing USA, 1987, p. 396.)

pounded by the "soft" thoracic wall that is pulled in as the diaphragm descends. Progressive atelectasis and reduced lung compliance then lead to a train of events as depicted in Figure 10–10, resulting in a protein-rich, fibrin-rich exudation into the alveolar spaces with the formation of hyaline membranes. The fibrin-hyaline membranes constitute barriers to gas exchange, leading to CO_2 retention and hypoxemia. The hypoxemia itself further impairs surfactant synthesis, and a vicious cycle ensues.

Surfactant synthesis is modulated by a variety of hormones, including cortisol, insulin, prolactin, and thyroxine. The role of glucocorticoids is particularly important. Corticosteroids induce the formation of surfactant lipids and apoprotein in fetal lung.[27,31] Surfactant synthesis may be suppressed

by the infants of diabetic mothers' compensatory high blood levels of insulin, which counteracts the effects of steroids. This may explain why infants of diabetic mothers have a higher risk of developing RDS.

MORPHOLOGY. The lungs are distinctive on gross examination. Although of normal size, they are solid, airless, reddish purple like the liver, and they usually sink in water. On microscopic examination the alveoli are poorly developed, and those that are present are collapsed. The atelectasis results from the clearance of fluid without its replacement by air. When the infant dies early in the course of the disease, necrotic cellular debris is present in the terminal bronchioles and alveolar ducts. Later, the necrotic material becomes incorporated within pink hyaline membranes that line the respiratory bronchioles, alveolar ducts, and random alveoli, mostly the proximal alveoli (Fig. 10–11). The membranes are largely made up of fibrinogen and fibrin admixed with cell debris derived chiefly from necrotic alveolar-lining pneumocytes. The sequence of events that leads to the formation of hyaline membranes was depicted in Figure 10–10. To this sequence can be added necrosis of alveolar lining cells owing to hypoxia, a lesion that develops early

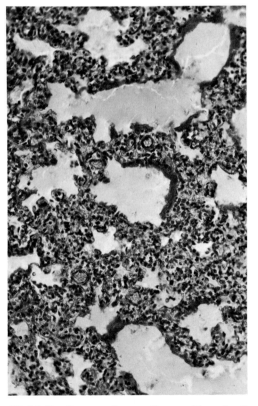

Figure 10–11. Hyaline membrane disease. There is alternating atelectasis and dilatation of the alveoli, and many airspaces are filled with fluid and lined by thick hyaline membranes.

and may be quite prominent. There is a remarkable paucity of inflammatory reaction associated with these membranes. The lesions of hyaline membrane disease are never seen in stillborn infants or in those live-born babies who die within a few hours of birth.

In infants who survive more than 48 hours reparative changes are seen in the lungs. The alveolar epithelium proliferates under the surface of the membrane, which may be desquamated into the airspace, where it may undergo partial digestion or phagocytosis by macrophages.

CLINICAL COURSE. Although a classic clinical presentation was described earlier, the actual clinical course and prognosis for neonatal respiratory distress syndrome are difficult to predict on a case-by-case basis—much depends on the maturity and birth weight of the infant, the therapy employed, and the promptness of institution of the therapy. A major thrust in the control of RDS focuses on prevention, either by delaying labor till the fetal lung reaches maturity or by inducing maturation of the lung in the fetus at risk. Critical to these objectives is the ability to assess fetal lung maturity accurately. Because pulmonary secretions are discharged into the amniotic fluid, analysis of amniotic fluid phospholipids provides a good estimate of the level of surfactant in the alveolar lining.

Once the infant is delivered, the major threat to life is inadequate pulmonary exchange of oxygen and carbon dioxide, and with it a metabolic acidosis. Overall, the mortality rate is approximately 20 to 30%, reaching levels exceeding 50% in infants in the range of 1000 gm of body weight. The cornerstone of treatment is the delivery of oxygen to these severely hypoxic infants, usually accomplished by a variety of ventilatory assistance methods in combination with surfactant replacement therapy.[32] Prophylactic administration of surfactant at birth to extremely premature infants (gestational age less than 26 weeks) and symptomatic administration of surfactant to infants born at 27 to 30 weeks of gestation appear to be beneficial in some cases.

In uncomplicated cases, recovery begins to occur within 3 or 4 days. However, therapy carries with it the now well-recognized hazard of *oxygen toxicity* caused by oxygen-derived free radicals. High concentrations of oxygen administered for prolonged periods have been proved to cause retrolental fibroplasia in the eyes and toxic changes in the lungs. Mechanical ventilation and oxygen toxicity may give rise to a subacute or chronic fibrosing condition called *bronchopulmonary dysplasia* (BPD). Clinically, BPD is characterized by persistence of respiratory distress for up to 3 to 6 months. Pathologically, the larger airways show epithelial hyperplasia and squamous metaplasia.

Alveolar walls are thickened, and there is peribronchial as well as interstitial fibrosis. If oxygen toxicity is avoided and the infant can be kept alive for about 3 or 4 days, recovery can be anticipated without permanent sequelae.

Infants who recover from RDS are at increased risk for developing a variety of other complications as well. Most important among these are *patent ductus arteriosus, intraventricular hemorrhage*, and *necrotizing enterocolitis*. Thus, although the high technology of today saves many infants with RDS, it also brings to the surface the exquisite fragility of the immature neonate.

ERYTHROBLASTOSIS FETALIS —HEMOLYTIC DISEASE OF NEWBORN

Erythroblastosis fetalis is defined as a hemolytic disease in the newborn caused by blood-group incompatibility between mother and child. When the fetus inherits red cell antigenic determinants from the father that are foreign to the mother, a maternal immune reaction may occur, leading to hemolytic disease in the infant. Basic to such a phenomenon are leakage of fetal red cells into the maternal circulation and, in turn, transplacental passage of the maternal antibodies into the fetus. Any of the numerous red cell antigenic systems may theoretically be involved, but the major antigens known to induce clinically significant immunologic disease are the ABO and certain of the Rh antigens. The resultant fetal hemolytic reaction may cause mild-to-severe disease in the newborn, or even death. The incidence of Rh erythroblastosis in urban populations has declined remarkably, owing largely to the current methods of preventing Rh immunization in "at-risk" mothers. Nevertheless, it is necessary to discuss Rh hemolytic disease because successful prophylaxis of this disorder has resulted directly from an understanding of its pathogenesis.

ETIOLOGY AND PATHOGENESIS. To explain the pathogenesis of Rh hemolytic disease (Fig. 10–12A), a few details of the Rh antigenic system will be reviewed. Of the numerous Rh antigens, the D antigen is the major cause of Rh incompatibility. It is estimated that 15% of whites and 7% of blacks do not possess the D antigen and so are said to be Rh negative. Thus, among whites there is an approximately 12% chance (85% of 15%) of a mating between an Rh-positive male and an Rh-negative female. However, the frequency of manifest Rh erythroblastosis is much lower because several factors influence the maternal immune response to Rh-positive fetal cells. *Concurrent ABO incompati-*

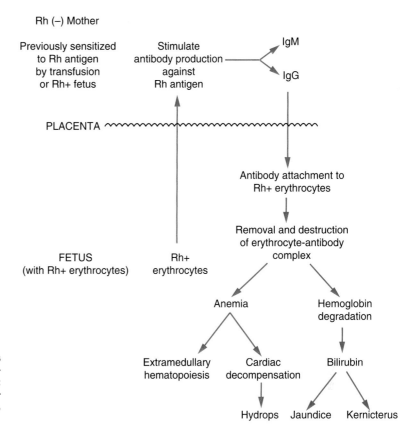

Rh (−) Mother

Previously sensitized to Rh antigen by transfusion or Rh+ fetus

Stimulate antibody production against Rh antigen

IgM

IgG

PLACENTA

Antibody attachment to Rh+ erythrocytes

Removal and destruction of erythrocyte-antibody complex

FETUS (with Rh+ erythrocytes)

Rh+ erythrocytes

Anemia

Hemoglobin degradation

Extramedullary hematopoiesis

Cardiac decompensation

Bilirubin

Hydrops   Jaundice   Kernicterus

Figure 10–12. Pathogenesis of erythroblastosis fetalis. (Redrawn with permission from Stevenson, R.E., Hall, J.G., and Goodman, R.M. (eds.): Human Malformations and Related Anomalies, Vol. 1. New York, Oxford University Press, 1993, p. 163.)

bility protects the mother against immunization, presumably because leaked fetal red cells are promptly coated by circulating isohemagglutinins and then removed from the circulation by the mononuclear phagocytic system. Another critical factor that determines the magnitude of the antibody response is the *dose of the immunizing antigen.* Hemolytic disease develops in the newborn only when the mother has experienced a significant transplacental "bleed." In the great majority of pregnancies, transplacental hemorrhages of such magnitude occur only during delivery or abortions. *Previous sensitization* significantly alters the risk of developing erythroblastosis fetalis. The first exposure to Rh antigens initially stimulates an increase in IgM antibodies that do not cross the placenta. Subsequently, there is a rise in IgG antibodies, small enough to cross the placenta. Because primary immunization usually occurs during labor, hemolytic disease rarely occurs during the first pregnancy unless from a previous abortion or stillbirth of an Rh-positive fetus might induce prior sensitization. The greatest risk is encountered in second and subsequent pregnancies of Rh-positive infants because in presensitized women even a small transplacental bleed could trigger a brisk secondary IgG response. Anti-D immunoglobulin administered to Rh-negative women within 72 hours before the birth of an Rh-positive infant prevents sensitization of the maternal lymphoid

system and therefore subsequent Rh hemolytic disease in later pregnancies.

Owing to the remarkable success achieved in prevention of Rh hemolytic disease by such therapy, *fetomaternal ABO incompatibility is currently the most common cause of erythroblastosis fetalis.* However, although ABO incompatibility occurs in approximately 20 to 25% of pregnancies, laboratory evidence of hemolytic disease occurs only in 1 in 10 of such infants and the hemolytic disease is severe enough to require treatment in only 1 in 200 cases.[33] Several factors account for this. First, most anti-A and anti-B antibodies are of the IgM type and hence do not cross placenta. Second, neonatal red cells express blood group antigens A and B poorly. Third, many cells other than red cells express A and B antigens and thus sop up some of the transferred antibody. ABO hemolytic disease occurs almost exclusively in infants born to group O mothers, because some have IgG anti-A and anti-B antibodies without obvious sensitization.

There are two consequences of excessive destruction of red blood cells in the neonate (Fig. 10–12). One is *anemia,* and the other is the accumulation of bilirubin (*jaundice*). However, the severity of these changes varies considerably, depending on the degree of hemolysis and the maturity of the infant organ systems. Extramedullary hematopoiesis in the liver and spleen may suffice to maintain normal red cell levels if the he-

Table 10–5. GENERAL CAUSES OF HYDROPS FETALIS

DISEASE ENTITY	EST. PERCENTAGE
Cardiovascular	26
Malformations	
Tachyarrhythmia	
High-output failure	
Chromosome abnormality	10
45, X	
Trisomy 21	
Thoracic	9
Cystic adenomatoid malformation	
Chondrodysplasia	
Diaphragmatic hernia	
Twin-twin transfusion	8
Anemia	6
Alpha thalassemia	
Fetomaternal transfusion	
Isoimmunization	
Fetal infection	4
Cytomegalovirus	
Bacteria	
Toxoplasma	
Urinary tract malformation	3
Urethral obstruction	
Prune belly syndrome	
Miscellaneous	11
Not determined	22

Only some of the most common entities under major categories are listed.

Adapted from Machin, G.A.: Hydrops revisited, literature review of 1,414 cases published in the 1980's. Am. J. Med. Genet. 34:366, 1989; copyright © 1989 John Wiley & Sons. Reprinted by permission of Wiley-Liss, A Division of John Wiley & Sons, Inc.)

molysis is mild. If the hemolytic reaction is marked, anemia associated with jaundice and the presence of unconjugated bilirubin occurs. As unconjugated bilirubin is water insoluble and has an affinity for lipids, it binds to lipids in the brain owing to the poorly developed blood-brain barrier in the infant, resulting in serious damage to the central nervous system, termed *kernicterus*. In addition, the anemia may be associated with hypoxic injury to the heart and liver, resulting in circulatory and hepatic failure and edema. If severe, plasma protein levels may drop to as low as 2.0 to 2.5 gm/dl because of reduced hepatic synthesis. *This decrease in oncotic pressure within the circulation, combined with a secondary increase in venous capillary pressure due to cardiac failure, results in generalized edema and ascites* (anasarca). This latter condition is referred to as *hydrops fetalis*.

A few additional comments on the causes of *hydrops fetalis* are in order at this time. The list of disorders reported to be associated with hydrops fetalis is extensive, including both immune (as in the case of erythroblastosis fetalis) and nonimmune conditions.[34] The latter group includes structural anomalies and hamartomas of the fetus, chromosomal abnormalities, inherited metabolic disease, and intrauterine infection (Table 10–5). In addition, approximately 10% of cases of nonimmune hydrops may be related to monozygous twin pregnancies and twin-twin transfusion occurring through anastomoses between the two circulations.

MORPHOLOGY. The anatomic findings in erythroblastosis fetalis vary with the severity of the hemolytic process. Infants may be stillborn, die within the first few days, or recover completely. In its mildest form, the anemia may be only slight, and the child may survive without further complication. More severe hemolysis gives rise to jaundice and other features associated with hemolytic anemias. In some cases, hydrops fetalis develops. In most cases the liver and spleen are enlarged, the degree depending on the severity of the hemolytic processes and the compensatory extramedullary erythropoiesis. Extensive extramedullary hematopoiesis within the liver may compromise intrahepatic circulation, further compromising hepatocyte function, which may already be tenuous.

The most serious threat in erythroblastosis is central nervous system damage known as **kernicterus**.[35] In jaundiced infants, the unconjugated bilirubin appears to be particularly toxic to the brain tissue. The brain is enlarged and edematous and, when sectioned, is found to have a bright yellow pigmentation (kernicterus), particularly in the basal ganglia, thalamus, cerebellum, cerebral gray matter, and spinal cord. This pigmentation is evanescent and fades within 24 hours despite prompt fixation. The precise blood level of bilirubin that induces kernicterus is unpredictable, but neural damage rarely occurs if the serum bilirubin concentration is below 20 mg/dl. At lower levels, premature infants especially are at risk.

Histologically, the diagnosis of erythroblastosis fetalis depends on the identification of abnormally increased erythropoietic activity in the infant. The red cell series in the marrow is hyperactive, and extramedullary hematopoiesis is almost invariably present in the liver (Fig. 10–13), spleen, and possibly other tissues, such as the lymph nodes, kidneys, lungs, and even the heart. This hematopoietic activity is sufficiently striking to account for increased numbers of reticulocytes, normoblasts, and erythro-

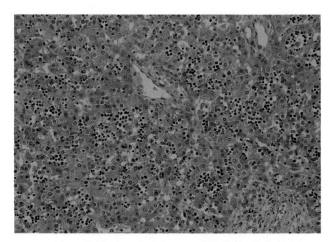

Figure 10–13. Numerous islands of extramedullary hematopoiesis (small blue cells) are scattered among mature hepatocytes in this infant with erythroblastosis fetalis.

blasts in the circulating blood. Evidence of subcutaneous and visceral edema is present in the hydrops syndrome along with fluid in the peritoneal, pleural, and pericardial cavities.

CLINICAL FEATURES. The clinical manifestations of erythroblastosis vary with the severity of the disease and can be predicted from the preceding discussion. Minimally affected infants display pallor, possibly accompanied by hepatosplenomegaly (to which may be added jaundice with more severe hemolytic reactions), whereas the most gravely ill neonates present with intense jaundice, widespread edema, and signs of neurologic involvement in the pattern referred to as hydrops fetalis. These latter infants may be supported by a variety of measures, including phototherapy (visual light oxidizes toxic unconjugated bilirubin to harmless, readily excreted, water-soluble dipyrroles) and, in severe cases, total exchange transfusion of the infant.

As mentioned previously, ABO incompatibility is the most common cause of hemolytic disease of the newborn. However, it should be kept in mind that approximately 2% of women at risk for Rh incompatibility fail to benefit from immunoprophylaxis and develop anti-D antibodies in the last trimester or within 72 hours after labor. Some of these cases may result from unrecognized previous Rh-positive abortions, but many are believed to be due to significant transplacental bleeds during the early part of the third trimester.[36] Therefore, anti-D immunoglobulin administered during the last trimester as well as after birth further reduces the risk of Rh disease. There is no effective protection against ABO reactions.

INBORN ERRORS OF METABOLISM

The number of now well-characterized inborn errors of metabolism has become astronomic and far beyond the scope of this chapter.[37,38] Most of these conditions are exceedingly rare. Some were discussed earlier, in Chapter 5. Only two, phenylketonuria (PKU) and galactosemia, are selected for inclusion here because, in both, prompt recognition during the first days of life permits the institution of an appropriate dietary regimen that can prevent early death or, even worse, survival with mental retardation.

PHENYLKETONURIA (PKU)

There are several variants of this inborn error of metabolism. The most common form, referred to as classic PKU, is quite common in persons of Scandinavian descent and is distinctly uncommon in blacks and Jews.

Homozygotes with this autosomal recessive disorder classically have a severe lack of phenylalanine hydroxylase, leading to hyperphenylalaninemia and PKU. Affected babies are normal at birth but within a few weeks develop a rising plasma phenylalanine level, which in some way impairs brain development. Usually by six months of life severe mental retardation becomes all too evident; fewer than 4% of untreated phenylketonuric children have IQ values greater than 50 or 60. About one-third of these unfortunate children are never able to walk, and two-thirds cannot talk. Seizures, other neurologic abnormalities, decreased pigmentation of hair and skin, and eczema often accompany the mental retardation in untreated children. Hyperphenylalaninemia and the resultant mental retardation can be avoided by restriction of phenylalanine intake early in life. Hence a number of screening procedures are routinely used for detection of PKU in the immediate postnatal period.

Many clinically normal female PKU patients who were treated with diet early in life have now reached childbearing age. Most of them have discontinued dietary treatment and have marked hyperphenylalaninemia. Children born to such women are profoundly mentally retarded and have multiple congenital anomalies, even though the infants themselves are heterozygotes. This syndrome, termed *maternal PKU*,[39] results from the teratogenic effects of phenylalanine that crosses the placenta and affects the developing fetus. Hence, *it is imperative that maternal phenylalanine levels be lowered by dietary means prior to conception.*

The biochemical abnormality in PKU is an inability to convert phenylalanine into tyrosine. In normal children, less than 50% of the dietary intake of phenylalanine is necessary for protein synthesis. The rest is converted to tyrosine by the phenylalanine hydroxylase system, which has several components in addition to the enzyme phenylalanine hydroxylase (Fig. 10–14). With a block in phenylalanine metabolism due to lack of phenylalanine hydroxylase, minor shunt pathways come into play, yielding phenylpyruvic acid, phenyllactic acid, phenylacetic acid, and o-hydroxyphenylacetic acid, which are excreted in large amounts in the urine in PKU. Some of these abnormal metabolites are excreted in the sweat, and phenylacetic acid in particular imparts a strong musty or mousy odor to affected infants. It is believed that excess phenylalanine or its metabolites contribute to the brain damage in PKU.

At the molecular level, several mutant alleles of the phenylalanine hydroxylase gene have been identified.[39a] It seems that only those mutations that result in severe deficiency of the enzyme result in classic PKU. In those with a partial deficiency of phenylalanine hydroxylase, only modest elevations of phenylalaine levels occur, without any neurologic damage. This condition, referred to as *benign hyperphenylalaninemia*, is important to recognize because the affected individuals may

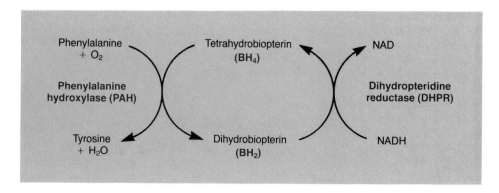

Figure 10-14. The phenylalanine hydroxylase system.

well test "positive" in the widely utilized Guthrie screening test but will not develop the stigmata of classic PKU. Measurement of serum phenylalanine levels is necessary to differentiate benign hyperphenylalaninemia and PKU.

As alluded to earlier, a number of variant forms of PKU have been identified. They account for 3 to 10% of all cases of PKU and result from deficiencies of enzymes other than phenylalanine hydroxylase. For instance, some patients lack dihydropteridine reductase (DHPR; see Fig. 10–14). Like those with classic PKU, they are also unable to metabolize phenylalanine, but in addition they have associated abnormalities of tyrosine and tryptophan metabolism, since DHPR is required for hydroxylation of these two amino acids. The concomitant impairment of tyrosine and tryptophan hydroxylation leads to disturbance in the synthesis of neurotransmitters, and neurologic damage is not arrested despite normalization of phenylalanine levels. *It is clinically important to recognize these variant forms of PKU because they cannot be treated by dietary control of phenylalanine levels.*

GALACTOSEMIA

Galactosemia is an autosomal recessive disorder of galactose metabolism. Normally, lactose, the major carbohydrate of mammalian milk, is split into glucose and galactose in the intestinal microvilli by lactase. Galactose is then converted to glucose in three steps (Fig. 10–15). *Two variants of galactosemia have been identified. In the more common variant there is a total lack of galactose-1-phosphate uridyl transferase (GALT) involved in reaction 2. The rare variant arises from a deficiency of galactokinase, involved in reaction 1.* Because galactokinase deficiency leads to a milder form of the disease not associated with mental retardation, it is not considered in our discussion. As a result of the transferase lack, galactose-1-phosphate accumulates in many locations, including the liver, spleen, lens of the eye, kidneys, heart muscle, cerebral cortex, and erythrocytes. Alternative metabolic pathways are activated, leading to the production of galactitol, which also accumulates in the tissues. Hetero-

zygotes may have a mild deficiency but are spared the clinicomorphologic consequences of the homozygous state.

The clinical picture is variable, probably reflecting the heterogeneity of mutations in the GALT gene leading to galactosemia.[40] The liver, eyes, and brain bear the brunt of the damage. The early-to-develop *hepatomegaly* is due largely to fatty change, but in time widespread scarring that closely resembles the cirrhosis of alcohol abuse may supervene (Fig. 10–16). *Opacification of the lens (cataracts)* develops, probably because the lens absorbs water and swells as galactitol, produced by alternative metabolic pathways, accumulates and increases its tonicity. *Nonspecific alterations appear in the central nervous system,* including loss of nerve cells, gliosis, and edema, particularly in the dentate nuclei of the cerebellum and the olivary nuclei of the medulla. Similar changes may occur in the cerebral cortex and white matter.

There is still no clear understanding of the mechanism of injury to the liver and brain. Toxicity has been imputed to galactose-1-phosphate. Alternatively, galactitol has been indicted as the toxic product. It is also possible that the abnormal galactose metabolism interferes with the formation of galactose-containing cerebral lipids.

Almost from birth these infants *fail to thrive. Vomiting* and *diarrhea* appear within a few days of milk ingestion. *Jaundice* and *hepatomegaly* usually become evident during the first week of life and may seem to be a continuation of the physiologic jaundice of the newborn. The *cataracts* develop within a few weeks, and within the first 6 to 12 months of life mental retardation may be detected. Even in untreated infants the mental deficit is usually not as severe as that with PKU. Accumulation of galactose and galactose-1-phosphate in the kidney impairs amino acid transport, resulting in aminoaciduria. There is an increased frequency of fulminant *Escherichia coli* septicemia.

Most of the clinical and morphologic changes can be prevented by early removal of galactose from the diet for at least the first two years of life. Control instituted soon after birth prevents the cataracts and liver damage and permits almost normal mental development. The diagnosis can be sus-

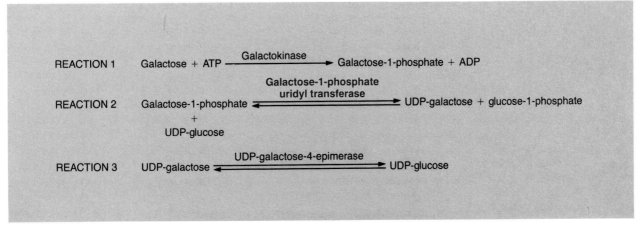

REACTION 1   Galactose + ATP $\xrightarrow{\text{Galactokinase}}$ Galactose-1-phosphate + ADP

REACTION 2   Galactose-1-phosphate $\underset{\xrightarrow{\hspace{2cm}}}{\xleftarrow{\text{Galactose-1-phosphate uridyl transferase}}}$ UDP-galactose + glucose-1-phosphate
  +
  UDP-glucose

REACTION 3   UDP-galactose $\underset{\xrightarrow{\hspace{2cm}}}{\xleftarrow{\text{UDP-galactose-4-epimerase}}}$ UDP-glucose

Figure 10–15. Pathways of galactose metabolism.

pected by the demonstration in the urine of a reducing sugar other than glucose, but tests that directly identify the deficiency of the transferase in leukocytes and erythrocytes are more reliable. Antenatal diagnosis is possible in cultured fibroblasts from amniotic fluid.

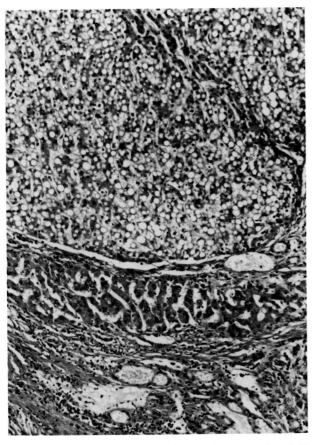

Figure 10–16. Galactosemia. Liver shows extensive fatty change and a delicate fibrosis. (Courtesy of Dr. Joe Rutledge, University of Texas Southwestern Medical School, Dallas.)

CYSTIC FIBROSIS (MUCOVISCIDOSIS)

Among the genetic pediatric disorders, cystis fibrosis (CF) is the most important. It is very common and often fatal in childhood and young adult life.[41] It is fundamentally a *widespread disorder in the secretory process of all exocrine glands affecting both mucus-secreting and eccrine sweat glands throughout the body.* The abnormally viscid mucous secretions lead to obstruction of organ passages, resulting in most of the clinical features of this disorder, for example, recurrent pulmonary infections leading to chronic lung disease, pancreatic insufficiency, steatorrhea, malnutrition, hepatic cirrhosis, intestinal obstruction, and male infertility. These manifestations may appear at any point in life from before birth to much later in childhood or even in adolescence.

With an incidence of 1 in 2000 live births, *CF is the most common lethal genetic disease that affects white populations.* It is uncommon among Asians and blacks. Cystic fibrosis follows simple autosomal recessive transmission, and homozygotes express this syndrome fully. Heterozygotes have no recognizable clinical symptoms. On the basis of the frequency of affected homozygotes in the white population, it is estimated that 1 in 20 individuals must be heterozygous carriers.

ETIOLOGY AND PATHOGENESIS. Although a large number of abnormalities have been described in CF, it is now agreed that *the primary defect is in the regulation of epithelial chloride transport.*[42] In normal duct epithelia, chloride is transported by plasma membrane channels *(chloride channels).* Opening of these channels is mediated by agonist-induced increases in cAMP, followed by activation of a protein kinase A that phosphorylates the channel. In sweat gland ducts, a defect in chloride transport leads to decreased reabsorption of sodium chloride (NaCl) from the lumen and thus increased sweat chloride (Fig. 10–17, *left).* This

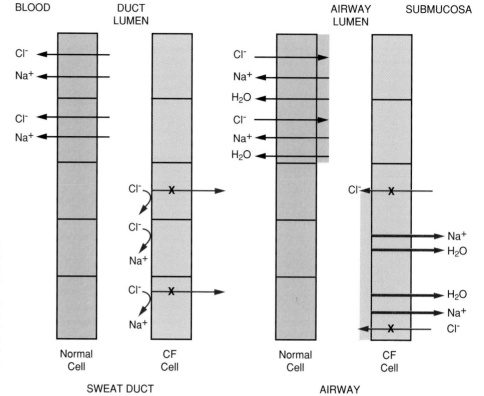

Figure 10-17. Chloride channel defect in the sweat duct of cystic fibrosis causes increased chloride and sodium concentration in sweat. In the airway, cystic fibrosis patients have decreased chloride secretion, increased sodium and water reabsorption leading to dehydration of the mucus layer coating epithelial cells, defective mucociliary action, and mucus plugging of airways.

forms the basis of the clinical diagnosis of CF: *an increased concentration of chloride in sweat.* In the *airway epithelium* the chloride channel defect in cystic fibrosis results in loss or reduction of chloride secretion into the airways (Fig. 10-17, *right*). Active sodium absorption is also increased in cystic fibrosis, and both of these ion changes increase water reabsorption from the lumen,[42a] *lowering the water content of the mucus blanket coating mucosal cells.* This dehydration of the mucus layer leads to defective mucociliary action and the accumulation of hyperconcentrated, viscid secretions that obstruct the air passages and predispose to recurrent pulmonary infections.[43]

The CF gene is located on chromosome 7 (band q31-32),[44] *and encodes a protein that serves as a chloride channel.*[45] The protein, named CFTR (cystic fibrosis transmembrane conductance regulator), has two transmembrane domains, two nucleotide binding domains (NBD), and a regulatory domain (R domain) that contains protein kinase A and C phosphorylation sites (Fig. 10-18). Almost 200 mutations of the CF gene have been identified, with 70% of cases bearing a deletion of three nucleotides coding for phenylalanine at amino acid position 508 (ΔF508).[46] The ΔF508 mutation results in defective processing of the protein from the endoplasmic reticulum to the Golgi apparatus; the protein does not become fully glycosylated and is instead degraded before it reaches the cell surface (see Fig. 10-18, *bottom*). Other mutations affect the nucleotide binding domains and the R do-

mains required for phosphorylation of CFTR, or the membrane-spanning domains essential for conduction.[47]

In general, the severity of the resulting disease correlates with the degree to which the mutation affects chloride transport. On one end of the spectrum is the ΔF508 homozygous mutation, which is associated with practically absent membrane CFTR, early pancreatic insufficiency, and various degrees of pulmonary deficiency.[48] In the middle are certain ΔF508 heterozygotes, (R117/Δ508) who may have good long-term pancreatic function but are not protected from lung injury.[49] On the other end are mutations in the membrane-spanning domains, which have relatively normal chloride transport; patients with such mutations may have male sterility as the only manifestation of the disease.[47] Exceptions abound, however, and in particular, there is a great deal of variability in the magnitude of pulmonary disease within similar genotypes. Defects in additional chloride channels, or in transport of other ions as well, or involvement of alternative pathogenetic mechanisms may account for these discrepancies.

Secondary pathogenetic mechanisms clearly play a role in CF. In the lung, for example, defective mucociliary action due to deficient hydration of the mucus results in inability of the airways to clear bacteria (see Chapter 15).[43] *Pseudomonas aeruginosa* species, in particular, colonize the lower respiratory tract, first intermittently, then chronically. Concurrent viral infections predispose

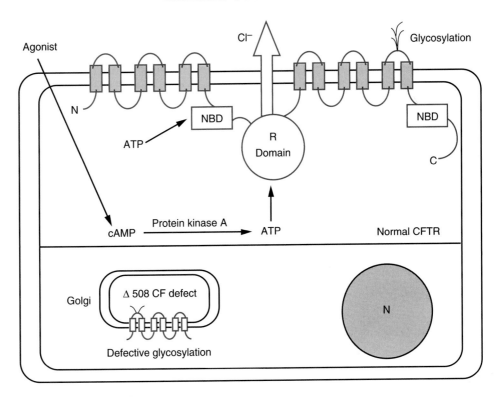

Figure 10–18. *Top,* Normal CFTR structure and activation. CFTR consists of two transmembrane domains, two nucleotide binding domains (NBD), and a regulatory R domain. Agonists (e.g., acetylcholine) bind to epithelial cells, increase cAMP, which activates protein kinase A, the latter phosphorylating the CFTR at the R domain, resulting in opening of the chloride channel. *Bottom,* The most common mutation in the CFTR gene results in defective protein glycosylation in the Golgi/ER and degradation of CFTR before it reaches the cell surface.[47]

to such colonization. In chronic infections, Pseudomonas species express abundant amounts of *alginate*, endowing the organisms with mucoid growth into microcolonies that are protected from antibodies or antibiotics, thus favoring persistence of the infection. Antibody and cell-mediated reactions induced by the organisms then result in further tissue destruction that characterizes the lung lesions in CF.

MORPHOLOGY. The anatomic changes are highly variable and depend on which glands are affected and on the severity of this involvement. In some infants, the disease is quite mild and does not seriously disturb their growth and development, and they readily survive into adolescence or adulthood. In others, the pancreatic involvement is severe and impairs intestinal absorption because of the pancreatic achylia, and so malabsorption, inanition, and stunted development not only seriously hamper life but also shorten survival. In others, the mucus secretion defect leads to defective mucociliary action, obstruction of bronchi and bronchioles, and crippling fatal pulmonary infections (Fig. 10–19). Thus, cystic fibrosis may be compatible with long life or may cause death in infancy. Significantly, the sweat glands, producing a watery secretion, are morphologically unaffected.

Pancreatic abnormalities are present in approximately 85 to 90% of patients. In the milder cases, there may be only accumulations of mucus in the small ducts with some dilatation of the exocrine glands. In more advanced cases, usually seen in older children or adolescents, the ducts are totally plugged, causing atrophy of the exocrine glands and progressive fibrosis (see Fig. 10–20). Total atrophy of the exocrine portion of the pancreas may occur, leaving only the islets within a fibrofatty stroma. The total loss of pancreatic exocrine secretion impairs fat absorption, and so avitaminosis A may contribute to squamous metaplasia of the lining epithelium of the ducts in the pancreas, which are already injured by the inspissated mucus secretions. Thick viscid plugs of mucus may also be found in the small intestine of infants. Sometimes these cause small bowel obstruction, known as **meconium ileus.**

The **liver involvement** follows the same basic pattern. Bile canaliculi are plugged by mucinous material. When this is of long duration, biliary cirrhosis (see Chapter 18) with its diffuse hepatic nodularity may develop. Such severe hepatic involvement is encountered in only approximately 5% of patients.

The **salivary glands** are frequently involved, with histologic changes similar to those described in the pancreas: progressive dilatation of ducts, squamous metaplasia of the lining epithelium, and glandular atrophy followed by fibrosis.

The **pulmonary changes** are seen in almost every case and are the most serious complications of this disease. These stem from the viscous mucous secretions of the submucosal glands of the

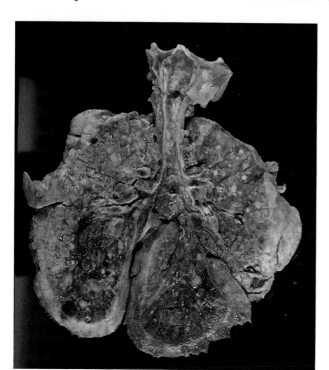

Figure 10–19. Lungs of a patient dying of cystic fibrosis. There is extensive mucus plugging and dilation of the tracheobronchial tree. The pulmonary parenchyma is consolidated by a combination of both secretions and pneumonia—the green color associated with Pseudomonas infections. (Courtesy of Dr. Eduardo Yunis, Children's Hospital of Pittsburgh).

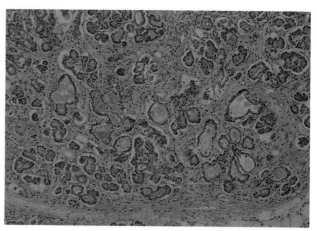

Figure 10–20. Mild to moderate cystic fibrosis changes in the pancreas. Ducts are dilated and plugged with eosinophilic mucin, and parenchymal glands are atrophic and replaced by fibrous tissue.

respiratory tree with secondary obstruction and infection of the air passages. The bronchioles are often distended with thick mucus associated with marked hyperplasia and hypertrophy of the mucus-secreting cells. Superimposed infections give rise to severe chronic bronchitis and bronchiectasis (see Chapter 15). In many instances, lung abscesses develop. *Staphylococcus aureus* and *Pseudomonas aeruginosa* are the two most common organisms responsible for lung infections. As mentioned previously, a mucoid form of *P. aeruginosa* is particularly frequent and causes chronic reactions. Even more sinister is the increasing frequency of infection with another pseudomonad, *P. cepacia*. This opportunistic bacterium is particularly hardy, and infection with this organism has been associated with fulminant illness.

A variety of other morphologic changes may be present; important among these is *the obstruction of the epididymis and vas deferens, which is responsible for azoospermia and infertility in 95% of the males who survive to adulthood.*

CLINICAL COURSE. Few childhood diseases are as protean as CF in clinical manifestations. The symptomatology is extremely varied and ranges from mild to severe, from onset at birth to onset years later. Approximately 5 to 10% of the cases come to

clinical attention at birth or soon after because of an attack of meconium ileus. More commonly, manifestations of malabsorption (e.g., large, foul stools; abdominal distention; and poor weight gain) appear during the first year of life. The faulty fat absorption may induce deficiency states of the fat-soluble vitamins, resulting in manifestations of avitaminosis A, D, or K. If the child survives these hazards, pulmonary problems, such as chronic cough, persistent lung infections, obstructive pulmonary disease, and cor pulmonale, may make their appearance. Persistent pulmonary infections are responsible for 80 to 90% of the deaths. With improved control of infections, more patients are now surviving to adulthood; the median life expectancy is approximately 26 years.

The diagnosis of CF is based on clinical findings and the biochemical abnormalities in sweat. A properly administered and interpreted sweat test is crucial to the diagnosis. An increase in sweat electrolytes (often the mother makes the diagnosis because her baby tastes salty) along with one or more major clinical features is necessary for diagnosis.

In addition to the implications of the discovery of the CF gene to the detection of CF, advances in therapy are now being explored. Transfer of the CFTR gene corrects the chloride defect in cells from CF patients *in vitro*, and it has been possible to efficiently deliver the CFTR gene to lung epithelial cells in experimental animals. These findings raise the hope that gene therapy may eventually be clinically effective in the treatment of CF.

SUDDEN INFANT DEATH SYNDROME (SIDS)

A panel convened by the National Institute of Child Health and Human Development recently defined the sudden infant death syndrome as "the sudden death of an infant under one year of age which remains unexplained after a thorough case investigation, *including performance of a complete autopsy, examination of the death scene, and review of the clinical history.*"[49] An aspect of SIDS that is not stressed in the definition is that the infant usually dies while asleep, hence the pseudonyms of "crib death" or "cot death."

INCIDENCE AND EPIDEMIOLOGY. SIDS is estimated to account for about 8000 deaths annually in the United States. As infantile deaths due to nutritional problems and microbiologic infections have come under control in countries enjoying higher standards of living, SIDS has assumed greater importance and in many countries, including the United States, is the most common cause of mortality in postnatal infants. Around the world, it causes from 1 to 5 deaths per 1000 live births.

Approximately 90% of all SIDS deaths occur during the first six months of life, most between the ages of two and four months. This narrow window of peak susceptibility is a unique characteristic that is independent of other risk factors (to be described) and the geographic locale. Most of these infants die at home, usually during the night after a period of sleep. Only rarely is the catastrophic event observed, but even when seen it is reported that the apparently healthy infant suddenly turns blue, stops breathing, and becomes limp without emitting a cry or struggling. Most have had minor manifestations of an upper respiratory infection preceding the fatal event. In recent years the term "near-SIDS" has been applied to those infants who could be resuscitated after such an episode. Although this term is diagnostically imprecise and many such infants have definable underlying diseases, some of the apparently normal "near-misses" have been reported to succumb later to SIDS. The circumstances surrounding SIDS have been explored in great detail.[49a] There appears to be an increased risk of SIDS in infants sleeping in a prone position, prompting the American Academy of Pediatrics to recommend placing healthy infants in a supine position when laying them down to sleep.[50] In addition, based on epidemiologic studies, a composite of factors that are associated with an increased risk of SIDS has been identified. These factors relate to both the mother and the infant, as summarized in Table 10–6. It is worth noting, however, that a number of these factors are features of infant deaths in general.

MORPHOLOGY. At autopsy a variety of findings have been reported.[50a] They are usually subtle and of uncertain significance and are not present in all cases. Within the respiratory system, there may be some histologic evidence of recent infection (correlating with the clinical symptoms), although the changes are generally considered not to be of

Table 10–6. FACTORS ASSOCIATED WITH SIDS

MATERNAL	INFANT
Young (younger than 20 years of age)	Prematurity
Unmarried	Low birth weight
Short intergestational intervals	Male sex
Low socioeconomic group	Product of a multiple birth
Smoking	
Drug abuse (e.g., methadone)	Not the first sibling
Risk greater for American blacks than whites (?socioeconomic)	SIDS in a prior sibling

lethal significance. The central nervous system shows astrogliosis of the brain stem. Nonspecific findings include frequent persistence of hepatic extramedullary hematopoiesis and periadrenal "brown" fat, and an increased volume of adrenal chromaffin cells. It is tempting to speculate that many of these findings relate to chronic hypoxemia, retardation of normal development, and chronic stress. An increase in the thickness of small pulmonary arteries, cardiac right ventricular hypertrophy, and histologic abnormalities in the myocardial conduction system (in particular the bundle of His and the sinoatrial node) have been reported by some authors, although the observations have not been confirmed by others. Finally, petechiae in the pleura and epicardium as well as pulmonary congestion and edema compatible with hypoxic death are often found, but these could be agonal changes. Thus, autopsy fails to provide a clear cause of death, and this may well be related to the possibility that SIDS is not a single entity.

PATHOGENESIS. Although the cause of SIDS remains unknown, extensive studies over the last 10 years have begun to shed some light on this family tragedy. A wide array of theories, many subsequently disproved or discarded, have been proposed regarding the pathogenesis of SIDS. It is therefore not surprising that many believe that SIDS is a heterogenous entity, an idea supported by the diagnosis of specific disorders, such as a *deficiency in medium-chain acyl-CoA dehydrogenase,* in some infants clinically presenting with sudden, unexpected death. It has been estimated that approximately 10% of SIDS cases are due to an inborn error in metabolism.

There is currently agreement on two issues. One is that some of the hypothetical events thought to explain SIDS, such as *apnea* and *abnormal temperature control,* may be related to the other neonatal risk factors cited, including prematurity, and birth weight. The other is that the underlying pathophysiology in many cases may originate *in utero.* This latter concept has led to the postulate that there may be a group of infants with subtle developmental abnormalities who are subsequently at risk for sudden death during the first six months of life, a time when integration of numerous, complex autonomic functions is being accomplished. Because of the anatomic finding of astrogliosis in the brain stem, as well as its importance in integrating cardiopulmonary function and arousal mechanisms, some of the studies focus on abnormalities in this region.[51] It is postulated that a neural developmental delay may be a critical and possibly common abnormality in the pathophysiology of SIDS.[51a]

The litany of speculative hypotheses could be continued, but suffice it to say that none of these theories, alone or in combination, can at present explain these unexpected deaths. As mentioned at the outset, it is likely that SIDS is a heterogeneous, multifactorial disorder. Thus, it might be expected that further investigations will allow an increasing number of patients to be moved from the "unexplained" to the "explained" category, permitting fewer "maybe's."

TUMORS AND TUMOR-LIKE LESIONS OF INFANCY AND CHILDHOOD

Only 2% of all malignant tumors occur in infancy and childhood; nonetheless, cancer (including leukemia) is the leading cause of death from disease in the United States in children over the age of 4 and up to 14 years of age. Neoplastic disease accounts for approximately 9% of all deaths in this cohort; only accidents cause significantly more deaths. Benign tumors are even more common than cancers. Most benign tumors are of little concern, but on occasion they cause serious disease by virtue of their location or rapid increase in size.

It is difficult to segregate, on morphologic grounds, true tumors or neoplasms from tumor-like lesions in the infant and child. Displaced cells and masses of tissue may be present from birth that are histologically normal in appearance but nonetheless grow at approximately the same rate as the fetus and infant. Indeed, few neoplasms grow as rapidly as the normal embryo. The question is whether such displaced cells and masses should be construed as new growths or simply as malformations that enlarge along with the child. Moreover, a period of rapid growth may be followed by spontaneous regression and disappearance in a significant minority of these lesions, a scenario almost never observed in tumors occurring in older patients. In recognition of these intergrades between normal tissue growth and true neoplasia, several special categories of tumor-like lesions have been created.

The term *heterotopia* (or *choristoma*) is applied to microscopically normal cells or tissues that are present in abnormal locations. Examples of heterotopias include a rest of pancreatic tissue found in the wall of the stomach or small intestine, or a small mass of adrenal cells found in the kidney, lungs, ovaries, or elsewhere. The heterotopic rests are usually of little significance, but they can be confused clinically with neoplasms. Rarely, they are sites of origin of true neoplasms, producing the paradox of an adrenal carcinoma arising in the ovary.

The term *hamartoma* refers to an excessive but focal overgrowth of cells and tissues native to the organ in which it occurs. Although the cellular elements are mature and identical to those found in the remainder of the organ, they do not reproduce the normal architecture of the surrounding tissue. Hamartomas can be thought of as the linkage between malformations and neoplasms—the line of demarcation between a hamartoma and a benign neoplasm is frequently tenuous and is variously interpreted. Hemangiomas, lymphangiomas, rhabdomyomas of the heart, adenomas of the liver, and developmental cysts within the kidneys, lungs, or pancreas are interpreted by some as hamartomas and by others as true neoplasms. The frequency of these lesions in infancy and childhood and their clinical behavior give credence to the belief that many are developmental aberrations. However, their unequivocally benign histology does not preclude bothersome and rarely life-threatening clinical problems in some cases.

BENIGN TUMORS AND TUMOR-LIKE LESIONS

Reference has already been made to the difficulty in distinguishing benign tumors from hamartomas. The benign neoplasms are far more common in infancy and childhood than are cancers. Virtually any tumor may be encountered, but within this wide array hemangiomas, lymphangiomas, fibrous lesions, and teratomas deserve special mention. They are described in greater detail in appropriate chapters, but here a few comments will be made about their special features in childhood.

Hemangiomas (see Chapter 11) are the most common tumors of infancy. Architecturally they do not differ from those encountered in adults. In children most are located in the skin, particularly on the face and scalp, where they produce flat-to-elevated, irregular, red-blue masses; some of the flat, larger lesions (considered by some to represent vascular ectasias; see Chapter 11) are referred to as "port-wine stains." Hemangiomas may enlarge along with the growth of the child, but in many instances they spontaneously regress (Fig. 10–21). In addition to their cosmetic significance, they can represent one facet of the hereditary disorder, von Hippel–Lindau disease (see Chapter 20). Very rarely, vascular tumors, particularly

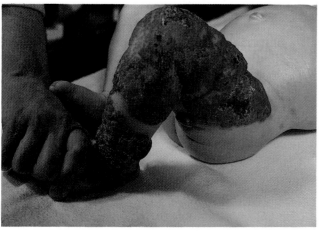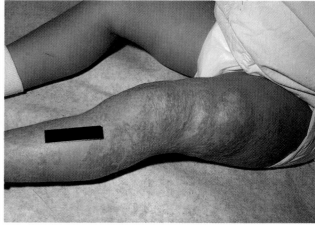

A   B

Figure 10-21. Congenital capillary hemangioma. At birth (A), and at two years of age (B) after undergoing spontaneous regression. (Courtesy of Dr. Eduardo Yunis, Children's Hospital of Pittsburgh.)

those in the liver and soft tissues, become malignant.

A wide variety of lesions are of lymphatic origin. Some of them—*lymphangiomas*—are hamartomatous or neoplastic in origin, whereas others appear to represent abnormal dilations of pre-existing lymph channels known as *lymphangiectasis*. The lymphangiomas are usually characterized by cystic and cavernous spaces. Lesions of this nature may occur on the skin but, more important, are encountered in the deeper regions of the neck, axilla, mediastinum, retroperitoneal tissue, and elsewhere. Although histologically benign, they tend to increase in size after birth, both by the collection of fluid and by the budding of pre-existing spaces. In this manner they encroach on vital structures, such as those in the mediastinum or nerve trunks in the axilla, to constitute serious clinical problems. Lymphangiectasis, in contrast, usually presents as a diffuse swelling of part or all of an extremity; considerable distortion and deformation may result as a consequence of the spongy, dilated subcutaneous and deeper lymphatics. However, the lesion is not progressive and does not extend beyond its original location. Nonetheless, it gives rise to difficult corrective cosmetic problems.

Fibrous tumors occurring in infants and children range from sparsely cellular proliferations of spindle-shaped cells (designated as *fibromatosis*) to richly cellular lesions indistinguishable from fibrosarcomas occurring in adults. Biologic behavior cannot be predicted based on histology alone, however, as some of the lesions (including the cellular fibromatoses or infantile fibrosarcomas) may spontaneously regress. In some of these soft tissue fibrous lesions, a variable proportion of the cells acquire a moderate amount of pink cytoplasm and express muscle-specific actin. These *myofibromatoses* present in infants and younger children, and although usually solitary, they may be multifocal,

involving any organ. Solitary lesions are benign, but multifocal lesions may result in significant morbidity and mortality when they involve vital organs.

Teratomas (see Chapter 7) illustrate the relationship of histologic maturity to biologic behavior. They may occur as benign well-differentiated cystic lesions or as solid malignant (immature) teratomas. They exhibit two peaks in incidence: the first at approximately two years of age and the second in late adolescence or early adulthood. The first peak represents congenital neoplasms; the later-occurring lesions may also be of prenatal origin but more slowly growing. *Most teratomas of infancy and childhood arise in the sacrococcygeal region.* Other sites include the gonads and various midline locations, such as the mediastinum, retroperitoneum, and head and neck.

Sacrococcygeal teratomas occur in 1 in 20,000 to 40,000 live births, four times more frequently in females than in males (Fig. 10-22). Occasionally diagnosed by prenatal imaging studies, these tumors may be associated with nonimmune hydrops fetalis or polyhydramnios and, depending on their size, may necessitate cesarean section delivery. In view of the overlap in the mechanisms underlying teratogenesis and oncogenesis, it is interesting that approximately 10% of sacrococcygeal teratomas are associated with congenital anomalies, primarily defects of the hindgut and cloacal region and other midline defects (meningocele, spina bifida), not believed due to the local effects of the tumor. Approximately 75% of these tumors are histologically mature (see Chapter 23) with a benign course, and about 12% are unmistakably malignant (containing endodermal sinus tumor) and lethal. The remainder are designated as immature teratomas and their malignant potential correlates with the amount of immature tissue elements present. Most of the benign teratomas are encoun-

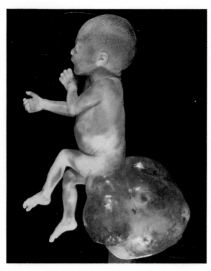

Figure 10-22. Sacrococcygeal teratoma. Note the size of the lesion compared to that of the infant.

Table 10-7. COMMON MALIGNANT NEOPLASMS OF INFANCY AND CHILDHOOD

0 TO 4 YEARS	5 TO 9 YEARS	10 TO 14 YEARS
Leukemia	Leukemia	
Retinoblastoma	Retinoblastoma	
Neuroblastoma	Neuroblastoma	
Wilms' tumor		
Hepatoblastoma	Hepatocarcinoma	Hepatocarcinoma
Soft tissue sarcoma (especially rhabdomyo-sarcoma)	Soft tissue sarcoma	Soft tissue sarcoma
Teratomas		
Central nervous system tumors	Central nervous system tumors	
	Ewing's tumor	
	Lymphoma	Osteogenic sarcoma
		Thyroid carcinoma
		Hodgkin's disease

tered in younger infants (below the age of four months), whereas children with malignant lesions tend to be somewhat older.

MALIGNANT TUMORS

Cancers of infancy and childhood differ biologically and histologically from their counterparts occurring later in life. The main differences, some of which have been alluded to above, include the following:

- Incidence and type of tumor[52]
- Relatively frequent demonstration of a close relationship between abnormal development (teratogenesis) and tumor induction (oncogenesis)
- Prevalence of underlying familial or genetic aberrations
- Tendency of fetal and neonatal malignancies to spontaneously regress or cytodifferentiate[53]
- Improved survival or cure of many childhood tumors, so that more attention is now being paid to minimizing the adverse delayed effects of chemotherapy and radiotherapy in survivors, including the development of second malignancies.

INCIDENCE AND TYPES. The most frequent childhood cancers arise in the hematopoietic system, nervous tissue (including the central and sympathetic nervous system, adrenal medulla, and retina), soft tissues, bone, and kidney. This is in sharp contrast to adults, in whom the skin, lung, breast, prostate, and colon are the most common sites of tumors.

Neoplasms that exhibit sharp peaks in incidence in children younger than ten years of age include (1) leukemia (principally acute lympho-blastic leukemia), (2) neuroblastoma (see Fig. 10-23), (3) Wilms' tumor, (4) hepatoblastoma, (5) retinoblastoma, (6) rhabdomyosarcoma, (7) teratoma, (8) Ewing's sarcoma and finally, posterior fossa neoplasms—principally (9) juvenile astrocytoma, (10) medulloblastoma, and (11) ependymoma. Other forms of cancer are also common in childhood but do not have the same striking early peak. The age distribution of these cancers is roughly indicated in Table 10-7. Within this large array, leukemia alone accounts for more deaths in children younger than 15 years of age than all the other tumors collectively.

Histologically, many of the malignant pediatric neoplasms are unique. In general, they tend to have a more primitive (embryonal) rather than pleomorphic-anaplastic microscopic appearance and frequently exhibit features of organogenesis specific to the site of tumor origin. Because of this latter characteristic, these tumors are frequently designated by the suffix -blastoma, for example, nephroblastoma (Wilms' tumor), hepatoblastoma, and neuroblastoma.

Because of their primitive histologic appearance, many childhood tumors have been collectively referred to as *small round blue cell tumors (SRBCTs)*. These are characterized by sheets of cells with small, round nuclei. The differential diagnosis of such tumors includes neuroblastoma, lymphoma, rhabdomyosarcoma, Ewing's sarcoma (peripheral neuroectodermal tumor), and, occasionally, Wilms' tumor. Rendering a definitive diagnosis is usually possible on histologic examination alone, but when necessary, clinical and radiographic findings combined with ancillary studies, such as chromosome analysis, immunoperoxidase stains, and electron microscopy, are used. The diagnostic features associated with the more common childhood neoplasms are summarized in Table 10-8. Three of these tumors are particularly illus-

Table 10–8. GENETIC AND OTHER USEFUL MARKERS OF SMALL ROUND CELL TUMORS OF CHILDHOOD

	GENETIC MARKERS	OTHER DIAGNOSTICALLY USEFUL FEATURES
Neuroblastoma	1p deletion,* n-*myc* amplification* DNA hyperdiploidt	Clinical elevation in level of urinary catecholamines Neurosecretory granules by electron microscopy
Ewing's sarcoma/PNET	t(11;22)	MIC2 gene expression
Rhabdomyosarcoma	t(2;13)—alveolar rhabdomyosarcoma	Desmin immunohistochemical positivity Alternating thick and thin filaments by electron microscopy
Burkitt's lymphoma	t(8;14)	B cell; most commonly expressing IgM, kappa light chains
Lymphoblastic lymphoma/ acute lymphoblastic leukemia	DNA hyperdiploidt* Various translocations, including t(9;22)*	T cell
Wilms' tumor	11p13 deletion/mutation 11p15.5 deletion/mutation 16q13 deletion (probable)	
Retinoblastoma	13q14 deletion/mutation	
Medulloblastoma	Isochromosome 17q	

* Generally associated with a poorer prognosis.
t Generally associated with a better prognosis.
PNET = Peripheral neuroectodermal tumor.

trative and will be discussed here: neuroblastoma, retinoblastoma, and Wilms' tumor.

Neuroblastoma and Ganglioneuroma

Neuroblastoma is one of the most common childhood extracranial solid tumors. Alone, it accounts for about 15% of all childhood cancer death.[54] A great deal is known about the molecular biology and genetics of this neoplasm. Studies strongly suggest that there are at least two, possibly three, clinicobiologic subsets of neuroblastoma, ranging from those that rarely kill, however hopeless the clinical situation may appear to be, to those that rapidly cause death despite all therapeutic efforts.

Thirty-five per cent of these tumors appear during the first year of life, 20% during the second year. Altogether, 85 to 90% are found in children younger than five years of age. Most occur sporadically, but in about 20% of instances there is strong evidence of a hereditary predisposition, probably in the form of inheritance of a germline mutation rendering the individual vulnerable to a second somatic "hit" (see section on clinical features).

MORPHOLOGY. In childhood, about 25 to 35% of neuroblastomas arise in the adrenal medulla. The remainder occur anywhere along the sympathetic chain, with the second most common location being the paravertebral region of the posterior mediastinum. Closely following is the paravertebral region in the lower abdomen, but tumors may arise in numerous other sites, including the pelvis and neck and within the brain. By contrast, rare neuroblastomas in adults are found in the head, neck, and legs.

Macroscopically, neuroblastomas range in size from minute nodules (the "in situ lesions") to large masses more than 1 kg in weight (Fig. 10–23). In situ neuroblastomas are reported to be 40 times more frequent than overt tumors. The great preponderance of these lesions spontaneously regress leaving only a focus of fibrosis or calcification in the adult. Indeed, some clinically overt neuroblastomas have regressed or, alternatively, have undergone differentiation and maturation into a relatively benign ganglioneuroma. Some neuroblastomas are sharply demarcated and may appear encapsulated, but others are far more infiltrative and invade surrounding structures, such as the kidneys, renal vein, and vena cava, and envelope the aorta. On transection, they are composed of soft, gray, "brain-like" tissue. Larger tumors have areas of necrosis, cystic softening, and hemorrhage. Occasionally, foci of calcification can be palpated.

Histologically, there is a considerable range of differentiation among these neoplasms. Most are composed of small, primitive-appearing cells with dark nuclei, scant cytoplasm, and poorly defined cell borders growing in solid sheets. Such tumors may be very difficult to differentiate from other "small blue round cell tumors." In characteristic lesions, rosettes (Homer-Wright pseudorosettes) can be found in which the tumor cells are arranged

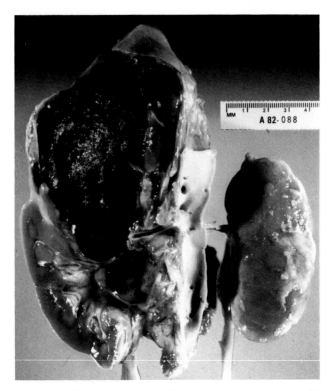

Figure 10–23. Adrenal neuroblastoma in a six-month-old child. The hemorrhagic, partially encapsulated tumor has displaced the opened left kidney and is impinging on the aorta and left renal artery. (Courtesy of Dr. Joe Rutledge, University of Texas Southwestern Medical School, Dallas.)

about a central space filled with fibrillar extensions of the cells (Fig. 10–24).

Some neoplasms reveal some level of differentiation. Clusters or scattered larger cells having more abundant cytoplasm with large vesicular nuclei and a prominent nucleolus may be found in tumors composed largely of primitive neuroblasts.

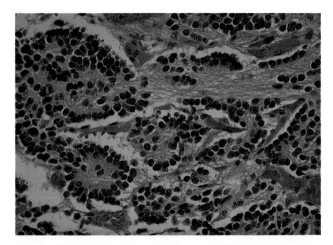

Figure 10–24. Adrenal neuroblastoma. This tumor is composed of small cells embedded in a finely fibrillar matrix.

Even better differentiated lesions may contain many more large cells resembling neurons; such neoplasms merit the designation **ganglioneuroma.**

Metastases, when they develop, appear early and widely. In addition to local infiltration and lymph node spread, there is a pronounced tendency to spread through the bloodstream to involve the liver, lungs, and bones. A staging system for this tumor is as follows:

- Stage I. Tumor is confined to the organ of origin.
- Stage II. Tumor extends in continuity beyond organ of origin but does not cross the midline; ipsilateral lymph nodes may or may not be involved.
- Stage III. Tumor extends in continuity beyond the midline; ipsilateral beyond the midline; ipsilateral lymph nodes may or may not be involved.
- Stage IV. Metastatic disease to the viscera, distal lymph nodes, soft tissue, and skeleton.
- Stage IV-S (Special). Patients whose disease would be classified as stage I or II but who have distant disease of the liver, skin, or bone marrow (without evidence of bony destruction).

The staging system is of particular importance with neuroblastomas, as will become evident.

CLINICAL COURSE AND BIOLOGIC FEATURES. In young children, under two years of age, neuroblastomas generally present with very large abdominal masses, fever, and possibly weight loss. In older children, they may not come to attention until metastases produce manifestations, such as bone pain, respiratory symptoms, or gastrointestinal complaints. The course of these neoplasms is extremely variable, and, as indicated earlier, there appear to be distinctive subsets based on many variables.[55]

- *Age and stage* are important determinants of outcome. Infants younger than one year of age have an excellent prognosis irrespective of the stage of the neoplasm. Most often in this age group, the neoplasms are stage I or II. At this early age, even when metastases are present, in about half the spread is limited to the liver, bone marrow, and skin (stage IV-S), and such infants have at least an 80% 5-year survival with only minimal therapy. Even when the dissemination is more widespread in the first year of life, the survival is greater than 50%. At this age with stages I or II therapy yields a 95 to 98% survival. On the other hand, children older than one year of age with stages III and IV tumor have only a 10% survival despite all forms of treatment.
- *Deletion of the short arm of chromosome 1 distal to band p32* (determined either karyotypically or by loss of heterozygosity) modifies the outlook significantly (Fig. 10–25). This is the most characteristic cytogenetic abnormality in these neoplasms and implies loss of a suppressor gene for neuroblastoma (see Chapter 7). Recent studies

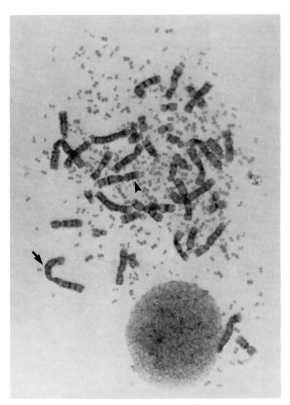

Figure 10–25. Karyotype of a neuroblastoma with poor prognosis. Arrows point to both copies of chromosome 1—one *(arrowhead)* with deletion of most of the distal short arm. The small fragments of material in the background are double minutes. (Courtesy of Dr. Jonathan Fletcher, Brigham and Women's Hospital, Boston.)

indicate that in a few cases there is alternatively or concomitantly loss of heterozygosity from the long arm of chromosome 13 or 14. The meaning of such genetic heterogeneity is not clear.

- *Amplification of N-myc oncogenes*, producing double minutes (Fig. 10–25) and homogeneously staining regions (HSRs) are additional and adverse alterations. Up to 300 copies of N-*myc* have been observed in some tumors; the greater the number of copies, the greater the number of double minutes and HSRs and the worse the prognosis. However, some patients with a single copy follow a rapid downhill course, and so it is not simply the copy number, but rather the level of gene expression.

- *Ploidy* of the tumor cells also affects prognosis. All manner of hyperdiploidy and aneuploidy may be encountered. Near diploid or near tetraploid contents of DNA are associated with an intermediate or poor prognosis.

- The *differentiation* of primitive neuroblasts into more benign ganglionic cells appears to be at least partially effected by nerve growth factor (NGF). The NGF receptor is encoded by a Trk proto-oncogene. There is a high degree of correlation between the *level of expression of the Trk*

gene and a favorable outcome—the greater the expression the longer the survival.[56]

Retinoblastoma

Retinoblastoma is the most common malignant eye tumor of childhood and is responsible for approximately 1% of all deaths from cancer in the age group of newborn to 15 years. From a pathologic as well as from a clinical standpoint, retinoblastoma is unusual in several aspects when compared with most other solid tumors. Retinoblastoma can be multifocal and bilateral; it undergoes spontaneous regression; patients have a high incidence of second primary tumors; and retinoblastoma frequently occurs as a congenital tumor. The condition is hereditary in a significant number of cases. The incidence decreases with age, with the great majority of cases being diagnosed before the age of four years.

Retinoblastomas occur in both familial and sporadic patterns. Familial cases typically develop multiple tumors that are bilateral, although they may be unifocal and unilateral. Of the sporadic *nonheritable* tumors, all are unilateral and unifocal.

PATHOGENESIS. As detailed in Chapter 7, retinoblastoma serves as a prototype of a diverse group of human cancers associated with recessive loss-of-function mutations at distinct genetic loci harboring suppressor cancer genes. The Rb gene, located on chromosome 13q14, was the first isolated human gene governing cancer predisposition.[58] It encodes a nuclear protein that functions as a block to exit from G1 in the cell cycle[59] (Fig. 7–28, Chapter 7) and also appears to be important in differentiation. In familial cases, infants are born with one normal and one defective Rb gene, the latter either through the inheritance of a mutant allele from a carrier parent or as a new germinal mutation. The second mutation in the retina is somatic. In contrast, in sporadic cases, both the mutations are somatic and occur in retinal cells. Since the retinal cell that gives rise to a nonhereditary retinoblastoma must acquire two somatic mutations, and since the somatic mutation rate is low, all patients with sporadic retinoblastoma have only a single focus of tumor formation.

Patients with familial retinoblastoma are also at increased risk for developing osteosarcoma and other soft tissue tumors, and Rb inactivation has also been found in small cell carcinoma of the lung and in carcinoma of the bladder, breast, and prostate.[60]

MORPHOLOGY. Retinoblastoma is believed to arise from a cell of neuroepithelial origin, usually in the posterior retina. The tumors tend to be nodular masses, often with satellite seedings. On light microscopic examination, undifferentiated areas of these tumors are composed of small round cells with large hyperchromatic nuclei and scant cytoplasm, resembling undifferentiated retinoblasts.

Differentiated structures are found within many retinoblastomas, the most characteristic of these being the rosettes described by Flexner and Wintersteiner **(Flexner-Wintersteiner rosettes;** Fig. 10–26). These structures consist of clusters of cuboidal or short columnar cells arranged around a central lumen. The nuclei are displaced away from the lumen, which by light microscopy appears to have a limiting membrane resembling the external limiting membrane of the retina. Photoreceptor-like elements protrude through the membrane, and some taper into fine filaments.

Tumor cells may disseminate through the choroidal vasculature or may spread beyond the eye through the optic nerve or subarachnoid space. In advanced cases, the tumor may penetrate through the sclera and grow in the orbit. Metastases to the preauricular and cervical lymph nodes commonly follow overt extraocular extension. The most common sites of distant metastases are the central nervous system, skull, distal bones, and lymph nodes.

Spontaneous necrosis or regression of a retinoblastoma is marked by calcification and severe inflammation. The mechanism responsible for spontaneous regression is unknown.

CLINICAL FEATURES. The tumor may be present at birth but most commonly presents at two years of age. The presenting findings include poor vision, strabismus, a whitish hue to the pupil, and pain and tenderness in the eye. About 90% of cases are sporadic, and of those most (75 to 80%) are unilateral. Six to ten per cent of cases are familial, the majority being bilateral or multifocal. Untreated the tumors are usually fatal, but with early treatment by enucleation, chemotherapy and radiotherapy survival is the rule. As noted earlier some tumors spontaneously regress and patients with retinoblastoma are at increased risk for developing osteosarcoma and other soft tissue tumors.

Wilms' Tumor

Wilms' tumor is the most common primary renal tumor of childhood, usually diagnosed between the ages of two and five years. Its biology and histology illustrate many of the important concepts of childhood neoplasia: the relationship between malformations and neoplasia; premalignant lesions and the two-hit theory of oncogenesis; the similarity between tumor and developmental histology; and, finally, the potential for treatment modalities to dramatically affect prognosis and outcome.

PATHOGENESIS AND GENETICS. The risk of Wilms' tumor is increased in association with at least three recognizable groups of congenital malformations[61] exhibiting defects in at least two distinct chromosomal loci.[62] The first group have the *WAGR syndrome* characterized by *a*niridia, *g*enital anomalies, and mental *r*etardation and have a 33% chance of developing Wilms' tumor. Studies of these patients led to the identification of an autosomal dominant gene for aniridia within band p13 on chromosome 11. Slightly proximal to this, also within band p13, is the Wilms' tumor–associated gene, WT-1 (Table 10–9; see also Chapter 7). Many cases of infants with WAGR syndrome have a sporadic deletion of genetic material at 11p13 that includes both of these loci. It has already been noted in the discussion of congenital malformations that the WT-1 protein is expressed within the kidney and gonads of the developing human fetus, and that transgenic mice lacking both copies of the WT-1 locus have renal agenesis.

A second group of patients at risk for Wilms' tumor have the *Denys-Drash syndrome*, which is characterized by gonadal dysgenesis (male pseudohermaphroditism) and nephropathy leading to renal failure. The majority of these patients develop Wilms' tumors. As in patients with WAGR, the genetic abnormality in these children has also been mapped to chromosome 11, band p13. However, in patients with Denys-Drash syndrome, the genetic abnormality is a dominant negative mutation in the WT-1 gene that affects its DNA binding properties, rather than a deletion.[63] It is not surprising that there may be some clinical overlap between these two groups of patients, depending on the size and nature of the 11p13 deletion or mutation.

Clinically distinct from these previous two groups of patients but also having an increased risk of developing Wilms' tumor are those children with *Beckwith-Wiedemann syndrome*, characterized by enlargement of body organs, hemihypertrophy, renal medullary cysts, and abnormal large cells in adrenal cortex (adrenal cytomegaly). The genetic locus that is involved in these patients is in band p15.5 of chromosome 11 distal to the WT-1 locus. The function of this second Wilms' tumor gene (WT-2) is unknown. Selected loss of maternal alleles in this group of Wilms' tumors, combined with the demonstration of uniparental paternal disomy for 11p15.5 in a few sporadic cases of Beckwith-Wiedemann syndrome, suggests a role for *genomic imprinting* at the WT-2 locus. In addition, patients with Beckwith-Wiedemann syndrome are also at increased risk for developing hepatoblastoma, adrenocortical tumors, rhabdomyosarcomas, and pancreatic tumors.

A few familial cases of Wilms' tumors not associated with identifiable deletions or mutations involving either the WT-1 or the WT-2 gene suggest that there may be another locus that plays a role in

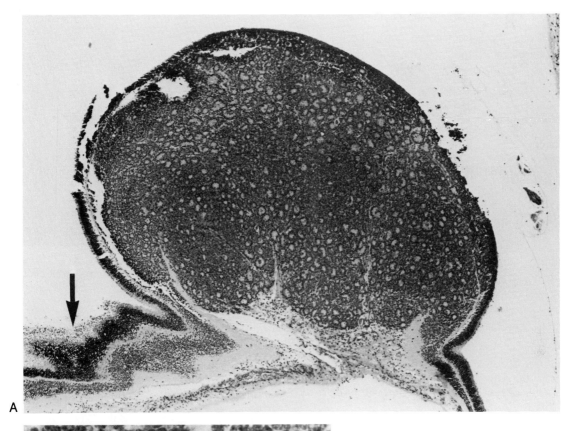

A

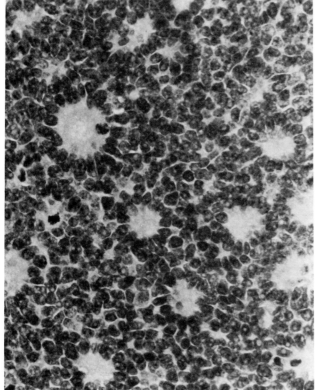

B

Figure 10–26. *A,* Focus of retinoblastoma arising from retina *(arrow). B,* Higher power view of retinoblastoma showing differentiated rosettes (Flexner-Wintersteiner rosettes). (Courtesy of Drs. Daniel Albert and Theodore Dryja.)

Table 10–9. THE WILMS' TUMOR–ASSOCIATED GENE WT-1

Location:	Chromosome 11p13
Protein/function:	Transcription factor

Embryonic expression:	Early
	  Intermediate mesoderm
	  Mesenchyme of metanephros
	  Epithelial cells of nephric tubules
	Later
	  Mesothelium, spinal cord, brain
	  Derivatives of urogenital ridge

Developmental anomalies:	WT-1 homozygous deletion
	  Renal agenesis (mice)
	Heterozygous gross deletions
	  WAGR syndrome: *Wilms'*
	  tumor susceptibility,
	  aniridia, genitourinary
	  malformations, mental
	  retardation
	Dominant point mutations
	  Denys-Drash syndrome:
	  ambiguous genitalia,
	  streak gonads, renal
	  failure, ↑susceptibility
	  to Wilms' tumor

Cancer:	Wilms' tumor

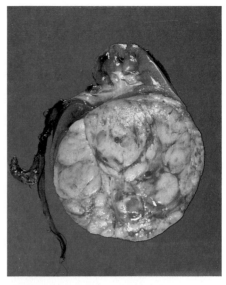

Figure 10–27. Wilms' tumor in lower pole of kidney with the characteristic tan to gray color and well-circumscribed margins.

some tumors. Studies demonstrating a loss of heterozygosity on the long arm of chromsome 16 point to the potential identification of a critical gene in this region.[64]

Related to the molecular genetic and corresponding heterogeneity of Wilms' tumor is the recognition of a "premalignant" or precursor lesion in many of these cases—*nephroblastomatosis.* This term refers to multicentric or diffuse foci of immature nephrogenic elements within areas of otherwise non-neoplastic kidney parenchyma.[65] Recognition of this lesion is important, as its presence implies a substantially increased risk of developing a Wilms' tumor.

MORPHOLOGY. Grossly, Wilms' tumor tends to present as a large, solitary, well-circumscribed mass, although 10% are either bilateral or multicentric at the time of diagnosis. On cut section, the tumor is soft, homogeneous, and tan to gray with occasional foci of hemorrhage, cyst formation, and necrosis (Fig. 10–27).

Microscopically, Wilms' tumors are characterized by recognizable attempts to recapitulate different stages of nephrogenesis. The classic triphasic combination of blastemal, stromal, and epithelial cell types is observed in the vast majority of lesions, although the percentage of each component is variable (Fig. 10–28). Epithelial "differentiation" is usually in the form of abortive tubules or glomeruli. Stromal cells are usually fibrocytic or myxoid in nature, although skeletal muscle "differentiation" is not uncommon. Rarely, other heterologous elements are identified, including squamous

or mucinous epithelium, smooth muscle, adipose tissue, cartilage, and osteoid and neurogenic tissue. Approximately 5% of tumors contain foci of anaplasia (cells with large, hyperchromatic, pleomorphic nuclei and abnormal mitoses), the only histologic feature correlating with prognosis.[66]

CLINICAL FEATURES. Most children with Wilms' tumors present with a large abdominal mass that may be unilateral or, when very large, may extend across the midline and down into the pelvis. Hematuria, pain in the abdomen following some hemorrhagic incident, intestinal obstruction, and the appearance of hypertension are other patterns of presentation. In a considerable number of these

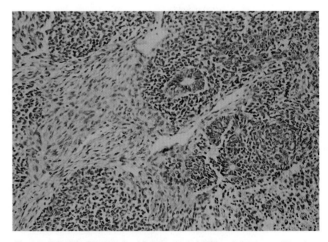

Figure 10–28. Triphasic histology of Wilms' tumor with stromal, less cellular area on the left, with spindle-shaped cells, epithelial (one clear tubule in the center) and blastemal (tightly packed blue cells) elements.

patients, pulmonary metastases are present at the time of primary diagnosis.

Up to the mid-1960s, the 5-year survival rate of these patients was tragically low (10 to 40%), a tragedy rendered the more poignant because of the age of the patients. However, the combined use of chemotherapy, radiotherapy, and surgery has produced dramatic results in patients whose lesions were previously thought to be inoperable. Most large centers now report 90% long-term survival rates if the tumors are available for primary treatment with the three modalities mentioned. Even recurrences can be successfully treated.

Acknowledgment. We wish to thank Drs. Daniel Albert and Theodore Dryja for the use of text and figure related to retinoblastoma from the fourth edition.

1. Koops, B.L., et al.: Neonatal mortality risk in relation to birth weight and gestational age: Update. J. Pediatr. 101:969, 1982.
2. Palo, P., and Erkkola, R.: Risk factors and deliveries associated with preterm, severely small for gestational age fetuses. Am. J. Perinatol. 10:88, 1993.
3. Pearce, J.K., and Campbell, S.: Intrauterine growth retardation. Birth Defects 21:109, 1985.
4. Kalousek, D.: Confined placental mosaicism and intrauterine development. Pediatr. Pathol. 10:69, 1990.
5. Levene, M.I., and Dubowitz, V.: Intrauterine growth retardation. In Stern, L., and Vert, P. (eds.): Neonatal Medicine, New York, Masson Publishing USA, Inc., 1987, p. 107.
6. Apgar, V.: A proposal for a new method of evaluation of the newborn infant. Curr. Res. Anesth. Analg. 32:260, 1953.
7. Drage, J.S., and Berendes, H.: Apgar scores and outcome of the newborn. Pediatr. Clin. North Am. 13:635, 1966.
8. Jepson, H.A., et al.: The Apgar score: Evolution, limitations, and scoring guidelines. Birth 18(2):83, 1991.
9. Gresham, E.L.: Birth trauma. Pediatr. Clin. North Am. 22:317, 1975.
10. Andre, M., and Vert, P.: Birth injury. In Stern, L., and Vert, P. (eds.): Neonatal Medicine. New York, Masson Publishing USA, Inc., 1987, p. 176.
11. Shepard, T.H.: Human teratogenicity. Adv. Pediatr. 33:225, 1986.
12. Rosenthal, N., and Abramowsky, C.R.: The causes of morbidity and mortality among infants born at term. Arch. Pathol. Lab. Med. 112:178, 1988.
13. Stevenson, R.E., et al. (eds.): Human Malformations and Related Anomalies, Vol. 1. New York, Oxford University Press, 1993.
14. Nyhan, W.L.: Structural abnormalities: A systematic approach to diagnosis. Clin. Symp. 42:1, 1990.
15. Stevenson, R.E.: The environmental basis of human anomalies. In Stevenson, R.E., et al. (eds.): Human Malformations and Related Anomalies, Vol. 1. New York, Oxford University Press, 1993.
16. Beckman, D.A., and Brent, R.L.: Mechanism of known environmental teratogens: Drugs and chemicals. Clin. Perinatol. 13:649, 1986.
17. Jones, K.L.: The Fetal Alcohol Syndrome. Growth Genet. Horm. 4:1, 1988.
18. Lyons, K.M., and Hogan, B.L.M.: The DVR gene family in embryonic development. In Robertson, L.J., et al. (eds.): Cell-Cell Signaling in Vertebrate Development. New York, Academic Press, 1993.
19. Ardinger, H.H., et al.: Association of genetic variation in TGFX gene in the cleft lip and palate. Am. J. Hum. Genet. 45:348, 1990.
20. Kreidberg, J.A., et al.: WT-1 is required for early kidney development. Cell 74:679, 1993.
20a. George, E., et al.: Defects in mesoderm, neural tube, and vascular development in mouse embryos lacking fibronectin. Development 119:1079, 1993.
21. Redline, R.W., et al.: Homeobox genes and congenital malformations. Lab. Invest. 66:659, 1992.
22. Dolle, P., et al.: Disruption of the Hoxd-13 gene induces localized heterochrony leading to mice with neotenic limbs. Cell 75:431, 1993.
23. Tabin C.: Retinoids, homeobox genes, and genetic factors. Cell 66:199, 1991.
23a. Riddle R., et al.: Sonic Hedgehog mediates the polarizing activity of the ZPA. Cell 75(7):1401, 1993.
24. Morris-Kay B.: Retinoic acid receptors in normal growth and development. Cancer Surv. 14:181, 1992.
24a. Kessel, M.: Respecification of vertebral identities by retinoic acid. Development 115:487, 1992.
25. Lammer, E.J., et al.: Retinoic acid embryopathy. N. Engl. J. Med. 313(14):837, 1985.
25a. Maulbecker, C.C., and Gruss, P.: The oncogenic potential of Pax genes. EMBO J. 12:2361, 1993.
26. Morey, A.L., et al.: Clinical and histopathological features of parvovirus B19 infection in the human fetus. Br. J. Obstet. Gynaecol. 99:556, 1992.
27. Stark, A.R., and Frantz, I.D.: Respiratory distress syndrome. Pediatr. Clin. North Am. 33:533, 1986.
28. Editorial: Born before their time into this breathing world. Br. Med. J. 2:1403, 1976.
29. Oh, W., and Stern, L.: Respiratory diseases of the newborn. In Stern, L., and Vert, P. (eds.): Neonatal Medicine. New York, Masson Publishing USA, Inc., 1987, p. 395.
30. Jobe, A.H.: Lung development, surfactant, and respiratory distress syndrome. Acta Paediatr. Jpn. 32(5):1, 1990.
31. Ballard, P.L., et al.: Regulation of pulmonary surfactant apoprotein SP28-36 gene in fetal human lung. Proc. Natl. Acad. Sci. U.S.A. 83:9527, 1986.
32. Gortner, L.: Natural surfactant for neonatal respiratory distress syndrome in very premature infants: A 1992 update. J. Perinat. Med. 20(6):409, 1992.
33. Cherry, S.H.: Current concepts in hemolytic disease and blood group incompatibility. Mt. Sinai J. Med. 47:454, 1980.
34. Machin, G.A.: Hydrops revisited, literature review of 1,414 cases published in the 1980's. Am. J. Med. Genet. 34:366, 1989.
35. Harper, R.G., et al.: Kernicterus. Clin. Perinatol. 7:75, 1980.
36. Tovey, L.A.D.: Hemolytic disease of the newborn: The changing scene. Br. J. Obstet. Gynaecol. 93:960, 1986.
37. Burton, B.K.: Inborn errors of metabolism: The clinical diagnosis in early infancy. Pediatrics 79:359, 1987.
38. Scriver, C.R., et al.: (eds.): The Metabolic Basis of Inherited Disease, 6th ed. New York, McGraw-Hill, 1989.
39. Medical Research Council Working Party on Phenylketonuria: Phenylketonuria due to phenylalanine hydroxylase deficiency: An unfolding story. Br. Med. J. 306(6870):115, 1993.
39a. Eisensmith, R.C. and Woo, S.L.: Molecular basis of phenylketonuria and related hyperphenylalaninemias: Mutation and polymorphisms in the human phenylalanine hydroxylase gene. Hum. Mutat. 1(1):13, 1992.
40. Reichardt, J.K.: Genetic basis of galactosemia. Hum. Mutat. 1(3):190, 1992.
41. Davis, P.B.: Cystic fibrosis from bench to bedside. N. Engl. J. Med. 325:757, 1991.
42. Sperra, T.J., and Collins, F.S.: The molecular basis of cystic fibrosis. Annu. Rev. Med. 44:133, 1993.
42a. Jiaūg C., et al.: Altered fluid transport across airway epithelium in cystic fibrosis. Science 262:424, 1993.
43. Koch, C., and Hoiby, N.: Pathogenesis of cystic fibrosis. Lancet 341:1065, 1993.
44. Rommens, J.M., et al.: Identification of the cystic fibrosis gene: Cloning and characterization of the complementary DNA. Science 245:1066, 1989.

45. Bear, C.E., et al.: Purification and functional reconstruction of the cystic fibrosis transmembrane conductance regulator (CFTR). Cell 68:809, 1992.

46. Tsui, L.C.: Mutations and sequence variations detected in the cystic fibrosis transmembrane conductance regulator (CFTR) gene: A report from the cystic fibrosis genetic analysis consortium. Hum. Mutat. 1:197, 1992.

47. Welsh, M.J., and Smith, A.E.: Molecular mechanisms of CFTR chloride channel dysfunction in cystic fibrosis. Cell 73:1251, 1993.

48. The Cystic Fibrosis Genotype Phenotype Consortium: The relation between genotype and phenotype with cystic fibrosis: Analysis of the most common mutation (ΔF508). N. Engl. J. Med. 329:1308, 1993.

49. Willinger, M., et al.: Defining the sudden infant death syndrome (SIDS): Deliberations of an expert panel convened by the National Institute of Health and Human Development. Pediatr. Pathol. 11:677, 1991.

49a. Hoffman, J.H., et al.: Risk factors for SIDS: Results of the National Institute of Child Health and Human Development SIDS Cooperative Epidemiologic Study. Ann. N.Y. Acad. Sci. 533:13, 1988.

50. AAP Task Force on Infant Positioning and SIDS: Positioning and SIDS. Pediatrics 89:1120, 1992.

50a. Valdes-Dapena, M.: The sudden infant death syndrome: Pathologic findings. Clin. Perinatol. 19:701, 1992.

51. Becker, L.E.: Neural maturational delay as a link in the chain of events leading to SIDS. Can. J. Neurol. Sci. 17:361, 1990.

51a. Kinney, H.C., et al.: The neuropathology of the sudden infant death syndrome: A review. J. Neuropathol. Exp. Neurol. 51:115, 1992.

52. Isaacs, H., Jr.: Perinatal (congenital and neonatal) neoplasms: A report of 110 cases. Pediatr. Pathol. 3:165, 1985.

53. Bolande, R.P.: Models and concepts derived from human teratogenesis and oncogenesis in early life. J. Histochem. Cytochem. 32(8):878, 1984.

54. Woods, W.G., et al.: Neuroblastoma represents distinct clinical-biologic entities: A review and perspective from the Quebec neuroblastoma screening project. Pediatrics 89:114, 1992.

55. Shimada, H.: Neuroblastoma: Pathology and biology. Acta Pathol. Jpn. 42:229, 1992.

56. Nakagawara, A., et al.: TRK expression in neuroblastoma: Association between high levels of expression of the TRK gene and favorable outcome in human neuroblastoma. N. Engl. J. Med. 328:847, 1993.

57. Zimmerman, L.E.: Retinoblastoma and retinocytoma. In Spencer, W.H. (ed.): Ophthalmic Pathology: An Atlas and Textbook, Vol. 2, 3rd ed. Philadelphia, W.B. Saunders Co., 1985, pp. 1292–1351.

58. Friend, S.H., et al.: A human DNA segment with properties of the gene that predisposes to retinoblastoma and osteosarcoma. Nature 323:643, 1986.

59. Livingston, D.M., et al.: Q in X structural and functional contributions to the G1 blocking action of the retinoblastoma protein (The 1992 Gordon Hamilton Fairley Memorial Lecture). Br. J. Cancer 68(2):264, 1993.

60. Wiman, K.G.: The retinoblastoma gene: Role in cell cycle control and cell differentiation. FASEB J. 7(10):841, 1993.

61. Clericuzio, C.L.: Clinical phenotypes and Wilms' tumor. Med. Pediatr. Oncol. 21:182, 1993.

62. Knudson, A.G.: Introduction to the genetics of primary renal tumors in children. Med. Pediatr. Oncol. 21:193, 1993.

63. Hastie, N.D.: Dominant negative mutations in the Wilms' tumor (WT1) gene cause Denys-Drash syndrome: Proof that a tumour-suppressor gene plays a crucial role in normal genitourinary development. Hum. Molec. Genet. 1(5):293, 1992.

64. Coppes, M.J., et al.: Loss of heterozygosity mapping in Wilms' tumor indicates the involvement of three distinct regions and a limited role for nondisjunction or mitotic recombination. Genes Chromosom. Cancer 5(4):326, 1992.

65. Beckwith, J.B.: Wilms' tumor and other renal tumors of childhood. Major Probs. Pathol. 18:313, 1986.

66. Beckwith, J.B., et al.: Nephrogenic rests, nephroblastomatosis, and the pathogenesis of Wilms' tumor. Pediatr. Pathol. 10:1, 1990.

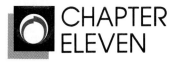

CHAPTER ELEVEN

Blood Vessels

FREDERICK J. SCHOEN, M.D., Ph.D.

Although blood vessels can be secondarily affected by lesions in adjacent structures, primary vascular disease is the major concern of this chapter. In general, vascular abnormalities cause clinical disease by (1) progressively narrowing the lumina of vessels and producing ischemia of the tissue perfused by that vessel; (2) provoking intravascular thrombosis, causing acute obstruction or embolism (or both); or (3) weakening the walls of vessels, thereby leading to dilatation or rupture. To facilitate the understanding of the pathogenesis of the diseases that affect blood vessels, we first consider some of the anatomic and functional characterstics of these structures.

NORMAL

Arteries and veins have distinctive structures. Arterial walls are generally thicker than their venous counterparts, to withstand the higher blood pressures in arteries. The thickness of the arterial walls gradually diminishes as the vessels become smaller, but at the same time the wall-to-lumen ratio becomes greater. Veins have a larger overall diameter, a larger lumen, and a narrower wall than corresponding arteries.

467

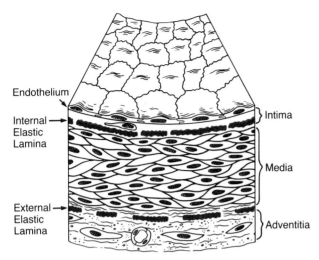

Endothelium

Internal Elastic Lamina

External Elastic Lamina

Intima

Media

Adventitia

Figure 11–1. Diagrammatic representation of the main components of the vascular wall, seen here in a muscular artery. (Redrawn with permission from Ross, R., and Glomset, J.A.: The pathogenesis of atherosclerosis. The New England Journal of Medicine, 295:369, 1976.)

Three basic structural constituents make up the walls of blood vessels: endothelium, smooth muscle, and connective tissue, including elastic elements. They are arranged in concentric layers (or *tunicas*)—an *intima*, a *media,* and an *adventitia*—most clearly distinguished in the larger vessels (Fig. 11–1). The relative amount and configuration of the basic structural constituents vary along the circulatory system. At some sites, local adaptations to mechanical or metabolic requirements may necessitate that some components are newly added, augmented, reduced, or omitted.

Arteries are divided into three types, based on their size and certain histologic features: (1) large or elastic arteries, including the aorta and its major branches; (2) medium-sized or muscular arteries (such as the coronary or renal arteries), also referred to as distributing arteries; and (3) small arteries (usually less than 2 mm in diameter) that course, for the most part, within the substance of tissues and organs.

In normal arteries, the *intima* is composed of the lining endothelial cells with minimal underlying subendothelial connective tissue. It is separated from the media by a dense elastic membrane *(internal elastic lamina),* which is interrupted by fenestrae, through which smooth muscle cells may migrate from the media into the intima. The outer limit of the media of most arteries is marked by a well-defined external elastic lamina that is usually somewhat less well developed and delineated than the internal membrane. In the large and medium-sized arteries, the smooth muscle cell layers of the media that are near the vessel lumen depend primarily on direct diffusion from the vessel lumen for their nutritional needs. Because diffusion of oxygen from the lumen to the outer layers of the media is inadequate in the largest vessels, small

arterioles arising in the adventitia from exiting branches course through the adventitia and send vascular twigs into the outer one-half to two-thirds of the media, a region not perfused from the lumen. Such vessels that perfuse the vascular walls are called *vasa vasorum,* literally "vessels of the vessels." Beyond the media is the adventitia, a poorly defined layer of investing connective tissue in which nerve fibers and the vasa vasorum are dispersed.

The *media* varies among different vessels. In the larger *elastic arteries* (i.e., aorta and innominate, subclavian, common carotid, iliac, and pulmonary arteries), the media is rich in elastic fibers, disposed in fairly compact, fenestrated layers separated by alternating layers of smooth muscle cells. The elastic components of the aorta allow it to expand during systole, thereby storing some of the energy of the heart beat. Between cardiac contractions (diastole), elastic recoil of the vascular wall propels blood through the peripheral vascular system. During aging, the aorta loses elasticity, and these vessels expand less readily, particularly when blood pressure is increased. Thus the arteries often become progressively tortuous and dilated in older individuals (called *ectasia*).

Muscular arteries are branches of elastic arteries (e.g., coronary or renal arteries) in which the media is composed predominantly of circularly or spirally arranged smooth muscle cells and the extracellular matrix they produce. Local blood flow and blood pressure are regulated by changes in lumen size through smooth muscle cell contraction *(vasoconstriction)* or relaxation *(vasodilatation),* controlled in part by the autonomic nervous system and in part by local metabolic factors and cellular interactions. Because the resistance of a blood vessel to fluid flow is inversely proportional to the fourth power of the diameter (i.e., halving the diameter increases resistance 16-fold), small changes in the lumen size of small blood vessels by vasoconstriction or plaque can have a profound flow-limiting effect.

Arterioles, the smallest branches of the arteries (generally 20 to 100 μm in diameter, having primarily a smooth muscle cell–containing media), regulate blood flow into capillary beds. Under autonomic and local control the medial smooth muscle of arterioles is capable of making dramatic adjustments in lumen diameter that regulate systemic arterial blood pressure and significantly influence local blood flow distribution among the various capillary beds. Thus arterioles are the principal points of normal resistance to blood flow, inducing both a sharp reduction in pressure and a change from pulsatile to steady flow, as blood passes from arterioles to capillaries. Moreover, the small arteries and the arterioles bear the brunt of blood pressure elevations; these abnormal stresses alter their structure (to be detailed later).

Each of the three types of arteries (elastic,

muscular, arteriole) tends to be involved in specific disease processes and to have its own pattern of pathologic lesions. Thus *atherosclerosis* is a disease largely of elastic and muscular arteries, whereas *hypertension* is associated with functional and structural changes in the small muscular arteries and arterioles. Specific types of vasculitis involve certain vascular segments.

The term *capillary* is restricted to those vessels that have approximately the diameter of a red blood cell (7 to 8 μm). The cumulative surface area of capillaries in the entire human body is extensive, approximately 700 m² (more than that of two tennis courts). Lined by endothelial cells, capillaries are supported on the outside by a thin basement membrane, composed mostly of type IV collagen. In some capillaries (and venules), *pericytes* reside outside the endothelial cells but enveloped in their own basal lamina that may fuse with the endothelial basement membrane. Slow flow, very large surface area, and walls only one cell thick render capillaries ideally suited to the rapid exchange of diffusible substances between blood and extravascular tissue.

Capillaries in different sites have different structures. There are three general types, distinguished by the degree of continuity of endothelium and of basement membrane. Muscle, heart, lung, skin, and nervous system capillaries have a *continuous endothelial layer*; this allows the permeability of these capillaries to be highly regulated through control of transport across and between endothelial cells. Indeed, closed interendothelial junctions provide the structural basis for the relative impermeability to large molecules, such as plasma proteins. In contrast, endocrine glands, renal glomeruli, and some vessels of the gastrointestinal tract have fenestrated (i.e., interrupted) endothelia, which allow more rapid transport of larger molecules and fluid (e.g., hormones or the glomerular filtrate) than do capillaries with a continuous endothelium. Some capillary vascular channels (called *sinusoids*) have a discontinuous endothelium with partial or no basement membrane, as in the liver, spleen, and bone marrow. Such structures facilitate the passage of cells across the walls.

Blood returning to the heart from capillary beds flows initially into the *postcapillary venules* and then sequentially through collecting venules and small, medium, and large veins. Postcapillary venules are an important point of interchange between the lumen of the vessels and the surrounding tissues. Because the pressure in the venules is lower than that in the capillary bed, as well as lower than interstitial tissue pressure, fluid can enter the circulation from the tissue surrounding the venules. Moreover, as we have seen, both vascular leakage and leukocytic exudation occur preferentially in venules in many types of inflammation (see Chapter 3).

Veins are thin-walled vessels with relatively large lumina. The intima is composed of an endothelial lining adherent to a scant connective tissue layer, bounded by a poorly defined internal elastic membrane. The media of veins is not as well developed as that in arteries and provides relatively poor support. Veins are thus predisposed to abnormal irregular dilation, compression, and easy penetration by tumors and inflammatory processes. The valves found in many veins, particularly those in the extremities, serve to eliminate back flow.

Lymphatics are identified in tissue sections as collapsed, thin-walled, endothelium-lined channels devoid of blood cells. Although the major function of the lymphatics is as a protective drainage system returning interstitial tissue fluid to the blood, they also constitute an important pathway for disease dissemination through transport of bacteria and tumor cells to distant sites.

VASCULAR WALL CELLS AND THEIR RESPONSE TO INJURY

Endothelium and smooth muscle cells, the main cellular components of the walls of blood vessels, play an important role in vascular pathology. Much has been learned about the properties of these cells over the last decade, and a few points are highlighted here.

ENDOTHELIAL CELLS

Endothelial cells (ECs) form a monolayer that lines the entire vascular system (Fig. 11–2). ECs are polygonal, elongated cells that have many pinocytotic vesicles and form junctional complexes with their neighbors. They uniquely contain *Weibel-Palade bodies*, 0.1 μm wide, 3 μm long membrane-bound structures that represent the storage organelle for von Willebrand's factor (vWF). ECs are identified immunohistochemically with antibody to vWF and other endothelial antigens.

The structural and functional integrity of *endothelial cells* (collectively called *endothelium*) is a fundamental requirement for maintenance of vessel wall homeostasis and circulatory function. Vascular endothelium is a versatile multifunctional tissue having many synthetic and metabolic properties (Table 11–1). As a semipermeable membrane, endothelium controls the transfer of small and large molecules into the arterial wall and through the walls of capillaries and venules. In most regions, the intercellular junctions are normally impermeable to such molecules, but the relatively labile junctions between ECs may widen under the influence of hemodynamic factors (e.g., high blood

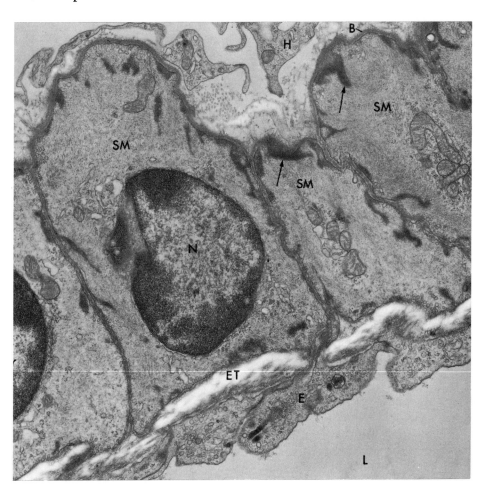

Figure 11-2. Wall of small artery in the myocardium. Continuous endothelium (E) is separated from smooth muscle layer (SM) by a thin elastica (ET)—unstained. Note peripheral bands in smooth muscle cells (arrows) and prominent external basement membrane (B). L = lumen; H = perivascular fibroblast; N = nucleus.

pressure) and vasoactive agents (e.g., histamine in inflammation; see Chapter 3). Moreover, ECs serve a role in the maintenance of a nonthrombogenic blood-tissue interface (see Chapter 4), the modulation of blood flow and vascular resistance, the metabolism of hormones, the regulation of immune and inflammatory reactions, the modification of lipoproteins during transport in the artery wall, and the growth regulation of other cell types, particularly smooth muscle cells. Thus the endothelium is an active participant in the interaction between blood and tissues. Besides contributing to the formation of thrombi, endothelial injury may be responsible, at least in part, for the initiation of atherosclerosis and the vascular lesions of hypertension and other disorders, as we shall see.

ENDOTHELIAL DYSFUNCTION

With the several antithrombotic properties of ECs, it is not surprising that mechanical denudation of

Table 11-1. ENDOTHELIAL CELL PROPERTIES AND FUNCTIONS

Maintenance of permeability barrier	Modulation of blood flow and vascular reactivity
Elaboration of anticoagulant and antithrombotic molecules	Vasconstrictors: endothelin, ACE
Prostacyclin	Vasodilators: NO/EDRF, prostacyclin
Thrombomodulin	Regulation of inflammation and immunity
Plasminogen activator	IL-1, IL-6, IL-8
Heparin-like molecules	Adhesion molecules
Elaboration of prothrombotic molecules	Histocompatibility antigens
Von Willebrand factor (Factor VIIIa)	Regulation of cell growth
Tissue factor	Growth stimulators: PDGF, CSF, FGF
Plasminogen activator inhibitor	Growth inhibitors: heparin, TGF-β
Extracellular matrix production (collagen, proteoglycans)	Oxidation of LDL

ACE = angiotensin converting enzyme (AI → AII); NO/EDRF = nitric oxide/endothelium-derived relaxing factor; IL = Interleukin; PDGF = platelet-derived growth factor; CSF = colony-stimulating factor; FGF = fibroblast growth factor; TGF-β = transforming growth factor beta.

the endothelial lining with exposure of blood to subendothelial connective tissue initiates thrombosis. An important conceptual advance, however, is the realization that *structurally intact ECs can respond to various abnormal stimuli by adjusting some of the constitutive functions and by expressing some newly acquired (induced) properties. The term endothelial dysfunction is often used to describe several types of potentially reversible changes in the functional state of ECs that occur as a response to environmental stimuli.*[1,2] *Two functional alterations of endothelium deserve comment. Endothelial stimulation* denotes a rapid (within minutes), reversible response that is independent of new protein synthesis. Examples are the EC contraction induced by histamine, serotonin, and other vasoactive mediators that cause intracellular gaps in venules and the expression of adhesive glycoprotein P-selectin (see Chapter 3) by thrombin or histamine-stimulated ECs. In contrast to stimulation, *endothelial activation* depends on new (or altered) protein synthesis and thus requires hours or even days to occur. This response is most frequently induced by inflammatory cytokines, exemplified by induction of endothelial leukocyte adhesion molecule-1 (ELAM-1) by interleukin-1 (IL-1), and tumor necrosis factor (TNF) and class II major histocompatibility complex (MHC) molecules by interferon gamma (IFN-γ).

A wide variety of specific surface and metabolic properties of ECs are subject to physiologic regulation and pathologic change. Immunoregulatory cytokines and other humoral mediators can induce the loss of normal EC nonthrombogenic functions through stimulation of expression of prothrombotic surface molecules (e.g., tissue factor) that activate coagulation. In some situations, EC dysfunction also comprises loss of surface heparin-like proteoglycan molecules that prevent thrombus formation and inhibit smooth muscle cell growth, thereby promoting thrombosis and intimal thickening, and depressed release of EC-derived relaxing factors, leading to abnormal vasoconstriction. These changes can result in acute occlusion of a vessel by spasm or a localized thrombotic event and may contribute to atherosclerosis. There is currently increasing scrutiny of the molecular entities involved in endothelial perception of injury, in the regulation of gene expression by various stimuli, and how acute alterations in endothelial phenotype contribute to chronic disease.[3] The relationship of endothelial dysfunction to atherosclerosis is discussed in detail later in this chapter.

VASCULAR SMOOTH MUSCLE CELLS

Vascular smooth muscle cells (SMCs) are capable of many functions, including vasoconstriction and dilatation in response to normal or pharmacologic stimuli; synthesis of various types of collagen, elastin, and proteoglycans; elaboration of growth factors and cytokines; and migration and proliferation. Normally the predominant cellular element of the vascular media, SMCs are an important element of vascular reparative processes and proliferative diseases. For example, SMS proliferation and production of extracellular matrix components contribute to atherosclerotic plaque. Resting vascular SMCs are spindle-shaped, with single, elongated nuclei, resembling fibroblasts. The contractile function of SMCs is mediated by cytoplasmic filaments that contain actin and myosin. The most characteristic ultrastructural feature of SMCs is a basal lamina around each individual cell membrane.

INTIMAL THICKENING—A RESPONSE TO VASCULAR INTIMAL INJURY

Smooth muscle proliferation is one important response to vascular wall injury. Healing of the damaged intima of blood vessels comprises SMC proliferation in and migration from the media to the intima, subsequent multiplication of intimal cells and synthesis and deposition of extracellular matrix (Fig. 11–3). Injuries that cause only focal endothelial loss without frank denudation can often be repaired by migration and proliferation of neighboring ECs so the subendothelium remains covered. A more extensive or chronic injury induces a more complex repair sequence.[4]

The reaction is potentiated by accompanying injury to the SMCs of the media. During the healing response, SMCs undergo changes that resemble dedifferentiation.[5] In conjunction with losing the capacity to contract, gaining the capacity to divide, and increasing synthesis of extracellular matrix molecules, SMCs in the intima lose their thick, myosin-containing filaments and greatly increase the amount of organelles involved with protein synthesis, such as rough endoplasmic reticulum and Golgi apparatus. This is often called a shift from the "contractile" phenotype to the "proliferative-synthetic" phenotype. The degree of proliferation can be striking. Although only a rare SMC is dividing in the normal arterial wall, approximately 15 to 40% of cells have undergone mitosis within 48 hours after experimental arterial injury.[6] Intimal SMCs may return to a nonproliferative state when either the overlying endothelial layer is re-established or the abnormal chronic endothelial stimulation ceases.

The migratory and proliferative activity of SMCs is physiologically regulated by both growth promoters and inhibitors. Promoters include platelet-derived growth factor (PDGF) derived from not only platelets but also endothelial cells and macrophages, basic fibroblast growth factor (bFGF), and IL-1. Inhibitors include heparan sulfates, nitric oxide (NO)/endothelial-derived relaxing

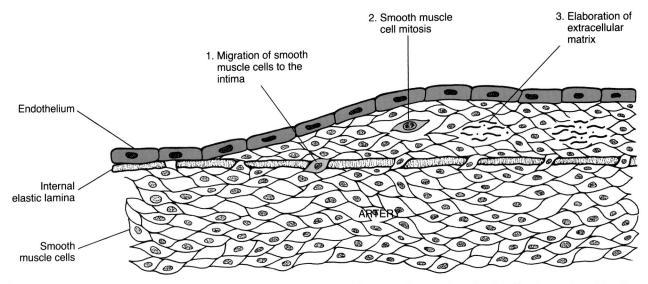

Figure 11-3. Schematic mechanism for intimal thickening, emphasizing smooth muscle cell migration to, and proliferation and extracellular matrix elaboration in, the intima. (Modified and redrawn from Schoen, F.J.: Interventional and Surgical Cardiovascular Pathology: Clinical Correlations and Basic Principles. Philadelphia, W.B. Saunders Co., 1989, p. 254.)

factor (EDRF), interferon-gamma, and transforming growth factor-beta (TGF-β). Some promoters and inhibitors are endogenous to the vascular wall (e.g., PDGF, heparan sulfates, and TGF-β); others, such as IL-1, are not. *In essence, vascular injury stimulates smooth muscle cell growth by disrupting the physiologic balance between SMC growth inhibition and growth stimulation.*

Reconstitution of the damaged vascular wall, including endothelium, comprises a physiologic healing response with the formation of a *neointima.* Under certain circumstances, intimal thickening as a healing response becomes exaggerated, resulting in *intimal thickening–hyperplasia,* which can cause stenosis or occlusion of small and medium-sized blood vessels or vascular grafts. Intimal hyperplasia of SMCs is a generic pathobiologic process, in which SMC migration, proliferation, and elaboration of extracellular matrix are the common mechanisms that cause or contribute to many well-known, important clinical vascular disorders. The initial injurious stimulus in these disorders varies from predominantly mechanical (angioplasty restenosis) to predominantly immunologic (transplant arteriosclerosis) to multifactorial (atherosclerosis).[7]

VASCULAR DISEASES

Vascular diseases affect primarily arteries, and of these, the most prevalent, clinically significant problem is *atherosclerosis.* In the course of time, this disorder affects nearly every individual to some degree. Other arterial diseases are less common but, in individual instances, may be responsible for considerable disability and even death. Although certain of the venous disorders, such as varicose veins, are also commonly encountered in clinical practice, diseases of veins are more noteworthy for the disability they produce than for their importance as causes of death. Many are disabling to the point of being crippling, and certain disorders, such as phlebothrombosis, may lead to death by thromboembolism. Diseases of arteries, veins, and lymphatics are discussed separately.

CONGENITAL ANOMALIES

Many aberrations of the usual anatomic pattern of branching and anastomosing may be found, but most are of importance only in surgical operative technique; prior recognition of the deviation avoids the risk of disrupting an unexpected vessel. Occasionally, however, minor anomalies have significance in potentiating or even preventing disease. For example, a double renal arterial supply may prevent infarction of a kidney when one of the vessels is occluded by a thrombus or embolus. Maldevelopment of a major coronary branch may predispose the myocardium to infarction or may cause sudden death. Among these diverse vascular anomalies, two have particular importance: *developmental* or *berry aneurysm,* and *arteriovenous fistulas or aneurysms.* Berry aneurysms involve cerebral vessels and are discussed in Chapter 29.

ARTERIOVENOUS FISTULA. Abnormal communications between arteries and veins can arise as developmental defects, from rupture of an arterial aneurysm into the adjacent vein, from penetrating injuries that pierce the walls of artery and vein and produce an artificial communication, or from inflammatory necrosis of adjacent vessels. The connection between artery and vein may consist of a well-formed vessel, a vascular channel formed by the canalization of a thrombus, or an aneurysmal sac. Such lesions are rare and usually small. Nevertheless, they are often of clinical significance because they short-circuit blood from the arterial to the venous side, causing the heart to pump additional volume. This can induce cardiac failure (high-output failure). Moreover, they can rupture and cause hemorrhage, especially in the brain. In contrast, intentionally created AV fistulas are used to provide vascular access for chronic hemodialysis.

ATHEROSCLEROSIS AND OTHER FORMS OF ARTERIOSCLEROSIS

Arteriosclerosis literally means "hardening of the arteries"; more accurately, however, it refers to a group of disorders that have in common thickening and loss of elasticity of arterial walls. Three distinctive morphologic variants are included within the term arteriosclerosis: *atherosclerosis*, characterized by intimal thickening and lipid deposition; *Monckeberg's medial calcific sclerosis*, characterized by calcification of the media of muscular arteries; and *arteriolosclerosis*, marked by proliferative or hyaline thickening of the walls of small arteries and arterioles. Because atherosclerosis is by far the most common and important form of arteriosclerosis, it is discussed first and in detail.

ATHEROSCLEROSIS

Atherosclerosis overwhelmingly accounts for more death and serious morbidity in the Western world than any other disorder. Global in distribution, it has reached epidemic proportions in economically developed societies. Although any artery may be affected, the aorta and the coronary and cerebral systems are the prime targets, and so *myocardial infarction, cerebral infarction, and aortic aneurysms* are the major consequences of this disease. Atherosclerosis also takes a toll through other consequences of acutely or chronically diminished arterial perfusion, such as *gangrene of the legs, mesenteric occlusion, sudden cardiac death, chronic ischemic heart disease,* and *ischemic encephalopathy.* Despite a reduction in mortality from myocardial infarction and other forms of ischemic heart disease, nearly 50% of all deaths in the United

States continue to be attributed to atherosclerosis-related diseases. Although not usually clinically evident until middle age or later, when the arterial lesions precipitate organ injury (Fig. 11–4), atherosclerosis is a slowly progressive disease that begins in childhood.[8]

DEFINITION. Atherosclerosis is a disease primarily of the elastic arteries (e.g., aorta, carotid, and iliac arteries) and large and medium-sized muscular arteries (e.g., coronary and popliteal arteries). *The basic lesion—the atheroma, or fibrofatty plaque—consists of a raised focal plaque within the intima, having a core of lipid (mainly cholesterol and cholesterol esters) and a covering fibrous cap.* Atheromas are sparsely distributed at first, but as the disease advances, they become more and more numerous, sometimes covering the entire circumference of severely affected arteries. As the plaques increase in size, they progressively encroach on the lumen of the artery as well as on the subjacent media. *Consequently, in small arteries, plaques are occlusive, compromising blood flow to distal organs and causing ischemic injury, but in large arteries they are destructive, weakening the affected vessel wall, causing aneurysms or rupture or favoring thrombosis. Moreover, extensive atheromas are friable, often yielding emboli of their grumous contents into the distal circulation (atheroemboli), most commonly noted in the kidneys.*

EPIDEMIOLOGY AND RISK FACTORS. The variable occurrence and severity of atherosclerosis among individuals and groups may provide important clues to its pathogenesis. Epidemiologic data are expressed largely in terms of the *incidence of or the number of deaths caused by ischemic heart disease (IHD)* (see Chapter 12).

Deaths from cardiovascular disease in the United States rose from 14% of all deaths in 1937 to 54% in 1968, almost all cases being related to atherosclerosis. Happily, they appeared to plateau in the late 1960s, and by 1975, for the first time, the rate showed a statistically significant decline, which has been maintained since. The downward trend is believed to be mediated largely by a reduction in atherosclerosis influenced by changes in diet and lifestyle, better control of hypertension, and improved therapy for myocardial infarction and other complications of IHD.

Nevertheless, the death rate related to atherosclerosis in the United States is still among the highest in the world, lower than for Finland and Scotland, but above that of other well-developed, affluent countries, such as Canada, France, and the other Scandinavian countries. The rates are remarkably low in Asia, Africa, and South and Central America. For example, death rates from IHD in Japan are one-sixth of those in the United States. Japanese who migrate to the United States, how-

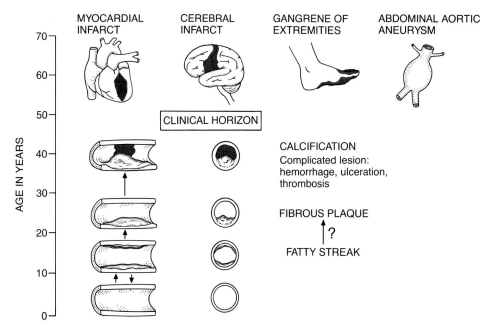

Figure 11–4. The natural history of atherosclerosis. Plaques usually develop slowly and insidiously over many years, beginning in childhood or shortly thereafter. As described in the text, they may progress from a fatty streak to a fibrous plaque and then to a complicated plaque that is likely to lead to clinical effects. (Modified by permission from McGill, H.C., Jr., et al.: Natural history of human atherosclerotic lesions. *In* Sandler, M., and Bourne, G.H. (eds.): Atherosclerosis and Its Origin. New York, Academic Press, 1963, p. 42; *and* Wissler, R.M.: *In* Braunwald, E. (ed.): Heart Disease. Philadelphia, W.B. Saunders Co., 1984, p. 1188.)

ever, and adopt the lifestyles and dietary customs of their new home acquire the predisposition to atherosclerotic diseases of the American population.

Epidemiologic studies also indicate that increased age, male gender, and certain genetic factors increase the risk of atherosclerosis. Clinically overt atherosclerosis, as evidenced by death rates from IHD, rises with each decade except in the very aged. Death rates from IHD are significantly higher in men; myocardial infarction is particularly uncommon in premenopausal women. Naturally, other risk factors, described below, influence the relative risk of IHD in women. Some families suffer an increased frequency of heart attacks at an early age. This *familial predisposition* is most likely polygenic. In particular, hyperlipidemia (including genetic defects in lipoprotein metabolism; see Chapter 5), hypertension and diabetes tend to be familial. Although the aforementioned factors are unchangeable in an individual, *other risk factors, particularly diet, lifestyle, and personal habits important in the pathogenesis and progression of this disease, are to a large extent potentially reversible.*

The risk factors that predispose to atherosclerosis and resultant IHD have been identified by means of a number of prospective studies in well-defined population groups, most notably the famed Framingham (Massachusetts) Study and others (e.g., the Multiple Risk Factor Intervention Trial [MRFIT])[9,10] (Table 11–2 and Figs. 11–5 and 11–6). *Of the various risk factors, four are most significant: (1) hyperlipidemia, (2) hypertension, (3) cigarette smoking, and (4) diabetes.*

Hyperlipidemia. Hypercholesterolemia and other abnormalities in lipid metabolism contribute a major risk factor in atherosclerosis. The evidence linking hypercholesterolemia and atherosclerosis takes many forms:

- Atherosclerotic plaques are rich in cholesterol and cholesterol esters, which are derived largely from lipoproteins in blood.
- Lesions of atherosclerosis can be induced in many experimental animals, including subhuman primates, by feeding them diets that raise the plasma cholesterol level.
- Genetic disorders causing severe hypercholesterolemia (e.g., congenital absence of either LDL receptors or HDL cholesterol) lead to premature atherosclerosis, often fatal in childhood, despite the absence of any other risk factor. Acquired diseases that cause hypercholesterolemia, such as the nephrotic syndrome and hypothyroidism, also increase the risk of IHD.
- With few exceptions, populations having relatively high levels of blood cholesterol have higher mortality from IHD, and the Framingham and other studies indicate increasing risk with increasing serum cholesterol concentrations.

Table 11–2. RISK FACTORS FOR ATHEROSCLEROSIS

MAJOR
Diet and hyperlipidemia (hypercholesterolemia, hypertriglyceridemia)
Hypertension
Cigarette smoking
Diabetes

MINOR
Obesity
Physical inactivity
Male gender
Increasing age
Family history
Stress ("type A" personality)
Oral contraceptives
High carbohydrate intake
Hyperhomocysteinemia

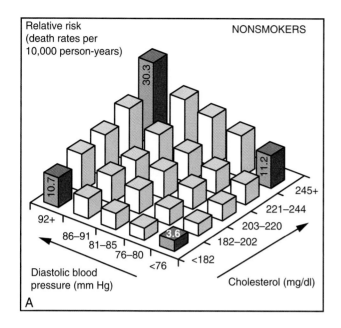

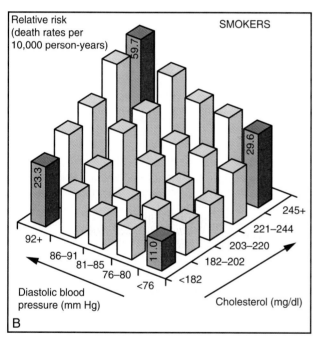

Figure 11–5. Age-adjusted coronary heart disease death rates per 10,000 person-years by level of serum cholesterol and diastolic blood pressure (DBP) for nonsmokers *(A)* and cigarette smokers *(B)* screened in the Multiple Risk Factor Intervention Trial (MRFIT). Rates per 10,000 person-years are noted on some bars; the height of the bars reflects the level of risk. (Modified and redrawn by permission from Neaton, J.D., et al.: Serum cholesterol, blood pressure, cigarette smoking, and death from coronary heart disease. Arch. Intern. Med. *152:*56–64, 1992. Copyright 1992, American Medical Association.)

- Finally, prospective studies, such as the Lipids Research Clinics Coronary Primary Prevention Trial,[11] have shown that treatment with diet and cholesterol-lowering drugs reduces cardiovascular mortality in selected patients with hypercho-

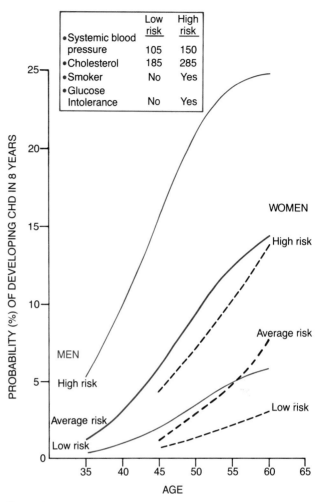

Figure 11–6. Graph depicting the influence of added risks. Probability of developing coronary heart disease in 8 years according to age, sex, and risk category (The Framingham Heart Study). (With permission from Braunwald, E. (ed.): *Heart Disease: A Textbook of Cardiovascular Medicine.* Philadelphia, W.B. Saunders Co., 1984, p. 1209.)

lesterolemia. A randomized, controlled trial of a similar treatment in patients with familial hypercholesterolemia yielded regression of coronary arterial lesions in both men and women.[12]

No single level of plasma cholesterol identifies those at risk. The higher the level, the higher the risk, although the risk rises more steeply once a plateau level of approximately 200 mg/dl is exceeded (5.2 mmol/liter). *The most striking association is with elevated levels of low-density lipoprotein (LDL),* the lipoprotein moiety richest in cholesterol; however, *hypertriglyceridemia* with increased concentrations of very low–density lipoprotein (VLDL) also appears to increase risk. In contrast, serum levels of high-density lipoprotein (HDL) are *inversely* related to risk: the higher the level, the lower the risk. Thus HDL is often called the "good cholesterol."

High dietary intake of cholesterol and saturated fats, such as those present in egg yolk, animal fats, and butter, raises the plasma cholesterol level. Conversely, a diet low in cholesterol and low in the ratio of saturated-to-polyunsaturated fats lowers plasma cholesterol levels. Paradoxically, Greenland Eskimos, who have a high dietary fat consumption, have low rates of IHD. This is thought to be due to the high content of omega-3 fatty acids in their diets (present in fish and fish oils). Such fatty acids have a number of antiatherogenic effects, including the lowering of plasma LDL, increasing plasma HDL, and modifying production by blood and vascular cells of mediators that affect platelet function and inflammation (e.g., prostaglandins and leukotrienes)[13] (see Chapter 3).

Hypertension. Although the mechanism is not entirely clear, elevated blood pressure unequivocally accelerates atherogenesis and increases the incidence of IHD and cerebrovascular disease.[14] The higher the blood pressure, the greater the risk. Both diastolic and systolic hypertension are deleterious. In the MRFIT study, increased death rates were associated with systolic blood pressure above 110 mm Hg and diastolic pressure greater than 70 mm Hg. After age 45 years, hypertension is a stronger risk factor than hypercholesterolemia. Antihypertensive therapy reduces the incidence of strokes and IHD.

Cigarette Smoking. Smoking is firmly established as a risk factor in diseases caused by atherosclerosis.[15] Smoking is the dominant cause of the increased incidence of IHD in women, increases the incidence of sudden death among victims of heart attacks, and increases the degree of aortic and coronary atherosclerosis at autopsy. Cessation of cigarette smoking in high-risk individuals is followed within a few years by a reduction in the risk of dying of IHD.

Diabetes. There is a twofold increase in incidence of myocardial infarction in diabetics compared with nondiabetics, an increased tendency toward cerebral thrombosis and infarction, and an 8-fold to 150-fold increased frequency of gangrene of the lower extremities. The complex mechanisms of increased atherosclerosis in diabetes are discussed in Chapter 19.[16]

Other Risk Factors. These are sometimes referred to as minor, or "soft," risk factors because they are associated with a less pronounced and difficult to quantitate risk. These include (1) insufficient regular physical activity, (2) competitive stressful lifestyle with "type A" personality behavior (although this is controversial), (3) obesity, (4) the use of oral contraceptives, (5) hyperuricemia, (6) high carbohydrate intake, and (7) hyperhomocysteinemia.[17]

Each of the major risk factors noted earlier contributes individually to the possible development of clinically significant atherosclerosis, but multiple factors exert a synergistic (more than additive) effect (see Figs. 11–5 and 11–6). Nevertheless, some patients with atherosclerosis-related diseases have no obvious risk factors. Moreover, demonstration of an epidemiologic association does not necessarily prove a pathogenetic (causal) relationship. For these reasons and because of the overall importance of atherosclerosis, its causes and pathogenesis remain subjects of lively speculation and controversy. In preparation for a discussion of pathogenesis, however, it is desirable first to understand the morphology of the lesions.

MORPHOLOGY. The key morphologic abnormalities in atherosclerosis are focal intimal thickenings and lipid accumulations, producing the characteristic **atheromatous plaques.** By far the most important lesions, being the principal cause of arterial narrowing in adults, these are discussed first. Discussed subsequently is the **fatty streak,** present nearly universally in children and important mainly as a possible precursor of the atheromatous plaque.

Atheromatous Plaque. Also called the fibrous, fibrofatty, lipid, or fibrolipid plaque, atheromatous plaques appear white to whitish yellow and impinge on the lumen of the artery. They vary in size from 0.3 to 1.5 cm in diameter but sometimes coalesce to form larger masses (Fig. 11–7). On section, the superficial portion of these lesions at the luminal surface tends to be firm and white (the **fibrous cap**) and the deep portions yellow or whitish yellow and soft. The centers of larger plaques may contain a yellow, grumous debris, called an **atheroma,** a name derived from the Greek word for gruel.

The distribution of atherosclerotic plaques in humans is characteristic. The abdominal aorta is much more involved than the thoracic aorta, and aortic lesions tend to be much more prominent around the ostia of its major branches. In descending order (after the lower abdominal aorta), the most heavily involved vessels are the coronary arteries (usually within the first 6 cm), the popliteal arteries, the descending thoracic aorta, the internal carotid arteries, and the vessels of the circle of Willis. Vessels of the upper extremities are usually spared, as are the mesenteric and renal arteries, except at their ostia. Nevertheless, in an individual case, the severity of atherosclerosis in one artery does not predict the severity in another. Atherosclerotic lesions usually involve the arterial wall only partially around its circumference ("eccentric" lesions) and are patchy and variable along the vessel length.

Atherosclerotic plaques have three principal components: (1) cells, including smooth muscle cells, macrophages, and other leukocytes; (2) connective tissue extracellular matrix, including collagen, elastic fibers, and proteoglycans; and (3) intracellular and extracellular lipid deposits (Fig. 11–8). These three components occur in varying proportions in different plaques, giving

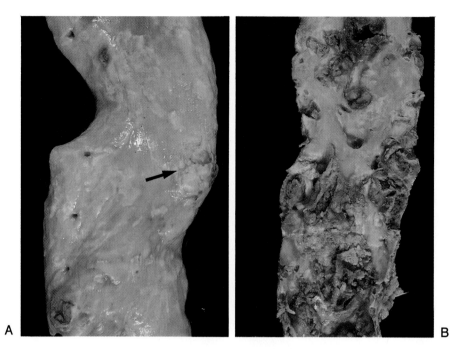

Figure 11-7. Atherosclerosis in the aorta, gross photographs. *A,* Mild atherosclerosis composed of fibrous plaques, one of which is denoted by the arrow. *B,* Severe disease with diffuse complicated lesions.

rise to a spectrum of lesions. Typically, the superficial fibrous cap is composed of smooth muscle cells with a few leukocytes and relatively dense connective tissue; a cellular area beneath and to the side of the cap (the "shoulder"), consisting of a mixture of macrophages, smooth muscle cells, and T lymphocytes; and a deeper necrotic **core,** in which there is a disorganized mass of lipid material, cholesterol clefts, cellular debris, lipid-laden **foam cells,** fibrin, thrombus in various stages of organization, and other plasma proteins (Fig. 11–9). The lipid is primarily cholesterol and cholesterol esters. Current studies indicate that foam cells predominantly derive from blood monocytes (to become macrophages), but SMCs also imbibe lipid to become foam cells. Finally, particularly around the periphery of the lesions, there is usually evidence of neovascularization (proliferating small blood vessels). Not considered atherosclerosis, diffuse lipid-free thickening of the intima of the coronary arteries to a thickness approximately equal to that of the media, common in adults, is a normal response of the vessel wall to hemodynamic and other stresses.

Variations of the histologic features of plaques involve the relative numbers of SMCs and macrophages, the amount and distribution of collagen, other extracellular matrix, and lipid. Typical atheromas contain relatively abundant lipid. Nevertheless, many so-called fibrous plaques are composed

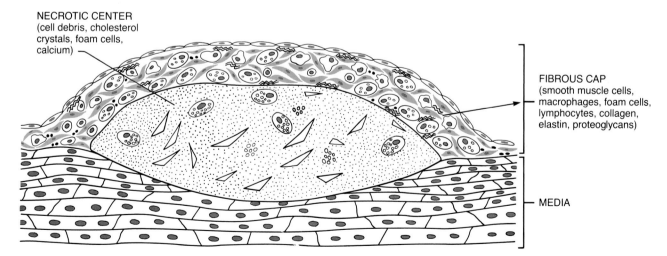

NECROTIC CENTER
(cell debris, cholesterol crystals, foam cells, calcium)

FIBROUS CAP
(smooth muscle cells, macrophages, foam cells, lymphocytes, collagen, elastin, proteoglycans)

MEDIA

Figure 11-8. Major components of well-developed atheromatous plaque: fibrous cap composed of proliferating smooth muscle cells, macrophages, lymphocytes, foam cells, and extracellular matrix. The necrotic core consists of necrotic debris, extracellular lipid with cholesterol crystals and foamy macrophages.

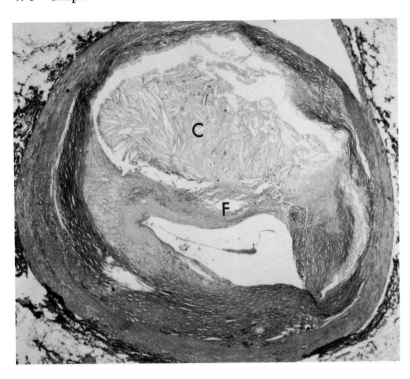

Figure 11-9. Histologic section of an atheromatous plaque. F = fibrous cap; C = central lipid core with typical cholesterol clefts. The lumen has been narrowed considerably. Note also that the media of the artery is thinned under the most advanced plaque.

mostly of SMCs and fibrous tissue. In advanced atherosclerosis, progressive fibrosis may convert the fatty atheroma to a fibrous scar.

The "complicated lesion" of atherosclerosis, defined by the following changes, has the most clinical significance:

• Almost always, atheromas in advanced disease undergo patchy or massive **calcification.** Arteries may be converted to virtual pipe stems, and the aorta may assume an eggshell brittleness. Using calcification as a marker, new technology, such as intravascular ultrasound or ultrafast computed tomographic scanning, may provide an accurate noninvasive means for aiding in diagnosis (and therapy).[18]

• Focal **rupture** or gross **ulceration,** or both, of the luminal surface of atheromatous plaques may result in exposure of highly thrombogenic substances that induce thrombus formation (see Fig. 12-3) or discharge of the debris into the bloodstream, producing microemboli **(cholesterol emboli** or **atheroemboli).**

• Superimposed **thrombosis,** the most feared complication, usually occurs on fissured or ulcerated lesions. Thrombi may partially or completely occlude the lumen; they may become incorporated within the intimal plaque by organization (see Fig. 11-9).

• **Hemorrhage** into a plaque may occur, especially in the coronary arteries, from rupture of either the overlying fibrous cap or the thin-walled capillaries that vascularize the plaque. A contained hematoma may induce plaque rupture.

• Although atherosclerosis is initially an intimal disease, in severe cases, particularly in larger vessels, the underlying media undergoes considerable pressure or ischemic atrophy with loss of elastic tissue, causing sufficient weakness to permit **aneurysmal dilation,** discussed later.

Fatty Streak. Fatty streaks are not significantly raised and thus do not cause any disturbance in blood flow. They may be precursors, however, of the more ominous atheromatous plaques. The streaks begin as multiple yellow, flat spots less than 1 mm in diameter that coalesce into elongated streaks, 1 cm long or longer. Fatty streaks (Fig. 11-10) are composed of lipid-filled foam cells. T lymphocytes and extracellular lipid are present in smaller amounts than in plaques, and proteoglycans, collagen, and elastic fibers are found in variable amounts.

Fatty streaks appear in the aortas of some children younger than one year of age and all children older than ten years, regardless of geography, race, sex, or environment. Coronary fatty streaks are less common than aortic but begin to form in adolescence, and they occur at the same anatomic sites that are later prone to develop plaques.[19] They subsequently decrease in number as atherosclerotic plaques become more prevalent.

The relationship of fatty streaks to atherosclerotic plaques is controversial. Fatty streaks occur early in life, often in areas of the vasculature that are not particularly susceptible to developing atheromas later in life. Moreover, they frequently affect individuals in geographic locales and populations in which atherosclerotic plaque is uncommon. Thus, not all fatty streaks are destined to be-

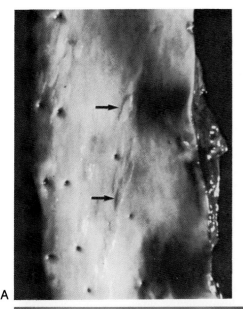

A

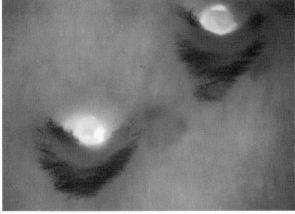

B

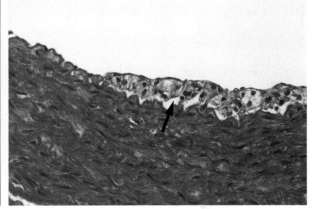

C

Figure 11–10. Fatty streak—an intimal collection of foam cells. *A,* Aorta from patient with fatty streaks *(arrows)* seen on reflected light. They are associated largely with the ostia of branch vessels. *B,* Close-up photograph of fatty streaks from aorta of experimental hypercholesterolemic rabbit shown following staining with Sudan red, a lipid-soluble dye, illustrating relationship of lesions to branch vessel ostia. *C,* Photomicrograph of fatty streak in experimental hypercholesterolemic rabbit, demonstrating intimal macrophage-derived foam cells *(arrow).* (*B* Courtesy of Myron I. Cybulsky, M.D., Brigham and Women's Hospital, Boston.)

come fibrous plaques or more advanced lesions. Fatty streaks, however, are also related to the known risk factors of atherosclerosis in adults (especially serum lipoprotein cholesterol concentrations and smoking). Some experimental evidence also supports the concept of the evolution of fatty streaks into plaques. **Thus, whatever the fate of a specific fatty streak, the prevalence of these lesions in the aorta and coronaries early in life emphasizes that atherosclerosis has its roots early in life.**

PATHOGENESIS. Historically, two hypotheses for atherogenesis were dominant: One emphasized cellular proliferation in the intima as a reaction to insudation of plasma proteins and lipids from the blood, whereas the other postulated that organization and repetitive growth of thrombi resulted in plaque formation. The contemporary view of the pathogenesis of atherosclerosis incorporates elements of both older theories and is called the *response to injury hypothesis.* Formulated in 1973 and modified in 1986 and 1993,[20, 21] it states that *the lesions of atherosclerosis are initiated as a response to some form of injury to arterial endothelium.* The injury postulated is a form of endothelial dysfunction without necessary denudation, which increases permeability to plasma constituents, including lipids, and permits blood *monocytes* and eventually platelets to adhere to endothelium. Monocytes adhere and subsequently enter the intima, transform into macrophages, and accumulate lipid to become foam cells, contributing to the evolution of the lesion. Factors released from activated platelets at the surface or monocytes then cause migration of SMCs from media into the intima, followed by proliferation and synthesis of extracellular matrix components by SMCs, leading to the accumulation of collagen and proteoglycans. Single or short-lived injurious events can be followed by restoration of endothelial function and regression of the lesion. Repeated or chronic injury, however, results in the development of an atheromatous plaque, probably by permitting continuing increased permeability, ingress of mono-

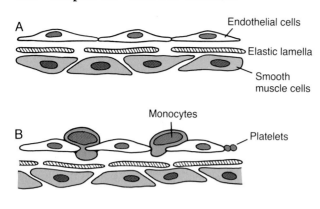

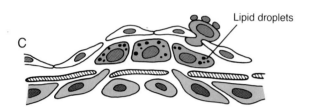

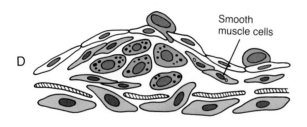

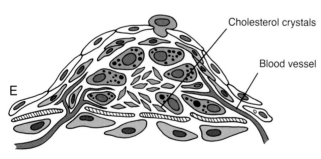

Figure 11–11. Processes in the response to injury hypothesis. *A,* Normal. *B,* Endothelial injury with adhesion of monocytes and platelets (latter to denuded endothelium). *C,* Migration of monocytes (from lumen) and smooth muscle cells (from media) into intima. *D,* Smooth muscle cell proliferation in the intima. *E,* Well-developed plaque.

cytes, or perhaps platelet interactions. These events are summarized in Figure 11–11. We now examine the various component processes of this hypothesis and how they may explain plaque progression.

Role of Endothelial Injury. There is considerable experimental support for *endothelial damage* as a major factor in atherogenesis. Endothelial injury

induced in experimental animals by mechanical denudation, hemodynamic forces (AV fistula), immune complex deposition, irradiation, and chemicals causes intimal smooth muscle proliferation and, in the presence of high-lipid diets, typical atheromas. *It should be stressed, however, that early lesions develop at sites of morphologically intact endothelium* (Fig. 11–12), and thus some form of endothelial dysfunction is thought to initiate the process. Three manifestations of such dysfunction appear to be most important: increased endothelial permeability, increased monocyte adhesion, and increased EC replication. All of these are early events in experimental hypercholesterolemia.

Blood monocyte adherence to ECs is probably mediated by the induction of specific receptor molecules on the surface of activated ECs. Indeed, the expression of vascular cell adhesion molecule (VCAM-1), the EC-leukocyte adhesion molecule (see Chapter 3), was noted as an early molecular marker of lesion-prone areas as a response to experimental hypercholesterolemia.[22] In humans, intercellular adhesion molecule (ICAM-1) and VCAM-1 expression is increased in the endothelium of atherosclerotic plaques.[23]

Risk factors such as hypertension and cigarette smoking may also cause endothelial damage or increased endothelial permeability. Endothelial alterations induced by hemodynamic forces (shear stress or turbulent flow) can possibly explain the distribution of plaques at branch and fork points of arteries and in portions of the abdominal aorta. The molecular mechanisms by which the various risk factors cause induction of endothelial-leukocyte adhesion molecules and other changes in the endothelium are currently being explored. One postulated common pathway is related to injury-induced activation of a specific family of transcription factors (NF-κB) that regulate expression of inducible EC genes.[24]

Role of Macrophages and Other Inflammatory/ Immunologic Mechanisms. Following adherence to endothelium early in the course of experimental hypercholesterolemia, monocytes emigrate into the intima and subsequently accumulate LDL. The directed migration of monocytes into the subendothelial space is presumably in response to a gradient of chemotactic factors produced in the intima including oxidized lipids (see later), fragments of tissue matrix proteins, or inflammatory cytokines, such as monocyte chemotactic protein-1 (MCP-1) and macrophage colony-stimulating factor (M-CSF). Macrophages also proliferate in the intima.

Most importantly, however, macrophages ingest lipid to produce *foam cells.* Although monocytes/macrophages express the LDL receptor, the rate at which they take up native LDL is too low to generate foam cells. They can, however, take up a modified form of LDL (not recognized by the LDL receptor). The modification is oxidative damage, induced by endothelial cell, platelet, and

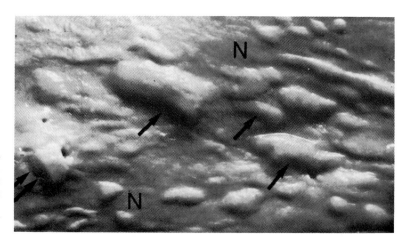

Figure 11–12. Scanning electron photomicrograph of an early atherosclerotic plaque, demonstrating that the endothelium covering such a plaque is intact. (With permission from Benditt, E.P.: The origin of atherosclerosis. Sci. Am. 236:74, 1977. Copyright ©1977 by Scientific American, Inc. All rights reserved.)

white blood cell enzymes. The specific receptor on macrophages for *oxidized LDL* is called the *scavenger receptor* (see Chapter 5). Foam cells may therefore be considered to be specialized macrophages. They are present in variable numbers in all stages of human atheromatous plaques; indeed, recall that fatty streaks, probably the most elementary lesions of atherosclerosis, are collections of macrophage-derived foam cells.

The precise stimuli for recruitment and the role of the T lymphocytes (both CD4+ and CD8+) found within progressing atheromas are uncertain.

In view of the large number of secretory products and biologic activities of macrophages, detailed in our discussion of inflammation (see Chapter 3), it is likely that they play a role in the progression of atherosclerotic lesions.[25] For example, macrophages produce IL-1 and TNF (which increase adhesion of leukocytes) as well as chemotactic factors for leukocytes (e.g., MCP-1 and M-CSF) that may further recruit leukocytes into the plaque. They produce toxic oxygen species that also cause *oxidation of the LDL* in the lesions; recall that oxidized LDL is recognized by the scavenger receptor (see Chapter 5). Finally, growth stimulators and growth inhibitors elaborated by macrophages (e.g., PDGF, FGF, and TGF-β) may modulate the proliferation of smooth muscle cells and the deposition of extracellular matrix in the lesions.

Role of Smooth Muscle Cell Proliferation. In addition to lipid accumulation (to be discussed subsequently), *SMC proliferation and extracellular matrix deposition in the intima are the major processes that account for the progressive growth of atherosclerotic lesions*. The proliferating SMCs originate from cells migrating from the media and possibly also in some cases from pre-existing myointimal cells. A number of SMC mitogens and chemotactic agents derived from cells found in atherosclerotic lesions or serum have been implicated in such proliferation. Principal among these are PDGF, present in the platelet alpha granules and released after platelet adhesion

to foci of injury, but also produced by macrophages, ECs, and SMCs; FGF, and other cytokines that may be produced by ECs, monocytes, macrophages, T lymphocytes and the SMCs themselves, especially IL-1; and transforming growth factor-alpha (TGF-α). In addition, growth stimulation can also be theoretically accomplished by loss of growth inhibitors, such as heparin-like molecules elaborated by both ECs and SMCs, or TGF-β produced by macrophages or ECs. SMCs also elaborate and remodel the extracellular components of the atheromatous plaque, and growth factors are also involved in such processes. Furthermore, SMCs can accumulate large amounts of cholesterol and cholesterol esters and, together with infiltrating macrophages, also give rise to the foam cells in the plaque.

Role of Hyperlipidemia. The pathways of cholesterol metabolism are discussed in detail in Chapter 5, in the context of familial hypercholesterolemia; for the purposes of the present discussion, it is worthwhile to recall that all lipids in plasma circulate in combination with protein. The plasma lipoproteins are complexes of lipid and protein assembled as globular particles, each consisting of a core of neutral lipid (primarily triglycerides and cholesterol esters) surrounded by a coat composed of polar lipids (phospholipid and free cholesterol) and apolipoproteins (also called apoproteins). Lipoprotein transport is also controlled by the lipoprotein-processing proteins (lecithin-cholesterol acyltransferase [LCAT], lipoprotein lipase, hepatic lipase, and cholesterol ester transfer protein) and the lipoprotein receptors that recognize lipoproteins and mediate their cellular uptake and catabolism (LDL receptor, chylomicron remnant receptor, and the scavenger receptor). In the past decade, nearly all the genes that code for these proteins have been isolated, sequenced, and mapped in the human genome; abnormalities in them may explain premature atherosclerosis in some cases.

The abnormality common to most syndromes of premature atherosclerosis is hyperlipoproteinemia. A number of genetic and acquired derange-

Table 11-3. THE HYPERLIPOPROTEINEMIAS AND THEIR GENETIC BASIS

ELECTROPHORETIC PHENOTYPE	INCREASED LIPOPROTEIN CLASS(ES)	INCREASED LIPID CLASS(ES)	KNOWN UNDERLYING GENETIC DEFECTS
1	Chylomicrons	Triglycerides	Mutation in lipoprotein lipase gene
2a	LDL	Cholesterol	Mutation in LDL receptor gene or in apolipoprotein B gene
2b	LDL and VLDL	Cholesterol and triglycerides	Mutation in LDL receptor gene or in apolipoprotein B gene
3	Remnants (chylomicrons) and IDL	Triglycerides and cholesterol	Mutation in apolipoprotein E gene
4	VLDL	Triglycerides	Unknown
5	VLDL and chylomicrons	Triglycerides and cholesterol	Mutation in apolipoprotein CII gene

LDL = Low-density lipoprotein; VLDL = very-low-density lipoprotein; IDL = intermediate-density lipoprotein.
Courtesy of Robert S. Lees, M.D., Boston Heart Foundation and Harvard-MIT Program in Health Sciences and Technology.

ments influence both exogenous and endogenous pathways of cholesterol metabolism and can result in hyperlipoproteinemia. Hyperlipoproteinemias can be due to either primary genetic defects in lipid metabolism (Table 11–3) or secondary to some other underlying disorder, such as the nephrotic syndrome, alcoholism, hypothyroidism, or diabetes mellitus. Four types of lipoprotein abnormality are frequently found in the population (and, indeed, one or more are present in 50 to 80% of myocardial infarction survivors): (1) increased LDL cholesterol levels, (2) decreased HDL cholesterol levels, (3) increased chylomicron remnants and IDL, and (4) increased levels of an abnormal lipoprotein Lp(a) (see later).

The most well-studied example of genetically induced hyperlipoproteinemia causing severe atherosclerosis in young individuals is familial hypercholesterolemia caused by defects in the LDL receptor; this leads to inadequate hepatic uptake of LDL, markedly increasing circulating LDL (see Chapter 5). *Genetic defects in apoproteins may also be associated with hyperlipoproteinemia and accelerated atherosclerosis.*[26] For example, increased LDL cholesterol levels in one syndrome are due to the presence of a genetically variant apoprotein E that fails to bind properly to the LDL receptor. This defect has been traced to a single amino acid substitution (e.g., arginine to cysteine at residue 158) in the receptor binding site of the apoprotein E molecule, which reduces binding activity to 1 to 2% of normal. Mutations producing defective apo B-100 cause similar binding abnormalities, resulting in increased serum LDL. Indeed, apolipoprotein genetic variability may play a role in atherosclerosis susceptibility in the general population. With the availability of transgenic mice deficient in apo E that develop atherosclerosis with cholesterol feeding, an animal model may now be used to evaluate the combined effects of genes and environmental influences in atherogenesis.[27]

A number of mechanisms have been postulated to account for the role of lipids in lesion formation:

- Increases in plasma levels of LDL or some component of hyperlipidemic serum may *increase the rate of lipid penetration into the artery wall.*
- Local modification of LDL may render it more atherogenic.[28] In addition to being readily ingested by macrophages through the scavenger receptor (see Chapter 5), oxidized LDL could accelerate atherogenesis by other mechanisms: (1) It is chemotactic for circulating monocytes; (2) it increases monocyte adhesion; (3) it inhibits the motility of macrophages already in lesions, thus favoring the recruitment and retention of macrophages in the lesions; (4) it stimulates release of growth factors and cytokines; (5) it is cytotoxic to ECs and SMCs; and (6) it is immunogenic. This suggests that antioxidants (e.g., vitamin E) might be efficacious in preventing atherosclerosis by reducing LDL oxidative modification.[29]
- *Hyperlipoproteinemia may directly alter EC function*, without leading to denudation, through focal EC death (see earlier), increased permeability, increased replication, or increased monocyte adhesion.

Role of Thrombosis. Thrombosis is a complication of late-stage atherosclerosis, and organization of thrombi may contribute to plaque formation and their encroachment on the lumen. Although platelets generally do not adhere to the arterial wall without prior severe injury or endothelial denudation, more subtle biochemical disruptions of the normal EC could render it thrombogenic.

Lipoprotein(a) (lp[a]) is an altered form of LDL that contains the apolipoprotein B-100 portion of the LDL linked to apolipoprotein(a) (apo[a]), itself a large glycoprotein molecule sharing a high degree of structural homology to plasminogen (a key protein in fibrinolysis). Lp(a) could be atherogenic by various mechanisms, including interference with both LDL and plasminogen metabolism[30] or promotion of SMC proliferation.[31] Indeed, epidemiologic studies have shown a significant correlation between increased blood levels of lp(a) and coronary and cerebral vascular disease, independent of the level of total cholesterol or LDL.

Other Theories of Atherogenesis. *The development of the atheromatous plaque could also be explained if SMC proliferation were in fact the primary event.* For example, the *monoclonal hypothesis* of atherogenesis was based on the observation that some human plaques are monoclonal or, at the most, oligoclonal. This was interpreted by Benditt and Benditt as evidence that plaques may be equivalent to benign monoclonal neoplastic growths (such as leiomyomas), perhaps induced by

an exogenous chemical (e.g., cholesterol or some of its oxidized products) or an oncogenic virus.[32] Although the universal monoclonal nature of plaques has been questioned, there is evidence in animals that certain viruses (e.g., the agent of Marek's disease in chickens) cause plaques in the aorta, and both herpesvirus and cytomegalovirus have been detected in human atheromatous plaques.[33]

Figure 11–13 summarizes the major proposed mechanism of atherogenesis. *The current trend is to consider that atherosclerosis is a chronic inflammatory response of the vascular wall to a variety of initiating events that can occur early in life. Multiple pathogenic mechanisms contribute to the plaque formation and progression, including endothelial dysfunction, monocyte adhesion and infiltration, smooth muscle proliferation, extracellular matrix deposition, lipid accumulation, and thrombosis.*

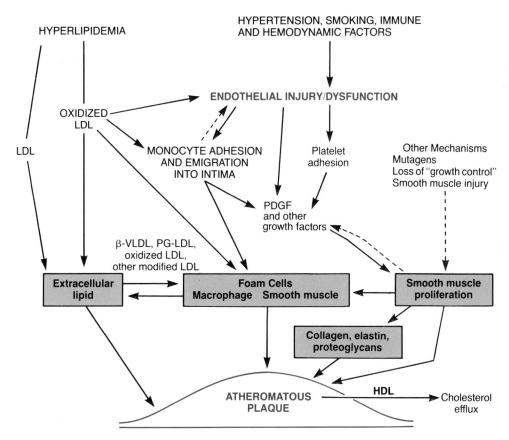

Figure 11–13. Schematic diagram of hypothetical sequence of events and cellular interactions in atherosclerosis. Hyperlipidemia, as well as other risk factors, is thought to cause endothelial injury resulting in adhesion of platelets and monocytes and release of growth factors, including platelet-derived growth factor (PDGF), which lead to smooth muscle cell migration and proliferation. Smooth muscle cells produce large amounts of collagen and proteoglycans, contributing to the atheromatous plaque. Foam cells of atheromatous plaques are derived from both macrophages and smooth muscle cells — from macrophages via the β-VLDL receptor and LDL modifications recognized by scavenger receptors (e.g., oxidized LDL), and from smooth muscle cells by less certain mechanisms. Extracellular lipid is derived from insudation from the lumen, particularly in the presence of hypercholesterolemia, and also from degenerating foam cells. Cholesterol accumulation in the plaque should be viewed as reflecting an imbalance between influx and efflux, and it is possible that HDL helps clear cholesterol from these accumulations. The diagram also depicts other postulated mechanisms for smooth muscle cell proliferation, bypassing primary endothelial injury; the action of mutagens, loss of growth control, indirect smooth muscle cell injury (such as by oxidized LDL). PG = proteoglycan. (Modified with permission from Cotran, R.S., and Munro, J.M.: Pathogenesis of atherosclerosis: Recent concepts. *In* Grundy, S.M., and Bearn, A.G. (eds.): The Role of Cholesterol in Atherosclerosis: New Therapeutic Opportunities. Philadelphia, Hanley and Belfus, 1988, p. 5.)

CLINICAL SIGNIFICANCE. The clinical manifestations of atherosclerosis are as varied as the vessels affected and the extent and configuration of the atheromatous change. Atherosclerotic lesions cause clinical disease by the following:

- Slow, insidious narrowing of the vascular lumina, resulting in ischemia of tissues perfused by the involved vessels
- Sudden occlusion of the lumen by superimposed thrombosis or hemorrhage into an atheroma, producing ischemia and, if severe and prolonged, infarction of the tissues in the perfusion zone
- Providing a site for thrombosis and then embolism
- Weakening the wall of a vessel, causing an aneurysm or rupture

In larger vessels, such as the aorta, the important complications of these plaques are large mural thrombi that may dislodge and yield peripheral emboli, aneurysmal dilation due to destructive impingement of the atheromatous plaques on the media, or rupture of cholesterol emboli into the bloodstream. In smaller arteries, however, the narrowing of the lumen by atheromatous plaques, especially if accompanied by thrombosis or hemorrhage, can lead to occlusion, causing myocardial infarction or stroke. Although any organ or tissue in the body may theoretically be so involved, *symptomatic atherosclerotic disease is most often localized to the arteries supplying the heart, brain, kidneys, lower extremities, and small intestine.*

Given the fact that atherosclerosis and IHD are virtually epidemic in affluent populations, potential methods of control are understandably major concerns, and many clinical trials of prevention have been instituted. A review of clinical trials is beyond the scope of this book. Suffice it to say here that the evidence is good that control of hypertension and cigarette smoking diminishes the risk of IHD. Moreover, treatment of hypercholesterolemia with diet and drugs reduces mortality from IHD, and *dietary* reduction of plasma cholesterol and cholesterol LDL levels would likely retard the progression of atherosclerosis. Thus, experts on all sides of the controversy advocate a reduction in fat intake, avoidance of obesity, moderation of salt intake, cessation of smoking, and the pursuit of physical activity to reduce overall risk. Moreover, there is now substantial evidence that experimentally induced fatty streaks and fibrous plaques can regress and that even advanced lesions in patients can regress when plasma cholesterol levels are reduced for sufficient periods of time.

Moreover, atherosclerosis develops at an early age. The ongoing Pathologic Determinants of Atherosclerosis in Youth Study (PDAY) demonstrated that serum lipoprotein cholesterol concentrations and smoking are important determinants of the early stages of atherosclerosis noted at autopsy in adolescents and young adults.[34] These data provide justification for efforts directed toward risk factor reduction in young persons.

MONCKEBERG'S ARTERIOSCLEROSIS (MEDIAL CALCIFIC SCLEROSIS)

Medial sclerosis is characterized by ring-like calcifications within the media of medium-sized to small muscular arteries of obscure cause. The calcification is not associated with any inflammatory reaction, and the intima and adventitia are largely unaffected. *The calcific deposits do not narrow the lumen.* Commonly bone and even marrow form within the calcific masses. Although Monckeberg's medial calcific sclerosis may occur together with atherosclerosis in the same individual or even in the same vessel (e.g., in the arteries of the legs of aged individuals), *the two disorders are totally distinct.* The vessels most affected are the femoral, tibial, radial, and ulnar arteries and the arterial supply of the genital tract of both sexes, almost exclusively in individuals older than 50 years of age. Of relatively little clinical significance, this disorder accounts for roentgenographic densities in the vessels of the extremities in aged individuals.

HYPERTENSIVE VASCULAR DISEASE AND ARTERIOSCLEROSIS

Hypertension is a disease largely of the vasculature. The pathogenesis of hypertension is likely due, in part, to functional and perhaps structural changes in blood vessels. Moreover, the primary consequences of hypertension consist of pathologic vascular changes, including accelerated atherosclerosis and hyaline and hyperplastic arteriolosclerosis as well as arteriolitis in some cases of severe hypertension. In this section, we discuss mechanisms of hypertension, followed by the pathologic changes of the vasculature that it causes.

HYPERTENSION

Elevated blood pressure is a staggering health problem for three major reasons: It is very common, its consequences are widespread and sometimes devastating, and it remains asymptomatic until late in its course.[35] Hypertension has been identified as one of the most important risk factors in both coronary heart disease and cerebrovascular accidents; it may also lead to congestive heart failure (hypertensive heart disease), aortic dissection, and renal failure. The detrimental effects of blood

Table 11-4. CLASSIFICATION OF BLOOD PRESSURE IN ADULTS

BLOOD PRESSURE RANGE (mm Hg)	CATEGORY
Diastolic	
<85	Normal blood pressure
85–89	High-normal blood pressure
90–104	Mild hypertension
105–114	Moderate hypertension
≥ 115	Severe hypertension
Systolic, when diastolic <90 mm Hg	
<140	Normal blood pressure
140–159	Borderline isolated systolic hypertension
≥ 160	Isolated systolic hypertension

Classification based on the average of two or more readings on two or more occasions.

Modified with permission from 1988 Joint National Committee: The 1988 report of the Joint National Committee on Detection, Evaluation, and Treatment of High Blood Pressure. Arch. Intern. Med. *148*:1023, 1989; and Kaplan, N.M.: Systemic hypertension: Mechanisms and diagnosis, In: Braunwald, E. (ed.): Heart Disease, 4th ed. W.B. Saunders Co., Philadelphia, 1992.

Table 11-5. MAIN CAUSES AND POSSIBLE FACTORS IN THE PATHOGENESIS OF HYPERTENSION

ESSENTIAL HYPERTENSION
Genetic defect in renal sodium excretion
Genetic defect in sodium/calcium transport in vascular smooth muscle
Variation in genes encoding angiotensinogen and other proteins in renin-angiotensin system
Other increased vasoconstrictive influences: behavioral, neurogenic, hormonal

SECONDARY HYPERTENSION
Renal disease: increased renin secretion, sodium and fluid retention, decreased vasodilator (vasodepressor) secretion
Endocrine causes: aldosteronism, oral contraceptives, pheochromocytoma, thyrotoxicosis
Vascular causes: coarctation of the aorta, vasculitis
Neurogenic causes: psychogenic, increased intracranial pressure

pressure increase continuously as the pressure increases, and there is no rigidly defined threshold of blood pressure above which an individual is considered at risk for the complications of hypertension and below which he or she is safe. Nevertheless, a sustained diastolic pressure greater than 90 mm Hg or a sustained systolic pressure in excess of 140 mm Hg are generally considered to constitute hypertension. The classification of blood pressure in adults is shown in Table 11-4. By these criteria, screening programs reveal that 25% of persons in the general population are hypertensive. The prevalence increases with age. In older age groups, the disease is likely to be relatively mild; hypertension in young adults tends to be more severe. Blacks are affected by hypertension about twice as often as whites and seem more vulnerable to its complications.

About 90 to 95% of hypertension is idiopathic and apparently primary (essential hypertension). Of the remaining 5 to 10%, most is secondary to renal disease or, less often, to narrowing of the renal artery, usually by an atheromatous plaque (renovascular hypertension). Infrequently, secondary hypertension is the result of adrenal disorders, such as primary aldosteronism, Cushing's syndrome, or pheochromocytoma (Table 11-5). *Both essential and secondary hypertension may be either benign or malignant, according to the clinical course.* In most cases, hypertension remains at a modest level and fairly stable over years to decades and, unless a myocardial infarction or cerebrovascular accident supervenes, is compatible with long life. This form of the disorder is termed *benign hypertension.* Although a benign course is most characteristic of idiopathic or essential hypertension, it may also be seen with the secondary disorder. About 5% of

hypertensive persons show a rapidly rising blood pressure, which, if untreated, leads to death within a year or two. This is called *accelerated* or *malignant hypertension.* The full-blown clinical syndrome of malignant hypertension includes severe hypertension (diastolic pressure over 120 mm Hg), renal failure, and retinal hemorrhages and exudates, with or without papilledema. *This form of hypertension may develop in previously normotensive persons but more often is superimposed on pre-existing benign hypertension, either essential or secondary.* In its pure form, malignant hypertension typically develops in the fourth decade of life.

PATHOGENESIS OF HYPERTENSION

Blood pressure is a complex trait that is determined by the interaction of multiple genetic and environmental factors. Therefore it should not be surprising that the pathogenesis of hypertension remains an enigma. Because the potential mechanisms of hypertension constitute aberrations of normal regulatory processes, the physiologic regulation of blood pressure is discussed next, followed by pathologic considerations.

Regulation of Normal Blood Pressure

The magnitude of the arterial pressure depends on two fundamental hemodynamic variables: *cardiac output* and *total peripheral resistance* (Fig. 11-14). For the most part, total peripheral resistance is accounted for by resistance of the arterioles, predominantly related to lumen size. This in turn is determined by the thickness of the arteriolar wall and the effects of neural and hormonal influences that either constrict or dilate these vessels. Vasoconstricting agents are angiotensin II, catechol-

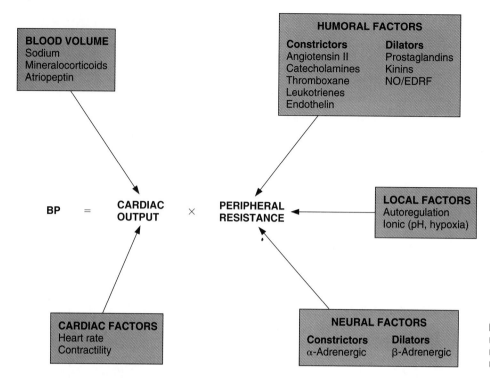

Figure 11-14. Blood pressure regulation. NO/EDRF denotes nitric oxide/endothelium-derived growth factor.

amines, thromboxane, leukotrienes, and endothelin. Vasodilators include kinins, prostaglandins, and nitric oxide. These mediators act by binding specific receptors on the surfaces of smooth muscle cells. Certain metabolic products (such as lactic acid, hydrogen ions, and adenosine) and hypoxia are also local vasodilators. An important property intrinsic to resistance vessels is *autoregulation*, a process by which increased blood flow to such vessels leads to vasoconstriction. An essentially adaptive mechanism that protects from hyperperfusion, autoregulation is probably mediated by the local levels of adenosine; the resultant vasoconstriction leads to increased cardiac workload, reduction of cardiac output, and correction of hyperperfusion. *Arterial hypertension can best be considered a disease dependent on factors that may alter the relationship between blood volume and total arteriolar resistance.*

The kidneys play an important role in blood pressure regulation by at least three mechanisms:

1. *Renin-angiotensin system* (Fig. 11-15). Through the elaboration of renin, the kidney eventually forms *angiotensin II*, which alters blood pressure by increasing both peripheral resistance and blood volume. The former effect is achieved largely by its ability to cause vasoconstriction through direct action on vascular smooth muscle, the latter by stimulation of aldosterone secretion, which increases distal tubular reabsorption of sodium and thus of water.

2. *Sodium homeostasis.* The kidney is intimately involved in the complex process of sodium homeostasis. In addition to the renin-angiotensin system mechanism, two other renal factors have important bearing on sodium homeostasis: the *glomerular filtration rate (GFR)* and *GFR-independent natriuretic factors.* When blood volume is reduced, the GFR falls; this in turn leads to increased reabsorption of sodium by proximal tubules in an attempt to conserve sodium and expand blood volume. GFR-independent factors include *atrial natriuretic factor (ANF)*, or *atriopeptin*, a group of peptides secreted by heart atria in response to volume expansion, which inhibit sodium reabsorption in distal tubules and cause vasodilation.

3. *Renal vasodepressor substances,* The kidney produces a variety of vasodepressor or antihypertensive substances that presumably counterbalance the vasopressor effects of angiotensin. These include the prostaglandins, a urinary kallikrein-kinin system, platelet-activating factor, and nitric oxide.

Abnormalities in these renal mechanisms are implicated in the pathogenesis of hypertension in a variety of renal diseases (see Chapter 20), but they no doubt play a role in essential hypertension.

Mechanisms of Essential Hypertension

Although the cause of most cases of hypertension is unknown (hence the term "essential"), speculations abound, and the subject is a source of lively controversy. Indeed, there is now agreement that a single defect is unlikely to account for essential hypertension. At the most elemental level, the cause must be related to either a primary increase

RENIN-ANGIOTENSIN SYSTEM

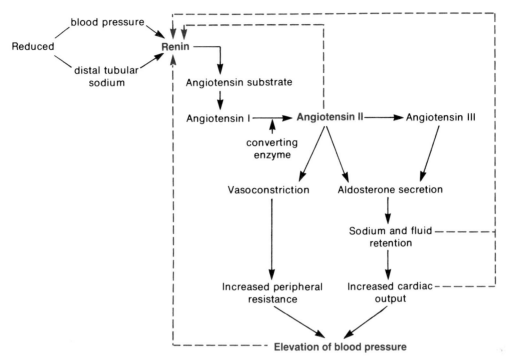

Figure 11–15. Role of renin-angiotensin system in the regulation of blood pressure. Solid lines represent positive interactions; broken lines show negative interactions or feedback inhibition.

in cardiac output or an increase in peripheral resistance, and the several theories of the origin of hypertension stress one or the other event (see Fig. 11–14).

Those who advocate a primary increase in cardiac output suggest that the basic nonstructural, probably genetic defect is reduced renal sodium excretion in the presence of normal arterial pressure (defective pressure natriuresis). As illustrated in Figure 11–16, decreased sodium excretion would lead to an increase in fluid volume and a rise in cardiac output. In the face of increasing cardiac output, peripheral vasoconstriction (due to autoregulation, discussed earlier) occurs to prevent overperfusion of tissues, which would result from an unchecked increase in cardiac output. Autoregulation, however, leads to increased peripheral resistance and along with it an elevation of blood pressure. At the higher setting of blood pressure, enough additional sodium can be excreted by the kidneys to equal intake and prevent fluid retention. Thus, an altered but steady state of sodium excretion is achieved ("resetting of pressure natriuresis").

The second hypothesis implicates vasoconstrictive influences as the primary events. These could be (1) behavioral or neurogenic factors, as shown by the reduction of blood pressure that can be achieved by meditation (the relaxation response); (2) increased release of vasoconstrictor agents

(e.g., renin, catecholamines, endothelin); or (3) a primary increased sensitivity of vascular smooth muscle, caused by a genetic defect in cell membrane transport of sodium and calcium, leading to increased intracellular calcium and contraction in the smooth muscle cells.

Both hereditary and environmental factors have been implicated in hypertension. When both parents are hypertensive, the children have a much increased risk of developing hypertension. Studies on twins and familial aggregations support a role for the genetic constitution in the causation of hypertension. If heredity is involved, how is the genetic defect manifested? Defects relating to renal sodium reabsorption or sodium and calcium transport in vascular smooth muscle have been suggested, which could lead to hypertension by the mechanisms described previously.

Nevertheless, although it is unlikely that a single gene defect causes essential hypertension,[36] evidence suggests that inherited variations in blood pressure may depend in part on genetically determined heterogeneity in the renin-angiotensin system. For example, a genetic linkage study has shown a predisposition to essential hypertension associated with specific molecular variants of the gene encoding angiotensinogen, the physiologic substrate for renin.[37] In this study, increased concentrations of plasma angiotensin were present in hypertensive subjects carrying a common angio-

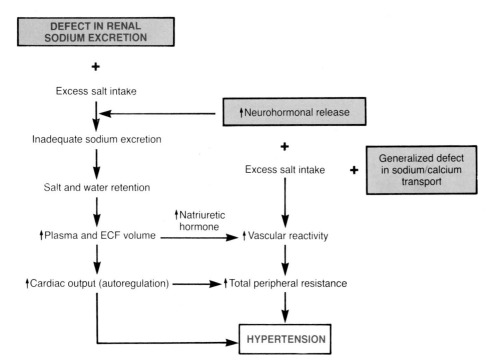

Figure 11-16. Hypothetical schema for pathogenesis of essential hypertension implicating genetic defects in renal sodium excretion, or in sodium-calcium transport, or causing increased neurohormonal release—coupled with excess salt intake. Increased cardiac output and increased total peripheral resistance contribute to the hypertension.

tensinogen gene variant that had a strong association with hypertension.

It is likely that environmental factors are also involved in the expression of the genetic abnormalities. The role of environment is illustrated by the lower incidence of hypertension in Chinese people living in their native country as compared with persons of Chinese descent living in the United States. Environmental factors implicated in the causation of hypertension include stress, obesity, smoking, inactivity, and heavy consumption of salt. The evidence linking the level of dietary sodium intake with the prevalence of hypertension in different population groups is impressive. It must be stressed that in both of the major hypotheses discussed, heavy sodium intake augments the hypertension.

Essential hypertension is thus a complex disorder that may have more than one cause. It may be initiated by a disturbance in any of the factors that control normal blood pressure, many of which are environmental (stress, salt intake, estrogens) but act in the genetically predisposed individual. In established hypertension, both increased blood volume and increased peripheral resistance contribute to the increased pressure.

Vascular Pathology in Hypertension

Hypertension accelerates atherogenesis and causes changes in the structure of the walls of blood vessels that potentiate both aortic dissection and cerebrovascular hemorrhage. In addition, hypertension is associated with two forms of small blood vessel disease: hyaline arteriolosclerosis and hyperplastic arteriolosclerosis (Fig. 11–17). Both lesions are clearly related to elevations of blood pressure, but other causes may also be involved.

HYALINE ARTERIOLOSCLEROSIS. This condition is encountered frequently in elderly patients, whether normotensive or hypertensive, but it is more generalized and more severe in patients with hypertension. The condition is also seen commonly in diabetes and forms part of the microangiography characteristic of diabetic disease (see Chapter 19). Whatever the clinical setting, the vascular lesion consists of a homogeneous, pink, hyaline thickening of the walls of arterioles with loss of underlying structural detail and with narrowing of the lumen.

It is believed that the lesions reflect leakage of plasma components across vascular endothelium and increasing extracellular matrix production by smooth muscle cells. Presumably, the chronic hemodynamic stress of hypertension or a metabolic stress in diabetes accentuates endothelial injury, thus resulting in leakage and hyaline deposition (see Fig. 11–17A). The narrowing of the arteriolar lumina causes impairment of the blood supply to affected organs, particularly well exemplified in the kidneys. Thus, **hyaline arteriolosclerosis is a major morphologic characteristic of benign nephrosclerosis,** in which the arteriolar narrowing causes diffuse renal ischemia and symmetric contraction of the kidneys (see Chapter 20).

HYPERPLASTIC ARTERIOLOSCLEROSIS. The hyperplastic type of arteriolosclerosis is generally related

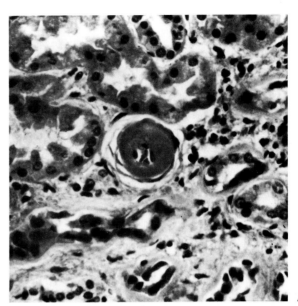

Figure 11-17. Arteriolosclerosis and arteriolitis. *A*, Hyaline arteriolosclerosis. Arteriolar wall is hyalinized, and lumen is markedly narrowed. Note also interstitial fibrosis and tubular atrophy. *B*, Hyperplastic arteriolosclerosis of malignant hypertension (onionskinning). *C*, Necrotizing arteriolitis of malignant nephrosclerosis with fibrinoid degeneration of walls of arterioles and small arteries.

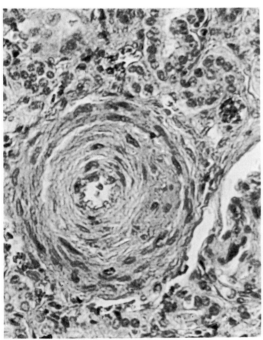

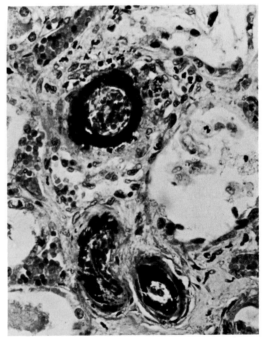

to more acute or severe elevations of blood pressure and is therefore characteristic of malignant hypertension (diastolic pressures usually over 110 mm Hg). This form of arteriolar disease can be identified with the light microscope by virtue of its onionskin, concentric, laminated thickening of the walls of arterioles with progressive narrowing of the lumina (see Fig. 11–17B). With the electron microscope, these reduplicated cells have the appearance of smooth muscle cells. The basement membrane is likewise thickened and reduplicated. Frequently, but not invariably, these hyperplastic changes are accompanied by deposits of fibrinoid and acute necrosis of the vessel walls, referred to as **necrotizing arteriolitis** (see Fig. 11–17C). The

arterioles in all tissues throughout the body may be affected, favored sites being the kidney (see Chapter 20), periadrenal fat, gallbladder, and peripancreatic and intestinal arterioles.

INFLAMMATORY DISEASE — THE VASCULITIDES

Vascular inflammatory injury, often with necrosis of blood vessels *(vasculitis)*, is encountered in diverse diseases and clinical settings. The terms arteritis, vasculitis, and angiitis are used interchange-

Table 11–6. CLASSIFICATION OF VASCULITIS BASED ON PATHOGENESIS

INFECTIOUS
Bacterial (e.g., Neisseria)
Rickettsial (e.g., Rocky Mountain spotted fever)
Spirochetal (e.g., syphilis)
Fungal (e.g., aspergillosis)
Viral (e.g., herpes)

IMMUNOLOGIC
Immune complex–mediated
  Henoch-Schönlein purpura
  Essential cryoglobulinemic vasculitis
  Serum sickness vasculitis
  Lupus vasculitis
  Hepatitis B microscopic polyarteritis
Direct antibody attack–mediated
  Goodpasture's syndrome (antibasement membrane antibodies)
  Kawasaki disease (antiendothelial antibodies)
ANCA associated (possibly ANCA mediated)
  Wegener's granulomatosis
  Microscopic polyangiitis (microscopic polyarteritis)
  Churg-Strauss syndrome
Cell-mediated
  Allograft organ rejection

UNKNOWN
Giant cell (temporal) arteritis
Takayasu's arteritis
Polyarteritis nodosa (classic polyarteritis nodosa)

ANCA = Antineutrophil cytoplasmic antibodies.
Courtesy of J.C. Jennette, M.D., University of North Carolina.

ably because veins and capillaries may be involved in some of the conditions. The two most common mechanisms are direct injury to vessels by infectious pathogens and immune-mediated inflammation (Table 11–6). In a particular patient, it is critically important to distinguish between these two mechanisms because the treatment approaches differ widely (e.g., the immunosuppressive therapy appropriate for immune-mediated vasculitis would be contraindicated for infectious vasculitis). Moreover, physical and chemical injury, such as irradiation, mechanical trauma, and toxins, can also cause vascular damage. The so-called *noninfectious systemic necrotizing vasculitides* are segregated into a number of distinctive clinicopathologic syndromes affecting multiple organ systems. Many of these entities have an immunologic basis, as was pointed out in the previous consideration of systemic lupus erythematosus (SLE) and other connective tissue disorders.

PATHOGENESIS OF VASCULITIS. Several pathogenetic mechanisms that may be common to many vasculitides are discussed here.

Immune Complexes. Many types of vasculitis are thought to be induced by immune complexes; the evidence can be summarized as follows:

- The vascular lesions resemble those found in experimental immune complex–mediated conditions, such as the local Arthus phenomenon and serum sickness.
- DNA–anti-DNA immune complexes and complement are present in the vascular lesions of SLE-associated vasculitis.
- In patients with mixed cryoglobulinemia, IgG, IgM, and complement components have been seen in involved vessels.
- In some patients, viruses and other antigens have been localized in the lesions, together with immunoglobulin and complement, and immune complexes are found in the circulation.
- The most impressive evidence is the demonstration of a high incidence of hepatitis B antigen (HBsAg) and HBsAg–anti-HBsAg immune complexes in the sera and, with complement, in the vascular lesions of some patients with vasculitis. Moreover, recent studies have found that chronic hepatitis C virus (HCV) infection was associated with glomerulonephritis. In such patients, HCV RNA was detected in the serum, and cryoprecipitates contained IgG anti-HCV antibodies, suggesting deposition within glomeruli of HCV–anti-HCV immune complexes as the cause.[38]

Whether complexes accrue in vessel walls by deposition from the circulation, by *in situ* formation, or by a combination of these mechanisms is not known (see Chapter 20). Moreover, immune complexes cannot account for many forms of inflammatory vasculitis.[39]

Antineutrophil Cytoplasmic Antibodies. In many patients with vasculitis, the serum reacts with cytoplasmic antigens in neutrophils by immunofluorescence and immunochemical assays, indicating the presence of *antineutrophil cytoplasmic autoantibodies (ANCA)*.[40,41] Two relatively distinct patterns of neutrophil immunofluorescence are observed: perinuclear (called *P-ANCA*) and cytoplasmic (called *C-ANCA*). P-ANCA are directed largely toward *myeloperoxidase* in the primary granules of neutrophils. One of the neutrophil antigens involved in C-ANCA is a potentially tissue-destructive, neutral leukocyte protease (proteinase 3).

There is some correlation between the type of ANCA and the specific vasculitis syndrome. The C-ANCA pattern is detected in the majority of patients with active Wegener's granulomatosis and microscopic polyangiitis but infrequently in other vasculitides. In contrast, P-ANCA is uncommon in Wegener's granulomatosis but is observed frequently in patients with polyarteritis nodosa (PAN) and primary glomerular disease.

ANCA are proving to be useful diagnostic indicators in the study of vasculitis; their presence and titers usually correlate with disease activity. What triggers their induction, however, and whether they play a pathogenetic role is still unclear. One postulated sequence is that these anti-

Table 11–7. CLASSIFICATION AND CHARACTERISTICS OF VASCULITIS

LARGE VESSEL VASCULITIS

Giant cell (temporal) arteritis	Granulomatous arteritis of the aorta and its major branches, with a predilection for the extracranial branches of the carotid artery. *Often involves the temporal artery. Usually occurs in patients older than 50 and often is associated with polymyalgia rheumatica*
Takayasu's arteritis	Granulomatous inflammation of the aorta and its major branches. *Usually occurs in patients younger than age 50.*

MEDIUM-SIZED VESSEL VASCULITIS*

Polyarteritis nodosa (classic polyarteritis nodosa)	Necrotizing inflammation of medium-sized or small arteries without glomerulonephritis or vasculitis in arterioles, capillaries, or venules
Kawasaki disease	Arteritis involving large, medium-sized, and small arteries and associated with mucocutaneous lymph node syndrome. *Coronary arteries are often involved. Aorta and veins may be involved. Usually occurs in children*

SMALL VESSEL VASCULITIS

Wegener's granulomatosis‡	Granulomatous inflammation involving the respiratory tract and necrotizing vasculitis affecting small to medium-sized vessels, e.g., capillaries, venules, arterioles, and arteries. *Necrotizing glomerulonephritis is common*
Churg-Strauss syndrome†	Eosinophil-rich and granulomatous inflammation involving the respiratory tract and necrotizing vasculitis affecting small to medium-sized vessels and associated with asthma and blood eosinophilia
Microscopic polyangiitis (microscopic polyarteritis)†	Necrotizing vasculitis with few or no immune deposits affecting small vessels, i.e., capillaries, venules, or arterioles. *Necrotizing arteritis involving small and medium-sized arteries may be present. Necrotizing glomerulonephritis is common. Pulmonary capillaritis often occurs*
Henoch-Schönlein purpura	Vasculitis with IgA-dominant immune deposits affecting small vessels, i.e., capillaries, venules, or arterioles. *Typically involves skin, gut, and glomeruli and associated with arthralgias or arthritis*
Essential cryoglobulinemic vasculitis	Vasculitis with cryoglobulin immune deposits affecting small vessels, i.e., capillaries, venules, or arterioles, and associated with cryoglobulins in serum. *Skin and glomeruli are often involved.*
Cutaneous leukocytoclastic angiitis	Isolated cutaneous leukocytoclastic angiitis without systemic vasculitis or glomerulonephritis.

* Note that some small and large vessel vasculitides may involve medium-sized arteries, but large and medium-sized vessel vasculitides do not involve vessels smaller than arteries.

† Strongly associated with antineutrophil cytoplasmic autoantibodies, usually P-ANCA.

‡ Strongly associated with antineutrophil cytoplasmic autoantibodies, almost always C-ANCA.

Modified with permission from Jennette J.C., et al.: Nomenclature of systemic vasculitides: The proposal of an international consensus conference. *Arthr. Rheum. 37*:187–192, 1994.

bodies activate neutrophils, causing a respiratory burst and degranulation, thereby stimulating the release of toxic oxygen free radicals and lytic enzymes from neutrophils and resulting in EC and tissue damage. Such neutrophil activation is potentiated by the cytokines associated with these diseases, possibly triggered by intercurrent infections. In addition, there is evidence that antibodies to proteinase 3 inhibit α_1-antitrypsin activity, thus potentiating tissue damage. Of interest is that antibodies against myeloperoxidase injected into rats produce glomerulonephritis and granulomatous vasculitis of small vessels.[42]

Other Mechanisms of Vasculitis. Other immunologic and nonimmunologic pathogenetic mechanisms should be considered.[43] Defects in immunoregulation, well described in SLE (see Chapter 6), may predispose to the development of vasculitis owing to cytotoxic antibodies to normal ECs, seen in patients with active SLE. Antibodies to ECs "activated" by cytokines may contribute to the vasculitis of Kawasaki's disease. The presence of a mononuclear inflammatory cellular infiltrate rich in T cells and of granulomas in some vasculitides suggests that cell-mediated immunity directed against foreign antigens or endogenous components of the vessel wall may play a role. Finally, it should be remembered that vasculitis may be caused by direct action of infectious organisms on the vessel wall.

CLASSIFICATION. Most classifications of systemic vasculitis depend on the size of the involved blood vessels, the anatomic site, the histologic characteristics of the lesion, and the clinical manifestations. There is considerable clinical and pathologic overlap among these disorders. The nomenclature used here is that developed at the Chapel Hill Consensus Conference on the Nomenclature of Systemic Vasculitides (Table 11–7 and Fig. 11–18),[44] and the sequence of entities discussed follows that in Table 11–7.

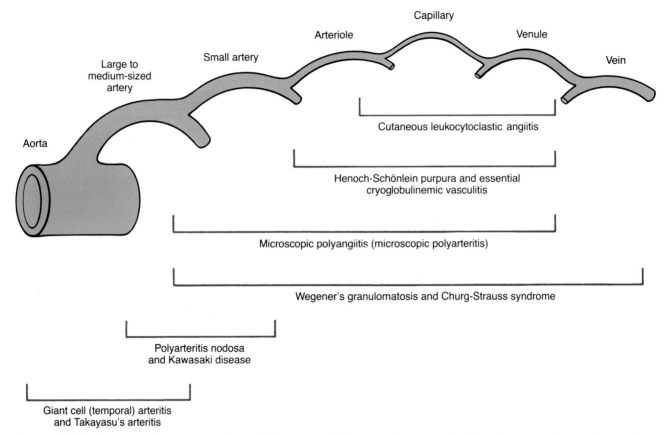

Figure 11-18. Diagrammatic representation of the lesions of the vasculature involved by the major forms of vasculitis. (Reproduced by permission from Jennette, J.C., et al.: Nomenclature of systemic vasculitides: The proposal of an international consensus conference. Arthritis Rheum. 37:187, 1994.)

GIANT CELL (TEMPORAL) ARTERITIS

Giant cell (temporal) arteritis, the most common of the vasculitides, is a focal granulomatous inflammation of arteries of medium size and small size that affects principally the cranial vessels, especially the temporal arteries in older individuals (rare before age 50) but also the vertebral and ophthalmic arteries. In other expressions of this disorder, lesions have been found in arteries throughout the body, and in some cases the aortic arch has been involved to produce so-called *giant cell aortitis.* There is a genetic predisposition, as evidenced by an increased prevalence of HLA-DR4 antigen in these patients, and occasional familial clustering.

The cause of this relatively common disease remains unknown. The morphologic alterations suggest an immunologic reaction against a component of the arterial wall, such as elastin. Some support for such a concept is provided by the finding of cell-mediated immunity to arterial antigen in some patients and by the clinical improvement that is almost always achieved by corticosteroid treatment.

MORPHOLOGY. The histologic changes in arteries are quite variable and fall into three general pat-

terns: (1) granulomatous lesions replete with giant cells; in temporal arteritis, these are often in relation to fragments of a fragmented internal elastic membrane (Figure 11-19); (2) nonspecific white cell infiltration (lymphocytes and eosinophils) throughout the arterial wall; and (3) intimal fibrosis, usually with no morphologically apparent disruption of the internal elastic lamina. Giant cells are

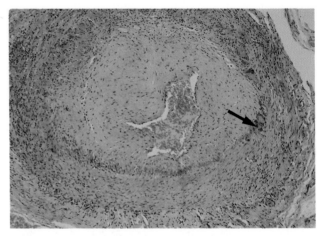

Figure 11-19. Temporal (giant cell) arteritis. Circumferential giant cells (GC) mark location of degenerated internal elastic membrane *(arrow)*. L = lumen.

present in only two-thirds of cases of temporal arteritis, and many histologic sections may have to be examined before one is detected. Thrombus formation commonly occurs in affected vessels and may be followed by either obliteration of the lumina or organization and recanalization. In healed phases, the artery has considerable scarring that may be difficult to distinguish from aging changes, and it may be a fibrous cord with the lumen obliterated.

Temporal arteritis may be insidious and vague in onset or may be heralded by the sudden onset of headache, tenderness or severe throbbing pain (or both) over the artery, swelling and redness in the overlying skin, visual loss, and facial pain. Almost half the patients have systemic involvement and the syndrome of *polymyalgia rheumatica*, a flu-like syndrome with joint stiffness. There is often claudication of the jaw. Visual symptoms that vary from blurred or double vision to the sudden onset of blindness occur in 40% of patients.

The erythrocyte sedimentation rate (ESR) is markedly elevated in most cases. Biopsy may be diagnostic. Approximately one-third of biopsy results of the temporal artery, however, are negative in patients with classic manifestations of this disease, and it must be assumed that the lesions were focal and missed on biopsy. In the absence of morphologic confirmation, it is often necessary to institute therapy on clinical grounds alone. When the disease is of acute and almost calamitous onset, corticosteroid therapy must be instituted promptly to prevent visual impairment. Involvement of visceral vessels may give rise to manifestations of myocardial ischemia, gastrointestinal disturbances, or neurologic derangements.

TAKAYASU'S ARTERITIS

This granulomatous vasculitis of medium and larger arteries was described in 1908 by Takayasu as a *clinical syndrome characterized principally by ocular disturbances and marked weakening of the pulses in the upper extremities (pulseless disease), related to fibrous thickening of the aortic arch with narrowing or virtual obliteration of the origins of the great vessels arising in the arch.* Most common in Asia, it has been reported in most areas of the world, including the United States. The illness is seen predominantly in females 15 to 40 years old. The cause and pathogenesis are unknown.

MORPHOLOGY. Although Takayasu's arteritis classically involves the aortic arch, in one-third of cases, it also affects the remainder of the aorta and its branches, and in some it is limited to the descend-

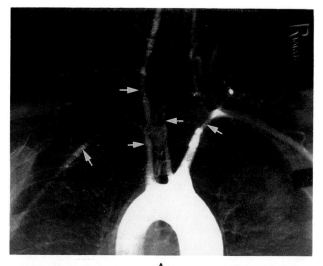

A

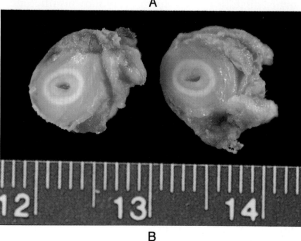

B

Figure 11-20. Takayasu's arteritis. *A,* Aortic arch angiogram showing narrowing of brachiocephalic, carotid, and subclavian arteries *(arrows). B,* Gross photograph of two cross-sections of the right carotid artery taken at autopsy of patient shown in *A,* demonstrating marked intimal thickening with minimal residual lumen.

ing thoracic and abdominal aorta. The gross morphologic changes comprise, in most cases, irregular thickening of the aortic wall with intimal wrinkling. When the aortic arch is involved, the orifices of the major arteries to the upper portion of the body may be markedly narrowed or even obliterated by intimal thickening, accounting for the designation "pulseless disease" (Fig. 11-20). Histologically, the early changes consist of an adventitial mononuclear infiltrate with perivascular cuffing of the vasa vasorum. Later, there may be intense mononuclear inflammation in the media, in some cases accompanied by granulomatous changes, replete with Langhans' giant cells and central necrosis. The morphologic changes of Takayasu's arteritis may be indistinguishable from those in giant cell (temporal) arteritis.[45] Thus, the distinction between active giant cell lesions of the aorta is based largely on clinical data, including the age of the patient. Moreover, the description Takayasu's is currently being used widely to designate most giant cell lesions of the aorta in young patients. Later stages show extensive fibrosis of the media and marked thickening of the intima by smooth muscle cells and associated extracellular matrix.

The salient clinical features include weakening of the pulses of the upper extremities with markedly lower blood pressure in the upper extremities; ocular disturbances, including visual defects, retinal hemorrhages, and total blindness; hypertension; and various neurologic deficits, ranging from dizziness and focal weakness to complete hemiparesis. Unusual patients have identical histologic features of aortitis but with the clinical features of aortic dilatation and aortic valvular insufficiency. The course of the disease is quite variable.

POLYARTERITIS NODOSA GROUP

This group is characterized by systemic involvement with the vasculitic process and includes the *classic* type of vasculitis, also called the *macroscopic* form of PAN, as well as certain variants. *Classic PAN* is manifested by necrotizing inflammation of small or medium-sized muscular arteries, typically involving renal and visceral vessels and sparing the pulmonary circulation. Neither glomerulonephritis nor vasculitis of arterioles, capillaries, or venules is present.

MORPHOLOGY. The primary targets of PAN are the main visceral arteries (e.g., renal, coronary, hepatic, and mesenteric). Thus the most frequent sites of involvement in autopsy series are the kidneys (85%), heart (75%), liver (65%), and gastrointestinal tract (50%). Grossly, the individual lesions involve sharply localized segments of vessel with a predilection for branching points and bifurcations. Intravascular thrombosis is a frequent sequela to the acute vasculitis. Segmental erosion with weakening of the arterial wall due to the inflammatory process may cause aneurysmal dilatation or localized rupture that is perceived clinically as a palpable nodule and can be demonstrated by arteriography. Impairment of perfusion causing ulcerations, infarcts, ischemic atrophy, or hemorrhages in the areas supplied by these vessels may provide the first clue to the existence of the underlying disorder.

Microscopically, the changes in the vessels may be divided into acute, healing, and healed stages (Fig. 11–21). Acute lesions are characterized by fibrinoid necrosis, which may extend to involve the full thickness of the arterial wall, particularly in small arteries. Necrosis is most often localized to a portion of the circumference rather than its entirety. Numerous leukocytes, including neutrophils, eosinophils, and mononuclear cells, may be present in and often around the vessel wall.

Healing lesions are characterized by transmural scarring in addition to the continuing necrotizing process. At this stage, the leukocytic infiltrate has large numbers of macrophages and plasma cells, thrombosis becomes organized, and the fibrosis may extend into the surrounding adventitia. Healed lesions have marked fibrotic thickening of the affected arterial wall. Elastic tissue stains often demonstrate loss or fragmentation of the internal elastic lamina and its replacement by fibrous tissue.

All stages may coexist, either within the same vessel or in different vessels. Indeed, only rarely are all lesions at one stage of inflammatory activity.

CLINICAL COURSE. Classic PAN is a disease of young adults, although it may occur in children and older individuals. The course may be acute, subacute, or chronic and is frequently remittent, with long symptom-free intervals. Because the vascular involvement is widely scattered, the clinical signs and symptoms of this disorder may be varied and puzzling. The most common manifestations are fever of unknown cause and weight loss; hypertension, usually developing rapidly; abdominal pain and melena (bloody stool) due to vascular lesions in the alimentary tract; diffuse muscular aches and pains; and peripheral neuritis, which is predominantly motor. Because small vessel involvement is absent, however, there is no glomerulonephritis. About 30% of patients with PAN have hepatitis B antigen in their serum, and, as mentioned earlier, P-ANCA are often present in the serum and correlate with disease activity.

The diagnosis can usually be definitely established by the identification of necrotizing arteritis on tissue biopsy specimens, particularly *medium-sized* arteries of clinically involved tissue, such as kidney and nodular skin lesions. Angiography shows vascular aneurysms or occlusions of main visceral arteries in 50% of cases. Untreated, the disease is fatal in most cases, either during an acute fulminant attack or following a protracted course, but therapy with corticosteroids and cyclophosphamide results in remissions or cures in 90%. Effective treatment of the hypertension is a prerequisite for a favorable prognosis.

In *allergic granulomatosis and angiitis* (the Churg-Strauss syndrome), the vascular lesions may be histologically identical to those of classic PAN. There is a strong association, however, with bronchial asthma and eosinophilia and pulmonary and splenic vessels, and peripheral nerves and skin are frequently involved by intravascular and extravascular granulomas. Infiltration of vessels and perivascular tissues by eosinophils is striking. P-ANCA are present in 75% of patients.

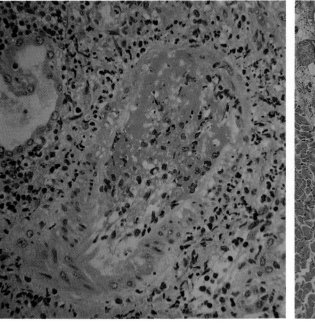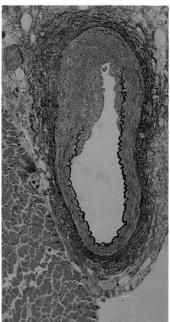

Figure 11-21. Polyarteritis nodosa. *A,* Polyarteritis nodosa with segmental fibrinoid necrosis and thrombotic occlusion of the lumen of this small renal artery. Note that part of the vessel wall at the bottom right is uninvolved. *B,* Elastic tissue stain of artery showing healed polyarteritis. At upper left corner, the internal elastic lamina is destroyed, and there is intimal and medial thickening. The vessels shown in both *A* and *B* were removed from a single patient simultaneously.

A

B

KAWASAKI SYNDROME (MUCOCUTANEOUS LYMPH NODE SYNDROME)

Kawasaki syndrome is an arteritis involving large, medium-sized, and small arteries (often the coronary arteries) that is associated with the mucocutaneous lymph node syndrome, usually in young children and infants (80% younger than four years old). The acute illness is manifested by fever, conjunctival and oral erythema and erosion, edema of the hands and feet, erythema of the palms and soles, a skin rash often with desquamation, and enlargement of cervical lymph nodes. It is usually self-limited.[46] Epidemic in Japan, the disease has also been reported in Hawaii and increasingly in the United States. Approximately 20% of patients develop cardiovascular sequelae, with a range of severity from asymptomatic coronary artery ectasia or aneurysm formation to giant coronary artery aneurysms (7 to 8 mm) with rupture or thrombosis, myocardial infarction, or sudden death. It is the leading cause of acquired heart disease in children in the United States. Acute fatalities occur in 1 to 2% of patients owing to coronary arteritis with superimposed thrombosis or ruptured coronary artery aneurysm. Pathologic changes outside the cardiovascular system are rarely significant.

MORPHOLOGY. Although the vasculitis resembles that of PAN, with necrosis and pronounced inflammation affecting the entire thickness of the vessel wall, fibrinoid necrosis is usually less prominent in Kawasaki syndrome. Coronary artery lesions range from severe destruction of all constituents of the wall by a segmental necrotizing process, with moderate fibrinoid changes and dense infiltrate of inflammatory cells, to mild changes involving the intima only.[47] As with PAN, severe lesions can result in weakening of the vessel wall with thrombosis, aneurysm formation, and rarely rupture. The large and medium-sized extramural branches of the coronary arteries are much more severely involved than the small intramyocardial branches. The inflammatory infiltrate is composed mainly of lymphoid cells and neutrophils, although eosinophils may be seen. The proposed sequence begins with swelling and proliferation of endothelial cells, progresses to inflammatory involvement of the full thickness of the vessel wall, and ends with healing and scar formation.

The clinical and epidemiologic characteristics suggest an infectious etiology; however, the specific cause is unknown. Once the disease is evolving, patients have a number of immunoregulatory disturbances, including T-cell activation, polyclonal B-cell activation, and circulating immune complexes. Lytic autoantibodies to cytokine-activated endothelial cells reported in patients with acute disease disappear in convalescence; they may contribute to the vascular injury in this disorder. Intravenous gamma globulin administered with aspirin appears to reduce the prevalence of long-term coronary artery abnormalities.[48]

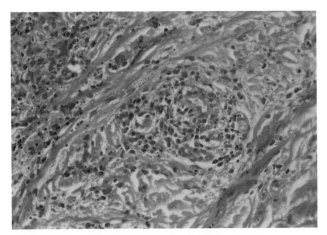

Figure 11–22. Leukocytoclastic vasculitis in skin biopsy. Note fragmentation of neutrophil nuclei in and around vessel walls.

MICROSCOPIC POLYANGIITIS (MICROSCOPIC POLYARTERITIS, HYPERSENSITIVITY (LEUKOCYTOCLASTIC) ANGIITIS)

This type of necrotizing vasculitis generally affects smaller vessels than PAN (arterioles, capillaries, and venules). In a single patient, all lesions tend to be of the same age. It typically involves the skin, mucous membranes, lungs, brain, heart, gastrointestinal tract, kidneys, and muscle. Necrotizing glomerulonephritis and pulmonary capillaritis are particularly common. The major resultant clinical features are hemoptysis, hematuria, and proteinuria; bowel pain or bleeding; and muscle pain or weakness. Cutaneous vasculitis is manifested by palpable purpura. In many cases, an immunologic reaction to an antigen such as drugs (e.g., penicillin), microorganisms (e.g., streptococci), heterologous proteins, and tumor antigens can be traced as the precipitating cause, but *there are few or no demonstrable immune deposits in this type of vasculitis.*

MORPHOLOGY. In contrast to PAN, muscular and large arteries are spared; thus, macroscopic infarcts similar to those seen in PAN are uncommon. Histologically, segmental fibrinoid necrosis of the media may be present, but in some lesions the change is limited to infiltration with neutrophils, which become fragmented as they follow the vessel wall **(leukocytoclasia).** The term **leukocytoclastic angiitis** is given to such lesions, most commonly found in postcapillary venules (Fig. 11–22). Immunoglobulins and complement components are often present in the vascular lesions of the skin, especially if these are examined within 24 hours of development, but in general, there is a paucity of immunoglobulin demonstrable by immunofluorescence microscopy ("pauci-immune injury").

With the exception of those who develop widespread renal or brain involvement, most patients respond well simply to removal of the offending agent. P-ANCA are present in 70% of patients. Disseminated vascular lesions of hypersensitivity angiitis may also appear in a number of relatively distinct syndromes, including Henoch-Schönlein purpura, essential mixed cryoglobulinemia, vasculitis associated with some of the connective tissue disorders, and vasculitis associated with malignancy. They are discussed with the specific entities elsewhere in this book.

WEGENER'S GRANULOMATOSIS

This form of necrotizing vasculitis is characterized by (1) *acute necrotizing granulomas* of the upper and lower respiratory tract (nose, sinuses, and lung); (2) *focal necrotizing vasculitis* affecting small to medium-sized vessels (e.g., capillaries, venules, arterioles, and arteries), most prominent in the lungs and upper airways but affecting other sites as well; and (3) renal disease in the form of focal or diffuse necrotizing glomerulitis.[49] Some patients who do not manifest the full triad are said to have "limited" Wegener's granulomatosis.

MORPHOLOGY. The vasculitis affects small arteries and veins and has been described in virtually every vessel and organ of the body, most commonly respiratory tract, kidneys, and spleen. Involvement of the respiratory tract takes the form of focal acute necrosis in the nasal and oral cavities, paranasal sinuses, larynx, or trachea as well as focal lesions scattered throughout the lung parenchyma. Almost identical with those of the acute phase of PAN (Fig. 11–23), these lesions often contain granulomas, which may be within, adjacent to, or clearly separated from the vessel wall. These areas are generally surrounded by a zone of fibroblastic proliferation with giant cells and leukocytic infiltrate and may become cavitary, creating a more than superficial resemblance to a tubercle. Thus the major pathologic differential is mycobacterial or fungal infection. Lesions may ultimately undergo progressive fibrosis and organization.

The renal lesions are of two types (see Chapter 20). In milder forms, or early in the disease, there is acute focal proliferation and necrosis in the glomeruli, with thrombosis of isolated glomerular capillary loops (focal necrotizing glomerulonephritis). More advanced glomerular lesions are characterized by diffuse necrosis, proliferation, and crescent formation (crescentic glomerulonephritis). Patients with focal lesions may have only hematuria and proteinuria responsive to therapy, whereas those

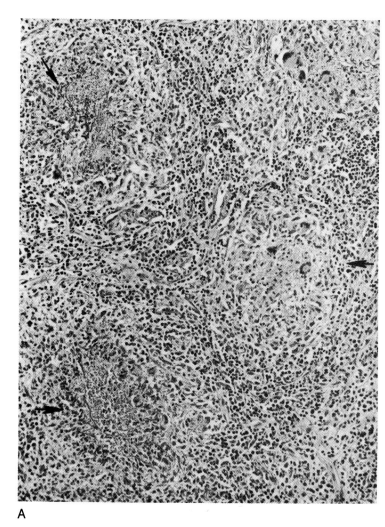

A

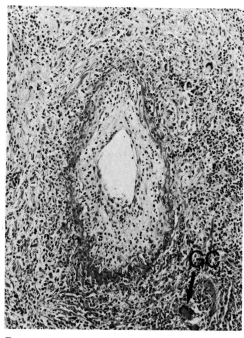

B

Figure 11-23. Wegener's granulomatosis. A, Multiple granulomas in lungs (arrows). Note central necrosis and multinucleated giant cells. B, Involved small artery demonstrating markedly thickened, fibrotic wall infiltrated with leukocytes. There is perivascular inflammation and a giant cell (GC).

with diffuse disease can develop rapidly progressive renal failure.

The peak incidence is in the fifth decade. Typical clinical features include persistent pneumonitis with bilateral nodular and cavitary infiltrates (95%), chronic sinusitis (90%), mucosal ulcerations of the nasopharynx (75%), and evidence of renal disease (80%). Other features include skin rashes, muscle pains, articular involvement, mononeuritis, or polyneuritis, and fever. Untreated, the course of the disease is malignant; 80% of patients die within 1 year. This grim prognosis is improved dramatically by the use of immunosuppressive-cytotoxic drugs, such as cyclophosphamide; up to 90% of patients demonstrate significant improvement with such therapy.

The striking resemblance to PAN and serum sickness suggests that Wegener's granulomatosis may represent some form of hypersensitivity, possibly to an inhaled infectious or other environmental agent, but this is unproved. Immune complexes have been seen in the glomeruli and vessel walls in occasional patients. The presence of granulomas and dramatic response to cyclophosphamide also strongly suggest an immunologic mechanism, perhaps of the cell-mediated type. C-ANCA is found in up to 93% of patients with active generalized disease, and this appears to be a good marker for disease activity. During treatment, a rising titer of ANCA suggests a relapse; most patients in remission have a negative test or the titer falls significantly.

Sometimes difficult to differentiate from Wegener's granulomatosis is a condition called *lymphomatoid granulomatosis*, characterized by pulmonary infiltration by nodules of lymphoid and plasmacytoid cells, often with cellular atypia. Although these infiltrates invade vessels, giving the histologic appearance of a vasculitis, they do not constitute a true vasculitis. About one-third of patients eventually show similar lesions in the kidneys, liver, brain, and other organs. Lymphomatoid granulomatosis likely represents an evolving lymphoproliferative disorder because up to 50% develop a lymphoid malignancy, most commonly non-Hodgkin's lymphoma.

THROMBOANGIITIS OBLITERANS (BUERGER'S DISEASE)

Thromboangiitis obliterans (Buerger's disease) is a distinctive disease characterized by segmental, thrombosing, acute and chronic inflammation of intermediate and small arteries and sometimes veins of the extremities.[50] The condition had occurred almost exclusively in men who were heavy cigarette smokers. Regrettably, there has been an increase in reported cases in women, probably reflecting increases in smoking by women in the past several decades. Buerger's disease begins before the age of 35 years in most patients and before 20 years in some. In many cases, it affects the arms as well as the legs.

The relationship to cigarette smoking is one of the most consistent aspects of this disorder. Several possibilities have been postulated for this association, including direct endothelial cell toxicity induced by hypersensitivity to some tobacco products, vasoconstriction induced by disturbances in catecholamine metabolism, and hypercoagulability leading to thrombosis. None of these is proved.

MORPHOLOGY. The lesions are sharply segmental and usually begin in arteries of small and medium size. It should be noted that, in contrast to atherosclerosis, Buerger's disease affects predominantly the medium and small arteries of upper and lower extremities and only occasionally the larger arteries. Veins and adjacent nerves accompanying arteries are often secondarily affected, leading to progressive fibrous encasement of these structures.

The acute involvement of either artery or vein is characterized by polymorphonuclear infiltration of all coats of the vessel wall, together with mural or occlusive thrombosis of the lumen. **Small mi-croabscesses within the thrombus create a pattern quite distinct from the bland thrombosis of atherosclerosis** (Figure 11-24). These abscesses have a central focus of polymorphonuclear leukocytes surrounded by a wall of granulomatous inflammation. In time, the thrombus undergoes organization and recanalization.

The early manifestations are a superficial nodular phlebitis, cold sensitivity of the Raynaud type (see below) in the hands, and pain in the instep of the foot induced by exercise (so-called "instep claudication"). Eventually, patients suffer from vascular insufficiency that often leads to excruciating pain and ultimately gangrene of the extremities. Remissions and relapses correlate with cessation or resumption of smoking.

VASCULITIS ASSOCIATED WITH OTHER DISORDERS

Vasculitis may sometimes be associated with an underlying disorder, such as an immunologic connective tissue disease, a malignancy, or systemic illnesses such as mixed cryoglobulinemia and Henoch-Schönlein purpura. Usually of the hypersensitivity angiitis pattern, it may resemble classic PAN in some cases. Of the *connective tissue disorders*, rheumatoid arthritis and SLE, as pointed out earlier, commonly manifest a vasculitis (Fig. 11-25). *Rheumatoid vasculitis* usually affects small and medium-sized arteries in multiple organs and may thereby result in life-threatening visceral infarction but also may cause a clinically significant aortitis.[51] It occurs predominantly after long-standing rheumatoid arthritis in patients who also exhibit rheumatoid nodules, hypocomplementemia, and high

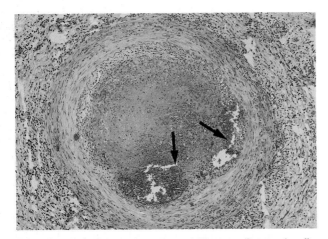

Figure 11-24. Thromboangiitis obliterans (Buerger's disease). Lumen is occluded by a thrombus containing two abscesses *(arrows)*. Vessel wall is infiltrated with leukocytes.

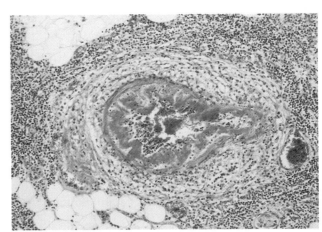

Figure 11-25. Vasculitis with fibrinoid necrosis in a patient with active systemic lupus erythematosus.

titers of rheumatoid factor. *Malignancies* associated with vasculitis are commonly of the lymphoproliferative type.

INFECTIOUS ARTERITIS

Nonsystemic arteritis is most frequently caused by the direct invasion of infectious agents—usually bacteria or fungi, particularly aspergillosis and mucormycosis. Vascular lesions frequently accompany bacterial pneumonia, or occur adjacent to caseous tuberculous reactions, in the neighborhood of abscesses, or in the superficial cerebral vessels in cases of meningitis. Much less commonly, they arise from the hematogenous spread of bacteria, in cases of septicemia or embolization from infective endocarditis. Vascular infections may weaken the arterial wall and result in the formation of a *mycotic aneurysm* (see below).

Clinically, infectious arteritis may be important on several counts. By inducing thrombosis, it adds an element of infarction to tissues that are already the seat of an inflammatory reaction and worsen the initial infection. In bacterial meningitis, for example, inflammation of the superficial vessels of the brain may predispose to vascular thromboses, with subsequent infarction of the brain substance and extension of the subarachnoid infection into the brain tissue.

RAYNAUD'S DISEASE

Raynaud's disease refers to paroxysmal pallor or cyanosis of the digits of the hands or feet, and infrequently the tips of the nose or ears (acral parts). It is caused by intense vasospasm of local small arteries or arterioles, principally of young, otherwise healthy women. Characteristically, the fingers change color in the sequence white—blue—red. *No organic changes are present in the arterial walls except late in the course, when intimal proliferation can appear*. Of uncertain cause, Raynaud's disease reflects an exaggeration of normal central and local vasomotor responses to cold or emotion.

In contrast, *Raynaud's phenomenon* refers to arterial insufficiency of the extremities *secondary to the arterial narrowing induced by various conditions, including systemic lupus erythematosus, systemic sclerosis (scleroderma), atherosclerosis, or Buerger's disease (see above)*. Indeed, Raynaud's phenomenon may be the first manifestation of any of these conditions.

The course of Raynaud's disease is usually benign, but long-standing, chronic cases can have atrophy of the skin, subcutaneous tissues, and muscles. Ulceration and ischemic gangrene are rare.

ANEURYSMS AND DISSECTION

An *aneurysm* is a *localized abnormal dilatation of any vessel*. Aneurysms may occur in any artery or vein of the body, most commonly the aorta. Aneurysms can be either "true" or "false." A *true aneurysm* is bounded by generally complete but often attenuated arterial wall components, with quantitatively or qualitatively (or both) altered structure. The blood within a true aneurysm remains within the confines of the circulatory system. Atherosclerotic, syphilitic, and congenital aneurysms are of this type. In contrast, a *false aneurysm* (also called *pseudoaneurysm* or "pulsating hematoma") is an extravascular hematoma that communicates with the intravascular space. The vascular wall has been breached, and the wall of the aneurysmal sac consists of only outer arterial layers or periarterial tissue. A leak at the junction *(anastomosis)* of a vascular graft with a natural artery produces this type of lesion. Arterial dissections, usually of the aorta (sometimes inadvisedly called *dissecting aneurysms*), arise when blood enters the wall of the artery, dissecting between its layers and creating a cavity within the vessel wall itself.

The two most important causes of true aortic aneurysms are atherosclerosis and cystic medial degeneration. Syphilis also causes aortic aneurysms. Arterial aneurysms can also be caused by PAN, Kawasaki syndrome and other vasculitides, trauma leading to AV aneurysms, or congenital defects, such as that producing berry aneurysms in the brain (see Chapter 29).

Aneurysms are often classified by macroscopic shape and size. A *berry* aneurysm is a small, spherical dilatation, rarely exceeding 1 to 1.5 cm in diameter, that is most frequent in the brain. *Saccular* aneurysms are essentially spherical (involving only a portion of the vessel wall) and vary in size from 5 to 20 cm in diameter, often partially or completely filled by thrombus. A *fusiform* aneurysm is a gradual, progressive dilation of the complete circumference of the vessel. Fusiform aneurysms vary in diameter (up to 20 cm) and in length; many involve the entire ascending and transverse portions of the aortic arch, whereas others may involve large segments of the abdominal aorta or even the iliacs.

Infection of a major artery that significantly weakens its walls is called a *mycotic aneurysm*. A mycotic aneurysm can be either "true" or "false"; thrombosis and rupture are possible complications. Mycotic aneurysms may originate either (1) from lodgment of a septic embolus at some point within a vessel, usually as a complication of infective endocarditis, (2) as an extension of an adjacent suppurative process; or (3) by circulating organisms directly infecting the arterial wall.

Atherosclerosis, the most frequent etiology of aneurysms, causes arterial wall thinning through medial destruction secondary to plaque that originates in the intima. *Atherosclerotic aneurysms usually occur in the abdominal aorta, most frequently between the renal arteries and the iliac bifurcation, or in the common iliac arteries,* but the arch and descending parts of the thoracic aorta can be involved.

ABDOMINAL AORTIC ANEURYSMS

Aneurysms in the abdominal aorta give rise to clinical symptoms by various effects: (1) rupture into the peritoneal cavity or retroperitoneal tissues with massive or fatal hemorrhage (Fig. 11–26); (2) impingement on an adjacent structure, such as compression of a ureter or erosion of vertebrae; (3) occlusion of a vessel by either direct pressure or mural thrombus formation, particularly of the vertebral branches that supply the spinal cord; (4) embolism from the atheroma or mural thrombus; and (5) creation of an abdominal mass that simulates a tumor.

Large aneurysms materially shorten longevity, primarily owing to rupture, a danger directly related to the size of the aneurysm. The risk of rupture for a small abdominal aortic aneurysm (less than approximately 4 cm) is about 2%; aneurysms larger than 5 cm are the most dangerous, with a risk 5 to 10% per year.[52] Thus, large aneurysms are usually surgically replaced by prosthetic grafts. Timely surgery is key; operative mortality for unruptured aneurysms is approximately 5%, whereas emergency surgery after rupture carries a mortality rate of more than 50%.

PATHOGENESIS. Atherosclerosis is a major etiologic factor in abdominal aortic aneurysms, but an evolving view based on observations suggests a multifactorial causation. Abdominal aortic aneurysms rarely develop before the age of 50 and are much more common in men. Aortic aneurysms have been shown to be familial (beyond the familial/genetic predisposition to atherosclerosis or hypertension), and genetic defects different from those associated with increased risk of atherosclerosis increase their frequency. Clearly, as discussed subsequently, genetic defects in structural components of the aorta can themselves produce aneurysms and dissections. One school of thought holds that such genetic defects in a connective tissue component responsible for the strength of blood vessels could provide a particularly susceptible substrate on which atherosclerosis or hypertension, or both, could act to weaken the aortic wall.[53,54] Hemodynamic factors may also play a role.

MORPHOLOGY. Abdominal aortic aneurysms are usually positioned below the renal arteries and above the bifurcation of the aorta (see Fig. 11–26). Not infrequently, they are accompanied by smaller fusiform or saccular dilatations of the iliac arteries. The aneurysm often contains atheromatous ulcers covered by mural thrombi, with consequent thinning and destruction of the media, prime sites for the formation of atheroemboli that lodge in the vessels of the kidneys or lower extremities. Sometimes the entire aneurysmal dilatation is filled with laminated thrombus (see Fig. 11–26A). Occasionally

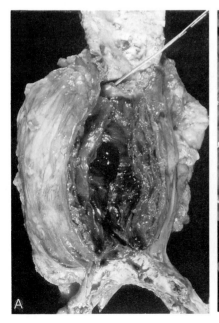
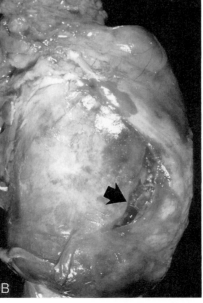

Figure 11–26. Gross photographs of abdominal aortic aneurysm that ruptured. *A*, Opened aneurysm, showing location of rupture indicated by a probe. The wall of the aneurysm is exceedingly thin, and the aneurysm itself is filled by a large quantity of unorganized thrombus. *B*, An external view of the rupture site *(arrow)*.

the aneurysm may affect the origins of the renal, superior, and inferior mesenteric arteries, either by producing direct pressure on these vessels or by narrowing or occluding their ostia with mural thrombi.

Two variants of abdominal aortic aneurysm merit special mention. *Inflammatory abdominal aortic aneurysms* are characterized by dense periaortic fibrosis containing an abundant lymphoplasmacytic inflammatory reaction with many macrophages and often giant cells.[55] Their cause is uncertain. *Mycotic abdominal aneurysms* are abdominal aortic aneurysms that have become infected by lodgment of circulating organisms in the wall, particularly in bacteremia from a primary Salmonella gastroenteritis. In such cases, suppuration further destroys the media, potentiating rapid dilatation and rupture.

It is important to keep in mind that abdominal aortic aneurysms (and indeed peripheral arterial disease in general) is generally accompanied by widespread systemic and coronary atherosclerosis; patients with such aneurysms are at significant risk for other complications of atherosclerosis. Indeed, patients with atherosclerotic aortic or peripheral vascular disease have a high incidence (a risk of more than five times normal) of IHD and other cardiovascular disease.[56]

SYPHILITIC (LUETIC) ANEURYSMS

Syphilitic aneurysms are almost always confined to the thoracic aorta and usually involve the arch. The ascending and transverse portions of the arch are favored sites, but the dilation may extend distally to the level of the diaphragm and, even more important, proximally to the level of the aortic valve. At one time, syphilis accounted for the majority of aneurysms of the thoracic aorta, but with the decline in cases of tertiary syphilis, the disorder is uncommon.

MORPHOLOGY. The development of such aneurysms is based on the medial destruction characteristic of tertiary syphilis. Inflammatory involvement begins in the adventitia of the aorta, particularly involving the vasa vasorum with the production of obliterative endarteritis rimmed by an infiltrate of lymphocytes and plasma cells. The narrowing of the lumina of the vasa causes ischemic injury of the aortic media, with patchy uneven loss of the medial elastic fibers and muscle cells followed by inflammation, scarring, and frequently vascularization of the damaged media. Aneurysmal dilatation can occur secondarily. Dissection is unusual owing to medial scarring. Contraction of fibrous scars may lead to wrinkling of intervening segments of aortic intima, called "tree-barking." Luetic involvement of the aorta favors the development of superimposed atherosclerosis, inducing sometimes florid atheromatosis of the aortic root (an unusual location for "garden variety" atherosclerosis), which can occlude the coronary ostia.

Luetic aortitis may also cause aortic valve ring dilation, resulting in valvular insufficiency through circumferential stretching of the valve cusps and widening of the commissures between the cusps. Over the course of time, the regurgitant turbulence produces thickening and rolling of the free margins, worsening the valvular incompetence. As a consequence, the left ventricular wall undergoes volume overload hypertrophy, sometimes producing a massively enlarged heart (that can reach 1000 gm, about three times normal weight), descriptively referred to as "cor bovinum" ("cow's heart").

Whether of luetic or atherosclerotic etiology, thoracic aortic enlargements give can rise to signs and symptoms referable to (1) encroachment on mediastinal structures, (2) respiratory difficulties due to encroachment on the lungs and airways, (3) difficulty in swallowing due to compression of the esophagus, (4) persistent cough due to irritation of or pressure on the recurrent laryngeal nerves, (5) pain caused by erosion of bone (i.e., ribs and vertebral bodies), (6) cardiac disease as the aortic aneurysm leads to dilation of the aortic valve or narrowing of the coronary ostia, and (7) rupture of the aneurysm.

AORTIC DISSECTION (DISSECTING HEMATOMA)

Aortic dissection is a catastrophic illness characterized by dissection of blood along the laminar planes of the aortic media, with the formation of a blood-filled channel within the aortic wall (Figs. 11–27 and 11–28) that often ruptures, causing massive hemorrhage. In contrast to atherosclerotic and syphilitic aneurysms, aortic dissection is not usually associated with marked dilatation of the aorta. For this reason, the older term "dissecting aneurysm" is discouraged. Aortic dissection occurs principally in two groups of patients: One is most commonly men 40 to 60 years of age, in whom hypertension is almost invariably an antecedent (more than 90% of cases of dissection). The second major group of patients has a systemic or localized abnormality of connective tissue that affects the aorta (e.g., Marfan's syndrome, discussed subsequently and in Chapter 5). Dissection can also be a complication of arterial cannulation (e.g., during diagnostic catheterization or cardiopulmonary bypass). Rarely, for unknown reasons, aortic dissection occurs during pregnancy. In contrast, dissection is

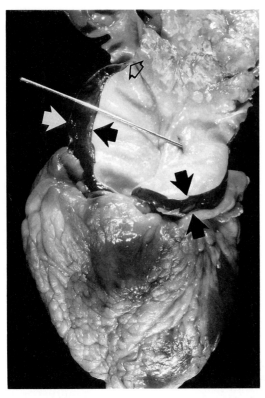

Figure 11–27. Aortic dissection. Gross photograph demonstrating small, oblique intimal tear in proximal aorta (demarcated by probe), exposing the media and allowing blood to enter its internal portions, creating an intramural hematoma *(between arrows)*. Note that the intimal tear has occurred in a region largely free from atherosclerotic plaque, and that propagation of the intramural hematoma is arrested at the site more distally where atherosclerosis begins *(open arrow)*.

unusual in the face of substantial atherosclerosis. Arteries other than the aorta may also be involved.

MORPHOLOGY. There is usually, but not always, an intimal tear that extends into but not through the media of the ascending aorta, usually within 10 cm of the aortic valve (see Fig. 11–27). Presumably, this is the origin of dissection. Such tears are usually transverse or oblique, 1 to 5 cm in length, with sharp but jagged edges. The dissection can extend proximally toward the heart as well as distally along the aorta to variable distances, sometimes all the way into the iliac and femoral arteries. In some instances, the blood reruptures into the lumen of the aorta, producing a second or distal intimal tear and a new vascular channel within the media of the aortic wall that connects the proximal and distal intimal tears. It is assumed that in these "double-barreled" aortas, the two intimal tears have permitted the establishment of through-and-through blood flow and thus averted a fatal extra-aortic hemorrhage. In the course of time, such false channels may become endothelialized.

The most common precipitating cause of death is rupture of the dissection into any of the three body cavities (i.e., pericardial, pleural, or peritoneal). Other vascular complications that frequently correlate with clinical manifestations include extension of the dissection into the great arteries of the neck or into the coronary, renal, mesenteric, or iliac arteries, causing critical vascular obstruction. Retrograde dissection into the aortic root can cause disruption of the aortic valvular apparatus. Thus common clinical manifestations include cardiac tamponade, aortic insufficiency, and myocardial infarction; compression of spinal arteries may cause transverse myelitis.

The hemorrhage (actually a **dissecting intramural hematoma**) in the aorta or other arterial vessel occurs quite characteristically between the middle and outer thirds of the media (see Fig. 11–28). In most patients with aortic dissection, the media shows a variety of histologic changes that could conceivably weaken the wall, but uncertainty exists about the specificity of these lesions and their role in causing dissection. These degenerative changes range from only mild fragmentation of elastic tissue (the most easily recognized abnormality) to overt *cystic medial degeneration* (sometimes called "cystic medial necrosis," an inaccurate term because true necrosis is not present). The characteristic microscopic lesion of cystic medial degeneration includes not only elastic tissue fragmentation and disruption, but also focal separation of the elastic and fibromuscular elements of the tunica media by small cleft-like or cystic spaces filled with amorphous material resembling the ground substance (amorphous extracellular matrix) of connective tissue and ultimately large-scale loss of elastic laminae (Fig. 11–29). Inflammation is absent. Cystic medial degeneration of the aorta frequently accompanies Marfan syndrome. Haphazardly distributed throughout the thickness of the media, elastic tissue defects **are also frequently found incidentally at autopsy of patients who are free from dissection,** increasing in severity with age and possibly the presence of hypertension. Moreover, many patients with dissection have minimal histologic abnormality.

PATHOGENESIS. Some dissections are related to the inherited connective tissue disorder Marfan syndrome, an autosomal dominant disease of connective tissue fibrillin characterized by skeletal, cardiovascular, and ocular manifestations (see Chapter 5). The serious cardiovascular complications of the Marfan syndrome include aortic dissection, dilatation of the aortic root (called *annuloaortic ectasia*) and mitral valve prolapse.

Regardless of the underlying etiology, the trigger for intimal tear and intramural aortic hemorrhage is unknown in most cases of dissection. Since, as stated above, there is not a good correlation between dissection and the presence of medial

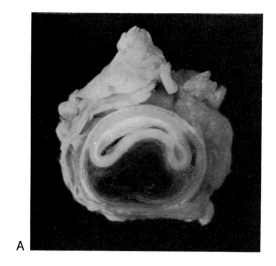

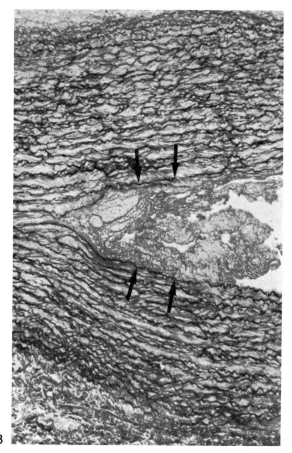

Figure 11-28. Aortic dissection, detailed features. *A,* Cross-section of common carotid artery with extension of aortic dissection causing collapse of vessel lumen. *B,* Photomicrograph of aortic dissection demonstrating advancing dissecting hematoma *(arrows)* cleaving the media.

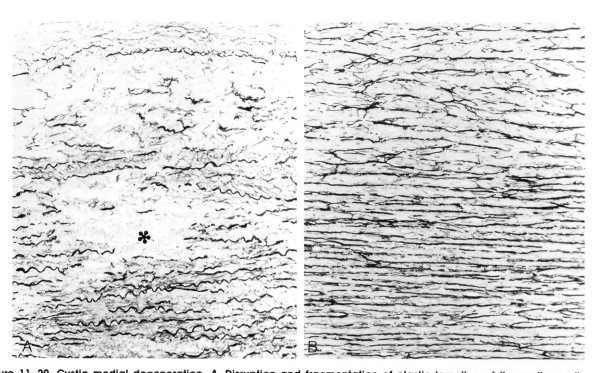

Figure 11-29. Cystic medial degeneration. *A,* Disruption and fragmentation of elastic lamellae of the aortic media, with formation of areas devoid of elastin *(asterisk),* that resemble cystic spaces, from a patient with Marfan syndrome. *B,* Normal media for comparison, showing the regular layered pattern of elastic tissue. Both photographs are of tissue stained with the elastic tissue stain, highlighting elastin as black.

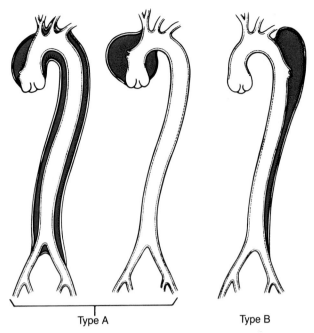

Type A   Type B

Figure 11–30. Classification of dissection into types A and B. Type A (proximal) involves the ascending aorta, whereas type B (distal) does *not* involve the ascending aorta.

structural lesions, abnormal medial histology is not critical to the development of dissection. The precise role of hypertension, clearly the major risk factor in aortic dissection overall, is uncertain, but it may damage the aortic media. Certainly, once the tear has occurred, the increased blood pressure must enhance the progression of dissection within the vessel wall. Indeed, aggressive antihypertensive therapy is often effective in limiting an evolving dissection.

CLINICAL COURSE. The risk and nature of serious complications of dissection depend strongly on the level of the aorta affected. Thus aortic dissections are generally classified into two types: (1) the more common (and dangerous) *proximal* lesions, involving either the ascending portion only or both the ascending and the descending aorta (types I and II of DeBakey's classification, often collectively called type A), and (2) *distal lesions not involving the ascending part* and usually beginning distal to the subclavian artery (DeBakey type III, often called type B) (Fig. 11–30). The classic clinical symptoms of aortic dissection are the sudden onset of excruciating pain, usually beginning in the anterior chest, radiating to the back, and moving downward as the dissection progresses. This intense pain can be readily confused with that of acute myocardial infarction. The antemortem diagnosis of aortic dissection and the differentiation of the various types are based largely on aortic angiography, but the noninvasive techniques, two-dimensional cardiac ultrasound (especially transesophageal echocardiography), computed to-

mography (CT), and magnetic resonance imaging (MRI), are increasingly useful.[57]

At one time, aortic dissection was almost invariably fatal, but the prognosis has markedly improved. The development of surgical procedures involving plication of the aortic wall and the early institution of intensive antihypertensive therapy permit salvage of 65 to 75% of patients with dissections.

VEINS AND LYMPHATICS

Varicose veins and phlebothrombosis/thrombophlebitis together account for at least 90% of clinical venous disease. In general, varicose veins have narrowing or abnormal dilation with subsequent incompetence of the venous valves causing venous stasis. Thrombosis may occur, but embolism is rare. In contrast, pulmonary embolism and infarction are potential serious sequelae of thrombophlebitis.

VARICOSE VEINS

Varicose veins are abnormally dilated, tortuous veins produced by prolonged, increased intraluminal pressure. The *superficial veins* of the leg are the preponderant site of involvement. Much less common, but more important, however, portal hypertension (usually due to cirrhosis of the liver) leads to varices in the esophageal and hemorrhoidal veins (see Chapter 18).

It is estimated that 10 to 20% of the general population eventually develop varicose veins in the lower legs. The condition is much more common over age 50, in obese persons, and in women, a reflection of the elevated venous pressure in the lower legs caused by pregnancy.

A *familial tendency* toward the development of varicosities is postulated to be due to defective development of the walls of veins. The most important influence on intraluminal venous blood pressure is posture; when the legs are dependent for long periods of time, venous pressures in these sites are markedly elevated (up to ten times normal). Therefore occupations that require long periods of standing and long automobile or airplane rides frequently lead to marked venous stasis and pedal edema, even in normal individuals with essentially normal veins *(simple orthostatic edema)*.

MORPHOLOGY. Veins affected by varicosities are dilated, tortuous, elongated, and scarred. There is marked variation in the thickness of the wall, with thinning at the points of maximal dilation. Intraluminal thrombosis and valvular deformities (thickening, rolling, and shortening of the cusps) are frequently discovered when these vessels are

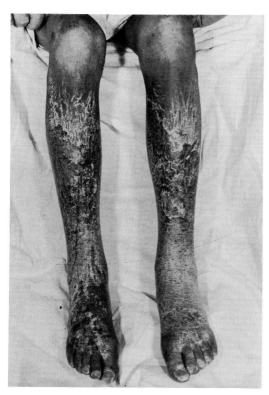

Figure 11-31. Stasis dermatitis in varicose veins of lower extremities.

opened. Microscopically, the changes consist of variations in the thickness of the vein wall caused by dilation on the one hand and by compensatory hypertrophy of the smooth muscle and subintimal fibrosis on the other hand. Frequently there is elastic tissue degeneration and spotty calcifications within the media **(phlebosclerosis).**

CLINICAL COURSE. Varicose dilation of veins renders the valves incompetent and leads to venous stasis, congestion, edema, and thrombosis. *Despite thrombosis of superficial varicose veins, embolism is very rare. This is in sharp contrast to the relatively frequent thromboembolism that arises from thrombosed deep veins (see subsequently),* in which contraction of surrounding muscles tends to "milk" the contents loose from their attachments to the vein walls. In the legs, distention of the veins is often painful, but most patients have no symptoms until marked venous stasis and edema develop. *Some of the most disabling sequelae are the development of persistent edema in the extremity and trophic changes in the skin that lead to stasis dermatitis and ulcerations* (Fig. 11–31). Because of the impaired circulation, the tissues of the affected part are extremely vulnerable to injury. Wounds and infections heal slowly or tend to become chronic *varicose ulcers.*

THROMBOPHLEBITIS AND PHLEBOTHROMBOSIS

Because venous thrombosis inevitably leads to inflammatory changes within the vein wall, *thrombophlebitis* and *phlebothrombosis* are two designations for a single entity. Predisposing factors have already been considered in the general discussion of thrombosis (see Chapter 4). It need simply be reemphasized now that *cardiac failure, neoplasia, pregnancy, obesity, the postoperative state, and prolonged bed rest or immobilization are the most important clinical settings predisposing to venous thrombosis.*

MORPHOLOGY. The deep leg veins account for more than 90% of cases of thrombophlebitis. Specific mention should be made of the periprostatic venous plexus in the male and the pelvic veins in the female as additional sites for the appearance of thrombi. The large veins in the skull and the dural sinuses are possible sites of thrombosis when these channels become inflamed by bacterial infections of the meninges, middle ears, or mastoids. Similarly, infections in the abdominal cavity, such as peritonitis, acute appendicitis, acute salpingitis, and pelvic abscesses, may lead to inflammation and thrombosis of the portal vein or its tributaries.

Thrombi in the legs tend, on the whole, to arise insidiously and to produce in the early stages few, if any, signs or symptoms. Local manifestations, including edema distal to the occluded vein, dusky cyanosis, dilatation of superficial veins, heat, tenderness, redness, swelling, and pain, may be absent in a bedridden patient. In some cases, however, pain can be elicited by pressure over affected veins, squeezing the calf muscles or forced dorsiflexion of the foot (Homan's sign). There are now several noninvasive methods (iodine-labeled fibrinogen, ultrasonography, plethysmography) that aid in the diagnosis, but venous angiography may have to be performed in some cases to establish the presence of deep vein thrombosis.

Not infrequently, the first manifestation of thrombophlebitis is the development of an embolic episode. Indeed, pulmonary embolism is a common and serious clinical problem, particularly in hospitalized patients (see Chapter 15), that strongly influences the management of all cardiac, postpartum, and postoperative cases. All such patients are urged to move about constantly in bed, perform muscle exercises to stimulate the venous flow in the legs, and become ambulatory as soon as is clinically feasible. In particularly vulnerable individuals, anticoagulant therapy may be administered when long-term bed rest is mandatory.

Two special variants of primary phlebothrombosis are phlegmasia alba dolens and migratory thrombophlebitis. *Phlegmasia alba dolens* (painful white leg) refers to iliofemoral venous thrombosis occurring usually in pregnant women in the third trimester or immediately following delivery (aptly also called "milk leg"). It is postulated that the thrombus initiates a phlebitis, and the perivenous inflammatory response induces lymphatic blockage with painful swelling. The predisposition to thrombosis here is attributed to the stasis of flow caused by the pressure of the gravid uterus and to the development of a hypercoagulable state during pregnancy. *Migratory thrombophlebitis* is a term given to the appearance of venous thrombi, often multiple, which classically disappear at one site to reappear elsewhere. This is encountered predominantly as one of the paraneoplastic syndromes (see Chapter 7) in patients having a deep-seated visceral cancer, particularly arising from pancreas, lung, or colon.

LYMPHANGITIS AND LYMPHEDEMA

Bacterial infections may spread into and through the lymphatics to create acute inflammatory involvements in these channels. The most common etiologic agents are the group A beta-hemolytic streptococci, although any virulent pathogen may be responsible for an acute lymphangitis. Anatomically, the affected lymphatics are dilated and filled with an acute exudate, chiefly of neutrophils and histiocytes, that usually extends through the wall into the perilymphatic tissues and may in severe cases produce cellulitis or focal abscesses. The lymph nodes of drainage often have acute lymphadenitis.

Clinically, lymphangitis is recognized by painful subcutaneous red streaks that extend along the course of lymphatics, with painful enlargement of the regional lymph nodes. If the lymph nodes fail to block the spread of bacteria, drainage into the venous system initiates a bacteremia or septicemia.

Any occlusion of lymphatic vessels is followed by the abnormal accumulation of interstitial fluid in the affected part, referred to as *obstructive lymphedema*. The most common causes of such lymphatic blockage are (1) spread of malignant tumors with obstruction of either the lymphatic channels or the nodes of drainage, (2) radical surgical procedures with removal of regional groups of lymph nodes (e.g., the axillary dissection of radical mastectomy), (3) postirradiation fibrosis, (4) filariasis, and (5) postinflammatory thrombosis and scarring of lymphatic channels. The morphologic changes consist of dilatation of lymphatics up to the points of obstruction, accompanied by increases of interstitial fluid. Persistence of the edema leads to an increase of subcutaneous interstitial fibrous tissue, with consequent enlargement of the affected part, brawny induration, "peau

d'orange" appearance of the skin, and skin ulcers. *Chylous ascites, chylothorax,* and *chylopericardium* are caused by rupture of obstructed, dilated lymphatics into the peritoneum, pleural cavity, and pericardium. Almost invariably, this is due to obstruction of lymphatics by an infiltrating tumor mass.

TUMORS

Vascular tumors constitute a spectrum—from the benign hemangiomas to intermediate lesions that are locally aggressive but infrequently metastasize, to relatively rare, highly malignant angiosarcomas. In addition, congenital malformations, such as those that occur in the Sturge-Weber syndrome, may present as tumor-like lesions, as do some nonneoplastic inflammatory vascular proliferations, such as the *granuloma pyogenicum* of pregnancy. For these reasons, vascular neoplasms are difficult to categorize clinically and histologically. Here we describe only those lesions that are common or clinically important.

Vascular neoplasms are divided into benign, intermediate, and malignant based on two major anatomic characteristics: (1) the degree to which the neoplasm is composed of well-formed vascular channels and (2) the extent and regularity of the endothelial cell proliferation (Table 11–8). In general, benign neoplasms are made up largely of well-formed vessels with well-differentiated endothelial cell proliferation; in contrast, frankly malignant tumors are solidly cellular and anaplastic, with scant numbers of only poorly developed vascular channels. The endothelial nature of neoplastic proliferations that do not form distinct vascular lumina can sometimes be confirmed by endothelial cell–specific markers such as vWF by immunohistochemical techniques (see earlier in this chapter). Be-

Table 11–8. TUMORS AND TUMOR-LIKE CONDITIONS OF BLOOD VESSELS

BENIGN
  Hemangioma
    Capillary
    Cavernous
    Epithelioid
    Granuloma pyogenicum
    Deep soft tissue hematoma
  Glomus tumor
  Vascular ectasias

INTERMEDIATE
  Hemangioendothelioma
  Epithelioid hemangioendothelioma

MALIGNANT
  Angiosarcoma
  Hemangiopericytoma
  Kaposi's sarcoma

cause these lesions constitute abnormalities of unregulated vascular proliferation, a particularly exciting possibility is that of controlling such growth by agents that inhibit blood vessel formation (antiangiogenic factors).[58]

BENIGN TUMORS AND TUMOR-LIKE CONDITIONS

Hemangioma

Hemangiomas are extremely common tumors, particularly in infancy and childhood, constituting 7% of all benign tumors. Although they are for convenience called tumors, it is yet unknown whether such masses are true neoplasms (hamartomas) or developmental abnormalities. There are several histologic and clinical variants (Fig. 11–32).

CAPILLARY HEMANGIOMA. *Capillary hemangiomas* are composed of blood vessels that resemble capillaries—narrow, thin-walled, and lined by relatively thin endothelium. Usually occurring in the skin, subcutaneous tissues, and mucous membranes of the oral cavities and lips, they may also occur in internal viscera, such as the liver, spleen, and kidneys.

MORPHOLOGY. Varying in size from a few millimeters up to several centimeters in diameter, they are bright red to blue, level with the surface of the skin or slightly elevated, with intact covering epithelium (see Fig. 11–32A). Occasionally, pedunculated lesions are formed, attached by a broad-to-slender stalk. The "strawberry type" of capillary hemangioma (juvenile hemangiomas) of the skin of newborns grows rapidly in the first few months, begins to fade when the child is one to three years old, and regresses by age five in 80% of cases.

Histologically, capillary hemangiomas are usually well-defined but unencapsulated aggregates of closely packed, thin-walled capillaries, usually blood-filled, separated by scant connective tissue stroma (see Fig. 11–32C). The lumina may be partially or completely thrombosed and organized. Rupture of vessels causes scarring and accounts for the hemosiderin pigment occasionally found.

CAVERNOUS HEMANGIOMA. *Cavernous hemangiomas* are distinguished by the formation of large, cavernous vascular channels. Often occurring in childhood, they have a predilection for the skin of the head and neck and mucosal surfaces of the body but are also found in many viscera, particularly the liver, spleen, pancreas, and occasionally the brain. In one rare systemic entity, *von Hippel–Lindau disease* (discussed in Chapter 29), cavernous hemangiomas occur within the cerebellum or brain stem and eye grounds, along with similar angiomatous lesions or cystic neoplasms in the pancreas and liver as well as other visceral neoplasms.

MORPHOLOGY. Grossly, the usual cavernous hemangioma is a red-blue, soft, spongy mass 1 to 2 cm in diameter. Quite rarely, giant forms occur that affect large subcutaneous areas of the face, extremities, or other regions of the body. Histologically, the mass is sharply defined, but not encapsulated, and made up of large, cavernous vascular spaces, partly or completely filled with blood separated by a scant connective tissue stroma (Fig. 11–32D). Intravascular thrombosis or rupture of channels can occur.

In most situations, the tumors are of little clinical significance; however, they can be a cosmetic disturbance, and when present in the brain, they are a potential source of increased intracranial pressure or hemorrhage.

GRANULOMA PYOGENICUM (GRANULATION TISSUE-TYPE HEMANGIOMA). Of uncertain neoplastic nature and currently considered a polypoid form of capillary hemangioma, these masses appear as exophytic red nodules on the skin and gingival or oral mucosa and are often ulcerated (see Fig. 11–32B). One-third of lesions develop after trauma, growing rapidly to reach a maximum size of 1 to 2 cm within a few weeks. Histologically, the proliferating capillaries are separated by extensive edema and an acute and chronic inflammatory infiltrate, with a striking resemblance to exuberant granulation tissue. Most do not recur after excision. *Pregnancy tumor* (granuloma gravidarum) is a granuloma pyogenicum occurring in the gingiva of 1 to 5% of pregnant women that regresses after delivery.

Glomus Tumor (Glomangioma)

A *glomangioma* is a benign but exquisitely painful tumor that arises from the modified smooth muscle cells of the glomus body, a neuromyoarterial receptor that is sensitive to variations in temperature and regulates arteriolar flow. Glomus bodies may be located anywhere in the skin but *are most commonly found in the distal portion of the digits*, especially under the fingernails.

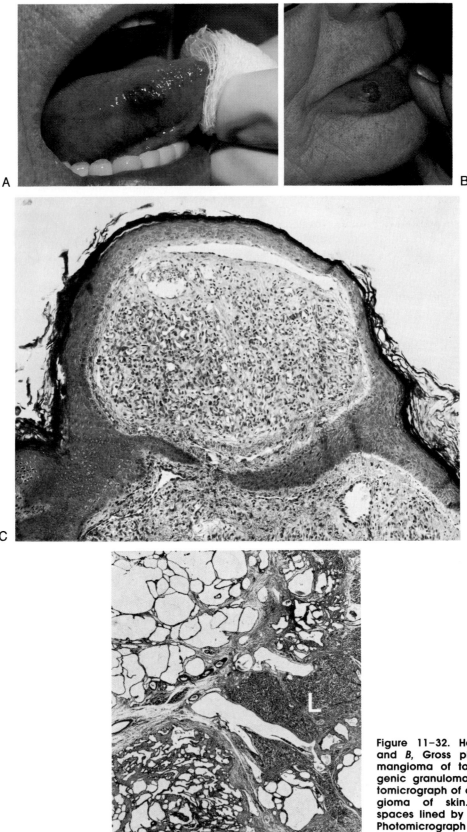

Figure 11–32. Hemangiomas. *A* and *B*, Gross photographs, hemangioma of tongue and pyogenic granuloma of lip. *C*, Photomicrograph of capillary hemangioma of skin. Note slit-like spaces lined by endothelium. *D*, Photomicrograph of cavernous hemangioma of liver. The dilated spaces are lined by endothelium. L = liver parenchyma. (*A* and *B* courtesy of John Sexton, M.D., Beth Israel Hospital, Boston.)

MORPHOLOGY. Grossly, the lesions are usually under 1 cm in diameter, and many are less than 3 mm. When present in the skin, they are slightly elevated, rounded, red-blue, firm, exquisitely painful nodules. Under the nail, they appear as minute foci of fresh hemorrhage. Histologically, **two components are present:** branching vascular channels separated by a connective tissue stroma that contains the second element—**aggregates, nests, and masses of the specialized glomus cells.** The individual cells are usually regular in size, round or cuboidal, and have scant cytoplasm and on electron microscopy have features typical of smooth muscle cells.

Vascular Ectasias (Telangiectases)

The term *telangiectasis* designates a group of abnormally prominent capillaries, venules, and arterioles that creates a small focal red lesion, usually in the skin or mucous membranes. Telangiectases probably represent congenital anomalies or acquired exaggerations of pre-existing vessels and are therefore not true neoplasms.

NEVUS FLAMMEUS. This is a "ten-dollar" term for the ordinary birthmark. Most commonly on the head and neck, they range in color from light pink to deep purple and are ordinarily flat. Histologically, they show only dilatation of vessels in the dermis. The vast majority ultimately fade and regress.

A special form of nevus flammeus, the so-called *port-wine stain,* may grow proportionately with a child, thicken the skin surface, and become unsightly. Port-wine stains in the distribution of the trigeminal nerve may be associated with the *Sturge-Weber syndrome* (also called *encephalotrigeminal angiomatosis*). An extremely uncommon congenital disorder attributed to faulty development of certain mesodermal and ectodermal elements, it is characterized by venous angiomatous masses in the leptomeninges over the cortex and by ipsilateral port-wine nevi of the face. Because it is often associated with mental retardation, seizures, hemiplegia, and radiopacities in the skull, a large vascular malformation in the face may well be more than a coincidence in a child who exhibits some evidence of mental deficiency.

SPIDER TELANGIECTASIS. The *spider telangiectasis* consists of a focal minute network of subcutaneous small arteries or arterioles arranged in a radial fashion about a central core. It is usually found on the upper parts of the body, particularly the face, neck, and upper chest, and is most common in *pregnant women* or in patients with liver disease, particularly *cirrhosis of the liver*. The high circulating levels of estrogen found in these two conditions in some way probably evokes these vascular changes. Because these are composed of arterial vessels, they frequently pulsate.

HEREDITARY HEMORRHAGIC TELANGIECTASIA (OSLER-WEBER-RENDU DISEASE). *Osler-Weber-Rendu disease* is characterized by multiple small aneurysmal telangiectases distributed over the skin and mucous membranes, present from birth and apparently of hereditary origin. It is a rare disorder, transmitted as a dominant Mendelian trait by either the male or the female and affecting both sexes equally. About 20% of cases, however, lack a family history.

The small (less than 5 mm) lesions are found directly beneath the skin or mucosal surfaces of the oral cavity, lips, alimentary tract, respiratory tract, and urinary tract as well as in the liver, brain, and spleen. Nosebleeds and bleeding into the intestinal, urinary, or respiratory tract are common clinical manifestations. Although this hemorrhagic tendency becomes more pronounced with increasing age, and severe hemorrhage may necessitate transfusions, patients with this condition have a normal life expectancy.

Bacillary Angiomatosis

Bacillary angiomatosis is a potentially fatal infectious disease that causes a distinct non-neoplastic proliferation of small blood vessels in the skin, lymph nodes, and visceral organs of patients with human immunodeficiency virus (HIV) infection and other states of immunocompromise. Grossly, cutaneous bacillary angiomatosis is marked by one to numerous red papules and nodules or rounded subcutaneous masses. Histologically, there is a tumor-like growth pattern with proliferation of capillaries having protuberant endothelial cells, which have nuclear atypia and mitoses. The key features in differentiating this from pyogenic granuloma, or the vascular neoplasm Kaposi's sarcoma or angiosarcoma that it resembles (see later), include numerous neutrophils, nuclear dust, and purplish granular material that proves to consist of rickettsia-like bacteria, the underlying cause of bacillary angiomatosis[59] (closely related to *Rickettsiae quintana*, transmitted by the body louse and the cause of trench fever). Treatment of the cutaneous infection with erythromycin cures the condition.

INTERMEDIATE-GRADE TUMORS

Hemangioendothelioma

Hemangioendothelioma is used to denote a true neoplasm of vascular origin composed predominantly of masses of endothelial cells growing in and

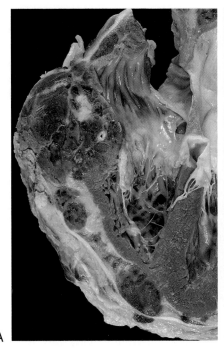

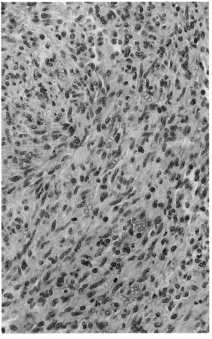

Figure 11–33. Angiosarcoma. A, Gross photograph of angio-sarcoma of heart (right ventri-cle). B, Photomicrograph of this tumor, which has some histologic features of malig-nancy, including moderate anaplasia.

A

B

about vascular lumina. *The hemangioendothelioma represents an intermediate grade between the well-differentiated hemangiomas and the frankly ana-plastic, totally cellular angiosarcomas (see later). It is most frequently encountered in the skin but may affect the spleen and liver.* Histologically, vascular channels are evident, with masses and sheets of spindle-shaped cells, occasionally with mitotic fig-ures and some pleomorphism. The chief impor-tance of this tumor lies in its differentiation from the more ominous angiosarcoma. The clinical set-ting is critical. Borderline lesions that are present at birth often mature eventually, but in the setting of chronic lymphedema they should cause concern.

Epithelioid hemangioendothelioma is a unique vascular tumor occurring around medium-sized and large veins in the soft tissue of adults. In such tumors, well-defined vascular channels are incon-spicuous, and the tumor cells are plump and often cuboidal, thus resembling epithelial cells. Occur-ring in the lung as a so-called *intravascular bron-choalveolar tumor,* such a tumor can be misdiag-nosed as metastatic carcinoma. Clinical behavior is variable; most are cured by excision, but up to 40% recur, and 20% eventually metastasize.

MALIGNANT TUMORS

Angiosarcoma (Hemangiosarcoma)

Hepatic angiosarcomas are rare but of interest be-cause they are associated with distinct carcinogens, including arsenic (exposure to arsenical pesticides),

Thorotrast (a radioactive contrast medium previ-ously widely used in radiology), and polyvinyl chloride (PVC) (widely used in plastics). The in-creased frequency of angiosarcomas among workers in the PVC industry is one of the truly well-documented instances of chemical carcinogen-esis in humans. With all three agents, there is a very long latent period of many years between exposure and the development of tumors. The tumors are often multicentric and may arise con-comitantly in the spleen.

MORPHOLOGY. Angiosarcoma is a malignant neo-plasm of vascular origin, characterized by masses of endothelial cells displaying the cellular atypia and anaplasia characteristic of malignancy (Fig. 11–33). It may occur in both sexes and at all ages, anywhere in the body (see Fig. 11–33A) but most often in the skin, soft tissue, breast, and liver. Grossly, cutaneous angiosarcoma may begin as deceptively small, sharply demarcated, asympto-matic, often multiple red nodules, but eventually most angiosarcomas become large, fleshy masses of pale gray-white, soft tissue. The margins blend imperceptibly with surrounding structures. Central softening and areas of necrosis and hemorrhage are frequent.

Microscopically, **all degrees of differentiation of these tumors may be found,** from those that are largely vascular with plump, anaplastic but recog-nizable endothelial cells to tumors that are quite undifferentiated, produce no definite blood ves-sels, and are markedly atypical (see Fig. 11–33B). In this more malignant variant, pleomorphism, tumor giant cells, and mitoses are characteristic.

Clinically, angiosarcomas have all the usual features of a malignancy, with local invasion and distal metastatic spread. Some patients survive only weeks to months, whereas others may live for many years.

Hemangiopericytoma

Hemangiopericytoma, a rare neoplasm, may occur anywhere in the body but is most common on the lower extremities and in the retroperitoneum. Electron microscopic studies clearly trace the origin of these tumors to pericytes. Most of these neoplasms are small, but rarely they achieve a diameter of 8 cm. They consist of numerous capillary channels surrounded by and enclosed within nests and masses of spindle-shaped cells, which occasionally can be ovoid or even round. Silver impregnation can be used to confirm that these cells are outside the basement membrane of the endothelium and hence are pericytes rather than ECs. The tumors may recur, and as many as 50% metastasize to lungs, bone, and liver. Regional lymph nodes are sometimes affected.

Kaposi's Sarcoma

Long considered to be an obscure tumor with an interesting epidemiology and an unknown histogenesis, Kaposi's sarcoma has come to the forefront because of its frequent occurrence in patients with acquired immunodeficiency syndrome (AIDS). Four forms of the disease are recognized:

1. *The classic, or European form*, first described by Kaposi in 1862, was endemic to older men of Eastern European (especially Ashkenazic Jews) or Mediterranean descent but uncommon in the United States. Clinically, this form consists of multiple red to purple skin plaques or nodules primarily in the lower extremities, slowly increasing in size and number and spreading to more proximal sites. The tumors frequently remain asymptomatic and localized to the skin and subcutaneous tissue but are locally aggressive, with an erratic course of lapses and remissions. Rarely do they involve visceral organs or cause the death of the patient.

2. *African Kaposi's* is clinically similar to the European form but occurs in children and younger men in equatorial Africa. It has a very high prevalence in these regions, representing up to 10% of all tumors. In young children, the disease is often associated with generalized involvement of lymph nodes, resembling lymphoma.

3. *Transplant-associated Kaposi's sarcoma* occurs in organ transplant recipients who receive high doses of immunosuppressive therapy. Lesions are either localized to the skin or widely metastatic but often regress when immunosuppressive therapy is discontinued.

4. *AIDS-associated Kaposi's sarcoma* is found in approximately one-third of AIDS patients, and it is more common in male homosexuals than in other risk groups. Cutaneous Kaposi's sarcoma lesions have no site of predilection but tend to disseminate widely early in the course. The tumors respond to cytotoxic chemotherapy and to therapy with alpha-interferon. Most patients eventually succumb to the infectious complications of AIDS rather than directly to the consequences of Kaposi's sarcoma. About one-third of these patients with Kaposi's sarcoma, however, subsequently develop a second malignancy, usually lymphoma, leukemia, or myeloma.

MORPHOLOGY. Kaposi's sarcoma represents a spectrum of lesions consisting of red-purple coalescent macules, papules, and plaques (Fig. 11–34). The earliest lesions may at first resemble a petechia or may be a red papulonodule and later compose spongy nodular tumors measuring 7 cm or more in diameter (Fig. 11–34A). In disseminated disease (aggressive forms), mucosal surfaces, lymph nodes, salivary glands, and viscera may be involved. Bleeding from intestinal involvement is a common, serious complication. Histologically, all types of Kaposi's sarcoma are essentially similar. The early, or "patch," stage is characterized by jagged, thin-walled, dilated vascular spaces in the epidermis, with interstitial inflammatory cells and extravasated red cells (with hemosiderin deposition), a picture that may be difficult to distinguish from granulation tissue. The more characteristic features are seen in the later nodular lesions and consist of plump, spindle-shaped stromal cells containing irregular, angulated, slit-like spaces filled with red cells and lined by recognizable endothelium, intertwined with normal vascular channels (see Fig. 11–34B). The angiomatous elements tend to blend imperceptibly with the neoplastic stromal cells, and thus the lesions eventually may resemble angiosarcomas or fibrosarcomas. Kaposi's sarcoma associated with AIDS cannot be reliably distinguished by histologic features from the form not associated with immune deficiency.

The pathogenesis of Kaposi's sarcoma is unknown. Epidemiologic features suggest a viral etiology. HIV itself is a cofactor in patients with AIDS, as suggested by the induction of Kaposi's sarcoma–like lesions in transgenic mice with the HIV transactivating *(tat)* gene. The data suggest that growth factors released by T lymphocytes and the HIV tat protein released (activated) by retrovirus-infected CD4+ T lymphocytes act together to

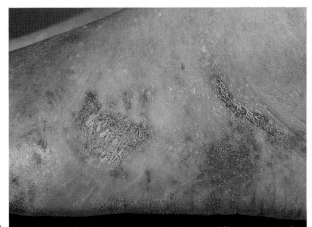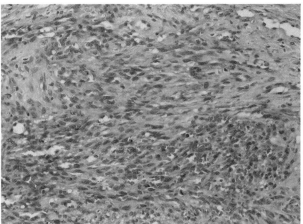

A   B

Figure 11-34. Kaposi's sarcoma. A, Gross photograph. B, Photomicrograph showing vascular channels filled with red blood cells and spindle-shaped stromal cells.

induce the proliferation of Kaposi's sarcoma spindle cells, of as yet undetermined mesenchymal origin.[60,61] Cytokines produced by the activated lymphoid cells permit continued self-renewal, activation and proliferation of non-neoplastic endothelial cells, smooth muscle cells, and fibroblasts to cause blood vessel formation.

TUMORS OF LYMPHATICS

Lymphangioma

Lymphangiomas are the lymphatic analog of the hemangiomas of blood vessels.

SIMPLE (CAPILLARY) LYMPHANGIOMA. These masses, composed of small lymphatic channels, tend to occur subcutaneously in the head and neck region and in the axilla. Rarely, they are found in the trunk, within internal organs, or in the connective tissue in and about the abdominal or thoracic cavities.

On body surfaces, they are slightly elevated or sometimes pedunculated lesions, 1 to 2 cm in diameter. Histologically, they are composed of a network of endothelium-lined lymph spaces that can be *differentiated from capillary channels only by the absence of blood cells.* Sometimes the lining cells hypertrophy, become cuboidal, and take on the appearance of glandular epithelium. These tumors are completely benign clinically.

CAVERNOUS LYMPHANGIOMA (CYSTIC HYGROMA). These benign lymphatic tumors are composed of cavernous lymphatic spaces and therefore are analogous to the cavernous hemangioma. Almost invariably occurring in children in the neck or axilla and only rarely retroperitoneally, they occasionally achieve considerable size, up to 15 cm in diameter. Such large masses may fill the axilla or pro-

duce gross deformities in and about the neck. The tumors are made up of massively dilated cystic spaces lined by endothelial cells and separated by a scant intervening connective tissue stroma. The margins of the tumor are not discrete, and these lesions are not encapsulated. Their removal is therefore difficult, and when bits of tumor are left in surgical resections, recurrence may be expected.

Lymphangiosarcoma (Lymphedema-Associated Angiosarcoma)

Lymphangiosarcoma is a rare tumor that develops after prolonged lymphatic obstruction with lymphedema.[62] Most cases occur in the edematous arms of patients treated by radical mastectomy for carcinoma of the breast. Clinically the edematous arm may undergo acute swelling followed by the appearance of subcutaneous nodules, hemorrhage, and skin ulceration. The nodules are frequently multiple, but they later become confluent, forming a large mass. On the average, they appear about 10 years after the mastectomy and have a very poor prognosis. They may also develop after prolonged lymphedema in the lower legs. Histologically, the tumor is composed of channels lined by anaplastic endothelial cells.

PATHOLOGY OF THERAPEUTIC INTERVENTIONS IN VASCULAR DISEASE

Characteristic additional morphologic changes are associated with current modes of therapy, such as thrombolysis, percutaneous balloon angioplasty, and vascular replacement, including coronary artery bypass graft surgery. Some key morphologic considerations of each of these and related interventions are discussed briefly.

THROMBOLYSIS

Dissolution of a clot in an unwanted location, *thrombolysis*, was originally used for the treatment of deep vein thrombosis and pulmonary embolism but is now also used for treating acute peripheral arterial thrombosis and embolism and for thrombosed prosthetic heart valves, catheters, and shunts.[63] Thrombolytic agents used currently act directly or indirectly as plasminogen activators.

Persistence of total occlusion with failure of clot lysis occurs in approximately 30% of patients undergoing thrombolytic therapy. The major complications of thrombolytic therapy that lessen enthusiasm for its use in patients with occlusive vascular disorders include hemorrhage due to the systemic fibrinolytic state (15% of patients) and thrombotic reocclusion (15 to 35% of patients). Reocclusion is related to the continued presence of the factors responsible for the original thrombus initiation. *Thus, although thrombolytic therapy reestablishes antegrade flow in the infarct-related coronary artery, it does not reverse factors responsible for initiating the original thrombus, such as ad-* *vanced atherosclerotic plaques, intimal rupture, enhanced platelet adhesiveness, or coronary or other arterial spasm.*

BALLOON ANGIOPLASTY AND RELATED TECHNIQUES

Balloon angioplasty (dilatation of an atheromatous stenosis of an artery by a balloon catheter) is being used extensively. Although done in the peripheral arteries in many cases, angioplasty has been studied most extensively following coronary arterial dilatation *(percutaneous transluminal coronary angioplasty)*. The process of balloon dilatation of an atherosclerotic vessel characteristically causes plaque fracture, often with accompanying localized hemorrhagic dissection of the adjacent arterial wall[64] (Fig. 11–35). The plaque splits at its weakest point, which is not necessarily the area most severely obstructed. *The key elements of luminal expansion in angioplasty are plaque rupture, medial dissection, and stretching of the media of the dissected segment,* leading to local flow abnormalities and generation of new, potentially thrombogenic blood-contacting surfaces. *Thus an atherosclerotic plaque following angioplasty is "unstable," having many features of the disrupted plaque associated with the acute coronary syndromes and other complications of atherosclerosis.*

Uncommonly, *abrupt reclosure* follows the angioplasty. This usually occurs as a result of compression of the lumen by an extensive dissection. Nevertheless, most patients improve symptomatically following angioplasty, thereby avoiding the need for aortocoronary bypass graft surgery at that

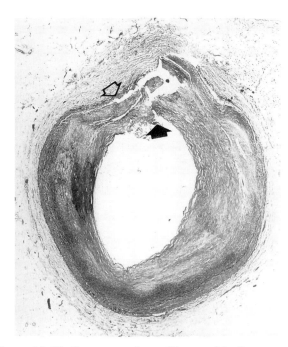

Figure 11–35. Coronary artery with recent balloon angioplasty, in low-power photomicrograph showing intimal-medial split *(solid arrow)* and partial circumferential dissection *(open arrow)*.

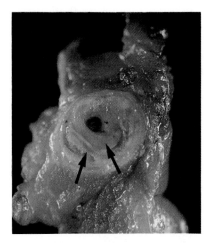

Figure 11–36. Gross photograph of restenosis following balloon angioplasty, demonstrating residual atherosclerotic plaque *(left arrow)* and new, glistening proliferative lesion *(right arrow)*.

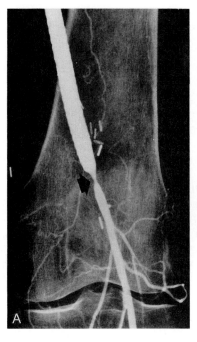
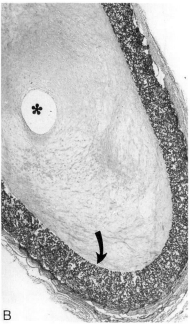

Figure 11–37. Anastomotic hyperplasia at the distal anastomosis of synthetic femoropopliteal graft. A, Angiogram demonstrating constriction *(arrow)*. B, Photomicrograph demonstrating Gore-Tex graft *(arrow)* with prominent intimal proliferation and very small residual lumen *(asterisk)*. (A courtesy of Anthony D. Whittemore, M.D., Brigham and Women's Hospital, Boston.)

time. The long-term success of angioplasty is limited by the development of *proliferative restenosis* that occurs in approximately 30 to 40% of patients within the first 4 to 6 months following angioplasty. The factors causing restenosis are complex but probably relate primarily to endothelial cell and smooth muscle cell injury, plaque inflammatory cell elaboration of cytokines and growth factors, local thrombosis, and vasoconstriction.[65] The end result is an occlusive, rapidly progressive fibrous lesion that contains abundant smooth muscle cells and extracellular matrix (Fig. 11–36).

VASCULAR REPLACEMENT

Many patients now receive synthetic or autologous grafts that replace a segment of vessel or bypass diseased arteries. The clinical performance of a vascular graft depends primarily on its type and location. Large-diameter (>10 cm) Dacron grafts in current use function well in high-flow, low-resistance locations such as the aorta. In contrast, small-diameter fabric vascular grafts (<6 to 8 mm in diameter) perform less well.

The most widely used small vessel replacements are *autologous saphenous vein* (the patient's own vein, dissected free, reversed in direction, and transplanted to a different site) and *expanded-polytetrafluoroethylene* (ePTFE, essentially a spongy Teflon fabric). Failure of small-diameter vascular prostheses (<6 mm diameter) is most frequently due to thrombotic occlusion or intimal fibrous hyperplasia, either generalized (in vein grafts) or anastomotic (in synthetic grafts) (Fig. 11–37).

Healing of a vascular graft depends on the mi-

gration and proliferation of endothelial cells and smooth muscle cells, derived from adjacent artery at the anastomosis. The ability to endothelialize cardiovascular prostheses is limited in humans, and full endothelialization of clinical grafts is unusual. Luminal coverage develops relatively slowly and incompletely; formation of *neointima* (a surface covered by endothelial cells) is generally restricted to a 10- to 15-mm zone near the anastomosis, and the remainder of the graft surface constitutes a *pseudointima* (thrombus or cells other than endothelial cells).

Coronary Artery Bypass Graft Surgery

Coronary artery bypass graft surgery (aortocoronary bypass) is one of the most frequently performed major surgical procedures in the United States (more than 230,000 per year). Bypasses are done using grafts of either autologous reversed saphenous vein or internal mammary artery (usually the left internal mammary artery is used owing to proximity to the heart). The long-term patency of saphenous vein grafts is 60% or less at 10 years, owing to pathologic changes, including thrombosis (usually occurs early), intimal thickening (which usually occurs several months to several years postoperatively), and atherosclerosis in the graft, sometimes with superimposed plaque rupture, thrombi, or aneurysms (usually more than 2 to 3 years).[66] In contrast, the internal mammary artery has a greater than 90% patency at 10 years.

1. Pober, J., and Cotran, R.S.: Cytokines and endothelial cell biology. Physiol. Rev. 70:427, 1990.

2. Simionescu, M.: Endothelial cell response to normal and abnormal stimuli, modulation, dysfunction, injury; adaptation, repair, death. *In* Simionescu, N., and Simionescu, M. (eds.): Endothelial Cell Dysfunctions. New York, Plenum Press, 1992, p. 3.

3. Gerritsen, M.E., and Bloor, C.M.: Endothelial gene expression in response to injury. F.A.S.E.B. J. 7:523, 1993.

4. Casscells, W.: Migration of smooth muscle and endothelial cells. Critical events in restenosis. Circulation 86:723, 1992.

5. Kocher, O., et al.: Phenotypic features of smooth muscle cells during the evolution of experimental carotid artery intimal thickening. Lab. Invest. 65:459, 1991.

6. Clowes, A.W., et al.: Regulation of smooth muscle cell growth in injured artery. J. Cardiovasc. Pharmacol. 14:S12, 1989.

7. Schoen, F.J.: Interventional and Surgical Cardiovascular Pathology: Clinical Correlations and Basic Principles. Philadelphia, W.B. Saunders Co., 1989, p. 33.

8. Strong, J.P.: The natural history of atherosclerosis in childhood. Ann. N.Y. Acad. Sci. 623:9, 1991.

9. Neaton, J.D., and Wentworth, D.: Serum cholesterol, blood pressure, cigarette smoking, and death from coronary heart disease. Overall findings and differences by age for 316,099 white men. Arch. Intern. Med. 152:56, 1992.

10. Kannel, W.B.: Contributions of the Framingham Study to the conquest of coronary artery disease. Am. J. Cardiol. 62:1109, 1988.

11. Lipid Research Clinics Program: The lipid research clinics coronary primary prevention trial results. I. Reduction in incidence of coronary heart disease. J.A.M.A. 251:351, 1984.

12. Kane, J.P., et al.: Regression of coronary atherosclerosis during treatment of familial hypercholesterolemia with combined drug regimens. J.A.M.A. 264:3007, 1990.

13. Knapp, H.R., et al.: In-vivo indexes of platelet and vascular function during fish-oil administration in patients with atherosclerosis. N. Engl. J. Med. 314:937, 1986.

14. Chobanian, A.V.: The influence of hypertension and other hemodynamic factors in atherogenesis. Prog. Cardiovasc. Dis. 26:177, 1983.

15. McGill, H.: The cardiovascular pathology of smoking. Am. Heart J. 115:250, 1988.

16. Bierman, E.L.: Atherogenesis in diabetes. Atheroscler. Thromb. 12:647, 1992.

17. Clarke, R., et al.: Hyperhomocysteinemia: An independent risk factor for vascular disease. N. Engl. J. Med. 324:1149, 1991.

18. Mintz, G.S., et al.: Target lesion calcification in coronary artery disease: An intravascular ultrasound study. J. Am. Coll. Cardiol. 20:1149, 1992.

19. Berenson, G.S., et al.: Atherosclerosis of the aorta and coronary arteries and cardiovascular risk factors in persons aged 6 to 30 years and studied at necropsy (The Bogalusa Heart Study). Am. J. Cardiol. 70:851, 1992.

20. Ross, R.: The pathogenesis of atherosclerosis. An update. N. Engl. J. Med. 314:488, 1986.

21. Ross, R.: The pathogenesis of atherosclerosis: A perspective for the 1990s. Nature 362:801, 1993.

22. Cybulsky, M.I., and Gimbrone, M.A.: Endothelial expression of a mononuclear leukocyte adhesion molecule during atherogenesis. Science 251:788, 1991.

23. Poston, R.N., et al.: Expression of intercellular adhesion molecule-1 in atherosclerotic plaques. Am. J. Pathol. 140:665, 1992.

24. Collins, T.: Endothelial nuclear factor-κB and the initiation of the atherosclerotic lesion. Lab. Invest. 68:499, 1993.

25. Libby, P., and Hansson, G.K.: Involvement of the immune system in human atherogenesis: Current knowledge and unanswered questions. Lab. Invest. 64:5, 1991.

26. Breslow, J.L.: The genetic basis of lipoprotein disorders. J. Int. Med. 231:627, 1992.

27. Plump, A.S., et al.: Severe hypercholesterolemia and atherosclerosis in apolipoprotein E-deficient mice created by homologous recombination in ES cells. Cell 71:343, 1992.

28. Witztum, J.L., and Steinberg, D.: Role of oxidized low density lipoprotein in atherogenesis. J. Clin. Invest. 88:1785, 1991.

29. Steinberg, D.: Antioxidant vitamins and coronary heart disease. N. Engl. J. Med. 318:1487, 1993.

30. Nachman, R.L.: Thrombosis and atherogenesis: Molecular connections. Blood 79:1897, 1992.

31. Grainger, D.J., et al.: Proliferation of human smooth muscle cells promoted by lipoprotein (a). Science 260:1655, 1993.

32. Benditt, E.P.: Implications of the monoclonal character of human atherosclerotic plaques. Am. J. Pathol. 86:693, 1977.

33. Hajjar, D.P.: Viral pathogenesis of atherosclerosis. Impact of molecular mimicry and viral genes. Am. J. Pathol. 139:1195, 1991.

34. Strong, J.P.: Atherosclerotic lesions. Natural history, risk factors, and topography. Arch. Pathol. Lab. Med. 116:1268, 1992.

35. Kaplan, N.M.: Systemic hypertension: Mechanisms and diagnosis. *In* Braunwald, E. (ed.): Heart Disease, 4th ed. Philadelphia, W.B. Saunders Co., 1992, p. 817.

36. Kurtz, T.W., and Spence, M.A.: Genetics of essential hypertension. Am. J. Med. 94:77, 1993.

37. Jeunemaitre, X., et al.: Molecular basis of human hypertension: Role of angiotensinogen. Cell 71:169, 1992.

38. Johnson, R.J., et al.: Membranoproliferative glomerulonephritis associated with hepatitis C virus infection. N. Engl. J. Med. 328:465, 1993.

39. Cotran, R.S., and Pober, J.S.: Recent insights into the mechanisms of vascular injury. Implications for the pathogenesis of vasculitis. *In* Simionescu, N., and Simionescu, M. (eds.): Endothelial Cell Dysfunctions. New York, Plenum Press, 1992, p. 183.

40. Jennette, J.C.: Antineutrophil cytoplasmic autoantibody-associated disease: A pathologist's perspective. Am. J. Kidney Dis. 18:164, 1991.

41. Ewert, B.H., et al.: The pathogenic role of antineutrophil cytoplasmic autoantibody. Am. J. Kidney Dis. 18:188, 1991.

42. Brouwer, E., et al.: Antimyeloperoxidase-associated proliferative glomerulonephritis: An animal model. J. Exp. Med. 177:905, 1993.

43. Cotran, R.S.: Pathogenesis of vasculitis. An update. Adv. Pathol. 3:301, 1990.

44. Jennette, J.C., et al.: Nomenclature of systemic vasculitides: The proposal of an international consensus conference. Arthr. Rheum. 37:187, 1994.

45. Hall, S., et al.: Takayasu arteritis. A study of 32 North American patients. Medicine 64:89, 1985.

46. Rowley, A.H., et al.: Kawasaki syndrome. Curr. Probl. Pediatr. 21:387, 1991.

47. Naoe, S., et al.: Kawasaki disease. With particular emphasis on arterial lesions. Acta Pathol. Jpn. 41:785, 1991.

48. Dajani, A.S., et al.: Diagnosis and therapy of Kawasaki disease in children. Circulation 87:1776, 1993.

49. Hoffman, G.S., et al.: Wegener granulomatosis: An analysis of 158 patients. Ann. Intern. Med. 116:488, 1992.

50. Joyce, J.W.: Buerger's disease (thromboangiitis obliterans). Rheum. Dis. Clin. North Am. 16:463, 1990.

51. Gravallese, E.M., et al.: Rheumatoid aortitis: A rarely recognized but clinically significant entity. Medicine 68:95, 1989.

52. Ernst, C.B.: Abdominal aortic aneurysms. N. Engl. J. Med. 328:1167, 1993.

53. Kuivaniemi, H., et al.: Genetic causes of aortic aneurysms. Unlearning at least part of what the textbooks say. J. Clin. Invest. 88:1441, 1991.

54. Prockop, D.: Mutations in collagens as a cause of connective tissue diseases. N. Engl. J. Med. 326:540, 1992.

55. Sterpetti, A.V., et al.: Inflammatory aneurysms of the abdominal aorta: Incidence, pathologic, and etiologic considerations. J. Vasc. Surg. 9:643, 1989.

56. Criqui, M.H., et al.: Mortality over a period of 10 years in patients with peripheral arterial disease. N. Engl. J. Med. 326:381, 1992.
57. Cigarra, J.E., et al.: Diagnostic imaging in the evaluation of suspected aortic dissection. N. Engl. J. Med. 328:35, 1993.
58. Ezekowitz, R.A., et al.: Interferon alpha-2a therapy for life-threatening hemangiomas of infancy. N. Engl. J. Med. 326:1456, 1992.
59. Relman, D.A., et al.: The agent of bacillary angiomatosis. An approach to the identification of uncultured pathogens. N. Engl. J. Med. 323:1573, 1990.
60. Ensoli, B., et al.: Pathogenesis of AIDS-associated Kaposi's sarcoma. Hemat. Oncol. Clin. North Am. 5:281, 1991.
61. Chandran-Nair, B., et al.: Identification of a major growth factor for AIDS-Kaposi's sarcoma cells as oncostatin M. Science 255:1430, 1992.
62. Case records of the Massachusetts General Hospital. Case 18, 1993. N. Engl. J. Med. 328:1337, 1993.
63. Marder, V.J.: Thrombolytic therapy: Current status. N. Engl. J. Med. 318:1512, 1585, 1988.
64. Waller, B.F.: Morphology of percutaneous transluminal coronary angioplasty used in the treatment of coronary heart disease. In Virmani, R., et al. (eds.): Cardiovascular Pathology. Philadelphia, W.B. Saunders Co., 1991, p. 100.
65. Libby, P., et al.: A cascade model for restenosis. A special case of atherosclerosis progression. Circulation 86:III-47, 1992.
66. Virmani, R., et al.: Aortocoronary saphenous vein bypass grafts. In Waller, B.F. (ed.): Contemporary Issues in Cardiovascular Pathology. Philadelphia, F.A. Davis Co., 1988, p. 41.

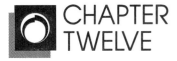

CHAPTER TWELVE

The Heart

FREDERICK J. SCHOEN, M.D., Ph.D.

NORMAL

Expected heart weight varies with height and skeletal structure; it averages approximately 250 to 300 gm in females and 300 to 350 gm in males. Normally the thickness of the free wall of the right ventricle is 0.3 to 0.5 cm and that of the left ventricle 1.3 to 1.5 cm. Greater weight or ventricular thickness indicates *hypertrophy*, and enlarged chamber size implies *dilatation.* An apparently normal (or less than normal) left ventricular thickness, however, may be found in a markedly heavy, hypertrophied heart that has dilated before death. Increased weight or size of the heart is known as *cardiomegaly.*

VALVES

The four cardiac valves respond passively to pressure and flow changes within the heart. They function as loose flaps (leaflets or cusps) that seal the valvular orifices against regurgitation of blood when closed but fold out of the way when the valve is open, to provide an obstruction-free orifice. During the closed phase, the three cusps of the *semilunar* valves (aortic and pulmonic) overlap along an area (the *lunula*) between the free edge and a line marked by a white ridge on the ventricular surface of the cusp (linea alba). The overlap is substantial; in the aortic valve, for example, the total cuspal area is about 40% greater than the valve orifice area. Because only the portion of the cusps below the linea alba separates aortic from left ventricular cavity blood, defects or fenestra-

517

tions of the cusp in the lunula usually do not compromise valve competence. Each aortic cusp has a small nodule (nodules of Arantius or Morgagni's nodules) in the center of the free edge, which facilitates closure. On gross inspection, normal valve leaflets appear thin and translucent.

The free margins of the *atrioventricular* (AV) valves (mitral and tricuspid) are tethered to the ventricular wall by many delicate chordae tendineae, attached to papillary muscles, which are contiguous with the underlying ventricular walls. Each of the two mitral valve leaflets is connected by chordae to both left ventricular papillary muscles.

Thus normal mitral valve function depends on the coordinated actions of cusps, chordae tendineae, papillary muscles, and associated left ventricular wall (collectively the *mitral apparatus*). Tricuspid valve function depends on analogous structures. In a similar fashion, the function of semilunar valves depends on the integrity and coordinated movements of the cusps and their attachments. Thus dilatation of the aortic root in hypertension or syphilis can keep the aortic valve cusps from coming together during closure, just as left ventricular dilatation or a ruptured chorda or papillary muscle can keep the mitral valve from complete closure, each resulting in regurgitant flow.

The cardiac valves are endothelium lined; all have a similar, layered architecture consisting predominantly of a dense collagenous core *(fibrosa)* close to the outflow surface and continuous with valvular supporting structures and loose connective tissue *(spongiosa)* near to the inflow surface. In general, normal valve leaflets and cusps do not have blood vessels because they are thin enough to be nourished by diffusion from blood inside the heart.

MYOCARDIUM

The human heart is remarkably efficient, durable, and reliable. Basic to this function is the near-indefatigable cardiac muscle, the *myocardium,* a collection of branching and anastomosing fibers composed of individual cells *(cardiac myocytes).* The cardiac myocyte is divided into structural and functional subunits, the *sarcomeres,* that have partially overlapping myosin (thick) and actin (thin) filaments and whose lengths range from 1.6 to 2.2 μm, depending on the state of contraction. Cardiac contraction involves collective shortening of sarcomeres by sliding of the actin filaments between the myosin filaments toward the center of each sarcomere. Shorter sarcomeres have considerable overlap of actin filaments in their centers, even during diastole, and consequent reduction in contractile force, whereas longer lengths, to a degree, enhance contractility (Frank-Starling mechanism). Thus moderate ventricular dilatation increases the force of contraction. There is a point, however, with progressive dilatation at which overlap of the actin and myosin filaments is reduced, and the force of contraction turns sharply downward, as occurs in heart failure.

Although nearly the entire volume of the myocardium is occupied by cardiac muscle cells, myocytes compose only approximately 25% of the total number of cells. The remainder are endothelial cells, associated with capillaries, and connective tissue cells. Inflammatory cells are generally rare, and collagen is sparse in the normal myocardium.

In addition, specialized excitatory and conducting myocytes containing only a few contractile myofilaments are involved in the regulation of the rate and rhythm of the heart *(Purkinje cells).* These myofibers are plentiful in (1) the sinoatrial (SA) pacemaker of the heart, *the SA node,* located at the junction of the right atrial appendage with the opening of the superior vena cava; (2) the *AV node,* located at the junction of the medial wall of the right atrium with the interventricular septum; and (3) the *bundle of His,* which courses down the interventricular septum toward the apex to divide into right and left branches that further arborize in the respective ventricles. Lesions involving these specialized structures underlie many of the disturbances in cardiac rhythm.

BLOOD SUPPLY

Most of the coronary arterial blood flow to the myocardium occurs during diastole, when the pressure in the aortic root is high and the microcirculation is not compressed by the cardiac contraction. The coronary arterial circulation consists of long vessels that run along the outside surface of the heart *(epicardial coronary arteries)* and short but narrow distal vessels that course through the myocardium (intramural arteries). Knowledge of the areas of supply *(perfusion)* of the three major coronary arteries helps to explain the correlation between sites of vascular lesions and regions of myocardial infarction. Most commonly, the anterior descending branch of the left coronary artery supplies most of the apex of the heart, the anterior surface of the left ventricle, and the anterior two-thirds of the interventricular septum; the right coronary artery supplies the entire right ventricular free wall, the adjacent half of the posterior wall of the left ventricle, and the posterior third of the interventricular septum. Whichever coronary vessel becomes the posterior descending coronary artery and thereby perfuses the posterior third of the septum is called "dominant." In a *right dominant circulation,* present in approximately four-fifths of individuals, the circumflex branch of the left coronary artery generally perfuses only a portion of the lateral aspect of the left ventricle. *Thus occlusions of the right as well as the left coronary artery and their major branches can cause left ventricular damage.* At the cellular level, individual muscle fibers are almost always adjacent to several capillaries. In hypertrophied hearts, enlarged fibers may outgrow their blood supply.

Functionally the right and left coronary arteries behave as end arteries, although anatomically there are numerous intercoronary anastomoses in most normal hearts (called *collaterals*). Although little blood courses through these channels in the normal heart, when one trunk is narrowed, blood flows from the high to the low pressure system, and simultaneously the channels enlarge. Progressive development of these anastomoses stimulated by ischemia may play a role in supporting the blood flow to areas of the myocardium deprived of adequate perfusion. However, when blood flow is compromised, collateral blood flow is less effective in the subendocardium, the area therefore most susceptible to ischemic damage.

EFFECTS OF AGING ON THE HEART

With an increasing number of persons surviving into their eighth decade and beyond, knowledge of changes in the cardiovascular system that are expected to occur with aging is important. Changes occur in the myocardium, chamber cavities, valves, epicardial coronary arteries, conduction system, pericardium, and aorta (Table 12–1).[1,2] *Brown atrophy* is a term used to describe a small, brown heart with extensive lipofuscin deposits in the muscle cells, and the term *basophilic degeneration* describes the accumulation within cardiac myocytes of a gray bluish material, likely glucan, a probable byproduct of glycogen metabolism. With advancing age, the amount of subepicardial fat increases, particularly over the anterior surface of the right ventricle.

Compared with "younger" myocardium, elderly myocardium also has fewer myocytes, increased collagenized connective tissue, and a variable deposition of amyloid. Moreover, associated with increasing age is a reduction in the size of the left ventricular cavity, particularly in the base-to-apex dimension, in part owing to a generally lower cardiac output. This chamber alteration, accompanied by a rightward shift and tortuosity of a dilated ascending aorta, causes the basal ventricular septum to bend leftward, bulging into the left ventricular outflow tract. The configuration, termed a *sigmoid septum,* can simulate the obstruction to blood leaving the left ventricle that often occurs with hypertrophic cardiomyopathy (HCM) (see discussion later).

Several changes of the valves are noted, in-

Table 12–1. CHANGES IN THE AGING HEART

MYOCARDIUM (WALLS)
Increased mass
Lipofuscin deposition
Brown atrophy
Basophilic degeneration
Increased subepicardial fat
Amyloid deposits

CHAMBERS
Increased left atrial cavity size
Decreased left ventricular cavity size
Sigmoid-shaped ventricular septum

VALVES
Aortic valve calcific deposits
Mitral-valve annular calcific deposits
Fibrous thickening of leaflets
Buckling of mitral leaflets toward the left atrium
Lambl's excrescences

EPICARDIAL CORONARY ARTERIES
Tortuosity
Increased cross-sectional luminal area
Calcific deposits
Atherosclerotic plaque

AORTA
Dilated ascending aorta with rightward shift
Elongated (tortuous) thoracic aorta
Sinotubular junction calcific deposits
Elastic fragmentation and collagen accumulation
Atherosclerotic plaque

cluding calcification of the mitral annulus (unusually of clinical importance) and aortic valve (frequently leading to aortic stenosis [see discussion later]). In addition, the valves develop fibrous thickening, and the mitral leaflets tend to buckle back toward the left atrium during ventricular systole, simulating a prolapsing (myxomatous) mitral valve (see discussion later). Moreover, small filiform processes *(Lambl's excrescences)* are on the closure lines of aortic and mitral valves in nearly all subjects older than 60 years of age. Lambl's excrescences are wear-and-tear lesions that arise from small thrombi on the valve contact margins.

Although the morphologic changes described are common in elderly patients at necropsy and may mimic disease, only in a minority are they associated with clinical cardiac dysfunction.

PRINCIPLES OF CARDIAC DYSFUNCTION

A large spectrum of disease processes can involve the heart and blood vessels,[3–5] but dysfunction of the heart or the overall cardiovascular system can only occur by one of the following mechanisms (Table 12–2): (1) Disruption of the continuity of the circulatory system (e.g., a gunshot wound

Table 12–2. CAUSES OF CARDIOVASCULAR DYSFUNCTION

Loss of blood
Irregular heartbeat
Obstructed flow
Regurgitant or misdirected flow
Pump failure
    Contractile dysfunction (systolic failure)
    Inadequate filling (diastolic failure)

through the thoracic aorta) that permits blood to escape; in such cases, the heart cannot fill, and the resistance against which it pumps is lost. (2) Disorders of cardiac conduction (e.g., heart block) or arrhythmias owing to generation of impulses in an uncoordinated manner (e.g., ventricular fibrillation), which leads to contractions of the muscular walls that are not uniform and efficient. (3) A lesion preventing valve opening or one narrowing the lumen of a vessel (e.g., aortic valvular stenosis or coarctation), which obstructs blood flow and overworks the pump behind the obstruction. (4) Regurgitant flow (e.g., mitral or aortic valvular regurgitation) that causes some of the output from each contraction to reflux backward; this necessarily forces portions of the pump to expel the same blood several times and thereby induces substantial myocardial stress. (5) Failure of the pump itself. In the most frequent circumstance, damaged muscle itself contracts weakly or inadequately, and the chambers cannot empty properly. In some conditions, however, the muscle cannot relax sufficiently, the left ventricular chamber cannot dilate during diastole, and the heart cannot properly fill.

CONGESTIVE HEART FAILURE

Any one of the causes mentioned above, when sufficiently severe or advanced, may ultimately impair cardiac function and render the heart unable to maintain an output sufficient for the metabolic requirements of the tissues and organs of the body, producing congestive heart failure (CHF). As stated, *CHF occurs either because of a decreased myocardial capacity to contract or because of an inability to fill the cardiac chambers with blood.* Most instances of heart failure are the consequence of progressive deterioration of myocardial contractile function *(systolic dysfunction)*, as often occurs with ischemic injury, pressure or volume overload, or dilated cardiomyopathy.[6] Sometimes, however, failure results from an inability of the heart chambers to expand sufficiently during diastole to accommodate an adequate ventricular blood volume *(diastolic dysfunction)*, as can occur with massive left ventricular hypertrophy, myocardial fibro-

sis, deposition of amyloid, or constrictive pericarditis.[7] Whatever its basis, CHF is characterized by diminished cardiac output (sometimes called forward failure) or damming back of blood in the venous system (so-called backward failure), or both.

CARDIAC HYPERTROPHY: PATHOPHYSIOLOGY AND PROGRESSION TO FAILURE

Central to any consideration of CHF is a discussion of *cardiac hypertrophy*, the compensatory response of the myocardium to increased work. Myocardial hyperfunction induces increased myocyte size (cellular hypertrophy through addition of sarcomeres, the contractile elements) that causes an increase in the overall mass and size of the heart. The diameters of cardiac myocytes can increase from the normal 15 μm to 25 μm or more in hypertrophy. Because adult cardiac myocytes cannot divide, augmentation of myocyte number *(hyperplasia)* cannot occur in the adult heart.

The pattern of hypertrophy reflects the stimulus.[8] Pressure-overloaded ventricles (e.g., hypertension or aortic stenosis) develop *concentric hypertrophy*, with an increased ratio of wall thickness to cavity radius. In contrast, volume-overloaded ventricles (e.g., mitral regurgitation) develop hypertrophy with dilatation *(eccentric hypertrophy)*, with proportionate increases in ventricular radius and wall thickness.

The structural/biochemical/molecular basis for myocardial contractile failure is obscure in many cases. In some instances (e.g., myocardial infarction), there is obvious death of myocytes and loss of vital elements of the "pump"; the remaining, noninfarcted regions of cardiac muscle are overworked. In contrast, in valvular heart disease, increased pressure or volume work affects the chamber wall globally. The increased myocyte size that occurs in cardiac hypertrophy is usually accompanied by decreased capillary density, increased intercapillary distance, and deposition of fibrous tissue.[9]

Moreover, the molecular changes in hypertrophied hearts that initially mediate enhanced function may contribute to the development of heart failure.[10] With prolonged hemodynamic overload, gene expression is altered, leading to re-expression of a pattern of protein synthesis analogous to that seen in fetal cardiac development; other changes are analogous to events that occur during mitosis of normally proliferating cells. Thus proteins related to contractile elements, excitation-contraction coupling, and energy utilization may be significantly altered through production of different isoforms that either may be less functional than normal or may be reduced or increased in amount.

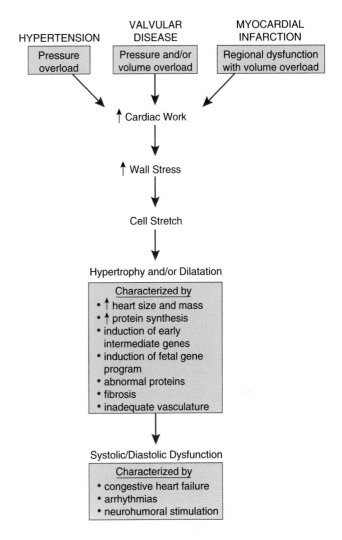

Figure 12-1. Schematic representation of the sequence of events in hypertrophy and heart failure, emphasizing cardiac cellular and extracellular changes.

Other proposed but not established mechanisms potentiating CHF include reduced adrenergic drive, decreased calcium availability, impaired mitochondrial function, and microcirculatory spasm.

This discussion indicates that geometry, structure, and composition (cells and extracellular matrix) of the hypertrophied heart are not normal. *Clearly cardiac hypertrophy constitutes a tenuous balance between adaptive characteristics (including new sarcomeres) and potentially deleterious structural and biochemical/molecular alterations (including decreased capillary to myocyte ratio, increased fibrous tissue, and synthesis of abnormal, perhaps dysfunctional, proteins). It should not be surprising therefore that cardiac hypertrophy often evolves to cardiac failure.* A proposed sequence of events that compose the response to increased cardiac work is summarized in Figure 12–1. Besides predisposing to CHF, left ventricular hypertrophy is an independent risk factor for cardiac mortality and morbidity, especially for sudden death and ischemic heart disease.[11] Interestingly, and in contrast to *pathologic hypertrophy* just discussed, hypertrophy that is induced by exercise *(physiologic hypertrophy)* seems to have minimal or no deleterious effect.

Whatever the underlying basis for CHF, a variety of compensatory mechanisms come into play when the hypertrophied heart can no longer accommodate the increased demand. The heart begins to dilate, as discussed earlier, thereby stretching the sarcomeres and increasing the force of contraction and secondarily the stroke volume. Increased stretching of myocytes, however, leads to further hypertrophy. Simultaneously there is expansion of the blood volume, further augmenting stroke volume. Eventually, however, the compensatory mechanisms themselves constitute an added burden. Myocardial hypertrophy may become increasingly detrimental because of the increased metabolic requirements of the enlarged muscle mass. Indeed, muscle mass and wall tension (see previously) are major determinants of the oxygen consumption of the heart; the other major factors are heart rate and contractility (inotropic state, or force of contraction). Increased blood volume, which supports the cardiac output in the short term, also imposes an additional load on the failing heart.

Ultimately, the primary cardiac disease and the superimposed compensatory burdens further encroach on the myocardial reserve until cardiac dilatation progresses beyond the point at which adequate myocardial tension can be generated. Then begins the downward slide of stroke volume and cardiac output that often ends in death. Thus at autopsy, the heart of patients having CHF is generally characterized by increased weight, progressive wall thinning, chamber dilatation, and microscopic changes of hypertrophy, but the extent of these changes varies from one patient to the next.

It is impossible from morphologic examination of the heart to differentiate a damaged but compensated heart from one that has decompensated. *Moreover, many of the significant adaptations and morphologic changes noted in CHF are distant from the heart and are produced by the hypoxic and congestive effects of the failing circulation on other organs and tissues.*[12] It is important to recall, however, that hypoxic or congestive changes, or both, may be produced in peripheral tissues and organs by states of circulatory insufficiency of noncardiac origin (e.g., hemorrhagic or septic shock). During shock, many organs suffer injury because of hypoperfusion (see Chapter 4).

To some extent, the right and left sides of the heart act as two distinct anatomic and functional units. Under various pathologic stresses, one side or even one chamber may fail, so from the clinical standpoint, left-sided and right-sided failure can occur separately. Nevertheless, because the vascular system is a closed circuit, failure of one side cannot exist for long without eventually producing excessive strain on the other, terminating in total heart failure. Despite this interdependency, the clearest understanding of the pathologic physiology and anatomy is derived from a consideration of failure of each side separately.

LEFT-SIDED HEART FAILURE

As discussed here, left-sided heart failure is most often caused by (1) ischemic heart disease, (2) hypertension, (3) aortic and mitral valvular diseases (particularly calcific aortic stenosis and rheumatic heart disease), and (4) myocardial diseases. Except with obstruction at the mitral valve or other processes that restrict the size of the left ventricle, this chamber is usually hypertrophied and often dilated, sometimes quite massively. Secondary enlargement of the left atrium is frequently present. Atrial fibrillation (i.e., uncoordinated, chaotic contraction of the atrium) often results; this may either compromise stroke volume or cause blood stasis and possible thrombus formation (particularly

in the appendages). A fibrillating left atrium carries an increased risk of embolic stroke.[13] The distant effects of left-sided failure are manifested most prominently in the lungs, although the function of the kidneys and brain may also be markedly impaired.

LUNGS. With the progressive damming of blood within the pulmonary circulation, pressure in the pulmonary veins mounts and is ultimately transmitted retrogradely to the capillaries. The result is pulmonary congestion and edema, with heavy, wet lungs as described in detail in Chapter 15. It is sufficient to note here that the lung changes include, in sequence, (1) a perivascular and interstitial transudate, particularly in the interlobular septa; (2) progressive edematous widening of alveolar septa; and (3) accumulation of edema fluid in the alveolar spaces. Transferrin in edema fluid and hemoglobin from erythrocytes, which leak from congested capillaries, are phagocytosed by macrophages and converted to hemosiderin. Hemosiderin-containing macrophages in the alveoli (called *heart failure cells*) denote previous episodes of pulmonary edema (see Fig. 4–4).

These anatomic changes produce striking clinical manifestations. *Dyspnea* (breathlessness), usually the earliest and the cardinal complaint of patients in left-sided heart failure, is an exaggeration of the normal breathlessness that follows exertion. With further impairment, there is *orthopnea*, which is dyspnea on lying down that is relieved by sitting or standing. Thus the orthopneic patient needs to sleep sitting upright. *Paroxysmal nocturnal dyspnea* is an extension of orthopnea that consists of attacks of extreme dyspnea bordering on suffocation, usually occurring at night. Cough is a common accompaniment of left-sided failure.

KIDNEYS. With left-sided heart failure, the decreased cardiac output causes a reduction in renal perfusion, which activates the renin-angiotensin-aldosterone system, inducing retention of salt and water with consequent expansion of the interstitial fluid and blood volumes. This compensatory reaction contributes to the pulmonary edema in left-sided heart failure. In kidneys already suffering from hypoperfusion, the reduced cardiac output may lead to ischemic acute tubular necrosis (see Chapter 20). If the perfusion deficit of the kidney becomes sufficiently severe, impaired excretion of nitrogenous products may cause azotemia, known as *prerenal azotemia*.

BRAIN. In far-advanced CHF, cerebral hypoxia may give rise to *hypoxic encephalopathy* (see Chapter 29), with irritability, loss of attention span, and restlessness, which may even progress to stupor and coma.

RIGHT-SIDED HEART FAILURE

Right-sided heart failure occurs in pure form in only a few diseases. Usually it is a consequence of left-sided failure because any increase in pressure in pulmonary circulation incident to left-sided failure inevitably produces an increased burden on the right side of the heart. The causes of right-sided failure then must include all those that induce left-sided heart failure.

Pure right-sided failure most often occurs with *cor pulmonale*, i.e., right ventricular pressure overload induced by intrinsic disease of the lungs or pulmonary vasculature (see the section on pulmonary [right-sided] hypertensive heart disease later in this chapter). In these cases, the right ventricle is burdened by increased resistance within the pulmonary circulation; dilatation is generally confined to the right ventricle and atrium. This can be acute with right-sided dilatation and thinning in massive pulmonary embolism. In chronic right-sided overload (e.g., owing to chronic obstructive pulmonary disease), right ventricular hypertrophy is usually present. Clinically constrictive pericarditis simulates right-sided failure by restricting filling of the heart that dams blood back into the systemic venous system, although the right ventricle itself may be structurally normal.

The major morphologic and clinical effects of pure right-sided failure differ from those of left-sided failure in that pulmonary congestion is minimal, whereas engorgement of the systemic and portal venous systems is pronounced. The major organs affected by right-sided heart failure are the liver, spleen, kidneys, subcutaneous tissues, and brain as well as the entire portal area of venous drainage.

LIVER. The liver is usually slightly increased in size and weight; a cut section displays the prominent "nutmeg" pattern of *chronic passive congestion* of the liver (see Fig. 4–5). This is composed of congested red centers of the liver lobules surrounded by the paler, sometimes fatty, peripheral regions. In some instances, especially when left-sided failure is also present, the severe central hypoxia produces *centrilobular necrosis* along with the sinusoidal congestion. If the right-sided failure is severe and rapidly developing, rupture of sinusoids produces *central hemorrhagic necrosis.* With long-standing severe right-sided cardiac failure, the central areas in time can become fibrotic, creating the so-called *cardiac sclerosis.*

KIDNEYS. Congestion of the kidneys is more marked with right-sided heart failure than with left-sided failure, leading to greater fluid retention, peripheral edema, and more pronounced azotemia.

PORTAL SYSTEM OF DRAINAGE. Right-sided heart failure leads to elevated pressure in the portal vein and its tributaries. Splenic congestion produces a tense, enlarged spleen. Microscopically there may be marked sinusoidal dilatation, accompanied by areas of recent hemorrhage. With long-standing congestion, the enlarged spleen may achieve a weight of 500 to 600 gm (normal, approximately 150 gm), and the long-standing edema may produce fibrous thickening of the sinusoidal walls, to create the firm organ characteristic of *congestive splenomegaly.* In addition, abnormal accumulations of transudate in the peritoneal cavity may give rise to *ascites.*

SUBCUTANEOUS TISSUES. Peripheral edema of dependent portions of the body, especially ankle edema, is a hallmark of right-sided failure. In severe or long-standing cases, edema may be quite massive and generalized, a condition termed *anasarca.*

PLEURAL AND PERICARDIAL SPACES. Effusions may appear, particularly in the right thoracic cavity.

BRAIN. Symptoms essentially identical to those described in left-sided failure may occur, representing venous congestion and hypoxia of the central nervous system.

The effects of pure left-sided heart failure are largely due to pulmonary congestion and edema. Right-sided heart failure induces essentially a systemic (and secondary portal) venous congestive syndrome, with hepatic and splenic enlargement, peripheral edema, pleural and pericardial effusions, and ascites. In contrast to left-sided failure, respiratory symptoms may be absent or quite insignificant in right-sided failure. *In many cases of frank chronic cardiac decompensation, however, the patient presents with the picture of full-blown CHF, encompassing the clinical syndromes of both right-sided and left-sided heart failure.*

TYPES OF HEART DISEASE

Heart disease is the predominant cause of disability and death in all industrialized nations. In the United States, it accounts currently for about 750,000 deaths annually, nearly half of the total mortality and more than 1½ times the number of deaths caused by all forms of cancer together. In the United States, the yearly economic burden of ischemic heart disease, the most prevalent subgroup, is estimated to be in excess of $100 billion.

Four categories of disease account for about 85 to 90% of all cardiac deaths: (1) ischemic heart disease; (2) hypertensive heart disease and pulmonary hypertensive heart disease (cor pulmonale); (3) certain valvular diseases—calcific aortic valve stenosis, mitral valve prolapse, infective endocarditis, and rheumatic heart disease; and (4) congenital heart disease. Ischemic heart disease is responsible for the great majority of these deaths and is considered first.

ISCHEMIC HEART DISEASE

Ischemic heart disease (IHD) is the generic designation for a group of closely related syndromes resulting from *ischemia*—an imbalance between the supply and demand of the heart for oxygenated blood. Ischemia comprises not only insufficiency of oxygen *(hypoxia, anoxia)*, but also reduced availability of nutrient substrates and inadequate removal of metabolites (see Chapter 1). Because coronary artery narrowing or obstruction owing to atherosclerosis underlies myocardial ischemia in the vast majority of cases, IHD is often termed *coronary artery disease* (CAD) or *coronary heart disease* (CHD).

The heart may suffer a deficiency of perfusion whenever an increase in demand (e.g., increased heart rate) outpaces the supply of blood, but *in more than 90% of cases, the cause is reduction in coronary blood flow.* Systemic hemodynamic deterioration (e.g., shock) or some form of nonatherosclerotic coronary disease can contribute to the perfusion deficit. Diminished oxygen transport of the blood (e.g., cyanotic congenital heart disease, severe anemia, or advanced lung disease) results in hypoxia but generally not ischemia. As implied earlier, pure hypoxia is a less deleterious condition than ischemia because perfusion (including metabolic substrate delivery and waste removal) is maintained in isolated hypoxia.

Depending on the rate of development and ultimate severity of the arterial narrowing(s) and the myocardial response, four ischemic syndromes may result: (1) *angina pectoris*, of which there are three variants, the most threatening being unstable angina; (2) *myocardial infarction*, the most important form of IHD, in which there can be substantial myocardial damage; (3) *chronic ischemic heart disease* with CHF; and (4) *sudden cardiac death*. Because there is usually a long period (decades) of silent, slowly progressive, coronary atherosclerosis, before any of these overt disorders become manifest, *the syndromes of IHD are only the late manifestations of coronary atherosclerosis that likely began during childhood* (see Chapter 11).

EPIDEMIOLOGY. IHD, in its various forms, is the leading cause of death in the United States and other industrialized nations, accounting for about 80% of all cardiac mortality. Annually IHD causes approximately 600,000 deaths (one-third of all deaths), and about 5 million Americans are diagnosed with IHD. Awesome as these data may be, they represent an improvement over those that prevailed several decades ago. Since 1968, the overall death rate from IHD has fallen in the United States by almost 40%, owing to both (1) prevention achieved by changed lifestyles that modify determinants of risk, such as smoking, elevated blood cholesterol, hypertension, and a sedentary lifestyle, and (2) therapeutic advances, for example, use of new medications, coronary care units, coronary bypass surgery, and improved control of arrhythmias.[14] Potentially there can be additional risk reduction associated with maintenance of normal blood glucose levels in diabetic patients, postmenopausal estrogen replacement therapy, and aspirin prophylaxis in middle-aged men.[15] Postinfarction thrombolysis and percutaneous transluminal coronary angioplasty (PTCA) are additional important therapeutic improvements (see Chapter 11), the long-term impact of which is not yet established.

OVERALL PATHOGENESIS. Although some instances may be related to increased myocardial demand or reduced oxygen-carrying capacity of the blood, *the dominant influence in the causation of the IHD syndromes is diminished coronary perfusion relative to myocardial demand, owing largely to a complex dynamic interaction among fixed atherosclerotic narrowing of the epicardial coronary arteries, intraluminal thrombosis overlying a ruptured or fissured atherosclerotic plaque, platelet aggregation, and vasospasm.* Although there are still some areas of uncertainty, the following observations are reasonably well established.

Role of Fixed Coronary Obstructions. More than 90% of patients with IHD have advanced stenosing coronary atherosclerosis ("fixed" obstructions). Most have one or more lesions causing at least 75% reduction of the cross-sectional area of at least one of the major epicardial arteries, a level of obstruction at which the augmented coronary flow provided by compensatory vasodilation is no longer sufficient to meet even moderate increases in myocardial demand.

Although only a single major coronary epicardial trunk may be affected, more often two or all three—left anterior descending (LAD), left circumflex (LCX), and right coronary (RC) arteries—are involved (Fig. 12–2). Clinically significant stenosing plaques may be located anywhere within the three major vessels but tend to predominate within the first 2 cm of the LAD and LCX arteries and the proximal and distal thirds of the RC artery. Sometimes the major secondary (but still epicardial) branches are also involved (i.e., diagonal branches of the LAD, obtuse marginal branches of the LCX, or posterior descending branch of the RC). *The hemodynamic impact of stenoses, however, and thus the onset and prognosis of IHD and other complications of atherosclerosis do not entirely depend on the extent and severity of fixed, chronic anatomic disease. Additionally, dynamic changes in*

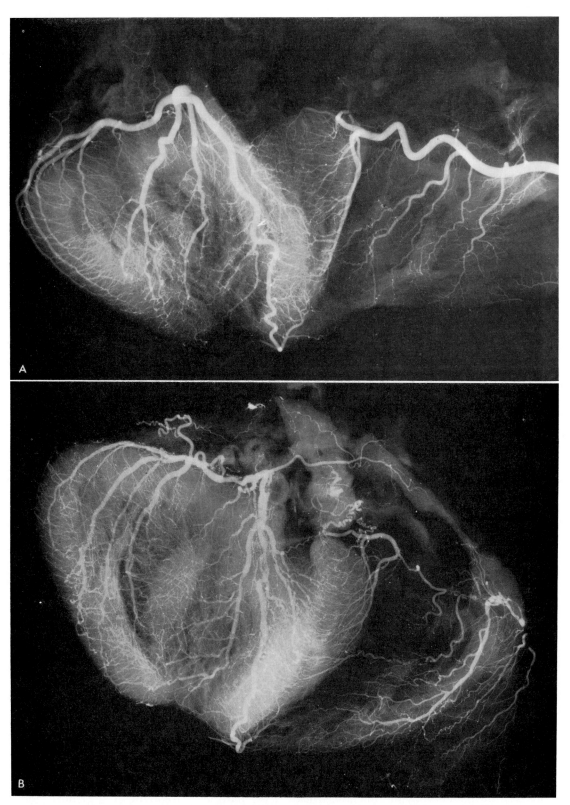

Figure 12–2. Angiographic appearance of coronary arteries without and with coronary artery disease. *A*, Angiogram (radiograph of heart injected via the coronary arteries with radiopaque dye) of open heart with normal coronary arteries filling completely with dye. On the right is the horizontal main right coronary artery coming from right to left, eventually becoming the vertical posterior descending coronary artery near the center of the photograph. At top left is the short left main coronary artery. The left anterior descending artery runs nearly vertically in the center of the photograph from the left main, ultimately anastomosing distally with the posterior descending coronary artery branch from the right. The horizontal branch running to the left from the left main is the left circumflex coronary artery. Between the anterior descending and the circumflex arteries are several large diagonal branches arising proximally from the left anterior descending. The vessels show progressively diminishing lumina with no irregular narrowings or obstruction. *B*, Angiogram of an open heart with coronary arteries severely narrowed by atherosclerosis. The right coronary artery fails to fill over much of its length, but twigs of this vessel are filled by retrograde anastomotic collaterals. There is uneven narrowing and tortuosity of both left anterior descending and circumflex coronary arteries. Compare with *A*.

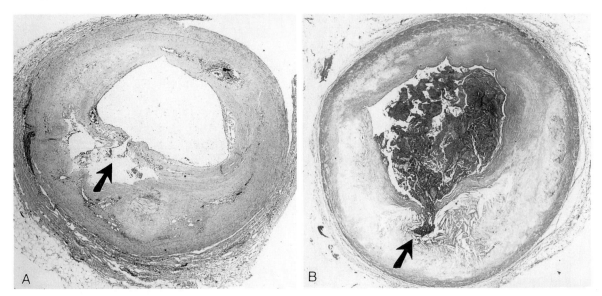

Figure 12–3. Atherosclerotic plaque rupture. *A,* Plaque rupture, without superimposed thrombus, in patient having sudden cardiac death. *B,* Acute coronary thrombosis superimposed on a ruptured atherosclerotic plaque, triggering fatal myocardial infarction. In both *A* and *B,* an arrow points to the site of plaque rupture. (*B,* reproduced from Schoen, F.J.: Interventional and Surgical Cardiovascular Pathology: Clinical Correlations and Basic Principles. Philadelphia, W.B. Saunders Co., 1989, p. 61.)

coronary plaque morphology (to be discussed) play a critical role in the natural history.

Role of Acute Plaque Change. *Acute myocardial ischemia is often precipitated by disruption of previously only partially stenosing atherosclerotic plaques with hemorrhage, fissuring, or ulceration. Such vascular injury is fundamental to the development of the acute coronary syndromes—unstable angina, acute myocardial infarction, or sudden ischemic death—in most patients* (Figs. 12–3 and 12–4).[16-18] High-grade but slowly developing occlusions probably stimulate well-developed collateral vessels over time that may protect against infarction. *Thus in many patients, acute ischemic events are a complication not of the most complete stenoses but result from a catastrophic disruption of a moderately stenotic (usually 50 to 75%), lipid-rich plaque, which itself was insufficient to induce stable angina before disruption. This is often followed by mural or total thrombosis.*

Accumulating evidence indicates that the intraluminal thrombotic process resulting from plaque disruption is dynamic and repetitive. Fissuring of coronary atherosclerotic plaque was present in 9% of patients dying of noncardiac causes in one study.[19] Indeed, subsequent fibrotic organization of the fragmented plaque and overlying thrombosis is an important mechanism of progression and growth of atherosclerotic lesions in many cases. Most fissures probably reseal and incorporate thrombus at the same time but do not produce clinical symptoms.

The factors that trigger acute plaque change are uncertain, but influences both extrinsic and in-

trinsic to the plaque are likely important. An episode of vasospasm that fractures a calcific plaque, tachycardia imposing physical stresses, hypercholesterolemia, and intraplaque hemorrhage are possible contributors. Interestingly there is a pronounced circadian periodicity for the time of onset of acute myocardial infarction and other acute coronary syndromes, with a peak incidence at 9 to 11 A.M., concurrent with a surge in blood pressure and immediately following heightened platelet reactivity.[20] Stresses produced by blood flow or coronary intraluminal pressure or tone in areas of stenosis may also contribute to tearing of the plaque.

The structural features of plaques may contribute to the propensity to disruption. Lesions that rupture characteristically have a markedly eccentric configuration (in which the plaque is not uniform around the vessel circumference), a large, soft core of necrotic debris and lipid, covered by a thin fibrous cap. Fissures frequently occur at the junction of the fibrous cap with the adjacent normal arterial wall (plaque-free segment), a location associated with high circumferential stress.[21]

Role of Coronary Thrombus. Coronary thrombosis, partial or total, plays a critical role in acute coronary syndromes. In myocardial infarction, the added thrombus converts a disrupted, partially stenotic plaque to a complete stenosis. In unstable angina, transient mural thrombosis occurs close to the time of chest pain, and there is a temporal relation between chest pain and measured increases in the transcardiac concentrations of thromboxane A_2 and other platelet contents. This indicates transient or labile platelet activation, se-

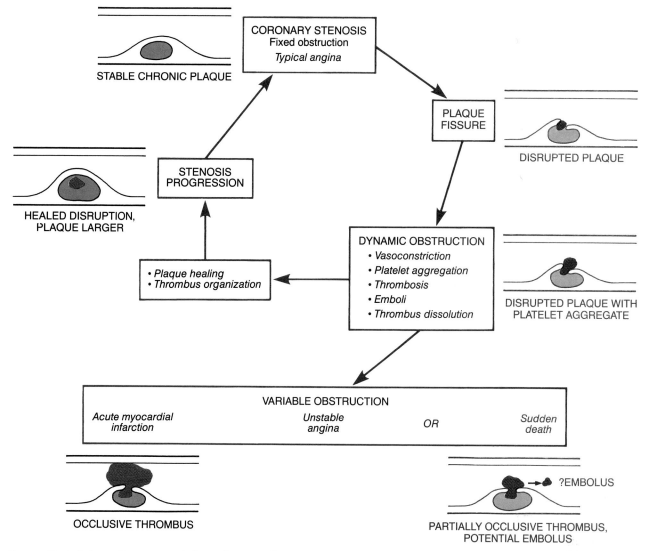

Figure 12–4. Schematic representation of sequential progression of coronary artery lesion morphology, beginning with stable chronic plaque responsible for typical angina and leading to the various acute coronary syndromes. (Modified and redrawn from Schoen, F.J.: Interventional and Surgical Cardiovascular Pathology: Clinical Correlations and Basic Principles. Philadelphia, W.B. Saunders Co., 1989, p. 63.)

cretion, and aggregation[22] and suggests increased thromboxane A_2 and other mediators at sites of plaque disruption, probably promoting further platelet aggregation and vasoconstriction. In unstable angina, thrombus has actually been observed directly through angioscopes, fiberoptic catheters that are threaded into the coronary arteries.[23] In such patients, small fragments of thrombotic material are found in the distal intramyocardial circulation with associated microinfarcts frequently noted, suggesting that intermittent fragmentation of thrombus can lead to embolic vascular occlusion in some patients. Thus mural thrombus not only encroaches into the vessel lumen to impair flow, but also can serve as a powerfully thrombogenic substrate and can embolize. Finally, thrombus is a potent activator of multiple growth-related signals in smooth muscle cells; both platelet-mediated and

smooth muscle cell–mediated events contribute to the growth of atherosclerotic lesions (see Chapter 11).

Role of Vasoconstriction. Transient vasoconstriction may be induced at a site of plaque disruption and thrombosis. This occurs in large part because normal endothelial cell elaboration of relaxing factors may be impaired relative to secretion of contracting factors.

Thus, as summarized here and in Table 12–3, the acute coronary syndromes of unstable angina, acute myocardial infarction, and sudden death (discussed later) share a common pathophysiologic basis, with coronary atherosclerotic plaque rupture as the pathologic hallmark and associated intraluminal platelet-fibrin thrombus. Typical angina com-

Table 12-3. CORONARY ARTERY PATHOLOGY IN ISCHEMIC HEART DISEASE

SYNDROME	PATHOLOGY
Stable angina	>75% stenoses
Unstable angina	Plaque rupture with mural thrombus, often thromboemboli
Myocardial infarction	Plaque rupture, complete thrombosis
Sudden death	Severe multivessel disease, often plaque rupture, often thrombus or thromboemboli

monly results from increases in myocardial oxygen demand that outstrip the ability of markedly stenosed coronary arteries to increase oxygen delivery. In unstable angina, a relatively small fissure or disruption of an atherosclerotic plaque may lead to a sudden change in plaque morphology, with platelet aggregation or mural thrombus and frequently vasoconstriction leading to transient reduction in coronary blood flow. In some cases, distal microinfarcts occur secondary to thromboemboli. Moreover, in myocardial infarction, plaque disruption induces thrombotic occlusion. Sudden coronary death frequently involves a rapidly progressing coronary lesion, in which plaque disruption and often partial thrombus (and possibly embolization) lead to regional myocardial ischemia that induces a fatal ventricular arrhythmia.

ANGINA PECTORIS

Angina pectoris is a symptom complex of IHD characterized by paroxysmal attacks of substernal or precordial chest discomfort (variously described as constricting, squeezing, choking, or knife-like) caused by transient (15 seconds to 15 minutes) myocardial ischemia that falls short of inducing the cellular necrosis that defines infarction. There are three overlapping patterns of angina pectoris: (1) stable or typical angina, (2) Prinzmetal's or variant angina, and (3) unstable or crescendo angina. They are caused by varying combinations of increased myocardial demand and decreased myocardial perfusion, owing to fixed stenosing plaques, disrupted plaques, vasospasm, thrombosis, platelet aggregation, and embolization. Episodes occur in a specific patient at various levels of exertion at different times. Moreover, it is being increasingly recognized that not all ischemic events are perceived by patients, even though such events may have adverse prognostic implications (silent ischemia).[24]

Stable angina, the most common form and therefore called typical angina pectoris, is characteristically associated with electrocardiographic ST segment depression because ischemia is most intense in the poorly perfused subendocardial region of the left ventricular myocardium. The pathogenesis of typical angina pectoris appears to be the reduction of coronary perfusion to a critical level by chronic stenosing coronary atherosclerosis; this renders the heart vulnerable to further ischemia whenever there is increased demand, such as that produced by physical activity, emotional excitement, or any other cause of increased cardiac workload. Typical angina pectoris is generally relieved by rest (thereby decreasing demand) or nitroglycerin, a strong vasodilator (thereby increasing supply). In particular instances, vasospasm may contribute to the imbalance between supply and demand.

Prinzmetal's variant angina refers to a pattern of episodic angina that occurs at rest and has been documented to be due to coronary artery spasm. Usually there is elevation of the ST segment (in contrast to the ST segment depression in typical angina), indicative of transmural ischemia. Although individuals with this form of angina may well have significant coronary atherosclerosis, the anginal attacks are generally unrelated to physical activity, heart rate, or blood pressure. Prinzmetal's angina generally responds promptly to vasodilators, such as nitroglycerin and calcium channel blockers.

Unstable or crescendo angina refers to a pattern of pain that occurs with progressively increasing frequency, is precipitated with progressively less effort, often occurs at rest, and tends to be of prolonged duration. The ischemia that occurs in unstable angina falls precariously short of inducing infarction, and so this syndrome is sometimes referred to as preinfarction angina or acute coronary insufficiency.

In most patients, unstable angina is induced by fissuring, ulceration, or rupture of an atherosclerotic plaque with superimposed partial (mural) thrombosis and possibly embolization or vasospasm (or both). Although ischemia is usually transient and incomplete and involves only a small region of myocardium, microinfarcts may occur. As discussed earlier, platelet activation and aggregation are largely responsible by causing thrombus formation and potentiating vasospasm. Moreover, unstable angina forewarns of the possibility of subsequent acute myocardial infarction. Thus in the spectrum of IHD, unstable angina lies intermediate between stable angina on the one hand and myocardial infarction on the other.

MYOCARDIAL INFARCTION

Acute myocardial infarction, also known as "heart attack," is overwhelmingly the most important form of IHD in industrialized nations and alone is the leading cause of death in the United States and elsewhere. About 1.5 million individuals in the United States suffer an acute myocardial infarction annually, of which approximately 500,000 are hospitalized.

TRANSMURAL VERSUS SUBENDOCARDIAL INFARCTION. *There are two types of myocardial infarction, each having differing morphology and clinical significance.* The more common type is the *transmural infarct,* in which the ischemic necrosis involves the full or nearly full thickness of the ventricular wall in the distribution of a single coronary artery. This pattern of infarction is usually associated with coronary atherosclerosis, plaque rupture, and superimposed thrombosis. In contrast, *subendocardial (nontransmural) infarct* constitutes an area of ischemic necrosis limited to the inner one-third or at most one-half of the ventricular wall, often extending laterally beyond the perfusion territory of a single coronary artery. As previously pointed out, the subendocardial zone is normally the least well-perfused region of myocardium and therefore most vulnerable to any reduction in coronary flow. In the great majority of subendocardial infarcts, there is diffuse stenosing coronary atherosclerosis and global reduction of coronary flow but *neither* plaque rupture *nor* superimposed thrombosis. The two types of infarcts, however, are closely interrelated because, in experimental models and likely in humans, the transmural infarct begins with a zone of subendocardial necrosis that extends in a "wave-front" across the full thickness of the ventricular wall (see later). Therefore a subendocardial infarct can occur as a result of a plaque rupture followed by coronary thrombus that becomes lysed before myocardial necrosis extends across the major thickness of the wall.

In the past, an acute myocardial infarct diagnosed by enzyme elevation or other clinical criteria in which Q waves failed to develop on the electrocardiogram was considered a subendocardial infarct. The presence or absence of Q waves, however, does not reliably predict the distinction between transmural and subendocardial myocardial infarction, as determined at autopsy. Many patients with transmural infarcts have no Q waves and vice versa. Nevertheless, there is a useful prognostic distinction between acute myocardial infarction with or without Q waves. The acute mortality in patients with non–Q wave infarcts (which tend to be smaller and only infrequently are associated with total occlusions of the infarct-related vessel) is half that in patients with Q-wave infarcts. Despite a low early mortality rate, however, patients with non–Q wave infarcts have a risk of later infarction and a high late mortality rate. Thus the non–Q wave infarct can be an unstable rather than a completely benign condition.

INCIDENCE AND RISK FACTORS. The risk factors for atherosclerosis, the major underlying cause of IHD in general, are discussed in Chapter 11 and are not reiterated here. Suffice it to say that *myocardial infarction may occur at virtually any age, but the frequency rises progressively with increasing age.* Myocardial infarction may occur in the very

elderly as well as in younger individuals, even in the first three decades of life, particularly when such predispositions to atherosclerosis as hypertension, cigarette smoking, diabetes mellitus, genetic hypercholesterolemia, and other causes of hyperlipoproteinemia are present. Five per cent of myocardial infarcts occur in people under age 40 years, and 45% occur under age 65. Blacks and whites are affected equally often. Throughout life, men are at significantly greater risk of myocardial infarction than women, the differential progressively declining with advancing age. *Except for those having some predisposing atherogenic condition, women are remarkably protected against myocardial infarction during reproductive life.* The use of oral contraceptives, *as formulated in the past,* increased the risk of myocardial infarction, especially in smokers older than age 35. Newer formulations have markedly reduced estrogen content with consequent reduced risk at all ages. Moreover, epidemiologic evidence strongly suggests that estrogen replacement therapy protects postmenopausal women against myocardial infarction through favorable adjustment of risk factors.[25]

PATHOGENESIS. We now consider the basis for and subsequent consequences of myocardial ischemia, particularly as they relate to the transmural infarct.

Coronary Arterial Occlusion. *As previously described, at least 90% of transmural acute myocardial infarcts are caused by an occlusive intracoronary thrombus overlying an ulcerated or fissured stenotic plaque.* In addition, increased myocardial demand, as with tachycardia, or hemodynamic compromise, such as a drop in blood pressure, can worsen the situation and frequently constitutes the final blow in an already precarious situation. Recall that occlusive thrombosis may occur in markedly atherosclerotic coronary arteries without inducing infarction, owing to intercommunications between major epicardial trunks and their ramifications *(collateral circulation),* which may expand to provide perfusion from a relatively unobstructed trunk. Despite all these variables, *until proved otherwise in a specific case, behind every acute transmural myocardial infarct, a dynamic interaction has occurred among several or all of the following: severe coronary atherosclerosis, an acute atheromatous plaque change (fissuring, ulceration), superimposed thrombosis, platelet activation, and vasospasm.*

In the typical case, the following sequence of events can be proposed:

- The initial event is a sudden change in the morphology of an atheromatous plaque, i.e., intraplaque hemorrhage, ulceration, or fissuring.
- Platelets are exposed to subendothelial collagen and necrotic plaque contents, leading to adhesion, aggregation, activation, and release of adenosine diphosphate (ADP), a potent platelet

aggregator, with buildup of a platelet mass. The platelet mass may give rise to emboli or potentiate occlusive thrombosis.

- Simultaneously tissue thromboplastin is released, activating the extrinsic pathway of coagulation.
- Adherent activated platelets release thromboxane A_2, serotonin, and platelet factors 3 and 4, predisposing to coagulation, favoring vasospasm, and adding to the bulk of the thrombus.
- Frequently within minutes, the thrombus evolves to become completely occlusive.

DeWood and coworkers demonstrated that when coronary angiography was performed within 4 hours of the onset of apparent myocardial infarction, a thrombosed coronary artery was found in almost 90% of cases.[26] The incidence of acute occlusion, however, fell to about 60% when angiography was delayed until 12 to 24 hours after onset. Thus with the passage of time, at least some occlusions appear to clear spontaneously because of lysis of the thrombus or relaxation of spasm or a combination of the two. Numerous subsequent studies of therapeutic thrombolysis using intravenous or intracoronary infusion of fibrinolysins have implied the presence of thrombi by restoring flow to obstructed vessels in 75 to 95% of recent myocardial infarcts.[27] Thus there can be little doubt about the importance of thrombosis in the induction of most acute myocardial infarcts, and nearly all thrombi are initiated by acute plaque changes.

In the approximately 10% of cases of transmural acute myocardial infarction unassociated with atherosclerotic thrombosis, mechanisms other than thrombotic occlusion may be involved:

- In about one-third of these cases, the coronary arteries are free of atherosclerosis by angiography.
- Vasospasm with or without coronary atherosclerosis may induce the acute perfusion deficit, perhaps in association with platelet aggregation.
- Emboli from a left-sided mural thrombosis or vegetative endocarditis or paradoxic emboli from the right side of the heart or the peripheral veins (through a patent foramen ovale) could cause coronary occlusion.

Myocardial Response. *Occlusion of a major coronary artery results in ischemia throughout the anatomic region supplied by that artery (called area at risk), most pronounced in the subendocardium* (Fig. 12–5). Acutely ischemic myocardium undergoes progressive biochemical, functional, and morphologic changes, the outcome of which largely depends on the severity and duration of flow deprivation. The principal biochemical consequence of myocardial ischemia is the onset of anaerobic glycolysis within seconds, leading to inadequate production of high-energy phosphates (e.g., creatine phosphate and adenosine triphosphate [ATP]) and accumulation of potentially noxious breakdown products (such as lactic acid). Myocardial function

is exceedingly sensitive to severe ischemia; striking loss of contractility is evident within 60 seconds of onset. Ultrastructural changes develop within a few minutes after onset of ischemia (e.g., cell and mitochondrial swelling, glycogen depletion). These early changes are reversible, and cell death is not immediate. As demonstrated experimentally in the dog, only severe ischemia lasting at least 20 to 40 minutes or longer leads to irreversible damage (necrosis) of some cardiac myocytes. Ultrastructural evidence of *irreversible* myocyte injury (primarily structural defects in the sarcolemmal membrane) develops after 20 to 40 minutes in severely ischemic myocardium (with blood flow of 10% or less of normal).[28] Microvascular injury follows. This time frame is summarized in Table 12–4.

Thus, although function becomes strikingly abnormal within 1 minute after onset of ischemia, myocardial coagulation necrosis occurs only after 20 to 40 minutes of severe ischemia (i.e., function is more sensitive to ischemia than myocyte viability). Classic acute myocardial infarction with extensive necrosis occurs when the perfusion of the myocardium is reduced severely below its needs for an extended interval (hours), causing profound, prolonged ischemia and resulting in permanent loss of function through cell death by coagulation necrosis. In contrast, if restoration of myocardial blood flow (i.e., *reperfusion*) follows briefer periods of flow deprivation (less than 20 minutes in the most severely ischemic myocardium), loss of cell viability generally does not result. Myocardial ischemia also contributes to arrhythmias. Sudden death, a leading cause of mortality in IHD patients, is usually due to ventricular fibrillation caused by myocardial irritability induced by ischemia or infarction. Interestingly, studies of resuscitated survivors of "sudden death" show that the majority do not develop acute myocardial infarction; in such cases, ischemia owing to severe chronic coronary arterial stenosis, and in many cases, acute plaque change with minimal thrombus presumably led directly to the fatal arrhythmia.

The progression of ischemic necrosis in the myocardium is summarized in Figure 12–6. Irreversible injury of ischemic myocytes occurs first in the subendocardial zone. With more extended ischemia, a *wavefront* of cell death moves through the myocardium to involve progressively more of the transmural thickness of the ischemic zone. The precise location, size, and specific morphologic features of an acute myocardial infarct depend on (1) the location, severity, and rate of development of coronary atherosclerotic obstructions; (2) the size of the vascular bed perfused by the obstructed vessels; (3) the duration of the occlusion; (4) the metabolic/oxygen needs of the myocardium at risk; (5) the extent of collateral blood vessels; (6) the presence, site, and severity of coronary arterial spasm; and (7) other factors, such as alterations in blood pressure, heart rate, and cardiac rhythm.

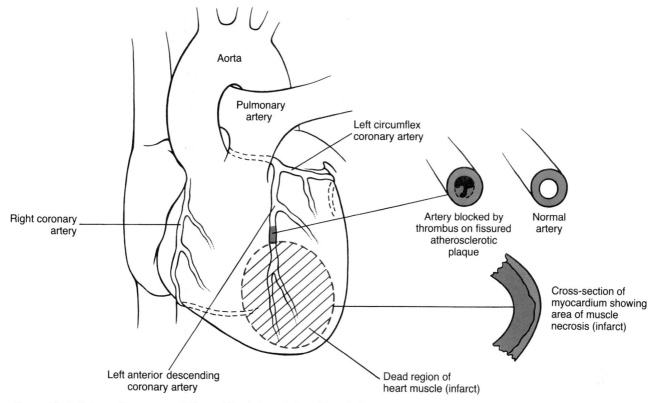

Labels in figure:
Aorta
Pulmonary artery
Left circumflex coronary artery
Artery blocked by thrombus on fissured atherosclerotic plaque
Normal artery
Right coronary artery
Cross-section of myocardium showing area of muscle necrosis (infarct)
Left anterior descending coronary artery
Dead region of heart muscle (infarct)

Figure 12–5. Schematic representation of the inter-relationship of chronic atherosclerotic obstruction *(pink)*, acute plaque change, superimposed thrombus *(black)*, and myocardial injury in acute myocardial infarction.

The extent of necrosis is largely complete within 3 to 6 hours in experimental models, involving nearly all of the ischemic myocardial bed at risk supplied by the occluded coronary artery. Progression of necrosis, however, frequently follows a more protracted course in humans, in whom the coronary arterial collateral system, stimulated by chronic ischemia, is probably better developed and thereby more effective.

MORPHOLOGY. Virtually all transmural infarcts involve at least a portion of the left ventricle (including the interventricular septum).[29] About 15 to 30% of those that affect the posterior free wall and posterior portion of the septum transmurally extend into the adjacent right ventricular wall. Isolated infarction of the right ventricle, however, occurs in only 1 to 3% of cases. Atrial infarction can be found in 5 to 10% of cases of acute myocardial infarction, most often in conjunction with a large posterior left ventricular infarct.

Transmural infarcts usually encompass nearly the entire perfusion zone of the occluded coronary artery but may involve the entire circumference of the left ventricle. Almost always there is a narrow rim (approximately 0.1 mm) of preserved subendocardial myocardium sustained by diffusion of oxygen/nutrients from the lumen. In the unusual instance that the coronary arteries may appear entirely normal despite careful analysis, it is presumed that the causal mechanism was vasospasm or a lysed thrombus. The frequencies of critical narrowing (and thrombosis) of each of the three main arterial trunks and the corresponding sites of myocardial lesions (in the typical right dominant heart) are as follows:

Left anterior descending coronary artery (40 to 50%) — Anterior wall of left ventricle near apex; anterior two-thirds of interventricular septum

Table 12–4. APPROXIMATE TIME OF ONSET OF KEY EVENTS IN ISCHEMIC CARDIAC MYOCYTES

FEATURE	TIME
Onset of ATP depletion	Seconds
Loss of contractility	< 2 min
ATP reduced	
to 50% of normal	10 min
to 10% of normal	40 min
Irreversible cell injury	20–40 min
Microvascular injury	>1 hr

ATP = Adenosine triphosphate.

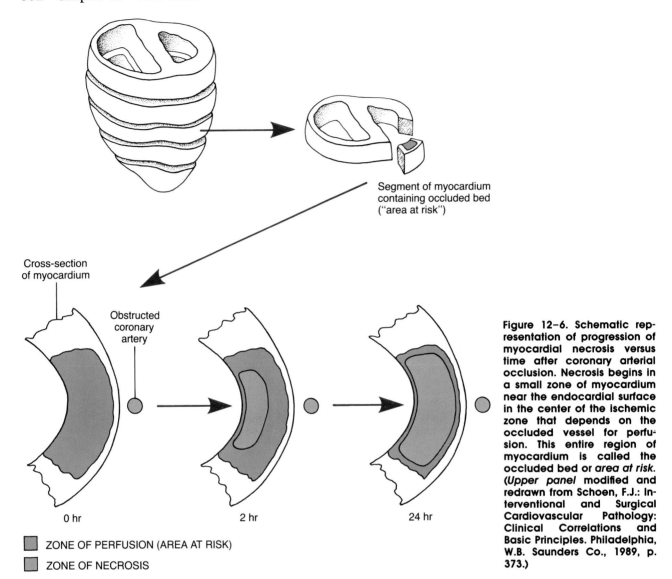

Segment of myocardium
containing occluded bed
("area at risk")

Cross-section
of myocardium

Obstructed
coronary
artery

0 hr   2 hr   24 hr

ZONE OF PERFUSION (AREA AT RISK)

ZONE OF NECROSIS

Figure 12–6. Schematic representation of progression of myocardial necrosis versus time after coronary arterial occlusion. Necrosis begins in a small zone of myocardium near the endocardial surface in the center of the ischemic zone that depends on the occluded vessel for perfusion. This entire region of myocardium is called the occluded bed or *area at risk.* **(***Upper panel* **modified and redrawn from Schoen, F.J.: Interventional and Surgical Cardiovascular Pathology: Clinical Correlations and Basic Principles. Philadelphia, W.B. Saunders Co., 1989, p. 373.)**

Right coronary artery (30 to 40%)	Inferior/posterior wall of left ventricle; posterior one-third of interventricular septum; posterior right ventricular free wall in some cases
Left circumflex coronary artery (15 to 20%)	Lateral wall of left ventricle

Other locations of critical coronary arterial lesions causing infarcts are sometimes encountered, such as the left mainstem coronary artery or the secondary branches (e.g., diagonal branches of the left anterior descending artery or marginal branches of the circumflex artery). In contrast, stenosing atherosclerosis or thrombosis of a penetrating intramyocardial branch of the epicardial trunks is almost never encountered. Occasionally

the observation of multiple severe stenoses or thromboses in the absence of myocardial infarction indicates that intercoronary collaterals likely provided sufficient flow to prevent ischemic necrosis.

Several infarcts of varying age in the same heart are frequently found. Repetitive necrosis of adjacent regions yields progressive **extension** of an individual infarct over a period of days to weeks— "stuttering infarct." Examination of the heart in such cases often reveals a central zone of infarction that is days to weeks older than a peripheral margin of more recent ischemic necrosis. An initial infarct may extend because of retrograde propagation of a thrombus, more proximal vasospasm, impaired cardiac contractility that renders flow through moderate stenoses critically insufficient, the development of platelet-fibrin microemboli, or the appearance of an arrhythmia that impairs cardiac function.

Areas of damage undergo a progressive se-

Table 12–5. RECOGNITION OF ACUTE MYOCARDIAL NECROSIS BY PATHOLOGIC METHODS

FEATURE	ONSET
Ultrastructural features of irreversible damage	20–40 min
Wavy fibers	1–3 hr
Staining defect with tetrazolium dye	2–3 hr
Classic histologic features of necrosis	4–12 hr
Gross alterations	12–24 hr

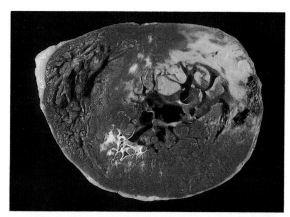

Figure 12–7. Acute myocardial infarct, predominantly of the posterolateral left ventricle, demonstrated histochemically by a lack of staining by the triphenyltetrazolium chloride stain in areas of necrosis. The staining defect is due to the enzyme leakage that follows cell death. The infarct is of approximately 4 days' duration, and transmural. Note the myocardial hemorrhage at one edge of the infarct that was associated with cardiac rupture, and the anterior scar (lower left), indicative of old infarct.

quence of changes that consist of typical ischemic coagulative necrosis, followed by inflammation and repair that parallels that occurring after injury at other, noncardiac sites. The appearance of an infarct at autopsy depends on the duration of survival of the patient following myocardial infarction onset.

Early recognition of acute myocardial infarcts by pathologists is a difficult problem, particularly when death has occurred within minutes to a few hours after the onset of the ischemic injury, because diagnostic morphologic changes lag behind the actual injury (Table 12–5). Myocardial infarcts less than 6 to 12 hours old are usually inapparent on gross examination. It is often possible, however, to highlight the area of necrosis by histochemical changes that first become apparent after 2 to 3 hours. Immersion of tissue slices in a solution of triphenyltetrazolium chloride (TTC) imparts a brick-red color to intact, noninfarcted myocardium where the dehydrogenase enzymes are preserved. Because dehydrogenases are depleted in the area of ischemic necrosis (i.e., they leak out through the damaged cell membranes), an infarcted area is revealed as an unstained pale zone (especially apparent after fixation, when unstained myocardium appears light brown) (Fig. 12–7). Thereafter the evolution of lesions is visible grossly. By 18 to 24 hours, the lesion can be identified in routinely fixed gross slices (including those not stained with TTC) because of either pallor or a red-blue hue owing to the stagnated, trapped blood. Progressively thereafter the infarct becomes a more sharply defined, yellow, somewhat softened area that by 10 days to 2 weeks is rimmed by a hyperemic zone of highly vascularized granulation tissue. Over the succeeding weeks, the injured region evolves to a fibrous scar.

The histopathologic changes also have a more or less predictable sequence (summarized in Fig. 12–8). Using light microscopy of sections stained by routine tissue stains, the typical microscopic changes of coagulative necrosis are not detectable for at least the first 4 to 12 hours. "Wavy fibers" may be present at the periphery of the infarct; it is thought that these changes result from the forceful systolic tugs by the viable fibers immediately adjacent to the noncontractile dead fibers, stretching and buckling them. An additional ischemic change

may be seen in the margins of infarcts: so-called vacuolar degeneration or **myocytolysis** comprising large vacuolar spaces within cells, containing water. This potentially reversible alteration is particularly frequent in the thin zone of viable subendocardial cells. Subendocardial myocyte vacuolization may be noted in the absence of an infarct, in which case it often signifies severe chronic ischemia.

The necrotic muscle elicits acute inflammation (typically most prominent at 2 to 3 days); thereafter macrophages remove the necrotic myocytes (most notable 5 to 10 days), and the damaged zone is progressively replaced by the ingrowth of highly vascularized granulation tissue (most prominent at 2 to 4 weeks), which progressively becomes less vascularized and more fibrous. In most instances, scarring is well advanced by the end of the sixth week, but the efficiency of repair depends on the size of the original lesion. A large infarct may not heal as readily as a small one. Once a lesion is well healed, it is impossible to distinguish its age (i.e., an 8-week-old and a 10-year-old lesion can look similar). The morphologic changes in myocardial infarction are summarized in Table 12–6.

The morphology of the subendocardial infarct is analogous qualitatively to that of transmural lesions. By definition, however, the areas of necrosis are limited to the inner third of the left ventricular wall. The lesion may be multifocal, cover an arc of the circumference of the left ventricle, or sometimes totally encircle it. The temporal sequence of macroscopic and microscopic changes already described for transmural myocardial infarctions follows, save that the changes in gross appearance may not be as sharply defined as in larger lesions.

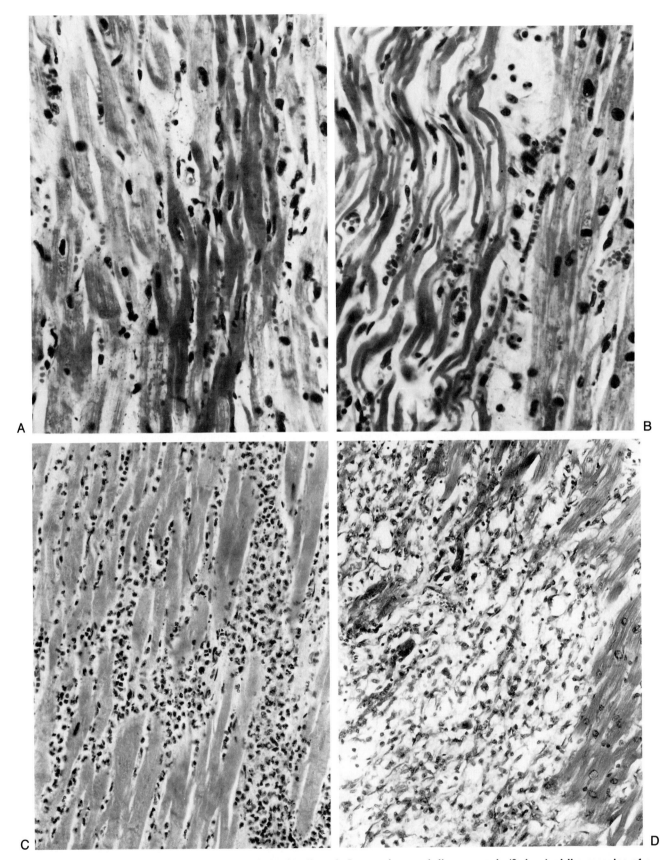

Figure 12–8. Microscopic features of myocardial infarction. *A,* Focus of coagulation necrosis (2 days) at the margins of a large infarct. Dark coagulated myofibers with preserved outlines contrast with surrounding viable normal myocardial cells. *B,* Wavy fibers in a 1-day-old infarct showing coagulative changes, elongation, and narrowing, compared with adjacent normal fibers. Widened spaces between the dead fibers contain edema fluid and scattered neutrophils. *C,* Dense polymorphonuclear leukocytic infiltrate in area of acute myocardial infarction of 3 to 4 days' duration. *D,* Nearly complete removal of necrotic myocytes by phagocytosis (approximately 7 to 10 days)

Illustration continued on following page

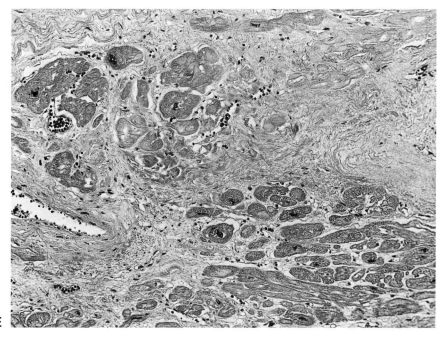

Figure 12–8. *(Continued)*. *E*, Well-healed myocardial infarct with replacement of the necrotic fibers by dense collagenous scar. A few residual cardiac muscle cells are present.

Morphologic complications following myocardial infarction include cardiac rupture, pericarditis, mural thrombosis, and aneurysm. These are discussed later in the context of clinical consequences.

INFARCT MODIFICATION BY THROMBOLYSIS. Thrombolytic therapy with various fibrinolytic agents such as streptokinase or tissue-type plasminogen activator (tPA) is often used (approximately 15% of all myocardial infarcts) in an attempt to dissolve the thrombus that initiated the infarct, to re-establish blood flow to the area at risk for infarction, and possibly to rescue the ischemic (but not yet necrotic) heart muscle (see Chapter 11). Thrombolysis re-establishes the patency of the occluded coronary artery in about 70%

of cases and significantly improves the survival rate. *Thrombolysis, however, can at best remove a thrombus occluding a coronary artery; insignificant changes take place in the underlying atherosclerotic plaque that initiated it.*

Because severe ischemia does not cause immediate cell death, even in the most severely affected regions of myocardium, and because not all regions of myocardium are equally ischemic, the outcome of reperfusing previously ischemic myocardium is complex. Reperfusion of myocardium sufficiently early (within 15 to 20 minutes) after onset of ischemia may prevent all necrosis. Reperfusion after a longer interval can salvage (i.e., prevent necrosis of) at least some myocytes that would have died with more prolonged or permanent ischemia.

Figure 12–9 illustrates the gross appearance of an infarct that has been reperfused. A partially completed then reperfused infarct is hemorrhagic

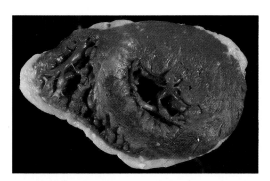

Figure 12–9. Gross appearance of myocardium modified by reperfusion. Large, densely hemorrhagic, anterior wall acute myocardial infarct from patient with left anterior descending (LAD) artery thrombus treated with streptokinase intracoronary thrombolysis (triphenyltetrazolium chloride (TTC)–stained heart slice).

535

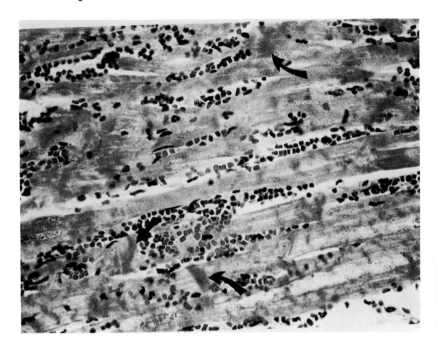

Figure 12-10. Myocardial necrosis with hemorrhage and contraction bands *(arrow)*, visible as dark bands spanning the myofibers. This is the characteristic appearance of reperfused, previously markedly ischemic myocardium.

Table 12-6. SEQUENCE OF CHANGES IN MYOCARDIAL INFARCTION

TIME	ELECTRON MICROSCOPE	HISTOCHEMISTRY	LIGHT MICROSCOPE	GROSS CHANGES
0–½ hr	*Reversible injury* Mitochondrial swelling; distortion of cristae; relaxation of myofibrils	↓Dehydrogenases ↓Oxidases ↓Phosphorylases ↓Glycogen ↓K and ↑ Na^+ and Ca^{++}		
1–2 hr	*Irreversible injury* Sarcolemmal disruption; mitochondrial amorphous densities		Waviness of fibers at border	
4–12 hr	Margination of nuclear chromatin		Beginning coagulation necrosis; edema; hemorrhage; beginning neutrophilic infiltrate	
18–24 hr			Continuing coagulation necrosis; pallor (pyknosis of nuclei, shrunken eosinophilic cytoplasm), marginal contraction band necrosis	Pallor
24–72 hr			Total coagulative necrosis with loss of nuclei and striations; heavy interstitial infiltrate of neutrophils	Pallor, sometimes hyperemia
3–7 days			Beginning disintegration of dead myofibers and resorption of sarcoplasm by macrophages; onset of marginal fibrovascular response	Hyperemic border, central yellow-brown softening
10 days			Well-developed phagocytosis; prominent granulation tissue with fibrovascular reaction in margins	Maximally yellow and soft vascularized margins, red-brown and depressed
7th wk				Scarring complete

because some vasculature injured during the period of ischemia becomes leaky on restoration of flow. Moreover, morphologic disintegration of myocytes that were critically damaged by the preceding ischemia is accentuated or accelerated by reperfusion. With early reperfusion of an area of ischemia, irreversibly injured myocytes often have *necrosis with contraction bands* (Fig. 12–10). Contraction bands are intensely eosinophilic transverse bands that span the involved myofibers. They are produced by hypercontraction of myofibrils in the dying cell that has damaged membranes after ischemia due to exposure to plasma calcium ions. Thus *reperfusion not only salvages reversibly injured cells, but also alters the morphology of cells already lethally injured at the time of reflow.*

Data suggest that the consequences of reperfusion can be altered by certain conditions in the myocardium that exist at reflow and that reperfusion of ischemic myocardium can result in some *new* cellular damage that blunts the beneficial effect of reperfusion itself.[30] Such damage is called *reperfusion injury* (defined as cell death induced by reperfusion of myocytes that were still viable before reperfusion—not accelerated disintegration by reperfusion of already dead myocytes). Reflow-mediated injury is most likely linked, at least in part, to the early generation of oxygen free radicals during reperfusion and is separate from the ischemic damage that occurs during the period of coronary artery occlusion.

Although most of the viable myocardium existing at the time of reflow ultimately recovers after alleviation of ischemia, critical abnormalities in cellular biochemistry and function of myocytes salvaged by reperfusion may persist for several days (prolonged postischemic ventricular dysfunction, or "stunned myocardium").[31] Recall that following the onset of ischemia, function becomes abnormal long before viability is lost (i.e., function is more sensitive to ischemia than viability). Although normal function is ultimately recovered, stunned myocardium may not be capable of sustaining life, and patients with large regions of dysfunctional myocardium may require mechanical circulatory assistance to survive until myocardium that was stunned regains adequate function. The several potential outcomes of irreversible and reversible ischemic myocardial injury are summarized in Figure 12–11.

CONSEQUENCES AND COMPLICATIONS OF MYOCARDIAL INFARCTION. The clinical diagnosis of acute myocardial infarction is mainly based on three sets of data: (1) symptoms, (2) electrocardiographic (ECG) changes, and (3) elevations of specific serum enzymes, although other diagnostic modalities are available (see subsequently). Typi-cally the onset is sudden and devastating with severe, substernal or precordial pain that often radiates to the left shoulder, arm, or jaw, often accompanied by sweating, nausea, vomiting, or breathlessness. Occasionally the clinical manifestations consist only of burning substernal or epigastric discomfort that is misinterpreted as "indigestion" or "heartburn." In about 10 to 15% of patients, the onset is entirely asymptomatic and the disease is discovered only later by ECG changes, usually consisting of new Q waves.

As mentioned earlier, soluble cytoplasmic enzymes leak out of fatally damaged myocardial cells. Elevations of serum enzymes, particularly creatine phosphokinase (CPK) and lactate dehydrogenase (LDH), are sensitive and reliable indicators of myocardial infarction. The CPK serum level rises above baseline within 4 to 8 hours and may peak very early or not for several days, falling to baseline in about 4 days. Substantial elevation of the MB isoenzyme of CPK (CPK-MB) is quite specific for myocardial infarction. Although trace amounts of CPK-MB are present in the small intestine, tongue, diaphragm, uterus, and prostate, diseases in these organs that might cause slight elevations of the MB isoenzyme are not likely to be confused with a myocardial infarction. The LDH level does not begin to rise until about 24 hours, peaks in 3 to 6 days, and may not return to normal until the end of the second week. Other diagnostic modalities such as echocardiography (for visualization of abnormalities of regional wall motion), radioisotopic studies (such as radionuclide angiography [for chamber configuration], perfusion scintigraphy [for regional perfusion]), and magnetic resonance imaging (for structural characterization) sometimes provide additional anatomic, biochemical, and functional data.

After the onset of an acute ischemic event, one of several pathways may be followed. Regrettably one is brief and marked by sudden cardiac death (SCD) within 1 to 2 hours (20% of patients), accounting for about half of all IHD deaths. If the patient with acute myocardial infarction reaches the hospital, the likelihood of the most serious complications is as follows:

- Uncomplicated cases (10 to 20% of cases).
- Complicated cases (80 to 90% of cases).

  - Cardiac arrhythmias (75 to 95% of complicated cases).
  - Left ventricular congestive failure and mild-to-severe pulmonary edema (60%).
  - Cardiogenic shock (10 to 15%).
  - Rupture of free wall, septum, or papillary muscle (1 to 5%).
  - Thromboembolism (15 to 40%).

Some important complications following myo-

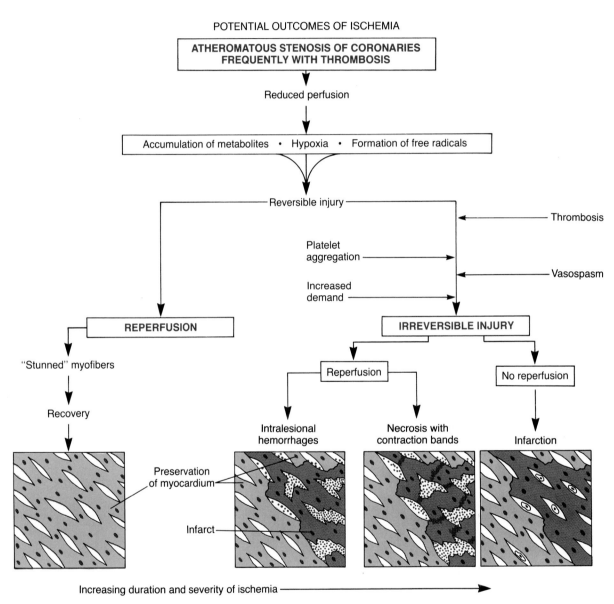

POTENTIAL OUTCOMES OF ISCHEMIA

Figure 12-11. Several potential outcomes of reversible and irreversible ischemic injury to the myocardium.

cardial infarction are illustrated in Figure 12–12. *Myocardial infarcts produce abnormalities in left ventricular function approximately proportional to their size.* Most often, there is some degree of left ventricular failure with hypotension, pulmonary vascular congestion, and transudation into the interstitial pulmonary spaces. Failure may be mild and transient or may progress to pose a serious threat when pulmonary edema causes marked respiratory embarrassment. Severe "pump failure" *(cardiogenic shock)*, which occurs in 10 to 15% of patients following myocardial infarction, generally indicates a large infarct (often greater than 40% of the left ventricle). Cardiogenic shock has a nearly 70% mortality rate and accounts for two-thirds of in-hospital deaths.

Many patients have conduction disturbances and myocardial irritability following myocardial infarction, which undoubtedly are responsible for many sudden deaths. They take the form of heart block, sinus bradycardia, sinus tachycardia, ventricular premature contractions or ventricular tachycardia, ventricular fibrillation, or asystole. Prompt intervention by mobile and hospital coronary care units has succeeded in controlling potentially lethal arrhythmias in many patients.

Were these hazards not enough, patients still confront the risks of myocardial rupture and mural thrombosis with peripheral embolization. Myocardial rupture frequently has catastrophic consequences. The *cardiac rupture syndromes* result from the mechanical weakening that occurs in necrotic and subsequently inflamed myocardium and include (1) rupture of the ventricular free wall (most commonly), usually with hemopericardium and cardiac tamponade (see Fig. 12–12A); (2) rupture of the interventricular septum (less commonly), leading to a left-to-right shunt; and (3) papillary muscle rupture (least commonly), resulting in the acute onset of severe acute mitral regurgitation. Cardiac rupture may occur at almost anytime after myocardial infarction but is most frequent approximately 4 to 7 days after onset. Mitral regurgitation after myocardial infarction is also frequently due to early ischemic dysfunction of a papillary muscle and underlying myocardium without rupture and later to papillary muscle fibrosis and shortening or ventricular dilatation.

A fibrinous or fibrinohemorrhagic *pericarditis* usually develops about the second or third day. It is most often localized to the region overlying the necrotic area and usually resolves with healing of the infarct. Pericarditis is the epicardial manifestation of the inflammation elicited by a direct underlying transmural infarct. Infarction of the right ventricular myocardium adjacent to the posterior left ventricle can yield serious functional impairment.

Infarct *extension*, defined by new necrosis adjacent to an existing infarct, discussed previously, should be distinguished from infarct *expansion*, defined by disproportionate stretching, thinning, and dilatation of the infarct region (often associated with mural thrombus). *Ventricular aneurysm* is a late complication that most commonly results from a large anteroseptal, transmural infarct that heals into a large area of thin scar tissue that paradoxically bulges during systole (see Fig. 12–12B). Early myocardial infarct expansion likely provides the substrate for scar thinning and late aneurysm formation. With any infarct, the combination of a local myocardial abnormality in contractility (causing stasis) with endocardial damage (causing a thrombogenic surface) can potentiate mural thrombosis (see Chapter 4) and thromboembolism.

The propensity toward specific complications and the prognosis after infarction depend primarily on myocardial infarct size, site, and transmural extent (i.e., the fractional thickness of the myocardial wall that is damaged—subendocardial or transmural). Large transmural infarcts yield a higher probability of cardiogenic shock, arrhythmias, and late congestive heart failure. Patients with anterior transmural infarcts are at greatest risk for regional dilatation, mural thrombi, and rupture and thus have a substantially worse clinical course than those with inferior (posterior) infarcts. In contrast, posterior transmural infarcts are more likely to be complicated by serious conduction blocks, right ventricular involvement, or both. Although mural thrombi may form on the endocardial surface of subendocardial infarcts, pericarditis, rupture, and ventricular aneurysms rarely occur.

Multiple dynamic structural changes maintain cardiac output after infarction.[32] Initially there is compensatory hypertrophy of noninfarcted myocardium, which is hemodynamically beneficial. Late decreases in ventricular performance, however, with depression of regional and global contractile function may occur owing to degenerative changes in viable myocardium (see section on cardiac hypertrophy, earlier in this chapter).

Short-term and long-term prognosis after myocardial infarction depends on many factors, the most important of which are the residual quality of left ventricular function and the extent of vascular obstructions in vessels that perfuse viable myocardium. The overall total mortality within the first year is about 35%, including those victims who die before reaching the hospital. The early mortality rate during hospitalization is approximately 10 to 15% and in the year following infarction is another 7 to 10%. Thereafter there is a 3 to 4% mortality among survivors with each passing year. Attempts to prevent infarction in those who have never ex-

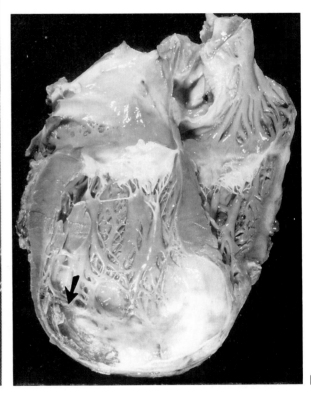

Figure 12-12. Complications of myocardial infarction. *A*, Anterior myocardial rupture in an acute infarct. *B*, Apical aneurysm with laminated mural thrombus *(arrow)* in remote infarct. In *B*, the left ventricle is on the left.

perienced a myocardial infarction through control of risk factors *(primary prevention)* or prevent reinfarction in those who have recovered from an acute myocardial infarction *(secondary prevention)* are active.

CHRONIC ISCHEMIC HEART DISEASE

The designation chronic ischemic heart disease (CIHD) is used here for the hearts in patients, often but not exclusively elderly, who insidiously develop CHF, sometimes fatal, as a consequence of ischemic myocardial damage. In most instances, there has been a history of angina and usually prior episodes of myocardial infarction, often as remote as 5 to 10 years before the onset of the CHF. In some individuals, however, progressive myocardial damage is entirely silent, and the first indication of IHD is CHF. Most cases of CIHD constitute simply

postinfarction cardiac decompensation based on inadequate or exhausted hypertrophy of noninfarcted viable myocardium that is itself in jeopardy of ischemic injury. The term *ischemic cardiomyopathy* is often used clinically to describe CIHD. Whatever the terminology, a significant number of individuals suffering from CIHD eventually die.

MORPHOLOGY. The pericardial surface of the heart in CIHD may have adhesions as a result of healing of pericarditis associated with past myocardial infarcts. Invariably there is moderate to severe stenosing atherosclerosis of the coronary arteries and sometimes total occlusions resulting from organized thrombi. Discrete, gray-white scars of healed previous infarcts are usually present. The mural endocardium is generally normal except for some superficial, patchy, fibrous thickenings. The major microscopic findings include diffuse myocardial atrophy and subendocardial vacuolization; diffuse, interstitial and patchy replacement fibrous tissue; and large healed scars of previous acute infarcts.

The clinical diagnosis of CIHD is made largely by the insidious onset of CHF in patients who have past episodes of myocardial infarction or anginal attacks. In some instances, CHF is the first manifestation of the progressive atherosclerotic encroachment on the cardiac reserve, and the diagnosis rests largely on the exclusion of other forms of cardiac involvement in patients of advanced age.

SUDDEN CARDIAC DEATH

Most commonly sudden cardiac death (SCD) is defined as unexpected death from cardiac causes early (usually within 1 hour) after or without the onset of symptoms. In the vast majority of cases in adults, SCD is a complication and often the first clinical manifestation of IHD. Less frequently SCD is caused by a congenital structural abnormality, aortic valve stenosis, hereditary or acquired abnormalities of the cardiac conduction system, mitral valve prolapse, myocarditis, or idiopathic dilated or hypertrophic cardiomyopathy. It is estimated that in the United States this catastrophe strikes about 300,000 to 400,000 individuals annually.

MORPHOLOGY. Marked coronary atherosclerosis with critical (greater than 75%) stenosis involving more than one of the three major vessels is present in 80 to 90% of victims; only 10 to 20% of cases are of nonatherosclerotic origin. Usually there are high-grade stenoses (greater than 90%). The precise frequency of **acute coronary changes** (i.e., thrombosis, plaque fissuring, intraplaque hemorrhage) has varied among the many relevant reports, but they were common (75 to 80%) in some.[33] A healed myocardial infarct is present in about 40%, but in those who have been rescued by prompt therapy from sudden cardiac arrest, new myocardial infarction is found in 25% or less.

The ultimate mechanism of death is almost always a lethal arrhythmia (e.g., asystole, ventricular fibrillation). Long-standing coronary atherosclerosis with diffuse myocardial atrophy, interstitial fibrosis, and possibly healed infarcts can impinge on the conduction system and create electromechanical cardiac instability. In most cases, however, acute myocardial ischemia with or without plaque fissuring or myocardial infarction induces irritability of myocardium distant from the conduction system and triggers the fatal arrhythmia, unrelated to the conduction system per se.

Data suggest that increased sympathetic stimulation may contribute to the triggering of SCD.[34] It thus appears that *SCD is a multifactorial catastrophe involving in most instances myocardial ischemia, often induced by an acute coronary artery change superimposed on the substrate of advanced coronary atherosclerosis, and complicated by other factors favoring generation of a serious arrhythmia in severely ischemic myocardium.*

HYPERTENSIVE HEART DISEASE

Hypertensive heart disease (HHD) is the response of the heart to the increased demands induced by systemic or pulmonary hypertension.

SYSTEMIC (LEFT-SIDED) HYPERTENSIVE HEART DISEASE

The minimal criteria for the diagnosis of systemic HHD are the following: (1) left ventricular hypertrophy (usually concentric) in the absence of other cardiovascular pathology that might have induced it and (2) a history of hypertension.[35] In addition, because hypertension strongly predisposes to atherosclerosis, most patients with elevated blood pressure have coronary atherosclerosis. Notwithstanding, the Framingham Study established unequivocally that even mild hypertension (levels only slightly above 140/90 mm Hg), if sufficiently prolonged, induces left ventricular hypertrophy. Approximately 25% of the population of the United States suffers from hypertension of this degree, making systemic HHD the second most common form of cardiac disease. The pathogenesis of hypertension is discussed in Chapter 11. In hypertension, hypertrophy of the heart is an adaptive response to pressure overload but can lead to myocardial dysfunction, cardiac dilatation, and ultimately CHF (see section on cardiac hypertrophy, earlier in this chapter).

MORPHOLOGY. Because systemic hypertension induces left ventricular pressure overload, the essential morphologic evidence of compensated left-sided HHD is hypertrophy without dilatation (concentric hypertrophy) of the left ventricle without other lesions that might account for it (e.g., aortic valve stenosis or coarctation of the aorta). The thickening of the left ventricular wall is symmetric, increases the ratio of wall thickness to radius of ventricular chamber, and increases the weight of the heart disproportionately to the increase in overall size (Fig. 12–13). The left ventricular wall thickness may exceed 2.0 cm and the heart weight exceed 500 gm. In time, the in-

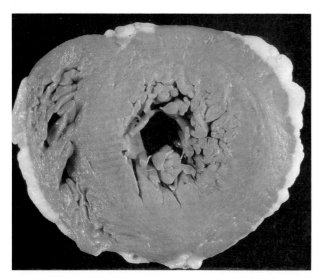

Figure 12–13. Hypertensive heart disease, with marked concentric thickening of the left ventricular wall causing reduction of the size of the lumen.

creased thickness of the left ventricular wall imparts a stiffness that impairs diastolic filling. There is usually no obstruction to left ventricular outflow. The onset of decompensation is usually accompanied by dilatation of the ventricular chamber, thinning of the wall, and enlargement of the external dimensions of the heart.

Microscopically the earliest changes of systemic HHD are myocyte enlargement with an increase in transverse diameters, which are difficult to appreciate on routine microscopy. At a more advanced stage, the cellular and nuclear enlargement becomes somewhat more irregular, with variation in cell size among adjacent cells, loss of myofibrils, and increased interstitial fibrosis. The biochemical, molecular, and morphologic changes that occur in hypertensive hypertrophy are similar to those noted in other conditions of myocardial overload (see section on cardiac hypertrophy, earlier in this chapter).

Compensated systemic HHD may be asymptomatic and suspected only in the appropriate clinical setting by ECG or echocardiographic indications of left ventricular enlargement. As already emphasized, other causes for such hypertrophy must be excluded. In many patients, however, it comes to attention by the onset of atrial fibrillation (owing to left atrial enlargement) or CHF with cardiac dilatation, or both. Depending on the severity of the hypertension, its duration, the adequacy of therapeutic control, and the underlying basis for the hypertension, the patient may enjoy normal longevity and die of unrelated causes, may develop progressive IHD owing to the effects of hypertension in potentiating coronary atherosclerosis, may suffer progressive renal damage or cerebrovascular stroke, or may experience progressive heart fail-

ure. The risk of SCD is also increased. There is substantial evidence that effective control of hypertension in time can lead to regression of cardiac hypertrophy.

PULMONARY (RIGHT-SIDED) HYPERTENSIVE HEART DISEASE (COR PULMONALE)

Pulmonary (right-sided) HHD constitutes the right ventricular enlargement secondary to pulmonary hypertension caused by disorders that affect the lungs or pulmonary vasculature (Table 12–7). Thus *cor pulmonale*, as pulmonary HHD is frequently called, is the right-sided counterpart of left-sided (systemic) HHD. *Right ventricular dilatation and thickening caused by diseases of the left side of the heart and congenital heart diseases are excluded by this definition of cor pulmonale.*

Based on the suddenness of development of the pulmonary hypertension, cor pulmonale may be acute or chronic. *Acute cor pulmonale* refers to the right ventricular dilatation that follows massive pulmonary embolism. *Chronic cor pulmonale* usually implies right ventricular hypertrophy (and later dilatation) secondary to prolonged pressure overload owing to obstruction of the pulmonary arteries or arterioles or compression or obliteration of septal capillaries (e.g., owing to emphysema).

MORPHOLOGY. In acute cor pulmonale, there is marked dilatation of the right ventricle. On cross section, the normal sickle shape of the right ventri-

Table 12–7. DISORDERS PREDISPOSING TO COR PULMONALE

DISEASES OF THE LUNGS
Chronic obstructive pulmonary disease
Diffuse pulmonary interstitial fibrosis
Extensive persistent atelectasis
Cystic fibrosis

DISEASES OF PULMONARY VESSELS
Pulmonary embolism
Primary pulmonary vascular sclerosis
Extensive pulmonary arteritis (e.g., Wegener's granulomatosis)
Drug-, toxin-, or radiation-induced vascular sclerosis
Extensive pulmonary tumor micrometastases

DISORDERS AFFECTING CHEST MOVEMENT
Kyphoscoliosis
Marked obesity (pickwickian syndrome)
Neuromuscular diseases

DISORDERS INDUCING PULMONARY ARTERIOLAR CONSTRICTION
Metabolic acidosis
Hypoxemia
    Chronic altitude sickness
    Obstruction to major airways
    Idiopathic alveolar hypoventilation

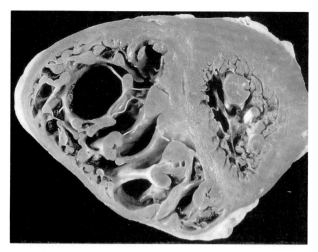

Figure 12-14. Chronic cor pulmonale. Transection of heart revealing a markedly dilated and hypertrophied right ventricle *(to the left)*, with thickened free wall and hypertrophied trabeculae. The transected left ventricle *(to the right)* has been compressed and dwarfed by the right ventricular enlargement.

cle is transformed to a dilated ovoid cavity possibly with thinning of the right ventricular wall (normal thickness, 0.3 to 0.5 cm). In chronic cor pulmonale, the ventricular wall thickens, sometimes up to 1.0 cm or more, and may even come to approximate that of the left ventricle (Fig. 12–14). More subtle stages of right ventricular hypertrophy may be revealed by thickening of the muscle bundles in the outflow tract, immediately below the pulmonary valve, or of the moderator band, the muscle bundle that connects the septum to the anterior right ventricular papillary muscle. Sometimes there is secondary compression of the left ventricular chamber. Rarely, secondary tricuspid regurgitation leads to slight fibrous thickening of this valve, but otherwise the remainder of the heart is essentially unchanged.

Chronic cor pulmonale is a surprisingly common condition because of its association with such widespread disorders as chronic bronchitis and emphysema (COPD), which affect perhaps 40 million or more individuals in the United States alone. In most instances, however, clinical effects of the pulmonary impairment overshadow those of the heart.

VALVULAR HEART DISEASE

Disorders that are characterized principally by valvular involvement and dysfunction include calcific aortic valve stenosis, calcification of the mitral annulus, mitral valve prolapse, rheumatic heart disease, three forms of vegetative endocarditis (including infective endocarditis, nonbacterial thrombotic endocarditis, and endocarditis of systemic lupus erythematosus), and carcinoid heart disease. Before these disorders are presented, a discussion of a few general principles is in order.

The functional disturbances engendered by valvular disease are stenosis and insufficiency. *Stenosis is the failure of a valve to open completely,* thereby impeding forward flow. *Insufficiency or regurgitation, in contrast, results from failure of a valve to close completely,* thereby allowing reversed flow. These abnormalities can be either *pure,* when only stenosis *or* regurgitation is present, or *mixed,* when both stenosis *and* regurgitation are present in a single valve. Stenosis and insufficiency often coexist in the same valve, but one of these defects usually predominates. *Isolated* disease refers to disease affecting one valve. More than one valve may be dysfunctional (*combined* disease). *Functional regurgitation* results when a valve becomes incompetent owing to dilatation of the ventricle, which causes the right or left ventricular papillary muscles to be pulled down and outward, thereby preventing coaptation of otherwise intact leaflets during systole.

Abnormalities of flow often produce abnormal heart sounds *(murmurs).* Valvular dysfunction can vary in degree from slight and physiologically unimportant to severe and rapidly fatal. The clinical consequences depend on the valve involved, the degree of impairment, and the rate of its development. At one end of the spectrum, sudden destruction of an aortic valve cusp by infection (as in infective endocarditis; see later) may cause rapidly fatal cardiac failure owing to massive regurgitation. In contrast, hemodynamically significant mitral stenosis is usually remarkably well tolerated. Depending on degree, duration, and etiology, valvular stenosis or insufficiency, like other forms of heart disease, often produces secondary changes in the heart, blood vessels, and other organs, both proximal and distal to the valvular lesion. One change in the heart frequently seen is a patch of endocardial thickening at the point where a jet lesion impinges, such as the focal endocardial fibrosis in the left atrium secondary to a regurgitant jet of mitral insufficiency. Other important alterations include myocardial hypertrophy and pulmonary and systemic changes discussed earlier.

Valvular abnormalities may be caused by congenital disorders (see later) or by a variety of acquired diseases. *Valvular insufficiency may result from either intrinsic disease of the valve cusps or damage to or distortion of the supporting structures (e.g., the aorta, mitral annulus, chordae tendineae, papillary muscles, ventricular free wall) without primary changes in the cusps. It may appear acutely as with rupture of chordae or chronically with leaflet scarring and retraction. In contrast, valvular stenosis almost always is due to a primary cuspal abnormality and is virtually always a chronic process.* The most important causes of acquired heart valve dys-

Table 12-8. MAJOR ETIOLOGIES OF ACQUIRED HEART VALVE DISEASE

MITRAL VALVE DISEASE	AORTIC VALVE DISEASE
Mitral Stenosis	***Aortic Stenosis***
Postinflammatory scarring (rheumatic heart disease)	Postinflammatory scarring (rheumatic heart disease)
	Senile calcific aortic stenosis
	Calcification of congenitally deformed valve
Mitral Regurgitation	***Aortic Regurgitation***
Abnormalities of leaflets and commissures	Intrinsic valvular disease
Postinflammatory scarring	Postinflammatory scarring (rheumatic heart disease)
Infective endocarditis	Infective endocarditis
Mitral valve prolapse	Aortic disease
Abnormalities of tensor apparatus	Degenerative aortic dilatation
Rupture of papillary muscle	Syphilitic aortitis
Papillary muscle dysfunction (fibrosis)	Ankylosing spondylitis
Rupture of chordae tendineae	Rheumatoid arthritis
Abnormalities of left ventricular cavity and/or anulus	Marfan syndrome
LV enlargement (myocarditis, congestive cardiomyopathy)	
Calcification of mitral ring	

LV = Left ventricular.
Modified from Schoen, F.J.: Surgical pathology of removed natural and prosthetic valves. Hum. Pathol. *18:*558, 1987.

function are summarized in Table 12–8[36] and are discussed in the specific sections following. In contrast to the many potential causes of valvular insufficiency, only a relatively few conditions produce acquired valvular stenosis.

DEGENERATIVE CALCIFIC AORTIC VALVE STENOSIS

Aortic stenosis is the most frequent valve abnormality; it can be congenital (when the valvular obstruction is present from birth) or acquired. The definition of *congenital aortic stenosis* excludes congenital bicuspid and the rare unicuspid valves that do not cause functional stenosis at birth but have enhanced susceptibility to superimposed damage that later can cause stenosis. *Acquired aortic stenosis* is usually the consequence of calcification induced by "wear and tear" of either congenitally bicuspid (or unicuspid) valves (see later) or calcification of aortic valves with previous normal anatomy in aged individuals. With the decline in the incidence of rheumatic fever, rheumatic aortic stenosis now accounts for less than 10% of cases of acquired aortic stenosis. Therefore the overwhelming majority of cases represent age-related degenerative calcification and come to clinical attention

primarily in the sixth to seventh decades of life with pre-existing bicuspid valves (see later) but not until the eighth and ninth decades with previously normal valves.

MORPHOLOGY. The morphologic hallmark of nonrheumatic, calcific aortic stenosis (with either tricuspid or bicuspid valves) is heaped-up calcified masses within the aortic cusps that ultimately protrude through the outflow surfaces into the sinuses of Valsalva, preventing the opening of the cusps. The calcific deposits distort the cuspal architecture, primarily at the bases; the free cuspal edges are usually not involved (Fig. 12–15). Distinct from atherosclerosis, the calcific process begins in the valvular fibrosa, at the points of maximal cusp flexion (the margins of attachment), and the microscopic layered architecture is largely preserved. The process is primarily dystrophic calcification without lipid deposition or cellular proliferation distinct from atherosclerosis (see Chapter 1). An earlier, hemodynamically insignificant, stage of the calcification process is called **aortic valve sclerosis.**

Notably, in contrast to rheumatic aortic stenosis (see later), there is no commissural fusion in degenerative aortic stenosis. By the time these changes are seen at surgical resection or postmortem examination, however, the cusps are often

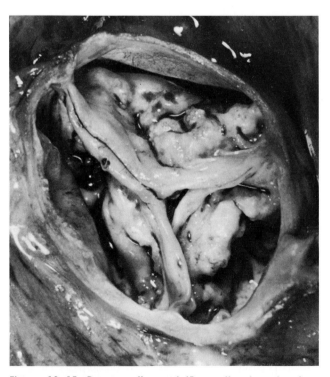

Figure 12–15. Degenerative calcific aortic stenosis of a previously normal valve having three cusps (view from aortic aspect of valve). Nodular masses of calcium are heaped up within sinuses of Valsalva. Note that the commissures are not fused, as in postrheumatic aortic valve stenosis (see Fig. 12–19C).

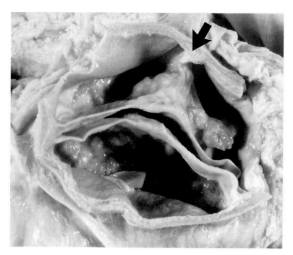

Figure 12–16. Calcific aortic stenosis superimposed on a congenitally bicuspid valve. As is common, one cusp has a partial fusion at its center, called a *raphe (arrow)*.

heavily fibrosed and thickened. The mitral valve is generally normal in patients with calcific aortic stenosis, other than primary mitral annular calcification or direct extension of aortic valve calcific deposits onto the mitral anterior leaflet. In contrast, virtually all patients with rheumatic aortic stenosis have concomitant structural abnormalities of the mitral valve (see later).

Congenitally Bicuspid Aortic Valve

In approximately 1 to 2% of the population, the aortic valve is congenitally bicuspid. The two cusps are usually of unequal size, with the larger cusp having a midline *raphe*, resulting from the incomplete separation of two cusps; less frequently the cusps are of the same size. Valves that become bicuspid owing to an acquired deformity (e.g., post-inflammatory commissural fusion in rheumatic valve disease) have an enlarged composite cusp containing the fused commissure.

Bicuspid aortic valves are generally neither stenotic nor symptomatic at birth or throughout early life, but they are predisposed to progressive calcification, similar to that occurring in aortic valves with initially normal anatomy (Fig. 12–16). The raphe that composes the incomplete commissure is frequently a major site of calcific deposits. With or without calcification, bicuspid aortic valves may also become incompetent or be complicated by infective endocarditis.

Regardless of whether the underlying valve with aortic stenosis has two or three cusps, the obstruction to left ventricular outflow caused by massive calcification leads to a gradually increasing pressure gradient across the calcified valve, which may reach 75 to 100 mm Hg in severe cases. Left

ventricular pressure must consequently rise to 200 mm Hg or more in such instances, and cardiac output is maintained by the development of concentric left ventricular (pressure overload) hypertrophy. Eventually as the stenosis worsens, angina or syncope may appear. Angina is probably a consequence of impaired microcirculatory perfusion of the hypertrophied myocardium. The basis of syncope is poorly understood, but there is an increased risk of sudden death. Eventually, cardiac decompensation with CHF may ensue. The onset of such symptoms (angina, syncope, or CHF) in aortic stenosis heralds the exhaustion of compensatory cardiac hyperfunction and therefore carries a poor prognosis if not treated by surgery (death in more than 50% within 3 years). Patients with aortic stenosis are often drastically improved by surgical aortic valve repair or replacement. Because valvular obstructions can progress rapidly, the new noninvasive technique Doppler echocardiography (which measures flow velocities as well as structure) can be used repetitively to examine the progression of disease with time.[37]

MITRAL ANNULAR CALCIFICATION

In elderly individuals, especially women, degenerative calcific deposits can develop in the ring (*annulus*) of the mitral valve. They can often be visualized on gross inspection as irregular, stony hard nodules (2 to 5 mm in thickness) that lie behind the leaflets. Inflammatory change is absent. The process generally does not affect valvular function but, in unusual cases, may lead to regurgitation by interference with systolic contraction of the mitral valve ring or to stenosis by impairing opening of the mitral leaflets. Occasionally the calcium deposits may penetrate sufficiently deeply to impinge on the atrioventricular conduction system and produce arrhythmias (and occasionally sudden death). Because calcific nodules may provide a site for thrombi that can embolize, patients with mitral annular calcification have an increased risk of stroke.[38] The calcific nodules can also be the nidus for infective endocarditis. Heavy calcific deposits are sometimes visualized on echocardiography or seen as a distinctive, ring-like opacity on chest radiographs.

MITRAL VALVE PROLAPSE (MYXOMATOUS DEGENERATION OF THE MITRAL VALVE)

In this valvular abnormality, one or both mitral leaflets are enlarged, redundant, or "floppy" and *prolapse*, or balloon back, into the left atrium during systole. On auscultation, only a midsystolic click or clicks may be heard, corresponding to

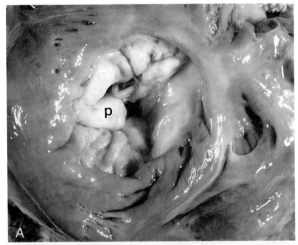

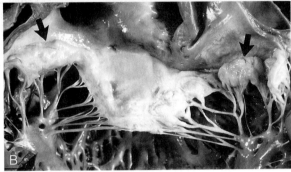

Figure 12-17. Myxomatous degeneration of the mitral valve. A, Left atrial aspect. B, Opened mitral valve. Both show pronounced hooding of the posterior mitral leaflet (p in A; arrows in B). (From Schoen, F.J.: Interventional and Surgical Cardiovascular Pathology: Clinical Correlations and Basic Principles. Philadelphia, W.B. Saunders Co., 1989, p. 119.)

tion of the fibrosa layer of the valve, on which the structural integrity of the cusp depends, accompanied by marked thickening of the spongiosa layer. Normally the thickness of the fibrosa and spongiosa are approximately equal; in the well-defined myxomatous valve, the thickness of the spongiosa far exceeds that of the fibrosa. The collagenous structure of the chordae tendineae is also attenuated.

Secondary changes reflect the stresses and injury incident to the billowing leaflets: (1) fibrous thickening of the valve leaflets, particularly where they rub against each other; (2) linear fibrous thickening of the left ventricular endocardial surface where abnormally long chordae snap against it; (3) thickening of the mural endocardium of the left ventricle or atrium as a consequence of friction-induced injury by the prolapsing leaflets; (4) thrombi on the atrial surfaces of the leaflets, particularly in the recesses behind the ballooned cusps; and (5) focal calcifications at the base of the posterior mitral leaflet. Recall that slight degrees of hooding are normal, particularly in elderly individuals.

snapping or tensing of an everted cusp, scallop, or chorda tendineae. Often, however, the valve becomes incompetent, and the mitral regurgitation induces an accompanying late systolic or sometimes holosystolic murmur. This is an extremely common condition, thought to be present in about 5 to 10% of the population of the United States, most often young women. Usually it is an incidental finding on physical examination, but it may have serious import in a small fraction of those affected.

MORPHOLOGY. The essential anatomic change in mitral valve prolapse is interchordal ballooning (hooding) of the mitral leaflets or portion of the leaflets (Fig. 12-17).[39] Frequently the chordae tendineae in myxomatous degeneration are elongated or thinned, and occasionally they are ruptured. Concomitant involvement of the tricuspid valve is present in 20 to 40% of cases, and the aortic or pulmonic valve (or both) may also be affected. Commissural fusion, characteristic of rheumatic heart disease, is absent.

Histologically the essential change is attenua-

The basis for the changes within the valve leaflets and associated structures is unknown. Favored is the proposition of a developmental anomaly perhaps involving connective tissue throughout the body because this valvular abnormality is one common feature of Marfan syndrome (see Chapter 5) and occasionally occurs with other hereditary disorders of connective tissues. Even in the absence of these well-defined conditions, there are hints of extracardiac systemic structural abnormalities in some individuals with the floppy mitral valve syndrome, such as scoliosis, straight back, and high arched palate.

Most patients with mitral valve prolapse are asymptomatic, and the condition is discovered only on routine examination by the presence of a midsystolic click. Echocardiography reveals mitral valve prolapse. A minority of patients have chest pain mimicking angina, dyspnea, and fatigue or, curiously, psychiatric manifestations, such as depression, anxiety reactions, and personality disorders. Although the great majority of patients with mitral valve prolapse have no untoward effects, approximately 3% develop one of four serious complications[40]:

- *Infective endocarditis*, manyfold more frequent in these patients than in the general population.
- *Mitral insufficiency*, either slow onset attributed to cuspal deformity, dilatation of the mitral annulus or chordal lengthening, or sudden owing to chordal rupture.
- *Stroke or other systemic infarct*, resulting from embolism of leaflet thrombi.
- *Arrhythmias*, both ventricular and atrial can de-

velop. Sudden death is uncommon. The mechanism of ventricular arrhythmia is unknown in most cases.

RHEUMATIC FEVER AND RHEUMATIC HEART DISEASE

Rheumatic fever (RF) is an acute, often recurrent, inflammatory disease principally of children that generally follows a pharyngeal (but not skin) infection with group A beta-hemolytic streptococci. Evidence strongly suggests that RF is the result of an immune response to streptococcal antigens inciting either a cross reaction to tissue antigens or a streptococcal-induced autoimmune reaction to normal tissue antigens.

RF is characterized by fever; arthralgia; and a constellation of findings that includes (major manifestations) (1) migratory polyarthritis of the large joints, (2) carditis, (3) subcutaneous nodules, (4) erythema marginatum of the skin, and (5) Sydenham's chorea—a neurologic disorder with involuntary purposeless, rapid movements. The diagnosis is established by the Jones criteria: evidence of a preceding group A streptococcal infection, with the presence of two major manifestations or of one major and one minor manifestation (including fever, arthralgia, or elevated acute phase reactants).[41] Although the acute attack may induce arthritis and sometimes myocarditis, both usually resolve. In contrast, the chronic sequelae of the cardiac valve involvement can be disabling. *Chronic rheumatic heart disease (RHD) is characterized principally by deforming fibrotic valvular disease (particularly mitral stenosis), which produces permanent dysfunction and severe, sometimes fatal, cardiac failure decades later.*

INCIDENCE. The incidence of RF and therefore of RHD has steadily declined in the United States and other developed countries. In 1940, the mortality rate from RHD in the United States was 20.6 per 100,000 population; in 1982, it was 2.2. This decline in morbidity and mortality from RF has been related to improved socioeconomic living conditions, better control of streptococcal infections by penicillin, and some apparent overall reduction in the virulence of the causative organisms. Nonetheless, the disease continues to be a global problem, with an estimated 15 to 20 million new cases a year, and there is an occasional resurgence of RF in localized areas of the United States. During the 1980s, there were major outbreaks in Salt Lake City, Pittsburgh, and other large U.S. cities; reemergence of particularly virulent strains of the group A streptococcus has been suggested as the cause.[42]

ETIOLOGY AND PATHOGENESIS. *RF is a postinfectious, immunologic disease that results either from (1) heightened immunologic reactivity to streptococcal antigens that evoke antibodies cross reactive with human tissue antigens or (2) some form of autoimmune reaction incited by a streptococcal infection.*[43,44] The evidence is as follows:

- Initial attacks of RF follow some weeks after streptococcal infection; the time interval (1 to 5 weeks) is appropriate for generation of and damage from an immune response.
- Depending on the time interval between the pharyngitis and RF, elevated serum titers of antibodies to streptolysin O (ASO) and hyaluronidase (both elaborated by the streptococcal organism) are almost always present.
- The tissue lesions of RF and RHD are sterile and do not result from direct bacterial invasion.
- Recurrent acute RF is preceded by a streptococcal infection.

What determines which individual will develop RF (and RHD) after a provocative streptococcal infection remains unknown, as do the precise antigenic tissue targets of the putative cross-reactive antibodies. More severe and longer lasting bouts of streptococcal pharyngitis increase the likelihood of RF. The attack rate is approximately 3% following streptococcal pharyngitis (i.e., only a minority suffer the immunologic sequelae of the infection). Individual susceptibility may be related to genetically determined immune response genes to streptococcal antigens. Potential antigenic targets include (1) heart valve glycoproteins that cross-react with the hyaluronate capsule of the streptococcus, itself identical to human hyaluronate; (2) myocardial and smooth muscle sarcolemma that are cross-reactive with streptococcal membrane antigens; and (3) cardiac myosin (that shares antigenic determinants with streptococcal M protein, the chief virulence factor of group A streptococci). It is proposed that streptococcal infection in some way activates an autoimmune reaction to heart tissues, but direct evidence for *autoimmunity* and the specific cause of RF and RHD is not firmly established. The proposed pathogenetic sequence and the morphologic features of acute RF are summarized in Figure 12-18.

MORPHOLOGY. During acute RF, widely disseminated, focal, inflammatory lesions are found in various sites. Most distinctive within the heart, they are called **Aschoff bodies.** They constitute foci of fibrinoid necrosis surrounded by lymphocytes, macrophages, an occasional plasma cell, and plump "activated" histiocytes called Anitschkow cells or Aschoff cells. These distinctive cells have abundant amphophilic cytoplasm and central round-to-ovoid nuclei in which the chromatin is disposed in a cen-

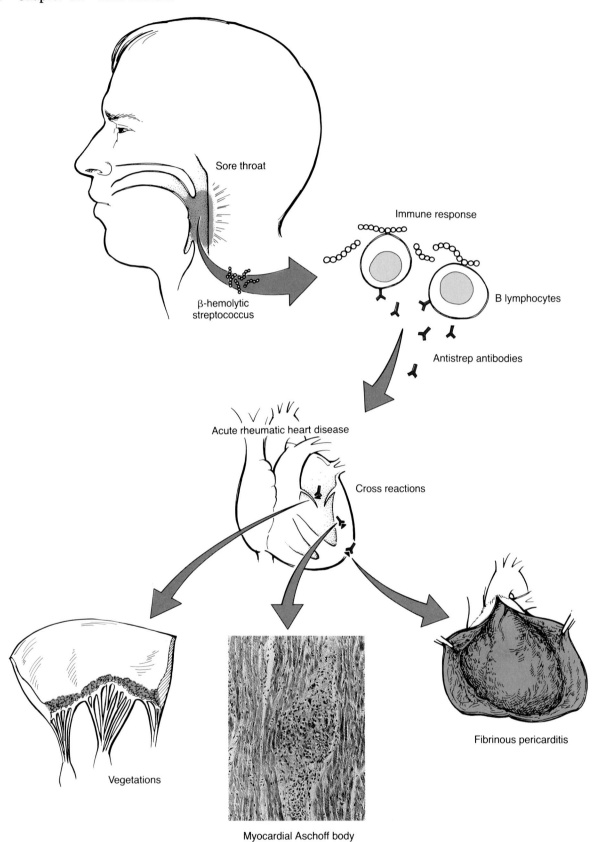

Figure 12–18. The pathogenetic sequence and key morphologic features of acute rheumatic heart disease and an Aschoff body in the interstitium of the myocardium. Acute rheumatic fever frequently causes mitral valvulitis, with a linear array of small vegetations along the line of closure of the leaflets.

tral, slender, wavy ribbon resembling a caterpillar (hence the designation "caterpillar cells"). Some of the larger altered histiocytes are multinucleated to form Aschoff giant cells. **This varied inflammatory infiltrate about the central focus of fibrinoid necrosis constitutes the full-blown Aschoff body that is pathognomonic of RF.**

During acute RF, Aschoff bodies may be found in any of the three layers of the heart—pericardium, myocardium, or endocardium—hence a **pancarditis.** In the pericardium, they are located in the subserosal fat and fibrous tissue and are accompanied by a fibrinous or serofibrinous pericardial exudate, described as a "bread-and-butter" pericarditis, which generally resolves without sequelae. The myocardial involvement takes the form of scattered Aschoff bodies within the interstitial connective tissue, often perivascular. Adjacent myocytes may be damaged.

There is usually concomitant involvement of the endocardium and the left-sided valves by inflammatory foci not characteristic of Aschoff bodies. Typically there are foci of fibrinoid necrosis within the cusps or along the chordae tendineae on which sit small (1 to 2 mm) friable vegetations —**verrucae**—along the lines of closure. These irregular, warty projections probably result from the precipitation of fibrin at sites of erosion of inflamed endocardial surfaces where the leaflets impinge on each other. These acute valvular changes cause little disturbance in cardiac function and usually resolve or induce only minimal fibrosis, with little if any functional deficit. Chronic valvular involvement, however, is the most ominous aspect of rheumatic carditis, being responsible for the disability decades later. Subendocardial lesions, perhaps exacerbated by regurgitant jets, may induce irregular thickenings called **MacCallum's plaques,** usually in the left atrium.

Chronic RHD is characterized by organization of the acute endocardial inflammation and subsequent deforming fibrosis; the valvular leaflets become thickened and retracted, causing permanent deformity. **In chronic disease, the mitral valve is virtually always deformed, but involvement of another valve, such as the aortic, may be the most clinically important in some cases. The cardinal anatomic changes of the mitral (or tricuspid) valve are leaflet thickening, commissural fusion and shortening, thickening and fusion of the chordae tendineae** (Fig. 12–19). Microscopically there is diffuse fibrosis and neovascularization that obliterate the originally layered and avascular leaflet architecture. Aschoff bodies are replaced by fibrous scar; diagnostic forms are rarely seen in surgical specimens or autopsy tissue from patients with chronic RHD.

RF is overwhelmingly the most frequent cause of mitral stenosis. The mitral valve alone is involved in 65 to 70% of the cases, mitral and aortic in about 25%; similar but generally less severe fibrous thickenings and stenoses can occur in the tricuspid valve and rarely in the pulmonic. Fibrous bridging across the valvular commissures and calcification create "fish mouth" or "buttonhole" stenoses. With tight mitral stenosis, the left atrium and sometimes also the right atrium progressively dilate. The long-standing congestive changes in the lungs may induce pulmonary vascular and parenchymal changes and in time lead to right ventricular hypertrophy. Thrombi may form within the auricular appendages. The clinically important consequences of chronic RHD usually do not appear until at least several decades after the acute attack.

Joints. The likelihood of acute arthritis increases with age at the time of the attack, appearing in about 90% of adults and less commonly in children. The large joints, such as the knees, are most often affected. The changes are transitory and resolve without sequelae.

Skin. Lesions of the skin take the form of **subcutaneous nodules** or **erythema marginatum** and are present in 10 to 60% of cases, more often in children. Subcutaneous nodules, essentially giant Aschoff bodies, are most often located overlying the extensor tendons of the extremities at the wrists, elbows, ankles, and knees. Erythema marginatum begins as flat to slightly elevated, slightly reddened maculopapules with reddened and elevated erythematous margins that progressively enlarge; it tends to have a "bathing-suit" distribution but may also occur over the thighs, lower extremities, and face.

CLINICAL COURSE. Acute RF appears most often in children between the ages of 5 and 15 years. Both younger and older individuals, however, may be affected; about 20% of first attacks occur in middle to later life. Attacks often begin with migratory polyarthritis accompanied by fever. Typically, one joint after another becomes painful and swollen for a period of days and then subsides spontaneously, leaving no residual disability. Acute carditis develops in about 50 to 75% of children but only about 35% of adults having a single acute attack of RF. Should a pericardial friction rub appear, it usually clears in the course of days to weeks and leaves no sequelae. During the initial acute attack, myocarditis is the most threatening cardiac problem. Myocarditis induces arrhythmias, particularly atrial fibrillation; fibrillation potentiates atrial thrombi that constitute potential sources of emboli. Moreover, myocarditis may lead to cardiac dilation and resultant functional mitral insufficiency, causing murmurs; cardiac failure may ensue in some cases, representing the major cause of death during acute RF. After the acute attack, the insufficiency usually resolves as the myocardium heals. Overall the prognosis for the primary

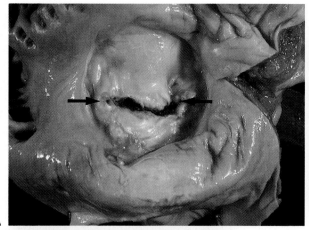

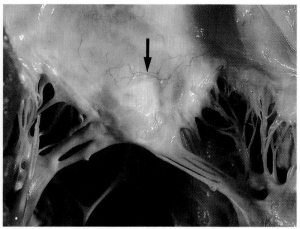

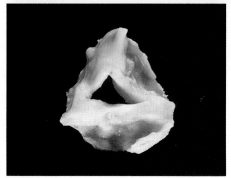

Figure 12-19. Chronic rheumatic heart disease. A and B, Mitral stenosis illustrating diffuse fibrous thickening and distortion of cusps, intercommissural fusion and thickening and shortening of the chordae tendineae. There is marked dilatation of the left atrium. A, Left atrial view of mitral stenosis (commissural fusion noted by *arrows*). B, Opened valve. Note neovascularization of valve leaflet *(arrow)*. C, Surgically removed specimen of rheumatic aortic stenosis, with thickening and distortion of the cusps and intercommissural adhesions. (C, reproduced from Schoen, F.J., and St. John Sutton, M.: Contemporary issues in the pathology of valvular heart disease. Human Pathol. *18*:568, 1987.)

attack is generally good, and only 1% of patients die from fulminant RF.

After an initial attack, there is increased vulnerability to reactivation of the disease with subsequent pharyngeal infections, and the same manifestations are likely to appear with each recurrent attack. Carditis is likely to be reactivated and to worsen with each recurrence; damage is cumulative. Because of the threat of recurrent disease, it is now standard practice to administer prophylactic long-term antistreptococcal therapy to anyone who has had RF. Other hazards include embolization from mural thrombi, primarily within the atria or their appendages, and infective endocarditis superimposed on chronically deformed valves. For unexplained reasons, females appear to be more vulnerable to mitral valve stenosis than males. Despite damaged valves, the heart may remain compensated for the duration of a long life, but usually over the span of decades, decompensation and eventual full-blown cardiac failure develop. This course can now be altered by surgical repair or replacement of damaged valves.

INFECTIVE ENDOCARDITIS

Infective endocarditis (IE), one of the most serious of all infections, is characterized by colonization or invasion of the heart valves or the mural endocar-dium by a microbiologic agent, leading to the formation of bulky, friable *vegetations* laden with organisms. Not only the valves, but also the aorta (infective endoaortitis), aneurysmal sacs, or other blood vessels can also become infected. Virtually every form of microbiologic agent, including fungi, rickettsiae (Q fever), and chlamydiae, has at one time or another been responsible for these infections, but most cases are bacterial, hence the usual term, *bacterial endocarditis*. Prompt diagnosis and effective treatment of IE can significantly alter the outlook for the patient.

Traditionally IE has been classified on clinical grounds into acute and subacute forms. This subdivision expresses the range of severity of the disease and its tempo, determined in large part by the virulence of the infecting microorganism and the presence of underlying cardiac disease. *Acute endocarditis* describes a destructive, tumultuous infection, usually of a previously normal heart valve with a highly virulent organism, that leads to death within days to weeks of more than 50% of patients. In a previously abnormal heart, organisms of low virulence can cause infection, particularly on deformed valves; in such cases, the disease may appear insidiously and, even untreated, pursue a protracted course of weeks to months *(subacute endocarditis)*. In contrast to the high mortality of acute IE, most patients with subacute IE recover after appropriate therapy.

The vegetations found in the heart in both

clinical variants of the disease are composed of fibrin, inflammatory cells, and organisms. Nevertheless, the highly virulent organisms of acute endocarditis tend to produce necrotizing, ulcerative, invasive valvular infections, whereas the lower virulence organisms of subacute disease are less destructive, and the vegetations often show evidence of healing. Both the clinical and the morphologic patterns, however, are points along a spectrum, and a clear delineation between acute and subacute disease does not exist in all cases.

EPIDEMIOLOGY AND PATHOGENESIS. As stated previously, IE may develop in previously normal hearts, but a variety of cardiac abnormalities predispose to this form of infection. In years past, RHD was the major contributor, but now more common is congenital heart disease (particularly anomalies that have small shunts or tight stenoses creating high-velocity jet streams [e.g., a small interventricular septal defect], patent ductus arteriosus, or tetralogy of Fallot), myxomatous mitral valve, degenerative calcific valvular stenosis, bicuspid aortic valve (whether calcified or not), and artificial valves and vascular grafts. Equally important as predisposing influences are neutropenia, immunodeficiency (including patients infected with human immunodeficiency virus [HIV]), therapeutic immunosuppression (as in organ transplant recipients), indwelling vascular catheters, diabetes mellitus, and alcohol or intravenous drug abuse. Sterile platelet-fibrin deposits that accumulate at sites of impingement of jet streams created by preexisting cardiac disease or catheters may also be important in the development of subacute endocarditis.

More than half of cases are attributable to various streptococci—most prominently the viridans group (not the group responsible for RF). They are the dominant cause of subacute disease, and as organisms of relatively low virulence, they generally gain a foothold only in hearts having some underlying disease or predisposition. In contrast, the highly virulent *Staphylococcus aureus* accounts overall for about 20 to 30% of cases; it can infect normal valves and is the leading cause of acute endocarditis. Other significant etiologic agents include *Streptococcus pneumoniae*, gram-negative enteric bacilli, and fungi. Several different organisms may involve a valve simultaneously. In intravenous drug abusers, left-sided lesions predominate, but right-sided valves are commonly affected; the major organism is *S. aureus*.[45] In about 5 to 20% of all cases of endocarditis, no organism can be isolated from the blood ("culture-negative" endocarditis) because of prior antibiotic therapy, because of difficulties in isolation of the offending agent, or because organisms become deeply embedded within the enlarging vegetation and are not released into the blood.

Foremost among the factors predisposing to the development of endocarditis is seeding of the blood with microbes. In subacute endocarditis, the portal of entry of the agent into the bloodstream may be overt, as with an established infection elsewhere, drug addiction, or a previous dental or surgical procedure. Covert, transient bacteremias, however, emanate frequently from the gut, oral cavity, and trivial injuries, seeding the blood with organisms that are usually of low virulence (e.g., *Streptococcus viridans*, *Streptococcus faecalis*, *Escherichia coli*).

The influences surrounding the development of acute IE are less well understood. Sometimes they are well defined, as when the blood is seeded by highly virulent organisms such as *S. aureus* in intravenous drug abuse with repeated contamination of the blood, indwelling vascular catheters, or prosthetic valves that constitute foreign bodies inviting the localization of blood-borne agents. Direct attachment of bacteria to valvular endothelial cells may also be important in the pathogenesis of acute endocarditis.

MORPHOLOGY. The diagnostic findings in both the subacute and acute forms of the disease are friable, bulky, usually bacteria-laden fibrinous vegetations most commonly on the heart valves. They may occur singly or multiply on one or more valves on either side of the heart, are up to several centimeters in greatest dimension, and are readily fragmented (Fig. 12–20). The vegetations in acute endocarditis are situated more often on previously normal valves, cause perforation or erosion of the underlying valve leaflet, and sometimes erode into the underlying myocardium to produce an abscess cavity **(ring abscess)**, one of several important complications (Fig. 12–21). In contrast, in the subacute form of the disease, vegetations are smaller and less often erode or perforate the cusps. With nonvalvular congenital defects, the vegetations tend to be located on the "downstream" margin of the jet stream (e.g., on the right ventricular margins of a ventricular septal defect). Infections associated with valve prostheses are discussed later. Figure 12–22 compares the gross appearance of the vegetations of infective endocarditis with those of acute RF, nonbacterial thrombotic endocarditis (NBTE) (see below), and the endocarditis of systemic lupus erythematosus, called Libman-Sacks endocarditis (see later).

With treatment, the vegetations sometimes undergo progressive sterilization, organization, and fibrosis and can eventually become calcified, leaving only irregular heaped-up fibrocalcific nodular excrescences on the valve leaflets ("healed endocarditis"). A residual perforation that occurred during the active phase may be noted. Valves with healed endocarditis frequently show neovascularity, particularly in the spongiosa of the nonscarred areas.

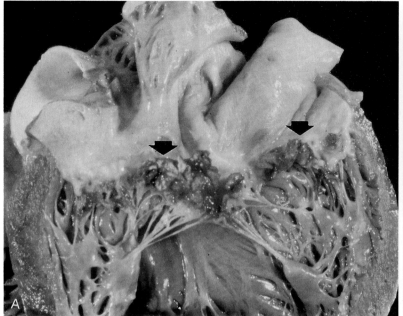
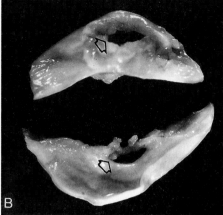
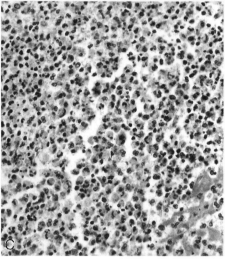

Figure 12-20. Bacterial infective endocarditis. *A,* Endocarditis (bacterial) of mitral valve with extensive friable vegetations, denoted by *arrows. B,* Endocarditis of a bicuspid aortic valve with perforations of two cusps, denoted by *arrows. C,* Histologic appearance of vegetation in endocarditis with extensive acute inflammatory cells and fibrin. Bacterial organisms were demonstrated by tissue Gram stain. (*B,* reproduced from Schoen, F.J.: Surgical pathology of removed natural and prosthetic heart valves. Hum. Pathol. *18:*558–567, 1987.)

CLINICAL COURSE. Fever is the most consistent sign of IE. With subacute disease, particularly in the elderly, however, fever may be slight or absent, and the only manifestations are nonspecific fatigue, loss of weight, and a flu-like syndrome. Murmurs are present in 90% of patients with left-sided lesions but may merely relate to the pre-existent cardiac abnormality predisposing to IE. Petechiae, subungual hemorrhages, and Roth's spots in the eyes (secondary to microemboli), have now become uncommon clinical findings owing to the shortened clinical course of the disease as a result of antibiotic therapy.

In contrast, acute endocarditis has a stormy onset with rapidly developing fever, chills, weakness, and lassitude. Complications generally begin within the first weeks of the onset of the disease. A murmur is likely because of the large size of the vegetations or leaflet destruction. The vegetations are also more likely to fragment and embolize.

Sometimes complications involving the heart or extracardiac sites call attention to the endocarditis. They include the following:

- *Cardiac complications:*

  - Valvular insufficiency or stenosis with cardiac failure
  - Myocardial ring abscess, with possible perforation of aorta, interventricular septum or free wall or invasion of the conduction system
  - Suppurative pericarditis
  - Partial dehiscence of artificial valves, often with paravalvular leak

- *Embolic complications* (leading to infarcts or metastatic infection):

  - With left-sided lesions—to the brain (cerebral abscess, meningitis), spleen (abscess), kidneys (abscess), other sites
  - With right-sided lesions—to the lungs (abscess, pneumonia)

- *Renal complications:*

  - Embolic infarction
  - Focal glomerulonephritis (due to microemboli), which may lead to nephrotic syndrome or renal failure or both (see Chapter 20)
  - Diffuse glomerulonephritis (due to antigen-an-

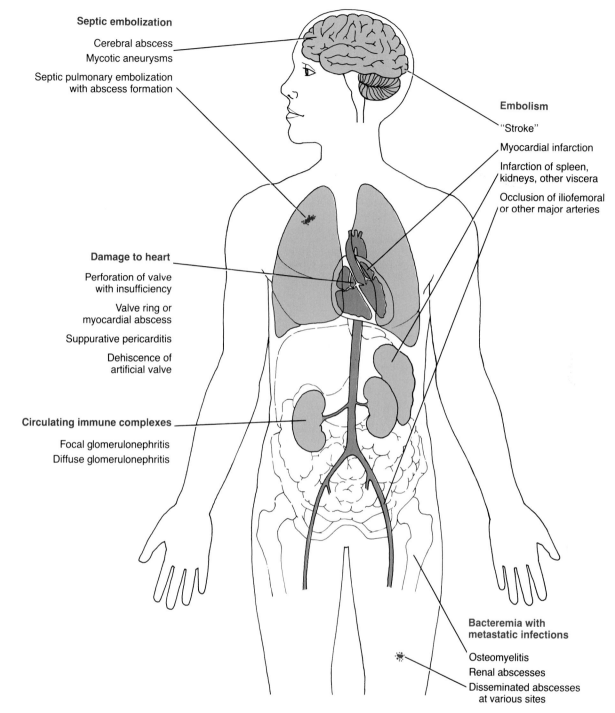

Figure 12–21. Schematic representation of the potential complications of infective endocarditis. (Modified by permission from Bisno, A.L.: Staphylococcal endocarditis and bacteremia. Hosp. Pract. 21:139, 1986.) (Illustration by Susan Tilberry.)

Labels in figure:

Septic embolization
Cerebral abscess
Mycotic aneurysms
Septic pulmonary embolization with abscess formation

Embolism
"Stroke"
Myocardial infarction
Infarction of spleen, kidneys, other viscera
Occlusion of iliofemoral or other major arteries

Damage to heart
Perforation of valve with insufficiency
Valve ring or myocardial abscess
Suppurative pericarditis
Dehiscence of artificial valve

Circulating immune complexes
Focal glomerulonephritis
Diffuse glomerulonephritis

Bacteremia with metastatic infections
Osteomyelitis
Renal abscesses
Disseminated abscesses at various sites

tibody complex deposition), which can lead to renal failure (see Chapter 20)
• Multiple abscesses—with acute staphylococcal endocarditis

Although the diagnosis can be suspected based on the appearance of one or more of the complications mentioned, a positive blood culture is required for confirmation. With repeated blood sam-ples, positive cultures can be obtained in 80 to 95% of cases. More important than the diagnosis of IE is its prevention by the prophylactic use of anti-biotics in the patient with some form of cardiac anomaly or artificial valve who is about to have a dental or surgical procedure or other form of inva-sive intervention. With early diagnosis and appro-priate treatment, the overall 5-year survival is in the range of 50 to 90%, being best for streptococ-

Comparison of vegetations

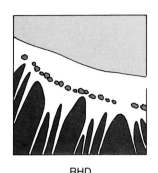 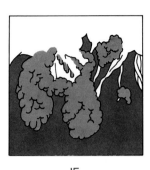 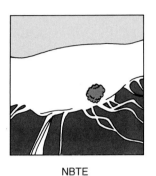 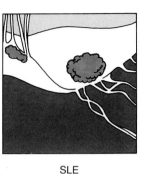

RHD   IE   NBTE   SLE

Figure 12–22. Diagrammatic comparison of the lesions in the four major forms of vegetative endocarditis. The rheumatic fever phase of RHD (rheumatic heart disease) is marked by a row of warty, small vegetations along the lines of closure of the valve leaflets. IE (infective endocarditis) is characterized by large irregular masses on the valve cusps that can extend onto the chordae (see Fig. 12–20). NBTE (nonbacterial thrombotic endocarditis) typically exhibits small, bland vegetations, usually attached at the line of closure. One or many may be present (see Fig. 12–23). SLE (Libman-Sacks endocarditis) has small or medium-sized vegetations on either or both sides of the valve leaflets.

cus-induced subacute disease and worst for staphylococcal or fungal acute endocarditis. Emboli, intractable cardiac failure owing to valvular destruction, and uncontrolled infection owing to a ring abscess are indications for surgical valve replacement.

NONBACTERIAL THROMBOTIC ENDOCARDITIS

Nonbacterial thrombotic endocarditis (NBTE) is a form of vegetative endocarditis most often encountered in debilitated patients, such as those with cancer or sepsis—hence the previously used term *marantic endocarditis.*

MORPHOLOGY. NBTE, previously called marantic endocarditis, is characterized by the deposition of small, sterile masses of fibrin and other blood elements on the valve leaflets of either side of the heart, usually on previously normal valves. In contrast to IE, the vegetations of NBTE do not contain organisms, are nondestructive, tend to be small (1 to 5 mm), and occur singly or multiply along the line of closure of the leaflets or cusps (Fig. 12–23). Histologically, they are composed of bland thrombus without accompanying inflammatory reaction, organization, or induced valve damage.

NBTE frequently occurs concomitantly with venous thromboses or pulmonary embolism, suggesting *a common origin in a hypercoagulable state*

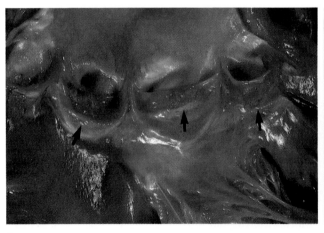 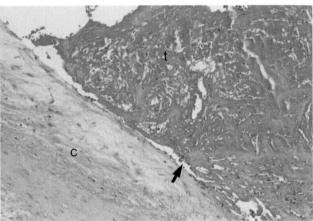

A   B

Figure 12–23. Nonbacterial thrombotic endocarditis (NBTE). A, Nearly complete row of thrombotic vegetations is noted along the line of closure of the aortic valve cusps (arrows). B, Photomicrograph of such a lesion shows bland thrombus. There is virtually no inflammation in the valve cusp (c) or thrombotic deposit (t), and the thrombus is only loosely attached at their junction (arrow).

with systemic activation of blood coagulation. This may be related to some underlying disease, such as cancer, and, in particular, mucinous adenocarcinomas of the pancreas, gastrointestinal tract, or ovary. The striking association with mucinous adenocarcinomas in general may relate to the procoagulant effect of circulating mucin. Lesions of NBTE, however, are also seen occasionally in association with nonmucin-producing tumors, such as promyelocytic leukemia, and in other debilitating diseases or conditions (e.g., hyperestrogenic states) promoting hypercoagulability. Endocardial trauma as from an indwelling catheter is also a well-recognized predisposing condition.

Although the local effect on the valves is unimportant, NBTE may achieve clinical significance by producing emboli and resultant infarcts in the brain, heart, or elsewhere. For inexplicable reasons, although these bland vegetations could provide a soil for the implantation of microorganisms, IE forming on pre-existing NBTE is unusual.

ENDOCARDITIS OF SYSTEMIC LUPUS ERYTHEMATOSUS (LIBMAN-SACKS DISEASE)

In systemic lupus erythematosus, mitral and tricuspid valvulitis is occasionally encountered and leads to the development of small, sterile vegetations.

MORPHOLOGY. The lesions are small, usually ranging from 1 to 4 mm in diameter, sterile, granular pink vegetations that may be single or multiple. Most frequently the lesions are located on the undersurfaces of the atrioventricular valves, but they may be scattered on the valvular endocardium, on the chordae tendineae, and on the mural endocardium of atria or ventricles. Histologically the verrucae consist of a finely granular, fibrinous eosinophilic material that may contain hematoxylin bodies (the tissue equivalent of the lupus erythematosus cell of the blood and bone marrow; see Chapter 6). An intense valvulitis is present, characterized by fibrinoid necrosis of the valve substance that is often contiguous with the vegetation. The small vegetations on the valve leaflets can sometimes be confused with the much larger friable vegetations of IE or with NBTE. Subsequent fibrosis and serious deformity can result that requires surgery.

CARCINOID HEART DISEASE

In patients with carcinoid tumors, cardiac involvement, principally of the endocardium and valves of the right heart, is one of the major sequelae of the *carcinoid syndrome* (see Chapter 17). The syndrome is characterized by *distinctive episodic flushing of the skin and cramps, nausea, vomiting, and diarrhea in almost all patients; bronchoconstrictive episodes resembling asthma in about one-third of patients; and cardiac lesions in about one-half.* The carcinoid syndrome is encountered in about 1% of all patients who have carcinoid tumors (argentaffinomas) whatever the primary site and in 10% of those with gastrointestinal carcinoid tumors with hepatic metastases.

MORPHOLOGY. The cardiovascular lesions associated with the carcinoid syndrome are distinctive, comprising fibrous intimal thickenings on the inside surfaces of the cardiac chambers and valvular leaflets, mainly in the right ventricle and tricuspid and pulmonic valves, and occasionally the major blood vessels (Fig. 12–24). The endocardial plaque-like thickenings are composed predominantly of smooth muscle cells and sparse collagen fibers embedded in an acid mucopolysaccharide-rich matrix material in the endocardial lining. Elastic fibers are not present in the plaque. Underlying structures are otherwise unremarkable, including the subendocardial elastic tissue layer. Occasionally left-sided lesions are also encountered.

The clinical and pathologic findings relate to the elaboration by these tumors of a variety of bioactive products, including serotonin (5-hydroxytryptamine), kallikrein, bradykinin, histamine, prostaglandins, and newly described tachykinins. Which of the secretory products induces the syndrome or the cardiac pathology is still not clear. Although serotonin is accorded greatest importance, there is a rough correlation between the plasma levels of the tumor-derived tachykinins, neuropeptide K and substance P, and urinary excretion of the serotonin metabolite 5-hydroxyindoleacetic acid (HIAA) and the severity of the right heart lesions.[46]

The fact that the cardiac changes are largely right-sided is explained by inactivation of both serotonin and bradykinin in the blood during passage through the lungs by the monoamine oxidase found in the pulmonary vascular endothelium. In the absence of hepatic metastases, gastrointestinal carcinoids (which have venous drainage via the portal system) do not usually induce the syndrome because there is rapid metabolism of serotonin during passage of blood through the liver. In contrast, argentaffinomas primary in organs outside of the portal system of venous drainage (e.g., ovary or lung), whose venous drainage bypasses the liver, may induce the carcinoid syndrome without antecedent hepatic metastases. Left-sided lesions can occur when blood containing the responsible mediator enters the left heart owing to incomplete inactivation of very high blood levels or with a pul-

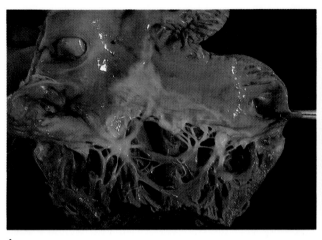
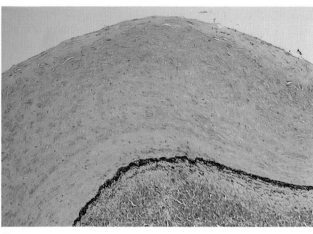

A   B

Figure 12–24. Carcinoid heart disease. *A,* Characteristic endocardial fibrotic lesion involving the right ventricle and tricuspid valve. *B,* Microscopic appearance of carcinoid heart disease with intimal thickening. Movat stain shows underlying myocardial elastic tissue black and acid mucopolysaccharides blue-green.

monary carcinoid or patent foramen ovale with right to left flow. Rarely similar left-sided plaques are found in patients who receive methysergide therapy for migraine headaches; this compound is metabolized to serotonin as it passes through the pulmonary vasculature.

COMPLICATIONS OF ARTIFICIAL VALVES

Replacement of damaged cardiac valves with prostheses has now become a common and often life-saving mode of therapy. Artificial valves fall primarily into two categories—*mechanical prostheses* using different types of occluders, such as caged balls, tilting disks, or hinged flaps, and tissue valves, usually *bioprostheses* consisting of chemically treated animal tissue, especially porcine aortic valve tissue, which has been preserved in a dilute glutaraldehyde solution and subsequently mounted on a prosthetic frame (called a "stent"). Mechanical valves are composed of nonphysiologic biomaterials that employ one or two rigid, mobile poppet occluder(s), whereas tissue valves are flexible, trileaflet valves that function somewhat like natural valves.

Approximately 60% of substitute valve recipients have a serious prosthesis-related problem within 10 years postoperatively.[47] The most frequent valve-related complications include (1) thromboembolism (local occlusion of the prosthesis by thrombus or distant thromboemboli), (2) partial dehiscence (separation) of the suture line anchoring the valve leading to a paravalvular leak, (3) infective endocarditis, (4) durability problems caused by structural deterioration, and (5) intrinsic (design-related) obstruction to forward flow (Table

12–9).[48] Although the *frequency* of prosthetic valve-related events is similar among valve types, the *nature* of these complications differs among types.

- *Thromboembolic complications* constitute the major problem with mechanical valves (Fig. 12–25). This necessitates long-term anticoagulation in patients with these devices. Hemorrhagic complications, however, such as stroke or gastrointestinal bleeding, may arise secondarily in patients who receive long-term anticoagulation.
- *Infective endocarditis* is an infrequent but serious potential complication developing in about 6% of patients within 5 years of valve replacement. Always with mechanical valves and frequently with bioprostheses, endocarditis is located at the prosthesis-tissue interface, causing a ring abscess. Indeed, with extension of the infection, a paravalvular perforation may develop, producing a regurgitant blood leak—or worse, the entire prosthesis may be dislocated from its attachments. In addition, bioprosthetic valves may develop vegetations that directly involve the prosthetic valvular cusps themselves. As with other forms of endocarditis, vegetations can embolize. The major organisms causing such infections are

Table 12–9. CAUSES OF FAILURE OF CARDIAC VALVE PROSTHESES

Thrombosis/thromboembolism
Anticoagulant-related hemorrhage
Prosthetic valve endocarditis
Structural deterioration (intrinsic)
   Wear, fracture, poppet escape, cuspal tear, calcification
Nonstructural dysfunction
   Pannus, suture/tissue entrapment, paravalvular leak, disproportion, hemolytic anemia, noise

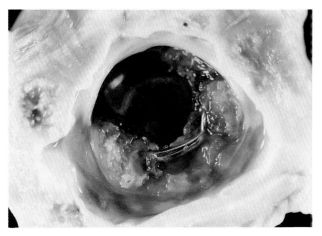

Figure 12–25. Thrombosis of a mechanical prosthetic heart valve.

staphylococcal skin contaminants (e.g., *S. aureus, S. epidermidis*) early (less than 1 month) postoperatively and streptococci later.

- *Structural deterioration* uncommonly causes failure of contemporary mechanical valves, but it is a major failure mode of bioprostheses. Within 10 years postoperatively (Fig. 12–26), at least 30% of tissue valves require replacement for calcification, often with tearing.

- Other complications, such as hemolysis induced by high blood shear, mechanical obstruction to flow inherent in all artificial valves, and dysfunction owing to ingrowth of fibrous tissue, may be serious in some cases.

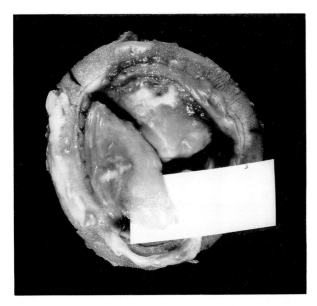

Figure 12–26. Calcification with secondary tearing of a porcine bioprosthetic heart valve. (Reproduced from Schoen, F.J.: Surgical pathology of removed natural and prosthetic heart valves. Hum. Pathol. 18:558–567, 1987.)

MYOCARDIAL DISEASE

Here our consideration is limited to two broad categories of myocardial involvement as detailed by the World Health Organization (WHO):[49] (1) *cardiomyopathy,* defined as "heart muscle disease of unknown cause," generally referred to as *primary* or *idiopathic cardiomyopathy,* and (2) *specific heart muscle disease,* defined as "heart muscle disease of known cause or associated with disorders of other systems." For example, patients who have a dilated heart of unclear etiology showing only nonspecific hypertrophy and fibrosis are said to have *idiopathic dilated cardiomyopathy,* whereas those with heart failure secondary to cardiac amyloid deposition are said to have *amyloid heart disease.* Some patients have *myocarditis,* characterized by an inflammatory reaction within the myocardium. Because myocarditis is generally considered to be due to a virus or other infective agent or to drug-induced or autoimmune injury (hypersensitivity), it is classified as specific heart muscle disease, even if the inciting virus or other cause is uncertain in a particular case.

Although not considered myocardial disease per se, myocardial dysfunction also occurs indirectly as a complication of ischemic, valvular, hypertensive (systemic and pulmonary), and congenital heart disease and some pericardial diseases. The morphologic changes and functional disturbances are generally nonspecific and are similar to those of idiopathic dilated cardiomyopathy. One important example is cardiac failure in a patient with severe coronary atherosclerosis and resultant myocardial damage, often called "ischemic cardiomyopathy" but more correctly termed *atherosclerotic coronary artery and ischemic heart disease with heart failure.* Clearly, although cardiomyopathy frequently causes profound and often fatal CHF, the term *cardiomyopathy is not synonymous with end-stage heart failure* because the latter has numerous causes, both known and unknown.

Without additional data, the clinician encountering a patient with myocardial disease is usually unaware of the etiology or whether the underlying process is idiopathic or secondary. The clinical picture is largely determined by one of the following three clinical, functional, pathologic patterns, each of which can have either a known or an unknown cause (Fig. 12–27):

- Dilated.
- Hypertrophic.
- Restrictive.

Among these three categories, the dilated form is most common (90% of cases), and the restrictive is least prevalent. Within these hemodynamic patterns of myocardial dysfunction, there is a spectrum of clinical severity, and overlap of clinical features often occurs between groups. Although

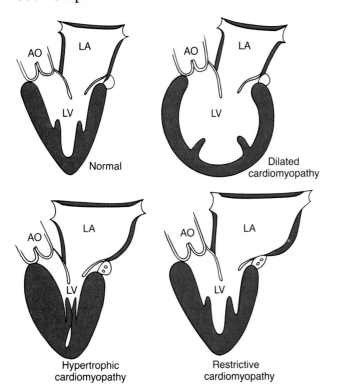

Figure 12-27. Representation of the three distinctive clinical-pathologic-functional forms of myocardial disease.

the right internal jugular vein, advancing it under fluoroscopic or echocardiographic guidance through the tricuspid valve toward the right side of the ventricular septum, and snipping a small piece of myocardium in its jaws. Each biopsy specimen is a 1- to 3-mm fragment of myocardium (including endocardium), most frequently derived from the apical half of the right side of the ventricular septum. Implicit in the use of right-sided biopsy is the assumption that this location has representative pathology. Because most myocardial diseases affect both ventricles, correlation between right-sided and left-sided findings is generally considered to be good. The multiple pieces of tissue obtained can be used for routine histologic studies; viral culture; electron microscopy, and immunohistochemical, biochemical, and molecular studies.

As discussed previously, we closely follow the WHO classification, in which *primary* or *idiopathic cardiomyopathy* refers to heart muscle diseases of unknown cause, and *specific heart muscle disease* refers to those myocardial disorders of known etiology, *excluding* ischemic, valvular, systemic, and pulmonary hypertensive, congenital, and pericardial involvements (summarized in Table 12–10).

CARDIOMYOPATHY

Dilated Cardiomyopathy

Idiopathic dilated cardiomyopathy (DCM) is characterized by the gradual development of cardiac failure associated with four-chamber hypertrophy and dilatation of the heart of unknown cause. Genetic influences have been documented in some cases of DCM, particularly when multiple members of a family are affected. DCM has a familial occurrence in approximately 20% of cases. Autosomal dominant, autosomal recessive, and X-linked inheritance have all been proposed for particular kindreds. No specific biochemical, functional, or structural abnormality of genetic origin can be identified in most cases. However, a recent study suggested localization of X-linked dilated cardio-

light microscopic and ultrastructural morphology generally reveal the cause of specific myocardial disease, the abnormal morphology is nonspecific in idiopathic cardiomyopathy. Moreover, in idiopathic dilated cardiomyopathy, the degree of abnormality of the morphologic changes does not necessarily reflect the degree of dysfunction or the patient's prognosis.

Because tissue biopsies are a valuable and often indispensable diagnostic tool to evaluate the morphology, biochemistry, and other characteristics of normal and abnormal tissues, a procedure to biopsy the heart muscle *(endomyocardial biopsy)* has been used widely in the diagnosis and management of patients with myocardial disease and cardiac transplant recipients.[50] Endomyocardial biopsy involves inserting a device (called a *bioptome*) into

Table 12-10. FUNCTIONAL PATTERNS OF CARDIOMYOPATHY, SPECIFIC HEART MUSCLE DISEASE, AND INDIRECT MYOCARDIAL DYSFUNCTION

FUNCTIONAL PATTERN	CARDIOMYOPATHY (IDIOPATHIC)	SPECIFIC (SECONDARY)	INDIRECT MYOCARDIAL DYSFUNCTION
Dilated (systolic disorder)	Dilated cardiomyopathy	Infective myocarditis; hemochromatosis; chronic anemia; alcohol; Adriamycin; sarcoidosis	Ischemic heart disease; valvular heart disease; hypertensive heart disease; congenital heart disease
Hypertrophic (diastolic disorder)	Hypertrophic cardiomyopathy	Friedreich's ataxia; glycogen storage disease; infants of diabetic mothers	Hypertensive heart disease, especially in aged individuals; aortic stenosis
Restrictive (diastolic disorder)	Restrictive cardiomyopathy	Amyloidosis; radiation-induced fibrosis	Pericardial constriction

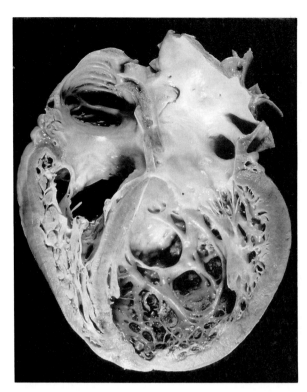

Figure 12–28. Idiopathic dilated cardiomyopathy. Four-chamber dilatation and hypertrophy are evident. There is granular mural thrombus at the apex of the left ventricle (on the right). The coronary arteries were unobstructed.

myopathy to the Duchenne muscular dystrophy (dystrophin) gene (see Chapter 28).[51]

Although DCM is in a sense a wastebasket term to describe dilated and failing hearts having no well-defined cause, there is a strong suspicion that many cases represent the common end point of a variety of remote insults to the myocardium. When first seen late in its course, the result of these various injuries is the same (i.e., the specific etiology cannot be determined). Although proof of a cause-and-effect relationship is lacking in nearly all cases, certain pathogenic pathways may be suspected in a given patient: (1) alcohol or other toxicity, (2) previous myocarditis, and (3) pregnancy-associated nutritional deficiency or immunologic reaction (see below). In DCM, the primary abnormality is impairment of left ventricular myocardial contractility (systolic failure); in the end stage, patients may have ejection fractions of less than 25% (normal, approximately 50 to 65%).

MORPHOLOGY. The heart of idiopathic DCM is usually heavy, weighing two to three times normal, and large and flabby, usually with dilatation of all chambers (Fig. 12–28). Nevertheless, because of the wall thinning that accompanies dilatation, the ventricular wall thickness may be less than, equal to, or more than normal. Mural thrombi are common, particularly near the apex of the left and right ventricles and in the atria, and may be a source of thromboemboli. There are no primary valvular alterations, and mitral regurgitation, when present, is primarily a result of left ventricular chamber dilatation **(functional mitral regurgitation).** The coronary arteries are usually but not always free of significant narrowing, but any coronary arterial obstructions and macroscopic myocardial scarring that do exist are insufficient to explain the degree of cardiac dysfunction that is present. The left ventricle often has patchy myocardial (mostly subendocardial) fibrous scars, some probably reflecting healed ischemic damage. These result from the imbalance of perfusion supply and demand caused by hypertrophy and dilatation, fixed coronary obstruction, or embolic damage. Additional superficial endocardial plaques largely represent fibrosis that accompanies and is secondary to the dilated ventricle. Specific heart muscle disease that induces a dilated pattern (e.g., myocarditis or iron overload) can have similar gross features.

The histologic changes of idiopathic DCM also are generally nonspecific and usually do not reflect an etiologic agent. The sizes of individual muscle cells vary; most are hypertrophied, but many are attenuated or stretched. The nuclei are usually enlarged throughout, indicating hypertrophy. Interstitial and endocardial fibrosis of variable degree is usually present, and small fibrous scars often replace individual cells or groups of cells (i.e., **replacement fibrosis,** reflecting healing of previous myocyte necrosis). Leukocytes are usually absent or are present in fibrous tissue only. Examination by transmission electron microscopy shows nonspecific changes of myofiber hypertrophy and degeneration.

DCM may occur at any age, including in childhood, but it usually affects those 20 to 60 years old. It presents with slowly developing CHF that is progressive and unremitting in most cases, but patients may slip precipitously from a compensated to a decompensated functional state. Fifty percent of patients die within 2 years, and only 25% of patients survive longer than 5 years. Death is usually attributable to progressive cardiac failure or arrhythmia. Embolism from dislodgment of an intracardiac thrombus may occur. Cardiac transplantation is frequently recommended.

A variant is *arrhythmogenic right ventricular cardiomyopathy* or *arrhythmogenic right ventricular dysplasia*, a sometimes familial disorder that is most commonly associated with right-sided and sometimes left-sided heart failure and various rhythm disturbances, particularly ventricular tachycardia.[52] Sudden death occurs frequently. Morphologically the right ventricular wall is severely thinned, with

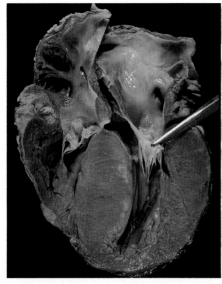
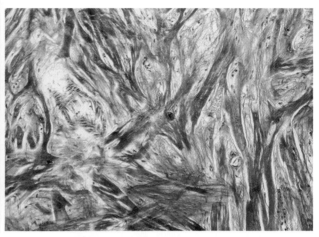

A B

Figure 12–29. Hypertrophic cardiomyopathy with asymmetric septal hypertrophy. *A*, The septal muscle bulges into the left ventricular outflow tract, and the left atrium is enlarged. The anterior mitral leaflet has been moved away from the septum to reveal a fibrous endocardial plaque (see text). *B*, Histologic appearance demonstrating disarray, extreme hypertrophy, and peculiar branching of myocytes as well as the interstitial fibrosis characteristic of hypertrophic cardiomyopathy (collagen is blue in this Masson trichrome stain).

extensive fatty infiltration, loss of myocytes, and interstitial fibrosis.

Hypertrophic Cardiomyopathy

Hypertrophic cardiomyopathy (HCM) is also known by such terms as *idiopathic hypertrophic subaortic stenosis* and *hypertrophic obstructive cardiomyopathy*. It is characterized by a heavy muscular *hyper*contracting heart, in striking contrast to the flabby, *hypo*contracting heart of DCM. It represents a diastolic rather than systolic disorder.

MORPHOLOGY. The essential anatomic feature of HCM is massive myocardial hypertrophy (Fig. 12–29).[53] The classic pattern is said to be disproportionate thickening of the ventricular septum as compared with the free wall of the left ventricle (with a ratio greater than 1.3), frequently termed **asymmetric septal hypertrophy.** In about 10% of cases, however, the hypertrophy is symmetric throughout the heart. On cross section, the ventricular cavity loses its usual round-to-ovoid shape and may be compressed into a "banana-like" configuration by bulging of the ventricular septum into the lumen (see Fig. 12–29A). Although disproportionate hypertrophy can involve the entire septum, it is usually localized to the subaortic (most common), midventricular, or apical region. When the basal septum is markedly thickened at the level of the mitral valve, the outflow of the left ventricle may be narrowed during systole. Sometimes also present are endocardial thickening or mural

plaque formation in the left ventricular outflow tract and thickening of the anterior mitral leaflet; both findings are a result of contact of the anterior mitral leaflet with the septum during ventricular systole (correlating with echocardiographic observation of systolic anterior motion of the mitral valve). These features correlate with functional left ventricular outflow tract obstruction during systole.

The most important histologic features of the myocardium in HCM are (1) extensive myocyte hypertrophy to a degree unusual in other conditions, with transverse myocyte diameters frequently more than 40 μm (normal approximately 15 μm); (2) haphazard disarray of bundles of myocytes, individual myocytes, and contractile elements in sarcomeres within cells **(myofiber disarray),** and (3) interstitial and replacement fibrosis (see Fig. 12–29B). Myofiber disarray typically involves 10 to 50% of the septum and somewhat less of the left ventricular free wall. Myofiber disarray, however, is not unique to HCM and may also be seen with other forms of myocardial hypertrophy, usually to a far lesser extent.

The differential diagnosis includes any disorder that can produce diastolic dysfunction or left ventricular outflow obstruction, with or without disproportionate thickening of the ventricular septum. The two most common diseases that must be distinguished from HCM are amyloidosis and HHD coupled with age-related subaortic septal hypertrophy (see earlier section on hypertensive heart disease). Occasionally valvular or congenital subvalvular aortic stenosis can also mimic HCM. In contrast to the hypertrophy induced by the increased workload of valvular, hypertensive, ischemic, and congenital heart diseases, that observed in HCM develops progressively *in the absence of an identifiable extrinsic inciting stress.*

HCM has been shown to have a genetic basis in many cases. In approximately half of patients, the disease is familial and the pattern of transmission is autosomal dominant with variable expression. Remaining cases appear to be sporadic; it is possible that some represent new mutations or are the result of autosomal recessive transmission with reduced gene penetrance. In some kindreds with HCM, missense mutations have been identified in the genes on chromosome 14 for isoforms of the heavy chain of cardiac myosin, the principal contractile protein in the thick filaments of muscle sarcomeres. However, both the genetic and the structural characteristics of the disease are heterogeneous.[54] The mechanism by which altered myosin heavy chains produce the phenotype of HCM is uncertain.

The course of HCM is extremely variable. Many patients remain the same over years of observation, and some improve. The major problems in HCM are atrial fibrillation with mural thrombus formation, embolization from the mural thrombi, IE on the mitral valve, intractable cardiac failure, and sudden death; the last is the most common cause of death and particularly likely in young males with familial HCM or with a family history of sudden death. The frequency of sudden death is 2 to 3% per year for adults and 4 to 6% per year for children. In HCM, cardiac failure is due to reduced chamber size and poor compliance with reduced stroke volume that results from decreased diastolic filling of the massively hypertrophied left ventricle. End-stage heart failure can be accompanied by dilatation. Interestingly, different specific responsible gene mutations carry vastly differing prognoses.

Although symptoms are not due solely to thickening of the ventricular septum or obstruction, thinning of the septum by surgery (i.e., myotomy/myectomy) is occasionally done. Most patients can be significantly helped by medical therapy that enhances ventricular relaxation.

Restrictive Cardiomyopathy

In the restrictive form of primary myocardial disease, diastolic relaxation and left ventricular chamber filling are impeded; the contractile (systolic) function of the left ventricle is usually unaffected. Thus the functional state can be confused with that of constrictive pericarditis or HCM.

MORPHOLOGY. In idiopathic **restrictive cardiomyopathy (RCM),** the ventricles are of approximately normal size or slightly enlarged, the cavities are not dilated, and the myocardium is firm. Biatrial dilatation is commonly observed. Microscopically there is patchy or diffuse interstitial fibrosis, which can vary from minimal to extensive, but the cause is unknown.

Any disorder that interferes with ventricular filling can mimic RCM, including secondary involvement by deposition disease (such as amyloid) or radiation fibrosis, and constrictive pericarditis or HCM. In many cases, distinct morphologic patterns indicative of specific heart muscle disease may be revealed by light or electron microscopy of endomyocardial biopsy or autopsy specimens; these include myocardial deposition of amyloid, sarcoid granulomas, metastatic tumor, or products of an inborn error of metabolism.

Several other restrictive conditions require brief mention. *Endomyocardial fibrosis* is principally a disease of children and young adults in Africa and other tropical areas, characterized by fibrosis of the ventricular endocardium and subendocardium that extends from the apex toward the inflow tract of the right or left ventricle, or both. It may also involve the tricuspid and mitral valves. The fibrous tissue markedly diminishes the volume and compliance of affected chambers and so induces a restrictive functional defect. Ventricular mural thrombi sometimes develop, and indeed there is a suggestion that the fibrous tissue results from the organization of mural thrombi. The etiology of this condition is unknown.

Loeffler's endomyocarditis is also marked by endomyocardial fibrosis typically with large mural thrombi similar to those seen in the tropical disease, but cases are unrestricted to a specific geographic area. Although the specific cause is unknown, eosinophils are considered important in the pathogenesis of this disease.[55] In addition to the cardiac changes, there is often an eosinophilic leukocytosis and sometimes frank eosinophilic leukemia, which can result in infiltration of other organs by eosinophils, and a rapidly fatal downhill course. In patients with eosinophilic endomyocardial disease, circulating eosinophils generally have measurable structural and functional abnormalities, and many are degranulated. The release of toxic products of eosinophils, especially major basic protein, is postulated to initiate endocardial damage, with subsequent foci of endomyocardial necrosis accompanied by an eosinophilic infiltrate, followed by scarring of the necrotic area and layering of the endocardium by thrombus, and finally organization of the thrombus. Untreated or medically treated eosinophilic endomyocardial disease has a poor prognosis, so surgical endomyocardial strippng (decortication) is often recommended.

Endocardial fibroelastosis is an uncommon heart disease of obscure etiology characterized by focal or diffuse, cartilage-like fibroelastic thickening usually involving the mural left ventricular endocardium. Most common in the first 2 years of life, it is often accompanied by some form of congenital cardiac anomaly, most often aortic valve obstruction in about one-third of all cases. The significance of endocardial fibroelastosis depends on the extent of involvement. When focal, it may have no functional importance; when diffuse, it may be responsible for rapid and progressive cardiac decompensation and death, particularly in children.

SPECIFIC HEART MUSCLE DISEASE

Of the many diseases of known cause or associated with disorders of other systems (*specific heart muscle disease*) summarized in Table 12–11, only sev-

Table 12–11. MAJOR ASSOCIATIONS OF SPECIFIC HEART MUSCLE DISEASE

CARDIAC INFECTIONS
  Viruses
  Chlamydia
  Rickettsia
  Bacteria
  Fungi
  Protozoa

TOXIC
  Alcohol
  Cobalt
  Catecholamines
  Carbon monoxide
  Lithium
  Hydrocarbons
  Arsenic
  Cyclophosphamide
  Doxorubicin (Adriamycin) and daunorubicin

METABOLIC
  Hyperthyroidism
  Hypothyroidism
  Hypokalemia
  Hyperkalemia
  Nutritional deficiency—protein, thiamine, other avitaminoses
  Hemochromatosis

NEUROMUSCULAR DISEASE
  Friedreich's ataxia
  Muscular dystrophy
  Congenital atrophies

STORAGE DISORDERS AND OTHER DEPOSITIONS
  Hunter-Hurler syndrome
  Glycogen storage disease
  Fabry's disease
  Amyloidosis

INFILTRATIVE
  Leukemia
  Carcinomatosis
  Sarcoidosis
  Radiation-induced fibrosis

IMMUNOLOGIC
  Myocarditis (several forms)
  Post-transplant rejection

eral will be discussed in detail. This group can cause any of the three main functional patterns described earlier. For example, myocarditis and toxicities can clinically mimic DCM. Although hemochromatosis (iron storage disease) usually causes a dilated heart with systolic dysfunction, other deposition diseases, such as amyloidosis, can cause a restrictive state with diastolic dysfunction.

Myocarditis

Myocarditis is best defined as an inflammatory involvement of the heart muscle characterized by a leukocytic infiltrate and resultant nonischemic necrosis or degeneration of myocytes. The clinical spectrum is broad, ranging from asymptomatic involvement that ultimately resolves completely, through acute or late onset of CHF, to SCD. It is difficult to be certain of the precise clinical incidence of this condition because often the diagnosis is based on indirect evidence (e.g., heart failure with fever and sudden appearance of ECG changes indicative of a diffuse myocardial lesion in the absence of other definable causes). Of all patients with the recent onset of unexplained CHF, chest pain, or life-threatening arrhythmias who have endomyocardial biopsy (see earlier), approximately 4 to 10% are demonstrated to have myocarditis. The causes of myocarditis include many microbiologic agents, various forms of immunologically mediated damage, toxicity, hypersensitivity reactions, and reactions to physical agents. The etiologic spectrum is presented in Table 12–12; in many cases, however, the cause remains undetermined.

Most cases of well-documented myocarditis are viral in origin. It may occur at any age; infants, immunosuppressed individuals, and pregnant

Table 12–12. MAJOR CAUSES OF MYOCARDITIS

INFECTIONS
  Viruses (e.g., coxsackievirus, ECHO, influenza, HIV, cytomegalovirus)
  Chlamydia (e.g., *C. psittaci*)
  Rickettsia (e.g., *R. typhi* (typhus fever))
  Bacteria (e.g., Corynebacterium (diphtheria), Neisseria (meningococcus), Borrelia (Lyme disease))
  Fungi (e.g., Candida)
  Protozoa (e.g., Trypanosoma (Chagas' disease), toxoplasmosis)
  Helminths (e.g., trichinosis)

IMMUNE-MEDIATED REACTIONS
  Postviral
  Poststreptococcal (rheumatic fever)
  Systemic lupus erythematosus
  Drug hypersensitivity (e.g., methyldopa, sulfonamides)
  Transplant rejection

UNKNOWN
  Sarcoidosis
  Giant cell myocarditis

HIV = human immunodeficiency virus.

women are particularly vulnerable. The most frequently implicated agents are Coxsackievirus A and B, ECHO, poliovirus, and influenza A and B viruses. In most instances, the cardiac involvement follows several days to a few weeks after a primary viral infection elsewhere, as in the lungs, upper respiratory tract, or neuromuscular system (such as poliomyelitis). Occasionally myocarditis is the sole or, at least, the major focus of infection and so is referred to as *primary myocarditis.* Documentation of a viral etiology is difficult, even with endomyocardial biopsy tissues. Most often, recourse is made to serologic demonstration of a rising antibody titer in the serum, but the polymerase chain reaction (PCR) technique has demonstrated viral DNA in the myocardium in some cases of myocarditis.[56]

There is still uncertainty about the mechanisms involved in the production of cardiac damage by viral agents. Two major possibilities exist.[57] There may be direct viral cytotoxicity, but this is considered infrequent. Increasing evidence suggests that immune mediation of myocardial inflammatory lesions occurs in most cases, probably through T cell–dependent mechanisms. Usually myocarditis induced by virus is a biphasic disease consisting of an initial, virus-mediated myocardial or extracardiac infection that is cleared by monocytes and the humoral immune system. This is followed by an immunologic phase mediated by T lymphocytes directed at either novel antigens that develop as a result of interaction between virus and myocardium or myocardial antigens that cross react with either the virus or tissue external to the heart that has been altered by the virus.

Less commonly, myocarditis is caused by a nonviral microbiologic agent or its products (i.e., a toxin). A particularly important form of direct cardiac infection is that caused by the protozoa *Trypanosoma cruzi* producing Chagas' disease. Although uncommon in the northern hemisphere, Chagas' disease affects up to one-half of the population in endemic areas of South America, and myocardial involvement is found in approximately 80% of infected individuals.[58] About 10% of patients die during an acute attack; others may enter a chronic immune-mediated phase and develop progressive signs of cardiac insufficiency 10 to 20 years later. Trichinosis is the most common helminthic disease with associated cardiac involvement. Traditionally considered a myocarditis, injury to the myocardium by the potent exotoxin of the bacterium *Corynebacterium diphtheriae* is characterized by patchy myocyte necrosis with only a sparse lymphocytic infiltrate.

Lyme disease is a systemic illness caused by the bacterial spirochete *Borrelia burgdorferi* that has dermatologic, neurologic, and rheumatologic manifestations. Myocarditis occurs in approximately two-thirds of patients with Lyme disease; spirochetes can be demonstrated in the myocardium of some.[59] Lyme myocarditis is usually mild

and reversible but occasionally requires a temporary pacemaker for AV block.

Myocarditis occurs in many patients with acquired immunodeficiency syndrome (AIDS).[60] Two types have been identified: (1) inflammation and myocyte damage without a clear etiologic agent and (2) myocarditis caused directly by HIV or by an opportunistic pathogen. Although HIV nucleic acid sequences have been detected in some patients who have died of AIDS,[61] the relationship of the HIV to the pathogenesis of AIDS-related myocarditis is uncertain.

There are also noninfectious causes of myocarditis. Myocarditis can be related to allergic reactions *(hypersensitivity)* to a particular drug, including some antibiotics, diuretics, and antihypertensive agents. Several forms of myocarditis are associated with systemic diseases of immune origin, such as RF and systemic lupus erythematosus. Cardiac sarcoidosis and rejection of a transplanted heart may also be considered to be forms of myocarditis.

Against this background we can turn to the anatomic changes seen in the major forms of myocarditis.

MORPHOLOGY. During the active phase of myocarditis, the heart may appear normal or enlarged with dilatation of either ventricle or all chambers. The lesions may be diffuse or patchy. The ventricular myocardium is typically flabby and often mottled by either pale foci or minute hemorrhagic lesions. The endocardium and valves are unaffected except that mural thrombi may be present in any chamber.

The histologic changes vary widely, and only some generalizations can be offered. During active disease, myocarditis is most frequently characterized by an interstitial mononuclear, predominantly lymphocytic inflammatory infiltrate and by injury (usually focal necrosis) to myocytes adjacent to the inflammatory cells, not typical of ischemic damage (Fig. 12–30).[62] Although endomyocardial biopsies are diagnostic in some cases, they can be spuriously negative because inflammatory involvement may be focal or patchy.

Importantly not all myocardial inflammation constitutes myocarditis. The mere presence of myocardial inflammatory cells (without associated myocyte damage) is generally considered an insufficient basis for diagnosis because focal collections of lymphocytes and monocytes are frequent in DCM (and in some other situations), generally but not always localized to areas of myocardial fibrous tissue. Moreover, focal aggregates of mononuclear cells (predominantly macrophages), occasionally with a necrotic myocyte (often with contraction bands) and sometimes with focal neutrophils, may be seen in the myocardium of patients who have been treated with high-dose pres-

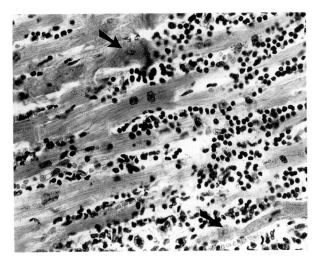

Figure 12-30. Myocarditis, with mononuclear inflammatory cell infiltrate and associated myocyte injury. (Reproduced from Schoen, F.J.: Interventional and Surgical Cardiovascular Pathology: Clinical Correlations and Basic Principles. Philadelphia, W.B. Saunders Co., 1989, p. 185.)

sor agents (such as dopamine) or who have elevated endogenous catecholamines (see discussion of pheochromocytoma in Chapter 25).

The histologic pattern of reaction to bacterial or fungal invasion depends on the specific causative organism but in general mirrors the changes produced by the same organism in extracardiac localizations, including a patchy, focal, suppurative reaction and sometimes microabscesses. Similarly, larger parasites produce their typical tissue reactions within the heart muscle. The myocarditis of Chagas' disease is rendered distinctive by parasitization of scattered myofibers by trypanosomes accompanied by an inflammatory infiltrate of neutrophils, lymphocytes, macrophages, and occasional eosinophils (Fig. 12–31). Hypersensitivity reactions that involve the myocardium induce interstitial infiltrates that are principally perivascular, composed of lymphocytes, macrophages, and a high proportion of eosinophils.

There remains a morphologically distinctive form of myocarditis of uncertain cause called **giant cell myocarditis** characterized by a widespread inflammatory cellular infiltrate containing multinucleate giant cells interspersed with lymphocytes, eosinophils, plasma cells, and macrophages and having at least focal but frequently extensive necrosis (**idiopathic giant cell myocarditis** or, in the past, Fiedler's myocarditis). The giant cells are of macrophage origin in some cases and of myocyte origin in others.

If the patient survives the acute phase of myocarditis, the inflammatory lesions either resolve, leaving no residual changes, or heal by progressive fibrosis, as mentioned earlier. Sometimes the persistent connective tissue is sufficiently scattered

and subtle to be virtually inapparent. With more severe damage, focal minute scars may remain; in extremely florid cases, they may become confluent and grossly visible.

CLINICAL COURSE. At one end of the clinical spectrum, the disease is entirely asymptomatic, and such patients recover completely without sequelae. At the other end of the spectrum, the myocarditis is manifested by the precipitous onset of CHF or arrhythmias. A systolic murmur may appear, related to dilatation of the left ventricle. Between these extremes are the many levels of involvement associated with such symptoms as fatigue, dyspnea, palpitations, and precordial discomfort, sometimes accompanied by fever when the myocarditis is of infectious origin. The clinical features of myocarditis can mimic those of acute myocardial infarction.[63] Occasionally, years later, when an attack of myocarditis is forgotten, the patient may be diagnosed as having DCM. The strongest support for the myocarditis-DCM link comes from patients that have been observed to progress from unequivocal myocarditis to unequivocal DCM on successive biopsy specimens.

Toxic, Metabolic, and Other Specific Causes

ALCOHOL. *Alcohol* or its metabolites (especially acetaldehyde) has a direct toxic effect on the myocardium. Although chronic alcohol damage clinically resembles DCM, "alcoholic CM" is really alcohol-related heart disease and is therefore excluded from the category of idiopathic disorders. Nevertheless, the cause-and-effect relationship with alcohol alone remains tenuous, and no morphologic features serve to distinguish alcohol-in-

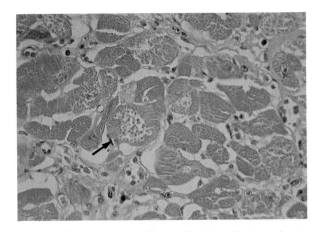

Figure 12–31. The myocarditis of Chagas' disease. A myofiber is distended with trypanosomes *(arrow)*. There is a surrounding inflammatory reaction and individual myofiber necrosis.

duced cardiac damage from idiopathic DCM. Moreover, chronic alcoholism may be associated with thiamine deficiency, introducing an element of beriberi heart disease (indistinguishable from DCM) (see Chapter 9).

ADRIAMYCIN AND OTHER DRUGS. The anthracycline chemotherapeutic agents doxorubicin (Adriamycin) and daunorubicin are well recognized causes of toxic myocardial injury. The hazard is dose dependent (cardiotoxicity usually requires a total dose greater than 500 mg/m^2) and attributed primarily to lipid peroxidation of myofiber membranes. Many other agents, such as lithium, phenothiazines, and cocaine, have been implicated in myocardial injury and sometimes SCD. Common threads running throughout the cardiotoxicity of many chemicals and drugs (including diphtheria exotoxin) are myofiber swelling and vacuolization, fatty change, individual cell lysis (myocytolysis), and sometimes patchy foci of necrosis.[64] Electron microscopy usually reveals cytoplasmic vacuolization and lysis of myofibrils, typified by Adriamycin cardiotoxicity. With discontinuance of the toxic agent, these changes may resolve completely, leaving no apparent sequelae. Sometimes, however, nonspecific hypertrophy with interstitial fibrosis or small focal replacement scars remain, and both the physiologic and morphologic patterns are indistinguishable from those of idiopathic DCM.

CATECHOLAMINES. Foci of myocardial necrosis with contraction bands are frequently observed in patients who have a pheochromocytoma (see Chapter 25), with its elaboration of catecholamines. This is considered to be a manifestation of "catecholamine effect" that appears in association with the administration of large doses of vasopressor agents such as dopamine. Cocaine also causes catecholamine-induced cell damage. The mechanism of catecholamine cardiotoxicity is uncertain, but it appears to relate either to direct toxicity of these agents to cardiac myocytes via calcium overload or to vasomotor constriction in the myocardial circulation in the face of an increased heart rate. In these cases, the mononuclear cell infiltrate is likely a secondary reaction to the foci of myocyte cell death.[65] A similar morphology may be encountered in patients who have recovered from hypotensive episodes or have been resuscitated from a frank cardiac arrest. In such cases, myocyte necrosis results from ischemia followed by reperfusion (see section on ischemic heart disease, earlier in this chapter), and inflammation follows. Curiously some patients with intracranial lesions associated with elevated cerebrospinal fluid pressure have focal myocardial necrosis with contraction bands.

PERIPARTUM STATE. *Peripartum cardiomyopathy* is the designation given to a globally dilated heart when it is discovered within several months before or after delivery. Although the mechanism behind this relationship is uncertain, pregnancy invokes the possibilities of hypertension, volume overload, nutritional deficiency, other metabolic derangement, or as yet poorly characterized immunologic reaction. Whatever the basis, in about half of these patients, proper function is restored, and dilatation of the heart disappears within months after delivery, in contrast to the classic course of DCM.

AMYLOIDOSIS. *Cardiac amyloidosis* (see Chapter 6) may appear along with systemic amyloidosis or may affect only the heart, particularly in the aged (so-called *senile isolated cardiac amyloidosis*). In the cardiovascular senile form of amyloidosis (isolated cardiac amyloidosis), the deposited proteins are known as senile amyloid (ASc) proteins, and two forms (ventricular and atrial) have been identified. The ventricular form has an amino acid sequence similar to that of serum prealbumin (transthyretin), but the protein in the more common atrial form is yet unknown. Clinically important amyloid deposits can occur in the hearts of patients with multiple myeloma (see Chapter 6). Most frequently cardiac amyloidosis produces restrictive hemodynamics, but it can be asymptomatic or can be manifested by CHF, arrhythmias, or features mimicking those of ischemic or valvular disease owing to deposits in the interstitium, conduction system, vasculature, and valves, respectively.

MORPHOLOGY. Grossly, the heart in cardiac amyloidosis varies from normal to firm, rubbery, and noncompliant with thickened walls. Usually the chambers are of normal size, but in some cases they are dilated. Numerous, small semitranslucent nodules may be seen at the atrial endocardial surface, particularly on the left. Amyloid deposits are extracellular and they may occur in the myocardial interstitium, conduction tissue, valves, endocardium, pericardium, and small intramural coronary arteries. In the interstitium, amyloid deposits often form rings around cardiac myocytes and capillaries. Intramural arteries may have sufficient amyloid in their walls to compress and occlude the lumina.

IRON OVERLOAD. *Iron overload* can occur in hereditary hemochromatosis and hemosiderosis owing to multiple blood transfusions. The heart is identical in each. Patients with iron storage disease present most commonly with a dilated pattern. Iron deposition is more prominent in ventricles than atria and in the working myocardium than in the conduction system. It is thought that iron causes dysfunction by interfering with metal-dependent enzyme systems.

MORPHOLOGY. Grossly, the myocardium of the iron-overloaded heart is rust-brown in color but is usually otherwise indistinguishable from that of idiopathic DCM. Microscopically, there is marked accumulation of hemosiderin within cardiac myocytes (contrast with the extracellular deposition of amyloid discussed previously), particularly in the perinuclear region, demonstrable with a Prussian blue stain. This is associated with varying degrees of cellular degeneration and replacement fibrosis. Ultrastructurally, cardiac myocytes contain abundant perinuclear siderosomes (iron-containing lysosomes).

HYPERTHYROIDISM AND HYPOTHYROIDISM. The cardiac effects of abnormal thyroid function exemplify the reaction to systemic metabolic disorders. Cardiac manifestations are among the earliest, most consistent features of hyperthyroidism and hypothyroidism. In *hyperthyroidism* (see Chapter 25), tachycardia, palpitations, and cardiomegaly are common; supraventricular arrhythmias occasionally appear. The cause of cardiomegaly is unknown. There is clear evidence, however, for direct as well as indirect effects of thyroid hormones on the cells of the heart, largely through stimulation of specific nuclear receptors, through activation of extranuclear sites, and by altering plasma membrane function.[66] Moreover, thyroid hormones alter responsiveness of cells to sympathetic stimulation by modulating adrenergic receptor function, density, or both. Cardiac failure occurs uncommonly, usually in the elderly superimposed on other cardiac diseases. Histologic features are those of nonspecific hypertrophy. In *hypothyroidism* (see Chapter 25), cardiac output is decreased, with reduced stroke volume and heart rate. Increased peripheral vascular resistance and decreased blood volume result in narrowing of the pulse pressure, prolongation of circulation time, and decreased flow to peripheral tissues. Reduced circulation in the skin accounts for the characteristic cold sensitivity. In well-advanced myxedema, the heart is flabby, enlarged, and dilated. Histologic features include myofiber swelling with loss of striations and basophilic degeneration, accompanied by interstitial mucopolysaccharide-rich edema fluid. A similar fluid sometimes accumulates within the pericardial sac. To these changes, the term *myxedema heart* has been applied.

PERICARDIAL DISEASE

Pericardial lesions are almost always associated with disease in other portions of the heart or surrounding structures or secondary to a systemic disorder; isolated pericardial disease is unusual. Despite the large number of etiologies of pericardial disease, there are relatively few anatomic forms of pericardial involvement.

ACCUMULATIONS OF FLUID IN THE PERICARDIAL SAC

Pericardial Effusion

Normally there is about 30 to 50 ml of thin, clear, straw-colored, translucent fluid in the pericardial space. Under a variety of circumstances, *pericardial effusions* may appear; because they accumulate slowly and are rarely larger than 500 ml, they are usually without clinical significance except for producing a characteristic globular enlargement of the heart shadow on x-ray film. Rarely a large volume or rapid accumulation of a lesser volume may embarrass diastolic filling of the heart, requiring withdrawal.

Serous effusion in cardiac failure is most common. The fluid is completely clear, or straw colored, and sterile; the serosal surfaces remain smooth and glistening. Serosanguineous (as in blunt chest trauma) and chylous effusions, containing lipid droplets, from lymphatic obstruction owing to benign or malignant mediastinal neoplasms, rarely achieve sufficient volume to have clinical significance.

Hemopericardium

Hemopericardium is the accumulation of pure blood in the pericardial sac, distinct from hemorrhagic pericarditis, a condition in which there is an inflammatory exudate containing blood mixed with pus. Hemopericardium is almost invariably due to rupture of the heart wall secondary to myocardial infarction, traumatic perforation, or rupture of the intrapericardial aorta. In such cases, blood rapidly fills the sac under greatly increased pressure, producing *cardiac tamponade*. Small amounts of blood may result from the trauma sustained during cardiopulmonary resuscitation; marked hemorrhage is unusual. As little as 200 to 300 ml of pericardial fluid (blood) may be sufficient to cause death when it accumulates rapidly.

PERICARDITIS

Inflammations of the pericardium are usually secondary to a variety of cardiac diseases, to systemic disorders, or to metastases from neoplasms arising in remote sites. Primary pericarditis is unusual and almost always of viral origin. The major causes of pericarditis are presented in Table 12–13. The various etiologies cited usually evoke an acute pericarditis, but a few, such as tuberculosis and fungi, produce chronic reactions. Because it is usually impossible from pathologic examination to determine the etiologic basis for the reaction, a morphologic classification follows, dividing the pericar-

Table 12–13. CAUSES OF PERICARDITIS

INFECTIOUS AGENTS
  Viruses
  Pyogenic bacteria
  Tuberculosis
  Fungi
  Other parasites

PRESUMABLY IMMUNOLOGICALLY MEDIATED
  Rheumatic fever
  Systemic lupus erythematosus
  Scleroderma
  Postcardiotomy
  Postmyocardial infarction (Dressler) syndrome
  Drug-hypersensitivity reaction

MISCELLANEOUS
  Myocardial infarction
  Uremia
  Following cardiac surgery
  Neoplasia
  Trauma
  Radiation

---

ditides into acute and chronic forms and further subdividing the acute reactions based on the character of the exudate.

Acute Pericarditis

SEROUS PERICARDITIS. Serous inflammatory exudates are characteristically produced by noninfectious inflammations, such as RF, systemic lupus erythematosus, scleroderma, tumors, and uremia. An infection in the tissues contiguous to the pericardium, for example, a bacterial pleuritis, may cause sufficient irritation of the parietal pericardial serosa to cause a sterile serous effusion. In time, however, infection may extend across the anatomic barrier, and the serous exudate is transformed into a frank suppurative reaction.

In some instances, a well-defined viral infection elsewhere—upper respiratory tract, pneumonia, parotitis—antedates the pericarditis and serves as the primary focus of infection. Occasionally the virus can be isolated from the exudate. Infrequently a viral pericarditis occurs as an apparent primary involvement, usually in young adults, that may accompany myocarditis *(myopericarditis)*. In many instances, however, the etiology of an apparent primary serous pericarditis remains unknown.

Morphologically whatever the cause, there is an inflammatory reaction in the epicardial and pericardial surfaces with scant numbers of polymorphonuclear leukocytes, lymphocytes, and histiocytes. Usually the volume of fluid is not large (50 to 200 ml) and accumulates slowly. Organization into fibrous adhesions rarely occurs.

FIBRINOUS AND SEROFIBRINOUS PERICARDITIS. These two anatomic forms are *the most frequent type of pericarditis* and represent essentially similar processes, a more or less serous fluid mixed with a fibrinous exudate. Common causes include acute myocardial infarction, the postinfarction (Dressler's) syndrome (likely an autoimmune condition, that appears several weeks after a myocardial infarction), uremia, chest radiation, RF, systemic lupus erythematosus, and trauma. Just as pneumonia or suppurative infections in the pleural cavities may produce serous pericarditis, in more severe cases, they may cause the outpouring of fibrin. A fibrinous reaction also follows routine cardiac surgery.

The gross morphologic alterations have already been described (see Fig 12–19*B*). As with all inflammatory exudates, *fibrin may be digested with resolution of the exudate, or it may become organized* (see Chapter 3).

From the clinical standpoint, *the development of a loud pericardial friction rub is the most striking characteristic of fibrinous pericarditis.* A collection of serous fluid may obliterate the rub by separating the two layers of the pericardium. Pain, systemic febrile reactions, and signs suggestive of cardiac failure may accompany the pathognomonic friction rub.

PURULENT OR SUPPURATIVE PERICARDITIS. This form of pericardial inflammation almost invariably denotes the invasion of the pericardial space by infective organisms. These organisms may reach the pericardial cavity by several routes: (1) direct extension from neighboring inflammations, such as an empyema of the pleural cavity, lobar pneumonia, mediastinal infections, or extension of a ring abscess through the myocardium or aortic root in infective endocarditis (see section on infective endocarditis, earlier in this chapter); (2) seeding from the blood; (3) lymphatic extension; or (4) direct introduction during cardiotomy. Immunosuppressive therapy potentiates all of these pathways.

The exudate ranges from a thin to a creamy pus of up to 400 to 500 ml in volume. The serosal surfaces are reddened, granular, and coated with the exudate (Fig. 12–32). Microscopically there is an acute inflammatory reaction. Sometimes the inflammatory process extends into surrounding structures to induce a so-called *mediastinopericarditis*.

The clinical findings are essentially the same as those present in fibrinous pericarditis, but signs of systemic infection are usually marked: for example, spiking temperatures, chills, and fever.

Organization is the usual outcome; resolution is infrequent. Because of the great intensity of the inflammatory response, the organization frequently produces *constrictive pericarditis*, a serious consequence (see later).

HEMORRHAGIC PERICARDITIS. An exudate composed of blood mixed with a fibrinous or suppurative effusion is most commonly caused by tuberculosis or by direct malignant neoplastic involvement of the pericardial space. It may also be found in

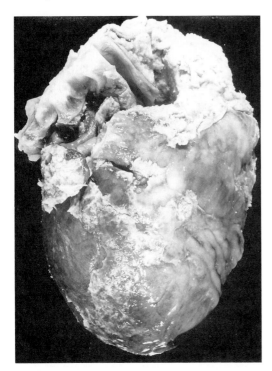

Figure 12-32. Acute suppurative pericarditis caused by *Staphylococcus aureus* infection. Extensive purulent exudate is evident.

bacterial infections or in cases of pericarditis occurring in patients with uremia or some underlying bleeding diathesis. Hemorrhagic pericarditis often follows cardiac surgery and sometimes is responsible for significant blood loss or even tamponade, requiring a "second-look" operation.

If the underlying cause is a tumor, neoplastic cells may be present in the effusion, so cytologic examination of fluid removed through a pericardial tap may yield the specific cause. The clinical significance is similar to that of fibrinous or suppurative pericarditis.

CASEOUS PERICARDITIS. Caseation within the pericardial sac is, until proved otherwise, tuberculous in origin; infrequently mycotic infections evoke a similar pattern. The pericardium is usually involved by direct spread from tuberculous foci within the tracheobronchial nodes. The anatomic changes are typical of tuberculous infections elsewhere and need no further description. Caseous pericarditis is the most frequent antecedent of disabling, fibrocalcific, chronic constrictive pericarditis.

Chronic or Healed Pericarditis

Chronic pericarditis is a misnomer that is applied to the healed stage of the various forms of pericardial inflammation already described. In some cases, organization merely produces plaque-like fibrous thickenings of the serosal membranes ("soldier's plaque") or thin, delicate adhesions of obscure origin that are observed fairly frequently at autopsy and rarely cause impairment of cardiac function. In other cases, organization results in complete obliteration of the pericardial sac. This fibrosis yields a delicate, stringy type of adhesion between parietal and visceral pericardium called *adhesive pericarditis*, which rarely hampers or restricts cardiac action. In some cases, however, healed pericarditis can be clinically important, especially when it takes the form of adhesive mediastinopericarditis or constrictive pericarditis.

ADHESIVE MEDIASTINOPERICARDITIS. This form of pericardial fibrosis may follow a suppurative or caseous pericarditis, previous cardiac surgery, or irradiation to the mediastinum. Only rarely is it a sequel to simple fibrinous exudation. The pericardial sac is obliterated, and adherence of the external aspect of the parietal layer to surrounding structures produces a great strain on cardiac function. With each systolic contraction, the heart is pulling not only against the parietal pericardium, but also against the attached surrounding structures. Systolic retraction of the rib cage and diaphragm, pulsus paradoxus, and a variety of other characteristic clinical findings may be observed. *The increased workload causes cardiac hypertrophy and dilatation, which may be quite massive in more severe cases, mimicking idiopathic DCM (see earlier).*

CONSTRICTIVE PERICARDITIS. The heart may be encased in a dense, fibrous, or fibrocalcific scar that limits diastolic expansion and seriously restricts cardiac output. Sometimes there is a well-defined history of a previous suppurative, hemorrhagic, or caseous (tuberculous) pericarditis, but more often the cause is uncertain. In constrictive pericarditis, the pericardial space is obliterated, and the heart is surrounded by a dense, adherent layer of scar or calcification, often 0.5 to 1.0 cm thick, that can resemble a plaster mold in extreme cases *(concretio cordis)*.

Although the signs of cardiac failure may resemble those produced by adhesive mediastinopericarditis, the local findings in the heart are quite different. *Cardiac hypertrophy and dilatation cannot occur because of the dense enclosing scar, and the heart is consequently quiet with reduced output.* The major therapy is surgical removal of the shell of constricting fibrous tissue *(pericardiectomy).*

RHEUMATOID HEART DISEASE

Rheumatoid arthritis is mainly a disorder of the joints, but it is also associated with many nonarticular involvements (e.g., subcutaneous rheumatoid nodules, acute vasculitis, and Felty's syndrome [see

Chapter 27]). The heart is also involved in 20 to 40% of cases of severe prolonged rheumatoid arthritis. The most common finding is a fibrinous pericarditis that may progress to fibrous thickening of the visceral and parietal pericardium with dense fibrous adhesions. In the early stages of this process, rheumatoid inflammatory granulomatous nodules resembling those that occur subcutaneously may be identifiable deep to the pericardial surfaces. Much less frequently, rheumatoid nodules involve the myocardium, endocardium, valves of the heart, and root of the aorta. Rheumatoid valvulitis can lead to marked fibrous thickening and secondary calcification of valve cusps, producing changes resembling those of chronic rheumatic valvular disease, but intercommissural adhesion is rarely present. Amyloid involving the heart can also occur secondary to rheumatoid arthritis.

NEOPLASTIC HEART DISEASE

Primary tumors of the heart are rare; in contrast, metastatic tumors to the heart occur in about 5% of patients dying of cancer. The most common primary tumors, in descending order of frequency, are myxomas, fibromas, lipomas, papillary fibroelastomas, rhabdomyomas, angiosarcomas, and other sarcomas. The five most common all are benign and account collectively for 80 to 90% of primary tumors of the heart.[67]

PRIMARY CARDIAC TUMORS

MYXOMA. *Myxomas* are the most common primary tumor of the heart in adults (Fig. 12–33).[68] Although they may arise in any of the four chambers or, rarely, on the heart valves, about 90% are located in the atria, with a left-to-right ratio of approximately 4:1 *(atrial myxomas).*

MORPHOLOGY. The tumors are almost always single, but rarely several occur simultaneously. The region of the fossa ovalis in the atrial septum is the favored site of atrial origin. Myxomas range from small (less than 1 cm) to large (up to 10 cm) sessile or pedunculated masses (see Fig. 12–33A) that vary from globular and hard lesions mottled with hemorrhage to soft, translucent, papillary, or villous lesions having a myxoid appearance. The pedunculated form is frequently sufficiently mobile to move into or sometimes through the AV valves during systole, causing intermittent and often position-dependent obstruction. Sometimes such mobility exerts a "wrecking-ball" effect, causing damage to the valve leaflets.

Histologically, myxomas are composed of stellate or globular myxoma cells, endothelial cells, mature or immature smooth muscle cells, and a variety of intermediate forms embedded within an abundant acid mucopolysaccharide ground substance and covered by endothelium (see Fig. 12–33B). Peculiar structures that variably resemble poorly formed glands or vessels are characteristic. Some inflammation is usually present.

It has long been questioned whether cardiac myxomas are hamartomas or organized thrombi, but the weight of evidence is on the side of benign neoplasia. All the tumor cell types present are thought to derive from differentiation of primitive multipotential mesenchymal cells.

The major clinical manifestations are due to valvular "ball-valve" obstruction, embolization, or a syndrome of constitutional symptoms, such as fever and malaise. Sometimes fragmentation with systemic embolization calls attention to these lesions. Constitutional symptoms are likely due to the elaboration by some myxomas of the cytokine interleukin-6, a major mediator of the acute phase response of the systemic inflammatory reaction. Echocardiography provides the opportunity to identify these masses noninvasively. Surgical removal is usually curative, although rarely the neoplasm recurs months to years later.

LIPOMA. *Lipomas* may occur in the subendocardium, subepicardium, or within the myocardium, as localized, poorly encapsulated masses, which may be asymptomatic, can create ball-valve obstructions as with myxomas, or produce arrhythmias. They are most often located in the left ventricle, right atrium, or atrial septum and are not necessarily neoplastic. In the atrial septum, the depositions are called "lipomatous hypertrophy."

PAPILLARY FIBROELASTOMA. *Papillary fibroelastomas* are curious, usually incidental lesions, most often identified at autopsy.

MORPHOLOGY. Generally they are located on valves, particularly the ventricular surfaces of semilunar valves and the atrial surfaces of AV valves. They constitute a distinctive cluster of hair-like projections up to 1 cm in diameter, covering up to several centimeters in diameter of the endocardial surface. Histologically, they are covered by endothelium, deep to which is myxoid connective tissue containing abundant mucopolysaccharide matrix and elastic fibers. Although called neoplasms, it is possible that fibroelastomas represent organized thrombi, similar to the much smaller, usually trivial, heaped up **Lambl's excrescences** that are frequently found on the aortic valves of older individuals.

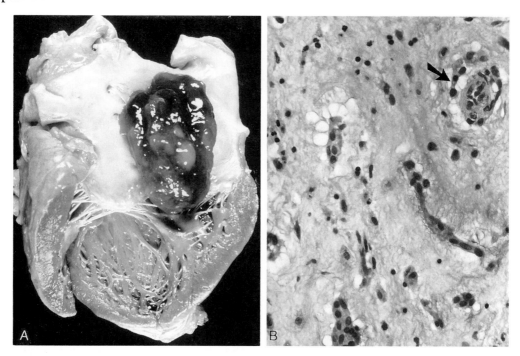

Figure 12–33. Left atrial myxoma. *A,* Gross photograph showing large pedunculated lesion arising from the region of the fossa ovalis. *B,* Microscopic appearance, with abundant ground substance in which are scattered mononuclear leukocytes and abnormal vascular formations *(arrow). (B* reproduced from Schoen, F.J.: Interventional and Surgical Cardiovascular Pathology: Clinical Correlations and Basic Principles. Philadelphia, W.B. Saunders Co., 1989, p. 209.)

RHABDOMYOMA. *Rhabdomyomas* are the most frequent primary tumor of the heart in infants and children and are frequently discovered in the first years of life because of obstruction of a valvular orifice or cardiac chamber.

MORPHOLOGY. They are generally small, gray-white myocardial masses up to several centimeters in diameter located on either the left or the right side of the heart, protruding into the ventricular chambers. Histologically they are composed of a mixed population of cells, the most characteristic of which are large, rounded, or polygonal cells containing numerous glycogen-laden vacuoles separated by strands of cytoplasm running from the plasma membrane to the more or less centrally located nucleus, the so-called **spider cells.** These cells can be shown to have myofibrils. That rhabdomyomas are hamartomas or malformations rather than true neoplasms is supported by a high frequency of tuberous sclerosis (see Chapter 29) in patients with cardiac rhabdomyomas.

SARCOMA. Cardiac *angiosarcomas* and other sarcomas are not distinctive from their counterparts in other locations (see Chapter 11) and so require no further comment here.

CARDIAC EFFECTS OF NONCARDIAC NEOPLASMS

With enhanced patient survival due to diagnostic and therapeutic advances, significant cardiovascular effects of noncardiac neoplasms and their therapy are now commonly recognized clinically[69] (Table 12–14). Effects may be due directly to local infiltration of tumor tissue or indirectly to circulating mediators. Some neoplasms, such as carcinoid tumors, have cardiac consequences that may be

Table 12–14. CARDIOVASCULAR EFFECTS OF NONCARDIAC NEOPLASMS

DIRECT CONSEQUENCES OF TUMOR
  Pericardial and myocardial metastases
  Large vessel obstruction
  Pulmonary tumor emboli

INDIRECT CONSEQUENCES OF TUMOR—COMPLICATIONS OF CIRCULATING MEDIATORS
  Nonbacterial thrombotic endocarditis (NBTE)
  Carcinoid heart disease
  Pheochromocytoma-associated heart disease
  Myeloma-associated amyloidosis

EFFECTS OF TUMOR THERAPY
  Chemotherapy
  Radiation therapy

Modified from Schoen, F.J., et al.: Cardiac effects of non-cardiac neoplasms. Cardiol. Clin. 2:657, 1984.

Table 12-15. THE SPECTRUM OF DIRECT EFFECTS OF TUMORS ON THE HEART AND PERICARDIUM

SITE OF METASTASIS	FUNCTIONAL CONSEQUENCES	MOST LIKELY PRIMARY TUMOR
Myocardium via hematogenous route	Arrhythmias Obstruction Restriction Infarction Dyskinesia	Any
Pericardium	Effusion Restriction	Lung or breast carcinoma, leukemia, lymphoma
Right atrial chamber	Obstruction	Renal adenocarcinoma, hepatoma, lung
Lung (multiple tumor emboli)	Cor pulmonale	Gastric or breast carcinoma, hepatoma

Modified from Schoen, F.J., et al.: Cardiac effects of noncardiac neoplasms. Cardiol. Clin. 2:657, 1984.

more life-threatening than local effects. Occasionally the cardiac complication represents the dominant feature of the presentation of a noncardiac malignant tumor. Moreover, chemotherapy and radiation manifest their own distinct cardiovascular side effects and toxicities.

The direct effects of cardiac metastases on the heart are varied (Table 12-15). Carcinomas of the lung and breast, melanomas, leukemias, and lymphomas most frequently involve the heart. Metastases can reach the heart and pericardium by retrograde lymphatic extension (most carcinomas), by hematogenous seeding (many tumors), by direct contiguous extension (primary carcinoma of the lung, breast, or esophagus), or by direct contiguous venous extension (tumors of the kidney or liver). Clinical symptoms are most often associated with pericardial spread, by either of two major mechanisms. Most commonly, there is only modest tumor bulk, but a pericardial effusion that causes tamponade; less commonly, there is sufficient tumor bulk to directly restrict cardiac filling. Myocardial metastases are usually clinically silent or have nonspecific features, such as a generalized defect in ventricular contractility or compliance. Bronchogenic carcinoma or malignant lymphoma may infiltrate the mediastinum extensively, causing encasement, compression, or invasion of the superior vena cava with resultant obstruction to blood coming from the head and upper extremities (*superior vena cava syndrome*). Renal cell carcinoma, because of its high propensity to invade the renal vein, can grow in the lumen of the renal vein into and along the inferior vena cava, blocking venous return to the heart. Tumor may extend into the right atrium. Microscopic pulmonary tumor emboli can cause unexplained progressive dyspnea, even in the face of grossly normal lungs.

Of the indirect cardiac effects of noncardiac tumors, NBTE, carcinoid heart disease, pheochromocytoma-associated myocardial damage and amyloidosis are discussed earlier in this chapter.

The effects of chemotherapy are primarily associated with Adriamycin and related compounds (see section on specific heart muscle disease, earlier in this chapter). With the use of radiotherapy techniques permitting cure of mediastinal neoplasms, the effects of radiation on the heart are clinically important in some cases. The spectrum of radiation heart disease includes pericarditis, pericardial effusion, myocardial fibrosis, and chronic pericardial disorders most commonly. Other cardiac effects of radiotherapy include accelerated CAD and mural and valvular endocardial fibrosis.

CONGENITAL HEART DISEASE

Congenital heart disease is a general term used to describe abnormalities of the heart or great vessels that are present from birth. Most such disorders arise from faulty embryogenesis, during gestational weeks 3 through 8, when major cardiovascular structures undergo development. Although some severe anomalies may be incompatible with intrauterine survival, most are associated with live births. Some may produce manifestations soon thereafter, frequently accompanying the change from fetal to postnatal circulatory patterns (with reliance on the lungs, rather than placenta, for oxygenation). Others, however, do not necessarily become evident until adulthood (e.g., aortic coarctation or atrial septal defect [ASD]). Immense strides have been made in the diagnosis and therapy of congenital heart defects, allowing extended survival for many children.[70,71] Most forms are now amenable to surgical repair with good results.

INCIDENCE. Congenital heart disease is the most common type of heart disease among children. Although figures vary, a generally accepted incidence is 6 to 8 per 1000 live-born, full-term births. The incidence is higher in premature infants and in stillborns. Twelve disorders account for about 85% of cases, with approximate frequencies presented in Table 12-16. These anomalies are described below.

ETIOLOGY. The cause of congenital heart disease is unknown in more than 90% of patients. Multifactorial genetic and environmental inputs, however, are suspected, including chromosomal defects, viruses, chemicals, and radiation. There is a twofold to tenfold increase in the incidence of congenital heart disease in siblings of an affected child or

Table 12–16. FREQUENCIES OF CARDIAC MALFORMATIONS IN 1000 CONSECUTIVE CHILDREN*

MALFORMATION	% OF CONGENITAL HEART DISEASE
Ventricular septal defect (VSD)	33
Patent ductus arteriosus (PDA)	10
Tetralogy of Fallot	9
Aortic stenosis (AS)	8
Pulmonary stenosis (PS)	10
Coarctation of aorta	5
Atrial septal defect (ASD)	5
Transposition of great arteries	5
Atrioventricular septal defect	4
Truncus arteriosus	1
Tricuspid atresia	1
Total anomalous pulmonary venous connection (TAPVC)	1

* Combinations of lesions tabulated with dominant malformation. Data modified from Moller, J.H.: 1000 Consecutive children with a cardiac malformation with 26- to 37-year follow-up. Am. J. Cardiol. 70:661, 1992.

children of an affected parent, pointing to genetic influences, and there is a well-defined gender preponderance toward males for certain specific defects. Interestingly monozygotic twins, despite having identical genes, have only a 10% concordance for ventricular septal defects (VSDs), clearly indicating that more than genetics are involved. Nevertheless, identifiable chromosomal abnormalities compose about 5% of cases, specifically +14q-; trisomies 21, 18, 13, 22, and 9 (mosaic); and Turner's syndrome (XO).

Fewer than 1% of cases can be definitively attributed to environmental influences. The best documented external influence is maternal rubella infection in the first trimester of pregnancy. In addition to cataracts, deafness, and microcephaly, maternal rubella may result in patent ductus arteriosus (PDA), pulmonary valvular or arterial stenosis or both, aortic stenosis, tetralogy of Fallot, and VSD, either singly or in combination. A large number of other cardiac teratogenic influences have been identified in animals, such as hypoxia, ionizing radiation, and various drugs; in humans, there is substantial evidence implicating the drug thalidomide, alcohol consumption, and, less strongly, cigarette smoking.

That the cause of congenital heart disease is in most cases multifactoral is important to genetic counseling. Because environmental insults cause damage during a specific vulnerable period of embryogenesis and because most cardiovascular abnormalities of genetic origin are associated with well-defined multisystem syndromes, parents of an affected child having neither of these predispositions can be reassured that the increased risk for defects in subsequent children is small (probably below 5%). When more than one member of a family is affected, however, the risk rises sharply.

CLINICAL CONSEQUENCES. *The varied structural anomalies in hearts with congenital defects fall primarily into two major categories: shunts or obstructions. A shunt* is an abnormal communication between chambers or blood vessels (or both). Abnormal channels permit the flow of blood from left to right or the reverse, depending on pressure relationships. When blood from the right side of the heart enters the left side *(right-to-left shunt)*, a dusky blueness of the skin and mucous membranes *(cyanosis)* results because poorly oxygenated blood enters the systemic circulation. Congenital heart defects that produce right-to-left shunts from early infancy are known as *cyanotic congenital heart disease* (e.g., tetralogy of Fallot, transposition of the great arteries [TGA], persistent truncus arteriosus, tricuspid atresia, and total anomalous pulmonary venous connection [TAPVC]). One consequence of these abnormal communications is that bland or septic emboli arising in peripheral veins can bypass the normal filtration action of the lungs and thus enter the systemic circulation *(paradoxical embolism)*; brain infarction and abscess are potential consequences.

In contrast, left-to-right shunts are not initially associated with cyanosis, but these can result in progressive pulmonary hypertension and right ventricular overload with hypertrophy. Although the foramen ovale and the ductus arteriosus functionally close soon after birth, rendering the pulmonary vascular bed a low-pressure, low-resistance system, the presence of a shunt may expose the pulmonary circulation to increased volume or pressure in congenital heart disease. Shunts associated with increased pulmonary blood flow include ASDs, and shunts associated with both increased pulmonary blood flow and pressure include VSDs and PDA. The muscular pulmonary arteries (less than 1 mm diameter) first respond to increased pressure by medial hypertrophy and vasoconstriction, which maintains relatively normal distal pulmonary capillary and venous pressures, helping to prevent pulmonary edema. Prolonged pulmonary arterial vasoconstriction, however, stimulates the development of irreversible obstructive intimal lesions. Consequently the pressure on the right side of the heart can rise to exceed that on the left, eventually reversing the shunt to right-to-left and creating what is called *late cyanotic congenital heart disease* or *Eisenmenger's syndrome* (e.g., in cases of VSD, ASD, AV septal defect, and PDA).

Once significant irreversible pulmonary hypertension develops, the structural defects of congenital heart disease are considered irreparable. The secondary pulmonary vascular changes eventually lead to the patient's death. This is the rationale for *early* surgical or nonsurgical intervention. In contrast to left-to-right shunts (which tend to increase pulmonary blood flow), congenital hypoplasia of the right ventricular outflow tract or pulmonary arteries (e.g., tetralogy of Fallot) may result in greatly decreased pulmonary blood flow.

Clinical findings frequently associated with severe, long-standing cyanosis include clubbing of the tips of the fingers and toes (hypertrophic osteoarthropathy) and polycythemia. Cerebral thrombosis in very young children sometimes occurs in these settings, presumably related to the polycythemia and consequently increased blood viscosity and perhaps triggered by a febrile illness inducing dehydration.

Some developmental anomalies of the heart produce obstructions to flow because of abnormal narrowings of chambers, valves, or blood vessels. Prime examples are valvular stenoses (partial narrowings) or artresias (complete obstructions) and therefore are called *obstructive congenital heart disease* (e.g., coarctation of the aorta, aortic valvular stenosis, and pulmonary valvular stenosis).

In congenital heart disease, altered hemodynamics usually cause cardiac dilatation or hypertrophy (or both). A decrease in the volume and muscle mass of a cardiac chamber is called *hypoplasia* if it occurs before birth and *atrophy* if it develops after birth. Moreover, congenital anomalies produce jet streams, and therefore endothelial injury where the jet impinges, and pose a particular risk for IE (e.g.,VSD, PDA, tetralogy of Fallot, and tight aortic stenosis). Children with significant congenital cardiac defects may also fail to thrive, may suffer from retarded development, and are at greater risk of developing the usual diseases of childhood.

LEFT-TO-RIGHT SHUNTS — LATE CYANOSIS

Atrial Septal Defect

An ASD represents an abnormal opening in the atrial septum that allows free communication of blood between the right and left atria (not to be confused with a patent foramen ovale, present in up to one-third of normal individuals and of no significance unless right-sided pressures are elevated [see later]). An ASD is the most common congenital cardiac anomaly that may first come to clinical attention in adults.

During fetal life, pressure in the right atrium is higher than that in the left, and oxygenated placental blood in the right atrium flows across the foramen ovale and into the left atrium. With birth and opening of the pulmonary circulation, however, the pressure relationships are reversed, but left-to-right blood flow is prevented by the flap valve covering the foramen ovale. Fusion of this

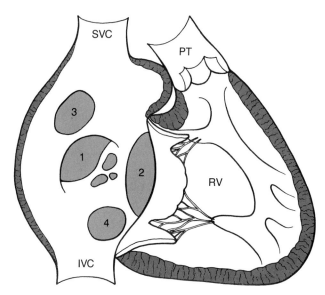

Figure 12–34. Locations of atrial septal defect. 1 = secundum; 2 = primum; 3 = sinus venosus; 4 = coronary sinus (rare). (IVC = inferior vena cava; PT = pulmonary trunk; RV = right ventricle; SVC = superior vena cava.) (Courtesy of William D. Edwards, M.D., Mayo Clinic, Rochester, MN.)

valve to the limbus of the fossa ovalis normally follows in about two-thirds of infants. A nonfunctional oblique slit known as a *patent foramen ovale* persists in about one-third of individuals, but it permits little or no flow because of the flap valve.

MORPHOLOGY. The three major types of ASDs, classified according to their location in the septum, are secundum, primum, and sinus venosus (Fig. 12–34). The **secundum-type ASD** represents approximately 90% of all ASDs, most of which are isolated. The defect results from a deficiency or fenestration of the embryonic septum primum, deficiency of septum secundum, or both and involves the valve or limbus of the fossa ovalis. When associated with another defect, such as PDA, VSD, pulmonary stenosis, TGA, or tetralogy of Fallot, the other defect is usually hemodynamically dominant. The atrial aperture may be of any size and may be single, multiple, or fenestrated. A large secundum defect creates essentially one common atrial chamber. The term **common** atrium or ventricle implies that most of the septum is absent.

Primum anomalies represent only about 5% of ASDs. They occur low in the atrial septum, anteroinferior to the fossa ovalis and adjacent to the AV valves, and are usually associated with a cleft anterior mitral leaflet. This combination is known as a partial atrioventricular septal defect (see later).

Sinus venosus defects are located high in the atrial septum, posterior to the fossa ovalis, near the entrance of the superior vena cava, which may straddle the defect. They account for about 5% of

ASDs and are commonly accompanied by anomalous connections of right pulmonary veins to the superior vena cava or right atrium.

ASDs result in a left-to-right shunt, largely because pulmonary vascular resistance is considerably less than systemic vascular resistance and because the compliance (distensibility) of the right ventricle is much greater than that of the left. Pulmonary blood flow may be 2 to 4 times normal. Although some neonates may be in profound CHF with an isolated ASD, ASDs are well tolerated if small (less than 1 cm in diameter). Even larger defects do not usually constitute serious problems during the first decades of life, when the flow is from left-to-right. An isolated large ASD usually does not become symptomatic in a patient before 30 years of age, whereas a small ASD is virtually always asymptomatic. A murmur is often present; it arises as a result of excessive flow through the pulmonary valve. Eventually volume hypertrophy of the right atrium and right ventricle develop.

Irreversible pulmonary hypertension develops in fewer than 10% of subjects with an isolated unoperated ASD because the lungs usually tolerate an increase in flow, in contrast to an increase in pressure (see VSD, next). Cyanosis, respiratory difficulties, and cardiac failure ensue progressively in those with severe pulmonary hypertension, however. IE is rare with ASDs because of the low-pressure gradients and sluggish flow, but paradoxic embolism or brain abscess can occur when the flow is reversed.

The objectives of surgical closure of an ASD are the reversal of the hemodynamic abnormalities and the prevention of complications, including heart failure, paradoxic embolization, and irreversible pulmonary vascular disease. Mortality is low, and postoperative survival is comparable to that of a normal population.[72]

Ventricular Septal Defect

An abnormal opening in the ventricular septum that allows free communication between right and left ventricles is the most common congenital cardiac anomaly. Frequently VSD is associated with (or is an integral part of) other structural defects, particularly tetralogy, transposition, and truncus, but also PDA, ASD, and aortic coarctation. About 30% occur as isolated anomalies. Depending on the size of the defect, it may produce difficulties virtually from birth or, with smaller lesions, may not be recognized until later or may even spontaneously close.

MORPHOLOGY. VSDs are classified according to size and location. They range from probe paten-

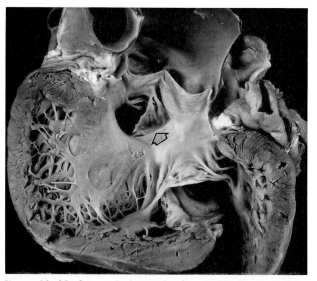

Figure 12–35. Gross photograph of a ventricular septal defect (membranous type) observed from the left side; defect denoted by *arrow*. (Courtesy of William D. Edwards, M.D., Mayo Clinic, Rochester, MN.)

cies to lesions sufficiently large to create virtually a common ventricle. About 90% involve the region of the membranous septum (membranous VSD) and are therefore close to the AV (His) bundle of the conduction system (Fig. 12–35). The remainder lie below the pulmonary valve (infundibular, supracristal, or subarterial) or are located within the muscular septum. Although most often single, VSDs in the muscular septum may be multiple (so-called "Swiss-cheese septum").

The functional significance of a VSD depends on the size of the defect and the presence or absence of pulmonary stenosis; these determine pulmonary vascular pressure and resistance. Small defects (less than 0.5 cm in diameter) are known as Roger's disease, and most are muscular. About 50% close spontaneously, and the remainder are generally well tolerated for years. They induce a loud murmur, however, heard throughout systole, sometimes accompanied by a systolic thrill. Large defects are usually membranous or infundibular, and they generally remain patent and permit a significant left-to-right flow. Aortic insufficiency may also be present owing to inadequate annular support adjacent to the VSD, resulting in focal prolapse. Right ventricular hypertrophy and pulmonary hypertension are present from birth. Over time, irreversible pulmonary vascular disease develops in all patients with large unoperated VSDs, leading to shunt reversal, cyanosis, clubbing, and polycythemia.

Large defects may become manifest virtually at birth because of signs of cardiac failure accompanying the murmur. A particular risk in those with small or moderate-sized defects is superimposed IE at the site of the jet lesion, a complication rarely encountered with large defects. Surgical closure of incidental VSDs is generally not attempted during infancy, in hope of spontaneous closure. Correction, however, is indicated in older children with large defects, before pulmonary hypertension and obstructive pulmonary vascular disease develops and renders the lesion inoperable.

Patent Ductus Arteriosus

PDA results when the ductus arteriosus, a normal aortopulmonary vascular channel during intrauterine life, remains open after birth. After birth, with left-to-right flow, the increased levels of oxygen and changes in prostaglandin metabolism stimulate ductal muscular contraction, and in a full-term infant, the ductus usually closes functionally within the first day or two of life. In contrast, in premature infants and in infants with respiratory distress syndrome at birth (hypoxemia), the ductus may remain patent. In full-term infants with PDA, there may be a true structural defect in the wall.

About 85 to 90% of PDAs occur as isolated defects. The remainder are most often associated with VSD, coarctation, or pulmonary or aortic stenosis. The length and diameter of the ductus vary widely from only a slight defect between the closely approximated pulmonary artery and aorta to several centimeters in length and from several micrometers to 1 cm in diameter.

Most often PDA does not produce functional difficulties at birth. Indeed a narrow ductus may have no effect on growth and development during childhood. Its existence, however, can generally be detected by a continuous harsh murmur, described as "machinery-like." Often it is accompanied by a systolic thrill. Because the shunt is at first left-to-right, there is no cyanosis. Obstructive pulmonary vascular disease eventually ensues, however, with ultimate reversal of flow and all its associated consequences, including cyanosis, clubbing, polycythemia, and right ventricular failure. At this point, the lesion becomes inoperable.

There is generally agreement that a PDA should be closed as early in life as is feasible. Up to the recent past, operative closure was recommended. Currently large-scale studies of pharmacologic closure (indomethacin to suppress vasodilatory prostaglandin E synthesis) have proved promising. Preservation of ductal patency (by administering prostaglandin E) assumes great importance in the survival of infants with various forms of congenital heart disease with obstructed pulmonary or systemic blood flow, such as pulmonary or aortic valve atresia, or TGA. Ironically the ductus may be either life-threatening or life-saving.

Atrioventricular Septal Defect

AV septal defects result from abnormal development of the embryologic AV canal, in which the superior and inferior endocardial cushions fail to fuse adequately, resulting in incomplete closure of the AV septum and inadequate formation of the septal tricuspid and anterior mitral leaflets. Four potential lesions are possible, including primum ASD, inlet (subtricuspid) VSD, cleft anterior mitral leaflet, and widened anteroseptal tricuspid commissure. The two most common combinations are *partial* AV septal defect (consisting of a primum ASD and a cleft anterior mitral leaflet, causing mitral insufficiency) and *complete* AV septal defect (consisting of a large combined AV septal defect and a large common AV valve—essentially a hole in the center of the heart). In the complete form, all four cardiac chambers freely communicate, inducing volume hypertrophy of each. More than one-third of all patients with the complete AV septal defect have Down syndrome. Surgical repair is possible.

RIGHT-TO-LEFT SHUNTS— EARLY CYANOSIS

Tetralogy of Fallot

The four features of Fallot's tetralogy, the most common form of cyanotic congenital heart disease, are (1) VSD, (2) obstruction to the right ventricular outflow tract (subpulmonary stenosis), (3) an aorta that overrides the VSD, and (4) right ventricular hypertrophy (Fig. 12–36). All of the features result embryologically from anterosuperior displacement of the infundibular septum. Even untreated, patients with tetralogy often survive into adult life. Indeed, in an analysis of a large series of patients with this condition but never having had cardiac surgery, about 10% were alive at 20 years and 3% at 40 years. The clinical consequences of tetralogy of Fallot depend primarily on the severity of subpulmonary stenosis.

MORPHOLOGY. The heart is often enlarged and may be "boot-shaped" owing to marked right ventricular hypertrophy, particularly of the apical region. The VSD is usually large and approximates the diameter of the aortic orifice. The aortic valve forms its superior border, thereby overriding the defect and both ventricular chambers. The obstruction to right ventricular outflow is most often due to narrowing of the infundibulum (subpulmonic stenosis) but often accompanied by pulmonary valvular stenosis. Sometimes there is complete atresia of the pulmonary valve and variable portions of the

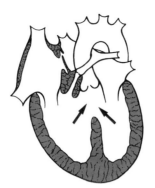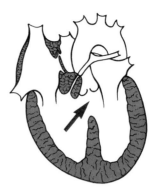

Mild
Subpulmonary Stenosis.
Left-to-Right Shunt

Moderate
Subpulmonary Stenosis.
Bidirectional Shunt

Severe
Subpulmonary Stenosis.
Right-to-Left Shunt

Figure 12–36. Tetralogy of Fallot. Diagrammatic representation of anatomic variants, indicating that the direction of shunting across the VSD depends on the severity of the subpulmonary stenosis. Arrows indicate the direction of the blood flow. (Courtesy of William D. Edwards, M.D., Mayo Clinic, Rochester, MN.)

pulmonary arteries, such that blood flow through a patent ductus or dilated bronchial arteries, or through both, is necessary for survival. Aortic valve insufficiency or ASD may also be present, and a right aortic arch is present in about 25%.

The severity of obstruction to right ventricular outflow determines the direction of blood flow. If the subpulmonary stenosis is mild, the abnormality resembles an isolated VSD, and the shunt may be left-to-right, without cyanosis (so-called "pink tetralogy"). *As the obstruction increases in severity, there is commensurately greater resistance to right ventricular outflow. As it approaches the level of systemic vascular resistance, right-to-left shunting predominates and, along with it, cyanosis.* With increasing severity of subpulmonic stenosis, the pulmonary arteries are progressively smaller and thinner walled (hypoplastic), and the aorta is progressively larger in diameter. As the child grows and the heart increases in size, the pulmonic orifice does not expand proportionally, making the obstruction ever worse. Thus most infants with tetralogy are cyanotic from birth or soon thereafter. The subpulmonary stenosis, however, protects the lungs from pressure overload, and right ventricular failure is rare because the right ventricle is decompressed into the left ventricle and aorta. Complete surgical repair is possible for classic tetralogy but is more complicated for patients with pulmonary atresia and dilated bronchial arteries.

Transposition of Great Arteries

Transposition implies ventriculoarterial discordance, such that the aorta arises from the right ventricle, and the pulmonary artery emanates from the left ventricle (Fig. 12–37). In the so-called complete form (to be described), the AV connections are

normal (concordant), with right atrium joining right ventricle and left atrium emptying into left ventricle. Transposition may be associated with AV discordance (so-called corrected transposition) or double inlet left ventricle, but these are beyond the scope of this chapter. Transposition associated with tricuspid atresia is discussed with the latter anomaly.

The essential embryologic defect in complete transposition is abnormal formation of the truncal and aortopulmonary septa. *The aorta arises from the right ventricle and lies anterior and to the right of the pulmonary artery (in contrast, in the normal heart, the aorta is posterior and to the right).* The result is separation of the systemic and pulmonary circulations, a condition incompatible with postnatal life, unless a shunt exists for adequate mixing of blood. This malformation, particularly common in offspring of diabetic mothers, causes cyanosis from birth. Patients with transposition and a VSD (about

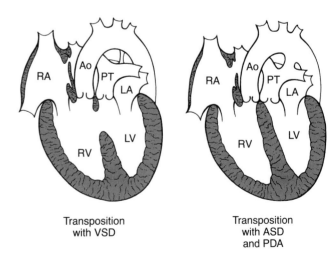

Transposition
with VSD

Transposition
with ASD
and PDA

Figure 12–37. Diagrammatic representation of transposition of the great vessels. (Ao = aorta; LA = left atrium; LV = left ventricle; PT = pulmonary trunk; RA = right atrium; RV = right ventricle.) (Courtesy of William D. Edwards, M.D., Mayo Clinic, Rochester, MN.)

35%) have a stable shunt. Those with only a patent foramen ovale or PDA (about 65%), however, have unstable shunts that tend to close and therefore require immediate intervention to open a right-left communication (such as balloon atrial septostomy) within the first few days of life. Right ventricular hypertrophy becomes prominent as this chamber functions as the systemic ventricle. Concurrently the left ventricle becomes thin-walled (atrophic) as it supports the low-resistance pulmonary circulation.

The outlook for infants with transposition of the great vessels depends on the degree of "mixing" of the blood, the magnitude of the tissue hypoxia, and the ability of the right ventricle to maintain the systemic circulation. Without surgery, most patients die within the first months of life. Rare survivals into young adult life without surgery have been reported, usually when there is an associated large interatrial defect, a VSD with some pulmonic stenosis, or a single ventricle.

Truncus Arteriosus

The persistent truncus arteriosus anomaly arises from a developmental failure of separation of the embryologic truncus arteriosus into the aorta and pulmonary artery. This results in a single great artery that receives blood from both ventricles, accompanied by an underlying VSD, and that gives rise to the systemic, pulmonary, and coronary circulations. The truncal valve usually resembles a tricuspid aortic valve but may have two, four, or even five cusps in some cases. Truncus arteriosus is associated with a large number of concomitant defects, including right aortic arch (30%), hypoplastic pulmonary arteries, absence of the ductus arteriosus, or coronary artery abnormalities and, as mentioned, various defects in the truncal valve, from gross insufficiency to stenosis. Because blood from the right and left ventricles mixes, there is early systemic cyanosis as well as increased pulmonary blood flow. If irreversible pulmonary hypertension develops, the defects are inoperable. Consequently, surgical correction is attempted at an early age, often with gratifying results.

Tricuspid Atresia

Complete occlusion of the tricuspid valve orifice is known as *tricuspid atresia*. It results embryologically from unequal division of the AV canal, and thus the mitral valve is larger than normal. This lesion is almost always associated with underdevelopment (hypoplasia) of the right ventricle. The circulation is maintained by a right-to-left shunt through an interatrial communication (ASD or patent foramen ovale). A VSD is also present and affords communication between the left ventricle and the great artery that arises from the hypoplastic right ventricle. Two subtypes of tricuspid atresia are important clinically: one with normally related great arteries and the other with transposed great arteries. Cyanosis is present virtually from birth, and there is a high mortality in the first weeks or months of life. Palliative or reparative surgery is usually possible.

Total Anomalous Pulmonary Venous Connection

TAPVC, in which no pulmonary veins directly join the left atrium, results embryologically when the common pulmonary vein fails to develp or becomes atretic, causing primitive systemic venous channels from the lungs to remain patent. TAPVC may drain into the right atrium, superior vena cava, azygous vein, innominate veins, coronary sinus, inferior vena cava, hepatic veins, portal vein, left gastric vein, or ductus venosus. In more than half of cases, the anomalous pulmonary veins join either to the left innominate vein or to the coronary sinus. Either a patent foramen ovale or an ASD is always present, allowing pulmonary venous blood to enter the left atrium. There may be obstruction of the pulmonary veins, particularly when the connection is subdiaphragmatic.

Consequences of TAPVC include volume and pressure hypertrophy of the right atrium and right ventricle, and these chambers and the pulmonary trunk are dilated. The left atrium is hypoplastic, but the left ventricle is usually normal in size. Cyanosis may be present, owing to mixing of well-oxygenated and poorly oxygenated blood at the site of anomalous pulmonary venous connection and owing to a large right-to-left shunt at the ASD.

OBSTRUCTIVE CONGENITAL ANOMALIES

Coarctation of Aorta

Coarctation (narrowing, constriction) of the aorta ranks high in frequency among the common structural anomalies. Males are affected three to four times more often than females, although females with Turner's syndrome (see Chapter 10) frequently have a coarctation. Two classic forms have been described: (1) an "infantile" form with tubu-

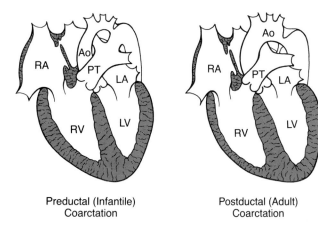

Figure 12-38. Diagram showing preductal and postductal coarctations of the aorta. (Ao = aorta; LA = left atrium; LV = left ventricle; PT = pulmonary trunk; RA = right atrium; RV = right ventricle.) (Courtesy of William D. Edwards, M.D., Mayo Clinic, Rochester, MN.)

lar hypoplasia of the aortic arch proximal to a patent ductus that is often symptomatic in early childhood and (2) an "adult" postductal form in which there is a discrete ridge-like infolding of the aorta, just opposite the closed ductus arteriosus (ligamentum arteriosum) (Fig. 12–38). Encroachment on the aortic lumen is of variable severity, sometimes leaving only a small channel or at other times producing only minimal narrowing. Clinical manifestations depend almost entirely on the severity of the narrowing and the patency of the ductus arteriosus. Although coarctation may occur as a solitary defect, it is accompanied by a bicuspid aortic valve in 50% of cases and may also be associated with congenital aortic stenosis, ASD, VSD, mitral regurgitation, and Berry aneurysms of the circle of Willis. Rarely, narrowing of the aorta may occur at other sites along its length.

Preductal coarctation usually leads to manifestations early in life, and indeed, it may cause signs and symptoms immediately after birth. Many infants with this anomaly do not survive the neonatal period without surgical intervention. Patency of the ductus arteriosus is critical to supply sufficient blood to the aorta to sustain the circulation to the lower parts of the body. With preductal coarctation, right ventricular failure may appear very early. In such cases, the delivery of unsaturated blood through the ductus arteriosus produces cyanosis in the lower half of the body, whereas the head and arms are unaffected because their blood supply derives from vessels having origins proximal to the ductus.

The outlook is different with *postductal coarctation,* unless it is very severe. Most of the children are asymptomatic, and the disease may go unrecognized until well into adult life. Typically there is hypertension in the upper extremities, but there are weak pulses and a lower blood pressure in the lower extremities, associated with manifestations of arterial insufficiency (i.e., claudication and coldness). Particularly characteristic in adults is the development of collateral circulation between the precoarctation arterial branches and the postcoarctation arteries. Thus the intercostal and internal mammary arteries may become enlarged and may cause radiographically visible erosions ("notching") of the undersurfaces of the ribs.

With all significant coarctations, murmurs are often present throughout systole, and sometimes a thrill is present. Similarly, there is cardiomegaly owing to left ventricular hypertrophy. Ultimately aortography is definitive. With uncomplicated coarctation, surgical resection and end-to-end anastomosis or replacement of the affected aortic segment by a prosthetic graft yields excellent results. Postoperative persistent hypertension is a complication in some patients. Untreated, the mean duration of life is about 40 years, and deaths are usually caused by CHF, intracranial hemorrhage, infective aortitis at the point of narrowing, and rupture or dissection of the precoarctation aorta related to the hypertension and degenerative structural changes in the aortic wall.

Pulmonary Stenosis or Atresia with Intact Ventricular Septum

This relatively frequent malformation represents an obstruction at the pulmonary valve. It may occur as an isolated defect in which the valve is almost always a dome-shaped acommissural valve or as part of a more complex anomaly, either tetralogy of Fallot or transposition, in which the valve is usually bicuspid but occasionally unicommissural or dysplastic tricuspid. When the valve is entirely atretic, the anomaly is commonly associated with a hypoplastic right ventricle and an ASD.

With atresia, there is no communication between the right ventricle and lungs, and so flow bypasses the right ventricle through an ASD, entering the lungs through a PDA. Pulmonary stenosis may be mild to severe. Right ventricular hypertrophy often develops, and there is sometimes poststenotic dilatation of the pulmonary artery owing to jet-stream injury to the wall. With coexistent subpulmonary stenosis (as in tetralogy), the high ventricular pressure is not transmitted to the valve, and the pulmonary trunk is not dilated and may in fact be hypoplastic.

Mild stenosis may be asymptomatic and compatible with long life. The smaller the valvular orifice, the more severe is the cyanosis and the earlier its appearance. Isolated valvular stenosis is easily corrected with surgery or in some cases by balloon valvuloplasty. When these lesions are associated with right ventricular hypoplasia, the surgical options are more complex and risky.

Aortic Stenosis and Atresia

As stated earlier, the aortic valvular orifice may be narrowed or stenosed by acquired disease (RHD, degenerative calcific aortic stenosis), by anomalous development (atresia or stenosis), or by a combination of both (calcification of a congenitally malformed valve). The most common congenital anomaly is a bicuspid aortic valve, which is usually of little functional significance early in life but is predisposed to calcification in adult life (see earlier). Rarely there is a single cusp, which surprisingly is compatible with survival.

Here we are concerned with the narrowings and obstructions of the aortic valve present from birth. In severe congenital aortic stenosis or atresia, obstruction of the left ventricular outflow tract leads to underdevelopment (hypoplasia) of the left ventricle and ascending aorta. There may be dense, procelain-like left ventricular endocardial fibroelastosis (see section on restrictive cardiomyopathy, earlier in this chapter). The ductus must be open to allow blood flow to the aorta and coronary arteries. This constellation of findings, called the *hypoplastic left heart syndrome*, is nearly always fatal in the first week of life, when the ductus closes. Surgical repair is possible but carries a relatively high mortality rate.

Less severe degrees of congenital aortic stenosis may be compatible with long survival. There are three major types of stenosis: valvular, subvalvular and supravalvular. With *valvular aortic stenosis*, the cusps may be hypoplastic (small), dysplastic (thickened, nodular), or abnormal in number (acommissural, unicommissural, bicuspid). *Subaortic stenosis* represents either a thickened ring (discrete type) or collar (tunnel type) of dense endocardial fibrous tissue below the level of the cusps. With the exception of coarctation of the aorta and PDA, other associated anomalies are uncommon; aortic stenosis is an isolated lesion in 80% of cases. Pressure hypertrophy of the left ventricle develops as a consequence of the obstruction to blood flow. Sometimes poststenotic dilatation of the aortic root develops. *Supravalvular aortic stenosis* represents an inherited form of aortic dysplasia in which the ascending aortic wall is greatly thickened, causing luminal constriction. It may be related to a developmental disorder affecting multiple organ systems, including the vascular system, which includes hypercalcemia of infancy (Williams' syndrome). Studies suggest that mutations in the elastin gene can cause supravalvular aortic stenosis.[73]

A prominent systolic murmur is usually detectable and sometimes a thrill, which does not distinguish the site of stenosis. In general, congenital stenoses are well tolerated unless very severe. Mild stenoses can be managed conservatively with antibiotic prophylaxis and avoidance of strenuous activity, but the threat of sudden death with exertion always looms. Surgical correction is usually eventually indicated, for both mild and severe stenosis, largely for hemodynamic reasons and to lessen the chance of IE.

CONGENITAL HEART DISEASE IN ADULTS

The adult congenital heart disease patient population includes those who have never had cardiac surgery, those who have had reparative cardiac surgery and require no further operation, those who have had incomplete or palliative surgery, and those who are inoperable, apart from organ transplantation. The number of adults with congenital heart disease is increasing rapidly as a direct result of advances in diagnostic methods and in the surgical and medical care of infants and children with congenital heart disease.[74] More than 85% of the estimated 25,000 infants born annually with congenital malformations of the heart are likely to reach adulthood.

An understanding of prognosis and potential problems after cardiac surgery or interventional catheterization requires not only knowledge of the preoperative congenital malformation, but also the nature and effects of the therapeutic interventions and the postoperative or postinterventional residual lesions and sequelae.[75] Many patients with congenital heart disease have an increased risk of endocarditis; those with cyanotic congenital heart disease may have specific difficulties owing to hyperviscosity, abnormal hemostasis, and abnormal renal function and urate metabolism. With certain congenital cardiac malformations, childbearing imposes a formidable threat to maternal survival, and pregnancy is therefore proscribed for those individuals. In addition, maternal congenital heart disease exposes the fetus to immediate risks that threaten its intrauterine viability and to other risks that present as congenital and developmental malformations.

Unavoidable residual lesions may exist after reparative surgery for congenital heart disease, including abnormal valves and an increased risk of arrhythmias. Valves may be congenitally malformed, intrinsically normal but damaged by the original disease, or residually incompetent or stenotic malformed valves for which complete repair has not been possible. In addition, there may be residual abnormalities in the intrinsic ventricular morphology or ventricular mass or function. Prosthetic patches, valves, and conduits can have sequelae and potential complications that vary with the physical and hemodynamic characteristics of the biomaterials and devices. Moreover, preoperative structural changes of the pulmonary vascular bed, especially obstructions of the resistance vessels due to pulmonary hypertension, markedly affect prognosis.

CARDIAC TRANSPLANTATION

Transplantation of cardiac allografts (approximately 2500 per year worldwide)[76] is now frequently performed for severe, intractable heart failure of diverse causes, the two most common of which are DCM and IHD. Three major factors contribute to the widespread success of cardiac transplantation: (1) better selection of candidates, (2) improved maintenance immunosuppression (including the use of cyclosporine A, along with steroids and azathioprine), and (3) early histopathologic diagnosis of acute allograft rejection by sequential endomyocardial biopsy.

Allograft rejection is a major postoperative problem; endomyocardial biopsy is the only reliable means of diagnosing acute cardiac rejection before substantial myocardial damage (and clinical recognition) has occurred and at a stage that is reversible in the majority of instances. Rejection is characterized by interstitial lymphocytic inflammation that in its more advanced stages damages adjacent myocytes (Fig. 12–39). When myocardial injury is not extensive, the "rejection episode" is usually successfully reversed by increased immu-

nosuppressive therapy. The more severe stages, however, are accompanied by extensive myocyte necrosis and frequently inflammatory injury to the vasculature that may lead to precipitous interstitial edema or hemorrhage. Advanced rejection may be irreversible and fatal.

Other postoperative problems include infection and development of malignancies, particularly lymphomas (generally related to Epstein-Barr virus in the presence of profound chronic therapeutic immunosuppression). The major current limitation to the long-term success of cardiac transplantation is late, progressive, diffuse stenosing intimal proliferation of the coronary arteries (graft arteriosclerosis). This is a particularly vexing problem because it may lead to silent myocardial infarction (particularly difficult to diagnose because these patients, with denervated hearts, do not experience chest pain); in this situation, CHF or sudden death is the usual outcome.[77] Despite these problems, the outlook is good, with a 1-year survival of 70 to 80% and 5-year survival of more than 60%.

1. Waller, B.F., and Morgan, R.: The very elderly heart. In Waller, B.F. (ed.): Contemporary Issues in Cardiovascular Pathology. Philadelphia, F.A. Davis Co., 1988, p. 361.
2. Wei, J.Y.: Age and the cardiovascular system. N. Engl. J. Med. 327:1735, 1992.
3. Schoen, F.J.: Interventional and Surgical Cardiovascular Pathology: Clinical Correlations and Basic Principles. Philadelphia, W.B. Saunders Co., 1989.
4. Virmani, R., et al. (eds.): Cardiovascular Pathology. Philadelphia, W.B. Saunders Co., 1991.
5. Silver, M.D. (ed.): Cardiovascular Pathology, 2nd ed. New York, Churchill Livingstone, 1991.
6. Katz, A.M.: Cardiomyopathy of overload. A major determinant of prognosis in congestive heart failure. N. Engl. J. Med. 322:100, 1990.
7. Grossman, W.: Diastolic dysfunction in congestive heart failure. N. Engl. J. Med. 325:1552, 1992.
8. Oparil, S.: Pathogenesis of ventricular hypertrophy. J. Am. Coll. Cardiol. 5:56B, 1985.
9. Weber, K.T., et al.: Remodeling and reparation of the cardiovascular system. J. Am. Coll. Cardiol. 20:3, 1992.
10. Schwartz, K., et al.: Switches in cardiac muscle gene expression as a result of pressure and volume overload. Am. J. Physiol. 262:R364, 1992.
11. Frohlich, E.D.: Left ventricular hypertrophy, cardiac diseases and hypertension: Recent experiences. J. Am. Coll. Cardiol. 14:1587, 1989.
12. Just, H.: Peripheral adaptations in congestive heart failure: A review. Am. J. Med. 90:23S, 1991.
13. Ezekowitz, M.D., et al.: Warfarin in the prevention of stroke associated with nonrheumatic atrial fibrillation. N. Engl. J. Med. 327:1406, 1992.
14. Kirshenbaum, J.M.: Therapy for acute myocardial infarction: An update. Heart Dis. Stroke 1:211, 1992.
15. Manson, J.E., et al.: The primary prevention of myocardial infarction. N. Engl. J. Med. 326:1406, 1992.
16. Fuster, V., et al.: The pathogenesis of coronary artery disease and the acute coronary syndromes. N. Engl. J. Med. 326:242, 310, 1992.
17. Falk, E.: Why do plaques rupture? Circulation 86:III-30, 1992.
18. MacIsaac, A.I., et al.: Toward the quiescent coronary plaque. J. Am. Coll. Cardiol. 22:1228, 1993.
19. Davies, M.J.: A macro and micro view of coronary vas-

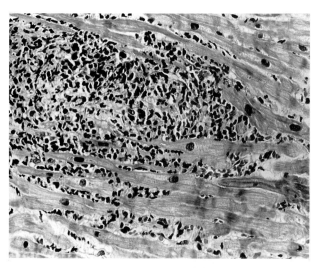

Figure 12–39. Histologic features of cardiac allograft rejection, demonstrating lymphatic infiltrate, with associated damage to the cardiac myocytes.

cular insult in ischemic heart disease. Circulation 82:II-38, 1990.

20. Muller, J.E., et al.: Circadian variation and triggers of onset of acute cardiovascular disease. Circulation 79:733, 1989.

21. Richardson, P.D., et al.: Influence of plaque configuration and stress distribution on fissuring of coronary atherosclerotic plaques. Lancet 2:941, 1989.

22. Chesebro, J.H., et al.: Plaque disruption and thrombosis in unstable angina pectoris. Am. J. Cardiol. 68:9C, 1991.

23. Mizuno, K., et al.: Angioscopic evaluation of coronary artery thrombi in acute coronary syndromes. N. Engl. J. Med. 326:287, 1992.

24. Cohn, P.F.: Mechanisms of myocardial ischemia. Am. J. Cardiol. 70:14G, 1992.

25. Nabulsi, A.A., et al.: Association of hormone-replacement therapy with various cardiovascular risk factors in postmenopausal women. N. Engl. J. Med. 328:1069, 1993.

26. DeWood, M.A., et al.: Prevalence of total coronary occlusion during the early hours of transmural myocardial infarction. N. Engl. J. Med. 303:897, 1980.

27. Marder, V.J., and Sherry, S.: Thrombolytic therapy: Current status. N. Engl. J. Med. 318:1512, 1585, 1988.

28. Jennings, R.B., et al.: Development of cell injury in sustained acute ischemia. Circulation 82:II-2, 1990.

29. Edwards, W.D.: Pathology of myocardial infarction and reperfusion. In Gersh, B.J., and Rahimtoola, S.H. (eds.): Acute Myocardial Infarction. New York, Elsevier, 1991, p. 14.

30. Virmani, R., et al.: Reperfusion injury in the ischemic myocardium. Cardiovasc Pathol 1:117, 1992.

31. Bolli, R.: Myocardial "stunning" in man. Circulation 86:1671, 1992.

32. Braunwald, E., and Pfeffer, M.A.: Ventricular enlargement and remodeling following acute myocardial infarction: Mechanisms and management. Am. J. Cardiol. 68:1D, 1991.

33. Davies, M.J., and Thomas, A.: Thrombosis and acute coronary artery lesions in sudden cardiac ischemic death. N. Engl. J. Med. 310:1137, 1984.

34. Willich, S.N., et al.: Sudden cardiac death. Support for a role of triggering in causation. Circulation 87:1442, 1993.

35. Frohlich, E.D., et al.: The heart in hypertension. N. Engl. J. Med. 327:998, 1992.

36. Schoen, F.J., and St. John Sutton, M.: Contemporary issues in the pathology of valvular heart disease. Human Pathol. 18:568, 1987.

37. Faggiano, P., et al.: Rate of progression of valvular aortic stenosis in adults. Am. J. Cardiol. 70:229, 1992.

38. Benjamin, E.J., et al.: Mitral annular calcification and the risk of stroke in an elderly cohort. N. Engl. J. Med. 327:374, 1992.

39. Virmani, R., et al.: Mitral valve prolapse. In Virmani, R., et al. (eds.): Cardiovascular Pathology. Philadelphia, W.B. Saunders, Co., 1991, p. 419.

40. Chesler, E., and Gornick, C.C.: Maladies attributed to myxomatous mitral valve. Circulation 82:328, 1991.

41. Dajani, A.S., et al.: Guidelines for the diagnosis of rheumatic fever: Jones criteria, updated 1992. Circulation 87:302, 1993.

42. Klein, J.O.: Reemergence of virulent group A streptococcal infections. Pediatr. Infect. Dis. J. 10:S3, 1991.

43. Bisno, A.L.: Group A streptococcal infections and acute rheumatic fever. N. Engl. J. Med. 325:783, 1991.

44. Stollerman, G.H.: Rheumatogenic streptococci and autoimmunity. Clin. Immunol. Immunopathol. 61:131, 1991.

45. Dressler, F.A., and Roberts, W.C.: Modes of death and types of cardiac diseases in opiate addicts: Analysis of 168 necropsy cases. Am. J. Cardiol. 64:909, 1989.

46. Lundin, L., et al.: Carcinoid heart disease: Relationship of circulating vasoactive substances to ultrasound-detectable cardiac abnormalities. Circulation 77:264, 1988.

47. Hammermeister, K.E., et al.: A comparison of outcomes in men 11 years after heart-valve replacement with a mechanical valve or bioprosthesis. N. Engl. J. Med. 328:1289, 1993.

48. Schoen, F.J., et al.: Pathological considerations in replacement cardiac valves. Cardiovasc. Pathol. 1:29, 1992.

49. Edwards, W.D.: Cardiomyopathies. In Virmani, R. (ed.): Cardiovascular Pathology. Philadelphia, W.B. Saunders Co., 1991, p. 257.

50. Hauck, A.J., and Edwards, W.D.: Histopathologic examination of tissues obtained by endomyocardial biopsy. In Fowles, R.E. (ed.): Cardiac Biopsy. New York, Futura Publishing Co., 1992, p. 95.

51. Towbin, J.A.: X-linked dilated cardiomyopathy: Molecular genetic evidence of linkage to the Duchenne muscular dystrophy (dystrophin) gene at the Xp21 locus. Circulation 87:1854, 1993.

52. Nava, A., et al.: Familial occurrence of right ventricular dysplasia: A study involving nine families. J. Am. Coll. Cardiol. 12:1222, 1988.

53. Maron, B.J., et al.: Hypertrophic cardiomyopathy. Interrelations of clinical manifestations, pathophysiology, and therapy. N. Engl. J. Med. 316:780, 844, 1987.

54. Solomon, S.D.: Left ventricular hypertrophy and morphology in familiar hypertrophic cardiomyopathy associated with mutations of the beta-myosin heavy chain gene. J. Am. Coll. Cardiol. 22:498, 1993.

55. Weller, P.R.: The immunobiology of eosinophils. N. Engl. J. Med. 324:1110, 1991.

56. Jin, O., et al.: Detection of enterovirus RNA in myocardial biopsies from patients with myocarditis and cardiomyopathy using gene amplification by polymerase chain reaction. Circulation 82:8, 1990.

57. Huber, S.A.: Viral myocarditis. A tale of two diseases. Lab. Invest. 66:1, 1992.

58. Morris, S.A., et al.: Pathophysiological insights into the cardiomyopathy of Chagas' disease. Circulation 82:1900, 1990.

59. de Koning, J., et al.: Demonstration of spirochetes in cardiac biopsies of patients with Lyme disease. J. Infect. Dis. 160:150, 1989.

60. Baroldi, G., et al.: Focal lymphocytic myocarditis in acquired immunodeficiency syndrome (AIDS): A correlative morphologic and clinical study in 26 consecutive fatal cases. J. Am. Coll. Cardiol. 12:463, 1988.

61. Grody, W.W., et al.: Infection of the heart by the human immunodeficiency virus. Am. J. Cardiol. 66:203, 1990.

62. Aretz, H.T., et al.: Myocarditis. A histopathologic definition and classification. Am. J. Cardiovasc. Pathol. 1:3, 1986.

63. Dec, G.W., et al.: Viral myocarditis mimicking acute myocardial infarction. J. Am. Coll. Cardiol. 20:85, 1992.

64. Van Vleet, J.F., et al.: Cardiovascular and skeletal muscle systems. In: Handbook of Toxicologic Pathology. New York, Academic Press, 1991, p. 539.

65. Kloner, R.A., et al.: The effects of acute and chronic cocaine use on the heart. Circulation 85:407, 1992.

66. Polikar, R., et al.: The thyroid and the heart. Circulation 87:1435, 1993.

67. Tazelaar, H.D., et al.: Pathology of surgically excised primary cardiac tumors. Mayo Clin. Proc. 67:957, 1992.

68. Wold, L.E., and Lie, J.T.: Cardiac myxomas. A clinicopathologic profile. Am. J. Pathol. 101:217, 1980.

69. Schoen, F.J., et al.: Cardiac effects of noncardiac neoplasms. Cardiol. Clin. 2:657, 1984.

70. Morris, C.D., and Menashe, V.D.: 25-year mortality after surgical repair of congenital heart defect in childhood. J.A.M.A. 266:3447, 1991.

71. Moller, J.H., and Kaplan, E.L.: Forty years of cardiac disease in children. Progress and problems. Minn. Med. 74:26, 1991.

72. Murphy, J.G., et al.: Long-term outcome after surgical repair of isolated atrial septal defect. N. Engl. J. Med. 323:1645, 1990.

73. Curan, M.E., et al.: The elastin gene is disrupted by a translocation associated with supravalvular aortic stenosis. Cell *73*:159, 1993.

74. Perloff, J.K.: Congenital heart disease in adults. A new cardiovascular subspecialty. Circulation *84*:1881, 1991.

75. Edwards, W.D.: Congenital heart disease. *In* Schoen, F.J.: Interventional and Surgical Cardiovascular Pathology: Clinical Correlations and Basic Principles. Philadelphia, W.B. Saunders Co., 1989, p. 281.

76. O'Connell, J.B., et al.: Cardiac transplantation: Recipient selection, donor procurement, and medical follow-up. Circulation *86*:1061, 1992.

77. Schoen, F.J., and Libby, P.: Cardiac transplant graft arteriosclerosis. Trends Cardiovasc. Med. *1*:216, 1991.

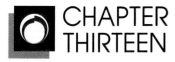

CHAPTER THIRTEEN

Diseases of Red Cells and Bleeding Disorders

The bone marrow, lymph nodes, and spleen all are involved in hematopoiesis. Traditionally, these organs and tissues have been divided into *myeloid tissue*, which includes the bone marrow and the cells derived from it (e.g., erythrocytes, platelets, granulocytes, and monocytes), and *lymphoid tissue*, consisting of thymus, lymph nodes, and spleen. This subdivision is artificial with respect to both the normal physiology of hematopoietic cells and the diseases affecting them. For example, although bone marrow is not the site where most of the mature lymphoid cells are found, it is the source of lymphoid stem cells. Similarly, leukemias, which are neoplastic disorders of the leukocytes, originate within the bone marrow but involve the lymph nodes and spleen quite prominently. Some red cell disorders (hemolytic anemias) result from the formation of autoantibodies, signifying a primary disorder of the lymphoid tissues. Thus, it is not possible to draw neat lines between diseases involving the myeloid and lymphoid tissues. Recognizing this difficulty, we have somewhat arbitrarily divided diseases of the hematopoietic tissues

into two chapters. In the first, we shall consider diseases of red cells and those affecting hemostasis. In the second, we shall discuss diseases affecting the leukocytes and the lymph nodes and disorders affecting primarily the spleen.

NORMAL

A complete discussion of normal hematopoiesis is beyond our scope, but certain features are helpful to an understanding of the diseases of blood.

NORMAL DEVELOPMENT OF BLOOD CELLS

In the human embryo, clusters of stem cells, called "blood islands," appear in the yolk sac in the third week of fetal development. At about the third month of embryogenesis some of these cells migrate to the liver, which then becomes the chief site of blood cell formation until shortly before birth. Beginning in the fourth month of development, hematopoiesis commences in the bone marrow. At birth, all the marrow throughout the skeleton is active and is virtually the sole source of blood cells. In the full-term infant, hepatic hematopoiesis has dwindled to a trickle but may persist in widely scattered small foci, which become inactive soon after birth. Up to the age of puberty, all the marrow throughout the skeleton is red and hematopoietically active. Usually by 18 years of age only the vertebrae, ribs, sternum, skull, pelvis, and proximal epiphyseal regions of the humerus and femur retain red marrow, the remaining marrow becoming yellow, fatty, and inactive. Thus, in adults, only about one-half of the marrow space is active in hematopoiesis.

Several features of this normal sequence should be emphasized. By the time of birth, the bone marrow is virtually the sole source of all forms of blood cells, and a major source of lymphocyte precursors. In the premature infant, foci of hematopoiesis are frequently evident in the liver, and, rarely, in the spleen, lymph nodes, or thymus. However, significant postembryonic extramedullary hematopoiesis is abnormal in the full-term infant. With an increased demand for blood cells in the adult, the fatty marrow may become transformed to red, active marrow. Moreover, this is accompanied by increased productive activity throughout the marrow. These adaptive changes are capable of increasing red cell production (erythropoiesis) seven- to eight-fold. Thus, if the marrow precursor cells are not destroyed by metastatic cancer or irradiation, for example, and necessary substrate is available (e.g., adequate amounts of iron, protein, requisite vitamins), such loss of red cells as may occur in hemolytic disorders produces anemia only when the marrow compensatory mechanisms are outstripped. Under these circumstances, extramedullary hematopoiesis may reappear, first within the liver and then in the spleen and lymph nodes.

ORIGIN AND DIFFERENTIATION OF HEMATOPOIETIC CELLS

There is little doubt that the formed elements of blood—erythrocytes, granulocytes, monocytes, platelets, and lymphocytes—have a common origin in a pluripotent hematopoietic stem cell.[1] This common precursor then gives rise to lymphoid stem cells and the trilineage myeloid stem cells, which are committed to produce lymphocytes and the myeloid cells, respectively (Fig. 13–1). The lymphoid stem cell, which has not been identified definitively, is believed to be the origin of precursors of T cells (pro–T cells), B cells (pro–B cells),

and possibly natural killer (NK) cells. The details of lymphoid differentiation will not be discussed here, but it is worth pointing out that, unlike myeloid differentiation, there are no distinctive, morphologically recognizable stages. For definition, reliance must be placed on the detection of differentiation-specific antigens by monoclonal antibodies (see Chapter 14). From the multipotent myeloid stem cell arise at least three types of *committed stem cells* capable of differentiating along the erythroid/megakaryocytic, eosinophilic, and granulocyte-macrophage pathways. The committed stem cells have been called colony-forming units (CFU) because they give rise to colonies of differentiated progeny *in vitro* (see Fig. 13–1). From the various committed stem cells, intermediate stages are derived, and ultimately the morphologically recognizable precursors of the differentiated cell lines, that is, proerythroblasts, myeloblasts, megakaryoblasts, monoblasts, and eosinophiloblasts. These in turn give rise to mature progeny. Since the mature blood elements have a finite life span, it follows that their numbers must be constantly replenished. This can be realized if the stem cells possess the capacity not only to differentiate but also to renew themselves. *Thus, self-renewal is an important property of stem cells.* The pluripotent stem cells have the greatest capacity for self-renewal, but normally most of them are not in cell cycle. As commitment proceeds, self-renewal ability becomes limited, but a greater fraction of the stem cells are found to be in cycle. For example, very few trilineage myeloid stem cells are normally in cell cycle, but up to 50% of CFU-GM (the precursors of granulocytes and macrophages) are synthesizing DNA. This suggests that normally the pool of differentiated cells is replenished mainly by the proliferation of restricted stem cells. It is interesting to note that, although the earliest recognizable precursors (e.g., myeloblasts or proerythroblasts) are in active cell division, they cannot self-replicate, that is, they differentiate and "die." By definition, then, they are not stem cells.

Since most forms of marrow failure or neoplastic disorders (e.g., aplastic anemias, leukemias, polycythemia) are disorders of stem cells, much interest is centered on the physiologic mechanisms that regulate the proliferation and differentiation of progenitor cells. Involved in these processes are soluble factors as well as stromal cells of the bone marrow. Among the hematopoietic growth factors, stem cell factor (also called c-*kit* ligand) acts on the most immature stem cell. Others, such as the granulocyte-macrophage colony-stimulating factor (GM-CSF), act on CFU-GM. Because genes for most of the growth factors have been cloned, large amounts of recombinant proteins can be generated. Some recombinant factors are currently being utilized to stimulate hematopoiesis. Included in this group are erythropoietin, GM-CSF, and G-CSF.

NORMAL ANATOMY AND MORPHOLOGY OF BONE MARROW. The bone marrow not only is a

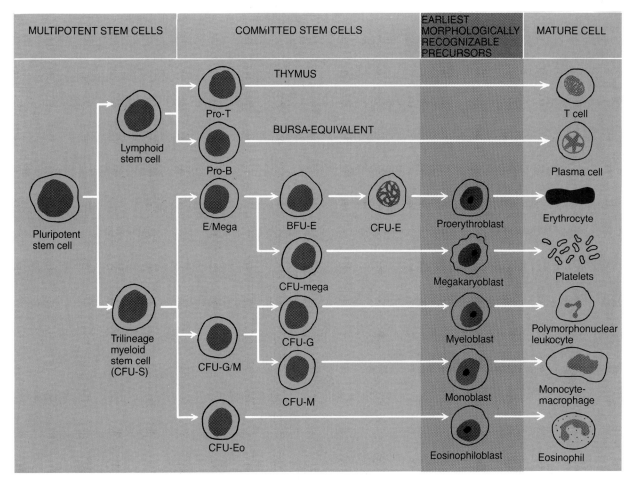

| MULTIPOTENT STEM CELLS | COMMITTED STEM CELLS | EARLIEST MORPHOLOGICALLY RECOGNIZABLE PRECURSORS | MATURE CELL |

THYMUS

BURSA-EQUIVALENT

Pluripotent stem cell

Lymphoid stem cell

Pro-T

Pro-B

T cell

Plasma cell

E/Mega

BFU-E

CFU-E

Proerythroblast

Erythrocyte

CFU-mega

Megakaryoblast

Platelets

Trilineage myeloid stem cell (CFU-S)

CFU-G/M

CFU-G

Myeloblast

Polymorphonuclear leukocyte

CFU-M

Monoblast

Monocyte-macrophage

CFU-Eo

Eosinophiloblast

Eosinophil

Figure 13–1. Differentiation of hematopoietic cells. (Modified from Wyngaarden, J.B., Smith, L.H., and Bennett, J.C. (eds.): Cecil Textbook of Medicine, 19th ed. Philadelphia, W.B. Saunders Co., 1992, p. 820.)

reservoir of stem cells but also provides a unique microenvironment in which the orderly proliferation and differentiation of precursor cells takes place. In addition, it regulates the release of fully differentiated cells into the circulation. Under the electron microscope, the marrow cavity appears to be a vast network of thin-walled sinusoids lined by a single layer of endothelial cells. Basement membrane and adventitial cells are present, but they form a discontinuous layer outside the endothelium. In between the sinusoidal network lie clusters of hematopoietic cells and fat cells. Differentiated blood cells enter the sinusoids by transcellular migration through the endothelial cells. That this process is finely regulated is attested to by the fact that when hematopoiesis takes place at extramedullary sites, for example the spleen (see Chapter 14), the peripheral blood contains all forms of abnormal as well as primitive blood cells that do not enter the blood in normal medullary hematopoiesis.

MORPHOLOGY. Although the morphology of the hematopoietic cells within the bone marrow is best studied in smears of marrow aspirates, useful infor-

mation can also be obtained by studying the histology of bone marrow biopsies. For example, a reasonable estimate of marrow activity may be obtained by examining the ratio of fat cells to hematopoietic elements in bone marrow biopsies. In normal adults this ratio approaches 1:1, but with marrow hypoplasia (e.g., aplastic anemia) the proportion of fat cells is greatly increased, and conversely, fat cells may virtually disappear in diseases characterized by increased hematopoiesis (e.g., leukemias). When subjected to fixatives and tissue staining methods, the cells of the bone marrow and peripheral blood differ in appearance from those in air-dried Giemsa- or Wright-stained preparations. The maturational sequence of various cell types and their specific names are described in specialized texts. The earliest identifiable myeloid cells, that is, pronormoblasts, myeloblasts, and monoblasts, all are moderately large (10 to 20 μm in diameter), having abundant, deeply basophilic cytoplasm; round nuclei with coarsely clumped chromatin; and prominent nucleoli. It is extremely difficult, if not impossible, to differentiate in tissue sections the various "blast" forms. Often, tentative identification must be made on the basis of "the company they keep." Thus, a primitive cell found in relation to a focus of granulocytes is likely to be a myeloblast.

The relative proportion of cells in the bone marrow is almost always deranged in diseases of the blood and bone marrow. Normally, the marrow contains about 60% granulocytes and their precursors; 20% erythroid precursors; 10% lymphocytes and monocytes and their precursors; and 10% unidentified or disintegrating cells. Thus, the normal myeloid-to-erythroid ratio is 3:1. The dominant cell types in the myeloid compartment include myelocytes, metamyelocytes, and granulocytes. In the erythroid compartment the dominant forms are polychromatophilic and orthochromic normoblasts.

We now turn to consider the various disorders of the red blood cells.

PATHOLOGY

ANEMIAS

The function of red cells is the transport of oxygen into tissues. In physiologic terms, therefore, anemia may be defined as a reduction in the oxygen transport capacity of the blood. Since in most instances the reduced oxygen-carrying capacity of blood results from a deficiency of red cells, *anemia may be defined as a reduction below normal limits of the total circulating red cell mass*. This value is not easily measured, however, and therefore anemia has been defined as a reduction below normal in the volume of packed red cells, as measured by the hematocrit, or a reduction in the hemoglobin concentration of the blood. It hardly needs pointing out that fluid retention may expand plasma volume and fluid loss may contract plasma volume, creating spurious abnormalities in clinically measured values.

Innumerable classifications of anemia have been proposed. A highly acceptable one based on the underlying mechanism is presented in Table 13–1. Whatever the nature of anemia, the reduction in red cell mass and oxygen transport, when sufficiently severe, leads to certain changes throughout the body.

MORPHOLOGY. The skin is pale and usually becomes thin and inelastic as the epidermis and dermis atrophy. Frequently, the nails become brittle and lose their normal convexity to assume a concave spoon-shape (koilonychia), particularly in iron deficiency anemia. Cells that are particularly vulnerable to hypoxia may undergo fatty change or

Table 13–1. CLASSIFICATION OF ANEMIA ACCORDING TO UNDERLYING MECHANISM

I. BLOOD LOSS
  A. Acute: Trauma
  B. Chronic: Lesions of GI tract, gynecologic disturbances

II. INCREASED RATE OF DESTRUCTION (HEMOLYTIC ANEMIAS)
  A. Intrinsic (intracorpuscular) abnormalities of red cells
    Hereditary
    1. Red cell membrane disorders
      a. Disorders of membrane cytoskeleton: Spherocytosis, elliptocytosis
      b. Disorders of lipid synthesis: Selective increase in membrane lecithin
    2. Red cell enzyme deficiencies
      a. Glycolytic enzymes: Pyruvate kinase deficiency, hexokinase deficiency
      b. Enzymes of hexose monophosphate shunt: G6PD, glutathione synthetase
    3. Disorders of hemoglobin synthesis
      a. Deficient globin synthesis: Thalassemia syndromes
      b. Structurally abnormal globin synthesis (hemoglobinopathies): Sickle cell anemia, unstable hemoglobins
    Acquired
    1. Membrane defect: Paroxysmal nocturnal hemoglobinuria
  B. Extrinsic (extracorpuscular) abnormalities
    1. Antibody-mediated
      a. Isohemagglutinins: Transfusion reactions, erythroblastosis fetalis
      b. Autoantibodies: Idiopathic (primary), drug-associated, SLE, malignancies, mycoplasma infection
    2. Mechanical trauma to red cells
      a. Microangiopathic hemolytic anemias: Thrombotic thrombocytopenic purpura, DIC
      b. Cardiac traumatic hemolytic anemia
    3. Infections: Malaria
    4. Chemical injury: Lead poisoning
    5. Sequestration in mononuclear phagocyte system: Hypersplenism

III. IMPAIRED RED CELL PRODUCTION
  A. Disturbance of proliferation and differentiation of stem cells: Aplastic anemia, pure red cell aplasia, anemia of renal failure, anemia of endocrine disorders
  B. Disturbance of proliferation and maturation of erythroblasts
    1. Defective DNA synthesis: Deficiency or impaired utilization of vitamin B_{12} and folic acid (megaloblastic anemias)
    2. Defective hemoglobin synthesis
      a. Deficient heme synthesis: Iron deficiency
      b. Deficient globin synthesis: Thalassemias
    3. Unknown or multiple mechanisms: Sideroblastic anemia, anemia of chronic infections, myelophthisic anemias due to marrow infiltrations

even ischemic necrosis. Such damage is most frequently encountered in the muscle cells of the myocardium, the epithelial cells of the proximal convoluted tubules of the kidney, the centrilobular hepatic cells, and the sensitive ganglion cells of the cortex and basal ganglia.

The increased demand for erythropoiesis in anemia causes the fatty marrow to become active and red if the marrow is capable of response. In some anemic states, such as aplastic anemia, the marrow cannot react. When the need is great, extramedullary hematopoiesis ensues, reverting to the fetal patterns of blood formation. Other more specific changes may also appear, determined by the particular type of anemia.

CLINICAL FEATURES. Attendant on the deranged physiology and morphologic alterations described, many nonspecific clinical signs and symptoms are seen in patients with anemia. Classically, these patients are pale and many have the nail deformity described. Weakness, malaise, and easy fatigability are common complaints. The lowered oxygen content of the circulating blood leads to dyspnea on mild exertion. If the fatty changes in the myocardium are sufficiently severe, cardiac failure may develop and compound the respiratory difficulty caused by reduced oxygen transport. Occasionally, the myocardial hypoxia manifests itself as angina pectoris, particularly when a pre-existing vascular disease has already rendered the myocardium partially ischemic. With acute blood loss and shock, oliguria and anuria may develop in the shock kidney. Central nervous system hypoxia may be evidenced by headache, dimness of vision, and faintness.

ANEMIAS OF BLOOD LOSS

Acute Blood Loss

The clinical and morphologic reactions to blood loss depend on the rate of hemorrhage and whether the blood is lost externally or internally. With acute blood loss, the alterations reflect principally the loss of blood volume rather than the loss of hemoglobin. Shock and death may follow. If the patient survives, the blood volume is rapidly restored by shift of water from the interstitial fluid compartment. The resulting hemodilution lowers the hematocrit. Reduction in the oxygenation of tissues triggers the production of erythropoietin, and the marrow responds by increasing erythropoiesis. When the blood is lost internally, as into the peritoneal cavity, the iron can be recaptured, but if the blood is lost externally, the adequacy of the red cell recovery may be hampered by iron deficiency when insufficient reserves are present.

Soon after the acute blood loss the red blood cells appear normal in size and color (normocytic, normochromic). However, as the marrow begins to regenerate, changes occur in the peripheral blood. *Most striking is an increase in the reticulocyte count, reaching 10 to 15% after 7 days.* The reticulocytes are seen as polychromatophilic macrocytes in the usual blood smear. These changes of red cell regeneration can sometimes be mistaken for an underlying hemolytic process. Mobilization of plate-

lets and granulocytes from the marginal pools leads to thrombocytosis and leukocytosis in the period immediately following acute blood loss.

Chronic Blood Loss

Chronic blood loss induces anemia only when the rate of loss exceeds the regenerative capacity of the erythroid precursors or when iron reserves are depleted. In addition to chronic blood loss, any cause of iron deficiency such as malnutrition, malabsorption states, or an increased demand above the daily intake as occurs in pregnancy will lead to an identical anemia, discussed later.

HEMOLYTIC ANEMIAS

The hemolytic anemias all are characterized by (1) shortening of the normal red cell life span, that is, premature destruction of red cells; (2) accumulation of the products of hemoglobin catabolism; and (3) a marked increase in erythropoiesis within the bone marrow, in an attempt to compensate for the loss of red cells. These and some other general features will be briefly discussed before we describe the features of specific hemolytic anemias.

As is well known, the physiologic destruction of senescent red cells takes place within the mononuclear phagocytic cells of the spleen. In hemolytic anemias, too, the premature destruction of red cells occurs predominantly within the mononuclear phagocyte system (extravascular hemolysis). In only a few cases does lysis of red cells within the vascular compartment (intravascular hemolysis) predominate.

Intravascular hemolysis occurs when normal erythrocytes are damaged by mechanical injury, complement fixation to red cells, or exogenous toxic factors. Trauma to red cells may be caused by mechanical cardiac valves or by thrombi within the microcirculation. Complement fixation may occur on antibody-coated cells during transfusion of mismatched blood. Toxic injury is exemplified by falciparum malaria (see Chapter 8) and clostridial sepsis.

Whatever the mechanism, *intravascular hemolysis is manifested by (1) hemoglobinemia, (2) hemoglobinuria, (3) methemalbuminemia, (4) jaundice, and (5) hemosiderinuria.* When hemoglobin escapes into the plasma, it is promptly bound by an $alpha_2$ globulin (haptoglobin) to produce a complex that prevents excretion into the urine, since the complexes are rapidly cleared by the reticuloendothelial system. *A decrease in serum haptoglobin level is characteristically seen in all cases of intravascular hemolysis.* When the haptoglobin is depleted, the unbound or free hemoglobin is in part rapidly oxidized to methemoglobin, and both he-

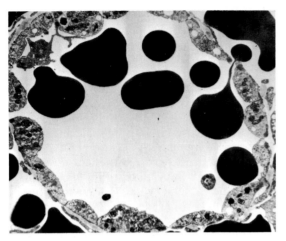

Figure 13–2. Splenic sinus (electron micrograph). An erythrocyte is in process of squeezing from cord into sinus lumen. Note degree of deformability required for red cell to pass through wall of sinus. (With permission from Enriquez, P., and Neiman, R.S.: The Pathology fo the Spleen: A Functional Approach. Chicago, The American Society of Clinical Pathologists, 1976, p. 7.)

moglobin and methemoglobin are excreted through the kidneys, imparting a red-brown color to the urine—hemoglobinuria and methemoglobinuria. The renal proximal tubular cells may reabsorb and catabolize much of this filtered hemoglobin, but some passes out with the urine. Within the tubular cells, iron released from the hemoglobin produces hemosiderosis of the renal tubular epithelium, and shedding of such cells into the urine (where they can be identified by iron stains) constitutes the basis of the *hemosiderinuria*. Concomitantly, the heme groups derived from the complexes are catabolized within the mononuclear phagocyte system, leading ultimately to jaundice. In hemolytic anemias, the serum bilirubin is unconjugated and the level of hyperbilirubinemia depends on the functional capacity of the liver as well as on the rate of hemolysis. With a normal liver, the jaundice is rarely severe. Excessive bilirubin excreted by the liver into the gastrointestinal tract leads eventually to increased formation and fecal excretion of urobilin (see Chapter 18).

Extravascular hemolysis takes place whenever red cells are injured, are rendered "foreign," or become less deformable. For example, in hereditary spherocytosis an abnormal membrane cytoskeleton decreases the deformability of the red cell. Analogously, in sickle cell anemia, the abnormal hemoglobin "gels" or "crystallizes" within the erythrocyte, deforming it and reducing its plasticity. Since extreme alterations in shape are required for red cells to navigate the splenic sinusoids successfully, reduced deformability makes the passage difficult and leads to sequestration within the cords, followed by phagocytosis (Fig. 13–2). This is believed to be an important pathogenetic mechanism of extravascular hemolysis in a variety of

hemolytic anemias. With extravascular hemolysis it is obvious that hemoglobinemia, hemoglobinuria, and the related intravascular changes do not appear. However, the catabolism of erythrocytes in the phagocytic cells induces anemia and jaundice that are otherwise indistinguishable from those caused by intravascular hemolysis. Furthermore, since some hemoglobin manages to escape from the phagocytic cells, plasma haptoglobin levels are invariably reduced. The morphologic changes that follow are identical to those in intravascular hemolysis, except that the erythrophagocytosis generally causes hypertrophy of the mononuclear phagocyte system of cells, and this may lead to splenomegaly.

MORPHOLOGY. Certain morphologic changes are standard in the hemolytic anemias, whether caused by intravascular or extravascular mechanisms. The anemia and lowered tissue oxygen tension stimulate increased production of erythropoietin, leading to **a marked increase in the numbers of normoblasts in the marrow** (Fig. 13–3); sometimes the expansion leads to extramedullary hematopoiesis. The accelerated compensatory erythropoiesis leads to a **prominent reticulocytosis in the peripheral blood.** The elevated levels of bilirubin, when excreted through the liver, promote the formation of pigment gallstones (cholelithiasis). With chronicity, the phagocytosed red cells or hemoglobin will eventually lead to hemosiderosis, usually confined to the mononuclear phagocyte system. Thus, whatever the basis of the hemolysis, when sufficiently chronic, a common sequence of morphologic changes may be anticipated.

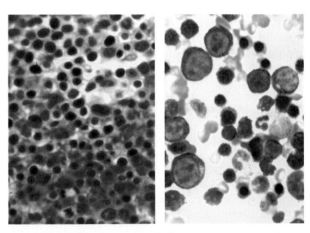

Figure 13–3. Marrow section *(left)* and smear *(right)* from a patient with hemolytic anemia. The marrow is markedly hypercellular, owing to proliferation of normoblasts, seen more clearly in the smear. (Courtesy of Dr. Jose Hernandez, Department of Pathology, University of Texas Southwestern Medical School, Dallas.)

The hemolytic anemias can be classified in a variety of ways. One has already been suggested, namely division into intravascular and extravascular hemolytic disorders. However, since the number of disorders with predominantly intravascular hemolysis is limited, this classification is not entirely satisfactory. A pathogenetic classification could be based on whether the underlying cause of red cell destruction is extrinsic (extracorpuscular mechanism) or a defect inherent in the red cell (intracorpuscular defect). These anemias can also be divided into hereditary and acquired disorders. *In general, hereditary disorders are due to intracorpuscular defects and the acquired disorders to extrinsic factors such as autoantibodies.* Each of the classifications has value, but here we shall follow the intrinsic-extrinsic outline given in Table 13–1, limiting consideration to the more common entities.

Hereditary Spherocytosis (HS)

This inherited disorder is characterized by an intrinsic defect in the red cell membrane that renders erythrocytes spheroidal, less deformable, and vulnerable to splenic sequestration and destruction. The prevalence of HS is highest in people of northern European extraction, in whom rates of 1 in 5000 have been reported. In approximately 75% of cases the inheritance follows an autosomal dominant pattern. Most of the remaining patients have an autosomal recessive form of the disease.

PATHOGENESIS. The spheroidal shape of the erythrocyte appears to result from a fundamental defect in the skeleton of the red cell membrane.[2] Spectrin, the major protein of the membrane cytoskeleton, consists of two polypeptide chains, alpha and beta, which are intertwined (helical) dimers, lying "flat" on the cytoplasmic aspect of the cell membrane (Fig. 13–4). The individual spectrin dimers are like segments of an extensive cable network that are linked to each other head to head to form tetramers. Lateral connections between spectrin tetramers are established through two additional proteins, actin and protein 4.1. The two-dimensional spectrin cable meshwork so formed is tethered to the inner surface of the cell membrane by yet another protein, called ankyrin, which forms a bridge between spectrin and the transmembrane ion transporter, called protein 3. This bridge is stabilized by protein 4.2. Another linkage of spectrin to the plasma membrane glycophorin occurs via protein 4.1. Together these proteins are responsible for maintenance of the normal shape, strength, and flexibility of the red cell membrane. Although a deficiency of any one of the membrane skeletal proteins could adversely affect the red cells, *a deficiency of spectrin seems to be the most common abnormality in patients with all forms of HS.* The spectrin content of these cells varies from 60 to 90% of normal, and correlates closely with the severity of spherocytosis.

The molecular basis of spectrin deficiency is quite varied. A primary defect in spectrin molecules is found in some patients, but much more common is a *mutation in the ankyrin gene.* The resultant reduced synthesis of ankyrin leads, in turn, to a secondary reduction in the assembly of spectrin on the membrane.[3] In addition, primary defects in protein 3 have also been detected in some kindreds. Regardless of the primary molecular defect, *spectrin deficiency is associated with reduced membrane stability and spontaneous loss of red cell membrane* (Fig. 13–5). The resulting reduction in cell surface-to-volume ratio "forces" the cells to assume the smallest possible diameter for a given volume, namely a sphere.

Although much remains to be learned about the molecular defects in HS, the travails of the spherocytic red cells are fairly well defined. In the life of the "portly" (and therefore inflexible) spherocyte, the spleen acts as the villain. Red cells must undergo extreme deformation to leave the cords of Billroth and enter the sinusoids. Because of their spheroidal shape and reduced membrane plasticity, spherocytes have great difficulty in leaving the cords. Reduced deformability of spheroidal red cells has been aptly compared to the difficulties encountered by an "obese man attempting to bend at the waist."[4] As an increasing number of spherocytes are trapped in the spleen, the already sluggish circulation of the cords stagnates further and the environment around the cells becomes progressively more hostile. Lactic acid accumulates and the extracellular pH falls, which in turn inhibits glycolysis and generation of ATP. Loss of ATP impairs the ability to extrude sodium, adding an element of osmotic injury. Stagnation in the cords also promotes contact with macrophages, which are plentiful, and eventually the hapless spherocytes fall prey to the appetite of phagocytic cells. *The cardinal role of the spleen in the premature demise*

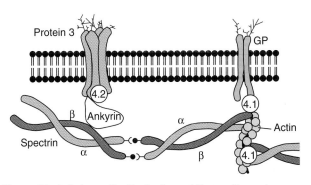

Figure 13–4. Schematic illustration of the erythrocyte membrane skeleton proteins and their interactions: α- and β-spectrin, ankyrin, protein 3 (the anion exchanger), protein 4.1, protein 4.2, actin, and GP (glycophorin). (Modified and redrawn from Gallagher, P.G., and Forget, B.G.: Spectrin genes in health and disease. Semin. Hematol. 30:4, 1993.)

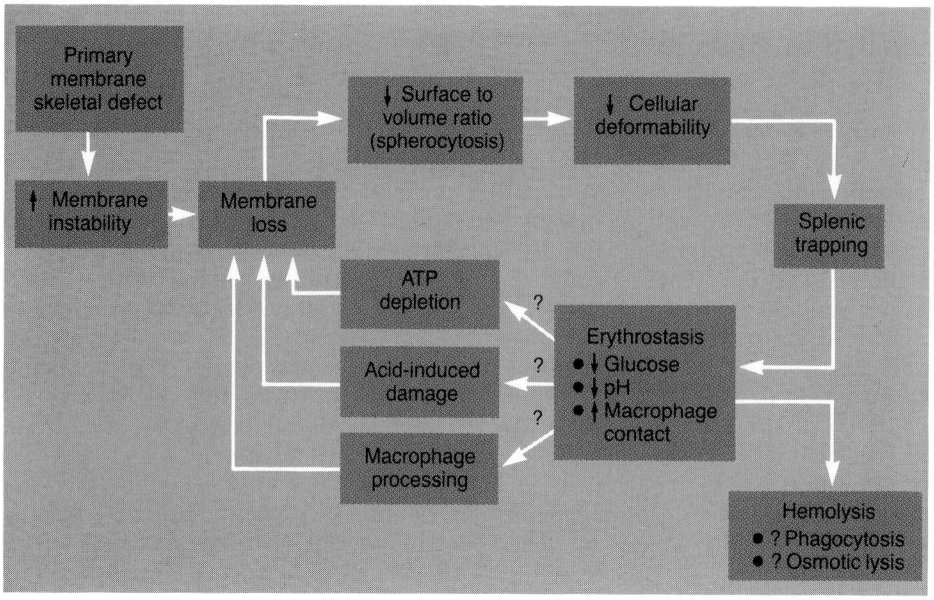

Figure 13-5. Model of the pathophysiology of hereditary spherocytosis. (Adapted from Wyngaarden, J.B., Smith, L.H., and Bennett, J.C. (eds.): Cecil Textbook of Medicine, 19th ed. Philadelphia, W.B. Saunders Co., 1992, p. 859.)

of the spherocytes is proved by the invariably beneficial effect of splenectomy. The spherocytes persist, but the anemia is corrected.

MORPHOLOGY. Perhaps the most outstanding morphologic feature of this disease is the spheroidal shape of the red cells, apparent on smears as abnormally small cells lacking their central zone of pallor (Fig. 13-6). Spherocytosis, although distinctive, is not pathognomonic, since it is also seen in autoimmune hemolytic anemias. In addition to reticulocytosis and the general features of all hemolytic anemias, as previously detailed, certain alterations are fairly distinctive. Moderate splenic enlargement is characteristic of hereditary spherocytosis (500 to 1000 gm); in few other hemolytic anemias is the spleen enlarged as much or as often. It results from marked congestion of the cords of Billroth, leaving the sinuses virtually empty. Erythrophagocytosis can be seen within the congested cords. Typically present are the associated changes found in all hemolytic anemias, including increased erythropoiesis, bone changes, and hemosiderosis. Cholelithiasis (pigment stones) occurs in 40 to 50% of the affected adults.

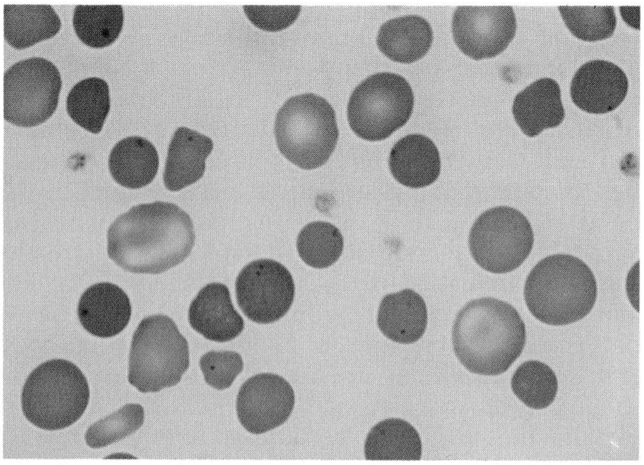

CLINICAL COURSE. The characteristic clinical features are anemia, splenomegaly, and jaundice.[5] The severity of the disease varies greatly from one patient to another. It may make its appearance at birth with marked jaundice, requiring exchange transfusion. In others, the mild red cell destruction is readily compensated for by increased erythropoiesis. Only when this compensatory reaction is outpaced do symptomatic patients have a chronic hemolytic anemia, usually of mild-to-moderate severity. However, this more or less stable clinical course may be punctuated by "crises" of two kinds, often triggered by intercurrent infections. A *hemolytic crisis* may develop, characterized by the sudden onset of a wave of massive hemolysis accompanied by fever, abdominal pain, increasing jaundice, low blood pressure, and even shock. Alternatively, an *aplastic crisis* (triggered usually by a parvovirus infection of the marrow red cell precursors) may appear. It is characterized by temporary suppression of red cell production, manifested by sudden worsening of the anemia, and the disappearance of reticulocytes from the peripheral blood. Transfusions may be necessary to support the patient, but eventually both these crises remit

Figure 13-6. Peripheral smear from a patient with hereditary spherocytosis. Note the anisocytosis and several dark-appearing spherocytes with no central pallor. (Courtesy of Dr. Robert W. McKenna, Department of Pathology, University of Texas Southwestern Medical School, Dallas.)

in most instances. Gallstones, found in many patients, may also produce symptoms. Diagnosis of HS is based on family history, hematologic findings, and laboratory evidence of spherocytosis, manifested by osmotic fragility. The spherocytes are particularly vulnerable to osmotic lysis, induced *in vitro* by solutions of hypotonic salt, since there is little margin for expansion of red cell volume without rupture.

Hemolytic Disease Due to Erythrocyte Enzyme Defects: Glucose-6-Phosphate Dehydrogenase Deficiency

The erythrocyte and its membrane are vulnerable to injury by exogenous and endogenous oxidants. Normally, intracellular reduced glutathione (GSH) inactivates such oxidants. *Abnormalities in the hexose monophosphate shunt or in glutathione metabolism resulting from deficient or impaired enzyme function reduce the ability of red cells to protect themselves against oxidative injuries and lead to hemolytic disease.* The most important of these enzyme derangements is a hereditary deficiency of glucose-6-phosphate dehydrogenase (G6PD) activity involved in the hexose monophosphate shunt pathway. G6PD reduces NADP to NADPH while oxidizing glucose-6-phosphate. NADPH then provides the reducing power that converts oxidized glutathione to reduced glutathione.

Several hundred G6PD genetic variants have been identified, but fortunately most evoke no clinical disorder or hemolytic anemia. Two variants, designated G6PD A⁻ and G6PD Mediterranean, lead to clinically significant hemolysis.[6] The A⁻ type is present in about 10% of American blacks; G6PD Mediterranean, as the name implies, is found largely in populations in the Middle East.

In the A⁻ type of deficiency, the activity of the enzyme is normal in reticulocytes, indicating that there is no defect in synthesis. However, the mutant enzyme is unstable, with a half-life of 13 days (normal 62 days). As a result, older red cells are markedly deficient in enzyme activity. Exposure to an oxidant, therefore, tends to induce hemolysis of older red cells but not younger ones. In the Mediterranean variant, the deficiency is far more severe because there is both impaired synthesis and reduced stability of the enzyme.

Inheritance of the mutant gene is X-linked. Thus, the defect is expressed in all erythrocytes of the affected male. In the heterozygous female, two populations of red cells, some deficient, others normal, are present owing to random inactivation of the X chromosomes. It follows that males are more vulnerable to oxidant injury than females. It might be noted that the prevalence of such deleterious genes is thought to have been maintained

because a deficiency of G6PD may protect against malaria due to *Plasmodium falciparum.*

Numerous oxidant drugs may trigger hemolytic crises, principally the antimalarials — primaquine and quinacrine (Atabrine) — in addition to sulfonamides, nitrofurans, and others. *Even more important are infections that presumably act by the generation of oxidant free radicals in macrophages.*

The pathophysiology of hemolysis seems to involve the following sequence. Infection or exposure to oxidant drugs causes oxidation of GSH to GSSG, presumably through the production of H_2O_2. Since the regeneration of GSH is impaired in G6PD-deficient cells, hydrogen peroxide accumulates and causes oxidation of the sulfhydryl groups of the globin chains. This leads to denaturation of hemoglobin and formation of precipitates (Heinz bodies) within the cell. The peripheral blood smear shows Heinz bodies within the red cells as dark inclusions when stained with crystal violet. When attached to the cell membrane, Heinz bodies decrease erythrocyte deformability. As the inclusion-bearing red cells pass through the splenic cords, macrophages pluck out the Heinz bodies, giving rise to red cells that appear to have a bite of cytoplasm removed ("bite" cells) (Fig. 13–7). The resultant loss of membrane leads to further membrane damage and simultaneously induces the formation of spherocytes. All these changes predispose the red cells to become trapped in splenic cords and destroyed by erythrophagocytosis.

The clinical features of G6PD deficiency may be surmised from this discussion. Persons with the deficient enzyme do not have hemolysis unless exposed to the oxidant injuries alluded to above. After a variable lag period of 2 to 3 days, acute intravascular hemolysis, characterized by hemoglo-

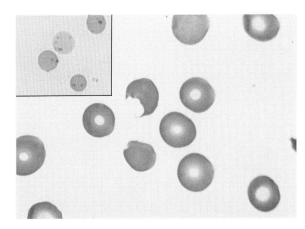

Figure 13–7. Peripheral blood smear from a patient with G6PD deficiency following exposure to an oxidant drug. *Inset,* Red cells with precipitates of denatured globin (Heinz bodies) revealed by supravital staining. As the splenic macrophages pluck out these inclusions, "bite cells" like the one in this smear are produced. (Courtesy of Dr. Robert W. McKenna, Department of Pathology, University of Texas Southwestern Medical School, Dallas.)

binemia, hemoglobinuria, and decreased hematocrit levels, is triggered. Since only senescent red cells are lysed, the episode is self-limited and hemolysis stops when only the younger red cells remain in the circulation (despite continued administration of the oxidant drug). Because patients with the Mediterranean variant have much lower levels of G6PD, their anemia is more severe.

The recovery phase is heralded by reticulocytosis, as in the case of other hemolytic anemias. Since hemolytic episodes related to deficiencies of G6PD occur only when there is oxidant injury, the morphologic changes encountered in most chronic hemolytic anemias are rarely present.

Sickle Cell Disease

Sickle cell disease is the prototype of *hereditary hemoglobinopathies, characterized by the production of a structurally abnormal hemoglobin.* Hemoglobin, as you recall, is a tetramer of four globin chains, comprising two pairs of similar chains, each with its own heme group. The hemoglobin in the adult is composed of 96% HbA ($\alpha_2\beta_2$), 3% hemoglobin A$_2$ ($\alpha_2\delta_2$), and 1% fetal hemoglobin (HbF, $\alpha_2\gamma_2$). The clinically significant variant hemoglobins involve beta-chain abnormalities. Sickle cell anemia results from a point mutation that leads to substitution of valine for glutamic acid at the sixth position of the beta-globin chain. The resultant hemoglobin, HbS, has abnormal physiochemical properties that lead to sickle cell disease. Several hundred abnormal hemoglobins have been identified in which there is either a point mutation or a deletion in one of the globin chains.

About 8% of black Americans are heterozygous for hemoglobin S. If an individual is homozygous for the sickle mutation, almost all the hemoglobin in the erythrocyte is HbS. In the heterozygote, only about 40% is HbS, the remainder being normal hemoglobins. Where malaria is endemic, as many as 30% of black Africans are heterozygous. This frequency may be related in part to the slight protection against falciparum malaria afforded by HbS.

PATHOGENESIS. On deoxygenation the HbS molecules undergo aggregation and polymerization. This change converts hemoglobin from a freely flowing liquid to a viscous gel, leading ultimately to distortion of the red cells, which acquire a sickle or holly-leaf shape (Fig. 13–8).

Sickling of red cells is initially a reversible phenomenon; with oxygenation, HbS returns to the depolymerized state. However, with repeated episodes of sickling and unsickling, membrane damage ensues and the cells become irreversibly sickled. These deformed cells retain their abnormal shape even when fully oxygenated and despite deaggregation of HbS. Sickled cells lose potassium and water and at the same time gain calcium, which normally is rigorously excluded. They have difficulty in maintaining normal intracellular volume, and consequently intracellular hemoglobin concentration increases and the cells become denser.[7] The formation of HbS has two major consequences: (1) a chronic hemolytic anemia, and (2) occlusion of small blood vessels, resulting in ischemic tissue damage (Fig. 13–9).

A number of factors affect the rate and degree of sickling.

- *Perhaps most important of all is the amount of HbS and its interaction with the other hemoglobin chains in the cell.* In heterozygotes approximately 40% of the hemoglobin is HbS, the rest being HbA, which interacts only weakly with HbS during the processes of gelation. Therefore, the het-

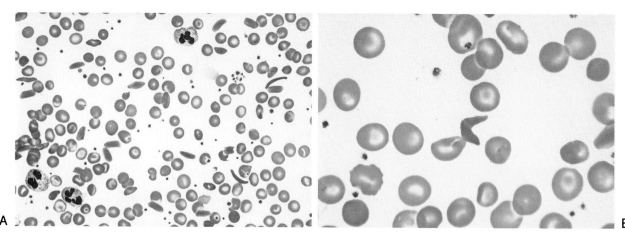

Figure 13–8. Peripheral blood smear from a patient with sickle cell anemia. *A,* Low magnification shows sickle cells, anisocytosis, and poikilocytosis. *B,* Higher magnification shows an irreversibly sickled cell in the center. (Courtesy of Dr. Robert W. McKenna, Department of Pathology, University of Texas Southwestern Medical School, Dallas.)

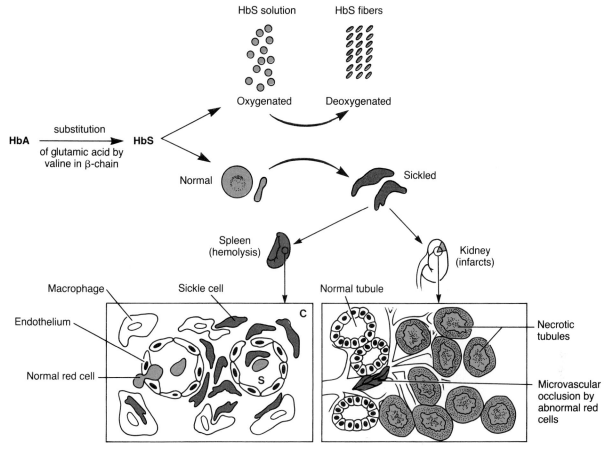

Figure 13-9. Pathophysiology and morphologic consequences of sickle cell anemia. S = splenic sinusoids; C = splenic cords.

erozygote has little tendency to sickle, except under conditions of severe hypoxia. Such an individual is said to have the *sickle cell trait*, and unless exposed to marked hypoxia has no hemolysis of red cells, nor an anemia. In contrast, the homozygote, with virtually undiluted hemoglobin of the S type, has full-blown *sickle cell anemia*. Beta-globin chains other than the normal HbA and other non-alpha globins influence the crystallization of HbS and the severity of sickle cell anemia. For example, fetal hemoglobin (HbF) with its gamma-globin chains does not interact with HbS, and hence newborns do not manifest the disease until they are five to six months of age, when the amount of HbF in the cells begins to approach adult levels. The modulating effect of beta-globin chains is seen also with other mutant hemoglobins, such as HbC and HbD. Either of these may be present along with HbS in red cells of a double heterozygote for HbS and the variant globin gene. When HbC is present along with HbS, the clinical features are less severe (than in patients homozygous for HbS), since HbS copolymerizes with HbC to a lesser extent than with other HbS molecules.

• *The rate of HbS polymerization is also signifi-* *cantly affected by the hemoglobin concentration per cell*, that is, the mean corpuscular hemoglobin concentration (MCHC). The higher the HbS concentration within the cell, the greater are the chances of contact and interaction between HbS molecules. Thus, *dehydration, which increases the MCHC, greatly facilitates sickling and vascular occlusion* (see below). Conversely, for a given amount of HbS per cell, conditions that decrease the MCHC reduce disease severity. This is most clearly illustrated in patients with homozygous sickle cell anemia and coexistent α-thalassemia. These patients have milder disease because thalassemia is characterized by reduced globin synthesis, which limits the total hemoglobin concentration per cell.

• Finally, *a fall in pH*, by reducing the oxygen affinity of hemoglobin, can increase sickling since it enhances the amount of deoxygenated HbS.

Irreversibly sickled cells (ISC) have very rigid and nondeformable cell membranes and have difficulty in negotiating the splenic sinusoids. They become sequestered in the spleen, where they are destroyed by the mononuclear phagocyte system. Some intravascular hemolysis may also occur owing to increased mechanical fragility of the severely damaged cells. *The average red cell survival correlates with the percentage of ISC in circulation* and is shortened to approximately 20 days. This finding supports the concept that the hemolysis results primarily from the lysis of ISC.

The pathogenesis of microvascular occlusions, a clinically important component of sickle cell anemia, is much less certain. For a long time it had been assumed that occlusion of small blood vessels was caused by impaction of nondeformable, sickled cells in capillaries and venules. However, there is no correlation between the frequency of irreversibly sickled cells and the frequency or severity of ischemic episodes. Hence it is believed that microvascular occlusion is initiated by cells that contain HbS but are not obviously sickled. In this regard, several abnormalities of charge and organization of phospholipids have been noted in red cells of patients with sickle cell anemia. These changes increase the adhesiveness of the red cells to the endothelium *in vitro;* indeed cells that are not irreversibly sickled are the most adherent to cultured endothelial cells. Furthermore, it has been demonstrated that adherence of red cells to capillary endothelium *in vitro* correlates with the severity of vaso-occlusive episodes *in vivo.* On the basis of these findings it is proposed that red cells that are not irreversibly sickled, but whose cell membranes have been altered by repeated cycles of reversible sickling, adhere to the endothelium and cause narrowing of microvessels. This leads secondarily to trapping of the more rigid, sickled cells and subsequent vaso-occlusion.[8]

MORPHOLOGY. The anatomic alterations are based on the following three characteristics of sickle cell anemia: increased destruction of the sickled red cells with the development of anemia, increased release of hemoglobin and formation of bilirubin, and capillary stasis and thrombosis. The consequences of the increased red cell destruction and anemia have already been detailed in the general consideration of all hemolytic anemias. Briefly, these involve pallor of the skin, systemic iron overload, and fatty changes in the heart, liver, and tubules of the kidney. The bone marrow is hyperplastic. This increased activity is due to expansion of normoblasts. The white cells and megakaryoctyes are unaffected. The expansion of the marrow may lead to resorption of bone with secondary new bone formation to produce the roentgenographic appearance in the skull of the "crew haircut." Extramedullary hematopoiesis may appear in the spleen or liver, and, rarely, in other sites.

In children, during the early phase of the disease, the spleen is commonly enlarged up to 500 gm. Histologically, there is marked congestion of the red pulp, due mainly to the trapping of sickled red cells in the splenic cords and sinuses (Fig. 13–10). This erythrostasis in the spleen leads to thrombosis and infarction or at least to marked tissue hypoxia. Continued scarring causes progressive shrinkage of the spleen so that by adolescence or early adulthood only a small nubbin of fibrous tissue may be left; this is called **autosplenectomy** (Fig. 13–11). Infarction secondary to vascular occlusions and anoxia occurs also in the bones, brain, kidney, liver, and retina. Thrombotic occlusions have also been described in the pulmonary vessels, and many patients have cor pulmonale. Vascular stagnation in the subcutaneous tissue leads to leg ulcers in adult patients but is rare in children. The increased release of hemoglobin leads to pigment gallstones in some individuals, and all patients develop hyperbilirubinemia during periods of active hemolysis.

CLINICAL COURSE. *From the description of the disease to this point, it is evident that these patients are beset with problems stemming from (1) severe anemia, (2) vaso-occlusive complications, and (3) chronic hyperbilirubinemia.* Increased susceptibility to infections is another threat, the basis of which is not entirely clear. In children splenic function is impaired, even though splenomegaly is present. Perhaps extensive erythrophagocytosis causes a blockade of the mononuclear phagocyte system. Later, splenic infarcts significantly reduce the size and function of this organ. The *"functional splenectomy"* predisposes to blood-borne infections, in particular by encapsulated organisms such as *Streptococcus pneumonia* and *Haemophilus influenzae.* Septicemia and meningitis caused by these two organisms are the most common causes of death in children with sickle cell anemia.

Chronic hemolysis induces a fairly severe anemia, with hematocrit values ranging between 18 and 30%. The hemolysis is associated with striking reticulocytosis and hyperbilirubinemia. Irreversibly sickled cells ranging in frequency from 5 to 15% can usually be seen in the peripheral smear. This protracted course is frequently punctuated by a variety of "crises." *Vaso-occlusive crises*, also called *painful crises*, represent episodes of hypoxic injury and infarction. Usually no predisposing causes can be identified, although an association with infection, dehydration, and acidosis (all of which favor sickling) has been noted. The pain can be extreme and may be referred to the abdomen, chest, or joints, depending on the site of vascular insufficiency. Sites most commonly involved by vaso-occlusive episodes are the bones, lungs, liver, brain, spleen, and penis. *In children, painful bone crises are extremely common and often difficult to distinguish from acute osteomyelitis.* Similarly, chest pain may be confused with infections, which are also common. Central nervous system hypoxia may produce manifestations of a seizure or stroke. Al-

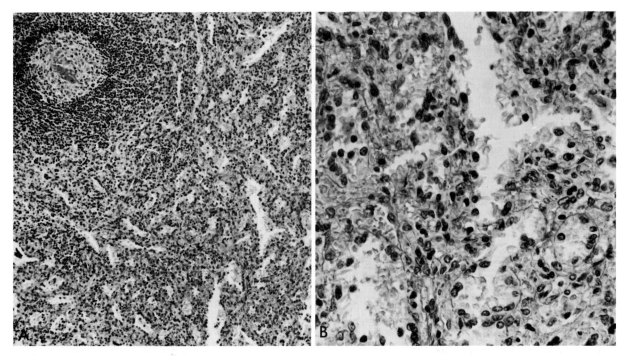

Figure 13–10. *A,* Spleen in sickle cell anemia (low power). White pulp on upper left is normal. Red pulp with its cords and sinusoids is markedly congested. *B,* Under high power, splenic cords are prominent owing to trapping of sickled red cells, which can also be seen in sinusoids. (Courtesy of Dr. Jose Hernandez, Department of Pathology, University of Texas Southwestern Medical School, Dallas.)

though such crises are frequently reversible, they may be fatal. Leg ulcers are an additional reflection of the vaso-occlusive tendency. An *aplastic crisis* represents a temporary cessation of bone marrow activity, usually triggered by parvovirus infection of erythroid progenitor cells. Reticulocytes disappear from the peripheral blood, and there is sudden and rapid worsening of anemia. A so-called *sequestration crisis* may appear in children with splenomegaly. Massive sequestration of deformed red cells leads to rapid splenic enlargement, hypovolemia, and sometimes shock. With transfusion, this can be reversed. Male patients may suddenly develop painful priapism owing to vascular engorgement of the penis. Chronic hypoxia causes a generalized impairment of growth

and development as well as organ damage affecting spleen, heart, and lungs.

Diagnosis usually is readily made from the clinical findings and the appearance of the peripheral blood smear. It can be confirmed by various tests for sickling that, in general, are based on mixing a blood sample with an oxygen-consuming reagent, such as metabisulfite, to induce sickling. Hemoglobin electrophoresis demonstrates hemoglobin S on the basis of specific mobility. Prenatal diagnosis is possible by analysis of fetal DNA obtained by amniocentesis or chorionic biopsy (see Chapter 5). Despite improvement in therapy, sickle cell anemia still markedly shortens longevity; many patients die within the first 3 years of life owing to overwhelming infections. Those who

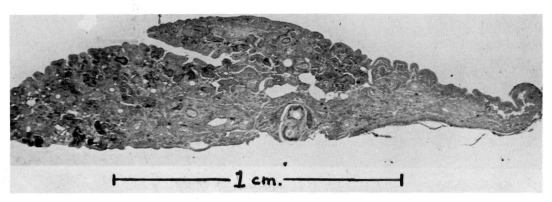

Figure 13–11. Sickle cell anemia. Cross-section of a totally fibrotic spleen—autosplenectomy.

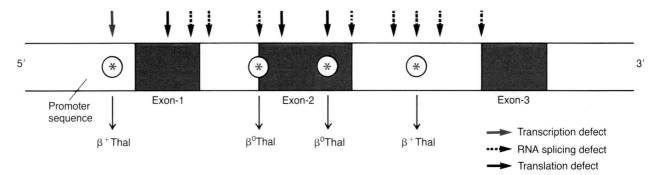

Figure 13–12. Diagrammatic representation of the beta-globin gene, and some sites where point mutations giving rise to β thalassemia have been localized. (Modified from Wyngaarden, J.B., Smith, L.H., and Bennett, J.C. (eds.): Cecil Textbook of Medicine, 19th ed. Philadelphia, W.B. Saunders Co., 1992.)

cross these early hurdles may live up to the fourth or fifth decade.

Thalassemia Syndromes

The thalassemia syndromes are a heterogeneous group of mendelian disorders, all characterized by a lack of or decreased synthesis of either the alpha- or the beta-globin chain of hemoglobin A ($\alpha_2\beta_2$). *β-thalassemia is characterized by deficient synthesis of the beta chain, whereas α-thalassemia is characterized by deficient synthesis of the alpha chain. The hematologic consequences of diminished synthesis of one globin chain derive not only from the low intracellular hemoglobin (hypochromia) but also from the relative excess of the other chain.* For example, in β-thalassemia there is an excess of alpha chains. As a consequence, free alpha chains tend to aggregate into insoluble inclusions within erythrocytes and their precursors, causing premature destruction of maturing erythroblasts within the marrow *(ineffective erythropoiesis)* as well as lysis of mature red cells in the spleen *(hemolysis)*.

β-Thalassemias

The abnormality common to all β-thalassemias is a total lack or a reduction in the synthesis of structurally normal beta-globin chains with unimpaired synthesis of alpha chains. However, the clinical severity of the anemia as well as the biochemical and genetic basis of beta-globin chain deficiency is quite varied. We shall begin our discussion with the molecular lesions in β-thalassemia and then integrate the clinical variants with the underlying molecular defects.

MOLECULAR PATHOGENESIS. The adult hemoglobin, or HbA, contains two alpha chains and two beta chains. The beta chains are coded by two beta-globin genes each located on one of the two number 11 chromosomes. In contrast, two pairs of functional alpha-globin genes are located on each number 16 chromosome.

β-thalassemia syndromes can be classified into two categories: (1) *β⁰-thalassemia*, associated with total absence of beta-globin chains in the homozygous state; and (2) *β⁺-thalassemia*, characterized by reduced (but detectable) beta-globin synthesis in the homozygous state. Sequencing of cloned beta-globin genes obtained from thalassemia patients has revealed approximately 100 different mutations responsible for β⁰- or β⁺-thalassemia.[9] Most of these result from point mutations. Unlike α-thalassemia, to be discussed later, gene deletions are uncommon in β-thalassemia. Details of these mutations and their effects on beta-globin synthesis can be found in specialized texts.[10] A few illustrative examples will be cited (Fig. 13–12).

- *Promoter region mutations.* Several point mutations within the promoter sequences reduce binding of RNA polymerase and thereby reduce the transcription rate by 75 to 80%. Since some beta-globin is synthesized, the patients develop β⁺-thalassemia.
- *Chain terminator mutations.* Two types of mutations can cause premature termination of mRNA translation. A point mutation in one of the exons can lead to the formation of a stop codon; in other cases, single nucleotide substitutions or small deletions alter mRNA reading frames and introduce stop codons downstream that terminate protein synthesis (frame shift mutations; see Chapter 5). Premature chain termination by either of these two mechanisms generates nonfunctional fragments of the beta-globin gene, leading to β⁰-thalassemia.
- *Splicing mutations. Mutations that lead to aberrant splicing are the most common cause of β-thalassemia.* Most of these affect introns, but some have been located within exons. If the mutation alters the normal splice junctions, splicing does not occur and all of the mRNA formed is abnormal. Unspliced mRNA is degraded within the nucleus, and β⁰-thalassemia results. However, some mutations affect the introns at locations away from the normal intron-exon splice junction. These mutations create new sites sensitive to the action of splicing enzymes at abnormal

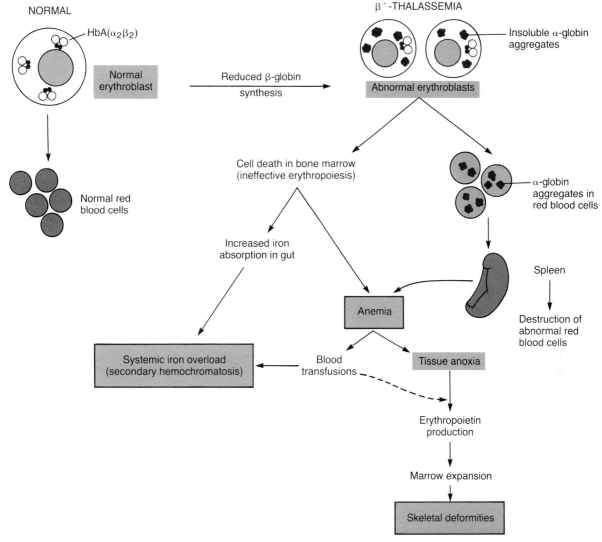

Figure 13–13. Pathogenesis of β-thalassemia major. Note that aggregates of excess of alpha-globins are not visible on routine blood smears. Blood transfusions, on the one hand, correct the anemia and reduce stimulus for erythropoietin secretion and deformities induced by marrow expansion; on the other hand, they add to systemic iron overload.

locations—within an intron, for example. Because normal splice sites remain unaffected, both normal and abnormal splicing occurs, giving rise to normal as well as abnormal beta-globin mRNA. These patients develop β+-thalassemia.

Impaired beta-globin synthesis contributes to the pathogenesis of anemia by two mechanisms (Fig. 13–13). The primary effect, of course, is lack of adequate HbA formation, so that the overall concentration of Hb in the cells (MCHC) is lower and the cells are hypochromic. Much more important is the effect on red cell survival, resulting from an imbalance between alpha- and beta-chain synthesis. Since synthesis of alpha-globin chains continues unimpaired, most of the chains produced cannot find complementary beta chains to bind. The free alpha chains form highly unstable aggregates that precipitate within the red cell precursors

in the form of insoluble inclusions. *A variety of untoward effects follow, the most important being cell membrane damage leading to a loss of K+ and impaired DNA synthesis. The net effect is destruction of the red cell precursors within the bone marrow, a phenomenon called ineffective erythropoiesis.* It is estimated that approximately 70 to 85% of the marrow normoblasts are destroyed in severely affected patients. The inclusion-bearing red cells derived from the precursors that escape intramedullary death are at increased risk for sequestration and destruction in the spleen. The inclusions damage the cell membranes, reduce their plasticity, and render them a "happy meal" for phagocytes in the spleen. The hemolytic component leads to a considerable shortening of red cell survival.

In severe β-thalassemia, marked anemia produced by ineffective erythropoiesis and hemolysis leads to several additional problems. Erythropoietin secretion is stimulated, which leads to extensive expansion of the erythropoietic elements in the bone marrow and often at extramedullary sites. Massive erythropoiesis within the bones invades the bony cortex, impairs bone growth, and produces other skeletal abnormalities, described later. Extramedullary hematopoiesis involves the liver and spleen and in extreme cases produces extraosseous masses in the thorax, abdomen, and pelvis. *Another disastrous effect seen in severe β-thalassemia (as well as in other causes of ineffective erythropoiesis) is excessive absorption of dietary iron.* This, coupled with the iron accumulation due to repeated blood transfusions required by these patients, leads to a severe state of iron overload. Secondary injury to parenchymal organs, particularly the iron-laden liver, often follows and sometimes induces secondary hemochromatosis (see Chapter 18).

CLINICAL SYNDROMES. The clinical classification of β-thalassemias is based on the severity of the anemia, which in turn is based on the type of genetic defect (β^+ or β^0) as well as the gene dosage (homozygous or heterozygous).[11] In general, individuals who are homozygous for the β-thalassemia genes (β^+ or β^0) have very severe, transfusion-dependent anemia and are said to have *β-thalassemia major.* The presence of one normal gene in the heterozygotes usually leads to enough normal beta-globin chain synthesis so that the affected individuals are usually asymptomatic with only a mild anemia. This condition is referred to as *β-thalassemia minor* or *β-thalassemia trait.* A third clinical variant is characterized by an intermediate degree of severity, the so-called *β-thalassemia intermedia.* These patients have severe anemia, but not enough to require regular blood transfusions. Genetically, intermedia disorders are heterogeneous and include mild variants of homozygous β^+-thalassemia, some severe variants of heterozygous β-thalassemia (β^0/β or β^+/β), and double heterozygosity for the β^+ and β^0 genes (genotype β^+/β^0). The clinical and morphologic features of thalassemia intermedia will not be described separately but may be surmised from the following discussions of thalassemia major and minor.

Thalassemia Major. The β-thalassemia genes are most frequent, and thalassemia major is most common, in Mediterranean countries and parts of Africa and Southeast Asia. In the United States, the incidence is highest in immigrants from these areas. As indicated in Table 13–2, the genotype of these patients is usually β^+/β^+ or β^0/β^0. In some cases it is β^0/β^+ (double heterozygotes, if the two parents are carriers of β^+ and β^0). With all these genotypes the anemia is very severe and first becomes manifest 6 to 9 months after birth, as hemoglobin synthesis switches from HbF to HbA. In untransfused patients, Hb levels range between 3 and 6 gm/dl. The peripheral blood smear shows severe abnormalities; there is marked anisocytosis (variation in size) with many small and virtually colorless (microcytic, hypochromic) red cells. Abnormal forms, including target cells (so called because the small amount of hemoglobin collects in the center), stippled red cells, and fragmented red cells, are common. Inclusions representing aggregated alpha chains are usually not seen unless the spleen has been removed. The reticulocyte count is elevated, but because of ineffective erythropoiesis it is lower than would be predicted from the severity of anemia. Variable numbers of poorly hemoglobinized normoblasts are seen in the peripheral blood. The red cells contain either no HbA at all (β^0/β^0 genotype) or very small amounts (β^+/β^+ genotype). HbF is markedly increased and indeed constitutes the major hemoglobin of red cells. HbA_2 levels may be normal, low, or high.

MORPHOLOGY. The major morphologic alterations, in addition to those characteristic of all hemolytic anemias, involve the bone marrow and spleen. In the typical patient there is striking expansion of the red marrow that can lead to thinning of the cortical bone, with new bone formation on the external aspect (Fig. 13–14). These changes are particularly evident in the maxilla and frontal bones of the face, sparing the mandible since it usually contains little marrow. Marked splenomegaly and hepatomegaly result both from reticuloendothelial cell hyperplasia secondary to active erythrophagocytosis and from extramedullary hematopoiesis. The spleen may increase up to 1500 gm in weight.

Hemosiderosis and even sometimes secondary hemochromatosis appear, related to a number of factors. Many of these patients have received numerous transfusions, providing a ready explanation for the iron overload. Ineffective erythropoiesis and possibly the chronic tissue hypoxia lead to increased intestinal absorption of iron. In any event, the hemosiderosis may have secondary consequences when the iron pigment accumulates in the myocardium, liver, or pancreas to induce organ injury (see Chapter 18).

The clinical course of β-thalassemia major is generally brief because, unless supported by transfusions, children suffer from growth retardation and die at an early age from the profound effects of anemia. Blood transfusions not only improve the anemia but also suppress secondary features related to excessive erythropoiesis. The clinical manifestations can be deduced largely from the hematologic and morphologic changes. In those who survive long enough the face becomes overlarge and somewhat distorted. Since the mandible is unaffected there is often malocclusion. Hepatosplenomegaly is usually present; the tissue hypoxia and systemic hemosiderosis may lead to delayed sexual

Table 13–2. CLINICAL AND GENETIC CLASSIFICATION OF THALASSEMIAS

CLINICAL NOMENCLATURE	GENOTYPE	DISEASE	MOLECULAR GENETICS
A. β-Thalassemias			
I. Thalassemia major	1. Homozygous β^0-thalassemia (β^0/β^0) 2. Homozygous β^+-thalassemia (β^+/β^+)	Severe, requires blood transfusions regularly	1. Rare gene deletions in β^0/β^0 2. Defects in transcription, processing, or translation of beta-globin mRNA
II. Thalassemia intermedia	β^0/β β^+/β^+	Severe, but does not require regular blood transfusions	
III. Thalassemia minor	β^0/β β^+/β	Asymptomatic with mild or absent anemia; red cell abnormalities seen	
B. α-Thalassemias			
I. Silent carrier	$-\alpha/\alpha\alpha$	Asymptomatic; no red cell abnormality	Gene deletions mainly
II. α-Thalassemia trait	1. $--/\alpha\alpha$ (Asian) 2. $-\alpha/-\alpha$ (black African)	Asymptomatic, like β-thalassemia minor	
III. HbH disease	$--/-\alpha$	Severe, resembles β-thalassemia intermedia	
IV. Hydrops fetalis	$--/--$	Lethal *in utero*	

development secondary to regressive changes in the gonads and other endocrine organs. Cardiac disease resulting from progressive iron overload and secondary hemochromatosis (see Chapter 18) is an important cause of death even in patients who can otherwise be supported by blood transfusions. To reduce the amount of iron overload, most patients also receive iron chelators. With transfusions and iron chelation many patients survive into the third decade, but the overall outlook continues to be grim. Currently, bone marrow transplantation from an HLA-identical sibling is the only therapy that offers a cure.[12] Prenatal diagnosis is possible by molecular analysis of DNA.

Thalassemia Minor. This is much more common than thalassemia major and understandably affects the same ethnic groups. In most cases these pa-

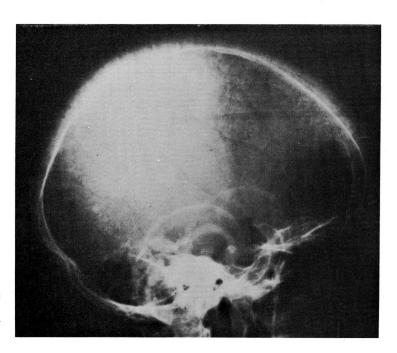

Figure 13–14. Thalassemia. X-ray film of skull showing new bone formation on outer table, producing perpendicular radiations characterized as a "crew haircut."

tients are heterozygotes for the β^+ or β^0 gene. Thalassemia trait is believed to offer resistance against falciparum malaria, accounting for its prevalence in those parts of the world where malaria is endemic. Almost invariably, individuals with the thalassemia trait are asymptomatic, and anemia is very mild, if present. The peripheral blood smear usually shows some abnormalities affecting the red cells, including hypochromia, microcytosis, basophilic stippling, and target cells. Mild erythroid hyperplasia is seen in the bone marrow. The red cell survival may be slightly shortened or normal. A characteristic finding on hemoglobin electrophoresis is an increase in HbA$_2$, which may constitute 4 to 8% of the total hemoglobin (normal $2.5 \pm 0.3\%$). HbF levels may be normal or slightly increased. Recognition of β-thalassemia trait is important on two counts: (1) its differentiation from the hypochromic microcytic anemia of iron deficiency and (2) genetic counseling. The importance of differentiating thalassemia trait from iron deficiency lies in the fact that the latter is benefited by iron therapy, whereas the former may be worsened. The distinction can usually be made by measurement of serum iron, total iron-binding capacity, and serum ferritin (see Iron Deficiency Anemia). Hemoglobin electrophoresis is also helpful.

α-Thalassemias

These disorders are characterized by reduced synthesis of alpha-globin chains. Since there are normally four alpha-globin genes, the severity of the clinical syndromes shows a great variation, depending on the number of defective alpha-globin genes. As in the case of β-thalassemias, the anemia stems both from lack of adequate hemoglobin and from the effects of excess unpaired non-alpha chains (β, γ, δ). However, the situation is somewhat complicated by the fact that normally different non-alpha-chains are synthesized at different times of development. Thus, in the newborn with α-thalassemia, there is an excess of unpaired gamma-globin chains, resulting in the formation of gamma$_4$-tetramers called Hb Barts, whereas in adults the excess beta-globin chains aggregate to form tetramers called HbH. Since the non-alpha chains in general form more soluble and less toxic aggregates than those derived from alpha chains, the hemolytic anemia and ineffective erythropoiesis tend to be less severe than with β-thalassemias of similar degree of chain imbalance. A variety of molecular lesions have been detected in α-thalassemia. Unlike β-thalassemia, however, the most common cause of reduced alpha-chain synthesis seems to be the deletion of alpha-globin genes.

CLINICAL SYNDROMES. These are classified on the basis of the number and position of the alpha-globin genes deleted, which in turn determine the clinical syndrome. It will be useful at this point to recall that alpha-globin genes occur in linked pairs on each of the two chromosomes 16. Each alpha gene normally contributes approximately 25% of the alpha-globin chains and may be deleted independently of the other alpha-globin genes. The terminology of α-thalassemias is best considered along with Table 13–2, in which clinical terms and their genetic equivalents are presented along with the salient clinical features. Capsule descriptions follow.

Silent Carrier State. This is characterized by the deletion of a single alpha-globin gene and barely detectable reduction in alpha-globin chain synthesis. These individuals carrying three normal alpha-globin genes are completely asymptomatic and do not have anemia.

α-Thalassemia Trait. This is characterized by deletion of two alpha-globin genes. The involved genes may be from the same chromosome (with the other chromosome carrying the two normal genes), or one alpha-globin gene may be deleted from each of the two chromosomes (see Table 13–2). The former genotype is more common among Asian populations, whereas the latter is seen in those of African origin. Both of these genetic patterns produce similar quantitative deficiencies of alpha-globin chains and therefore are identical clinically, but the position of deleted genes makes a big difference to the likelihood of severe α-thalassemia (HbH disease or hydrops fetalis) in the offspring. As is evident from Table 13–2, in black African populations, in whom the two alpha genes are deleted from two separate chromosomes, mating of two individuals with the α-thalassemia trait would not result in progeny with HbH disease or hydrops fetalis.

The clinical picture in α-thalassemia trait is identical to that described for β-thalassemia minor, that is, minimal or no anemia and no abnormal physical signs.

Hemoglobin H Disease. This is associated with deletion of three of the four alpha-globin genes. As already discussed, HbH disease is seen mainly in Asian populations and rarely in those of African origin. With only one normal alpha-globin gene, the synthesis of alpha chains is markedly reduced and tetramers of excess beta globin, called HbH, are formed. HbH has extremely high oxygen affinity and therefore is not useful for oxygen exchange. Hence the patient's anemia appears disproportionate to the level of Hb. Inclusions of HbH can be demonstrated by incubation of red cells with brilliant cresyl blue *in vitro*. Oxidized HbH is precipitated by this procedure, since it is unable to withstand oxidative stress. This property of HbH is the major cause of anemia, since older red cells with precipitates of oxidized HbH are removed by the spleen. These patients have a moderately severe anemia; the clinical picture resembles that of β-thalassemia intermedia.

Hydrops Fetalis. This is the most severe form of α-thalassemia, resulting from the deletion of all four alpha-globin genes. In the fetus, excess gamma-globin chains form tetramers (Hb Barts) that have extremely high oxygen affinity but are unable to deliver the oxygen to tissues. Severe tissue anoxia associated with this condition invariably leads to intrauterine fetal death. The fetus shows severe pallor, generalized edema, and massive hepatosplenomegaly similar to that seen in erythroblastosis fetalis (see Chapter 10).

Paroxysmal Nocturnal Hemoglobinuria (PNH)

Despite its rarity, this disorder has fascinated hematologists and immunologists because of the elusive nature of the underlying molecular abnormality. It is now known that PNH results from a somatic mutation affecting a pluripotent stem cell. The clonal progeny of the mutant stem cell (red cells, white cells, platelets) are deficient in a family of proteins that are attached to the cell membrane by a glycosyl phosphatidyl inositol (GPI) anchor. Because several GPI-linked proteins inactivate complement, their absence renders blood cells unusually sensitive to lysis by endogenous complement.

Three GPI-linked proteins that regulate complement activity—decay-accelerating factor, or CD55; membrane inhibitor of reactive lysis, or CD59; and a C8 binding protein—are deficient in PNH. Of these, CD59 is perhaps the most important because it limits spontaneous *in vivo* activation of the alternative complement pathway by rapid inactivation of C3 convertase. The membrane defect in PNH is not limited to red blood cells; platelets and granulocytes are also more sensitive to lysis by complement.[13]

Patients classically have intravascular hemolysis, which is paroxysmal and nocturnal in only 25% of cases. Most of the remaining patients have chronic hemolysis without dramatic hemoglobinuria. Over the long course of the disease, hemosiderinuria with loss of iron eventually leads to iron deficiency (Fig. 13–15). The other clinical manifestations include multiple episodes of venous thromboses in the hepatic, portal, or cerebral veins, which are fatal in 50% of cases. Infection related to granulocytopenia or abnormal leukocyte function is also prominent. The course of this disease is chronic, with a median survival of 10 years. Because PNH is an acquired clonal disorder of stem cells it sometimes evolves into other stem cell disorders, such as aplastic anemia and acute leukemia.

Immunohemolytic Anemia

Hemolytic anemias in this category are caused by extracorpuscular mechanisms. Although these disorders are commonly referred to as autoimmune hemolytic anemias (AHAs), the designation *immunohemolytic anemias* is preferred because in some instances the immune reaction is initiated by drug ingestion.[14] The immunohemolytic disorders have been classified in various ways but most commonly on the basis of the specific nature of antibody involved (Table 13–3).

Whatever the antibody, the differentiation of immunohemolytic anemias from other forms of hemolytic anemia depends on demonstration of the anti–red cell antibodies. The major diagnostic criterion is the *Coombs' antiglobulin test,* which relies on the capacity of the antibodies prepared in animals against human globulins to agglutinate red cells if these globulins are present on red cell surfaces. The temperature dependence of the autoantibody further helps to specify the type of antibody. Quantitative immunologic methods to

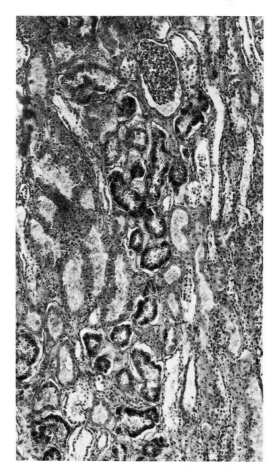

Figure 13–15. Paroxysmal nocturnal hemoglobinuria. Dark renal tubules are heavily laden with hemosiderin in a 37-year-old patient with multiple recurrent hemolytic episodes.

Table 13–3. CLASSIFICATION OF IMMUNE HEMOLYTIC ANEMIAS

I. WARM ANTIBODY TYPE
The antibody is of the IgG type, does not usually fix complement, and is active at 37°C.
   A. *Primary* or idiopathic
   B. *Secondary* to:
      1. Lymphomas and leukemias
      2. Other neoplastic diseases
      3. Autoimmune disorder (particularly SLE)
      4. Drugs

II. COLD AGGLUTININ TYPE
The antibodies are IgM and are most active *in vitro* at 0–4°C. Antibodies dissociate at 30°C or above. The antibody fixes complement at warmer temperatures, but agglutination of cells by IgM and complement occurs only in the peripheral cool parts of the body.
   A. *Acute* (mycoplasmal infection, infectious mononucleosis)
   B. *Chronic*
      1. Idiopathic
      2. Associated with lymphoma

III. COLD HEMOLYSINS (Paroxysmal Cold Hemoglobinuria)
IgG antibodies bind to red cells at low temperature, fix complement, and cause hemolysis when the temperature is raised to 30°C.

SLE = systemic lupus erythematosus.

measure these autoantibodies directly are now available.

WARM ANTIBODY HEMOLYTIC ANEMIA. This is the most common form of immune hemolytic anemia. In about 60% of patients, the condition is idiopathic and primary; in the remaining 40% there is an underlying predisposing condition (see Table 13–3), or some drug exposure to thus produce a secondary form of immune hemolytic anemia. The vast majority of autoantibodies are of the IgG class; only sometimes are IgA antibodies found. Most of the red cell destruction in this form of hemolytic disease is not due to intravascular hemolysis.[14] Instead, IgG-coated red cells are bound to Fc receptors on monocytes and splenic macrophages and undergo spheroidal transformation. This process results from a partial loss of the red cell membrane by attempted phagocytosis of the IgG-coated cell. *The spherocytes are then sequestered and removed in the spleen, the major site of red cell destruction in this disorder. Thus, moderate-to-severe splenomegaly is characteristic of this form of anemia.*

As is the case with most forms of autoimmunity, the cause of autoantibody formation is largely unknown. Surprisingly, in many cases the antibodies are directed against the Rh blood group antigens. The mechanisms of drug-induced hemolysis are better understood. Three different immunologic mechanisms have been implicated.[15]

- *Hapten model.* The drugs—exemplified by penicillin and cephalosporins—act as a hapten and combine with the red cell membrane to induce antibody directed against the red cell–drug complex, resulting in the destructive sequence cited above. This form of hemolytic anemia is usually caused by large intravenous doses of the antibiotic and occurs 1 to 2 weeks after onset of therapy.
- *Immune complex model.* The drug serving as a hapten binds to a plasma protein and the drug-protein complex evokes IgG or IgM antibodies. The resultant immune complexes nonspecifically attach to the red blood cell membrane, fixing complement and causing severe intravascular lysis. Here the red cells are "innocent bystanders." The red cell destruction, however, may also be extravascular if the antibody cannot fix complement. Quinidine and phenacetin are prototype drugs responsible for this form of hemolysis.
- *Autoantibody model.* The drug, such as the antihypertensive agent α-methyldopa, in some manner initiates the production of antibodies that are directed against intrinsic red cell antigens, in particular the Rh blood group antigens. Approximately 10% of patients taking methyldopa develop autoantibodies that can be detected in the Coombs' test. However, only 1% develop clinically significant hemolysis.

COLD AGGLUTININ IMMUNE HEMOLYTIC ANEMIA. This form of immune hemolytic anemia is caused by IgM antibodies that bind avidly to red cells at low temperatures (0 to 4°C).[16] Because they agglutinate red cells at low temperatures, they are referred to as cold agglutinins. These antibodies occur *acutely* during the recovery phase of certain infectious disorders such as mycoplasmal pneumonia and infectious mononucleosis. This form of hemolytic anemia is self-limited and rarely induces clinical manifestations of hemolysis. *Chronic* cold agglutinins occur with lymphoproliferative disorders and as an idiopathic condition. The antibodies produced are monoclonal, suggesting that the underlying basis is similar to that of other monoclonal gammopathies (see Chapter 14). The clinical symptoms result from an *in vivo* agglutination of red cells and fixation of complement in distal body parts, where the temperature may drop to below 30°C. Thus there may be intravascular hemolysis. In most cases, however, the IgM bound to red cells is released when the cells return to 37°C. This leaves C3, specifically C3b, bound to the cell membrane, making it susceptible to phagocytosis by mononuclear phagocytes in the liver and spleen. The hemolytic anemia usually is of variable severity. In addition, vascular obstruction caused by red cell agglutinates results in pallor, cyanosis of the body parts exposed to cold temperatures, and Raynaud's phenomenon (see Chapter 11).

COLD HEMOLYSIN HEMOLYTIC ANEMIA. These autoantibodies are characteristic of the disease *paroxysmal cold hemoglobinuria* (PCH), which is noted for acute intermittent massive hemolysis, frequently with hemoglobinuria, following exposure of the affected patient to cold. Lysis is clearly complement-dependent. The autoantibodies are IgG in nature and are directed against the P blood group antigen; they attach to the red cells and bind complement at low temperatures. When the temperature is elevated, the hemolytic action is mediated by the activation of the lytic complement cascade. The antibody is also known as the Donath-Landsteiner (DL) antibody, previously associated with syphilis. Today, most cases of PCH follow various infections such as mycoplasmal pneumonia, measles, mumps, and some ill-defined viral and "flu" syndromes. The mechanisms responsible for the production of such autoantibodies are unknown.

Hemolytic Anemia Resulting from Trauma to Red Cells

Fragmentation of red blood cells when exposed to physical trauma may be severe enough to give rise to significant intravascular hemolysis. Clinically important are the hemolytic anemias associated with insertion of valve prostheses and diffuse deposition of fibrin in the microvasculature. In addition to immediate rupture, a wide variety of erythrocytic abnormalities are produced and are recognized in the peripheral blood film as burr cells, helmet cells, and triangle cells, as well as fragments of erythrocytes (schistocytes) (Fig. 13–16). *Hemolysis due to narrowing or obstructions in the microvasculature is called microangiopathic hemolytic anemia.* This form of anemia is encountered in disseminated intravascular coagulation (DIC), thrombotic thrombocytopenic purpura (TTP), the hemolytic-uremic syndrome, malignant hypertension, renal

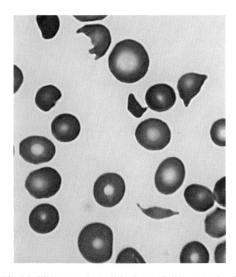

Figure 13–16. Microangiopathic hemolytic anemia. The peripheral blood smear from a patient with hemolytic-uremic syndrome shows several fragmented red cells. (Courtesy of Dr. Robert W. McKenna, Department of Pathology, University of Texas Southwestern Medical School, Dallas.)

cortical necrosis, systemic lupus erythematosus (SLE), and metastatic adenocarcinoma. The common denominator is the presence of some vascular lesion. In DIC, the microthrombi constitute the point of impaction. In malignant hypertension, it is the markedly narrowed arterioles. In SLE, it is the necrotizing arteritis and arteriolitis. In patients with *prosthetic heart valves* (particularily aortic valves), the red cells are damaged by the shear stress resulting from the turbulent blood flow and abnormal pressure gradients (see also Chapter 12). Hemolysis can also occur in patients with severe aortic stenosis without prosthetic valves.

In most of these settings, the hemolysis is only a minor part of the clinical problem, and these patients rarely exhibit the morphologic changes encountered in the more chronic hemolytic diseases discussed earlier.

ANEMIAS OF DIMINISHED ERYTHROPOIESIS

Diminished erythropoiesis may result from a deficiency of some vital substrate necessary for red cell formation. Included in this group are iron deficiency anemias, in which heme synthesis is impaired, and anemia of vitamin B_{12} and folate deficiency, characterized by defective DNA synthesis (megaloblastic anemias). Other causes of decreased erythropoiesis include anemia of chronic disease and "marrow stem cell failure." The latter embraces such conditions as aplastic anemia, pure red cell aplasia, and anemia of renal failure.

Megaloblastic Anemias

The following discussion will attempt first to characterize the major features of these anemias and then to discuss the two principal types of megaloblastic anemia: (1) pernicious anemia (PA), the major form of vitamin B_{12} deficiency anemia; and (2) folate deficiency anemia.

The megaloblastic anemias constitute a diverse group of entities, having in common impaired DNA synthesis and distinctive morphologic changes in the blood and bone marrow. As the name implies, the erythroid precursors and erythrocytes are abnormally large, thought to be related to impairment of cell maturation and division. The precise basis of these changes is not fully understood.

Some of the metabolic roles of vitamin B_{12} and folate will be considered later, but for now it suffices that vitamin B_{12} and folic acid are coenzymes in the DNA synthetic pathway. A deficiency of these vitamins or impairment in their utilization results in deranged or inadequate synthesis of

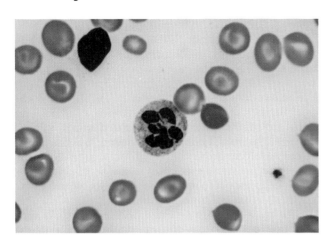

Figure 13-17. Peripheral blood smear from a patient with megaloblastic anemia shows a neutrophil with a six-lobed nucleus (macropolycyte). (Courtesy of Dr. Robert W. McKenna, Department of Pathology, University of Texas Southwestern Medical School, Dallas.)

DNA. The synthesis of RNA and protein is unaffected, however, so there is cytoplasmic enlargement not matched by DNA synthesis, which appears to delay or block mitotic division. Thus there appears to be asynchronism between the cytoplasmic maturation and nuclear maturation.

MORPHOLOGY. Certain morphologic features are common to all forms of megaloblastic anemia. The peripheral blood reveals marked variation in the size and shape of red cells (anisocytosis), which are nonetheless normochromic. **Many erythrocytes are macrocytic and oval shaped (macro-ovalocytes), with mean corpuscular volumes (MCVs) over 100 μm³ (normal 82 to 92).** Because they are thicker than normal and well filled with hemoglobin, most macrocytes lack the central pallor of normal red cells and may even appear "hyperchromic," but the mean corpuscular hemoglobin concentration (MCHC) is not elevated. The reticulocyte count is lower than normal and, occasionally with severe anemia, nucleated red cells appear in the circulating blood. **Neutrophils too are larger than normal (macropolymorphonuclear) and are hypersegmented, that is, have five to six or more nuclear lobules** (Fig. 13-17). The marrow is hypercellular, and the megaloblastic change is detected in all stages of red cell development. The most primitive cells (promegaloblasts) are large, with a deeply basophilic cytoplasm and a distinctive fine chromatin pattern in the nucleus (Fig. 13-18, cell A). The nucleoli are large. As these cells differentiate and begin to acquire hemoglobin, the nucleus retains its finely distributed chromatin and thus fails to undergo the chromatin clumping typical of the normoblast. For example, orthochromatic megaloblasts have a large amount of pink, well-hemoglobinized cytoplasm, but the

nucleus, instead of becoming pyknotic, remains relatively large and immature, creating an apparent dissociation between cytoplasmic and nuclear maturation. Because DNA synthesis is impaired in all proliferating cells, the granulocytic precursors also reveal nuclear-cytoplasmic asynchrony, yielding giant metamyelocytes and band forms and hypersegmentation of the neutrophils, as previously mentioned. Megakaryocytes, too, may be abnormally large and have bizarre, multilobate nuclei, but sometimes they appear relatively normal. With increased cellularity, much or all of the normally fatty marrow may be converted to red marrow. The erythroid-to-myeloid ratio, normally 1:3, may be transformed to 1:1. Nuclear-cytoplasmic asynchrony becomes apparent in all cells having a relatively rapid turnover, so megaloblastic and other cytologic alterations appear in the mucosal epithelium of the gastrointestinal tract, principally within the stomach.

Because of these maturational derangements there is an accumulation of megaloblasts in the bone marrow, yielding too few erythrocytes; hence the anemia. Two concomitant processes further aggravate the anemia: (1) ineffective erythropoiesis and (2) increased hemolytic destruction of red cells. Ineffective erythropoiesis results from intramedullary destruction of megaloblasts, which undergo autohemolysis more readily than do nor-

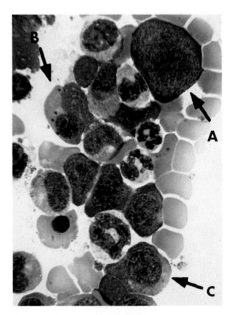

Figure 13-18. Marrow smear from a patient with megaloblastic anemia. A to C, Megaloblasts in various stages of differentiation. Note that the orthochromatic megaloblast (B) is hemoglobinized (as evidenced by cytoplasmic color), but in contrast to an orthochromatic normoblast the nucleus is not pyknotic. The granulocytic precursors are also large. (Courtesy of Dr. Jose Hernandez, Department of Pathology, University of Texas Southwestern Medical School, Dallas.)

Table 13-4. CAUSES OF MEGALOBLASTIC ANEMIA

VITAMIN B$_{12}$ DEFICIENCY

Decreased intake	Inadequate diet
	Impaired absorption
	Intrinsic factor deficiency
	Pernicious anemia
	Gastrectomy
	Malabsorption states
	Diffuse intestinal disease—e.g., lymphoma, systemic sclerosis
	Ileal resection, ileitis
	Competitive parasitic uptake
	Fish tapeworm infection
	Bacterial overgrowth in blind loops and diverticula of bowel
Increased requirement	Pregnancy, hyperthyroidism, disseminated cancer

FOLIC ACID DEFICIENCY

Decreased intake	Inadequate diet—alcoholism, infancy
	Impaired absorption
	Malabsorption states
	Intrinsic intestinal disease
	Anticonvulsants, oral contraceptives
Increased loss	Hemodialysis
Increased requirement	Pregnancy, infancy, disseminated cancer, markedly increased hematopoiesis
Impaired utilization	Folic acid antagonists

UNRESPONSIVE TO VITAMIN B$_{12}$ OR FOLIC ACID THERAPY

	Metabolic inhibitors, e.g., mercaptopurines, fluorouracil, cytosine
	Unexplained disorders
	Pyridoxine- and thiamine-responsive megaloblastic anemia
	Acute erythroleukemia (M6) (Di Guglielmo's syndrome)

Modified from Beck, W.S.: Megaloblastic anemias. *In* Wyngaarden, J.B., and Smith, L.H. (eds.): Cecil Textbook of Medicine, 18th ed. Philadelphia, W.B. Saunders Co., 1988, p. 900.

moblasts and are more vulnerable to phagocytosis by mononuclear phagocytic cells in the marrow than are normal erythroid precursors. Premature destruction of granulocytic and platelet precursors also occurs, resulting in leukopenia and thrombocytopenia. The basis of the increased hemolysis of the mature erythrocytes is not entirely clear. Both an intracorpuscular defect, related perhaps to the defective red cells, and a poorly characterized plasma factor are believed to contribute. As in other hemolytic states, accelerated destruction of the red cells may lead to anatomic signs of mild-to-moderate iron overload after several years (see Chapter 18).

Anemias of Vitamin B$_{12}$ Deficiency: Pernicious Anemia (PA)

The major causes of megaloblastic anemia are listed in Table 13-4. As mentioned at the outset, pernicious anemia is an important cause of vitamin B$_{12}$ deficiency. *The feature that sets pernicious anemia apart from the other vitamin B$_{12}$ deficiency megaloblastic anemias is the cause of the vitamin B$_{12}$ malabsorption: atrophic gastritis with failure of production of intrinsic factor (IF).*

It is well to discuss first the economy of vitamin B$_{12}$ in the body in order to place PA in per-spective relative to the other forms of vitamin B$_{12}$ deficiency anemia.

Etiology of Vitamin B$_{12}$ Deficiency. Vitamin B$_{12}$ is a complex organometallic compound known as cobalamin. It is composed of a corrin ring (similar to the porphyrin ring) to which a cobalt atom is attached. The synthetic therapeutic form of vitamin B$_{12}$ is a stable cyanocobalamin. Under normal circumstances, humans are totally dependent on dietary animal products for their vitamin B$_{12}$ requirement. Microorganisms are the ultimate origin of cobalamin in the food chain. Plants and vegetables contain very little cobalamin save that contributed by microbial contamination; strictly vegetarian or macrobiotic diets then do not provide adequate amounts of this essential nutrient. The daily requirement is of the order of 2 to 3 μg, and the normal balanced diet contains significantly larger amounts. The reserves in the body, when fully maintained, are sufficient for years.

Absorption of vitamin B$_{12}$ requires IF, which is secreted by the parietal cells of the fundic mucosa along with HCl (Fig. 13-19). Initially the vitamin is released from its protein-bound form in animal foods by the action of pepsin in the acidic environment of the stomach. After peptic digestion of vitamin B$_{12}$-containing foods, the liberated vitamin is bound to salivary vitamin B$_{12}$-binding proteins

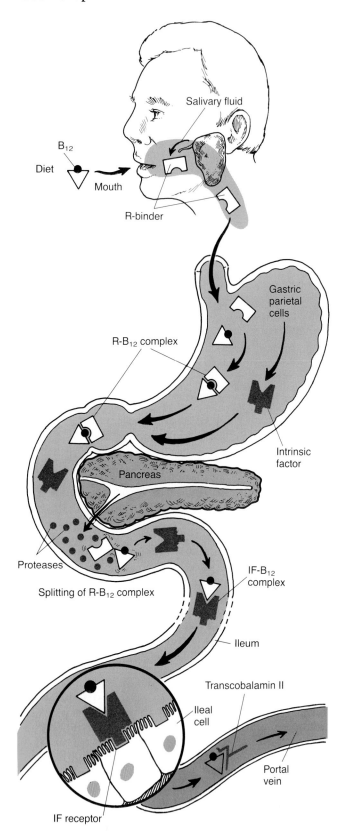

Figure 13–19. Schematic illustration of vitamin B₁₂ absorption.

(cobalophilins), also referred to as rapid (R) binders because of their electrophoretic mobility. Only a small amount is bound directly to IF. The R-B₁₂ complexes are transported to the duodenum, where they are broken down by the action of pancreatic proteases, and the released vitamin B₁₂ then attaches to IF. In this form, IF–vitamin B₁₂ complex is transported to the ileum, where it adheres to IF-specific receptors on the ileal cells. Vitamin B₁₂ then traverses the plasma membrane to enter the mucosal cell. It is picked up from the cell by a plasma protein, transcobalamin II, which is capable of delivering it to the liver and other cells of the body, particularly the rapidly proliferating pool in the bone marrow and mucosal lining of the gastrointestinal tract.

With this background we can consider the various causes of vitamin B₁₂ deficiency (Table 13–4). Inadequate diet is obvious but must be present for many years to deplete reserves. The absorption of vitamin B₁₂ may be impaired by disruption of any one of the steps outlined earlier. With achlorhydria and loss of pepsin secretion (which occurs in some elderly individuals), vitamin B₁₂ is not readily released from its protein-bound form. With gastrectomy and PA, IF is not available for transport to the ileum. With loss of exocrine pancreatic function, vitamin B₁₂ deficiency occurs because the vitamin cannot be released from the R-B₁₂ complexes. Ileal resection or diffuse ileal disease can remove or damage the site of IF–vitamin B₁₂ complex absorption. Tapeworm infestation, by competing for the nutrient, can induce a deficiency state. Under some circumstances, for example, pregnancy, hyperthyroidism, and disseminated cancer, the demand for vitamin B₁₂ can be so great as to produce a relative deficiency, even with normal absorption.

BIOCHEMICAL FUNCTIONS OF VITAMIN B₁₂. There are only two reactions in humans known to require vitamin B₁₂. *Methylcobalamin is an essential cofactor for the enzyme N⁵-methyltetrahydrofolate-homocysteine methyltransferase, involved in the conversion of homocysteine to methionine* (Fig. 13–20). In the process, methylocobalamin yields its methyl group and is regenerated from N⁵-methyltetrahydrofolic acid (N⁵-methyl-FH₄), the principal form of folic acid in plasma, which is thus converted to tetrahydrofolic acid (FH₄). The FH₄ is crucial, since it is required (through its derivative N⁵,¹⁰-methylene FH₄) for the conversion of deoxyuridine monophosphate (dUMP) to deoxythymidine monophosphate (dTMP), which is an immediate precursor of DNA. It has been postulated that the fundamental cause of impaired DNA synthesis in vitamin B₁₂ deficiency is the reduced availability of tetrahydrofolic acid, since most of it is "trapped" as N⁵-methyl-FH₄. In addition to the trapping of tetrahydrofolic acid in its methylated form, the "internal" folate deficiency resulting from the lack of

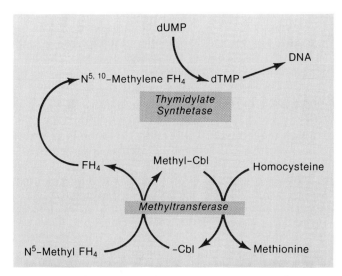

Figure 13-20. Diagram of relationship between N⁵-methyl FH₄: homocysteine methyltransferase and thymidylate synthetase. In cobalamin deficiency, folate is sequestered as N⁵-methyl FH₄. This ultimately deprives thymidylate synthetase of its folate coenzyme (N⁵,¹⁰-methylene FH₄) and thereby impairs DNA synthesis. (With permission from Wyngaarden, J.B., Smith, L.H., and Bennett, J.C. (eds.): Cecil Textbook of Medicine, 19th ed. Philadelphia, W.B. Saunders Co., 1992.)

vitamin B_{12} may also be caused by a failure to synthesize the metabolically active polyglutamate forms of folates.[17,17a] The synthesis of folate polyglutamates requires the single carbon formate groups derived from methionine, which in turn is generated by a vitamin B_{12}–dependent reaction (see Fig. 13-20). Whatever the mechanism of internal folate deficiency, the hypothesis that lack of folate is the proximate cause of anemia in vitamin B_{12} deficiency is supported by the observation that the anemia improves with the administration of folic acid.

Neurologic complications appear with vitamin B_{12} deficiency but are an even greater enigma.[18] Since the administration of folic acid, which relieves the megaloblastic anemia of vitamin B_{12} deficiency, fails to improve the neurologic deficit, internal folate deficiency must not be involved. It was stated earlier that only two reactions are known to require vitamin B_{12}. In addition to the transmethylation reaction discussed previously, cobalamin is involved in the *isomerization of methylmalonyl coenzyme A to succinyl coenzyme A, requiring adenosyl cobalamin as a prosthetic group on the enzyme methylmalonyl-CoA mutase.* A deficiency of vitamin B_{12} thus leads to increased levels of methylmalonate, excreted in the urine as methylmalonic acid. Interruption of the succinyl pathway with the build-up of increased levels of methylmalonate and propionate (a precursor) could lead to the formation of abnormal fatty acids that may be incorporated into neuronal lipids. This biochemical abnormality may predispose to myelin breakdown and thereby produce some of the neurologic complications of vitamin B_{12} deficiency (see Chapter 29).

With this overview of vitamin B_{12} metabolism we can now turn our attention to pernicious anemia.

INCIDENCE. Although somewhat more prevalent in Scandinavian and "English-speaking" populations, PA occurs in all racial groups, including, in the United States, blacks and Hispanics. It is a disease of older age, generally diagnosed in the fifth to eighth decades of life. A genetic predisposition is strongly suspected, but no definable genetic pattern of transmission has been discerned. As discussed next, these patients probably inherit a predisposition to forming autoantibodies.

PATHOGENESIS. Pernicious anemia is believed to result from immunologically mediated, possibly autoimmune, destruction of gastric mucosa. The resultant *chronic atrophic gastritis* is marked by a loss of parietal cells, a prominent infiltrate of lymphocytes and plasma cells, and megaloid and atypical nuclear changes in the mucosal cells similar to those found in the bone marrow. A number of immunologic reactions are associated with these morphologic changes. *Three types of antibodies are present in many, but not all, patients with PA.* About 75% of patients have an antibody that blocks vitamin B_{12}–IF binding, referred to as a *blocking antibody.* In the serum these are predominantly IgG, but may also be IgA. These are also found in the gastric juice, but here IgA antibodies predominate.[19] A second type, known as *binding antibody,* reacts with both IF and IF–vitamin B_{12} complex and is found in about 50% of patients. It is present in the serum and gastric juice and can also be identified by immunofluorescence techniques in plasma cells in the gastric mucosa. It does not occur in the absence of the blocking antibody. The third type of antibody, present in 85 to 90% of patients, localizes in the microvilli of the canalicular system of the gastric parietal cell, sometimes referred to as *parietal canalicular antibody.* It is directed against the alpha and beta subunits of the gastric proton pump.[20]

Despite the presence of these autoantibodies it is not established that they are the primary cause of gastric mucosal injury. It is suspected that an autoreactive T-cell response initiates gastric mucosal injury, which then triggers the formation of autoantibodies. These antibodies cause further mucosal injury, and after the mass of IF-secreting cells falls below a threshold (and the reserves of stored vitamin B_{12} are depleted), anemia develops. In an animal model of autoimmune gastritis, the disease is mediated by CD4+ T cells, and a pattern of autoantibodies resembling that seen in PA develops.[20] The possibility that PA is an autoimmune disease is also supported by the well-known association of this disease with autoimmune thyroiditis and adrenalitis. Conversely, patients with other organ-specific autoimmune disease have a predisposition to developing autoantibodies against **IF.**

It should be pointed out, however, that parietal canalicular antibodies are not absolutely specific for **PA** or other autoimmune diseases. They can be found in up to 50% of elderly patients with idiopathic chronic gastritis not associated with **PA.** Conceivably, they result from gastric injury, rather than cause it.

MORPHOLOGY. The major specific changes in PA are found in the bone marrow, alimentary tract, and central nervous system. Widespread nonspecific alterations incident to the generalized tissue hypoxia and abnormal hemolysis of blood may be present. The changes in the bone marrow and blood are similar to those described earlier for all megaloblastic anemias.

In the **alimentary system,** abnormalities are regularly found in the tongue and stomach. The tongue is shiny, glazed, and "beefy" **(atrophic glossitis).** The changes in the stomach are those of type A chronic gastritis (see Chapter 17). The most characteristic histologic alteration is the atrophy of the fundic glands, affecting both chief cells and parietal cells. The parietal cells are virtually absent. The glandular lining epithelium is replaced by mucus-secreting goblet cells that resemble those lining the large intestine. Such metaplasia is referred to as **intestinalization.** Some of the cells as well as their nuclei may increase to double the normal size. Presumably, these enlargements reflect the megaloid alterations discussed earlier. As will be seen, patients with pernicious anemia have a higher incidence of gastric cancer. The gastric changes are primary and are not the effect of the vitamin B_{12} deficiency, hence parenteral administration of vitamin B_{12} corrects the bone marrow changes, but gastric atrophy and achlorhydria persist.

Central nervous system lesions are found in approximately three-quarters of all cases of fulminant pernicious anemia, but it should be noted that in some cases neuronal involvement may occur in the absence of megaloblastic anemia. **The principal alterations involve the spinal cord, where there is myelin degeneration of the dorsal and lateral tracts,** sometimes followed by loss of axons. These changes give rise to spastic paraparesis, sensory ataxia, and severe paresthesias in the lower limbs. Less frequently, degenerative changes occur in the ganglia of the posterior roots and in the peripheral nerves (see Chapter 29). Because both sensory and motor pathways are involved, the term "subacute combined degeneration" or "combined system disease" is sometimes used to designate the neurologic changes associated with vitamin B_{12} deficiency.

The hemolytic tendency and ineffective erythropoiesis in all megaloblastic anemias may give rise to hemosiderosis seen in the liver, spleen, and bone marrow and in other elements of the mononuclear phagocyte system, but the spleen and liver usually are not significantly enlarged.

CLINICAL COURSE. Pernicious anemia is characteristically insidious in onset, so that by the time the patient seeks medical attention the anemia is usually quite marked. The usual course is progressive unless halted by therapy.

Diagnostic features include (1) a moderate-to-severe megaloblastic anemia; (2) leukopenia with hypersegmented granulocytes; (3) mild-to-moderate thrombocytopenia; (4) neurologic changes related to involvement of the posterolateral spinal tracts; (5) achlorhydria even after histamine stimulation; (6) inability to absorb an oral dose of cobalamin (assessed by urinary excretion of radiolabeled cyanocobalamin given orally, called the Schilling test); (7) low serum levels of vitamin B_{12}; (8) excretion of methylmalonic acid in the urine; and (9) a striking reticulocytic response and improvement in hematocrit levels following parenteral administration of vitamin B_{12}.

The cytologic aberrations in the gastric mucosa are associated with an increased risk of gastric cancer (see Chapter 17). In addition, cardiac failure incident to hypoxic injury to the myocardium and intercurrent infections are hazards. However, with parenteral vitamin B_{12} the anemia can be cured and the peripheral neurologic changes reversed, or at least halted in their progression. Overall longevity may be restored virtually to normal.

Anemia of Folate Deficiency

A deficiency of folic acid, more properly pteroylmonoglutamic acid, results in a megaloblastic anemia having the same characteristics as those encountered in vitamin B_{12} deficiency. However, the neurologic changes seen in vitamin B_{12} deficiency do not occur. Megaloblastic anemia secondary to folate deficiency is not common, but precarious folate levels in the body are surprisingly common: among the economically deprived of all countries who live on marginal diets; among pregnant women, in whom dietary inadequacies combine with increased metabolic requirements; and among alcoholics and drug addicts, with their well-known grossly inadequate diet. *The prime function of folic acid, specifically tetrahydrofolate (FH_4) derivatives, is to act as an intermediate in the transfer of one-carbon units such as formyl and methyl groups to various compounds* (Fig. 13–21). In this process, FH_4 acts as an acceptor of one-carbon fragments from compounds such as serine and formiminoglutamic acid (FIGlu), and the FH_4 derivatives so generated donate the acquired one-carbon fragments for the synthesis of biologically active molecules. FH_4, then, may be viewed as the biologic "middleman"

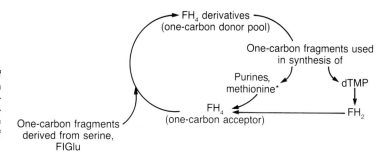

Figure 13-21. Schematic illustration of the role of folate derivatives in the transfer of one-carbon fragments for synthesis of biologic macromolecules. FH_4 = tetrahydrofolic acid; FH_2= dihydrofolic acid; FIGlu = formiminoglutamate; dTMP = deoxythymidylate monophosphate. *Synthesis of methionine also requires vitamin B_{12}.

in this trade. The most important metabolic processes dependent on such one-carbon transfers are (1) the synthesis of purines; (2) the synthesis of methionine from homocysteine, a reaction that also requires vitamin B_{12}; and (3) the synthesis of deoxythymidylate monophosphate (dTMP). In the first two reactions, FH_4 is regenerated from its one-carbon carrier derivatives and is available to accept another one-carbon fragment and re-enter the donor pool. In the synthesis of thymidylate, a dihydrofolate is produced that has to be reduced by dihydrofolate reductase to FH_4 to re-enter the pool. The reductase step is significant, since this enzyme is susceptible to inhibition by various drugs. Among the biologically active molecules whose synthesis is dependent on folates, thymidylate is perhaps the most important. As discussed earlier in relation to pernicious anemia, dTMP is required for DNA synthesis. It should be apparent from our discussion that suppressed synthesis of DNA, the common denominator of folic acid and vitamin B_{12} deficiency, is the immediate cause of megaloblastosis. A clinically insignificant biochemical effect of folate deficiency is the failure to metabolize formiminoglutamic acid (FIGlu), a breakdown product of histidine. With a deficiency of folate, FIGlu accumulates and is excreted in the urine, providing a useful clinical indicator of folate deficiency.

ETIOLOGY. Humans are entirely dependent on dietary sources for their folic acid requirement, which is of the order of 50 to 200 μg daily. Most normal diets contain ample amounts, the richest sources being green vegetables such as lettuce, spinach, asparagus, and broccoli. Certain fruits (e.g., lemons, bananas, melons) and animal proteins (e.g., liver) contain lesser amounts. The folic acid in these foods is largely in the form of folylpolyglutamates. *Despite their abundance in raw foods, polyglutamates (depending on the specific form) are very sensitive to heat; boiling, steaming, or frying of foods for 5 to 10 minutes may destroy up to 95% of the folate content.* Intestinal conjugases split the polyglutamates into monoglutamates that are readily absorbed in the proximal jejunum. During intestinal absorption they are modified so that only 5-methyltetrahydrofolate enters the circulation as

the normal transport form of folate. The bodily reserves of folate are relatively modest, and a deficiency may arise with months of a negative balance. There are three major causes of folic acid deficiency: (1) decreased intake, (2) increased requirements, and (3) impaired utilization (see Table 13-4).

Decreased intake can result from either a nutritionally inadequate diet or impairment of intestinal absorption. A normal daily diet contains folate in excess of the minimal daily adult requirement. Inadequate dietary intakes are almost invariably associated with grossly deficient diets, particularly those lacking vitamins such as the "B group." *Such dietary inadequacies are most frequently encountered in chronic alcoholics, the indigent, and the very elderly.* In alcoholics with cirrhosis, other mechanisms of folate deficiency such as trapping of folate within the liver, excessive urinary loss, and disordered folate metabolism have also been implicated. Under these circumstances, the megaloblastic anemia is often accompanied by general malnutrition and manifestations of other avitaminoses, including cheilosis, glossitis, and dermatitis. Malabsorption syndromes such as nontropical and tropical sprue may lead to inadequate absorption of this nutrient. Similarly, diffuse infiltrative disease of the small intestine (e.g., lymphoma) may impair intestinal absorption. In addition, certain drugs, particularly the anticonvulsant phenytoin and oral contraceptives, impair absorption.

Despite adequate intake of folic acid, a *relative deficiency* can be encountered in states of increased requirement, such as pregnancy, infancy, hematologic derangements associated with hyperactive hematopoiesis (hemolytic anemias), and disseminated cancer. In all these circumstances, the demands of active DNA synthesis render normal intake inadequate.

Folic acid antagonists, such as methotrexate, 6-mercaptopurine, and cyclophosphamide, inhibit dihydrofolate reductase and lead to a deficiency of tetrahydrofolate. With inhibition of folate function, all rapidly growing cells are affected, thus leading to ulcerative lesions within the gastrointestinal tract as well as megaloblastic anemia. Owing to their growth-inhibitory actions, these antimetabolites are used in cancer therapy.

As mentioned at the outset, *the megaloblastic anemia resulting from a deficiency of folic acid is identical to that encountered in vitamin B₁₂ deficiency.* Thus, the recognition of folate deficiency requires the demonstration of (1) decreased folate levels in the serum or red cells and (2) increased excretion of FIGlu after an administered dose of histidine.

Although prompt hematologic response heralded by the appearance of a reticulocytosis follows the administration of folic acid, it should be cautioned that even in patients with a vitamin B₁₂ deficiency anemia, a similar reticulocytosis may be produced by folic acid therapy. However, folic acid has no effect on the progression of the neurologic changes typical of the vitamin B₁₂ deficiency states, and therefore the hematologic response to folate therapy cannot be used to rule out vitamin B₁₂ deficiency.

Iron Deficiency Anemia

Deficiency of iron is probably the most common nutritional disorder in the world. Although the prevalence of iron deficiency anemia is higher in the developing countries, this form of anemia is also common in the United States. The factors underlying the iron deficiency differ somewhat in various population groups and can be best considered in the context of normal iron metabolism.

IRON METABOLISM. Normally, the total body iron content is in the range of 2 gm in women and up to 6 gm in men. As indicated in Table 13–5, it is divided into functional and storage compartments. Approximately 80% of the functional iron is found in hemoglobin; myoglobin and iron-containing enzymes such as catalase and the cytochromes contain the rest. The storage pool represented by hemosiderin and ferritin contains approximately 15 to 20% of total body iron. It should be noted that even healthy young females have substantially smaller stores of iron than do males. They are therefore in much more precarious iron balance and are accordingly more vulnerable to excessive losses or increased demands associated with menstruation and pregnancy.

Table 13–5. IRON DISTRIBUTION IN HEALTHY YOUNG ADULTS (mg)

	MEN	WOMEN
Total	3450	2450
Functional		
Hemoglobin	2100	1750
Myoglobin	300	250
Enzymes	50	50
Storage		
Ferritin, hemosiderin	1000	400

All storage of iron is in the form of either ferritin or hemosiderin. *Ferritin is essentially a protein-iron complex* that can be found in all tissues but particularly in liver, spleen, bone marrow, and skeletal muscles. In the liver, most of the ferritin is stored within the parenchymal cells, whereas in other tissues, such as spleen and bone marrow, it is mainly in the mononuclear phagocytic cells. The iron within the hepatocytes is derived from plasma transferrin, whereas the storage iron in the mononuclear phagocytic cells, including that in Kupffer's cells, is obtained largely from the breakdown of red blood cells. Within cells, ferritin is located both in the cell sap and in lysosomes, in which the protein shells of the ferritin are degraded and iron is aggregated into *hemosiderin* granules. With the usual cellular stains, hemosiderin appears in cells as golden-yellow granules. The iron is chemically reactive, and when hemosiderin is exposed to potassium ferrocyanide (Prussian blue reaction) in tissue sections the granules turn blue-black. With normal iron stores only trace amounts of hemosiderin are found in the body, principally in reticuloendothelial cells in the bone marrow, spleen, and liver. In iron-overloaded cells, most of the iron is stored in the form of hemosiderin.

Very small amounts of ferritin normally circulate in the plasma. *Since the plasma ferritin is derived largely from the storage pool of body iron, its level is a good indicator of the adequacy of body iron stores.* In iron deficiency, serum ferritin is always below 12 μg/liter, whereas in iron overload very high values approaching 5000 μg/liter may be obtained. It should be noted, however, that the relationship between the degree of overload and serum ferritin levels is not linear. There are three circumstances under which serum ferritin cannot be used as a measure of body iron stores: in liver damage, in inflammatory states, and with some tumors. In these states, serum ferritin levels may be extremely high despite normal body iron stores. The physiologic importance of the storage iron pool is that it is readily mobilizable in the event of an increase in body iron requirements, as may occur following loss of blood.

Iron is transported in the plasma by an iron-binding glycoprotein called transferrin (Fig. 13–22), which is synthesized in the liver. In the normal individual, transferrin is about 33% saturated with iron, yielding serum levels that average 120 μg/dl in men and 100 μg/dl in women. Thus, the total iron-binding capacity of serum is in the range of 300 to 350 μg/dl. The major function of plasma transferrin is to deliver iron to the cells, including erythroid precursors, where iron is required for hemoglobin synthesis. Immature red cells possess high-affinity receptors for transferrin, and iron is transported into erythroblasts by receptor-mediated endocytosis.[21]

The absorption of iron and its regulation are

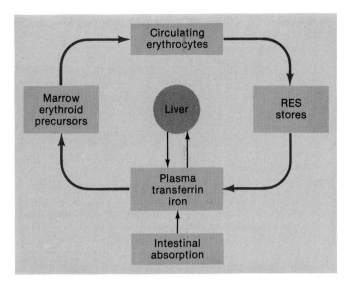

Figure 13-22. The internal iron cycle. In the plasma, iron bound to transferrin is transported to the marrow, where it is transferred to developing red blood cells and incorporated into hemoglobin. The mature red blood cells are released into the circulation and, after 120 days, are ingested by macrophages in the reticuloendothelial system (RES). Here the iron is extracted from hemoglobin and returned to the plasma, completing the cycle. (With permission from Wyngaarden, J.B., Smith, L.H., and Bennett, J.C. (eds.): Cecil Textbook of Medicine, 19th ed. Philadelphia, W.B. Saunders Co., 1992, p. 841.)

cells, heme is enzymatically degraded to release iron. In contrast, only 1 to 2% of nonheme iron is absorbed, by mechanisms that are complex and poorly understood. According to recent studies, three proteins are involved in the transfer of inorganic (nonheme) iron from the lumen of the gut to cytosol. At first, *luminal mucins* bind iron at the acid pH of the stomach. This complex keeps iron soluble and available for absorption in the more alkaline pH of the duodenum. At the surface of the duodenal mucosal cell, iron binds to an *integrin-like* molecule that somehow facilitates its passage across the cell membrane. A cytosolic protein called *mobilferrin* accepts iron within the cell and delivers it to ferritin or transferrin[22] (see Fig. 13–23).

After absorption, both heme and nonheme iron appear to enter a common pool in the mucosal cell. Normally, a fraction of the iron that enters the cell is rapidly delivered to plasma transferrin. Most, however, is deposited as ferritin, some to be transferred more slowly to plasma transferrin, and some to be lost with exfoliation of mucosal cells. The extent to which the mucosal iron is distributed along these various pathways depends largely on the body's iron requirements. When the body is replete with iron, formation of ferratin within the mucosal cells is maximal, whereas in iron deficiency transport into plasma is enhanced.

Since body losses of iron are limited, iron balance is maintained largely by regulating the absorptive intake (mucosal block). The factors that regulate the absorption of available iron into the mucosal cell are largely unknown. It is, however, known that the rate and level of absorption are dependent on total body iron content and erythropoietic activity, more specifically the iron needs of the erythroid precursors. As body stores rise, the percentage of iron absorbed falls, and vice versa. Some signal must be delivered to the mucosal cell, modifying its uptake and transfer of iron, and al-

complex and poorly understood. The most active site of iron absorption is the doudenum, but the stomach, ileum, and colon may also participate to a small degree.

Mucosal uptake of iron occurs by two distinct pathways (Fig. 13–23). Approximately 25% of the heme iron derived from hemoglobin, myoglobin, and other animal proteins is absorbed. Released from its apoproteins by gastric acids, heme is taken up directly by the mucosal cells. Once inside the

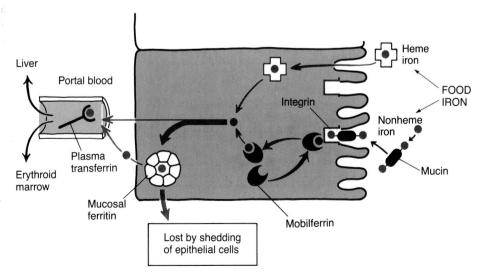

Figure 13-23. Diagrammatic representation of iron absorption. Mucosal uptake of heme and nonheme iron is depicted. When the storage sites of the body are replete with iron and erythropoietic activity is normal, most of the absorbed iron is lost into the gut by shedding of the epithelial cells. Conversely, when body iron needs increase or when erythropoiesis is stimulated, a greater fraction of the absorbed iron is transferred into plasma transferrin, with a concomitant decrease in iron loss through mucosal ferritin.

though there are many hypotheses, the nature of the signal remains unknown.

ETIOLOGY. With this background of normal iron metabolism, we can discuss the causes and effects of iron deficiency.[23]

Iron requirements are best understood in the context of the fixed daily losses of iron, ranging between 1 and 1.5 mg. Thus to maintain a normal iron balance, approximately 1 mg of iron must be absorbed from the diet every day. Because only 10 to 15% of the ingested iron is absorbed, the daily iron requirement for adult males is 5 to 10 mg and for adult females 7 to 20 mg. Since the average daily dietary intake of iron in the Western world is about 15 to 20 mg, most men ingest more than adequate iron, whereas many women consume just enough or marginally adequate amounts of iron.

The bioavailability of dietary iron is as important as the overall content. Heme iron is much more absorbable than inorganic iron. The absorption of the latter is influenced by other dietary contents. Ascorbic acid, citric acid, amino acids, and sugars in the diet enhance absorption of inorganic iron, but tannates (as in tea), carbonates, oxalates, and phosphates inhibit its absorption.

An iron deficiency may result from (1) dietary lack, (2) impaired absorption, (3) increased requirement, or (4) chronic blood loss.

Dietary lack is a rare cause of iron deficiency in industrialized countries having abundant food supplies (including meat) and where about two-thirds of the dietary iron is in the readily assimilable heme form. The situation is quite different in developing countries, where food is less abundant and diets are predominantly vegetarian, containing poorly absorbable inorganic iron. However, dietary inadequacy is still encountered in privileged societies under the following circumstances:

- *The elderly* often have very restricted diets with little meat for economic reasons or because of poor dentition.
- *The very poor,* often minority group, individuals are at risk for obvious reasons.
- *Infants* are also at high risk because the diet, predominantly milk, contains very small amounts of iron. Human breast milk, for example, provides only about 0.3 mg/liter of iron, which, however, has better bioavailability than cow's milk, which contains about twice as much iron but has poor bioavailability.
- *Children,* especially during the early years of life, have a critical need for dietary iron to accommodate growth and expansion of the blood volume.

Impaired absorption is encountered in sprue, other causes of intestinal steatorrhea, and chronic diarrhea. Gastrectomy impairs iron absorption by decreasing hydrochloric acid and transit time through the duodenum. Specific items in the diet,

as is evident from the preceding discussion, may also affect absorption.

Increased requirement is an important potential cause of iron deficiency. Growing infants and children, adolescents, and premenopausal (particularly pregnant) women have a much greater requirement for iron than do nonmenstruating adults. Particularly at risk are economically deprived women having multiple, frequent pregnancies.

Chronic blood loss is the most important cause of iron deficiency in the Western world. Bleeding within the tissues or cavities of the body may be followed by total recovery and recycling of the iron. However, external hemorrhage depletes the reserves of iron. Such depletion may occur from the gastrointestinal tract (e.g., peptic ulcers, hemorrhagic gastritis, gastric carcinoma, colonic carcinoma, hemorrhoids, or hookworm or pinworm disease), from the urinary tract (e.g., renal, pelvic, or bladder tumors), or from the genital tract (e.g., menorrhagia, uterine cancer).

When all the potential causes of an iron deficiency are taken into consideration, *deficiency in adult males and postmenopausal women in the Western world should be considered to be caused by gastrointestinal blood loss until proven otherwise. To prematurely ascribe an iron lack in such individuals to any of the other possible origins is to run the risk of missing an occult gastrointestinal cancer or other bleeding lesion.*

Whatever the basis, iron deficiency induces a hypochromic microcytic anemia. Simultaneously, depletion of essential iron-containing enzymes in cells throughout the body may cause other changes, including koilonychia, alopecia, atrophic changes in the tongue and gastric mucosa, and intestinal malabsorption. Uncommonly, esophageal webs may appear, to complete the triad of major findings in the *Plummer-Vinson syndrome:* (1) microcytic hypochromic anemia, (2) atrophic glossitis, and (3) esophageal webs (see Chapter 17).

At the outset of chronic blood loss or other states of negative iron balance, the reserves in the form of ferritin and hemosiderin may be adequate to maintain normal hemoglobin and hematocrit levels as well as normal serum iron and transferrin saturation. Progressive depletion of these reserves will eventually lower the serum iron and transferrin saturation levels but still may not give rise to anemia. Up to this stage of blood loss there is increased erythroid activity in the bone marrow. Thereafter, anemia will appear when all iron stores are depleted, now accompanied by low levels of serum iron and transferrin saturation as well as low serum ferritin.

MORPHOLOGY. The bone marrow reveals increased erythropoietic activity, manifested by increased numbers of normoblasts. Specificity is lent to these

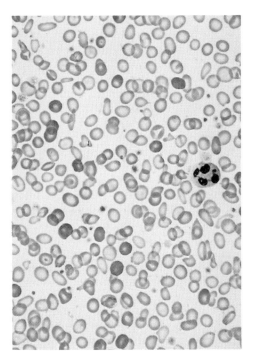

Figure 13-24. Hypochromic microcytic anemia of iron deficiency. Note the small red cells containing a narrow rim of hemoglobin at the periphery. Contrast with the scattered fully hemoglobinized cells derived from a recent blood transfusion given to the patient. (Courtesy of Dr. Robert W. McKenna, Department of Pathology, University of Texas Southwestern Medical School, Dallas.)

changes by the disappearance of stainable iron from the reticuloendothelial cells in the bone marrow. In the peripheral blood smear, red cells appear smaller (microcytic) and much paler (hypochromic) than normal. In many cells, hemoglobin is seen only in the form of a narrow peripheral rim (Fig. 13-24).

The clinical manifestations related to the anemia are nonspecific and were detailed earlier. Frequently, the dominating signs and symptoms relate to the underlying cause of the anemia, for example, gastrointestinal or gynecologic disease, malnutrition, pregnancy, and malabsorption. The atrophic glossitis may be responsible for difficulty in swallowing. Gastrointestinal disturbances may be present, associated with the disorder that led to the chronic blood loss (e.g., bleeding peptic ulcer or gastric carcinoma, diverticulitis, colonic cancer) or may emanate from the development of the atrophic gastritis.

The diagnosis of iron deficiency anemia ultimately rests on laboratory studies. Both hemoglobin and hematocrit are depressed, usually to moderate levels, and are associated with hypochromia, microcytosis, and some poikilocytosis. *The serum iron and serum ferritin are low, and the total plasma iron-binding capacity (reflecting transferrin concentration) is high. Low serum iron with increased iron-binding capacity results in a reduction of transferrin saturation levels to below 15%.* Reduced heme synthesis leads to elevation of free erythrocyte protoporphyrin. Usually the leukocytes and platelets are not affected. The alert clinician who investigates an unexplained iron deficiency anemia occasionally discovers an occult lesion or cancer and thereby saves a life.

Anemia of Chronic Disease

Impaired red cell production associated with chronic diseases is perhaps the most common cause of anemia among hospitalized patients in the United States.[24] It is associated with defective iron utilization and may therefore mimic iron deficiency. The chronic illnesses associated with this form of anemia can be grouped into three categories:

- Chronic microbial infections, such as osteomyelitis, bacterial endocarditis, and lung abscess
- Chronic immune disorders, such as rheumatoid arthritis and regional enteritis
- Neoplasms, such as Hodgkin's disease and carcinomas of the lung and breast.

The common features that characterize anemia in these diverse clinical settings are *low serum iron and reduced total iron-binding capacity in association with abundant stored iron in the mononuclear phagocytic cells.* This combination suggests that there is a defect in the reutilization of iron due to some impediment in the transfer of iron from the storage pool to the erythroid precursors. The basis of this defect is not clear, but increased secretion of cytokines, such as interleukin-1 (IL-1), has been implicated. In addition, defects in erythropoietin production and shortened red cell survival have also been documented. The anemia is usually mild, and the dominant symptoms are those of the underlying disease. The red blood cells may be normocytic and normochromic or may be hypochromic and microcytic as in anemia of iron deficiency. *The presence of increased storage iron in the marrow macrophages, a high serum ferritin level, and reduced total iron-binding capacity readily rule out iron deficiency as the cause of anemia.* Treatment of the underlying condition corrects the anemia.

Aplastic Anemia

This somewhat misleading term is applied to pancytopenia, characterized by (1) anemia, (2) neutropenia, and (3) thrombocytopenia. The basis for these changes is a failure or suppression of multi-

Table 13–6. MAJOR CAUSES OF
APLASTIC ANEMIA

A. ACQUIRED
    I. Idiopathic
        Primary stem cell defect
        Immune mediated
    II. Chemical agents
        Dose related
            Alkylating agents
            Antimetabolites
            Benzene
            Chloramphenicol
            Inorganic arsenicals
        Idiosyncratic
            Chloramphenicol
            Phenylbutazone
            Organic arsenicals
            Methylphenylethylhydantoin
            Streptomycin
            Chlorpromazine
            Insecticides: e.g., DDT, parathion
    III. Physical agents (e.g., whole-body radiation)
    IV. Viral infections
        Non-A, non-B hepatitis
        CMV infections
        EBV infections
        Herpes varicella-zoster
    V. Miscellaneous
        Infrequently, many other drugs and chemicals

B. INHERITED
    I. Fanconi's anemia

CMV = cytomegalovirus; EBV = Epstein-Barr virus.

potent myeloid stem cells, with inadequate production or release of the differentiated cell lines.

ETIOLOGY. The major circumstances under which aplastic anemia may appear are listed in Table 13–6.

Most cases of aplastic anemia of so-called known etiology follow exposure to chemicals and drugs. With some agents the marrow damage is predictable, dose related, and, in most instances, reversible when the use of the offending agent is stopped. Best documented as known myelotoxins are benzene, chloramphenicol, alkylating agents, and antimetabolites (e.g., 6-mercaptopurine, vincristine, and busulfan). In other instances, the pancytopenia appears as an apparent idiosyncratic reaction to very small doses of known myelotoxins, e.g., chloramphenicol, or following the use of such drugs as phenylbutazone, methylphenylethylhydantoin, streptomycin, and chlorpromazine, which are generally without effect in other individuals. In such idiosyncratic reactions the aplasia may be severe and sometimes irreversible and fatal.

Whole-body *irradiation* is an obvious mechanism for destruction of hematopoietic stem cells. The effects of radiation are dose related. Persons at risk are those who receive therapeutic irradiation, and individuals exposed to nulcear explosions or nuclear plant accidents.

Although aplastic anemia may appear following a variety of *infections* (including HIV), it most commonly follows viral hepatitis of the non-A,

non-B type.[25] Why certain individuals develop this hematologic complication in the course of their infection is not understood, but it is not related to the severity of infection.

Fanconi's anemia is a rare autosomal recessive disorder characterized by defects in DNA repair (see Chapter 7). In these patients the marrow hypofunction becomes evident early in life and is accompanied by multiple congenital anomalies, such as hypoplasia of the kidney and spleen and hypoplastic anomalies of bone, particularly involving the thumbs or radii.

Despite all these possible causal influences, in fully 50% of the cases no provocating factor can be identified, and hence they are lumped into the *idiopathic* category.[26]

PATHOGENESIS. Although we speak of myelotoxic chemicals, drugs, and infections as causes of aplastic anemia, the precise mechanism of stem cell failure in these settings is poorly understood. Idiopathic cases are even more mysterious. Both immunologically mediated suppression and a primary abnormality of stem cells have been invoked. Each of these is considered next.

Because there is growing evidence that T cell–derived cytokines are intimately involved in the regulation of normal hematopoiesis, much attention has focused on the possibility that idiopathic aplastic anemia may result from immunologically mediated suppression of hematopoiesis. In support of the suppressor cell hypothesis is cited the ability of T lymphocytes from aplastic anemia patients to inhibit the *in vitro* growth of normal myeloid (CFU-GM) or erythroid stem cells (BFU-E) obtained from healthy individuals.[27] The recovery of autologous marrow in some cases by administration of antilymphocyte globulin therapy is also consistent with an immunologic causation of aplastic anemia.[28] The notion that aplastic anemia results from a fundamental stem cell abnormality is supported by recent studies that indicate that in many cases of aplastic anemia, cells in the peripheral blood are clonal descendants of a single stem cell.[30] Presumably some forms of marrow insult cause genetic damage that results in the generation of stem cells with poor proliferative and differentiative capacity. If one such altered stem cell dominates, the resultant picture is that of aplastic anemia. The occasional transformation of aplastic anemia into acute leukemia lends further credence to this hypothesis. It has been suggested that even in cases with immunologic derangements there is a primary abnormality of stem cells, which secondarily evokes an immune response against self. If the immune response is vigorous, the altered stem cells are depleted, and aplasia occurs.[29]

MORPHOLOGY. The bone marrow is markedly hypocellular and is composed largely of empty

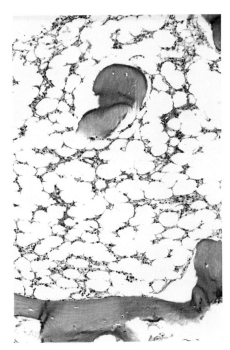

Figure 13–25. Aplastic anemia—bone marrow. The marrow is markedly hypocellular, composed largely of fat cells. (Courtesy of Dr. Robert W. McKenna, Department of Pathology, University of Texas Southwestern Medical School, Dallas.)

marrow spaces populated by fat cells, fibrous stroma, and scattered or clustered foci of lymphocytes and plasma cells (Fig. 13–25). In less extreme instances, scattered precursor cells are found. Megakaryocytes are either absent or scant. A number of additional morphologic changes may accompany these marrow failures. They are related to bacterial infections or hemorrhagic diatheses secondary to the granulocytopenia or thrombocytopenia, respectively. The toxic drug or agent may injure not only the bone marrow but also the liver, the kidneys, and other structures. Benzene, for example, may cause fatty changes in the liver and kidneys. In some patients, especially those with multiple transfusions, systemic hemosiderosis is present.

CLINICAL COURSE. Aplastic anemia may occur at any age and in either sex. Usually the onset is gradual, but in some cases the disorder strikes with suddenness and great severity. The initial manifestations vary somewhat, depending on the cell line predominantly affected. Anemia may cause the progressive onset of weakness, pallor, and dyspnea. Petechiae and ecchymoses may herald thrombocytopenia. Granulocytopenia may manifest itself only by frequent and persistent minor infections or by the sudden onset of chills, fever, and prostration. *Splenomegaly is characteristically absent, and if present, the diagnosis of aplastic anemia should be seriously questioned.* Typically, the red cells are

normocytic and normochromic, although occasionally slight macrocytosis is present; *reticulocytosis is absent.*

The diagnosis rests on examination of bone marrow biopsy and peripheral blood. It is important to distinguish aplastic anemia from other causes of pancytopenia, such as "aleukemic" leukemia and myelodysplastic syndromes (see Chapter 14). Since pancytopenia is common to all these conditions, their clinical manifestations are often indistinguishable. However, with aplastic anemia the marrow is hypocellular owing to stem cell failure, whereas in leukemia and myelodysplasia the marrow is populated by abnormal and immature myeloid cells. The prognosis of marrow aplasia is quite unpredictable. As mentioned earlier, withdrawal of toxic drugs may lead to recovery in some cases. The idiopathic form has a poor prognosis. There is increasing use of bone marrow transplantation to replace the defective stem cells, and in selected cases this is an effective form of therapy.[31] Benefit may also be derived from immunosuppressive therapy with antithymocyte globulin, which presumably neutralizes the marrow-suppressive effect of immune cells.

Pure Red Cell Aplasia (PRCA)

Pure red cell aplasia is a rare form of marrow failure resulting from a specific aplasia of erythroid elements while granulopoiesis and thrombopoiesis remain normal.[32] PRCA may be primary, without any associated disease, or secondary to some neoplasm, particularly a thymic tumor (thymoma, see Chapter 25). The latter association raises the question of some thymus-related immunologic mechanism, and, indeed, in about half the patients, resection of the primary tumor is followed by hematologic improvement. In all likelihood the primary form is also related to autoimmunity against erythroid precursors, and in such patients immunosuppressive therapy may be beneficial. Plasmapheresis has also been used with success in refractory cases.

Other Forms of Marrow Failure

Space-occupying lesions that destroy significant amounts of bone marrow or perhaps disturb the marrow architecture depress its productive capacity. This form of marrow failure is referred to as *myelophthisic anemia.* As would be anticipated, all the formed elements of blood are concomitantly affected. However, characteristically immature forms of the red and white cells appear in the peripheral blood, a phenomenon attributed to a poorly defined "irritation effect." The most common cause of myelophthisic anemia is metastatic cancer, arising most often from a primary lesion in the breast, lung, prostate, thyroid, or adrenals. Multiple myeloma, leukemia, osteosclerosis, and lymphomas are less commonly implicated. Myelophthisic anemia has also been observed with myelofibrosis, a diffuse fibrosis of the marrow. Such cases are variants of the myeloproliferative syndrome (see Chapter 14).

Diffuse liver disease, whether it be toxic, infectious, or a form of cirrhosis, is for obscure reasons often associated with an anemia attributed to bone marrow failure. Other contributing factors include folate deficiency and iron deficiency due to gastrointestinal blood loss (varices, hemorrhoids). In most of these instances, there is a pure erythropoietic depression and the red cells are normocytic, but if folate deficiency is significant, they are macrocytic. Depression of the white cell count and platelets has been described but is infrequent.

Chronic renal failure, whatever its cause, is almost invariably associated with anemia that tends to be roughly proportional to the severity of the uremia. The basis of the anemia is multifactorial. There is evidence of an extracorpuscular defect inducing chronic hemolysis. Some patients have an iron deficiency secondary to the bleeding tendency often encountered in uremia. Concomitantly, there is reduced red cell production, related most likely to advanced destruction of the kidneys, with inadequate formation of erythropoietin. Not surprisingly, therefore, administration of recombinant erythropoietin results in significant improvement of anemia in patients with renal failure.

POLYCYTHEMIA

Polycythemia, or *erythrocytosis,* as it is sometimes referred to, denotes an increased concentration of red cells, usually with a corresponding increase in hemoglobin level. Such an increase may be *relative,* when there is hemoconcentration due to decreased plasma volume, or *absolute,* when there is an increase in total red cell mass. *Relative polycythemia* results from any cause of dehydration, such as deprivation of water, prolonged vomiting, diarrhea, or excessive use of diuretics. It is also associated with an obscure condition of unknown etiology called stress polycythemia, or Gaisböck's syndrome. *Absolute polycythemia* is said to be *primary* when the increase in red cell mass results from an intrinsic abnormality of the myeloid stem cells, and *secondary* when the red cell progenitors are normal but proliferate in response to increased levels of erythropoietin. Primary polycythemia (polycythemia vera) is one of several expressions of clonal, neoplastic proliferation of myeloid stem cells and is therefore best considered with other myeloproliferative disorders (see Chapter 14). Secondary polycythemias may be caused by an increase in erythropoietin secretion that is physio-

Table 13–7. PATHOPHYSIOLOGIC CLASSIFICATION OF POLYCYTHEMIA

RELATIVE	Reduced plasma volume (hemoconcentration)
ABSOLUTE	
Primary:	Abnormal proliferation of myeloid stem cells, normal or low erythropoietin levels (polycythemia vera)
Secondary:	Increased erythropoietin levels
	Appropriate: lung disease, high-altitude living, cyanotic heart disease
	Inappropriate: erythropoietin-secreting tumors (e.g., renal cell carcinoma, hepatoma, cerebellar hemangioblastoma)

logically appropriate or by an inappropriate (pathologic) secretion of erythropoietin (Table 13–7).

BLEEDING DISORDERS — HEMORRHAGIC DIATHESES

Excessive bleeding may result from (1) increased fragility of vessels, (2) platelet deficiency or dysfunction, (3) derangements in the coagulation mechanism, and (4) combinations of these. Each of these categories is treated in successive sections.

BLEEDING DISORDERS CAUSED BY VESSEL WALL ABNORMALITIES

Disorders within this category, sometimes called nonthrombocytopenic purpuras, are relatively common but do not usually cause serious bleeding problems. Most often, they induce small hemorrhages (petechiae and purpura) in the skin or mucous membranes, particularly the gingivae. On occasion, however, more significant hemorrhages may occur into joints, muscles, and subperiosteal locations or take the form of menorrhagia, nosebleeds, gastrointestinal bleeding, or hematuria. *The platelet count, bleeding time, and coagulation time are usually normal.*

The varied clinical conditions in which hemorrhages can be related to abnormalities in the vessel wall include the following:

- *Many infections* induce petechial and purpuric hemorrhages, but especially implicated are meningococcemia, other forms of septicemia, severe measles, and several of the rickettsioses. The involved mechanism is presumably microbiologic damage (vasculitis) to the microvasculature or disseminated intravascular coagulation.
- *Drug reactions* sometimes induce abnormal

bleeding. In many instances the vascular injury is mediated by the formation of drug-induced antibodies and the deposition of immune complexes in the vessel walls, with the production of a hypersensitivity (leukocytoclastic) vasculitis (see Chapter 11).

- *Scurvy and the Ehlers-Danlos syndrome* represent examples of predisposition to hemorrhage related to impaired formation of the collagenous support of vessel walls. Essentially the same mechanism may be encountered in the very elderly, in whom atrophy of collagen is implicated. Similar is the predisposition to skin hemorrhages in *Cushing's syndrome*, in which the protein-wasting effects of excessive corticosteroid production cause loss of perivascular supporting tissue.
- *Henoch-Schönlein purpura* is a systemic hypersensitivity disease of unknown cause characterized by a purpuric rash, colicky abdominal pain (presumably due to focal hemorrhages into the gastrointestinal tract), polyarthralgia, and acute glomerulonephritis (see Chapter 20). All these changes are thought to result from the deposition of circulating immune complexes within vessels throughout the body and within the glomerular mesangial regions.
- *Hereditary hemorrhagic telangiectasia* is an autosomal dominant disorder characterized by dilated, tortuous blood vessels that have thin walls and hence bleed readily. Bleeding may occur anywhere in the body but is most common under the mucous membranes of the nose (epistaxis), tongue, mouth, and eyes.

In most of these conditions, the hemorrhagic diathesis does not cause massive bleeding but more often calls attention to the underlying disorder.

BLEEDING RELATED TO REDUCED PLATELET NUMBER: THROMBOCYTOPENIA

Reduction in platelet number constitutes an important cause of generalized bleeding. Platelet counts normally range between 150,000 to 300,000/mm³, and a count below 100,000/mm³ is generally considerd to constitute thrombocytopenia. However, spontaneous bleeding does not become evident until the count falls below 20,000/mm³. Platelet counts in the range of 20,000 to 50,000/mm³ are associated with post-traumatic bleeding.

The important role of platelets in hemostasis was discussed in an earlier chapter (see Chapter 4). It hardly needs reiteration that they are vital to hemostasis in that they form temporary plugs and participate in the clotting reaction. Thus, thrombocytopenia is characterized principally by bleeding, most often from small vessels. The common sites of such hemorrhage are the skin and mucous mem-

Table 13–8. CAUSES OF THROMBOCYTOPENIA

I. DECREASED PRODUCTION OF PLATELETS
Generalized diseases of bone marrow
  Aplastic anemia: congenital and acquired (Table 13–6)
  Marrow infiltration: leukemia, disseminated cancer
Selective impairment of platelet production
  Drug-induced: alcohol, thiazides, cytotoxic drugs
  Infections: measles, HIV
Ineffective megakaryopoiesis
  Megaloblastic anemia
  Paroxysmal nocturnal hemoglobinuria

II. DECREASED PLATELET SURVIVAL
Immunologic destruction
  Autoimmune: idiopathic thrombocytopenic purpura, SLE
  Isoimmune: post-transfusion and neonatal
  Drug-associated: quinidine, heparin, sulfa compounds
  Infections: infectious mononucleosis, HIV infection, CMV
Nonimmunologic destruction
  Disseminated intravascular coagulation
  Thrombotic thrombocytopenic purpura
  Giant hemangiomas
  Microangiopathic hemolytic anemias

III. SEQUESTRATION
Hypersplenism

IV. DILUTIONAL

SLE = systemic lupus erythematosus; HIV = human immunodeficiency virus; CMV = cytomegalovirus.

branes of the gastrointestinal and genitourinary tracts, where the bleeding is usually associated with the development of small petechiae. Intracranial bleeding is another danger in thrombocytopenic patients with markedly depressed platelet counts.

The many causes of thrombocytopenia can be classified into the four major categories cited in Table 13–8.

A few comments about the less common causes are in order before we turn to the more common forms of thrombocytopenia.

- Generalized *diseases of bone marrow* may compromise the number of megakaryocytes. Thus, thrombocytopenia is seen in aplastic anemia and in the leukemias.
- Thrombocytopenia due to *ineffective megakaryopoiesis* can occur in megaloblastic anemias resulting from a deficiency of folate or vitamin B_{12}.
- As with hemolytic anemias, thrombocytopenia may be related to *increased destruction of platelets* following drug ingestion or infections. The drugs most commonly involved are quinine, quinidine, methyldopa, thiazide diuretics, and heparin. Immune reactions implicated in these drug reactions are essentially similar to those underlying drug-induced hemolytic anemias.[33]
- *Thrombocytopenia is one of the most common hematologic manifestations of AIDS.* It may occur early in the course of HIV infection and is be-

lieved to be multifactorial. Involved mechanisms include immune-complex–mediated injury of platelets, formation of antiplatelet antibodies due to molecular mimicry, and HIV-mediated suppression of megakaryocytes.[34]

- An acute postviral thrombocytopenia (sometimes called *acute idiopathic thrombocytopenic purpura*) may develop in children following recovery from a viral exanthem or upper respiratory tract infection. For reasons not entirely clear these and some other viruses induce the formation of antiplatelet antibodies, leading to platelet autoimmunity. Unlike idiopathic autoimmune thrombocytopenia (to be described later), the disease is self-limited and resolves spontaneously in 4 to 6 weeks.

- Just as red cells can be destroyed by *mechanical injury* in microangiopathic hemolytic anemia, so platelets may be destroyed by prosthetic heart valves, the narrowed microcirculation in malignant hypertension, and arterial disease associated with significant roughening of the endothelial surface.

- Thrombocytopenia may appear unpredictably in any patient who has marked splenomegaly, or what has been referred to as *hypersplenism* (see Chapter 14). Normally the spleen sequesters 30 to 40% of the mass of circulating platelets and, when enlarged, sequestrates as much as 90% of all platelets. Should the thrombocytopenia constitute an important part of the clinical problem, it can be cured by splenectomy.

- Masssive *transfusions* may produce a dilutional thrombocytopenia. Blood stored for longer than 24 hours contains virtually no viable platelets; thus, plasma volume and red cell mass are reconstituted by transfusion, but the number of circulating platelets is relatively reduced.

Neonatal and Post-transfusion (Isoimmune) Thrombocytopenia

These disorders result from the development of antibodies directed against a platelet isoantigen. In addition to HLA and ABO antigens, platelets possess several antigenic determinants not present in other blood cells. These include the Duzo, PL, and Bak antigen systems. The pathophysiology of *neonatal thrombocytopenia* is similar to that of the hemolytic reaction in erythroblastosis fetalis (see Chapter 10). A PL^{A1} antigen–negative mother carrying an antigen-positive fetus develops IgG antibodies against the PL^{A1} antigen, and the resulting antibodies cross the placenta to cause thrombocytopenia in the newborn. Anti-PL^{A1} antibodies are also believed to be responsible for the purpura associated with *post-transfusional thrombocytopenia*. In most cases the patient is PL^{A1}-negative and has been sensitized to PL^{A1}-positive blood by either a previous transfusion or pregnancy.

Idiopathic Thrombocytopenic Purpura (ITP)

In this chronic autoimmune disorder, platelets are destroyed by the formation of antiplatelet antibodies. It should be noted that immunologically mediated destruction of platelets (immune thrombocytopenia) occurs in many different settings, including systemic lupus erythematosus, AIDS, following viral infections, and as a complication of drug therapy. These secondary forms of immune thrombocytopenia can sometimes mimic the idiopathic autoimmune variety, and hence the diagnosis of this disorder should be made only after exclusion of other known causes of thrombocytopenia. Particularly important in this regard is systemic lupus erythematosus (SLE), a multisystem autoimmune disease (see Chapter 6) that can present with thrombocytopenia.

PATHOGENESIS. Although it has been known for some time that ITP is caused by antibody-mediated destruction of platelets, the nature of the autoantigens was for a long time a mystery. Recent studies, however, firmly implicate two platelet glycoprotein complexes, IIb/IIIa and Ib/IX, as the target antigens.[35] Antibodies against these membrane glycoproteins can be demonstrated in the plasma as well as bound to the platelet surface (platelet-associated immunoglobulins) in approximately 80% of patients with ITP. In the overwhelming majority of cases, the platelet autoantibodies are of the IgG class, but in approximately 40% IgM antibodies coexist.

The mechanism of platelet destruction is similar to that seen in autoimmune hemolytic anemias. Opsonized platelets are rendered susceptible to phagocytosis by the cells of the mononuclear phagocytic system. About 75 to 80% of patients are remarkably improved or sometimes cured following splenectomy, which suggests that the spleen is the major site of removal of sensitized platelets. Since it is also the major site of autoantibody synthesis, the beneficial effects of splenectomy may in part derive from removal of the source of autoantibodies. Although destruction of sensitized platelets is the major mechanism of thrombocytopenia, there is some evidence that megakaryocytes may be attacked as well, since some antiplatelet antibodies also react with megakaryocytes. In most cases, however, the megakaryocyte injury is not significant enough to deplete their numbers. Because platelet glycoproteins play an important role in hemostasis, antibody coating of these molecules can also interefere with the formation of a hemostatic plug.

MORPHOLOGY. The principal morphologic lesions of thrombocytopenic purpura are found in the spleen and bone marrow. The secondary changes related to the bleeding diathesis may be found in any tissue or structure in the body.

The spleen is normal in size. Histologically, there is congestion of the sinusoids and hyperactivity and enlargement of the splenic follicles, manifested by the formation of prominent germinal centers. In many instances, megakaryocytes are found within the sinuses and sinusoidal walls. These splenic findings are not distinctive and cannot be considered as pathognomonic of this disorder.

The alterations in the bone marrow are equally nonspecific. Most often the bone marrow appears quite normal and contains the usual numbers and types of erythropoietic and leukopoietic cells. An increased number of megakaryocytes is usually seen. Some are apparently immature with large, nonlobulated, single nuclei. These findings are not characteristic of ITP but merely represent accelerated thrombopoiesis. As such, they are seen in most forms of thrombocytopenia resulting from increased platelet destruction. The importance of the bone marrow examination is to rule out thrombocytopenias resulting from bone marrow failure. A decrease in the number of megakaryocytes virtually rules out the diagnosis of ITP.

The secondary changes relate to the hemorrhages that are dispersed throughout the body. The skin, serosal linings of the body cavities, epicardium and endocardium, lungs, and mucosal lining of the urinary tract are favorite sites for such petechial and ecchymotic hemorrhage (Fig. 13–26). Hemorrhages are also prone to occur in the brain, joint spaces, nasopharynx, and gastrointestinal tract.

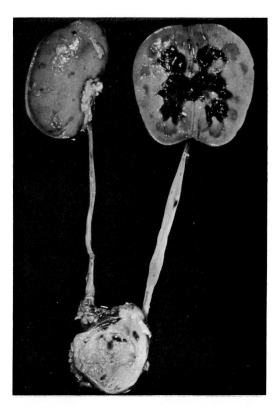

Figure 13-26. Thrombocytopenic purpura. Urinary tract with intrapelvic hemorrhages in kidneys and focal mucosal hemorrhages in urinary bladder.

ITP occurs most commonly in adults, particularly in women of childbearing age. The clinical manifestations of this disease are quite variable and nonspecific, and they can occur in thrombocytopenia from other causes. Occasionally, the disease begins with a sudden shower of petechial hemorrhages into the skin without apparent antecedent injury or disease. More frequently, there is a long history of easy bruising, nosebleeds, bleeding from the gums, and extensive hemorrhages into soft tissues from relatively minor trauma. Also, the disease may become manifest first by the appearance of melena, hematuria, or excessive menstrual flow. Subarachnoid hemorrhage and intracerebral hemorrhage are serious consequences of thrombocytopenic purpura but, fortunately, are rare in patients treated with steroids. Splenomegaly and lymphadenopathy are extremely uncommon in ITP, and their presence should lead one to consider other possible diagnoses.[36]

The diagnosis can be only suspected by clinical features and must be supported by demonstration of thrombocytopenia with normal or increased megakaryocytes in the bone marrow. Accelerated thrombopoiesis also leads to the formation of abnormally large platelets (megathrombocytes), detected easily in a blood smear. The bleeding time is prolonged, but tests for clotting are normal or near normal. Tests for platelet autoantibodies are not yet widely available. *Therefore, a diagnosis of ITP should be made only after all the possible known causes for platelet deficiencies, such as those listed in Table 13–8, have been ruled out.*

Thrombotic Microangiopathies: Thrombotic Thrombocytopenic Purpura (TTP) and Hemolytic-Uremic Syndrome (HUS)

The term "thrombotic microangiopathies" encompasses a spectrum of clinical syndromes that includes TTP and HUS. Traditionally, TTP has been characterized by its occurrence in adult females and the pentad of fever, thrombocytopenia, microangiopathic hemolytic anemia, transient neurologic deficits, and renal failure.[32] HUS, like TTP, is also associated with microangiopathic hemolytic anemia and thrombocytopenia but is distinguished from it by the absence of neurologic symptoms, the dominance of acute renal failure, and onset in childhood. Recent studies have tended to blur these distinctions because many adult patients with

TTP lack one or more of the five criteria and some patients with HUS have fever and neurologic dysfunction.[38] Further evidence of overlap is provided by the occurrence of TTP and HUS in the setting of HIV infection. Fundamental to both of these conditions is widespread formation of hyaline thrombi in the microcirculation, which are composed primarily of dense aggregates of platelets that are surrounded by fibrin.

The pathogenesis of thrombotic microangiopathies is obscure. According to some investigators, *perturbation of the endothelium* is of primary importance.[38] In support of this, several abnormalities, including reduced synthesis of prostacyclin and impaired generation of nitrous oxide, both of which prevent platelet aggregation and cause vasodilatation, have been documented. The possible mechanisms of endothelial damage are discussed in Chapter 20. Endothelial damage is also postulated to be responsible for the release of unusually large multimers of factor VIII–von Willebrand complex into the circulation. These large multimers may cause pathologic aggregation of platelets and predispose to microvascular thrombosis. The development of myriad platelet aggregates induces *thrombocytopenia,* and the intravascular thrombi provide a rational explanation for *a microangiopathic form of hemolytic anemia* and widespread organ dysfunction. At one time these conditions were uniformly fatal, but with recent improvements in treatment including plasma exchange, approximately 80% survival can be expected.[39] It should be noted that despite some similarities with disseminated intravascular coagulation (DIC), the two conditions are thought to be separate and distinct. Unlike in DIC, activation of the clotting system is not of primary importance.

BLEEDING DISORDERS RELATED TO DEFECTIVE PLATELET FUNCTIONS

Qualitative defects of platelet function may be congenital or acquired. Several congenital disorders characterized by prolonged bleeding time and normal platelet count have been described. The discussion of these rare diseases is warranted by the fact that they provide excellent model systems for investigating the molecular mechanisms of platelet functions.[40]

Congenital disorders of platelet function may be classified into three groups on the basis of the predominant functional abnormality: (1) *defects of adhesion,* (2) *defects of aggregation,* and (3) *disorders of platelet secretion (release reaction).*

- Bleeding resulting from defective adhesion of platelets to the subendothelial collagen is best illustrated by the autosomal recessive *Bernard-Soulier syndrome.* In this disorder there is an inherited deficiency of a platelet membrane glyco-

protein complex (GpIb/IX). This glycoprotein is a receptor for von Willebrand's factor and is essential for normal platelet adhesion to collagen (see Chapter 4).
- Bleeding due to *defective platelet aggregation* is exemplified by *thrombasthenia,* which is also transmitted as an autosomal recessive trait. Thrombasthenic platelets fail to aggregate with ADP, collagen, epinephrine, or thrombin, owing to a deficiency of GpIIb/IIIa, the fibrinogen receptor. In normal platelets these glycoproteins favor aggregation by creating fibrinogen "bridges" between adjacent platelets (see Chapter 4).
- *Disorders of platelet secretion* are characterized by normal initial aggregation with collagen or ADP, but the subsequent responses, such as secretion of prostaglandins and release of granule-bound ADP, are impaired. The underlying biochemical defects of the so-called *storage pool disease* are varied, complex, and beyond the scope of our discussion.

Among the *acquired defects* of platelet function, two are clinically significant.[41] The first is related to *ingestion of aspirin* and other nonsteroidal anti-inflammatory drugs, which may significantly prolong the bleeding time. Aspirin is a potent inhibitor of the enzyme cyclooxygenase and can suppress the synthesis of prostaglandins (see Chapter 3), which are known to be involved in platelet aggregation and the subsequent platelet release reaction (see Chapter 4). The antiplatelet effect of aspirin forms the basis of its use in the management of recurrent myocardial infarction (see Chapter 12). In approximately 10% of healthy normal subjects, ingestion of even 1 gm of aspirin may prolong the bleeding time significantly and lead to increased bruisability. Clinically significant postoperative oozing may occur in such patients if aspirin is used as an analgesic. It is suspected that these individuals have minor platelet function defects that are magnified by the intake of aspirin. *Uremia* (see Chapter 20) is the other condition that exemplifies an acquired defect in platelet functions. Although the pathogenesis of bleeding in uremia is complex and poorly understood, several abnormalities of platelet function have been found.

HEMORRHAGIC DIATHESES RELATED TO ABNORMALITIES IN CLOTTING FACTORS

A deficiency of every one of the known clotting factors has been reported at one time or another as the cause of a bleeding disorder. The bleeding in these conditions differs somewhat from that encountered in platelet deficiencies. The apparent spontaneous appearance of petechiae or purpura is uncommon. More often *the bleeding manifests as the development of large ecchymoses or hematomas following an injury, or as prolonged bleeding after a laceration or any form of surgical procedure.* Bleeding into the gastrointestinal and urinary tracts, and particularly into weight-bearing joints, is a common manifestation. Typical stories describe the patient who continues to ooze for days following a tooth extraction or who develops a hemarthrosis after a relatively trivial stress on a knee joint. History may well have been changed by the presence of a hereditary coagulation defect in the intermarried royal families of Great Britain and Europe. Clotting abnormalities may occur as acquired defects, or, as mentioned, may be hereditary in origin.

Acquired disorders are usually characterized by multiple clotting abnormalities. Vitamin K deficiency (see Chapter 9) results in depressed synthesis of factors II, VII, IX and X and protein C. Since the liver makes virtually all the clotting factors, severe parenchymal liver disease may be associated with a hemorrhagic diathesis. Disseminated intravascular coagulation produces a deficiency of multiple coagulation factors.

Hereditary deficiencies have been identified for each of the clotting factors. Deficiencies of factor VIII (hemophilia A) and of factor IX (Christmas disease, or hemophilia B) are transmitted as sex-linked recessive disorders. Most of the others follow autosomal patterns of transmission. *Typically, these hereditary disorders involve a single clotting factor.*

The details of the diagnostic tests used to identify the special clotting factor deficiency are beyond our scope and are readily available in specialized texts. In most cases, four screening procedures will localize the hemostatic abnormality: (1) bleeding time, (2) platelet count, (3) the prothrombin time, and (4) the partial thromboplastin time. Against this background we can turn to the more common of the coagulation disorders.

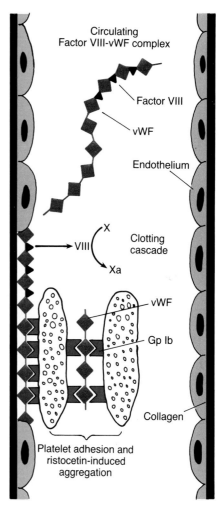

Figure 13–27. Structure and function of factor VIII—von Willebrand's factor (vWF) complex. Factor VIII is synthesized by the liver, and vWF in the endothelial cells. The two circulate as a complex in the circulation. Factor VIII takes part in the coagulation cascade by activating factor X. vWF causes adhesion of platelets to subendothelial collagen via the GpIb platelet receptor. Ristocetin activates GpIb receptors *in vitro* and causes platelet aggregation if vWF is present.

Deficiencies of Factor VIII–vWF Complex

Hemophilia A and von Willebrand's disease, two of the most common inherited disorders of bleeding, are caused by qualitative or quantitative defects involving the factor VIII–vWF complex. Before we can discuss these disorders it is essential to review the structure and function of these proteins.[42,43]

Plasma factor VIII–vWF is a complex made up of two separate proteins (factor VIII and vWF factor), *which can be distinguished by functional, biochemical, and immunologic criteria.* One component, which is required for the activation of factor X in the intrinsic coagulation pathway, is called *factor VIII procoagulant protein,* or *factor VIII*

(Fig. 13–27, and Chapter 4). Deficiency of factor VIII gives rise to hemophilia A. Through noncovalent bonds, factor VIII is linked to a much larger protein called *von Willebrand's factor* (vWF). The latter, which forms approximately 99% of the complex, is not a discrete protein but exists in the form of a series of multimers that contain up to 100 subunits with molecular weight exceeding 20×10^6 daltons. Von Willebrand's factor can also bind several other proteins that are involved in hemostasis, including collagen, heparin, and platelet membrane glycoproteins (GpIb and IIb/IIIa). GpIb serves as the major receptor for vWF, and it is believed that it is through this receptor that vWF bridges collagen and platelets (Fig. 13–27). Indeed, *the most important function of vWF in vivo is to facilitate the adhesion of platelets to subendothelial collagen.* vWF is crucial to the normal process of hemostasis, (see Chapter 4) and its absence in von Willebrand's disease leads to a bleeding diathesis.

In addition to its function in platelet adhesion, vWF serves as a carrier for factor VIII and is important for its stability. The half-life of factor VIII in the circulation is 12 hours if vWF is present but only 2.4 hours if the latter is lacking (as in patients with von Willebrand's disease).

Von Willebrand's factor can be assayed by immunologic techniques or by the so-called *ristocetin aggregation test.* Ristocetin (once used as an antibiotic) binds to platelets *in vitro* and activates vWF receptors on their surface. This leads to platelet aggregation if vWF is available to "bridge" the platelets (Fig. 13–27). Thus, ristocetin-induced platelet aggregation can be used as a bioassay for vWF.

The two components of the factor VIII–vWF complex are coded by separate genes and are synthesized by different cells. Von Willebrand's factor is produced by endothelial cells and megakaryocytes, and it can be demonstrated in platelet alpha-granules. *Endothelial cells are the major source of plasma vWF.* Factor VIII can be synthesized by several tissues, but in the absence of liver disease, hepatocytes are the major source of this protein. To summarize, *the two components of factor VIII–vWF complex, synthesized separately, come together and circulate in the plasma as a unit that serves to promote the clotting as well as the platelet–vessel wall interactions necessary to ensure hemostasis.* With this background we can discuss the diseases resulting from deficiencies of factor VIII–vWF complex.

von Willebrand's Disease (vWD)

With an estimated frequency of 1%, vWD is believed to be one of the most common inherited disorders of bleeding in humans. According to some, it is even more common than hemophilia A. Clinically, it is characterized by spontaneous bleeding from mucous membranes, excessive bleeding from wounds, menorrhagia, and a prolonged bleeding time in the presence of a normal platelet count. In most cases it is transmitted as an autosomal dominant disorder, but several rare autosomal recessive variants have been identified.

More than 20 variants of vWD have been described, and they can be grouped into two major categories:

• Types I and III vWD are associated with a *reduced quantity of circulating vWF.* Type I, an autosomal dominant disorder, accounts for approximately 70% of all cases and is relatively mild. Type III (an autosomal recessive disorder) is associated with extremely low levels of vWF, and correspondingly the clinical manifestations are severe. Fortunately it is much less common than type I. The molecular basis of reduced vWF levels in these two variants remains to be determined.

• Type II vWD, characterized by a qualitative defect in vWF, is inherited as an autosomal dominant disorder. Because of point mutations or sometimes deletions, the vWF that is formed is abnormal, and multimer assembly is defective. Large and intermediate multimers, representing the most active forms of vWF, are missing from plasma. Type II vWD accounts for 10 to 15% of all cases and is associated with mild to moderate bleeding.[44]

Because vWF stabilizes factor VIII by binding to it, a deficiency of vWF gives rise to a secondary decrease in factor VIII levels. *To summarize, patients with von Willebrand's disease have a compound defect involving platelet function and the coagulation pathway.* However, except in the most severely affected (e.g., homozygous) patients, effects of factor VIII deficiency such as bleeding into the joints, which characterize hemophilia, are uncommon.

Hemophilia A (Factor VIII Deficiency)

Hemophilia A is the most common *hereditary disease with serious bleeding.* It is caused by a reduction in the amount or activity of factor VIII. This protein serves as a cofactor for the activation of factor X in the coagulation cascade (see Chapter 4). Hemophilia A is inherited as an X-linked recessive trait, and thus it occurs in males and in homozygous females. However, excessive bleeding has been described in heterozygous females, presumably caused by extremely "unfavorable lyonization" (inactivation of the normal X chromosome in most of the cells). Approximately 30% of the patients have no family history; presumably their disease is caused by new mutations.

Hemophilia A exhibits a wide range of clinical severity that correlates well with the level of factor VIII activity. Those with less than 1% of normal activity develop severe disease; levels between 2 to 5% of normal are associated with moderate disease; and patients with 6 to 50% of activity develop mild disease.

The variable degrees of deficiency in the level of factor VIII procoagulant are related to the type of mutation in the factor VIII gene. As with β-thalassemias, several genetic lesions (deletions, nonsense mutations that create stop codons, splicing errors) have been documented.[45] Patients with deletions and point mutations that create stop codons have no detectable factor VIII and hence develop the severe form of disease. In a minority of patients, the mutations do not affect the synthesis of factor VIII, but the functional domains are altered. In such cases levels of factor VIII appear normal by bioassay, but the protein is inactive. Approximately 15% of severely affected patients with low or absent factor VIII have antibodies against factor VIII that can complicate replacement therapy. The basis of formation of these antibodies is not clear.

In all symptomatic cases there is a tendency toward massive hemorrhage following trauma or operative procedures. In addition, "spontaneous" hemorrhages are frequently encountered in regions of the body normally subject to trauma, particularly the joints, where they are known as hemarthroses. Recurrent bleeding into the joints leads to progressive deformities that may be crippling. *Petechiae and ecchymoses are characteristically absent.*

Typically, patients with hemophilia A have normal bleeding time and platelet counts, with prolonged partial thromboplastin time. Factor VIII assays are required for diagnosis.

Treatment of hemophilia A involves infusion of factor VIII, currently derived from human plasma. Replacement therapy, however, is not an unalloyed blessing. It carries with it the risk of transmission of viral diseases. Until the mid-1980s, before routine screening of blood for HIV antibodies was instituted, thousands of hemophiliacs received factor VIII concentrates containing HIV, and many have developed AIDS (see Chapter 6). With current blood banking practices, the risk of HIV transmission has been virtually eliminated, but the threat of other undetected infections remains. Ultimately, the only safe factor VIII will be one derived from the cloned factor VIII gene. Clinical trials of replacement therapy with recombinant factor VIII are now in progress. Efforts to develop somatic gene therapy for hemophilia are also underway.

Hemophilia B (Christmas Disease, Factor IX Deficiency)

Severe factor IX deficiency is a disorder that is clinically indistinguishable from hemophilia A. Moreover, it is also inherited as an X-linked recessive trait and may occur asymptomatically or with associated hemorrhage. In about 14% of these patients, factor IX is present but nonfunctional. As with hemophilia A, *the partial thromboplastin time is prolonged, and bleeding time is normal.* Identification of Christmas disease (named after the first patient with this condition and not the holiday) is possible only by assay of the factor levels.

DISSEMINATED INTRAVASCULAR COAGULATION (DIC)

Disseminated intravascular coagulation is an acute, subacute, or chronic thrombohemorrhagic disorder occurring as a secondary complication in a variety of diseases. It is characterized by activation of the coagulation sequence that leads to the formation of microthrombi throughout the microcirculation of the body, but often in a quixotically uneven distribution. Sometimes the coagulopathy is localized to a specific organ or tissue. *As a consequence of the thrombotic diathesis, there is consumption of platelets, fibrin, and coagulation factors and, secondarily, activation of fibrinolytic mechanisms.* Thus, DIC may present with signs and symptoms relating to tissue hypoxia, and infarction caused by the myriad microthrombi, or as a hemorrhagic disorder related to depletion of the elements required for hemostasis (hence the term "consumption coagulopathy" is sometimes used to describe DIC). Activation of the fibrinolytic mechanism aggravates the hemorrhagic diathesis.

ETIOLOGY AND PATHOGENESIS. At the outset it must be emphasized that DIC is not a primary disease. It is a coagulopathy that occurs in the course of a variety of clinical conditions. In discussing the general mechanisms underlying DIC, it is useful to review briefly the normal process of blood coagulation and clot removal discussed earlier (see Chapter 4). It suffices here to recall that clotting may be initiated by either of two pathways: (1) the *extrinsic pathway,* which is triggered by the release of tissue factor ("tissue thromboplastin"); and (2) the *intrinsic pathway,* which involves the activation of factor XII by surface contact with collagen or other negatively charged substances. Both pathways, through a series of intermediate steps, result in the generation of thrombin, which in turn converts fibrinogen to fibrin. This process is regulated by *clot-inhibiting influences,* which include the activation of fibrinolysis involving generation of plasmin; the clearance of activated clotting factors by the mononuclear phagocyte system or by the liver; and activation of endogenous anticoagulants such as protein C.

From this brief review, it may be concluded that DIC may result from pathologic activation of the extrinsic and/or intrinsic pathways of coagulation or impairment of clot-inhibiting influences. Since the latter rarely constitute primary mechanisms of DIC, we will focus our attention on the abnormal initiation of clotting.[46]

There are two major mechanisms that trigger DIC: (1) release of tissue factor or thromboplastic substances into the circulation; and (2) widespread injury to the endothelial cells. Tissue thromboplastic substances may be derived from a variety of sources, such as placenta in obstetric complications

Table 13–9. MAJOR DISORDERS ASSOCIATED WITH DIC

OBSTETRIC COMPLICATIONS
Abruptio placentae
Retained dead fetus
Septic abortion
Amniotic fluid embolism
Toxemia

INFECTIONS
Gram-negative sepsis
Meningococcemia
Rocky Mountain spotted fever
Histoplasmosis
Aspergillosis
Malaria

NEOPLASMS
Carcinomas of pancreas, prostate, lung, and stomach
Acute promyelocytic leukemia

MASSIVE TISSUE INJURY
Traumatic
Burns
Extensive surgery

MISCELLANEOUS
Acute intravascular hemolysis, snakebite, giant hemangioma, shock, heat stroke, vasculitis, aortic aneurysm, liver disease

DIC = disseminated intravascular coagulation.

(Table 13–9) and the granules of leukemic cells in acute promyelocytic leukemia. Mucus released from certain adenocarcinomas can also act as a thromboplastic substance by directly activating factor X, independent of factor VII. In gram-negative sepsis (an important cause of DIC), bacterial endotoxins cause increased synthesis, membrane exposure, and release of tissue factor from monocytes. Furthermore, activated monocytes release IL-1 and tumor necrosis factor-alpha (TNF-α), both of which increase the expression of tissue factor on endothelial cell membranes and simultaneously decrease the expression of thrombomodulin. The latter, you may recall, activates protein C, an anticoagulant. The result is both activation of the clotting system and inhibition of coagulation control. TNF-α is an extremely important mediator of DIC in septic shock. In addition to the effects previously mentioned, TNF-α upregulates the expression of adhesion molecules on endothelial cells and thus favors adhesion of leukocytes, which in turn damage endothelial cells by releasing oxygen-derived free radicals and preformed proteases.[47]

Endothelial injury, the other major trigger, can initiate DIC by causing release of tissue factor, promoting platelet aggregation, and activating the intrinsic coagulation pathway. Even subtle endothelial injury can unleash procoagulant activity by enhancing membrane expression of tissue factor. Widespread endothelial injury may be produced by deposition of antigen-antibody complexes (e.g., SLE), temperature extremes (e.g., heat stroke, burns), or microorganisms (e.g., meningococci, rickettsiae).

Several disorders associated with DIC are listed in Table 13–9. Of these, DIC is most likely to follow *obstetric complications, malignancy, sepsis,* and *major trauma.* The initiating factors in these conditions are often multiple and inter-related. For example, in infections, particularly those caused by gram-negative bacteria, endotoxins released by the bacteria may activate both the intrinsic and the extrinsic pathways by producing endothelial cell injury and release of thromboplastins from inflammatory cells; furthermore, endotoxins inhibit the anticoagulant activity of protein C by suppressing thrombomodulin expression on endothelium. Endothelial cell damage may also be produced directly by meningococci, rickettsiae, and viruses. Antigen-antibody complexes formed during the infection can activate the classic complement pathway, and the complement fragments can secondarily activate both platelets and granulocytes. Endotoxins as well as other bacterial products are also capable of directly activating factor XII. In *massive trauma, extensive surgery,* and *severe burns,* the major mechanism of DIC is believed to be autoinfusion of tissue thromboplastins. In *obstetric* conditions thromboplastins derived from the placenta, dead retained fetus, or amniotic fluid may enter the circulation. However, hypoxia, acidosis, and shock, which often coexist with the surgical and obstetric conditions, can also cause widespread endothelial injury. Supervening infection may complicate the problems further. Among cancers, acute promyelocytic leukemia and carcinomas of the lung, pancreas, colon, and stomach are most frequently associated with DIC. These tumors are associated with the release of a variety of thromboplastic substances, including tissue factors, proteolytic enzymes, mucin, and other undefined tumor products.

The consequences of DIC are twofold. First, there is widespread deposition of fibrin within the microcirculation. This may lead to ischemia of the more severely affected or more vulnerable organs, and to a hemolytic anemia resulting from fragmentation of red cells as they squeeze through the narrowed microvasculature (microangiopathic hemolytic anemia). Second, a hemorrhagic diathesis may dominate the clinical picture. This results from consumption of platelets and clotting factors as well as activation of plasminogen. Plasmin not only can cleave fibrin but also can digest factors V and VIII, thereby reducing their concentration further. In addition, fibrinolysis leads to the formation of fibrin degradation products, which inhibit platelet aggregation and fibrin polymerization, and have antithrombin activity. All these influences lead to the hemostatic failure seen in DIC (Fig. 13–28).

MORPHOLOGY. In general, thrombi are found in the following sites in decreasing order of frequency: brain, heart, lungs, kidneys, adrenals, spleen, and

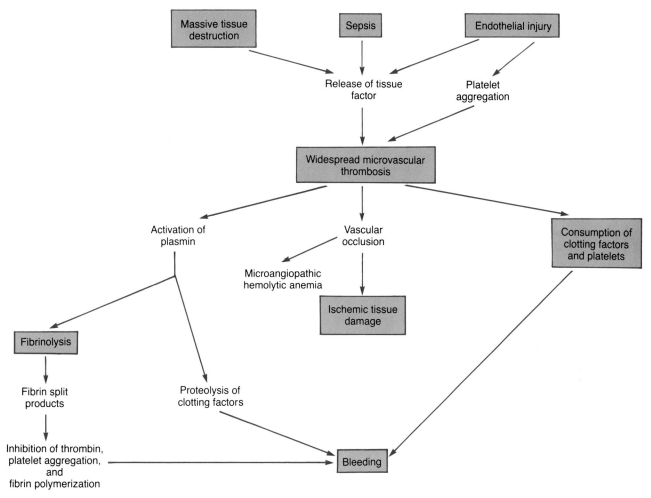

Figure 13–28. Pathophysiology of disseminated intravascular coagulation (DIC).

liver. However, no tissue is spared, and occasionally thrombi are found in only one or several organs without affecting others. In giant hemangiomas, for example, they are localized to the neoplasm. In this condition they are believed to result from local stasis and recurrent trauma to the poorly supported blood vessels. The affected kidneys may reveal small thrombi in the glomeruli (Fig. 13–29) that may evoke only a reactive swelling of endothelial cells; however, in severe cases, microinfarcts or even bilateral renal cortical necrosis may result. Numerous fibrin thrombi may be found in the alveolar capillaries, sometimes associated with pulmonary edema and exudation of fibrin, to create "hyaline membranes" reminiscent of ARDS (see Chapter 15). In the central nervous system, microinfarcts may be caused by the fibrin thrombi, occasionally complicated by simultaneous fresh hemorrhage. Such changes are the basis for the bizarre neurologic signs and symptoms sometimes observed in this syndrome. The manifestations of DIC in the endocrine glands are of considerable

interest. In meningococcemia, the massive adrenal hemorrhages of the Waterhouse-Friderichsen syndrome (see Chapter 25) are probably related to fibrin thrombi within the microcirculation of the adrenal cortex. Similarly, Sheehan's postpartum pituitary necrosis (see Chapter 25) may be one of the expressions of DIC. In toxemia of pregnancy (see Chapter 23), the placenta exhibits widespread microthrombi, providing a plausible explanation for the premature atrophy of the cytotrophoblast and syncytiotrophoblast encountered in this condition.

The bleeding manifestations of DIC are not dissimilar to those encountered in the hereditary and acquired disorders affecting the hemostatic mechanisms discussed earlier.

CLINICAL COURSE. The onset may be fulminant, as in endotoxic shock or amniotic fluid embolism, or it may be insidious and chronic, as in cases of carcinomatosis or retention of a dead fetus. Overall, about 50% of individuals with **DIC** are obstetric patients having complications of pregnancy. In this

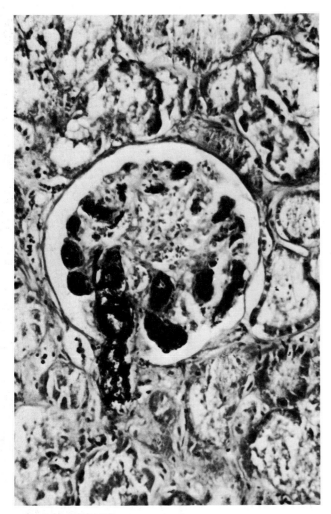

Figure 13–29. Disseminated intravascular coagulation (DIC). An affected glomerulus shows multiple darkly stained thrombi. (Courtesy of Dr. Patrick Ward, Department of Pathology and Laboratory Medicine, University of Minnesota School of Medicine, Duluth.)

vation and laboratory studies are necessary for the diagnosis. It is usually necessary to monitor the following: fibrinogen, platelets, prothrombin time, partial thromboplastin time, and fibrin degradation products.

The prognosis is highly variable and depends, to a considerable extent, on the underlying disorder. The management of these cases requires meticulous maneuvering between the Scylla of the thrombotic tendency and the Charybdis of the bleeding diathesis. Thus is posed the dilemma of whether to attempt to block coagulation or to control bleeding by the administration of coagulants. Each patient must be treated individually, and, depending on the clinical picture, potent anticoagulants such as heparin and antithrombin III or coagulants in the form of fresh-frozen plasma may be administered. Platelet transfusions may sometimes be necessary. DIC is another of the therapeutist's nightmares.

setting, the disorder tends to be reversible with delivery of the fetus. About 33% of the patients have carcinomatosis. The remaining cases are associated with the various entities previously listed.

It is almost impossible to detail all the potential clinical presentations, but a few common patterns may be cited. A microangiopathic hemolytic anemia may appear. Respiratory symptoms such as dyspnea, cyanosis, and extreme respiratory difficulty may predominate. Neurologic signs and symptoms including convulsions and coma represent another pattern. Renal changes such as oliguria and acute renal failure may dominate. Circulatory failure and shock may appear suddenly or develop progressively. In general, *acute DIC, associated for example with obstetric complications or major trauma, is dominated by bleeding diathesis, whereas chronic DIC, such as may occur in a patient with cancer, tends to present initially with thrombotic complications.* Accurate clinical obser-

1. Spangude, G.J.: Hematopoietic stem cell differentiation. Curr. Opin. Immunol. 3:171, 1991.
2. Becker S.E., and Lux S.: Disorders of the red cell membrane. In Nathan, D.G., and Oski, F.A. (eds.): Hematology of Infancy and Childhood, 4th ed. Philadelphia, W.B. Saunders Co., 1993, p. 529.
3. Hanspal, M., et al.: Molecular basis of spectrin and ankyrin deficiencies in severe hereditary spherocytosis: Evidence indicating a primary defect in ankyrin. Blood 77:165, 1991.
4. Jandl, J.H., et al.: Red cell filtration and the pathogenesis of certain hemolytic anemias. Blood 18:33, 1961.
5. Becker, P.S., and Lux, S.E.: Hereditary spherocytosis and related disorders. Clin. Hematol. 14:15, 1985.
6. Beutler, E.: Glucose-6-phosphate dehydrogenase deficiency. N. Engl. J. Med. 324:169, 1991.
7. Plott, O.S., and Glover, G.J.: Sickle cell disease. In Nathan, D.G., and Oski, F.A. (eds.): Hematology of Infancy and Childhood, 4th ed. Philadelphia, W.B. Saunders Co., 1993, p.732.
8. Fabry, M.E., et al.: Demonstration of endothelial adhesion of sickle cells in vivo: A distinct role for deformable sickle discocytes. Blood 79:1602, 1992.
9. Kazazian, H.J., Jr.: The thalassemia syndromes: Molecular basis and prenatal diagnosis. Semin. Hematol. 27:209, 1990.
10. Lukens, J.H.: The thalassemias and related disorders: Quantitative disorders of hemoglobin synthesis. In Lee, G.R., et al. (eds.): Wintrobe's Clinical Hematology, 9th ed. Philadelphia, Lea & Febiger, 1993, p.1102.
11. Giardina, P.J., and Hilgartner, M.W.: Update on thalassemia. Pediatr. Rev. 13:55, 1992.
12. Lucarelli, G., et al.: Bone marrow transplantation in patients with thalassemia. N. Engl. J. Med. 322:417, 1990.
13. Rosse, W.F.: Paroxysmal nocturnal hemoglobinuria. Curr. Top. Microbiol. Immunol. 178:163, 1992.
14. Engelfreit, C.P., et al.: Autoimmune hemolytic anemia. Semin. Hematol. 29:3, 1992.
15. Petz, L.D.: Drug-induced hemolysis. N. Engl. J. Med. 313:510, 1985.
16. Nydegger, U.E., Kazatchkine, M.D., and Meischer, P.A.: Immunopathologic and clinical features of hemolytic anemia due to cold agglutinins. Semin. Hematol. 28:66, 1991.
17. Chanarin, I. et al.: Cobalamin and folate: Recent developments. J. Clin. Pathol. 45:277, 1992.
17a. Tefferi, A., and Pruthi, R.K.: The biochemical basis of cobalamin deficiency. Mayo Clin. Proc. 69:181, 1994.

18. Beck, W.S.: Cobalamin and the nervous system. N. Engl. J. Med. *318*:1752, 1988.
19. Taylor, K.B., et al.: Gastrointestinal and liver diseases. *In* Stites, D.P., et al. (eds.): Basic and Clinical Immunology, 6th ed. Los Altos, Appleton & Lange, 1987, p. 462.
20. Gleeson, P.A., and Toh, B.H.: Molecular targets in pernicious anemia. Immunol. Today *12*:233, 1991.
21. Seligman, P.A., et al.: Molecular mechanisms of iron metabolism. *In* Stamatoyannopoulos, G., et al. (eds.): Molecular Basis of Blood Diseases. Philadelphia, W.B. Saunders Co., 1987, p. 219.
22. Conrad, M.E., and Umbreit, J.N.: A concise review: Iron absorption—the mucin-mobilferrin-integrin pathway: A competitive pathway for metal absorption. Am. J. Hematol. *42*:67, 1993.
23. Scrimshaw, N.S.: Iron-deficiency and its functional consequences. Compr. Ther. *11*:40, 1985.
24. Sears, D.A.: Anemia of chronic disease. Med. Clin. North Am. *76*:567, 1992.
25. Young, N.S., and Mortimer, P.P.: Viruses and bone marrow failure. Blood *63*:729, 1984.
26. Thomas, E.D., and Storb, R.: Acquired aplastic anemia: Progress and perplexity. Blood *64*:325, 1984.
27. Mangan, K.F., et al.: In vitro evidence for disappearance of erythroid progenitor T suppressor cells following allogeneic bone marrow transplantation for severe aplastic anemia. Blood *71*:144, 1988.
28. Marsh, J.C.W., et al.: Survival after anti-lymphocyte globulin therapy for aplastic anemia depends on disease severity. Blood *70*:1046, 1987.
29. Nissen, C.: The pathophysiology of aplastic anemia. Semin. Hematol. *28*:313, 1991.
30. Young, N.S.: The problem of clonality in aplastic anemia: Dr. Dameshek's riddle, restated. Blood *29*:1385, 1992.
31. Speck, B.: Allogeneic bone marrow transplantation for severe aplastic anemia. Semin. Hematol. *28*:319, 1991.
32. Dessypris, E.N.: The biology of pure red cell aplasia. Semin. Hematol. *28*:275, 1991.
33. Salama, A., and Mueller-Eckhardt, C.: Immune-mediated blood dyscrasias related to drugs. Semin. Hematol. *29*:54, 1992.
34. Kaplan, C., et al.: Virus-induced autoimmune thrombocytopenia and neutropenia. Semin. Hematol. *29*:34, 1992.
35. Kiefel, V., et al.: Serologic, biochemical, and molecular aspects of platelet autoantigens. Semin. Hematol. *29*:26, 1992.
36. Waters, A.H.: Autoimmune thrombocytopenia: Clinical aspects. Semin. Hematol. *29*:18, 1992.
37. Kwaan, H.S.: Clinicopathologic features of thrombotic thrombocytopenic purpura. Semin. Hematol. *24*:71, 1987.
38. Ruggenenti, P., and Remuzzi, G.: Thrombotic microangiopathies. Crit. Rev. Oncol. Hematol. *11*:243, 1991.
39. Thompson, C.E., et al.: Thrombotic microangiopathies in the 1980s: Clinical features, response to treatment, and the impact of human immunodeficiency virus epidemic. Blood *80*:1890, 1992.
40. Beardsley, D.S.: Platelet abnormalities in infancy and childhood. *In* Nathan, D.G., and Oski, F.A. (eds.): Hematology of Infancy and Childhood, 4th ed. Philadelphia, W.B. Saunders Co., 1993, p.1589.
41. Bick, R.L.: Acquired platelet function defects. Hematol. Oncol. Clin. North Am. *6*:1203, 1992.
42. Ginsburg, D.: Biology of inherited coagulopathies: Von Willebrand factor. Hematol. Oncol. Clin. North Am. *6*:1011, 1992.
43. White, G.C., and Shoemaker, C.B.: Factor VIII gene and hemophilia A. Blood *73*:1, 1989.
44. Ginsburg, D., and Bowie, E.J.W.: Molecular genetics of von Willebrand disease. Blood *79*:2507, 1992.
45. Gitschier, J.: The molecular basis of hemophilia A. Ann. N.Y. Acad. Sci. *614*:89, 1991.
46. Moake, J.L.: Hypercoagulable states. Adv. Intern. Med. *35*:235, 1990.
47. Risberg, B., et al.: Disseminated intravascular coagulation. Acta Anesthiol. Scand. *35*(Suppl. 95):60, 1991.

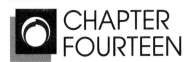

CHAPTER FOURTEEN

Diseases of White Cells, Lymph Nodes, and Spleen

White Cells and Lymph Nodes

NORMAL

The origin and differentiation of white cells (granulocytes, monocytes, and lymphocytes) were briefly discussed in Chapter 13 along with the other formed elements of blood. Lymphocytes and monocytes not only circulate in the blood and lymph but also accumulate in discrete and organized masses, the so-called lymphoreticular system. Components of this system include lymph nodes, thymus, spleen, tonsils, adenoids, and Peyer's patches. Less discrete collections of lymphoid cells occur in the bone marrow, lungs, and gastrointestinal tract and other tissues. Lymph nodes are the most widely distributed and easily accessible component of the lymphoid tissue and are hence frequently examined for the diagnosis of lymphoreticular disorders. It would therefore be advantageous to review the normal morphology of lymph nodes.

Lymph nodes are discrete structures surrounded by a capsule composed of connective tissue and a few elastic fibrils. The capsule is perforated at various points by afferent lymphatics that empty into the peripheral sinus subjacent to the capsule. Situated in the cortex or peripheral portion of the node are spherical aggregates of lymphoid tissue, the so-called primary follicles, which represent the B-cell areas. On antigenic stimulation, the primary follicles enlarge and develop pale-staining germinal centers composed of follicular center cells. Surrounding these germinal centers are mantles of small unchallenged B cells. The T cells occupy the parafollicular regions. The

629

medullary cords, occupying the central portion of the node, contain predominantly plasma cells and some lymphocytes.

The morphologic description of the lymph node just given is highly idealized and falsely static. The size and morphology of lymph nodes are modified by immune responses. As secondary lines of defense, they are constantly responding to stimuli, even in the absence of clinical disease. Trivial injuries and infections effect subtle changes in lymph node histology. More significant bacterial infections inevitably produce enlargement of nodes and sometimes leave residual scarring. For this reason, lymph nodes in the adult are almost never "normal," and they usually bear the scars of previous events, rendering the inguinal nodes particularly inappropriate for evaluative biopsies. Except in the child, it is difficult to find a "normal" node, and in histologic evaluations it is often necessary to distinguish changes secondary to past experience from those related to present disease.

PATHOLOGY

Disorders of white cells may be classified into two broad categories, *proliferative* and those characterized by a deficiency of leukocytes, that is, *leukopenias*. Proliferations of white cells and lymph nodes may be reactive or neoplastic. Since their major function is host defense, reactive proliferation in response to an underlying primary, often microbial, disease is fairly common. Neoplastic disorders, although less frequent, are much more important. In the following discussion, we shall describe first the leukopenic states and summarize the common reactive disorders, and then consider in some detail malignant proliferations of the white cells that in many instances arise in the nodes.

LEUKOPENIA

The number of circulating white cells may be markedly decreased in a variety of disorders. An abnormally low white cell count *(leukopenia)* usually results from reduced numbers of neutrophils *(neutropenia, granulocytopenia)*. *Lymphopenias* are much less common, and in addition to the congenital immunodeficiency diseases (see Chapter 6), they are associated with specific clinical syndromes (e.g., Hodgkin's disease, nonlymphocytic leukemias, following corticosteroid therapy, and occasionally in chronic diseases). Only the more common leukopenias involving granulocytes will be discussed here.

NEUTROPENIA — AGRANULOCYTOSIS

Reduction in the number of granulocytes in the peripheral blood—*neutropenia*—may be seen in a wide variety of circumstances. A marked reduction in neutrophil count has serious consequences by predisposing to infections. When of this magnitude, it is referred to as *agranulocytosis*.

PATHOGENESIS. A reduction in circulating granulocytes will occur if (1) there is reduced or ineffective production of neutrophils or (2) there is accelerated removal of neutrophils from the circulating blood.

Inadequate or ineffective granulopoiesis may be encountered with (1) suppression of myeloid stem cells, as occurs in aplastic anemia (see Chapter 13) and a variety of leukemias and lymphomas—in these conditions, granulocytopenia is accompanied by anemia and thrombocytopenia; (2) suppression of the committed granulocytic precursors, which occurs after exposure to certain drugs, as discussed below; or (3) megaloblastic anemias, due to vitamin B_{12} or folate deficiency (see Chapter 13), in which defective DNA synthesis produces abnormal granulocytic precursors, rendering them susceptible to intramedullary death (ineffective granulopoiesis).

Accelerated removal or destruction of neutrophils is encountered with (1) immunologically mediated injury to the neutrophils, which may be idiopathic with no other abnormality, associated with a well-defined immunologic disorder (e.g., Felty's syndrome; see Chapter 27), or produced by exposure to drugs; (2) splenic sequestration, in which excessive destruction occurs secondary to enlargement of the spleen, associated also with excessive destruction of red cells and platelets; and (3) increased peripheral utilization, as may occur in overwhelming bacterial, fungal, or rickettsial infections.

Among the many associations mentioned, *the most significant neutropenias (agranulocytoses) are produced by drugs*. Certain drugs, such as alkylating agents and antimetabolites used in cancer treatment, produce agranulocytosis in a predictable, dose-related fashion. They cause a generalized suppression of the bone marrow, and therefore other cells are also affected (aplastic anemia). Agranulocytosis may also be encountered as an idiosyncratic reaction to a large variety of agents. The roster of implicated drugs includes aminopyrine, chloramphenicol, sulfonamides, chlorpromazine, thiouracil, and phenylbutazone. The neutropenia induced by chlorpromazine and related phenothiazines is believed to result from the suppression of granulocytic precursors in the bone marrow.

Agranulocytosis following administration of aminopyrine, thiouracil, and certain sulfonamides is believed to result from immunologically mediated destruction of mature neutrophils. The immunologic mechanisms are similar to those involved in

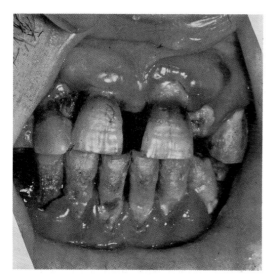

Figure 14-1. Agranulocytosis. Gingival margins show chronic suppurative necrotizing infection due to loss of protective white cells in circulation.

drug-induced hemolytic anemias (see Chapter 13). In many cases, no antecedent cause of neutropenia can be detected, but autoimmunity is suspected, since serum antibodies directed against neutrophil-specific antigens can be detected.[1] Severe neutropenia may also occur in association with polyclonal or monoclonal proliferations of CD8+ large granular lymphocytes.[2] The mechanism of this neutropenia is not clear, but suppression of granulocytic progenitors in the bone marrow is considered most likely.

MORPHOLOGY. The anatomic alterations in the bone marrow depend on the underlying basis of the neutropenia. When it is caused by excessive destruction of the mature neutrophils, the marrow may be hypercellular with increased numbers of immature granulocytic precursors. Hypercellularity is also seen with ineffective granulopoiesis, as occurs in megaloblastic anemias. Agranulocytosis caused by agents that affect the granulocytic precursors is understandably associated with hypocellular marrow, resulting from greatly decreased leukopoietic elements.

Infections are a characteristic feature of agranulocytosis. Ulcerating necrotizing lesions of the gingiva, floor of the mouth, buccal mucosa, pharynx, or anywhere within the oral cavity (agranulocytic angina) are quite characteristic of agranulocytosis (Fig. 14-1). These ulcers are typically deep, undermined, and covered by gray to green-black necrotic membranes from which numerous bacteria or fungi can be isolated. Similar ulcerations may occur in the skin, vagina, anus, or gastrointestinal tract, but these sites are much less frequently involved. Severe necrotizing infections are also encountered, but less prominently, in the lungs, urinary tract, and kidneys. All these sites of infection are characterized by massive growth of bacteria (or other agents) with relatively poor leukocytic response. In many instances, the bacteria grow in colony formation (botryomycosis) as though they were cultured on nutrient media. The regional lymph nodes draining these infections are enlarged and inflamed. The spleen and liver are rarely enlarged.

CLINICAL COURSE. The symptoms and signs of neutropenias are those of bacterial infections. They include malaise, chills, and fever, followed in sequence by marked weakness and fatigability. In severe agranulocytosis with virtual absence of neutrophils, these infections may become so overwhelming as to cause death within a few days.

Characteristically, the total white cell count is reduced to 1000 cells per mm³ of blood, and when counts fall below 500 per mm³ serious infections tend to occur. In addition to control of bacterial infections, current treatment efforts are directed toward increasing the production of neutrophils by administration of recombinant human granulopoietic factors such as granulocyte-macrophage colony-stimulating factor (GM-CSF) and G-CSF.

REACTIVE (INFLAMMATORY) PROLIFERATIONS OF WHITE CELLS AND NODES

Leukocytosis

Leukocytosis is a common reaction in a variety of inflammatory states. The particular white cell series affected varies with the underlying cause. In Chapter 3 we discussed *polymorphonuclear leukocytosis* (granulocytosis), which accompanies acute inflammation. Pyogenic infections are common causes of neutrophilic leukocytosis, but it may also result from nonmicrobial stimuli, such as tissue necrosis caused by burns or myocardial infarction. In patients with severe, life-threatening sepsis, in addition to leukocytosis there may be morphologic changes in the neutrophils, such as toxic granulations and cytoplasmic vacuoles. *Toxic granules* are coarse and darker than the normal neutrophilic granules. Although their precise origin is not entirely clear, they are believed to represent abnormal forms of azurophilic granules.

Eosinophilic leukocytosis is characteristic of allergic disorders, such as bronchial asthma, hay fever, parasitic infections, and some diseases of the skin. The skin diseases include pemphigus, eczema, and dermatitis herpetiformis, all of which are probably immunologic in origin. In hospitalized adult patients the most likely cause of eosinophilia is an allergic drug reaction. *Elevations in monocyte count* may be seen in several chronic infections, including tuberculosis, bacterial endocarditis, brucellosis, rickettsiosis, and malaria. Certain collagen vascular diseases, such as systemic lupus erythematosus (SLE) and rheumatoid arthritis, are associated with monocytosis, as are inflammatory bowel diseases, such as ulcerative colitis and Crohn's disease. *Lymphocytosis* may accompany monocytosis in chronic inflammatory states such as brucellosis and tuberculosis, representing in these instances a sustained activation of the immune response. The lymphocyte count may also be increased in acute viral infections such as viral hepatitis, in cytomegalovirus infections, and particularly in infectious mononucleosis (see Chapter 8).

In most instances, reactive leukocytosis is easy to distinguish from neoplastic proliferation of the white cells (i.e., leukemias) by the rarity of immature cells in the blood. However, in some inflammatory states, many immature white cells may appear in the blood and a picture of leukemia may be simulated *(leukemoid reaction)*. The distinction from leukemias may then be difficult, as discussed later.

Infections and other inflammatory stimuli may not only cause leukocytosis but also involve the lymph nodes, which act as defensive barriers. The infections that lead to lymphadenitis are numerous. Some that produce distinctive morphologic patterns are described in other chapters. In most instances, however, the lymphadenitis is entirely nonspecific, designated acute or chronic nonspecific lymphadenitis.

Acute Nonspecific Lymphadenitis

Lymph nodes undergo reactive changes whenever challenged by microbiologic agents or their toxic products, or by cell debris and foreign matter introduced into wounds or into the circulation, as in drug addiction.

Acutely inflamed nodes are most commonly caused by direct microbiologic drainage and are seen most frequently in the cervical area in association with infections of the teeth or tonsils, or in the axillary or inguinal regions secondary to infections in the extremities. Similarly, acute lymphadenitis is found in those nodes draining acute appendicitis, acute enteritis, or any other acute infection. Generalized acute lymphadenopathy is characteristic of viral infections and bacteremia, particularly in children. The nodal reactions in the abdomen —mesenteric adenitis—may induce acute abdominal symptoms closely resembling acute appendicitis, a differential diagnosis that plagues the surgeon.

MORPHOLOGY. Macroscopically, the nodes become swollen, gray-red, and engorged. Histologically, there is prominence of the lymphoid follicles, with large germinal centers containing numerous mitotic figures. Histiocytes often contain particulate debris of bacterial origin or derived from necrotic cells. When pyogenic organisms are the cause of the reaction, the centers of the follicles may undergo necrosis; indeed, the entire node may sometimes be converted into a suppurative mass. With less severe reactions, there is sometimes a neutrophilic infiltrate about the follicles, and numerous neutrophils can be found within the lymphoid sinuses. The cells lining the sinuses become hypertrophied and cuboidal and may undergo hyperplasia.

Clinically, nodes with acute lymphadenitis are enlarged because of the cellular infiltration and edema. As a consequence of the distention of the capsule, they are tender to touch. When abscess formation is extensive, they become fluctuant. The overlying skin is frequently red, and sometimes penetration of the infection to the skin surface produces draining sinuses, particularly when the nodes have undergone suppurative necrosis. As might be expected, healing of such lesions is associated with scarring.

Chronic Nonspecific Lymphadenitis

Chronic reactions assume one of three patterns, depending on their causation.

MORPHOLOGY. Follicular hyperplasia is caused by chronic infections with microbes that activate B cells. It is distinguished by prominence of the large germinal centers, which appear to bulge against the surrounding collar of small B lymphocytes (Fig. 14–2). Prominent within these germinal centers are lymphocytes in varying stages of "blast" transformation and large numbers of histiocytes containing phagocytized debris of bacterial or cellular origin. Plasma cells, histiocytes, and occasionally neutrophils or eosinophils may be found in the parafollicular regions, and there generally is striking hyperplasia of the mononuclear phagocytic cells lining the lymphatic sinuses. Some specific causes of follicular hyperplasia include disorders such as rheumatoid arthritis, toxoplasmosis, and early stages of human immunodeficiency virus (HIV) infection.

This form of lymphadenitis may be confused morphologically with follicular (nodular) lymphomas (see later discussion of non-Hodgkin's lymphomas). It is beyond our scope to go into all the subtle morphologic features in this differential diagnosis, but several points may be noted. Favoring reactive follicular hyperplasia are (1) preservation of the

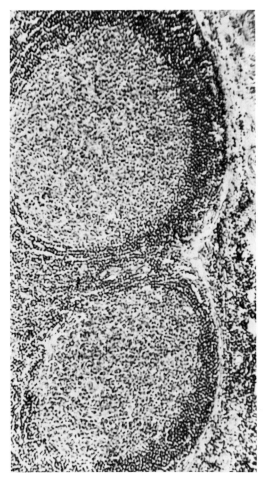

Figure 14-2. Chronic follicular hyperplasia, demonstrating marked enlargement and prominence of germinal centers.

lymph node architecture with presence of normal lymphoid tissue between germinal centers; (2) marked variation in the shape and size of lymphoid nodules; (3) a mixed population of lymphocytes in different stages of differentiation and histiocytes within germinal centers, that is, reactive follicles are pleomorphic, whereas lymphomatous nodules tend to be monomorphic; and (4) prominent phagocytic activity in germinal centers.

Paracortical lymphoid hyperplasia is characterized by reactive changes within the T-cell regions of the lymph node that encroach on, and sometimes appear to efface, the germinal follicles. In these regions, the T cells undergo progressive transformation to immunoblasts. In addition, there is hypertrophy of the sinusoidal and vascular endothelial cells and a mixed cellular infiltrate, principally of macrophages and sometimes of eosinophils. Such changes are encountered particularly often in immunologic reactions induced by drugs (especially Dilantin) or following smallpox vaccination. Similar reactions have been described after the use of other vaccines.

Sinus histiocytosis refers to distention and prominence of the lymphatic sinusoids, encountered in lymph nodes draining cancers, particularly carcinoma of the breast. The lining endothelial cells are markedly hypertrophied, and the sinuses may be virtually engorged with histiocytes. This pattern of reaction has been thought to represent an immune response on the part of the host against the tumor or its products.

Characteristically, lymph nodes in chronic reactions are not tender, because they are not under increased pressure. Chronic lymphadenitis is particularly common in inguinal and axillary nodes. Both groups drain relatively large areas of the body and so are frequently challenged, for which reason these lymph nodes are inappropriate as biopsy specimens in the study of hematologic and lymphomatous disorders.

NEOPLASTIC PROLIFERATIONS OF WHITE CELLS

Malignant proliferative diseases constitute the most important white cell disorders. The several categories of these diseases can be briefly defined as follows:

1. *Malignant lymphomas* take the form of cohesive tumorous lesions, composed mainly of lymphocytes and rarely of histiocytes, that arise in lymphoid tissue anywhere in the body, most commonly within lymph nodes.

2. *Leukemias and myeloproliferative disorders* are neoplasms of the hematopoietic stem cells arising in the bone marrow that secondarily flood the circulating blood or other organs with transformed cells.

3. *Plasma cell dyscrasias and related disorders,* usually arising in the bones, take the form of localized or disseminated proliferations of antibody-forming cells. Thus, this category is marked by the appearance in the peripheral blood of abnormal levels of complete immunoglobulins or the light or heavy chains of the immunoglobulins.

4. The *histiocytoses* represent proliferative lesions of histiocytes that include rare histiocytic neoplasms that present as malignant lymphomas, mentioned above. A special category of histiocytes referred to as Langerhans' cells gives rise to a spectrum of disorders, some of which behave as disseminated malignant tumors, and others as localized benign proliferations. This group is called Langerhans' cell histiocytoses.

As can be seen, the neoplastic disorders of the white cells are extremely varied. In the following sections, each of the categories is treated separately.

MALIGNANT LYMPHOMAS

Lymphomas are malignant neoplasms characterized by the proliferation of cells native to the lymphoid tissues, that is, lymphocytes, histiocytes, and their precursors and derivatives. The term "lymphoma" is something of a misnomer, since these disorders are lethal unless controlled or eradicated through therapy. There are no "benign" lymphomas.

Within the broad group of malignant lymphomas, *Hodgkin's disease* (Hodgkin's lymphoma) is segregated from all other forms, which constitute the *non-Hodgkin's lymphomas*. Although both have their origin in the lymphoid tissues, Hodgkin's disease is set apart by the presence of a distinctive unifying morphologic feature, the Reed-Sternberg giant cell. In addition, the nodes contain non-neoplastic inflammatory cells, which in most cases outnumber the neoplastic element represented by the Reed-Sternberg cell. Therefore, we shall discuss non-Hodgkin's lymphomas and Hodgkin's disease separately.

NON-HODGKIN'S LYMPHOMAS (NHL)

The usual presentation of NHL is as a localized or generalized lymphadenopathy. However, in about one-third of cases it may be primary in other sites where lymphoid tissue is found, for example, in the oropharyngeal region, gut, bone marrow, and skin. Lymph node enlargement due to lymphomatous disease must be differentiated from that caused by the more frequent infectious and inflammatory disorders. Lymphomatous involvement often produces marked nodal enlargement, which is almost always nontender (Fig. 14–3). Although variable, all forms of lymphoma have the potential to spread from their origin in a single node or chain of nodes to other nodes, and eventually to disseminate to the spleen, liver, and bone marrow. Some, after becoming widespread, spill over into the blood, creating a leukemia-like picture in the peripheral blood.

Although we speak of NHL as a group, we should recognize that it encompasses a wide spectrum of disorders, differing in patient age at onset, the cells of origin, and response to therapy. It is therefore necessary to classify NHL into various subgroups.

Few areas of pathology have evoked as much controversy and confusion as the classification of NHL. Regrettably, even among expert "lymphomaniacs" there has been no unanimity regarding the best approach, and until the recent past there were more classifications than experts. In 1982, an international panel of hematopathologists decided to stem the growing tide of classifications by proposing yet another, possibly the ultimate, classification, entitled the Working Formulation of Clinical Usage,[3] which is now widely accepted. Before the Working Formulation is discussed, some important principles relevant to the classification of NHL need to be emphasized.

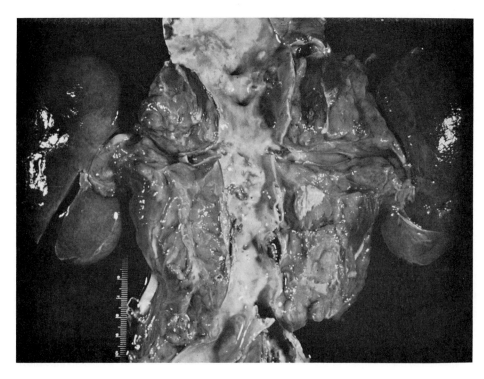

Figure 14–3. Lymphoma involving periaortic nodes.

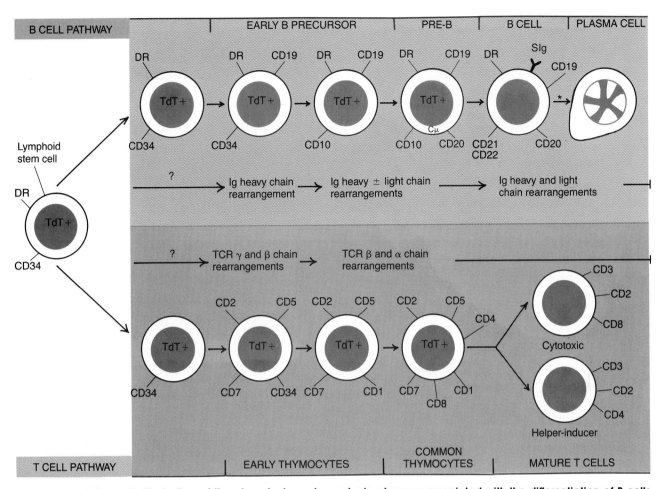

Figure 14–4. Schematic illustration of the phenotypic and genotypic changes associated with the differentiation of B cells and T cells. Not shown are some CD4+, CD8+ cells (common thymocytes) that also express CD3. *Stages between resting B cells and plasma are not depicted. CD = cluster designation; TdT = terminal deoxynucleotidyl transferase; Ig = immunoglobulin; TCR = T-cell receptor.

- As tumors of the immune system, NHLs may originate in T cells, B cells, or histiocytes; distinction can be made on the basis of phenotypic and molecular characteristics of the tumor cells. The vast majority of NHLs (80 to 85%) are of B-cell origin; the remainder are in large part T-cell tumors. Tumors of histiocytes or macrophages are quite uncommon. Tumors of T and B cells may represent cells arrested at any stage along their differentiation pathways (Fig. 14–4). This figure also illustrates the genotypic and phenotypic characteristics of differentiating T and B cells that are useful in subdividing this group of tumors. Some additional cell surface markers useful in the study of lymphomas and leukemias are listed in Table 14–1.[4]

- Histologically, the lymphoma cells exhibit two different growth patterns: *they are either clustered into identifiable nodules (nodular lymphoma) or spread diffusely throughout the node (diffuse lymphoma)* (Figs. 14–5 and 14–6). With either pattern the normal lymph node architecture is completely destroyed. The distinction between nodular and diffuse lymphomas, proposed initially by Rappaport, has proved to be an important and reliable indicator of tumor behavior. In general, *nodular (or follicular) architecture is associated with a significantly superior prognosis to that of diffuse pattern.*

- It may be recalled that normal B cells form follicles within lymph nodes; malignant B cells tend to recapitulate this behavior with nodule formation. *Not surprisingly, therefore, nodular lymphomas are composed exclusively of B cells.* Lukes first pointed out that during antigen-induced differentiation within germinal centers of lymph nodes normal B cells undergo a series of morphologic changes, diagrammed in Figure 14–7. Such transformation of small B cells to activated immunoblasts is characterized by changes in cell and nuclear size and in nuclear configuration (clefts or folds). One suggested sequence of changes is as follows: small cleaved cell to large cleaved cell to small noncleaved cell to large noncleaved cell. Nodular lymphomas that arise from these follicular center cells are composed of any of these differentiation patterns, as though they had been arrested at a particular stage of

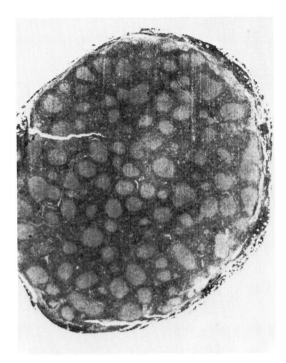

Figure 14-5. Non-Hodgkin's lymphoma, nodular pattern. Nodular aggregates of lymphoma cells are present throughout lymph node and in perinodal fat. (Courtesy of Dr. José Hernandez, Department of Pathology, University of Texas Southwestern Medical School, Dallas.)

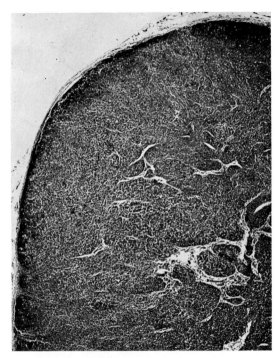

Figure 14-6. Non-Hodgkin's lymphoma, diffuse pattern. Nodal architecture is replaced by a diffuse sea of neoplastic lymphoid cells.

transformation. It should be remembered, however, that neoplastic follicular center cells can also spread diffusely in the lymph nodes and therefore give rise to diffuse lymphomas as well. Morphologically, some of the large follicular center cells have an uncanny resemblance to histiocytes. In the past, this gave rise to the erroneous impression that tumors composed of large follicular center cells were of histiocytic origin.

With this background we can discuss the Working Formulation for Clinical Usage. Under this scheme *NHLs are divided into three prognostic groups, designated as low-, intermediate-, and high-grade, based on survival statistics* (Table 14–2). The 10-year survival rates for tumors classified as low-grade, intermediate-grade, and high-grade lymphomas, respectively, are approximately 45, 26, and 23%. Within each prognostic group are several morphologic categories based on the architecture (follicular or diffuse) and the cytologic appearance of cells. No attempt is made to classify malignancies by their cell of origin, since in general immunophenotyping has not proved to have significant prognostic value. The Working Formulation also contains a miscellaneous group to encompass the rare histiocytic tumors and two unusual forms of T-cell neoplasia. The individual tumors within the working formulation are described below.

Low-Grade Lymphomas

This category includes three tumors: small lymphocytic lymphoma; follicular, predominantly small cleaved cell lymphoma; and follicular, mixed (small cleaved and large cell) lymphoma. The two follicular lymphomas will be discussed together, since they form a distinct clinicopathologic group.

Small Lymphocytic Lymphoma (SLL)

This pattern makes up approximately 4% of all NHLs and is the only low-grade lymphoma that does not have a follicular architecture.

MORPHOLOGY. SLL consists of compact, small, apparently unstimulated lymphocytes with dark-staining round nuclei, scanty cytoplasm, and little variation in size (Fig. 14–8). Mitotic figures are rare, and there is little or no cytologic atypia. **Involvement of bone marrow is present in almost all cases, and in about 60% of patients the neoplastic cells spill over into blood, evoking a chronic lymphocytic leukemia–like picture.** Indeed, SLL is considered to be the solid (lymphomatous) counterpart of chronic lymphocytic leukemia (CLL), which is described later.

Clinically, SLL and the related CLL occur primarily in the sixth and seventh decades. Typically,

Table 14–1. SOME IMMUNE CELL ANTIGENS DETECTED BY MONOCLONAL ANTIBODIES

ANTIGEN DESIGNATION	COMMENTS
Primarily T Cell–Associated	
CD1	Expressed on cortical thymocytes
CD2	Present on all T cells: thymic and peripheral, and NK cells
CD3	Expressed initially in thymus and retained on all peripheral T cells
CD4	Expressed on the helper subset of peripheral T cells
CD5	Expressed on all T cells, and a small subset of B cells
CD7	Expressed on all T cells
CD8	Expressed on the cytotoxic subset of peripheral T cells, and some NK cells
Primarily B Cell–Associated	
CD10	Expressed on developing B cells; also called CALLA
CD19	Present on developing and mature B cells but not on plasma cells
CD20	Expressed on developing B cells after CD19 and retained on mature B cells
CD21	EBV receptor; present on all resting B cells
CD22	Present on all resting B cells
Primarily Monocyte- or Macrophage-Associated	
CD13	Expressed on immature and mature monocytes and granulocytes
CD14	Expressed on all monocytes
CD15	Expressed on all granulocytes
CD33	Expressed on myeloid progenitors and monocytes
Primarily NK Cell–Associated	
CD16	Present on all NK cells and granulocytes
CD56	Present on all NK cells and a subset of T cells
Primarily Stem Cell and Progenitor Cell–Associated	
CD34	Expressed on pluripotent stem cells and progenitor cells of many lineages
Present on All Leukocytes	
CD45	
CD11a	

CD = cluster designation; NK = natural killer; CALLA = common acute lymphoblastic leukemia antigen; EBV = Epstein-Barr virus.

these patients have generalized lymphadenopathy with mild-to-moderate enlargement of the liver and spleen; the associated symptoms are mild, and prolonged survival is usual. Approximately 20% of patients have a monoclonal gammopathy; others have hypogammaglobulinemia with increased susceptibility to bacterial infections.

Phenotypically, these tumors resemble a rare subset of B cells. Like mature B cells, they express surface immunoglobulin (Ig), CD19, CD20, and CD21. However, they also express CD5, a molecule found on all T cells and a very small subset of normal B cells.

Follicular Lymphomas

There are two cytologic subgroups of low-grade follicular lymphomas: follicular small cleaved cell and follicular mixed cell type. *Follicular small cleaved cell lymphoma* is the archetype of follicular lymphomas and the most common form of follicular NHL.

MORPHOLOGY. The neoplastic B cells tend to recapitulate normal lymphoid follicles, and hence they resemble the cells seen within normal germinal centers (Fig. 14–9). Small cleaved cells are slightly larger than normal lymphocytes, with scanty cytoplasm. **The most distinctive feature that differentiates the tumor cells from small normal lymphocytes is their irregular "cleaved" nuclear contour, characterized by prominent clefts, indentations, and linear infoldings.** The nuclear chromatin is coarse and condensed, and nucleoli are indistinct. Mitoses are infrequent. In addition to the small cleaved lymphocyte, there may be scattered large cleaved or noncleaved cells within the nodule, but they account for no more than 20% of the cells. **When the frequency of large cells exceeds 20% but is less than 50%, the term "follicular mixed small cleaved and large cell" is used.** Follicular, mixed lymphomas constitute a small proportion of all follicular center cell tumors.

Immunophenotypically, as might be expected from their morphologic similarity to germinal center cells, the neoplastic B cells in all follicular lymphomas express surface Ig and other B cell antigens, such as CD10, CD19, CD20, and CD21. In most cases, the cells also express B-cell activation antigens, such as CD17 and CD25. Unlike in SLL, CD5 is not expressed.

Clinically, the low-grade follicular lymphomas form a distinct clinicopathologic group that differs in several respects from the more aggressive large cell lymphomas. They constitute approximately 40% of adult NHLs in the United States and are characterized by the following features.[5]

- They occur predominantly in older individuals (rarely in persons younger than 40 years of age). The median age at diagnosis is 50 to 60 years.
- They affect males and females equally.
- They present with painless lymphadenopathy, which is frequently generalized. Nodal masses do not usually invade adjacent soft tissues. Involvement of extranodal sites, such as the gastrointestinal tract, central nervous system, or testis, is quite uncommon. However, bone marrow is frequently involved (75% of cases) at the time of diagnosis.
- Peripheral blood involvement in the form of frank leukemia is less common than in SLL, but small clonal B-cell populations can be detected in most cases by flow cytometry or molecular techniques.
- In the majority of patients (about 85%), tumor cells reveal a characteristic translocation, t(14;18). The breakpoint on chromosome 18 in-

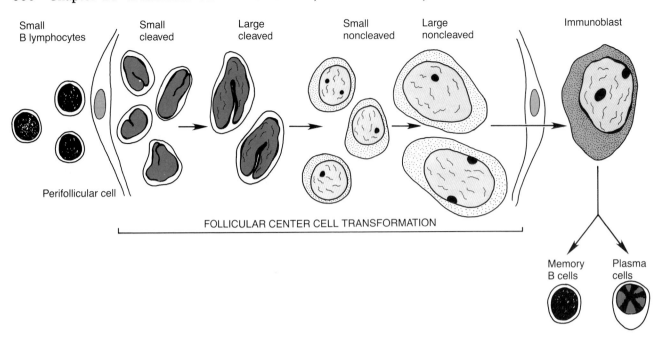

Figure 14-7. Schematic representation of normal antigen-induced transformation of B cells in the germinal centers of lymphoid follicles. (Drawn after Lukes, R.J., et al.: Immunologic approach to non-Hodgkin's lymphoma and related leukemias: Analysis of the result of multiparameter studies of 425 cases. Semin. Hematol. *15*:322, 1978.) Some authors (Weisenburger, D.D., et al.: Pathol. Annu. *25*:99, 1990) consider noncleaved cells to be the precursors of cleaved cells.

volves 18q21, where the *bcl*-2 gene has been mapped. The significance of this translocation was discussed previously (see Chapter 7).

• Follicular lymphomas have a long natural history (median survival 7 to 9 years) that appears to be largely unaffected by treatment. It seems virtually impossible to eradicate these indolent tumors.

• In time, follicular lymphomas progress to a diffuse high-grade histologic type, with or without treatment. Such a transition usually occurs in approximately 30% of cases, especially in those with a high proportion of large cells, and most likely represents the emergence of an aggressive

Table 14-2. A WORKING FORMULATION OF NON-HODGKIN'S LYMPHOMAS FOR CLINICAL USAGE

WORKING FORMULATION

Low-Grade
Small lymphocytic
Follicular, predominantly small cleaved cell
Follicular, mixed small cleaved and large cell

Intermediate-Grade
Follicular, predominantly large cell
Diffuse, small cleaved cell
Diffuse, mixed small and large cell
Diffuse, large cell

High-Grade
Large cell, immunoblastic
Lymphoblastic
Small noncleaved cell

Miscellaneous

subclone of the neoplastic B cells. Median survival is less than 1 year after such transformation.[6]

Intermediate-Grade Lymphomas

There are four tumors in this category of the Working Formulation, one with a follicular architecture and the other three with a diffuse pattern. The diffuse intermediate-grade lymphomas are distinguished on the basis of their cellular composition.

Follicular, Predominantly Large Cell Lymphoma

This is an uncommon tumor and represents less than 15% of all follicular NHLs.

MORPHOLOGY. In contrast to the low-grade follicular lymphomas, the majority of the neoplastic cells are large, with cleaved or noncleaved nuclei. Mitotic figures are also more numerous.

Clinically these tumors are very prone to evolving into diffuse large cell lymphomas early in their course and have a poorer prognosis than the vast majority of follicular lymphomas.

Diffuse Small Cleaved Cell Lymphoma

This type is composed of small cleaved cells that are morphologically and phenotypically similar to

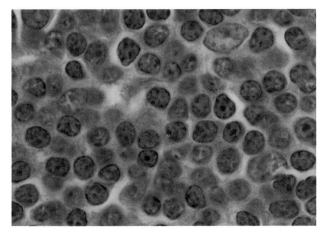

Figure 14–8. Non-Hodgkin's lymphoma, small lymphocytic type. Cytology is that of mature, uniform, unstimulated lymphocytes. (Courtesy of Dr. José Hernandez, Department of Pathology, University of Texas Southwestern Medical School, Dallas.)

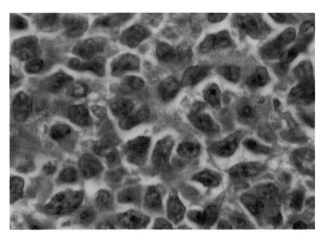

Figure 14–9. Non-Hodgkin's lymphoma, follicular small cleaved cell type. At this magnification the follicular architecture is not seen. Nuclei are irregular with indentations and marked angularity. (Courtesy of Dr. José Hernandez, Department of Pathology, University of Texas Southwestern Medical School, Dallas.)

those that are present in the follicular small cleaved cell lymphoma. They express sIg, pan B-cell antigens, and, in many cases, CD10. In contrast to follicular lymphomas of similar histologic type, these tumors have a higher male-to-female ratio and a median survival in the range of 2 to 4 years rather than 7 to 9 years. As compared with that in the United States, the incidence of these tumors is higher in Europe, particularly in Italy.

In recent years a phenotypically and genetically distinct subgroup of diffuse small cleaved cell lymphomas, variously called "centrocytic lymphoma," "mantle zone lymphoma," and "intermediately differentiated lymphocytic lymphoma," has been identified. This tumor is believed to arise from the mantle zone of lymphoid follicles rather than from follicular center cells. These tumors express pan B-cell antigens, but they can be distinguished from follicular center cells by the absence of CD10 and the presence of CD5 antigens. Further distinctiveness is conferred by the frequent occurrence of a t(11;14) translocation involving the Ig locus on chromosome 14 and the *bcl*-1 or *PRAD*-1 locus on chromosome 11. This locus encodes cyclin D1, a proto-oncogene involved in the regulation of cell cycle.[7]

Diffuse Mixed Small and Large Cell Lymphoma

This is an uncommon form of intermediate-grade lymphoma.

MORPHOLOGY. These tumors contain a mixture of small cleaved cells already described and large cells that may be cleaved or noncleaved. The nuclei of **large cleaved cells** are irregular in contour, indented, and larger than nuclei of normal histio-

cytes or endothelial cells (often used as a reference in evaluating size). The nuclear chromatin is slightly more dispersed than in a normal small lymphocyte, and nucleoli are inconspicuous. The cytoplasm is scant and pale. **Large noncleaved cells** are up to four times the size of normal lymphocytes, with a round or oval nucleus and one to two prominent nucleoli (Fig. 14–10). The nuclear chromatin is vesicular, and mitoses are prominent. The amount of cytoplasm is greater than in large cleaved cells and stains pale blue.

Diffuse Large Cell Lymphoma

This variant is the most common of intermediate-grade lymphomas. Morphologically, these tumors

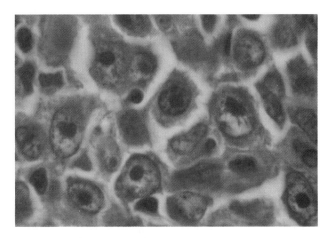

Figure 14–10. Non-Hodgkin's lymphoma, diffuse large cell type. Tumor cells have large nuclei (compare with Figures 14–8 and 14–9) and prominent nucleoli. (Courtesy of Dr. José Hernandez, Department of Pathology, University of Texas Southwestern Medical School, Dallas.)

contain predominantly large cells of the cleaved and noncleaved types described above. It should be noted that the distinction between diffuse large cell lymphomas and the diffuse mixed variant is difficult and somewhat arbitrary. The two are merely different morphologic expressions within the spectrum of large cell lymphomas. Although classified as intermediate-grade lymphomas, the clinical and immunophenotypic features of these two variants are akin to those of the high-grade large cell immunoblastic lymphoma and will therefore be described in the next section.

High-Grade Lymphomas

Three fairly distinct lymphomas fall into this category: (1) large cell immunoblastic lymphomas; (2) lymphoblastic lymphoma, a tumor that occurs in adolescents and is associated with a characteristic clinical presentation; and (3) small noncleaved lymphomas, which include Burkitt's lymphoma and related B-cell neoplasms. Of these, large cell immunoblastic lymphomas are clinically indistinguishable from the diffuse mixed small and large cell lymphomas, and diffuse large cell lymphomas. The remaining two are quite distinct from each other as well as from the rest of the aggressive lymphomas.

Large Cell Immunoblastic Lymphoma

These lymphomas display a wide range of morphologic features.

> **MORPHOLOGY.** In some cases the tumor cells have **plasmacytoid features.** These cells are four to five times larger than small lymphocytes and have a round or oval large nucleus that appears vesicular owing to margination of chromatin at the nuclear membrane. One or two centrally placed prominent nucleoli are usually seen. In other cases, the tumor cells may contain **large multilobated (polymorphous) nuclei,** or the nucleus may be round with a **clear cytoplasm.** Although features such as plasmacytoid appearance and clear cytoplasm or polymorphous nucleus are suggestive of B and T immunoblasts, respectively, these distinctions are not absolute.

Phenotypically, immunoblastic lymphomas and the related diffuse mixed large and small cell lymphomas and diffuse large cell lymphomas are heterogeneous. Approximately 80% are of B-cell origin; most of the remaining are T-cell tumors. Only rare tumors have markers of macrophages. As expected, all B-cell tumors in this group express sIg and the pan B-cell markers CD19 and CD20, but the expression of B-cell activation antigens is variable. The T-cell tumors express CD3, CD2, and either CD4 or CD8. They lack the immature T-cell marker CD1.

Large cell immunoblastic lymphomas and the diffuse large cell and mixed lymphomas described earlier share several clinicopathologic features that differentiate them from follicular lymphomas. Collectively they are sometimes referred to as diffuse large cell lymphomas.

- They constitute 40 to 50% of adult NHLs; approximately one-half have the diffuse large cell morphology. There is a slight male predominance, with a median age of about 60 years. However, the age range is much wider than in follicular lymphomas, and diffuse NHLs constitute about 20% of childhood lymphomas.
- In contrast to patients with follicular lymphomas, patients with these tumors typically present with a rapidly enlarging, often symptomatic mass at a single nodal or extranodal site. Localized disease and extranodal manifestations are more common than in follicular lymphomas. Indeed, involvement of the gastrointestinal tract, skin, bone, or brain may be the presenting feature. The Waldeyer's ring of oropharyngeal lymphoid tissue is involved in about 50% of these cases.
- Involvement of liver and spleen is not common at the time of diagnosis, but when it occurs, the lymphoma cells form large destructive masses, rather than forming the uniform miliary nodules that involve B-cell areas in low-grade follicular lymphomas.
- Bone marrow involvement is relatively uncommon in these patients, especially at the time of diagnosis. With progressive disease, however, the marrow may be involved, and, rarely, a leukemic picture may emerge.
- Approximately 50% of B-immunoblastic lymphomas are associated with a previous history of an immunologic disorder such as Sjögren's syndrome or Hashimoto's thyroiditis or with states of immunosuppression as in renal allograft recipients and patients with acquired immunodeficiency syndrome (AIDS). These monoclonal neoplasms seem to evolve from polyclonal B-cell proliferations.
- These three diffuse lymphomas are aggressive tumors that are rapidly fatal if untreated. However, with intensive combination chemotherapy, complete remission can be achieved in 60 to 80% of the patients, and approximately 50% remain free from disease for several years and may be considered cured. This favorable response is related to the fact that these tumors have a high growth fraction, and most anticancer agents act on cells that are actively dividing (see Chapter 7). In contrast, it should be recalled that although follicular lymphomas follow an indolent course, they are very difficult to cure.
- Despite impressive advances in accurate identification of the cell of origin and morphologic subclassification of these lymphomas, most studies have failed to show any significant correlation

between cytologic subtype, immunologic phenotype, and response to therapy.

Lymphoblastic Lymphoma (LL)

This is a distinct clinicopathologic entity closely related to T-cell acute lymphoblastic leukemia (T-ALL).

> **MORPHOLOGY.** The tumor cells resemble the lymphoblasts of ALL. They are fairly uniform in size, with scanty cytoplasm and nuclei that are somewhat larger than those of small lymphocytes. The nuclear chromatin is delicate and finely stippled, and nucleoli are either absent or inconspicuous. In many, but not all, cases the nuclear membrane shows deep subdivision, imparting a convoluted (lobulated) appearance. In keeping with its aggressive growth, the tumor shows a high rate of mitosis, and as with other tumors having a high mitotic rate (e.g., Burkitt's lymphomas), a "starry sky" pattern is produced by the interspersed benign macrophages.

Lymphoblastic lymphoma predominantly affects males (2:1); most patients are younger than 20 years of age; however, adults with this disease have been described. Although it constitutes less than 5% of all NHLs, approximately 40% of cases of childhood lymphoma fall into this category. A very characteristic clinical feature is the presence of a prominent mediastinal mass in 50 to 70% of patients at the time of diagnosis, suggesting a thymic origin. The disease is rapidly progressive, and early dissemination to the bone marrow and thence to blood and meninges leads to the evolution of a picture resembling T-ALL. Until recently, the prognosis was grim, but recent attempts to treat this tumor aggressively by utilizing protocols effective in ALL have produced encouraging results.

In keeping with their thymic origin, the phenotype of the tumor cells resembles intrathymic T cells. Terminal deoxynucleotidyl transferase, an enzyme associated with primitive lymphoid cells, is expressed in all cases. In some patients the cells are CD1+, CD2+, CD5+, and CD7+, as are early thymocytes, whereas in others CD4 and CD8 are coexpressed on tumor cells (see Fig. 14–4). The latter is noteworthy because CD4 and CD8 are never expressed together on mature peripheral T cells. In many cases surface CD3 expression is lacking, but cytoplasmic CD3 is present.

Small Noncleaved Cell Lymphoma

Within this category fall Burkitt's lymphoma, endemic in Africa, and related tumors seen outside Africa. Histologically, the African and nonendemic diseases are identical, although there are clinical and virologic differences. The relationship of these disorders to the Epstein-Barr virus (EBV) is discussed in Chapter 7.

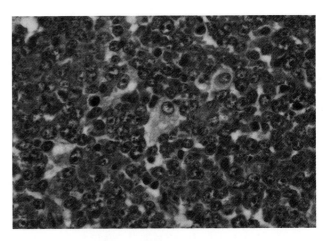

Figure 14–11. Burkitt's lymphoma. Tumor cells have multiple small nucleoli and high mitotic index. The lack of significant variation in nuclear shape and size lends a monotonous appearance interrupted by pale-staining, benign tissue macrophages, which impart a "starry sky" appearance better appreciated at a lower magnification. (Courtesy of Dr. José Hernandez, Department of Pathology, University of Texas Southwestern Medical School, Dallas.)

> **MORPHOLOGY.** These tumors consist of a sea of strikingly monotonous cells, 10 to 25 μm in diameter, with round or oval nuclei containing two to five prominent nucleoli. The nuclear size approximates that of benign macrophages within the tumor. There is a moderate amount of faintly basophilic or amphophilic cytoplasm, which also is intensely pyroninophilic and often contains small, lipid-filled vacuoles (better appreciated on stained imprints of the tumor). A high mitotic index is very characteristic, as is cell death, accounting for the presence of numerous tissue macrophages with ingested nuclear debris. Since these benign macrophages, which are diffusely distributed among the tumor cells, are often surrounded by a clear space, they create a "starry sky" pattern (Fig. 14–11).

These B-cell tumors resemble activated germinal center B cells. They express surface IgM, pan B-cell markers, and CD10. The African cases are CD21 positive, whereas the majority of the sporadic cases are CD21 negative. Both the African and the non-African cases are found largely in children or young adults, accounting for approximately 30% of childhood NHLs in the United States. In both forms, the disease rarely arises in the lymph nodes. In African cases, involvement of the maxilla or mandible is the common mode of presentation (Fig. 14–12), whereas abdominal tumors (bowel, retroperitoneum, ovaries) are more common in cases seen in America. Leukemic transformation of Burkitt's lymphoma is uncommon, especially in African cases. These tumors respond well to aggressive chemotherapy, and long remissions have been reported. Although relapse occurs

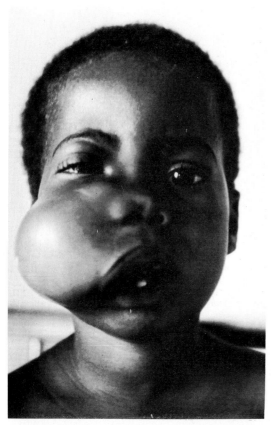

Figure 14–12. Burkitt's lymphoma in a nine-year-old child. The maxillary tumor mass is a characteristic presentation of this disease in Africa.

in many cases, many long-term survivors can be expected with present methods of treatment.

Miscellaneous

This group includes several tumors such as the rare true histiocytic lymphomas and some that cannot be readily assigned to any one of the other categories. Only two, both of which are of T-cell origin, will be described here because each is associated with a rather distinct clinical presentation.

Mycosis Fungoides and Sézary Syndrome

These tumors of peripheral CD4+ T cells are characterized by the involvement of skin and therefore belong to the group of *cutaneous T cell lymphomas.*

Clinically, the cutaneous lesions of *mycosis fungoides* show three somewhat distinct stages, discussed later (see Chapter 26). Briefly, mycosis fungoides presents with an inflammatory premycotic phase and progresses through a plaque phase to a tumor phase. *Histologically, there is infiltration of the epidermis and upper dermis by neoplastic T cells, which have an extremely unusual cerebriform nucleus,* characterized by marked infolding of the

nuclear membrane. In most patients with progressive disease, extracutaneous manifestations, characterized by nodal and visceral dissemination, appear. *Sézary syndrome* is a related condition in which skin involvement is manifested clinically as a generalized exfoliative erythroderma, but *in contrast to mycosis fungoides, the skin lesions rarely proceed to tumefaction.* Instead, there is an associated leukemia of "Sézary" cells that have the same cerebriform appearance noted in the tissue infiltrates of mycosis fungoides. Circulating Sézary cells can also be identified in up to 25% of cases of mycosis fungoides in the plaque or tumor phase, indicating that the two diseases have much in common. These are indolent tumors with a median survival rate of 8 to 9 years. A relationship between mycosis fungoides and HTLV-1 and HTLV-2 infection has been suggested but has not yet been widely confirmed.[8]

Adult T-Cell Leukemia/Lymphoma

This T-cell neoplasm caused by infection with a retrovirus, human T-cell leukemia virus type 1 (HTLV-1), is endemic in southern Japan and the Caribbean basin, but similar cases have been found sporadically elsewhere, including the southeastern United States. The pathogenesis of this tumor was discussed in Chapter 7. It should be noted that in addition to causing lymphoid malignancies, HTLV-1 infection can also give rise to a progressive demyelinating disease that affects the central nervous system and the spinal cord (see Chapter 29).

Adult T-cell leukemia/lymphoma is characterized by skin lesions, generalized lymphadenopathy, hepatosplenomegaly, hypercalcemia, and an elevated leukocyte count with multilobed CD4+ lymphocytes. The leukemic cells constitutively express high levels of receptors for interleukin 2 (IL-2). Therefore, targeting of the IL-2 receptor with antibody-toxin conjugates is being tested as a therapeutic approach to this malignancy. In the vast majority of cases this is an extremely aggressive disease, with a median survival time of about 8 months. Approximately 15 to 20% of patients follow a chronic course: their disease is clinically indistinguishable from cutaneous T-cell lymphomas.

DIAGNOSIS AND STAGING. The diagnosis of NHLs can be suspected from the clinical features, but *histologic examination of the node is required for diagnosis.* Definite assignment of lymphomas to T- or B-cell lineage is accomplished by immunotyping and by analysis of T- and B-receptor gene rearrangements.[9] DNA hybridization studies also aid in the distinction between monoclonal (neoplastic) and polyclonal (reactive) proliferations of lymphocytes. Because neoplastic lymphocytes are associated with unique (clonal) gene rearrangements, the pattern of rearrangement can be used as a clonal tumor marker. This can be exploited to de-

Table 14–3. CLINICAL STAGES OF HODGKIN'S AND NON-HODGKIN'S LYMPHOMAS (ANN ARBOR CLASSIFICATION)*

STAGE	DISTRIBUTION OF DISEASE
I	Involvement of a single lymph node region (I) or involvement of a single extralymphatic organ or site (I_E).
II	Involvement of two or more lymph node regions on the same side of the diaphragm alone (II) or with involvement of limited contiguous extralymphatic organ or tissue (II_E).
III	Involvement of lymph node regions on both sides of the diaphragm (III), which may include the spleen (III_S) and/or limited contiguous extralymphatic organ or site (III_E, III_ES).
IV	Multiple or disseminated foci of involvement of one or more extralymphatic organs or tissues with or without lymphatic involvement.

* All stages are further divided on the basis of the absence (A) or presence (B) of the following systemic symptoms: significant fever, night sweats, and/or unexplained weight loss of greater than 10% of normal body weight.

From Carbone, P.T., et al.: Symposium (Ann Arbor): Staging in Hodgkin's disease. Cancer Res. 31:1707, 1971.

tect minimal residual disease after treatment or recurrences before they become clinically manifest.[10]

A form of clinical staging developed for Hodgkin's disease (see Table 14–3) is often used for NHL. However, it is much less useful in NHL, since the correlation between the anatomic extent of the disease and the prognosis is less well established. For example, small lymphocytic lymphoma (SLL) is generally disseminated when the patient is first seen, but the prognosis in this case is excellent. Furthermore, the pattern of spread of NHL, unlike that in Hodgkin's disease, is less predictable, and hence the utility of clinical staging is diminished.

A summary of the salient clinicopathologic features of NHLs is presented in Table 14–4.

HODGKIN'S DISEASE

Hodgkin's disease, like NHL, is a disorder involving primarily the lymphoid tissues.[11] It arises almost invariably in a single node or chain of nodes and spreads characteristically to the anatomically contiguous nodes. Nevertheless, it is separated from NHL for several reasons. First, it is characterized morphologically by the presence of distinctive neoplastic giant cells called Reed-Sternberg (RS) cells, admixed with a variable inflammatory infiltrate. Second, it is often associated with somewhat distinctive clinical features, including systemic manifestations such as fever. Finally, the target cell of neoplastic transformation has yet to be identified with certainty. It accounts for 0.7% of all new cancers in the United States (which amounts to approximately 7400 new cases per

year). Although overall it is an uncommon form of cancer, its importance stems from the fact that it is one of the most common forms of malignancy in young adults, with an average age at diagnosis of 32 years. Happily, tremendous progress has been made in the treatment of this disease in the last two decades, and it is now considered to be curable in most cases.

CLASSIFICATION. According to the widely used Rye classification there are four subtypes of Hodgkin's disease: (1) *lymphocyte predominance*, (2) *mixed cellularity*, (3) *lymphocyte depletion*, and (4) *nodular sclerosis*. Before delineating them, however, we should describe the common denominator among all—the RS cell—and the method used to characterize the extent of the disease in a patient —namely, the staging system.

MORPHOLOGY. A distinctive tumor giant cell known as the Reed-Sternberg (RS) cell is considered to be the essential neoplastic element in all forms of Hodgkin's disease, and its identification is essential for the histologic diagnosis. **Classically, it is a large cell (15 to 45 μm in diameter), most often binucleate or bilobed, with two halves often appearing as mirror images of each other** (Fig. 14–13). **At other times there are multiple nuclei, or the single nucleus is multilobate and polypoid. The nucleus is enclosed within an abundant amphophilic cytoplasm. Prominent within the nuclei are large, inclusion-like, "owl-eyed" nucleoli generally surrounded by a clear halo.** In typical RS cells the nucleoli are acidophilic or, at the least, amphophilic, and react strongly with RNA stains. Several variant forms of RS cells, including uninucleate cells and multinucleate giant cells, have been described, but they are not diagnostic. One variant, the so-called **lacunar cell,** is encountered primarily within one of the distinctive patterns of Hodgkin's disease, called nodular sclerosis.

It is somewhat anticlimactic to report that cells closely simulating or identical with RS cells have been identified in conditions other than Hodgkin's disease. RS-like cells have been found in infectious mononucleosis and in solid tissue cancers, mycosis fungoides, lymphomas, and other conditions. Thus, although RS cells are requisite for the diagnosis, they must be present in an appropriate background of non-neoplastic inflammatory cells (lymphocytes, plasma cells, eosinophils). Stated another way, **the RS cell is necessary but not sufficient for the diagnosis.**

The *staging of Hodgkin's disease* (see Table 14–3) is of great clinical importance, since the course, choice of therapy, and prognosis all are intimately related to the distribution of the disease. Staging involves not only a careful physical examination but also several investigative procedures,

Table 14–4. SUMMARY OF NON-HODGKIN'S LYMPHOMAS

LYMPHOMA TYPE OR GROUP	% (IN ADULTS)	SALIENT MORPHOLOGY	IMMUNOPHENOTYPE	COMMENTS
Small Lymphocytic Lymphoma (SLL)	3–4	Small unstimulated lymphocytes in a diffuse pattern	>95% B cells	Occurs in old age; generalized lymphadenopathy with marrow involvement and blood picture resembling CLL; indolent course with prolonged survival
Follicular Lymphomas	40	Germinal center cells arranged in a follicular pattern	B cells	Follicular small cleaved cell type most common; occur in older patients; generalized lymphadenopathy; associated with t(14;18); leukemia less common than in SLL; indolent course but difficult to cure
*Diffuse Lymphomas**	40–50	Various cell types; predominantly large germinal center cells; some mixed with smaller cells; others with immunoblastic morphology	~80% B cells ~20% post-thymic T cells	Occur in older patients as well as pediatric age group; greater frequency of extranodal, visceral disease; marrow involvement and leukemia very uncommon at diagnosis and poor prognostic sign; aggressive tumors but up to 60% are curable
Lymphoblastic Lymphoma	4	Cells somewhat larger than lymphocytes; in many cases nuclei markedly lobulated; high mitotic rate	>95% immature intrathymic T cells	Occurs predominantly in children (40% of all childhood lymphomas); prominent mediastinal mass; early involvement of bone marrow and progression to T-cell ALL; very aggressive
Small Noncleaved (Burkitt's) Lymphoma	<1	Cells intermediate in size between small lymphocytes and immunoblasts; prominent nucleoli; high mitotic rate	B cells	Endemic in Africa, sporadic elsewhere; predominantly affects children; extranodal visceral involvements presenting features; rapidly progressive but responsive to therapy; t(8;14) translocation characteristic
Mycosis Fungoides and Sézary Syndrome	Uncommon	Medium to large cells with markedly convoluted (cerebriform) nucleus	CD4+ T cells	Occur in older males; proclivity for involvement of skin in both forms; tumorous masses in mycosis fungoides; Sézary syndrome is leukemic variant
Adult T-Cell Leukemia/ Lymphoma	Rare	Very variable; cells may have cerebriform nuclei	CD4+ T cells	Associated with HTLV-1 infection; endemic in Japan and the Caribbean; cutaneous lesions, leukemia, spleen and lymph node involvement; rapidly fatal

* Includes diffuse large cell, diffuse mixed, and large cell immunoblastic lymphomas of the Working Formulation. Other NHLs with diffuse pattern, e.g., lymphoblastic lymphomas, that form distinct clinicopathologic categories not included.
  CLL = chronic lymphocytic leukemia; ALL = acute lymphoblastic leukemia.

including lymphangiography (or computed tomography of abdomen and pelvis), chest radiograph, biopsy of the bone marrow, and ultrasonography of liver and spleen. Staging laparotomy, which allows direct visualization of the intra-abdominal nodes, liver biopsy, and removal of the spleen, is now used infrequently.[12] The more aggressive the variant of the disease, the greater the probability that it will be in a more advanced stage at the time of diagnosis.

With this background we can turn to the morphologic classification of Hodgkin's disease into its subgroups and point out some of the salient clinical features of each. Later the manifestations common to all will be presented. The essential morphologic feature that serves to differentiate three subgroups

(lymphocyte predominance, mixed cellularity, and lymphocyte depletion) is the frequency of the neoplastic elements (RS cells) relative to the reactive elements, represented by small lymphocytes. The natural history of untreated Hodgkin's disease appears to be related to the ratio of RS cells to lymphocytes. The fourth subgroup, nodular sclerosis, appears to represent a special expression of the disease and has distinctive clinicopathologic features. The relative frequency of the four histologic subtypes may be gleaned from Table 14–5.

LYMPHOCYTE PREDOMINANCE HODGKIN'S DISEASE.
This uncommon variant, accounting for approximately 6% of all cases, is characterized by a dif-

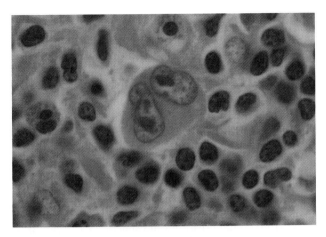

Figure 14–13. Hodgkin's disease. A binucleate Reed-Sternberg cell with prominent inclusion-like nucleoli is surrounded by dark-staining lymphocytes. (Courtesy of Dr. José Hernandez, Department of Pathology, University of Texas Southwestern Medical School, Dallas.)

Figure 14–14. Hodgkin's disease, lymphocyte-predominance type. A low-power view shows that numerous lymphocytes have diffusely infiltrated the node. (Courtesy of Dr. José Hernandez, Department of Pathology, University of Texas Southwestern Medical School, Dallas.)

fuse or sometimes vaguely nodular infiltrate of mature lymphocytes admixed with variable numbers of benign histiocytes (Fig. 14–14). Typical RS cells are extremely difficult to find. More common are variant cells that have a delicate, multilobed, puffy nucleus that has been likened in appearance to popcorn ("popcorn cell") or to elephant feet.[13] Other cells such as eosinophils, neutrophils, and plasma cells are scanty or absent, and there is little evidence of necrosis or fibrosis. A majority of patients are males, usually younger than 35 years of age, and they present with limited disease (Table 14–5). The prognosis is excellent.

The nodular form of the lymphocyte predominance pattern has more than a superficial resemblance to nodular NHLs; indeed, as discussed later, many cases of lymphocyte predominance are actually tumors of B cells.[14]

MIXED CELLULARITY HODGKIN'S DISEASE. This is the second most common form of Hodgkin's disease. It occupies an intermediate clinical position between the lymphocyte predominance and the lymphocyte depletion patterns. Typical RS cells are plentiful, but there are fewer lymphocytes than in lymphocyte predominance disease. The involvement of the lymph nodes is almost always diffuse. This pattern of Hodgkin's disease is rendered distinctive by its heterogeneous cellular infiltrate, which includes eosinophils, plasma cells, and benign histiocytes. Small areas of necrosis and fibrosis may be present, but they are usually not as prominent as in the lymphocyte depletion type. The mixed cellularity form of Hodgkin's disease is also more common in males.

Although the disease may be diagnosed in any of the clinical states, as compared with the lymphocyte predominance pattern, more patients present with disseminated disease, and these patients more often have systemic manifestations (see Table 14–5).

LYMPHOCYTE DEPLETION HODGKIN'S DISEASE. This least common form of Hodgkin's disease is characterized by a paucity of lymphocytes and a relative abundance of RS cells or their pleomorphic variants. It presents in two morphologic forms, the so-called **diffuse fibrosis** and the **reticular variants.** In the former, the node is hypocellular and is replaced largely by a proteinaceous fibrillar material. Pleomorphic histiocytes, a few typical and atypical RS cells, and some lymphocytes are scattered within the fibrillar material (Fig. 14–15). The reticular variant is much more cellular and is composed of highly anaplastic, large, pleomorphic cells that resemble RS cells. Only a few typical RS cells can be recognized. A majority of patients with the lymphocyte depletion pattern are older males, have disseminated involvement (see Table 14–5), present with systemic manifestations, and have an aggressive form of the disease.

Table 14–5. PERCENTAGE OF PATIENTS IN EACH PATHOLOGIC STAGE ACCORDING TO HISTOLOGIC SUBTYPE

| HISTOLOGIC SUBTYPE | NUMBER OF PATIENTS | PATHOLOGIC STAGE (%) | | |
		I and II	III	IV
Lymphocyte predominance	55	76	22	2
Mixed cellularity	215	44	47	9
Lymphocyte depletion	21	19	62	19
Nodular sclerosis	628	60	35	5

From Desforges, J.F., et al.: Hodgkin's disease. N. Engl. J. Med. *301*:1212, 1979. Reprinted by permission of the New England Journal of Medicine.

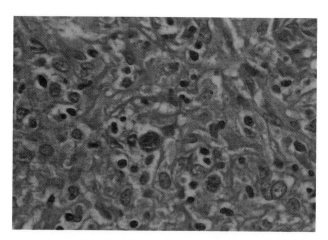

Figure 14-15. Hodgkin's disease, lymphocyte-depletion type. All cellular elements are greatly diminished. An atypical Reed-Sternberg cell is present in the center of the field. (Courtesy of Dr. José Hernandez, Department of Pathology, University of Texas Southwestern Medical School, Dallas.)

NODULAR SCLEROSIS HODGKIN'S DISEASE. This is the most common form of Hodgkin's disease. It is distinct from the other three forms, both clinically and histologically, and is characterized morphologically by two features. The first is the presence of a particular variant of the RS cell, the **lacunar cell** (Fig. 14-16). This cell is large and has a single hyperlobated nucleus with multiple small nucleoli and an abundant, pale-staining cytoplasm with well-defined borders. In formalin-fixed tissue, the cytoplasm of these cells often retracts, giving rise to the appearance of cells lying in clear spaces, or "lacunae." The other distinctive feature seen in most cases is the collagen bands that divide the lymphoid tissue into circumscribed nodules (see Fig. 14-16). The fibrosis may be scant or abundant, and the cellular infiltrate may show varying proportions of lymphocytes, eosinophils, and lacunar cells. Classic RS cells are infrequent.

Clinically, nodular sclerosis Hodgkin's disease has several distinctive features: It is the only form more common in women, and it has a striking propensity to involve the lower cervical, supraclavicular, and mediastinal lymph nodes. Most of the patients are adolescents or young adults, and they have an excellent prognosis, especially when seen in clinical stages I and II.

It is apparent that Hodgkin's disease spans a wide range of histologic patterns and that certain forms, with their characteristic fibrosis, eosinophils, neutrophils, and plasma cells, come deceptively close to simulating an inflammatory reactive process. **The diagnosis, then, of Hodgkin's disease rests solely on the unmistakable identification of RS cells in most variants and of the lacunar cells in the nodular sclerosis pattern.**

In all forms, involvement of the spleen, liver, bone marrow, and other organs and tissues may appear in due course and take the form of irregular, tumor-like nodules of tissue resembling that present in the nodes. At times the spleen is greatly enlarged and the liver is moderately enlarged by these nodular masses. At other times, the involvement is more subtle and becomes evident only on microscopic examination.

ETIOLOGY AND PATHOGENESIS. The origins of Hodgkin's disease are unknown. In the past it was believed that Hodgkin's disease was an unusual inflammatory reaction (possibly to an infectious agent) that behaved like a neoplasm. However, it is now widely accepted that Hodgkin's disease is a neoplastic disorder and that the RS cells or their variants represent the transformed cells. In all likelihood the inflammatory cells accumulate in response to cytokines secreted by the RS cells. Indeed, many cytokines, including IL-5, IL-4, tumor necrosis factor-alpha (TNF-α), GM-CSF, and transforming growth factor-beta (TGF-β), have been detected in Hodgkin's tissue. Of these, IL-5 secretion correlates with eosinophil accumulation (a feature of mixed cellularity and nodular sclerosis subtypes). TGF-β, a fibrogenic cytokine, is found almost exclusively in the nodular sclerosis variant, where it is produced by eosinophils.[15] It is of interest that despite the abundance of eosinophils in the mixed cellularity histologic type, there is little fibrosis, and TFG-β mRNA is not detected in the eosinophils. Thus it appears that the specific histologic pattern of Hodgkin's disease may be determined by the unique combination of cytokines secreted by RS cells and the non-neoplastic cellular infiltrate.

Although the neoplastic nature of RS cells seems to be accepted, the origin of these cells remains an enigma. Despite extensive histochemical, flow cytometric, and molecular studies no single immune cell has been incriminated as the target of transformation in all cases.[16] The body of information on this subject can be summarized as follows:

- Immunoenzymatic staining of RS cells has revealed staining with antigens specific for T cells (CD3, CD5, T-cell receptor-beta [TCR-β], and CD2), or, in some cases, specific for B cells (CD19 and CD20). In general, cells within the lymphocyte predominance type tend to stain with B-cell antigens, and these B cells reveal restricted light chain expression, suggesting monoclonality.
- Molecular analysis of T-cell receptor (TCR) and Ig gene rearrangements has revealed a similar dichotomy. In some cases, RS cells and cell lines derived from these cells show clonal rearrangements of Ig genes; in others, TCR-β and TCR-γ gene arrangements have been described.

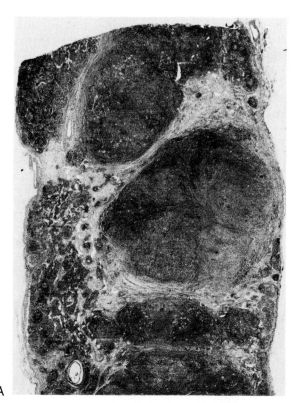
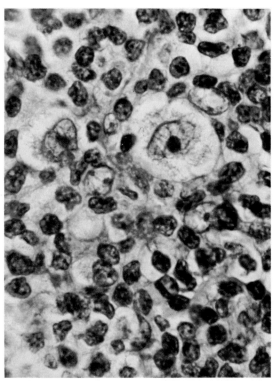

A   B

Figure 14–16. Hodgkin's disease—nodular sclerosis. *A*, Low-power view shows well-defined bands of collagen enclosing nodules of abnormal lymphoid tissue. *B*, High-power view shows the distinctive lacunar cell, so called because the cell appears to lie within a cleared space. (Low-magnification photograph courtesy of Dr. José Hernandez, Department of Pathology, University of Texas Southwestern Medical School, Dallas.)

- In virtually all cases of Hodgkin's disease, RS cells express lymphocyte activation antigens, such as HLA-DR, CD30, CD25, and CDw70.

The general consensus from these studies seems to be that Hodgkin's disease is histogenetically heterogeneous, arising in some cases from activated B cells and in others from T cells, but virtually never from cells of the mononuclear phagocyte series.

Given that lymphoid cells are the target of transformation, what causes the neoplastic change? For years EBV has been suspected as an etiologic agent on the basis of epidemiologic and serologic studies. Thus patients with a history of infectious mononucleosis or with elevated titers of antibodies against EBV antigens incur a slightly higher risk of Hodgkin's disease. The seroepidemiologic evidence has been bolstered by recent molecular studies.[17,18] EBV genomes can be identified in RS cells in 40 to 50% of cases, and in some parts of the world EBV RNA can be identified in virtually all cases.[19] More important, the EBV DNA is present in a clonal pattern, making it very unlikely that the virus infected RS cells after clonal expansion. Footprints of this virus are found most commonly in the mixed cellularity subtype and almost never in the lym-

phocyte predominance variant. While these studies provide considerable evidence for an association between EBV and Hodgkin's disease, they do not prove that EBV causes this disorder. Viral infection may be one of several steps involved in the pathogenesis of Hodgkin's disease.

To summarize, the accumulated phenotypic and molecular studies suggest that Hodgkin's disease is heterogeneous with respect to both the cell type involved and the etiologic agent(s). The nodular form of lymphocyte predominance type is clearly a B-cell neoplasm; others may arise from B cells or T cells. Evidence of EBV infection is present in some but not all cases. EBV-negative Hodgkin's disease may be linked to an as yet unidentified (microbial?) agent.

CLINICAL COURSE. Hodgkin's disease, like NHLs, usually presents with a painless enlargement of lymph nodes. Although a definitive distinction between Hodgkin's disease and NHLs can be made only by examination of a lymph node biopsy, several clinical features favor the diagnosis of Hodgkin's disease (Table 14–6). Younger patients, with the more favorable histologic types, tend to present in clinical stage I or II (see Table 14–5) and are usually free from systemic manifestations. Patients with disseminated disease (stages III and

Table 14–6. CLINICAL DIFFERENCES BETWEEN HODGKIN'S AND NON-HODGKIN'S LYMPHOMAS

HODGKIN'S DISEASE	NON-HODGKIN'S LYMPHOMA
More often localized to a single axial group of nodes (cervical, mediastinal, para-aortic)	More frequent involvement of multiple peripheral nodes
Orderly spread by contiguity	Noncontiguous spread
Mesenteric nodes and Waldeyer's ring rarely involved	Waldeyer's ring and mesenteric nodes commonly involved
Extranodal involvement uncommon	Extranodal involvement common

IV) are more likely to present with systemic complaints, such as fever, unexplained weight loss, pruritus, and anemia. As mentioned earlier, these patients generally have the histologically less favorable variants. Cutaneous anergy resulting from depressed cell-mediated immunity is seen in most cases. The basis of this immune dysfunction is poorly understood.

With modern treatment protocols tumor burden (i.e., stage) rather than histologic type is the most important prognostic variable. Currently the 5-year survival rate of patients with stages I and IIA is close to 90%, and many can be cured. Even with advanced disease (stages IVA and IVB), 60 to 70% 5-year disease-free survival can be achieved.[12]

Progress in the treatment of Hodgkin's disease has created a new set of problems. Long-term survivors of chemotherapy and radiotherapy have an increased risk of developing second cancers. Acute nonlymphocytic leukemia and lung cancer lead the list of second malignancies, but also included are NHL, breast cancer, gastric cancer, and malignant melanoma.[20] The many therapeutic steps forward, in the light of this unhappy byproduct, may involve a few steps backward.

LEUKEMIAS AND MYELOPROLIFERATIVE DISEASES

The leukemias are malignant neoplasms of the hematopoietic stem cells characterized by diffuse replacement of the bone marrow by neoplastic cells. In most cases, the leukemic cells spill over into the blood, where they may be seen in large numbers. These cells may also infiltrate the liver, spleen, lymph nodes, and other tissues throughout the body. Although the presence of excessive numbers of abnormal cells in the peripheral blood is the most dramatic manifestation of leukemia, it should be remembered that the leukemias are primary

disorders of the bone marrow. Indeed, some patients with a diffusely infiltrated bone marrow may present with leukopenia rather than leukocytosis.

CLASSIFICATION. Traditionally, leukemias are classified on the basis of the cell type involved and the state of maturity of the leukemic cells. Thus, *acute leukemias* are characterized by the presence of very immature cells (called blasts) and by a rapidly fatal course in untreated patients. On the other hand, *chronic leukemias* are associated, at least initially, with well-differentiated (mature) leukocytes and with a relatively indolent course. Two major variants of acute and chronic leukemias are recognized: *lymphocytic* and *myelocytic* (myelogenous). Thus, a simple classification would have four patterns of leukemia: acute lymphocytic leukemia (ALL), chronic lymphocytic leukemia (CLL), acute myelocytic (myeloblastic) leukemia (AML), and chronic myelocytic leukemia (CML). This simple and time-honored classification raises several difficulties when dealing with "chronic leukemias." Acute leukemias, despite differences in their cell of origin, share important morphologic and clinical features. They are associated with replacement of normal marrow elements by a sea of proliferating "blast cells" that do not seem to undergo normal maturation. Consequently, there is a loss of mature myeloid elements such as red cells, granulocytes, and platelets, and hence clinical features of acute leukemias are dominated by anemia, infections, and hemorrhages.

In contrast, the grouping together of chronic lymphocytic and myelogenous leukemias is problematic. A characteristic shared by these two disorders is that they are not rapidly fatal, but the clinical and morphologic features that seem to unite the acute leukemias are lacking. Furthermore, this traditional grouping of chronic leukemias has become less tenable with the knowledge that *chronic myelogenous leukemia (CML), polycythemia vera, essential thrombocytopenia, and myeloid metaplasia are related disorders that represent clonal, neoplastic proliferations of the multipotent myeloid stem cells* (see Fig. 13–1). If the erythrocytic precursors dominate, the resulting clinical disorder is classified as *polycythemia vera;* on the other hand, the dominance of granulocytic series is manifested as *chronic myeloid leukemia.* It seems that the term *chronic myeloproliferative disorders,* coined by Dameshek almost 50 years ago, best describes these neoplasms of the myeloid stem cell. Although the individual chronic myeloproliferative disorders have distinctive clinical features, interconversions and overlaps between members of this group are well known and further attest to their relatedness. For example, a patient may present initially with polycythemia vera, but over the years this may "convert" to myeloid metaplasia with myelofibrosis.

In analogy with chronic myeloproliferative disorders, it is possible to segregate chronic lympho-proliferative disorders. This group would include *chronic lymphocytic leukemia* and *hairy cell leukemia*, both representing neoplastic proliferations of lymphoid cells, most often of B-cell lineage. It will be apparent that as proliferative disorders of lymphoid cells, they are related to the non-Hodgkin's lymphomas already discussed. Indeed, as already mentioned, there is very little clinical or anatomic difference between CLL and small lymphocytic lymphomas.

Despite the conceptually appealing distinctions between myeloproliferative and lymphoproliferative disorders, in the ensuing discussion we shall follow a clinically oriented approach of segregating the acute and chronic leukemias from the chronic myeloproliferative disorders, such as polycythemia vera and myeloid metaplasia. Our discussion will focus initially on the distinctive pathophysiologic and clinical features of different forms of leukemias; it will be followed by the description of morphologic changes that are common to most leukemias, and, finally, a discussion of the etiology and pathogenesis of leukemias and lymphomas.

ACUTE LEUKEMIAS

As with all leukemias, the acute ones have their origin in neoplastic monoclonal proliferation of hematopoietic stem cells.

PATHOPHYSIOLOGY. Morphologic and cell kinetic studies have indicated that in acute leukemias there is a block in differentiation of leukemic stem cells and that the leukemic blasts have a prolonged rather than shortened generation time. *Thus, the accumulation of leukemic blasts in acute leukemia results from clonal expansion of transformed stem cells as well as a failure of maturation into functional end cells.* As the leukemic precursor cells (blasts) accumulate in the marrow, they suppress normal hematopoietic stem cells by physical replacement as well as by other, poorly understood mechanisms. Suppression of normal hematopoietic stem cells in acute leukemia has two important clinical implications: (1) the major manifestations result from the paucity of normal red cells, white cells, and platelets; and (2) therapeutically the aim is to reduce the population of the leukemic clone enough to allow recovery of normal stem cells. Another therapeutic approach, applicable to some leukemias, is to induce the differentiation of the leukemic blasts.

Leukemic transformation may affect any stage during the differentiation of pluripotent hematopoietic stem cells (see Fig. 13–1). Involvement of the lymphoid series gives rise to ALL, whereas neoplastic transformation of myeloid progenitor cells is expressed in the form of AML. Each of these two major subtypes is considered separately after a brief review of the clinical and laboratory features common to most forms of acute leukemias.

CLINICAL FEATURES. The acute leukemias have the following characteristics:

- *Abrupt stormy onset:* Most patients present within 3 months of the onset of symptoms.
- *Symptoms related to depression of normal marrow function:* fatigue due mainly to anemia; fever, reflecting an infection due to absence of mature leukocytes; bleeding (petechiae, ecchymoses, epistaxis, gum bleeding) secondary to thrombocytopenia.
- *Bone pain and tenderness,* resulting from marrow expansion with infiltration of the subperiosteum.
- *Organ infiltration, manifested by generalized lymphadenopathy, splenomegaly, and hepatomegaly.* They occur in all acute leukemias, but more commonly in ALL. Testicular involvement is also particularly common in ALL.
- *Central nervous system manifestations,* such as headache, vomiting, and nerve palsies resulting from meningeal spread; these features are more common in children than in adults, and more common in ALL than in AML.

LABORATORY FINDINGS. Anemia is almost always present. The white blood cell count is variably elevated, sometimes to more than 100,000 cells per microliter, but in about 50% of the patients is less than 10,000 cells per microliter. Much more important is the identification of immature white cells, including blast forms, in the circulating blood and the bone marrow, where they make up 60 to 100% of all the cells. The platelet count is usually depressed to less than 100,000 per microliter. Uncommonly, there is pancytopenia with few blast cells in the blood (aleukemic leukemia), but the bone marrow is nonetheless flooded with blasts, ruling out aplastic anemia. With this review we can turn to specific forms of acute leukemia.

Acute Lymphoblastic Leukemia (ALL)

Acute lymphoblastic leukemia is primarily a disease of children and young adults. Approximately 2500 new cases are diagnosed each year in the United States in individuals younger than 15 years of age; this constitutes 80% of childhood acute leukemias. ALL occurs in adults, but much less frequently. Childhood ALL has a peak incidence at approximately four years of age. It is almost twice as common in whites as in nonwhites and is slightly more frequent in boys than in girls.[21]

MORPHOLOGY. ALL can be subdivided by morphologic and immunologic criteria. Morphologic subtypes designated L1, L2, and L3 have been

Table 14–7. FAB CLASSIFICATION OF ACUTE LYMPHOBLASTIC LEUKEMIAS

CYTOLOGIC FEATURES*	L1	L2	L3
Cell Size	Small cells predominate	Large, heterogeneous in size	Large and homogeneous
Amount of Cytoplasm	Scant	Variable, often moderately abundant	Moderately abundant
Nucleoli	Not visible, or small and inconspicuous	One or more present, often large	One or more present, often prominent
Nuclear Chromatin	Homogeneous in any one case	Variable, heterogeneous in any one case	Finely stippled and homogeneous
Nuclear Shape	Regular, occasional clefting or indentation	Irregular, clefting and indentation	Regular, oval to round
Basophilia of Cytoplasm	Variable	Variable	Intensely basophilic
Cytoplasmic Vacuolation	Variable	Variable	Prominent

* The first three criteria are most useful for separating the two common classes of ALL, L1 and L2. Nuclear shape and chromatin characteristics are less useful because there is significant overlap between L1 and L2 in these parameters. Basophilia of cytoplasm and cytoplasmic vacuolation are especially useful in the identification of the least common type of ALL, L3.

defined in the French-American-British (FAB) classification of acute leukemias (Table 14–7). In approximately 85% of children with ALL, lymphoblasts are predominantly of the L1 subtype; fewer than 15% have L2 morphology, a subtype more commonly seen in adults. L3 ALL usually equates with leukemic manifestation of Burkitt's lymphoma and makes up approximately 1 to 2% of the lymphoblastic leukemias in children.

In addition to the morphologic features described in Table 14–7, it should be noted that leukemic lymphoblasts (in contrast to myeloblasts) do not contain peroxidase-positive granules but rather contain large aggregates of periodic acid–Schiff (PAS)–positive material. Staining for terminal deoxytransferase (TdT), a DNA polymerase, is also useful in differentiating ALL from AML because it is present in 95% of cases of ALL but only 5% of AML cases. TdT-negative ALLs are typically of the L3 type.

Immunologic subtypes are based on the origin of the leukemic lymphoblasts and their stage of differentiation. Because immunophenotyping has prognostic implications, it is detailed in Table 14–8 and summarized below:

- While the leukemic blasts express surface Ig in less than 2% of the patients, the vast majority of ALLs (80%) have proved to be of B cell origin.
- The leukemic blasts of almost every patient with B-cell ALL express the pan B-cell antigen CD19. In some patients with early precursor B-cell ALL, CD19 is the only B-cell specific marker on the leukemic cells.
- T lymphoblasts in patients with T-cell ALL seem to be arrested at early intrathymic stages of maturation. Thus, T-cell ALL is related to lympho-

blastic lymphoma but distinct from other T-cell neoplasms, such as adult T-cell leukemia/lymphoma and Sézary syndrome, in which the neoplastic cells express the mature peripheral T-cell phenotype. Like lymphoblastic lymphoma, T-cell ALL is often associated with a prominent mediastinal (thymic) mass.

- Except for mature B-cell ALL, which is typically associated with L3 morphology, there is no correlation between the morphologic and immunologic subtypes.

KARYOTYPIC CHANGES. Approximately 90% of patients with ALL have numerical or structural changes in the chromosomes of the leukemia cells. The more common changes and their clinical associations are listed in Table 14–9. In general, hyperdiploidy is a good prognostic indicator; all translocations are associated with poor prognosis, even when they occur in phenotypically favorable subgroups such as early pre–B-cell ALL. Hence such karyotypic information is considered valuable in designing therapeutic strategies.[22]

PROGNOSIS. Dramatic advances have been made in the treatment of ALL. With modern chemotherapy (which includes prophylactic kill of leukemic cells that find sanctuary in the CNS), more than 90% of children with ALL achieve complete remission, and approximately two-thirds can be considered cured. The prognosis is influenced by several factors, including age, immunophenotype, and cytogenetic changes as discussed. Briefly, ALL in children between two and ten years of age with early pre-B phenotype and hyperdiploidy in the range of 51 to 60 chromosomes has the most favorable outcome. Adults (with any phenotype) and children with the mature B phenotype or T-cell disease fare much less well. The presence of translocation worsens the prognosis in all groups. Allo-

Table 14–8. MAJOR IMMUNOLOGIC SUBTYPES OF ACUTE LYMPHOBLASTIC LEUKEMIA AND ASSOCIATED PROGNOSIS

SUBTYPE	PHENOTYPE	MORPHOLOGY	APPROXIMATE FREQUENCY (%)	PROGNOSIS*
Early pre-B		L1 or L2		Very good
CALLA (CD10) negative	DR+, sIg−, Cμ−, CD19+, CD10−		5–10	
CALLA positive	DR+, sIg−, Cμ−, CD19+, CD10+		55–60	
Pre-B	DR+, sIg−, Cμ+, CD19+, CD10+	L1 or L2	20	Intermediate
Mature B	DR+, sIg+, Cμ−, CD19+, CD10±	L3	1–2	Poor
Immature T	DR−, sIg−, CD19−, CD10−, T+	L1 or L2	15	Intermediate

* In all cases, the prognosis is worsened if there is an associated chromosomal translocation (see Table 14–9).

DR = HLA-DR (class II) antigens; sIg = surface immunoglobulin; Cμ = cytoplasmic μ chains; T = T-cells-associated antigens, e.g., CD2, CD5, CD7. CALLA = common acute lymphoblastic leukemia antigen, synonymous with CD10.

geneic bone marrow transplantation offers hope for those in poor prognostic categories.

Acute Myeloblastic Leukemia (AML)

Acute myeloblastic leukemias affect primarily adults between the ages of 15 and 39 years. They constitute only 20% of childhood leukemias. AML is extraordinarily heterogeneous, reflecting the complexities of myeloid cell differentiation.

MORPHOLOGY. In most cases myeloblasts can be readily distinguished from lymphoblasts in the usual Wright-Giemsa stain. Myeloblasts reveal delicate nuclear chromatin, three to five nucleoli, and fine, azurophilic, **myeloperoxidase-positive** granules in the cytoplasm (Fig. 14–17). Distinctive red-staining rod-like structures **(Auer rods)** are present in some cases, more often in the promyelocytic variant (Fig. 14–18). Monocytic differentiation is associated with staining for lysosomal nonspecific esterases. TdT is present in less than 5% of cases.

CLASSIFICATION. Acute myeloblastic leukemias are of diverse origin. Some arise by transformation of multipotent (trilineage) myeloid stem cells (see Fig. 13–1), as evidenced by common cytogenetic abnormalities in granulocytic and erythroid precursors, even though myeloblasts dominate the blood and bone marrow. In others the common granulocyte-monocyte precursor is involved, giving rise to myelomonocytic disease (Fig. 14–19). In the revised FAB classification (Table 14–10), AML is divided into eight categories.[23] This scheme takes into account both the degree of maturation (M0 to M3) and the predominant line of differentiation of the leukemic stem cells (M4 to M7). In view of the marked heterogeneity of this group of leukemias, some authorities prefer to use the term "acute nonlymphocytic leukemia" to encompass the varied morphologic expressions. Monoclonal antibodies that recognize determinants on various myelomonocytic cells are useful in the diagnosis of AML, especially when morphologic and histochemical features are equivocal (see Table 14–1).[24]

CHROMOSOMAL ABNORMALITIES. Special high-resolution banding techniques have revealed chromosomal abnormalities in approximately 90% of all

Table 14–9. SELECTED KARYOTYPIC CHANGES IN ACUTE LYMPHOBLASTIC LEUKEMIA AND ASSOCIATED FEATURES

NUMERIC CHANGES

Hyperdiploidy (>50 chromosomes)   Found in 25–30% of all childhood ALL, less common in adults with ALL; associated with favorable clinical features such as lower leukocyte counts, white race, age 2 to 10 years, and early pre-B phenotype

Pseudoploidy (46 chromosomes but with structural rearrangements)   Found in approximately 40% of children with ALL, and a higher precentage of adults with ALL; patients have high white cell counts, less frequent early pre-B phenotype and relatively poor prognosis

STRUCTURAL CHANGES

t(9;22)(q34;q11) Philadelphia chromosome   Found in 2–5% of childhood ALL and a higher percentage of adults with ALL; patients have high white cell counts, older age at presentation, and CNS involvement; prognosis is unfavorable; no association with any particular phenotype

t(8;14)(q24;q32) or variations   Found in 1–3% of all ALL and in 80–90% of sIg+ mature B-cell ALL, with L3 morphology; patients have high white cell count, CNS disease, and poor prognosis

t(1;19)(q23;p13)   Found in 5–6% of childhood ALL; associated with pre-B (cytoplasmic μ+) phenotype; translocation-bearing patients with pre-B ALL have poor prognosis

t(4;11)(q21;q23) and other rearrangements of 11q23   Found in approximately 5% of childhood ALL, usually in association with early pre-B, CALLA-negative phenotype; usually seen in very young children; carries poor prognosis

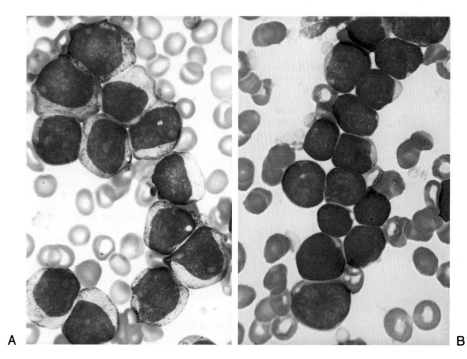

Figure 14-17. Acute leukemia. *A,* Acute myeloblastic leukemia (M1). Myeloblasts have delicate nuclear chromatin, prominent nucleoli, and fine azurophilic granules in the cytoplasm. *B,* Acute lymphoblastic leukemia (L1). Lymphoblasts have fewer nucleoli than do myeloblasts, and the nuclear chromatin is more condensed. Cytoplasmic granules are absent. (Courtesy of Dr. Robert W. McKenna, Department of Pathology, University of Texas Southwestern Medical School, Dallas.)

AML patients. In 50 to 70% of the cases, the karyotypic changes can be detected by standard cytogenetic techniques. Many of the nonrandom chromosomal abnormalities have prognostic implications that are independent of other clinical prognostic factors;[25] these are summarized in Table 14-11. The t(15;17) translocation characteristic of acute promyelocytic leukemia (M3) is of particular

interest because it results in the fusion of a truncated retinoic acid receptor-α (RAR-α) gene on chromosome 17 to a transcription unit called PML (for *promyelocytic leukemia*) on chromosome 15. Analogous to the *abl-bcr* fusion in chronic myeloid leukemia, the RAR-α–PML rearrangement produces a hybrid mRNA that can be detected in virtually all cases of M3 leukemia. The fused gene encodes an abnormal retinoic acid receptor that in

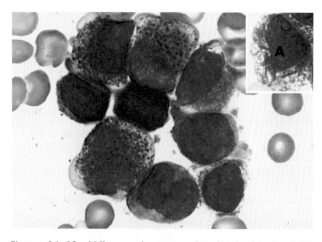

Figure 14-18. AML—acute promyelocytic leukemia (M3). Peripheral blood smear shows hypergranular promyelocytes. Cell in the inset (labeled A) shows prominent Auer rods. (Courtesy of Dr. José Hernandez, Department of Pathology, University of Texas Southwestern Medical School, Dallas.)

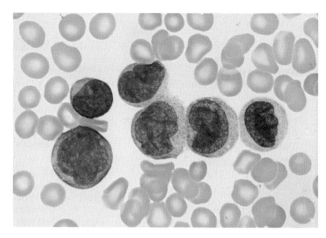

Figure 14-19. AML—acute monocytic leukemia (M5). Peripheral smear shows one monoblast and five promonocytes with folded nuclear membranes. (Courtesy of Dr. Robert W. McKenna, Department of Pathology, University of Texas Southwestern Medical School, Dallas.)

Table 14–10. REVISED FAB CLASSIFICATION OF ACUTE MYELOBLASTIC (MYELOCYTIC) LEUKEMIAS

	CLASS	INCIDENCE (% OF AML)	MARROW MORPHOLOGY/COMMENTS
M0	Minimally differentiated AML	2–3%	Blasts lack definitive cytologic and cytochemical markers of myeloblasts (e.g., myeloperoxidase negative) but express myeloid lineage antigens and resemble myeloblasts ultrastructurally
M1	AML without differentiation	~20%	Very immature but ≥3% are peroxidase positive; few granules or Auer rods and little maturation beyond the myeloblast stage
M2	AML with maturation	30–40%	Full range of myeloid maturation through granulocytes; Auer rods present in most cases; presence of t(8;21) defines a prognostically favorable subgroup
M3	Acute promyelocytic leukemia	5–10%	Majority of cells are hypergranular promyelocytes often with many Auer rods per cell; patients are younger (median age 35–40 yrs) and often develop DIC; the t(15;17) translocation is characteristic.
M4	Acute myelomonocytic leukemia	15–20%	Myelocytic and monocytic differentiation evident; myeloid elements resemble M2; monocytic cells positive for nonspecific esterases; the presence of chromosome 16 abnormalities defines a subset with eosinophils in the marrow and excellent prognosis
M5	Acute monocytic leukemia	~10%	Monoblasts (peroxidase-negative, nonspecific esterase-positive) and promonocytes predominate; tends to occur in older patients and characterized by very high incidence of organomegaly, lymphadenopathy, and tissue infiltration; gingival hypertrophy and skin infiltration common
M6	Acute erythroleukemia	~5%	Abnormal erythroblasts (some megaloblastoid, others with giant or multiple nuclei) predominate, some myeloblasts present; affected persons are of advanced age
M7	Acute megakaryocytic leukemia	~1%	Blasts of megakaryocytic lineage predominate; react with platelet-specific antibodies directed against GPIIb/IIIa or vWF; myelofibrosis or increased marrow reticulin in most cases

DIC = disseminated intravascular coagulation; vWF = von Willebrand's factor.

some manner blocks cell differentiation.[26] It is interesting to note that high doses of the vitamin A derivative *all-trans-retinoic* acid are able to overcome this block in differentiation both *in vitro* and *in vivo*, and this agent has been successfully used to induce remission in patients with M3 AML. This is the first example in which the molecular pathogenesis of a malignant tumor can be correlated with specific therapy.[27]

PROGNOSIS. AML is a difficult disease to treat. Approximately 60% of the patients achieve complete remission with chemotherapy, but only 15 to 30% of these remain free from disease for five

Table 14–11. SELECTED KARYOTYPIC ABNORMALITIES AND THEIR IMPACT ON PROGNOSIS IN ACUTE MYELOBLASTIC LEUKEMIA

CYTOGENETIC ABNORMALITY	FAB SUBGROUP AND FREQUENCY	PROGNOSIS/COMMENT
t(9;22)(q34;q11) Ph chromosome	10–15% of M1	Poor; bcr-c-abl fusion gene formed
t(8;21)(q22;q22)	20–25% of M2	Favorable
t(15;17)(q22;q21)	70–80% of M3	Intermediate; unique to M3; RAR-α–PML fusion gene formed
Abnormalities of chromosome 16, e.g., inv(16)(p13q22),del(16)(q22)	20–25% of M4	Favorable
Abnormalities of chromosome 11, e.g., t(variable;11), and 11q− with breakpoint at 11q23	30–40% of M5	Poor
Absence or deletions of chromosomes 5 or 7 (−7; del 7q; −5; del 5q)	Varied	Poor; most commonly seen in secondary leukemias associated with exposure to environmental or occupational carcinogens

RAR-α = retinoic acid receptor-α.

years. For this reason, an increasing number of patients are being treated with allogeneic bone marrow transplantation, and in some studies 50 to 60% of those who undergo transplantation in first remission appear to be cured.

MYELODYSPLASTIC SYNDROMES

This term refers to a group of clonal stem cell disorders characterized by maturation defects resulting in ineffective hematopoiesis and an increased risk of transformation to acute myeloblastic leukemias. In patients with this syndrome, bone marrow is partly or wholly replaced by the clonal progeny of a mutant pluripotent stem cell that retains the capacity to differentiate into red cells, granulocytes, and platelets, but in a manner that is both ineffective and disordered. As a result, the bone marrow is usually *hypercellular or normocellular,* but the peripheral blood shows *pancytopenia.* The abnormal stem cell clone in the bone marrow is genetically unstable, with a tendency to accumulate mutations and give rise to an acute leukemia.

MORPHOLOGY. Myelodysplastic syndromes are characterized by disordered (dysplastic) differentiation affecting all three lineages (erythroid, myeloid, and megakaryocytic). The cytologic features include megaloblastoid erythroid precursors, hypogranular myeloid precursors, increased proportion of blast cells in the marrow, micromegakaryocytes, agranular platelets, and unilobed or bilobed neutrophils.

On the basis of specific morphologic features in the marrow and peripheral blood, the myelodysplastic syndromes are divided into five categories, which will not be detailed here. It should be pointed out, however, that the clinical and morphologic distinction of AML from myelodysplasia may be difficult. If the bone marrow contains more than 30% myeloblasts, a diagnosis of AML is made. Cytogenetic studies reveal chromosomal abnormalities in up to two-thirds of patients.[29] Some of the more common ones are del(5q); +8; −7,der(11q); −5,der(12p); and −Y.

Myelodysplastic syndrome affects older individuals, between 60 and 70 years of age. As in acute leukemia, patients with this disorder present with weakness, infections, and hemorrhages, all due to pancytopenia. Approximately half of the patients are asymptomatic, and the disease is discovered following incidental blood tests. Ten to forty percent of the patients progress to frank AML, hence myelodysplasia may be regarded as a preleukemic condition, others are constantly threatened by infections and hemorrhages. The median survival is influenced by the specific form of mye-lodysplasia and by karyotypic abnormalities and varies from 9 to 29 months.[30]

CHRONIC MYELOID LEUKEMIA (CML)

This form of leukemia accounts for 15 to 20% of all cases of leukemia. It is a disease primarily of adults between the ages of 25 and 60 years, with the peak incidence in the fourth and fifth decades of life.

PATHOPHYSIOLOGY. CML arises by neoplastic transformation and clonal expansion of a pluripotent stem cell. Although virtually all hematopoietic lineages (myeloid, erythroid, megakaryocytic, B lymphocytic, and in some cases T lymphocytic) are involved in this disease, the granulocytic precursors constitute the dominant cell line.[31] As mentioned earlier, CML is one of the four chronic myeloproliferative disorders. It is distinguished from other members of this group by the presence of a distinctive cytogenetic and molecular abnormality. In more than 90% of cases the Ph chromosome, usually representing the reciprocal translocation t(9;22)(q34;q11), can be identified in the dividing progeny of stem cells. This translocation results in the formation of the *bcr-c-abl* fusion gene, which encodes a 210-kd fusion protein with potent tyrosine kinase activity (see Chapter 7). Transfection of the fusion gene into murine bone marrow cells gives rise to a syndrome resembling human CML, and hence the formation of the *bcr-c-abl* gene is considered a critical event in the pathogenesis of CML. Indeed, most authorities consider the presence of *bcr-c-abl* mRNA and protein as the *sine qua non* of CML. The minority of CML patients who are Ph negative by cytogenetic analysis also reveal *bcr-c-abl* rearrangements. It may be recalled that some patients with ALL also have Ph chromosome and *bcr-c-abl* rearrangements. However, molecular analysis reveals that in ALL, the translocation leads to the formation of a smaller, 190-kd fusion protein.

Cell kinetic and culture techniques reveal that there is a 10- to 20-fold increase in the mass of granulocytic precursors in the marrow. These neoplastic precursor cells coexist with a smaller number of *bcr-c-abl* negative (normal) progenitor cells.[32] The basis of expansion of the Ph-positive precursor cells is not clear. It has been reported that Ph-positive progenitor cells have reduced adherence to the stromal matrix of the bone marrow. Presumably this allows a premature release of these cells from the marrow and thereby disrupts the normal stroma-dependent proliferation-maturation sequence.

CLINICAL FEATURES. The onset of CML is usually slow, and the initial symptoms may be quite nonspecific. They are caused by anemia or by hyper-

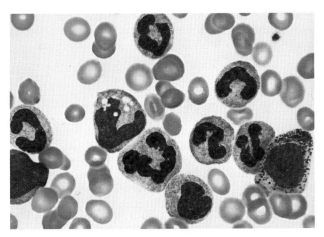

Figure 14-20. Chronic myeloid leukemia. Peripheral blood smear shows many mature neutrophils, some metamyelocytes, and a myelocyte. (Courtesy of Dr. Robert W. McKenna, Department of Pathology, University of Texas Southwestern Medical School, Dallas.)

metabolism due to increased cell turnover and include easy fatigability, weakness, weight loss, and anorexia. Sometimes the first symptom is a dragging sensation in the abdomen caused by the extreme splenomegaly characteristic of this condition. Usually, there is marked elevation of the leukocyte count, commonly exceeding 100,000 cell per mm³ (Fig. 14–20). The circulating cells are predominantly neutrophils and metamyelocytes, but basophils and eosinophils are also prominent. A small number of myeloblasts (<10%) can usually be detected in the peripheral blood. Because CML originates from the stem cells, it is not surprising that up to 50% of patients have thrombocytosis early in the course of their disease. A characteristic finding in CML is the almost total lack of alkaline phosphatase in granulocytes. This can be used to distinguish CML from a leukemoid reaction, which is also associated with a striking elevation of the granulocyte count in response to infection, stress, chronic inflammation, and certain neoplasms. However, the diagnostic feature of CML is the presence of Ph chromosome and bcr-c-abl rearrangements.

The course of CML is one of slow progression, and even without treatment a median survival of 3 years can be expected. After a variable period averaging 3 years, approximately 50% of patients enter an "accelerated phase," during which there is a gradual failure of response to treatment, increasing anemia and thrombocytopenia, acquisition of additional cytogenetic abnormalities, and finally, transformation into a picture resembling acute leukemia ("blast crisis"). In the remaining 50%, blast crises occur abruptly without an intermediate accelerated phase. In 70% of patients the blasts have the morphologic and cytochemical features of myeloblasts, whereas in the remaining 30% of patients the blasts contain the enzyme TdT and ex-

press B-lineage antigens, such as CD10 and CD19. This observation supports the notion that the target cell for transformation in CML is a pluripotent stem cell capable of both myeloid and lymphoid differentiation.

The treatment of CML is unsatisfactory. Although it is possible to induce remissions with chemotherapy, the median survival (3 to 4 years) is unaltered. Bone marrow transplantation is the only curative treatment, and hence it is being increasingly utilized as the definitive form of therapy. After the development of blast crisis, all forms of treatment become virtually ineffective.

CHRONIC LYMPHOCYTIC LEUKEMIA (CLL)

CLL is perhaps the most indolent of all leukemias. It accounts for 25% of all cases of leukemia in the United States and Europe, and occurrs typically in persons over 50 years (median age 60 years); males are affected twice as commonly as females. It is distinctly uncommon in Japan and other Asian countries.

PATHOPHYSIOLOGY. CLL shows considerable overlap with small lymphocytic lymphoma. Like most other lymphoid malignancies, CLL is a neoplastic disorder of B cells. T-cell CLL is rare (<5% of all cases) in the United States but fairly common in Japan and other Asian countries.

The transformed B cells in CLL show the following characteristics:

- They express the pan B-cell antigens (CD19, CD20) but do not contain TdT or express the early B-cell antigen CD10. Thus, their phenotype is quite distinct from the lymphoblasts seen in most cases of ALL. They do express CD5, a T-cell–associated antigen that is expressed on a very small subset of normal B cells.
- They express surface Ig (IgM and IgD), but the number of immunoglobulin molecules on the cells is so low that they may appear to be sIg negative by immunofluorescence. They express either λ or κ light chains, indicating monoclonality.
- They are long-lived but are unable to differentiate into antibody-secreting plasma cells *in vivo*.

Very little is known about the molecular pathogenesis of CLL. Rearrangements of bcl-2 occur in 10 to 15% of cases, and the bcl-1 gene is mutated in less than 5%.[33] Because bcl-2 overexpression prevents apoptosis, failure of programmed cell death may account for the accumulation of B cells, at least in some cases.

CHROMOSOMAL ABNORMALITIES. Approximately 50% of the patients with CLL have abnormal karyotypes. Trisomy 12 is the most common, being

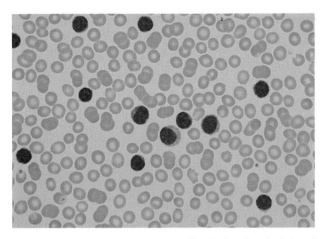

Figure 14–21. Chronic lymphocytic leukemia. Peripheral blood smear is flooded with transformed B cells that have the appearance of unstimulated small or medium-sized lymphocytes. (Courtesy of Dr. José Hernandez, Department of Pathology, University of Texas Southwestern Medical School, Dallas.)

seen in about one-third of the patients; abnormalities of 13q are seen in 25 to 40% of cytogenetically abnormal cases; less frequently, abnormalities of chromosomes 14 and 6 are noted. Patients with trisomy 12 carry a poor prognosis, but the presence of 13q abnormalities do not seem to influence the clinical course. In general, however, patients with cytogenetic changes require early treatment and have a significantly shorter survival.

CLINICAL FEATURES. Patients with CLL are often asymptomatic. When symptoms are present, they are nonspecific and include easy fatigability, loss of weight, and anorexia. Generalized lymphadenopathy and hepatosplenomegaly are present in 50 to 60% of the cases. Total leukocyte count may be increased only slightly or may reach 200,000 per mm³. In all cases there is absolute lymphocytosis of small, mature-looking lymphocytes (Fig. 14–21). Only a small fraction of lymphocytes are large ones with indented nuclei and nucleoli. Smudge cells (crushed nuclei of lymphocytes) are commonly seen in peripheral smears. Because the leukemic B cells fail to respond to antigenic stimulation, these patients often have hypogammaglobulinemia and increased susceptibility to bacterial infections. Paradoxically, some 10 to 15% of patients develop autoantibodies directed against red blood cells or platelets, resulting in autoimmune hemolytic anemia or thrombocytopenia. It is interesting to note that the CD5+ subset of B cells has been incriminated as the source of autoantibodies in several autoimmune diseases. Presumably in some cases the neoplastic CD5+ B cells retain the ability to secrete autoantibodies.

The course and prognosis of CLL are extremely variable and depend primarily on the clinical stage. Overall, the median survival is 4 to 6 years. Whether the prognostic value of cytogenetic changes is independent of the clinical stage is not yet established. Unlike in CML, transformation to acute leukemia with blast crisis is not common.

HAIRY CELL LEUKEMIA

This is a rare but distinctive form of chronic B-cell leukemia that derives its picturesque name from the appearance of the leukemic cells—fine hair-like projections, best recognized under the phase contrast microscope but also visible in routine blood smears.[34] A cytochemical feature that is quite characteristic of hairy cell leukemia is the presence of tartrate-resistant acid phosphatase (TRAP) in neoplastic B cells. The hairy cells express the pan B-cell markers CD19 and CD20, and the monocyte-associated antigen CD11c. In addition, plasma cell–associated antigen-1 (PCA-1) is also present on the leukemic cells. Normal B cells with this cluster of antigens have not been found.

Hairy cell leukemia occurs mainly in older males, and *its manifestations result largely from infiltration of bone marrow, liver, and spleen. Splenomegaly,* often massive, is the most common and sometimes the only abnormal physical finding. *Hepatomegaly* is less common and not as marked, and lymphadenopathy is distinctly rare. *Pancytopenia,* resulting from marrow failure and splenic sequestration, is seen in more than half the cases. *Leukocytosis* is not a common feature, being present in only 25% of patients. Hairy cells can be identified in the peripheral blood smear in most cases. Splenectomy is of benefit in approximately two-thirds of the patients. Until recently this disease could not be cured, and the median survival was less than 5 years. However, treatment with interferon-α and newer chemotherapeutic agents has led to lasting remissions and possibly cures.

MORPHOLOGY OF ALL LEUKEMIAS. There are two aspects to the morphologic features of leukemias: (1) the specific cytologic details of the leukemic cells seen in peripheral blood smears and bone marrow aspirates, and (2) the tissue changes produced by infiltrations of leukemic cells. The cytologic features specific for each form of leukemia have already been described. The tissue alterations produced by various leukemias are often similar and may be separated into primary changes, attributed directly to the abnormal overgrowth or accumulation of white cells; and secondary changes, caused both by the destructive effects of masses of these cells and by their relative ineffectiveness in protecting against infection. **Although the leukemic cells may infiltrate any tissue or organ of the body, the most striking changes are seen in the bone marrow, spleen, lymph nodes, and liver.** In the full-blown case, the bone marrow develops a muddy, red-brown to

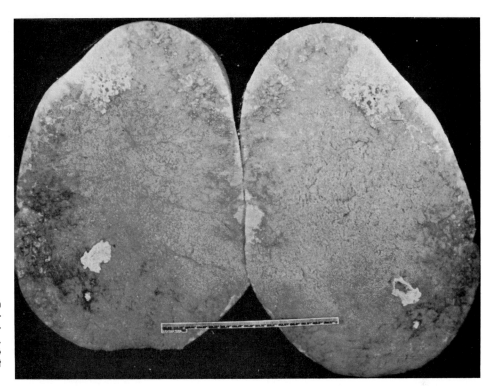

Figure 14–22. Spleen in chronic myelogenous leukemia. The massive enlargement dwarfs the 15-cm rule. Numerous small infarcts are dispersed through the cut surface.

gray-white color as the normal marrow is diffusely replaced by masses of white cells. Sometimes these infiltrates extend into previously fatty marrow and encroach on and erode the cancellous and cortical bone.

Massive **splenomegaly** is associated with CML and hairy cell leukemia. Splenic weights of 5000 gm or more are not unusual. Such spleens may virtually fill the abdominal cavity and extend into the pelvis. With CLL, enlargement of the spleen is less striking, and the acute forms of leukemia produce only moderate splenomegaly. When the splenomegaly is massive, as is most characteristic of CML, numerous areas of pale infarction may appear throughout the substance, caused presumably by infiltration and compression of vessels by leukemic cells (Fig. 14–22). In minimally enlarged spleens, the histologic appearance may be of focal leukemic infiltrates, with a background of fairly well-preserved normal architecture. In the lymphocytic forms, the white pulp is primarily involved. With more severe involvement the infiltrates become more diffuse and destroy the normal splenic architecture.

Whereas splenomegaly is more prominent with myelogenous than with lymphocytic leukemia, extreme **lymph node enlargement** is more characteristic of the lymphocytic forms (Fig. 14–23). Nevertheless, some degree of lymph node involvement is commonly present with all forms of leukemia. The affected nodes remain discrete, rubbery, and homogeneous. The cut section is soft and gray-white and tends to bulge above the level of the capsule. On histologic examination the nodes are flooded by the neoplastic cells, which may extend into the capsule and perinodal tissue. With CLL, the histologic picture is identical to that of a small lymphocytic lymphoma.

Enlargement of the liver is somewhat more prominent with lymphocytic than with myelogenous leukemia. Histologically, the lymphocytic infiltrates are characteristically confined to the portal areas (Fig. 14–24), whereas infiltrates of myelogenous leukemia are not well defined and are present within the sinusoids throughout the lobule.

In addition to the principal sites of involvement, other tissues and organs, such as the kidneys, adrenals, thyroid, myocardium, and testes, may be infiltrated. Of particular importance is the infiltration of the central nervous system by leukemic cells. This occurs most commonly in ALL. **Infiltrates in the gingiva are particularly characteristic of monocytic leukemia (M5).** Patients with this disorder have swelling and hypertrophy of the gingival margins, often with secondary infections.

The **secondary changes of all forms of leukemia** derive in large part from the pancytopenia that results from inhibition of normal hematopoiesis by leukemic cells. Anemia and thrombocytopenia are characteristic, especially of acute leukemia. Many times, the bleeding diathesis caused by the thrombocytopenia is the most striking clinical and anatomic feature of the disease. Petechiae and ecchymoses are seen in the skin. Hemorrhages also occur into the serosal linings of the body cavities and into the serosal coverings of the viscera, particularly of the heart and lungs. Mucosal hemorrhages into the gingivae and urinary tract are

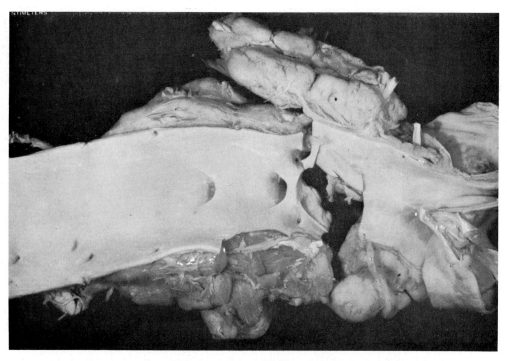

Figure 14-23. Periaortic lymph node enlargement in chronic lymphocytic leukemia.

common. Disseminated intravascular coagulation, so common in acute promyelocytic leukemia (M3), also leads to widespread bleeding. Infections are a prominent feature, especially in acute leukemias. They are particularly common in the oral cavity, skin, lungs, kidneys, urinary bladder, and colon, and they are often caused by "opportunists" such as fungi, Pseudomonas, and commensals.

ETIOLOGY AND PATHOGENESIS OF LEUKEMIAS AND LYMPHOMAS. As with many other forms of cancer, several environmental agents have been implicated in the causation of leukemias and lymphomas.[35] Well-established influences include ionizing radiation and chemicals. Exposure to radiation—occupational, therapeutic, or accidental—increases the incidence of several leukemias (with the curious exception of CLL). The increased risk of leukemias and NHLs following treatment with alkylating agents is also well established. The risk is even greater if both irradiation and chemotherapy have been used, as for example in the treatment of Hodgkin's disease.

Two viruses, HTLV-1 and EBV, have been associated with acute T-cell leukemia/lymphoma and Burkitt's lymphoma, respectively. Recent studies have implicated HTLV-1 and HTLV-2 in the causation of mycosis fungoides as well.[8] The possible mechanisms of transformation by these viral agents were discussed earlier (see Chapter 7).

Finally, it should be recalled that with high-resolution banding techniques nonrandom karyo-typic abnormalities, most commonly translocations, are noted in the majority of all leukemias and lymphomas. In addition to having prognostic implications, study of such abnormalities has provided important insights into the molecular basis of cancer. Several oncogenes located near the breakpoints are dysregulated by the translocations.[36] Those of particular relevance to the pathogenesis of leukemias and lymphomas include *bcl-1*, *bcl-2*, c-*myc*, c-*abl*, and RAR-α. All of these were discussed earlier.

MYELOPROLIFERATIVE DISORDERS

The concept that myeloproliferative disorders result from clonal neoplastic proliferations of the multipotent myeloid stem cells is well established. It was mentioned previously that four disorders—chronic myeloid leukemia, polycythemia vera, myeloid metaplasia with myelofibrosis, and essential thrombocythemia—are included in this group. CML was discussed along with other leukemias. Of the remaining three, only polycythemia vera and myeloid metaplasia with myelofibrosis will be presented here. Essential thrombocythemia occurs too infrequently to merit further discussion.

Polycythemia Vera

Like all other myeloproliferative disorders, polycythemia vera is associated with excessive proliferation of erythroid, granulocytic, and megakaryocytic elements, all derived from clonal expansion of a

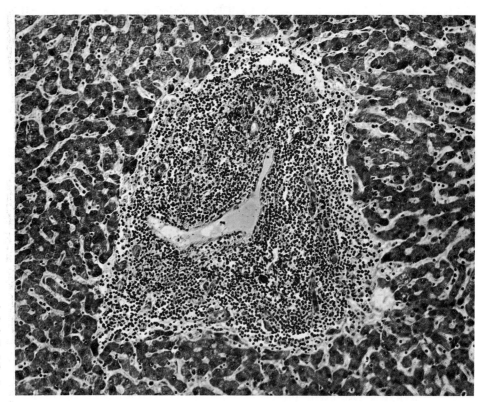

Figure 14–24. Chronic lymphocytic leukemia in liver. High-power detail of a periportal infiltrate. (With permission from Jackson, H.J., Jr., and Parker, F., Jr. (eds.): Hodgkin's Disease and Allied Disorders. New York, Oxford University Press, 1947.)

pluripotent stem cell. However, in *polycythemia vera the erythroid precursors dominate, and hence there is an absolute increase in red cell mass.* This should be contrasted with relative polycythemia, resulting from hemoconcentration (see Chapter 13). Furthermore, unlike other forms of absolute polycythemia that result from an increased secretion of erythropoietin, polycythemia vera is associated with virtually undetectable levels of serum erythropoietin.[37]

In vitro culture of hematopoietic stem cells has provided important insights into the pathophysiology of polycythemia vera. In the blood and bone marrow of these patients there is an increase in the number of proliferating myeloid stem cells that seem to require extremely small amounts of erythropoietin and other hematopoietic growth factors.[38] Although the basis of the increased sensitivity of hematopoietic progenitor cells to growth factors is not known, it could explain the profound marrow hyperplasia seen in this disorder.

MORPHOLOGY. The major anatomic changes stem from the increase in blood volume and viscosity brought about by the erythrocytosis. Plethoric congestion of all tissues and organs is characteristic of polycythemia vera. The liver is enlarged and frequently contains foci of myeloid metaplasia. The spleen is also slightly enlarged, up to 250 to 300 gm, and quite firm. The major blood vessels are uniformly distended with thick, viscous blood.

Consequent to the increased viscosity and vascular stasis, thromboses and infarctions are common. Hemorrhages occur in about a third of these patients, probably owing to excessive distention of blood vessels and abnormal platelet function. They usually affect the gastrointestinal tract, oropharynx, or brain. Although these hemorrhages are said on occasion to be spontaneous, more often they follow some minor trauma or surgical procedure. Peptic ulceration has been described in about a fifth of these patients.

The basic changes occur in the bone marrow, which is markedly hypercellular. Hematopoiesis expands markedly to replace fatty marrow; such extension can be detected by magnetic resonance imaging. Typically, the marrow demonstrates hyperplasia of erythroid, granulocytic, and megakaryocytic elements. At the time of diagnosis, moderate to marked increase in marrow reticulin is seen in approximately 10% of the patients. As the disease changes its course, the marrow reflects the alterations and may become progressively fibrotic (myelofibrosis) or may be replaced by blasts (leukemic transformation), as discussed below.

CLINICAL COURSE. Polycythemia vera appears insidiously, usually in late middle age (median age at onset, 60 years).[37] Males are affected somewhat more often than females, and whites are more vulnerable than blacks. The major clinical features stem from the increased blood volume and viscosity, vascular stasis, thrombotic tendency, and hemorrhagic diathesis. Most of the excess blood is trapped in the venous circulation, which is greatly distended. Classically, therefore, patients are plethoric and somewhat cyanotic owing to stagnation and deoxygenation of blood in peripheral vessels. Headache, dizziness, gastrointestinal symptoms, hematemesis, and melena are common. There is usually intense pruritus and an increased tendency to peptic ulceration, both possibly the result of an increased release of histamine from basophils. High cell turnover gives rise to hyperuricemia, and symptomatic gout is seen in 5 to 10% of cases.

The diagnosis is usually made in the laboratory. Hemoglobin concentration ranges from 14 to 28 gm/dl with hematocrit values of 60% or more. Because there is hyperplasia of granulocytic precursors as well as megakaryocytes in the bone marrow, the white cell count is elevated, ranging between 12,000 and 50,000 cells per mm³, and the platelet count is often greater than 500,000 cells per mm³. In contrast to CML, granulocyte alkaline phosphatase levels are above normal. The platelets usually exhibit morphologic and functional abnormalities manifested as giant forms and megakaryocytic fragments and defective aggregation.

About 30% of patients develop some thrombotic complications, affecting usually the brain or heart. Hepatic vein thrombosis may give rise to the Budd-Chiari syndrome. Minor hemorrhages (epistaxis, bleeding gums) are common. Life-threatening hemorrhages occur in 5 to 10% of cases.

In patients who receive no treatment, death resulting from these vascular episodes occurs within months after diagnosis. However, if the red cell mass can be maintained at nearly normal levels by phlebotomies, median survival of 10 years can be achieved.

Extended survival with treatment has revealed that the *natural history of polycythemia vera involves a gradual transition to a "spent phase," during which clinical and anatomic features of myeloid metaplasia with myelofibrosis develop.* Approximately 15 to 20% of patients undergo such a transformation after an average period of 10 years. This transition is brought about by creeping fibrosis in the bone marrow (myelofibrosis) and a shift of hematopoiesis to the spleen, which enlarges markedly. This is perhaps the most striking example of conversion of one myeloproliferative disorder to another. As with CML, certain patients with polycythemia vera develop a terminal acute myeloblastic leukemia. However, the incidence of this transition is much lower than in CML. It is estimated to be about 2% in patients who are treated with phlebotomy alone[39] and about 15% in those who receive myelosuppressive treatment with chlorambucil or marrow irradiation with radioactive phosphorus. Presumably, the increase is related to the mutagenic effects of these therapeutic agents.

Myeloid Metaplasia with Myelofibrosis

In this chronic myeloproliferative disorder the proliferation of the neoplastic myeloid stem cells occurs principally in the spleen *(myeloid metaplasia)*, and in the fully developed syndrome the bone marrow is hypocellular and fibrotic *(myelofibrosis)*.[40] Sometimes polycythemia vera and, less often, CML "burn out," as it were, and terminate in a myelofibrotic pattern. In many patients, however, extramedullary hematopoiesis in the spleen and marrow fibrosis arise insidiously without an identifiable preceding syndrome; hence the term *agnogenic (idiopathic) myeloid metaplasia* is sometimes used to describe this condition.

Although the marrow is flooded with proliferating fibroblasts, it is clear that the fibroblasts are not clonal descendants of the neoplastic stem cell. Instead, fibrosis seems to be secondary to an inappropriate release of growth factors from neoplastic megakaryocytes.[41] Two growth factors have been implicated: platelet-derived growth factor (PDGF) and TFG-β. They are synthesized by megakaryocytes and released into the surrounding tissues either by leakage from the abnormal (neoplastic) cells or following intramedullary death of these cells. Both PDGF and TGF-β are fibroblast mitogens; in addition TGF-β promotes the deposition of extracellular matrix by increasing the expression of genes that encode collagens, fibronectin, and proteoglycans. TGF-β is also a powerful angiogenic factor, and capillary proliferation is prominent in myelofibrosis. The central role of megakaryocytes in myelofibrosis is supported by several observations: (1) early in the course of the disease there is hyperplasia of morphologically abnormal megakaryocytes; (2) fibroblast proliferation is most pronounced around areas of megakaryocyte necrosis; and (3) functional and morphologic abnormalities of megakaryocytes and platelets are more pronounced in myelofibrosis than in the other myeloproliferative disorders.[42] It is widely believed that the proliferation of neoplastic stem cells begins within the marrow and there is subsequent seeding of the spleen and other organs, such as the liver. As the disease progresses, marrow fibrosis occurs secondary to the elaboration of the fibroblast growth factors mentioned above. By the time the patient comes to clinical attention, fibroblasts have already taken over the marrow, and the spleen remains the major site of myeloproliferation.

MORPHOLOGY. The principal site of the extramedullary hematopoiesis is the **spleen,** which is usually markedly enlarged, sometimes up to 4000 gm (Fig.

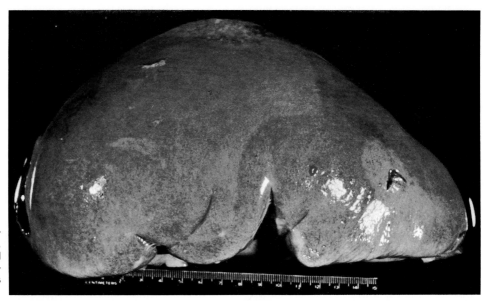

Figure 14-25. Myeloid metaplasia with myelofibrosis. Spleen is markedly enlarged and dwarfs the 15-cm rule. Irregular shading of capsule is an artifact.

14-25). On section, it is firm, red to gray, and very similar to spleens with myelogenous leukemia. As with CML, multiple subcapsular infarcts may be present. Histologically, **there is trilineage proliferation affecting normoblasts, granulocyte precursors, and megakaryocytes; however, megakaryocytes are usually prominent owing to their large size and nuclear morphology** (Fig. 14-26). Sometimes disproportional activity of any one of the three major cell lines is seen. Initially the extramedullary hematopoiesis is confined to the sinusoids, but later it may extend to involve the cords.

The **liver** may be moderately enlarged, with foci of extramedullary hematopoiesis. The lymph nodes are only rarely the site of blood cell formation and usually are not enlarged.

Early in the course of disease the marrow is often hypercellular with trilineage proliferation. Morphologically, the erythroid and granulocytic precursors appear normal, but megakaryocytes are large and dysplastic, and they tend to occur in nests. During this cellular phase, fibrosis is minimal. With progression, the marrow becomes hypocellular and diffusely fibrotic. Even at this stage clusters of atypical megakaryocytes may be found in the sea of fibrosis.

CLINICAL COURSE. Myeloid metaplasia is uncommon in individuals younger than 60 years of age. Except when preceded by polycythemia vera or CML, it usually comes to clinical attention because of either progressive anemia or marked splenic enlargement, producing a dragging sensation in the left upper quadrant. Nonspecific symptoms such as fatigue, weight loss, and night sweats result from increased metabolism associated with the expanded mass of myeloid cells. Owing to a high rate of cell turnover, hyperuricemia and secondary gout may complicate the picture.

Most striking are the laboratory findings. There is usually a moderate-to-severe normochromic normocytic anemia. Red cells show all manner of variation in size and shape, but *particularly characteristic are teardrop-shaped erythrocytes (poikilocytes)* (Fig. 14-27). In addition, numerous normoblasts and basophilic stippled red cells appear in the peripheral blood. The white cell count may be normal, reduced, or markedly elevated (80,000 to 100,000 cells per mm³), with a shift to the left. Basophils are usually prominent. Typically, myeloblasts, myelocytes, and metamyelocytes constitute a small fraction of the white cell popula-

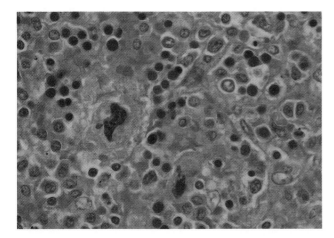

Figure 14-26. Myeloid metaplasia with myelofibrosis. Microscopic section of the spleen shows a megakaryocyte with a large irregular nucleus, small clusters of normoblasts with dark compact nuclei, and immature myeloid cells with somewhat larger, vesicular nuclei. (Courtesy of Dr. José Hernandez, Department of Pathology, University of Texas Southwestern Medical School, Dallas.)

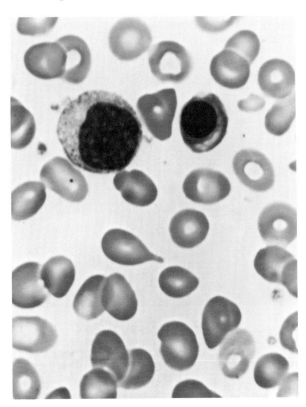

Figure 14–27. Myeloid metaplasia with myelofibrosis. Peripheral blood smear shows a teardrop red cell in the center field. An immature myeloid cell (left) and a nucleated red cell (right) are seen. (Courtesy of Dr. José Hernandez, Department of Pathology, University of Texas Southwestern Medical School, Dallas.)

tion on peripheral smear. The platelet count is usually normal or elevated at the time of diagnosis, but thrombocytopenia supervenes as the disease progresses. Morphologic abnormalities of the platelets (giant forms) are frequent, and sometimes fragments of megakaryocytes may be detected in the peripheral blood. *To summarize, teardrop poikilocytes, leukoerythroblastosis, and abnormal platelets in the peripheral smear are highly suggestive of myeloid metaplasia with myelofibrosis. Biopsy of the marrow to detect the early deposition of reticulin or the more advanced fibrosis is essential for diagnosis.*

In some cases, the clinical and hematologic features may resemble those of CML, but the Ph chromosome and *bcr-c-abl* rearrangements are absent. An equally difficult differential diagnosis is myelophthisic anemia secondary to an identifiable cause of marrow injury. In such cases the diagnosis can be established only by careful history-taking to elicit the cause of marrow injury or by morphologic detection of the underlying cause (e.g., cancer) in the marrow biopsy.

The course of this disease is difficult to predict. In different series median survival time has varied from 1 to 5 years.[40] Threats to life are intercurrent infections, thrombotic episodes or bleeding related to platelet abnormalities, and in 5 to 20% of cases, transformation to acute myeloid leukemia.

PLASMA CELL DYSCRASIAS AND RELATED DISORDERS

The plasma cell dyscrasias have in common the *expansion of a single clone of immunoglobulin-secreting cells and a resultant increase in serum levels of a single homogeneous immunoglobulin or its fragments.* In many, but not all, cases, these dyscrasias behave as malignant diseases. Collectively, these disorders account for about 15% of deaths from malignant white cell disease. As neoplasms of B cells, plasma cell dyscrasias are related to the non-Hodgkin's B-cell lymphomas. They differ, however, from the B-cell lymphomas by virtue of the fact that, in plasma cell disorders, the neoplastic B cells are differentiated enough to secrete immunoglobulins, and in most cases the clinical features are not dominated by lymphadenopathy. However, there are overlaps, as in the case of Waldenström's macroglobulinemia, to be described later.

The monoclonal immunoglobulin identified in the blood is referred to as an M component in reference to *m*yeloma. Since complete M components have molecular weights of 160,000 or higher, they are restricted largely to circulating plasma and extracellular fluid. However, they may appear in the urine when there is some form of glomerular damage with heavy proteinuria. In some of these dyscrasias, excess light (L) or heavy (H) chains are also synthesized along with complete immunoglobulins. Occasionally, only L chains or H chains are produced, without complete Ig. The *free L chains, known as Bence Jones proteins,* are sufficiently small to be rapidly excreted in the urine, and so may be totally cleared from the blood or persist only at very low levels. However, with renal failure or massive synthesis, they may appear in the blood in significant concentrations. Thus, *the common thread throughout this diverse group of entities is the appearance of excessive levels of complete or incomplete immunoglobulins in the plasma and/or urine. Hence, a variety of alternative designations have been applied to these dyscrasias, such as gammopathies, monoclonal gammopathies, dysproteinemias, and paraproteinemias.*[43]

A variety of clinicoanatomic patterns can be differentiated among these gammopathies.

• *Multiple myeloma (plasma cell myeloma)* is the most important and most common syndrome. It is characterized by multiple neoplastic tumorous masses of plasma cells scattered throughout the skeletal system. *Solitary myeloma, or solitary plasmacytoma,* is an infrequent variant consisting of a solitary neoplastic mass of plasma cells found in bone or some soft tissue site.

- *Waldenström's macroglobulinemia* is characterized by the synthesis of IgM and the presence of a diffuse infiltrate of neoplastic B cells throughout the bone marrow as well as lymph nodes, liver, and spleen. Hence there is associated lymphadenopathy and hepatosplenomegaly, but the lytic bone lesions typical of myeloma are not present.
- *Heavy-chain disease* is a rare gammopathy distinguished by neoplastic medullary and extramedullary infiltrates of plasma cells, and precursors that synthesize only heavy chains.
- *Primary or immunocyte-associated amyloidosis* results from a monoclonal proliferation of plasma cells, with excessive production of free light chains that are deposited as amyloid.
- *Monoclonal gammopathy of undetermined significance* (MGUS) refers to instances in which M components are identified in the blood of patients having no symptoms or signs of any of the better-characterized monoclonal gammopathies.

Against this background we can turn to some of the specific clinicoanatomic entities. Primary amyloidosis was discussed along with other disorders of the immune system in Chapter 6.

MULTIPLE MYELOMA

Multiple myeloma is a plasma cell cancer that originates in the bone marrow and is characterized by involvement of the skeleton at multiple sites. It may also spread to many extraosseous sites. As pointed out, the neoplastic plasma cells synthesize complete and/or incomplete immunoglobulins. It is the most common of the gammopathies.

ETIOLOGY AND PATHOGENESIS. Although cells with mature plasma cell morphology and function dominate the lesions, phenotypic studies indicate that multiple myeloma is a disease of hematopoietic stem cells.[44] Myeloma cells may express not only plasma cell–associated antigens such as PCA-1 (and in some cases the early B-cell antigen CD10) but also antigens typically associated with myelomonocytic cells (CD33), megakaryocytes (GpIIa/IIIa), and erythroid cells. Thus, it seems that myeloma arises from the transformation of a pluripotent stem cell that differentiates predominantly along the B cell–plasma cell pathway.

The proliferation and differentiation of myeloma cells seem to be dependent on several cytokines, most notably IL-6. Serum levels of this cytokine are increased in patients with active disease, and indeed it appears that high serum IL-6 levels are associated with a poor prognosis.[45] IL-6 seems to be produced by tumorous plasma cells themselves as well as by fibroblasts and macrophages in the surrounding stroma. It is believed that stromal cells, induced to secrete IL-6 under the influence of tumor-derived cytokines such as IL-1, are the major source of IL-6. These observations have spurred some investigators to initiate therapeutic trials of antibodies directed against IL-6 in patients with aggressive disease.[46]

In addition to causing the growth of myeloma cells, cytokines also mediate bone destruction — the major pathologic feature of multiple myeloma. Loss of bone is in large part due to osteoclastic reabsorption induced by the tumor. A variety of cytokines produced by the tumor cells, including TNF-β, IL-1, IL-6, and M-CSF, have been implicated as osteoclast-activating factors.[47]

MORPHOLOGY. Multiple myeloma presents most often as multifocal destructive bone lesions throughout the skeletal system. Although any bone may be affected, the following distribution was found in a large series of cases: vertebral column, 66%; ribs, 44%; skull, 41%; pelvis, 28%; femur, 24%; clavicle, 10%; and scapula, 10%. These focal lesions generally begin in the medullary cavity, erode the cancellous bone, and progressively destroy the cortical bone. Pathologic fractures are often produced by plasma cell lesions; they are most common in the vertebral column but may affect any of the numerous bones suffering erosion and destruction of their cortical substances. On section, the bony defects are typically filled with soft, red, gelatinous tissue. Most commonly, the lesions appear radiographically as punched-out defects, usually 1 to 4 cm in diameter (Fig. 14–28), but in some of the cases only diffuse demineralization is evident. Microscopic examination of the marrow reveals an increased number of plasma cells, constituting 10 to 90% of all cells in the marrow. The neoplastic plasma cells may resemble normal mature plasma cells or sometimes take the form of undifferentiated blast cells that may be large and pleomorphic (see Fig. 14–28). With progressive disease, plasma cell infiltrations of soft tissues may be encountered in the spleen, liver, kidneys, lungs, and lymph nodes, or more widely.

Renal involvement, generally called **myeloma nephrosis,** is one of the more distinctive features of multiple myeloma. Grossly, the kidneys may be normal in size or color, slightly enlarged and pale, or shrunken and pale because of interstitial scarring. The most characteristic features are microscopic. Interstitial infiltrates of abnormal plasma cells may be encountered. Even in the absence of these, proteinaceous casts are prominent in the distal convoluted tubules and collecting ducts. Most of these casts are made up of Bence Jones proteins, but they may also contain complete immunoglobulins, Tamm-Horsfall protein, and albumin. Some casts have tinctorial properties of amyloid. This is not surprising in view of the fact that AL amyloid is

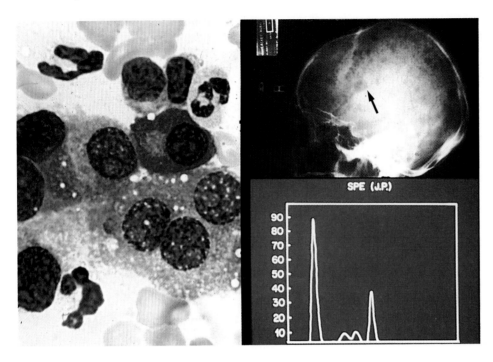

Figure 14-28. Multiple myeloma—a composite of characteristic features. Plasma cells in the bone marrow (left), lytic lesions in the skull and other bones (top right), and a monoclonal immunoglobulin spike seen in serum protein electrophoresis (bottom right). (Courtesy of Dr. José Hernandez, Department of Pathology, University of Texas Southwestern Medical School, Dallas.)

derived from Bence Jones proteins. The casts are usually surrounded by multinucleate giant cells derived from fusion of infiltrating macrophages. Very often the cells lining tubules containing casts become necrotic or atrophic. It is believed that free light chains (Bence Jones proteins), which are filtered by the glomerulus and then reabsorbed by the tubular cells, are toxic to the tubule cells. Metastatic calcification may be encountered within the kidney because of the hypercalcemia that frequently accompanies multiple myeloma. When complicated by amyloidosis, typical glomerular lesions associated with renal amyloidosis are present. Pyelonephritis may occur owing to the increased susceptibility of these patients to infections.

CLINICAL COURSE. The peak age incidence of multiple myeloma is between 50 and 60 years. Both sexes are affected equally. As previously stated, the *clinical features of myeloma stem from the effects of (1) infiltration of organs, particularly bones, by the neoplastic plasma cells; and (2) the production of excessive immunoglobulins, which often have abnormal physicochemical properties.*

Infiltration of bones is manifested by pain and pathologic fractures. Hypercalcemia resulting from bone resorption may give rise to neurologic manifestations such as confusion, weakness, lethargy, constipation, and polyuria. It also contributes to renal disease. *Recurrent infections with bacteria such as* Streptococcus pneumoniae, Staphylococcus aureus, *and* E. coli, *resulting from severe suppression of normal immunoglobulins, also pose a major clinical problem.* Cellular immunity is relatively

unaffected. The loss of humoral immunity in multiple myeloma seems to result from induction of suppressor macrophages.

In 99% of patients with multiple myeloma, electrophoretic analysis reveals increased levels of immunoglobulins in the blood and/or light chains (Bence Jones proteins) in the urine. Monoclonal immunoglobulins ("M component") of the IgG type are found in 55% of patients; in 25% of cases the myeloma cells produce IgA. The other immunoglobulins (i.e., IgM, IgD, and IgE) are rarely increased. Bence Jones proteinuria along with plasma M component occurs in 60 to 70% of all myeloma patients. However, in approximately 20% of cases Bence Jones proteinuria without an increase in complete immunoglobulin molecules in the serum is noted. Excessive production and aggregation of myeloma proteins may lead to the hyperviscosity syndrome in approximately 7% of patients, particularly in those with the IgA myeloma. Manifestations of the hyperviscosity syndrome, including retinal hemorrhages, prolonged bleeding, and neurologic changes, are much more common with Waldenström's macroglobulinemia and are therefore discussed later.

Of great significance is renal insufficiency, which is second only to infections as a cause of death. The pathogenesis of renal failure, which may occur in up to 50% of patients, is multifactorial and is discussed in Chapter 20. The most important factor appears to be Bence Jones proteinuria, since the excreted light chains are believed to be directly toxic to the tubular epithelial cells. *Amyloidosis of the AL type occurs in some patients* owing to excessive production of immunoglobulin light chains.

The clinical diagnosis of multiple myeloma rests on radiographic and laboratory findings. The radiographic changes are so distinctive that a reasonably certain diagnosis can usually be made. *Classically, the individual lesions appear as sharply punched-out defects having a rounded soap-bubble appearance on x-ray film, but generalized osteoporosis may also be seen.* Marrow examination reveals aggregates of plasma cells that suppress and replace normal hematopoietic elements. The resultant marrow failure gives rise to a normocytic normochromic anemia, sometimes accompanied by moderate leukopenia and thrombocytopenia. Rarely, neoplastic plasma cells flood the peripheral blood, giving rise to *plasma cell leukemia.* Identification of monoclonal immunoglobulins in the blood and urine constitutes one of the most important diagnostic features of this disease. The monoclonal immunoglobulins produce a high spike when serum or urine is subjected to electrophoresis (see Fig. 14–28). Immunoelectrophoresis is used to identify the nature of monoclonal immunoglobulins. Quantitative analyses of monoclonal immunoglobulins usually reveal more than 3 gm of Ig per dl of serum and more than 6 mg of Bence Jones proteins per dl of urine.

The prognosis for this condition depends on the stage at the time of diagnosis. Patients with multiple bony lesions, if untreated, rarely survive for more than 6 to 12 months. Chemotherapy in the form of alkylating agents induces remission in 50 to 70% of patients, but the median survival is still a dismal 3 years. Autologous and allogeneic bone marrow transplantation after intensive chemotherapy offers the promise of cure.[48]

Solitary Myeloma (Plasmacytoma)

About 3 to 5% of monoclonal gammopathies consist of a solitary plasmacytic lesion, in either bone or soft tissue. The bony lesions tend to occur in the same locations as in multiple myeloma. Extraosseous lesions are often located in the lungs, oronasopharynx, or nasal sinuses. Modest elevations of M proteins in the blood or urine may be found in a minority of patients.

When patients with such localized disease are followed, *progression to classic multiple myeloma becomes manifest in most patients with osseous plasmacytoma, whereas extraosseous primaries rarely disseminate.* It appears that the solitary plasmacytoma involving the bones is an early stage of multiple myeloma, but in some individuals it may be present for 10 to 20 years without progression. Extraosseous plasmacytomas, particularly those involving the upper respiratory tract, represent limited disease that can usually be cured by local resection.

WALDENSTRÖM'S MACROGLOBULINEMIA

This dyscrasia, constituting about 5% of monoclonal gammopathies, *is marked by a diffuse, leukemia-like infiltration of the bone marrow by lymphocytes, plasma cells, and hybrid forms that synthesize a monoclonal IgM immunoglobulin, leading to macroglobulinemia.* The disease may best be viewed as a cross between multiple myeloma and small lymphocytic lymphoma. As in myeloma, the neoplastic B cells secrete a monoclonal immunoglobulin. However, unlike myeloma but similar to lymphoma, the tumor cells diffusely infiltrate the lymphoid tissues, including bone marrow, spleen, and lymph nodes.

MORPHOLOGY. Typically, there is a diffuse, sparse-to-heavy infiltrate in the bone marrow of lymphocytes, plasma cells, lymphocytoid plasma cells, and other variants on this theme. The infiltrate is rarely as heavy as that encountered in leukemia and does not occur in the tumorous masses that are characteristic of plasma cell myeloma. Thus, there is no bone erosion or characteristic radiographic finding. A similar infiltrate may be present in the lymph nodes, spleen, or liver in patients having disseminated disease. Infiltration of the nerve roots, meninges, and cerebral substance by proliferating cells may also occur.

CLINICAL COURSE. Waldenström's macroglobulinemia is a disease of old age, presenting between the sixth and the seventh decades. The dominant presenting complaints are weakness, fatigability, and weight loss—all nonspecific symptoms. Approximately half the patients have lymphadenopathy, hepatomegaly, and splenomegaly. The specific complaints stem largely from the abnormal physicochemical properties of the macroglobulins. Because of their large size and increased concentration in blood, the macroglobulins tend to form large aggregates that greatly increase the viscosity of blood, giving rise to the hyperviscosity syndrome. This is characterized by the following features:

- *Visual impairment* resulting from the striking tortuosity and distention of retinal veins; retinal hemorrhages and exudates may also contribute to the visual problems.
- *Neurologic problems* such as headaches, dizziness, deafness, and stupor, stemming from sluggish blood flow and sludging.
- *Bleeding* related to the formation of complexes between macroglobulins and clotting factors as well as interference with platelet functions.
- *Cryoglobulinemia* resulting from precipitation of macroglobulins at low temperatures produces

symptoms such as Raynaud's phenomenon and cold urticaria.

Like multiple myeloma, Waldenström's macroglobulinemia is a progressive disease with a median survival of about 4 years.

HEAVY-CHAIN DISEASE

These extremely rare monoclonal gammopathies will be discussed only briefly. Three variants have been described, each characterized by elevated levels in the blood or urine of a specific heavy chain of immunoglobulins. *Gamma-chain disease*, encountered most often in the elderly, resembles a malignant lymphoma. The manifestations consist of lymphadenopathy, anemia, and fever, often accompanied by malaise, weakness, and hepatomegaly or splenomegaly. The course can be rapidly downhill to death within a few months or may be protracted for years.

Alpha-chain disease, the most common in this group, is a disorder of IgA-producing cells involving mainly the sites of normal IgA synthesis. It occurs mainly in young adults, most commonly in the Mediterranean area, and is characterized by massive infiltration of the lamina propria of the intestine and abdominal lymph nodes by lymphocytes, plasma cells, and histiocytes. Villous atrophy and severe malabsorption with diarrhea, steatorrhea, and hypocalcemia are consequences of the infiltrate. Like other monoclonal gammopathies, alpha-chain disease is progressive and fatal.

Mu-chain disease is the rarest of these entities, most often encountered in patients with chronic lymphocytic leukemia. Hepatomegaly and splenomegaly are usually present, but in contrast to the usual case with CLL, peripheral lymphadenopathy is inconspicuous.

MONOCLONAL GAMMOPATHY OF UNDETERMINED SIGNIFICANCE

M proteins can be identified in the serum of 1% of asymptomatic healthy persons older than 50 years of age and in 3% older than 70 years of age. *To this dysproteinemia without associated disease, the term "monoclonal gammopathy of undetermined significance" (MGUS) is applied.* MGUS is the most common monoclonal gammopathy.

Approximately 20% of patients with MGUS develop a well-defined plasma cell dyscrasia (myeloma, Waldenström's macroglobulinemia, or amyloidosis) over a period of 10 to 15 years. The diagnosis of MGUS should be made with caution and after careful exclusion of all other specific forms of monoclonal gammopathies. In general, patients with MGUS have less than 3 gm/dl of monoclonal protein in the serum and no Bence Jones proteinuria.

Whether a given patient with MGUS will follow a benign course, as most do, or develop a well-defined plasma cell neoplasm cannot be predicted, and hence periodic assessment of serum M component levels and Bence Jones proteinuria is warranted.

LANGERHANS' CELL HISTIOCYTOSIS

The term "histiocytosis" is an umbrella designation for a variety of proliferative disorders of histiocytes or macrophages. Some, such as the rare histiocytic lymphomas mentioned earlier, are clearly malignant, whereas others, such as the reactive histiocytic proliferations in lymph nodes, are clearly benign. Between these two extremes is a small cluster of conditions characterized by proliferation of a special type of histiocyte called the Langerhans' cell (see Chapter 6). These Langerhans' cell histiocytoses are associated with tumor-like proliferations, but there is insufficient evidence to consider them truly neoplastic. The general consensus seems to be that these are reactive disorders in which the proliferation of Langerhans' cells results from disturbances in immunoregulation. A variety of disturbances in T cells have been described, but it is difficult to determine whether they are primary or coincidental.[49] In the past these disorders were referred to as histiocytosis X and subdivided into three categories: Letterer-Siwe syndrome, Hand-Schüller-Christian disease, and eosinophilic granuloma. These three conditions are now believed to represent different expressions of the same basic disorder. The proliferating cell in all forms is the Langerhans' cell of marrow origin, which is normally found in the epidermis. These cells, believed to be part of the mononuclear phagocyte system, are HLA-DR positive and express the CD1 antigen.[50] They have abundant, often vacuolated cytoplasm, with vesicular oval or indented nuclei. *Characteristic is the presence of HX bodies (Birbeck granules) in the cytoplasm. Under the electron microscope these are seen to have a pentalaminar, rod-like, tubular structure, with characteristic periodicity and sometimes a dilated terminal end (tennis-racket appearance)* (Fig. 14–29).

Langerhans' cell histiocytosis presents as three clinicopathologic entities:

Acute disseminated Langerhans' cell histiocytosis (Letterer-Siwe disease) occurs most frequently before two years of age but occasionally may affect adults. The dominant clinical feature is the development of cutaneous lesions that resemble a seborrheic eruption secondary to infiltrations of Langerhans' histiocytes over the front and back of the

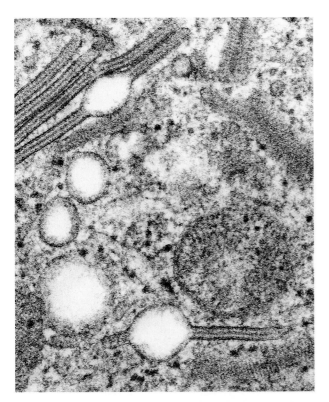

Figure 14-29. Langerhans' cell histiocytosis. An electron micrograph shows rod-like Birbeck granules with characteristic periodicity and dilated terminal end. (Courtesy of Dr. George Murphy, University of Pennsylvania School of Medicine, Philadelphia.)

trunk and on the scalp. Most of those affected have concurrent hepatosplenomegaly, lymphadenopathy, pulmonary lesions, and, eventually, destructive osteolytic bone lesions. Extensive infiltration of the marrow often leads to anemia, thrombocytopenia,

and predisposition to recurrent infections such as otitis media and mastoiditis. The course of untreated disease is rapidly fatal. With intensive chemotherapy 50% of patients survive 5 years.

Unifocal and multifocal Langerhans' cell histiocytosis (unifocal and multifocal eosinophilic granuloma). Both of these variants are characterized by expanding, erosive accumulations of Langerhans' cells, usually within the medullary cavities of bones. Histiocytes are variably admixed with eosinophils, lymphocytes, plasma cells, and neutrophils. The eosinophilic component ranges from scattered mature cells to sheetlike masses of cells.

Virtually any bone in the skeletal system may be involved, most commonly the calvarium, ribs, and femur. Similar lesions may be found in the skin, lungs, or stomach, either as unifocal lesions or as components of the multifocal disease.

Unifocal lesions usually affect the skeletal system. They may be asymptomatic or may cause pain and tenderness and, in some instances, pathologic fractures. This is an indolent disorder that may heal spontaneously or be cured by local excision or irradiation.

Multifocal Langerhans' cell histiocytosis usually affects children, who present with fever; diffuse eruptions, particularly on the scalp and in the ear canals; and frequent bouts of otitis media, mastoiditis, and upper respiratory tract infections. An infiltrate of Langerhans' cells may lead to mild lymphadenopathy, hepatomegaly, and splenomegaly. In about 50% of patients, involvement of the posterior pituitary stalk of the hypothalamus leads to diabetes insipidus. The combination of calvarial bone defects, diabetes insipidus, and exophthalmos is referred to as the Hand-Schüller-Christian triad. Many patients experience spontaneous regression; others can be treated with chemotherapy.

Spleen

SPLENOMEGALY	NEOPLASMS
Nonspecific Acute Splenitis	**CONGENITAL ANOMALIES**
Congestive Splenomegaly	**RUPTURE**
Splenic Infarcts	

NORMAL

The spleen is to the circulatory system as the lymph nodes are to the lymphatic system. Among its functions are filtration from the bloodstream of

all "foreign" matter, including obsolescent and damaged blood cells, and participation in the immune response to all blood-borne antigens. Designed ingeniously for these functions, the spleen is a major repository of mononuclear phagocytic cells in the red pulp and of lymphoid cells in the white pulp. Normally in the adult it weighs about 150 gm and measures some 12 cm in length, 7 cm in

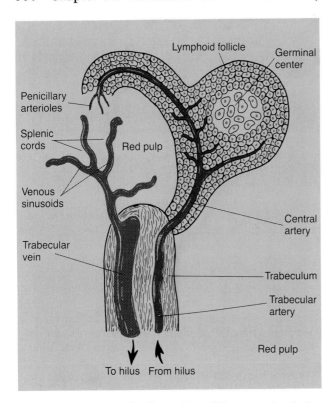

Figure 14-30. Schematic illustration of the normal splenic architecture. (Modified from Faller, D.V.: Diseases of the spleen. *In* **Wyngaarden, J.B., and Smith, L.H. (eds.): Cecil Textbook of Medicine, 18th ed. Philadelphia, W.B. Saunders Co., 1988, p. 1036.)**

endothelial lining of the sinusoid is of the open or discontinuous type, providing passage of blood cells between the sinusoids and cords. The splenic cords are spongelike and consist of a labyrinth of macrophages loosely connected through long dendritic processes to create both a physical and a functional filter through which the blood can slowly seep.

It is widely believed that the blood, as it traverses the red pulp, takes two routes to reach the splenic veins.[51] Some of the capillary flow is into the splenic cords and is then gradually filtered out into the surrounding splenic sinusoids to reach the veins; this is the so-called open circulation, which is functionally the slow compartment. The other pathway involves direct passage from the capillaries to the splenic veins without the intervening stage of passage through the cords. This, the "closed circuit," is understandably the more rapid compartment. According to current views, only a small fraction of the blood entering the spleen at any given time pursues the "open" route. Nevertheless, during the course of a day the total volume of blood passes through the filtration beds of the splenic cords, where it is exposed to the remarkably sensitive and effective phagocytic macrophages, which are able to screen the blood.

Most anatomic disorders of the spleen are secondary to some systemic disorder and thus are the consequence of normal splenic function. These can be segregated into four categories.

1. *Filtration of unwanted elements from the blood* by phagocytosis in the splenic cords is a major function of the spleen.[52] As you know, $\frac{1}{120}$ of all red cells are destroyed daily by phagocytosis in the reticuloendothelial system. Engulfment by splenic macrophages accounts for approximately half this removal of obsolescent red cells from the circulation. The splenic phagocytes are also remarkably efficient in "culling" damaged red cells and leukocytes and red cells rendered foreign by antibody coating, as well as the abnormal red cells encountered in several of the anemias (e.g., hereditary spherocytosis, sickle cell anemia). As discussed earlier (see Chapter 13), the red cells have to undergo extreme deformation during passage from the cords into the sinusoids. In several hemolytic anemias, the reduced plasticity of the red cell membrane leads to trapping of the abnormal red cells within the cords and subsequent phagocytosis by the cordal macrophages. In addition to removal of the red cells, splenic macrophages are also involved in "pitting" of red cells, by which inclusions such as Heinz bodies are neatly excised without destruction of the erythrocytes. The phagocytes are also active in removal of other particulate matter from the blood, such as bacteria, cell debris, and abnormal macromolecules produced in some of the inborn errors of metabolism (e.g., Gaucher disease, Niemann-Pick disease).

width, and 3 cm in thickness. It is enclosed within a thin, glistening connective tissue capsule that appears slate gray and through which the dusky red, friable parenchyma of the splenic substance can be seen. The cut surface of the spleen is dotted with gray specks, the splenic, or malpighian, follicles that constitute the white pulp. In three dimensions this white pulp forms periarterial sheaths of lymphoid cells around the arteries, most abundant about the larger branches and progressively more attenuated as the arterial supply penetrates the splenic substance. A cross section of such an arrangement reveals a central artery surrounded eccentrically by a collar of T lymphocytes, the so-called periarteriolar lymphatic sheath. At intervals the lymphatic sheaths expand, usually on one side of the artery, to form lymphoid nodules composed principally of B lymphocytes (Fig. 14-30). On antigenic stimulation, typical germinal centers form within these B-cell areas. Eventually, the arterial system terminates in fine penicilliary arterioles, which at first are enclosed within a thin mantle of lymphocytes but which then enter the red pulp, leaving behind their "fellow-travelers."

The red pulp of the spleen is traversed by numerous thin-walled vascular sinusoids, separated by the splenic cords, or "cords of Billroth." The

2. The spleen is a *major secondary organ in the immune system.* The reticular network in the periarterial lymphatic sheaths traps antigen, permitting it to come into contact with effector lymphocytes.

3. The spleen is a *source of lymphoreticular cells and sometimes hematopoietic cells.* Splenic hematopoiesis normally ceases before birth, but in severe anemia, extramedullary splenic hematopoiesis may be reactivated.

4. Because of its rich vascularization and phagocytic function, the spleen also constitutes a *reserve pool and storage site.* In humans, the normal spleen harbors only about 30 to 40 ml of erythrocytes, but with splenomegaly this reservoir is greatly increased. The normal spleen also stores approximately 30 to 40% of the total platelet mass in the body. With splenomegaly this platelet storage may markedly increase, sometimes to up to 80 to 90% of the total platelet mass. Similarly, the enlarged spleen may trap a sufficient number of white cells to induce leukopenia.

In view of all these functions it is no wonder that the spleen becomes secondarily involved in a wide variety of systemic disorders.

PATHOLOGY

As the largest unit of the mononuclear phagocyte system, the spleen is involved in all systemic inflammations and generalized hematopoietic disorders and many metabolic disturbances. It is rarely the primary site of disease. When the spleen is involved in systemic disease, splenic enlargement usually develops, and therefore splenomegaly is a major manifestation of disorders of this organ.

SPLENOMEGALY

Splenic enlargement may be an important diagnostic clue to the existence of an underlying disorder, but the condition itself may cause problems. When sufficiently enlarged, the spleen may cause a dragging sensation in the left upper quadrant and, through pressure on the stomach, cause discomfort after eating. In addition, its storage function may lead to the sequestration of significant numbers of blood elements, giving rise to a syndrome known as *hypersplenism,* which is characterized by the triad of (1) splenomegaly; (2) a reduction of one or more of the cellular elements of the blood, leading

Table 14-12. DISORDERS ASSOCIATED WITH SPLENOMEGALY

I. INFECTIONS
Nonspecific splenitis of various blood-borne infections (particularly infective endocarditis)
Infectious mononucleosis
Tuberculosis
Typhoid fever
Brucellosis
Cytomegalovirus
Syphilis
Malaria
Histoplasmosis
Toxoplasmosis
Kala-azar
Trypanosomiasis
Schistosomiasis
Leishmaniasis
Echinococcosis

II. CONGESTIVE STATES RELATED TO PORTAL HYPERTENSION
Cirrhosis of liver
Portal or splenic vein thrombosis
Cardiac failure (right-sided)

III. LYMPHOHEMATOGENOUS DISORDERS
Hodgkin's disease
Non-Hodgkin's lymphomas
Histiocytoses
Multiple myeloma
Myeloproliferative syndromes (chronic myelogenous leukemia, polycythemia vera, myeloid metaplasia with myelofibrosis)
Chronic lymphocytic leukemia
Acute leukemias (inconstant)
Hemolytic anemias (autoimmune hemolytic anemia, hereditary spherocytosis, hemoglobinopathies)
Thrombocytopenic purpura

IV. IMMUNOLOGIC-INFLAMMATORY CONDITIONS
Rheumatoid arthritis
Felty's syndrome
Systemic lupus erythematosus

V. STORAGE DISEASES
Gaucher disease
Niemann-Pick disease
Mucopolysaccharidoses

VI. MISCELLANEOUS
Amyloidosis
Primary neoplasms and cysts
Secondary neoplasms

to anemia, leukopenia, thrombocytopenia, or any combination of these, in association with hyperplasia of the marrow precursors of the deficient cell type; and (3) correction of the blood cytopenia(s) by splenectomy. The precise cause of this syndrome is still uncertain, but increased sequestration of the cells and the consequent enhanced lysis by the splenic macrophages seem to be the likely explanation for the cytopenias.

A listing, by no means exhaustive, of the disorders associated with splenomegaly is provided in Table 14-12. The splenomegaly in virtually all the conditions mentioned has been discussed elsewhere. There remain only a few disorders that require consideration.

Nonspecific Acute Splenitis

Enlargement of the spleen, sometimes also called acute splenic tumor, occurs in any blood-borne infection. The nonspecific splenic reaction in these infections may be caused not only by the microbiologic agents themselves but also by the products of the inflammatory disease.

MORPHOLOGY. The spleen is enlarged (up to 200 to 400 gm) and soft. The splenic substance is often diffluent and may be sufficiently soft to literally flow out from the cut surface. Microscopically, the major change is acute congestion of the red pulp, which may encroach on and sometimes virtually efface the lymphoid follicles. An infiltrate of neutrophils, plasma cells, and occasionally eosinophils is sometimes present throughout the white and red pulp. At times there is acute necrosis of the centers of the splenic follicles, particularly when the causative agent is a hemolytic streptococcus. Rarely, abscess formation occurs.

Congestive Splenomegaly

Persistent or chronic venous congestion may cause enlargement of the spleen, referred to as *congestive splenomegaly*. The venous congestion may be systemic in origin, may be caused by intrahepatic derangement of portal venous drainage, or may be due to obstructive venous disorders in the portal or splenic veins. All these disorders ultimately lead to portal or splenic vein hypertension. *Systemic, or central venous, congestion* is encountered in cardiac decompensation involving the right side of the heart, as may occur in tricuspid or pulmonic valvular disease or chronic cor pulmonale or following left-sided heart failure. Such systemic passive congestion produces only moderate enlargement of the spleen, so that it rarely exceeds 500 gm in weight.

The only common causes of striking congestive splenomegaly are the various forms of cirrhosis of the liver. The diffuse fibrous scarring of alcoholic cirrhosis and pigment cirrhosis evokes the most extreme enlargements. Other forms of cirrhosis are less commonly implicated.

Congestive splenomegaly is also caused by obstruction of the extrahepatic portal vein or splenic vein. The venous obstruction may be due to *spontaneous portal vein thrombosis*, which is usually associated with some intrahepatic obstructive disease or may be initiated by inflammatory involvement of the portal vein *(pylephlebitis)*, such as follows intraperitoneal infections. Thrombosis of the splenic vein itself may be initiated by the pressure of tumors in neighboring organs, for example, carcinoma of the stomach or pancreas.

MORPHOLOGY. Long-standing congestive splenomegaly produces marked enlargement of the spleen (1000 gm or more); the organ is firm and becomes increasingly so the longer the congestion lasts. The weight may reach 5000 gm. The capsule may be thickened and fibrous but is otherwise uninvolved. The cut surface has a meaty appearance and varies from gray-red to deep red, depending on the amount of fibrosis. Often the malpighian corpuscles are indistinct. Microscopically, the pulp is suffused with red cells during the early phases but becomes increasingly more fibrous and cellular with time. The increased portal venous pressure causes deposition of collagen in the basement membrane of the sinusoids, which appear dilated owing to the rigidity of their walls. The resulting impairment of blood flow from the cords to the sinusoids prolongs the exposure of the blood cells to the cordal macrophages, resulting in excessive destruction (hypersplenism).[53] Foci of recent or old hemorrhage may be present with deposition of hemosiderin in histiocytes. Organization of these focal hemorrhages gives rise to Gandy-Gamna nodules —foci of fibrosis containing deposits of iron and calcium salts encrusted on connective tissue and elastic fibers.

Splenic Infarcts

Splenic infarcts are comparatively common lesions. Caused by occlusion of the major splenic artery or any of its branches, they are almost always due to emboli that arise in the heart. The spleen, along with kidneys and brain, ranks as one of the most frequent sites of localization of systemic emboli. The infarcts may be small or large, multiple or single, and sometimes involve the entire organ. They are usually of the bland, anemic type. Septic infarcts are found in infective endocarditis of the valves of the left side of the heart.

MORPHOLOGY. Infarcts are characteristically pale and wedge-shaped, with their bases at the periphery where the capsule is often covered with fibrin (Fig. 14–31). Septic infarction modifies this appearance as frank suppurative necrosis develops. In the course of healing of these splenic infarcts, large, depressed scars may develop.

NEOPLASMS

Neoplastic involvement of the spleen is rare except in tumors of the lymphohematopoietic system. When present they induce splenomegaly.

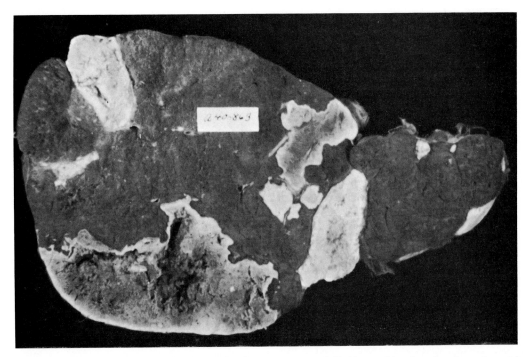

Figure 14–31. Splenic infarcts. Multiple wedge-shaped lesions are present, the largest having developed cystic softening.

The following types of benign tumors may arise in the spleen: fibromas, osteomas, chondromas, lymphangiomas, and hemangiomas. The two last-named are the most common and are often cavernous in type. Undoubtedly, some of the hemangiomas are better classified as hamartomas than as neoplasms. Splenic involvement occurs in a variety of leukemias and lymphomas, as already discussed.

CONGENITAL ANOMALIES

Complete absence of the spleen is rare and is usually associated with other congenital abnormalities such as situs inversus and cardiac malformations. *Hypoplasia* is a more common finding.

Accessory spleens (spleniculi) are common and have been encountered singly or multiply in one-fifth to one-third of all postmortem examinations. They are usually small spherical structures that are histologically and functionally identical with the normal spleen, reacting to various stimuli in the same manner. They are generally situated in the gastrosplenic ligament or the tail of the pancreas, but are sometimes located in the omentum or mesenteries of the small or large intestine. Accessory spleens may have great clinical importance. In some hematologic disorders such as hereditary spherocytosis, thrombocytopenic purpura, and hypersplenism, splenectomy is a standard method of

treatment. If a large accessory spleen is overlooked, the benefit from the removal of the definitive spleen may be lost.

RUPTURE

Rupture of the spleen is usually caused by a crushing injury or severe blow. Much less often, it is encountered in the apparent absence of trauma; this event is designated as spontaneous rupture. It is a clinical maxim that the normal spleen never ruptures spontaneously. In all instances of apparent nontraumatic rupture, some underlying condition should be suspected as the basis for the enlargement or weakening of this organ. Spontaneous rupture is encountered most often in infectious mononucleosis, malaria, typhoid fever, leukemia, and the other types of acute splenitis. Rupture is usually followed by extensive, sometimes massive, intraperitoneal hemorrhage. The condition usually must be treated by prompt surgical removal of the spleen to prevent death from loss of blood and shock.

1. Shastri, K.A., and Logue, G.L.: Autoimmune neutropenia. Blood 81:1984, 1993.
2. McKenna, R., et al.: Granulated T lymphocytosis with neutropenia: Malignant or benign chronic lymphoproliferative disorder? Blood 66:259, 1985.
3. National Cancer Institute: Sponsored study of classifica-

tion of non-Hodgkin's lymphomas: Summary and description of Working Formulation for Clinical Usage. Cancer *49*:2112, 1982.

4. Vaickus, L., et al.: Immune markers in hematologic malignancies. Crit. Rev. Oncol. Hematol. *11*:267, 1991.

5. O'Reilly, S.E., and Conners, J.M.: Non-Hodgkin's lymphoma I: Characterization and treatment. Br. Med. J. *304*:1682, 1992.

6. Freedman, A.S., and Nadler, L.M.: Non-Hodgkin's lymphomas. *In* Holland, J.F., et al. (eds.): Cancer Medicine, 3rd ed. Philadelphia, Lea & Febiger, 1993, p. 2028.

7. Swerdlow, S.H., and Williams, M.E.: Centrocytic lymphoma—a distinct clinicopathologic, immunophenotypic, and genotypic entity. Pathol. Annu. *28*(2):171, 1993.

8. Zucker, F., et al.: Human lymphotropic retroviruses associated with mycosis fungoides. Blood *80*:1537, 1992.

9. Chen, Y.-T., et al.: Immunohistochemistry and gene rearrangement studies in the diagnosis of malignant lymphomas: A comparison of 152 cases. Hum. Pathol. *22*:1249, 1991.

10. Cossman, J., et al.: Molecular genetics and the diagnosis of lymphoma. Arch. Pathol. Lab. Med. *112*:117, 1988.

11. Takvorian, T., and Canellos, G.: Hodgkin's disease. *In* Holland, J.F., et al. (eds.): Cancer Medicine, 3rd ed. Philadelphia, Lea & Febiger, 1993, p. 1998.

12. Carde, P.: Hodgkin's disease. I. Identification and classification. Br. Med. J. *305*:99, 1992.

13. Poppema, S.: Lymphocyte-predominance Hodgkin's disease. Semin. Diagn. Pathol. *9*:257, 1992.

14. Schmid, C., et al.: L and H cells of nodular lymphocyte predominant Hodgkin's disease show immunoglobulin light chain restriction. Am. J. Pathol. *139*:1281, 1991.

15. Kadin, M., et al.: Eosinophils are the major source of transforming growth factor-β1 in nodular sclerosing Hodgkin's disease. Am. J. Pathol. *142*:11, 1993.

16. Stein, H., and Hummel, M.: What is the origin of the malignant cell in Hodgkin's disease? Leuk. Lymph. *10*(Suppl.):99, 1993.

17. Jarrett, R., and Onions, D.: Viruses and Hodgkin's disease. Leukemia *6*:(Suppl. 1), 1992.

18. Weiss L. M., and Chang, K. L.: Molecular biologic studies of Hodgkin's disease. Semin. Diagn. Pathol. *9*:272, 1992.

19. Chang, K. L., et al.: High prevalence of Epstein-Barr virus in Reed-Sternberg cells of Hodgkin's disease in Peru. Blood *81*:496, 1993.

20. Tucker, M.A., et al.: Risk of second cancers after treatment of Hodgkin's disease. N. Engl. J. Med. *318*:76, 1988.

21. Trigg, M.E.: Acute lymphoblastic leukemia in children. *In* Holland, J.F., et al. (eds.): Cancer Medicine, 3rd ed. Philadelphia, Lea & Febiger, 1993, p. 2153.

22. Raimondi, S.C.: Current status of cytogenetic research in childhood acute lymphoblastic leukemia. Blood *81*:2237, 1993.

23. Bennett, J.M., et al.: Proposal for recognition of minimally differentiated acute myeloid leukemia (AML-M0). Br. J. Hematol. *78*:325, 1991.

24. Hirsch-Ginsberg, C., et al.: Recent advances in the diagnosis of acute leukemia. Cancer Bull. *45*:64, 1993.

25. Schiffer, C.A.: Acute myeloid leukemia in adults. *In* Holland, J.F., et al. (eds.): Cancer Medicine, 3rd ed. Philadelphia, Lea & Febiger, 1993, p. 1907.

26. Divero, D., et al.: Identification of DNA rearrangements in the retinoic acid receptor-α (RAR-α) locus in all patients with acute promyelocytic leukemia (APL) and mapping of APL breakpoints within the RAR-α second intron. Blood *79*:3331, 1992.

27. Degos, L.: Retinoic acid in acute promyelocytic leuke-

mia: A model for differentiation therapy. Curr. Opin. Oncol. *2*:45, 1992.

28. Kouides, P.A., and Bennett, J.M.: Morphology and classification of myelodysplastic syndromes. Hematol. Oncol. Clin. North Am. *6*:485, 1992.

29. Mecucci, C., and Van den Berghe, H.: Cytogenetics. Hematol. Oncol. Clin. North Am. *6*:523, 1992.

30. Ganser, A., and Hoelzer, D.: Clinical course of myelodysplastic syndromes. Hematol. Oncol. Clin. North Am. *6*:607, 1992.

31. Kantarjian, H.M.: Chronic myelogenous leukemia: A concise update. Blood *82*:691, 1993.

32. Leemhuis, T., et al.: Identification of BCR/ABL negative primitive hematopoietic progenitor cells within chronic myeloid leukemia marrow. Blood *81*:801, 1993.

33. Keating, M.J.: Chronic lymphoproliferative disorders: Chronic lymphocytic leukemia and hairy cell leukemia. Curr. Opin. Oncol. *5*:35, 1993.

34. Chang, K.L., et al.: Hairy cell leukemia. Current status. Am. J. Clin. Pathol. *97*:719, 1992.

35. Vogel, V.G., and Fisher, R.E.: Epidemiology and etiology of leukemia. Curr. Opin. Oncol. *5*:26, 1993.

36. Cline, M.J.: The molecular basis of leukemia. N. Engl. J. Med. *330*:328, 1994.

37. Murphy, S.: Polycythemia vera. Disease-A-Month *38*:167, 1992.

38. Dai, C.H., et al.: Polycythemia vera. II. Hypersensitivity of bone marrow erythroid, granulocyte macrophage, and megakaryocytic progenitor cells to interleukin-3 and granulocyte-macrophage colony stimulating factor. Blood *80*:891, 1992.

39. Ellis, J.T., et al.: Studies of the bone marrow in polycythemia vera and the evolution of myelofibrosis and second hematologic malignancies. Semin. Hematol. *23*:144, 1986.

40. Hasselbalch, H.C.: Idiopathic myelofibrosis. Dan. Med. Bull. *40*:39, 1993.

41. Reilly, J.T., et al.: Characterization of an acute micro-mega-karyocytic leukemia: Evidence for the pathogenesis of myelofibrosis. Br. J. Hematol. *83*:58, 1993.

42. Reilly, J.T.: Pathogenesis of idiopathic myelofibrosis: Role of growth factors. J. Clin. Pathol. *45*:461, 1992.

43. Osserman, E.F., et al.: Multiple myeloma and related plasma cell dyscrasias. J.A.M.A. *258*:2930, 1987.

44. Mandelli, F., et al.: Biology and treatment of multiple myeloma. Curr. Opin. Oncol. *4*:73, 1992.

45. Kelin, B., and Bataille, R.: Cytokine network in human myeloma. Hematol. Oncol. Clin. North Am. *6*:273, 1992.

46. Klein, B., et al.: Murine anti-interleukin 6 monoclonal antibody therapy for a patient with plasma cell leukemia. Blood *78*:1198, 1991.

47. Bataille, R., et al.: Mechanisms of bone lesions in multiple myeloma. Hematol. Oncol. Clin. North Am. *6*:285, 1992.

48. Gahrton, G., et al.: Allogeneic bone marrow transplantation in multiple myeloma. N. Engl. J. Med. *325*:1267, 1991.

49. Lukens, J.N.: Langerhans cell histiocytosis. *In* Less, G.R., et al. (eds.): Wintrobe's Clinical Hematology, 9th ed. Philadelphia, Lea & Febiger, 1993, p. 1640.

50. Ben-Ezra, J.M., and Koo, C.E.: Langerhans cell histiocytosis and malignancies of the M-PIRE system. Am. J. Clin. Pathol. *99*:464, 1993.

51. Weiss, L.: Red pulp of the spleen: Structural basis of blood flow. Clin. Hematol. *12*:375, 1983.

52. Rosse, W.F.: Spleen as a filter. N. Engl. J. Med. *317*:704, 1987.

53. Bishop, M.B., and Lansing, L.S.: The spleen: A correlative overview of normal and pathologic anatomy. Hum. Pathol. *13*:334, 1982.

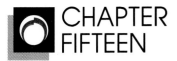

CHAPTER FIFTEEN

The Lung

LESTER KOBZIK, M.D., and FREDERICK J. SCHOEN, M.D., Ph.D.

NORMAL

The lungs are ingeniously constructed to carry out their cardinal function, the exchange of gases between inspired air and the blood.[1,2] The right lung is divided into three lobes; the left lung has only two lobes, its middle lobe equivalent being the *lingula*. The lung airways—the main right and left bronchi—arise from the trachea and then branch dichotomously, giving rise to progressively smaller airways. The right main stem bronchus is more vertical and more directly in line with the trachea than is the left. As a consequence, aspirated foreign material, such as vomitus, blood, and foreign bodies, tends to enter the right lung rather than the left. Accompanying the branching airways is the double arterial supply to the lungs, that is, the pulmonary and bronchial arteries. In the absence of significant cardiac failure, the bronchial arteries of aortic origin can often sustain the vitality of the pulmonary parenchyma when pulmonary arterial supply is shut off, as by emboli.

Progressive branching of the bronchi forms *bronchioles*, which are distinguished from bronchi by the lack of cartilage and submucosal glands within their walls. Further branching of bronchioles leads to the *terminal bronchioles*, which are less than 2 mm in diameter. The part of the lung distal to the terminal bronchiole is called the *acinus*, or the *terminal respiratory unit*; it is approximately spherical in shape, with a diameter of about 7 mm. Acini contain alveoli and are thus the site of gas exchange. As illustrated in Figure 15–8A, an acinus is composed of *respiratory bronchioles* (emanating from the terminal bronchiole),

673

which give off from their sides several alveoli; these bronchioles then proceed into the *alveolar ducts*, which immediately branch and empty into the *alveolar sacs*—the blind ends of the respiratory passages whose walls are formed entirely of alveoli. It is important to note that the alveoli open into the ducts through large mouths. In the correct plane of section, therefore, all alveoli are open and have incomplete walls. A cluster of three to five terminal bronchioles, each with its appended acini, is usually referred to as the pulmonary *lobule*. As will be seen, this lobular architecture assumes importance in distinguishing the major forms of emphysema.

From the microscopic standpoint, it is well to remember that except for the vocal cords, which are covered by stratified squamous epithelium, nearly the entire respiratory tree, including the larynx, trachea, and bronchioles, is lined by pseudostratified, tall, columnar, ciliated epithelial cells, heavily admixed in the cartilaginous airways with mucus-secreting goblet cells. The bronchial mucosa also contains neuroendocrine cells that exhibit neurosecretory-type granules and contain serotonin, calcitonin, and gastrin-releasing peptide (bombesin). Numerous submucosal, mucus-secreting glands are dispersed throughout the walls of the trachea and bronchi (but not the bronchioles).

The microscopic structure of the alveolar walls (or alveolar septa) consists, from blood to air, of the following (Fig. 15–1).

1. The *capillary endothelium* lining the intertwining network of anastomosing capillaries.

2. A *basement membrane and surrounding interstitial tissue* separating the endothelial cells from the alveolar lining epithelial cells. In thin portions of the alveolar septum, the basement membranes of epithelium and endothelium are fused, whereas in thicker portions they are separated by an interstitial space *(the pulmonary interstitium)* containing fine elastic fibers, small bundles of collagen, a few fibroblast-like interstitial cells, smooth muscle cells, mast cells, and rarely lymphocytes and monocytes.

3. The alveolar epithelium comprises a continuous layer of two principal cell types: flattened, plate-like pavement *type I pneumocytes* (or membranous pneumocytes) covering 95% of the alveolar surface, and rounded *type II pneumocytes*. Type II cells are important for at least two reasons: (a) they are the source of *pulmonary surfactant*,[3] contained in osmiophilic *lamellar bodies* seen with electron microscopy, and (b) they are the main cell type involved in the repair of alveolar epithelium after destruction of type I cells. Loosely attached to the epithelial cells or lying free within the alveolar spaces are the *alveolar macrophages*, derived from blood monocytes and belonging to the mononuclear phagocyte system. Often they are filled with carbon particles and other phagocytosed materials. The alveolar walls are not solid but are

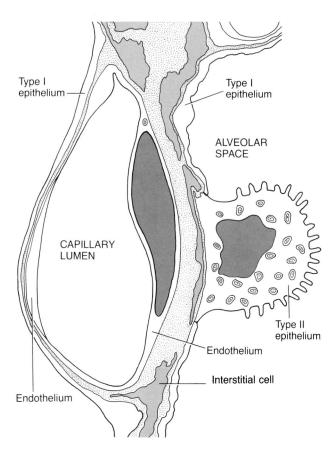

Figure 15–1. Microscopic structure of alveolar wall. Note that the basement membrane (stippled) is thin on one side and widened where it is continuous with the interstitial space. Portions of interstitial cells are shown.

perforated by numerous *pores of Kohn*, which permit the passage of bacteria and exudate between adjacent alveoli (see Fig. 15–21).

Adjacent to the alveolar cell membrane is the pulmonary surfactant layer (discussed in Chapter 10 in the section on respiratory distress syndrome in newborns).

PATHOLOGY

It is impossible to overemphasize the importance of lung disease in the overall perspective of pathology and clinical medicine. Primary respiratory infections, such as bronchitis, bronchopneumonia, and other forms of pneumonia, are commonplace in clinical and pathologic practice. In this day of cigarette smoking and air pollution, chronic bronchitis and emphysema have become rampant. Malignancy of the lungs has risen steadily in incidence, particularly in women, until it is now the most common lethal visceral malignancy in both males and females, surpassing even breast cancer in women. Moreover, the lungs are secondarily involved in almost all forms of terminal disease, so that at virtually every autopsy some degree of pulmonary edema, atelectasis, or bronchopneumonia is found. In the present consideration of the lung, emphasis will be placed on primary diseases that affect this important organ. For detailed descriptions of less common conditions, the reader is referred to current comprehensive books of pulmonary disease.[4,5]

CONGENITAL ANOMALIES

Developmental defects of the lung[6] include (1) agenesis or hypoplasia of both lungs, one lung, or single lobes; (2) tracheal and bronchial anomalies; (3) vascular anomalies; (4) congenital lobar overinflation (emphysema); (5) congenital cysts; and (6) intralobar and extrapulmonary lobar sequestrations. The last two anomalies are seen more frequently and are discussed here.

Congenital cysts represent an abnormal detachment of a fragment of primitive foregut, and most consist of *bronchogenic cysts.* Bronchogenic cysts may occur anywhere in the lungs as single or, on occasion, multiple cystic spaces from microscopic size to more than 5 cm in diameter. They are usually found adjacent to bronchi or bronchioles but may or may not have demonstrable connections with the airways. They are lined by bronchial-type epithelium and are usually filled with mucinous secretions or with air. Complications include infection of the secretions, with suppuration, lung abscess, or rupture into bronchi, causing hemorrhage and hemoptysis; or rupture into the pleural cavity, with pneumothorax or interstitial emphysema.

Bronchopulmonary sequestration refers to the presence of lobes or segments of lung tissue *without a normal connection to the airway system.* Blood supply to the sequestered area arises not from the pulmonary arteries but from the aorta or its branches. *Intralobar sequestrations* are found within the lung substance and are usually associated with recurrent localized infection or bronchiectasis. *Extralobar sequestrations* are external to the lung and may be found anywhere in the thorax or mediastinum. Found most commonly in infants as abnormal mass lesions, they may be associated with other congenital anomalies.

ATELECTASIS

Atelectasis refers either to incomplete expansion of the lungs or to the collapse of previously inflated lung substance, producing areas of relatively airless pulmonary parenchyma. Significant atelectasis re-

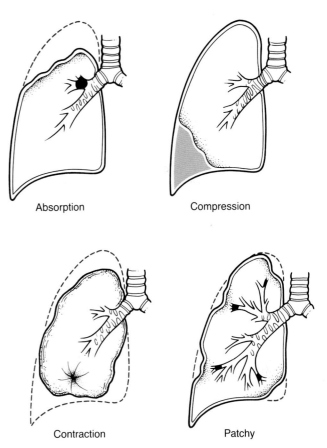

Figure 15-2. Illustration of the various forms of atelectasis in the adult.

duces oxygenation and predisposes to infection. Acquired atelectasis, encountered principally in adults, may be divided into *obstructive* (or *absorptive*), *compressive,* contraction (from scarring), and *patchy atelectasis* (Fig. 15-2).

Obstructive atelectasis is the consequence of complete obstruction of an airway, which in time leads to *absorption* of the oxygen trapped in the dependent alveoli, without impairment of blood flow through the affected alveolar walls. Since lung volume is diminished, the mediastinum may shift *toward* the atelectatic lung. Obstructive atelectasis is caused principally by excessive secretions or exudates within smaller bronchi and is therefore most often found in bronchial asthma, chronic bronchitis, bronchiectasis, and postoperative states and with aspiration of foreign bodies. Although bronchial neoplasms can cause atelectasis, in most instances they cause subtotal obstruction and produce localized emphysema.

Compressive atelectasis results whenever the pleural cavity is partially or completely filled by fluid exudate, tumor, blood, or air (the last-mentioned constituting *pneumothorax*), or with *tension pneumothorax,* when air pressure impinges on and threatens the function of lung and mediastinum, especially the major vessels. Compressive atelectasis is most commonly encountered in patients in cardiac failure who develop pleural fluid and in patients with neoplastic effusions within the pleural cavities. Similarly, abnormal elevation of the diaphragm, such as that which follows peritonitis or subdiaphragmatic abscesses or which occurs in seriously ill postoperative patients, will induce basal atelectasis. With compressive atelectasis, the mediastinum shifts *away* from the affected lung. *Patchy atelectasis* develops when there is loss of pulmonary surfactant, as in neonatal and adult respiratory distress syndromes.

Because the collapsed lung parenchyma can be re-expanded, *atelectasis is a reversible disorder.* However, atelectatic parenchyma is prone to developing superimposed infections.

DISEASES OF VASCULAR ORIGIN

PULMONARY CONGESTION AND EDEMA

A general consideration of edema is in Chapter 4, and pulmonary congestion and edema were described briefly in the context of congestive heart failure (see Chapter 12). Pulmonary edema can result from *hemodynamic* disturbances *(hydrodynamic or cardiogenic pulmonary edema)* or from direct *increases in capillary permeability*, owing to microvascular injury (Table 15–1).

Hemodynamic Pulmonary Edema

The most common *hemodynamic* mechanism of pulmonary edema is that attributable to *increased hydrostatic pressure*, as occurs in left-sided congestive heart failure. Accumulation of fluid in this setting can be accounted for by Starling's law of capillary interstitial fluid exchange (see Chapter 4).

Whatever the clinical setting, pulmonary congestion and edema are characterized by heavy, wet lungs. Fluid accumulates initially in the basal regions of the lower lobes, since hydrostatic pressure is greater in these sites. Histologically, the alveolar capillaries are engorged and an intra-alveolar granular pink precipitate is seen. Alveolar microhemorrhages and hemosiderin-laden macrophages *(heart failure cells)* may be present. In long-standing cases of pulmonary congestion, such as those seen in mitral stenosis, hemosiderin-laden macrophages are abundant, and fibrosis and thickening of the alveolar walls cause the soggy lungs to become firm and brown *(brown induration)*. These changes not only impair normal respiratory function but also predispose to infection.

Table 15–1. CLASSIFICATION AND CAUSES OF PULMONARY EDEMA

HEMODYNAMIC EDEMA
  Increased Hydrostatic Pressure
    Left-sided heart failure
    Mitral stenosis
    Volume overload
    Pulmonary vein obstruction
  Decreased Oncotic Pressure
    Hypoalbuminemia
      Nephrotic syndrome
      Liver disease
      Protein-losing enteropathies
  Lymphatic Obstruction

EDEMA DUE TO MICROVASCULAR INJURY
  Infectious agents: viruses, Mycoplasma, other
  Inhaled gases: oxygen, sulfur dioxide, cyanates, smoke
  Liquid aspiration: gastric contents, near-drowning
  Drugs and chemicals
    Chemotherapeutic agents: bleomycin, other
    Other medications: amphotericin B, colchicine, gold
    Other: heroin, kerosene, paraquat
  Shock, trauma, and sepsis
  Radiation
  Miscellaneous
    Acute pancreatitis; extracorporeal circulation; massive fat, air, or amniotic fluid embolism; uremia; heat; diabetic ketoacidosis; thrombotic thrombocytopenic purpura (TTP); disseminated intravascular coagulation (DIC)

EDEMA OF UNDETERMINED ORIGIN
  High altitude
  Neurogenic

Edema Due to Microvascular Injury

The second mechanism leading to pulmonary edema is *injury to the capillaries of the alveolar septa.* Here the pulmonary capillary hydrostatic pressure is usually not elevated, and hemodynamic factors play a secondary role. The edema results from primary injury to the vascular endothelium or damage to alveolar epithelial cells (with secondary microvascular injury). This results in leakage of fluids and proteins first into the interstitial space and, in more severe cases, into the alveoli. When the edema remains localized, as it does in most forms of pneumonia, it is overshadowed by the manifestations of infection. When diffuse, however, alveolar edema is an important contributor to a serious and often fatal condition, the *adult respiratory distress syndrome (ARDS)*, which will be discussed next.

ADULT RESPIRATORY DISTRESS SYNDROME (ARDS, DIFFUSE ALVEOLAR DAMAGE)

ARDS and its many synonyms (including adult respiratory failure, shock lung, diffuse alveolar damage [DAD], acute alveolar injury, and traumatic wet

Table 15–2. COMMON CLINICAL ASSOCIATIONS IN ADULT RESPIRATORY DISTRESS SYNDROME

Diffuse pulmonary infections
Inhalation of oxygen, smoke or other irritant gas
Drug toxicity or idiosyncratic reaction
Aspiration of gastric fluid
Near-drowing (salt or fresh water)
Massive air, fat, or amniotic fluid embolism
Radiation therapy
Shock
Sepsis
Extensive surface burns
Massive fractures and other trauma
Disseminated intravascular coagulation (DIC) and other
    blood disorders
Acute pancreatitis
Hemodialysis and cardiopulmonary bypass
Uremia, diabetic ketoacidosis, and other metabolic disorders

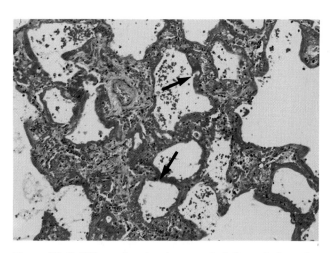

Figure 15–3. Diffuse alveolar damage (adult respiratory distress syndrome), shown in photomicrograph. Some of the alveoli are collapsed, others distended. Many contain dense proteinaceous debris, desquamated cells, and hyaline membranes *(arrows)*.

lungs) are descriptive terms for a syndrome caused by diffuse alveolar capillary damage and characterized clinically by the rapid onset of severe life-threatening respiratory insufficiency, cyanosis, and severe arterial hypoxemia that is refractory to oxygen therapy, and that frequently progresses to extrapulmonary multisystem organ failure. In most patients there is evidence of severe pulmonary edema (often called *noncardiogenic, low-pressure,* or *high-permeability pulmonary edema*), with chest radiographs showing a diffuse alveolar infiltration. Although hyaline membranes are a characteristic histologic feature of both ARDS and the respiratory distress syndrome of newborns (see Chapter 10), the pathogenetic mechanisms are distinct (see following).

ARDS is a well-recognized complication of numerous and diverse conditions, including both direct injuries to the lungs and systemic disorders (Table 15–2). Direct lung injuries causing ARDS include *diffuse* pulmonary and other viral infections, oxygen toxicity, inhalation of toxins and other irritants, and aspiration of gastric contents. Systemic conditions causing ARDS include septic shock, shock associated with trauma, hemorrhagic pancreatitis, burns, complicated abdominal surgery, narcotic overdose and other drug reactions, hypersensitivity reactions to organic solvents, hemodialysis, and cardiac surgery involving extracorporeal pumps. In many cases, a combination of the foregoing conditions is present (e.g., shock, oxygen therapy, and sepsis).

MORPHOLOGY. In the acute edematous stage, the lungs are heavy, firm, red, and boggy. They exhibit congestion, interstitial and intra-alveolar edema, and inflammation. In addition to the congestion, and edema, there is fibrin deposition. The alveolar walls become lined with waxy **hyaline membranes** that are similar to those seen in hyaline membrane disease of neonates (see Chapter 10) (Fig. 15–3). Alveolar hyaline membranes consist of fibrin-rich edema fluid mixed with the cytoplasmic and lipid remnants of necrotic epithelial cells. Subsequently, type II epithelial cells undergo proliferation in an attempt to regenerate the alveolar lining; resolution is unusual; more commonly, there is organization of the fibrin exudate, with resultant intra-alveolar fibrosis. Marked thickening of the alveolar septa ensues, caused by proliferation of interstitial cells and deposition of collagen. Fatal cases often have superimposed bronchopneumonia.

PATHOGENESIS. ARDS is best viewed as the clinical and pathologic end result of acute alveolar injury caused by a variety of insults and probably initiated by different mechanisms.[7] The final common pathway is *diffuse damage to the alveolar capillary walls;* this is followed by a relatively nonspecific and often predictable series of morphologic and physiologic alterations leading to respiratory failure. *In contrast, the mechanism of the respiratory distress syndrome of newborns is a deficiency in pulmonary surfactant.* In ARDS, the initial injury is to either capillary endothelium (most frequently) or alveolar epithelium (occasionally), but eventually both are clearly affected. Damage to these cells leads to increased capillary permeability, interstitial and then intra-alveolar edema, fibrin exudation, and formation of hyaline membranes. Importantly, the exudate and diffuse tissue destruction that occur with ARDS cannot be easily resolved, and the result is generally organization with scarring, producing severe chronic changes, in contrast to the transudate of cardiogenic pulmonary edema that usually resolves.

The immediate (but not the sole) cause of poor

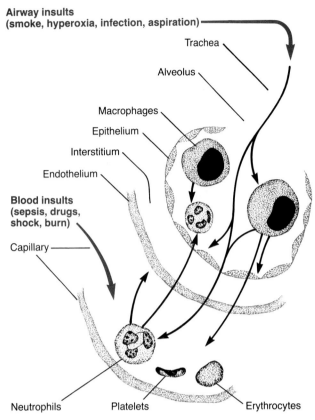

Airway insults
(smoke, hyperoxia, infection, aspiration)

Trachea

Alveolus

Macrophages

Epithelium

Interstitium

Endothelium

Blood insults
(sepsis, drugs,
shock, burn)

Capillary

Neutrophils   Platelets   Erythrocytes

Figure 15–4. Schematic pathogenesis of adult respiratory distress syndrome (diffuse alveolar damage). (Redrawn with permission from Repine, J.E.: Scientific perspectives on adult respiratory distress syndrome. Lancet 339:466, 1992. © The Lancet Ltd, 1992.)

lung aeration in ARDS is pulmonary edema due to a generalized defect in capillary-membrane permeability. The capillary defect is believed to be produced by an interaction of inflammatory cells and mediators, including leukocytes, cytokines, oxygen radicals, complement, and arachidonate metabolites, that damages the endothelium and allows fluid and proteins to leak across it (Fig. 15–4). Endotoxin is also important in many cases (see below).

Neutrophils play a key role in the pathogenesis of ARDS, being aggregated in the lung microvessels of most patients with this condition and having the capacity to injure pulmonary endothelial cells through release of toxic oxygen metabolites and destructive enzymes. In some situations, such as hemodialysis and cardiopulmonary bypass, neutrophil accumulation in the lung is induced by extrapulmonary activation of complement via the alternative pathway, as a result of blood contact with the membranes of these devices. Sepsis also causes nonspecific activation of complement. However, ARDS can also develop in the face of systemic neutropenia and without pulmonary neutrophilic aggregates.

Macrophages are an alternative source of in-

jury in patients with ARDS. Macrophages, you may recall (see Chapter 3), can generate toxic oxygen products, proteases, arachidonic acid metabolites, platelet-activating factor (PAF), and cytokines that regulate inflammation. Indeed, to some extent, neutrophilic inflammation in ARDS may be driven by macrophage-derived peptide cytokines, for example, interleukin-8 (IL-8). Additional physiologic effects of these mediators include vasoconstriction and platelet aggregation, both of which may decrease blood flow to aerated regions of the lungs.

Endotoxin is likely an important stimulus to the initiation of ARDS, amplifying complement-mediated responses of neutrophils, especially intrapulmonary leukocyte accumulation and subsequent damage to endothelial cells. Endotoxin induces the release of proinflammatory cytokines from macrophages and can increase endothelial expression of adhesion molecules for leukocytes.

CLINICAL COURSE. Patients who develop ARDS are usually hospitalized for one of the predisposing conditions listed earlier, and initially they may have no pulmonary symptoms. ARDS is heralded by profound dyspnea and tachypnea, but the chest radiograph is initially normal. Subsequently, there is increasing cyanosis and hypoxemia, respiratory failure, and the appearance of diffuse bilateral infiltrates on x-ray examination. Hypoxemia can then become unresponsive to oxygen therapy, and respiratory acidosis can develop.

The functional abnormalities in ARDS are not homogeneously distributed throughout the lungs. The lungs are focally stiff and have a decrease in functional volume. In essence, patients' lungs can be divided into areas that are infiltrated, consolidated, or collapsed (and thus poorly aerated and poorly compliant) and regions that have nearly normal levels of compliance and ventilation. Although blood is diverted away from poorly aerated regions in healthy lungs, lungs with ARDS continue to have perfusion of poorly aerated regions, contributing to ventilation-perfusion mismatching and hypoxemia. Inhaled nitric oxide, a potent vasodilator (see Chapter 3), decreases pulmonary artery pressure and pulmonary vascular resistance, which are usually elevated in ARDS, while not changing systemic arterial pressure and systemic vascular resistance.[8]

Therapy is difficult, and ARDS is frequently fatal. The high concentrations of oxygen that are required to treat ARDS can themselves contribute to perpetuation of the damage (oxygen toxicity). The usual cause of death is either respiratory failure or multiorgan dysfunction (due to the systemic effects of the same mediators that are produced in the lung). Progression from one phase to the next can be rapid (a few hours), but some patients recover with resorption of the edema fluid and reexpansion of atelectatic areas. However, despite improvements in supportive respiratory therapy, the mortality rate among the 150,000 ARDS cases seen yearly in the United States is still about 60%.

PULMONARY EMBOLISM, HEMORRHAGE, AND INFARCTION

Occlusions of the pulmonary arteries by blood clot are almost always embolic in origin. Large-vessel *in situ* thromboses are rare and develop only in the presence of pulmonary hypertension, pulmonary atherosclerosis, and heart failure. The usual source of these emboli (thrombi in the deep veins of the leg in more than 95% of cases) and the magnitude of the clinical problem were discussed in Chapter 4, where the disturbing frequency of pulmonary embolism (PE) and infarction was emphasized. Suffice it to say here that PE causes more than 50,000 deaths in the United States each year. Its incidence at autopsy has varied from 1% in the general population of hospital patients to 30% in patients dying after severe burns, trauma, or fractures to 65% of hospitalized patients in one study in which special techniques were applied to discover emboli at autopsy. It is the sole or a major contributing cause of death in about 10% of adults dying acutely in hospitals.

MORPHOLOGY. The morphologic consequences of embolic occlusion of the pulmonary arteries depend on the size of the embolic mass and the general state of the circulation. Large emboli may impact in the main pulmonary artery or its major branches or lodge at the bifurcation as a saddle embolus (Fig. 15–5). Sudden death often ensues, owing largely to the blockage of blood flow through the lungs. Death may also be caused by acute dilation of the right side of the heart (acute cor pulmonale). Smaller emboli can travel out into the more peripheral vessels, where they may or may not cause infarction. In patients with adequate cardiovascular function, the bronchial artery supply can often sustain the lung parenchyma despite obstruction to the pulmonary arterial system. Under these circumstances, hemorrhages may occur, but there is no infarction of the underlying lung parenchyma. Only about 10% of emboli actually cause infarction. Although the underlying pulmonary architecture may be obscured by the suffusion of blood, hemorrhages are distinguished by the preservation of the pulmonary alveolar architecture; in such cases resorption of the blood permits reconstitution of the pre-existing architecture.

PE usually causes infarction only when the circulation is already inadequate, namely, in patients with heart or lung disease. For this reason, pulmonary infarcts tend to be uncommon in the young. About three fourths of all infarcts affect the lower lobes, and in over half they occur multiply. They vary in size from lesions barely visible to the naked eye to massive involvement of large parts of an entire lobe. Characteristically, they extend to the periphery of the lung substance as a wedge with the apex pointing toward the hilus of the lung. In many cases an occluded vessel can be identified near the apex of the infarct.

The pulmonary infarct is classically hemorrhagic and appears as a raised, red-blue area in the early stages (Fig. 15–6). Often the apposed pleural surface is covered by a fibrinous exudate. The red cells begin to lyse within 48 hours, and the infarct becomes paler and eventually red-brown as hemosiderin is produced. With the passage of time, fibrous replacement begins at the margins as a gray-white peripheral zone and eventually converts the infarct into a contracted scar. Histologically, the diagnostic feature of acute pulmonary infarction is the ischemic necrosis of the lung substance within the area of hemorrhage, affecting the alveolar walls, bronchioles, and vessels. If the infarct is caused by an infected embolus, the infarct is modified by a more intense neutrophilic exudation and more intense inflammatory reaction. Such lesions are referred to as **septic infarcts,** and indeed some convert to abscesses.

CLINICAL COURSE. PE is a complication principally in patients already suffering from some underlying disorder, such as cardiac disease or cancer, or who are immobilized for long periods. Hypercoagulable states, either *primary* (e.g., antithrombin III or protein C deficiencies, defective fibrinolysis, and, paradoxically, the presence of lupus anticoagulant) or *secondary* (e.g., obesity, recent surgery, cancer, oral contraceptive use, pregnancy), frequently contribute to the original deep vein thrombus. Indwelling central venous lines can be a nidus for right atrial thrombus, which can be a source of PE.

The pathophysiologic response and clinical significance of PE depend on the extent to which the pulmonary artery blood flow is obstructed, size of the occluded vessel(s), number of emboli, overall status of the cardiovascular system, and release of vasoactive factors, for example, thromboxane A_2 (TxA_2), from platelets that accumulate at the site of thrombus. Emboli result in two main pathophysiologic consequences: *respiratory compromise* due to the nonperfused, although ventilated segment, and *hemodynamic compromise* due to increased resistance to pulmonary blood flow engendered by the embolic obstruction. The latter leads to pulmonary hypertension and can cause acute failure of the right ventricle.

A large PE is one of the few causes of virtually instantaneous death. During cardiopulmonary resuscitation in such instances, the patient frequently is said to have "electromechanical dissociation," in which the electrocardiogram has a rhythm, but no pulses are palpated, because of the massive block-

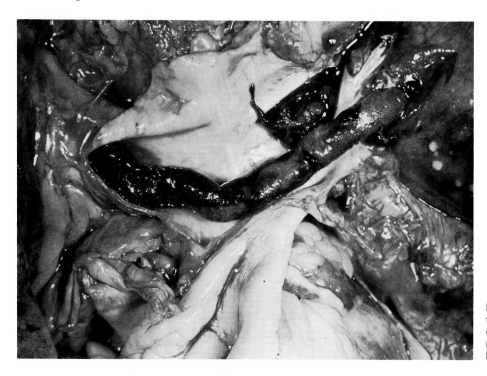

Figure 15-5. Large embolus from deep femoral vein lying at bifurcation of main pulmonary arteries, extending into left and right branches.

age of blood in the systemic venous circulation. However, if survival occurs following a sizable PE, the clinical syndrome may mimic myocardial infarction, with severe chest pain, dyspnea, shock, elevation of temperature, and increased levels of serum lactose dehydrogenase (LDH). Usually, however, *small emboli* induce only transient chest pain and cough or possibly pulmonary hemorrhages without infarction in persons with a normal cardiovascular system. Only in the predisposed in whom the bronchial circulation itself is inadequate will small emboli cause small infarcts. Such patients manifest dyspnea, tachypnea, fever, chest pain, cough, and hemoptysis. An overlying fibrinous pleuritis may produce a pleural friction rub.

The chest radiograph may disclose a pulmonary infarct, usually 12 to 36 hours after it has occurred, as a wedge-shaped infiltrate. Emboli can also be detected by pulmonary perfusion lung scanning after parenteral injection of macroaggregates of albumin labeled with radionuclides, such as technetium-99m. Pulmonary angiography is the most definitive diagnostic technique but entails more risk to the patient than do perfusion scans.

After the initial acute insult, emboli often resolve via contraction and fibrinolysis, particularly in the relatively young. Unresolved, multiple small emboli over the course of time may lead to pulmonary hypertension, pulmonary vascular sclerosis, and chronic cor pulmonale. Perhaps most important is the fact that a small embolus may presage a larger one. In the presence of an underlying predisposing factor, patients with a PE have a 30% chance of developing a second embolus.

Prevention of PE constitutes a major clinical problem for which there is no easy solution. Prophylactic therapy includes early ambulation in postoperative and postpartum patients, elastic stockings and isometric leg exercises for bedridden patients, and preventive anticoagulation in high-risk individuals. It is sometimes necessary to resort to insertion of a screen ("umbrella") into the inferior vena cava or ligation of this vein, not small procedures in an already serious ill patient. Treatment of existing PE often includes anticoagulation, preceded by thrombolysis in some cases.

PULMONARY HYPERTENSION AND VASCULAR SCLEROSIS

The pulmonary circulation is normally one of low resistance, and pulmonary blood pressure is only about one-eighth of systemic blood pressure. Pul-

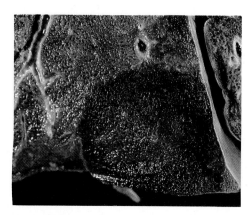

Figure 15-6. Recent, small, roughly wedge-shaped hemorrhagic pulmonary infarct.

monary hypertension (when mean pulmonary pressure reaches one-fourth of systemic levels) is most frequently *secondary* to structural cardiopulmonary conditions that increase pulmonary blood flow and/or pressure, pulmonary vascular resistance, or left heart resistance to blood flow. These include (1) chronic obstructive or interstitial lung diseases, (2) antecedent congenital or acquired heart disease, or (3) recurrent PEs. Pulmonary vascular resistance is also increased by vasoconstriction, an initially reversible, functional change that can be induced by hypoxia and other conditions (see later). For example then, patients with emphysema have hypoxia as well as destruction of lung parenchyma and hence have fewer alveolar capillaries. This causes increased pulmonary arterial resistance and, secondarily, pressure. Pulmonary hypertension occurs in patients with mitral stenosis, for example, because of an increase in left atrial pressure that leads to an increase in pulmonary venous pressure and, consequently, to an increase in pulmonary artery pressure. Patients with pulmonary thromboembolism may have pulmonary hypertension primarily owing to a reduction in the functional cross-sectional area of the pulmonary vascular bed brought about by the obstructing emboli, which in turns leads to an increase in pulmonary vascular resistance. Uncommonly, pulmonary hypertension is encountered in patients in whom all known causes of increased pulmonary pressure are excluded, and this is referred to as *primary*, or *idiopathic, pulmonary hypertension.*

PATHOGENESIS. The endothelial cells in the lungs contribute in important ways to the dynamic regulation of pulmonary blood flow and pulmonary vascular resistance. Dysfunction of pulmonary vascular endothelial cells plays a central part in the vascular responses of both idiopathic (primary) and secondary pulmonary hypertension.[9]

In *secondary forms of pulmonary hypertension,* endothelial cell dysfunction is produced by the process initiating the disorder, such as the increased shear and mechanical injury associated with left-to-right shunts or the biochemical injury produced by fibrin in thromboembolism. In *primary pulmonary hypertension,* endothelial dysfunction and injury (idiopathic in most cases, but sometimes associated with autoimmune disorders, toxic substances, and perhaps specific genetic determinants) may be causal. Decreased elaboration of prostacyclin, decreased production of nitric oxide, and increased release of endothelin all promote pulmonary vasoconstriction. Also, decreased elaboration of prostacyclin and nitric oxide promotes platelet adhesion and activation. Moreover, decreased expression of thrombomodulin, decreased synthesis of heparin sulfate, increased release of plasminogen-activator inhibitor type I, decreased release of tissue-type plasminogen activator, and possibly increased expression of tissue factor all

can promote the formation and persistence of fibrin. Finally, production and release of growth factors and cytokines induce the migration and replication of vascular smooth muscle cells and elaboration of extracellular matrix.

Some patients with pulmonary hypertension have a vasospastic component; in such patients, pulmonary vascular resistance can be rapidly decreased with vasodilators. Pulmonary hypertension has also been reported after ingestion of certain plants or medicines, including the leguminous plant, *Crotalaria spectabilis*, indigenous to the tropics and used medicinally in "bush tea," the appetite depressant agent *aminorex*, and adulterated olive oil. It has been suggested that such substances may act through endothelial injury, as described earlier.

MORPHOLOGY. A variety of vascular lesions occur in pulmonary hypertension.[10] Although they are not always specific and frequently overlap between primary and secondary forms, specific histologic appearances have diagnostic and prognostic implications.[11] The presence of many organizing or recanalized thrombi favors recurrent PE as the cause, and the coexistence of diffuse pulmonary fibrosis, or severe emphysema and chronic bronchitis, points to chronic hypoxia as the initiating event. The vessel changes can involve the entire arterial tree, from the main pulmonary arteries down to the arterioles (Fig. 15–7). In the most severe cases, atheromatous deposits form in the pulmonary artery and its major branches, resembling (but being lesser in degree than) systemic atherosclerosis. The arterioles and small arteries (40 to 300 μm in diameter) are most prominently affected, with striking increases in the muscular thickness of the media (medial hypertrophy) and intimal fibrosis, sometimes narrowing the lumina to pinpoint channels. These changes are present in all forms of pulmonary hypertension but are best developed in the primary form. One extreme of the spectrum of pathologic changes, present most prominently in primary pulmonary hypertension or congenital heart disease with left-to-right shunts, is **plexogenic pulmonary arteriopathy,** so-called because a tuft of capillary formations is present, producing a network, or web, that spans the lumina of dilated thin-walled arteries. Biopsy of the lung may be done in some cases to grade the degree of pulmonary hypertensive vascular abnormalities and thereby aid therapeutic decision making, especially in congenital heart disease, in which severe secondary pulmonary vascular changes may preclude surgical repair of the underlying cardiac anomaly (see Chapter 12).

CLINICAL COURSE. Although secondary forms can occur at any age, primary pulmonary hypertension is most common in women of 20 to 40 years and is

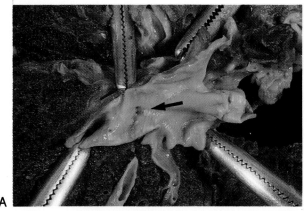

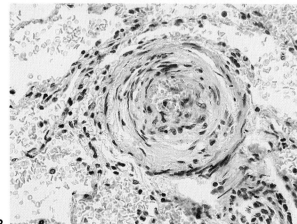

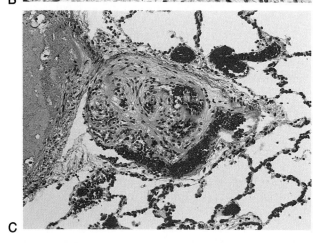

Figure 15–7. Vascular changes in pulmonary hypertension.
A, Gross photograph of atheroma formation, a finding that is usually limited to large vessels. *B,* Marked medial hypertrophy. *C,* Plexogenic lesion characteristic of advanced pulmonary hypertension seen in small arteries and arterioles.

also seen occasionally in young children. Clinical signs and symptoms of both the primary and the secondary forms of vascular sclerosis become evident only with advanced arterial disease. In cases of primary disease, the presenting features are

usually dyspnea and fatigue, but some patients have chest pain of the anginal type. In the course of time, severe respiratory distress, cyanosis, and right ventricular hypertrophy occur, and death from decompensated cor pulmonale, often with superimposed thromboembolism and pneumonia, usually ensues within 2 to 5 years in 80% of patients.[12] However, continuous therapy with vasodilators (e.g., calcium channel blockers or inhaled nitric oxide [NO] as a substitute for endogenous endothelium-derived relaxing factor [EDRF]/NO) and antithrombotic medications (e.g., warfarin, prostacylin, and thromboxane receptor blockers) appears to improve the outcome. Heart-lung transplantation is occasionally done.

OBSTRUCTIVE VERSUS RESTRICTIVE PULMONARY DISEASE

Pulmonary physiologists have popularized the classification of *diffuse* pulmonary diseases into two categories: (1) *obstructive disease* (or *airway disease*), characterized by an increase in resistance to air flow owing to partial or complete obstruction at any level, from the trachea and larger bronchi to the terminal and respiratory bronchioles; and (2) *restrictive disease,* characterized by reduced expansion of lung parenchyma, with decreased total lung capacity. Although many conditions have both obstructive and restrictive components, distinction between the two patterns of pulmonary dysfunction is useful in correlating the results of pulmonary function tests with the radiologic and histologic findings in individual patients.

The major obstructive disorders (excluding tumor or inhalation of a foreign body) are *emphysema, chronic bronchitis, bronchiectasis,* and *asthma.* In patients with these diseases, pulmonary function tests show increased pulmonary resistance and limitation of maximal expiratory air flow rates during forced expiration. Expiratory airflow obstruction may result either from *anatomic airway narrowing,* such as is classically observed in asthma, or from *loss of elastic recoil of the lung,* which characteristically occurs in emphysema.

In contrast, restrictive diseases are identified by a reduced total lung capacity. The restrictive defect occurs in two general conditions: (1) *chest wall disorders in the presence of normal lungs* (e.g., neuromuscular diseases such as poliomyelitis, severe obesity, pleural diseases, and kyphoscoliosis) and (2) *acute or chronic interstitial and infiltrative diseases.* The classic acute restrictive disease is the adult respiratory distress syndrome (ARDS, see earlier in this chapter). Chronic restrictive diseases include the dust diseases, or pneumoconioses, and most of the infiltrative conditions, discussed later.

CHRONIC OBSTRUCTIVE PULMONARY DISEASE

The term "chronic obstructive pulmonary disease" (COPD) refers to a group of conditions that share a major symptom—dyspnea—and are accompanied by chronic or recurrent obstruction to air flow within the lung. Because of the increase in environmental pollutants, cigarette smoking, and other noxious exposures, the incidence of COPD has increased dramatically in the past few decades and now ranks as a major cause of activity-restricting or bed-confining disability in the United States.

In their prototypical forms, these individual disorders—chronic bronchitis, bronchiectasis, asthma, emphysema—have distinct anatomic and clinical characteristics (Table 15–3). For example, patients with predominant emphysema and those with predominant bronchitis form distinct clinical categories, as shown in Table 15–4. However, many patients have overlapping features of damage at both the acinar (emphysema) and the bronchial (bronchitis) levels, almost certainly because one pathogenic mechanism—cigarette smoking—is common to both, as we shall see. Add the frequent component of reversible airway hyper-reactivity (asthma) in these patients, and one can understand the utility and popularity of the broad "umbrella" term COPD.

EMPHYSEMA

Emphysema is a condition of the lung characterized by *abnormal permanent enlargement of the airspaces distal to the terminal bronchiole, accompanied by destruction of their walls, and without obvious fibrosis.*[13] In contrast, the enlargement of airspaces unaccompanied by destruction is termed *overinflation,* for example, the distention of airspaces in the opposite lung following unilateral pneumonectomy.

Types of Emphysema

Not only can emphysema be defined in terms of the *anatomic nature* of the lesion, but also it can be further classified according to its *anatomic distribution* within the lobule. Recall that the lobule is a cluster of acini, the alveolated terminal respiratory units. Although the term "emphysema" is sometimes loosely applied to diverse conditions, there are four types: (1) centriacinar, (2) panacinar, (3) paraseptal, and (4) irregular. Of these, the first two are the most important clinically (Fig. 15–8).

CENTRIACINAR (CENTRILOBULAR EMPHYSEMA). The distinctive feature of this type of emphysema is the pattern of involvement of the lobules; **the central or proximal parts of the acini, formed by respiratory bronchioles, are affected, whereas distal alveoli are spared** (Fig. 15–9A). Thus, both emphysematous and normal airspaces exist within the same acinus and lobule. The lesions are more common and usually more severe in the upper lobes, particularly in the apical segments. The walls of the emphysematous spaces often contain large amounts of black pigment. Inflammation around bronchi and bronchioles and in the septa is common. In severe centriacinar emphysema, the distal acinus may be involved, and differentiation from panacinar emphysema becomes difficult. Moderate-to-severe degrees of emphysema occur predominantly in heavy smokers, often in association with chronic bronchitis. In addition, some lesions of so-called coal workers' pneumoconiosis (see later in this chapter) bear a striking resemblance to centriacinar emphysema. These points suggest an im-

Table 15–3. DISORDERS ASSOCIATED WITH AIRFLOW OBSTRUCTION: THE SPECTRUM OF COPD

CLINICAL TERM	ANATOMIC SITE	MAJOR PATHOLOGIC CHANGES	ETIOLOGY	SIGNS/SYMPTOMS
Chronic bronchitis	Bronchus	Mucus gland hyperplasia, hypersecretion	Tobacco smoke, air pollutants	Cough, sputum production
Bronchiectasis	Bronchus	Airway dilatation and scarring	Persistent or severe infections	Cough; purulent sputum; fever
Asthma	Bronchus	Smooth muscle hyperplasia, excess mucus, inflammation	Immunologic or undefined causes	Episodic wheezing, cough, dyspnea
"Small airway disease," bronchiolitis	Bronchiole	Inflammatory scarring/obliteration	Tobacco smoke, air pollutants, misc.	Cough, dyspnea
Emphysema	Acinus	Airspace enlargement; wall destruction	Tobacco smoke	Dyspnea

Table 15–4. EMPHYSEMA AND CHRONIC BRONCHITIS

	PREDOMINANT BRONCHITIS	PREDOMINANT EMPHYSEMA
Appearance	"Blue bloater"	"Pink puffer"
Age	40–45	50–75
Dyspnea	Mild; late	Severe; early
Cough	Early; copious sputum	Late; scanty sputum
Infections	Common	Occasional
Respiratory insufficiency	Repeated	Terminal
Cor pulmonale	Common	Rare; terminal
Airway resistance	Increased	Normal or slightly increased
Elastic recoil	Normal	Low
Chest radiograph	Prominent vessels; large heart	Hyperinflation; small heart

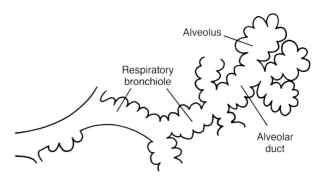

A   NORMAL ACINUS

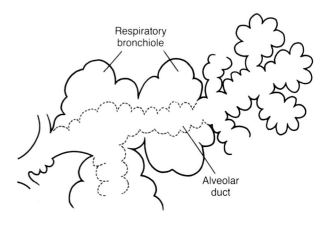

B   CENTRILOBULAR EMPHYSEMA

portant role for tobacco products and coal dust in the genesis of this type of emphysema.

PANACINAR (PANLOBULAR) EMPHYSEMA. In this type the **acini are uniformly enlarged from the level of the respiratory bronchiole to the terminal blind alveoli** (see Fig. 15–9B). It is important to emphasize that the prefix **pan-** refers to the entire acinus but not to the entire lung. In contrast to centriacinar emphysema, panacinar emphysema tends to occur more commonly in the lower zones and in the anterior margins of the lung, and it is usually most severe at the bases. This type of emphysema is associated with **alpha₁-antitrypsin deficiency** (see Chapter 18).

PARASEPTAL (DISTAL ACINAR) EMPHYSEMA. In this type the **proximal portion of the acinus is normal, but the distal part is dominantly involved.** The emphysema is more striking adjacent to the pleura, along the lobular connective tissue septa, and at the margins of the lobules. It occurs adjacent to areas of fibrosis, scarring, or atelectasis and is usually more severe in the upper half of the lungs. The characteristic findings are of multiple, continuous, enlarged airspaces from less than 0.5 mm to more than 2.0 cm in diameter, sometimes forming cyst-like structures. This type of emphysema probably underlies many of the cases of spontaneous pneumothorax in young adults.

IRREGULAR EMPHYSEMA. Irregular emphysema, so named because the acinus is irregularly involved, is almost invariably associated with scarring. Thus, it may be the most common form of emphysema, as careful search of most lungs at autopsy shows one or more scars from a healed inflammatory process. In most instances, these foci of irregular emphysema are asymptomatic.

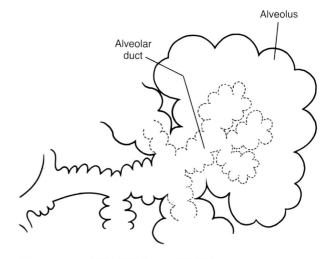

C   PANACINAR EMPHYSEMA

Figure 15–8. Forms of emphysema. A, Diagram of normal structures within the acinus, the fundamental unit of the lung. B, Centrilobular (centriacinar) emphysema with dilatation that principally affects the respiratory bronchioles, at least at the outset. C, Panacinar emphysema with initial distention of the peripheral structures (i.e., alveolus and alveolar duct); the disease later extends to affect the respiratory bronchioles. Normal anatomy is stippled in B and C.

INCIDENCE. Emphysema is a common disease. Thurlbeck reports a 50% combined incidence of panacinar and centriacinar emphysema at autopsy.

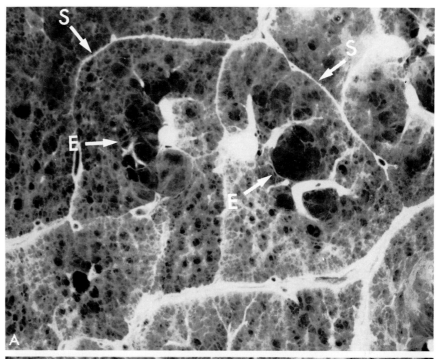

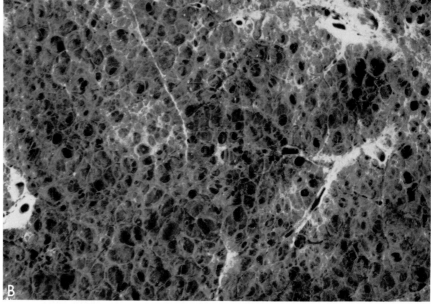

Figure 15–9. *A*, Centrilobular emphysema (magnification ×5). The pulmonary arteries contain a mass of injected barium gelatin. The emphysematous foci (E) abut on blood vessels and spare the septa (S) where the alveolar spaces cluster. *B*, Panacinar emphysema (×5) involving the entire pulmonary architecture. Compare with *A*. (With permission from Bates, D.V., et al.: Respiratory Function in Disease, 2nd ed. Philadelphia, W.B. Saunders Co., 1971.)

He considers the pulmonary disease to be responsible for the death of 6.5% of these patients.[14] *There is a clear-cut association between heavy cigarette smoking and emphysema,* and the most severe type occurs in males who smoke heavily. Although the emphysema does not become disabling until the fifth to eighth decades of life, it is well known clinically that ventilatory deficits may make their first appearance decades earlier in those destined to develop the full-blown disease.

PATHOGENESIS. While details of the genesis of the two common forms of emphysema—centriacinar and panacinar—remain unsettled, *the most plausi-*

ble hypothesis to account for the destruction of alveolar walls is the protease-antiprotease mechanism.

This hypothesis is based on two important observations, one clinical and one experimental. The first is that homozygous patients with a genetic deficiency of the enzyme alpha$_1$-antitrypsin (α_1-AT) have a markedly enhanced tendency to develop pulmonary emphysema,[15] which is compounded by smoking. α_1-AT (which is present in serum, tissue fluids, and macrophages) is a major inhibitor of proteases (particularly elastase) secreted by neutrophils during inflammation (see Chapter 18). The α_1-AT is specified by the *proteinase inhibitor (Pi)* locus on chromosome 14 and is transmitted codominantly. Because of significant polymorphism, some 70 phenotypes of α_1-AT have been identified. The normal phenotype, called PiMM, is present in 90% of the population. Of the several phenotypes associated with α_1-AT deficiency, PiZZ is the most common, being present in 0.012% of the United States population. More than 80% of PiZZ phenotypes develop symptomatic emphysema which occurs at an earlier age and with greater severity if the individual smokes. Therefore, the most important therapeutic intervention in α_1-AT deficiency is cessation of smoking. The second observation bearing on the protease-antiprotease hypothesis is experimental in that intratracheal instillation of the proteolytic enzyme papain, which degrades elastin, causes emphysema in experimental animals.[16]

The *protease-antiprotease theory* holds that alveolar wall destruction results from an imbalance between proteases (mainly elastase) and antiproteases in the lung. The principal antielastase activity in serum and interstitial tissue is α_1-AT (other protease inhibitors are secretory leukoprotease inhibitor[17] [SLPI] in bronchial mucus and serum alpha$_1$-macroglobulin), and the principal cellular elastase activity is derived from neutrophils (other elastases are formed by macrophages, mast cells, pancreas, and bacteria). Neutrophil elastase is capable of digesting human lung, and this digestion can be inhibited by α_1-AT. Such elastase induces emphysema when instilled into the trachea of experimental animals.[18] Thus, the following sequence is postulated to explain the effect of α_1-AT deficiency on the lung: neutrophils are normally sequestered in the lung (more in the lower zones than in the upper), and a few gain access to the alveolar space. Any stimulus that increases either the number of leukocytes (neutrophils and macrophages) in the lung or the release of their elastase-containing granules increases elastolytic activity. Stimulated neutrophils also release oxygen free radicals, which, as previously noted, inhibit α_1-AT activity. With low levels of serum α_1-AT, the process of elastic tissue destruction is unchecked, with consequent emphysema. *Thus, emphysema is seen to result from the destructive effect of high protease activity in subjects with low antiprotease activity.* The primacy of the neutrophil is accepted for patients with α_1-AT deficiency, but in the more common smoking-related emphysema, recent evidence emphasizes the role of proteases from both macrophages and neutrophils and their function within the microenvironment at sites where inflammatory cells adhere to lung matrix.[19]

The protease-antiprotease hypothesis also explains the deleterious effect of cigarette smoking because both increased elastase availability and decreased antielastase activity occur in smokers (Fig. 15–10).

1. Smokers have greater numbers of neutrophils and macrophages in their alveoli. The in-

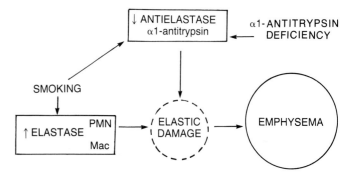

Figure 15–10. Protease-antiprotease mechanism of emphysema. Smoking inhibits antielastase and favors the recruitment of leukocytes and release of elastase. PMN = polymorphonuclear leukocytes; Mac = alveolar macrophages.

creased recruitment of neutrophils into the lung is likely to result, in part, from the release by activated alveolar macrophages of *neutrophil chemotactic factors (e.g., IL-8),* this release being stimulated by smoking. In addition, nicotine is chemotactic for neutrophils, and cigarette smoke activates the alternative complement pathway.

2. Smoking stimulates release of elastase from neutrophils.

3. Smoking enhances elastolytic protease(s) activity in macrophages; macrophage elastase is not inhibited by α_1-AT and, indeed, can proteolytically digest this enzyme.

4. Oxidants in cigarette smoke and oxygen free radicals secreted by neutrophils inhibit α_1-AT and thus decrease net antielastase activity in smokers.

It is thus postulated that impaction of smoke particles in the small bronchi and bronchioles, with the resultant influx of neutrophils and macrophages, and increased elastase and decreased α_1-AT activity, causes the centriacinar emphysema seen in smokers.

MORPHOLOGY. The diagnosis and classification of the emphysemas are based on naked eye (or hand lens) examination of lungs fixed in a state of inflation. Panacinar emphysema, when well developed, produces voluminous lungs, often overlapping the heart and hiding it when the anterior chest wall is removed. The macroscopic features of centriacinar emphysema are less impressive. The lungs may not appear particularly pale or voluminous unless the disease is well advanced. Generally, the upper two-thirds of the lungs are more severely affected. Large apical blebs or bullae are more characteristic of irregular emphysema secondary to scarring.

Microscopic examination is necessary to visualize the abnormal fenestrations in the walls of the alveoli, the complete destruction of septal walls, and the distribution of damage within the pulmonary lobule. With advance of the disease, adjacent alveoli fuse, producing even larger abnormal airspaces and possibly blebs or bullae. Often the respiratory bronchioles and vasculature of the lung are deformed and compressed by the emphysematous distortion of the airspaces, and, as mentioned, there may or may not be evidence of bronchitis or bronchiolitis.

CLINICAL COURSE. The clinical manifestations of emphysema do not appear until at least one-third of the functioning pulmonary parenchyma is incapacitated. Dyspnea is usually the first symptom; it begins insidiously but is steadily progressive. In some patients, cough or wheezing is the chief complaint, easily confused with asthma. Cough and expectoration are extremely variable and depend on the extent of the associated bronchitis. Weight loss is common and may be so severe as to suggest a hidden malignant tumor. Classically, the patient is barrel-chested and dyspneic, with obviously prolonged expiration, and sits forward in a hunched-over position, attempting to squeeze the air out of the lungs with each expiratory effort. These unfortunate persons have a pinched face and breathe through pursed lips. *The only reliable and consistently present finding on physical examination is slowing of forced expiration.*

In patients with severe emphysema, cough is often slight, overdistention is severe, diffusing capacity is low, and blood gas values are relatively normal. Such patients may overventilate and remain well oxygenated and, therefore, are euphoniously if somewhat ingloriously designated as *"pink puffers"* (see Table 15–4). On the other hand, patients with chronic bronchitis more often have a history of recurrent infection, abundant purulent sputum, hypercapnia, and severe hypoxemia, prompting the equally inglorious designation of *"blue bloaters."* A hazard in severe bronchitis, in addition to the respiratory difficulties, is the development of cor pulmonale and eventual congestive heart failure, related to secondary pulmonary vascular hypertension. Death in most patients with COPD is due to (1) respiratory acidosis and coma, (2) right-sided failure, and (3) massive collapse of the lungs secondary to pneumothorax.

Other Types of Emphysema

Now we come to some conditions in which the term "emphysema" is applied less stringently and to some closely related conditions.

COMPENSATORY EMPHYSEMA (COMPENSATORY HYPERINFLATION). This term is sometimes used to designate dilation of alveoli but not destruction of septal walls in response to loss of lung substance elsewhere. It is best exemplified by the hyperexpansion of the residual lung parenchyma that follows surgical removal of a diseased lung or lobe.

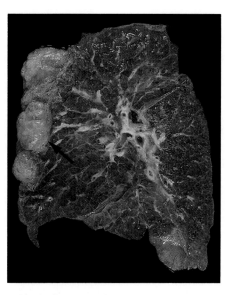

Figure 15–11. Bullous emphysema with large subpleural bullae (arrow).

SENILE EMPHYSEMA. Senile emphysema refers to the overdistended, sometimes voluminous lungs found in the aged. These changes result from age-related alterations of the internal geometry of the lung—**larger alveolar ducts** and **smaller alveoli**—that occur without loss of elastic tissue or destruction of lung substance.

OBSTRUCTIVE OVERINFLATION. Obstructive overinflation refers to the condition in which the lung expands because air is trapped within it. A common cause is subtotal obstruction by a tumor or foreign object. A classic example is **congenital lobar overinflation** in infants, probably resulting from hypoplasia of bronchial cartilage and sometimes associated with other congenital cardiac and lung abnormalities. Overinflation in obstructive lesions occurs either (1) because of a ball-valve action of the obstructive agent, so that air enters on inspiration but cannot leave on expiration; or (2) because the bronchus may be totally obstructed, but ventilation through "collaterals" may bring in air from behind the obstruction. These collaterals are the **pores of Kohn** and other direct accessory **bronchioloalveolar connections** (the canals of Lambert). Obstructive overinflation can be a life-threatening emergency because the affected portion extends sufficiently to compress the remaining normal lung.

BULLOUS EMPHYSEMA. Bullous emphysema refers merely to any form of emphysema that produces large subpleural blebs or bullae (spaces more than 1 cm in diameter in the distended state) (Fig. 15–11). They represent localized accentuations of one of the four forms of emphysema, are most often subpleural, and occur near the apex, sometimes in relation to old tuberculous scarring. On occasion rupture of the bullae may give rise to pneumothorax.

INTERSTITIAL EMPHYSEMA. The entrance of air into the connective tissue stroma of the lung, mediastinum, or subcutaneous tissue is designated interstitial emphysema. In most instances, alveolar tears in pulmonary emphysema provide the avenue of entrance of air into the stroma of the lung, but rarely a wound of the chest that allows air to be sucked in or a fractured rib that punctures the lung substance may underlie this disorder. Alveolar tears usually occur when there is a combination of coughing plus some bronchiolar obstruction, producing sharply increased pressures within the alveolar sacs. Children with whooping cough and bronchitis, patients with obstruction to the airways (by blood clots, tissue, or foreign bodies) or being artificially ventilated, and individuals who suddenly inhale irritant gases provide classic examples.

Progressive accumulation of air may dissect through the fibrous connective tissue of the alveolar walls and into and along the fibrous septa of the lung to reach the mediastinum, and thence possibly the subcutaneous tissues. If the collection of air is small, it usually has no clinical importance. However, extensive insufflation of the lung may encroach on the small blood vessels, creating serious impairment of blood flow through the lungs. When the interstitial air treks into the subcutaneous tissue, the patient may literally blow up into an alarming, although usually harmless, appearance with marked swelling of the head and neck and crackling crepitation all over the chest. In most instances such air is promptly resorbed as soon as the point of entrance is sealed.

CHRONIC BRONCHITIS

This disorder, so common among habitual smokers and inhabitants of smog-laden cities, is not nearly so trivial as was once thought. When persistent for years, it may (1) be associated with chronic obstructive airway disease, as discussed earlier; (2) lead to cor pulmonale and heart failure; and (3) cause atypical metaplasia and dysplasia of the respiratory epithelium, providing a possible soil for cancerous transformation. The widely accepted definition of chronic bronchitis is a clinical one—*chronic bronchitis is present in any patient who has persistent cough with sputum production for at least 3 months in at least 2 consecutive years.* In *simple chronic bronchitis,* patients have a productive cough but no physiologic evidence of airflow obstruction. Some individuals may demonstrate hyper-reactive airways with intermittent bronchospasm and wheezing. This condition is called *chronic asthmatic bronchitis.* Finally, some patients, especially heavy smokers, develop chronic airflow

obstruction, usually with evidence of associated emphysema, and are classified as showing *obstructive chronic bronchitis.* Ten to twenty per cent of the urban adult population have chronic bronchitis; country dwellers have a lower incidence.[14]

PATHOGENESIS. Two sets of factors are important in the genesis of chronic bronchitis: (1) chronic irritation by inhaled substances, and (2) microbiologic infections. Both sexes and all ages may be affected, but chronic bronchitis is most frequent in middle-aged men. Cigarette smoking remains the paramount influence. Chronic bronchitis is four to ten times more common in heavy smokers irrespective of age, sex, occupation, and place of dwelling.

The hallmark and earliest feature of chronic bronchitis is *hypersecretion of mucus* in the large airways, and it is associated with hypertrophy of the submucosal glands in the trachea and bronchi.[20] As chronic bronchitis persists, there is also *a marked increase in goblet cells of small airways— small bronchi and bronchioles*—leading to excessive mucus production that contributes to airway obstruction. It is thought that both the submucosal gland hypertrophy and the increase in goblet cells are caused by tobacco smoke or other pollutants (e.g., sulfur dioxide, nitrogen dioxide); similar changes can be produced experimentally by inhalation of a variety of irritants. Mucosal secretion is under autonomic (vagal) control, but whether airway irritants cause mucus hypersecretion by stimulating neurohormonal pathways remains unproven.

Although mucus hypersecretion in large airways is the cause of sputum overproduction, it is now thought that accompanying *alterations in the small airways of the lung* (small bronchi and bronchioles, less than 2 to 3 mm in diameter) *can result in physiologically important and early manifestations of the chronic airway obstruction.*[21,22] Histologic studies of the small airways in young smokers disclose (1) goblet cell metaplasia with mucous plugging of the lumen, (2) clustering of pigmented alveolar macrophages, (3) inflammatory infiltration, and (4) fibrosis of the bronchiolar wall (in a somewhat older group of patients).[23,24] It is postulated that smoking and other irritants, which cause the hypertrophy of mucous glands characteristic of chronic bronchitis, also cause *bronchiolitis,* also known as *small airway disease.* Certain physiologic studies suggest that this respiratory bronchiolitis is an important component in early and relatively mild airflow obstruction. *However, when bronchitis is accompanied by moderate to severe airflow obstruction, coexistent emphysema is the dominant lesion.*[22]

The role of *infection* appears to be secondary. It is not responsible for the initiation of chronic bronchitis but is probably significant in maintaining it and may be critical in producing acute exacerbations. Cigarette smoke predisposes to infection in

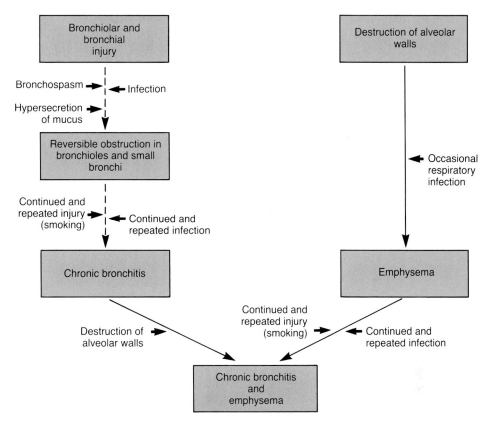

Figure 15–12. Schematic representation of evolution of chronic bronchitis *(left)* and of emphysema *(right)*. Although both can culminate in chronic bronchitis and emphysema, the pathways are different, and either one may predominate. Dashed arrows on left indicate that, in the natural history of chronic bronchitis, it is not known whether there is a predictable progression from obstruction in small airways to chronic (obstructive) bronchitis. (With permission from Fishman, A.P.: The spectrum of chronic obstructive disease of the airways. *In* Fishman A.P. (ed.): Pulmonary Diseases and Disorders, 2nd ed. New York, McGraw-Hill, 1988, p. 1164.)

more than one way: it interferes with ciliary action of the respiratory epithelium, may cause direct damage to airway epithelium, and inhibits the ability of bronchial and alveolar leukocytes to clear bacteria. Viral infections can also cause exacerbations of chronic bronchitis.

Following this review of the pathogenesis of both emphysema and chronic bronchitis, reference should be made to Figure 15–12, which attempts to follow the evolution of both conditions into chronic obstructive airway disease.

MORPHOLOGY. Grossly, there may be hyperemia, swelling, and bogginess of the mucous membranes, frequently accompanied by excessive mucinous to mucopurulent secretions layering the epithelial surfaces. Sometimes, heavy casts of secretions and pus fill the bronchi and bronchioles.

The characteristic histologic feature of chronic bronchitis is enlargement of the mucus-secreting glands of the trachea and bronchi. Although the numbers of goblet cells increase slightly, the **major increase is in the size of the mucous glands.** This increase can be assessed by the ratio of the thickness of the mucous gland layer to the thickness of the wall between the epithelium and the cartilage **(Reid index).** The Reid index (normally <0.4) is increased in chronic bronchitis, usually in proportion to the severity and duration of the disease. The bronchial epithelium may exhibit squamous metaplasia and dysplasia. There is marked narrowing of

bronchioles caused by goblet cell metaplasia, mucous plugging, inflammation, and fibrosis. In the most severe cases there may be obliteration of lumina **(bronchiolitis obliterans).** As discussed earlier, these bronchiolar changes probably contribute to the obstructive features in bronchitis patients.

The clinical *sine qua non* of chronic bronchitis is a persistent cough productive of copious sputum. For many years, no other respiratory functional impairment is present, but eventually dyspnea on exertion develops. With the passage of time, and usually with continued smoking, other elements of COPD may appear, including hypercapnia, hypoxemia, and mild cyanosis. Differentiation of pure chronic bronchitis from that associated with emphysema can be made in the classic case (see Table 15–3), but, as mentioned, many patients with COPD have both conditions. Long-standing severe chronic bronchitis commonly leads to cor pulmonale with cardiac failure. Death may also result from further impairment of respiratory function incident to acute intercurrent bacterial infections.

BRONCHIAL ASTHMA

Asthma is a disease characterized by hyper-reactive airways, leading to episodic, reversible bronchoconstriction, owing to increased responsiveness of the tracheobronchial tree to various stimuli.[25,26] Some

Table 15–5. TYPES OF ASTHMA

TYPES OF ASTHMA	PRECIPITATING FACTORS*	MECHANISM OR IMMUNOLOGIC REACTION
Extrinsic		
Atopic (allergic)	Specific allergens	Type I (IgE) immune reaction
Occupational	Chemical challenge	Type I immune reactions
Allergic bronchopulmonary aspergillosis	Antigen (spores) challenge	Type I and III immune reactions
Intrinsic		
Nonreaginic	Respiratory tract infection	Unknown; hyperreactive airways
Pharmacologic (e.g., aspirin-sensitive)	Aspirin	Decreased prostaglandins, increased leukotrienes

* All types may be precipitated by cold, stress, exercise. All have hyper-reactive airways.

of these stimuli would have little or no effect on nonasthmatics with normal airways.

Those afflicted experience unpredictable disabling attacks of severe dyspnea, coughing, and wheezing triggered by sudden episodes of bronchospasm. Between the attacks, patients may be virtually asymptomatic, but in some persons chronic bronchitis or cor pulmonale often supervenes. Rarely, a state of unremitting attacks *(status asthmaticus)* proves fatal; usually such unfortunate patients have had a long history of asthma. In some cases, the attacks are triggered by exposure to an allergen to which the patient has previously been sensitized, but often no allergic trigger can be identified.

Asthma has traditionally been divided into two basic types—extrinsic (allergic, reagin-mediated, atopic) and intrinsic (idiosyncratic). *Extrinsic asthma* is initiated by a type I hypersensitivity reaction induced by exposure to an extrinsic antigen. Subtypes include *atopic (allergic) asthma, occupational asthma* (many forms), and *allergic bronchopulmonary aspergillosis* (bronchial colonization with Aspergillus organisms followed by development of IgE antibodies). In contrast, *intrinsic asthma* is initiated by diverse, nonimmune mechanisms, including aspirin, pulmonary infections, especially those caused by viruses, cold, inhaled irritants (pollutants such as sulfur dioxide), stress, and exercise. Table 15–5 lists the various groups, the precipitating factors, and the possible mechanisms involved in each group. As with other classification schemes, patients often ignore categories and manifest overlapping characteristics. For example, the patient with extrinsic asthma and increased airway hyper-reactivity is also more likely to manifest bronchospasm after exposure to one of the agents associated with intrinsic asthma.

PATHOGENESIS. *Chronic airway inflammation involving many cell types and inflammatory mediators accompanies the bronchial hyper-responsiveness of asthma.*[25,27] Nevertheless, the precise relationship of the inflammatory cells and their mediators to airway hyper-reactivity is not fully understood. The mechanistic details have been best studied in allergic asthma, so this will be considered first.

Atopic, or Allergic, Asthma. This most common type of asthma usually begins in childhood. The disease is triggered by environmental antigens such as dusts, pollens, animal dander, and foods, but potentially any antigen is implicated (Fig. 15–13). A positive family history of atopy is common, and asthmatic attacks are often preceded by allergic rhinitis, urticaria, or eczema. Serum IgE levels are usually elevated. A skin test with the offending antigen results in an immediate wheal-and-flare reaction, *a classic example of type I IgE-mediated hypersensitivity reaction* (see Chapter 6). IgE-mediated sensitivity elicits an *acute immediate response and a late-phase reaction.*

Recall that exposure of presensitized IgE-coated mast cells to the same or a cross-reacting antigen stimulates the release of chemical mediators from these cells. In the case of airborne antigens, the reaction occurs first on sensitized mast cells *on the mucosal surface* (see Fig. 15–13); the resultant mediator release opens the mucosal intercellular tight junctions and enhances penetration of antigen to the more numerous submucosal mast cells. In addition, direct stimulation of *subepithelial vagal* (parasympathetic) *receptors* provokes bronchoconstriction through both central and local reflexes (including those mediated by unmyelinated sensory C-fibers). This occurs within minutes after stimulation and is called the *acute,* or *immediate, response.* As detailed in Chapter 6, the mediators of IgE-triggered reactions include both primary and secondary mediators. The primary mediators include (1) histamine, which causes bronchoconstriction by direct and cholinergic reflex actions, increased venular permeability, and increased bronchial secretions; and (2) eosinophilic and neutrophilic chemotactic factors (e.g., *leukotriene B_4),* which selectively attract eosinophils and neutrophils. Histamine is probably important in the first few minutes of an asthmatic attack. The secondary mediators include (1) *leukotrienes C_4, D_4, and E_4,* extremely potent mediators that cause prolonged bronchoconstriction as well as increased vascular permeability and increased mucus secretion; (2) *prostaglandin D_2 (PGD_2),* which elicits bronchoconstriction and vasodilatation; (3) *platelet-activating factor (PAF),* which causes aggregation of platelets and release of histamine and serotonin from their granules; and (4) cytokines, such as IL-1, tumor necrosis factor (TNF), and IL-6, some of which have been found to exist in a preformed state within the mast cell granules.[28] The acute

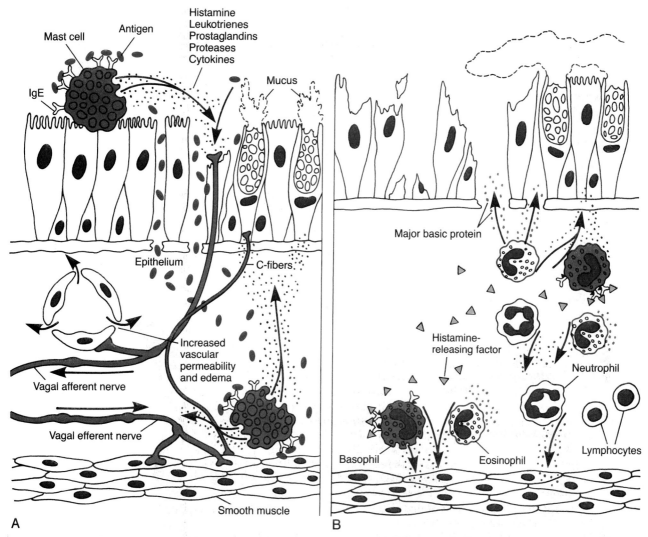

Figure 15–13. A model for immediate and late stages of allergic asthma. *A,* The immediate reaction is triggered by antigen (Ag)-induced cross-linking of IgE bound to IgE receptors (FcRϵ) on mast cells (and possibly FcRϵ-expressing eosinophils and macrophages) in the airways. These cells release preformed mediators that open tight junctions between epithelial cells. Antigen can then enter the mucosa to activate mucosal mast cells and eosinophils, which in turn release additional mediators. Collectively, the mediators, either directly or via neuronal reflexes, induce bronchospasm, increased vascular permeability, and mucus production as well as recruit additional mediator-releasing cells from the blood. *B,* The arrival of recruited cells signals the initiation of the late stage of asthma, in which residual antigen binding to IgE (not shown) may trigger a fresh round of mediator release. Factors, particularly from eosinophils, may also stimulate release of mediators from other inflammatory cells and cause damage to the epithelium. (Modified and redrawn with permission from Lichtenstein, L.: The nasal late phase response: An in vivo model. *Hospital Practice 23(1):*121, 1988. Illustrations by Ilil Arbel.)

reaction is thus associated with bronchoconstriction, edema, mucus secretion, flushing, and, in certain instances, hypotension. This is followed by the *late-phase reaction,* which starts 4 to 8 hours later and may persist for 12 to 24 hours.

The *late-phase reaction* is mediated in part by a swarm of leukocytes—*neutrophils, eosinophils,* and *lymphocytes*—recruited by the chemotactic factors and cytokines[29] derived from mast cells during the acute-phase response, or by other mediators produced by the chronic inflammatory cells already present in asthmatics suffering a recurrent attack. These leukocytes release a second wave of mediators that stimulate the late reaction. Histamine-re-

leasing factors, produced by various cell types, induce release of histamine from basophils, causing bronchoconstriction and edema. In addition, neutrophils cause further inflammatory injury, and the *major basic protein of eosinophils causes epithelial damage*[30] *and airway constriction.*[31] The presence of both immediate and delayed reactions in IgE-mediated events helps explain the prolonged manifestations of asthma and similar allergies.

Nonatopic Asthma. The second large group is the *nonatopic,* or *nonreaginic,* variety of asthma, which is most frequently triggered by respiratory tract infection. Viruses (e.g., rhinovirus, parainfluenza virus) rather than bacteria are the most common provokers.[32] A positive family history is uncommon, serum IgE levels are normal, and there are no other associated allergies. In these patients, skin test results are usually negative, and although hypersensitivity to microbial antigens may play a role, present theories place more stress on hyper-irritability of the bronchial tree. *It is thought that virus-induced inflammation of the respiratory mucosa lowers the threshold of the subepithelial vagal receptors to irritants.* Inhaled air pollutants, such as sulfur dioxide, ozone, and nitrogen dioxide, may also contribute to the chronic airway inflammation and hyper-reactivity present in some cases.

Drug-Induced Asthma. Several pharmacologic agents provoke asthma. *Aspirin-sensitive asthma* is a somewhat fascinating type, occurring in patients with recurrent rhinitis and nasal polyps. These individuals are exquisitely sensitive to very small doses of aspirin, and they experience not only asthmatic attacks but also urticaria. It is probable that aspirin triggers asthma in these patients by inhibiting the cyclooxygenase pathway of arachidonic acid metabolism without affecting the lipoxygenase route, thus tipping the balance toward elaboration of the bronchoconstrictor leukotrienes.

Occupational Asthma. This form of asthma is stimulated by fumes (epoxy resins, plastics), organic and chemical dusts (wood, cotton, platinum), gases (toluene), and other chemicals (formaldehyde, penicillin products). Very minute quantities of chemicals are required to induce the attack, which usually occurs after repeated exposure. The underlying mechanisms vary according to stimulus and include type I IgG-mediated reactions, direct liberation of bronchoconstrictor substances, and hypersensitivity responses of unknown origin.

MORPHOLOGY. The morphologic changes in asthma have been described principally in patients dying of status asthmaticus, but it appears that the pathology in nonfatal cases is similar. Grossly, the lungs are overdistended because of overinflation, and there may be small areas of atelectasis. The most striking macroscopic finding is occlusion of bronchi and bronchioles by thick, tenacious **mucous plugs.** Histologically, the mucous plugs contain whorls of shed epithelium, which give rise to the well-known **Curschmann's spirals.** Numerous eosinophils and Charcot-Leyden crystals are present; the latter are collections of crystalloid made up of eosinophil membrane protein. The other characteristic histologic findings of asthma (Fig. 15–14) include (1) thickening of the basement membrane of the bronchial epithelium; (2) edema and an inflammatory infiltrate in the bronchial walls, with a prominence of eosinophils, which form 5 to 50% of the cellular infiltrate; (3) an increase in size of the submucosal glands; and (4) hypertrophy of the bronchial wall muscle, a reflection of prolonged bronchoconstriction. Emphysematous changes sometime occur, and if chronic bacterial infection has supervened, bronchitis (described earlier) may appear.

CLINICAL COURSE. The classic asthmatic attack lasts up to several hours and is followed by prolonged coughing; the raising of copious mucous secretions provides considerable relief of the respiratory difficulty. In some patients, these symptoms persist at a low level all the time. In its most severe form, *status asthmaticus,* the severe acute paroxysm persists for days and even weeks, and, under these circumstances, ventilatory function may be so impaired as to cause severe cyanosis and even death. The clinical diagnosis is aided by the demonstration of an elevated eosinophil count in the peripheral blood and the finding of eosinophils, Curschmann's spirals, and Charcot-Leyden crystals in the sputum. In the usual case, with intervals of freedom from respiratory difficulty, the disease is more discouraging and disabling than lethal. With appropriate therapy to relieve the attacks, patients with asthma are able to maintain a productive life. Occasionally, the disease disappears spontaneously. In the more severe forms, the progressive hyperinflation may eventually produce emphysema. Superimposed bacterial infections may lead to chronic persistent bronchitis, bronchiectasis, or pneumonia. In some cases, cor pulmonale and heart failure eventually develop.

BRONCHIECTASIS

Bronchiectasis is a chronic necrotizing infection of the bronchi and bronchioles leading to or associated with abnormal dilation of these airways. It is manifested clinically by cough, fever, and the expectoration of copious amounts of foul-smelling, purulent sputum. To be considered bronchiectasis, the dilation should be permanent; reversible bronchial dilation often accompanies viral and bacterial pneumonia. Bronchiectasis has many origins and usually develops in association with the following conditions:[33]

1. *Bronchial obstruction,* due to tumor, foreign bodies, and occasionally mucous impaction, in which the bronchiectasis is localized to the obstructed lung segment; or due to diffuse obstructive airway diseases, most commonly atopic asthma and chronic bronchitis.

2. *Congenital or hereditary conditions,* including *congenital bronchiectasis* (caused by a defect in the development of bronchi), *cystic fibrosis* (see Chapter 10), *intralobar sequestration of the lung* (see earlier in this chapter), *immunodeficiency states,* and *immotile cilia* and *Kartagener's syndromes* (see below).

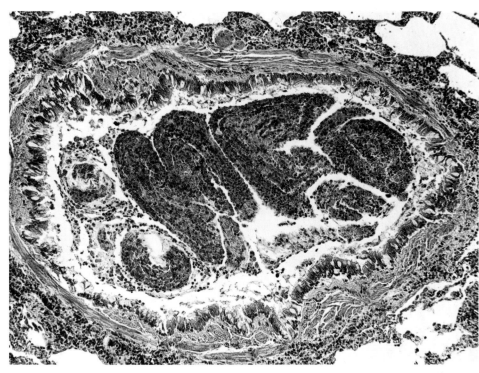

Figure 15–14. Bronchial asthma, histologic appearance. A small bronchus containing plugs of mucin secretion as well as inflammatory cells within lumen. Note hypertrophy of mucin-secreting lining cells, hypertrophy of smooth muscle, and the peribronchial inflammatory infiltrate.

3. *Necrotizing pneumonia*, most often caused by the tubercle bacillus or staphylococci or mixed infections.

ETIOLOGY AND PATHOGENESIS. *Obstruction* and *infection* are the major influences associated with bronchiectasis, and it is likely that both are necessary for the development of full-fledged lesions. After bronchial obstruction (e.g., by tumors or foreign bodies), air is resorbed from the airways distal to the obstruction, with resultant atelectasis. Often accompanying atelectasis are early bronchial wall inflammation and the presence of intraluminal secretions that result in dilatation of the walls of those airways that are patent. These changes are reversible. *However, the changes become irreversible (1) if the obstruction persists*, especially during periods of growth, because the airways will not be able to develop normally; and *(2) if there is added infection.* Infection plays a role in the pathogenesis of bronchiectasis in two ways: (a) it produces bronchial wall inflammation, with weakening, and further dilation; and (b) the extensive bronchial and bronchiolar damage causes endobronchial obliteration, with atelectasis distal to the obliteration and subsequent bronchiectasis around atelectatic areas, as described earlier.

These mechanisms—infection and obstruction —are most readily apparent in the severe form of bronchiectasis associated with cystic fibrosis (see Chapter 10). In this disorder, there is squamous metaplasia of the normal respiratory epithelium with impairment of normal mucociliary action, infection, necrosis of the bronchial and bronchiolar walls, and subsequent bronchiectasis. In younger children, the changes take the form of bronchiolitis (occlusion of the bronchioles by granulation tissue), but older children tend to develop full-blown bronchiectasis.

In *Kartagener's syndrome* (bronchiectasis, sinusitis, and situs inversus) there is a *defect in ciliary motility, associated with structural abnormalities of cilia, most commonly absent or irregular dynein arms*—the structures on the microtubular doublets of cilia that are responsible for the generation of ciliary movement. The lack of ciliary activity interferes with bacterial clearance, predisposes the sinuses and bronchi to infection, and also affects cell motility during embryogenesis, resulting in the situs inversus. Males with this condition tend to be infertile, owing to ineffective mobility of the sperm tail. The syndrome is inherited as an autosomal recessive trait and is variable, as about half the patients with defective cilia have no situs inversus for uncertain reasons. In some groups of patients the cilia are not immobile but have abnormal movement (ciliary dyskinesia). More may be involved in the genesis of this syndrome than ciliary abnormalities, since some abnormal cilia may be found in otherwise normal individuals or in patients with viral illnesses and bronchial inflammation.[34]

MORPHOLOGY. Bronchiectasis usually affects the lower lobes bilaterally, particularly those air passages that are most vertical, and is most severe in the more distal bronchi and bronchioles. When

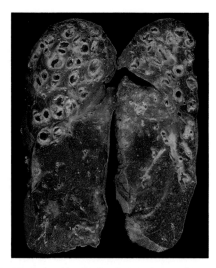

Figure 15–15. Bronchiectasis. Cut surface of lung showing transected, markedly distended peripheral bronchi, in this case predominantly in upper lobes—an unusual localization.

tumors or aspiration of foreign bodies leads to bronchiectasis, the involvement may be sharply localized to a single segment of the lungs. **The airways are dilated, sometimes up to four times normal size.** These dilations may produce long, tube-like enlargements **(cylindroid bronchiectasis)** or, in other cases, may cause **fusiform** or even sharply saccular distention **(saccular bronchiectasis).**

Characteristically, the bronchi and bronchioles are sufficiently dilated that they can be followed, on gross examination, directly out to the pleural surfaces and may produce an almost cystic pattern to the cut surface of the lung (Fig. 15–15). By contrast, in the normal lung, the bronchioles cannot be followed by ordinary gross dissection beyond a point 2 to 3 cm removed from the pleural surfaces.

The histologic findings vary with the activity and chronicity of the disease. In the full-blown, active case, there is an intense acute and chronic inflammatory exudation within the walls of the bronchi and bronchioles, associated with desquamation of the lining epithelium and extensive areas of necrotizing ulceration. There may be pseudostratification of the columnar cells or squamous metaplasia of the remaining epithelium. In some instances, the necrosis completely destroys the bronchial or bronchiolar walls and forms a lung abscess. Fibrosis of the bronchial and bronchiolar walls and peribronchiolar fibrosis develop in the more chronic cases.

CLINICAL COURSE. Bronchiectasis causes severe, persistent cough; expectoration of foul-smelling, sometimes bloody sputum; and dyspnea and or-

thopnea in severe cases. A systemic febrile reaction may occur when powerful pathogens are present. These symptoms are often episodic and are precipitated by upper respiratory tract infections or the introduction of new pathogenic agents. In the full-blown case, the cough is paroxysmal in nature. Such paroxysms are particularly frequent when the patient rises in the morning, and the changes in position lead to drainage into the bronchi of the collected pools of pus. Obstructive ventilatory insufficiency can lead to marked dyspnea and cyanosis. Cor pulmonale, metastatic brain abscesses, and amyloidosis are less frequent complications of bronchiectasis.

PULMONARY INFECTIONS

Respiratory tract infections are more frequent than infections of any other organ and account for the largest number of workdays lost in the general population. The vast majority are upper respiratory tract infections caused by viruses, but viral, mycoplasmal, bacterial, and fungal infections of the lung (pneumonia, bronchopneumonias, lung abscesses, and tuberculosis) still account for an enormous amount of morbidity and rank among the major immediate causes of death.[35] Many of these infections have been described in detail in Chapter 8. Here we shall review only those aspects of the pathology of pulmonary infections that need further discussion.

BACTERIAL PNEUMONIA

Bacterial invasion of the lung parenchyma evokes exudative solidification *(consolidation)* of the pulmonary tissue known as bacterial pneumonia. Many variables, such as the specific etiologic agent, the host reaction, and the extent of involvement, determine the precise form of pneumonia. Thus, classification may be made according to etiologic agent (e.g., pneumococcal or staphylococcal pneumonia), the nature of the host reaction (e.g., suppurative, fibrinous), or the gross anatomic distribution of the disease (lobular bronchopneumonia vs. lobar pneumonia; Fig. 15–16).

Patchy consolidation of the lung is the dominant characteristic of bronchopneumonia (Fig. 15–17). This parenchymal infection usually represents an extension of a pre-existing bronchitis or bronchiolitis. It is an extremely common disease that tends to occur in the more vulnerable two extremes of life —infancy and old age. In the young, there is little previous experience with pathogenic organisms, rendering these patients susceptible to organisms of even low virulence. Resistance likewise falls in the aged, particularly in those already suffering from some serious disorder. Bronchopneumonia, a

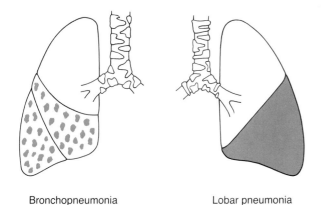

Figure 15-16. Comparison of bronchopneumonia and lobar pneumonia.

common finding on postmortem examinations, frequently terminates a long course of progressive heart failure or disseminated tumor.

Lobar pneumonia is an acute bacterial infection of a large portion of a lobe or of an entire lobe (see Fig. 15–20). Classic lobar pneumonia is now infre-

quent, owing to the effectiveness with which antibiotics abort these infections and prevent the development of full-blown lobar consolidation.

These anatomic but still classic categorizations are often difficult to apply in the individual case, because patterns overlap. The lobular involvement may become confluent, producing virtually total lobar consolidation; in contrast, effective antibiotic therapy for any form of pneumonia may limit involvement to a subtotal consolidation. Moreover, the same organisms may produce lobular pneumonia in one patient, whereas in the more vulnerable individual a full-blown lobar involvement develops. *Most important, from the clinical standpoint, are identification of the causative agent and determination of the extent of disease.*

PATHOGENESIS. Each day, our respiratory airways and alveoli are exposed to more than 10,000 liters of air containing hazardous dusts, chemicals, and microorganisms. The fates of inhaled particles depend on their sizes. Thus, particles larger than 10 μm are deposited largely in the turbulent air flow of the nose and upper airways; particles of 3 to 10

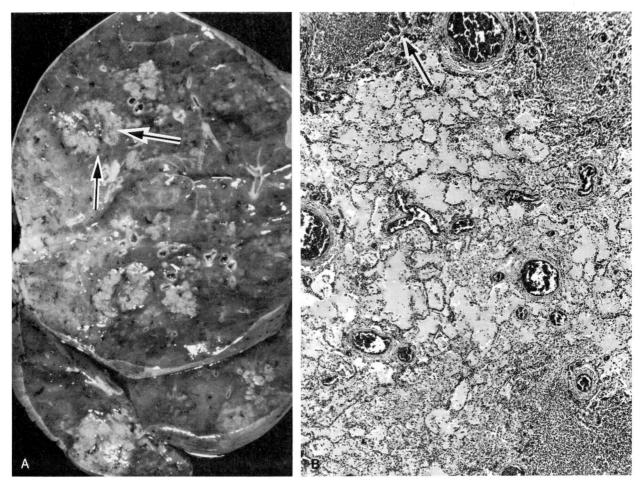

Figure 15–17. Bronchopneumonia. *A,* Gross section of lung showing patches of gray, purulent consolidation *(arrows). B,* Histologic section illustrating patchiness of inflammatory reaction. Note the edema fluid in less involved alveoli. Arrow points to bronchus with inflammation and ulceration.

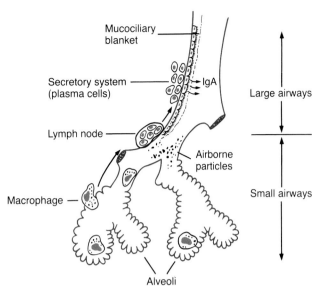

Mucociliary
blanket

Secretory system
(plasma cells)

IgA

Large airways

Lymph node

Airborne
particles

Macrophage

Small airways

Alveoli

Figure 15-18. Components of lungs' defenses: mucociliary escalator in proximal bronchi and alveolar macrophages in distal airways. Arrows indicate possible routes alveolar macrophages may take in eliminating airborne particles. (From Daniele, R.P.: Immune defenses of the lung. *In* Fishman, A.P. (ed.): Pulmonary Diseases and Disorders. New York, McGraw-Hill, 1988, p. 589. Used by permission of McGraw-Hill Book Company.)

μm lodge in the trachea and bronchi by impaction; and smaller particles, about the size of most bacteria, 1 to 5 μm, are deposited in the terminal airways and alveoli. Smaller particles (less than 1 μm) may remain suspended in the inspired air and can be exhaled.

However, the normal lung is free from bacteria. A number of potent defense mechanisms clear or destroy any bacteria inhaled with air or fortuitously deposited in the airway passages as follows (Fig. 15–18):

1. *Nasal clearance.* Particles, including aerosolized droplets carrying microorganisms deposited near the front of the airway on the nonciliated epithelium, are normally removed by sneezing and blowing, whereas those deposited posteriorly are swept over the mucus-lined ciliated epithelium to the nasopharynx, where they are swallowed.

2. *Tracheobronchial clearance.* This is accomplished by mucociliary action: the beating motion of cilia moves a film of mucus continuously from the lung toward the oropharynx; particles deposited on this film are eventually either swallowed or expectorated.

3. *Alveolar clearance.* Bacteria or solid particles deposited in the alveoli are phagocytosed by *alveolar macrophages.* A particle is either digested or carried to the ciliated bronchioles. From here the macrophage is propelled to the oropharynx and then swallowed. Alternatively, the particle-laden macrophage may move through the interstitial space and either re-enter the bronchioles or enter

lymphatic capillaries. If the particle load is heavy and macrophage transport to the surface and alveolar pathways is overwhelmed, some particles may eventually reach the regional lymph nodes and, via the bloodstream, be carried elsewhere in the body.

Pneumonia can result whenever these defense mechanisms are impaired or whenever the resistance of the host in general is lowered. Factors that affect resistance in general include chronic diseases, immunologic deficiency, treatment with immunosuppressive agents, leukopenia, and unusually virulent infections. The clearing mechanisms can be interfered with by many factors, such as the following:

1. *Loss or suppression of the cough reflex,* as a result of coma, anesthesia, neuromuscular disorders, drugs, or chest pain. This may lead to *aspiration* of gastric contents.

2. *Injury to the mucociliary apparatus,* by either impairment of ciliary function or destruction of ciliated epithelium, due to cigarette smoke, inhalation of hot or corrosive gases, viral diseases, or genetic disturbances (e.g., the immotile cilia syndrome).

3. *Interference with the phagocytic or bactericidal action of alveolar macrophages,* by alcohol, tobacco smoke, anoxia, or oxygen intoxication.

4. *Pulmonary congestion and edema.*

5. *Accumulation of secretions* in conditions such as cystic fibrosis and bronchial obstruction.

Several other points need to be emphasized. First, one type of pneumonia sometimes predisposes to another, especially in debilitated patients. For example, the most common cause of death in viral influenza epidemics is bacterial pneumonia. Second, although the portal of entry for most pneumonias is the respiratory tract, hematogenous spread from one focus to other foci can occur, and secondary seeding of the lungs may be difficult to distinguish from primary pneumonia. Finally, many patients with chronic diseases acquire terminal pneumonias while hospitalized *(nosocomial infection).* Bacteria common to the hospital environment may have acquired resistance to antibiotics; opportunities for spread are increased; invasive procedures such as intubations and injections are common; and bacteria may contaminate equipment used in respiratory care units.

ETIOLOGY. For bronchopneumonia, the common agents are staphylococci, streptococci, pneumococci, *Haemophilus influenzae, Pseudomonas aeruginosa,* and the coliform bacteria, although virtually any lung pathogen may also produce this pattern. In the case of lobar pneumonia, 90 to 95% are caused by pneumococci *(Streptococcus pneumoniae).* Most common are types 1, 3, 7, and 2. Type 3 causes a particularly virulent form of lobar pneumonia. Occasionally, *Klebsiella pneumoniae,* staphylocci, streptococci, *Haemophilus influenzae,*

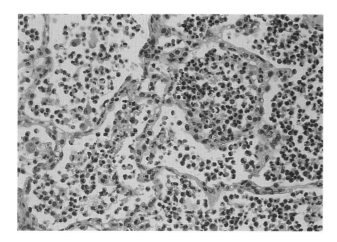

Figure 15-19. Acute pneumonia. The stage of early red hepatization with congested septal capillaries and extensive white cell exudation into alveoli. Fibrin nets have not yet formed.

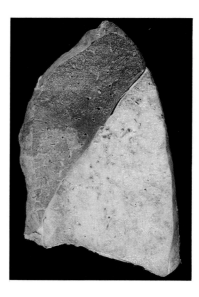

Figure 15-20. Lobar pneumonia—gray hepatization, gross photograph. The lower lobe is uniformly consolidated.

and (in this day of antibiotic resistance) some of the gram-negative organisms, such as the Pseudomonas and Proteus bacilli, are also responsible for lobar involvement. A lobar distribution appears merely to be a function of the virulence of the organism and the vulnerability of the host. Heavy contamination by virulent pathogens may evoke this pattern in healthy adults, whereas organisms of lower virulence may accomplish the same in the predisposed patient. In lobar pneumonia, there is more extensive exudation that leads to spread through the pores of Kohn. Moreover, the copious mucoid encapsulation produced by the pneumococci protects the organisms against immediate phagocytosis and thus favors their spread.

MORPHOLOGY. Lobar pneumonia is a widespread fibrinosuppurative consolidation of large areas and even whole lobes of the lung. Four stages of the inflammatory response have classically been described: congestion, red hepatization, gray hepatization, and resolution. Present-day effective antibiotic therapy frequently slows or halts the progression.

In the first stage of **congestion** the lung is heavy, boggy, and red. It is characterized by vascular engorgement, intra-alveolar fluid with few neutrophils, and often the presence of numerous bacteria. The stage of **red hepatization** that follows is characterized by massive confluent exudation with red cells (congestion) and neutrophils and fibrin filling the alveolar spaces (Fig. 15–19). On gross examination, the lobe now appears distinctly red, firm, and airless with a liver-like consistency, hence the term "hepatization." The stage of **gray hepatization** follows with progressive disintegration of red cells and the persistence of fibrinosuppurative exudate, giving the gross appearance of a grayish-brown, dry surface (Fig. 15–20). In the final

stage of **resolution** the consolidated exudate within the alveolar spaces undergoes progressive enzymic digestion to produce a granular, semifluid debris that is resorbed, ingested by macrophages, or coughed up. Pleural fibrinous reaction to the underlying inflammation, often present in the early stages if the consolidation extends to the surface **(pleuritis),** may similarly resolve. More often it undergoes organization, leaving fibrous thickening or permanent adhesions.

Foci of **bronchopneumonia** are consolidated areas of acute suppurative inflammation. The consolidation may be patchy through one lobe but is more often multilobar and frequently bilateral and basal, because of the tendency of secretions to gravitate into the lower lobes. Well-developed lesions are usually 3 to 4 cm in diameter, slightly elevated, dry, granular, gray-red to yellow, and poorly delimited at their margins (see Fig. 15–17A). Histologically, the reaction usually comprises a suppurative, neutrophil-rich exudate that fills the bronchi, bronchioles, and adjacent alveolar spaces (see Figs. 15–17B and 15–19). Occasionally, consolidation of lung secondary to obstructive lesions (or rarely, aspiration of mineral oils) causes a predominance of **lipid-laden foamy macrophages** and is designated **lipid pneumonia.**

Complications of pneumonia include (1) tissue destruction and necrosis, causing **abscess formation** (particularly common with type 3 pneumococci or Klebsiella infections); (2) spread of infection to the pleural cavity, causing the intrapleural fibrinosuppurative reaction known as **empyema;** (3) **organization** of the exudate, which may convert a portion of the lung into solid tissue (Fig. 15–21); and (4) **bacteremic dissemination** to the heart valves, pericardium, brain, kidneys, spleen, or

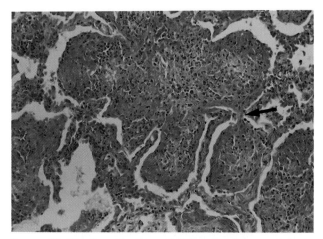

Figure 15–21. Organization of intra-alveolar exudate in lobar pneumonia, seen in areas to be streaming through pores of Kohn *(arrow).*

joints, causing metastatic abscesses, endocarditis, meningitis, or suppurative arthritis.

CLINICAL COURSE. The major symptoms of pneumonia are malaise, fever, and cough productive of sputum. When fibrinosuppurative pleuritis is present, it is accompanied by pleuritic pain and pleural friction rub. The characteristic radiologic appearance of lobar pneumonia is that of a radiopaque, usually well-circumscribed lobe, while bronchopneumonia shows focal opacities.

The clinical picture is dramatically modified by the administration of antibiotics. Treated patients may be relatively afebrile with few clinical signs 48 to 72 hours after the initiation of antibiotics. The identification of the organism and the determination of its antibiotic sensitivity are the keystones to appropriate therapy. Fewer than 10% of patients with pneumonia now succumb, and in most such instances, death may be attributed either to a complication, such as empyema, meningitis, endocarditis, or pericarditis, or to some predisposing influence, such as debility or chronic alcoholism.

VIRAL AND MYCOPLASMAL PNEUMONIA (PRIMARY ATYPICAL PNEUMONIA)

The term *"primary atypical pneumonia"* (PAP) was initially applied to an acute febrile respiratory disease characterized by patchy inflammatory changes in the lungs, largely confined to the alveolar septa and pulmonary interstitium. The term "atypical" denotes the lack of alveolar exudate, but a much more accurate designation is *interstitial pneumonitis.* The pneumonitis is caused by a variety of organisms, the most common being *Mycoplasma pneumoniae.* Other etiologic agents are viruses,

including influenza virus types **A** and **B**, the respiratory syncytial viruses (RSV), adenovirus, rhinoviruses, rubeola and varicella viruses; Chlamydia (psittacosis); and *Coxiella burnetii* (Q fever).[36] In some cases, the cause cannot be determined.

Any one of these agents may cause merely an upper respiratory tract infection, recognized as the common cold, or a more severe lower respiratory tract infection. The circumstances that favor such extension of the infection are often mysterious but include malnutrition, alcoholism, and underlying debilitating illnesses.

MORPHOLOGY. All causal agents produce essentially similar morphologic patterns. Because patients with mild cases recover, our understanding of the anatomic changes is necessarily largely based on the more severe, fatal expressions of these infections. The pneumonic involvement may be quite patchy or may involve whole lobes bilaterally or unilaterally. The affected areas are red-blue, congested, and subcrepitant. **There is no obvious consolidation such as is encountered in lobar pneumonia.** The pleura is smooth, and pleuritis or pleural effusions are infrequent.

The histologic pattern depends on the severity of the disease. **Predominant is the interstitial nature of the inflammatory reaction, virtually localized within the walls of the alveoli.** The alveolar septa are widened and edematous and usually have a mononuclear inflammatory infiltrate of lymphocytes, histiocytes, and occasionally plasma cells. In very acute cases, neutrophils may also be present. The alveoli may be free from exudate, but in many patients there are intra-alveolar proteinaceous material, a cellular exudate, and characteristically pink hyaline membranes lining the alveolar walls, similar to those seen in hyaline membrane disease of infants. These changes reflect **alveolar damage** similar to that seen diffusely in the adult respiratory distress syndrome (see Fig. 15–3). Subsidence of the disease is followed by reconstitution of the native architecture.

Superimposed bacterial infection modifies the histologic picture by causing ulcerative bronchitis and bronchiolitis, and may yield the anatomic changes already described in the section on bacterial pneumonia. Some viruses, such as herpes simplex, varicella, and adenovirus, may be associated with necrosis of bronchial and alveolar epithelium and acute inflammation. Epithelial giant cells with intranuclear or intracytoplasmic inclusions may be present in cytomegalic inclusion disease. Other viruses produce cytopathic changes, as described in Chapter 8.

CLINICAL COURSE. The clinical course is extremely varied. Many cases masquerade as severe upper respiratory tract infections or as "chest colds." Even patients with well-developed atypical pneumonia have few localizing symptoms. Cough may well be absent, and the major manifestations may consist only of fever, headache, muscle aches, and pains in the legs. The edema and exudation are both strategically located to cause an alveolocapillary block and thus evoke symptoms out of proportion to the scanty physical findings. One of the useful laboratory aids in differentiating viral atypical pneumonia from the *M. pneumoniae* form is detection of elevated cold agglutinin titers in the serum. These are present in about half of patients with Mycoplasma and in 20% of adenovirus infections and are absent in other viral pneumonias.

The ordinary sporadic form of the disease is usually mild with a low mortality rate, below 1%. However, interstitial pneumonia may assume epidemic proportions with intensified severity and greater mortality, as all too grimly documented in the highly fatal influenzal pandemics of 1915 and 1918 and the many smaller epidemics since then. Secondary bacterial infection by staphylococci or streptococci is common in such circumstances.

LUNG ABSCESS

The term "pulmonary abscess" describes a local suppurative process within the lung characterized by necrosis of lung tissue. Oropharyngeal surgical procedures, sinobronchial infections, dental sepsis, and bronchiectasis play important roles in their development.

ETIOLOGY AND PATHOGENESIS. Although under appropriate circumstances any pathogen may produce an abscess, the commonly isolated organisms include aerobic and anaerobic streptococci, *Staphylococcus aureus*, and a host of gram-negative organisms. Mixed infections occur very often because of the important causal role that inhalation of foreign material plays.[37] *Anaerobic organisms* normally found in the oral cavity, including members of the Bacteroides, Fusobacterium, and Peptococcus species, are the exclusive isolates in about 60% of cases. The causative organisms are introduced by the following mechanisms:

1. *Aspiration of infective material* (the most frequent cause). This is particularly common in acute alcoholism, coma, anesthesia, sinusitis, gingivodental sepsis, and debilitation in which the cough reflexes are depressed. Aspiration of gastric contents is serious because the gastric acidity adds to the irritant role of the food particles and, in the course of aspiration, mouth organisms are inevitably introduced.

2. *Antecedent primary bacterial infection.* Postpneumonic abscess formations are usually associated with *Staphylococcus aureus, Klebsiella pneumoniae*, and the type 3 pneumococcus. Fungal infections and bronchiectasis are additional antecedents to lung abscess formation. Post-transplant or otherwise immunosuppressed individuals are at special risk for this complication.

3. *Septic embolism.* Infected emboli from thrombophlebitis in any portion of the systemic venous circulation or from the vegetations of infective bacterial endocarditis on the right side of the heart are trapped in the lung.

4. *Neoplasia.* Secondary infection is particularly common in the bronchopulmonary segment obstructed by a primary or secondary malignancy *(postobstructive pneumonia)*.

5. *Miscellaneous.* Direct traumatic penetrations of the lungs; spread of infections from a neighboring organ, such as suppuration in the esophagus, spine, subphrenic space, or pleural cavity; and hematogenous seeding of the lung by pyogenic organisms all may lead to lung abscess formation.

When all these causes are excluded, there are still cases in which no reasonable basis for the abscess formation can be identified. These are referred to as *"primary cryptogenic"* lung abscesses.

MORPHOLOGY. Abscesses vary in diameter from lesions of a few millimeters to large cavities of 5 to 6 cm. They may affect any part of the lung and may be single or multiple. Pulmonary abscesses due to aspiration are more common on the right (the more vertical main bronchus) and are most often single. Abscesses that develop in the course of pneumonia or bronchiectasis are usually multiple, basal, and diffusely scattered. Septic emboli and pyemic abscesses, by the haphazard nature of their genesis, are multiple and may affect any region of the lungs.

The cavity may or may not be filled with suppurative debris, depending on the presence or absence of a communication with one of the air passages. When such communications exist, the contained exudate may be partially drained to create an air-containing cavity. Superimposed saprophytic infections are prone to flourishing within the already necrotic debris of the abscess cavity. Continued infection leads to large, fetid, greenblack, multilocular cavities with poor demarcation of their margins, designated **gangrene of the lung.** The **cardinal histologic change in all abscesses is suppurative destruction of the lung parenchyma within the central area of cavitation** (Fig. 15–22). In chronic cases, considerable fibroblastic proliferation produces a fibrous wall.

CLINICAL COURSE. The manifestations of pulmonary abscesses are much like those of bronchiectasis and are characterized principally by cough, fever, and copious amounts of foul-smelling purulent or sanguineous sputum. Fever, chest pain, and weight loss are common. Clubbing of the fingers and toes may appear within a few weeks after onset of an abscess. Diagnosis of this condition can be suspected only from the clinical findings and

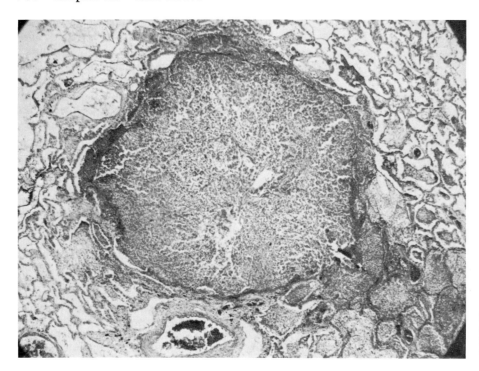

Figure 15–22. Pyemic lung abscess with complete destruction of underlying parenchyma within focus of involvement.

must be confirmed by roentgenography and bronchoscopy. Whenever an abscess is discovered, it is important to rule out an underlying carcinoma, as this is present in 10 to 15% of cases.

The course of abscesses is variable. With antimicrobial therapy, most resolve with no major sequelae. Complications include extension of the infection into the pleural cavity, hemorrhage, the development of *brain abscesses* or *meningitis* from septic emboli, and (rarely) reactive secondary amyloidosis (type AA).

PULMONARY TUBERCULOSIS

A general discussion of tuberculosis appears in Chapter 8. Here we shall only briefly describe the effects of this infection on the lungs.

As indicated earlier, the overwhelming preponderance of tuberculous infections affect the lungs and, indeed, begin there. Pulmonary involvement is still the major cause of tuberculosis morbidity and mortality. The prevention and control of these pulmonary infections account for tuberculosis' being a relatively uncommon cause of death today in the United States. However, the incidence of this infection in the United States began to increase again in the past decade, primarily reflecting infections in patients with acquired immunodeficiency syndrome (AIDS).[38] A further grim aspect of the resurgence of tuberculosis is the emergence of highly drug-resistant strains.[39] Moreover, in many parts of the world, underprivileged populations still suffer from death rates 20 times those of industrialized nations, and indeed high-incidence

pockets of infection are found among the poor in the most affluent countries.

Primary Pulmonary Tuberculosis

Except for the rare intestinal (bovine) tuberculosis, and the even more uncommon skin, oropharyngeal, and lymphoidal primary sites, the lungs are the usual location of primary infections. As detailed earlier (see Chapter 8), the initial focus of primary infection is the *Ghon complex,* which consists of (1) a parenchymal subpleural lesion, often just above or just below the interlobar fissure between the upper and the lower lobes, and (2) enlarged caseous lymph nodes draining the parenchymal focus (Fig. 15–23).

The course and fate of this initial infection are variable, but in most cases patients are asymptomatic and the lesions undergo fibrosis and calcification. Exceptionally, particularly in infants and children or immunodeficient adults, *progressive spread with cavitation, tuberculous pneumonia, or miliary tuberculosis* may follow a primary infection.

Secondary (Reactivation) Pulmonary Tuberculosis

Most cases of secondary pulmonary tuberculosis represent reactivation of an old, possibly subclinical infection. Recall that during primary infection bacilli may disseminate, without producing symptoms, and establish themselves in sites with high oxygen tension, particularly the lung apices. Reactivation in such sites occurs in no more than 5 to

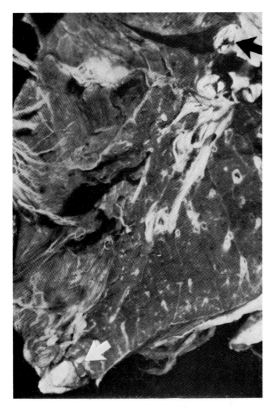

Figure 15–23. Primary pulmonary tuberculosis. Parenchymal focus of white caseation is present in lower left corner *(white arrow)*, and caseated lymph nodes of drainage can be seen in upper right *(black arrow)*.

10% of the cases of primary infection. However, secondary tuberculosis tends to produce more damage to the lungs than does primary tuberculosis. The immunopathogenesis of tuberculous lesions is complex (see Chapter 8).[40]

MORPHOLOGY. The **secondary pulmonary tuberculous lesion** is located in the apex of one or both lungs (Fig. 15–24). It begins as **a small focus of consolidation, usually less than 3 cm in diameter.** Less commonly, initial lesions may be located in other regions of the lung, particularly about the hilus. In almost every case of reinfection, the regional nodes develop foci of similar tuberculous activity. In the favorable case, the initial parenchymal focus develops a small area of caseation necrosis that does not cavitate, because it fails to communicate with a bronchus or bronchiole. The usual course is one of progressive fibrous encapsulation, leaving only fibrocalcific scars that depress and pucker the pleural surface and cause focal pleural adhesions. Sometimes, these fibrocalcific scars become secondarily blackened by anthracotic pigment.

Histologically, **coalescent granulomas are present, composed of epithelioid cells surrounded by a zone of fibroblasts and lymphocytes that**

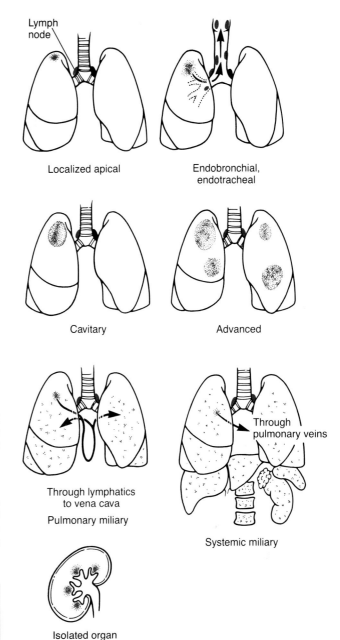

Figure 15–24. Diagrammatic representation of the many patterns of secondary tuberculosis, ranging from initial apical localization to miliary dissemination to isolated involvement of an organ (kidney).

usually contains Langhans' giant cells. Some necrosis (caseation) is usually present in the centers of these tubercles, the amount being entirely dependent on the sensitization of the patient and the virulence of the organisms (Fig. 15–25).

As the lesions progress, more tubercles coalesce to create a confluent area of consolidation. In the favorable case, either the entire area is eventually converted to a fibrocalcific scar, or the residual caseous debris becomes totally and heavily walled off by hyaline collagenous connective

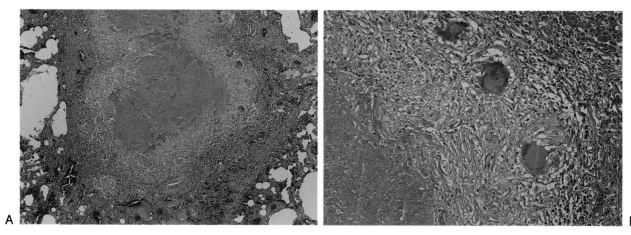

Figure 15–25. Characteristic tubercle at low magnification (*A*), and in detail (*B*), to illustrate central granular caseation and epithelioid and multinucleated giant cells.

tissue. In these late lesions, the multinucleate giant cells tend to disappear.

In cases of suspected tuberculous tissue changes, the diagnosis is confirmed by histologic staining, smears, and cultures of acid-fast organisms. Tubercle bacilli can be demonstrated in the early exudative and caseous phases, but it is usually impossible to find them in the late fibrocalcific stages. Lesions with sparse organisms can be highly infective; one can estimate that finding a single acid-fast bacillus in a routine histologic sample from a 1-cm³ granuloma indicates that a total of at least 2000 organisms are present within the granuloma! Hence, it cannot be assumed that their absence in histologic sections is tantamount to their total destruction, because in many of these instances culture of the lesions or inoculation of this material into guinea pigs yields the organisms.

The subsequent course of the secondary lesions is variable. They either may heal spontaneously or with therapy, resulting in a fibrocalcific nodule, or may progress along the many pathways, discussed next.

Progressive Pulmonary Tuberculosis

A variable number of active lesions continue to progress over a period of months or years, causing further pulmonary and even distant organ involvement. The resultant clinicopathologic consequences include cavitary fibrocaseous tuberculosis (apical and advanced), miliary tuberculosis, and tuberculous bronchopneumonia (see Fig. 15–24).

CAVITARY FIBROCASEOUS TUBERCULOSIS. The name fairly well describes this stage of disease. By erosion into a bronchiole, drainage of the caseous focus transforms it into a cavity. Growth and multi-plication of the tubercle bacilli under these conditions are favored by the increased oxygen tension.

In most cases, the cavity remains localized to the apex (apical cavitary fibrocaseous tuberculosis). The cavity is lined by a yellow-gray caseous material and is more or less walled off by fibrous tissue. Not uncommonly, thrombosed arteries may traverse these cavities to produce apparent fibrous bridging bands. When such cavitation occurs in the apices, the pathways for further dissemination of the tuberculous infection are prepared. The infective material may now disseminate through the airways to other sites in the lung or upper respiratory tract. Spread may also occur to the lymph nodes via the lymphatics and thence retrogressively through other lymphatics to other areas of the lung or other organs. Miliary dissemination through the blood is a further hazard. Cavitary fibrocaseous tuberculosis may affect one, many, or all lobes of both lungs in the form of isolated minute tubercles, confluent caseous foci, or large areas of caseation necrosis **(advanced fibrocaseous tuberculosis).**

In the progress of this disease, the pleura is inevitably involved, and, depending on the chronicity of the disease, serous pleural effusions, frank tuberculous empyema, or massive obliterative fibrous pleuritis may be found. In the course of extensive fibrocaseous tuberculosis, it is almost inevitable that tubercle bacilli become implanted on the mucosal linings of the air passages to produce **endobronchial and endotracheal tuberculosis.** These lesions may later become ulcerated and produce irregular, ragged, necrotic, mucosal ulcers. Accompanying the endobronchial tuberculosis, **laryngeal seeding and intestinal tuberculosis** may occur. Fortunately, these complications of tuberculosis are now uncommon.

MILIARY TUBERCULOSIS. Lymphohematogenous dissemination may give rise to miliary tuberculosis, confined only to the lungs or involving other

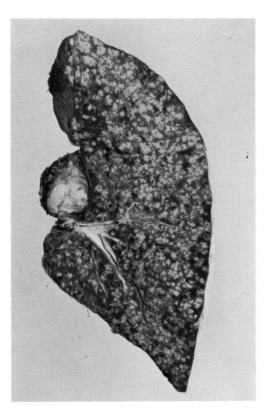

Figure 15–26. Advanced miliary tuberculosis of lung. Foci of caseation have coalesced to produce large nodules of consolidation.

organs also. The distribution of miliary lesions depends on the pathways of dissemination. Tuberculous infection may drain via the lymphatics through the major lymphatic ducts into the right side of the heart, and thence spread into a diffuse, blood-borne pattern throughout the lungs *alone*. Despite their small size, most of the bacilli are usually filtered out by the alveolar capillary bed. Therefore, the infective material may not reach the arterial systemic circulation. However, such limitation to the lungs usually is not complete, and some bacilli pass through the capillaries or through lymphatic-vascular anastomoses to enter the systemic circulation and produce distant organ seedings. Favored targets for miliary seeding are the bone marrow, liver, spleen, and retina, providing sites for biopsy or direct visualization of disease (retina). Occasionally, isolated organ involvement is found (e.g., kidneys, adrenals, testes).

In the miliary type of distribution, individual lesions vary from one to several millimeters in diameter and are distinct, yellow-white, firm areas of consolidation that usually do not have grossly visible central caseation necrosis or cavitation at the time of examination (Fig. 15–26). Histologically, however, these present the characteristic pattern of individual or multiple confluent tubercles having microscopic central caseation.

TUBERCULOUS BRONCHOPNEUMONIA. In the highly susceptible, highly sensitized individual, the tuberculous infection may spread rapidly throughout large areas of lung parenchyma and produce a diffuse bronchopneumonia, or lobar exudative consolidation, at one time descriptively referred to as "galloping consumption." Sometimes, with such overwhelming disease, well-developed tubercles do not form, and it may be difficult to establish on histologic grounds the tuberculous nature of the pneumonic process. However, numerous bacilli are usually present in such exudates.

CLINICAL COURSE. The clinical course of pulmonary tuberculosis is extremely variable and depends entirely on the activity, extent, and pattern of distribution of the tuberculous pulmonary infection (Chapter 8). The great majority of cases respond to present-day chemotherapeutic measures unless the disease is very advanced, the organisms are resistant to conventional therapies, or intercurrent problems such as diabetes mellitus, AIDS, or reactive amyloidosis complicate the outlook.

PNEUMONIA IN THE IMMUNOCOMPROMISED HOST

The appearance of a pulmonary infiltrate and signs of infection (e.g., fever) is one of the most common and serious complications in patients whose immune and defense systems are suppressed by disease, immunosuppression for organ transplants and tumors, or irradiation.[41] A wide variety of so-called opportunistic infectious agents, many of which rarely cause infection in normal hosts, can cause these pneumonias, and often more than one agent is involved. Mortality from these opportunistic infections is high. In the case of AIDS, nearly 100% of patients will suffer from an opportunistic infection, most commonly caused by *Pneumocystis carinii*.[42] Table 15–6 lists some of the opportunistic agents according to their prevalence and to whether they cause local or diffuse pulmonary infiltrates. It is well to remember that such infiltrates may also be due to drug reactions or to involvement of the lung by tumor. The specific infections are discussed in Chapter 8.

DIFFUSE INTERSTITIAL (INFILTRATIVE, RESTRICTIVE) DISEASES

This heterogeneous group of diseases is characterized predominantly by diffuse and usually chronic involvement of the pulmonary connective tissue,

Table 15–6. CAUSES OF PULMONARY INFILTRATES IN IMMUNOCOMPROMISED HOSTS

DIFFUSE INFILTRATE	FOCAL INFILTRATE
Common	**Common**
Cytomegalovirus	Gram-negative rods
Pneumocystis carinii	*Staphylococcus aureus*
Drug reaction	Aspergillus
	Candida
	Malignancy
Uncommon	**Uncommon**
Bacteria	Cryptococcus
Aspergillus	Mucor
Cryptococcus	*Pneumocystis carinii*
Malignancy	*Legionella pneumophila*

Modified from Fanta, C. H., and Pennington, J. L.: Fever and new lung infiltrates in the immunocompromised host. Clin. Chest Med. 2:19, 1981.

principally the most peripheral and delicate interstitium in the alveolar walls. Recall that the interstitium consists of the basement membrane of the endothelial and epithelial cells (fused in the thinnest portions), collagen fibers, elastic tissue, proteoglycans, fibroblasts, mast cells, and occasionally lymphocytes and monocytes.

There is no uniformity regarding terminology and classification of these disorders. Many of the entities are of unknown cause and pathogenesis, some have an intra-alveolar as well as an interstitial component, and there is frequent overlap in histologic features among the different conditions. Nevertheless, their similar clinical signs, symptoms, radiologic alterations, and pathophysiologic changes justify their consideration as a group. These disorders account for about 15% of noninfectious diseases seen by pulmonary physicians.

In general, the clinical and pulmonary functional changes are those of *restrictive rather than obstructive lung disease* (see the previous section on obstructive versus restrictive pulmonary dis-

ease). Patients have dyspnea, tachypnea, and eventual cyanosis, without wheezing or other evidence of airway obstruction. The classic physiologic features are reductions in oxygen-diffusing capacity, lung volumes, and compliance. *Chest radiographs show diffuse infiltration by small nodules, irregular lines, or "ground-glass" shadows,* hence the term "infiltrative." Eventually, secondary pulmonary hypertension and right-sided heart failure with cor pulmonale may result. Although the entities can often be distinguished in the early stages, the advanced forms are hard to differentiate, as they result in scarring and gross destruction of the lung, often referred to as "end-stage lung" or "honeycomb lung."

Diffuse infiltrative diseases are categorized into those with known causes and those of unknown cause (Table 15–7), some of which can be defined either as clinicopathologic syndromes or as having characteristic histology.[43] Many of these entities are discussed in other sections of this book. Here we shall briefly review current concepts of pathogenesis that may be common to all and discuss those in which lung involvement is the primary or a major problem. In terms of frequency, the most common associations are environmental diseases (24%), sarcoidosis (20%), idiopathic pulmonary fibrosis (15%), and the collagen-vascular diseases (8%). The remainder have more than 100 different causes and associations.

PATHOGENESIS. It is now thought that regardless of the type of interstitial disease or specific cause, the earliest common manifestation of most of the interstitial diseases is *alveolitis*,[44,45] that is, an accumulation of inflammatory and immune effector cells within the alveolar walls and spaces (Fig. 15–27). Under normal conditions these cells account for no more than 7% of the total lung cell population and consist of macrophages (93%), lymphocytes (7%), and neutrophils and eosinophils (less

Table 15–7. DIFFUSE INTERSTITIAL LUNG DISEASES

KNOWN CAUSE	UNKNOWN CAUSE

1. Occupational and environmental inhalants
   a. Inorganic dusts—silicosis, asbestos, coal workers' pneumoconiosis
   b. Organic dusts (hypersensitivity pneumonitis)
   c. Gases, fumes, aerosols (oxygen toxicity, sulfur dioxide, toluene)
2. Drugs and toxins
   Chemotherapeutic agents (busulfan, bleomycin)
   Antibiotics (nitrofurantoin)
   Antiarrhythmics (amiodarone)
   Other drugs (gold, penicillamine)
   Toxins (paraquat)
3. Infections
   Viral (influenza, cytomegalovirus)
   Bacterial (widespread tuberculosis)
   Fungal
   Parasitic (*Pneumocystis carinii*)
	1. Sarcoidosis
	2. Associated with collagen-vascular disorders and vasculitis (e.g., rheumatoid arthritis, systemic lupus erythematosus, Wegener's granulomatosis)
	3. Goodpasture's syndrome
	4. Idiopathic pulmonary hemosiderosis
	5. Eosinophilic pneumonia
	6. Histiocytosis X
	7. Alveolar proteinosis
	8. Desquamative interstitial pneumonitis
	9. Idiopathic pulmonary fibrosis

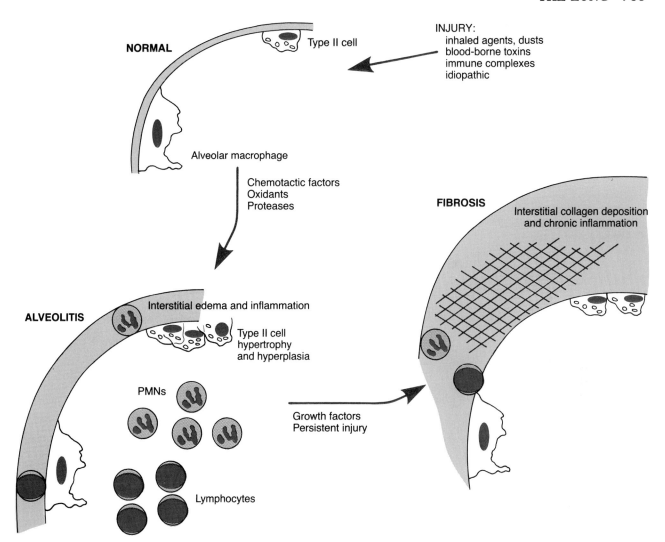

NORMAL

Type II cell

INJURY:
inhaled agents, dusts
blood-borne toxins
immune complexes
idiopathic

Alveolar macrophage

Chemotactic factors
Oxidants
Proteases

FIBROSIS

Interstitial collagen deposition
and chronic inflammation

Interstitial edema and inflammation

ALVEOLITIS

Type II cell
hypertrophy
and hyperplasia

PMNs

Growth factors
Persistent injury

Lymphocytes

Figure 15–27. Current concepts of the pathogenesis of chronic pulmonary fibrosis, in which alveolar injury by inhaled or blood-borne agents may be the initial trigger to macrophage and neutrophil accumulation and activation. In other conditions, T cell–mediated reactions may predominate. The end result is lung damage and fibrosis. PMNs = polymorphonuclear neutrophils.

than 1%). In alveolitis there is a marked increase in the number of these cells and a change in their relative proportions. The accumulation of leukocytes has two consequences: it distorts the normal alveolar structures *and* results in the release of mediators that can injure parenchymal cells and stimulate fibrosis. The final result is an end-stage fibrotic lung in which the alveoli are replaced by cystic spaces separated by thick bands of connective tissue interspersed with inflammatory cells.

The initial stimuli for alveolitis are as heterogeneous as the causes outlined in Table 15–5. Some of these stimuli, such as oxygen-derived free radicals and some chemicals, are directly toxic to endothelial cells, epithelial cells, or both. But beyond direct toxicity, a critical event is the *recruitment and activation of inflammatory and immune effector cells.* Neutrophil recruitment can be caused by complement activation in some disorders,[46] but in addition the alveolar macrophages, which increase in number in all interstitial diseases, release *chemotactic factors* for neutrophils (e.g., IL-8,[47] leukotriene B_4[48]). Some chemotactic agents also "activate" the neutrophils, causing them to secrete proteases and toxic oxygen free radicals, which contribute further to tissue damage and provide a mechanism for maintenance of the alveolitis. In diseases such as sarcoidosis, *cell-mediated immune reactions* result in the accumulation of monocytes and T lymphocytes and in the formation of granulomas. It is thought that interactions among lymphocytes and macrophages and the release of lymphokines and monokines are responsible for the slowly progressive pulmonary fibrosis that ensues. The alveolar macrophage, in particular, plays a central role in the development of fi-

Table 15–8. AIR POLLUTANT LUNG DISEASES

AGENT	DISEASE	EXPOSURE
Mineral Dusts		
Coal dust	Anthracosis	Coal mining (particularly hard coal)
	Macules	
	Progressive massive fibrosis	
	Caplan's syndrome	
Silica	Silicosis	Foundry work, sandblasting, hard-rock
	Caplan's syndrome	mining, stone cutting, others
Asbestos	Asbestosis	Mining, milling, and fabrication, installa-
	Pleural plaques	tion and removal of insulation
	Caplan's syndrome	
	Mesothelioma	
	Carcinoma of the lung, larynx, stomach, colon	
Beryllium	Acute berylliosis	Mining, fabrication
	Beryllium granulomatosis	
	?Bronchogenic carcinoma	
Iron oxide	Siderosis	Welding
Barium sulfate	Baritosis	Mining
Tin oxide	Stannosis	Mining
Organic Dusts That Induce Hypersensitivity Pneumonitis		
Moldy hay	Farmer's lung	Farming
Bagasse	Bagassosis	Manufacturing wallboard, paper
Bird droppings	Bird-breeder's lung	Bird handling
Organic Dusts That Induce Asthma		
Cotton, flax, hemp	Byssinosis	Textile manufacturing
Red cedar dust	Asthma	Lumbering, carpentry
Chemical Fumes and Vapors		
Nitrous oxide, sulfur dioxide ammonia, benzene, certain insecticides (e.g., cyanate gases)	Bronchitis	Occupational and accidental exposure
	Asthma	
	Pulmonary edema	
	Respiratory distress syndrome	
	Injury to exposed mucosa	
	Fulminant poisoning	

brosis, as reviewed in the discussion of chronic inflammation (see Chapter 3).

PNEUMOCONIOSES

The term *"pneumoconiosis"* was originally coined to describe the non-neoplastic lung reaction to inhalation of mineral dusts (e.g., coal dust [anthracosis], silica [silicosis], asbestos [asbestosis], and beryllium [berylliosis]) commonly encountered in the workplace. Less common mineral dust pneumoconioses include siderosis (iron dust), stannosis (tin dust), and baritosis (barium dust). The use of the term "pneumoconiosis" has been broadened to include diseases induced by organic as well as inorganic particulates and chemical fumes and vapors. A simplified classification is presented in Table 15–8. For all pneumoconioses, regulations limiting worker exposure have resulted in a decreased incidence of dust-associated diseases.

Although the pneumoconioses result from well-defined occupational exposure to specific airborne agents, there are also deleterious effects of particulate air pollution for the general population. A recent study indicated that the incidence not only of pneumoconioses and pulmonary fibrosis but also of asthma, chronic bronchitis, and lung cancer rises with increasing ambient air particulate exposure in the general population.[49]

The specific changes caused by the more important dusts are presented in succeeding sections; however, certain pathogenetic principles apply to all. *The development of a pneumoconiosis is dependent on (1) the amount of dust retained in the lung and airways; (2) the size, shape, and therefore buoyancy of the particles; (3) particle solubility and physiochemical reactivity; and (4) the possible additional effects of other irritants (e.g., concomitant tobacco smoking).*

The amount of dust retained in the lungs is determined by the dust concentration in the ambient air, the duration of the exposure, and the effectiveness of clearance mechanisms. Recall (from the discussion of bacterial pneumonia in this chapter) that (1) any influence, such as cigarette smoking, that affects the integrity of the mucociliary apparatus significantly predisposes to the accumulation of dust and (2) *the most dangerous particles range* from 1 to 5 μm in diameter because they may reach the terminal small airways and air sacs and settle in their linings. Under normal conditions there is always a small pool of intra-alveolar macrophages that is expanded by recruitment of more macrophages when dust reaches the alveolar spaces. However, the protection provided by phagocytosis of particles can be overwhelmed by the large dust burden deposited in occupational exposures and by specific chemical interactions of the particles with cells.

The solubility and cytotoxicity of particles, influenced to a considerable extent by their size, modify the nature of the pulmonary response. In general, the smaller the particle, the higher the surface area–to–mass ratio, and the more likely and the more rapidly toxic levels will appear in the pulmonary fluids (depending, of course, on the solubility of the agent). Larger particles resist dissolution and so may persist within the lung parenchyma for years. These tend to evoke fibrosing collagenous pneumoconioses, such as is characteristic of silicosis. The reaction to crystalline silica illustrates how the physiochemical reactivity of particles contributes to pathogenesis. Quartz (a form of crystalline silica) can cause direct injury to tissue and cell membranes by interaction with free radicals and other chemical groups on the particle surface. The resulting membrane damage may ultimately cause cell death. However, of more importance is the ability of silica to trigger macrophages to release a number of products that mediate an inflammatory response and initiate fibroblast proliferation and collagen deposition.[50,51] Proinflammatory and fibrosing mediators are also critical in the pathogenesis of the pulmonary reaction to asbestos.[52] Indeed, many of the same mediators and cytokines discussed earlier in the pathogenesis of diffuse interstitial fibrosis are likely to play a role in the pathogenic response to inhaled particulates (details below).

Some of the particles may be taken up by epithelial cells or may cross the epithelial cell lining and interact directly with fibroblasts and interstitial macrophages. Some may reach the lymphatics either by direct drainage or within migrating macrophages and thereby initiate an immune response to components of the particulates and/or to self-proteins, modified by the particles. This then leads to an amplification and extension of the local reaction. Although tobacco smoking worsens the effects of all inhaled mineral dusts, the effects of asbestos are particularly magnified by smoking.

Coal Workers' Pneumoconiosis — Simple and Complicated (Progressive Massive Fibrosis)

Coal, a form of combustible carbon, has long been mined for fuel. The spectrum of lung findings in coal workers is wide, varying from (1) asymptomatic anthracosis, in which pigment accumulates without a perceptible cellular reaction, to (2) simple coal workers' pneumoconiosis (CWP), in which accumulations of macrophages occur with little to no pulmonary dysfunction, to (3) complicated CWP, or progressive massive fibrosis (PMF), in which fibrosis is extensive and lung function is compromised.[53] Fortunately, dust reduction measures in the coal mines around the globe have drastically reduced the incidence of coal dust–induced disease. Although statistics vary, it appears that fewer than 10% of cases of simple CWP progress to PMF. It should be noted that PMF is a generic term that applies to a confluent, fibrosing reaction in the lung that can be a complication of any pneumoconiosis, although it is most common in CWP and silicosis.

The pathogenesis of complicated CWP, and, particularly, what causes the lesions of simple CWP to progress to PMF, is incompletely understood. Contaminating silica in the coal dust can favor progressive disease. However, evidence suggests that in most cases carbon dust itself is the major culprit, and studies have shown that complicated lesions contain considerably more dust than simple lesions.

MORPHOLOGY. Anthracosis is the most innocuous coal-induced pulmonary lesion in coal miners and is also commonly seen in all urban dwellers and tobacco smokers. Inhaled carbon pigment is engulfed by alveolar or interstitial macrophages, which then accumulate in the connective tissue along the lymphatics, including the pleural lymphatics, or in organized lymphoid tissue along the bronchi or in the lung hilus. At autopsy, linear streaks and aggregates of anthracotic pigment readily identify pulmonary lymphatics and mark the pulmonary lymph nodes.

Simple CWP is characterized by **coal macules** (1 to 2 mm in diameter) and the somewhat larger **coal nodules.** The coal macule consists of carbon-laden macrophages; the nodule also contains small amounts of a delicate network of collagen fibers. Although these lesions are scattered throughout the lung, the upper lobes and upper zones of the lower lobes are more heavily involved. They are located primarily adjacent to respiratory bronchioles, the site of initial dust accumulation. In due course, dilatation of adjacent alveoli occurs, a condition sometimes referred to as centrilobular emphysema. However, recall that by definition emphysema is associated with destruction of alveolar septa, and whether this occurs in primary CWP is not yet certain.

Complicated CWP (PMF) occurs on a background of simple CWP and generally requires many years to develop. It is characterized by intensely blackened scars larger than 2 cm, sometimes up to

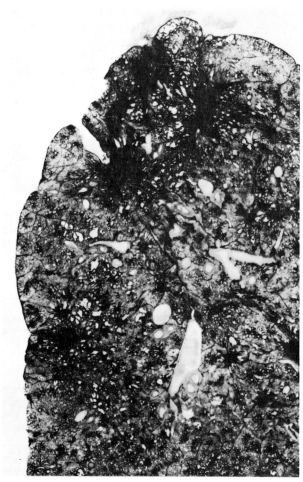

Figure 15–28. Progressive massive fibrosis superimposed on coal workers' pneumoconiosis. The large, blackened scars are located principally in the upper lobe. Note extensions of scars into surrounding parenchyma and retraction of adjacent pleura. (Courtesy of Dr. Werner Laquer, Dr. Jerome Kleinerman, and the National Institute of Occupational Safety and Health, Morgantown, WV.)

10 cm in greatest diameter. They are usually multiple (Fig. 15–28). Microscopically, the lesions consist of dense collagen and pigment. The center of the lesion is often necrotic, resulting most likely from local ischemia.

Caplan's syndrome is defined as the coexistence of rheumatoid arthritis with a pneumoconiosis, leading to the development of distinctive nodular pulmonary lesions that develop fairly rapidly. Like rheumatoid nodules (see Chapter 27), the nodular lesions in Caplan's syndrome have central necrosis surrounded by fibroblasts, macrophages, and collagen. This syndrome can also occur in asbestosis and silicosis.

CLINICAL COURSE. CWP is usually a benign disease that causes little decrement in lung function. Even mild forms of complicated CWP fail to demonstrate abnormalities of lung function. However, in a minority of cases PMF develops, leading to increasing pulmonary dysfunction, pulmonary hypertension, and cor pulmonale. Once PMF develops, it may become progressive even if further exposure to dust is prevented. The incidence of clinical tuberculosis is increased in persons with CWP, but whether this reflects a greater vulnerability to infection or, instead, socioeconomic factors inherent in the life of miners is unclear. There is also some evidence that exposure to coal dust increases the incidence of chronic bronchitis and emphysema, independent of smoking, thus complicating the management of the patient with CWP. However, to date, there is no compelling evidence that CWP in the absence of smoking predisposes to cancer.

Silicosis

Silicosis is a lung disease caused by inhalation of crystalline silicon dioxide (silica).[54] *Currently the most prevalent chronic occupational disease in the world,* silicosis usually presents, after decades of exposure, as a slowly progressing, nodular, fibrosing pneumoconiosis. As shown in Table 15–8, workers in a large number of occupations are at risk, especially sandblasters and many mine workers. Less commonly, very heavy exposure over months to a few years can result in acute silicosis, a lesion characterized by the generalized accumulation of a lipoproteinaceous material within alveoli (identical morphologically to alveolar proteinosis).

Silica occurs in both crystalline and amorphous forms, but crystalline forms (including quartz, crystobalite, and tridymite) are much more fibrogenic, revealing the importance of the physical form and surface properties in pathogenesis. Of these, quartz is most commonly implicated in silicosis. Following inhalation, the particles interact with epithelial cells and macrophages to initiate injury and cause fibrosis. The mechanisms of tissue and cell injury by crystalline silica are thought to be based on the chemical reactivity of the particle surface. SiOH groups on the surface form bonds (hydrogen and electrostatic) with membrane proteins and phospholipids, which leads to denaturation of membrane proteins and damage to the lipid membranes. In addition, surface free radicals (which decay as a result of vigorous reactivity, with a half-life of 30 hours) are generated during the cleavage of silica (as occurs during crushing of stone in mining). This initially high surface chemical reactivity makes freshly ground silica substantially more cytotoxic *in vitro* than its aged counterpart.

Although lung macrophages that ingest the silica particles may ultimately succumb to the toxic effects described earlier, silica causes activation and release of mediators by viable macrophages. Mediators identified include interleukin-1, TNF, fibronectin, lipid mediators, oxygen-derived free radicals, and fibrogenic cytokines.[54] Especially compelling is evidence that anti-TNF monoclonal antibodies can block lung collagen accumulation in mice given silica intratracheally.[55] Animals exposed to silica demonstrate a steady recruitment of macrophages and lymphocytes to the alveolus and interstitium. These cells may further amplify the process.

As with CWP (discussed above), the initial lesions tend to localize in the upper lung zones, although the reasons for this distribution are obscure. In contrast with CWP, however, early lesions of silicosis are more fibrotic and less cellular. An interesting, perhaps related phenomenon is that quartz, when mixed with other minerals, has a reduced fibrogenic effect. This is of practical importance because quartz in the workplace is rarely pure. Thus miners of the iron-containing ore hematite may have more quartz in their lungs than some quartz-exposed workers and yet have relatively mild lung disease because the hematite provides a protective effect. This may reflect interaction of the other minerals with charged groups on the silica crystalline surface, dampening this component of the toxic interaction of silica and cell membranes. In the earth, much of the silicon combines with oxygen and other elements to form silicates. Although amorphous silicates are biologically less active than crystalline silica, heavy lung burdens of these minerals may also produce lesions. Talc, vermiculite, and mica are examples of noncrystalline silicates that are less common causes of pneumoconioses.

CLINICAL COURSE. The disease is usually detected when routine chest radiography is performed on an asymptomatic worker. The radiographs typically show a fine nodularity in the upper zones of the lung, but pulmonary functions are either normal or only moderately affected. Most patients do not develop shortness of breath until late in the course, after PMF is present. At this time, the disease may be progressive, even if the patient is no longer exposed. The disease is slow to kill, but impaired pulmonary function may severely limit activity. Despite persistent controversy, there is no clear association of silica and the development of lung cancer in humans.[56,57]

Asbestos-Related Diseases

Asbestos is a family of crystalline hydrated silicates that form fibers. Based on epidemiologic studies, *occupational exposure* to asbestos is linked to (1) localized fibrous plaques or, rarely, diffuse pleural fibrosis; (2) pleural effusions; (3) parenchymal interstitial fibrosis *(asbestosis)*; (4) bronchogenic carcinoma; (5) mesotheliomas; and (6) laryngeal and perhaps other extrapulmonary neoplasms, including colon carcinomas.[58] An increased incidence of asbestosis-related cancer in family members of as-

MORPHOLOGY. Silicosis is characterized grossly in its early stages by tiny, barely palpable, discrete pale to blackened (if coal dust is also present) nodules in the upper zones of the lungs. As the disease progresses, these nodules may coalesce into **hard collagenous scars** (Fig. 15–29). Some nodules may undergo central softening and cavitation. This may be due to superimposed tuberculosis or to ischemia. The intervening lung parenchyma may be compressed or overexpanded, and a honeycomb pattern may develop. Fibrotic lesions may also occur in the hilar lymph nodes and pleura. Sometimes, thin sheets of calcification occur in the lymph nodes and are appreciated radiographically as "eggshell" calcification (e.g., calcium surrounding a zone lacking calcification). If the disease continues to progress, expansion and coalescence of lesions produce PMF. Histologically, the nodular lesions consist of concentric layers of hyalinized collagen surrounded by a dense capsule of more condensed collagen (Fig. 15–30). Examination of the nodules by polarized microscopy reveals the birefrigent silica particles.

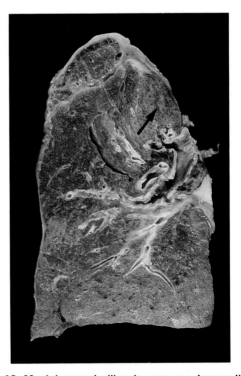

Figure 15–29. Advanced silicosis seen on transection of lung. Scarring has contracted the upper lobe into a small dark mass *(arrow)*. Note dense pleural thickening. (Courtesy of Dr. John Godleski, Brigham and Women's Hospital, Boston.)

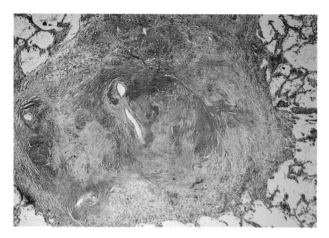

Figure 15-30. Several coalescent collagenous silicotic nodules (Courtesy of Dr. John Godleski, Brigham and Women's Hospital, Boston.)

bestos workers has alerted the general public to the potential hazards of asbestos in the environment. The proper public healthy policy toward low-level exposures that might be encountered in old buildings or schools is controversial, with some experts questioning the wisdom of expensive asbestos abatement programs for environments with airborne fiber counts that are up to 100-fold lower than allowed by occupational standards.

PATHOGENESIS. Concentration, size, shape, and solubility of the different forms of asbestos dictate whether disease will occur. There are two distinct geometric forms of asbestos: *serpentine* (curly and flexible fibers) and *amphibole* (straight, stiff, and brittle fibers). The serpentine chrysotile chemical form accounts for most of the asbestos used in industry. Amphiboles include crocidolite, amosite, tremolite, anthophyllite, and actinolyte. This confusing array of terms is important because amphiboles, even though less prevalent, are more pathogenic than chrysotiles, particularly with respect to induction of malignant pleural tumors (mesotheliomas). Indeed, some studies of mesotheliomas have shown the link is almost always to amphibole exposure. The relatively few cases of mesotheliomas arising in chrysotile workers are in all likelihood due to contamination of chrysotile with the amphibole tremolite.

The greater pathogenicity of straight and stiff amphiboles is apparently related to their aerodynamic properties and solubility. Chrysotiles, with their more flexible, curled structure, are likely to become impacted in the upper respiratory passages and removed by the mucociliary elevator. Furthermore, once trapped in the lungs, chrysotiles are gradually leached from the tissues because they are more soluble than amphiboles. In contrast, the straight, stiff amphiboles may align themselves in the airstream and thus be delivered deeper into the lungs, where they can penetrate epithelial cells and reach the interstitium. The length of amphibole fibers also plays a role in pathogenicity, those longer than 8 mm and thinner than 0.5 mm being more injurious than shorter, thicker ones. Nevertheless, both amphiboles and serpentines are fibrogenic, and increasing doses are associated with a higher incidence of all asbestos-related diseases, except that only amphibole exposure correlates with mesothelioma. Experimental studies have indicated that, in contrast to other inorganic dusts that induce cellular and fibrotic lung reactions, asbestos can also act as both a tumor initiator and a tumor promoter. However, potentially toxic chemicals adsorbed onto the asbestos fibers undoubtedly contribute to the oncogenicity of the fibers. *For example, the adsorption of carcinogens in tobacco smoke onto asbestos fibers may well be important in the remarkable synergy between tobacco smoking and the development of bronchogenic carcinoma in asbestos workers* (e.g., one study of asbestos workers found a 5-fold increase of bronchogenic carcinoma for asbestos exposure alone, while asbestos exposure and smoking together led to a 55-fold increase in the risk of lung cancer!).[59]

Asbestosis, like the other pneumoconioses, depends on the interaction of inhaled fibers with lung macrophages and other parenchymal cells. The initial injury occurs at bifurcations of small airways and ducts, where the stiff fibers land and penetrate. Macrophages both alveolar and interstitial attempt to ingest and clear the fibers and are activated to release chemotactic factors and fibrogenic mediators that amplify the response. Chronic deposition of fibers and persistent release of mediators eventually leads to generalized interstitial pulmonary inflammation and interstitial fibrosis. Specific fibrogenic cytokines that have been identified in the response of lung macrophages to asbestos include fibronectin, PDGF, and insulin-like growth factor I (IGF-I). It is not completely understood why silicosis is a nodular fibrosing disease and asbestosis a diffuse interstitial process. The more diffuse distribution may be related to the ability of asbestos to reach alveoli more consistently or its ability to penetrate epithelial cells, or to both.

MORPHOLOGY. Asbestosis is marked by **diffuse pulmonary interstitial fibrosis.** These changes are indistinguishable from those resulting from other causes of diffuse interstitial fibrosis, except for the presence of **asbestos bodies.** Asbestos bodies appear as **golden brown, fusiform or beaded rods with a translucent center and consist of asbestos fibers coated with an iron-containing proteinaceous material** (Fig. 15-31). They arise when macrophages attempt to phagocytose asbestos fibers; the iron is presumably derived from phagocyte ferritin. Other inorganic particulates may become coated with similar iron protein complexes, and the term "ferruginous bodies" is better used where there is no evidence of an asbestos core. It should be noted that asbestos bodies can sometimes be found in the lungs of normal persons, but usually in much lower concentrations and without an accompanying interstitial fibrosis.

Asbestosis begins as fibrosis around respiratory bronchioles and alveolar ducts and extends to involve adjacent alveolar sacs and alveoli. The fibrous tissue distorts the native architecture, creating enlarged airspaces enclosed within thick fibrous walls; eventually the affected regions become honeycombed. In contrast to CWP and silicosis, asbestosis begins in the lower lobes and subpleurally, but the middle and upper lobes of the lungs become affected as fibrosis progresses. Simultaneously, the visceral pleura undergoes fibrous thickening and sometimes binds the lungs to the chest wall. Large parenchymal nodules typical of Caplan's syndrome may appear in a few patients who have concurrent rheumatoid arthritis. The scarring may trap and narrow pulmonary arteries and arterioles, causing pulmonary hypertension and cor pulmonale.

Pleural plaques, the most common manifestation of asbestos exposure, are well-circumscribed plaques of dense collagen (Fig. 15–32), often containing calcium. They develop most frequently on the anterior and posterolateral aspects of the **parietal pleura** and over the domes of the diaphragm. They do not contain asbestos bodies and only rarely do they occur in persons who have no history or evidence of asbestos exposure. Uncommonly, asbestos exposure induces pleural effusions, which are usually serous but may be bloody. Rarely, diffuse visceral pleural fibrosis may occur and, in advanced cases, bind the lung to the thoracic cavity wall.

Both bronchogenic carcinomas and mesotheliomas (pleural and peritoneal) develop in workers exposed to asbestos. The risk of bronchogenic carcinoma is increased about fivefold for as-

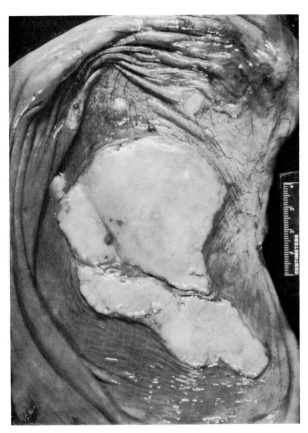

Figure 15–32. Asbestos exposure evidenced by severe, discrete, characteristic fibrocalcific plaques on pleural surface of diaphragm. (Courtesy of Dr. John Godleski, Brigham and Women's Hospital, Boston.)

bestos workers; the relative risk of mesotheliomas, normally a very rare tumor (2 to 17 cases per 1,000,000 persons), is more than a 1000-fold greater. Concomitant cigarette smoking greatly increases the risk of bronchogenic carcinoma, but not that of mesothelioma. These asbestos-related tumors are morphologically indistinguishable from cancers of other causes and are described later in this chapter.

CLINICAL COURSE. The clinical findings in asbestosis are indistinguishable from those of any other diffuse interstitial lung disease (see earlier in this chapter). Dyspnea is usually the first manifestation: at first it is provoked by exertion, later it is present even at rest. These manifestations rarely appear less than 10 years following first exposure and are more common after 20 years or more. The dyspnea is usually accompanied by a cough associated with production of sputum. The disease may remain static or progress to congestive heart failure, cor pulmonale, and death. Chest films reveal irregular linear densities, particularly in both lower lobes. With advancement of the pneumoconiosis, a honeycomb pattern develops. Pleural plaques are usu-

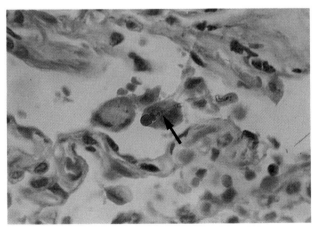

Figure 15–31. A high-power detail of an asbestos body, revealing the typical beading and knobbed ends (arrow).

ally asymptomatic and are detected on radiographs as circumscribed densities. Asbestosis complicated by lung or pleural cancer is associated with a particularly grim prognosis.

Berylliosis

Heavy exposure to airborne dusts or to fumes of metallic beryllium or its oxides, alloys, or salts may induce acute pneumonitis; more protracted low-dose exposure may cause pulmonary and systemic granulomatous lesions that closely mimic sarcoidosis (see following section). Recognition of the hazards of beryllium exposure in the workplace and enactment in the late 1940s of standards for limiting worker exposure resulted in the disappearance of acute berylliosis. Currently, workers in the nuclear and aerospace industries working with beryllium alloys are at highest risk for exposure, but new cases of chronic berylliosis are reported only occasionally.

Chronic berylliosis is caused by induction of cell-mediated immunity.[60] Because only 2% of exposed workers develop disease, it appears that genetic susceptibility is necessary for the initiation of an immune response. The development of delayed hypersensitivity leads to the formation of noncaseating granulomas in the lungs and hilar nodes or, less commonly, in the spleen, liver, kidney, adrenals, and distant lymph nodes. The pulmonary granulomas become progressively fibrotic, giving rise to irregular, fine nodular densities detected on chest radiographs. Hilar adenopathy is present in about half the cases.

Chronic berylliosis often does not result in clinical manifestations until many years after exposure, when the patient presents with dyspnea, cough, weight loss, and arthralgias. Some cases stabilize, other remit and relapse, still others progress to pulmonary failure. Epidemiologic evidence links heavy beryllium exposure to an increased incidence of lung cancer.

SARCOIDOSIS

Sarcoidosis is a disease of unknown cause characterized by noncaseating granulomas in many tissues and organs. Since other diseases, including mycobacterial or fungal infections and berylliosis, can also produce noncaseating ("hard") granulomas, the histologic diagnosis of sarcoidosis must be made by exclusion. Sarcoidosis can involve many systems and organs and present many clinical patterns, but bilateral hilar lymphadenopathy or lung involvement is visible on chest radiographs in 90% of cases. Eye and skin lesions are next in frequency.

The prevalence of sarcoidosis is higher in females than in males but varies widely in different countries and populations. In the United States, the rates are highest in the southeastern states;

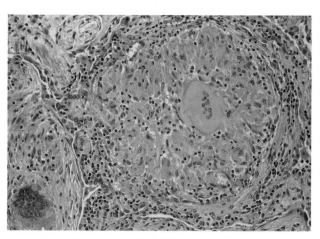

Figure 15–33. Characteristic sarcoid noncaseating granulomas in lung with many giant cells. (Courtesy of Dr. Ramon Blanco, Dept. of Pathology, Brigham and Women's Hospital, Boston.)

they are ten times higher in American blacks than in whites. By contrast, among Chinese and Southeast Asians, the disease is almost unknown.

ETIOLOGY AND PATHOGENESIS. The distinctive granulomatous tissue response seen in sarcoidosis suggests the presence of a persistent, poorly degradable antigen. Numerous intriguing immunologic abnormalities are present,[61] including increases in CD4+ lymphocytes within the lung and elevated levels of soluble IL-2 receptors in serum and lung lavage fluid. Alveolar macrophages also show an activated phenotype, with increased class II HLA expression and increased antigen-presenting capacity. The cytokines and factors secreted by these cells could well account for the influx of monocytes, alveolitis, and noncaseating granuloma formation in the lung and for the resulting progressive fibrosis, all characteristic features of pulmonary sarcoidosis. Like other T-cell responses to antigen, the T-cell proliferation in the sarcoid lung is oligoclonal, rather than a generalized, nonspecific response.[62] Nevertheless, numerous past efforts at identifying bacterial or viral agents or other inciting agents have failed. Two recent developments have reawakened interest in a possible role for mycobacteria in the pathogenesis of sarcoidosis. First is the observation of elevated circulating gamma-delta–T cells in some patients, a receptor subtype associated with response to mycobacterial antigens.[63] Second, the powerful polymerase chain reaction (PCR) technique is being applied to sarcoidal tissue in an attempt to detect minute amounts of mycobacterial DNA. True to its enigmatic self, sarcoid is providing conflicting results in these investigations.[64,65] and remains a disease of unknown etiology.

MORPHOLOGY. Histologically, all involved tissues show the classic **noncaseating granulomas** (Fig. 15–33), each composed of an aggregate of

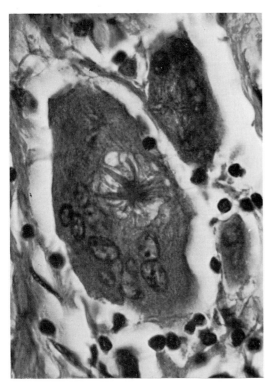

Figure 15–34. Characteristic asteroid body within a giant cell in sarcoidosis.

tightly clustered epithelioid cells, often with Langhans' or foreign body–type giant cells. Central necrosis is unusual. In chronic disease, the granulomas may become enclosed within fibrous rims or may eventually be replaced by hyaline fibrous scars. Two other microscopic features are often present in the granulomas: (1) laminated concretions composed of calcium and proteins known as Schaumann's bodies, and (2) stellate inclusions known as **asteroid bodies** enclosed within giant cells (Fig. 15–34), found in approximately 60% of the granulomas. Although characteristic, these microscopic features are not pathognomonic of sarcoidosis, because asteroid and Schaumann's bodies may be encountered in other granulomatous diseases (e.g., berylliosis) (see the preceding section on pneumoconiosis). Pathologic involvement of virtually every organ in the body has been cited at one time or another.

The **lungs** are common sites of involvement. Macroscopically, there is usually no demonstrable alteration, although at times the coalescence of granulomas may produce small nodules that are palpable or visible as 1- to 2-cm, noncaseating, noncavitated consolidations. Histologically, the lesions are distributed primarily along the lymphatics around bronchi and blood vessels, although alveolar lesions are also seen. The relative frequency of granulomas in the bronchial submucosa accounts for the high diagnostic yield of bronchoscopic biopsies. There appears to be a strong tendency for lesions to heal in the lungs, so varying stages of fibrosis and hyalinization are often found, causing interstitial pulmonary fibrosis. The pleural surfaces are sometimes involved.

Lymph nodes are involved in almost all cases, specifically the hilar and mediastinal nodes, but any other node in the body may be involved. Nodes are characteristically enlarged, discrete, and sometimes calcified. The tonsils are affected in about one-quarter to one-third of cases.

The **spleen** is affected microscopically in about three-quarters of the cases, but it is enlarged in only 18%. On occasion, granulomas may coalesce to form small nodules that are barely visible macroscopically. The capsule is not involved. The **liver** is affected slightly less often than the spleen. It may also be moderately enlarged and may contain scattered granulomas, more in portal triads than in the lobular parenchyma. Needle biopsy may permit the identification of these focal lesions. The **bone marrow** is an additional favored site of localization. Roentgenographic changes can be identified in about one-fifth of cases of systemic involvement. The radiologically visible bone lesions have a particular tendency to involve phalangeal bones of the hands and feet, creating small circumscribed areas of bone resorption within the marrow cavity, a diffuse reticulated pattern throughout the cavity, with widening of the bony shafts, and/or new bone formations on the outer surfaces.

Skin lesions are encountered in one-third to one-half of the cases. Sarcoidosis of the skin assumes a variety of macroscopic appearances (e.g., discrete subcutaneous nodules; focal, slightly elevated, erythematous plaques; or flat lesions that are slightly reddened and scaling and resemble those of lupus erythematosus). Lesions may also appear on the mucous membranes of the oral cavity, larynx, and upper respiratory tract. Involvement of the **eye, its associated glands, and the salivary glands** occurs in about one-fifth to one-half of the cases. The ocular involvement takes the form of iritis or iridocyclitis, either bilaterally or unilaterally. As a consequence, corneal opacities, glaucoma, and total loss of vision may occur. These ocular lesions are frequently accompanied by inflammations in the lacrimal glands, with suppression of lacrimation. Bilateral sarcoidosis of the parotid, submaxillary, and sublingual glands completes the **combined uveoparotid involvement designated as Mikulicz's syndrome** (see Chapter 16).

Sarcoid granulomas occasionally occur in the heart, kidneys, central nervous system, and endocrine glands, particularly in the pituitary, as well as in other body tissues.

CLINICAL COURSE. Because of its varying severity and the inconstant distribution of the lesions, sarcoidosis is a protean clinical disease. Sarcoidosis may be discovered unexpectedly on routine chest films as bilateral hilar adenopathy or may have peripheral lymphadenopathy, cutaneous lesions, eye involvement, splenomegaly, or hepatomegaly as a presenting manifestation. In the great majority of cases, however, patients seek medical attention because of the insidious onset of respiratory abnormalities (shortness of breath, cough, chest pain, hemoptysis) or of constitutional signs and symptoms (fever, fatigue, weight loss, anorexia, night sweats).

Sarcoidosis follows a fairly unpredictable course characterized by either progressive chronicity or periods of activity interspersed with remissions, sometimes permanent, that may be spontaneous or initiated by steroid therapy. Overall, 65 to 70% of affected patients recover with minimal or no residual manifestations. Twenty per cent have permanent loss of some lung function or some permanent visual impairment. Of the remaining 10%, some die of cardiac or central nervous system damage, but most succumb to progressive pulmonary fibrosis and cor pulmonale. Patients presenting with hilar lymphadenopathy alone (stage I) have the best prognosis, followed by those with adenopathy and pulmonary infiltrates (stage II). Surprisingly, it is those patients presenting with pulmonary disease and no adenopathy (stage III) who have few spontaneous remissions and are most likely to develop chronic pulmonary fibrosis.

IDIOPATHIC PULMONARY FIBROSIS

This term refers to a poorly understood pulmonary disorder characterized histologically by diffuse interstitial inflammation and fibrosis, which in the advanced case results in severe hypoxemia and cyanosis. There are at least 20 synonyms for this entity (e.g., chronic interstitial pneumonitis, Hamman-Rich syndrome), and in Britain it is known as *diffuse or cryptogenic (i.e., idiopathic) fibrosing alveolitis.* The term *usual interstitial pneumonitis (UIP)* is employed by some to differentiate this condition from the desquamative type (desquamative interstitial pneumonitis [DIP]), described later, and from other, rarer examples of so-called giant cell and lymphocytic interstitial pneumonitis.[66] It should be stressed that similar pathologic findings may occur as the result of well-defined entities, such as the pneumoconioses, hypersensitivity pneumonitis, oxygen toxicity pneumonitis, scleroderma, and irradiation injury. In about half the cases of interstitial fibrosis, however, there is no known underlying disease, and the term "idiopathic" is applied.

It is now thought that this disorder represents a stereotyped inflammatory response of the alveolar wall to injuries of different types, durations, and intensities. The proposed sequence of events,

described earlier, begins with some form of alveolar wall injury, which results in interstitial edema and accumulation of inflammatory cells (alveolitis). The type I membranous pneumocyte is particularly susceptible to injury. Subsequently, there is hyperplasia of type II pneumocytes in an attempt to regenerate the alveolar epithelial lining. Fibroblasts then proliferate, and progressive fibrosis of both the interalveolar septa and the intra-alveolar exudate result in obliteration of normal pulmonary architecture.

Immune mechanisms may trigger this sequence of events in some cases.[44] There are high levels of circulating immune complexes or cryoimmunoglobulins in the serum of some patients with idiopathic interstitial pneumonia, particularly in cases in which biopsy shows significant cellular infiltration rather than interstitial fibrosis. Granular deposits of IgG are sometimes seen in the alveolar walls, suggesting that immune complexes may play a pathogenetic role, but the nature of the antigens within the complexes is unknown.

MORPHOLOGY. The morphologic changes vary according to the stage of the disease. In early cases, the lungs are firm in consistency and microscopically show pulmonary edema, intra-alveolar exudation, hyaline membranes, and infiltration of the alveolar septa with mononuclear cells. There is hyperplasia of type II pneumocytes, which appear as cuboidal or even columnar cells lining the alveolar spaces. With advancing disease, there is organization of the intra-alveolar exudate by fibrous tissue, as well as thickening of the interstitial septa owing to fibrosis and variable amounts of inflammation. At this stage the lungs become solid, with alternating areas of fibrosis and more normal-appearing lung. In the end stages of the disorder, the lung consists of spaces lined by cuboidal or columnar epithelium and separated by inflammatory fibrous tissue (Fig. 15–35). This gives the typical appearance of the **honeycomb lung.** Small cysts are often seen, and there is also intimal thickening of the pulmonary arteries and lymphoid hyperplasia. As mentioned earlier, this advanced picture can result from any of the disorders listed in Table 15–7. Thus, it is necessary to exclude the known causes of interstitial fibrosis by clinical, radiologic, or serologic means before the diagnosis of idiopathic fibrosis is made.

As would be expected, patients exhibit varying degrees of respiratory difficulty and, in advanced cases, hypoxemia and cyanosis. The septal fibrosis constitutes a significant physiologic alveolocapillary block. Secondary pulmonary hypertension can be severe, and cor pulmonale and cardiac failure may result. The progression in an individual case is unpredictable, and in some patients the disease remits spontaneously. The process progresses in

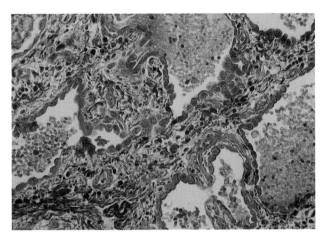

Figure 15-35. Diffuse interstitial fibrosis. Note marked interstitial fibrosis (highlighted blue in this Masson trichrome stain), focal chronic inflammation, and dilated spaces lined by cuboidal type II epithelial cells.

some very rapidly, leading to fibrosis in a matter of weeks, whereas in others it develops over many years. On average, death occurs in about 2 years.

DESQUAMATIVE INTERSTITIAL PNEUMONITIS (DIP)

In some patients with interstitial pneumonitis there is prominent aggregation of mononuclear cells (macrophages) within the alveoli, originally thought to be "desquamated" epithelial cells from the alveolar walls. These patients usually present with the slow development of cough and dyspnea, eventually leading to marked respiratory embarrassment, cyanosis, and clubbing of the fingers. Classically, the radiologic picture is that of bilateral lower-lobe ground-glass infiltrates.

MORPHOLOGY. The most striking histologic finding is the accumulation in the airspaces of a large number of macrophages containing lipid and periodic acid–Schiff (PAS)–positive granules. Some of the macrophages contain lamellar bodies (surfactant) within phagocytic vacuoles, presumably derived from necrotic type II pneumocytes. There is often an interstitial pneumonitis and an accompanying hyperplasia of the septal lining epithelial cells and desquamation of these cells into the airspaces (Fig. 15–36).

The cause is unknown. Patients benefit from steroid therapy, which often leads to clearing of the lungs. Some patients with DIP have or subsequently develop significant interstitial fibrosis; for this reason, many authors object to the term DIP and consider the entity an early stage of usual idiopathic interstitial fibrosis (discussed earlier).

Nevertheless, the presence of a prominent desquamative component has practical implications because such patients apparently have a better response to steroid therapy than those with the usual interstitial fibrotic pattern.[43]

HYPERSENSITIVITY PNEUMONITIS

The term "hypersensitivity pneumonitis" describes a spectrum of immunologically mediated, predominantly interstitial lung disorders caused by intense and often prolonged exposure to inhaled organic dusts and related occupational antigens.[67] Affected individuals have an abnormal sensitivity or heightened reactivity to the antigen, which, in contrast to that occurring in asthma, involves primarily the *alveoli. It is important to recognize these diseases early in their course, as progression to serious chronic fibrotic lung disease can be prevented by removal of the environmental agent.*

Most commonly, hypersensitivity results from the inhalation of organic dust containing antigens made up of spores of thermophilic bacteria, true fungi, animal proteins, or bacterial products. Numerous specifically named syndromes are described, depending on the occupation or exposure of the individual. *Farmer's lung* results from exposure to dusts generated from harvested, humid, warm hay that permits the rapid proliferation of the spores of thermophilic actinomycetes. *Pigeon breeder's lung* (bird fancier's disease) is provoked by proteins from serum, excreta, or feathers of the birds. *Humidifier* or *air-conditioner lung* is caused by thermophilic bacteria in heated water reservoirs. There is also mushroom picker's lung, maple bark disease, and duck fever (from duck feathers).

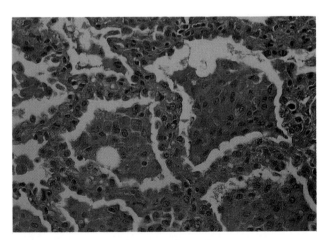

Figure 15-36. Desquamative interstitial pneumonitis. High-power detail of lung to demonstrate fibrous thickening of alveolar walls and accumulation of large numbers of mononuclear cells within alveolar spaces.

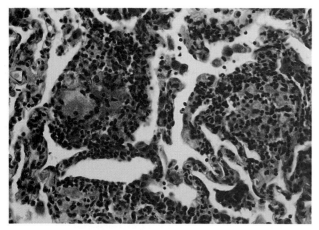

Figure 15-37. Hypersensitivity pneumonitis, histologic appearance. Loosely formed interstitial granulomas and chronic inflammation are characteristic.

MORPHOLOGY. Histologic information comes from biopsies of patients with subacute and chronic forms, rather than from those with acute attacks. The alterations (Fig. 15-37) include (1) interstitial pneumonitis consisting primarily of lymphocytes, plasma cells, and macrophages (some of the latter having a foamy cytoplasm), (2) interstitial fibrosis, (3) obliterative bronchiolitis, and (4) outright granuloma formation. In more than half the patients, there is also evidence of an intra-alveolar infiltrate.

The evidence from experimental and human studies strongly suggests a type III immune-complex pathogenesis for the early lesions, followed by a type IV delayed-hypersensitivity reaction for the granulomatous components.

The clinical manifestations are varied. Acute attacks, which follow inhalation of antigenic dust in sensitized patients, consist of recurring attacks of fever, dyspnea, cough, and leukocytosis. Diffuse and nodular infiltrates appear in the chest radiograph, and pulmonary function tests show an acute restrictive effect. Symptoms usually appear 4 to 6 hours after exposure. If exposure is continuous and protracted, a chronic form of the disease supervenes that no longer features the acute exacerbations on antigen re-exposure. Instead, there are signs of progressive respiratory failure, dyspnea, and cyanosis and a decrease in total lung capacity and compliance—a picture hard to differentiate from other forms of chronic interstitial disease.

Byssinosis is an occupational lung disease of textile workers that is apparently induced by the inhalation of airborne fibers of cotton, linen, and hemp. Acute effects include cough, wheezing, and airway obstruction, a picture that resembles bronchial asthma. Prolonged exposure leads to disabling chronic lung disease characterized by chronic bronchitis, emphysema, and interstitial granulomas.

Evidence for an immunologic hypersensitivity in this disorder is not as clear as that in the other conditions described in this section.

PULMONARY EOSINOPHILIA (PULMONARY INFILTRATION WITH EOSINOPHILIA)

A number of clinical and pathologic pulmonary entities are characterized by an infiltration of eosinophils likely of immunologic but incompletely understood origins.[68] The cause and pathogenesis of these disorders are diverse. They have been divided into the following categories: (1) *simple pulmonary eosinophilia*, or Löffler's syndrome; (2) *tropical eosinophilia*, caused by infection with *microfilariae*; (3) *secondary chronic pulmonary eosinophilia* (which occurs in a number of parasitic, fungal, and bacterial infections; in hypersensitivity pneumonitis; in drug allergies; and in association with asthma, allergic bronchopulmonary aspergillosis, or polyarteritis nodosa); and (4) so-called idiopathic *chronic eosophilic pneumonia*.

Löffler's syndrome is characterized by transient pulmonary lesions, eosinophilia in the blood, and a benign clinical course. Roentgenograms are often quite striking, with shadows of varying size and shape in any of the lobes, suggesting irregular intrapulmonary densities. The lungs show alveoli whose septa are thickened by an infiltrate composed of eosinophils and occasional interspersed giant cells, but there is no vasculitis, fibrosis, or necrosis.

Chronic eosinophilic pneumonia is characterized by focal areas of cellular consolidation of the lung substance distributed chiefly in the periphery of the lung fields. Prominent in these lesions are heavy aggregates of lymphocytes and eosinophils within both the septal walls and the alveolar spaces. Clinically, there is high fever, night sweats, and dyspnea, all of which respond to corticosteroid therapy. It is diagnosed when other causes of chronic pulmonary eosinophilia are excluded.

BRONCHIOLITIS OBLITERANS-ORGANIZING PNEUMONIA

This cumbersome designation refers to what is now recognized to be a common response to infectious or inflammatory injury of the lungs. Patients present with cough and dyspnea and often recall a recent respiratory tract infection. Patchy opacities or interstitial infiltrates are seen radiologically. Etiologies associated with bronchiolitis obliterans-organizing pneumonia (BOOP) include infections (viral, bacterial), inhaled toxins, drugs, collagen vascular disease, and bronchial obstruction.[69] The

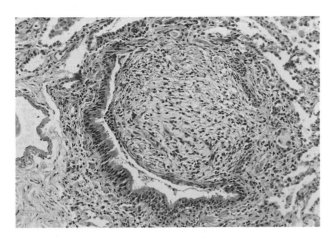

Figure 15–38. Bronchiolitis obliterans–organizing pneumonia (BOOP). Bronchiole showing plug of organizing exudate.

bronchiolar injury and repair distinguish this process from routine pneumonias. The major pathologic finding comprises polypoid plugs of loose, fibrous tissue filling bronchioles *(bronchiolitis obliterans)* and alveoli (Fig. 15–38). A variable chronic inflammatory cell infiltrate usually accompanies what appears to be a prolonged effort to resolve or organize the pulmonary injury. In most cases, patients improve gradually or with steroid therapy.

DIFFUSE PULMONARY HEMORRHAGE SYNDROMES

Hemorrhage from the lung is a dramatic complication of some interstitial lung disorders. Among these so-called *pulmonary hemorrhage syndromes*[70] are (1) Goodpasture's syndrome, (2) idiopathic pulmonary hemosiderosis, and (3) vasculitis-associated hemorrhage, which is found in conditions such as hypersensitivity angiitis, Wegener's granulomatosis, and lupus erythematosus (Fig. 15–39).

Goodpasture's Syndrome

Goodpasture's syndrome is an uncommon but intriguing condition characterized by the *simultaneous appearance of proliferative, usually rapidly progressive glomerulonephritis and a necrotizing hemorrhagic interstitial pneumonitis.* The evidence is quite substantial that the renal and pulmonary lesions are the consequence of antibodies evoked by antigens present in the glomerular and pulmonary basement membranes. The immunopathogenesis of the syndrome and the nature of the Goodpasture's antigens are described in Chapter 20, in the section on glomerulonephritis. Most cases

begin clinically with respiratory symptoms, principally hemoptysis, and radiographic evidence of focal pulmonary consolidations. Very soon, manifestations of glomerulonephritis appear, leading to rapidly progressive renal failure. The common cause of death is uremia. Most cases occur in the second or third decade of life, and there is a preponderance among males.

MORPHOLOGY. In the classic case, the lungs are heavy, with areas of red-brown consolidation. Histologically, there are acute focal necroses of alveolar walls associated with intra-alveolar hemorrhages, fibrous thickening of the septa, hypertrophy of lining septal cells, and (depending on the duration of the disease) organization of blood in the alveolar spaces. Often the alveoli contain hemosiderin-laden macrophages (see Fig. 15–39). Immunofluorescence studies reveal linear deposits of immunoglobulins along the basement membranes of the septal walls. The kidneys reveal the characteristic findings of focal proliferative glomerulonephritis in the early cases, or crescentic glomerulonephritis in patients with rapidly progressive glomerulonephritis. Linear deposits of immunoglobulins and complement are also seen by immunofluorescence studies along the glomerular basement membranes, similar to those in the alveolar septa.

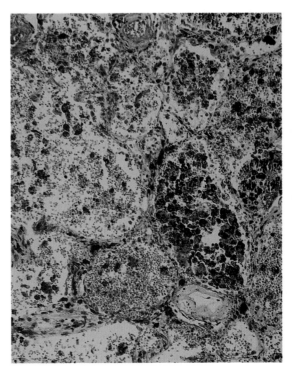

Figure 15–39. Acute intra-alveolar hemorrhage and hemosiderin-laden macrophages, reflecting past hemorrhage, are common features of the diffuse pulmonary hemorrhage syndromes (Prussian blue stain for iron).

The trigger initiating the anti–basement membrane antibodies is still unknown. In experimental animals, toxic pulmonary injury by toxic oxygen species or hydrocarbons increases fixation of antibodies onto basement membranes and induces pulmonary hemorrhage. In humans, virus infection, exposure to hydrocarbon solvents (used in the dry-cleaning industry), and smoking have been implicated as cofactors in the causation of the syndrome and may act by a similar mechanism.

The once dismal prognosis for this disease has been markedly improved by intensive *plasma exchange*. This procedure is thought to be beneficial by removing circulating anti–basement membrane antibodies as well as chemical mediators of immunologic injury. Simultaneous immunosuppressive therapy inhibits further antibody production. Both the lung hemorrhage and the glomerulonephritis improve with this form of therapy.

Idiopathic Pulmonary Hemosiderosis

Idiopathic pulmonary hemosiderosis is an uncommon pulmonary disease of obscure nature. It usually presents with an insidious onset of productive cough, hemoptysis, anemia, and weight loss associated with diffuse pulmonary infiltrations similar to Goodpasture's syndrome. However, it tends to occur in younger adults and children. The cause and pathogenesis are unknown, and no anti-basement membrane antibodies are detectable in serum or tissues.

> **MORPHOLOGY.** The lungs are moderately increased in weight, with areas of consolidation that are usually red-brown to red. The cardinal histologic features of pulmonary hemosiderosis are reported as "striking degeneration, shedding and hyperplasia of alveolar epithelial cells, and marked localized alveolar capillary dilatation." There are varying degrees of pulmonary interstitial fibrosis; hemorrhage into the alveolar spaces; and hemosiderosis, both within the alveolar septa and in macrophages lying free within the pulmonary alveoli.

Other Hemorrhagic Syndromes

A number of vasculitides involve small or large vessels within the lung, leading to acute hemorrhage and hemoptysis.[71] These include *Wegener's granulomatosis*, a necrotizing granulomatous inflammation considered in Chapter 11; allergic angiitis and granulomatosis (Churg-Strauss syndrome); and systemic lupus erythematosus and lupus-like reactions induced by drugs.

PULMONARY INVOLVEMENT IN COLLAGEN-VASCULAR DISORDERS

Diffuse interstitial fibrosis occurs classically in progressive systemic sclerosis *(scleroderma)*, discussed in Chapter 6. Less commonly, patchy and transient parenchymal infiltrates are noted in *lupus erythematosus*, and occasionally severe lupus pneumonitis may occur and may be one of the major clinical problems in such patients. In *rheumatoid arthritis*, pulmonary involvement is common and may occur in one of five forms: (1) chronic pleuritis, with or without effusion; (2) diffuse interstitial pneumonitis and fibrosis; (3) intrapulmonary rheumatoid nodules; (4) rheumatoid nodules with pneumoconiosis (Caplan's syndrome); and (5) pulmonary hypertension. Thirty to forty per cent of patients with classic rheumatoid arthritis have abnormalities in pulmonary function. In certain patients, the disorder progresses to end-stage lung disease.

PULMONARY ALVEOLAR PROTEINOSIS

This disease of obscure cause and pathogenesis is characterized radiologically by diffuse pulmonary opacification and histologically by accumulation in the intra-alveolar spaces of a dense granular material that contains abundant lipid and PAS-positive (carbohydrate-containing) material. Patients, for the most part, present with nonspecific respiratory difficulty of insidious onset, cough, and abundant sputum that often contains chunks of gelatinous material. Some have symptoms lasting for years, often with febrile illnesses. Progressive dyspnea, cyanosis, and respiratory insufficiency may occur, but some patients tend to have a benign course, with eventual resolution of the lesions. Pulmonary alveolar proteinosis does not usually progress to chronic fibrosis.

> **MORPHOLOGY.** The disease is characterized by a peculiar, homogeneous, granular precipitate within the alveoli, causing focal-to-confluent consolidation of large areas of the lungs, but without inflammatory reaction (Fig. 15–40). On section, turbid fluid exudes from these areas. As a consequence, there is a marked increase in the size and weight of the lung. The alveolar precipitate is PAS-positive and also contains finely divided lipid. Biochemically, the material is similar to surfactant but fails to show surfactant properties. By electron microscopy, the alveolar contents consist of necrotic alveolar macrophages and type II pneumocytes, amorphous precipitate, with considerable numbers of lamellar osmiophilic bodies morphologically resembling surfactant material. The involved alveoli are often lined with hyperplastic pneumocytes, and

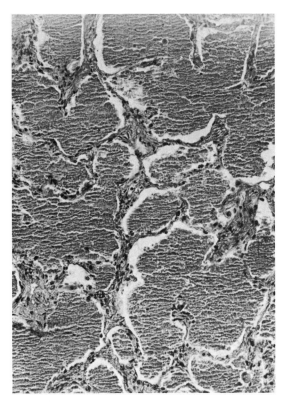

Figure 15–40. Pulmonary alveolar proteinosis, histologic appearance. Alveoli are filled with a dense, amorphous, protein-lipid granular precipitate.

focal areas of necrosis of these cells are seen with the light microscope.

Some patients suffering from this disease may have occupational exposure to irritating dusts (including silica dust) and other chemicals. This disease also occurs in immunosuppressed patients and in association with hematolymphoid malignancies and opportunistic infections. Theories of pathogenesis suggest either excessive production of surfactant-like material by hyperplastic type II epithelial cells or, more likely, a defect in the macrophage clearance of intra-alveolar accumulations of surfactant.

COMPLICATIONS OF THERAPIES

DRUG-INDUCED LUNG DISEASE

Drugs can cause a variety of alterations in respiratory structure and function, including bronchospasm, pulmonary edema, chronic pneumonitis with fibrosis, and hypersensitivity pneumonitis (Table 15–9). For example, cytotoxic drugs used in cancer therapy (e.g., bleomycin) cause pneumonitis and pulmonary fibrosis as a result of direct toxicity of the drug and by stimulating the influx of inflammatory cells into the alveoli. Amiodarone, a drug that controls resistant cardiac arrhythmias, is preferentially concentrated in the lung and causes significant pneumonitis in 5 to 15% of patients receiving it.

RADIATION-INDUCED LUNG DISEASE

Radiation pneumonitis is a well-known complication of therapeutic radiation of pulmonary or other thoracic tumors (esophageal, breast, mediastinal).[72] *Acute radiation pneumonitis* occurs in 1 to 6 months after therapy, manifested by fever, dyspnea, and radiologic infiltrates that correspond to an area of previous radiation. Morphologic changes are those of diffuse alveolar damage, including severe atypia of hyperplastic type II cells. Most patients respond to corticosteroid therapy. Some go on to manifest *chronic radiation pneumonitis*, with interstitial fibrosis in the affected area. Epithelial cell atypia and foam cells within vessel walls are also characteristic of radiation damage. The pathogenesis likely involves direct toxic injury to endothelial and epithelial cells from the radiation, with some blame going to additional injury from chemotherapeutic drugs or infections.

LUNG TRANSPLANTATION

Lung transplantation is the only effective treatment for a number of otherwise terminal lung diseases.[73] These are generally bilateral, diffuse irreversible conditions, including severe idiopathic pulmonary fibrosis, primary pulmonary hypertension, emphysema, and cystic fibrosis. While double-lung and heart-lung transplants are possible, in many cases a single lung transplant is performed, offering sufficient improvement in pulmonary function for each of two recipients from a single (and all too scarce) donor. When chronic infection is present (cystic fibrosis, bronchiectasis), both lungs of the recipient are removed and replaced to minimize potential

Table 15–9. EXAMPLES OF DRUG-INDUCED PULMONARY DISEASE

DRUG	PULMONARY DISEASE
Cytotoxic drugs:	
bleomycin	Pneumonitis and fibrosis
methotrexate	Hypersensitivity pneumonitis
Amiodarone	Pneumonitis and fibrosis
Nitrofurantoin	Hypersensitivity pneumonitis
Aspirin	Bronchospasm
Beta-antagonists	Bronchospasm

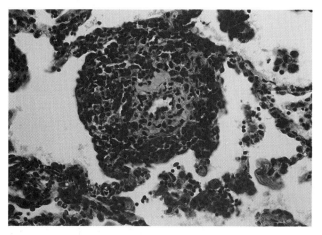

Figure 15–41. Acute rejection of a lung allograft is characterized by perivascular mononuclear cell infiltrates.

infectious complications related to immunosuppression.

MORPHOLOGY. The transplanted lung is subject to two major complications: infection and rejection.[74] Pulmonary infections in lung transplant patients are essentially those of any immunocompromised host, discussed earlier. They include bacterial and viral (especially cytomegalovirus) bronchopneumonias, pneumocystis pneumonia, and fungal infections. Moreover, despite routine immunosuppression postoperatively, rejection of the lung occurs to some degree in all patients. **Acute rejection** occurs during the early weeks to months after surgery, presenting as fever, dyspnea, cough, and radiologic infiltrates. Since these are the exact same clinical features seen with infections, diagnosis often relies on transbronchial biopsy. The morphologic features of acute rejection are primarily those of mononuclear cell infiltrates, either around small vessels (Fig. 15–41) or in the submucosa of airways, or both.[75] Treatment with increased corticosteroids or other immunosuppressive drugs is usually successful in reversing the clinical decline and radiologic infiltrates. **Chronic rejection** is a significant problem in 25 to 50% of all lung transplant patients. It is seen usually 6 to 12 months after surgery, manifested by cough and dyspnea. The major morphologic correlate of chronic rejection is **bronchiolitis obliterans,** the filling of small airways by an inflammatory-fibrous exudate. Evidence of ongoing cellular rejection around vessels is often also seen. While acute cellular airway rejection (the presumed forerunner of later, fibrous obliteration of these airways) is generally responsive to therapy, treatment of established bronchiolitis obliterans has been generally disappointing. Infrequent complications of lung transplantation include accelerated pulmonary arteriosclerosis in the graft and lymphoproliferative disease.

TUMORS

A variety of benign and malignant tumors may arise in the lung,[76,77] but the vast majority (90 to 95%) are bronchogenic carcinomas. About 5% are bronchial carcinoids, and 2 to 5% are mesenchymal and other miscellaneous neoplasms. The term "bronchogenic" refers to the origin of these tumors in the bronchial (and sometimes bronchiolar) epithelium.

BRONCHOGENIC CARCINOMA

In industrialized nations, "public enemy number one" among cancers is bronchogenic carcinoma. It is the most common visceral malignancy in males; it alone accounts for approximately one-third of all cancer deaths in males and over 7% of all deaths in both sexes. The incidence is increasing dramatically in women, and lung cancer has passed breast carcinoma as a cause of cancer death in women. Overall, lung cancer is the most frequent fatal malignancy.

The annual number of deaths from lung cancer in the United States increased from 18,000 in 1950 to an estimated 153,000 in 1994.[78] The age-adjusted death rate from cancer of the lung since 1950 has more than trebled in males, rising from 19.9 to an outstanding 74 per 100,000 population. The death rate in females since 1950 has risen from 4.5 to 31 per 100,000, almost certainly the delayed consequence of increased cigarette smoking among women. Cancer of the lung now accounts for 16% of all cancers in males and 13% in females. In 1994 there will be an estimated 150,000 new cases of lung cancer. Cancer of the lung occurs most often between ages 40 and 70 years, with a peak incidence in the sixth or seventh decade. Only 2% of all cases appear before the age of 40.

ETIOLOGY AND PATHOGENESIS

Role of Tobacco Smoking. The evidence provided by statistical and clinical observations establishing a positive relationship between tobacco smoking and lung cancer is incontrovertible.[79,80] Experimental data have also been pursued, but this approach is limited by species differences.

Statistical evidence is most compelling. In numerous retrospective studies of patients who died of bronchogenic carcinoma compared with control subjects, there was an invariable statistical association between the frequency of lung cancer and (1) the amount of daily smoking, (2) the tendency to inhale, and (3) the duration of the smoking habit. Compared with nonsmokers, average smokers of cigarettes have a tenfold greater risk of developing lung cancer, and heavy smokers (more than 40 cigarettes per day for several years) have at least a

20-fold greater risk. Eighty per cent of lung cancers occur in smokers. Cessation of smoking for 10 years reduces risk to control levels. Epidemiologic studies also show an association between cigarette smoking and the following cancers, in decreasing order of frequency: lip, tongue, floor of the mouth, pharynx, larynx, esophagus, urinary bladder, and pancreas.[80] Cigar and pipe smoking increase risk, although much more modestly than smoking of cigarettes.

Clinical evidence is obtained largely through observing histologic changes in the lining epithelium of the respiratory tract in smokers. A systematic study of the bronchial epithelium of smokers showed atypical and hyperplastic changes in about 10% of smokers, 1 to 2% of those smoking filter-tipped cigarettes, and 15% of patients who died of lung cancer. Nearly all (96.7%) of cigarette smokers showed some atypical cells in the bronchial tree, whereas 0.9% of control subjects had similar cells.[81,82]

Experimental work has comprised mainly attempts to induce cancer in experimental animals with extracts of tobacco smoke.[83] More than 1200 substances have been counted in cigarette smoke, and many of these are potential carcinogens. They include both initiators (polycyclic aromatic hydrocarbons such as benzo[a]pyrene) and promoters, such as phenol derivatives. Radioactive elements may also be found (polonium-210, carbon-14, potassium-40) as well as other contaminants, such as arsenic, nickel, molds, and additives. Protracted exposure of mice to these additives induces skin tumors. However, efforts to produce lung cancer by exposing animals to tobacco smoke have been unsuccessful. The few cancers that have been produced have been bronchioloalveolar carcinomas, a type of human tumor not strongly associated with smoking.

Role of Industrial Hazards. Certain industrial exposures increase the risk of developing lung cancer. All types of *radiation* may be carcinogenic.[84] There was an increased incidence of lung cancer among survivors of the Hiroshima and Nagasaki atomic bomb blasts. *Uranium* is weakly radioactive, but lung cancer rates among nonsmoking uranium miners are four times higher than those of the general population, and among smoking miners they are about ten times higher.

The risk of lung cancer is increased with *asbestos*. Indeed, lung cancer is the most frequent malignancy in persons exposed to asbestos, which has become a universally recognized carcinogen, particularly when coupled with smoking.[59] Asbestos workers who do not smoke have a five times increased risk, and those who smoke have a 50 to 90 times greater risk of developing lung cancer than do nonsmoking control subjects. The latent period before the development of lung cancer is 10 to 30 years. Among asbestos workers, one death

in five is due to bronchogenic carcinoma, one in ten to pleural or peritoneal mesotheliomas (see later in this chapter), and one in ten to gastrointestinal carcinomas.

There is also an increased risk of respiratory cancer among persons who work with *nickel, chromates, coal, mustard gas, arsenic, beryllium,* and *iron* and in newspaper workers, African gold miners, and haloether workers.

Role of Air Pollution. Unquestionably, we all "swim" in a sea of carcinogens, and it is conceivable that atmospheric pollutants may play some role in the increased incidence of bronchogenic carcinoma today. Recent attention has been drawn to the potential problem of "indoor" air pollution, especially by radon.[85,86] Radon is a ubiquitous radioactive gas linked epidemiologically to increased lung cancer in miners exposed to relatively high concentrations. The pathogenetic mechanism is believed to be inhalation and bronchial deposition of radioactive decay products that become attached to environmental aerosols. This has generated concern that low-level indoor exposure (e.g., in homes in areas of high radon in soil) may also lead to increased incidence of lung tumors, with some attributing the bulk of lung cancers in nonsmokers to this insidious carcinogen, also considered in Chapter 9. However, there remains substantial differences of opinion on the significance of the radon risk, with many skeptics awaiting more definitive studies.[87]

Role of Genetic Factors. Occasional familial clustering has suggested a genetic predisposition to lung cancer, as has the variable risk even among very heavy smokers. However, attempts at defining markers of genetic susceptibility have proved elusive.

The molecular basis of cancer has been discussed in Chapter 7. Recent studies have suggested a role for dominant oncogenes and the frequent loss or inactivation of recessive tumor suppressor genes in most lung cancers.[88] The dominant oncogenes include c-*myc* in small cell carcinomas and K-*ras* in adenocarcinomas.[89] The commonly deleted recessive genes include *p53*, the retinoblastoma gene, and an unknown gene or genes on the short arm of chromosome 3.[88]

Role of Scarring. Some lung cancers arise in the vicinity of pulmonary scars and are termed "scar cancers." Histologically, these tumors are usually adenocarcinomas. The scars incriminated are due to old infarcts, metallic foreign bodies, wounds, and granulomatous infections such as tuberculosis. In most cases, the scar is a desmoplastic response to the tumor,[90] but occasionally the scar has preceded the cancer.

Table 15-10. HISTOLOGIC CLASSIFICATION OF BRONCHOGENIC CARCINOMA

Squamous cell (epidermoid) carcinoma
Adenocarcinoma
   Bronchial derived
     (acinar; papillary; solid)
   Bronchioloalveolar
Small cell carcinoma
   Oat cell (lymphocyte-like)
   Intermediate cell (polygonal)
   Combined (usually with squamous)
Large cell carcinoma
   (undifferentiated; giant cell; clear cell)
Combined squamous cell carcinoma and adenocarcinoma

CLASSIFICATION. Numerous histologic classifications of bronchogenic carcinoma have been proposed, but the currently popular ones, based on classifications of the World Health Organization,[91] divide these tumors into four major categories: squamous cell carcinoma, and adenocarcinoma of approximately equal frequency, 25 to 40% each; small cell carcinoma, 20 to 25%; and large cell carcinoma, 10 to 15%. There may be mixtures of histologic patterns, even in the same cancer. Thus, combined types of squamous cell carcinoma and adenocarcinoma or of small cell and squamous cell carcinoma are not infrequent. Another classification in common clinical use is based on response to available therapies: *small cell carcinomas* (high initial response to chemotherapy) versus *non–small cell carcinomas* (less responsive). These histologic categories are summarized in Table 15–10. The strongest relationship to smoking is with squamous cell and small cell carcinoma.

From a histogenetic point of view, it seems most likely that all histologic variants of bronchogenic carcinoma, including small cell carcinoma as well as the bronchial carcinoid, to be described later, are derived from endoderm or a derivative —a view consistent with the frequency of tumors with mixed histologic patterns.[77,92]

MORPHOLOGY. Bronchogenic carcinomas arise most often in and about the hilus of the lung. About three-fourths of the lesions take origin from first-, second-, and third-order bronchi. A small number of primary carcinomas of the lung arise in the periphery of the lung substance from the alveolar septal cells or terminal bronchioles. These are predominantly adenocarcinomas, including those of the bronchioloalveolar type, to be discussed separately.

Carcinoma of the lung begins as an area of in situ cytologic atypia that, over an unknown interval of time, yields a small area of thickening or piling up of bronchial mucosa. With progression, this small focus, usually less than 1 cm² in area, assumes the appearance of an irregular, warty excrescence that elevates or erodes the lining epithelium (Fig. 15–42). The tumor may then follow a variety of paths. It may continue to fungate into the bronchial lumen to produce an intraluminal mass. It can also rapidly penetrate the wall of the bronchus to infiltrate along the peribronchial tissue (see Fig. 15–42) into the adjacent region of the carina or mediastinum. In other instances, the tumor grows along a broad front to produce a cauliflower-like intraparenchymal mass that appears to push lung substance ahead of it. In almost all patterns, the neoplastic tissue is gray-white and firm to hard. Especially when the tumors are bulky, focal areas of hemorrhage or necrosis may appear to produce yellow-white mottling and softening. Sometimes these necrotic foci cavitate.

Extension may occur to the pleural surface and then within the pleural cavity or into the pericardium. Spread to the tracheal, bronchial, and mediastinal nodes can be found in most cases. The frequency of nodal involvement varies slightly with the histologic pattern but averages over 50%.

More distant spread of bronchogenic carcinoma occurs through both lymphatic and hematogenous pathways. These tumors have a distressing habit of spreading widely throughout the body and at an early stage in their evolution. Often the metastasis presents as the first manifestation of the

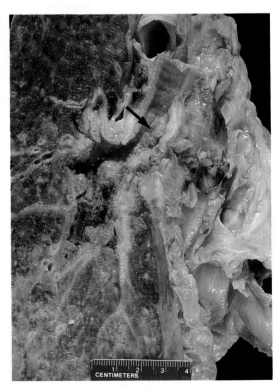

Figure 15-42. Bronchogenic carcinoma arising in mainstem bronchus. Note tumor *(arrow)* in the mucosa and nodular neoplasm invading bronchial wall and parenchyma.

underlying occult bronchogenic lesion. No organ or tissue is spared in the spread of these lesions, but the adrenals, for obscure reasons, are involved in more than half the cases. The liver (30 to 50%), brain (20%), and bone (20%) are additional favored sites of metastases.

Squamous Cell Carcinoma. This type is most commonly found in men and is **closely correlated with a smoking history.** The microscopic features are familiar in the form of production of keratin and intercellular bridges in the well-differentiated forms, but many less well-differentiated squamous cell tumors are encountered that begin to merge with the undifferentiated large cell pattern. This tumor arises in the larger, more central bronchi, tends to spread locally, and metastasizes somewhat later than the other patterns, but its rate of growth in its site of origin is usually more rapid than that of other types. Squamous metaplasia, epithelial dysplasia, and foci of frank carcinoma in situ are sometimes present in bronchial epithelium adjacent to the tumor mass.

Adenocarcinoma. Histologic classifications of adenocarcinomas include at least two forms: (1) the usual bronchial-derived adenocarcinoma; and (2) a somewhat distinctive type termed **bronchioloalveolar carcinoma,** which probably arises from terminal bronchioles or alveolar walls. There may be overlap between these two forms, but the bronchioloalveolar carcinoma has sufficiently distinctive gross, microscopic, and epidemiologic features to be discussed later.

Adenocarcinoma is the most common type of lung cancer in women and nonsmokers. The lesions are usually more peripherally located, tend to be smaller, and vary histologically from well-differentiated tumors with obvious glandular elements to papillary lesions resembling other papillary carcinomas, to solid masses with only occasional mucin-producing glands and cells. About 80% contain mucin. Adenocarcinomas grow more slowly than squamous cell carcinomas. Peripheral adenocarcinomas are sometimes associated with areas of scarring (see above). Adenocarcinomas, including bronchioloalveolar carcinomas, are less frequently associated with a history of smoking than are squamous or small cell carcinomas.

Small Cell Carcinoma. This highly malignant tumor has a distinctive cell type. The epithelial cells are generally small, have little cytoplasm and are round or oval and, occasionally, lymphocyte-like (although they are about twice the size of a lymphocyte). This is the classic **"oat cell"** (Fig. 15–43). Other small cell carcinomas have spindle-shaped or polygonal cells and may be thus classified (spindle or polygonal small cell carcinoma). The cells grow in clusters that exhibit neither glandular nor squamous organization.

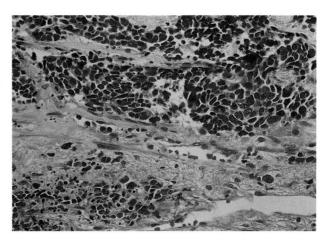

Figure 15–43. Small cell carcinoma, histologic appearance. Note islands of small, round, oval, or spindly, deeply basophilic cells with areas of necrosis in lower left.

Electron microscopic studies show dense-core neurosecretory granules in some of these tumor cells. The granules are similar to those found in the neuroendocrine argentaffin (Kulchitsky's) cells present along the bronchial epithelium, particularly in the fetus and neonate. The occurrence of neurosecretory granules, the ability of some of these tumors to secrete polypeptide hormones, and the presence (ascertained by immunohistochemical stains) of neuroendocrine markers such as neuron-specific enolase and parathormone-like and other hormonally active products suggest derivation of this tumor from neuroendocrine cells of the lining bronchial epithelium.

Small cell carcinomas have a strong relationship to cigarette smoking; only about 1% occur in nonsmokers. Most often hilar or central, they are the most aggressive of lung tumors, metastasize widely, and are virtually incurable by surgical means. They are the most common pattern associated with ectopic hormone production (see later).

Large Cell Carcinoma. This anaplastic carcinoma has larger, more polygonal cells and vesicular nuclei. Large cell carcinomas probably represent those squamous cell carcinomas and adenocarcinomas that are so undifferentiated that they can no longer be recognized. Some of these large cell carcinomas contain intracellular mucin, some exhibit larger numbers of multinucleate cells **(giant cell carcinoma),** some have cleared cells and are termed **clear cell carcinoma,** and some have a distinctly spindly histologic appearance **(spindle cell carcinoma).**

Secondary Pathology. Bronchogenic carcinomas cause related anatomic changes in the lung substance distal to the point of bronchial involvement. **Partial obstruction may cause marked focal em-**

Table 15–11. THE NEW INTERNATIONAL STAGING SYSTEM FOR LUNG CANCER

T1	Tumor ≤3 cm without pleural or mainstem bronchus involvement
T2	Tumor >3 cm or involvement of mainstem bronchus ≥2 cm from carina, or visceral pleura or lobar atelectasis
T3	Tumor with involvement of chest wall (including superior sulcus tumors), diaphragm, mediastinal pleura, pericardium, mainstem bronchus <2 cm from carina, or entire lung atelectasis
T4	Tumor with invasion of mediastinum, heart, great vessels, trachea, esophagus, vertebral body, or carina or with a malignant pleural effusion
N0	No demonstrable metastasis to regional lymph nodes
N1	Ipsilateral hilar or peribronchial nodal involvement
N2	Metastasis to ipsilateral mediastinal or subcarinal lymph nodes
N3	Metastasis to contralateral mediastinal or hilar lymph nodes, ipsilateral or contralateral scalene, or supraclavicular lymph nodes
M0	No (known) distant metastasis
M1	Distant metastasis present

	STAGE GROUPING		
Stage I	T1–2	N0	M0
Stage II	T1–2	N1	M0
Stage IIIa	T1–3	N2	M0
	T3	N0–2	M0
Stage IIIb	Any T	N3	M0
	T4	Any N	M0
Stage IV	Any T	Any N	M1

Modified with permission from Mountain, C.: Lung cancer staging classification. Clin. Chest Med. *14*:43, 1993.

physema; **total obstruction may lead to atelectasis.** The impaired drainage of the airways is a common cause for **severe suppurative or ulcerative bronchitis or bronchiectasis. Pulmonary abscesses** sometimes call attention to a silent carcinoma that has initiated the chronic suppuration. Compression or invasion of the superior vena cava can cause venous congestion, dusky head and arm edema, and, ultimately, circulatory compromise, the **superior vena cava syndrome.** Extension to the pericardial or pleural sacs may cause **pericarditis** (see Chapter 12) or **pleuritis** with significant effusions.

STAGING. A uniform TNM system for staging cancer according to its anatomic extent at the time of diagnosis is extremely useful for many reasons, chiefly for comparing treatment results from different centers. The staging system in current use[93] is presented in Table 15–11.

CLINICAL COURSE. Lung cancer is one of the most insidious and aggressive neoplasms in the whole realm of oncology. In the usual case, it is discovered in the sixth decade of life in patients whose symptoms are of approximately 7 months' duration. The major presenting complaints are cough (75%), weight loss (40%), chest pain (40%), and dyspnea (20%). Increased sputum production is common and often contains diagnostic tumor cells when examined as cytologic specimens (Fig. 15–44A). Similarly, cytologic examination of a fine-needle aspirate (FNA) of a tumor mass can often provide the diagnosis (see Fig. 15–44B). Some of the more common local manifestations of tumor and their pathologic bases are listed in Table 15–12. Not infrequently, the tumor is discovered by its secondary spread during the course of investigation of an apparent primary neoplasm elsewhere.

The outlook is poor for most patients with bronchogenic carcinoma. Despite all efforts at early diagnosis by frequent radioscopic examination of the chest, cytologic examination of sputum, bronchial washings or brushings, and the many improvements in thoracic surgery, radiotherapy, and chemotherapy, the overall 5-year survival rate is on the order of 9%. In many large clinics, not more than 20 to 30% of lung cancer patients have lesions sufficiently localized to permit even an attempt at resection. In general, the adenocarcinoma and squamous cell patterns tend to remain localized longer and have a slightly better prognosis than do the undifferentiated cancers, which usually are advanced lesions by the time they are discovered. The overall 5-year survival rate of males is approximately 10% for squamous cell carcinoma and adenocarcinoma, but only 3% for undifferentiated lesions. Surgical resection for *small cell carcinoma* is so ineffective that the diagnosis essentially precludes surgery. Untreated, the survival time for patients with small cell cancer is 6 to 17 weeks. But this cancer is particularly sensitive to radiation and chemotherapy, and indeed potential cure rates of 15 to 25% for limited disease have been reported in some centers. Unfortunately, most patients have distant metastases on diagnosis. Thus, even with treatment, the mean survival after diagnosis is about 1 year.

Despite this discouraging outlook, it must never be forgotten that many patients have been cured by lobectomy or pneumonectomy, emphasizing the continued need for early diagnosis and adequate prompt therapy. Indeed, in the uncommon but happy instance of *localized solitary tumors less than 4 cm in diameter, surgical resection results in up to 40% 5-year survival for patients with squamous cell carcinoma and 30% for patients with adenocarcinoma and large cell carcinoma.*

Bronchogenic carcinoma can be associated with a number of paraneoplastic syndromes[94] (see Chapter 7), some of which may antedate the development of a gross pulmonary lesion. The hormones or hormone-like factors elaborated include (1) *antidiuretic hormone (ADH)*, inducing hyponatremia due to inappropriate ADH secretion; (2) *adrenocorticotropic hormone (ACTH)*, producing Cushing's syndrome; (3) *parathormone, parathyroid hormone–related peptide, prostaglandin E, and some cytokines*, all implicated in the hypercalcemia often seen with lung cancer; (4) *calcitonin*, causing hypocalcemia; (5) *gonadotropins*, causing gyneco-

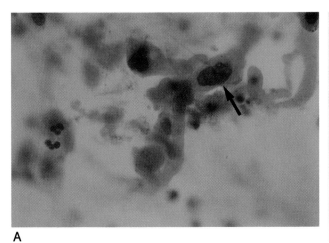

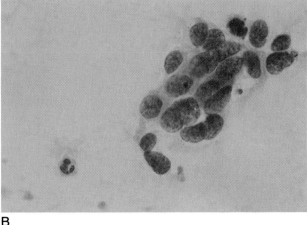

Figure 15–44. Cytologic diagnosis of lung cancer is often possible. *A,* A sputum specimen shows orangophilic, keratinized squamous carcinoma cell with a prominent hyperchromatic nucleus *(arrow). B,* Fine-needle aspirate of an enlarged lymph node shows clusters of tumor cells from a small cell carcinoma, with molding and nuclear atypia characteristic of this tumor (see also Fig. 15–43); note size of tumor cells compared with normal PMN in left lower corner.

mastia; and (6) *serotonin,* associated with the carcinoid syndrome. The incidence of clinically significant syndromes related to these factors ranges from 1 to 10% of all lung cancer patients, although a much higher proportion of patients will show elevated serum levels of these (and other) peptide hormones. Any one of the histologic types of tumors may occasionally produce any one of the hormones, but tumors producing ACTH and ADH are predominantly small cell carcinomas, whereas those producing hypercalcemia are mostly squamous cell tumors. The carcinoid syndrome is associated rarely with small cell carcinoma but is more common with the bronchial carcinoids, described later.

Other systemic manifestations of bronchogenic carcinoma include the *Lambert-Eaton myasthenic*

syndrome, where muscle weakness is caused by autoimmune antibodies (possibly elicited by tumor ionic channels) directed to the neuronal calcium channel;[94] *peripheral neuropathy,* usually purely sensory; dermatologic abnormalities, including *acanthosis nigricans* (see Chapter 26); hematologic abnormalities, such as *leukemoid reactions;* and finally a peculiar abnormality of connective tissue called *hypertrophic pulmonary osteoarthropathy,* associated with clubbing of the fingers.

Apical lung cancers in the superior pulmonary sulcus tend to invade the neural structures around the trachea, including the cervical sympathetic plexus, and produce a group of clinical findings that includes severe pain in the distribution of the ulnar nerve and *Horner's syndrome* (enophthalmos, ptosis, miosis, and anhidrosis) on the same side as the lesion. Such tumors are also referred to as *Pancoast's tumors.*

BRONCHIOLOALVEOLAR CARCINOMA

As the name implies, this form of lung cancer occurs in the pulmonary parenchyma in the terminal bronchioloalveolar regions. It represents, in various series, 1 to 9% of all lung cancers. Changes are very similar histologically to an apparently infectious disease of South African sheep known as *jagziekte.* However, numerous efforts to identify an infectious agent in humans or to transmit the disease to sheep with cell-free extracts of human carcinoma have been unavailing.

Table 15–12. LOCAL EFFECTS OF LUNG TUMOR SPREAD

CLINICAL FEATURE	PATHOLOGIC BASIS
Pneumonia/abscess/lobar collapse	Tumor obstruction of airway
Lipid pneumonia	Tumor obstruction; accumulation of cellular lipid in foamy macrophages
Pleural effusion	Tumor spread into pleura
Hoarseness	Recurrent laryngeal nerve invasion
Dysphagia	Esophageal invasion
Diaphragm paralysis	Phrenic nerve invasion
Rib destruction	Chest wall invasion
Superior vena caval (SVC) syndrome	SVC compression by tumor
Horner's syndrome*	Sympathetic ganglia invasion
Pericarditis/tamponade	Pericardial involvement

* Horner's syndrome = enophthalmos, ptosis, miosis and anhidrosis, unilateral.

MORPHOLOGY. Macroscopically, the tumor almost always occurs in the peripheral portions of the lung either as a single nodule or, more often, as multiple diffuse nodules that sometimes coalesce to produce a pneumonia-like consolidation. The parenchymal nodules have a mucinous, gray translucence when secretion is present and otherwise appear as solid, gray-white areas that can be confused with pneumonia on casual inspection.

Histologically, the tumor is characterized by distinctive, tall, columnar-to-cuboidal epithelial cells that line up along alveolar septa and project into the alveolar spaces in numerous branching papillary formations (Fig. 15–45). Tumor cells often contain abundant mucinous secretions. The degree of anaplasia is quite variable, but most tumors are well differentiated and tend to preserve the native septal wall architecture. Ultrastructurally, bronchioloalveolar carcinomas are a heterogeneous group, consisting of mucin-secreting bronchiolar cells, Clara cells, or, rarely, type II pneumocytes.

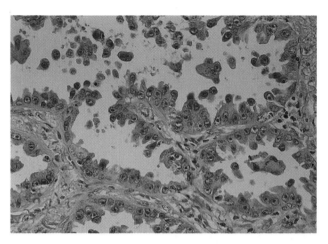

Figure 15–45. Terminal bronchioloalveolar carcinoma with characteristic tall, columnar cell papillary growth. Note loose tumor cells in alveoli, which may account for "aerogenous" spread of tumor often observed.

Clinically, these tumors occur in patients of all ages from the third decade to the advanced years of life. They are equally distributed among males and females. The symptoms, which usually appear late, are much like those of bronchogenic carcinoma, with cough, hemoptysis, and pain the major presenting findings. Because the tumor does not involve major bronchi, atelectasis and emphysema are infrequent. Occasionally, they may produce a picture of diffuse interstitial pneumonitis. Solitary lesions are surgically resectable, resulting in a 50 to 75% 5-year survival rate, but the overall survival rate is about 25%. Metastases are not widely disseminated or large, nor do they occur early. Eventually, however, they appear in up to 45% of cases.

NEUROENDOCRINE TUMORS

This designation describes pulmonary neoplasms that share morphologic and biochemical features with cells of the "dispersed neuroendocrine cell system (see Chapter 17)."[95] The normal lung contains neuroendocrine cells within the epithelium as single cells or as clusters, the neuroepithelial bodies.[1,95] Neoplasms of neuroendocrine cells in the lung include benign *tumorlets*, small, inconsequential hyperplastic neuroendocrine cells seen in areas of scarring or chronic inflammation; *carcinoids;* and the (already discussed) highly aggressive small cell carcinoma of the lung.

Bronchial Carcinoid

Bronchial carcinoids represent 1 to 5% of all lung tumors. They make up more than 90% of a group of bronchial tumors formerly classified as "bronchial adenoma" but now known to be often locally invasive or, occasionally, capable of metastasis. The

remaining 10% of the group includes *adenoid cystic carcinoma* and *mucoepidermoid carcinoma*—tumors with histologic patterns reminiscent of similar tumors in salivary glands (see Chapter 16). Most patients with carcinoid tumors are younger than 40 years of age, and the incidence is equal for both sexes. There is no known relationship to cigarette smoking or other environmental factors. Bronchial carcinoids show the neuroendocrine differentiation of the Kulchitsky's cells of bronchial mucosa and resemble intestinal carcinoids, described in detail in Chapter 17. They contain dense-core neurosecretory granules in their cytoplasm, secrete hormonally active polypeptides, and occasionally occur as part of multiple endocrine neoplasia.

MORPHOLOGY. On gross examination, the tumors grow as finger-like or spherical polypoid masses that commonly project into the lumen of the bronchus and are usually covered by an intact mucosa (Fig. 15–46A). They rarely exceed 3 to 4 cm in diameter. Most are confined to the main-stem bronchi. Others, however, produce little intraluminal mass but instead penetrate the bronchial wall to fan out in the peribronchial tissue, producing the so-called "collar-button" lesion.

Histologically, the tumor is composed of nests, cords, and masses of cells separated by a delicate fibrous stroma. In common with the lesions of the gastrointestinal tract, the individual cells are quite regular and have uniform round nuclei and infrequent mitoses (Fig. 15–46B). Occasional carcinoid tumors display variation in the size and shape of cells and nuclei and, along with this pleomorphism, tend to demonstrate a more aggressive and more invasive behavior. On electron microscopy the cells exhibit the dense-core granules characteristic of other neuroendocrine tumors and, by immunochemistry, are found to contain serotonin, neuron-specific enolase, bombesin, calcitonin, or other peptides.

The clinical manifestations of bronchial carcinoids emanate from their intraluminal growth, their capacity to metastasize, and the ability of some of the lesions to elaborate vasoactive amines. Persistent cough, hemoptysis, impairment of drainage or respiratory passages with secondary infections, bronchiectasis, emphysema, and atelectasis all are by-products of the intraluminal growth of these lesions.

Many carcinoids show infiltration or spread to local lymph nodes at the time of resection with apparently little ill effect on prognosis. Most interesting, albeit rare, are those functioning lesions of the argentaffinoma pattern capable of producing the classic carcinoid syndrome, that is, intermittent attacks of diarrhea, flushing, and cyanosis. Overall, most bronchial carcinoids do not have secretory activity and do not metastasize to distant sites but follow a relatively benign course for long periods and are therefore amenable to resection. The reported 5- to 10-year survival rates for typical carcinoids are 50 to 95%. A minority (≤10%) of tumors show cytologic atypia, necrosis, and aggressive behavior (50% recurrence or metastasis after 2 years) and are designated *atypical carcinoids*.

MISCELLANEOUS TUMORS

Lesions of the complex category of benign and malignant mesenchymal tumors, such as fibroma, fibrosarcoma, leiomyoma, leiomyosarcoma, lipoma, hemangioma, hemangiopericytoma, and chon-

droma, may occur but are rare. Benign and malignant lymphoreticular tumors and tumor-like conditions, similar to those described in other organs, may also affect the lung, either as isolated lesions or, more commonly, as part of a generalized disorder. These include non-Hodgkin's and Hodgkin's lymphoma, lymphomatoid granulomatosis, pseudolymphoma, and plasma cell granuloma.

A lung *hamartoma* is a relatively common lesion usually discovered as an incidental, rounded focus of radiopacity on a routine chest film, called a "coin lesion" (solitary nodule) by the roentgenologist. Any new solitary nodule in the lung requires clinical evaluation to determine whether a benign or malignant neoplasm has arisen. Pulmonary hamartomas are rarely over 3 to 4 cm in diameter and are composed mostly of mature (often calcified) cartilage. Occasionally, the cartilage contains cystic or cleft-like spaces, and these may be lined by characteristic respiratory epithelium. At other times, there are admixtures of fibrous tissue, fat, and blood vessels. Recall that hamartomas are overgrowths of mature, normal tissues, in abnormal proportions (see Chapter 7).

Tumors in the mediastinum either may arise in mediastinal structures or may be metastatic from the lung or other organs. They may also invade or compress the lungs. Table 15–13 lists the most common tumors in the various compartments of the mediastinum. Specific tumor types are discussed in appropriate sections of this book.

METASTATIC TUMORS

The lung is frequently the site of metastatic neoplasms. Both carcinomas and sarcomas arising anywhere in the body may spread to the lungs via the

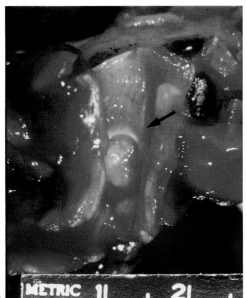

A

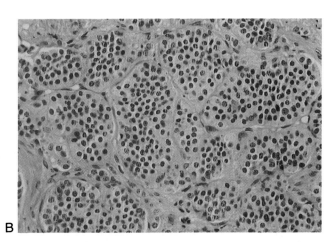

B

Figure 15–46. *A,* Bronchial carcinoid growing as a spherical, pale mass *(arrow)* protruding into lumen of bronchus. *B,* Histologic appearance of bronchial carcinoid, demonstrating small, rounded, uniform cells.

Table 15–13. MEDIASTINAL TUMORS AND
OTHER MASSES

SUPERIOR MEDIASTINUM	POSTERIOR MEDIASTINUM
Lymphoma	Neurogenic tumors
Thymoma	(schwannoma; neurofibroma)
Thyroid lesions	Lymphoma
Metastatic carcinoma	Gastroenteric hernia
Parathyroid tumors	
	MIDDLE MEDIASTINUM
ANTERIOR MEDIASTINUM	Bronchogenic cyst
Thymoma	Pericardial cyst
Teratoma	Lymphoma
Lymphoma	
Thyroid lesions	
Parathyroid tumors	

blood or lymphatics or by direct continuity.
Growth of contiguous tumors into the lungs occurs
most often with esophageal carcinomas and mediastinal lymphomas.

MORPHOLOGY. The pattern of metastatic growth
within the lungs is quite variable. In the usual case,
multiple discrete nodules are scattered throughout
all lobes (Fig. 15–47). These discrete lesions tend to
occur in the periphery of the lung parenchyma
rather than in the central locations of the primary
bronchogenic carcinoma.

As a second macroscopic variant, metastatic

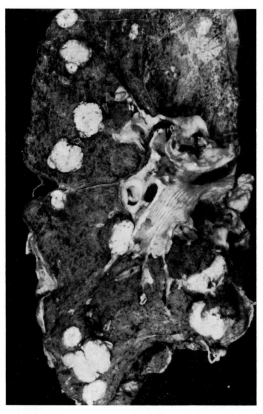

**Figure 15–47. Numerous metastases in lung from a breast
carcinoma in a 56-year-old woman.**

growth may confine themselves to peribronchiolar
and perivascular tissue spaces, presumably when
the tumor has extended to the lung through the
lymphatics. Here the lung septa and connective
tissue are diffusely infiltrated with the gray-white
tumor. The subpleural lymphatics may be outlined
by the contained tumor, producing a gross appearance referred to as *lymphangitis carcinoma-
tosa.* Least commonly, the metastatic tumor is
totally inapparent on gross examination and
becomes evident only on histologic section as
a diffuse intralymphatic dissemination dispersed
throughout the peribronchial and perivascular
channels. In certain instances, microscopic tumor
emboli fill the small pulmonary vessels and may result in life-threatening pulmonary hypertension.

PLEURA

Pathologic involvement of the pleura is, with rare
exceptions, a secondary complication of some underlying disease. Secondary infections and pleural
adhesions are particularly common findings at autopsy. Occasionally, the secondary pleural disease
assumes a dominant role in the clinical problem, as
occurs in bacterial pneumonia with the development of empyema. Important primary disorders include (1) primary intrapleural bacterial infections
that imply seeding of this space as an isolated focus
in the course of a transient bacteremia, and (2) a
primary neoplasm of the pleura—mesothelioma
(see later).

Pleural effusion is a common manifestation of
both primary and secondary pleural involvements.
Normally, no more than 15 ml of serous, relatively
acellular, clear fluid lubricates the pleural surface.
Increased accumulation of pleural fluid occurs in
five settings: (1) increased hydrostatic pressure, as
in right-sided congestive heart failure; (2) increased vascular permeability, as in pneumonia; (3)
decreased oncotic pressure, as in nephrotic syndrome; (4) increased intrapleural negative pressure, as in atelectasis; and (5) decreased lymphatic
drainage, as in mediastinal carcinomatosis. The
character of the pleural effusion can be divided,
for convenience, into inflammatory or noninflammatory, as summarized in Table 15–14.

INFLAMMATORY PLEURAL EFFUSIONS

Serous, *serofibrinous,* and fibrinous *pleuritis* all are
caused by essentially the same processes. Fibrinous
exudations generally reflect a later and more severe exudative reaction that, in an earlier developmental phase, might have presented as a serous or
serofibrinous exudate.

Table 15-14. PLEURAL SPACE FLUID ACCUMULATIONS

CONDITION	TYPE OF FLUID	COMMON ASSOCIATIONS
Inflammatory		
Serofibrinous pleuritis	Serofibrinous exudate	Inflammation in adjacent lung Collagen-vascular disease
Suppurative pleuritis (empyema)	Pus	Suppurative infection in adjacent lung
Hemorrhagic pleuritis	Bloody exudate	Tumor
Noninflammatory		
Hydrothorax	Transudate	Congestive heart failure (right-sided)
Hemothorax	Blood	Ruptured aortic aneurysm, trauma
Chylothorax	Chyle (lymph)	Tumor obstruction of normal lymphatics

The common causes of pleuritis are inflammatory diseases within the lungs, such as tuberculosis, pneumonia, lung infarcts, lung abscess, and bronchiectasis. Rheumatoid arthritis, disseminated lupus erythematosus, uremia, diffuse systemic infections, other systemic disorders, and metastatic involvement of the pleura can also cause serous or serofibrinous pleuritis. Radiation used in therapy for tumors in the lung or mediastinum often causes a serofibrinous pleuritis. In most instances, the serofibrinous reaction is only minimal, and the fluid exudate is resorbed with either resolution or organization of the fibrinous component. Accumulation of large amounts of fluid can sufficiently encroach on lung space to give rise to respiratory distress.

A purulent pleural exudate *(empyema)* usually results from bacterial or mycotic seeding of the pleural space. Most commonly, this occurs by contiguous spread of organisms from intrapulmonary infection, but occasionally it occurs through lymphatic or hematogenous dissemination from a more distant source. Rarely, infections below the diaphragm, such as the subdiaphragmatic or liver abscess, may extend by continuity through the diaphragm into the pleural spaces, more often on the right side.

Empyema is characterized by yellow-green, creamy pus composed of masses of neutrophils admixed with other leukocytes. Although it may be difficult to visualize microorganisms on smears of the exudate, it should be possible to demonstrate them by culture. Although empyema may accumulate in large volumes (up to 500 to 1000 ml), usually the volume is small. Empyema may resolve, but this fortunate outcome is less common than organization of the exudate, with the formation of dense, tough fibrous adhesions that frequently obliterate the pleural space or envelop the lungs; either can seriously embarrass pulmonary expansion.

True *hemorrhagic pleuritis* manifested by sanguineous inflammatory exudates is infrequent and is found in hemorrhagic diatheses, rickettsial diseases, and neoplastic involvement of the pleural cavity. The sanguineous exudate must be differentiated from hemothorax (see later). When hemorrhagic pleuritis is encountered, careful search should be made for the presence of exfoliated tumor cells.

NONINFLAMMATORY PLEURAL EFFUSIONS

Noninflammatory collections of serous fluid within the pleural cavities are called *hydrothorax.* The fluid is clear and straw colored. Hydrothorax may be unilateral or bilateral, depending on the underlying cause. The most common cause of hydrothorax is cardiac failure, and for this reason it is usually accompanied by pulmonary congestion and edema. In cardiac failure, hydrothorax is usually, but not invariably, bilateral. Transudates may collect in any other systemic disease associated with generalized edema and are therefore found in renal failure and cirrhosis of the liver. Isolated right-sided hydrothorax occurs in Meig's syndrome, an unusual combination of hydrothorax, ascites, and ovarian fibroma (see Chapter 23).

In most instances, hydrothorax is not loculated, but, in the presence of pre-existent pleural adhesions, local collections may be found walled off by bridging fibrous tissue. Except for these localized collections, the fluid usually collects basally, when the patient is in an upright position, and causes compression and atelectasis of the regions of the lung surrounded by fluid. If the underlying cause is alleviated, hydrothorax may be resorbed, usually leaving behind no permanent alterations. Relief of respiratory distress is accomplished by the withdrawal of large pleural transudates.

The escape of blood into the pleural cavity is known as *hemothorax.* It is almost invariably a fatal complication of a ruptured aortic aneurysm or vascular trauma. Pure hemothorax is readily identifiable by the large clots that accompany the fluid component of the blood. Because this calamity often leads to death within minutes to hours, it is uncommon to find any inflammatory response within the pleural cavity. Rarely, nonfatal leakage of smaller amounts may provide a stimulus to organization and the development of pleural adhesions.

Chylothorax is an accumulation of milky fluid, usually of lymphatic origin, in the pleural cavity. Chyle is milky-white because it contains finely emulsified fats. When it is allowed to stand, a creamy, fatty, supernatant layer separates. True chyle should by differentiated from turbid serous fluid, which does not contain fat and does not separate into an overlying layer of high fat content. Chylothorax may be bilateral but is more often confined to the left side. The volume of fluid is variable but rarely assumes the massive proportions of hydrothorax.

Chylothorax is most often caused by thoracic duct trauma or obstruction that secondarily causes rupture of major lymphatic ducts. This is encountered in malignant conditions arising within the thoracic cavity that cause obstruction of the major lymphatic ducts. More distant cancers may metastasize via the lymphatics and grow within the right lymphatic or thoracic duct to produce obstruction.

PNEUMOTHORAX

Pneumothorax refers to air or gas in the pleural cavities and may be spontaneous, traumatic, or therapeutic. Spontaneous pneumothorax may complicate any form of pulmonary disease that causes rupture of an alveolus. An abscess cavity that communicates either directly with the pleural space or with the lung interstitial tissue may also lead to the escape of air. In the latter circumstance, the air may dissect through the lung substance or back through the mediastinum (interstitial emphysema), eventually entering the pleural cavity. Pneumothorax is most commonly associated with emphysema, asthma, and tuberculosis. Traumatic pneumothorax is usually caused by some perforating injury to the chest wall, but sometimes the trauma pierces the lung and thus provides two avenues for the accumulation of air within the pleural spaces. Resorption of the pleural space air occurs slowly in spontaneous and traumatic pneumothorax, provided the original communication seals itself. Therapeutic pneumothorax was once a commonly practiced method of deflating the lung to favor the healing of tuberculous lesions.

Of the various forms of pneumothorax, the one that attracts greatest clinical attention is so-called *spontaneous idiopathic pneumothorax*. This entity is encountered in relatively young people; appears to be due to rupture of small, peripheral, usually apical subpleural blebs; and usually subsides spontaneously as the air is resorbed. Recurrent attacks are common and may be quite disabling.

Pneumothorax can be identified anatomically only by careful opening of the thoracic cavity under water to detect the escape of gas or air bubbles. Pneumothorax may have as much clinical significance as a fluid collection in the lungs, as it also causes compression, collapse, and atelectasis of the lung, and may be responsible for marked respiratory distress. Occasionally, the lung collapse is marked. When the defect acts as a flap valve and permits the entrance of air during inspiration but fails to permit its escape during expiration, it effectively acts as a pump that creates the progressively increasing pressures of *tension pneumothorax*, which may be sufficient to compress the vital mediastinal structures and the contralateral lung.

PLEURAL TUMORS

The pleura may be involved in primary or secondary tumors. Secondary metastatic involvement is far more common than are primary tumors. The most frequent metastatic malignancies arise from primary neoplasms of the lung and breast. Advanced mammary carcinomas frequently penetrate the thoracic wall directly to involve the parietal and then the visceral pleura. They may also reach these cavities through the lymphatics and, more rarely, the blood. In addition to these cancers, malignancy from any organ of the body may spread to the pleural spaces. Ovarian carcinomas, for example, tend to cause widespread implants in both the abdominal and the thoracic cavities. In most metastatic involvements, a serous or serosanguineous effusion follows that may contain desquamated neoplastic cells. For this reason, careful cytologic examination of the sediment is of considerable diagnostic value (Fig. 15–48).

Pleural Fibroma ("Benign Mesothelioma")

This benign pleural neoplasm, often called "benign mesothelioma," is a localized growth that is often attached to the pleural surface by a pedicle.[96] The tumor may be small (1 to 2 cm in diameter) or may reach an enormous size, but it always remains confined to the surface of the lung. These tumors do not usually produce a pleural effusion. Grossly, they consist of dense fibrous tissue with occasional cysts filled with viscid fluid; microscopically, the tumors show whorls of reticulin and collagen fibers among which are interspersed spindle cells resembling fibroblasts. For this reason, these mesotheliomas are also termed "fibromas." The benign pleural fibroma has no relationship to asbestos exposure.

Malignant Mesothelioma

Malignant mesotheliomas in the thorax arise from either the visceral or the parietal pleura.[97,98] Al-

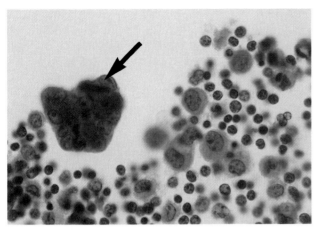

Figure 15–48. Metastatic adenocarcinoma (from breast primary) seen in cytologic examination of pleural effusion. Note the gland-like cluster of tumor cells and background of reactive mesothelial cells and leukocytes. (Courtesy of Dr. Edmund Cibas, Brigham and Women's Hospital; reproduced with permission from Atkinson, B.F. (ed.): Atlas of Diagnostic Cytopathology. Philadelphia, W.B. Saunders Co., 1992, p. 224.)

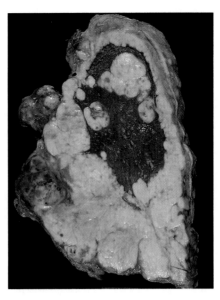

Figure 15–49. Malignant mesothelioma. Note thick, firm, white, pleural tumor tissue that ensheathes this bisected lung.

though uncommon, they have assumed great importance in the past few years because of their increased incidence among persons with heavy exposure to asbestos (see the section on pneumoconioses earlier in this chapter). In coastal areas with shipping industries in the United States and Great Britain, and in Canadian and South African mining areas, up to 90% of reported mesotheliomas are asbestos related. The lifetime risk of developing mesothelioma in heavily exposed individuals is as high as 7 to 10%. There is a long period of 25 to 45 years for the development of asbestos-related mesothelioma, and there seems to be no increased risk of mesothelioma in asbestos workers who smoke. *This is in contrast to the risk of asbestos-related bronchogenic carcinoma, already high, and is markedly magnified by smoking. Thus, for asbestos workers (particularly those who are also smokers), the risk of dying of lung carcinoma far exceeds that of developing mesothelioma.*

Asbestos bodies (see Fig. 15–31) are found in increased numbers in the lungs of patients with mesothelioma, and mesotheliomas can be induced readily in experimental animals by intrapleural injections of asbestos.[99] Another marker of *asbestos exposure,* the *asbestos plaque,* has been previously discussed. There is little doubt about the carcinogenicity of asbestos; the mechanisms of cancer induction are discussed in Chapter 7.

MORPHOLOGY. Malignant mesothelioma is a diffuse lesion that spreads widely in the pleural space and is usually associated with extensive pleural effusion and direct invasion of thoracic structures. The affected lung is ensheathed by a thick layer of soft, gelatinous, grayish-pink tumor tissue (Fig. 15–49).

Microscopically, malignant mesotheliomas consist of a mixture of two types of cells, either one of which might predominate in an individual case. Mesothelial cells have the potential to develop as either mesenchymal stromal cells or epithelium-like lining cells. The latter is the usual form of the mesothelium, an epithelium that lines the serous cavities of the body. The mesenchymal type of mesothelioma appears as a spindle cell sarcoma, resembling fibrosarcoma **(sarcomatoid type),** whereas the papillary type consists of cuboidal, columnar, or flattened cells forming a tubular and papillary structure **(epithelial type),** resembling adenocarcinoma (Fig. 15–50). Indeed, epithelial mesothelioma may at times be difficult to differen-

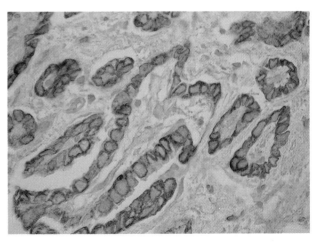

Figure 15–50. Malignant mesothelioma, epithelial type. Tumor cells are immunoperoxidase positive for keratin, as shown (brown), but would be CEA negative.

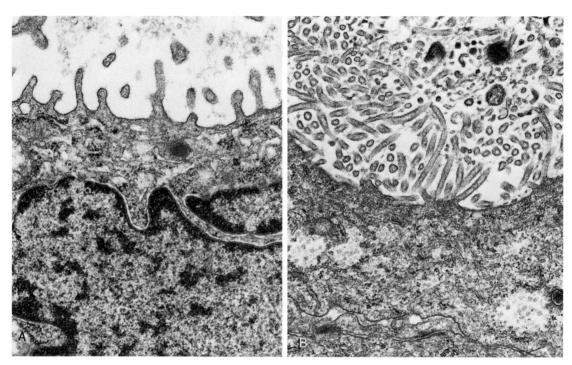

Figure 15-51. Ultrastructural features of pulmonary adenocarcinoma *(A)*, characterized by short, plump microvilli, contrasted with those of mesothelioma *(B)*, in which microvilli are numerous, long, and slender. (Courtesy of Dr. Noel Weidner, University of California, San Francisco, School of Medicine.)

tiate grossly and histologically from pulmonary adenocarcinoma. Special features that favor mesothelioma include the following: (1) positive staining for acid mucopolysaccharide, which is inhibited by previous digestion by hyaluronidase; (2) lack of staining for carcinoembryonic antigen (CEA) or the Leu-M1 antigen, two markers generally expressed by adenocarcinoma;[100] (3) strong staining for keratin proteins, with accentuation of perinuclear rather than peripheral staining (see Fig. 15-50); and, (4) on electron microscopy, the presence of lung microvilli and abundant tonofilaments, but absent microvillous rootlets and lamellar bodies (Fig. 15-51). The **mixed type** of mesothelioma contains both epithelial and sarcomatoid patterns.

The presenting complaints are chest pain, dyspnea, and, as noted, recurrent pleural effusions. Concurrent pulmonary asbestosis (fibrosis) is present in only 20% of patients with pleural mesothelioma. Fifty per cent of those with pleural disease die within 12 months of diagnosis, and very few survive longer than 2 years. The lung is invaded directly, and there is often metastatic spread to the hilar lymph nodes and, eventually, to the liver and other distant organs.

Mesotheliomas also arise in the peritoneum, pericardium, tunica vaginalis, and genital tract (benign adenomatoid tumor; see Chapter 22). *Peritoneal mesotheliomas* are particularly related to very heavy asbestos exposure; 50% of such patients also have pulmonary fibrosis. Although in about 50% of cases the disease remains confined to the abdominal cavity, intestinal involvement frequently leads to death from intestinal obstruction or inanition.

1. Wang, N.-S.: Anatomy. *In* Dail, D.H., and Hammar, S.P. (eds.): Pulmonary Pathology. New York, Springer-Verlag, 1993.
2. Murray, J.F.: The Normal Lung, 2nd ed. Philadelphia, W.B. Saunders Co., 1986.
3. Hamm, H., et al.: The surfactant system of the adult lung: Physiology and clinical perspectives. Clin. Invest. *70:*637, 1992.
4. Dail, D.H., and Hammar, S.P. (eds.): Pulmonary Pathology, 2nd ed. New York, Springer-Verlag, 1993.
5. Murray, J.F., and Nadel, J.A. (eds.): Textbook of Respiratory Medicine, 2nd ed. Philadelphia, W.B. Saunders Co., 1994.
6. Askin, F.B.: Pulmonary disorders in the neonate infant and child. *In* Thurlbeck, W.M. (ed.): Pathology of the Lung. New York, Thieme Med. Pubs., 1988, p. 115.
7. Rinaldo, J., and Christman, J.: Mechanisms and mediators of the adult respiratory distress syndrome. Clin. Chest Med. *11:*621, 1990.
8. Roissaint, R., et al.: Inhaled nitric oxide for the adult respiratory distress syndrome. N. Engl. J. Med. *328:*399, 1993.
9. Loscalzo, J.: Endothelial dysfunction in pulmonary hypertension. N. Engl. J. Med. *327:*117, 1992.
10. Burke, A., et al.: The pathology of primary pulmonary hypertension. Mod. Pathol. *4:*269, 1991.
11. Pietra, G.G., et al.: Histopathology of primary pulmonary hypertension: A qualitative and quantitative study of pulmonary blood vessels from 58 patients in the National Heart, Lung, and Blood Institute, Primary Pulmonary Hypertension Registry. Circulation *80:*1198, 1989.
12. Fuster, V., et al.: Primary pulmonary hypertension: Nat-

ural history and the importance of thrombus. Circulation 70:580, 1984.

13. Snider, G.L., et al.: The definition of emphysema: Report of the National Heart, Lung, and Blood Institute, Division of Lung Diseases Workshop. Am. Rev. Respir. Dis. 132:182, 1985.

14. Thurlbeck, W.M.: Chronic Airflow Obstruction in Lung Disease. Philadelphia, W.B. Saunders Co., 1976.

15. Laurell, C.B., and Eriksson, S.: The electrophoretic alpha₁-antitrypsin deficiency. Scand. J. Clin. Lab. Invest. 15:132, 1963.

16. Gross, P., et al.: Enzymatically produced pulmonary emphysema: A preliminary report. J. Occup. Med. 6:481, 1964.

17. Hubbard, R.C., and Crystal, R.G.: Antiproteases. In Crystal, R.G., et al. (eds.): The Lung: Scientific Foundations. New York, Raven Press, 1991, p. 1775.

18. Senior, R.M., et al.: The induction of pulmonary emphysema with human leukocyte elastase. Am. Rev. Respir. Dis. 116:469, 1977.

19. Campbell, E.J., and Senior, R.M.: Emphysema. In Fishman, A.P. (ed.): Update: Pulmonary Diseases and Disorders. New York, McGraw-Hill, 1992, p. 37.

20. Reid, L.: Chronic obstructive pulmonary diseases. In Fishman, A.P. (ed.): Pulmonary Diseases and Disorders, 2nd ed. New York, McGraw-Hill, 1988, p. 1247.

21. Wright, J.L., et al.: Diseases of the small airways. Am. Rev. Respir. Dis. 146:240, 1992.

22. Thurlbeck, W.M.: Pathology of chronic airflow obstruction. In Cherniack, N.S. (ed.): Chronic Obstructive Pulmonary Disease. Philadelphia, W.B. Saunders Co., 1991, p. 3.

23. Hogg, J.C., et al.: Site and nature of airway obstruction in chronic obstructive lung disease. N. Engl. J. Med. 278:1355, 1968.

24. Cosio, M.G., et al.: The relations between structural changes in small airways and pulmonary function tests. N. Engl. J. Med. 298:1277, 1979.

25. Barnes, P.J., et al. (ed.): Asthma: Basic Mechanisms and Clinical Management. London, Academic Press, 1992.

26. Markey, J.: Immunopharmacology of asthma. Immunol. Today 14:3179, 1993.

27. Litchfield, T., and Lee, T.: Asthma: Cells and cytokines. J. Asthma 29:181, 1992.

28. Gordon, J.R., and Galli, S.: Mast cells as a source of both preformed and immunologically inducible TNF-alpha/cachectin. Nature 346:274, 1990.

29. Galli, S.: New concepts about the mast cell. N. Engl. J. Med. 328:257, 1993.

30. Frigas, E., et al.: Cytotoxic effects of the guinea pig eosinophil major basic protein on tracheal epithelium. Lab. Invest. 42:35, 1980.

31. Gundel, R., et al.: Human eosinophil major basic protein induces airway constriction and airway hyperresponsiveness in primates. J. Clin. Invest. 87:1470, 1991.

32. Busse, W., et al.: The relationship of viral respiratory infections and asthma. Chest 101:385, 1992.

33. Davis, A.L., and Salzman, S.H.: Bronchiectasis. In Cherniack, N.S. (ed.): Chronic Obstructive Pulmonary Disease. Philadelphia, W.B. Saunders Co., 1991, p. 316.

34. Lieberman, J.: The immotile cilia syndrome. In Lieberman, J. (ed.): Inherited Diseases of the Lung. Philadelphia, W.B. Saunders Co., 1988, p. 31.

35. Pennington, J.E.: Respiratory Infections: Diagnosis and Management. New York, Raven Press, 1988.

36. Miller, R.: Mycoplasma, Chlamydia, and Coxiella infections of the respiratory tract. In Thurlbeck, W. (ed.): Pathology of the Lung. New York, Thieme Med. Pubs., 1988, p. 181.

37. Depaseo, W.: Aspiration pneumonia. Clin. Chest Med. 12:269, 1991.

38. Barnes, P.F., et al.: Tuberculosis in patients with human immunodeficiency virus infection. N. Engl. J. Med. 324:1644, 1991.

39. Snider, D.E., and Roper, W.: The new tuberculosis. N. Engl. J. Med. 326:703, 1992.

40. Dannenberg, A.: Delayed-type hypersensitivity and cell-mediated immunity in the pathogenesis of tuberculosis. Immunol. Today 12:228, 1991.

41. Rosenow, E.C.: Diffuse pulmonary infiltrates in the immunocompromised host. Clin. Chest Med. 11:55, 1990.

42. Ioachim, H.L.: Pathology of AIDS. Philadelphia, J.B. Lippincott Co., 1989.

43. Colby, T.V., and Carrington, C.B.: Infiltrative lung disease. In Thurlbeck, W. (ed.): Pathology of the Lung. New York, Thieme Med. Pubs., 1988, p. 425.

44. Sheppard, M.N., and Harrison, N.: Lung injury, inflammatory mediators, and fibroblast activation in fibrosing alveolitis. Thorax 47:1064, 1992.

45. Crouch, E.: Pathobiology of pulmonary fibrosis. Am. J. Physiol. 259:L159, 1990.

46. Ozaki, T., et al.: Neutrophil chemotactic factors in the respiratory tract of patients with chronic airway disease or idiopathic pulmonary fibrosis. Am. Rev. Respir. Dis. 145:85, 1992.

47. Lynch, J.P.I., et al.: Neutrophilic alveolitis in idiopathic pulmonary fibrosis: The role of interleukin-8. Am. Rev. Respir. Dis. 145:1433, 1992.

48. Martin, T.R., et al.: Relative contribution of leukotriene B₄ to the neutrophil chemotactic activity produced by the resident human alveolar macrophage. J. Clin. Invest. 80:1114, 1987.

49. Dockery, D.W., et al: An association between air pollution and mortality in six U.S. cities. N. Engl. J. Med. 329:1753, 1993.

50. Lapp, N., and Castranova, V.: How silicosis and coal workers' pneumoconiosis develop: A cellular assessment. Occup. Med. 8:35, 1993.

51. Weissner, J., et al.: The effect of chemical modification of quartz surfaces on particulate-induced pulmonary inflammation and fibrosis in the mouse. Am. Rev. Respir. Dis. 141:111, 1990.

52. Rom, W., et al.: Cellular and molecular basis of the asbestos-related diseases. Am. Rev. Respir. Dis. 143:408, 1991.

53. Green, F.: Coal-workers' pneumoconiosis and pneumoconiosis due to other carbonaceous dusts. In Churg, A., and Green, F. (eds.): Pathology of Occupational Lung Disease. New York, Igaku-Shoin Medical Publishers, Inc., 1988, p. 89.

54. Godleski, J.: The pneumoconioses: Silicosis and silicatosis. In Saldana, M. (ed.): Pathology of Pulmonary Disease. Philadelphia, J.B. Lippincott (in press).

55. Piguet, P., et al.: Requirement of tumor necrosis factor for development of silica-induced pulmonary fibrosis. Nature 344:245, 1990.

56. Pairon, J., et al.: Silica and lung cancer: A controversial issue. Eur. Respir. J. 4:730, 1991.

57. Hnizdo, E., and Slujis-Cremer, G.: Silica exposure, silicosis, and lung cancer: A mortality study of South African gold miners. Br. J. Ind. Med. 48:53, 1991.

58. Mossman, B., and Gee, J.: Asbestos-related diseases. N. Engl. J. Med. 320:1721, 1989.

59. Hammond, E., et al.: Asbestos exposure, cigarette smoking, and death rates. Ann. N.Y. Acad. Sci. 330:473, 1979.

60. Saltini, C., et al.: Maintenance of alveolitis in patients with chronic beryllium disease by beryllium-specific helper T cells. N. Engl. J. Med. 320:1103, 1990.

61. O'Connor, C., and Fitzgerald, M.: Speculations on sarcoidosis. Respir. Med. 86:277, 1992.

62. Moller, D., et al.: Bias toward use of specific T-cell receptor B-chain variable region in a subgroup of individuals with sarcoidosis. J. Clin. Invest. 82:1183, 1988.

63. Balbi, B., et al.: Increased numbers of T lymphocytes with gamma delta–positive antigen receptors in a subgroup of individuals with pulmonary sarcoidosis. J. Clin. Invest. 85:1353, 1990.

64. Bocart, D., et al.: A search for mycobacterial DNA in granulomatous tissues from patients with sarcoidosis using the polymerase chain reaction. Am. Rev. Respir. Dis. *1145:*142, 1992.

65. Saboor, S., et al.: Detection of mycobacterial DNA in sarcoidosis and tuberculosis with polymerase chain reaction. Lancet *339:*1012, 1992.

66. Flint, A., and Colby, T.V.: Surgical Pathology of Diffuse Infiltrative Lung Disease. Philadelphia, W.B. Saunders Co. (Grune & Stratton), 1987.

67. Fink, J.: Hypersensitivity pneumonitis. Clin. Chest Med. *13:*303, 1992.

68. Mayock, R.L., and Iozzo, R.: The eosinophilic pneumonias. *In* Fishman, A.P. (ed.): Pulmonary Diseases and Disorders, 2nd ed. New York, McGraw-Hill, 1988, p. 683.

69. Katzenstein, A.-L.A., and Askin, F.B.: Surgical Pathology of Non-Neoplastic Lung Disease, 2nd ed. Philadelphia, W.B. Saunders Co., 1990.

70. Müller, N., and Miller, R.R.: Diffuse pulmonary hemorrhage. Radiol. Clin. North Am. *29:*965, 1991.

71. Churg, A.: Vasculitis and mimics of vasculitis involving the lungs. *In* Churg, A., and Churg, J. (eds.): Systemic Vasculitides. New York, Igaku-Shoin, 1991, p. 121.

72. Davis, S., et al.: Radiation effects on the lung: Clinical features, pathology, and imaging findings. Am. J. Roentgenol. *159:*1157, 1992.

73. American Thoracic Society, Lung Transplantation. Report of the ATS Workshop on Lung Transplantation. Am. Rev. Respir. Dis. *147:*772, 1993.

74. Randhawa, P., and Yousem, S.A.: The pathology of lung transplantation. Pathol. Annu. *2:*247, 1992.

75. Yousem, S.A., et al.: A working formulation for the standardization of nomenclature of heart and lung rejection: Lung Rejection Study Group. J. Heart Transplant *9:*593, 1990.

76. Carter, D., and Eggleston, J.C.: Tumors of the lower respiratory tract. Atlas of Tumor Pathology. Second series, Fascicle 17. Washington, D.C., Armed Forces Institute of Pathology, 1980.

77. Mackay, B., et al.: Tumors of the Lung. Philadelphia, W.B. Saunders Co., 1991.

78. Boring, C.C., et al.: Cancer statistics, 1992. CA Cancer J. Clin. *42:*19, 1992.

79. Samet, J.M.: Epidemiology of lung cancer. Chest *103:*20, 1993.

80. Department of Health and Human Services: Smoking and Health—A National Status Report. A Report to Congress. Washington, DC, 1987.

81. Auerbach, O.: Changes in bronchial epithelium in relationship to sex, age, residence, smoking, and pneumonia. N. Engl. J. Med. *267:*111, 1962.

82. Auerbach, O.: Changes in bronchial epithelium in relationship to cigarette smoking, 1955–1960 vs. 1970–1977. N. Engl. J. Med. *300:*285, 1979.

83. Marchevsky, A.M.: Pathogenesis and experimental models of lung cancer. *In* Marchevsky, A.M. (ed.): Surgical Pathology of Lung Neoplasms. New York, Marcel Dekker, 1990, p. 7.

84. Cihak, R.W.: Radiation and lung cancer. Hum. Pathol. *25:*25, 1971.

85. Harley, N.H., and Harley, J.H.: Potential lung cancer risk from indoor radon exposure. CA Cancer J. Clin. *40:*265, 1990.

86. Samet, J.M.: Indoor radon and lung cancer: Estimating the risks. West. J. Med. *156:*25, 1992.

87. Abelson, P.H.: Uncertainties about health effects of radon (editorial). Science *250:*353, 1990.

88. Carbone, D.P., and Minna, J.D.: The molecular genetics of lung cancer. Adv. Intern. Med. *37:*153, 1992.

89. Rodenhuis, S., and Slebos, R.: Clinical significance of *ras* oncogene activation in human lung cancer. Cancer Res. *52:*2665, 1992.

90. Barsky, S.H., et al.: The extracellular matrix of pulmonary scar carcinomas is suggestive of a desmoplastic origin. Am. J. Pathol. *124:*412, 1986.

91. Yesner, R., et al. (eds.): International Histological Classification of Tumors, 2nd ed. Vol. 1. Geneva, World Health Organization, 1982.

92. Churg, A.: Tumors of the lung. *In* Thurlbeck, W. (ed.): Pathology of the Lung, New York, Thieme Med. Pubs., 1988, p. 311.

93. Mountain, C.: Lung cancer staging classification. Clin. Chest Med. *14:*43, 1993.

94. Patel, A., et al.: Paraneoplastic syndromes associated with lung cancer. Mayo Clin. Proc. *68:*278, 1993.

95. Gould, V.E., et al.: Neuroendocrine components of the bronchopulmonary tract: Hyperplasias, dysplasias, and neoplasms. Lab. Invest. *49:*519, 1983.

96. Steinetz, C., et al.: Localized fibrous tumor of the pleura: Correlation of histopathological, immunohistochemical, and ultrastructural features. Pathol. Res. Pract. *186:*344, 1990.

97. Corson, J.M.: Pathology of malignant mesothelioma. *In* Antman, K., and Aisner, J. (eds.): Asbestos-Related Malignancy. Philadelphia, W.B. Saunders Co. (Grune & Stratton), 1987, p. 179.

98. Churg, A.: Neoplastic asbestos-induced diseases. *In* Churg, A., and Green, F. (eds.): Pathology of Occupational Lung Disease. New York, Igaku-Shoin, 1988, p. 279.

99. Pott, F.: Neoplastic findings in experimental asbestos studies and conclusions for fiber carcinogenesis in humans. Ann. N.Y. Acad. Sci. *643:*205, 1991.

100. Sheibani, K., et al. Immunopathologic and molecular studies as an aid to the diagnosis of malignant mesothelioma. Hum. Pathol. *23:*107, 1992.

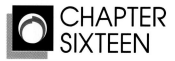

CHAPTER SIXTEEN

Head and Neck

Diseases of the head and neck range from the common cold to the uncommon neoplasms of the nose. Those selected for discussion are assigned, sometimes arbitrarily, to one of the following anatomic sites: (1) oral soft tissues, including the tongue; (2) upper airways, including the nose, pharynx, larynx, and nasal sinuses; (3) ears; (4) neck; and (5) salivary glands.

ORAL SOFT TISSUES

The oral cavity is a fearsome orifice guarded by ranks of upper and lower "horns" (lamentably, too subject to erosion), demanding constant gratification, and teeming with microorganisms, some of which are potentially harmful. Among the many disorders that affect its various parts, only the more important and/or frequent conditions involving the oral mucous membranes, lips, and tongue will be considered. Disorders of the teeth and those limited to the gingiva are left for specialized dental texts, and those of the jaws for Chapter 27, Skeletal System and Soft Tissue Tumors.

INFLAMMATIONS

The oral mucosa is highly resistant to its indigenous flora, having many defenses, including the competitive suppression of potential pathogens by organisms of low virulence, the elaboration of secretory immunoglobulin A (IgA) and other immunoglobulins by submucosal collections of lymphocytes and plasma cells, the antibacterial effects of saliva, and the diluting and irrigating effects of food and drink. Nonetheless, any lowering of these defenses, for example, with immunodeficiency or disruption of the microbiologic balance by antibacterial therapy, potentiates oral infection. Only the local, distinctive inflammations are considered here; the systemic disorders with oral manifestations (e.g., scarlet fever and measles) will be mentioned briefly in a subsequent section.

Herpes Simplex Virus (HSV) Infections

Most orofacial herpetic infections are caused by HSV type 1 (HSV-1). By contrast, HSV-2 most often involves the genital tract. In addition, HSV may produce a keratoconjunctivitis and, in neonates or immunocompromised individuals, may disseminate to induce severe keratitis or a highly lethal encephalitis (see Chapter 29). Most primary oral infections with HSV-1 are trivial "cold sores." Uncommonly, in children two to four years of age, they take the form of severe diffuse involvement of the oral and pharyngeal mucosa, the tongue, and the gingiva marked by fiery redness and swelling, soon followed by clusters of vesicles *(acute herpetic gingivostomatitis)*. Systemic manifestations are usually present.

> **MORPHOLOGY.** The vesicles range from lesions of a few millimeters to large bullae and, at first, are filled with a clear, serous fluid, but they often rupture to yield extremely painful, red-rimmed, shallow ulcerations. Microscopically, there is intra- and intercellular edema (acantholysis), yielding clefts that may become transformed into macroscopic vesicles. Individual epidermal cells in the margins of the vesicle or lying free within the fluid sometimes develop eosinophilic **intranuclear viral inclusions,** or several cells fuse to produce giant cells **(multinucleate polykaryons),** changes that permit the diagnostic Tzanck test based on microscopic examination of the vesicle fluid. The vesicles and shallow ulcers usually spontaneously clear within 3 to 4 weeks, but the virus treks along the regional nerves and eventually becomes dormant in the local ganglia (e.g., the trigeminal).

The great preponderance of adults harbor latent HSV-1, but in some individuals, usually young adults, the virus becomes reactivated to produce the common, but usually mild "cold sore." The influences predisposing to activation are poorly understood but are thought to include upper respiratory tract infections, excessive exposure to cold, wind, or sunlight, and allergic reactions.

Recurrent herpetic stomatitis (in contrast to acute gingivostomatitis) takes the form of groups of small (1 to 3 mm) vesicles frequently on the lips, about the nasal orifices, or on the buccal mucosa. They resemble those already described in the primary infections but are much more limited in duration, are milder, usually dry up in 4 to 6 days, and heal within a week or 10 days.

Aphthous Ulcers (Canker Sores)

These extremely common superficial ulcerations of the oral mucosa affect up to 40% of the population in the United States. They are more common in the first two decades of life, are painful and often recurrent, and tend to be prevalent within certain families.

The lesions appear as single or multiple, shal-

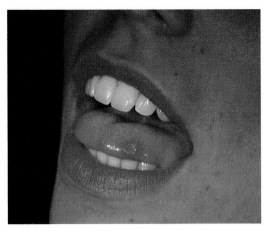

Figure 16–1. An aphthous ulcer of the tongue in a young woman. Doesn't it look painful? (Courtesy of Dr. John Sexton, Chief, Oral and Maxillofacial Surgery, Beth Israel Hospital, Boston.)

low, hyperemic ulcerations covered by a thin exudate and rimmed by a narrow zone of erythema. The underlying inflammatory infiltrate is at first largely mononuclear, but secondary bacterial infection introduces numerous neutrophils. The lesions may spontaneously clear within a week or be stubbornly persistent for weeks (Fig. 16–1).

The causation of these lesions is obscure, but sometimes they are associated with inflammatory bowel disease and Behçet's syndrome. Hypersensitivity, emotional stress, endocrine influences (pregnancy, menstruation), autoimmune reactions involving both cellular and humoral mechanisms, and a diversity of microbes have been suspected. Within the past few years attention has been drawn to *Streptococcus sanguis,* but the lesions do not respond to the usual antistreptococcal therapy.[1] Most ulcers are more painful than serious and require only symptomatic treatment.

Oral Candidiasis (Thrush)

The many localizations of candidal infection are fully described in Chapter 8, and so it suffices here to merely emphasize that oral lesions typically take the form of a superficial, curdy, gray to white inflammatory membrane composed of matted organisms enmeshed in a fibrinosuppurative exudate that can be readily scraped off to reveal an underlying erythematous inflammatory base. As was pointed out, this fungus is a normal inhabitant of the oral cavity and causes mischief only in individuals who are diabetic, neutropenic, immunoincompetent, as in those with acquired immunodeficiency syndrome (AIDS), have xerostomia, or are otherwise debilitated, or when the normal flora of the oral cavity is perturbed by antibiotic therapy.

Glossitis

Although the designation "glossitis" implies inflammation of the tongue, it is sometimes applied to the beefy-red tongue encountered in certain deficiency states that results from atrophy of the papillae of the tongue and thinning of the mucosa, exposing the underlying vasculature. In some instances, the atrophic changes do indeed lead to inflammation and even shallow ulcerations. Such changes may be encountered in deficiencies of vitamin B_{12} (pernicious anemia), riboflavin, niacin, or pyridoxine. Similar alterations are sometimes encountered with sprue and iron deficiency anemia possibly complicated by one of the vitamin B deficiencies mentioned. *The combination of iron deficiency anemia, glossitis, and esophageal dysphagia usually related to webs is known as the Plummer-Vinson or Paterson-Kelly syndrome.* Glossitis, characterized by ulcerative lesions (sometimes along the lateral borders of the tongue), may also be seen with jagged carious teeth, ill-fitting dentures, and rarely with syphilis, inhalation burns, or ingestion of corrosive chemicals.

Xerostomia

Xerostomia refers to dry mouth; this manifestation is a major feature of the autoimmune disorder Sjögren's syndrome in which it is usually accompanied by dry eyes (see Chapter 6). A lack of salivary secretions may also be a residual of radiation therapy or may be drug induced by a wide variety of anticholinergic agents. The oral cavity may merely reveal dry mucosa or atrophy of the papillae of the tongue, with fissuring and ulcerations or, in Sjögren's syndrome, concomitant inflammatory enlargement of the salivary glands.

Oral Manifestations of Systemic Disease

As oral clinicians are at pains to emphasize, the mouth is a part of the body. Not surprisingly, then, many systemic diseases are associated with oral lesions. Some of the more common are cited in Table 16–1, with a few words about the associated oral changes. Only one—hairy leukoplakia—is characterized in more detail.

Hairy leukoplakia is an uncommon oral lesion virtually restricted to patients with HIV infection. Sometimes it calls attention to the existence of the infection. It takes the form of white, confluent patches of fluffy ("hairy") hyperkeratotic thickening situated anywhere on the oral mucosa. Micro-

scopically, this distinctive appearance is attributable to piled-up layers of keratotic squames based on underlying mucosal acanthosis. Sometimes there is koilocytosis of the superficial, nucleated epidermal cells, indicative of human papillomavirus (HPV) infection. *In situ* hybridization has revealed HPV, Epstein-Barr virus (EBV), and sometimes also HIV in these lesions. In addition, there is sometimes superimposed candidal infection on the surface of the lesions, adding to the "hairiness." When the hairy leukoplakia is a harbinger of HIV infection, manifestations of AIDS-related complex (ARC; see definition in Chapter 6) or AIDS generally appear within 2 or 3 years.

Reactive Proliferations

Two lesions, sometimes loosely referred to as tumors—*irritation fibroma and reparative giant cell granuloma*—are reactive in nature and are not neoplasms. The former is a protruding fibrous nodule, usually of the gingivodental margin, at a site of chronic irritation. It is, in a sense, a focus of exaggerated inflammatory fibrosis. Although these lesions appear in both males and females, they are more common in females during pregnancy and are therefore referred to as "pregnancy tumors" (Fig. 16–2).

Analogously, the *giant cell granuloma* (also termed an *epulis*) is an unusual inflammatory lesion up to 1.5 cm in diameter that characteristically protrudes from the gingiva at some site of chronic inflammation. Generally, it is covered by intact gingival mucosa, but it may be ulcerated. Histologically, it is made up of a striking aggregation of multinucleate, foreign body–like giant cells separated by a fibroangiomatous stroma. Although not encapsulated, these lesions are usually well delimited and readily excised. Their major importance lies in their differentiation from true giant cell tumors generally found within the maxilla or the mandible, and from the histologically similar but frequently multiple reparative giant cell "brown tumors" seen in hyperparathyroidism (see Chapter 25).

TUMORS AND PRECANCEROUS LESIONS

Some common precancerous lesions and a variety of benign and malignant tumors occur in the oral soft tissues. Most of these tumors (e.g., hemangiomas, granular cell myoblastomas, lymphomas) also occur elsewhere and are described adequately in other sections, and so only the precancerous leu-

Table 16-1. ORAL MANIFESTATIONS OF SOME SYSTEMIC DISEASES

INFECTIONS

Scarlet fever	Fiery red tongue with prominent papillae—"raspberry tongue." White coated tongue through which hyperemic papillae project—"strawberry tongue"
Measles	A spotty enanthem in the oral cavity often precedes the skin rash. Ulcerations on the buccal mucosa about Stensen's duct produce Koplik's spots
Infectious mononucleosis	An acute pharyngitis and tonsillitis that may be coated with a gray-white exudative membrane. Enlargement of lymph nodes in the neck
Diphtheria	A characteristic dirty-white, fibrinosuppurative, tough, inflammatory membrane over the tonsils and retropharynx
Human immunodeficiency virus (HIV) infection—AIDS	Predisposition to opportunistic oral infections, particularly with herpes virus, Candida, and other fungi; sometimes oral lesions of Kaposi's sarcoma and hairy leukoplakia (described on the previous page)

DERMATOLOGIC CONDITIONS

Lichen planus	Reticulate, lace-like, white keratotic lesions that rarely become bullous and ulcerated. Seen in more than 50% of patients with cutaneous lichen planus and, rarely, is the sole manifestation
Pemphigus	Usually vulgaris. Vesicles and bullae prone to rupture, leaving hyperemic erosions covered with exudate
Bullous pemphigoid	Oral lesions resemble macroscopically those of pemphigus but can be differentiated histologically (see Chapter 26)
Erythema multiforme	A maculopapular, vesiculobullous eruption that sometimes follows an infection elsewhere, ingestion of drugs, development of cancer, or a collagen-vascular disease. When it involves the lips and oral mucosa, it is referred to as *Stevens-Johnson syndrome*

HEMATOLOGIC DISORDERS

Pancytopenia (agranulocytosis, aplastic anemia)	Severe oral infections in the form of gingivitis, pharyngitis, tonsillitis. May extend to cellulitis of the neck (*Ludwig's angina*)
Leukemia	With depletion of functioning neutrophils oral lesions may appear like those in pancytopenia
Monocytic leukemia	Leukemic infiltration and enlargement of the gingivae, often with accompanying periodontitis

MISCELLANEOUS

Melanotic pigmentation	May appear in Addison's disease, hemochromatosis, fibrous dysplasia of bone (Albright's syndrome), and Peutz-Jegher syndrome (gastrointestinal polyposis)
Phenytoin (Dilantin) ingestion	Striking fibrous enlargement of the gingivae
Pregnancy	A friable, red, pyogenic granuloma protruding from the gingiva ("pregnancy tumor")
Rendu-Osler-Weber syndrome	Autosomal dominant disorder with multiple aneurysmal telangiectases from birth beneath the skin or mucosal surfaces of the oral cavity, lips, gastrointestinal tract, respiratory tract, and urinary tract as well as in internal viscera

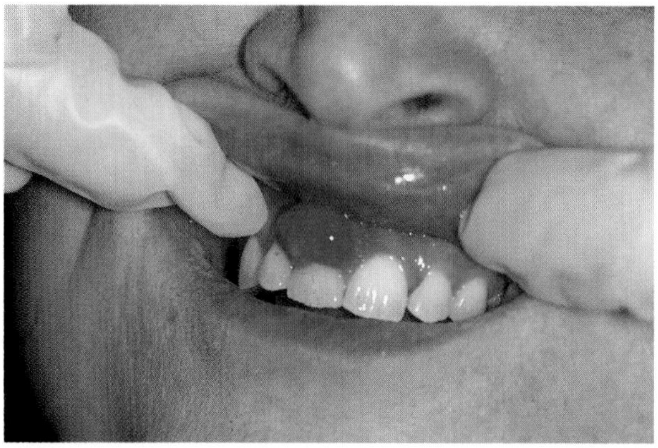

Figure 16-2. "Pregnancy tumor" protruding from the margin of the upper gingiva. (Courtesy of Dr. John Sexton, Chief, Oral and Maxillofacial Surgery, Beth Israel Hospital, Boston.)

koplakia, erythroplakia, papillomas, and squamous cell carcinoma will be considered here.

Leukoplakia and Erythroplakia

The term "leukoplakia" means simply "white plaque." It may be produced by several conditions, including epidermal proliferations—benign to malignant, tobacco or snuff-pouch keratosis, chronic cheek bite, lichen planus, palatitis nicotina, and candidiasis as well as other rarer lesions. However, 85 to 90% of all white plaques are caused by epidermal proliferations, and so most experts recommend the following definition: *Leukoplakia is a white plaque on the oral mucous membranes that cannot be removed by scraping and cannot be classified clinically or microscopically as another disease entity.*[2] All other white lesions are specified as to cause (e.g., lichen planus, candidal membrane). Thus defined, leukoplakic plaques range from completely benign epithelial thickenings to highly

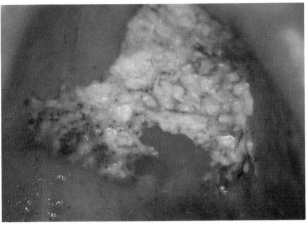

A

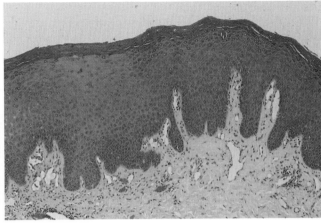

B

Figure 16–3. *A,* Leukoplakia of the hard palate. The numerous lesions have become virtually confluent. (Courtesy of Drs. E.E. Vokes, S. Lippman, et al., Department of Thoracic/Head and Neck Oncology, Texas Medical Center, Houston, and reprinted with permission from the New England Journal of Medicine, *328*:184, 1993.) *B,* Leukoplakia caused by marked epithelial thickening and hyperkeratosis.

atypical lesions with dysplastic changes that merge with carcinoma in situ. Thus, it must be emphasized that *leukoplakia is a clinical term; until proved otherwise it must be considered precancerous.*

Related to leukoplakia, but much less common and much more ominous, is *erythroplakia (dysplastic leukoplakia).* It represents a red, velvety, possibly eroded area within the oral cavity that usually remains level with or may be slightly depressed in relation to the surrounding mucosa. The epithelial changes in such lesions tend to be markedly atypical, incurring a much higher risk of malignant transformation than that with leukoplakia. Occasionally, intermediate forms are encountered that have the characteristics of both leukoplakia and erythroplakia, termed *speckled leukoerythroplakia.*

Both leukoplakia and erythroplakia may be encountered in adults at any age, but they are usually found between the ages of 40 and 70, with a 2-to-1 male preponderance. Although these lesions have multifactorial origins, the use of tobacco (cigarettes, pipes, cigars, and particularly chewing tobacco and buccal pouches) is the most common antecedent. Other potentiating influences are alcohol, ill-fitting dentures, and chronic exposure to persistent irritants (lovers of hot pizza take note). HPV sequences, particularly serotype 16, have been identified in more than half of these lesions.[3]

MORPHOLOGY. Leukoplakias may occur anywhere in the oral cavity (favored locations are buccal mucosa, floor of the mouth, ventral surface of the tongue, hard palate). They appear as solitary or multiple, white patches or plaques with indistinct or sharply demarcated borders (Fig. 16–3A). They may be slightly thickened and smooth, or wrinkled and indurated, or may appear as raised, sometimes corrugated, verrucose plaques. Histologically, they present an epithelial spectrum ranging from hyperkeratosis overlying a thickened, acanthotic but orderly mucosal epithelium (see Fig. 16–3B) to lesions with markedly dysplastic changes sometimes merging into carcinoma in situ. The more dysplastic or anaplastic the lesion, the more likely a subjacent inflammatory infiltrate of lymphocytes and macrophages.

The histologic changes in **erythroplakia** only rarely consist of orderly epidermal thickening; virtually all disclose superficial erosions with dysplasia, carcinoma in situ, or already developed carcinoma in the surrounding margins. An intense subepithelial inflammatory reaction with vascular dilatation accounts for the red appearance of the lesion.

The frequency of carcinoma in situ or overt cancerous changes in leukoplakia varies among reports from 1 to 16%, but a reasonable average is 5 to 6%.[4] Ominous features are a speckled appearance, warty or verrucous thickening, and occurrence in "high-risk sites" (e.g., floor of the mouth and ventral surface of the tongue); hence the need for biopsy of persistent lesions that fail to respond to such simple measures as avoidance of tobacco and alcohol. In the case of erythroplakia, the malignant transformation rate is about 50% (some would say higher).

Squamous Papilloma and Condyloma Acuminatum

These relatively innocuous benign lesions also occur on the skin and in the genital tract in both males and females (see Chapter 23). They are of interest because of their strong associations with HPV serotypes 6 and 11, which are rarely found in cancers arising in the oral cavity.

Squamous Cell Carcinoma

At least 95% of cancers of the oral cavity (including the tongue) are squamous cell carcinomas. The small residual includes adenocarcinomas (of mucous gland origin), melanomas, various carcinomas, and other rarities. The incidence of oral squamous cell cancers in the United States is about 4% for men and 2% for women, and so they are by no means uncommon. Although most are readily accessible to discovery and biopsy, it is disheartening that in 1989 in the United States they accounted for about 2% of all cancer deaths in men and 1% in women, indicating that 50% of these lesions prove fatal. Squamous cell carcinomas are most frequently diagnosed in persons between the ages of 50 and 70.

The genesis of these cancers is thought to be closely linked to the use of tobacco and alcohol. Nondrinking smokers have a 2- to 4-fold greater risk of developing these cancers than matched control subjects, which increases to 6- to 15-fold with both drinking and smoking. Moreover, there is a quantitative relationship between the amount of smoking and of alcohol consumption and the risk. Particularly implicated are chewing tobacco and buccal pouches. The use of marijuana has also been implicated. A major regional predisposing influence is the chewing of betel nuts and pan in India and parts of Asia. On the more pleasant side of the equation, several studies have reported that consumption of fruit and vegetables significantly reduces the risk.[5] Protracted irritation, as from ill-fitting dentures, jagged teeth, or chronic infections, is no longer thought to be an important direct antecedent to oral cancer, but nonetheless it may contribute to leukoplakia, which, as has already been noted, is an important subsoil for the development of oral cancer. In some studies, HPV-16 and closely related serotypes have been identified in almost half of the carcinomas of the tongue and floor of the mouth.[6] Actinic radiation (sunlight) and, particularly, pipe smoking are known predisposing influences to cancer of the lower lip.

All these possible environmental influences presumably act on a fertile genetic soil, and indeed a number of genotypic and molecular changes have been described in some but not all head and neck cancers. These include deletions of chromosome regions 18q, 10p, 8p, and 3p, mutations in p53 and overexpression of a mutated p53 protein, and amplification of the *int*-2 and *bcl*-1 oncogenes.[7] The large number of observed changes suggest a multistep origin of these cancers.

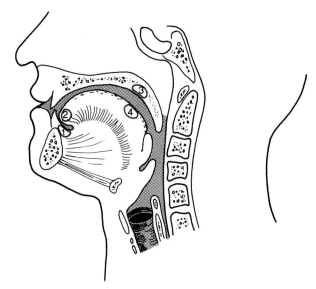

Figure 16-4. Schematic representation of the sites of origin of squamous cell carcinoma of the oral cavity, in numerical order of frequency.

MORPHOLOGY. Squamous cell carcinoma may arise anywhere in the oral cavity, but in large series, the favored locations are the floor of the mouth, tongue, hard palate, and base of tongue (Fig. 16-4). At one time, squamous cell carcinoma of the lips was quite common, but of recent date the frequency of this neoplasm has significantly diminished (perhaps with the disappearance of the clay pipe). In the early stages, cancers of the oral cavity appear either as raised, firm, pearly plaques or as irregular, roughened, or verrucose areas of mucosal thickening, possibly mistaken for leukoplakia. Either pattern may be superimposed on a background of apparent leukoplakia or erythroplakia. As these lesions enlarge, they create protruding masses (Fig. 16-5) or undergo central necrosis, forming an irregular, shaggy ulcer rimmed by elevated, firm, rolled borders.

Histologically, these cancers begin as *in situ* lesions sometimes with surrounding areas of epithelial atypicality or dysplasia, as described in leukoplakia and erythroplakia. They range from well-differentiated keratinizing neoplasms to anaplastic, sometimes sarcomatoid tumors, and from slowly to rapidly growing lesions. As a group, they tend, in time, to infiltrate locally before they metastasize to other sites. The routes of extension depend on the primary site. Favored sites of metastasis are mediastinal lymph nodes, lungs, liver, and bones. Unfortunately, such distant metastases are often occult at the time of discovery of the primary lesion.[8]

As with all cancers, early diagnosis is the paramount prognostic factor. The prognosis is best with lip lesions, the 5-year recurrence-free rate approximating 90%, and poorest with tumors in the floor

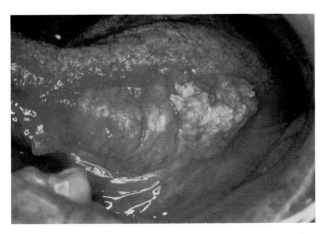

Figure 16–5. Carcinoma of the tongue. The tumor of the base of the tongue appears as a bulbous protruding mass. (Courtesy of Drs. E.E. Vokes, S. Lippman, et al., Department of Thoracic/Head and Neck Oncology, Texas Medical Center, Houston, and reprinted with permission from the New England Journal of Medicine, 328:184, 1993.)

of the mouth and at the base of the tongue, yielding only 20 to 30% 5-year recurrence-free rates. All squamous cell carcinomas of the oral cavity take months to years to progress from carcinoma in situ (after being preceded by leukoplakia) to invasive cancer, and so every death they cause must be viewed as a preventable tragedy.

UPPER AIRWAYS

The term "upper airways" is used here to include the nose, pharynx, and larynx and their related parts. Disorders of these structures are among the most common afflictions of humans, but fortunately the overwhelming majority are more nuisances than threats.

NOSE

Inflammatory diseases, mostly in the form of the common cold, as everyone knows, are the most common disorders of the nose and accessory air sinuses. Most of these inflammatory conditions are viral in origin, but often they are complicated by superimposed bacterial infections having considerably greater significance. Much less common are a few destructive inflammatory nasal diseases and tumors primary in the nasal cavity or paranasal sinuses.

Inflammations

Infectious *rhinitis,* the more elegant way of saying "common cold," is in most instances caused by one or more viruses. Major offenders are adenoviruses, echoviruses, and rhinoviruses. They evoke a profuse catarrhal discharge that is familiar to all and the bane of the kindergarten teacher. During the initial acute stages, the nasal mucosa is thickened, edematous, and red, the nasal cavities are narrowed, and the turbinates are enlarged. These changes may extend, producing a concomitant pharyngotonsillitis. Secondary bacterial infection enhances the inflammatory reaction and produces an essentially mucopurulent or sometimes frankly suppurative exudate. But as everyone knows, these infections soon clear up, usually in a week if appropriately treated but only after 7 days if ignored.

Allergic rhinitis (hay fever) is initiated by sensitivity reactions to one of a large group of allergens, perhaps most commonly the plant pollens. As is the case with asthma, allergic rhinitis is an Ige-mediated immune reaction with an early- and late-phase response (see section on type I hypersensitivity in Chapter 6). The allergic reaction is characterized by marked mucosal edema, redness, and mucous secretion, accompanied by a leukocytic infiltration in which eosinophils are prominent.

Recurrent attacks of nonspecific or allergic rhinitis eventually lead to focal protrusions of the mucosa, producing so-called *nasal polyps,* which may reach 3 to 4 cm in length. Histologically, these polyps are not neoplasms, but rather a focal collection of edematous mucosa having a loose stroma, often harboring hyperplastic or cystic mucous glands and infiltrated with a variety of inflammatory cells, including prominently neutrophils, eosinophils, and plasma cells with occasional clusters of lymphocytes (Fig. 16–6). In the absence of bacterial infection, the mucosal covering of these polyps is intact but, with chronicity, may become ulcerated or infected. When multiple or large, they may encroach on the airway and impair sinus drainage.

Chronic rhinitis is a sequel to repeated attacks of acute rhinitis, whether microbial or allergic in origin, with the eventual development of superimposed bacterial infection. A deviated nasal septum or nasal polyps with impaired drainage of secretions contribute to the microbial invasion. Frequently, there is superficial desquamation or ulceration of the mucosal epithelium and a variable inflammatory infiltrate of neutrophils, lymphocytes, and plasma cells subjacent to the epithelium. These suppurative infections sometimes extend into the air sinuses.

Acute sinusitis is most commonly preceded by acute or chronic rhinitis, but occasionally maxillary sinusitis arises by extension of a periapical infection through the bony floor of the sinus. The offending agents are usually inhabitants of the oral cavity, and the inflammatory reaction is entirely nonspecific. Impairment of drainage of the sinus by inflammatory edema of the mucosa is an important contributor to the process and, when complete,

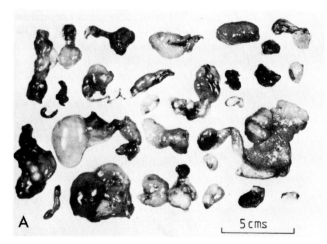
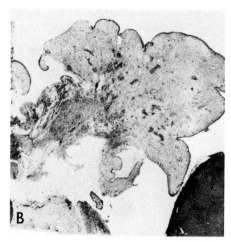

Figure 16–6. *A*, Multiple benign allergic polyps removed from the nose of an old man. *B*, Low-power histology of an allergic polyp exhibiting marked submucosal edema. (With permission from Friedman, I., and Osborn, D.A.: Pathology of Granulomas and Neoplasms of the Nose and Paranasal Sinuses. New York, Churchill Livingstone, 1982, p. 30.)

may impound the suppurative exudate, producing *empyema* of the sinus. Occasionally, obstruction of the outflow, most often of the frontal and next most often of the anterior ethmoid sinuses, leads to an accumulation of mucous secretions in the absence of direct bacterial invasion, producing a so-called *mucocele*. Acute sinusitis may, in time, give rise to *chronic sinusitis*, particularly when there is interference with drainage. Usually there is a mixed microbial flora, largely of normal inhabitants of the oral cavity. Particularly severe forms of chronic sinusitis are caused by fungi (e.g., mucormycosis), especially in diabetics. Very uncommonly, sinusitis is a component of *Kartagener's syndrome*, which also includes bronchiectasis and situs inversus. All these features are secondary to defective ciliary action. Although most instances of chronic sinusitis are more uncomfortable than disabling or serious, the infections have the ugly potential of spreading into the orbit or of penetrating into the enclosing bone and producing osteomyelitis or, even, into the cranial vault, causing septic thrombophlebitis of a dural venous sinus.

Necrotizing Lesions of the Nose and Upper Airways

Necrotizing ulcerating lesions of the nose and upper respiratory tract may be produced by (1) spreading mucormycotic infections, particularly in the diabetic; (2) Wegener's granulomatosis (discussed in Chapter 11); or (3) a once poorly understood condition called *lethal midline granuloma* or *polymorphic reticulosis*. Recent studies have proved that most (perhaps all) instances of this last mentioned entity represent a non-Hodgkin's lymphoma arising in an unusual location. Ulceration and superimposed bacterial infection frequently complicate the process, confusing the histologic changes by sometimes producing tumor-related granuloma-

tous inflammation. Concomitant lymphomatous lesions may be found in other organs and sites. At one time, these lesions were highly fatal, owing to uncontrolled growth of the lymphoma, possibly with penetration into the cranial vault, or because of tumor necrosis with secondary bacterial infection and blood-borne dissemination of the infection. Currently, the treatment of the lymphoma with the usual modalities has proved to be effective, in some cases, in bringing the destructive process under control.

NASOPHARYNX

Although the nasopharyngeal mucosa, related lymphoid structures, and glands may be involved in a wide variety of specific infections (e.g., diphtheria, infectious mononucleosis [discussed elsewhere]) as well as by neoplasms, the only disorders mentioned here are nonspecific inflammations; tumors are discussed separately later.

Inflammations

Pharyngitis and tonsillitis are frequent concomitants of the usual viral upper respiratory infections. Most often implicated are the multitudinous rhinoviruses, echoviruses and adenoviruses, and less frequently respiratory syncytial viruses, and the various influenzal strains. In the usual case there is reddening and slight edema of the nasopharyngeal mucosa, with reactive enlargement of the related lymphoid structures. Bacterial infections may be superimposed on these viral involvements, or the bacteria may be primary invaders. The most common offenders are the beta-hemolytic streptococci, but sometimes *Staphylococcus aureus* or other pathogens may be implicated. Particularly severe forms of pharyngitis and tonsillitis are seen in infants and children who have not yet developed any protective immunity to such agents and in adults rendered susceptible by neutropenia, some form of immunodeficiency, uncontrolled diabetes, or disruption of the normal oral flora by antibiotics. In these circumstances, microbial opportunists may be involved. The inflamed nasopharyngeal mucosa may be covered by an exudative membrane (pseudomembrane), and the nasopalatine and palatine tonsils may be enlarged and covered by exudate. A typical appearance is of enlarged, reddened tonsils (owing to reactive lymphoid hyperplasia) dotted by pinpoints of exudate emanating from the tonsillar crypts, so-called *follicular tonsillitis.*

The major importance of streptococcal "sore throats" lies in the possible development of post-streptococcal complications, for example, rheumatic fever (see Chapter 12) and glomerulonephritis (see Chapter 20). Whether recurrent episodes of acute tonsillitis favor the development of chronic tonsillitis (true chronic tonsillitis is extremely rare) is open to debate, but they may leave residual enlargement of the lymphoid tissue, inviting the tender mercies of the otolaryngologist. However, it should be noted that epidemiologic data suggest that excision of nasopharyngeal lymphoid structures significantly increases the risk of later developing Hodgkin's disease.

TUMORS OF THE NOSE, SINUSES, AND NASOPHARYNX

Tumors in these locations are infrequent but include the entire category of mesenchymal and epithelial neoplasms.[9] Brief mention may be made of somewhat distinctive types.

Nasopharyngeal angiofibroma is a highly vascular tumor that occurs almost exclusively in adolescent males. Despite its benign nature, it may cause serious clinical problems because of its tendency to bleed profusely during surgery.[10]

The *inverted papilloma* is a benign but locally aggressive neoplasm occurring in both the nose and the paranasal sinuses. As the name implies, the papillomatous proliferation of squamous epithelium, instead of producing an exophytic growth, extends into the mucosa, that is, is inverted (Fig. 16–7). If not adequately excised, it has a high rate of recurrence, with the potentially serious complication of invasion of the orbit or cranial vault; rarely, frank carcinoma may also develop.

Isolated plasmacytomas may arise in the lymphoid structures adjacent to the nose and sinuses. These may protrude within these cavities as

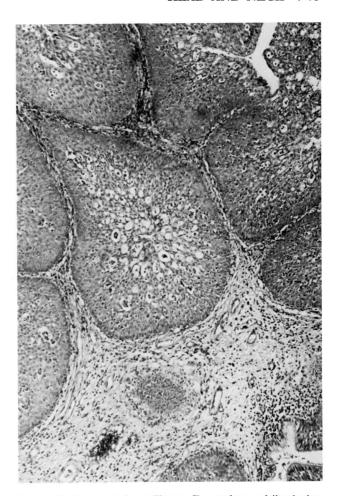

Figure 16–7. Inverted papilloma. The surface of the lesion is on the right. The masses of squamous epithelium are growing inward, hence the term "inverted." (Courtesy of Dr. Gilbert Brodsky, Brigham and Women's Hospital, Boston.)

polypoid growths, varying from 1 cm to several centimeters in diameter, covered usually by an intact overlying mucosa. The histology is that of a malignant plasma cell tumor and is identical to that described in Chapter 14. Only rarely do these lesions progress to multiple myeloma.

Olfactory neuroblastomas (esthesioneuroblastomas) are uncommon, highly malignant tumors composed of sheets of small round cells of neuroendocrine origin. They arise most often superiorly and laterally in the nose from the neuroendocrine cells dispersed in the olfactory mucosa. The differential anatomic diagnosis of these neoplasms includes all other small cell tumors, such as lymphoma, Ewing's sarcoma, and poorly differentiated carcinomas or sarcomas. Helpful is the demonstration by electron microscopy of neural processes and membrane-bound secretory granules as well as immunohistochemical techniques to disclose neuron-specific enolase, S-100 protein, and chromogranin. An 11-22 translocation has been found in most of these tumors, and also in Ewing's sarcoma of bone (see Chapter 27) and primitive neuroectodermal tumors, suggesting a common histogenesis of these small round cell tumors.[11] In addition, some of these small round cell tumors also reveal trisomy 8. Olfactory neuroblastomas tend to metastasize widely and, despite combinations of surgery, radiation, and chemotherapy, yield only a 20 to 60% 5-year survival rate.

Nasopharyngeal carcinomas take one of three patterns: (1) keratinizing squamous cell carcinomas (WHO-1), (2) nonkeratinizing squamous cell carcinomas (WHO-2), and (3) undifferentiated carcinomas that have an abundant non-neoplastic, lymphocytic infiltrate (WHO-3). The last pattern has often been called, erroneously, *lymphoepithelioma.* Three sets of influences apparently affect the origins of these neoplasms: (1) heredity, (2) age, and (3) infection with EBV. Nasopharyngeal carcinomas are particularly common in parts of Africa, where they are the most common childhood cancer. In contrast, in southern China, they are the most common cancer in adults but rarely occur in children. In the United States, they are extremely uncommon in both adults and children. Environment must play some role in this distribution, because migration from a high-incidence locale to a low-incidence locale is followed over the generations by a progressive decline in incidence. The Epstein-Barr virus genome has been identified in the tumor epithelial cells (not the lymphocytes) of most undifferentiated and nonkeratinizing squamous cell nasopharyngeal carcinomas, but no oncogenes are associated with the virus.[12] It is speculated that EBV may serve as a growth promoter, rendering the cells vulnerable to oncogenic events.

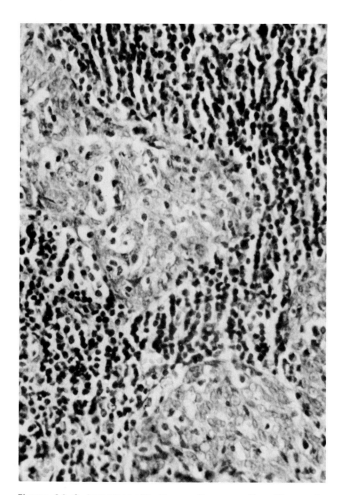

Figure 16–8. Lymphoepithelioma. The syncytium-like nests of epithelium are surrounded by masses of lymphocytes. (Courtesy of Dr. Gilbert Brodsky, Brigham and Women's Hospital, Boston.)

MORPHOLOGY. Histologically, the keratinizing and nonkeratinizing squamous cell lesions more or less resemble usual well differentiated and poorly differentiated squamous cell carcinomas arising in other locations. The undifferentiated variant is composed of large epithelial cells with oval or round vesicular nuclei, prominent nucleoli, and indistinct cell borders disposed in a syncytium-like array (Fig. 16–8). Admixed with the epithelial cells are abundant, mature, normal-appearing lymphocytes. The three histologic variants present as masses in the nasopharynx or sometimes in other locations, such as the tonsils, posterior tongue, or upper airways.

Nasopharyngeal carcinomas tend to grow silently until they have become unresectable and have often spread to cervical nodes or distant sites. Radiotherapy is the standard modality of treatment, yielding in most studies about a 50 to 70% 3-year survival rate. The undifferentiated carcinoma is the most radiosensitive, and the keratinizing the least radiosensitive.

LARYNX

The most common disorders that affect the larynx are inflammations. Tumors are uncommon but, when they occur, devastating because even though some are amenable to resection, it is often at the price of loss of the voice and sometimes a permanent tracheostomy.

Inflammations

Laryngitis may occur as the sole manifestation of allergic, viral, bacterial, or chemical insult, but more commonly it is part of a generalized upper respiratory tract infection or the result of heavy exposure to tobacco smoke. The larynx may also be affected in many systemic infectious diseases, such as tuberculosis and diphtheria. Although most nonspecific microbiologic involvements are self-limited, they may at times be serious, especially in infancy or childhood, when mucosal congestion, exudation, or edema may cause laryngeal obstruction. In particular, laryngoepiglottitis, caused by *Haemophilus influenzae* or beta-hemolytic streptococci in infants and young children with their small airways, may induce such sudden swelling of the epiglottis and vocal cords that a potentially lethal medical emergency is created. This form of disease is uncommon in adults owing to the larger size of the larynx and the stronger accessory muscles of respiration. *Croup* is the name given to laryngotracheobronchitis in children, in which the inflammatory narrowing of the airway produces the inspiratory stridor so frightening to parents. The most common form of laryngitis, encountered in heavy smokers, constitutes an important predisposition to the development of squamous epithelial changes in the larynx and sometimes overt carcinoma.

Reactive Nodules (Polyps)

Reactive nodules, also called "polyps," sometimes develop on the vocal cords, most often in heavy smokers or in individuals who impose great strain on their vocal cords *(singers' nodules)*. Adults, predominantly men, are most often affected. These nodules constitute smooth, rounded, sessile or pedunculated excrescences, generally only a few millimeters in greatest dimension, located usually on the true vocal cords. They are usually covered by squamous epithelium that may become keratotic, hyperplastic, or even slightly dysplastic. The core of the nodule is usually a loose myxoid connective tissue that sometimes is variably fibrotic or punctated by numerous, possibly ectatic, vascular channels. When nodules on opposing vocal cords impinge on each other, the mucosa may undergo ulceration.

Because of their strategic location, with corresponding greater inflammatory infiltration of the core of the lesion, they characteristically change the character of the voice and often cause progressive hoarseness. They virtually never give rise to cancers.

Hyperplasia, Keratosis, and Squamous Cell Carcinoma

MORPHOLOGY. The range of squamous epithelial changes encountered in leukoplakia, erythroplakia, and squamous cell carcinoma of the oral cavity are replicated in the larynx, yet for obscure reasons the terms "leukoplakia" and "erythroplakia" are seldom applied to the larynx. Instead, the spectrum of epithelial alterations are termed "hyperplasia," "keratosis," "dysplasia," "carcinoma in situ," and "invasive carcinoma."[13] By whatever name, the epithelial alterations range from smooth,

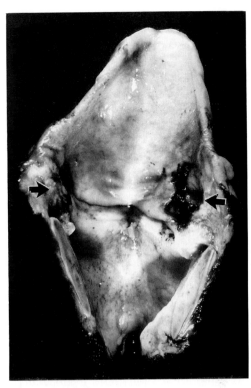

Figure 16-9. Laryngeal carcinoma. The posterior aspect of the larynx has been opened to reveal *(on the right and left arrows)* a bisected ulcerated carcinoma just above and partially involving the vocal cord.

white or reddened focal thickenings, sometimes roughened by keratosis, to irregular verrucose or ulcerated, white-pink lesions looking like cancer (Fig. 16-9). Histologically, these changes reflect a spectrum from orderly epithelial hyperplasia, with or without keratosis, to atypical hyperplasia, to dysplasia, to carcinoma in situ, to overt invasive cancer. Save for the rare adenocarcinoma arising in mucus-secreting glands, all are squamous cell carcinomas, most well differentiated.

When first seen, the orderly thickenings have almost no potential for malignant transformation, but the risk rises to 1 to 2% over the span of 5 to 10 years with mild dysplasia and 5 to 10% with severe dysplasia. In essence, **there are all gradations of epithelial hyperplasia of the true vocal cords, and the likelihood of the development of an overt carcinoma is directly proportional to the level of atypia when the lesion is first seen.** Only histologic evaluation can determine the gravity of the changes.[14]

The various changes described are most often related to tobacco smoke, the risk being proportional to the level of exposure. Indeed, up to the point of frank cancer, the changes often regress following cessation of smoking. However, other factors may also contribute. Epidemiologic evi-

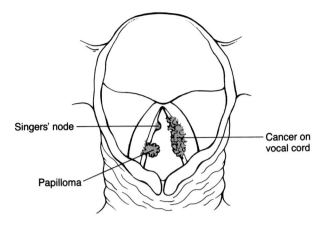

Figure 16–10. Diagrammatic comparison of a benign papilloma and an exophytic carcinoma of the larynx to highlight their quite different gross appearances.

dence suggests a dose-response relationship to asbestos inhalation, and to confound the issue further, the polymerase chain reaction has revealed HPV in some squamous cell carcinomas.[15] Multiple influences may then contribute, possibly in collaboration, in the production of carcinoma of the larynx.

The prognosis with overt carcinoma is strongly influenced by the location of the cancer within the larynx. The glottic tumors confined to the true vocal cords tend to be well differentiated, slowly growing, and late to metastasize. They are amenable to surgical excision and, if necessary, local radiotherapy. By contrast, those located above or below the vocal cords are often less well differentiated, tend to be more invasive, and spread earlier to regional nodes. About 30 to 50% of these patients have metastases at the time of diagnosis, but death is more often the consequence of local extension into some vital structure, such as the great vessels in the neck, or of infections in the lungs secondary to aspirated secretions and blood.

Papilloma and Papillomatosis

MORPHOLOGY. Solitary papillomas, usually occurring in adults, are true neoplasms that usually present as solitary, raspberry-like excrescences less than 1 cm in diameter on the true vocal cords (Fig. 16–10). Because of their fragility, the trauma of the opposite vocal cord may produce fragmentation and bleeding. Histologically, they have delicate, finger-like papillae with central cores of fibrous tissue covered by stratified squamous epithelium that is usually quite orderly. Trauma and repair may lead to some atypicality, but these lesions have virtually no malignant potential. They rarely recur after removal.

By contrast, in children, usually younger than six years of age, multiple papillomas, referred to as papillomatosis, may appear apparently in response to HPV infection (most often HPV-1). These childhood lesions often recur following removal and, in fact, may continue to recur into adult life. Rarely, protracted cases have been followed by overt carcinoma, raising the possibility of superinfection by one of the more ominous types of HPV.

EAR

Although disorders of the ear rarely shorten the quantity of life, many impair its quality. The most common aural disorders, in descending order of frequency, are (1) acute and chronic otitis (most often involving the middle ear and mastoid), sometimes leading to a cholesteatoma; (2) symptomatic otosclerosis; (3) aural polyps; (4) labyrinthitis; (5) carcinomas, largely of the external ear; and (6) paragangliomas, found mostly in the middle ear. Only those conditions that have distinctive morphologic features will be described. Paragangliomas will be discussed later. All these entities will be characterized here save for labyrinthitis, which has few distinctive morphologic changes.

INFLAMMATORY LESIONS

Inflammations of the ear, *otitis media, acute and/or chronic*, occur mostly in infants and children. They usually produce a serous exudate (when viral in origin) but may become suppurative when bacterial infection becomes superimposed. The most common offenders are *Streptococcus pneumoniae, H. influenzae,* and beta-hemolytic streptococci.

Repeated bouts of acute otitis media with failure of resolution lead to chronic disease. The causative agents of chronic disease are usually *Pseudomonas aeruginosa, Staphylococcus aureus,* or a fungus and, sometimes, a broadly mixed flora. Chronic infection has the potential to perforate the eardrum, encroaching on the ossicles or labyrinth, spreading into the mastoid spaces, and even penetrating into the cranial vault to produce there a temporal cerebritis or abscess. Otitis media in the diabetic person, when caused by *P. aeruginosa,* is especially aggressive and spreads widely (destructive necrotizing otitis media).

Cholesteatomas associated with chronic otitis media are not neoplasms, nor do they always contain cholesterol. Rather, they are cystic lesions 1 to 4 cm in diameter, lined by keratinizing squamous epithelium or metaplastic mucus-secreting epithelium, and filled with amorphous debris (derived largely from desquamated squames). Sometimes they contain spicules of cholesterol. The precise events involved in their development are not clear, but it is proposed that chronic inflammation and perforation of the eardrum with ingrowth of the squamous epithelium or metaplasia of the secretory epithelial lining of the middle ear are responsible for the formation of a squamous cell nest that becomes cystic. A chronic inflammatory reaction surrounds the keratinous cyst. Sometimes rupture not only enhances the inflammatory reaction but also induces the formation of giant cells that enclose partially necrotic squames and other particulate debris. These trivial lesions, by progressive enlargement, can erode into the ossicles, the labyrinth, the adjacent bone, or surrounding soft tissue and sometimes produce visible neck masses.

OTOSCLEROSIS

As the name implies, this condition refers to abnormal bone deposition in the middle ear about the rim of the oval window into which the footplate of the stapes fits. Both ears are usually affected. At first there is fibrous ankylosis of the footplate, followed in time by bony overgrowth anchoring it into the oval window. The degree of immobilization governs the severity of the hearing loss. This condition usually begins in the early decades of life; minimal degrees of this derangement are exceedingly common in the United States in young to middle-aged adults, but fortunately more severe symptomatic otosclerosis is relatively uncommon. In most instances it is familial, following autosomal dominant transmission with variable penetrance. The basis for the osseous overgrowth is completely obscure, but it appears to represent uncoupling of normal bone resorption and bone formation. Thus, it begins with bone resorption, followed by fibrosis and vascularization of the temporal bone in the immediate vicinity of the oval window, in time replaced by dense new bone anchoring the footplate of the stapes. In most instances, the process is slowly progressive over the span of decades, leading eventually to marked hearing loss.

TUMORS

The large variety of epithelial and mesenchymal tumors that arise in the ear—external, medial, internal—all are rare save for basal cell or squamous cell carcinomas of the pinna (external ear). These carcinomas tend to occur in elderly men and are thought to be associated with actinic radiation. By contrast, those within the canal tend to be squamous cell carcinomas, which occur in middle-aged to elderly women and are not associated with sun exposure. Morphologically, wherever they arise, they resemble their counterparts in other skin locations, beginning as papules that extend and eventually erode and invade locally. Neither the basal cell nor the squamous cell lesions of the pinna often extend beyond local invasion, but squamous cell carcinomas arising in the external canal may invade the cranial cavity or metastasize to regional nodes and, indeed, account for a 5-year mortality of about 50%.

NECK

Most of the conditions that involve the neck have been described elsewhere (e.g., squamous cell and basal cell carcinomas of the skin, melanocarcinomas, lymphomas), or they are only a component of a systemic disorder (e.g., generalized skin rashes, the lymphadenopathy of infectious mononucleosis or tonsillitis). What remains for consideration here are a few uncommon lesions unique to the neck.

BRANCHIAL CYST (LYMPHOEPITHELIAL CYST)

These benign cysts, usually appearing on the anterolateral aspect of the neck, arise either from remnants of the branchial arches or, as many believe, from developmental salivary gland inclusions within cervical lymph nodes. Whatever their origin, they are circumscribed cysts, 2 to 5 cm in diameter, with fibrous walls usually lined by stratified squamous or pseudostratified columnar epithelium underlaid by an intense lymphocytic infiltrate or, more often, well-developed lymphoid tissue with reactive follicles. The cystic contents may be clear, watery to mucinous fluid or may contain desquamated, granular cellular debris. The cysts enlarge only very slowly over the years, are rarely the site of cancerous transformation, and generally are readily excised. Similar lesions sometimes appear in the parotid gland or the oral cavity, beneath the tongue.

THYROGLOSSAL TRACT CYST

Embryologically, the thyroid anlage begins in the region of the foramen caecum at the base of the tongue, and as the gland develops it descends to its definitive location in the anterior neck. Remnants of this developmental tract may persist, producing cysts, 1 to 4 cm in diameter, that may be lined by stratified squamous epithelium when the cyst is near the base of the tongue or by pseudostratified columnar epithelium in lower locations. Obviously, transitional patterns are also encountered. The connective tissue wall of the cyst may harbor lymphoid aggregates or remnants of recognizable thyroid tissue. If the excision is not complete, stubborn recurrence can be expected. Malignant transformation within the lining epithelium has been reported but is rare.

PARAGANGLIOMA (CAROTID BODY TUMOR)

Paraganglia are clusters of neuroendocrine cells dispersed throughout the body, some connected with the sympathetic nervous system and others with the parasympathetic nervous system. The largest collection of these cells is found in the adrenal medulla, and the tumors of these cells are called pheochromocytomas (see section on adrenal medulla in Chapter 25). Tumors arising in extraadrenal paraganglia, such as the carotid body, are not surprisingly referred to as paragangliomas. Remarks here will be limited to the carotid body tumors, which are sometimes referred to as *chemodectomas*, as explained below. Those arising in paravertebral paraganglia (e.g., organs of Zuckerkandl) and rarely bladder have sympathetic connections, are chromaffin positive, and about half elaborate catecholamines, as do pheochromocytomas. Paraganglia arising in relation to the great vessels, the so-called aorticopulmonary chain, including the carotid bodies, aortic bodies, jugulotympanic ganglia, ganglion nodosum of the vagus nerve, and clusters located about the oral cavity, nose, nasopharynx, larynx, and orbit, are innervated by the parasympathetic nervous system, and their tumors are referred to as nonchromaffin paragangliomas. These tumors infrequently release catecholamines, but because the neuroendocrine cells that make up these lesions sense oxygen and carbon dioxide tensions within adjacent vessels, the tumors are sometimes referred to as *chemodectomas*.

MORPHOLOGY. The **carotid body tumor** is a prototype of a parasympathetic paraganglioma. It rarely exceeds 6 cm in diameter and arises close to or envelops the bifurcation of the common carotid artery. It is often thinly encapsulated and sometimes appears to lack a capsule. The tumor tissue is red-pink to brown and may be hemorrhagic. The microscopic features of all paragangliomas, wherever they arise, are remarkably uniform. They are composed of nests **(zellballen)** of polygonal chief cells enclosed by trabeculae of fibrous and sustentacular elongated cells.[16] The tumor cells have abundant, clear or granular, eosinophilic cytoplasm and rather uniform, round to ovoid, sometimes vesicular, nuclei (Fig. 16–11). Sometimes the cells are spindled. In most tumors there is little cell pleomorphism, and mitoses are scant. Electron microscopy often discloses well-demarcated neuroendocrine granules in paravertebral tumors, but they tend to be scant in nonfunctioning tumors.

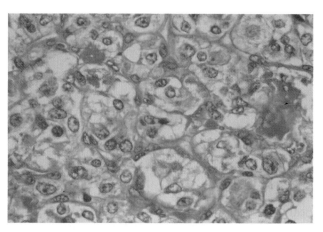

Figure 16–11. Microscopic detail revealing the tumor cells separated into clusters *(zellballen)* by elongated sustentacular cells.

However, the cells in most tumors are argyrophilic and by immunostains reveal neuron-specific enolase as well as possibly other bioactive products (e.g., serotonin, gastrin, somatostatin, bombesin).

Carotid body tumors (and paragangliomas in general) are rare. They occur slightly more often in females, usually in the sixth decade of life. They usually occur singly and sporadically but may be familial, with autosomal dominant transmission in the multiple endocrine neoplasia (MEN) II syndrome (see Chapter 25) and, in this case, are frequently multiple and sometimes bilaterally symmetric. Carotid body tumors frequently recur following incomplete resection, and despite their benign appearance many metastasize to local and distant sites. About 50% ultimately prove fatal largely because of infiltrative growth. Unfortunately, it is almost impossible histologically to judge the clinical course of a carotid body tumor —mitoses, pleomorphism, even vascular invasion are unreliable.[17]

SALIVARY GLANDS

There are three major salivary glands—parotid, submandibular, and sublingual—as well as innumerable minor salivary glands distributed throughout the mucosa of the oral cavity. All these glands, particularly the major ones, are subject to inflammation or to the development of neoplasms.

INFLAMMATION (SIALADENITIS)

Sialadenitis may be of viral, bacterial, or autoimmune origin. The most common form of viral sialadenitis is mumps, in which usually the major salivary glands, particularly the parotids, are affected (epidemic parotitis). Other glands (e.g., the pancreas and testes) may also be involved. Autoimmune disease underlies the inflammatory salivary changes of Sjögren's syndrome, discussed in Chapter 6. In this condition, the widespread involvement of the salivary glands and the mucus-secreting glands of the nasal mucosa induces *xerostomia* —dry mouth; associated involvement of the lacrimal glands produces dry eyes—*keratoconjunctivitis sicca.* The combination of salivary and lacrimal gland inflammatory enlargement with xerostomia is sometimes called *Mikulicz's syndrome,* a noncommittal term to include all forms of involvement of these glands, including sarcoidosis, leukemia, lymphoma, and other tumors, that are sometimes accompanied by xerostomia. Xerostomia may also be secondary to radiation-induced salivary gland atrophy or to drugs (e.g., antihistamines, phenothiazines).

SIALOLITHIASIS AND NONSPECIFIC SIALADENITIS.
Nonspecific bacterial sialadenitis most often involving the major salivary glands, particularly the submandibular glands, is an uncommon condition, usually secondary to ductal obstruction produced by stones *(sialolithiasis).* The common offenders are *Staphylococcus aureus* and *Streptococcus viridans.* The stone formation is sometimes related to obstruction of the orifices of the salivary glands by impacted food debris or by edema about the orifice following some injury. Frequently, the stones are of obscure origin. Dehydration with decreased secretory function may also predispose to secondary bacterial invasion, as sometimes occurs in patients receiving long-term phenothiazines that suppress salivary secretion. Perhaps dehydration with decreased secretion explains the development of bacterial suppurative parotitis in elderly patients with a recent history of major thoracic or abdominal surgery.

Whatever the origin, the obstructive process and bacterial invasion lead to a nonspecific inflammation of the affected glands that may be largely interstitial or, when induced by staphylococcal or other pyogens, may be associated with overt suppurative necrosis and abscess formation. Unilateral involvement of a single gland is the rule. The inflammatory involvement causes painful enlargement and sometimes a purulent ductal discharge.

NEOPLASMS

In view of their relatively undistinguished normal morphology, the salivary glands give rise to a surprising variety of benign and malignant tumors. A classification and the relative incidence of benign and malignant tumors are shown in Table 16–2.

Not included in the table are the rare benign and malignant mesenchymal tumors. As indicated in Table 16–2, only a relatively few epithelial neoplasms make up more than 90% of salivary gland tumors, and so our later consideration can be restricted to them. Overall, these neoplasms are relatively uncommon and represent fewer than 2% of tumors in humans. About 65 to 80% arise within the parotid, 10% in the submandibular gland, and the remainder in the minor salivary glands, including the sublingual glands. Fortunately, only a very small minority (about 15%) of tumors in the parotid glands are malignant, in contrast to about 40% in the submandibular glands and more than half in the minor salivary glands.[18] *The likelihood then of a salivary gland tumor being malignant is inversely proportional to the size of the gland.*

These tumors usually occur in adults, with a slight female predominance, but about 5% occur in children younger than 16 years of age. For unknown reasons, Warthin's tumors occur much more often in males. The benign tumors most often appear in the fifth to seventh decades of life. The malignant ones tend, on average, to appear somewhat later. Whatever the histologic pattern, neo-

Table 16–2. HISTOLOGIC CLASSIFICATION AND INCIDENCE OF BENIGN AND MALIGNANT TUMORS OF THE SALIVARY GLANDS

BENIGN	MALIGNANT

1. Pleomorphic adenoma (45.4%)	Mucoepidermoid carcinoma (15.7%)
	  i. Low grade
	  ii. High grade

2. Warthin's tumor (11%)	Adenoid cystic carcinoma (10%)
3. Lymphoepithelial lesion (0.6%)	Adenocarcinoma (8%)
4. Oncocytoma (0.7%)	Acinic cell carcinoma (3%)
5. Monomorphic adenoma (0.2%)	Malignant mixed tumor (5.7%)
6. Benign cyst (1%)	Epidermoid carcinoma (1.9%) Other anaplastic carcinomas (1.3%)

Data from Memorial Sloan-Kettering Cancer Center Tumor Registry (2807 patients). From Spiro, R.H.: Salivary neoplasms: Overview of a 35-year experience with 2807 patients. Head Neck Surg. 8:177–184, 1966. Copyright © 1966 John Wiley & Sons, reprinted by permission.

plasms in the parotid glands produce distinctive swellings in front of and below the ear. Generally, when first diagnosed, both benign and malignant lesions range from 4 to 6 cm in diameter and are mobile on palpation except in the case of neglected malignant tumors. Although benign tumors are known to have been present usually for many months to several years before coming to clinical attention, cancers seem to demand attention more promptly, probably because of their more rapid growth. Ultimately, however, there are no reliable criteria to differentiate, on clinical grounds, the benign from the malignant lesions, and morphologic evaluation is necessary.

Pleomorphic Adenoma

Because of their remarkable histologic diversity these neoplasms have also been called *mixed tumors*. They represent about 60% of tumors in the parotid, are less common in the submandibular glands, and are relatively rare in the minor salivary glands. In essence, they are composed of epithelial elements dispersed throughout a matrix of mucoid, myxoid, and chondroid tissue. In some tumors the epithelial elements predominate, and in others they are present only in widely dispersed foci.

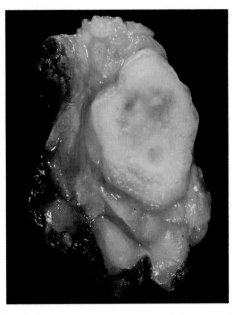

Figure 16–12. Pleomorphic adenoma of the parotid. The transected, sharply circumscribed, yellow-white tumor protrudes above the level of the surrounding glandular substance.

MORPHOLOGY. Most pleomorphic adenomas present as basically rounded, well-demarcated masses rarely exceeding 6 cm in greatest dimension (Fig. 16–12). Although they are encapsulated, in some instances the capsule is not fully developed, and expansile growth produces tongue-like protrusions into the surrounding gland, rendering enucleation of the tumor (in contrast with limited parotidectomy) hazardous. The cut surface is gray-white with variegated myxoid and blue translucent areas of chondroid.

The dominant histologic feature is the great heterogeneity mentioned. The epithelial elements resembling ductal cells or myoepithelial cells are disposed in duct formations, acini, irregular tubules, strands, or sheets of cells. These elements are typically dispersed within a mesenchyme-like background of loose myxoid tissue containing islands of chondroid and, rarely, foci of bone (Fig. 16–13). Sometimes the epithelial cells form well-developed apparent ducts lined by cuboidal to columnar cells underlaid by a layer of deeply chromatic, small myoepithelial cells. In other instances, there may be strands or sheets of myoepithelial cells. In the great majority of instances there is no epithelial dysplasia or evident mitotic activity. There is no difference in biologic behavior between the tumors composed largely of epithelial elements and those composed only of seemingly mesenchymal elements.

Little is known about the origins of these neoplasms save that radiation exposure increases the risk.[19] Equally uncertain is the histogenesis of the various components, but favored today is the view that all neoplastic elements, including those that appear mesenchymal, are of either myoepithelial or ductal reserve cell origin (hence the designation **pleomorphic adenoma**). The recurrence rate (perhaps months to years later) with adequate parotidectomy is about 4% but, with attempted enucleation, approaches 25% because of failure to recognize at surgery minute protrusions from the main mass.

Infrequently (2 to 3% of cases) a carcinoma arises in a pleomorphic adenoma, referred to variously as a *carcinoma ex pleomorphic adenoma* or a *malignant mixed tumor*. Most often there is a long history (10 years or more) of a salivary gland mass or prior attempts at excision. Usually the cancer takes the form of an adenocarcinoma or undifferentiated carcinoma, and often it virtually completely overgrows the last vestiges of the pre-existing pleomorphic adenoma, but to substantiate the diagnosis of carcinoma ex pleomorphic adenoma recognizable traces must be found. Save for an unusually long history of the mass, nothing is known about the influences that underlie this ominous turn of events, and it is not clear that prior surgery contributes. Regrettably, these cancers, when they appear, are among the most aggressive of all salivary gland malignancies, accounting for a 30 to 50% mortality in 5 years.

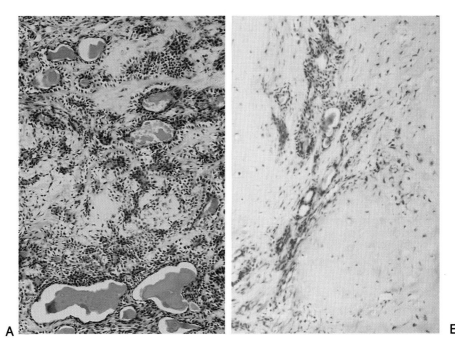

Figure 16–13. Microscopic appearance of a pleomorphic adenoma showing the architectural diversity. *A*, A more cellular area with gland formations and nests of epithelial cells separated by hyaline and collagenous stroma. *B*, A more myxoid area with a scant epithelial component. There is an island of apparent fibrocartilage at the bottom right.

Warthin's Tumor (Papillary Cystadenoma Lymphomatosum)

This curious benign neoplasm with its intimidating histologic name is the second most common salivary gland neoplasm. It arises almost always in the parotid gland (the only tumor virtually restricted to the parotid) and occurs five times more commonly in males than in females, usually in the fifth to seventh decades of life. About 10% are multifocal, and 10% bilateral.

MORPHOLOGY. Most Warthin's tumors (sometimes also called adenolymphomas) are round to oval, encapsulated masses, 2 to 5 cm in diameter, arising in the great majority of cases in the superficial parotid gland, where they are readily palpable. Transection reveals a pale gray surface punctuated by narrow cystic or cleft-like spaces filled with a mucinous or serous secretion. Microscopically, these spaces are lined by a double layer of epithelial cells resting on a dense lymphoid stroma sometimes bearing germinal centers (Fig. 16–14). Frequently the spaces are narrowed by polypoid projections of the lymphoepithelial elements. The double layer of lining cells is quite distinctive, with a surface palisade of columnar cells having an abundant, finely granular, eosinophilic cytoplasm, imparting an oncocytic appearance, resting on a layer of cuboidal to polygonal cells. Oncocytes are epithelial cells stuffed with mitochondria that impart to the cytoplasm the granular appearance. Secretory cells are dispersed in the columnar cell layer, accounting for the secretion within the lumina. Occasionally, there are foci of squamous metaplasia.

The histogenesis of these tumors has long been disputed. The occasional finding of small salivary gland rests in lymph nodes in the neck suggests that these tumors arise from the aberrant incorporation of similar inclusion-bearing lymphoid tissue in the parotids. Indeed, rarely, Warthin's tumors have arisen within cervical lymph nodes, a finding that should not be misconstrued to imply a metas-

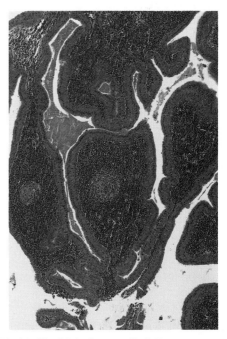

Figure 16–14. Warthin's tumor. Cleft-like spaces separate the lobules of tumor covered by a regular double layer of eosinophilic epithelial cells based on a lymphoid stroma bearing pale germinal centers.

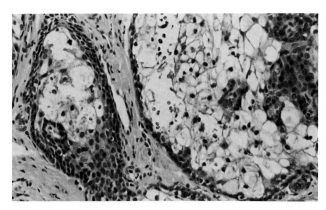

Figure 16–15. Mucoepidermoid carcinoma showing islands having squamous cells at the margins, gradually merging into central masses of mucous and clear cells.

tasis. These neoplasms are usually benign, but there are sporadic reports of malignant tumors.

Mucoepidermoid Carcinoma

These neoplasms are composed of variable mixtures of squamous cells, mucus-secreting cells, and intermediate hybrids. They represent about 10 to 15% of all salivary gland tumors, and while they occur preponderantly (60 to 70%) in the parotids, they account for a large fraction of salivary gland neoplasms in the other glands, particularly the minor salivary glands. Overall they are the most common form of *malignant* tumor primary in the salivary glands and are the most common radiation-induced neoplasm.

MORPHOLOGY. Mucoepidermoid carcinomas range up to 8 cm in diameter and, while apparently circumscribed, lack well-defined capsules and are often infiltrative at the margins. Pale gray-white on transection, they frequently reveal small, mucin-containing cysts. Histologically, the basic pattern is that of cords, sheets, or cystic configurations of squamous, mucous, or intermediate cells. The hybrid cell types often have squamous features, with small to large mucus-filled vacuoles, best seen when highlighted by the periodic acid–Schiff (PAS) stain (Fig. 16–15). The tumor cells may be quite regular and benign-appearing on one end of the spectrum or, alternatively, highly anaplastic and unmistakably malignant. Accordingly, mucoepidermoid carcinomas are subclassified into low, intermediate, or high grades. Low-grade lesions tend to be composed largely of mucus-secreting cells, often forming glandular spaces. On the other hand, high-grade tumors are composed largely of squamous cells with only a scattering of mucus-secreting cells.

The clinical course and prognosis depend on the grade of the neoplasm. Low-grade tumors may invade locally and recur in about 15% of cases, but only rarely do they metastasize and so yield a 5-year survival rate of over 90%. By contrast, high-grade neoplasms and, to a somewhat lesser extent, intermediate-grade tumors are invasive and difficult to excise and so recur in about 25 to 30% of cases and, in 30% of cases, disseminate to distant sites. The 5-year survival rate of these tumors is only 50%.

Other Salivary Gland Tumors

Two less common neoplasms merit brief description, adenoid cystic carcinoma and acinic cell tumor.

Adenoid cystic carcinoma is a relatively uncommon tumor in the parotids but is the most common neoplasm in the other salivary glands, particularly the minor salivary glands about the mouth. Similar neoplasms have been reported in the nose, sinuses, and upper airways and elsewhere.

MORPHOLOGY. Grossly, they generally are small, poorly encapsulated, infiltrative, gray-pink lesions. Histologically, they are composed of small cells having dark, compact nuclei and scant cytoplasm. These cells tend to be disposed in tubular, solid, or cribriform patterns reminiscent of cylindromas arising in the adnexa of the skin. The spaces between the tumor cells are often filled with a hyaline material thought to represent excess basement membrane (Fig. 16–16).

Although slowly growing, these are "sneaky," unpredictable tumors with a tendency to invade perineural spaces (making them the most painful salivary gland neoplasm), and they are stubbornly recurrent. Eventually, 50% or more disseminate widely to distant sites such as bone, liver, and brain, sometimes decades after attempted removal. Thus, although the 5-year survival rate is about 60 to 70%, it drops to about 30% at 10 years and 15% at 15 years. Neoplasms arising in the minor salivary glands have, on average, a poorer prognosis than those primary in the parotids.

The **acinic cell tumor** is composed of cells resembling the normal serous cells of salivary glands. They are relatively uncommon, representing only 2 to 3% of salivary gland tumors. The great majority arise in the parotids, and the small remainder in the submandibular glands. They rarely involve the minor glands, which normally have only a scant number of serous cells. Like Warthin's tumor, they are sometimes bilateral and/or multicentric. They are generally small, discrete lesions that may appear encapsulated. Histologically, they reveal a

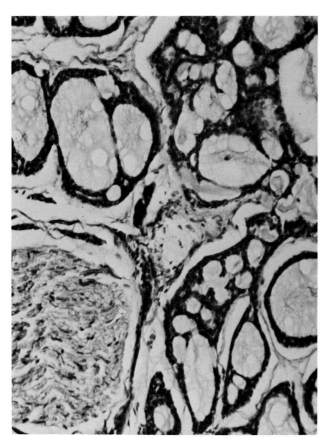

Figure 16–16. Adenoid cystic carcinoma in a salivary gland. The tumor cells have created a cribriform pattern enclosing secretions.

variable architecture and cell morphology. Most characteristically, the cells have apparent cleared cytoplasm, but sometimes the cells are solid or, at other times, vacuolated. The cells are disposed in sheets or microcystic, glandular, follicular, or papillary patterns. There is usually little anaplasia and few mitoses, but occasionally some tumors are slightly more pleomorphic.

The clinical course of these neoplasms is somewhat dependent on the level of pleomorphism. Overall, recurrence following resection is uncommon, but about 10 to 15% of these neoplasms metastasize to lymph nodes. The survival rate is in the range of 90% at 5 years and 60% at 20 years.

1. Hutton, K.P., and Rogers, R.S., III: Recurrent aphthous stomatitis. Dermatol. Clin. 5:761, 1987.
2. Silverman, S., and Shillitoe, E.J.: Etiology and predisposing factors. In Silverman, S. (ed.): Oral Cancer. New York, American Cancer Society, 1985, p. 2.
3. Maitland, M.J., et al.: Detection of human papillomavirus DNA in biopsies of human oral tissues. Br. J. Cancer 56:245, 1987.
4. Hogewind, W.F.C., et al.: Oral leukoplakia with emphasis on malignant transformation: A follow-up study of 46 patients. J. Craniomaxillofac. Surg. 17:128, 1989.
5. Boyle, P., et al.: Recent advances in the etiology and epidemiology of head and neck cancer. Curr. Opin. Oncol. 2:529, 1990.
6. Maitland, N.J., et al.: Detection of human papillomavirus genes in human oral tissue biopsies and cultures by polymerase chain reaction. Br. J. Cancer 59:698, 1989.
7. Cowan, J.M., et al.: Cytogenetic evidence of the multistep origin of head and neck squamous cell carcinoma. J. Natl. Cancer Inst. 84:793, 1992.
8. Carter, R.L.: Patterns and mechanisms of spread of squamous carcinomas of the oral cavity. Clin. Otolaryngol. 15:185, 1990.
9. Hyams, V.J., et al.: Tumors of the upper respiratory tract and ear. Atlas of Tumor Pathology. Second Series, Fascicle no. 25. Washington, DC, Armed Forces Institute of Pathology, 1988.
10. Jones, G.C., et al.: Juvenile angiofibroma. Arch. Otolaryngol. Head Neck Surg. 112:1191, 1986.
11. Whang-Penn, J., et al.: Translocation t (11:22) in esthesioneuroblastoma. Cancer Genet. Cytogenet. 1:155, 1987.
12. Hawkins, E.P., et al.: Nasopharyngeal carcinoma in children—a retrospective review and demonstration of Epstein-Barr viral genomes in tumor cell cytoplasm: A report of the Pediatric Oncology Group. Hum. Pathol. 21:805, 1990.
13. Crissman, J.D., and Zarbo, R.J.: Dysplasia, in situ carcinoma, and progression to invasive carcinoma of the upper aerodigestive tract. Am. J. Surg. Pathol. 13:5, 1989.
14. Barnes, L., and Gnepp, D.R.: Diseases of the larynx, hypopharynx, and esophagus. In Barnes, L. (ed.): Surgical Pathology of the Head and Neck. New York, Marcel Dekker, 1985, p. 156.
15. Hoshikama, T., et al.: Detection of human papillomavirus DNA in laryngeal squamous cell carcinomas by polymerase chain reaction. Laryngoscope 100:647, 1990.
16. Capella, C., et al.: Histopathology, cytology, and cytochemistry of pheochromocytomas and paragangliomas including chemodectomas. Pathol. Res. Pract. 186:176, 1988.
17. Wick, M.R., and Rosai, J.R.: Neuroendocrine tumors of the mediastinum. Semin. Diagn. Pathol. 8:35, 1991.
18. Shah, J.P., and Ihde, J.K.: Salivary gland tumors. Curr. Probl. Surg. 27:779, 1990.
19. Preston-Martin, S.: Prior x-ray therapy for acne related to tumors of the parotid gland. Arch. Dermatol. 125:921, 1989.

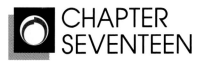

CHAPTER SEVENTEEN

The Gastrointestinal Tract

JAMES M. CRAWFORD, M.D., Ph.D.

Esophagus

NORMAL

The normal esophagus is a hollow, highly distensible muscular tube that extends from the pharynx, at about the level of the C-6 vertebra, to the gastroesophageal junction at the level of the T-11 or T-12 vertebra. Measuring between 10 and 11 cm in the newborn, it grows to a length of about 23 to 25 cm in the adult. Several points of luminal narrowing can be identified along its course—proximally at the cricoid cartilage, midway down in its course at the anterior crossing of the left main bronchus and left atrium, and distally where it pierces the diaphragm. Manometric recordings of intraluminal pressures in the esophagus have identified two high pressure areas that remain relatively contracted in the resting phase. A 3-cm segment in the proximal esophagus at the level of the cricopharyngeus muscle is referred to as the upper esophageal sphincter (UES); another 2- to 4-cm segment in the intra-abdominal portion just proximal to the anatomic gastroesophageal junction is referred to as the lower esophageal sphincter (LES).

In keeping with the structural organization of the gastrointestinal tract, the wall of the esophagus consists of mucosa, submucosa, muscularis propria, and an adventitia. The *mucosa* is composed of a nonkeratinizing stratified squamous epithelial layer that overlies a lamina propria. A small number of specialized cell types, such as melanocytes, endocrine cells, and Langerhans' cells (see Chapter 26), are present in the deeper portion of the epithelial layer.[1] The lamina propria is the nonepithelial portion of the mucosa, above the muscularis mucosa. It consists of areolar connective tissue and contains vascular structures, scattered inflammatory cells, and mucus-secreting glands. Finger-like extensions of the lamina propria, termed "papillae," extend into the epithelial layer. The muscularis mucosa is a delicate layer of longitudinally oriented smooth muscle bundles.

The *submucosa* consists of loose connective tissue containing blood vessels, a rich network of lymphatics, a sprinkling of inflammatory cells, occasional lymphoid follicles, nerve fibers (including the ganglia of Meissner's plexus), and submucosal glands. The submucosal glands are considered to be continuations of the minor salivary glands of the oropharynx and are scattered along the entire esophagus but are more concentrated in the upper and lower portions. The *muscularis propria*, as in

Thanks are given to Drs. Yogeshwar Dayal and Ronald A. DeLellis for the use of material from their chapter "The Gastrointestinal Tract" in the fourth edition of this book.

755

other portions of the gastrointestinal tract, consists of an inner circular and an outer longitudinal coat of smooth muscle with an intervening, well-developed myenteric plexus (Auerbach's plexus). The muscularis propria of the proximal 6 to 8 cm of the esophagus also contains striated muscle fibers from the cricopharyngeus. The relative proportion of these skeletal fibers decreases distally, and in the adult, they normally do not extend beyond the initial 10 to 12 cm. This feature explains why skeletal muscle disorders cause esophageal dysfunction.

In sharp contrast to the rest of the gastrointestinal tract, the esophagus is mostly devoid of a serosal coat. Only small segments of the intra-abdominal esophagus are covered by serosa; the thoracic esophagus is surrounded by fascia that condenses around the esophagus to form a sheath-like structure. In the upper mediastinum, the esophagus is supported in place by this fascial tissue, which forms a similar sheath around adjacent structures. This intimate anatomic proximity to important thoracic viscera is of significance in permitting the ready, widespread dissemination of infections and tumors of the esophagus into the posterior mediastinum. Spread is further facilitated by the rich network of mucosal and submucosal lymphatics that run longitudinally along the esophagus.

The functions of the esophagus, as is well known, are to conduct food and fluids from the pharynx to the stomach and to prevent reflux of gastric contents into the esophagus. These functions require coordinated motor activity: a wave of peristaltic contraction in response to swallowing or to esophageal distention, relaxation of the LES in anticipation of the peristaltic wave, and closure of the LES after the swallowing reflex. The mechanisms governing this motor function are strikingly complex, in part because of the gradation in esophageal muscle composition from proximal to distal. It suffices for our purposes that they involve both extrinsic and intrinsic innervation, myogenic properties, and humoral substances.

The control of the LES function is poorly understood but involves both active inhibition of the muscle by inhibitory neurons and cessation of tonic neural excitation to the sphincter. Although vagal fibers play a role in the maintenance of LES function, truncal or selective vagotomy has virtually no effect on LES tone or relaxation. Maintenance of sphincteric tone is necessary to prevent reflux of gastric contents, which are under positive pressure relative to the esophagus. Although many chemical agents (e.g., gastrin, acetylcholine, serotonin, prostaglandin $F_{2\alpha}$, motilin, substance P, histamine, and pancreatic polypeptide) increase LES tone, whether or not they play a role in normal physiologic function is uncertain. The rather banal anatomy of the esophagus and the LES belies their complex physiology.

PATHOLOGY

Lesions of the esophagus run the gamut from highly lethal cancers to the merely annoying "heartburn" that has affected many a partaker of a large, spicy meal. Esophageal varices, the result of cirrhosis and portal hypertension, are of major importance, because their rupture is frequently followed by massive hematemesis (vomiting of blood) and exsanguination. Esophagitis, achalasia, webs, and hiatal hernias are more frequent but less threatening to life. Distressing to the physician is that all disorders of the esophagus tend to produce similar symptoms.

Dysphagia (subjective difficulty in swallowing) is encountered both with deranged esophageal motor function and with diseases that narrow or obstruct the lumen. *Heartburn* (retrosternal burning pain) usually reflects regurgitation of gastric contents into the lower esophagus. *Pain* and *hematemesis* are sometimes evoked by esophageal disease, particularly by those lesions associated with inflammation or ulceration of the esophageal mucosa. The clinical diagnosis of esophageal disorders often requires specialized procedures, such as esophagoscopy, radiographic barium studies, and manometry.

CONGENITAL ANOMALIES
ATRESIA AND FISTULAS

Although developmental defects in the esophagus are uncommon, they must be corrected early because they are incompatible with life. Because they cause immediate regurgitation when feeding is attempted, they are usually discovered soon after birth. *Absence* (agenesis) of the esophagus is extremely rare; much more common are *atresia* and *fistula formation* (Fig. 17-1). In atresia, a segment of the esophagus is represented by only a thin, noncanalized cord, with a proximal blind pouch connected to the pharynx and a lower pouch leading to the stomach. Atresias are most commonly located at or near the tracheal bifurcation. Because the gut and respiratory tract begin as a single tube embryologically, it is not uncommon to have a fistula connecting the lower pouch with a bronchus or the trachea. Fistulas may less often involve the upper blind pouch. Often associated anomalies are congenital heart disease and malformations of other portions of the gastrointestinal tract. Aspiration and paroxysmal suffocation from food are obvious hazards; pneumonia and severe fluid and electrolyte imbalances also may occur.

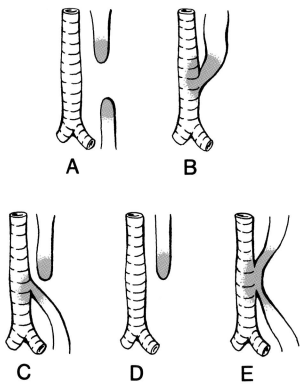

Figure 17-1. Esophageal atresia and tracheoesophageal fistula. Type C, in which the proximal esophagus ends in a blind pouch while the distal segment communicates with the trachea or a main stem bronchus, is the most common variety. (Adapted from Morson, B.C., and Dawson, I.M.P. (eds.): Gastrointestinal Pathology. Oxford, Blackwell Scientific Publications, 1972, p. 8.)

STENOSIS, WEBS, AND RINGS

Non-neoplastic constrictions *(stenoses)* of the esophagus may occur as developmental defects but most often are acquired as the result of severe esophageal injury, as from gastroesophageal reflux, radiation, scleroderma, or caustic injury. Stenosis usually develops in adulthood from inflammatory scarring of the esophagus and consists of fibrous thickening of the esophageal wall, particularly the submucosa, with atrophy of the muscularis propria. The lining epithelium is usually thin and sometimes ulcerated. In severe stenoses, virtually total obstruction may result. Progressive dysphagia, at first to solid foods but eventually to all foods, constitutes the major symptom.

Acquired constrictions caused by *mucosal rings* are uncommon, encountered mostly in women above 40 years of age. Those in the upper esophagus are often designated *webs*, and when the dysphagia is accompanied by anemia, the condition is referred to as the Paterson-Kelly or Plummer-Vinson syndrome. Those in the lower esophagus are designated *Schatzki's rings*, located at or just above

the squamocolumnar junction. Episodic dysphagia is the main symptom associated with webs and rings, usually provoked when an individual bolts solid food. Pain is infrequent. Well-developed webs and rings appear as smooth ledges, rarely protruding more than 5 mm into the lumen, with a thickness of 2 to 4 mm. Upper esophageal webs are covered by squamous mucosa and contain a vascularized fibrous tissue core; lower esophageal rings at the squamocolumnar junction have on their undersurface columnar gastric epithelium.

LESIONS ASSOCIATED WITH MOTOR DYSFUNCTION

Coordinated motor function is critical to proper function of the esophagus; gravity alone is not sufficient to move food from the pharynx to the stomach nor to prevent reflux of gastric contents—witness the blissful suckling of an infant while supine. Four major entities that are caused by or induce motor dysfunction of the esophagus are achalasia, hiatal hernia, diverticula, and lacerations of the esophagus.

ACHALASIA

Achalasia—failure of relaxation with consequent dilatation of the esophagus—is characterized clinically by progressive dysphagia and regurgitation. It usually becomes manifest in young adulthood but may appear in infancy or childhood. Manometric studies show three major abnormalities in the achalasia: (1) aperistalsis, (2) partial or incomplete relaxation of the LES with swallowing, and (3) increased resting tone of the LES.[2]

The pathogenesis of achalasia is poorly understood but may be the result of primary degenerative changes in neural innervation, the basis of which remains obscure. Secondary achalasia may arise from a more identifiable pathologic process. Chagas' disease, caused by *Trypanosoma cruzi*, causes destruction of the myenteric plexus of the esophagus, duodenum, colon, and ureter, with resultant dilatation of these structures. Diseases of the vagal dorsal motor nuclei, particularly polio or surgical ablation, can cause an achalasia-like illness. Other causes include diabetic autonomic neuropathy and infiltrative disorders, such as malignancy, amyloidosis, and sarcoidosis. *In most instances, however, achalasia occurs as a primary disorder of uncertain etiology.*

MORPHOLOGY. Classically, in primary achalasia there is progressive dilatation of the esophagus above the level of the LES. The wall of the esophagus may be of normal thickness, thicker than normal owing to hypertrophy of the muscularis, or markedly thinned out by dilatation. The myenteric ganglia are usually absent from the body of the esophagus but may or may not be reduced in number in the region of the lower sphincter. The mucosal lining may be unaffected, but sometimes inflammation, ulceration, or fibrotic thickening may be evident just above the lower sphincter.

The classic clinical symptom of achalasia is progressive dysphagia. Nocturnal regurgitation and aspiration of undigested food may occur. The most serious aspect of this condition is the hazard of developing esophageal squamous cell carcinoma, said to occur in about 5% of patients, typically at an earlier age than in those without this disease. Other complications include candidal esophagitis, lower esophageal diverticula (see later), and aspiration with pneumonia or airway obstruction.

HIATAL HERNIA

Hiatal hernia is characterized by separation of the diaphragmatic crura and widening of the space between the muscular crura and the esophageal wall. Two anatomic patterns are recognized (Fig. 17–2): the axial, or *sliding hernia* and the nonaxial, or *paraesophageal, hiatal hernia.* The sliding hernia constitutes 95% of cases; protrusion of the stomach above the diaphragm creates a bell-shaped dilatation, bounded below by the diaphragmatic narrowing. In paraesophageal hernias, a separate portion

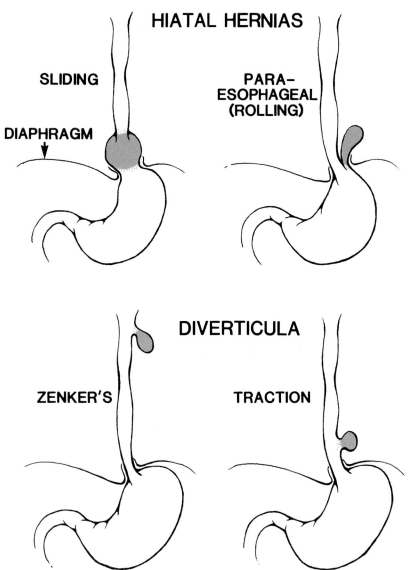

Figure 17–2. Comparison of various forms of hiatal hernias and esophageal diverticula.

of the stomach, usually along the greater curvature, enters the thorax through the widened diaphragmatic foramen.

The cause of hiatal hernia is unknown. Reflux esophagitis (discussed later) is frequently seen in association with sliding hernias, but compromise of the LES with regurgitation of peptic juices into the esophagus may be the result of, rather than the cause of, a sliding hernia. Traction on the esophagus, either during swallowing or as from long-standing inflammation, may accentuate a sliding hernia. Although usually sporadic, the uncommon paraesophageal hernias may be caused by previous surgery, including operations for sliding hernia.

Based on barographic studies, hiatal hernias are reported in 1 to 20% of adult subjects, increasing in incidence with age. Hiatal hernias, however, are well recognized in infants and children. Only about 9% of adults with a sliding hernia suffer from heartburn or regurgitation of gastric juices into the mouth. These symptoms are attributed to incompetence of the LES and are accentuated by positions favoring reflux (bending forward, lying supine) and obesity. Complications of hiatal hernias are numerous. Both types may ulcerate, causing bleeding and perforation. Paraesophageal hernias can become strangulated or obstructed, and early surgical repair has been advocated.

DIVERTICULA

As depicted in Figure 17-2, diverticular outpouchings may develop in the proximal or distal esophagus. Motor dysfunction is implicated in the genesis of the former. The potentially weak junctional area of pharyngeal constrictor muscles in the proximal esophagus is the site of the *pharyngeal (Zenker's) diverticulum*. This is classified as a "pulsion" diverticulum, although the role of increased intraluminal pressure is not established. The mucosal outpouching with submucosa and surrounding fibrous tissue may reach several centimeters in size and be the site of food accumulation with regurgitation (and aspiration) during sleep. More distal esophageal diverticula may develop from a fibrosing mediastinal reaction and are designated *traction diverticula*. Abnormal motility, however, can be demonstrated in the esophagus of most subjects with such diverticula, usually in the form of disordered peristalsis ("spasm").

LACERATIONS (MALLORY-WEISS SYNDROME)

Longitudinal tears in the esophagus at the esophagogastric junction are termed *Mallory-Weiss tears* and are believed to be the consequence of severe retching. They are encountered most commonly in alcoholics, attributed to episodes of excessive vomiting in the setting of toxic gastritis. Normally, a reflex relaxation of the musculature of the gastrointestinal tract precedes the antiperistaltic wave of contraction. During episodes of prolonged vomiting, it is speculated that this reflex relaxation fails to occur.[3] The refluxing gastric contents suddenly overwhelm the constriction of the musculature at the gastric inlet, and massive dilatation with tearing of the stretched wall ensues. Because these tears may occur in persons who have no history of vomiting, other mechanisms must exist; underlying inapparent hiatal hernias have been implicated.

MORPHOLOGY. The linear irregular lacerations are oriented in the axis of the esophageal lumen and are several millimeters to several centimeters in length. **They are usually found astride the esophagogastric junction or in the proximal gastric mucosa** (Fig. 17-3). The tears may involve only the mucosa or may penetrate deeply enough to perforate the wall. The histology is not distinctive. The early lesion is a nonspecific traumatic defect accompanied by fresh hemorrhage into the margins of the defect. A nonspecific inflammatory response follows. Infection of the defect may lead to an inflammatory ulcer or to mediastinitis.

Esophageal lacerations account for 5 to 10% of upper gastrointestinal bleeding episodes. Most often bleeding is not profuse and ceases without surgical intervention, although massive hematemesis may occur. Supportive therapy, such as vasoconstrictive medications, transfusions, and sometimes balloon tamponade, is usually all that is required. Healing is usually prompt, with minimal to no residua.

VARICES

Regardless of cause, portal hypertension, when sufficiently prolonged or severe, leads to the formation of collateral bypass channels wherever the portal and caval systems communicate. The pathogenesis of portal hypertension and the locations of these bypasses are considered in Chapter 18. Here we are concerned with the collaterals that develop in the region of the lower esophagus when portal flow is diverted through the coronary veins of the stomach into the plexus of esophageal subepithelial and submucosal veins, thence into the azygos veins, and eventually into the systemic circulation. The increased pressure in the esophageal plexus produces dilated tortuous vessels called varices. *Varices occur in approximately two-thirds of all cirrhotic patients and are most often associated with alcoholic cirrhosis.* They are less commonly found

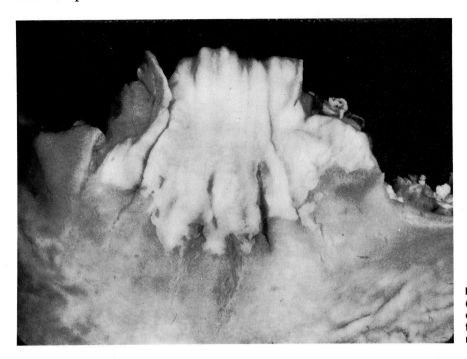

Figure 17-3. Esophageal laceration (Mallory-Weiss tears). Gross view demonstrating longitudinal lacerations extending from esophageal mucosa into stomach mucosa.

in association with other causes of cirrhosis and may be the presenting problem in patients with noncirrhotic portal hypertension, such as portal vein thrombosis (see Chapter 18).

MORPHOLOGY. Varices appear as tortuous dilated veins lying primarily within the submucosa of the distal esophagus and proximal stomach; venous channels directly beneath the esophageal epithelium may also become massively dilated. The net effect is irregular protrusion of the overlying mucosa into the lumen, although varices are collapsed in surgical or postmortem specimens (Fig. 17-4). When the varix is unruptured, the mucosa may be normal, but often it is eroded and inflamed because of its exposed position. **Variceal rupture produces massive hemorrhage into the lumen as well as suffusion of the esophageal wall with blood.** In this instance the overlying mucosa appears ulcerated and necrotic (Fig. 17-5). If rupture has occurred in the past, venous thrombosis and superimposed inflammation may be present.

Varices produce no symptoms until they rupture, when massive hematemesis ensues. Among patients with advanced cirrhosis of the liver, half the deaths result from rupture of a varix. Some patients die as a direct consequence of the hemorrhage, and others of the hepatic coma triggered by the hemorrhage. It must be remembered, however, that even when varices are present, they account for fewer than half of all episodes of hematemesis. Bleeding from concomitant gastritis, esophageal laceration, or peptic ulcer may also be profuse. Factors leading to rupture of a varix are unclear:

silent inflammatory erosion of overlying thinned mucosa, increased tension in progressively dilated veins, and vomiting with increased vascular hydrostatic pressure are likely to play roles. Once begun, the hemorrhage rarely subsides spontaneously, and endoscopic injection of thrombotic agents ("sclerotherapy") or balloon tamponade is

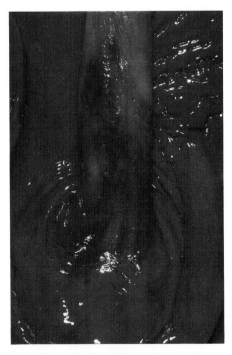

Figure 17-4. Esophageal varices. Gross view of everted esophagus and gastroesophageal junction, showing dilated submucosal veins (varices). The blue-colored varices have collapsed in this postmortem specimen.

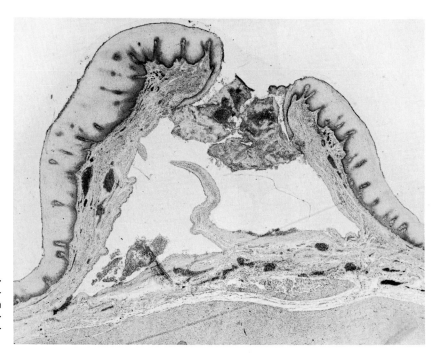

Figure 17–5. Esophageal varix. Low-power cross-section of a dilated submucosal varix that has ruptured through the mucosa. A small amount of thrombus is present within the point of rupture. (Hematoxylin and eosin.)

usually required. When varices bleed, 40% of all patients die during the first episode. Among those who survive, rebleeding occurs in more than half within 1 year, with a similar rate of mortality for each episode.

ESOPHAGITIS

Injury to the esophageal mucosa with subsequent inflammation is common worldwide. In northern Iran, the prevalence of esophagitis is more than 80%; it is also extremely high in regions of China. In the United States and other Western countries, esophagitis is present in about 10 to 20% of the adult population. The inflammation may have many origins, as follows:

- *Reflux esophagitis*, via reflux of gastric contents.
- Prolonged gastric intubation.
- Ingestion of irritants, such as alcohol, corrosive acids or alkalis (in suicide attempts), excessively hot fluids (i.e., hot tea in Iran), and heavy smoking.
- Cytotoxic anticancer therapy, with or without superimposed infection.
- Infection following bacteremia or viremia; herpes simplex viruses and cytomegalovirus are the more common offenders in the immunosuppressed.
- Fungal infection in debilitated or immunosuppressed patients or during broad-spectrum antimicrobial therapy. Candidiasis is the most common; mucormycosis and aspergillosis may occur.
- Uremia.

- Radiation.
- Systemic conditions associated with decreased LES tone, including hypothyroidism, systemic sclerosis, and pregnancy.
- In association with systemic desquamative dermatologic conditions, such as pemphigoid and epidermolysis bullosa.
- Graft-versus-host disease.

PATHOGENESIS. Among these conditions, *reflux of gastric contents (reflux esophagitis) is the first and foremost cause of esophagitis.* Many causative factors are implicated, less well characterized than the name implies:

- Decreased efficacy of esophageal antireflux mechanisms.
- Inadequate or slowed esophageal clearance of refluxed material.
- The presence of a sliding hiatal hernia.
- Increased gastric volume, contributing to the volume of refluxed material.
- Reduction in the reparative capacity of the esophageal mucosa by protracted exposure to gastric juices.

Any one of these influences may assume primacy in an individual case, but more than one is likely to be involved in most instances.

MORPHOLOGY. The anatomic changes depend on the causative agent and on the duration and severity of the exposure. Simple hyperemia may be the only alteration. In uncomplicated **reflux esophagitis**, three features are characteristic (Fig. 17–6):[4] eosinophils, with or without neutrophils, in the epithelial layer; basal zone hyperplasia; and

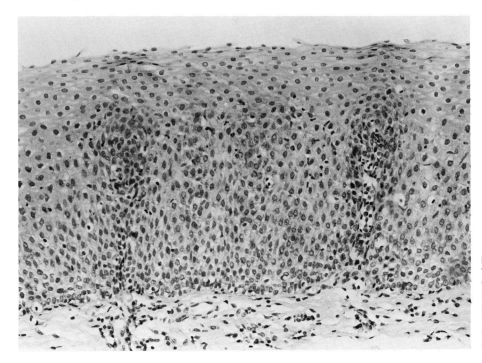

Figure 17–6. Reflux esophagitis. The expanded basal proliferative zone occupies more than half the epithelial thickness. The papillae also are elongated. Intraepithelial eosinophils are not evident at this magnification. (Hematoxylin and eosin.)

elongation of lamina propria papillae. Infiltrates of intraepithelial eosinophils are believed to be the earliest histologic abnormality because they occur even in the absence of basal zone hyperplasia. Intraepithelial neutrophils are markers of more severe injury, such as ulceration, rather than reflux esophagitis *per se.*

The many other causes of esophagitis exhibit their own characteristic features; the final common pathway for all is severe acute inflammation, superficial necrosis and ulceration with the formation of granulation tissue, accumulation of adherent purulent debris, and eventual fibrosis.

• In candidiasis, patches or all of the esophagus become covered by adherent, gray-white pseudomembranes teeming with densely matted fungal hyphae.

• Herpes and cytomegalovirus cause punched-out ulcers of the esophageal mucosa; the nuclear inclusions of herpesvirus are found in a narrow rim of degenerating epithelial cells at the margin of the ulcer, whereas cytomegalovirus inclusions tend to be found in capillary endothelium and stromal cells in the base of the ulcer.

• Pathogenic bacteria account for 10 to 15% of cases of infective esophagitis and cause bacterial invasion of the lamina propria with necrosis of the squamous epithelium.

• Following irradiation of the esophagus, submucosal and mural blood vessels exhibit marked intimal proliferation with luminal narrowing. The submucosa becomes severely fibrotic, and the mucosa exhibits atrophy, with flattening of the papillae and thinning of the epithelium.

• Chemically induced injury (lye, acids, detergents) may produce severe necrosis of the esophageal wall, with hemorrhage and severe inflammation. Localized esophageal ulceration may result from pharmaceutical tablets or capsules "sticking" in the esophagus.

• Graft-versus-host disease shares features with the skin, e.g., karyorrhexis of basal epithelial cells, atrophy, and fibrosis of the lamina propria with minimal inflammation.

Although largely limited to adults older than 40 years of age, reflux esophagitis is occasionally seen in infants and children. The clinical manifestations consist principally of dysphagia, heartburn, and sometimes regurgitation of a sour brash, hematemesis, or melena. *The severity of symptoms is not related closely to the presence and degree of esophagitis;* most people experience reflux symptoms without damage to the distal esophageal mucosa, owing to the short duration of the reflux. Anatomic damage appears best correlated with prolonged exposure of the lower esophagus to refluxed material. Rarely, chronic symptoms are punctuated by attacks of severe chest pain that may be mistaken for a "heart attack." The potential consequences of severe reflux esophagitis are bleeding, development of stricture, and a tendency to develop Barrett's esophagus with its attendant risks.

BARRETT'S ESOPHAGUS

Barrett's esophagus is a complication of long-standing gastroesophageal reflux, occurring in as many

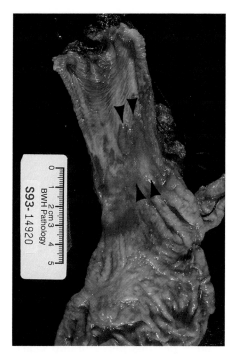

Figure 17-7. Barrett's esophagus. Gross view of distal esophagus *(top)* and proximal stomach *(bottom)*, showing granular zone of Barrett's esophagus *(arrowheads).*

lining. Healing occurs by re-epithelialization and ingrowth of pluripotent stem cells, which in the microenvironment of a low pH in the distal esophagus differentiate into a gastric type (cardiac or fundic) or intestinal type (specialized) epithelium that is more resistant to injury from refluxing gastric contents.

MORPHOLOGY. Barrett's esophagus is apparent as a red, velvety mucosa located between the smooth, pale pink esophageal squamous mucosa and the more lush, light brown gastric mucosa. It may exist as tongues extending up from the gastroesophageal junction, as an irregular circumferential band displacing the squamocolumnar junction cephalad, or as isolated patches (islands) in the distal esophagus (Fig. 17-7). **Microscopically, the esophageal squamous epithelium is replaced by metaplastic columnar epithelium,** as diagrammed in Figure 17-8. **Barrett's mucosa may be quite focal and variable from one site to the next.**

Critical to the pathologic evaluation of patients with Barrett's mucosa is the recognition of associated dysplasia, the presumed precursor of malignancy.[6] Dysplasia is recognized by the presence of cytologic and architectural abnormalities in glandular epithelium, consisting of enlarged, crowded, and stratified hyperchromatic nuclei and loss of intervening stroma between adjacent glandular structures. Dysplasia is classified as **low grade** or **high grade**, with the predominant distinction being a basal orientation of all nuclei in low-grade dysplasia versus nuclei reaching the apex of epithelial cells in high-grade dysplasia. Persistent high-grade dysplasia demands clinical intervention.

as 11% of patients with symptomatic reflux disease. *In Barrett's esophagus, the distal squamous mucosa is replaced by metaplastic columnar epithelium, as a response to prolonged injury.* Barrett's patients tend to have a long history of heartburn and other reflux symptoms and appear to have more massive reflux with more and longer reflux episodes than most reflux patients. It is unknown why the columnar epithelium develops in some patients with reflux and not in others.

The proposed pathogenesis of Barrett's esophagus is as follows:[5] Prolonged recurrent gastroesophageal reflux leads to inflammation and eventually to ulceration of the squamous epithelial

In addition to the symptoms of reflux esophagitis, the clinical significance of Barrett's esophagus relates to the secondary complications of local ulceration with bleeding and stricture. Of greatest

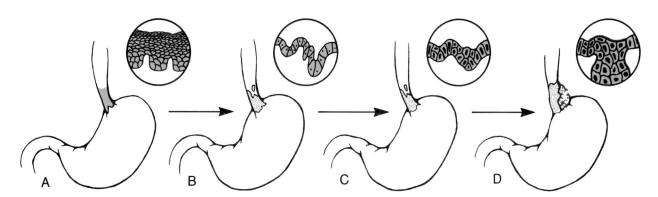

Figure 17-8. Schematic of Barrett's esophagus. The normal esophagus *(A)* is lined by a stratified squamous epithelium. Prolonged gastroesophageal reflux leads to a metaplastic replacement of the squamous epithelium in the distal esophagus by a columnar type of epithelium *(B)*, which is gastric, intestinal, or mixed in composition. In patients with long-standing Barrett's esophagus, the columnar epithelium may become dysplastic *(C)* and eventually lead to development of invasive adenocarcinoma *(D).*

importance is the development of adenocarcinoma, which occurs at an estimated 30-fold to 40-fold increased rate over the general population.

TUMORS

BENIGN TUMORS

Benign tumors of the esophagus are mostly mesenchymal in origin and mural in location, typified by the leiomyoma, which rarely exceeds 3 cm in diameter. Fibromas, lipomas, hemangiomas, neurofibromas, and lymphangiomas may arise. Mucosal polyps are usually composed of a combination of fibrous, vascular, or adipose tissue covered by an intact mucosa, aptly titled *fibrovascular polyps* or *pendunculated lipomas. Squamous papillomas* are sessile lesions with a central core of connective tissue and a hyperplastic papilliform squamous mucosa. In rare instances, a mesenchymal mass of inflamed granulation tissue, called an *inflammatory polyp,* may resemble a malignant lesion, hence its alternative name *inflammatory pseudotumor.*

MALIGNANT TUMORS

In the United States, carcinomas of the esophagus represent about 6% of all cancers of the gastrointestinal tract but cause a disproportionate number of cancer deaths.[7] They remain asymptomatic during much of their development and are often discovered too late to permit cure. With rare exception, malignant esophageal tumors arise from the epithelial layer. For many years, most esophageal cancers were of squamous cell origin, but there has been a declining incidence of these tumors coupled with a steadily increasing incidence of adenocarcinomas. Rare cancers (undifferentiated, carcinoid, malignant melanoma, and adenocarcinomas arising from the submucosal glands) are not discussed here.

Squamous Cell Carcinoma

Most squamous cell carcinomas occur in adults over age 50. The male-to-female ratio falls in the range of 2:1 to as high as 20:1. Although squamous cell carcinoma of the esophagus occurs throughout the world, its incidence varies widely among countries and within regions of the same country. Provinces of northern and eastern China exhibit annual incidence rates exceeding 100 per 100,000, with deaths from cancer of the esophagus constituting more than 20% of all cancer deaths. Other areas of high incidence include Puerto Rico, Iran, South Africa, and the republics of the former

Table 17–1. FACTORS ASSOCIATED WITH THE DEVELOPMENT OF SQUAMOUS CELL CARCINOMA OF THE ESOPHAGUS

DIETARY
Deficiency of vitamins (A, C, riboflavin, thiamine, pyridoxine)
Deficiency of trace metals (zinc, molybdenum)
Fungal contamination of foodstuffs
High content of nitrites/nitrosamines

LIFESTYLE
Alcohol consumption
Tobacco abuse

ESOPHAGEAL DISORDERS
Long-standing esophagitis
Achalasia
Plummer-Vinson syndrome

PREDISPOSING INFLUENCES
Long-standing celiac disease
Ectodermal dysplasia, epidermolysis bullosa
Tylosis
Genetic (racial) predisposition

Soviet Union. In the United States, it affects between 2 and 8 persons per 100,000 yearly and is predominantly a disease of men (male-to-female ratio = 4:1). Blacks throughout the world are at higher risk than are whites, with the incidence being fourfold higher for blacks in the United States.

ETIOLOGY AND PATHOGENESIS. The marked differences in epidemiology strongly implicate dietary and environmental factors (Table 17–1), with an ill-defined contribution from genetic predisposition. The presence of carcinogens, such as fungus-contaminated and nitrosamine-containing foodstuffs in China, may play a significant role in the extraordinary incidence of carcinoma in this region. Dietary deficiencies in vitamins and essential metals have been documented in China and South Africa. Alcohol consumption and smoking are strongly associated with esophageal cancer in Europe and the United States.[8] In the case of alcohol, the risk is related not only to the duration and severity of intake but also to the type of beverage consumed, being higher for hard liquor than for beer or wine. Some alcoholic drinks contain significant amounts of such carcinogens as polycyclic hydrocarbons, fusel oils, and nitrosamines along with other mutagenic compounds. Nutritional deficiencies associated with alcoholism may contribute to the process of carcinogenesis. Such influences cannot underlie the very high incidence of this tumor among the orthodox Muslims of Iran, who neither drink nor smoke. The potential role of human papillomavirus requires further exploration.

It appears that environmental and dietary factors perhaps act synergistically and that nutritional deficiencies possibly act as promoters or potentiators of the tumorigenic effects of carcinogens. Indeed, the chronic esophagitis so commonly observed in persons living in areas of high incidence

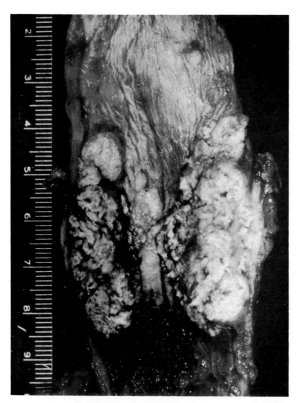

Figure 17-9. Squamous cell carcinoma of the esophagus, just above the gastroesophageal junction. The fungating mass has been transected anteriorly.

may itself be the result of chronic exposure to such carcinogens.[9] This chronic esophagitis results in an increased epithelial cell turnover, which, over a length of time in a continuously carcinogenic environment, progresses to dysplasia and eventually to carcinoma. The rate of progression along the chronic esophagitis-dysplasia-cancer sequence may well be modified or modulated by genetic or racial factors.

MORPHOLOGY. Like squamous cell carcinomas arising in other locations, those of the esophagus begin as apparent **in situ** lesions. When they become overt, about 20% of these tumors are located in the upper third, 50% in the middle third, and 30% in the lower third of the esophagus. Early overt lesions appear as small, gray-white, plaque-like thickenings or elevations of the mucosa. In months to years, these lesions become tumorous masses and may eventually encircle the lumen. Three morphologic patterns are described: **(1) protruded (60%)—a polypoid fungating lesion that protrudes into the lumen** (Fig. 17-9); **(2) flat (15%)—a diffuse, infiltrative form that tends to spread within the wall of the esophagus, causing thickening, rigidity, and narrowing of the lumen;** and **(3) excavated (25%)—a necrotic cancerous ulceration that excavates deeply into surrounding**

structures and may erode into the respiratory tree (with resultant fistula and pneumonia), or aorta (with catastrophic exsanguination), or may permeate the mediastinum and pericardium. The fortunate patient is found at the stage of **superficial esophageal carcinoma,** in which the malignant lesion is confined to epithelial layer (**in situ**) or is superficially invading the lamina propria or submucosa.

Most squamous cell carcinomas are moderately to well differentiated. Regardless of their degree of differentiation, most symptomatic tumors are quite large by the time they are diagnosed and have already invaded the wall or beyond. The rich lymphatic network in the submucosa promotes extensive circumferential and longitudinal spread, and intramural tumor cell clusters may often be seen several centimeters away from the main mass. Local extension into adjacent mediastinal structures occurs early and often in this disease (Fig. 17-10) and seriously limits the chance of curative resection. Tumors located in the upper third of the esophagus metastasize to cervical lymph nodes; those in the middle third spread to the mediastinal, paratracheal, and tracheobronchial nodes; and those in the lower third often spread to the gastric and celiac groups of nodes.

CLINICAL COURSE. Esophageal carcinoma is insidious in onset and produces dysphagia and obstruction gradually and late. Patients subconsciously adjust to their increasing difficulty in swallowing by progressively altering their diet from solid to liquid foods. Extreme weight loss and debilitation result from both the impaired nutrition and the effects of the tumor itself. Hemorrhage and sepsis may accompany ulceration of the tumor. Occasionally, the first alarming symptom is aspiration of food via a cancerous tracheoesophegeal fistula. Although the insidious growth of these neoplasms often leads to large lesions by the time a diagnosis is established, resectability rates have improved (from less than 50% to more than 80%) with the advent of endoscopic screening in patient populations at risk. The five-year survival rate in patients with superficial esophageal carcinoma is about 75%, compared with 25% in patients with more advanced lesions amenable to "curative" surgery, but only 5% for all patients with esophageal carcinoma. Local and distant recurrence after surgery are common. The presence of lymph node metastases at the time of resection significantly reduces the 5 year survival.

Adenocarcinoma

Because of confusion with gastric cancers arising at the gastroesophageal junction, true esophageal adenocarcinomas were thought to be unusual. With

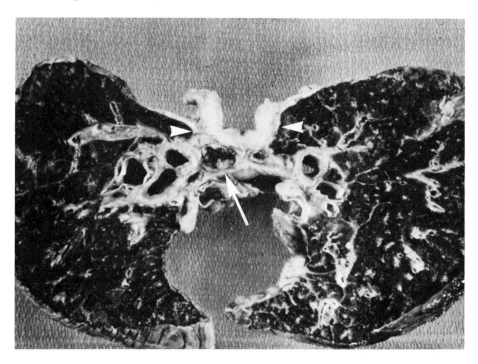

Figure 17–10. Esophageal carcinoma on transverse sectioning of esophagus and lungs. There is a diffuse thickening of the esophageal wall *(arrowheads)* by the infiltrating tumor. Tumor has extended into the tracheobronchial tree, leading to dense adhesions and expansion of the surrounding connective tissues. An anthracotic lymph node also contains metastatic tumor *(arrow).*

increasing recognition of Barrett's mucosa, it is apparent that many adenocarcinomas in the lower third of the esophagus are true esophageal cancers.[10] Accordingly, adenocarcinoma now represents one-quarter of all esophageal cancers reported in the United States and more than one-half of those in the distal third of the esophagus.

MORPHOLOGY. Adenocarcinomas arising in the setting of Barrett's esophagus are usually located in the distal esophagus and may invade the adjacent gastric cardia. Initially appearing as flat or raised patches of an otherwise intact mucosa, they may develop into large nodular masses up to 5 cm in diameter or may exhibit diffusely infiltrative or deeply ulcerative features. At the time of diagnosis, most tumors have invaded through the wall of the esophagus into adventitial tissue.

Microscopically, most tumors are mucin-producing glandular tumors with a histologic spectrum similar to gastric carcinomas (discussed later). The carcinomas may exhibit intestinal-type features or less often are made up of diffusely infiltrative signet-ring cells of a gastric type. The occasional development of squamous cell, adenosquamous, and adenocarcinoid carcinomas supports the concept that Barrett's epithelium arises from pluripotential cells.[11]

CLINICAL COURSE. Adenocarcinomas arising in Barrett's esophagus chiefly occur in patients older than 40 years of age, with a median age in the sixth decade. In keeping with Barrett's esophagus, adenocarcinoma is more common in men than in women, and whites are affected more frequently than are blacks, in contrast to squamous cell carcinomas. As in other forms of esophageal carcinoma, patients usually present because of dysphagia, progressive weight loss, bleeding, chest pain, and vomiting. Long-term symptoms of heartburn, regurgitation, and epigastric pain that are related to concurrent gastroesophageal reflux disease (and sliding hiatal hernias) are present in fewer than half of newly diagnosed patients.

The prognosis of esophageal adenocarcinoma is as poor as that for other forms of esophageal cancer, with a less than 15% 5-year survival rate. Early diagnosis with definitive resection improves 5-year survival to more than 50%. No medical therapy has been shown to decrease the risk of esophageal cancer in patients with Barrett's esophagus. In fact, medical therapy rarely if ever causes disappearance of Barrett's mucosa.[5] Although dysplasia appears to be a requisite precursor for the development of adenocarcinoma, patients with low-grade dysplasia may not progress to cancer over long periods of follow-up, and regression may occur.

Stomach

NORMAL

The stomach is a glandular digestive and endocrine organ that is divided into four major anatomic regions (Fig. 17–11).[12] The *cardia* is the narrow portion of the stomach immediately distal to the gastroesophageal junction. The portion of the proximal stomach that extends above the level of the gastroesophageal junction is called the *fundus,* and the remainder of the stomach proximal to the angle along the lesser curve *(incisuria angularis)* is the *body* or *corpus.* The stomach distal to this angle is the *antrum,* demarcated from the duodenum by the pyloric sphincter. The surface of the stomach exhibits coarse *rugae.* These infoldings of mucosa and submucosa extend longitudinally and are most prominent in the proximal stomach, flattening out when the stomach is distended. A finer, mosaic-like pattern is delineated by small furrows in the surface mucosa. The delicate texture of the mucosa is punctuated by gastric "pits," leading to the gastric glands.

The entire mucosal surface as well as the lining of the gastric pits is composed of surface "foveolar" cells. These tall, columnar, mucin-secreting cells have basal nuclei and crowded, small, relatively clear mucin-containing granules in the supranu-

clear region. Ultrastructurally, these surface cells have a rim of short microvilli around a central dome and a thin apical coating of fine filamentous glycocalyx. Deep within the gastric pits, into which the various glands empty, the surface epithelial cells are modified into so-called *neck cells.* These neck cells have a lower content of mucin granules and are thought to be the progenitors of both the surface epithelium and the cells of the gastric glands. Mitoses are extremely common in this region because the entire gastric mucosal surface is totally replaced every 2 to 6 days.

The *cardiac glands* in the gastric cardia are lined by mucinous cells indistinguishable from the neck cells of the gastric glands. The *gastric (oxyntic) glands* in the body and fundus are composed in the upper regions of mucous neck cells, blending into a zone rich in *parietal cells.* These are recognizable by their bright eosinophilia on hematoxylin and eosin preparations, attributable to their abundant mitochondria. The bases of the glands are a mixture of parietal cells and *chief cells,* the latter rendered distinctive by their large, basophilic, apically oriented zymogen granules. *Pyloric (antral) glands* are composed largely of mucous cells resembling those of the neck regions of the gastric glands. Scattered *neuroendocrine cells* (described later in this chapter) are present along the glandular epithelial layer and are more abundant in the antral region.

PARIETAL CELLS. The hallmark of gastric physiology is acid secretion in the form of hydrochloric acid. The normal human stomach contains approximately 1 billion parietal cells, which in their resting state contain large numbers of intracellular tubulovesicular structures derived from the endoplasmic reticulum. These membranes contain the hydrogen ion pump, a unique hydrogen-potassium-ATPase that pumps hydrogen across membranes in exchange for potassium ions. Within minutes of parietal cell stimulation, the tubulovesicular structures coalesce into an extensive intracellular canalicular network; fusion of this network with the apical membrane generates a vastly increased apically oriented surface for active extrusion of hydrogen ions, which

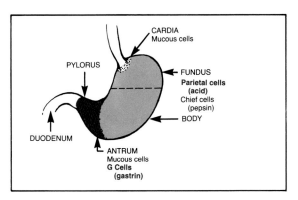

Figure 17–11. Anatomy of the stomach.

is coupled to chloride secretion.[13] *Stimulation of parietal cells can occur by several mechanisms: (1) neural—vagal stimulation; (2) endocrine— primarily gastrin (see later); and (3) local— histamine, released by mast cells.* Vagal and gastrin stimulation act by increasing intracellular calcium, whereas histamine stimulation activates cyclic adenosine monophosphate (cAMP) formation. Parietal cells also produce intrinsic factor, which binds with luminal vitamin B_{12} and facilitates ileal absorption of this vitamin.

CHIEF CELLS. The chief cells, concentrated at the base of gastric glands, are responsible for the secretion of the proteolytic enzymes *pepsinogen I and II*, in proenzyme form.[14] Ultrastructurally, they are classic protein-synthesizing cells, having extensive subnuclear rough endoplasmic reticulum, a prominent supranuclear Golgi apparatus, and numerous apical secretory granules.[12] On stimulation of chief cells by calcium and cAMP-mediated mechanisms similar to those for the parietal cell, the pepsinogens contained in the granules are released by exocytosis. These enzymes are activated by the low luminal pH and inactivated above pH 6 on entry into the duodenum.

STIMULATION OF GASTRIC ACID SECRETION

The process of gastric acid secretion is relevant to the later consideration of peptic ulcer disease. The capacity to secrete hydrochloric acid is directly proportional to the total number of parietal cells in the glands of the body and fundus of the stomach, that is, *the parietal cell mass*. The most important physiologic stimulus to these cells is food in the stomach, but its effect is mediated by humoral and neural mechanisms. *The secretory process is best considered by dividing it into three traditional phases—cephalic, gastric, and intestinal.* The cephalic phase is initiated by the sight, taste, smell, chewing, and swallowing of palatable food. This phase is largely mediated by direct vagal stimulation of gastrin release. The *gastric phase* involves stimulation of mechanical and chemical receptors in the gastric wall. Mechanical stimulation occurs with gastric distention and appears to be mediated by vagal impulses. The chemical stimuli, the most important of which are digested proteins and amino acids, induce the release of gastrin, the most potent mediator of acid secretion. Fat and glucose in the stomach do not stimulate gastric acid secretion. The *intestinal phase* is initiated when food containing digested protein enters the proximal small intestine. The stimulation of acid secretion that occurs at this time is thought to be related to the elaboration in the small intestine of a polypeptide quite distinct from gastrin.

Gastrin is produced by the G cells in the antral, pyloric, and duodenal mucosa. It occurs chiefly as a 17 or 34 amino acid peptide (G-17 and G-34). G-34 has a longer half-life in the circulation and so is the major form present in the blood. G-17, however, is the more potent stimulator of gastric acid secretion. *Histamine* is a potent acid secretagogue, although its importance as a physiologic stimulant of acid secretion remains uncertain. Nevertheless, although surgical interruption of vagal stimulation and thus gastrin release is a time-honored method for reducing peptic acid secretion, inhibition of histamine stimulation by blocking the H_2 receptor on the parietal cell membrane is a highly effective pharmaceutical maneuver. Directly blocking the K^+,H^+-ATPase activity is also quite effective.

GASTRIC MUCOSAL PROTECTION

How does the normal stomach resist the corrosive effects of acid-peptic-gastric secretion? At maximal secretory rates, the intraluminal concentration of hydrogen ion is *3 million times* greater than that of the blood and tissues. Several factors act to protect the gastric mucosa from autodigestion, collectively referred to as "the mucosal barrier."[15]

MUCUS SECRETION. Surface and mucous neck cells in the stomach and duodenum (as well as duodenal Brunner's glands) secrete a thin layer of mucus, which consists of a water-insoluble, viscoelastic gel, with a diffusion coefficient for H^+ that is one-fourth that of water. This gel is also impermeable to large molecules such as pepsin. Its production is stimulated by luminal acid and vagal stimulation, and its release from mucous cells is increased by prostaglandins.

BICARBONATE SECRETION. Both the stomach and the duodenum secrete bicarbonate into the boundary zone of adherent mucus, creating a relatively alkaline microenvironment immediately adjacent to the cell surface. Gastric bicarbonate secretion is about 5 to 10% of maximal acid secretion and is stimulated by luminal acid, mild irritants, vagal stimulation, and prostaglandins. Carbonic anhydrase is present not only in surface foveolar cells but also in parietal cells themselves, perhaps contributing to local protection at the apical cell surface of parietal cells.

EPITHELIAL BARRIER. Mucosal epithelial cells are bound to each other by intercellular tight junctions, providing a barrier to the back-diffusion of hydrogen ions. When the epithelium is disrupted, repair occurs rapidly by the process of *restitution*, in which existing cells migrate along the exposed basement membrane to fill in the defects created by the sloughing of cells.[16] Gastric epithelial cells also can replicate rapidly in response to injury.

MUCOSAL BLOOD FLOW. The gastric mucosa has a rich blood supply consisting of extensively arborizing capillaries. A rich blood flow is necessary to provide oxygen, bicarbonate, and nutrients to epithelial cells and to remove back-diffused acid. Mucosal blood flow is regulated by local vasoactive mediators, particularly endogenous nitric oxide (generated by endothelial cells), prostaglandins, and neuropeptides; increased blood flow occurs simultaneously with stimulation of acid secretion. Just as adequate blood flow is critical to mucosal function, mucosal ischemia may play a key role in promoting mucosal injury. Blood flow may be adversely affected by severe medical or surgical stress, exogenous agents, such as aspirin and alcohol, and entry into the lamina and propria of luminal agents, such as acid and pepsin.[17]

PROSTAGLANDIN PROTECTION. No topic is more controversial than the role of prostaglandins in mucosal function. Exogenous prostaglandins visibly protect the gastric mucosa from experimental alcohol-induced injury, but microscopic damage to surface epithelial cells is still extensive. Although several mechanisms may be operative, such as enhanced mucus secretion and bicarbonate output, the physiologic role of prostaglandin protection remains to be established.

NEURAL AND MUSCULAR COMPONENTS. Afferent neurons within the mucosa of the stomach and perhaps the duodenum can trigger a protective reflex vasodilatation when toxins or acid breach the epithelial barrier. In addition, the muscularis mucosa may serve to limit injury. Superficial damage, limited to the mucosa, can heal within hours to days. When damage extends into the submucosa, a minimum of several weeks is required for complete healing.

Imperfect as our understanding of these defensive mechanisms may be, they are clearly a physiologic marvel, or our gastric walls would suffer the same fate as a piece of swallowed meat.

PATHOLOGY

Gastric lesions are frequent causes of clinical disease. Peptic ulcers have become almost a hallmark of so-called civilized life and develop in up to 10% of the general population in North America. In this day of cigarette smoking, alcohol consumption, and stress, gastritis is one of the everyday causes of "indigestion." Gastric cancer, despite its decreasing incidence in the United States, still remains a leading cause of death from cancer.

CONGENITAL ANOMALIES

Heterotopic rests of normal tissue may be present at any site in the gastrointestinal tract, presumably arising from ectopic embryologic remnants. The most notable are *pancreatic heterotopia* and *gastric heterotopia*. Nodules of essentially normal pancreatic tissue may be present in the gastric or intestinal submucosa, in the muscle wall, or in a subserosal position and are rarely larger than 1 cm in size. When in the pylorus, localized inflammation may lead to pyloric obstruction. Conversely, small patches of ectopic gastric mucosa in the duodenum or in more distal sites may present as perplexing sources of bleeding, owing to peptic ulceration of adjacent mucosa.

DIAPHRAGMATIC HERNIAS

Weakness or partial-to-total absence of a region of the diaphragm, usually on the left, may permit the abdominal contents to herniate into the thorax during *in utero* development. These hernias differ from hiatal hernias (see earlier) in that the defect in the diaphragm does not involve the hiatal orifice. The hernial wall is most often composed only of peritoneum and pleura. Usually, the stomach or a portion of it insinuates into the pouch, but occasionally small bowel and even a portion of the liver accompany it, creating potentially lethal respiratory embarrassment in the newborn (Fig. 17–12). Occasionally, persistent weakness in the diaphragm may allow development of an asymptomatic diaphragmatic hernia in adults.

PYLORIC STENOSIS

Congenital hypertrophic pyloric stenosis is encountered in infants as a disorder that affects males three to four times more often than females, occurring in 1 in 300 to 900 live births. Regurgitation and persistent, projectile, nonbilious vomiting usually appear in the second or third week of life. Physical examination reveals visible peristalsis and a firm, ovoid palpable mass in the region of the pylorus or distal stomach, the result of hypertrophy and possibly hyperplasia of the muscularis propria of the pylorus. Edema and inflammatory changes in the mucosa and submucosa may aggravate the narrowing. Surgical muscle splitting is curative. The mode of inheritance is not firmly established, but multifactorial inheritance is suspected; monozygotic twins have a high rate of concordance of the condition.

Acquired pyloric stenosis in adults is one of the long-term risks of antral gastritis or peptic ulcers close to the pylorus. Gastric carcinomas, lymphomas, or adjacent carcinomas of the pancreas are

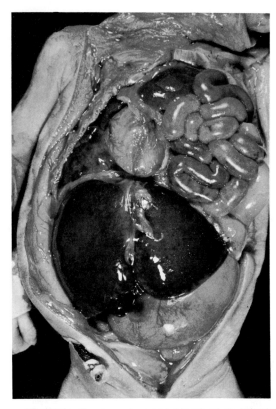

Figure 17–12. *In situ* view of opened trunk of an infant with a diaphragmatic hernia. Numerous loops of small bowel and portions of the colon are evident in the left pleural cavity. The markedly displaced lung can be seen at the very apex of the cavity.

more ominous causes. In these cases, inflammatory fibrosis or malignant infiltration narrows the pyloric channel, producing similar but less striking symptoms than in the infant. In rare instances, the appearance of pyloric stenosis in the absence of an underlying cause raises the possibility of the delayed appearance of the childhood pattern.

GASTRITIS

This diagnosis is both overused and often missed: overused when it is applied loosely to any transient upper abdominal complaint in the absence of validating evidence, and missed because most patients with chronic gastritis are asymptomatic. *Gastritis is simply defined as inflammation of the gastric mucosa.* Inflammation may be predominantly *acute*, with neutrophilic infiltration, or *chronic*, with lymphocytes or plasma cells predominating. Because there is no general agreement on the classification of gastritis,[18] we adhere to this simple distinction between types.

ACUTE GASTRITIS

Acute gastritis is an acute mucosal inflammatory process, usually of a transient nature. The inflammation may be accompanied by hemorrhage into the mucosa and, in more severe circumstances, by sloughing of the superficial mucosa. This severe erosive form of the disease is an important cause of acute gastrointestinal bleeding.

PATHOGENESIS. The pathogenesis is poorly understood, in part because normal mechanisms for gastric mucosal protection are not clear. Acute gastritis is frequently associated with:

- Heavy use of nonsteroidal anti-inflammatory drugs (NSAIDs), particularly aspirin
- Excessive alcohol consumption
- Heavy smoking
- Treatment with cancer chemotherapeutic drugs
- Uremia
- Systemic infections (e.g., salmonellosis)
- Severe stress (e.g., trauma, burns, surgery)
- Ischemia and shock
- Suicidal attempts, as with acids and alkali
- Gastric irradiation
- Mechanical trauma (e.g., nasogastric intubation)
- Following distal gastrectomy

One or more of the following influences are thought to be operative in these varied settings: increased acid secretion with back-diffusion, decreased production of bicarbonate buffer, reduced blood flow, disruption of the adherent mucus layer, and direct damage to the epithelium. Other potential mucosal insults have been identified, such as regurgitation of bile acids and lysolecithins from the proximal duodenum and inadequate mucosal synthesis of prostaglandins. It must be emphasized that a substantial portion of patients have idiopathic gastritis, with no associated disorders.

MORPHOLOGY. In its mildest form, the lamina propria exhibits only moderate edema and slight hyperemia. The surface epithelium is intact, and scattered neutrophils are present among mucosal epithelial cells. **The presence of neutrophils above the basement membrane (within the epithelial space) is abnormal and signifies active inflammation ("activity").** With more severe mucosal damage, erosion and hemorrhage develop. **"Erosion" denotes loss of the superficial epithelium, generating a defect in the mucosa that does not cross the muscularis mucosa. It is accompanied by a robust acute inflammatory infiltrate and extrusion of a fibrin-containing purulent exudate into the lumen.** Hemorrhage may occur independently, generating punctate dark spots in an otherwise hyperemic mucosa, or in association with erosion. Concurrent erosion and hemorrhage is termed **acute erosive hemorrhagic gastritis.** Large areas of the gastric mucosa may be denuded, but the involvement is superficial and rarely affects the entire depth of the mucosa. These lesions are but one step removed from stress ulcers, to be described later.

CLINICAL COURSE. Depending on the severity of the anatomic changes, acute gastritis may be entirely asymptomatic; may cause variable epigastric pain, nausea, and vomiting; or may present with overt hemorrhage, massive hematemesis, melena, and potentially fatal blood loss. Overall, it is one of the major causes of massive hematemesis, as in alcoholics. In particular settings, the condition is quite common. As many as 25% of persons who take daily aspirin as for example, for rheumatoid arthritis, develop acute gastritis, many with bleeding.

CHRONIC GASTRITIS

Chronic gastritis is defined as the presence of chronic mucosal inflammatory changes leading eventually to mucosal atrophy and epithelial metaplasia, usually in the absence of erosions. The epithelial changes may become dysplastic, and constitute a background for the development of carcinoma. Chronic gastritis is notable for distinct causal subgroups, location of disease in the stomach (e.g., antral, corporal), histology, and clinical features. Patterns of gastritis also vary in different parts of the world. The following discussion is based primarily on data from Western patient populations, in whom the prevalence of histologic chronic gastritis exceeds 50% in the later decades of life.[19]

PATHOGENESIS. The major etiologic associations of chronic gastritis are as follows:

- Immunologic, associated with pernicious anemia
- Chronic infection, especially *Helicobacter pylori*
- Toxic, as with alcohol consumption and cigarette smoking
- Postsurgical, especially following antrectomy and gastroenterostomy with reflux of bilious duodenal secretions
- Motor and mechanical, including obstruction, bezoars (luminal concretions), and gastric atony
- Radiation
- Granulomatous conditions (e.g., Crohn's disease; discussed later)
- Miscellaneous—graft-versus-host disease, amyloidosis, uremia

Autoimmune gastritis, also designated *diffuse corporal atrophic gastritis*, reflects the presence of autoantibodies to the gastric gland parietal cells and intrinsic factor. The antibodies to parietal cells include one against the acid-producing enzyme, H^+,K^+-ATPase.[20] Gland destruction and mucosal atrophy lead to loss of acid production. Also lost is production of intrinsic factor, leading to pernicious anemia, as further discussed in Chapter 13. This uncommon form of gastritis is seen in association with other autoimmune disorders, such as Hashimoto's thyroiditis and Addison's disease.

Most cases of chronic gastritis are unrelated to autoimmunity. *Chronic infection* now appears to be the major cause of chronic gastritis, for which *H. pylori* is accorded a major role.[21] This organism is a nonsporing, S-shaped, gram-negative rod measuring approximately 3.5×0.5 μm. *H. pylori* is present in a high percentage of patients with chronic gastritis affecting the antrum and corpus. *H. pylori* colonization rates increase with age, reaching 50% in asymptomatic American adults older than 50 years of age and representing the most common human gastrointestinal infection. In healthy human volunteers ingesting a large dose of *H. pylori*, gastritis developed with acute symptoms,[22] implicating this organism as a primary pathogen. More plausible is the theory that *H. pylori colonization of gastric mucosa damaged by other events leads to a state of retarded healing and chronic mucosal inflammation.* The pathogenic mechanisms remain unclear. Under investigation are the potential roles of alterations in the metabolic milieu, elaboration of bacterial toxins, and induction of a host inflammatory response. Patients with chronic gastritis and *H. pylori* usually improve when treated with antimicrobial agents, and relapses are associated with reappearance of this organism. *Most infected persons remain asymptomatic but are at increased risk for the development of peptic ulcer disease and, possibly, gastric cancer.*

MORPHOLOGY. Chronic gastritis may affect different regions of the stomach and exhibit varying degrees of mucosal damage. **Autoimmune gastritis is characterized by diffuse mucosal damage of the body-fundic mucosa, with less intense to absent antral damage. Gastritis in the setting of environmental etiologies (including infection by *H. pylori*) tends to affect antral mucosa predominantly or both antral and body-fundic mucosa.** Regardless of cause or location, the morphologic features are similar. By visual inspection, the mucosa is usually reddened and has a coarser texture than normal. There may be some flattening of the mucosa. Alternatively, the inflammation may create a boggy-appearing mucosa with thickened rugal folds, mimicking early infiltrative disease. With more severe chronic gastritis, the mucosa becomes more obviously thinned and flattened.

By microscopy, an inflammatory infiltrate of lymphocytes and plasma cells is present within the lamina propria. In the early stages, this infiltrate is usually limited to the upper third of the gastric mucosa **(chronic superficial gastritis; Fig. 17–13).** In more severe forms, the inflammatory infiltrate in-

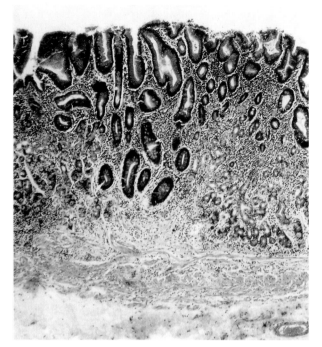

Figure 17–13. Chronic superficial gastritis. An intense chronic inflammatory infiltrate involves the upper portion of the mucosa, and there is regenerative change of glands with nuclear hyperchromasia. (Hematoxylin and eosin.)

volves the full thickness of the mucosa. Lymphoid aggregates, some with germinal centers, are frequently observed in the mucosa. Several additional histologic features are characteristic.

Activity. "Active" inflammation is signified by the presence of neutrophils within the surface and glandular epithelial layer.

Regenerative Change. The response of the epithelium to injury is increased mitotic activity in the neck region of the gastric glands. The less mature cells that populate the mucosa exhibit enlarged, hyperchromatic nuclei, and diminished to absent mucin vacuoles.

Metaplasia. Metaplastic columnar absorptive cells and mucous goblet cells of intestinal phenotype (primarily small intestine) may partially replace portions of the gastric mucosa. The body-fundic mucosa also may exhibit the simpler glands characteristic of the antral-pyloric region.

Atrophy. Atrophic change is evident by marked loss in glandular structures corresponding to the mucosal flattening observed grossly. Parietal cells, in particular, may be conspicuously absent in the autoimmune form, accompanied by compensatory hyperplasia of the gastrin-producing cells in the antral mucosa. Atrophy may be seen in persons of advanced age, without other features of gastritis.

H. pylori. **In chronic gastritis affecting the antrum or antrum and corpus, *H. pylori* is present in the superficial mucous layer and among the microvilli of epithelial cells in 95% of active cases and in 65% of quiescent cases.**[23] The organisms lie along the luminal surfaces of epithelial cells; they do not invade the mucosa. This is most easily demonstrated with Giemsa or Warthin-Starry stains (Fig. 17–14). The distribution of organisms can be patchy and irregular, with areas of heavy colonization adjacent to those with no organisms. Even in heavily colonized stomachs, **the organisms are absent from areas with intestinal metaplasia.**

Dysplasia. With long-standing chronic gastritis, the epithelium develops cytologic alterations, including variation in size, shape, and orientation of epithelial cells and nuclear enlargement and atypia. **Dysplastic alterations may become so severe as to constitute in situ carcinoma.** As such, they probably account for the increased incidence of gastric cancer observed in chronic gastritis, particularly the atrophic forms.

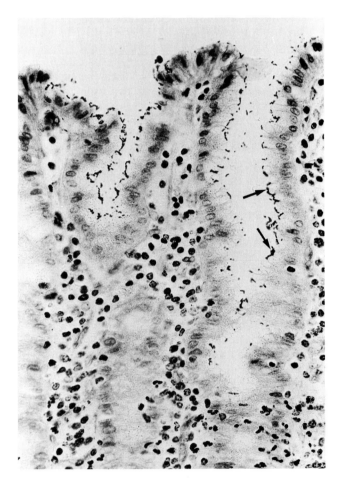

Figure 17–14. Helicobacter gastritis. A Warthin-Starry stain showing large numbers of Helicobacter organisms along the luminal surface of the gastric epithelial cells *(arrows).* Note that no tissue invasion is present.

CLINICAL FEATURES. Chronic gastritis usually causes few symptoms. Nausea, vomiting, and upper abdominal discomfort may occur. When severe parietal cell loss occurs in the setting of autoimmune gastritis, hypochlorhydria or achlorhydria and hypergastrinemia are characteristically present. Circulating gastric autoantibodies may be present or absent. A small subset of these patients (10%) may develop overt pernicious anemia after a period of years. The familial occurrence of pernicious anemia is well established; a high prevalence of gastric autoantibodies is also found in asymptomatic relatives of patients with pernicious anemia. The distribution suggests that the inheritance of autoimmune gastritis is autosomal dominant.[24]

Individuals with advanced antral or pangastritis associated with environmental etiologies are often hypochlorhydric, owing to parietal cell damage and atrophy of body-fundic mucosa. Because parietal cells are never completely destroyed, however, these patients do not develop achlorhydria or pernicious anemia. These patients do not have circulating antibodies to parietal cells or intrinsic factor, and have no associated autoimmune diseases.

Most important is the relationship of chronic gastritis to the development of peptic ulcer and gastric carcinoma (see later). Most patients with a peptic ulcer, whether duodenal or gastric, have antral or pangastritis that persists after the ulcer heals, suggesting that the gastritis is primary. The long-term risk of gastric carcinoma for persons with gastric atrophy is in the range of 2 to 4%, which is considerably greater than that for the normal population.

GASTRIC ULCERATION

Ulcers are defined as a breach in the mucosa of the alimentary tract, which extends through the muscularis mucosa into the submucosa or deeper. Although they may occur anywhere in the alimentary tract, none are as prevalent as the chronic peptic ulcers that occur in the duodenum and stomach. Acute gastric ulcers may also appear under conditions of severe systemic stress.

PEPTIC ULCERS

Peptic ulcers are chronic, most often solitary, lesions that occur in any portion of the gastrointestinal tract exposed to the aggressive action of acid-peptic juices. Both the acid and the pepsin are critical. The definition should be further qualified as in Table 17–2. The epidemiology and morphology of peptic ulcers are described, before addressing the putative causes.

Table 17–2. DISTINCTIVE FEATURES OF PEPTIC ULCERS

Usually a single lesion
Tends to be less than 4 cm in diameter
By definition, penetrates muscularis mucosa; may perforate gastric wall
Is frequently recurrent, with intermittent healing
Is located in the following sites, with decreasing frequency:
    Duodenum, first portion
    Stomach, usually antrum
    Within Barrett's mucosa
    In the margins of a gastroenterostomy (stomal ulcer)
    In the duodenum, stomach, or jejunum of patients with Zollinger-Ellison syndrome
    Within or adjacent to a Meckel's diverticulum that contains ectopic gastric mucosa

EPIDEMIOLOGY. In the United States, approximately 4 million people have peptic ulcers (duodenal and gastric), and 350,000 new cases are diagnosed each year. Around 100,000 patients are hospitalized yearly, and about 3000 people die each year as a result of peptic ulcer disease. The lifetime likelihood of developing a peptic ulcer is about 10% for American men and 4% for women.[25]

Peptic ulcers are remitting, relapsing lesions that are most often diagnosed in middle-aged to older adults, but they may first become evident in young adult life. They often appear without obvious precipitating influences and may then, after a period of weeks to months of active disease, heal with or without therapy. *Even with healing, however, the propensity to develop peptic ulcers remains.* Hence "once a peptic ulcer patient, always a peptic ulcer patient." Thus, it is difficult to obtain accurate data on the prevalence of active disease. Based on autopsy studies and population surveys, the best estimates indicate a prevalence of 6 to 14% for men and 2 to 6% for women. The male-to-female ratio for duodenal ulcers is about 3 : 1 and for gastric ulcers about 1.5 to 2 : 1. Women are most often affected at, or after, menopause. For unknown reasons, there has been a significant decrease in the prevalence of duodenal ulcers over the past decades but little change in the prevalence of gastric ulcers. No significant racial differences have been identified.

Genetic influences appear to play little or no role with peptic ulcer. *Duodenal ulcer is more frequent in patients with alcoholic cirrhosis, chronic obstructive pulmonary disease, chronic renal failure, and hyperparathyroidism.* In the last two conditions, we should note that hypercalcemia, whatever its cause, stimulates gastrin production and therefore acid secretion. The epidemiologic differences for duodenal and gastric ulcers raise the suspicion that these processes represent different diseases, sharing only ulceration as the final common pathway. The lack of a clear understanding of the basic pathogenesis of peptic ulcer disease, however, limits attempts to differentiate duodenal and gastric peptic ulcer disease further.

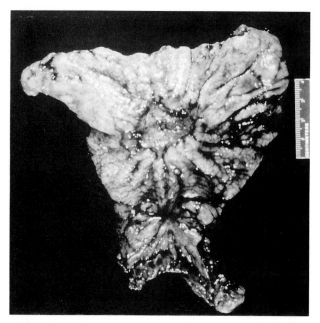

Figure 17–15. Peptic ulcer. A large, deeply excavated ulcer is present at the junction of the gastric antrum and body. The specimen has been opened along the greater curvature; the pylorus is in the lower portion of the field and has adherent blood clot.

MORPHOLOGY. At least 98% of peptic ulcers are located in the first portion of the duodenum or in the stomach, in a ratio of about 4:1. Most duodenal ulcers occur in the first portion of the duodenum, generally within a few centimeters of the pyloric ring. The anterior wall of the duodenum is more often affected than the posterior wall. Gastric ulcers are predominantly located along the lesser curvature, in or around the border zone between the corpus and the antral mucosa. Less commonly, they may occur on the anterior or posterior walls or along the greater curvature. Although the great majority of individuals have a single ulcer, in 10 to 20% of patients with gastric ulceration, there may be a coexistent duodenal ulcer.

Wherever they occur, chronic peptic ulcers have a fairly standard, virtually diagnostic gross appearance (Fig. 17–15). Small lesions (less than 0.3 cm) are most likely to be shallow erosions; those larger than 0.6 cm are likely to be ulcers. Although more than 50% of peptic ulcers have a diameter less than 2 cm, about 10% of benign ulcers are greater than 4 cm. Because carcinomatous ulcers may be less than 4 cm in diameter, **size does not differentiate a benign from a malignant ulcer.**

The classic peptic ulcer is a round-to-oval, sharply punched-out defect with relatively straight walls. The mucosal margin may overhang the base slightly, particularly on the upstream portion of the circumference. The margins are usually level with the surrounding mucosa or only slightly elevated (Fig. 17–16). Heaping-up of these margins is rare in the benign ulcer but is characteristic of the malignant lesion. The depth of these ulcers varies from superficial lesions involving only the mucosa and muscularis mucosa to deeply excavated ulcers having their bases on the muscularis propria. When the entire wall is penetrated, the base of the ulcer may be formed by adherent pancreas, omental

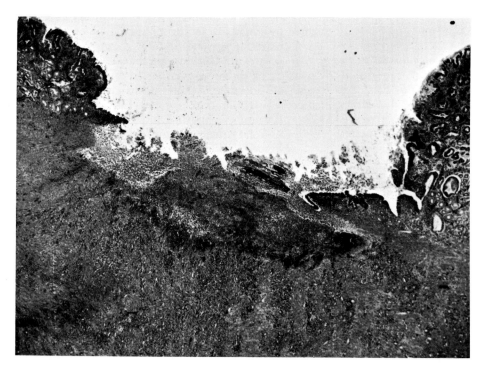

Figure 17–16. Low-power view of a peptic ulcer to illustrate depth of lesion. (Hematoxylin and eosin.)

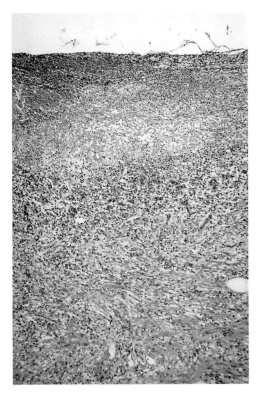

Figure 17–17. High-power detail of base of an ulcer, demonstrating some of the zones that constitute the inflammatory response. The lumen and zone of necrosis is above. (Hematoxylin and eosin.)

fat, or liver. Free perforation into the peritoneal cavity may occur.

The base of a peptic ulcer is smooth and clean to inspection, owing to peptic digestion of any exudate. At times, thrombosed or patent blood vessels (the source of life-threatening hemorrhage) are evident in the base of the ulcer. Scarring may involve the entire thickness of the stomach; puckering of the surrounding mucosa creates mucosal folds that radiate from the crater in a spoke-like fashion. The gastric mucosa surrounding a gastric ulcer is somewhat edematous and reddened, owing to the almost invariable gastritis.

The histologic appearance varies from active necrosis, to chronic inflammation and scarring, to healing. In active ulcers with ongoing necrosis, four zones are demonstrable: (1) The base and margins have a superficial thin layer of necrotic fibrinoid debris not visible to the naked eye; (2) beneath this layer is the zone of a nonspecific inflammatory infiltrate, with neutrophils predominating; (3) in the deeper layers, especially in the base of the ulcer, there is active granulation tissue infiltrated with mononuclear leukocytes; and (4) the granulation tissue rests on a more solid fibrous or collagenous scar (Fig. 17–17). Vessel walls within the scarred area are typically thickened by the surrounding inflammation and are occasionally thrombosed.

Chronic gastritis is virtually universal among patients with peptic ulcer disease, occurring in 85 to 100% of patients with duodenal ulcers and 65% with gastric ulcers. H. pylori infection is almost always demonstrable in these patients with gastritis.[21] Gastritis remains after the ulcer has healed; recurrence of the ulcer does not appear to be related to progression of the gastritis. This feature is helpful in distinguishing peptic ulcers from acute erosive gastritis or stress ulcers because gastritis in adjacent mucosa is generally absent in the latter two conditions.

PATHOGENESIS. The more that is written about a problem, the less is understood. Reams are devoted to the pathogenesis of peptic ulceration, but we are left only with the generalization that *peptic ulcers are produced by an imbalance between the gastroduodenal mucosal defense mechanisms and the damaging forces,* as diagrammed in Figure 17–18. Incorporation of the many countervailing influences into a unifying theory is not possible because pieces are missing from the puzzle. Moreover, there may be subsets of peptic ulcers involving different pathogenic pathways (e.g., duodenal versus gastric ulcers).

Gastric acid and pepsin are requisite for all peptic ulcerations.[26] *The importance of the acid is evidenced by the Zollinger-Ellison syndrome* (see section on carcinoid tumors, later in this chapter) *with its multiple peptic ulcerations, owing to excess gastrin secretion and acid production.* Nevertheless, only a minority of patients with duodenal ulcers have hyperacidity and only very few with gastric ulcers. The basis for the hyperacidity, when present, is not always clear. Possible causes are increased parietal cell mass, increased sensitivity to secretory stimuli, increased basal acid secretory drive, or impaired inhibition of stimulatory mechanisms such as gastrin release. In some patients with duodenal ulcers, there is too rapid gastric emptying, exposing the duodenal mucosa to an excessive acid load.

The apparent role of H. pylori in peptic ulceration cannot be overemphasized. H. pylori infection of gastric mucosa is present in 90 to 100% of patients with duodenal ulcer and 70% of those with gastric ulcer. Gastric ulcerogenesis presumably results from the action of bacterial *urease,* which generates ammonia, and *protease,* which breaks down glycoproteins in the gastric mucus. Damage to the protective mucus layer exposes the underlying epithelial cells to the damaging influence of acid-peptic digestion and may thus lead to inflammation. The chronically inflamed mucosa is more susceptible to acid-peptic injury and is thus more prone to peptic ulceration. This sequence of events may explain why gastric ulcers are so frequently located in the sites of chronic inflammation, such as the antrum. Gastric ulcers also develop fre-

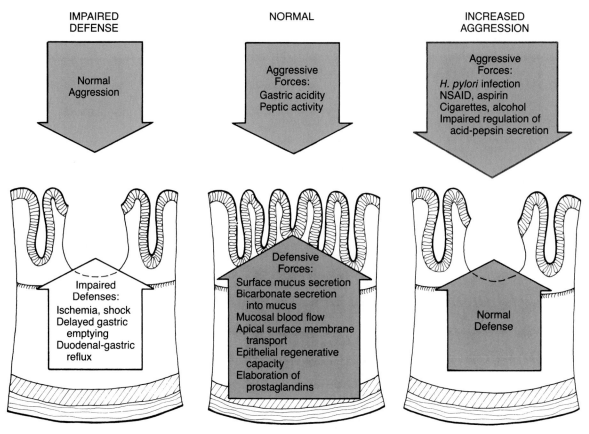

Figure 17–18. Diagram of aggravating causes of and defense mechanisms against peptic ulceration.

quently at the junction of antral and body-fundic mucosa, that is, the division between inflamed antral mucosa and normal acid-secreting mucosa. In the case of pangastritis, the more extensive the gastritis, the more proximal the gastric ulcer. Proximal gastric ulcers also occur with increased frequency in the elderly, coincident with the proximal migration of the antral-body mucosal junction with age. The mechanisms by which *H. pylori* promotes duodenal ulcerogenesis, and the reasons for the greater prevalence of *H. pylori* with this condition, remain a mystery, because the infectious process is limited to the gastric mucosa.

Impaired mucosal defense must be invoked in those ulcer patients with normal levels of gastric acid and pepsin and no demonstrable *H. pylori*. No specific defects in secretion of mucus and surface bicarbonate or in mucosal blood flow, however, can be clearly demonstrated in ulcer patients. Only with those patients chronically using NSAIDs, including aspirin, can a finger be pointed with some assurance at suppression of mucosal prostaglandin synthesis and a direct irritative, topical effect of the aspirin.[27] Nevertheless, effective treatment of peptic ulcers includes agents that increase mucus secretion, pointing out the importance of effective defense mechanisms.

Other possible ulcerogenic influences require mention. *Cigarette smoking* impairs healing and favors recurrence and so is suspected of being ulcerogenic, possibly by suppression of mucosal prostaglandin synthesis. *Alcohol* has not been proved to cause peptic ulceration directly,[17] but alcoholic cirrhosis is associated with an increased incidence of peptic ulcers. *Corticosteroids* in high dose and with repeated use have been implicated in promoting ulcers. Finally, there are compelling arguments that *personality* and *psychologic stress* are important contributing factors,[28] even though hard data on cause and effect are lacking. It is clear that we might well develop ulcers trying to fathom their cause(s).

CLINICAL COURSE. The great majority of peptic ulcers cause epigastric gnawing, burning, or aching pain. The pain tends to be worse at night and occurs usually 1 to 3 hours after meals during the day. Classically the pain is relieved by alkalis or food, but there are many exceptions. Occasionally, with penetrating ulcers the pain is referred to the back, the left upper quadrant, or chest. As with gastroesophageal reflux, the pain may be misinterpreted as being of cardiac origin. A significant minority first come to light with complications such as anemia, frank hemorrhage, or perforation. Nausea, vomiting, bloating, belching, and significant weight loss (raising the specter of some hidden malignancy) are additional manifestations. The

Table 17–3. COMPLICATIONS OF PEPTIC ULCER DISEASE

Bleeding
    Occurs in 25–33% of patients
    Most frequent complication
    May be life-threatening
    Accounts for 25% of ulcer deaths
    May be first indication of an ulcer
Perforation
    Occurs in about 5% of patients
    Accounts for two-thirds of ulcer deaths
    Rarely is first indication of an ulcer
Obstruction from edema or scarring
    Most often due to pyloric channel ulcers
    May also occur with duodenal ulcers
    Causes incapacitating, crampy abdominal pain
    Rarely may lead to total obstruction with intractable vomiting
Intractable pain

diagnosis rests ultimately on various imaging techniques and endoscopy. Collectively, these methods can accurately detect and diagnose more than 98% of peptic ulcers. Gastric analyses for acidity, endoscopic biopsy, and cytologic examinations of gastric aspirate or brushings help to establish the absence or presence of malignancy and chronic gastritis (both of which have treatment implications).

Peptic ulcers are notoriously chronic, recurring lesions. They more often impair the quality of life than shorten it. When untreated, the average individual requires 15 years for healing of either a duodenal or gastric ulcer.[29] With present-day therapies aimed at neutralization of gastric acid, promotion of mucus secretion, and inhibition of acid secretion (H_2 receptor antagonists and parietal cell H^+,K^+-ATPase inhibitors), most ulcer victims escape the surgeon's knife. The complications of peptic ulcer disease are shown in Table 17–3. Malignant transformation is unknown with duodenal ulcers and is extremely rare with gastric ulcers and is always open to the possibility that the seemingly benign lesion was from the outset a deceptive, ulcerative, gastric carcinoma. In addition, the underlying tendency to dysplasia and carcinoma relates primarily to the associated chronic gastritis, rather than to the ulcer *per se.*

ACUTE GASTRIC ULCERATION

Focal, acutely developing gastric mucosal defects may appear following severe stress, whatever its nature—hence the designation *stress ulcers.* Generally, there are multiple lesions located mainly in the stomach and occasionally in the duodenum. They range in depth from mere shedding of the superficial epithelium *(erosion)* to deeper lesions that involve the entire mucosal thickness *(ulceration).* The shallow erosions are, in essence, an extension of acute erosive gastritis (discussed earlier). The deeper lesions comprise well-defined ulcerations but are not precursors of chronic peptic ulcers, having a totally different pathobiology.

Stress erosions and ulcers are most commonly encountered in patients with shock, extensive burns, sepsis or severe trauma and conditions that raise intracranial pressure (such as head trauma or brain surgery) (Cushing's ulcers); and following intracranial surgery. Those occurring in the proximal duodenum and associated with severe burns or trauma are called *Curling's ulcers.* Drugs, particularly NSAIDs, also may cause acute gastric ulceration.

The genesis of the acute mucosal defects in these varied clinical settings is poorly understood. No doubt, many factors are shared with the less severe acute gastritis, such as impaired oxygenation. In the case of cranial lesions, direct stimulation of vagal nuclei by increased intracranial pressure (leading to hypersecretion of gastric acid) is proposed, but hyperacidity is not seen in other settings. Systemic acidosis, a common finding in these clinical settings, may contribute to mucosal compromise, presumably by lowering the intracellular pH of mucosal cells already rendered hypoxic by stress-induced splanchnic vasoconstriction.

MORPHOLOGY. Acute gastric ulcers are usually less than 1 cm in diameter, are circular and small, and rarely penetrate beyond the mucosa. The ulcer base is frequently stained a dark brown by the acid digestion of extruded blood. In contrast to chronic peptic ulcers, acute stress ulcers are found anywhere in the stomach. They may occur singly or, more often, multiply throughout the stomach and duodenum. The gastric rugal pattern is essentially normal, and the margins and base of the ulcer are not indurated. Microscopically, acute stress ulcers are abrupt lesions, with essentially unremarkable adjacent mucosa. Depending on the duration of the ulceration, there may be a suffusion of blood into the mucosa and submucosa and some inflammatory reaction. Conspicuously absent are scarring and thickening of blood vessels, as seen in chronic peptic ulcers. Healing with complete re-epithelialization occurs after the causative factors are removed. The time required for complete healing varies from days to several weeks.

CLINICAL COURSE. About 5 to 10% of patients admitted to hospital intensive care units acutely develop superficial gastric erosions or ulcers. These may be asymptomatic or may create a hemodynamic emergency because potentially lethal bleeding can occur. Although prophylactic antacid regimens and blood transfusions may blunt the impact of stress ulceration, *the single most important determinant of clinical outcome is the ability to correct underlying condition(s).* The gastric mucosa can recover completely if the patients do not succumb to the primary disease.

MISCELLANEOUS CONDITIONS

HYPERTROPHIC GASTROPATHY

This designation encompasses a group of uncommon conditions, all characterized by giant cerebriform enlargement of the rugal folds of the gastric mucosa (Fig. 17–19). The rugal enlargement is caused not by inflammation but by hyperplasia of the mucosal epithelial cells. *Three variants are recognized:*[30]

- *Ménètrier's disease,* resulting from profound hyperplasia of the surface mucous cells with accompanying glandular atrophy

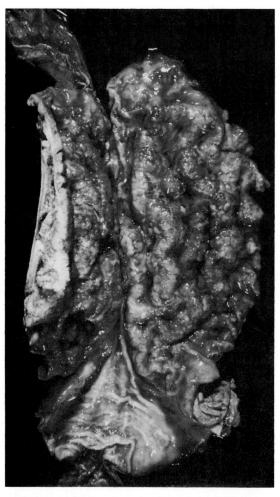

Figure 17–19. Hypertrophic gastropathy, sparing the antral region below. Marked thickening of rugal folds simulates diffuse neoplastic infiltration.

- *Hypertrophic-hypersecretory gastropathy,* associated with hyperplasia of the parietal and chief cells within gastric glands
- *Gastric gland hyperplasia secondary to excessive gastrin secretion,* in the setting of a gastrinoma (*Zollinger-Ellison syndrome*)

All three conditions are of clinical importance for two reasons: (1) *They may mimic infiltrative carcinoma or lymphoma of the stomach on radiographic examinations,* and (2) the enormous increase in acid secretions in the latter two conditions places patients at risk for peptic ulceration.

Ménètrier's disease, an idiopathic condition, is most often encountered in men (ratio 3 : 1) in the fourth to sixth decades of life but occasionally in children. Although the disorder may be asymptomatic, it often produces epigastric discomfort, diarrhea, weight loss, and sometimes bleeding related to superficial rugal erosions. The hypertrophic change may involve the body-fundus or antrum predominantly or affect the entire stomach. The gastric secretions contain excessive mucus and in many instances little to no hydrochloric acid owing to glandular atrophy. In some patients, there may be sufficient protein loss in the gastric secretions to produce hypoalbuminemia and peripheral edema, thus constituting a form of *protein-losing gastroenteropathy.* Infrequently, the mucosal hyperplasia becomes metaplastic, providing a soil for the development of gastric carcinoma.

GASTRIC VARICES

Gastric varices develop in the setting of portal hypertension[31] but less often than esophageal varices (discussed earlier). Most gastric varices lie within 2 to 3 cm of the gastroesophageal junction, arising from longitudinally placed submucosal veins. They often appear as mass-like nodular and tortuous winding elevations of the mucosa in the cardia or fundus. Owing to their deep submucosal or subserosal location and the normal color of the overlying mucosa, it may be difficult to distinguish varices from enlarged rugae or even malignancy. Because they rarely occur in the absence of esophageal varices, diagnosis can usually be made without resorting to potentially disastrous biopsy.

TUMORS

As with the remainder of the gastrointestinal tract, tumors arising from the mucosa predominate over mesenchymal and stromal tumors. These are broadly classified into polyps and carcinoma.

GASTRIC POLYPS

The term "polyp" is applied to any nodule or mass that projects above the level of the surrounding mucosa. Occasionally, a lipoma or leiomyoma arising in the wall of the stomach may protrude beneath the mucosa to produce an apparent polypoid lesion. *The use of the term "polyp" in the gastrointestinal tract, however, is generally restricted to mass lesions arising in the mucosa.* Gastric polyps are uncommon and are found in about 0.4% of adult autopsies and 3 to 5% of Japanese adults.[32] Although gastric polyps are usually found incidentally, dyspepsia or anemia resulting from blood loss may prompt the search for a gastrointestinal lesion.

The great majority of gastric polyps (more than 90%) are *non-neoplastic* and appear to be of an *inflammatory* or *hyperplastic* nature. Histologically, these polyps exhibit a mixture of hyperplastic pyloric-type glandular tissue, and intervening edematous lamina propria containing inflammatory cells and scant smooth muscle. Most hyperplastic polyps are small and sessile; some may approach several centimeters in diameter and have an apparent stalk. Multiplicity, sometimes numbering by the score, is observed in about 20 to 25% of cases. Hyperplastic polyps are seen most frequently in the setting of chronic gastritis.[33] They are regarded as having no malignant potential as such, but are nevertheless found in about 20% of stomachs resected for carcinoma. This is attributed to the tendency of chronically inflamed gastric mucosa both to form hyperplastic polyps and to undergo transformation into malignancy.

The adenoma of the stomach is a true neoplasm, representing 5 to 10% of the polypoid lesions in the stomach. *By definition, an adenoma contains proliferative dysplastic epithelium and thereby has malignant potential.* Adenomatous polyps are much more common in the colon (discussed later). Gastric adenomas may be *sessile* (without a stalk) or *pedunculated* (stalked). The most common location is the distal portion of the stomach, particularly the antrum. These lesions are usually single and may grow up to 3 to 4 cm in size before detection (Fig. 17–20). In contrast to the colon, adenomatous change may carpet a large region of flat gastric mucosa without forming a mass lesion.

As with the colonic counterpart, the incidence of gastric adenomas increases with age, particularly into and beyond the seventh decade of life. The male-to-female ratio is 2:1. Up to 40% of gastric adenomas contain a focus of carcinoma at the time of diagnosis,[34] and the risk of cancer in the adjacent gastric mucosa may be as high as 30%. In

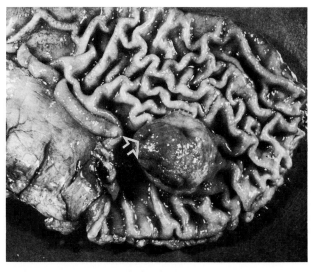

Figure 17–20. Adenomatous polyp of the stomach. Note the large size of the polyp and its lobulated configuration. A small ulceration *(arrow)* can be identified on its surface. (With permission from Kasimer, W., and Dayal, Y.: Gastritis, gastric atrophy, and gastric neoplasia. In Chopra, S., and May, R.J. (eds.): Pathophysiology of Gastrointestinal Disorders. Boston, Little, Brown, & Co., 1989.)

contrast to colonic adenomas, which usually arise from apparently normal mucosa, the usual substratum for gastric adenomas is chronic gastritis with prominent intestinal metaplasia. Colonic polyposis syndromes (discussed later) also have a particular propensity toward gastric adenoma formation.

GASTRIC CARCINOMA

Among the malignant tumors that occur in the stomach, carcinoma is overwhelmingly the most important and the most common (90 to 95%). Next in order of frequency are lymphomas (4%), carcinoids (3%), and malignant spindle cell tumors (2%).

EPIDEMIOLOGY. Gastric carcinoma is a worldwide disease. Its incidence, however, varies widely, being particularly high in Japan, Chile, Costa Rica, Colombia, China, Portugal, Iceland, Finland, and Scotland and considerably lower in the United States, United Kingdom, Canada, Australia, New Zealand, Greece, Honduras, and Sweden. In most countries, there has been a steady decline in both the incidence and the mortality of gastric cancer during the past six decades. Thus, since 1930, the annual mortality rate in the United States has dropped from about 38 to 7 per 100,000 population for men and from 28 to 4 per 100,000 for women.[7] Yet it remains among the leading killer cancers, representing 3% of all cancer deaths. This is attributable to its dismal 5-year survival rate,

Table 17-4. MAJOR FEATURES OF LAURENS' CLASSIFICATION OF GASTRIC CARCINOMA

| FEATURE | TYPE OF CARCINOMA | |
	Intestinal	*Diffuse*
Most common gross configuration	Polypoid; fungating	Ulcerative; infiltrating
Microscopic features		
Differentiation	Well-differentiated; gland-forming	Poorly differentiated; signet-ring cells
Mucin production	Limited: confined to gland lumens	Extensive: may be prominent in stroma around glands ("colloid" carcinoma)
Growth pattern	Expansile; inflammation often prominent	Noncohesive; infiltrative
Association with intestinal metaplasia	Almost universal	Less frequent
Clinical features		
Mean age (years)	55	48
Sex ratio (M:F)	2:1	approximately 1:1
Decreasing incidence in Western countries	Yes	No

Adapted from Antonioli, D.A.: Gastric carcinoma and its precursors. Monogr. Pathol. *31:*144, 1990.

which is less than 10% and has not changed appreciably in 60 years.

Some time ago, this form of neoplasia was divided by Laurens into intestinal and diffuse morphologic types (Table 17-4). The intestinal variant is thought to arise from gastric mucous cells that have undergone intestinal metaplasia. This pattern of cancer tends to be better differentiated and is the more common type in high-risk populations. *Intestinal-type carcinoma is the pattern that is progressively diminishing in frequency in the United States.* In contrast, the diffuse variant is thought to arise *de novo* from native gastric mucous cells, tends to be poorly differentiated, and now constitutes approximately half of gastric carcinomas in the United States. Most important, *the frequency of diffuse gastric carcinoma has not significantly changed in the last 60 years.* Although the intestinal-type carcinoma occurs primarily after age 50 years with a 2:1 male predominance and in the setting of chronic gastritis, the diffuse carcinoma occurs at an earlier age with no male predominance and has no particular association with chronic gastritis.[35] It would almost appear that there are two quite distinct forms of gastric carcinoma.

PATHOGENESIS. The major factors thought to affect the genesis of this form of cancer are summarized in Table 17-5. Environmental influences are thought to be the most important. When families migrate from high-risk to low-risk areas (or the reverse), successive generations acquire the level of risk that prevails in the new locales. Significantly, the altered risk results from a change in the incidence of the intestinal type of gastric carcinoma. The diet is suspected to be a primary offender, and adherence to certain culinary practices is associated with a high risk of gastric carcinoma. The presence of carcinogens, such as nitroso compounds and benzopyrene, appears to be particularly important. Thus, lack of refrigeration, common use of nitrite preservatives, water contamination with nitrates, and lack of fresh fruit and vegetables are common themes in high-risk areas. Specific foodstuffs that have been implicated in Japan

Table 17-5. FACTORS ASSOCIATED WITH INCREASED INCIDENCE OF GASTRIC CARCINOMA

DIET
Nitrites derived from nitrates (in food, drinking water, preservatives for prepared meats); undergo nitrosation to form nitrosamines and nitrosamides
Smoked and salted foods, pickled vegetables
Lack of fresh fruits and vegetables

HOST FACTORS
Chronic atrophic gastritis
  Hypochlorhydria: favors colonization with *H. pylori*
  Extensive intestinal metaplasia
Infection by *H. pylori*
  Present in most cases of intestinal-type carcinoma
Partial gastrectomy
  Favors reflux of bilious, alkaline intestinal fluid
Gastric adenomas
  40% harbor cancer at time of diagnosis
  30% have cancer in adjacent gastric mucosa at diagnosis

GENETIC
Slightly increased risk with blood group A
Close relatives have an above-average attack rate
Increased incidence in some racial groups

include pickled raw vegetables, salty sauces, and dried salted fish. Conversely, intake of green, leafy vegetables and citrus fruits, which contain antioxidants, is negatively correlated with gastric cancer.[36]

Acquired host factors are the second major area of scrutiny. An 18-fold increased risk of gastric carcinoma is reported in patients with chronic antral gastritis with atrophy: the cumulative cancer risk in patients older than 50 years is 7 to 10% within 10 years of diagnosis.[37] *Chronic corporal atrophic gastritis and overt pernicious anemia* also are associated with a threefold increased risk of gastric cancer. The gastric mucosa in each of these conditions shows glandular atrophy and intestinal metaplasia, and these histologic features may play a role in the increased risk of gastric cancer.[35] Patients who have had *partial gastrectomies* have a slightly higher risk of gastric cancer in the residual gastric stump, attributed to the hypochlorhydria, bile reflux, and chronic gastritis that occur in the postgastrectomy state. *Gastric adenomas* are known to turn malignant and may represent a final common pathway by which gastric carcinomas (at least of the intestinal type) arise.

Infection by H. pylori appears to serve as a cofactor in gastric carcinogenesis of the intestinal type.[38] In countries with regions of high and low mortality rates from gastric carcinoma, such as China, the incidence of *H. pylori* seroprevalence closely parallels that of gastric cancer. In high incidence countries, *H. pylori* infection is acquired earlier in life than in developed countries. It should be noted, however, that *most persons infected with H. pylori never develop gastric carcinoma.* Whether treatment of *H. pylori* infection will eventually lead to a reduction in the incidence of gastric carcinoma remains to be seen.

The role for genetic and racial factors remains less clear. Within the United States, blacks, Native Americans, and Hawaiians have a higher risk of developing gastric carcinoma. Because only about 4% of patients with gastric carcinoma have a family history of this disease, however, genetic factors are unlikely to be major influences. The molecular mechanisms underlying cancer promotion, from either genetic or environmental influences, have not yet been defined.

MORPHOLOGY. The location of gastric carcinomas within the stomach is as follows: pylorus and antrum, 50 to 60%; cardia, 25%; and the remainder in the body and fundus. The lesser curvature is involved in about 40% and the greater curvature in 12%. **Thus, a favored location is the lesser curvature of the antropyloric region.** Although less frequent, an ulcerative lesion on the greater curvature is more likely to be malignant.

Gastric carcinoma is classified based on (1) depth of invasion, (2) macroscopic growth pat-

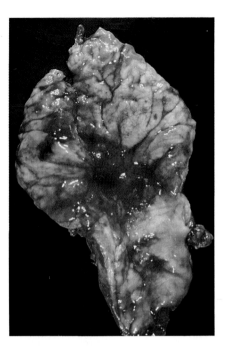

Figure 17–21. Gastric carcinoma of antral region, showing an ill-defined, excavated central ulcer surrounded by irregular, heaped-up borders.

tern, and (3) histologic subtype. The morphologic feature having the greatest impact on clinical outcome is the **depth of invasion. Early gastric carcinoma is defined as a lesion confined to the mucosa and submucosa, regardless of the presence or absence of perigastric lymph node metastases. Advanced gastric carcinoma is a neoplasm that has extended below the submucosa into the muscular wall** and has perhaps spread more widely. All cancers presumably begin as "early" lesions, which precede the development of "advanced" lesions.

The three macroscopic growth patterns of gastric carcinoma, which may be evident at both the early and the advanced stages, are (1) **exophytic,** with protrusion of a tumor mass into the lumen; (2) **flat or depressed,** in which no tumor mass is visibly obvious; and (3) **excavated,** when a shallow or deeply erosive crater is present (Fig. 17–21). Excavated cancers may closely mimic, in size and appearance, chronic peptic ulcers. In advanced cases, cancerous craters can be identified by their heaped-up, beaded margins and shaggy, necrotic bases as well as the overt neoplastic tissue extending into the surrounding mucosa and wall (Fig. 17–22). Uncommonly a broad region of the gastric wall or the entire stomach is extensively infiltrated by malignancy, creating a rigid, thickened "leather bottle," termed **linitis plastica.** Metastatic carcinoma, from the breast and lung, may generate a similar picture.

The histologic subtypes of gastric cancer have been variously subclassified, but **the two most im-**

EARLY GASTRIC CARCINOMA

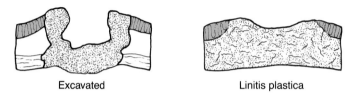

Exophytic   Flat or Depressed   Excavated

—— Mucosa
—— Submucosa
—— Muscularis Propria

ADVANCED GASTRIC CARCINOMA

Excavated   Linitis plastica

Figure 17–22. Diagram of growth patterns and spread of gastric carcinoma. In early gastric carcinoma, tumor is confined to the mucosa and submucosa and may exhibit an exophytic, flat or depressed, or excavated conformation. Advanced gastric carcinoma extends into the muscle wall and beyond. Exophytic and flat or depressed forms of advanced gastric carcinoma also can occur; these are not diagrammed.

portant types, as noted earlier, are the intestinal type and diffuse type of the Laurens classification (see Table 17–4).[39] **The intestinal variant is composed of neoplastic intestinal glands resembling those of colonic adenocarcinoma, which permeate the gastric wall but tend to grow along broad cohesive fronts in an "expanding" growth pattern.**[40] The neoplastic cells often contain apical mucin vacuoles, and abundant mucin may be present in gland lumina. **The diffuse variant is composed of gastric-type mucous cells, which generally do not form glands but rather permeate the mucosa and wall as scattered individual cells or small clusters in an "infiltrative" growth pattern.** In this variant, mucin formation expands the malignant cells and pushes the nucleus to the periphery, creating a "signet-ring" conformation (Fig. 17–23). Regardless of cell type, the amount of mucin formation varies and in poorly differentiated portions of the tumor may be absent. Conversely, excessive mucin production may generate large mucinous lakes that dissect tissue planes; isolated tumor cells or glands may be difficult to identify in such areas. Infiltrative tumors often evoke a strong mural desmoplastic reaction, in which the malignant cells are embedded; the ensuing fibrosis creates local rigidity of the wall, which provides a valuable clue to the presence of an infiltrative lesion.

Whatever the variant, all gastric carcinomas eventually penetrate the wall to involve the serosa and spread to regional and more distant lymph nodes. For obscure reasons, gastric carcinomas may metastasize to the supraclavicular sentinel (Virchow's) node as the first clinical manifestation of an occult neoplasm. Local invasion into the duodenum, pancreas, and retroperitoneum is charac-

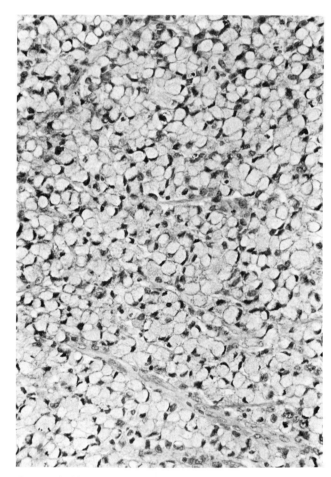

Figure 17–23. Diffuse infiltrating carcinoma of stomach. The uniform-sized tumor cells infiltrating the gastric wall show abundant mucin that pushes the nucleus to one side, giving the cells their typical "signet-ring" appearance. (Hematoxylin and eosin.) (From Kasimer, W., and Dayal, Y.: Gastritis, gastric atrophy, and gastric neoplasia. In Chopra, S., and May, R. J. (eds.): Pathophysiology of Gastrointestinal Disorders. Boston, Little, Brown & Co., 1989.)

teristic. At the time of death, widespread peritoneal seedings and metastases to the liver and lungs are common. A notable site of visceral metastasis is to one or both ovaries. Although uncommon, metastatic adenocarcinoma to the ovaries (from stomach, breast, pancreas, and even gallbladder) is so distinctive as to be called **Krukenberg tumor** (see Chapter 23).

CLINICAL COURSE. Gastric carcinoma is an insidious disease that is generally asymptomatic until late in its course. The symptoms include weight loss, abdominal pain, anorexia, vomiting, altered bowel habits, and less frequently dysphagia, anemic symptoms, and hemorrhage. Because these symptoms are essentially nonspecific, early detection of gastric cancer is difficult. The proportion of cancers diagnosed as early gastric carcinoma clearly depends on the intensity of the diagnostic effort to uncover asymptomatic disease. In Japan, where mass endoscopy screening programs are in place, early gastric carcinoma constitutes about 35% of all newly diagnosed gastric cancers. In Europe and the United States, where routine endoscopy is uncommon, this figure has remained at 10 to 15% over several decades.

The prognosis for gastric carcinoma depends mainly on depth of invasion and the extent of nodal and distant metastasis at the time of diagnosis; histologic type has no independent prognostic significance. The 5-year survival rate of surgically treated early gastric carcinoma is 90 to 95%, with only a small negative increment if lymph node metastases are present.[41] In contrast, the 5-year survival rate for advanced gastric cancer remains below 10%.

LESS COMMON GASTRIC TUMORS

Gastric *lymphomas* represent 5% of all gastric malignancies and are similar to intestinal lymphomas. *Neuroendocrine cell (carcinoid) tumors* are rare and tend to be infiltrative tumors that metastasize in about one-third of cases. Both of these tumors are described in detail in the section on tumors of the small and large intestines, later in this chapter. A wide variety of mesenchymal neoplasms, both benign and malignant, may arise in the stomach. These include stromal cell tumors, lipomas, and neurofibromas.

Metastatic involvement of the stomach is unusual. The most common sources of gastric metastases are leukemia and generalized lymphoma. Metastases of malignant melanoma and carcinomas tend to be multiple and may develop central ulceration. Breast and lung carcinoma may mimic diffuse gastric carcinoma by diffusely infiltrating the gastric wall to generate *linitis plastica*, as described earlier.

Small and Large Intestines

CONGENITAL ANOMALIES	**Necrotizing Enterocolitis**	**ABETALIPOPROTEINEMIA**	**TUMORS OF THE SMALL**
MECKEL'S DIVERTICULUM	**Antibiotic-Associated Colitis**	**IDIOPATHIC**	**AND LARGE INTESTINES**
CONGENITAL AGANGLIONIC	**(Pseudomembranous**	**INFLAMMATORY BOWEL**	**NON-NEOPLASTIC POLYPS**
MEGACOLON—	**Colitis)**	**DISEASE**	**NEOPLASTIC EPITHELIAL LESIONS**
HIRSCHSPRUNG'S DISEASE	**MISCELLANEOUS INTESTINAL**	**ETIOLOGY AND PATHOGENESIS**	**Adenomas**
ATRESIA AND STENOSIS	**INFLAMMATORY DISORDERS**	**CROHN'S DISEASE**	**Familial Adenomatous**
VASCULAR DISORDERS	**MALABSORPTION**	**ULCERATIVE COLITIS**	**Polyposis**
ISCHEMIC BOWEL DISEASE	**SYNDROMES**	**COLONIC DIVERTICULOSIS**	**Adenoma-Carcinoma**
ANGIODYSPLASIA	**CELIAC SPRUE**	**BOWEL OBSTRUCTION**	**Sequence**
HEMORRHOIDS	**TROPICAL SPRUE**	**HERNIAS**	**Colorectal Carcinoma**
ENTEROCOLITIS	**(POSTINFECTIOUS SPRUE)**	**ADHESIONS**	**Small Intestinal Neoplasms**
DIARRHEA AND DYSENTERY	**WHIPPLE'S DISEASE**	**INTUSSUSCEPTION**	**Carcinoid Tumors**
INFECTIOUS ENTEROCOLITIS	**BACTERIAL OVERGROWTH**	**VOLVULUS**	**GASTROINTESTINAL LYMPHOMA**
Viral Gastroenterocolitis	**SYNDROME**		**MESENCHYMAL TUMORS**
Bacterial Enterocolitis	**DISACCHARIDASE DEFICIENCY**		

NORMAL

The *small intestine* in the human adult is approximately 6 meters in length, and the *colon* (large intestine) is approximately 1.5 meters, ending in the *rectum*, which passes between the crura of the peroneal muscles before reaching the *anus*. The most distinctive feature of the small intestine is its mucosal lining, which is studded with innumerable *villi* (Fig. 17–24). These extend into the lumen as finger-like projections covered by epithelial lining cells. Between the bases of the villi are the pit-like crypts, which extend down to the mus-

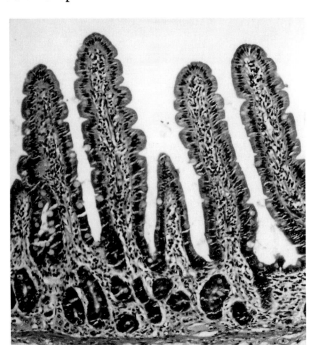

Figure 17-24. Normal small bowel histology, showing mucosal villi and crypts, lined by columnar cells. (Hematoxylin and eosin.)

cularis mucosa. In normal individuals, the villus-to-crypt height ratio is about 4 to 5:1. Within the duodenum are abundant submucosal mucous glands, termed *Brunner's glands.* These glands secrete bicarbonate ions, glycoproteins, and pepsinogen II and are virtually indistinguishable from the pyloric mucous glands.

The surface epithelium of the villi contains three cell types. *Columnar absorptive cells* are recognized by the dense array of *microvilli* on their luminal surface (the "brush border") and the underlying mat of intracellular microfilaments (the "terminal web"). Interspersed regularly between the absorptive cells are mucin-secreting *goblet cells* and a few *endocrine cells,* described later. Within the crypts reside *undifferentiated crypt cells,* goblet cells, more abundant endocrine cells, and scattered *Paneth cells;* the last cells mentioned have apically oriented bright eosinophilic granules and appear to play a role in the mucosal immune system.[42] *The villi are the sites for terminal digestion and absorption of foodstuffs by columnar absorptive cells. The crypts secrete ions and water, deliver immunoglobulin A (IgA) to the lumen, and serve as the site for cell division and renewal.* The mucous cells of both crypts and villi generate an adherent mucus coat, which both protects the surface epithelium and provides an ideal local milieu for uptake of nutrients.[43] Specific receptors for uptake of macromolecules also are present on the surface epithelial cells, such as those in the ileum for intrinsic factor–vitamin B_{12} complexes.

The small intestine accomplishes its absorptive function with a highly liquid luminal stream. *The purpose of the colon is to reclaim luminal water and electrolytes.* In contrast to the mucosa of the small intestine, *the colonic mucosa has no villi and is flat. The mucosa is punctuated by numerous straight tubular crypts that extend down to the muscularis mucosa* (Fig. 17-25). The surface epithelium is composed of columnar absorptive cells, which have shorter and less abundant microvilli than found in the small intestine, and goblet mucous cells. The crypts contain abundant goblet cells, endocrine cells, and undifferentiated crypt cells. Paneth cells are occasionally present at the base of crypts in the cecum and ascending colon.

The regenerative capacity of the intestinal epithelium is remarkable. Cellular proliferation is confined to the crypts; differentiation and luminal migration serve to replenish superficial cells lost to senescence and surface abrasion. Within the small intestine, cells migrate out of the crypts and upward to the tips of the villi, where they are shed into the lumen. This journey normally takes between 96 and 144 hours, leading to normal renewal of the epithelial lining every 4 to 6 days. Turnover of the colonic surface epithelium takes 3 to 8 days. The rapid renewal of intestinal epithelium provides a remarkable capacity for repair[44] but also renders the intestine particularly vulnerable to agents that interfere with cell replication, such as radiation and chemotherapy for cancer.

A diverse population of *endocrine cells* is scat-

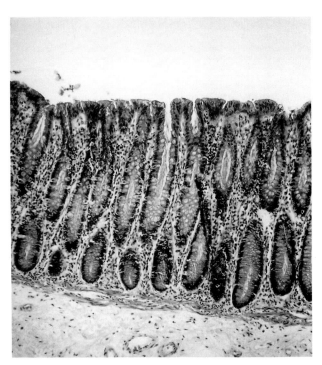

Figure 17-25. Normal colon histology, showing flat mucosal surface and abundant vertically oriented crypts. (Hematoxylin and eosin.)

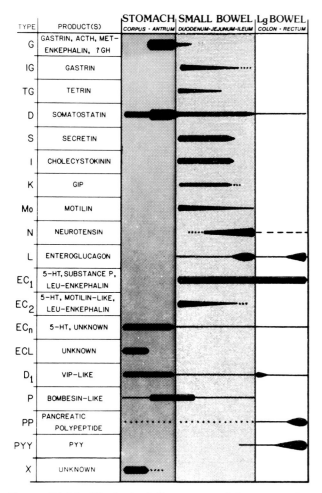

TYPE	PRODUCT(S)	STOMACH CORPUS · ANTRUM	SMALL BOWEL DUODENUM · JEJUNUM · ILEUM	Lg BOWEL COLON · RECTUM
G	GASTRIN, ACTH, MET-ENKEPHALIN, ?GH			
IG	GASTRIN			
TG	TETRIN			
D	SOMATOSTATIN			
S	SECRETIN			
I	CHOLECYSTOKININ			
K	GIP			
Mo	MOTILIN			
N	NEUROTENSIN			
L	ENTEROGLUCAGON			
EC₁	5-HT, SUBSTANCE P, LEU-ENKEPHALIN			
EC₂	5-HT, MOTILIN-LIKE, LEU-ENKEPHALIN			
ECₙ	5-HT, UNKNOWN			
ECL	UNKNOWN			
D₁	VIP-LIKE			
P	BOMBESIN-LIKE			
PP	PANCREATIC POLYPEPTIDE			
PYY	PYY			
X	UNKNOWN			

Figure 17–26. Chart depicting nomenclature, secretory products, and anatomic distribution of the various endocrine cells of the gastrointestinal tract. The width of the horizontal lines indicates their numbers relative to each other, and the extent of the lines depicts their presence in different segments of the gut. (Modified from O'Brian, D.S., and Dayal, Y.: The pathology of the gastrointestinal endocrine cells. In DeLellis, R.A. (ed.): Diagnostic Immunohistochemistry. New York, Masson Publishing U.S.A., Inc., 1982, p. 75.)

tered among the epithelial cells lining the gastric glands, small intestinal villi, and small and large intestinal crypts. Comparable cells are present in the epithelia lining the pancreas, biliary tree, lung, thyroid, and urethra. As a population, gut endocrine cells exhibit characteristic morphologic features. In most cells, the cytoplasm contains abundant fine eosinophilic granules, which harbor secretory products. The main portion of the cell is at the base of the epithelium, and the nuclei reside on the luminal side of the cytoplasmic granules. Finally, gut endocrine cells are generally positive by immunoperoxidase stains for chromogranin, synaptophysin, and neuron-specific enolase.

These cells are marked by the diversity of their secretory products and the distribution of cell subtypes (Fig. 17–26). Secretory granules are released at the basal surface of the endocrine cell or

along the basal part of its lateral surface; apical secretion (into the lumen) has never been observed. The various secretory products, some of which are present also in the mural autonomic neural plexus, act as chemical messengers and modulate normal digestive functions by a combination of endocrine, paracrine, and neurocrine mechanisms. Each endocrine cell type therefore exhibits a distribution tailored to meet the physiologic needs pertinent to a gut segment.[47]

Throughout the small intestine and colon are nodules of *lymphoid tissue*, which either lie within the mucosa or span the mucosa and a portion of the submucosa. They distort the surface epithelium to produce broad domes rather than villi; within the ileum, confluent lymphoid tissue becomes macroscopically visible as *Peyer's patches*. The surface epithelium over lymphoid nodules contains both columnar absorptive cells and *M (membranous) cells*, the latter found only in small and large intestinal lymphoid sites. M cells are able to transcytose antigenic macromolecules intact from the lumen to underlying lymphocytes, thus serving as an important afferent limb of the *intestinal immune system*. Throughout the intestines, T lymphocytes are scattered within the surface epithelium *(intraepithelial lymphocytes)*, generally of cytotoxic phenotype (CD8+). The lamina propria contains helper T cells (CD4+) and educated B cells. The lymphoid nodules and mucosal lymphocytes, together with isolated lymphoid follicles in the appendix and mesenteric lymph nodes, constitute the *Mucosa-Associated Lymphoid Tissue (MALT)*.[48]

A final comment pertains to *neuromuscular function*. Small intestinal peristalsis, both *anterograde* and *retrograde*, mixes the food stream and promotes maximal contact of nutrients with the mucosa. Colonic peristalsis prolongs contact of the luminal contents with the mucosa. Although intestinal smooth muscle cells are capable of initiating contractions, *both small and large intestinal peristalsis are mediated by intrinsic (myenteric plexus) and extrinsic (autonomic innervation) neural control*. The myenteric plexus consists of two neural networks: *Meissner's plexus* resides at the base of the submucosa, and *Auerbach's plexus* lies between the inner circumferential and outer longitudinal muscle layers of the muscle wall; lesser neural twigs extend between smooth muscle cells and ramify within the submucosa.

PATHOLOGY

Many conditions, such as infections, inflammatory diseases, and tumors, affect both the small and large intestines. These two organs are therefore considered together. Collectively, disorders of the intestines account for a large portion of human disease.

CONGENITAL ANOMALIES

In addition to such rarities as intestinal malrotation and developmental defects of the abdominal wall, several anomalies deserve separate mention.

MECKEL'S DIVERTICULUM

The vitelline duct, which connects the lumen of the developing gut to the yolk sac, normally involutes *in utero*, leaving behind a ligamentous cord. Persistence of the duct on the antimesenteric side of the bowel may give rise to a solitary diverticulum, usually within 30 cm of the ileocecal valve, termed *Meckel's diverticulum* (Fig. 17–27). *This is a true diverticulum, in that it contains all three layers of the normal bowel wall: mucosa, submucosa, and muscularis propria.* Meckel's diverticula may take the form of only a small pouch, or a blind segment having a lumen greater in diameter than that of the ileum and a length of up to 6 cm. Although the mucosal lining may be that of normal small intestine, *heterotopic rests of gastric mucosa (or pancreatic tissue) are found in about one-half of these anomalies.* Meckel's diverticula are present in an estimated 2% of the normal population, but most remain asymptomatic or are discovered incidentally. *When peptic ulceration occurs in the small intestinal mucosa adjacent to the gastric mucosa, mysterious intestinal bleeding or symptoms resembling those of acute appendicitis may result.* Alternatively, presenting symptoms may be related to intussusception, incarceration, or perforation.

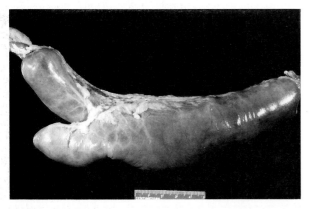

Figure 17–27. Meckel's diverticulum. Derived from an abnormal persistence of the vitelline duct, this diverticulum is most often located in the terminal ileum. Note that it is situated on the antimesenteric side of the bowel wall.

CONGENITAL AGANGLIONIC MEGACOLON — HIRSCHSPRUNG'S DISEASE

The enteric neuronal plexus develops from neural crest cells, which must migrate into the bowel wall during development, mostly in a cephalad-to-caudad direction. Congenital megacolon, or Hirschsprung's disease, results when the migration of neural crest cells arrests at some point before reaching the anus. Hence a *segment remains that lacks both Meissner's submucosal and Auerbach's myenteric plexuses. Loss of enteric neuronal coordination leads to functional obstruction and colonic dilatation proximal to the affected segment.*

MORPHOLOGY. Hirschsprung's disease is characterized by the absence of ganglion cells, and ganglia, in the muscle wall and submucosa of the affected segment. The rectum is always affected, with involvement of more proximal colon to variable extents. Most cases involve the rectum and sigmoid only, with longer segments in a fifth of cases and rarely the entire colon. Absence of mural ganglion cells is sometimes accompanied by thickening and hypertrophy of nonmyelinated nerve fibers, representing ramifications of the lumbosacral preganglionic fibers. **Proximal to the aganglionic segment, the colon undergoes progressive dilatation and hypertrophy, beginning with the descending colon. With time, the colon may become massively distended, sometimes achieving a diameter of 15 to 20 cm (megacolon).** When distention outruns the hypertrophy, the colonic wall becomes markedly thinned and may rupture, usually near the cecum. Mucosal inflammation or shallow **stercoral ulcers** produced by impacted, inspissated feces may appear.

Hirschsprung's disease occurs in approximately 1 out of 5000 to 8000 live births and is present with increased frequency (3.6%) in siblings of index cases. Males predominate 4:1. Short segment aganglionosis with megacolon is more common in males, whereas females predominate among patients with long affected segments. Ten per cent of all cases of Hirschsprung's disease occur in children with Down's syndrome, and serious neurologic abnormalities are present in another 5%, raising the possibility that this disease is only one feature of more generalized abnormal development of the neural crest.[49]

Hirschsprung's disease usually manifests itself in the immediate neonatal period by failure to pass meconium, followed by obstructive constipation. In those instances in which only a few centimeters of the rectum are affected, the buildup of pressure may permit occasional passage of stools or even intermittent bouts of diarrhea. Abdominal distention develops if a sufficiently large segment of colon is involved. The major threats to life in this disorder are superimposed enterocolitis with fluid and electrolyte disturbances and perforation of the colon or appendix with peritonitis.

Acquired megacolon is a condition of any age and may result from (1) *Chagas' disease* (see Chapter 8), in which the trypanosomes directly invade the bowel wall to destroy the enteric plexuses; (2) obstruction of the bowel as by a neoplasm or inflammatory stricture; (3) *toxic megacolon* complicating ulcerative colitis or Crohn's disease (see later); or (4) a functional psychosomatic disorder. Except for Chagas' disease, in which inflammatory involvement of the ganglia is evident, the remaining forms of megacolon are not associated with any deficiency of mural ganglia.

ATRESIA AND STENOSIS

Congenital intestinal obstruction is an uncommon but dramatic lesion that may affect any level of the intestines. Duodenal atresia is most common; the jejunum and ileum are equally involved and the colon virtually never. The obstruction may be complete *(atresia)* or incomplete *(stenosis)*. Atresia may take the form of an imperforate mucosal diaphragm or a string-like segment of bowel connecting intact proximal and distal intestine. Stenosis is less common and is due to a narrowed intestinal segment or a diaphragm with a narrow central opening. Single or multiple lesions appear to arise from developmental failure, intrauterine vascular accidents, or *intussusceptions* (telescoping of one intestinal segment within another) occurring after the intestine has developed. Failure of the cloacal diaphragm to rupture leads to an *imperforate anus*.

VASCULAR DISORDERS

Before considering vascular disorders of the intestines, a brief review of normal vasculature is in order. The superior and inferior mesenteric arterial supply of the intestine is characterized by progressive division of the vessels as they approach the gut, with rich arterial interconnections via arching mesenteric arcades. Numerous collaterals connect the mesenteric circulation with the celiac arterial axis proximally and the pudendal circulation distally. The venous drainage shares the proximal and distal anastomoses, the latter via the superior and inferior hemorrhoidal veins. The lymphatic drainage essentially parallels the vascular supply, without the intricate patterns of arcades. Because the colon is a retroperitoneal organ in the ascending

and descending portions, it derives considerable accessory arterial blood supply and lymphatic drainage from a wide area of the posterior abdominal wall.

ISCHEMIC BOWEL DISEASE

Ischemic lesions may be restricted to the small or large intestine or may affect both, depending on the particular vessel(s) affected. Acute occlusion of one of the three major supply trunks of the intestines—celiac and superior and inferior mesenteric arteries—may lead to infarction of several meters of intestine. *Insidious loss of one vessel may be without effect,* however, owing to the rich anastomotic interconnections. Lesions within the end-arteries, which penetrate the gut wall, produce small, focal ischemic lesions. The severity of injury ranges from (1) *transmural infarction* of the gut, involving all visceral layers; (2) *mural infarction* of the mucosa and submucosa; to (3) *mucosal infarction*, if the lesion extends no deeper than the muscularis mucosa.[50] *Almost always, transmural infarction implies mechanical compromise of the major mesenteric blood vessels. Mucosal or mural infarction more often results from hypoperfusion, either acute or chronic.* Mesenteric venous thrombosis is a less frequent cause of vascular compromise. The predisposing conditions for ischemia are as follows:

- *Arterial thrombosis:* severe atherosclerosis (usually at the origin of the mesenteric vessel), systemic vasculitis (e.g., polyarteritis nodosa; see Chapter 6), dissecting aneurysm, angiographic procedures, aortic reconstructive surgery, surgical accidents, hypercoagulable states, and oral contraceptives.
- *Arterial embolism:* cardiac vegetations, angiographic procedures, and aortic atheroembolism.
- *Venous thrombosis:* hypercoagulable states, oral contraceptives, antithrombin III deficiency, intraperitoneal sepsis, the postoperative state, invasive neoplasms (particularly hepatocellular carcinoma), cirrhosis, and abdominal trauma.
- *Nonocclusive ischemia:* cardiac failure, shock, dehydration, vasoconstrictive drugs (e.g., digitalis, vasopressin, propranolol).
- *Miscellaneous:* radiation injury, volvulus, stricture, and internal or external herniation.

Embolic arterial occlusion most often involves the branches of the superior mesenteric artery. The origin of the inferior mesenteric artery from the aorta is more oblique, and this may contribute to the relative sparing of this arterial axis from embolism. Despite the multiplicity of possible causes, there remains a significant percentage of cases in which no well-defined basis for the vascular insufficiency can be identified. Mesenteric vas-

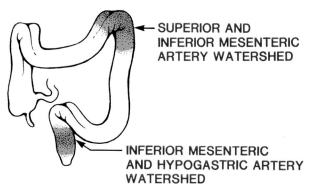

Figure 17-28. Ischemic disease of the colon. Although any area of the colon may be involved, the stippled area of the splenic flexure is more commonly affected because it is the watershed area between the major mesenteric arteries. The watershed area between the mesenteric and perineal circulation in the rectum also is prone to ischemic compromise.

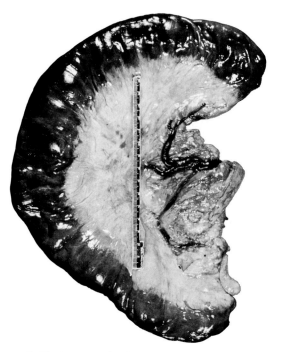

Figure 17-29. A loop of infarcted small intestine showing dark hemorrhagic discoloration. A large branching thrombus is evident in the arterial supply.

cular spasm has been invoked in some cases, without definitive proof.

MORPHOLOGY. The severity of vascular compromise and the time frame during which it develops are major determinants of the morphology of ischemic bowel disease. The most severe, acute lesions are considered first.

Transmural Infarction. Small intestinal infarction following sudden and total occlusion of mesenteric arterial blood flow may involve only a short segment but more often involves a substantial portion. Colonic infarction tends to occur at the splenic flexure, which represents the watershed between the distribution of the superior and inferior mesenteric arteries (Fig. 17-28). With mesenteric venous occlusion, antegrade and retrograde propagation of thrombus may lead to extensive involvement of the splanchnic bed. **Regardless of whether the arterial or venous side is occluded, the infarction appears hemorrhagic because of blood reflow into the damaged area.** In the early stages, the infarcted bowel appears intensely congested and dusky to purple-red (Fig. 17-29), with small and large foci of subserosal and submucosal ecchymotic discoloration. With time, the wall becomes edematous, thickened, rubbery, and hemorrhagic. The lumen commonly contains sanguinous mucus or frank blood. In arterial occlusions, the demarcation from normal bowel is usually sharply defined, but in venous occlusions, the area of dusky cyanosis fades gradually into the adjacent normal bowel. Histologically there is obvious edema, interstitial hemorrhage, and sloughing necrosis of the mucosa. Histologic features of the mural musculature become indistinct. There may be little inflammatory response. **Within 1 to 4 days, intestinal bacteria**

produce outright gangrene and sometimes perforation of the bowel.

Mural and Mucosal Infarction. Mural and mucosal infarction may involve any level of the gut from the stomach to anus. The lesions may be multifocal or continuous and widely distributed. Affected areas of the bowel may appear dark red or purple owing to the accumulated luminal hemorrhage. **Hemorrhage and an inflammatory exudate, however, are absent from the serosal surface.** On opening the bowel, there is hemorrhagic, edematous thickening of the mucosa, which may penetrate more deeply into the submucosa and muscle wall. Superficial ulceration may be present. In the mildest form of ischemic injury, the superficial epithelium of the colon, or the tips of small intestinal villi, may be necrotic or sloughed. Inflammation is absent, and there may only be mild vascular dilatation. With complete mucosal necrosis, epithelial sloughing leaves behind only the acellular scaffolding of the lamina propria (Fig. 17-30). When severe, there is extensive hemorrhage and necrosis of multiple tissue layers. Secondary acute and chronic inflammation is evident along the viable margins underlying and adjacent to the affected area. Bacterial superinfection and the formation of enterotoxic bacterial products may induce superimposed pseudomembranous inflammation, particularly in the colon. Thus, the mucosal changes may mimic enterocolitis of nonvascular origin.

Chronic Ischemia. With chronic vascular insufficiency to a region of intestine, mucosal inflamma-

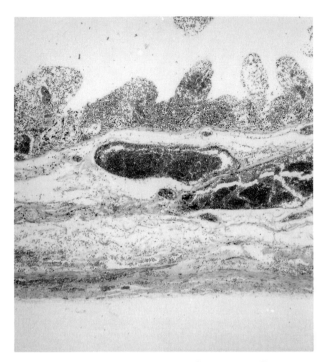

Figure 17-30. Mucosal infarction of small intestine, showing superficial sloughing of the epithelium with preservation of the villus architecture, and hemorrhagic suffusion of the lamina propria. There is edema and congestion in the submucosa. Note the absence of inflammation. (Hematoxylin and eosin.)

tion and ulceration may develop, mimicking both acute enterocolitis from other causes and idiopathic inflammatory bowel disease (see later). **Submucosal chronic inflammation and fibrosis may lead to stricture,** which typically occurs in the watershed area of the splenic flexure. **In both the small and the large intestines, chronic mucosal ischemia is notoriously segmental and patchy.**

CLINICAL CONSIDERATIONS. Bowel infarction is an uncommon but grave disorder that imposes a 50 to 75% death rate, largely because the window of time between onset of symptoms and perforation is small. It tends to occur in older individuals, when cardiac and vascular diseases are most prevalent. Pre-existent abdominal disease increases the risk of bowel infarction, owing to adhesions and torsion. Severe abdominal pain and tenderness develop suddenly in the setting of transmural infarction, sometimes accompanied by nausea, vomiting, and bloody diarrhea or grossly melanotic stool. Patients may progress to shock and vascular collapse within hours. Peristaltic sounds diminish or disappear, and spasm creates board-like rigidity of the abdominal wall musculature. Because there are far more common causes of these physical signs, such as acute appendicitis, perforated peptic ulcer, and acute cholecystitis, the diagnosis of intestinal gangrene may be delayed or missed, with disastrous consequences.

Mucosal and mural infarction, by themselves, may not be fatal, particularly if the cause of vascular compromise is corrected. A confusing array of nonspecific abdominal complaints, combined with intermittent bloody diarrhea, may be the only indication of nonocclusive enteric ischemia. Nevertheless, bowel embarassment may progress to more extensive infarction, and sepsis or serious blood loss may set in. Chronic ischemic colitis may present as an insidious inflammatory disease, with intermittent episodes of bloody diarrhea interspersed with periods of healing, mimicking inflammatory bowel disease (described later).

ANGIODYSPLASIA

Tortuous dilatations of submucosal and mucosal blood vessels are seen most often in the cecum or right colon, usually only after the sixth decade of life.[51] *Such lesions account for 20% of significant lower intestinal bleeding; intestinal hemorrhage may be chronic and intermittent or acute and massive.* Most angiodysplasias span the mucosa and submucosa, suggesting that they are ectatic nests of pre-existing veins, venules, and capillaries. The vascular channels may be separated from the intestinal lumen by only the vascular wall and a layer of attenuated epithelial cells, explaining the propensity toward bleeding.

The pathogenesis of angiodysplasia remains speculative but is attributed to mechanical factors operative in the colonic wall. Normal colonic distention and contraction may intermittently occlude the submucosal veins that penetrate the muscle wall. This then leads to focal dilatation and tortuosity of overlying submucosal and mucosal vessels. According to Laplace's law, tension in the wall of a cylinder is a function of intraluminal pressure and diameter. Because the cecum has the widest diameter of the colon, it develops the greatest wall tension, perhaps explaining the distribution of these lesions. Vascular degenerative changes related to aging also may play some role.

HEMORRHOIDS

Hemorrhoids are variceal dilatations of the anal and perianal venous plexuses. These extremely common lesions affect about 5% of the general population and develop in the setting of persistently elevated venous pressure within the hemorrhoidal plexus. The most frequent predisposing influences are constipation with straining at stool and the venous stasis of pregnancy. Except for pregnant women, they are rarely encountered in persons under the age of 30. More rarely but much more importantly, hemorrhoids may reflect collateral anastomotic channels that develop as a result of portal hypertension (see Chapter 18).

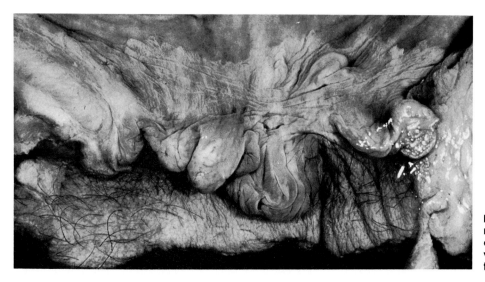

Figure 17-31. Internal hemorrhoids. Mucosal protrusions contain markedly dilated veins, at the rectoanal junction.

MORPHOLOGY. The varicosities may develop in the inferior hemorrhoidal plexus and thus are located below the anorectal line **(external hemorrhoids).** Alternatively they may develop from dilatation of the superior hemorrhoidal plexus and produce **internal hemorrhoids** (Fig. 17-31). Commonly both plexuses are affected, and the varicosities are referred to as combined hemorrhoids. Histologically these lesions consist only of thin-walled, dilated, submucosal varices that protrude beneath the anal or rectal mucosa. In their exposed, traumatized position, they tend to become thrombosed and, in the course of time, recanalized. Superficial ulceration, fissure formation, and infarction with strangulation may develop.

ENTEROCOLITIS

Diarrheal diseases of the bowel make up a veritable Augean stable of entities. Many are caused by microbiologic agents; others arise in the setting of malabsorptive disorders and idiopathic inflammatory bowel disease, discussed in subsequent sections. Consideration should first be given to the conditions known as *diarrhea* and *dysentery*.

DIARRHEA AND DYSENTERY

A typical adult human in the United States imbibes 2 liters of fluid per day, to which is added 1 liter of saliva; 2 liters of gastric juice; 1 liter of bile; 2 liters of pancreatic juice; and 1 liter of intestinal secretions. Of these 9 liters of fluid presented to the intestine, less than 200 gm of stool are excreted per day, of which 65 to 85% is water. Jejunal absorption of water amounts to 3 to 5 liters/day, ileal absorption 2 to 4 liters/day.[52] The colon normally absorbs 1 to 2 liters/day but is capable of absorbing almost 6 liters/day.

A precise definition of diarrhea is elusive, given the considerable variation in normal bowel habits. An increase in stool mass, stool frequency, or stool fluidity is perceived as diarrhea by most patients. For many individuals, this consists of daily stool production in excess of 250 gm, containing 70 to 95% water. More than 14 liters of fluid may be lost per day in severe cases of diarrhea, equivalent to the circulating blood volume. Diarrhea is often accompanied by pain, urgency, perianal discomfort, and incontinence. Low-volume, painful, bloody diarrhea is known as *dysentery*.

Diarrheal disorders are categorized as follows:

- *Secretory diarrhea:* net intestinal fluid secretion leads to the output of greater than 500 ml of fluid stool per day, which is isotonic with plasma and persists during fasting.
- *Osmotic diarrhea:* excessive osmotic forces exerted by luminal solutes lead to output of more than 500 ml of stool per day, which abates on fasting. Stool exhibits an osmotic gap (stool osmolality exceeds electrolyte concentration by 50 mOsm or more).
- *Exudative diseases:* purulent, bloody stools which persist during fasting; stools are frequent but may be small or large volume.
- *Deranged motility:* highly variable features regarding stool volume and consistency; other forms of diarrhea must be excluded.
- *Malabsorption:* long-term weight loss; voluminous, bulky stools with increased osmolarity owing to unabsorbed nutrients and excess fat (steatorrhea); usually abates on fasting.

The major causes of diarrhea are presented in Table 17-6. It is important to note that multiple mechanisms may be operative.

Table 17-6. MAJOR CAUSES OF DIARRHEAL ILLNESSES

SECRETORY DIARRHEA
Infectious: viral damage to surface epithelium
    Rotavirus
    Norwalk virus
    Enteric adenoviruses
Infectious: enterotoxin-mediated
    Vibrio cholerae
    Escherichia coli
    Bacillus cereus
    Clostridium perfringens
Neoplastic: tumor elaboration of secretogogues
    Thyroid medullary carcinoma (calcitonin, prostaglandin)
    Carcinoid (serotonin, prostaglandins)
    Pancreatic cholera syndrome (VIP, others)
    Ganglioneuroma, ganglioneuroblastoma, neurofibroma
      (VIP, prostaglandins)
    Villous adenoma in distal colon (nonhormone-mediated)
Excess laxative use
Defects in intraluminal digestion and absorption
    Bile salt malabsorption
    Excess delivery of free fatty acids to colon

OSMOTIC DIARRHEA
Disaccharidase deficiencies
Lactulose therapy (for hepatic encephalopathy, constipation)
Prescribed gut lavage ($NaSO_4$, polyethylene glycol)
Antacids ($MgSO_4$ and other magnesium salts)
Galactose-glucose malabsorption, fructose malabsorption
Mannitol, sorbitol ingestion (as from chewing gum)
Generalized malabsorption

EXUDATIVE DISEASES
Idiopathic inflammatory bowel disease
Infectious diarrhea
    Shigella
    Salmonella
    Campylobacter
    Entamoeba histolytica

DERANGED MOTILITY
Decreased intestinal transit time
    Pyloroplasty, hemigastrectomy
    Short-gut syndrome (following bypass or resection)
    Irritable bowel syndrome
    Colonic resection, ileocecal valve resection
    Hyperthyroidism
    Diabetic neuropathy
    Carcinoid syndrome
    Bowel irritation during active inflammation
Intestinal stasis
    Small intestinal diverticula
    Blind loop syndrome
    Bacterial overgrowth

MALABSORPTION

VIP = Vasoactive intestinal polypeptide.

INFECTIOUS ENTEROCOLITIS

Intestinal diseases of microbial origin are marked principally by diarrhea and sometimes ulceroinflammatory changes in the small or large intestine (or both). *Infectious enterocolitis is a global problem of staggering proportions, causing more than 12,000 deaths per day among children in developing countries and constituting one-half of all deaths before age 5 worldwide.*[53] *Although far less preva-* lent *in industrialized nations, in these populations attack rates for enterocolitis still approach one to two illnesses per person per year, second only to the common cold in frequency.* This results in an estimated 99 million acute cases of either vomiting or diarrhea per year in the United States, equivalent to 40% of the population.[54]

Among the most common offenders are rotavirus and Norwalk virus and enterotoxigenic *Escherichia coli.* Many pathogens, however, can cause diarrhea; the major offenders vary with the age, nutrition, immune status of the host, environment (living conditions, public health measures), and special predispositions, such as hospitalization, wartime dislocation, or foreign travel. In 40 to 50% of cases, the specific agent cannot be isolated.

Most of the implicated agents were discussed in detail in Chapter 8. Moreover, while viruses and bacteria are the predominant enteric pathogens in the United States, *parasitic disease and protozoal infections collectively affect more than one-half of the world's population on a chronic or recurrent basis.* These diseases also are covered in Chapter 8. Here our remarks will be limited to general principles and certain morphologic aspects of viral and bacterial illnesses.

Viral Gastroenterocolitis

Symptomatic human infection is caused by several distinct groups of viruses (Table 17–7). *Rotavirus* accounts for an estimated 140 million cases and 1 million deaths worldwide per year. The target population is children 6 to 24 months of age, but young infants and debilitated adults are susceptible to infection. *The minimal infective inoculum is approximately 10 particles, whereas an individual with rotavirus gastroenteritis typically sheds up to 10^{12} particles/ml stool.* Thus, outbreaks among pediatric populations in hospitals and daycare centers are legion. The clinical syndrome consists of an incubation period of approximately 2 days followed by vomiting and watery diarrhea for several days.

Small, round structured viruses, of which *Norwalk virus* is the prototype,[55] are responsible for the majority of cases of nonbacterial, food-borne epidemic gastroenteritis in older children and adults. Infection in young children is unusual. Outbreaks occur after exposure of multiple individuals to a common source. The clinical syndrome consists of an incubation period of 1 to 2 days, followed by 12 to 60 hours of nausea, vomiting, watery diarrhea, and abdominal pain.

Among the numerous types of *adenovirus*, the subtypes Ad40 and Ad41 of the subgenus F appear to be responsible for enteric infections. Adenovirus causes a moderate gastroenteritis with diarrhea and vomiting, lasting for a week to 10 days after an incubation period of approximately 1 week. *Calicivirus* and *astrovirus* primarily affect children and

Table 17-7. COMMON GASTROINTESTINAL VIRUSES

VIRUS	GENOME	SIZE (nm)	% U.S. CHILDHOOD HOSPITALIZATIONS	HOST AGE	MODE OF TRANSMISSION	PRODROME/ DURATION OF ILLNESS
Rotavirus (group A)	dsRNA	70	35–40	6–24 months	Person-to-person, food, water	2 days/3–8 days
Norwalk-like viruses	ssRNA*	27	Not applicable	School age, adult	Person-to-person, water, cold foods, raw shellfish	1–2 days/12–60 hours
Enteric adenoviruses	dsDNA	80	5–20	Child <2 years	Person-to-person	3–10 days/7+ days
Caliciviruses	ssRNA	35–40	3–5	Child	Person-to-person, water, cold foods, raw shellfish	1–3 days/4 days
Astroviruses	ssRNA	28	3–5	Child	Person-to-person, water, raw shellfish	24–36 hours/1–4 days

* Tentatively assigned to the Caliciviridae.
Adapted from Taterka, J. A., et al.: Viral gastrointestinal infections. Gastroenterol. Clin. North Am. 21:303–330, 1992.

have been responsible for a number of outbreaks. *Astrovirus* is better characterized and has a worldwide distribution. Those infected develop systemic symptoms of anorexia, headache, and fever.

MORPHOLOGY. During viral illness, the small intestinal mucosa usually exhibits modestly shortened villi and an infiltration of the lamina propria by lymphocytes. Vacuolization and loss of the microvillus brush border in surface epithelial cells may be evident, and the crypts appear hypertrophied. Viral particles may be present within surface epithelial cells by electron microscopy and in stool. In infants, rotavirus can produce a flat mucosa resembling celiac sprue (discussed later).

Although the mucosal damage resulting from viral gastroenteritis has been well documented,[56] insights into disease pathogenesis have been slow in coming. *Rotavirus selectively infects and destroys mature enterocytes in the small intestine, without infecting crypt cells.* The surface epithelium of the blunted villus is repopulated with immature secretory cells. With the loss of absorptive function and excess of secretory cells, there is net secretion of water and electrolytes, compounded by an osmotic diarrhea from incompletely absorbed nutrients.[57]

Bacterial Enterocolitis

Diarrheal illness may be caused by numerous bacteria (Table 17–8) and several pathogenic mechanisms, as mentioned in Chapter 8.

• *Ingestion of preformed toxin*, present in contaminated food. Major offenders are *Staphylococcus aureus*, Vibrios, and *Clostridium perfringens*.
• *Infection by toxigenic organisms*, which proliferate within the gut lumen and elaborate an enterotoxin.
• *Infection by enteroinvasive organisms*, which proliferate, invade, and destroy mucosal epithelial cells.

In the case of infection, key bacterial properties are *(1) the ability to adhere to the mucosal epithelial cells and replicate, (2) the ability to elaborate enterotoxins*, and *(3) the capacity to invade.*

BACTERIAL ADHESION AND REPLICATION. *In order to produce disease, ingested organisms must adhere to the mucosa; otherwise they will be swept away by the fluid stream.* Adherence of enterotoxigenic organisms such as *E. coli* and *Vibrio cholerae* is mediated by plasmid-coded adhesins. These proteins are expressed on the surface of the organism, sometimes in the form of fimbriae or *pili*, which are rigid or wiry surface projections. Adherence of enteropathogenic and enterohemorrhagic organisms, including *E. coli* and Shigella, also depends on plasmid-coded proteins, but their form is not known. Adherence causes effacement of the apical enterocyte membrane, with destruction of the microvillus brush border and changes in the underlying cell cytoplasm.[58] The factors regulating bacterial replication are not well understood, particularly because pathogenic organisms must compete with the normal bacterial flora to achieve a critical population density.

BACTERIAL ENTEROTOXINS. *Bacterial enterotoxins are polypeptides that cause diarrhea.*[59] Some *enterotoxins* cause intestinal secretion of fluid and electrolytes without causing tissue damage; this is accomplished by binding of the toxin to the epithelial cell membrane, entry of a portion of the toxin into the cell, and massive activation of electrolyte secretion accompanied by water. *Cholera toxin, elaborated by Vibrio cholerae, is the prototype secretagogue toxin,*[60] and is discussed in some detail in Chapter 8. *Strains of E. coli that produce heat-labile (LT) and heat-stable (ST) secretagogue toxins are the major cause of traveler's diarrhea.* Leukocytes are absent from the stool in these patients. A

Table 17–8. MAJOR CAUSES OF BACTERIAL ENTEROCOLITIS

ORGANISM	PATHOGENIC MECHANISM	SOURCE	CLINICAL FEATURES
Escherichia coli			Traveler's diarrhea, including:
ETEC	Cholera-like toxin, no invasion	Food, water	Watery diarrhea
EHEC	Shiga-like toxin, no invasion	Undercooked beef products	Hemorrhagic colitis, hemolytic uremic syndrome
EPEC	Attachment, enterocyte efface-ment, no invasion	Weaning foods, water	Watery diarrhea, infants and toddlers
EIEC	Invasion, local spread	Cheese, water, person-to-person	Fever, pain, diarrhea, dysentery
Salmonella	Invasion, translocation, lymphoid inflammation, dissemination	Milk, beef, eggs, poultry	Fever, pain, diarrhea or dysentery, bacteremia, extraintestinal infec-tion, common source outbreaks
Shigella	Invasion, local spread	Person-to-person, low-inoculum	Fever, pain, diarrhea, dysentery, epidemic spread
Campylobacter	?Toxins, invasion	Milk, poultry, animal contact	Fever, pain, diarrhea, dysentery, food sources, animal reservoirs
Yersinia entero-colitica	Invasion, translocation, lymphoid inflammation, dissemination	Milk, pork	Fever, pain, diarrhea, mesenteric adenitis, extraintestinal infection, food sources
Vibrio cholerae, other Vibrios	Enterotoxin, no invasion	Water, shellfish, person-to-person spread	Watery diarrhea, cholera, pandemic spread
Clostridium difficile	Cytotoxin, local invasion	Nosocomial environment	Fever, pain, bloody diarrhea, follow-ing antibiotic use, nosocomial acquisition
Clostridium perfringens	Enterotoxin, no invasion	Meat, poultry, fish	Watery diarrhea, food sources, "pigbel"
Mycobacterium tuberculosis	Invasion, mural inflammatory foci with necrosis and scarring	Contaminated milk, swallowing of coughed-up organisms	Chronic abdominal pain, complica-tions of malabsorption, stricture, perforation, fistulas, hemorrhage

ETEC = Enterotoxigenic *E. coli;* EHEC = enterohemorrhagic *E. coli;* EPEC = enteropathogenic *E. coli;* EIEC = enteroinvasive *E. coli.*

second group of enterotoxins are *cytotoxins,* exem-plified by Shiga toxin and toxins produced by en-terohemorrhagic *E. coli.* These toxins cause direct tissue damage through epithelial cell necrosis, and so fecal leukocytes are present.

BACTERIAL INVASION. Both enteroinvasive *E. coli* and Shigella possess a large virulence plasmid that confers the capacity for epithelial cell invasion, ap-parently by microbe-stimulated endocytosis. This is followed by intracellular proliferation, cell lysis, and cell-to-cell spread. Salmonellae quickly pass through intestinal epithelial cells via transcytosis with minimal epithelial damage; entry into the lamina propria leads to a 5 to 10% incidence of bacteremia. *Yersinia enterocolitica* penetrates the ileal mucosa and multiplies within Peyer's patches and regional lymph nodes.

MORPHOLOGY. Given the variety of bacterial path-ogens, the pathologic manifestations of enteric bacterial disease are quite variable.[61] Dramatic, even lethal, diarrhea may occur without a signifi-cant pathologic lesion, as in cholera resulting from *V. cholerae.* Characteristic histology may enable diagnosis with reasonable certainty, as with *Clos-tridium difficile*–induced pseudomembranous coli-tis (discussed later). **Most bacterial infections ex-hibit a general nonspecific pattern: damage of the surface epithelium; decreased epithelial cell maturation; an increased mitotic rate ("regenera-**tive change"); hyperemia and edema of the lam-ina propria; and variable neutrophilic infiltration into the lamina propria and epithelial layer.** In the small intestine, modest villus blunting may occur; in the colon, mucosal architecture is usually pre-served. With recovery, epithelial damage and neu-trophilic inflammation subside, leaving the residua of regenerative change and lymphoplasmacytic infiltration of the lamina propria. Alternatively pro-gressive destruction of the mucosa leads to ero-sion, ulceration, and severe submucosal inflamma-tion. Notable features of particular infections are summarized below:

- Salmonella (multiple species, including *S. typhi-murium* and *S. paratyphi*): primarily ileum and colon; blunted villi, vascular congestion, Peyer's patch involvement with swelling, congestion, and ulceration producing linear ulcers. With *S. typhi-murium*, bacteremia, fever, and systemic dissemi-nation constitute **"typhoid fever",** this may result in chronic infection of biliary tree, joints, bones, and meninges.
- Shigella: primarily distal colon; acute mucosal in-flammation and erosion, purulent exudate (Fig. 17–32).
- *Campylobacter jejuni* and other species: small in-testine, appendix, and colon; villus blunting, mul-tiple superficial ulcers, mucosal inflammation, pur-ulent exudate.
- *Yersinia enterocolitica* and *Y. pseudotuberculo-sis:* ileum, appendix, and colon; mucosal hemor-

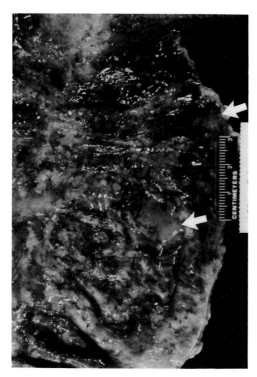

Figure 17–32. Infective enterocolitis. Segment of colon showing pale, granular, inflamed mucosa with patches of coagulated exudate *(white arrowhead)*. Compare with relatively normal mucosa *(white arrow)*.

rhage and ulceration; bowel wall thickening; Peyer's patch and mesenteric lymph node hypertrophy with necrotizing granulomas; systemic spread with peritonitis, pharyngitis, pericarditis.
- *V. cholerae:* essentially intact small intestinal mucosa, with mucus-depleted crypts.
- *C. perfringens:* usually similar to *V. cholerae* but with some epithelial damage; some strains produce a severe necrotizing enterocolitis with perforation ("pigbel").

CLINICAL CONSIDERATIONS. At the risk of oversimplification, bacterial enterocolitis takes the following forms:

- *Ingestion of preformed bacterial toxins:* Symptoms develop within a matter of hours; explosive diarrhea and acute abdominal distress herald an illness that passes within a day or so. Ingested systemic neurotoxins, as from *Clostridium botulinum,* may produce rapid, fatal respiratory failure.
- *Infection with enteric pathogens:* With ingestion of enteric pathogens, an incubation period of several hours to days is followed by *diarrhea and dehydration* if the primary pathogenic mechanism is a secretory enterotoxin, or *dysentery* if the primary mechanism is a cytotoxin or an enteroinvasive process. *Traveler's diarrhea* (e.g., Montezuma's revenge, *turista*) usually occurs fol-

lowing ingestion of fecally contaminated food or water; it begins abruptly and subsides within 2 to 3 days.
- *Insidious infection:* Yersinia and mycobacteria may present as subacute diarrheal illnesses mimicking Crohn's disease. All enteroinvasive organisms can mimic acute onset of idiopathic inflammatory bowel disease (discussed later).

The complications of bacterial enterocolitis are the logical consequences of massive fluid loss or destruction of the intestinal mucosal barrier, and include dehydration, sepsis, and perforation. Without quick intervention in severe cases, death ensues rapidly, particularly in the very young.

Necrotizing Enterocolitis

Necrotizing enterocolitis (NEC) is an acute, necrotizing inflammation of the small and large intestine and is the most common acquired gastrointestinal emergency of neonates, particularly those who are premature or of low birth weight.[62] It may occur at any time in the first 3 months of life, but its peak incidence is around the time when infants are started on oral foods (two to four days old). NEC is thought to result from a combination of ischemic injury, colonization by pathogenic organisms, excess protein substrate in the intestinal lumen, and functional immaturity of the neonatal gut. The higher prevalence of NEC in formula-fed infants, relative to breast-fed, suggests that the absence from commercial formulas of immunoprotective factors normally present in human breast milk may play a role.[63]

MORPHOLOGY. The disease primarily affects the terminal ileum and ascending colon, although in severe cases, the entire small and large bowel may be involved. In early phases, the mucosa exhibits edema, hemorrhage, and necrosis. As the disease progresses, the full thickness of the bowel wall becomes hemorrhagic, inflamed, and gangrenous. Necrotic inflammatory debris may adhere to the mucosal surface, and frank intraluminal hemorrhage may be present. Bacterial overgrowth and mural gas formation are inconstant features. Reparative change (epithelial regeneration, granulation tissue formation, and fibrosis) may be prominent, suggesting evolution of the injury for several days before clinical presentation.[64]

The disease may present as a mild gastrointestinal disturbance or as a fulminant illness with intestinal gangrene, perforation, sepsis, and shock. The typical patient has abdominal distention, tenderness, ileus, and diarrhea with occult or frank blood. Although treatment in the early stages involves maintenance of fluid and electrolyte balance and blood pressure, onset of gangrene and perforation requires prompt surgical intervention and usually massive resection. Long-term residua include short bowel syndrome and malabsorption owing to ileal resection, strictures, and recurrence of disease.

Antibiotic-Associated Colitis (Pseudomembranous Colitis)

This entity is *an acute colitis characterized by the formation of an adherent inflammatory "membrane" (pseudomembrane) overlying sites of mucosal injury.* It is usually caused by toxins of *C. difficile,* a normal gut commensal. This disease occurs most often in patients without a background of chronic enteric disease, following a course of broad-spectrum antibiotic therapy. Nearly all antibacterial agents have been implicated. Presumably toxin-forming strains flourish following alteration of the normal intestinal flora;[65] factors favoring the initiation of toxin production are not understood. The condition may rarely appear in the absence of antibiotic therapy, typically after surgery or superimposed on a chronic debilitating illness. Infrequently the small intestine is involved.

> **MORPHOLOGY. Pseudomembranous colitis derives its name from the plaque-like adhesion of fibrinopurulent-necrotic debris and mucus to damaged colonic mucosa—these are not true "membranes" because the coagulum is not an epithelial layer.** Pseudomembrane formation is not restricted to *C. difficile*–induced colitis: It also may occur following any severe mucosal injury, as in ischemic colitis, volvulus, and with necrotizing infections (staphylococci, shigella, candida, necrotizing enterocolitis). What is striking about *C. difficile* toxin–induced colitis is the microscopic lesion (Fig. 17–33). The surface epithelium is denuded, and the superficial lamina propria contains a dense infiltrate of neutrophils and occasional capillary fibrin thrombi. Superficially damaged crypts are distended by a mucopurulent exudate, which erupts out of the crypt to form a mushrooming cloud that adheres to the damaged surface—the coalescence of this "cloud" forms the pseudomembrane.

Antibiotic-associated colitis occurs primarily in adults as an acute or chronic diarrheal illness, although it has been recorded as a spontaneous infection in young adults without predisposing influences. Diagnosis is confirmed by the detection of the *C. difficile* cytotoxin in stool. Response to treatment is usually prompt, but relapse occurs in up to 25% of patients.

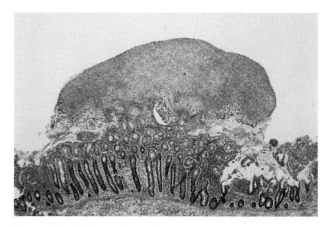

Figure 17–33. Pseudomembranous colitis. Low-power micrograph showing superficial erosion of the mucosa and an adherent "pseudomembrane" of fibrin, mucus, and inflammatory debris. (Hematoxylin and eosin.)

MISCELLANEOUS INTESTINAL INFLAMMATORY DISORDERS

Among the more unusual inflammatory disorders of the intestines,[68] two deserve particular mention.

The gastrointestinal manifestations of *human immunodeficiency virus* (HIV) infection are dominated by the presence of opportunistic pathogens, covered in Chapter 8. Some patients exhibit a malabsorptive syndrome with small intestinal villus atrophy or a colitic syndrome resembling ulcerative colitis (see later) in the absence of demonstrable pathogens. Most cases are probably due to microorganisms that have been missed or have not yet been identified as pathogens, but the concept of *acquired immunodeficiency syndrome (AIDS) enteropathy,*[66] attributable to direct mucosal damage by HIV infection, is an attractive but as yet unproven possibility.

Diarrhea is a significant complication of *bone marrow transplantation.* Pretransplant conditioning (by radiation or chemotherapy) may cause direct *toxic injury* to the small intestinal mucosa, evident as villus blunting, degeneration and flattening of crypt epithelial cells, decreased mitoses, and atypia of cell nuclei. Abrupt onset of severe watery diarrhea is a major feature of acute *graft-versus-host disease.* A distinctive histologic lesion is focal crypt cell necrosis, in which debris from necrotic cells occupies lacunae within the epithelial layer, with minimal to absent inflammatory cell response in the lamina propria.[67] In more advanced graft-versus-host disease, necrosis may become so severe as to lead to total sloughing of the mucosa. In addition to fluid and electrolyte derangements, the life-threatening complication of sepsis and intestinal hemorrhage may ensue. Alimentary tract symptoms are less evident in chronic graft-versus-host disease but may include dysphagia, secondary to esophageal involvement, and occasionally malabsorption owing to chronic intestinal injury.

MALABSORPTION SYNDROMES

Malabsorption is characterized by suboptimal absorption of fats, fat-soluble and other vitamins, proteins, carbohydrates, electrolytes and minerals, and water. At the most basic level, it is the result of disturbance of at least one of the following digestive functions:

1. *Intraluminal digestion,* in which proteins, carbohydrates, and fats are broken down into assimilable forms. The process begins in the mouth with saliva, receives a major boost from gastric peptic digestion, and continues in the small intestine, assisted by the emulsive action of bile salts (see Chapter 18).

2. *Terminal digestion,* which involves the hydrolysis of carbohydrates and peptides by disaccharidases and peptidases in the brush border of the small intestinal mucosa.

3. *Transepithelial transport,* in which nutrients, fluid, and electrolytes are transported across the epithelium of the small intestine for delivery to the intestinal vasculature. Absorbed fatty acids are converted to triglycerides and, with cholesterol, are assembled into chylomicrons for delivery to the intestinal lymphatic system.

Many diseases and disorders cause malabsorption (Table 17–9). The classification in Table 17–9 is most helpful for diseases in which there is a single, clear-cut abnormality. In many malabsorptive disorders, a defect in one pathophysiologic process predominates, but others may contribute. Although many causes of malabsorption can be established clinically, diagnosis frequently requires small intestinal mucosal biopsy (Table 17–10).

Clinically the malabsorption syndromes resemble each other more than they differ. The consequences of malabsorption affect many organ systems:[52]

- *Alimentary tract:* diarrhea—both from nutrient malabsorption and from excessive intestinal secretions, flatus, abdominal pain, weight loss, and mucositis resulting from vitamin deficiencies.
- *Hematopoietic system:* anemia from iron, pyridoxine, folate, or vitamin B_{12} deficiency and bleeding from vitamin K deficiency.
- *Musculoskeletal system:* osteopenia and tetany from calcium, magnesium, vitamin D, and protein malabsorption.
- *Endocrine system:* amenorrhea, impotence, infertility from generalized malnutrition, and hyperparathyroidism from protracted calcium and vitamin D deficiency.

Table 17–9. CLASSIFICATION OF MALABSORPTION SYNDROMES

DEFECTIVE INTRALUMINAL HYDROLYSIS OR SOLUBILIZATION
Primary pancreatic insufficiency
Secondary pancreatic insufficiency
Deficiency of intraluminal bile salts
Bacterial overgrowth
  Blind intestinal loops
  Multiple strictures and jejunal diverticula
  Fistulas
Postgastrectomy
Scleroderma and neuromuscular dysfunction

PRIMARY MUCOSAL CELL ABNORMALITIES
Disaccharidase deficiency and monosaccharide
  malabsorption
Abetalipoproteinemia
Vitamin B_{12} malabsorption
  Parietal cell loss (pernicious anemia)
  Ileal dysfunction or resection
Cystinuria and Hartnup's disease

REDUCED SMALL INTESTINAL SURFACE
Gluten-sensitive enteropathy (celiac sprue)
Refractory sprue
Whipple's disease
Short-gut syndrome
Crohn's disease
Allergic and eosinophilic gastroenteritis
Lymphoma-associated diffuse enteritis

INFECTION
Acute infectious enteritis
Parasitic infestation
Tropical sprue

LYMPHATIC OBSTRUCTION
Lymphoma
Tuberculosis and tuberculous lymphadenitis
Lymphangiectasia

IATROGENIC
Subtotal or total gastrectomy
Distal ileal resection or bypass
Radiation enteritis

DRUG-INDUCED
Cholestyramine
Colchicine
Irritant laxatives
Neomycin
p-Aminosalicylic acid
Phenindione

UNEXPLAINED
Hypogammaglobulinemia
Carcinoid syndrome
Diabetes mellitus
Mastocytosis
Hyperthyroidism, hypothyroidism, hypoadrenocorticism, and
  hypoparathyroidism

- *Skin:* purpura and petechiae from vitamin K deficiency; edema from protein deficiency; and dermatitis and hyperkeratosis from deficiencies of vitamin A, zinc, essential fatty acids, and niacin.
- *Nervous system:* peripheral neuropathy from vitamin A and B_{12} deficiencies.

The passage of abnormally bulky, frothy, greasy, yellow or gray stools is a prominent feature of malabsorption, accompanied by weight loss, ano-

Table 17-10. MALABSORPTION SYNDROMES—ABNORMALITIES IN SMALL INTESTINAL BIOPSY SPECIMENS

DISORDERS WITH CHARACTERISTIC FINDINGS

Diffuse lesions

Whipple's disease: lamina propria infiltrated with glycoprotein-containing macrophages, bacilli demonstrable in macrophages by ultrathin sections or electron microscopy, villus blunting

Abetalipoproteinemia: mucosal absorptive cells vacuolated by lipid inclusions, normal villus structure

Agammaglobulinemia: normal to flattened villi, absence to marked diminution of plasma cells in lamina propria, Giardia trophozoites often present

Discontinuous and patchy lesions

Intestinal lymphoma: variably flattened villi, malignant infiltrate of lymphoma cells in mucosa and submucosa, including infiltrate into surface epithelium

Intestinal lymphangiectasia: normal to blunted villi, dilated lymphatics in mucosa (lacteals) and submucosa

Parasitic infections: identification of parasite in biopsy specimens: giardiasis, strongyloidiasis, schistosomiasis, histoplasmosis, cryptosporidiosis, microsporidiosis, isosporiasis.

Eosinophilic and allergic gastroenteritis: normal to flattened villi, patchy infiltration of lamina propria and crypt epithelium with eosinophils and neutrophils

Mastocytosis: normal to flattened villi, patchy infiltration of lamina propria with mast cells, eosinophils, neutrophils

Amyloidosis: normal villus architecture, demonstration of amyloid in and about vessels of lamina propria

Crohn's disease: granulomas in mucosa and submucosa, patchy acute and chronic inflammation

Tuberculosis and tuberculous lymphadenitis: chance finding of caseating granuloma or margin of tuberculous ulcer

DISORDERS IN WHICH BIOPSY MAY BE ABNORMAL BUT IS NOT DIAGNOSTIC

Diffuse lesions

Celiac sprue (gluten-sensitive enteropathy): shortened to absent villi, hyperplastic crypts, severe damage of absorptive epithelial cells, chronic inflammation of lamina propria

Tropical sprue: shortened to absent villi and elongated crypts—similar to celiac sprue, absorptive cell damage mild, chronic inflammation of lamina propria

Variably continuous or patchy lesions

Viral gastroenteritis: indistinguishable from mild to moderate tropical sprue lesion

Intraluminal bacterial overgrowth: may be normal or indistinguishable from mild to moderate tropical sprue lesion

Folate or vitamin B_{12} deficiency, acute radiation enteritis: shortened villi, hypoplastic crypts, megalocytic epithelium, diminished mitoses, lamina propria inflammation

Systemic scleroderma: fibrosis of lamina propria and submucosa, distorted mucosal architecture

Lymphatic obstruction (e.g., from tumor, tuberculosis, Crohn's disease): variable dilatation of mucosal lymphatics

Lymphoma-associated lesion: indistinguishable from sprue, sometimes seen in patients harboring intestinal lymphoma

---

rexia, abdominal distention, borborygmi, and muscle wasting. *The malabsorptive disorders most commonly encountered in the United States are celiac sprue, chronic pancreatitis (see Chapter 19), and Crohn's disease (see later).*

CELIAC SPRUE

Celiac sprue is a chronic disease, in which there is a characteristic mucosal lesion of the small intestine and impaired nutrient absorption, which improves on withdrawal of wheat gliadins and related grain proteins from the diet.[69] This condition is known by a variety of names—*gluten-sensitive enteropathy, nontropical sprue, and celiac disease.* Celiac sprue occurs largely in whites and is rare or nonexistent among native Africans, Japanese, and Chinese. Its prevalence in the United States is not known accurately; in Europe, the prevalence is in the range of 1:2000 to 3000.

PATHOGENESIS. *The fundamental disorder in celiac sprue is a sensitivity to gluten, which contains the alcohol-soluble, water-insoluble protein component (gliadin) of wheat and closely related grains (oat, barley, and rye).* Although the host defect that leads to intestinal injury remains obscure, considerable evidence points to genetic susceptibility and immune-mediated intestinal injury.[70] Familial clustering is well documented. Ninety to 95% of patients express the DQw2 histocompatibility antigen on chromosome 6 and particularly a DQ alpha/beta heterodimer. Because the DQ locus is linked with HLA B8, as many as 80% of patients express this latter antigen as well. The small intestinal mucosa, when exposed to gluten, accumulates large numbers of B cells sensitized to gliadin. Antigliadin antibodies are detectable in the blood of most patients, particularly those under two years of age. An intriguing hypothesis invokes cross-reactivity of gliadin with a fragment of the E1b protein of type 12 adenovirus, raising the possibility that celiac disease results, in part, from environmental exposure to this virus.[71]

MORPHOLOGY. The mucosa appears flat or scalloped or may be visually normal. Biopsy specimens demonstrate a **diffuse enteritis,** with marked atrophy or total loss of villi (Fig. 17-34A). The surface epithelium shows vacuolar degeneration, loss of the microvillus brush border, and an increased number of intraepithelial lymphocytes. The crypts exhibit increased mitotic activity and are elongated, hyperplastic, and tortuous, so **the overall**

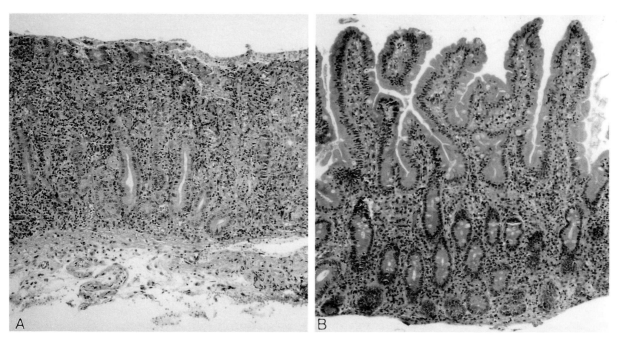

Figure 17–34. Celiac sprue (gluten-sensitive enteropathy). *A,* A jejunal peroral biopsy specimen of diseased mucosa showing severe atrophy and blunting of villi and a chronic inflammatory infiltrate of the lamina propria. *B,* Same patient as in *A* after 4 weeks on a gluten-free diet. (Hematoxylin and eosin.)

mucosal thickness remains the same. The lamina propria has an overall increase in plasma cells, lymphocytes, macrophages, eosinophils, and mast cells. All these structural changes are usually more marked in the proximal small intestine than in the distal because it is the duodenum and proximal jejunum that are exposed to the highest concentration of dietary gluten. Although these changes are characteristic of celiac sprue, they can be mimicked by other diseases, most notably tropical sprue. Mucosal histology usually reverts to normal or near-normal after a period of gluten exclusion from the diet (see Fig. 17–34*B*).

CLINICAL CONSIDERATIONS. The symptoms of celiac sprue vary tremendously from patient to patient. Symptomatic diarrhea and failure to thrive may be evident during infancy, yet adults may seek attention only in their fifth decade of life. The classic presentation includes diarrhea, flatulence, weight loss, and fatigue. Extraintestinal complications of malabsorption (cited earlier) may overshadow the intestinal symptoms. *Diagnosis requires (1) clinical documentation of malabsorption, (2) demonstration of the intestinal lesion by small bowel biopsy, and (3) unequivocal improvement in both symptoms and mucosal histology on gluten withdrawal from the diet.* If there is doubt about the diagnosis, gluten challenge followed by rebiopsy is indicated.[72]

Most patients with celiac sprue who adhere to a gluten-free diet remain well indefinitely and ultimately die of unrelated causes.[69] There is, however, a long-term risk of malignant disease, although it may be less than a twofold increase over the usual rate. More than half of these malignancies are intestinal lymphomas, including a disproportionately high number of T-cell lymphomas.[73] Other malignancies include gastrointestinal and breast carcinomas.

TROPICAL SPRUE (POSTINFECTIOUS SPRUE)

This condition is so named because this celiac-like disease occurs almost exclusively in people living in or visiting the tropics.[74] The disease is common in the Caribbean (but not in Jamaica), central and southern Africa, the Indian subcontinent and Southeast Asia, and portions of Central and South America. The disease may occur in endemic form, and epidemic outbreaks have occurred. No specific causal agent has been clearly associated with tropical sprue, but bacterial overgrowth by enterotoxigenic organisms (e.g., *E. coli* and Haemophilus) has been implicated.

MORPHOLOGY. Intestinal changes are extremely variable, ranging from near normal to severe diffuse enteritis. In contrast to celiac sprue, injury is seen at all levels of the small intestine. Patients frequently have folate or vitamin B_{12} deficiency, leading to markedly atypical enlargement of the nuclei of epithelial cells (megaloblastic change), reminiscent of changes seen in pernicious anemia.

Malabsorption usually becomes apparent in visitors to endemic locales within days or a few weeks of an acute diarrheal enteric infection and may persist if untreated. The mainstay of treatment is broad-spectrum antibiotics, supporting the concept of an infectious etiology. Intestinal lymphoma does not appear to be a hazard.

WHIPPLE'S DISEASE

Whipple's disease is a rare, systemic condition, which may involve any organ of the body but principally affects the intestine, central nervous system, and joints.

MORPHOLOGY. The hallmark of Whipple's disease is a small intestinal mucosa laden with distended macrophages in the lamina propria — the macrophages contain periodic acid–Schiff (PAS) positive granules and rod-shaped bacilli by electron microscopy (Fig. 17–35). In untreated cases, bacilli can be seen in neutrophils, in the extracellular space of the lamina propria, and even in epithelial cells. Accompanying these changes is involvement of mesenteric lymph nodes by the same process and lymphatic dilatation, suggesting lymphatic obstruction. Bacilli-laden macrophages also can be found in the synovial membranes of affected joints, the brain, cardiac valves, and elsewhere. **At each of these sites, inflammation is essentially absent.**[75]

Whipple's disease is principally encountered in whites in the fourth to fifth decades of life, with a strong male predominance of 10:1. It usually presents as a form of malabsorption with diarrhea and weight loss, sometimes of years' duration. Atypical presentations, with polyarthritis, obscure central nervous system complaints, and other symptom complexes, are common. Lymphadenopathy and hyperpigmentation are present in more than half of patients. The diagnosis rests on light microscopic changes of PAS-positive macrophages, which contain rod-shaped organisms by electron microscopy. This organism has been identified as a gram-positive actinomycete, named *Tropheryma whippelii*.[76] Although efforts to culture this organism have been uniformly unsuccessful, Whipple's disease nevertheless responds promptly and dramatically to antibiotic therapy. Some patients have a protracted course, and relapses occur.

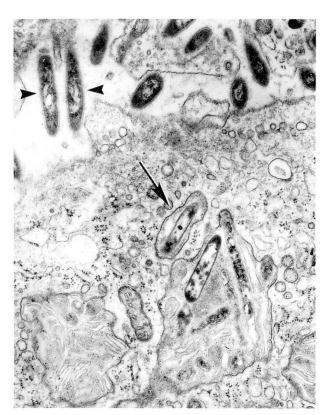

Figure 17–35. Whipple's disease. Electron micrograph of a lamina propria macrophage and its adjacent extracellular space *(top)* from a jejunal pretreatment biopsy specimen. Many bacilli are seen outside the macrophage *(arrowheads)*, and several disintegrating organisms are present within the macrophage *(arrow)*, contributing membranous material to intracellular granules. (With permission from Trier, J.S., et al.: Whipple's disease: Light and electron microscope correlation of jejunal mucosal histology with antibiotic treatment and clinical status. Gastroenterology 48:684–707, 1965.)

BACTERIAL OVERGROWTH SYNDROME

The proximal small bowel may be colonized by an abnormally large population of both aerobic and anaerobic organisms qualitatively similar to those present in the colon.[77] Although the small bowel lumen is not normally sterile, its bacterial population is held in check by the continuous peristaltic activity of the gut, normal gastric acidity, and the presence of immunoglobulins secreted into the lumen by the mucosal cells. Accordingly bacterial overgrowth can be expected to occur in patients with intestinal lesions that predispose to (1) *luminal stasis* — strictures, fistulas, diverticula, blind loops or pouches, reduplications, motility disorders, long afferent bowel loops following surgical reconstruction, and surgical denervation of bowel; (2) *hypochlorhydria or achlorhydria* — gastric mucosal atrophy, antacid therapy; and (3) *immune deficiencies or impaired mucosal immunity*. A wide spectrum of absorptive defects, including malabsorption of proteins, fats, carbohydrates, vitamins, water, and electrolytes, ensues.

The etiology of the malabsorption is multifactorial and related to bacterial deconjugation and dehydroxylation of luminal bile salts (necessary for luminal fat digestion), mucosal damage by bacterial enzymes, bacterial inactivation of luminal lipase, and competition for essential nutrients. Although small bowel biopsy specimens may show nonspecific increase in inflammatory infiltrates in the lamina propria, the mucosa may be virtually normal.[78] Demonstration of increased numbers of aerobic and anaerobic organisms in jejunal aspirates is a more pertinent diagnostic procedure. Treatment with appropriate antibiotics usually yields prompt clinical improvement.

DISACCHARIDASE DEFICIENCY

The disaccharidases, of which the most important is lactase, are located in the apical cell membrane of the villous absorptive epithelial cells. Congenital lactase deficiency is a rare condition, but acquired lactase deficiency is common, particularly among North American blacks. Incomplete breakdown of the disaccharide lactose into its monosaccharides, glucose and galactose, leads to osmotic diarrhea from the unabsorbed lactose. Bacterial fermentation of the unabsorbed sugars leads to increased hydrogen production, which is readily measured in exhaled air by gas chromatography.

When inherited as an enzyme deficiency, malabsorption becomes evident with the initiation of milk feeding. Infants develop explosive, watery, frothy stools and abdominal distention. Malabsorption is promptly corrected when exposure to milk and mild products is terminated. In the adult, lactase insufficiency may become apparent during viral and bacterial enteric infections. Neither light nor electron microscopy has disclosed abnormalities of the mucosal cells of the bowel in either the hereditary or acquired form of the disease.

ABETALIPOPROTEINEMIA

Inability to synthesize apolipoprotein B is a rare inborn error of metabolism that is transmitted by autosomal recessive inheritance.[79] It is characterized by a defect in the synthesis and export of lipoproteins from intestinal mucosal cells. Free fatty acids and monoglycerides resulting from hydrolysis of dietary fat enter the absorptive epithelial cells and are re-esterified in the normal fashion but cannot be assembled into chylomicrons. Consequently triglycerides are stored within the cells, creating lipid vacuolation, which is readily evident under the light microscope, particularly with special fat stains.[80] Concomitantly there is complete absence in plasma of all lipoproteins containing apolipoprotein B (chylomicrons, very low–density lipoproteins [VLDL], and low-density lipoproteins [LDL]). The failure to absorb certain essential fatty acids leads to systemic lipid membrane abnormalities readily evident in the characteristic acanthocytic erythrocytes ("burr cells"). The disease becomes manifest in infancy and is dominated by failure to thrive, diarrhea, and steatorrhea.

IDIOPATHIC INFLAMMATORY BOWEL DISEASE

Two inflammatory disorders of unknown etiology affecting the intestinal tract are Crohn's disease (CD) and ulcerative colitis (UC). These diseases share many common features and are collectively known as *inflammatory bowel disease (IBD)*. Both CD and UC are chronic, relapsing inflammatory disorders of obscure origin. CD is a granulomatous disease that may affect any portion of the gastrointestinal tract from mouth to anus but most often involves the small intestine and colon. UC is a nongranulomatous disease limited to colonic involvement. Before considering these diseases separately, the pathogenesis of IBD is considered.

ETIOLOGY AND PATHOGENESIS

The normal intestine is usually in a steady state of physiologic inflammation, representing a dynamic balance between (1) factors that activate the host immune system (e.g., luminal microbes, dietary antigens, endogenous inflammatory stimuli) and (2) host defenses that maintain the integrity of the mucosa and down-regulate inflammation.[81,82] The search for the cause(s) of loss of this balance in CD and UC has revealed many parallels, not the least of which is that *both diseases remain unexplained* and are thus best designated as *idiopathic*. Although CD and UC share important pathophysiologic features, it is important to remember that these two diseases may be partly or wholly distinct in their initial pathogenesis.

GENETIC PREDISPOSITION. Familial aggregations in IBD have been observed repeatedly; there is a tenfold increased risk for first-degree relatives, and concordance among twins for CD has been reported.[83] Extensive attempts to identify associations with HLA haplotypes have been largely unsuccessful except for the uniform presence of HLA-B27 in patients with IBD and ankylosing spondylitis and the association of the B5-DR2 HLA haplotype with UC in Japan.

INFECTIOUS CAUSES. The history of IBD research is littered with candidate pathogens, including viruses, chlamydia, atypical bacteria, and mycobacteria. The current champion for CD, at least, is *Mycobacterium paratuberculosis*,[84] but the data are ambiguous. It is important to recognize that many agents (Campylobacter, *E. coli*, Yersinia, Aeromonas, *C. difficile*) cause diseases that may be confused with IBD.[85]

STRUCTURAL CHANGES IN INTESTINAL MUCOSA. Many patients with CD and their relatives have increased intestinal permeability to polyethylene glycol. The permeability may reflect intrinsic differences in intestinal structure in susceptible patients or may be secondary to inflammatory activity. Alterations in mucin glycoproteins also have been documented in UC patients and family members, which persist independent of inflammatory activity.[86]

ABNORMAL HOST IMMUNOREACTIVITY. It is hypothesized that a primary disease process results in inappropriate exposure of the intestinal immune system to luminal or mucosal antigens, resulting in immune-mediated injury. Possible mechanisms for abnormal mucosal immunoreactivity include[87] (1) impaired function of small and large intestinal epithelial cells as antigen-presenting cells, (2) abnormal elaboration of cytokines, (3) abnormal function of natural killer lymphocytes, and (4) induction of cytotoxic antiepithelial antibodies. Finally, IBD-like colitis has been shown to occur in mice with genetically altered immune systems.[84] The fact that marked clinical improvement follows immunosuppressive therapy such as corticosteroids points toward an immune-mediated process, but the beneficial effect may merely reflect repression of epiphenomena. A satisfactory explanation for granuloma formation in CD is lacking.

INFLAMMATION AS THE FINAL COMMON PATHWAY. *Both the clinical manifestations of IBD and the diagnostic pathology are ultimately the result of activation of inflammatory cells whose products cause tissue injury.* Neutrophils are among the most important cellular sources of these mediators, with lesser contributions from eosinophils, mast cells, and fibroblasts. Infiltrating mononuclear cells (lymphocytes and macrophages) also contribute their share of inflammatory cytokines.[89] Most therapeutic agents act entirely or partly through nonspecific down-regulation of the immune system; more specific interventions are on the horizon.[90,91]

CROHN'S DISEASE

When first described in 1932, this idiopathic disorder was thought to be limited to the terminal ileum, hence the designation "terminal ileitis."[92] Recognition that sharply delineated bowel segments might be affected, with intervening unaffected ("skip") areas, led to the alternate name "regional enteritis." It is now clear that any level of the alimentary tract, including the colon, may be involved and that there are systemic manifestations; thus the eponymic name *Crohn's disease* is preferred. *When fully developed, CD is characterized pathologically by (1) sharply delimited and typically transmural involvement of the bowel by an inflammatory process with mucosal damage, (2) the presence of noncaseating granulomas, (3) fissuring and formation of fistulas, and (4) systemic manifestations in some patients.*

EPIDEMIOLOGY. CD occurs throughout the world but primarily in Western developed populations. Its annual incidence in the United States, United Kingdom, and Scandinavia is 1 to 3 per 100,000, which is slightly less frequent than UC.[81] It occurs at any age, from young childhood to advanced age, but peak ages of detection are the second and third decades of life with a minor peak in the sixth and seventh decades. Females are affected slightly more often than males. Whites appear to develop the disease two to five times more often than do nonwhites. In the United States, CD occurs three to five times more often among Jews than among non-Jews.

MORPHOLOGY. In CD, there is gross involvement of the small intestine alone in about 40% of cases, of small intestine and colon in 30%, and of the colon alone in about 30%. CD may involve the duodenum, stomach, esophagus, and even mouth, but these sites are distinctly uncommon. In diseased bowel segments, the serosa is granular and dull gray, and often the mesenteric fat wraps around the bowel surface **("creeping fat").** The mesentery of the involved segment also is thickened, edematous, and sometimes fibrotic. **The intestinal wall is rubbery and thick, the result of edema, inflammation, fibrosis, and hypertrophy of the muscularis propria.** As a result, the lumen almost always is narrowed; in the small intestine, this is evident on x-ray film as the "string sign," a thin stream of barium passing through the diseased segment. Strictures may occur in the colon but are usually less severe. **A classic feature of CD is the sharp demarcation of diseased bowel segments from adjacent uninvolved bowel. When multiple bowel segments are involved by "skip lesions," the intervening bowel is normal.**

A characteristic sign of early disease is focal mucosal ulcers resembling canker sores ("aphthous ulcers"), edema, and loss of the normal mucosal texture. With progressive disease, mucosal ulcers coalesce into long, serpentine "linear ulcers," which tend to be oriented along the axis of the bowel (Fig. 17–36). Because the intervening mucosa tends to be relatively spared, the mucosa acquires a coarsely textured, "cobblestone" ap-

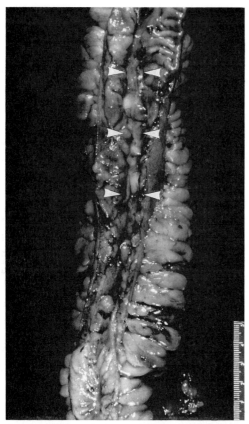

Figure 17-36. Crohn's disease of ileum, showing narrowing of the lumen, bowel wall thickening, serosal extension of mesenteric fat ("creeping fat"), and linear ulceration of the mucosal surface *(arrowheads).*

pearance. **Narrow fissures develop between the folds of the mucosa,** often penetrating deeply through the bowel wall and leading to bowel adhesions. Further extension of fissures leads to **fistula or sinus tract formation**—to an adherent viscus, to the outside skin or perineum, or into a blind cavity. Free perforation or localized abscesses also may develop.

The characteristic histologic features of CD are as follows.

Mucosal Inflammation. The earliest lesion in CD appears to be focal neutrophilic infiltration into the epithelial layer, particularly overlying mucosal lymphoid aggregates. As the disease becomes more established, **neutrophils infiltrate isolated crypts; when a sufficient number of neutrophils have traversed the epithelium of a crypt (both in the small and large intestine), a crypt abscess is formed,** usually with ultimate destruction of the crypt.

Ulceration. Ulceration is the usual outcome of severely active disease. Ulceration may be superficial, may undermine adjacent mucosa in a lateral fashion, or may penetrate deeply into underlying tissue layers. There is often an abrupt transition between ulcerated and adjacent normal mucosa.

Chronic Mucosal Damage. The hallmark of IBD, both CD and UC, is chronic mucosal damage. Architectural distortion is manifest in the small intestine as variable villus blunting (Fig. 17-37); in the

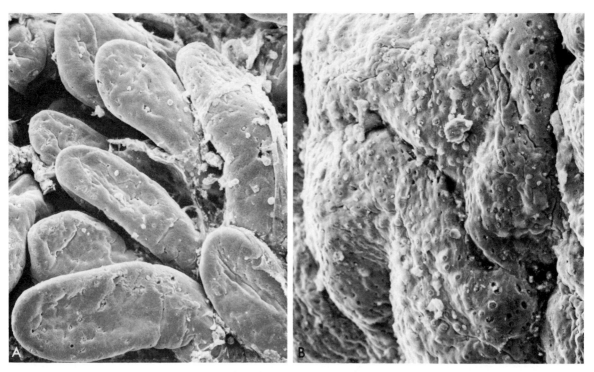

Figure 17-37. *A,* Scanning electron micrograph of normal ileal mucosa with thin, finger-shaped villi and mucous secretion exuding from goblet cell orifices. *B,* Uninvolved, nonulcerated mucosa of Crohn's disease with complete flattening and fusion of surface villi. More goblet cell orifices are visible, actively secreting mucus. (Courtesy of Dr. A. M. Dvorak, Beth Israel Hospital, Boston.)

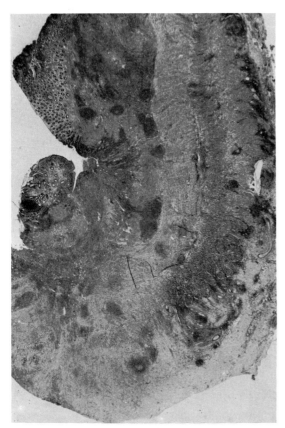

Figure 17-38. Crohn's disease. Low-power micrograph showing marked inflammation, thickening, and ulceration of bowel wall. Foci of mononuclear inflammatory cells (lymphoid aggregates) are evident at points distant from the ulceration. Note width of submucosa (Hematoxylin and eosin.)

colon, crypts exhibit irregularity and branching. Crypt destruction leads to progressive **atrophy,** particularly in the colon. The mucosa may undergo **metaplasia:** This may take the form of gastric antral-type glands **(pyloric metaplasia)** or as the development of Paneth cells in the distal colon, where they are normally absent **(Paneth cell metaplasia).**

Transmural Inflammation Affecting All Layers. Chronic inflammatory cells suffuse the affected mucosa and, to a lesser extent, all underlying tissue layers. **Lymphoid aggregates** are usually scattered throughout the bowel wall (Fig. 17-38).

Noncaseating Granulomas. Present in about half of cases, sarcoid-like granulomas may be present in all tissue layers, both within areas of active disease and in uninvolved regions of the bowel (Fig. 17-39). **Granulomas have been documented throughout the alimentary tract, from mouth to rectum, even in patients with CD limited to one bowel segment. Conversely, the absence of granulomas does not preclude the diagnosis of CD.**

Other Mural Changes. In diseased segments, the muscularis mucosa usually exhibits reduplication, thickening, and irregularity. Fibrosis of the submucosa, muscularis propria, and mucosa eventually leads to stricture formation. Less common findings are mucosal and submucosal lymphangiectasia, hypertrophy of mural nerve fibers, and localized vasculitis.

CLINICAL CONSIDERATIONS. The clinical manifestations of CD are extremely variable. The disease usually begins with intermittent attacks of relatively mild diarrhea, fever, and abdominal pain, spaced by asymptomatic periods lasting for weeks to many months. Although emotional influences are thought not to have any role in the initiation of the disease, attacks may be precipitated by periods of physical or emotional stress. In those with colonic involvement, occult or overt fecal blood loss may lead to anemia over the span of time, but massive bleeding is uncommon. In about one-fifth of patients, the onset is more abrupt, with acute right lower quadrant pain, fever, and diarrhea sometimes suggesting acute appendicitis or an acute bowel perforation. The course of the disease includes bouts of diarrhea with fluid and electrolyte losses, weight loss, and weakness.

During this lengthy, chronic disease, complica-

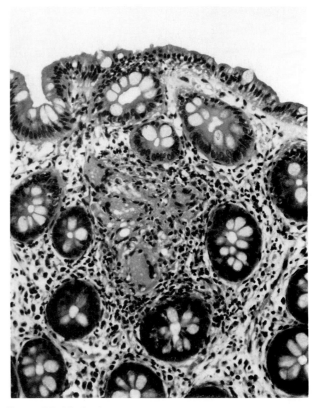

Figure 17-39. Crohn's disease. A noncaseating granuloma is present in the lamina propria of an uninvolved region of colonic mucosa. (Hematoxylin and eosin.)

tions may arise from *fibrosing strictures*, particularly of the terminal ileum, and *fistulas* to other loops of bowel, the urinary bladder, vagina, or perianal skin, or into a peritoneal abscess. Extensive involvement of the small bowel, including the terminal ileum, may cause *marked loss of albumin (protein-losing enteropathy), generalized malabsorption, specific malabsorption of vitamin B_{12} (with consequent pernicious anemia), or malabsorption of bile salts, leading to steatorrhea. Extraintestinal manifestations of this disease* include migratory polyarthritis, sacroiliitis, ankylosing spondylitis, erythema nodosum, or clubbing of the fingertips — these may even precede bowel involvement. Uveitis, nonspecific mild hepatic pericholangitis, and renal disorders secondary to trapping of the ureters in the inflammatory process sometimes develop. Systemic amyloidosis is a rare late consequence. There is an increased incidence of cancer of the gastrointestinal tract in patients with long-standing progressive CD, representing a fivefold to sixfold increased risk over age-matched populations.[93] The risk of cancer in CD, however, appears to be considerably less than that in chronic UC.

ULCERATIVE COLITIS

UC is an ulceroinflammatory disease limited to the colon and affecting only the mucosa and submucosa except in the most severe cases. In contrast to CD,

UC extends in a continuous fashion proximally from the rectum. Well-formed granulomas are absent. Similar to CD, UC is a systemic disorder associated in some patients with migratory polyarthritis, sacroiliitis, akylosing spondylitis, uveitis, hepatic involvement (pericholangitis and primary sclerosing cholangitis; see Chapter 18), and skin lesions.

EPIDEMIOLOGY. UC is global in distribution and varies in incidence relative to CD, supporting the concept that they are separate diseases. In the United States, United Kingdom, and Scandinavia, the incidence is about 4 to 6 per 100,000 population, which is slightly greater than CD. As with CD, the incidence of this condition has risen in recent decades.[94] In the United States, it is more common among whites than among blacks, and females are affected more often than males. The onset of disease peaks between the ages of 20 and 25 years, but the condition may arise in both younger and considerably older individuals. Individuals with UC and ankylosing spondylitis have an increased frequency of HLA-B27, but this association is related to the spondylitis and not to UC.

MORPHOLOGY. UC involves the rectum and extends proximally in a retrograde fashion to involve the entire colon ("pancolitis") in the more severe cases. It is a disease of continuity and

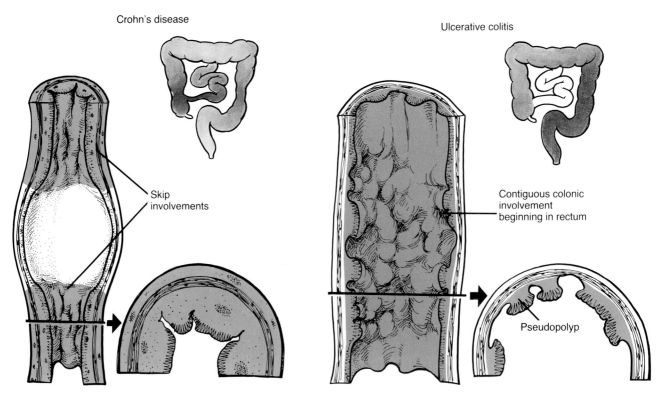

Figure 17–40. The distribution patterns of Crohn's disease and ulcerative colitis are compared as well as the different conformations of the ulcers and wall thickenings.

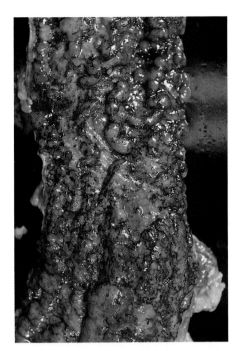

Figure 17–41. Ulcerative colitis. The pale, irregular regions comprise ulcerations that have in many instances coalesced, leaving virtual islands of residual mucosa. A tendency toward pseudopolyp formation is already evident. The darker material is adherent mucus stained by feces.

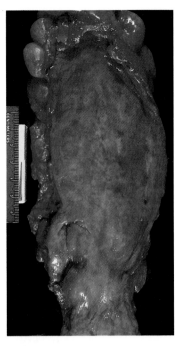

Figure 17–42. Ulcerative colitis, rectum. The markedly atrophic mucosa shows complete loss of mucosal folds and attenuation of mucosal thickness, exposing submucosal blood vessels through the translucent mucosa.

"skip" lesions such as occur in CD are not found (Fig. 17–40). In 10% of patients with severe pancolitis, the distal ileum may develop mild mucosal inflammation ("backwash ileitis"). The appendix may be involved with both CD and UC.

In the course of colonic involvement with UC, the mucosa may exhibit slight reddening and granularity with friability and easy bleeding. With fully developed severe, active inflammation, there may be extensive and broad-based ulceration of the mucosa in the distal colon or throughout its length (Fig. 17–41). Isolated islands of regenerating mucosa bulge upward to create **"pseudopolyps."** Often the undermined edges of adjacent ulcers interconnect to create tunnels covered by tenuous mucosal bridges. As with CD, the ulcers of UC are frequently aligned along the axis of the colon, but rarely do they replicate the linear serpentine ulcers of CD. With indolent chronic disease or with healing of active disease, progressive mucosal atrophy leads to a flattened and attenuated mucosal surface (Fig. 17–42). In contrast to CD, **mural thickening does not occur in UC, and the serosal surface is usually completely normal.** Only in the most severe cases of ulcerative disease (UC, CD, and other severe inflammatory diseases) does toxic damage to the muscularis propria and neural plexus lead to complete shutdown of neuromuscular function. In this instance, the colon progressively swells and becomes gangrenous (**toxic megacolon;** Fig. 17–43).

The mucosal features of UC are similar to those of colonic CD, with mucosal inflammation, chronic damage, and ulceration (Fig. 17–44). A diffuse mononuclear inflammatory infiltrate in the lamina propria, admixed with neutrophils and occasional eosinophils and mast cells, is almost universally present even at the time of clinical presentation.[95] In contrast to CD, **microscopic damage to the colonic mucosa is continuous from the rectum upward, and "skip" areas cannot be demonstrated** (Table 17–11). With healed disease, fibrosis is evident in the submucosa, and the muscularis mucosa

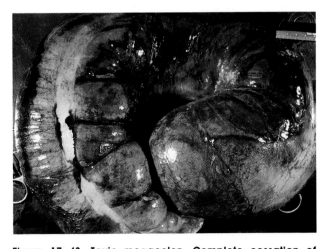

Figure 17–43. Toxic megacolon. Complete cessation of colon neuromuscular activity has led to massive dilatation of the colon, and black-green discoloration signifying gangrene and impending rupture.

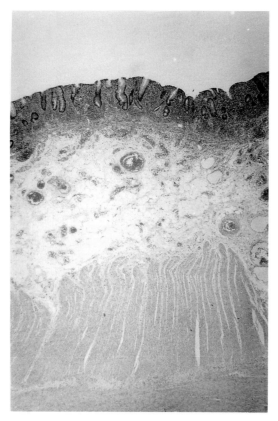

Figure 17–44. Ulcerative colitis. Low-power micrograph showing marked chronic inflammation of the mucosa with some spillover into submucosa. There is distortion of mucosal crypt architecture. The remainder of the bowel wall is essentially normal. (Hematoxylin and eosin.)

exhibits reduplication of fascicles and fibrosis over extended areas; stricture formation is rare.

Particularly significant in UC is the spectrum of epithelial changes signifying dysplasia and the progression to frank carcinoma.[96] Epithelial dysplasia is referred to as being **low grade** or **high grade**; pathologists are allowed some latitude in noting atypical changes **indefinite for dysplasia** because local inflammation may render identification of dysplasia extremely difficult.[97]

CLINICAL CONSIDERATIONS. UC typically presents as a relapsing disorder marked by attacks of bloody mucoid diarrhea that may persist for days, weeks, or months and then subside, only to recur after an asymptomatic interval of months to years or even decades. In the fortunate patient, the first attack is the last. At the other end of the spectrum, the explosive initial attack may lead to such serious bleeding and fluid and electrolyte imbalance as to constitute a medical emergency. Sudden cessation of bowel function with toxic dilatation (toxic megacolon) develops rarely with severe acute attacks. In most patients, bloody diarrhea containing stringy mucus, accompanied by lower abdominal pain and cramps usually relieved by defecation, is the first

manifestation of the disease. In a small number of patients, constipation may appear paradoxically, owing to disruption of normal peristalsis. Often the first attack is preceded by a stressful period in the patient's life. Spontaneously or more often after appropriate therapy, these symptoms abate in the course of days to weeks. Flareups, when they do occur, may be precipitated by emotional or physical stress and rarely concurrent intraluminal growth of enterotoxin-forming *C. difficile.*

The outlook for patients with UC depends on two factors: (1) the severity of active disease and (2) its duration. About 60% of patients have clinically mild disease, but almost all patients (97%) have at least one relapse during a 10-year period. About 30% of patients require colectomy within the first 3 years of onset owing to uncontrollable disease. On rare occasions, the disease runs a fulminant course; unless medically or surgically controlled, this toxic form of the disease can lead to death soon after onset.

The most feared long-term complication of UC is cancer. There is a tendency for dysplasia to arise in multiple sites, and the underlying inflammatory disease may mask the symptoms and signs of carcinoma. Historically the risk of cancer is highest in patients with pancolitis of 10 or more years' duration, in whom it exceeds by 20-fold to 30-fold that in a control population, equivalent to an absolute risk of colorectal cancer 35 years after diagnosis of 30%.[98] However, screening programs now indicate that *the rate of progression of UC to dysplasia and carcinoma is in fact quite low,* so the risk of cancer may be lower than previously thought.[99] Because great cost is involved in mass screening, the debate over the cost-effectiveness of repeated colonoscopies in patients with long-term inactive disease continues; the modest improvement in patient outcome may be related to better patient care, rather than identification of dysplasia *per se.*[100]

COLONIC DIVERTICULOSIS

A diverticulum is a blind pouch leading off the alimentary tract, lined by mucosa that communicates with the lumen of the gut. Congenital diverticula have all three layers of the bowel wall; the prototype is the *Meckel's diverticulum,* discussed earlier. Virtually all other diverticula are *acquired* and either lack or have an attenuated muscularis propria. Acquired diverticula may occur in the esophagus (see earlier), stomach, and duodenum; duodenal diverticula occur in more than 1% of adults, possibly reflecting defects from healed peptic ulcer disease. Multiple diverticula of the jejunum and ileum are rare, occurring in the setting of abnormalities in the muscle wall or myenteric plexus.[101] *Although colonic diverticula are unusual in persons under 30 years of age, in Western adult populations over the age of 60, the prevalence ap-*

Table 17-11. DISTINCTIVE FEATURES OF CROHN'S DISEASE AND ULCERATIVE COLITIS*

FEATURE	CROHN'S DISEASE — SI	CROHN'S DISEASE — C	ULCERATIVE COLITIS
Macroscopic			
Bowel region	Ileum ± colon	Colon ± ileum	Colon only
Distribution	Skip lesions	Skip lesions	Diffuse
Stricture	Early	Variable	Late/rare
Wall appearance	Thickened	Thin	Thin
Dilation	No	Yes	Yes
Microscopic			
Pseudopolyps	No to slight	Marked	Marked
Ulcers	Deep, linear	Deep, linear	Superficial
Lymphoid reaction	Marked	Marked	Mild
Fibrosis	Marked	Moderate	Mild
Serositis	Marked	Variable	Mild to none
Granulomas	Yes (50%)	Yes (50%)	No
Fistulas/sinuses	Yes	Yes	No
Clinical			
Fat/vitamin malabsorption	Yes	Yes, if ileum	No
Malignant potential	Yes	Yes	Yes
Response to surgery	Poor	Fair	Good

SI = Crohn's disease of the small intestine; C = Crohn's disease of the colon.
* Features not all present in a single case.

proaches 50%. Colonic diverticula generally occur multiply, and *so the condition is termed "diverticulosis."* They are much less frequent in nonindustrialized tropical countries and in Japan.

MORPHOLOGY. Most colonic diverticula are **small flask-like or spherical outpouchings, usually 0.5 to 1 cm in diameter** and located in the sigmoid colon (Fig. 17–45A). The descending colon or entire colon, however, may be affected. They tend to occur alongside the taeniae coli and are elastic, compressible, and easily emptied of fecal contents. As these sacs dissect into the appendices epiploicae, they may be missed on casual inspection. Histologically colonic diverticula have a thin wall composed of a flattened or atrophic mucosa, compressed submucosa, and attenuated or totally absent muscularis propria (see Fig. 17–45B). Hypertrophy of the circular layer of the muscularis propria in the affected bowel segment is usually seen; the taeniae coli are also unusually prominent.

Obstruction or perforation of diverticula leads to inflammation, which dissects into the immediately adjacent pericolic fat, generating **"diverticulitis."** In time, the inflammation may lead to marked fibrotic thickening in and about the colonic wall, sometimes producing narrowing sufficient to resemble a colonic cancer. Extension of diverticular infection may lead to pericolic abscesses, sinus tracts, and sometimes pelvic or generalized peritonitis.

PATHOGENESIS. The morphology of colonic diverticula strongly suggests that *two factors are important in their genesis: (1) focal weakness in the colonic wall and (2) increased intraluminal pressure.*[102] The colon is unique in that the longitudinal muscle coat is not complete but is gathered into three equidistant bands (the taeniae coli). Where nerves and arterial vasa recta penetrate the inner circular muscle coat alongside the taeniae, focal defects in the muscle wall are created. The connective tissue sheaths accompanying these perforating vessels provide points of weakness for herniations. *Exaggerated peristaltic contractions, with spasmodic sequestration of bowel segments, are the putative cause of increased intraluminal pressure.* It has been proposed that diets low in fiber reduce stool bulk, which in turn leads to increased peristaltic activity, particularly in the sigmoid colon. Exaggerated contractions sequester segments of bowel (segmentation); this deranged motility can lead to pain and cramps with no inflammation.

CLINICAL COURSE. Most individuals with diverticulosis remain asymptomatic throughout their lives —the lesions are most often discovered incidentally. Only about 20% of those affected ever develop manifestations: intermittent cramping or continuous lower abdominal discomfort, constipation, distention, and a sensation of never being able to empty the rectum completely. Patients sometimes experience alternating constipation and diarrhea. Occasionally there may be minimal chronic or intermittent blood loss or rarely massive hemorrhages.

Longitudinal studies have shown that diverticula can regress early in their development or may become more numerous and prominent with time. Whether a high-fiber diet prevents such progression or protects against superimposed diverticulitis is still unclear. Diets supplemented with high fiber may provide symptomatic improvement, but the treatment may seem worse than the disease. Even when diverticulitis supervenes, it most often resolves spontaneously. Relatively few patients re-

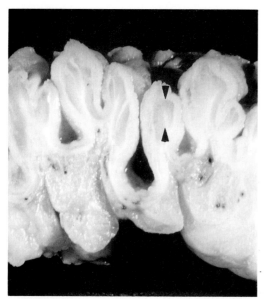

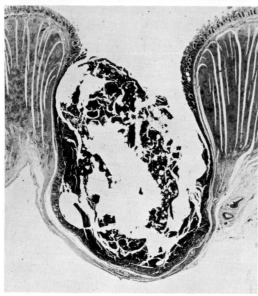

Figure 17–45. Diverticulosis. A, Section through sigmoid colon, showing multiple sac-like diverticula protruding through the muscle wall into the mesentery. The muscularis in between the diverticular protrusions is markedly thickened *(arrowheads)*. B, Low-power micrograph of diverticulum of colon, showing protrusion of mucosa and submucosa through the muscle wall, and contained fecal material. (Hematoxylin and eosin.)

quire surgical intervention for obstructive or inflammatory complications.

BOWEL OBSTRUCTION

Obstruction of the gastrointestinal tract may occur at any level, but the small intestine is most often involved owing to its narrow lumen. The causes of small and large intestinal obstruction are presented

Table 17–12. MAJOR CAUSES OF INTESTINAL OBSTRUCTION

MECHANICAL OBSTRUCTION
  Adhesions
  Hernias, internal or external
  Volvulus
  Intussusception
  Tumors
  Inflammatory strictures
  Obstructive gallstones, fecaliths, foreign bodies
  Congenital strictures; atresias
  Congenital bands
  Meconium in mucoviscidosis (cystic fibrosis)
  Imperforate anus

PSEUDO-OBSTRUCTION
  Paralytic ileus (e.g., postoperative)
  Vascular—bowel infarction
  Myopathies and neuropathies (e.g., Hirschsprung's disease)

in Table 17–12. Tumors and infarction, although the most serious, account for only about 10 to 15% of small bowel obstructions. Four of the entities — hernias, intestinal adhesions, intussusception, and volvulus—collectively account for 80%. The syndrome of intestinal obstruction is marked by abdominal pain and distention, vomiting, obstipation, and failure to pass flatus. If the obstruction is mechanical or vascular in origin, immediate surgical intervention is usually required.

HERNIAS

A weakness or defect in the wall of the peritoneal cavity may permit protrusion of a pouch-like, serosa-lined sac of peritoneum, called a *hernial sac.* The usual sites of such weakness are anteriorly at the inguinal and femoral canals, umbilicus, and in surgical scars. Rarely retroperitoneal hernias may occur, chiefly about the ligament of Trietz. *Hernias are of concern chiefly because segments of viscera frequently protrude and become trapped in them (external herniation).* This is particularly true with inguinal hernias because they tend to have narrow orifices and large sacs. The most frequent intruders are small bowel loops, but portions of omentum or large bowel also may become trapped. Pressure at the neck of the pouch may impair venous drainage of the trapped viscus. The resultant stasis and edema increase the bulk of the herniated loop, leading to permanent trapping, or *incarceration.* With time, compromise of arterial supply and venous drainage *(strangulation)* leads to infarction of the trapped segment.

ADHESIONS

Surgical procedures, infection, and even endometriosis often cause localized or more general peritoneal inflammation *(peritonitis)*. As the peritonitis heals, adhesions may develop between bowel segments or the abdominal wall and operative site. These fibrous bridges can create closed loops through which other viscera may slide and eventually become trapped *(internal herniation)*. The sequence of events following herniation—obstruction and strangulation—is much the same as with external hernias. Quite rarely, fibrous adhesions arise as congenital defects. Intestinal herniation must be considered then, even without a previous history of peritonitis or surgery.

INTUSSUSCEPTION

Intussusception occurs when one segment of the small intestine, constricted by a wave of peristalsis, suddenly becomes telescoped into the immediately distal segment of bowel. Once trapped, the invaginated segment is propelled by peristalsis farther into the distal segment, pulling its mesentery along behind it (Fig. 17–46). When encountered in infants and children, there is usually no underlying anatomic lesion or defect in the bowel, and the patient is otherwise healthy. Intussusception in adults, however, signifies an intraluminal mass or tumor as the point of traction. In both settings, intestinal obstruction ensues, and trapping of mesenteric vessels may lead to infarction.

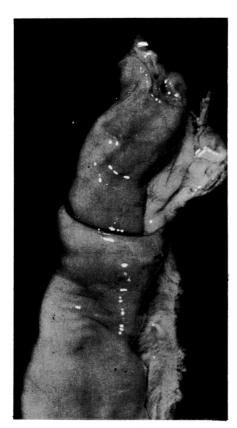

Figure 17–46. Intussusception of small intestine, viewed from external aspect.

VOLVULUS

Complete twisting of a loop of bowel about its mesenteric base of attachment also produces intestinal obstruction and infarction. This lesion occurs most often in large redundant loops of sigmoid, followed in frequency by the cecum, small bowel (all or portions), stomach, or (rarely) transverse colon. Recognition of this seldom encountered lesion demands constant awareness of its possible occurrence.

TUMORS OF THE SMALL AND LARGE INTESTINES

The classification of intestinal tumors is the same for the small and large bowel and is summarized in Table 17–13. In both segments, the majority of tumors are epithelial in origin. Of note, the colon (including the rectum) is one of the most common hosts of primary neoplasms in the body. Overall, colorectal cancer ranks second only to bronchogenic carcinoma among the cancer killers. Adenocarcinomas constitute the vast majority of colorectal cancers and represent 70% of all malignancies arising in the gastrointestinal tract.

Table 17–13. TUMORS OF THE SMALL AND LARGE INTESTINES

NON-NEOPLASTIC POLYPS
  Hyperplastic polyps
  Hamartomatous polyps
    Juvenile polyps
    Peutz-Jegher polyps
  Inflammatory polyps
  Lymphoid polyps

NEOPLASTIC EPITHELIAL LESIONS
  Benign polyps
    *Tubular adenoma**
    *Tubulovillous adenoma**
    *Villous adenoma**
  Malignant lesions
    *Adenocarcinoma**
    Carcinoid tumor
    Anal zone carcinoma

MESENCHYMAL LESIONS
  Benign lesions
    Leiomyoma
    Lipoma
    Neuroma
    Angioma
  Malignant lesions
    Leiomyosarcoma
    Liposarcoma
    Malignant spindle cell tumor
    Kaposi's sarcoma

LYMPHOMA (malignant)

* Italics denote the benign and malignant counterparts of the same neoplastic process.

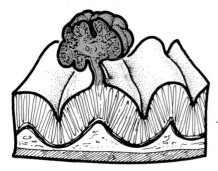

Hyperplastic polyp

Tubular adenoma

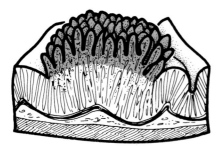

Villous adenoma

Figure 17–47. A diagrammatic representation of the three principal forms of colonic polyps. The hyperplastic polyp *(above)* **sits as a small, hemispheric dome on top of the mucosal fold. The tubular (pedunculated) adenoma** *(middle)* **has a slender stalk and a knobby, raspberry-like head. The sessile villous adenoma** *(below)* **has a broad base and myriad delicate papillae protruding into the lumen.**

Before embarking on our discussion, several concepts pertaining to terminology must be emphasized (Fig.17–47):

- A *polyp* is a tumorous mass that protrudes into the lumen of the gut; traction on the mass may create a stalked or *pedunculated* polyp. Alternatively the polyp may be *sessile*, without a definable stalk.
- Polyps may be formed as the result of abnormal mucosal maturation, inflammation, or architecture; these polyps are *non-neoplastic* and do not have malignant potential *per se*; an example is the hyperplastic polyp.
- Those epithelial polyps that arise as the result of proliferative *dysplasia* are termed *adenomatous polyps*, or *adenomas. They are true neoplastic lesions ("new growth") and are precursors of carcinoma.*
- Some polypoid lesions may be caused by submucosal or mural tumors. As with the stomach,

however, the term "polyp" applies primarily to lesions arising within the mucosa.

NON-NEOPLASTIC POLYPS

The overwhelming majority of intestinal polyps occur on a sporadic basis, particularly in the colon, and increase in frequency with age. Non-neoplastic polyps (mostly hyperplastic) represent about 90% of all epithelial polyps in the large intestine and are found in more than half of all persons age 60 years or older.[103] Inflammatory (pseudo-) polyps, representing nubbins of inflamed regenerating mucosa surrounded by ulceration, are seen in patients with long-standing inflammatory bowel disease (i.e., UC or CD). Lymphoid polyps are an essentially normal variant of the mucosal bumps containing intramucosal lymphoid tissue. Three forms of non-neoplastic polyps deserve separate mention.

MORPHOLOGY

Hyperplastic Polyps. These are small (less than 5 mm in diameter) epithelial polyps, which may arise at any age but are usually discovered in the sixth and seventh decades. They appear as nipple-like, hemispheric, smooth, moist protrusions of the mucosa, usually positioned on the tops of mucosal folds. They may occur singly but more often are multiple, and more than half are found in the rectosigmoid. Histologically they are composed of well-formed glands and crypts lined by non-neoplastic epithelial cells showing differentiation into mature goblet or absorptive cells, with scant lamina propria. Delayed shedding of otherwise normal surface epithelial cells leads to infoldings of the crowded epithelial cells, creating a serrated epithelial profile.[104] Although large hyperplastic polyps may rarely contain foci of adenomatous change, **the usual small, hyperplastic polyp has virtually no malignant potential.**

Juvenile Polyps. These lesions represent focal hamartomatous malformations of the mucosal elements. They may occur sporadically or be associated with the rare autosomal dominant **juvenile polyposis syndrome.** The vast majority occur in children below the age of five years. Nearly 80% occur in the rectum, but they may be scattered throughout the colon. Juvenile polyps tend to be large (1 to 3 cm in diameter), rounded, smooth or slightly lobulated lesions with stalks up to 2 cm in length. Histologically lamina propria constitutes the bulk of the polyp, enclosing abundant cystically dilated glands. Inflammation is common, and the surface may be congested or ulcerated. Generally they occur singly and, being hamartomatous lesions, have no malignant potential. There is a risk of adenomas, however, and hence adenocarcinoma may arise in patients with the juvenile polyposis syndrome. Smaller, isolated hamartomatous polyps may be identified in the colon of adults and are referred to as **retention polyps.**

Peutz-Jeghers Polyps. Hamartomatous lesions also may occur singly or multiply in the **Peutz-Jeghers syndrome.** This rare autosomal dominant syndrome is characterized by multiple hamartomatous polyps scattered throughout the entire gastrointestinal tract and melanotic mucosal and cutaneous pigmentation around the lips, oral mucosa, face, genitalia, and palmar surfaces of the hands. Peutz-Jeghers polyps tend to be large and pedunculated with a firm lobulated contour. Histologically an arborizing network of connective tissue and well-developed smooth muscle extends into the polyp and surrounds normal abundant glands lined by normal intestinal epithelium rich in goblet cells. The distribution of polyps is reported as stomach, 25%; colon, 30%; and small bowel, 100%. **Although these hamartomatous polyps themselves do not have malignant potential, patients with the syndrome have an increased risk of developing carcinomas of the pancreas, breast, lung, ovary, and uterus.**[105] When gastrointestinal adenocarcinoma occurs, it arises from concomitant adenomatous lesions.

NEOPLASTIC EPITHELIAL LESIONS

Adenomas

Adenomatous polyps are neoplasms that range from small, often pedunculated lesions to large neoplasms that are usually sessile. The prevalence of colonic adenomas is about 20 to 30% before age 40, rising to 40 to 50% after age 60. Males and females are affected equally. There is a well-defined familial predisposition to sporadic adenomas, accounting for both a fourfold greater risk among first-degree relatives and a fourfold greater risk of colorectal carcinoma among family members.

Adenomatous polyps are segregated into three subtypes based on the epithelial architecture:

- *Tubular adenomas:* tubular glands.
- *Villous adenomas:* villous projections.
- *Tubulovillous adenoma:* a mixture of tubular glands and villous projections.

There is considerable overlap among these categories, so by convention, tubular adenomas exhibit more than 75% tubular architecture, villous adenomas contain more than 50% villous architecture, and tubulovillous adenomas contain 25 to 50% villous architecture. Tubular adenomas are by far the most common; about 5 to 10% of adenomas are tubulovillous, and only 1% are villous.

All adenomatous lesions arise as the result of epithelial proliferative dysplasia, which may range *from mild to so severe as to constitute carcinoma in situ. Furthermore, there is strong evidence that most, and perhaps all, invasive colorectal adenocarcinomas arise in pre-existing adenomatous polyps* (discussed later). Because all degrees of dysplasia (mild, moderate, and severe) may be encountered in an adenoma of any subtype, it is impossible from gross inspection of a polyp to determine its clinical significance. However:

- Most tubular adenomas are small and become pedunculated as they enlarge; conversely, most pedunculated polyps are tubular.
- Villous adenomas tend to be large and sessile, and sessile polyps usually exhibit villous features.

The malignant risk with an adenomatous polyp is correlated with three interdependent features: polyp size, histologic architecture, and severity of epithelial dysplasia, as follows:[106] (1) Cancer is rare in tubular adenomas smaller than 1 cm in diameter. (2) The risk of cancer is high (approaching 40%) in sessile villous adenomas more than 4 cm in diameter. (3) Severe dysplasia, when present, is often found in villous areas. (4) The period required for an adenoma to double in size is estimated at about 10 years. Thus, they are slow growing and must certainly have been present for many years before detection.

MORPHOLOGY

Tubular Adenomas. Most (90%) are found in the colon—half in the rectosigmoid, but they can occur in the stomach and small intestine. In about half of the instances, they occur singly; in the remainder, two or more lesions are distributed at random. The smallest tubular adenomas are smooth contoured and sessile; larger ones tend to be coarsely lobulated and are pedunculated, having slender stalks. Uncommonly they exceed 2.5 cm in diameter. Histologically the stalk is composed of fibromuscular tissue and prominent blood vessels (derived from the submucosa), and it is usually covered by normal, non-neoplastic mucosa. Adenomatous epithelium, however, may extend down the stalk and into adjacent regions of the mucosa, particularly in the stomach. The raspberry-like head is composed of neoplastic epithelium, forming branching glands lined by tall, hyperchromatic, somewhat disorderly cells, which may or may not show mucin secretion (Fig. 17–48). In the clearly benign tubular adenoma, the branching glands are well separated by lamina propria, and the level of dysplasia is mild. All degrees of dysplasia, however, may be encountered. **Severe dysplasia (carcinoma in situ) may merge with areas of overt malignant change confined to the mucosa (intramucosal carcinoma). Carcinomatous invasion into the submucosal stalk of the polyp constitutes invasive adenocarcinoma** (Fig. 17–49).

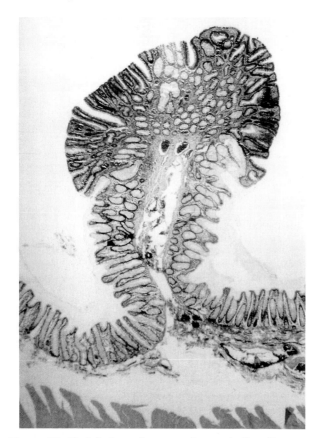

Figure 17-48. Tubular adenoma, demonstrating the neoplastic mucosa in the head of the polyp, and a slender stalk that is free from neoplastic epithelium. (Hematoxylin and eosin.)

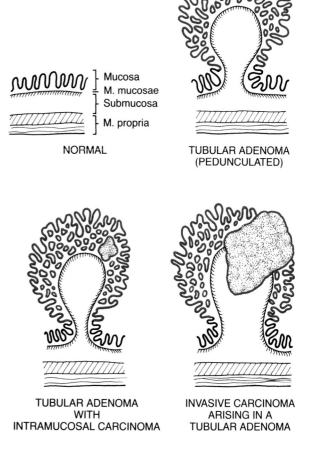

NORMAL

TUBULAR ADENOMA
(PEDUNCULATED)

Mucosa
M. mucosae
Submucosa
M. propria

TUBULAR ADENOMA
WITH
INTRAMUCOSAL CARCINOMA

INVASIVE CARCINOMA
ARISING IN A
TUBULAR ADENOMA

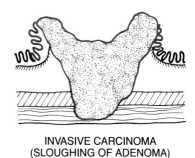

INVASIVE CARCINOMA
(SLOUGHING OF ADENOMA)

Figure 17-49. Schematic diagram of the progression of a pedunculated adenoma to invasive carcinoma.

Villous Adenomas. Villous adenomas have a propensity for the rectum and rectosigmoid, are generally sessile, and may be up to 10 cm in diameter. These velvety or cauliflower-like masses project about 1 to 3 cm above the surrounding normal mucosa. The finger-like papillae have at their cores a scant lamina propria and are covered by dysplastic columnar epithelium (Fig. 17-50). There may be considerable nuclear hyperchromasia and variation in nuclear size as well as all degrees of dysplasia. As noted earlier, the presence of invasive carcinoma (about 40%) correlates with the size of the polyp and the grade of dysplasia.

Tubulovillous Adenomas. Tubulovillous adenomas are typically intermediate between the tubular and villous lesions in terms of their frequency of having a stalk or being sessile, their size, and the general level of dysplasia found in such lesions. The risk of harboring in situ or invasive carcinoma generally correlates with the proportion of the lesion that is villous.

CLINICAL CONSIDERATIONS. Colorectal tubular (and tubulovillous) adenomas may be asymptomatic, but many are discovered during evaluation of anemia or occult bleeding. Villous adenomas are much more frequently symptomatic than the other patterns and often are discovered because of overt rectal bleeding. Rarely they may hypersecrete copious amounts of mucoid material rich in protein and potassium, leading to either hypoproteinemia or hypokalemia. Adenomas of the small intestine may be present with anemia and rarely with obstruction or intussusception; some are discovered incidentally during radiographic investigation or at postmortem examination.

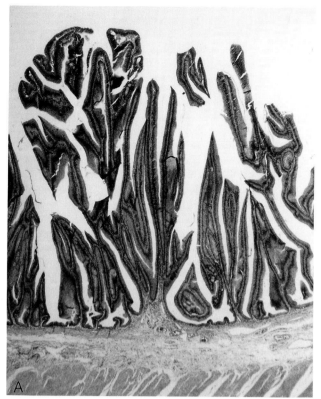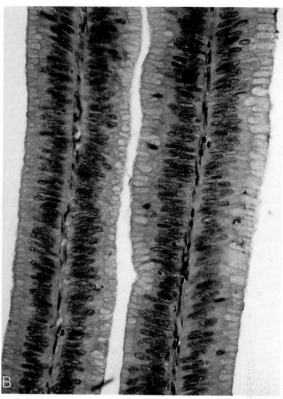

Figure 17-50. Villous adenoma. A, The frond-like villi form a sessile polyp that covers a broad area and lies directly on the muscularis mucosa and submucosa. B, Neoplastic epithelium characteristic of adenomas shows enlarged and hyperchromatic nuclei, some nuclear stratification, and mucin vacuoles. Note the scant lamina propria. (Hematoxylin and eosin.)

The clinical impact of malignant change in an adenoma depends on the following:[107,108]

- Severe dysplasia (carcinoma in situ) has not yet acquired the ability to metastasize and is still a benign lesion.
- Because lymphatic channels are largely absent in the colonic mucosa, intramucosal carcinoma also is regarded as having little to no metastatic potential.
- By crossing the muscularis mucosa into the submucosal space, invasive adenocarcinoma is a malignant lesion with metastatic potential. Nevertheless, endoscopic removal of a pedunculated adenoma is regarded as an adequate excision, provided that three histologic conditions are met: (1) The adenocarcinoma is superficial and does not approach the margin of excision across the base of the stalk; (2) there is no vascular or lymphatic invasion; and (3) the carcinoma is not poorly differentiated.
- Invasive adenocarcinoma arising in a sessile polyp cannot be adequately resected by polypectomy, and further surgery is required.
- Regardless of whether carcinoma is present, the only adequate treatment for a pedunculated or sessile adenoma is complete resection. If adenomatous epithelium remains behind in the patient, the patient is still considered to have a premalig-

nant lesion. In addition, invasive carcinoma may already be present in residual adenomatous tissue. Its presence cannot be excluded by histologic examination of the resected portion.

Familial Adenomatous Polyposis

Familial polyposis syndromes, the genetics of which are discussed in a later section, are uncommon autosomal dominant disorders that fall into two major categories. Peutz-Jeghers syndrome, described earlier, is characterized by hamartomatous polyps and a modestly increased risk of cancer, frequently in extragastrointestinal sites. Familial adenomatous polyposis (FAP) exhibits innumerable adenomatous polyps and has a frequency of progression to colon adenocarcinoma approaching 100%.[109]

FAP is the archetype of the adenomatous polyposis syndromes, in which patients typically develop 500 to 2500 colonic adenomas that carpet the mucosal surface (Fig. 17-51). Occasionally as few as 150 polyps are present; a minimum of 100 polyps is necessary for a diagnosis of FAP. Multiple adenomas may also be present elsewhere in the alimentary tract. Histologically the vast majority of polyps are tubular adenomas; occasional polyps

Figure 17–51. Familial adenomatous polyposis in an 18-year-old woman. The mucosal surface is carpeted by innumerable polypoid adenomas.

may have villous features. Some patients already have cancer of the colon or rectum at the time of diagnosis. Cancer-preventive measures include a prophylactic colectomy as soon as possible and the early detection of the disease in siblings and first-degree relatives at risk.

Gardner's syndrome is a variation of FAP, exhibiting intestinal polyps identical to those in FAP combined with multiple osteomas (particularly of the mandible, skull, and long bones), epidermal cysts, and fibromatosis. Less frequent are abnormalities of dentition, such as unerupted and supernumerary teeth, and a high frequency of duodenal and thyroid cancer. The syndrome is transmitted as an autosomal dominant trait with variable expressivity, and patients have the same high risk of developing colon cancer as those with FAP. Most workers believe that both FAP and Gardner's syndrome are variants of the same condition, with the wider spectrum of abnormalities seen in Gardner's syndrome representing variable penetrance of a common genetic mutation. *Turcot's syndrome* is a rare variant marked by the combination of adenomatous colonic polyposis and tumors of the central nervous system, mostly gliomas. An additional, rare familial syndrome with *flat adenomas* can give rise to deeply invasive carcinomas.[109]

The average age of onset of polyps in these adenomatous polyp syndromes is the second to third decade, followed by cancer within 10 to 15 years unless surgical resections interrupt the natural progression.

Adenoma-Carcinoma Sequence

The development of carcinoma from adenomatous lesions is referred to as the *adenoma-carcinoma sequence* and is documented by these observations:[110]

- Populations that have a high prevalence of adenomas have a high prevalence of colorectal cancer and vice versa.
- The distribution of adenomas within the colorectum is more or less comparable to that of colorectal cancer.
- The peak incidence of adenomatous polyps antedates by some years the peak for colorectal cancer.
- Tiny foci of cancer are relatively common within adenomatous polyps, but similar foci arising directly from nonpolypoid mucosa are extraordinarily rare.
- The risk of cancer is directly related to the number of adenomas and hence the virtual certainty of cancer in patients with familial polyposis syndromes.
- Programs that assiduously follow patients for the development of adenomas and removal of all that are suspicious reduce the incidence of colorectal cancer.

This compelling evidence is supported by the genetic alterations occurring in adenomas and colorectal cancer, for which the adenomatous polyposis syndromes serve as a paradigm.[109,111] These alterations were discussed in Chapter 7, and are summarized below:

- First, the gene associated with FAP and Gardner's syndromes has been mapped to chromosome 5q21. A candidate tumor suppressor gene has been identified, denoted APC (Adenomatous Polyposis Coli) or DP2.5. Mutation of APC also is an early event in the evolution of sporadic colon cancer.[112] Deletions in this chromosomal region also have been identified in gastric, esophageal, and lung carcinomas.
- Second, an early recognizable change in colonic neoplasms is loss of methyl groups in DNA (hypomethylation).
- Third, the *ras* gene is the most frequently observed activated oncogene in adenomas and colon cancers. It is mutated in fewer than 10% of adenomas under 1 cm in size, in 50% of adenomas larger than 1 cm, and in approximately 50% of carcinomas. Amplifications or alterations in other oncogenes, including *myc*, *myb*, *trk*, and *hst*, also have been found in colon cancer.
- Fourth, a common allelic loss in colon cancer is on 18q, termed DCC (Deleted in Colon Cancer). The encoded protein, a member of the cell adhesion family, is widely expressed in the colon mucosa; its expression is reduced or absent in 70 to 75% of colon cancers.

- Fifth, losses at 17p have been found in 70 to 80% of colon cancers, yet comparable losses are infrequent in adenomas. This region harbors the p53 suppressor gene encoding a phosphoprotein important in the cell cycle (see Chapter 7).
- Finally, instability of microsatellite DNA on chromosome 2 has been identified in patients with a genetic predisposition to colon cancer,[113] as has instability of microsatellite DNA on other chromosomes from tumors in patients with sporadic colon adenocarcinoma.[114] Such defects apparently lead to an inability to accurately copy DNA as a whole in colon cancer, leading to thousands of changes throughout the genome.

These considerations have led to the formulation of a multistage, "multi-hit" concept for colon cancer carcinogenesis, with potentially major contributions from genetic predisposition. A single sequence of events (e.g., steps one through five) does not necessarily appear to be operative; rather *cumulative alterations in the genome lead to progressive increases in size, level of dysplasia, and invasive potential of neoplastic lesions.*

Colorectal Carcinoma

Virtually 98% of all cancers in the large intestine are adenocarcinomas. They represent one of the prime challenges to the medical profession because they arise in polyps and produce symptoms relatively early and at a stage generally curable by resection. With an estimated 150,000 new cases per year and about 58,000 deaths, this disease accounts for nearly 15% of all cancer-related deaths in the United States.[7]

EPIDEMIOLOGY, ETIOLOGY, AND PATHOGENESIS. The peak incidence for colorectal carcinoma is age 60 to 70 years; fewer than 20% of cases occur under 50 years of age. When colorectal carcinoma is found in a young person, pre-existing UC or one of the polyposis syndromes must be suspected. With lesions in the rectum, the male-to-female ratio is 2 : 1; for more proximal tumors, there is no gender difference. Colorectal carcinoma has a worldwide distribution, with the highest incidence rates in the United States, Canada, Australia, Sweden and other affluent countries. Its incidence is substantially lower — up to 60-fold — in Japan, South America, and Africa. Environmental factors, particularly dietary practices, are implicated in these striking geographic contrasts. Japanese and Polish families that have migrated from their low-risk areas to the United States have acquired, over the course of 20 years, the attack rate prevailing in the new environment. It is noteworthy that both groups, for the most part, had turned to the dietary practices of their adoptive country.

The dietary factors receiving the most atten-

tion as predisposing to a higher incidence of cancer are[115] (1) a low content of unabsorbable vegetable fiber, (2) a corresponding high content of refined carbohydrates, (3) a high fat content (as from meat), and (4) decreased intake of protective micronutrients. It is theorized that reduced fiber content leads to decreased stool bulk, increased fecal transit time in the bowel, and an altered bacterial flora of the intestine. Potentially toxic oxidative byproducts of carbohydrate degradation by bacteria are therefore present in higher concentrations in the small stools and are held in contact with the colonic mucosa for longer periods of time. Moreover, high fat intake enhances the synthesis of cholesterol and bile acids by the liver, which in turn may be converted into potential carcinogens by intestinal bacteria. Refined diets also contain less of vitamins A, C, and E, which may act as oxygen radical scavengers. Intriguing as these dietary speculations may be, they remain unproven.

MORPHOLOGY. The distribution of the cancers in the colorectum appears to be changing in the United States: There is a well-defined shift toward the right colon, particularly in the elderly. Currently about 25% of carcinomas are located in the cecum or ascending colon and a similar proportion in the rectum and distal sigmoid. An additional 25% are located in the descending colon and proximal sigmoid; the remainder are scattered elsewhere. No longer are more than half of colorectal cancers readily detectable by digital or proctosigmoidoscopic examination. Most often carcinomas occur singly and have frequently obliterated their adenomatous origins. When multiple carcinomas are present, they are often at widely disparate sites in the colon. Although most cases occur sporadically, about 1 to 3% of colorectal carcinomas occur in patients with FAP or IBD.

Although almost all colorectal carcinomas begin as *in situ* lesions within adenomatous polyps, they evolve into different morphologic patterns. **Tumors in the proximal colon tend to grow as polypoid, fungating masses that extend along one wall of the capacious cecum and ascending colon** (Fig. 17–52). Obstruction is uncommon. **When carcinomas in the distal colon are discovered, they tend to be annular, encircling lesions that produce so-called napkin-ring constrictions of the bowel** (Fig. 17–53). The margins of the napkin ring are classically heaped up, beaded, and firm, and the midregion is ulcerated. The lumen is markedly narrowed, and the proximal bowel may be distended. Both forms of neoplasm directly penetrate the bowel wall over the course of time (probably years) and may appear as subserosal and serosal white, firm masses, frequently causing puckering of the serosal surface. Uncommonly, but particularly in association with UC, colorectal can-

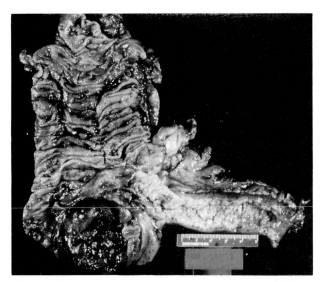

Figure 17–52. Carcinoma of the cecum. The fungating carcinoma projects into the lumen but has not caused obstruction.

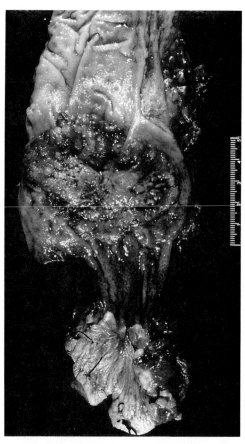

Figure 17–53. A carcinoma of the rectal canal. This nearly circumferential tumor has heaped-up edges and an ulcerated central portion. The resected anal skin is present in the lower portion of the specimen.

cers are insidiously infiltrative and difficult to identify radiographically and macroscopically. Such lesions tend to be exceedingly aggressive and infiltrative and spread at an early stage in their evolution.

In contrast to the gross pathology, **the microscopic characteristics of right-sided and left-sided colonic adenocarcinomas are similar.**[116] Differentiation may range from tall, columnar cells resembling their counterparts in adenomatous lesions (but are now invading the submucosa and muscularis propria; Fig. 17–54) to undifferentiated, frankly anaplastic masses. Invasive tumor incites a strong desmoplastic stromal response, leading to the characteristic firm, hard consistency of most colonic carcinomas. Many tumors produce mucin, which is secreted into the gland lumina or into the interstitium of the gut wall. Because this secretion dissects through the gut wall, it aids the extension of the malignancy and worsens the prognosis.

Certain exceptions should be noted. Foci of neuroendocrine differentiation may be found in about 10% of colorectal carcinomas. Alternatively in some cancers, the cells take on a signet-ring appearance. The small cell undifferentiated carcinoma appears to arise from neuroendocrine cells per se and elaborates a variety of bioactive secretory products. Some cancers, particularly in the distal colon, have foci of squamous cell differentiation and are therefore referred to as adenosquamous carcinomas. In contrast, carcinomas arising in the anorectal canal constitute a distinct subgroup of tumors, dominated by squamous cell carcinoma.

CLINICAL CONSIDERATIONS. Colorectal cancers remain asymptomatic for years; symptoms develop insidiously and frequently have been present for months, sometimes years, before diagnosis. Cecal and right colonic cancers are most often called to clinical attention by the appearance of fatigue, weakness, and iron-deficiency anemia. These bulky lesions bleed readily and may be discovered at an early stage, provided that the colon is examined thoroughly radiographically and during colonoscopy. Left-sided lesions come to attention by producing occult bleeding, changes in bowel habit, or crampy left lower quadrant discomfort. In theory, the chance for early discovery and successful removal should be greater with lesions on the left side because these patients usually have prominent disturbances in bowel function, such as melena, diarrhea, and constipation. Cancers of the rectum and sigmoid, however, tend to be more infiltrative at the time of diagnosis than proximal lesions and therefore have a somewhat poorer prognosis. It is a clinical maxim that iron-deficiency anemia in an older man means gastrointestinal cancer until proved otherwise. In women, the situation is less clear because menstrual losses, multiple pregnancies, or abnormal uterine bleeding may underlie such an anemia. Systemic manifestations, such as weakness, malaise, and weight loss, are ominous, in that they usually signify more extensive disease.

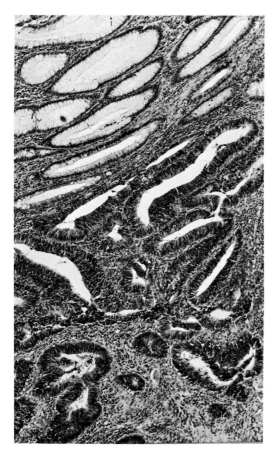

Figure 17–54. Transition zone between malignant glands of an adenocarcinoma of the colon and normal colonic epithelium. (Hematoxylin and eosin.)

Table 17–14. ASTLER-COLLER CLASSIFICATION OF CARCINOMA OF THE COLON AND RECTUM*

TUMOR STAGE	HISTOLOGIC FEATURES OF THE NEOPLASM
A	Limited to mucosa
B1	Extending into muscularis propria but not penetrating through it; uninvolved nodes
B2	Penetrating through muscularis propria; uninvolved nodes
C1	Extending into muscularis propria but not penetrating through it; involved nodes
C2	Penetrating through muscularis propria; involved nodes
D	Distant metastatic spread

* Incorrectly assigned eponyms: Dukes'; modified Dukes'; Dukes' Kirklin.
With permission from Astler, V.B., and Coller, F.A.: The prognostic significance of direct extension of carcinoma of the colon and rectum. Ann. Surg. *139:*846, 1954.

for a B2 lesion, 43% for a C1 lesion, and 23% for a C2 lesion. It is evident that the challenge is to discover these neoplasms when curative resection is possible, preferably when they are yet adenomatous polyps. Indeed each death from colonic cancer in the United States must be viewed as a preventable tragedy, and progress has been slow in coming.

Small Intestinal Neoplasms

Although the small bowel represents 75% of the length of the alimentary tract, its tumors account for only 3 to 6% of gastrointestinal tumors, with a slight preponderance of benign tumors. The most frequent benign tumors in the small intestine are leiomyomas, adenomas, and lipomas, followed by various neurogenic, vascular, and hamartomatous epithelial lesions. One of the enigmas of medicine is the rarity of malignant tumors of the small intestine—the annual U.S. death rate is under 1000, representing only about 1% of gastrointestinal malignancies. Small intestinal adenocarcinomas and carcinoids have roughly equal incidence, followed in order by lymphomas and sarcomas.

Adenocarcinomas of the small intestine grow in a napkin-ring encircling pattern or as polypoid fungating masses, in a manner similar to colonic cancers. Many small bowel carcinomas arise in the duodenum (including the ampulla of Vater) and may lead to obstructive jaundice early in their course. More typically, cramping pain, nausea, vomiting, and weight loss are the common presenting signs and symptoms, but such manifestations generally appear late in the course of these cancers. Most have already penetrated the bowel wall, invaded the mesentery or other segments of the gut, spread to regional nodes, and sometimes metastasized to the liver and more widely by the time of diagnosis. Despite these problems, wide

Laboratory diagnosis of colorectal carcinoma remains problematic, as discussed in Chapter 7.

All colorectal tumors spread by direct extension into adjacent structures and by metastasis through the lymphatics and blood vessels. In order of preference, the favored sites of metastatic spread are the regional lymph nodes, liver, lungs, and bones, followed by many other sites, including the serosal membrane of the peritoneal cavity, brain, and others. Generally the disease has spread beyond the range of curative surgery in 25 to 30% of patients. Anal region carcinomas are locally invasive and metastasize to regional lymph nodes and distant sites.

The single most important prognostic indicator of colorectal carcinoma is the extent of the tumor at the time of diagnosis. A widely used staging system is that described by Astler and Coller in 1954 (Table 17–14 and Fig. 17–55), which represents a modification of classifications proposed by Dukes and Kirklin.[117] *Staging can be applied only after the neoplasm has been resected and the extent of spread determined by surgical exploration and anatomic examination.* A patient with an Astler-Coller A lesion has a virtual 100% chance for 5-year survival after resection, falling to 67% for a B1 lesion, 54%

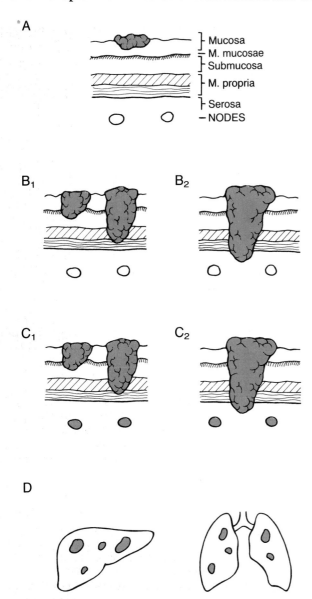

A

Mucosa
M. mucosae
Submucosa
M. propria
Serosa
NODES

B₁   B₂

C₁   C₂

D

Figure 17–55. Pathologic staging of colorectal cancer, according to the Astler-Coller system. Staging is based on the extent of local invasion and the presence of lymph node metastases (A through C) and the presence of distant visceral metastases (D).

"en bloc" excision of these cancers yields about a 70% 5-year survival rate.

Carcinoid Tumors

Neuroendocrine cells are normally dispersed along the length of the gastrointestinal tract mucosa as well as in many other organs, such as lung, pancreas, biliary tract, and elsewhere; tumors of these cells are called "carcinoids" on the basis of their slow growth pattern. The great preponderance of carcinoids arise in the gut, with a scattering of tumors in the pancreas or peripancreatic tissue,

lungs, biliary tree, and even liver. The peak incidence of these neoplasms is in the sixth decade, but they may appear at any age. As noted previously, almost half of small intestinal malignant tumors are carcinoids, whereas they constitute less than 2% of colorectal malignancies.

Although all carcinoids are potentially malignant tumors, the tendency for aggressive behavior correlates with the site of origin, the depth of local penetration, and the size of the tumor. First, *appendiceal and rectal carcinoids infrequently metastasize, even though they may show extensive local spread.* In contrast, ninety per cent of ileal, gastric, and colonic carcinoids that have penetrated halfway through the muscle wall have spread to lymph nodes and distant sites at the time of diagnosis.

HISTOGENESIS. The cells of carcinoid tumors resemble the neuroendocrine cells of the gut ultrastructurally and have a similar capacity to synthesize and secrete a variety of bioactive and hormonal products, as described earlier. For these reasons, the cell of origin is presumed to be the immature, functionally uncommited gut endocrine cell, which undergoes further differentiation during tumorigenesis.[118] *Although multiple bioactive products may be synthesized by a single tumor, most secrete a predominant product to produce a clinical syndrome called by that name, e.g., gastrinoma, somatostatinoma, VIPoma, and insulinoma.*

MORPHOLOGY. The appendix is the most common site of gut carcinoid tumors, followed by the small intestine (primarily ileum), rectum, stomach, and colon. **Those that arise in the stomach and ileum are frequently multicentric, but the remainder tend to be solitary lesions.** In the appendix, they appear as bulbous swellings of the tip, which frequently obliterate the lumen. Elsewhere in the gut, they appear as intramural or submucosal masses that create small, polypoid, or plateau-like elevations rarely more than 3 cm in diameter. The overlying mucosa may be intact or ulcerated, and the tumors may permeate the bowel wall to invade the mesentery. **A characteristic feature is a solid, yellow-tan appearance on transection.** The tumors are exceedingly firm owing to striking desmoplasia, and when these fibrosing lesions penetrate the mesentery of the small bowel, they may cause angulation or kinking sufficient to result in obstruction. When present, visceral metastases are usually small, dispersed nodules and rarely achieve the size seen with the primary lesions.

Histologically the neoplastic cells may form discrete islands, trabeculae, glands, or undifferentiated sheets. Whatever their organization, the tumor cells are monotonously similar, having a scant, pink, granular cytoplasm and a round-to-oval stippled nucleus. In most tumors, there is minimal variation in cell and nuclear size, and mitoses

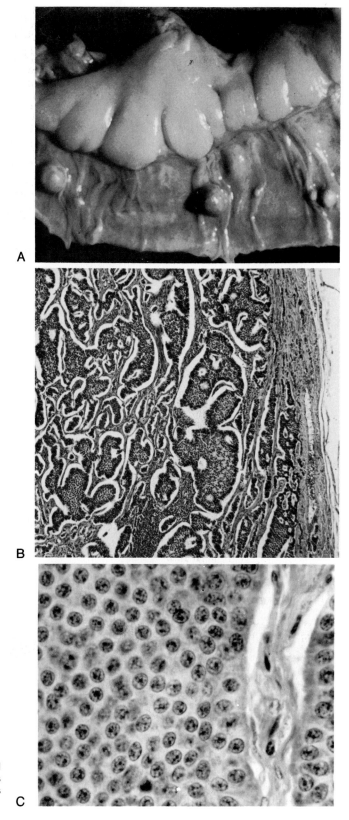

Figure 17–56. Carcinoid tumor. Multiple protruding ileal carcinoids (A), made up of nests and cords of cells invading the submucosa (B). The uniformity of the cells is evident (C). (Hematoxylin and eosin.)

Table 17–15. CLINICAL FEATURES OF CARCINOID SYNDROME

Vasomotor disturbances
  Cutaneous flushes and apparent cyanosis (most patients)
Intestinal hypermotility
  Diarrhea, cramps, nausea, vomiting (most patients)
Asthmatic bronchoconstrictive attacks
  Cough, wheezing, dyspnea (about one-third of patients)
Hepatomegaly
  Nodular, related to hepatic metastases (some cases)
Systemic fibrosis
  Cardiac involvement
    Pulmonic and tricuspid valve thickening and stenosis
    Endocardial fibrosis, principally in right ventricle
    (Bronchial carcinoids affect the left side)
  Retroperitoneal and pelvic fibrosis
  Collagenous pleural and intimal aortic plaques

are infrequent or absent (Fig. 17–56). In unusual cases, there may be more significant anaplasia and sometimes mucin secretion within the cells and gland formations. Rarely tumors arise resembling small cell carcinomas of the lung (see Chapter 15) or contain abundant psammoma bodies similar to those seen in papillary thyroid carcinomas (see Chapter 25). By electron microscopy, the cells in most tumors contain cytoplasmic, membrane-bound secretory granules with osmiophilic centers (dense-core granules). Most carcinoids can be shown to contain chromogranin A, synaptophysin, and neuron-specific enolase.

CLINICAL CONSIDERATIONS. Gastrointestinal carcinoids rarely produce local symptoms; many (especially rectal and appendiceal) are asymptomatic and are found incidentally. The secretory products of some carcinoids, however, may produce a variety of syndromes or endocrinopathies, depending on their anatomic site. Gastric, peripancreatic, and pancreatic carcinoids can release their products directly into the systemic circulation and can produce the *Zollinger-Ellison syndrome*, related to excess elaboration of gastrin; Cushing's syndrome, associated with adenocorticotropic hormone (ACTH) secretion; hyperinsulinism; and others. In some instances, these tumors may be under 1.0 cm in size and extremely difficult to find, even during surgical exploration.

Some neoplasms are associated with a distinctive *"carcinoid syndrome"* (Table 17–15); the cardiovascular ramifications of this syndrome are discussed in Chapter 12. The syndrome occurs in about 1% of all patients with carcinoids and in 20% of those with widespread metastases. Uncertainties remain about the precise origin of the carcinoid syndrome, but most manifestations are thought to arise from excess elaboration of serotonin (5-*hydroxytryptamine* [5HT]). Elevated levels of 5-HT and its metabolite, 5-*hydroxyindoleacetic acid* (5-HIAA), are present in the blood and urine

of most patients with the classic syndrome. 5-HT is degraded in the liver to functionally inactive 5-HIAA. Thus, with gastrointestinal carcinoids, hepatic metastases must be present for the development of the syndrome; not surprisingly, hepatic metastases are not necessary with extraintestinal carcinoids, such as those arising in the lungs or ovaries. The possibility that other secretory products of carcinoids, such as histamine, bradykinin, kallikrein, and prostaglandins, contribute to the manifestations of the carcinoid syndrome has not been excluded.

The overall 5-year survival rate for carcinoids (excluding appendiceal) is approximately 90%. Even with small bowel tumors with hepatic metastases, it is better than 50%. Widespread disease, however, usually causes death.

GASTROINTESTINAL LYMPHOMA

Any segment of the gastrointestinal tract may be secondarily involved by systemic dissemination of non-Hodgkin's lymphomas. Up to 40% of lymphomas, however, arise in sites other than lymph nodes, and the gut is the most common location. By definition, primary gastrointestinal lymphomas exhibit no evidence of liver, spleen, or bone marrow involvement at the time of diagnosis — regional lymph node involvement may be present. *Primary gastrointestinal lymphomas usually arise as sporadic neoplasms. They also occur more frequently in certain patient populations: chronic sprue-like malabsorption syndromes, natives of Mediterranean region, congenital immunodeficiency states, infection with HIV, and following organ transplantation with immunosuppression.*

(1) Sporadic lymphomas, also termed the *Western type,* are the most common form in the Western hemisphere. These B cell lymphomas appear to arise from the B cells of mucosa-associated lymphoid tissue (MALT; discussed earlier in the section on normal intestinal anatomy)[48] and differ from node-based lymphomas in that (1) many behave as focal tumors in their early stages and are amenable to surgical resection, (2) relapse may occur exclusively in the gastrointestinal tract, and (3) genotypic changes are different from those observed in nodal lymphomas. Unlike systemic lymphomas, translocations of t[14;18] and t[11;14] have not been found in gut "MALTomas," whereas *c-myc* rearrangements may be unusually prevalent. This type of gastrointestinal lymphoma usually affects adults, lacks a sex predilection, and may arise anywhere in the gut: stomach (55 to 60% of cases), small intestine (25 to 30%), proximal colon (10 to 15%), and distal colon (up to 10%). The appendix and esophagus are only rarely involved. Although sporadic lymphomas are not associated with other diseases, the concept has been advanced that lym-

phomas of MALT arise in the setting of chronic mucosal lymphoid activation, as may occur in Helicobacter-associated chronic gastritis.[119] The prognosis of sporadic B-cell lymphomas of the gut is generally better than lymphoma arising in other sites; 10-year survival for patients with localized disease may approach 85%.

(2) The *sprue-associated lymphoma* arises in some patients with a long-standing malabsorption syndrome that may or may not be a true gluten-sensitive enteropathy. It occurs in relatively young individuals (30 to 40 years of age), often following a 10- to 20-year history of symptomatic malabsorption. Alternatively a diffuse enteropathy with malabsorption may accompany the development of a lymphoma. This form of lymphoma arises most often in the proximal small bowel. As it is usually of T-cell origin, its overall prognosis is poor.

(3) *Mediterranean lymphoma* refers to an unusual intestinal B-cell lymphoma arising in children and young adults with Mediterranean ancestry, having a background of chronic diffuse mucosal plasmacytosis. The plasma cells synthesize abnormal alpha heavy chain, in which the variable portion has been deleted. A high proportion of patients have malabsorption preceding the development of the lymphoma. This condition, also referred to as *immunoproliferative small intestinal disease*, has a poor prognosis.[120]

MORPHOLOGY. Gastrointestinal lymphomas constitute 1 to 2% of all gastrointestinal malignancies and can assume a variety of gross appearances. Because all the gut lymphoid tissue is mucosal and submucosal, early lesions appear as plaque-like expansions of the mucosa and submucosa. Diffusely infiltrating lesions may produce full-thickness mural thickening, with effacement of the overlying mucosal folds and focal ulceration. Others may be polypoid, protruding into the lumen, or form large, fungating, ulcerated masses. Tumor infiltration into the muscularis propria splays the muscle fibers, gradually destroying them. Because of this feature, advanced lesions frequently cause motility problems with secondary obstruction. Large tumors sometimes perforate because of lack of stromal support; reduction in tumor bulk during chemotherapy also may lead to perforation.

In the earliest histologic lesions, atypical lymphoid cells may be seen infiltrating the mucosa, with effacement and loss of glands and massive expansion of lymphoid tissue. Extreme numbers of atypical lymphoid cells may populate the superficial epithelium (lymphoepithelial lesion). With established lymphomas, the mucosa, submucosa, and even muscle wall are replaced by a monotonous infiltrate of malignant cells, consisting of a mixture of small follicular center cells (both cleaved and uncleaved) and immunoblasts in varying proportion. Lymphoid follicles are occasionally formed. Most gut lymphomas are of B-cell type (over 95%) and are evenly split between low-grade and high-grade tumors. The small fraction of T-cell lymphomas occurring in the intestine are all high-grade lesions.

With gastrointestinal lymphoma, particularly of the sporadic type, early discovery is key to survival; thus, gastric lymphomas generally have a better outcome than those of the small or large bowel. Generally the depth of local invasion, size of the tumor, the histologic grade of the tumor, and extension into adjacent viscera are important determinants of prognosis.[121]

MESENCHYMAL TUMORS

Mesenchymal tumors may occur anywhere in the alimentary tract. Lipomas show a propensity for the submucosa of the small and large intestines, and lipomatous hypertrophy may occur in the ileocecal valve. A variety of spindle-cell lesions may arise in the muscle wall of any gut segment. Most of these tumors have been classified as smooth muscle lesions (leiomyomas and leiomyosarcomas). Immunohistochemical methods, however, have shown some to possess features of neural or histiocytic origin. Because these tumors are quite similar histologically as well as clinically, they are currently grouped under the umbrella of *gastrointestinal stromal tumors*.[122] Both benign and malignant

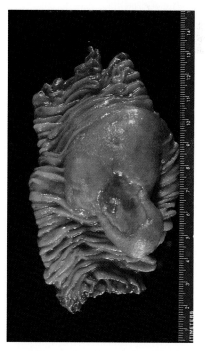

Figure 17–57. Colonic lipoma. Submucosal lipoma of transverse colon protrudes into the lumen, with ulceration of the overlying mucosa.

mesenchymal tumors may occur at any age and in either sex. Kaposi's sarcomas, which may involve the gut, are considered elsewhere (see Chapter 11).

MORPHOLOGY. Lipomas and benign stromal tumors are usually well-demarcated, firm nodules (almost always less than 4 cm in diameter) arising within the submucosa or muscularis propria. The overlying mucosa is stretched and attenuated. Rarely they grow to larger size and produce hemispheric elevation of the mucosa with ulceration over the dome of the tumor (Fig. 17–57). Malignant stromal tumors (primarily leiomyosarcoma) tend to produce large, bulky, intramural masses that eventually fungate and ulcerate into the lumen or project subserosally into the abdominal space. On cross section, they have a typical soft, fish-flesh appearance; are somewhat lobulated; and frequently have areas of hemorrhage, necrosis, or cystic softening.

Histologically lipomas, leiomyomas, and leiomyosarcomas resemble their counterparts encountered elsewhere (see Chapter 7). An uncommon form of mesenchymal tumor is the **leiomyoblastoma** of the stomach, in which larger, plump spindle cells display smooth muscle differentiation by immunohistochemical and ultrastructural criteria. Despite their aggressive appearance, these particular tumors possess a malignant potential intermediate between that of benign and malignant smooth muscle tumors.

Most mesenchymal tumors are asymptomatic. In the stomach, larger lesions (benign or malignant) may produce symptoms resembling those of peptic ulcer, particularly bleeding that is sometimes massive. Intestinal lesions may present with bleeding and, for the small intestine, rare obstruction or intussusception. Benign lesions are easily resectable. Surgical removal is usually possible for the malignant lesions as well because they tend to grow as cohesive masses. Five-year survival rate for leiomyosarcoma, for example, is 50 to 60%. Metastases, however, are present in about one-third of cases.

Appendix

NORMAL

Developmentally the appendix is an underdeveloped residuum of the otherwise voluminous cecum. The adult appendix averages 7 cm in length, is partially anchored by a mesenteric extension from the adjacent ileum, and has no known function. The appendix has the same four layers as the remainder of the gut and possesses a colonic-type mucosa. A distinguishing feature of this organ is the extremely rich lymphoid tissue of the mucosa and submucosa, which in young individuals forms an entire layer of germinal follicles and lymphoid pulp. This lymphoid tissue undergoes progressive atrophy during life to the point of complete disappearance in advanced age. In the elderly, the appendix, particularly the distal portion, sometimes undergoes fibrous obliteration.

PATHOLOGY

Diseases of the appendix loom large in surgical practice; appendicitis is the most common acute abdominal condition the surgeon is called on to treat. Appendicitis is one of the best-known medical entities and yet may be one of the most difficult diagnostic problems to confront the emergency physician. A differential diagnosis must include virtually every acute process that can occur within the abdominal cavity as well as some emergent conditions affecting organs of the thorax.

ACUTE APPENDICITIS

Inflammation in the right lower quadrant was considered a nonsurgical disease of the cecum (typhlitis or perityphlitis) until Fitz recognized acute appendicitis as a distinct entity in 1886.[123] Appendiceal inflammation is associated with obstruction in 50 to 80% of cases, usually in the form of a fecalith and, less commonly, a gallstone, tumor, or ball of worms *(oxyuriasis vermicularis)*. Continued secretion of mucinous fluid in the obstructed viscus presumably leads to a progressive increase in intraluminal pressure sufficient to cause eventual collapse of the draining veins. Ischemic injury then favors bacterial proliferation with additional inflammatory edema and exudation, further embarrassing the blood supply. Nevertheless, a significant minority of inflamed appendices have no demonstrable luminal obstruction, and the pathogenesis of the inflammation remains unknown.

MORPHOLOGY. At the earliest stages, only a scant neutrophilic exudate may be found throughout the mucosa, submucosa, and muscularis propria. Subserosal vessels are congested, and often there is a modest perivascular neutrophilic infiltrate. The inflammatory reaction transforms the normal glistening serosa into a dull, granular, red membrane; this transformation signifies **early acute appendicitis** for the operating surgeon. At a later stage, a prominent neutrophilic exudate generates a fibrinopurulent reaction over the serosa (Fig. 17–58). As the inflammatory process worsens, there is abscess formation within the wall, along with ulcerations and foci of suppurative necrosis in the mucosa. This state constitutes **acute suppurative appendicitis.** Further appendiceal compromise leads to large areas of hemorrhagic green ulceration of the mucosa and green-black gangrenous necrosis through the wall extending to the serosa, creating **acute gangrenous appendicitis,** which is quickly followed by rupture and suppurative peritonitis.

   The histologic criterion for the diagnosis of acute appendicitis is neutrophilic infiltration of the muscularis. Usually neutrophils and ulcerations are also present within the mucosa. Because drainage of an exudate into the appendix from alimentary tract infection (e.g., Campylobacter) may also induce a mucosal neutrophili infiltrate, evidence of muscular wall inflammation is requisite for the diagnosis.

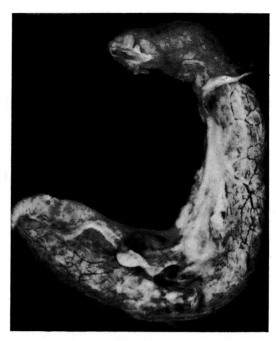

Figure 17–58. Acute appendicitis. A suppurative exudate covers the serosa of the appendix. Uneven dilatation is produced by impacted fecaliths.

   Acute appendicitis is mainly a disease of adolescents and young adults, but it may occur in any age group and affects males slightly more often than females. Classically acute appendicitis produces the following manifestations, in the sequence given: (1) pain, at first periumbilical but then localizing to the right lower quadrant; (2) nausea or vomiting; (3) abdominal tenderness, particularly in the region of the appendix; (4) mild fever; and (5) an elevation of the peripheral white blood cell count up to 15,000 to 20,000 cell/mm³. Regrettably this classic presentation is more often absent than present. Although pain, nausea, and vomiting usually develop, tenderness may be deceptively absent or maximal in atypical locations. In some cases, a retrocecal appendix may generate right flank or pelvic pain, whereas a malrotated colon may give rise to appendicitis in the left upper quadrant. The peripheral leukocytosis may be minimal or so high as to suggest alternative diagnoses. Nonclassic presentations are encountered more often in young children and in the very elderly, populations with a host of other plausible abdominal emergencies.

   There is general agreement that highly competent surgeons make false-positive diagnoses of acute appendicitis and remove normal appendices about 20 to 25% of the time.[124] *The discomfort and risks associated with an exploratory laparotomy and discovery of "no disease" are far outweighed by the morbidity and mortality (about 2%) associated with perforation.* Besides perforation, uncommon complications of appendicitis include pylephlebitis with thrombosis of the portal venous drainage, liver abscess, and bacteremia. In instances when the appendix is normal, most often no disease of any kind is found during abdominal exploration, leaving the surgeon mumbling about such vagaries as "cecitis" or "appendiceal colic." Definable conditions that mimic appendicitis are mesenteric lymphadenitis, usually secondary to an enterocolitis (often unrecognized) caused by Yersinia or a virus; systemic viral infection; acute salpingitis; ectopic pregnancy; "mittelschmerz" (pain caused by trivial pelvic bleeding at the time of ovulation); cystic fibrosis; and Meckel's diverticulitis.

True *chronic inflammation* of the appendix is rare as a pathologic entity, although occasionally granulation tissue and fibrosis associated with acute and chronic inflammation of the appendix suggest an organizing acute appendicitis. Much more frequently, recurrent acute attacks underly a seemingly chronic condition. Because in some individuals the appendix is a mere fibrous cord from birth, it cannot be assumed that appendiceal fibrosis is the result of a previous inflammation.

TUMORS OF THE APPENDIX

MUCOCELE AND PSEUDOMYXOMA PERITONEI

Dilatation of the appendiceal lumen by mucinous secretion is designated *mucocele* (Fig. 17–59). This transformation is caused by one of three patterns of epithelial proliferation:[125] (1) non-neoplastic epithelial hyperplasia indistinguishable from hyperplastic polyps of the colon, (2) mucinous cystadenoma (by far the most common form), or (3) mucinous cystadenocarcinoma.

> **MORPHOLOGY.** All three lesions are associated with appendiceal dilatation secondary to mucinous secretions. With **mucosal hyperplasia,** elongated but otherwise innocuous columnar mucous cells produce copious amounts of mucin, but there is no evidence of appendiceal rupture or of peritoneal mucinous implants. The histologic features of cystadenomas and cystadenocarcinomas closely mimic their ovarian counterparts (see Chapter 23). With **cystadenomas,** the luminal dilatation is associated with appendiceal perforation in 20% of instances, producing localized collections of mucus attached to the serosa of the appendix or lying free in the peritoneal cavity. Histologic examination of the mucus, however, reveals no neoplastic cells, and appendectomy is curative. **Mucinous cystadenocarcinomas** are one-fifth as common as cystadenomas. Macroscopically they produce mucin-filled cystic dilatation of the appendix indistinguishable from that seen with the benign tumors. Penetration of the appendiceal wall by neoplastic cells, however, and spread beyond the appendix in the form of peritoneal implants is frequently present. In its fully developed state, the peritoneal cavity becomes distended with tenacious, semisolid mucin —**pseudomyxoma peritonei**—in which anaplastic adenocarcinomatous cells can be found, distinguishing this process from mucinous spillage. The intraperitoneal spread of this mucin-secreting cancer is identical in appearance and lethal outcome to that of intraperitoneal ovarian mucinous cystadenocarcinoma (see Chapter 23).

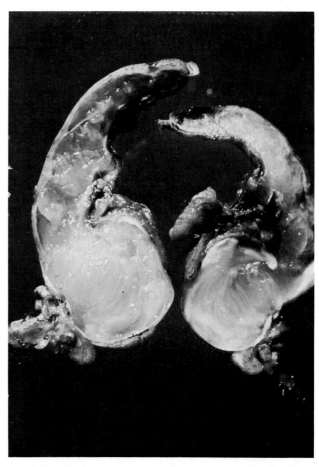

Figure 17–59. Hemisected mucocele of the appendix. Note the distention owing to the mucus accumulated in the lumen.

CARCINOMA AND OTHER TUMORS

The most common appendiceal tumor is the carcinoid, discussed earlier. This neoplasm most frequently involves the distal tip of the appendix, where it produces a solid bulbous swelling up to 2 to 3 cm in diameter. Although intramural and transmural extension may be evident, nodal metastases are infrequent, and distant spread is rare. On rare occasions, adenomas or nonmucin-producing adenocarcinomas of the appendix may cause a typical neoplastic enlargement of this organ. Benign and malignant mesenchymal growths resemble their counterparts in other areas.

Peritoneum

INFLAMMATION
PERITONEAL INFECTION
SCLEROSING RETROPERITONITIS
MESENTERIC CYSTS
TUMORS

INFLAMMATION

Peritonitis may result from bacterial invasion or chemical irritation. The most common causes of sterile peritonitis in order of frequency are bile, pancreatic enzymes, and surgically introduced foreign material.

Perforation or rupture of the biliary system evokes a highly irritating peritonitis. At first, the peritoneal exudate is bile-stained. Later, the biliary discoloration is masked by the progressive suppuration that ensues, concomitant with superimposed bacterial contamination.

Acute hemorrhagic pancreatitis is a calamitous disorder characterized by hemorrhage and necrosis of the pancreas (see Chapter 19). With leakage of pancreatic enzymes into the peritoneal cavity, proteolytic and lipolytic ferments evoke a striking peritoneal reaction. Digestion of adipose tissue produces fatty acids, leading to saponification with calcium to produce chalky white precipitates in areas of fat digestion and necrosis. Globules of free fat may be found floating in the peritoneal fluid that accumulates. After 24 to 48 hours, enzymatic damage and bacterial permeation of the bowel wall usually lead to a frank suppurative condition.

The reaction to surgically introduced foreign material such as talc is usually localized and minimal. No clinical symptoms ensue, although residual foreign body–type granulomas and fibrous tissue may develop. In contrast, abrasion of serosal surfaces during abdominal surgery, endometritis, and peritoneal infection (see later) may lead to fibrous adhesions between visceral structures. Although usually asymptomatic, occasionally internal herniation or intestinal obstruction may result.

Because the female genital tract opens into the peritoneal cavity, gynecologic processes also can produce a sterile peritonitis. Endometriosis may introduce blood into the peritoneal cavity, and ruptured dermoid cysts may invoke an intense peritoneal granulomatous reaction.

PERITONEAL INFECTION

Bacterial peritonitis is almost invariably secondary to extension of bacteria through the wall of a hollow viscus or to rupture of a viscus. The common disorders leading to such bacterial disseminations are *appendicitis, ruptured peptic ulcer, cholecystitis, diverticulitis, strangulation of bowel, acute salpingitis, abdominal trauma,* and *peritoneal dialysis.* Virtually every bacterial organism has been implicated, most commonly *E. coli,* alpha-hemolytic and beta-hemolytic streptococci, *Staphylococcus aureus,* enterococci, gram-negative rods, and *Clostridium perfringens.* The last organism is a frequent inhabitant of the gut and contributor to peritonitis but rarely causes gas gangrene in the abdominal cavity. Gynecologic infections may introduce gonococcus and chlamydia.

Spontaneous bacterial peritonitis may develop in the absence of an obvious source of contamination. It is an uncommon disorder seen most often in children, particularly those with the nephrotic syndrome. Among adults, 10% of cirrhotic patients with ascites develop spontaneous bacterial peritonitis during the course of their illness. The usual causal agents of the latter are *E. coli* and pneumococci, but the manner by which they invade the peritoneal cavity is unknown, possibly blood-borne.

MORPHOLOGY. Depending on the duration of the peritonitis, the membranes show the following changes. Approximately 2 to 4 hours after initiation, there is loss of the gray, glistening quality of the peritoneal surface, and it becomes dull and lusterless. At this time, there is a small accumulation of essentially serous or slightly turbid fluid. Later, the exudate becomes creamy and obviously suppurative. In some cases, it may be extremely thick and plastic and even inspissated, especially in dehydrated patients. The volume of exudates varies enormously. In many cases, it may be localized by the omentum and viscera to a small area of the abdominal cavity. In generalized peritonitis, it is important to remember that an exudate may accumulate under and above the liver to form **subhepatic** and **subdiaphragmatic abscesses.** Collections in the lesser omental sac may likewise create residual persistent foci of infection.

The inflammatory process is typical of an acute bacterial infection anywhere and produces the characteristic neutrophilic infiltration with fibrinopurulent exudation. The reaction usually remains superficial and does not penetrate deeply into the visceral structures or abdominal wall. **Tuberculous peritonitis** tends to produce a plastic exudate studded with minute, pale granulomas.

These inflammatory processes can heal either spontaneously or with therapy. In the course of healing, the following may obtain: *(1) the exudate may be totally resolved, leaving no residual fibrosis. (2) Residual, walled-off abscesses may persist, eventually to heal or serve as foci of new infection. (3) Organization of the exudate may occur, with the formation of fibrous adhesions that may be delicate or quite dense.*

SCLEROSING RETROPERITONITIS

Dense fibromatous overgrowth of the retroperitoneal tissues may sometimes develop, designated sclerosing retroperitonitis or retroperitoneal fibromatosis. In some instances, the mesentery also is involved. The fibrous overgrowth is entirely nondistinctive and, although infiltrative, does not display anaplasia. There is usually an accompanying inflammatory infiltrate of lymphocytes, plasma cells, and neutrophils, suggesting inflammatory rather than neoplastic disease. The fibrosis may encroach on the ureters to produce hydronephrosis. Alternatively fibrous tissue may surround retroperitoneal organs and extend into the mesentery. In some ways this process is an analogue of the desmoid tumor (see Chapter 7). The cause of this curious condition is obscure; in some instances, there is a history of intake of the drug methysergide, an ergot derivative used for migraine. Most cases, however, have no obvious cause. Similar fibrotic changes seen in other sites (mediastinal fibrosis, sclerosing cholangitis, and Riedel's [fibrosing] thyroiditis) suggest that the disorder is autoimmune and systemic in origin, preferentially involving the retroperitoneum.

MESENTERIC CYSTS

Large-to-small cystic masses are sometimes found within the mesenteries in the abdominal cavity or attached to the peritoneal lining of the abdominal wall. These cysts sometimes offer difficult clinical diagnostic problems because they present on palpation as abdominal masses. Many classifications have been attempted; the most widely used is based on pathogenetic origins: (1) those arising from sequestered lymphatic channels; (2) those derived from pinched-off enteric diverticula of the developing foregut and hindgut; (3) those derived from the urogenital ridge or its derivatives, i.e., the urinary tract and male and female genital tracts; (4) those derived from walled-off infections or following pancreatitis, more properly called *pseudocysts* (see Chapter 19); and (5) those of malignant origin, most often resulting from peritoneal involvement by intraabdominal adenocarcinomas.

TUMORS

Virtually all tumors of the peritoneum are malignant and can be divided into primary and secondary forms.

Primary tumors arising from the mesothelium of the peritoneum are extremely rare and are called mesotheliomas. These exactly duplicate mesotheliomas found in the pleura and the pericardium (see Chapter 15). Similar to the supradiaphragmatic tumors, peritoneal mesotheliomas are associated with asbestos exposure in at least 80% of cases. How inhaled asbestos induces a peritoneal neoplasm remains a mystery.

Secondary tumors of the peritoneum are, in contrast, quite common. In any form of advanced cancer, penetration to the serosal membrane or metastatic seeding (peritoneal carcinomatosis) may occur. The most common tumors producing diffuse serosal implantation and sometimes pseudomyxoma peritonei are ovarian and pancreatic carcinomas. Any type of intra-abdominal malignancy, however, may be implicated in peritoneal seeding and occasionally tumors from extra-abdominal locations.

Additional mention might be made of uncommon tumors that may arise from retroperitoneal tissues, i.e., fat, fibrous tissue, blood vessels, lymphatics, nerves, and the lymph nodes alongside the aorta. These native structures may give rise to benign or malignant tumors derived from any of the indigenous mesenchymal cell types, resembling their counterparts arising elsewhere in the body.

1. DeNardi, F.G., and Riddell, R.H.: The normal esophagus. Am. J. Surg. Pathol. 15:296, 1991.
2. Stuart, R.C., and Hennessy, T.P.J.: Primary disorders of oesophageal motility. Br. J. Surg. 76:1111, 1989.
3. Weiss, S., and Mallory, G.K.: Lesions of cardiac orifice of the stomach produced vomiting. J.A.M.A. 98:1353, 1932.
4. Jamieson, G.G., and Duranceau, A.: The pathology of gastroesophageal reflux. In Duranceau, A., and Jamieson, G.G. (eds.): Gastroesophageal Reflux. Philadelphia, W.B. Saunders Co., 1988, p. 46.

5. Spechler, S.J., and Goyal, R.K.: Barrett's esophagus. N. Engl. J. Med. 315:362, 1986.

6. Reid, B.J., et al.: Observer variation in the diagnosis of dysplasia in Barrett's esophagus. Hum. Pathol. 19:166, 1988.

7. Boring, C.C., et al.: Cancer statistics, 1993. CA Cancer J. Clin. 43:7, 1993.

8. Tuyas, A.J., et al.: Cancers of the digestive tract, alcohol and tobacco. Int. J. Cancer 30:9, 1982.

9. Oelette, G.J., et al.: Esophagitis in a population at risk for esophageal carcinoma. Cancer 57:2222, 1986.

10. Pra, M., et al.: Increasing incidence of adenocarcinoma of the esophagus and esophagogastric junction. Gastroenterology 104:510, 1993.

11. Smith, R.R.L., et al.: The spectrum of carcinoma arising in Barrett's esophagus. A clinicopathologic study of 26 patients. Am. J. Surg. Pathol. 8:563, 1984.

12. Antonioli, D.A., and Madara, J.L.: Functional anatomy of the gastrointestinal tract. In Ming, S.-C., and Goldman, H. (eds.): Pathology of the Gastrointestinal Tract. Philadelphia, W.B. Saunders Co., 1992, p. 14.

13. Mangeat, P., et al.: Acid secretion and membrane reorganization in single gastric parietal cell in primary culture. Biol. Cell 69:223, 1990.

14. Muller, M.J., et al.: Control of pepsinogen synthesis and secretion. Gastroenterol. Clin. North Am. 19:27, 1990.

15. Konturek, S.J.: Gastric cytoprotection. Scand. J. Gastroenterol. 20:543, 1985.

16. Silen, W.: Gastric mucosal defense and repair. In Johnson, L.R. (ed.): Physiology of the Gastrointestinal Tract. Vol. 2. New York, Raven Press, 1987, p. 1055.

17. Szabo, S.: Mechanisms of gastric mucosal injury and protection. J. Clin. Gastroenterol. 13(Suppl.):821, 1991.

18. Correa, P., and Yardley, J.H.: Grading and classification of chronic gastritis: One American response to the Sydney system. Gastroenterology 102:355, 1992.

19. Kreuning, J., et al.: Gastric and duodenal mucosa in "healthy" individuals. J. Clin. Pathol. 31:69, 1978.

20. Karisson, F.A., et al.: Major parietal cell antigen in autoimmune gastritis with pernicious anemia is the acid-producing H+,K+-adenosine triphosphatase of the stomach. J. Clin. Invest. 81:475, 1988.

21. Cover, T.L., and Blaser, M.J.: Helicobacter pylori and gastroduodenal disease. Annu. Rev. Med. 43:135, 1992.

22. Morris, A., and Nicholson, G.: Ingestion of Campylobacter pyloridis causes gastritis and raised fasting pH. Am. J. Gastroenterol. 82:192, 1987.

23. Blaser, M.J., et al.: Association of infection due to Helicobacter pylori with specific upper gastrointestinal pathology. Rev. Infect. Dis. 13(Suppl. 8):S704, 1991.

24. Strickland, R.G.: Gastritis. Springer Semin. Immunopathol. 12:203, 1990.

25. Grossman, M.I.: Peptic ulcer: Definition and epidemiology. In Rotter, J. (ed.): The Genetics and Heterogeneity of Common Gastrointestinal Disorders. New York, Academic Press, 1980, p. 21.

26. Soll, A.H.: Pathogenesis of peptic ulcer and implications for therapy. N. Engl. J. Med. 322:909, 1990.

27. Soll, A.H., et al.: Nonsteroidal anti-inflammatory drugs and peptic ulcer disease. Ann. Intern. Med. 114:307, 1991.

28. Feldman, M., et al.: Role of affect and personality in gastric acid secretion and serum gastrin concentration. Comparative studies in normal men and in male duodenal ulcer patients. Gastroenterology 102:175, 1992.

29. Fry, J.: Peptic ulcer: A profile. B.M.J. 2:809, 1964.

30. Komorowski, R.A., and Caya, J.G.: Hyperplastic gastropathy: Clinicopathologic correlation. Am. J. Surg. Pathol. 15:577, 1991.

31. Sarin, S.K., and Kumar, A.: Gastric varices: Profile, classification, and management. Am. J. Gastroenterol. 84:1244, 1989.

32. Ming, S.-C.: Epithelial polyps of the stomach. In Ming, S.-C., and Goldman, H. (eds.): Pathology of the Gastrointestinal Tract. Philadelphia, W.B. Saunders Co., 1992, p. 547.

33. Nakano, H., et al.: Study of the gastric mucosal background in patients with gastric polyps. Gastrointest. Endosc. 36:39, 1990.

34. Dekker, W., and Op den Orth, J.O.: Polyps of the stomach and duodenum: Significance and management. Dig. Dis. 10:199, 1992.

35. Craanen, M.E., et al.: Prevalence of subtypes of intestinal metaplasia in gastric antral mucosa. Dig. Dis. Sci. 36:1529, 1991.

36. Correa, P., et al.: Diet and gastric cancer: Nutrition survey in a high risk area. J. Natl. Cancer Inst. 70:673, 1983.

37. Sipponen, P.: Atrophic gastritis as a premalignant condition. Ann. Med. 21:287, 1989.

38. Parsonnet, J., et al.: Helicobacter pylori infection and the risk of gastric carcinoma. N. Engl. J. Med. 325:1127, 1991.

39. Lauren, P.: The two histological main types of gastric carcinoma: Diffuse and so-called intestinal-type carcinoma. Acta Path. Microbiol. Scand. 64:31, 1965.

40. Ming, S.-C.: Gastric carcinoma: A pathobiological classification. Cancer 39:2475, 1977.

41. Craanen, M.E., et al.: Early gastric cancer: A clinicopathologic study. J. Clin. Gastroenterol. 13:274, 1991.

42. Eisenhauer, P.B., et al.: Cryptdins: Antimicrobial defensins of the murine small intestine. Infect. Immun. 60:3556, 1992.

43. Specian, R.D., and Oliver, M.G.: Functional biology of intestinal goblet cells. Am. J. Physiol. Cell Physiol. 260:C183, 1991.

44. Nusrat, A., et al.: Intestinal epithelial restitution. Characterization of a cell culture model and mapping of cytoskeletal elements in migrating cells. J. Clin. Invest. 89:1501, 1992.

45. Pearse, A.G.E.: The APUD cell concept and its implications in pathology. Pathol. Annu. 9:27, 1974.

46. La Douarin, N.M.: The embryological origin of the endocrine cells associated with the digestive tract: Experimental analysis based on the use of a stable marking technique. In Bloom, S.R. (ed.): Gut Hormones. Edinburgh, Churchill Livingstone, 1978, p. 49.

47. Modlin, I.M., et al.: Biological markers of neuroendocrine tumors of the gastrointestinal tract and pancreas. Clinical review. Eur. J. Surg. 157:629, 1991.

48. Isaacson, P.G., and Spencer, J.: Malignant lymphoma of mucosa-associated lymphoid tissue. Histopathology 11:445, 1987.

49. Johnston, M.C., et al.: Neurocristopathy as a unifying concept: Clinical correlations. Adv. Neurol. 29:97, 1981.

50. Swerdlow, S.H., et al: Intestinal infarction: A new classification (Letter). Arch Pathol. Lab. Med. 106:218, 1981.

51. Mitsudo, S.M., et al.: Vascular ectasia of the right colon in the elderly: A distinct pathologic entity. Hum. Pathol. 10:587, 1979.

52. Chopra, S., and Trier, J.S.: Diarrhea and malabsorption. In Chopra, S., and May, R.J. (eds.): Pathophysiology of Gastrointestinal Diseases. Boston, Little, Brown, 1989, p. 125.

53. Guerrant, R.L., et al.: Diarrhea in developed and developing countries: Magnitude, special settings, and etiologies. Rev. Infect. Dis. 12(Suppl. 1):S41, 1990.

54. Garthright, W.E., et al.: Estimates of incidence and costs of intestinal infectious diseases in the United States. Pub. Health Rep. 103:107, 1988.

55. Lambden, P.R., et al.: Sequence and genome organization of a human small round-structured (Norwalk-like) virus. Science 259:516, 1993.

56. Schreiber, D.S., et al.: The mucosal lesion of the proximal small intestine in acute infectious nonbacterial gastroenteritis. N. Engl. J. Med. 288:1318, 1973.

57. Bass, D.M., and Greenberg, H.B.: Pathogenesis of viral gastroenteritis. In Field, M. (ed.): Diarrheal Diseases. New York, Elsevier, 1991, p. 139.

58. Knutton, S., et al.: Adhesion of enteropathogenic Escherichia coli to human intestinal enterocytes and cultured human intestinal mucosa. Infect. Immun. 55:69, 1987.

59. Schron, C.M., and Giannella, R.A.: Bacterial enterotoxins. In Field, M. (ed.) Diarrheal Diseases. New York, Elsevier, 1991, p. 115.

60. Lencer, W.I., et al.: Mechanism of cholera toxin action on a polarized human intestinal epithelial cell line: Role of vesicular traffic. J. Cell Biol. 117:1197, 1992.

61. Abrams, G.D.: Infectious disorders of the intestines. In Ming, S.-C., and Goldman, H. (eds.): Pathology of the Gastrointestinal Tract. Philadelphia, W.B. Saunders Co., 1992, p. 621.

62. Kliegman, R.M., and Fanaroff, A.A.: Necrotizing enterocolitis. N. Engl. J. Med. 310:1093, 1984.

63. Head, J.R.: Immunobiology of lactation. Semin. Perinatol. 1:195, 1977.

64. Ballance, W.A., et al.: Pathology of neonatal necrotizing enterocolitis: A ten-year experience. J. Pediatr. 117(Suppl.):S6, 1990.

65. Trnka, Y.M., and LaMont, J.T.: Clostridium difficile colitis. Adv. Intern. Med. 29:85, 1984.

66. Cummins, A.G.: Quantitative histological study of enteropathy associated with HIV infection. Gut 31:317, 1990.

67. Snover, D.C., et al.: A histopathologic study of gastric and small intestinal graft-versus-host disease following allogeneic bone marrow transplantation. Hum. Pathol. 16:387, 1985.

68. Jessurun, J., et al.: Microscopic and collagenous colitis: Different names for the same condition? Gastroenterology 91:1583, 1986.

69. Trier, J.S.: Celiac sprue. N. Engl. J. Med. 325:1709, 1991.

70. Marsh, M.N.: Gluten, major histocompatibility complex, and the small intestine. A molecular and immunobiologic approach to the spectrum of gluten sensitivity ('celiac sprue'). Gastroenterology 102:330, 1992.

71. Mantzaris, G.J., et al.: Cellular hypersensitivity to a synthetic dodecapeptide derived from human adenovirus 12 which resembles a sequence of A-gliadin in patients with coeliac disease. Gut 31:668, 1990.

72. Working Group of European Society of Paediatric Gastroenterology and Nutrition: Revised criteria for diagnosis of coeliac disease. Arch. Dis. Child. 65:909, 1990.

73. Spencer, J., et al.: Enteropathy-associated T cell lymphoma (malignant histiocytosis of the intestine) is recognized by a monoclonal antibody (HML-1) that defines a membrane molecule on human mucosal lymphocytes. Am. J. Pathol. 132:1, 1988.

74. Baker, S.J., and Mathan, V.I.: Syndrome of tropical sprue in South India. Am. J. Clin. Nutr. 21:984, 1968.

75. Ectors, N., et al.: Whipple's disease: A histological, immunocytochemical and electron microscopic study of the immune response in the small intestinal mucosa. Histopathology 21:1, 1992.

76. Relman, D.A., et al.: Identification of the uncultured bacillus of Whipple's disease. N. Engl. J. Med. 327:293, 1992.

77. Bjorneklett, A.: Small bowel bacterial overgrowth syndrome. Scand. J. Gastroenterol. 18(Suppl. 85):83, 1983.

78. Paulley, J.W.: Gut damage in human blind-loop syndrome. Gastroenterology. 81:195, 1981.

79. Isselbacher, K.J., Scheig, R., et al.: Congenital B-lipoprotein deficiency: An hereditary disorder involving a defect in the absorption and transport of lipids. Medicine 43:347, 1964.

80. Glickman, R.M., et al.: Immunofluorescence studies of apolipoprotein-B in intestinal mucosa. Gastroenterology 76:288, 1979.

81. Podolsky, D.K.: Inflammatory bowel disease (first of two parts). N. Engl. J. Med. 325:928, 1991.

82. Podolsky, D.K.: Inflammatory bowel disease (second of two parts). N. Engl. J. Med. 325:1008, 1991.

83. Lindberg, E., et al.: Antibodies (IgG, IgA, and IgM) to baker's yeast (Saccharomyces cerevisiae), yeast mannan, gliadin, ovalbumin and betalactoglobulin in monozygotic twins with inflammatory bowel disease. Gut 33:909, 1992.

84. Chiodini, R.J.: Crohn's disease and the Mycobacterioses: A review and comparison of two disease entities. Clin. Microbiol. Rev. 2:90, 1989.

85. Farmer, R.G.: Infectious causes of diarrhea in the differential diagnosis of inflammatory bowel disease. Med. Clin. North Am. 74:29, 1990.

86. Tysk, C., et al.: Colonic glycoproteins in monozygotic twins with inflammatory bowel disease. Gastroenterology 100:419, 1991.

87. Schreiber, S., et al.: The role of the mucosal immune system in inflammatory bowel disease. Gastroenterol. Clin. North Am. 21:451, 1992.

88. Sadlack, B., et al.: Ulcerative colitis–like disease in mice with a disrupted interleukin-2 gene. Cell 75:253, 1993.

89. Stevens, C., et al.: Tumor necrosis factor-α, interleukin-1β, and interleukin-6 expression in inflammatory bowel disease. Dig. Dis. Sci. 37:818, 1992.

90. Parkos, C.A., et al.: Neutrophil migration across a cultured intestinal epithelium. Dependence on a CD11b/CD18-mediated event and enhanced efficiency in physiologic direction. J. Clin. Invest. 88:1605, 1991.

91. Madara, J.L., et al.: 5'-AMP is the neutrophil derived paracrine factor that elicits chloride secretion from T84 intestinal epithelial cell monolayers. J. Clin. Invest. 91:2320, 1993.

92. Crohn, B.B., et al.: Regional ileitis: A pathologic and clinical entity. J.A.M.A. 99:1323, 1932.

93. Ekbom, A., et al.: Increased risk of large-bowel cancer in Crohn's disease with colonic involvement. Lancet 336:357, 1990.

94. Garland, C.F., et al.: Incidence rates of ulcerative colitis and Crohn's disease in 15 areas of the U.S. Gastroenterology 81:1115, 1981.

95. Nostrant, T.T., et al.: Histopathology differentiates acute self-limited colitis from ulcerative colitis. Gastroenterology 92:318, 1987.

96. Blackstone, M.O., et al.: Dysplasia-associated lesion or mass (DALM) detected by colonoscopy in long-standing ulcerative colitis: An indication for colectomy. Gastroenterology 80:366, 1981.

97. Riddell, R.H., et al.: Dysplasia in inflammatory bowel disease: Standardized classification with provisional clinical applications. Hum. Pathol. 14:931, 1983.

98. Ekbom, A., et al.: Ulcerative colitis and colorectal cancer—a population-based study. N. Engl. J. Med. 323:1228, 1990.

99. Nugent, F.W., et al.: Cancer surveillance in ulcerative colitis. Gastroenterology 100:1241, 1991.

100. Lashner, B.A., et al.: Colon cancer surveillance in chronic ulcerative colitis. Historical cohort study. Am. J. Gastroenterol. 85:1083, 1990.

101. Krishnamurthy, S., et al.: Jejunal diverticulosis: A heterogeneous disorder caused by a variety of abnormalities of smooth muscle or myenteric plexus. Gastroenterology 85:538, 1983.

102. Painter, N.S.: The cause of diverticular disease of the colon, its symptoms and its complications. J. R. Coll. Surg. (Edinburgh) 30:118, 1985.

103. Järvinen, H.J.: Other gastrointestinal polyps. World J. Surg. 15:50, 1991.

104. Bailar, J.C. III, and Smith, E. M.: Progress against cancer? N. Engl. J. Med. 314:1226, 1986.

105. Spigelman, A.D., et al.: Cancer and the Peutz-Jeghers syndrome. Gut 30:1588, 1989.

106. Winawer, S.J., et al.: Prevention of colorectal cancer by colonoscopic polypectomy. N. Engl. J. Med. 329:1977, 1993.

107. Cranley, J.P., et al.: When is endoscopic polypectomy adequate therapy for colonic polyps containing invasive carcinoma? Gastroenterology 91:419, 1986.

108. Haggitt, R.C., et al.: Prognostic factors in colorectal carcinomas arising in adenomas: Implications for lesions removed by endoscopic polypectomy. Gastroenterology 89:328, 1985.

109. Lynch, H.T., et al.: Colon cancer genetics. Cancer 70(Suppl.):1300, 1992.

110. Morson, B.C.: The polyp-cancer sequence in the large bowel. Proc. R. soc. Med. 67:451, 1974.

111. Rustgi, A.K., and Podolsky, D.K.: The molecular basis of colon cancer. Annu. Rev. Med. 43:612, 1992.

112. Powell, S.M., et al.: Molecular diagnosis of familial adenomatous polyposis. N. Engl. J. Med. 329:1982, 1993.

113. Peltomäki, P., et al.: Genetic mapping of a locus predisposing to human colorectal cancer. Science 260:810, 1993.

114. Thibodeau, S.N., et al.: Microsatellite instability in cancer of the proximal colon. Science 260:816, 1993.

115. Willett, W.C., et al.: Relation of meat, fat and fiber intake to the risk of colon cancer in a prospective study among women. N. Engl. J. Med. 323:1664, 1990.

116. Cooper, H.S., and Slemmer, J.R.: Surgical pathology of carcinoma of the colon and rectum. Semin. Oncol. 18:367, 1991.

117. Kyriakos, M.: The President's cancer, the Dukes classification, and confusion. Arch. Pathol. Lab. Med. 109:1063, 1985.

118. Solcia, E., et al.: Classification and histogenesis of gastroenteropancreatic endocrine tumours. Eur. J. Clin. Invest. 20(Suppl 1):S72, 1990.

119. Isaacson, P.G.: Extranodal lymphomas: The MALT concept. Verh. Dtsch. Ges. Path. 76:14, 1992.

120. Isaacson, P.G., et al.: Immunoproliferative small-intestinal disease: An immunohistochemical study. Am. J. Surg. Pathol. 13:1023, 1989.

121. Radaszkiewicz, T., et al.: Gastrointestinal malignant lymphomas of the mucosa-associated lymphoid tissue: Factors relevant to prognosis. Gastroenterology 102:1628, 1992.

122. Ueyama, T., et al.: A clinicopathologic and immunohistochemical study of gastrointestinal stromal tumors. Cancer 69:947, 1992.

123. Fitz, R.H.: Perforating inflammation of the vermiform appendix: With special references to its early diagnosis and treatment. Am. J. Med. Sci. 92:321, 1886.

124. Malt, R.A.: The perforated appendix (Editorial). N. Engl. J. Med. 315:1546, 1986.

125. Gray G.F., Jr., and Wackym, P.A.: Surgical pathology of the vermiform appendix. Pathol. Annu. 21:(Pt.2):111, 1986.

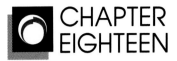

CHAPTER EIGHTEEN

The Liver and the Biliary Tract

JAMES M. CRAWFORD, M.D., Ph.D.

The Liver

NORMAL

Residing at the crossroads between the digestive tract and the rest of the body, the liver has the enormous job of maintaining the body's metabolic homeostasis. This includes the processing of dietary amino acids, carbohydrates, lipids, and vitamins; phagocytosis of particulate material in the splanchnic circulation; synthesis of serum proteins; biotransformation of circulating metabolites; and detoxification and excretion into bile of endogenous waste products and pollutant xenobiotics. Hepatic disorders therefore have far-reaching consequences, which are best understood from the perspective of normal structure and function.

The normal adult liver weighs 1400 to 1600 gm (2.5% of body weight). Incoming blood

831

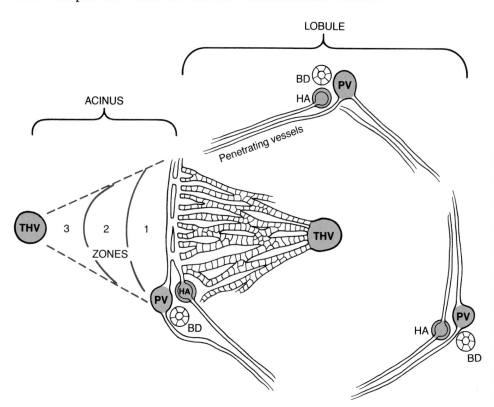

Figure 18–1. Microscopic liver architecture, depicted schematically. The classic hexagonal lobule is centered around a central vein (terminal hepatic venule), with portal triads at three of its six angles. The triangular acinus has as its base the penetrating vessels, which extend from portal veins and hepatic arteries to penetrate the parenchyma. The apex is formed by the terminal hepatic venule. Zones 1, 2, and 3 represent metabolic regions increasingly distant from the blood supply. PV = portal vein; HA = hepatic artery; BD = bile duct; THV = terminal hepatic venule.

arrives via the portal vein (60 to 70% of hepatic blood flow) and hepatic artery (30 to 40%) through the "gateway" of the liver, the *porta hepatis;* bile exits via the common hepatic bile duct. These three conduits ramify in parallel within the liver to form portal triads or *portal tracts.* The vast expanse of hepatic parenchyma is serviced via terminal branches of the portal vein and hepatic artery, which enter the parenchyma at intervals. Blood is collected into the hepatic vein, which exits by the "back door" of the liver into the inferior vena cava.

Classically the liver has been divided into 1- to 2-mm diameter hexagonal *lobules* oriented around the terminal tributaries of the hepatic vein *(terminal hepatic venules* or "central" *veins).* Because hepatocytes near the central vein are most remote from the blood supply, however, it has been argued that they are at the periphery of "metabolic lobules," referred to as *acini.* Conceptualized as roughly triangular, the acini have at their bases the terminal branches of hepatic artery and portal vein extending out from the portal tracts, and at their apices the terminal hepatic venules (Fig. 18–1).[1] The parenchyma of the hepatic acinus is divided into three zones, zone 1 being closest to the vascular supply, zone 3 abutting the terminal hepatic venule, and zone 2 being intermediate. This zonation is of considerable metabolic consequence because a lobular gradient of activity exists for many hepatic enzymes.[2] Moreover, many forms of hepatic injury exhibit a zonal distribution. Despite the many virtues of the acinar concept, the termi-

nology of the classic hepatic lobule persists in the practice of liver pathology (and in the writing of this chapter).

The hepatic parenchyma is organized into cribriform, anastomosing sheets or "plates" of hepatocytes, seen in microscopic sections as cords of cells radially disposed about the central vein. Hepatocytes immediately abutting the portal tract are referred to as the *limiting plate.* Hepatocytes exhibit minimal variation in overall size, but nuclei may vary in size, number, and ploidy, particularly with advancing age. Uninucleate, diploid cells tend to be the rule, but a significant fraction are binucleate, and the karyotype may range up to octaploidy.

Between the cords of hepatocytes are vascular sinusoids (Fig. 18–2). Hepatocytes are thus bathed on two sides by well-mixed portal venous and hepatic arterial blood, representing 25% of the cardiac output and placing hepatocytes among the most richly perfused cells in the body. The sinusoids are lined by fenestrated and discontinuous endothelial cells, which demarcate an extrasinusoidal *space of Disse,* into which protrude abundant microvilli of hepatocytes. Scattered *Kupffer cells* of the monocyte-phagocyte system are attached to the luminal face of endothelial cells, and occasional fat-containing lipocytes *(Ito cells)* of mesenchymal origin are found in the space of Disse. These lipocytes play a role in the storage and metabolism of vitamin A and contribute to collagen production in the normal and fibrotic liver.

Between abutting hepatocytes are *bile canalic-*

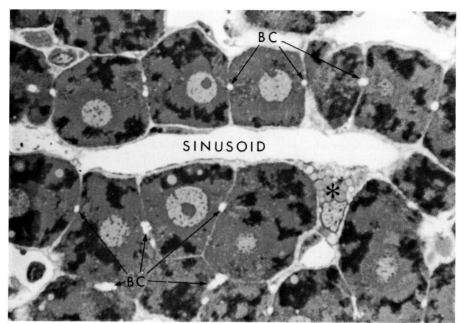

uli, which are channels 1 to 2 μm in diameter, formed by grooves in the plasma membranes of the facing cells and delineated from the vascular space by tight junctions. Numerous microvilli extend into these intercellular spaces, which constitute the outermost reaches of the biliary tree. Intracellular actin and myosin microfilaments surrounding the canaliculus help propel secreted biliary fluid along the canaliculi.[3] These channels begin in the centrilobular regions and progressively join to drain into the *canals of Hering* at the fringes of the portal tracts. In these canals, somewhat flattened biliary epithelial cells first appear. The biliary fluid enters into *interlobular bile ducts* within the portal tracts, which are lined by a mature cuboidal epithelium.

GENERAL PRINCIPLES

The liver is vulnerable to a wide variety of metabolic, toxic, microbial, circulatory, and neoplastic insults. In some instances, the disease is primary to the liver, as in viral hepatitis and hepatocellular carcinoma. More often the hepatic involvement is secondary, often to some of the most common diseases in humans, such as cardiac decompensation, disseminated cancer, alcoholism, and extrahepatic infections. The enormous functional reserve of the liver masks to some extent the clinical impact of early liver damage. With progression of diffuse disease or strategic disruption of bile flow, however, the consequences of deranged liver function become life-threatening. Before discussing specific disease processes, five general aspects of liver disease are reviewed: (1) morphologic patterns of injury; (2) general morphologic principles; (3) cirrhosis; and two common clinical signs of liver disease, (4) jaundice and (5) hepatic failure.

MORPHOLOGIC PATTERNS OF HEPATIC INJURY

MORPHOLOGY. The liver is an inherently simple organ, with a limited repertoire of responses to injurious events. Regardless of cause, five general reactions may occur.

Necrosis. Virtually any significant insult to the liver may cause hepatocyte necrosis. In ischemic necrosis, poorly stained mummified hepatocytes remain **(coagulative necrosis).** In necrosis that is toxic or immunologically mediated, isolated hepatocytes round up to form shrunken, pyknotic, and intensely eosinophilic **Councilman bodies** (a process known as **apoptosis**). Alternatively, hepatocytes may osmotically swell and rupture, so-called **hydropic degeneration.** Necrosis may be limited to scattered cells within the hepatic lobules **(focal necrosis)** or involve particular regions of the lobule **(zonal necrosis),** entire lobules **(submassive necrosis),** or the whole liver **(massive necrosis).** Focal necrosis is most characteristic of microbial infections, particularly smoldering forms of viral hepatitis. **Centrilobular necrosis** is characteristic of ischemic injury and many drug and toxic chemical reactions. **Midzonal necrosis** is a rare pattern, seen in yellow fever. Strictly **periportal necrosis** is seen primarily in phosphorus poisoning and eclampsia.

Massive necrosis is most commonly caused by severe chemical and drug toxicity or viral hepatitis. In other conditions, such as typhoid fever, tularemia, brucellosis, and herpes or adenovirus infection, expanding regions of the parenchyma are destroyed **(geographic necrosis).** With disseminated candidal or bacterial infection, macroscopic **abscesses** may occur.

Degeneration. **Short of outright necrosis, hepatocytes may take on a swollen, edematous appearance (ballooning degeneration) with irregularly clumped cytoplasm and large, clear spaces.** Alternatively, retained biliary material may impart a diffuse foamy swollen appearance to the hepatocyte **(cholestasis;** discussed shortly). Accumulation of specific substances in viable hepatocytes, such as iron, copper, and viral particles, may be of particular diagnostic value.

Inflammation. **Inflammation is defined as the influx of acute or chronic inflammatory cells into the liver and is termed hepatitis.** Although inflammation may be secondary to hepatocellular necrosis, lymphocytic attack of viable antigen-expressing liver cells is a common cause of liver damage. Inflammatory cells may be limited to the site of entry (portal tracts) or spill over into the parenchyma. In the case of focal hepatocyte necrosis, scavenger macrophages quickly generate scattered clumps of inflammatory cells in an otherwise innocuous parenchyma. Foreign bodies, organisms, and a variety of drugs may incite a granulomatous reaction.

Regeneration. **The liver has enormous reserve, and regeneration occurs in all but the most fulminant diseases.** Regeneration is signified by thickening of the hepatocyte cords (the result of hepatocyte proliferation) and some disorganization of the parenchymal structure. When massive hepatocellular necrosis occurs and leaves the connective tissue framework intact, almost perfect restitution can occur.

Fibrosis. **Fibrous tissue is formed in response to inflammation or direct toxic insult to the liver.** Deposition of collagen has lasting consequences on hepatic patterns of blood flow and perfusion of hepatocytes. In the initial stages, fibrosis may develop around portal tracts or the central vein or may be deposited directly within the space of Disse. **With continuing fibrosis, the liver is subdivided into nodules of regenerating hepatocytes surrounded by scar tissue, termed cirrhosis.**

CIRRHOSIS

Cirrhosis is among the top ten causes of death in the Western world, largely the result of alcohol abuse, chronic hepatitis, biliary disease, and iron overload. This end-stage form of liver disease is defined by three characteristics:[4]

- *Fibrosis* is present in the form of delicate bands (portal-central, portal-portal, central-central) or broad scars replacing multiple adjacent lobules.
- The *parenchymal architecture of the entire liver* is disrupted by interconnecting fibrous scars.
- Parenchymal *nodules* are created by regeneration of hepatocytes. The nodules may vary from micronodules (less than 3 mm in diameter) to macronodules (3 mm to several centimeters in diameter).

Several features should be underscored:

- *The parenchymal injury and consequent fibrosis are diffuse,* extending throughout the liver; focal injury with scarring does not constitute cirrhosis.
- *Nodularity is requisite for the diagnosis* and reflects the balance between regenerative activity and constrictive scarring.
- *The fibrosis, once developed, is generally irreversible;* some regression has been observed in humans with treated schistosomiasis and hemochromatosis.
- *Vascular architecture is reorganized* by the parenchymal damage and scarring, with the formation of abnormal interconnections between vascular inflow and hepatic vein outflow.[5]

There is no satisfactory classification of cirrhosis except for specification of the underlying etiology. The terms "micronodular" and "macronodular" should not be used as a primary classification, although the size of nodules may provide etiologic clues.[6] Many forms of cirrhosis (particularly alcoholic) are initially micronodular, but there is a tendency for nodules to increase in size with time,[7] counterbalanced by the constraints imposed by fibrous scarring.

The etiology of cirrhosis varies both geographically and socially; the following is the approximate frequency of etiologic categories in the Western world, most of which are discussed in detail later:[4]

Alcoholic liver disease	60–70%
Viral hepatitis	10%
Biliary diseases	5–10%
Primary hemochromatosis	5%
Wilson's disease	rare
Alpha$_1$-antitrypsin (AAT) deficiency	rare
Cryptogenic cirrhosis	10–15%

Infrequent types of of cirrhosis include (1) the cirrhosis developing in infants and children with galactosemia and tyrosinosis; (2) the desmoplastic reaction incited by a diffusely infiltrative cancer of the liver ("carcinomatous cirrhosis"); (3) drug-induced cirrhosis, as with alpha-methyldopa; and (4) syphilis. *Congenital syphilis,* now a rare disease, causes diffuse interstitial scarring of the liver that may mimic cirrhosis.[8] In the adult, *multiple hepatic gummas in tertiary syphilis* may, in time, give rise to contracted scars that produce deep creases in the surface of the liver. This pattern of involvement is called *hepar lobatum* but does not constitute a valid form of cirrhosis. Severe sclerosis can occur in the setting of cardiac disease ("cardiac cirrhosis"). After all the categories of cirrhosis of known causation have been excluded, a substantial number of cases remain. Referred to as *cryptogenic cirrhosis*, the magnitude of this "wastebasket" speaks eloquently to the difficulties in discerning the many origins of cirrhosis. *Once cirrhosis has developed, it is often impossible to establish an etiologic diagnosis on histologic grounds alone.*

All forms of cirrhosis may be clinically silent. When symptomatic, they lead to nonspecific clinical manifestations: anorexia, weight loss, weakness, and, in advanced disease, frank debilitation. Incipient or overt hepatic failure may develop, to be described shortly. The ultimate mechanism of most cirrhotic deaths is (1) progressive liver failure, (2) a complication related to portal hypertension (see later), or (3) the development of hepatocellular carcinoma.

PATHOGENESIS. Because progressive fibrosis is the central feature of cirrhosis, it is important to ask what initiates and drives the process. In the normal liver, interstitial collagens (types I and III) are concentrated in portal tracts, with occasional bundles in the space of Disse and around central veins. The collagen (reticulin) framework between hepatocytes is composed of delicate strands of type IV collagen in the space of Disse. In cirrhosis, types I and III collagen are deposited in all portions of the lobule, resulting in severe disruption of blood flow and impaired diffusion of solutes between hepatocytes and plasma. Collagenization of the space of Disse is accompanied by the loss of fenestrations in the sinusoidal endothelial cells. This further impairs the movement of proteins (e.g., albumin, clotting factors, lipoproteins) between hepatocytes and the plasma.[9] Indeed, hepatic failure can occur in the cirrhotic patient despite a liver of normal or even increased mass.

Although hepatocytes are capable of synthesizing collagen, the major source of excess collagen in cirrhosis appears to be the Ito cell.[10] While normally functioning as vitamin A fat-storage cells, during the development of cirrhosis they become activated, lose their retinyl ester stores, and transform into fibroblast-like cells. Ito cells also acquire contractile properties akin to myofibroblasts,[11] suggesting a role for these cells in the altered hemodynamics of the cirrhotic liver.

The stimuli for deposition of fibrous tissue are not yet clear, but several facts emerge, summarized in Figure 18–3.[12] (1) Most chronic inflammatory conditions of the liver are associated with an increased risk of cirrhosis. (2) Inflammatory me-

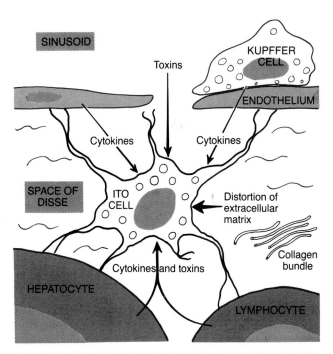

Figure 18–3. Proposed mechanisms for stimulation of collagen production by Ito cells in cirrhosis. Distortion of the extracellular matrix; secretion of cytokines from endothelial cells, Kupffer cells, hepatocytes, and inflammatory cells such as lymphocytes; and the direct action of toxins (or their metabolites) all have been proposed as possible stimuli for transforming Ito cells (lipocytes) into collagen-secreting myofibroblasts.

diators, particularly tumor necrosis factors alpha (TNF-α) and beta (TNF-β), and interleukin-1 (IL-1), may provide a direct link between hepatic inflammation and fibrosis. (3) Additional factors elaborated by Kupffer cells have a profound stimulatory effect on lipocytes. (4) Inflammatory disruption of the normal extracellular matrix may provide a stimulus for transformation of Ito cells into collagen-forming cells. Because fibrosis may develop in the absence of apparent inflammation, additional events, such as direct toxic stimulation of collagen deposition, must be postulated.

PORTAL HYPERTENSION

Increased resistance to portal blood flow may develop in a variety of circumstances, which can be divided into *prehepatic, intrahepatic, and posthepatic causes*. The major *prehepatic conditions* are obstructive thrombosis and narrowing of the portal vein before it ramifies within the liver. Prehepatic portal hypertension also may occur when massive splenomegaly shunts excessive blood into the splenic vein, which drains into the portal vein. The major *posthepatic causes* are severe right-sided heart failure, constrictive pericarditis, and hepatic vein outflow obstruction. The dominant *intrahepat-*

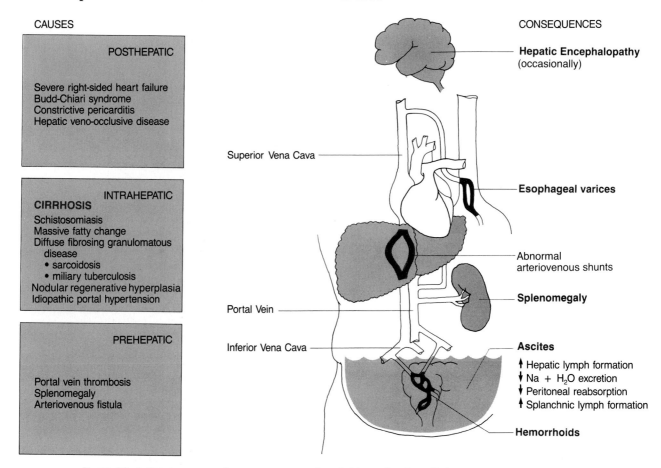

CAUSES

POSTHEPATIC

Severe right-sided heart failure
Budd-Chiari syndrome
Constrictive pericarditis
Hepatic veno-occlusive disease

INTRAHEPATIC
CIRRHOSIS
Schistosomiasis
Massive fatty change
Diffuse fibrosing granulomatous
    disease
    • sarcoidosis
    • miliary tuberculosis
Nodular regenerative hyperplasia
Idiopathic portal hypertension

PREHEPATIC

Portal vein thrombosis
Splenomegaly
Arteriovenous fistula

CONSEQUENCES

Hepatic Encephalopathy
(occasionally)

Superior Vena Cava

Esophageal varices

Abnormal
arteriovenous shunts

Splenomegaly

Portal Vein

Inferior Vena Cava

Ascites
↑ Hepatic lymph formation
↓ Na + H₂O excretion
↓ Peritoneal reabsorption
↑ Splanchnic lymph formation

Hemorrhoids

Figure 18–4. The causes and consequences of portal hypertension. Cirrhosis is the leading cause.

ic cause is cirrhosis, accounting for most cases of portal hypertension. Far less frequent are schistosomiasis; veno-occlusive disease (discussed later); massive fatty change; diffuse fibrosing granulomatous disease, such as sarcoidosis and miliary tuberculosis; and diseases affecting the portal microcirculation, exemplified by nodular regenerative hyperplasia (also discussed later).

Portal hypertension in cirrhosis results in part from increased resistance to portal flow at the level of the sinusoids and compression of central veins by perivenular fibrosis and expansile parenchymal nodules. However, anastomoses between the arterial and the portal systems within the scars also contribute to portal hypertension by imposing arterial pressure on the low-pressure portal venous system.[13] *The four major clinical consequences are (1) ascites, (2) the formation of portosystemic venous shunts, (3) congestive splenomegaly, and (4) hepatic encephalopathy (see later)* (Fig. 18–4).

Ascites

Ascites refers to the collection of excess fluid in the peritoneal cavity. It usually becomes clinically detectable when at least 500 ml has accumulated, but many liters may collect and cause massive abdominal distention. It is generally a serous fluid having less than 3 gm/dl of protein (largely albumin) as well as the same concentrations of solutes such as glucose, sodium, and potassium as in the blood. Thus, withdrawal of large volumes of ascitic fluid for relief of symptoms invokes a substantial loss of protein and solutes. The fluid may contain a scant number of mesothelial cells and mononuclear leukocytes. Influx of neutrophils suggests secondary infection, whereas red cells point to possible disseminated intra-abdominal cancer. With long-standing ascites, seepage of peritoneal fluid through transdiaphragmatic lymphatics may produce hydrothorax, more often on the right side.

The *pathogenesis of ascites* is complex, involving one or more of the following mechanisms:[14]

• *Sinusoidal hypertension,* altering Starling's forces and driving fluid into the space of Disse, which is then removed by hepatic lymphatics; this movement of fluid is also promoted by *hypoalbuminemia.*
• *Percolation of hepatic lymph from the liver capsule into the peritoneal cavity:* Normal thoracic duct lymph flow approximates 800 to 1000 ml/day. With cirrhosis, hepatic lymphatic flow may

approach 20 liters/day, exceeding thoracic duct capacity. Hepatic lymph is rich in proteins and low in triglycerides, which is reflected in the protein-rich ascitic fluid.
- *Renal retention of sodium and water,* despite a total body sodium that is greater than normal.

Portosystemic Shunts

With the rise in portal system pressure, bypasses develop wherever the systemic and portal circulation share common capillary beds. Principal sites are veins around and within the rectum (manifested as hemorrhoids), the cardioesophageal junction (esophagogastric varices), the retroperitoneum, and the falciform ligament of the liver (periumbilical and abdominal wall collaterals). Although hemorrhoidal bleeding may occur, it is rarely massive or life-threatening. *Much more important are the esophagogastric varices that appear in about 65% of patients with advanced cirrhosis of the liver and cause massive hematemesis and death in about half of them* (see esophageal varices, Chapter 17). Abdominal wall collaterals appear as dilated subcutaneous veins extending from the umbilicus toward the rib margins *(caput medusae);* they are an important clinical hallmark of portal hypertension.

Splenomegaly

Long-standing congestion may cause congestive splenomegaly. The degree of enlargement varies widely up to 1000 gm and is not necessarily correlated with other features of portal hypertension. Massive splenomegaly may secondarily induce a variety of hematologic abnormalities attributable to hypersplenism (see Chapter 13).

BILIRUBIN AND HEPATIC BILE FORMATION

Hepatic bile formation serves two major functions: (1) the emulsification of dietary fat in the lumen of the gut through the detergent action of bile salts and (2) the elimination of waste products. Bile constitutes the primary pathway for elimination of bilirubin, excess cholesterol, and xenobiotics which are insufficiently water-soluble to be excreted into urine. Because bile formation is one of the most sophisticated functions of the liver, it is also one of the most readily disrupted. Such disruption becomes clinically evident as yellow discoloration of the skin and sclerae (*jaundice* or *icterus*) owing to retention of pigmented bilirubin, and as *cholestasis,* defined as retention of not only bilirubin but also other solutes eliminated in bile.

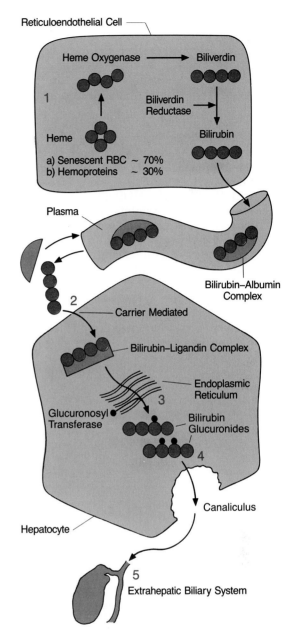

Figure 18-5. Schematic of bilirubin metabolism indicating types of derangements leading to jaundice: (1) excessive release of heme pigment (hemolytic anemia), (2) reduced hepatic uptake, (3) impaired conjugation of bilirubin, (4) deranged intrahepatic bilirubin excretion, (5) intrahepatic or extrahepatic biliary obstruction.

Bilirubin is the end product of heme degradation (Fig. 18-5). The majority of daily production (0.2 to 0.3 gm) is derived from breakdown of senescent erythroctyes by the mononuclear phagocytic system, especially in the spleen, liver, and bone marrow. Most of the remainder of bilirubin is derived from the turnover of hepatic heme or hemoproteins, e.g., the P_{450} cytochromes. A minor contribution comes from the premature destruction of newly formed erythrocytes in the bone marrow.

Bilirubin formed outside the liver is bound principally to serum albumin and transported to the liver. Albumin binding is necessary because bilirubin is virtually insoluble in aqueous solutions at physiologic pH. The small fraction of unbound bilirubin in plasma may increase in severe hemolytic disease or when protein-binding drugs displace bilirubin from albumin.

Hepatic processing of bilirubin involves (1) carrier-mediated uptake at the sinusoidal membrane; (2) intracellular binding, especially to ligandin; (3) delivery to the endoplasmic reticulum, possibly by rapid membrane-membrane transfer; (4) conjugation with one or two molecules of glucuronic acid by bilirubin UDP-glucuronosyltransferase (UGT); and (5) excretion of the water-soluble, nontoxic bilirubin glucuronides into bile. Most bilirubin glucuronides are deconjugated by bacterial beta-glucuronidases and degraded to colorless urobilinogens. The urobilinogens and the residue of intact pigment are largely excreted in feces. Approximately 20% of the urobilinogens formed are reabsorbed in the ileum and colon, returned to the liver, and promptly re-excreted into bile. The small amount that escapes this enterohepatic circulation is excreted in urine.

The brilliant yellow color of bilirubin makes it an easily identified component of hepatic bile formation. Bilirubin metabolism and excretion, however, are but a minor cog in the hepatic machinery that secretes 12 to 36 gm of bile acids into bile per day, mostly as taurine and glycine conjugates of cholic and chenodeoxycholic acid. The driving force for bile formation is the energy-dependent excretion of bile acids and inorganic electrolytes into the bile canaliculus; the electrolytes induce an osmotic gradient along which water flows. Approximately 10 to 20% of excreted bile acids are deconjugated in the intestines by bacterial action; virtually all conjugated and deconjugated bile acids are reabsorbed (especially in the ileum) and returned to the liver for uptake, reconjugation, and resecretion. Fecal loss of bile acids (0.2 to 0.6 gm/day) is matched by *de novo* hepatic synthesis of bile acids from cholesterol. The *enterohepatic circulation* of bile acids provides an efficient mechanism for maintaining a large endogenous pool of bile acids for digestive and excretory purposes.

JAUNDICE AND CHOLESTASIS

Clinical jaundice appears when bilirubin is elevated in blood and is deposited in tissues. Cholestasis refers to bile secretory failure per se, which is accompanied by the accumulation in blood of substances normally excreted in bile (bilirubin, bile salts, and cholesterol). Thus, jaundice and cholestasis frequently overlap; those conditions that produce jaundice in the absence of cholestasis are discussed presently.

Normal blood levels of bilirubin are less than

Table 18–1. CLASSIFICATION OF JAUNDICE

PREDOMINANTLY UNCONJUGATED HYPERBILIRUBINEMIA
Excess production of bilirubin
  Hemolytic anemias
  Resorption of blood from internal hemorrhage
    (e.g., alimentary tract bleeding, hematomas)
  Ineffective erythropoiesis syndromes
    (e.g., pernicious anemia, thalassemia)
Reduced hepatic uptake
  Drug interference with membrane carrier systems
  Possibly some cases of Gilbert's syndrome
Impaired bilirubin conjugation
  Physiologic jaundice of the newborn
    (decreased UGT activity, decreased excretion)
  Breast milk jaundice (?inhibition of UGT activity)
  Genetic deficiency of bilirubin UGT activity
    (Crigler-Najjar syndromes types I and II)
  Gilbert's syndrome (apparently mixed etiologies)
  Diffuse hepatocellular disease
    (e.g., viral or drug-induced hepatitis, cirrhosis)

PREDOMINANTLY CONJUGATED HYPERBILIRUBINEMIA
Decreased intrahepatic excretion of bilirubin
  Impaired canalicular transport of bilirubin glucuronides
    (Dubin-Johnson, Rotor's syndromes)
  Hepatocellular damage or toxicity
    (e.g., viral hepatitis, drug-induced hepatitis, total
    parenteral nutrition, systemic infection)
  Drug impairment of bilirubin excretion
    (e.g., oral contraceptives)
  Intrahepatic bile duct disease
    (e.g., primary biliary cirrhosis, primary sclerosing
    cholangitis, graft-versus-host disease, liver transplantation)
Extrahepatic biliary obstruction
  Gallstone obstruction of biliary tree
  Carcinomas of head of pancreas, extrahepatic bile ducts,
    ampulla of Vater
  Extrahepatic biliary atresia
  Biliary strictures and choledochal cysts
  Primary sclerosing cholangitis (extrahepatic)
  Fluke infestation

UGT = Uridine diphosphate-glucuronosyltransferase.

1.2 mg/dl. Jaundice becomes evident when bilirubin levels rise above 2.0 to 2.5 mg/dl; levels as high as 30 to 40 mg/dl can occur with severe disease. *Unconjugated bilirubin is not soluble in aqueous solution and is tightly complexed to albumin: As such, it cannot be excreted in urine even when the blood levels are high. The small amount of unbound pigment, when present in excess, may cause toxic damage to the neonatal brain (kernicterus) owing to immaturity of the blood-brain barrier. In contrast, conjugated bilirubin is water-soluble, nontoxic, and weakly associated with albumin. When present in excess, it is readily excreted in urine (bilirubinuria).* With both unconjugated and conjugated hyperbilirubinemia, pigmentation of the skin and sclerae is readily visible. Virtually all tissues (with the exception of the adult brain) are discolored to some degree.

Jaundice occurs when bilirubin production exceeds hepatic clearance capacity, via the following mechanisms (Table 18–1): *Excessive production of bilirubin, reduced hepatic uptake, and impaired he-*

patic conjugation produce unconjugated hyperbiliru-binemia. Decreased hepatic excretion of bilirubin conjugates and impaired extrahepatic bile flow produce conjugated hyperbilirubinemia. With prolonged conjugated hyperbilirubinemia, a portion of circulating pigment also may become covalently bound to albumin (the *delta fraction*). More than one mechanism may operate to produce jaundice in some diseases, but in general one mechanism predominates in a given disease state. Therefore, when a patient presents with jaundice, a knowledge of the predominant form of plasma bilirubin is of value in arriving at the possible cause of hyperbilirubinemia.

Cholestatic conditions, which may result from hepatocellular dysfunction or intrahepatic or extrahepatic biliary obstruction, may also present with jaundice. Alternatively, *pruritus* is a common presenting symptom, presumably related to the elevation in plasma levels of bile acids. Skin *xanthomas* sometimes appear, the result of hyperlipidemia and impaired excretion of cholesterol. A characteristic laboratory finding is elevated serum alkaline phosphatase, an enzyme present in bile duct epithelium and the canalicular membrane of hepatocytes. An isozyme is normally present in many other tissues such as bone, and so the increased levels must be verified as being hepatic in origin. Other manifestations of reduced bile flow relate to intestinal malabsorption, including deficiencies of the fat-soluble vitamins A, D, or K.

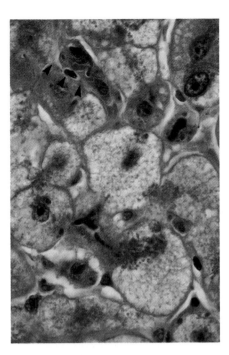

Figure 18–6. Cholestasis. Bile canaliculi are distended with inspissated bile, and Kupffer cells contain phagocytized bile *(arrowheads)*. Hepatocytes exhibit foamy degeneration and pigment accumulation. (Hematoxylin and eosin.)

MORPHOLOGY. The morphologic features of cholestasis depend somewhat on its severity, duration, and underlying cause. **Common to both obstructive and hepatocellular cholestasis is the accumulation of bile pigment within the hepatic parenchyma** (Fig. 18–6). Elongated green-brown plugs of bile are visible in dilated canaliculi, most prominent toward the centers of lobules (the most "upstream" portion of the biliary tree); this may become panlobular in the most severe cases. Rupture of canaliculi leads to extravasation of bile, which is quickly phagocytosed by Kupffer cells. Droplets of bile pigment also accumulate within hepatocytes, causing the cells to take on a wispy appearance (feathery or **foamy degeneration**). In the absence of bile duct disease, hepatocellular cholestasis per se does not lead to permanent liver damage.

Obstruction to the biliary tree, either intrahepatic or extrahepatic, induces distention of upstream bile ducts by bile; the bile stasis and backpressure induces proliferation of the duct epithelial cells.[15] **The resultant looping and reduplication of ducts is termed "bile duct proliferation" and is one of the most helpful features indicative of obstructive cholestasis.** The labyrinthine conduits further slow the flow of bile and favor the formation of concrements, which obstruct their lumina. Associated portal tract findings include edema and a periductular infiltrate of neutrophils. Primitive bile ductular structures also are formed along the interface between portal tract and parenchyma. Prolonged obstructive cholestasis leads not only to foamy change of centrilobular hepatocytes, but also focal destruction of the parenchyma. Coalescence of necrotic foci generates **bile lakes,** which are filled with cellular debris and pigment. **Unrelieved obstruction leads to portal tract fibrosis,** which initially extends into and subdivides the parenchyma with relative preservation of hepatic architecture. Ultimately an end-stage bile-stained, cirrhotic liver is created (biliary cirrhosis; discussed later).

Extrahepatic biliary obstruction is frequently amenable to surgical alleviation because it is most often produced by impaction of a gallstone in the common bile duct or ampulla of Vater (adults) or by extrahepatic biliary atresia (infants). In contrast, cholestasis resulting from diseases of the intrahepatic biliary tree or hepatocellular secretory failure (collectively termed *intrahepatic cholestasis*) cannot be benefited by surgery (short of transplantation), and the patient's condition may be worsened by an operative procedure. *There is thus considerable urgency in making a correct diagnosis of the cause of jaundice and cholestasis.* Cholestasis and jaundice are common to many hepatic diseases and are nonspecific clinical findings. It is appropriate, however, to consider those causes of hyperbilirubine-

Table 18-2. HEREDITARY HYPERBILIRUBINEMIAS

DISORDER	INHERITANCE	DEFECTS IN BILIRUBIN METABOLISM	LIVER PATHOLOGY	CLINICAL COURSE
Unconjugated Hyperbilirubinemia				
Crigler-Najjar syndrome type I	Autosomal recessive	Absent bilirubin UGT activity	Canalicular cholestasis	Fatal in neonatal period
Crigler-Najjar syndrome type II	Autosomal dominant with variable penetrance	Decreased bilirubin UGT activity	Normal	Generally mild, occasional kernicterus
Gilbert's syndrome	?Autosomal dominant	Decreased bilirubin UGT activity, with ?decreased hepatic uptake	Normal	Innocuous
Conjugated Hyperbilirubinemia				
Dubin-Johnson syndrome	Autosomal recessive	Impaired biliary excretion of bilirubin glucuronides: ?canalicular membrane-carrier defect	Pigmented cytoplasmic globules; ?epinephrine metabolites	Innocuous
Rotor's syndrome	Autosomal recessive	?Decreased hepatic uptake and storage ?Decreased biliary excretion	Normal	Innocuous

UGT = Uridine diphosphate-glucuronosyltransferase.

mia that are due to specific problems in bilirubin physiology before leaving this topic.

HEREDITARY HYPERBILIRUBINEMIAS

Three major conditions cause *unconjugated hyperbilirubinemia,* so-called because 80% or more of the serum bilirubin is unconjugated.

1. *Bilirubin overproduction.* Hemolytic disease is the most common cause. Resorption of major hemorrhages into the lungs, alimentary tract, or other tissues also may lead to excessive erythrocyte destruction. Because the normal liver can handle most of the load, the hyperbilirubinemia rarely exceeds 5 mg/dl. In disorders involving intramedullary hemolysis of abnormal erythrocytes (ineffective erythropoiesis), excessive bone marrow production of bilirubin assumes importance.

2. *Reduced hepatic uptake of bilirubin.* This is encountered in some cases of the genetic disorder called Gilbert's syndrome (discussed presently) and after administration of certain drugs such as rifampin.

3. *Impaired conjugation of bilirubin.* The activity of hepatocellular bilirubin UGT is low at birth and does not reach normal levels until about two weeks of age. Thus, almost every newborn develops transient and mild unconjugated hyperbilirubinemia, called *neonatal jaundice* or *physiologic jaundice of the newborn.* Breast-fed infants tend to exhibit jaundice with greater frequency, possibly the result of beta-glucuronidases present in maternal milk. Distinguishing these cases from newborns exhibiting jaundice owing to diffuse

hepatocellular disease or extrahepatic biliary obstruction is extremely important.

In rare cases, there may be a genetic lack of bilirubin UGT (Table 18-2). *Crigler-Najjar type I syndrome* is an extremely rare, almost invariably fatal form of severe unconjugated hyperbilirubinemia with complete lack of the enzyme, causing death within 18 months of birth secondary to kernicterus.[16] *Crigler-Najjar type II syndrome* is a less severe, nonfatal inherited disorder exhibiting a partial defect in bilirubin conjugation, the major consequence of which is having extraordinarily yellow skin. *Gilbert's syndrome* is a relatively common, benign, somewhat heterogeneous inherited condition presenting with a mild, fluctuating, often subclinical hyperbilirubinemia owing to decreased levels of bilirubin UGT.[17] Affecting up to 7% of the population, the hyperbilirubinemia may go undiscovered for years and is not associated with any liver pathology or functional derangements. When detected in adolescence or adult life, it is typically in association with stress, such as an intercurrent illness, strenuous exercise, or fasting. There is no clinical consequence of Gilbert's syndrome except for the anxiety that a jaundiced sufferer might justifiably experience with this otherwise innocuous condition.

In *conjugated hyperbilirubinemia,* more than half of the serum bilirubin is conjugated. This usually occurs in association with cholestasis, either intrahepatic or extrahepatic in origin. Isolated conjugated hyperbilirubinemia, however, occurs in *Dubin-Johnson syndrome,* in which excretion of bilirubin conjugates and other organic anions across the hepatocyte canalicular membrane is defective.

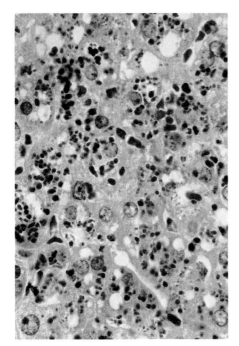

Figure 18–7. Dubin-Johnson syndrome, showing abundant pigmented inclusions in otherwise normal hepatocytes. (Hematoxylin and eosin.)

Apart from chronic or recurrent jaundice of fluctuating intensity, most patients are asymptomatic and have a normal life expectancy. The most distinctive feature of Dubin-Johnson syndrome is a gross black discoloration of the liver, caused by coarse pigmented granules within the cytoplasm of hepatocytes that can be resolved as lysosomes (Fig. 18–7)—the liver is otherwise normal. The pigment appears to be made of polymers of adrenaline

(epinephrine) metabolites[18] and appears to accumulate as a result of the hepatic defect.

Much less common than the Dubin-Johnson syndrome, *Rotor's syndrome* also represents a form of asymptomatic conjugated hyperbilirubinemia, but the liver is not pigmented. The nature of the metabolic defect is unclear, although derangements in hepatic uptake and storage of organic anions are suspected.

HEPATIC FAILURE

Just as jaundice heralds the loss of the liver's ability to form and secrete bile, hepatic failure reflects the destruction of overall hepatic function. This may come about through the insidious action of a chronic progressive disorder, by repetitive discrete bouts of parenchymal damage, or in some cases by sudden and massive obliteration. Whatever the sequence, loss of hepatic functional capacity must exceed 80 to 90% before hepatic failure ensues. In many cases, intercurrent disease, such as gastrointestinal bleeding, systemic infection, electrolyte disturbances, or severe stress (major surgery, heart failure), tips the balance toward decompensation when the functional reserve is precarious. In most cases of severe hepatic dysfunction, liver transplantation is the only hope for survival. A fortunate few can survive an acute event with conservative management until regeneration restores adequate hepatic function. Overall, mortality from hepatic failure is 70 to 95%.

Many disorders can lead to hepatic failure. The major disorders having such potential can be divided into three categories:

Table 18–3. MAJOR CLINICAL FEATURES OF HEPATIC FAILURE

CLINICAL FEATURE	BASIS
Jaundice	Total bilirubin metabolism is deranged, but hepatocyte excretion is rate-limiting, so conjugated hyperbilirubinemia predominates
Hypoalbuminemia	Reduced synthesis and secretion of albumin
Coagulopathy	Reduced synthesis and secretion of clotting factors (II, V, VII, IX, and X), worsened by malabsorption of vitamin K
Disseminated intravascular coagulation	Activation of Hageman factor, inadequate clearance of activated factors
Hyperammonemia	Defective urea cycle function
Fetor hepaticus	Inconstant; formation of mercaptans in gut
Increased serum levels of hepatic enzymes LDH; alanine aminotransferase/glutamic pyruvic transaminase (ALT/GPT); aspartate aminotransferase/glutamic oxaloacetic transaminase (AST/GOT)	Seen only with active liver cell necrosis; level of increase correlates with extent of liver destruction. LDH is relatively nonspecific
Gynecomastia, testicular atrophy, palmar erythema, and spider angiomas of the skin	Putatively related to impaired estrogen metabolism and consequent hyperestrogenism
Hepatic encephalopathy	To be discussed in text
Hepatorenal syndrome	To be discussed in text
Coma	Usually follows encephalopathy, precedes death

LDH = Lactate dehydrogenase.

- *Ultrastructural lesions that do not produce overt liver cell necrosis:* Reye's syndrome, acute fatty liver of pregnancy, tetracycline toxicity.
- *Chronic liver disease:* Relentless chronic hepatitis, cirrhosis, inherited metabolic disorders.
- *Massive hepatic necrosis:* Fulminant viral hepatitis; massive toxic damage as from acetaminophen, halothane, monoamine oxidase inhibitors used as antidepressants; industrial chemical agents such as carbon tetrachloride and phosphorus; and mushroom poisoning (e.g., Amanita species).

Whatever the underlying condition, the clinical features of hepatic failure are much the same, with characteristic signs and symptoms (Table 18–3). Hepatic encephalopathy and hepatorenal syndrome are given separate consideration below. Males exhibit *hypogonadism and gynecomastia,* related to impaired degradation of estrogens. *Palmar erythema* (from local vasodilatation) and telangiectasias of the skin ("spider angiomas") also are attributed to hyperestrinism but with little proof. Each angioma contains a central dilated arteriole from which small vessels radiate. *Ascites* is a particularly prominent feature of chronic liver failure in the setting of cirrhosis, as discussed earlier. *Weight loss, muscle wasting, hypoglycemia, prolongation of the prothrombin time, and a bleeding tendency* (because of impaired synthesis of blood clotting factors II, VII, IX, and X) also are frequent. *Fetor hepaticus* is a pungent, sour odor that can be detected in the exhaled breath of encephalopathic patients, attributed to volatile sulfur-containing compounds such as mercaptans. Laboratory tests that reflect deranged liver metabolism include elevated serum bilirubin, and decreased serum albumin and coagulation factors; these are useful for assessing the severity of liver dysfunction.

HEPATIC ENCEPHALOPATHY

Hepatic encephalopathy is a feared complication of acute and chronic liver failure. Patients exhibit a spectrum of disturbances in consciousness, ranging from subtle behavioral abnormalities to marked confusion and stupor to deep coma and death. These changes may progress over hours to days in fulminant hepatic failure or may emerge in the midst of a precipitating illness in a patient with marginal hepatic function. Associated findings include fluctuating neurologic signs, such as nonspecific electroencephalographic changes, limb rigidity and hyperreflexia, and rarely seizures. Particularly characteristic is *asterixis:* nonrhythmic, rapid extension-flexion movements of the head and extremities, best seen when the arms are held in extension with dorsiflexed wrists.

Hepatic encephalopathy is regarded as a metabolic disorder of the central nervous system and neuromuscular system. In the great majority of instances, there are only minor morphologic changes in the brain, such as edema and an astrocytic reaction. Two physiologic factors appear to be important in the genesis of this disorder: (1) shunting of blood around the liver, as occurs from spontaneous portosystemic connections that develop in the course of advanced cirrhosis or after surgical portocaval anastomosis, and (2) severe loss of hepatocellular function. The net result is exposure of the brain to an altered metabolic milieu, the specifics of which are not yet clear. Although this disorder appears to arise from impaired hepatic processing of endogenous metabolites, the exact pathogenesis of this disorder remains unclear.

HEPATORENAL SYNDROME

Hepatorenal syndrome refers to *the appearance of renal failure in patients with severe liver disease, in whom there are no intrinsic morphologic or functional causes for the renal failure.* Excluded by this definition are concomitant damage to both organs or instances of advanced cirrhosis in which circulatory collapse leads to acute tubular necrosis and renal failure. *Kidney function promptly improves if hepatic failure is reversed.* The appearance of this syndrome is typically heralded by a drop in renal output, associated with rising blood urea nitrogen (BUN) and creatinine. The ability to concentrate urine is retained, with a hyperosmolar urine devoid of proteins and abnormal sediment and surprisingly low in sodium (in contrast to renal tubular necrosis). Renal failure may rapidly progress to death in acute fulminant or advanced chronic hepatic disease. Alternatively, borderline renal insufficiency (serum creatinine 2 to 3 mg/dl) may persist for weeks to months, as in cirrhotic patients whose ascites is refractory to diuretic therapy. As with hepatic encephalopathy, the pathophysiology of renal failure remains unclear. The favored theory is reduction of renal blood flow, particularly to the cortex, the result of vasoconstriction. This is accompanied by a decreased glomerular filtration rate and avid renal retention of sodium.

After this general overview of pathologic features and clinical consequences of liver disease, we can now turn to specific types of disease.

PATHOLOGY

INFLAMMATORY DISORDERS

Inflammatory disorders of the liver dominate the clinical practice of hepatology. This is due in part to the fact that virtually any insult to the liver can kill hepatocytes and recruit inflammatory cells. In addition, inflammatory diseases are frequently chronic conditions that must be managed medically. Until recently there was little effective treatment for chronic hepatitis, and many patients would progress inexorably toward cirrhosis and hepatic failure. This bleak picture has now improved somewhat, making accurate diagnosis of the underlying etiology all the more important for patient management.

Among inflammatory disorders, infection ranks supreme. The liver is almost inevitably involved in blood-borne infections, whether systemic or arising within the abdomen. Although discussed elsewhere, those in which the hepatic lesion is prominent include miliary tuberculosis, malaria, staphylococcal bacteremia, the salmonelloses, candida, and amebiasis. The foremost primary hepatic infections are viral hepatitides.

VIRAL HEPATITIS

Systemic viral infections that can involve the liver include (1) infectious mononucleosis (Epstein-Barr virus), which may cause a mild hepatitis during the acute phase; (2) cytomegalovirus, particularly in the newborn or immunosuppressed patient; and (3) yellow fever, which has been a major and serious cause of hepatitis in tropical countries. Infrequently in children and immunosuppressed patients, the liver is affected in the course of rubella, adenovirus, herpes, or enterovirus infections.[19] *Unless otherwise specified, however, the term "viral hepatitis" is reserved for infection of the liver caused by a small (but growing) group of viruses having a particular affinity for the liver* (Table 18-4). Because these viruses cause similar clinicopathologic patterns of disease, the pathologic patterns of viral hepatitis are described together, after introducing each virus.

Hepatitis A Virus

Hepatitis A, long known as "infectious hepatitis," is a benign, self-limited disease with an incubation period of 14 to 45 days. *Hepatitis A virus (HAV) does not cause chronic hepatitis or a carrier state and only rarely causes fulminant hepatitis, and so the fatality rate associated with HAV is about 0.1%.*[20] HAV occurs throughout the world and is endemic in countries with substandard hygiene and sanitation, so the vast majority of native populations have detectable anti-HAV by the age of 10 years. Clinical disease tends to be mild or asymptomatic and rare after childhood. In developed countries, acute HAV tends to be a sporadic overt febrile illness.[21] In these countries, the prevalence of seropositivity increases gradually with age, reaching 50% by age 50 years in the United States. Overall, HAV accounts for about 25% of clinically evident acute hepatitis worldwide. HAV is spread by ingestion of contaminated water and foods (especially seafood) and is shed in the stool

Table 18-4. HEPATITIS VIRUSES

	HEPATITIS A VIRUS	HEPATITIS B VIRUS	HEPATITIS C VIRUS	HEPATITIS D VIRUS	HEPATITIS E VIRUS
Year of Identification	1973	1965	1989	1977	1980
Agent	27 nm icosahedral capsid, ssRNA	42 nm enveloped dsDNA	30–60 nm enveloped ssRNA	35 nm enveloped ssRNA; replication defective	32–34 nm unenveloped ssRNA
Classification	Picornavirus	Hepadnavirus	Flavivirus/pestivirus	Unknown	Caliciviridae
Transmission	Fecal-oral	Parenteral; close personal contact	Parenteral; close personal contact	Parenteral; close personal contact	Water-borne
Incubation Period (Days)	15–45	30–180	20–90	30–50 in superinfection	15–60
Fulminant Hepatitis	0.1–0.4%	1–4%	Rare	3–4% in coinfection	0.3–3%; 20% in pregnant women
Carrier State	None	0.1–1.0% of blood donors in U.S. and Western world	0.2–1.0% of blood donors in U.S. and Western world	1–10% in drug addicts and hemophiliacs	Unknown
Chronic Hepatitis	None	5–10% of acute infections	>50%	<5% coinfection, 80% superinfection	None
Hepatocellular Carcinoma	No	Yes	Yes	No increase above HBV	Unknown, but unlikely

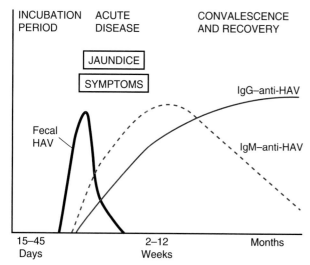

Figure 18–8. The sequence of serologic markers in acute hepatitis A infection.

for 2 to 3 weeks before and 1 week after the onset of jaundice. Thus, close personal contact with an infected individual or fecal-oral contamination during this period accounts for most cases, and explains the occurrence of outbreaks in institutional settings such as schools and nurseries. *Because the viremia of acute HAV is transient (during the relatively short incubation period and the first days of symptoms), this agent is rarely implicated in transfusion-acquired hepatitis.*

HAV is a small, nonenveloped, single-stranded RNA picornavirus that occupies its own genus, Hepatovirus. Ultrastructurally HAV is an icosahedral capsid 27 nm in diameter. In cell cultures of human and primate origin, HAV replicates and is released from infected cells without adverse effect on them. Furthermore, fecal shedding occurs before a rise in transaminases, indicative of copious release in bile without hepatic damage. Presumably hepatitis is caused by immunologic mechanisms, but this is far from established.

The pattern for HAV markers is shown in Figure 18–8. Specific antibody against HAV of the IgM type appears in blood at the onset of symptoms, constituting a reliable marker of acute infection. Fecal shedding of the virus ends as the IgM titer rises. The IgM response usually begins to decline in a few months and is followed by the appearance of IgG anti-HAV. The latter persists for years, perhaps for life, providing protective immunity against reinfection by all strains of HAV (and an impetus for development of a vaccine).[22]

Hepatitis B Virus

Hepatitis B virus (HBV), the cause of "serum hepatitis," is the most versatile of the hepatotropic viruses. *HBV can produce (1) acute hepatitis, (2)*

chronic nonprogressive hepatitis, (3) progressive chronic disease ending in cirrhosis, (4) fulminant hepatitis with massive liver necrosis, and (5) an asymptomatic carrier state with or without progressive disease. Furthermore, HBV plays an important role in the development of hepatocellular carcinoma (discussed later). The approximate frequencies of these outcomes are depicted in Figure 18–9. This agent also provides the backdrop for the defective delta hepatitis virus (discussed presently).

Globally, liver disease caused by **HBV** is an enormous problem, with an estimated worldwide carrier rate of 300 million; in the United States alone, there are 300,000 new infections per year. In contrast to HAV, HBV is present in blood for the last stages of the incubation period (30 to 180 days) and during active episodes of acute and chronic hepatitis and is present in all physiologic and pathologic body fluids, with the exception of stool. HBV is a hardy virus and can withstand extremes of temperature and humidity. Thus, although blood and body fluids are the primary vehicles of transmission, virus may also be spread by contact with body secretions, such as semen, saliva, sweat, tears, breast milk, and pathologic effusions. *Transfusion, blood products, dialysis, needle-stick accidents among health care workers, intravenous drug abuse, and homosexual activity constitute the primary risk categories for HBV infection;* in one-third of patients, the source of infection is unknown. In endemic regions, such as Africa and Southeast Asia, spread from an infected mother to a neonate during birth *(vertical transmission)* is common. These neonatal infections often lead to the carrier state for life.

HBV is a member of the *hepadnavirus* family, a group of DNA-containing viruses with strains causing hepatitis in humans, woodchucks, ground and tree squirrels, ducks, and other avian species.[23] The mature HBV virion is a 42-nm, spherical, double-layed "Dane particle," which has an outer surface envelope of protein, lipid, and carbohydrate enclosing an electron-dense, 28-nm, slightly hexagonal core. The genome of HBV is a partially double-stranded circular DNA molecule having 3200 nucleotides (Fig. 18–10). The organization of the HBV genome is unique,[24] in that all regions of the viral genome encode protein sequences, including the nucleocapsid (hepatitis B core antigen [HBcAg]), envelope glycoprotein (hepatitis B surface antigen [HBsAg]), DNA polymerase (a product of the P gene), and a protein from the X gene, which may play a role in replication. The DNA polymerase exhibits reverse transcriptase activity, and genomic replication occurs via an intermediate RNA template.[23] HBeAg is a polypeptide virtually identical to HBcAg, which contains a slightly longer "precore" region; this directs the HBeAg polypeptide toward secretion into blood. Infected hepatocytes are capable of synthesizing and secreting massive quantities of noninfective

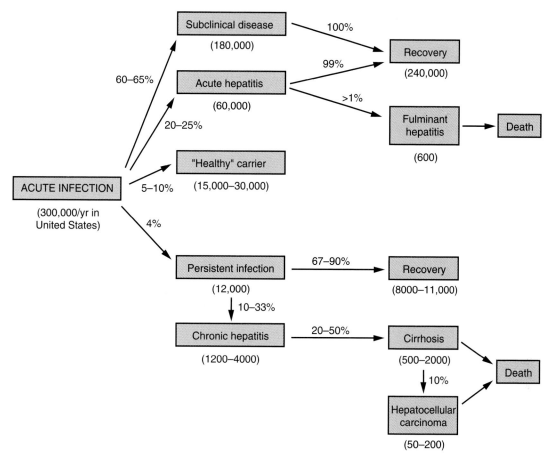

Figure 18–9. Schematic of the potential outcomes of hepatitis B infection in adults, with their approximate annual frequencies in the United States. (Population estimates courtesy of John L. Gollan, M.D., Ph.D., Brigham and Women's Hospital, Boston.)

surface protein (HBsAg), which appears in cells and the serum as spheres and tubules approximately 22 nm in diameter—this may occur with or without replication of infectious virions.

After exposure to the virus, there is a relatively long asymptomatic incubation period averaging 6 to 8 weeks (range 4 to 26 weeks), followed by acute disease lasting many weeks to months. The natural course of the disease can be followed by serum markers (Fig. 18–11):

- *HBsAg* appears before the onset of symptoms and peaks during overt disease. It usually declines to undetectable levels in 3 to 6 months.
- *HBeAg, HBV-DNA, and DNA polymerase* appear in the serum soon after HBsAg and are all markers of active viral replication. *Persistence of HBeAg is an important clinical indicator of continued active viral replication, continued infectivity, and probable progression to chronic hepatitis.*
- *Anti-HBe* is detectable shortly after the disappearance of HBeAg, implying that the acute infection has peaked and the disease is on the wane.
- *IgM anti-HBc* begins to be detectable in the

serum shortly before the onset of symptoms and concurrent with the onset of elevated transaminases (indicating hepatic injury). Over months, the IgM antibody is replaced by IgG anti-HBc, and so an elevated level of IgM anti-HBc indicates a recent acute infection.

- *Anti-HBs* does not rise until the acute disease is over and is usually not detectable for a few weeks to several months after the disappearance of HBsAg. This interval is referred to as the "window period," during which anti-HBc and anti-HBe are the only markers of the disease. Anti-HBs persists in the great majority of patients for life, conferring protection and forming the basis for current vaccination strategies.[25]

Immunologic mechanisms appear to be the primary cause of hepatocellular damage, specifically through the action of cytotoxic T cells.[26] A direct viral cytopathic effect is unlikely, given the absence of injury in "healthy" HBV carriers, despite the presence of hepatocytes containing complete virions or viral antigens. Instead the extraordinary variation in the course and outcome of HBV infections suggests the presence of modifying

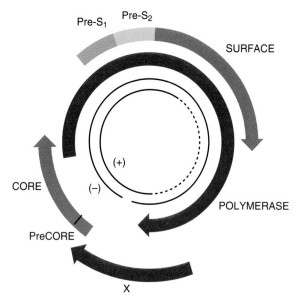

Figure 18-10. Diagrammatic representation of structure and transcribed components of the hepatitis B virion.

mation of complete virions and all associated antigens. Cellular expression of viral HBsAg and HBcAg in association with MHC class I molecules leads to activation of cytotoxic CD+8 T lymphocytes.

- An *integrative phase* follows, with incorporation of viral DNA into the genome of the host cell. With disappearance of viral replication and the appearance of antiviral antibodies, infectivity ends and liver damage subsides, but the risk of hepatocellular carcinoma persists.

Occasionally variant strains of HBV can emerge during active HBV infection with the wild-type strain.[29] Although most mutants cannot form infectious virions, some replicate successfully but are incapable of HBeAg expression, despite continued HBcAg production. The absence of a host antibody response to HBeAg is associated with fulminant hepatitis. A second ominous development is the emergence of vaccine-induced escape mutants, which appear to replicate in the presence of vaccine-induced immunity.[30]

influences, including genetic host responsiveness, antibody-mediated modulation of viral antigens, enhancement of the T-cell reaction by antibody-dependent cellular cytotoxicity, and possible concurrent infection with other viruses.[27] Despite such variability, several principles are operative:[28]

- HBV infections pass through two phases. The *proliferative phase* is a period during which HBV-DNA is present in episomal form, with for-

Hepatitis C Virus

For almost 20 years, parenterally transmitted, non-A, non-B (NANB) hepatitis has been known to cause 90 to 95% of cases of transfusion-associated hepatitis. The long search for the causative agent was rewarded in 1989 with the cloning of hepatitis C virus (HCV).[31] Serologic methods have now es-

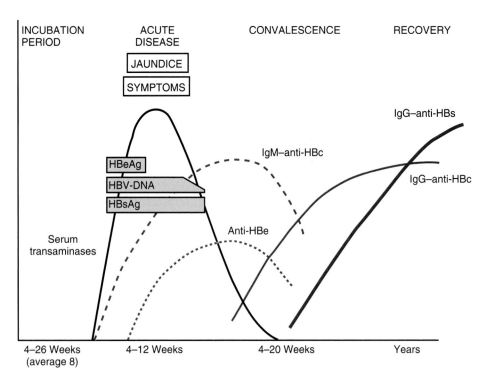

Figure 18-11. The sequence of serologic markers in acute hepatitis B infection, with resolution of active infection.

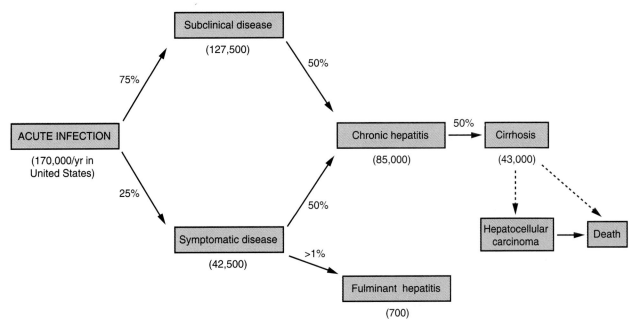

Figure 18–12. Schematic of the potential outcomes of hepatitis C infection in adults, with their approximate annual frequencies in the United States. (Population estimates courtesy of John L. Gollan, M.D., Ph.D., Brigham and Women's Hospital, Boston.)

tablished that HCV is a major cause of liver disease worldwide;[32] about 150,000 to 170,000 new cases of HCV are estimated to occur annually in the United States. The major routes of transmission are inoculations and blood transfusions. Vertical transmission has been documented; transmission by sexual contact appears to be extremely low. Sporadic hepatitis of unknown source accounts for 40% of cases. Seroprevalence in the United States population is 0.2 to 0.6%, and is about 8% in homosexuals and in house contacts, with higher levels in hemodialysis patients (8 to 24%), hemophiliacs (55 to 85%), and intravenous drug abusers (50 to 90%). Patients with unexplained cirrhosis and hepatocellular carcinoma have anti-HCV prevalence rates exceeding 50%. *In contrast to HBV, HCV has a high rate of progression to chronic disease and eventual cirrhosis, exceeding 50%* (Fig. 18–12). *Thus, although HBV is estimated to cause 30,000 new cases of chronic hepatitis annually in the United States, this figure is 85,000 for HCV.* Indeed, HCV may be the leading cause of chronic liver disease in the Western world.

HCV is a small, enveloped single-stranded RNA virus with a 30- to 60-nm diameter and similarities to the flavi/pesti viruses. The genome codes for a single polypeptide of approximately 3010 amino acids in one single open reading frame (Fig. 18–13); this is subsequently processed into functional proteins. The highly conserved region at the 5′ end encodes for the nucleocapsid protein. A hypervariable region encodes for the envelope (E1, E2/NS1) and five less conserved nonstructural regions, NS1 to NS5 toward the 3′ end. HCV virions have yet to be identified within hepatocytes, and the mechanism of liver injury is not established. Both cytocidal replication of HCV and immunologically mediated events have been implicated.[33]

The incubation period for HCV hepatitis ranges from 2 to 26 weeks, with a mean between 6 and 12 weeks. HCV RNA is detectable in blood for 1 to 3 weeks, coincident with elevations in serum

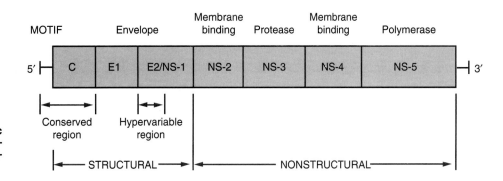

Figure 18–13. Diagrammatic representation of the genomic structure of the hepatitis C virus.

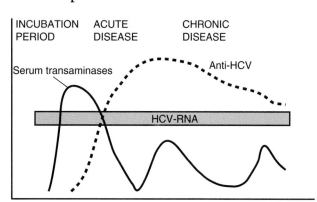

Figure 18-14. The sequence of serologic markers in acute hepatitis C infection, with progression to chronic infection.

transaminases (Fig. 18–14). Circulating RNA persists in many patients despite the presence of neutralizing antibodies,[34] including more than 90% of patients with chronic disease.[35] The clinical course of acute HCV hepatitis is likely to be milder than HBV, but individual cases may be severe and indistinguishable from HAV or HBV hepatitis. A clinical feature quite characteristic of HCV is episodic elevations in serum transaminases, with intervening normal or near-normal periods. Alternatively, transaminases may be persistently elevated or may remain normal.

Persistent infection and chronic hepatitis are the hallmarks of HCV infection, despite the generally asymptomatic nature of the acute illness. *Cirrhosis can be present at the time of diagnosis or may develop over 5 to 10 years.* Of particular concern is the finding that *the elevated titers of anti-HCV IgG following active infection do not seem to confer effective immunity to subsequent HCV infection, either from reactivation of an endogenous strain or by infection with a new strain.*[36] This may seriously hamper efforts to develop an effective HCV vaccine, particularly because HCV appears to be a relatively unstable virus, with continued alteration in envelope antigen expression.

Hepatitis D Virus

Also called the "delta agent" and "hepatitis delta virus," hepatitis D virus (HDV) is a unique RNA virus that is replication defective, causing infection only when it is encapsulated by HBsAg. Thus, *although taxonomically distinct from HBV, HDV is absolutely dependent on the genetic information provided by HBV for multiplication and causes hepatitis only in the presence of HBV.* Delta hepatitis thus arises in two settings.[37]

1. *Acute coinfection* occurs following exposure to serum containing both HDV and HBV. The HBV

must become established first to provide the HBsAg necessary for development of complete HDV virions.

2. *Superinfection* of a chronic carrier of HBV with a new inoculum of HDV results in disease about 30 to 50 days later. The carrier may have been previously "healthy " or may have had underlying chronic hepatitis.

Simultaneous coinfection with HBV and HDV results in hepatitis ranging from mild to fulminant, with fulminant disease more likely (about 3 to 4%) than with HBV alone. Chronicity rarely develops. When HDV is superimposed on chronic HBV infection, three possibilities arise (Fig. 18–15): (1) acute, severe hepatitis may erupt in a previously healthy HBV carrier; (2) mild HBV hepatitis may be converted into fulminant disease; or (3) chronic, progressive disease may develop (in 80% of patients), often terminating in cirrhosis.[38]

Infection by the delta agent is worldwide, but the prevalence varies greatly. In Africa, the Middle East, and southern Italy, 20 to 40% of HBsAg carriers have anti-HDV. In the United States, delta infection is uncommon and largely restricted to drug addicts and hemophiliacs, who exhibit prevalence rates of 1 to 10%. Other high-risk groups for HBV, such as homosexual men and health care workers, are at low risk for HDV infection for unclear reasons. Surprisingly, delta infection is uncommon in the large population of HBsAg carriers in Southeast Asia and China.

HDV is a 35-nm, double-shelled particle that by electron microscopy resembles the "Dane particle" of HBV. The external coat antigen of HBsAg surrounds an internal, 24-kd polypeptide, delta antigen (HDV Ag). Associated with HDV Ag is a small (1689 base pairs), circular molecule of single-stranded RNA, whose length is smaller than the genome of any known animal virus.[37] This RNA is considered "genomic," with the unique feature of three open reading frames on the negative (−) genomic strand and three on the transcribed "antigenomic" (+) strand. Although insights are few into HDV-induced liver diseaes, HDV itself does not appear to be directly pathogenic; HBV appears to be critical for the pathologic effects of HDV.

HDV RNA is detectable in the blood and liver just before and in the early days of acute symptomatic disease. IgM anti-HDV is the most reliable indicator of recent HDV exposure, although its appearance is late and frequently short-lived. Nevertheless, acute coinfection by HDV and HBV is best indicated by detection of IgM against both HDV Ag and HBcAg (the latter denoting new infection with hepatitis B). With chronic delta hepatitis arising from HDV superinfection, HBsAg is present in serum, and anti-HDV persists for months or longer. Future assays for serum HDV Ag and HDV RNA will greatly assist diagnosis of HDV infection.[37]

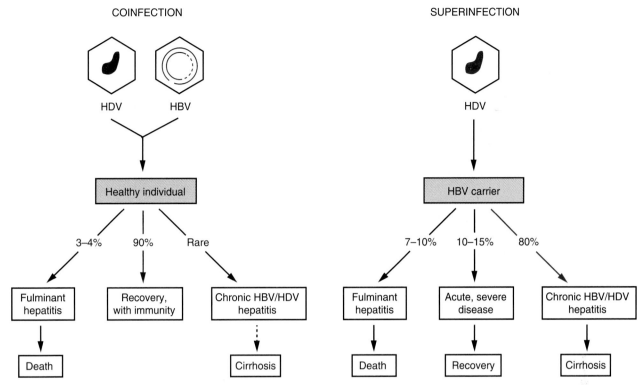

COINFECTION

HDV HBV

Healthy individual

3–4% 90% Rare

Fulminant hepatitis | Recovery, with immunity | Chronic HBV/HDV hepatitis

Death | Cirrhosis

SUPERINFECTION

HDV

HBV carrier

7–10% 10–15% 80%

Fulminant hepatitis | Acute, severe disease | Chronic HBV/HDV hepatitis

Death | Recovery | Cirrhosis

Figure 18–15. The differing clinical consequences of two patterns of combined hepatitis D virus and hepatitis B virus infection.

Hepatitis E Virus

Hepatitis E virus (HEV) hepatitis is an enterically transmitted, water-borne infection occuring primarily in young to middle-aged adults; sporadic infection and overt illness in children are rare.[39] Epidemics have been reported from Asia, the Indian subcontinent, sub-Saharan Africa, and Mexico. Sporadic infection seems to be uncommon and is seen mainly in travelers. *A characteristic feature of the infection is the high mortality rate among pregnant women, approaching 20%.* In most cases, the disease is self-limiting; HEV is not associated with chronic liver disease or persistent viremia.[40] The average incubation period after exposure is 6 weeks.

HEV is an unenveloped single-stranded RNA virus that is best characterized as a calicivirus.[40] Viral particles are 32 to 34 nm in diameter, and the RNA genome is approximately 7.6 kb in size. A specific antigen (HEV Ag) can be identified in the cytoplasm of hepatocytes during active infection. Diagnosis has been based on the detection by immune electron microscopy of virus-like particles in fecal specimens from acutely ill patients or by immunofluorescence methods to detect anti-HEV serologic activity.[39] With the recent propagation of HEV in tissue culture,[41] further insights may be forthcoming.

Clinicopathologic Syndromes

A number of clinical syndromes may develop after exposure to hepatitis viruses:

1. *Carrier state:* (a) without clinically apparent disease or (b) with chronic hepatitis.
2. *Asymptomatic infection:* serologic evidence only.
3. *Acute hepatitis:* (a) anicteric or (b) icteric.
4. *Chronic hepatitis:* (a) without or (b) with progression to cirrhosis.
5. *Fulminant hepatitis:* submassive to massive hepatic necrosis.

Not all of the hepatotropic viruses provoke each of these clinical syndromes: with rare exception, HAV and HEV do not generate a carrier state or cause chronic hepatitis. *Other infectious or noninfectious causes can lead to essentially identical syndromes,* particularly drugs and toxins. *Therefore serologic studies are integral to the diagnosis of viral hepatitis and the distinction between the various agents.*

Carrier State

The term "carrier" denotes an individual without manifest symptoms who harbors and therefore can transmit an organism. With hepatotropic viruses, there are those who (1) harbor one of the viruses but are suffering little or no adverse effects (a "healthy" carrier) and those who (2) have chronic

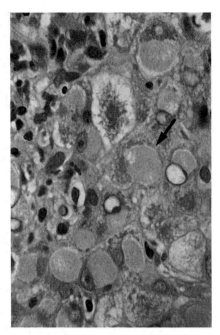

Figure 18-16. Ground-glass hepatocytes (arrows) in hepatitis B virus infection. (Hematoxylin and eosin.)

disease but are essentially free of symptoms or disability. Both constitute reservoirs of infection. The carrier state is best characterized for HBV. Infection early in life, particularly via vertical transmission during childbirth, produces a carrier state 90 to 95% of the time. In contrast, only 1 to 10% of adult infections yield a carrier state. *Individuals with impaired immunity are particularly likely to become carriers.* The situation is less clear with HDV, although there is a well-defined low risk of post-transfusion hepatitis D, indicative of a carrier state in conjunction with HBV.[42] HCV can clearly induce a carrier state, which is estimated at 0.2 to 0.6% of the general U.S. population.

MORPHOLOGY. In the "healthy" HBV carrier state, the liver biopsy is more or less normal. Viable isolated hepatocytes or clusters of cells have **"ground-glass," finely granular, eosinophilic cytoplasm** (Fig. 18–16) laden with HBsAg, which by electron microscopy is present as spheres and tubules. Other cells have **"sanded" nuclei** imparted by abundant HBcAg,[43] **indicating active viral replication.** In HBV/HDV carriers, HDV Ag is present in hepatocytes.[44] *In situ* hybridization techniques and cDNA probes are helpful in disclosing HBV viral DNA and HCV or HDV viral RNA sequences.[45] The chronic disease carrier is described later.

Acute Viral Hepatitis

Any one of the hepatotropic viruses can cause acute viral hepatitis. Whatever the agent, *the dis-*

ease is more or less the same and can be divided into four phases: (1) an incubation period, (2) a symptomatic preicteric phase, (3) a symptomatic icteric phase, and (4) convalescence. The incubation period for the different viruses is given earlier in Table 18–4. Peak infectivity occurs during the last asymptomatic days of the incubation period and the early days of acute symptoms. The *preicteric phase* is marked by nonspecific, constitutional symptoms. Malaise is the most characteristic initial complaint, followed in a few days by general fatigability, nausea, loss of appetite, and sometimes weight loss. Low-grade fever, headaches, muscle and joint aches, and pains and diarrhea are inconstant symptoms. About 10% of patients with acute hepatitis, most often those with hepatitis B, develop a serum sickness–like syndrome in the preicteric stage, consisting of fever, rash, and arthralgias. This is attributed to circulating immune complexes.[46] In anicteric cases, the illness may be dismissed as flu-like, unless its true nature is revealed by elevated serum aminotransferase levels.

The *icteric phase*, if it appears, is caused mainly by conjugated hyperbilirubinemia. *It is usual in adults (but not children) with HAV but is absent in about half the cases of HBV and the majority of cases of HCV.* In icteric patients, the urine turns darker (conjugated bilirubinuria), and the stools may become lighter owing to cholestasis. Retention of bile acids can cause distressing pruritus. The liver may be mildly enlarged and moderately tender to percussion. Laboratory findings include prolonged prothrombin time and hyperglobulinemia; the serum alkaline phosphatase is usually only mildly elevated. Curiously, with the onset of the icteric phase, the constitutional symptoms begin to clear, and the patient feels better. In a few weeks to perhaps several months, the jaundice and most of the other systemic symptoms clear as convalescence begins.

MORPHOLOGY. The morphologic changes in acute viral hepatitis are virtually the same regardless of the causative agent **and can be mimicked by drug reactions.** Grossly, the liver is slightly enlarged and more or less green depending on the phase of the acute disease and the degree of jaundice. Histologically **the major findings are (1) necrosis of random, isolated liver cells or small cell clusters; (2) diffuse liver cell injury; (3) reactive changes in Kupffer cells and sinusoidal lining cells and an inflammatory infiltrate in portal tracts; and (4) evidence of hepatocytic regeneration during the recovery phase.** Necrotic hepatocytes may be evident as fragmented, eosinophilic **Councilman bodies** or may be phagocytosed leading to the accumulation of clumps of lymphocytes and macrophages. Confluent necrosis may lead to **bridging necrosis** connecting portal-to-portal, central-to-

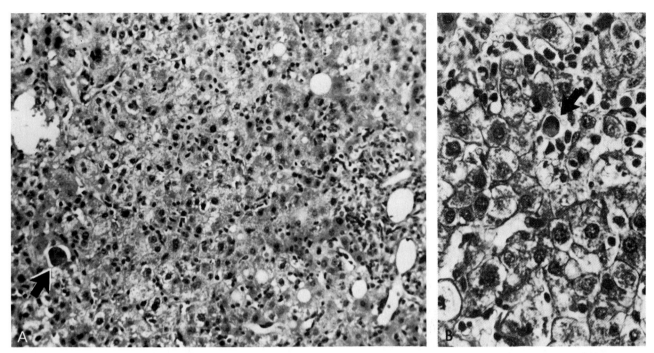

Figure 18–17. *A,* Acute viral hepatitis showing lobular disarray, mild periportal infiltrate at right, and Councilman body *(arrow). B,* High-power detail of acute viral hepatitis with cellular disarray, ballooning, inflammatory cells in sinusoids, and Councilman body *(arrow).* (Courtesy of the late Dr. Hans Popper, The Mount Sinai Medical Center, New York.)

central, or portal-to-central regions of adjacent lobules, signifying a more severe form of acute hepatitis.

Lobular disarray results from the cellular swelling (ballooning), necrosis, and regeneration of cells producing compression of the vascular sinusoids and loss of the normal, more or less radial array (Fig. 18–17). Fatty change is unusual except with HCV. An inconstant finding is **bile stasis** within the lobule. Inflammation is a characteristic, usually prominent feature of acute hepatitis. **Kupffer cells and sinusoidal lining cells undergo hypertrophy and hyperplasia** and are often laden with lipofuscin pigment owing to phagocytosis of hepatocellular debris. **The portal tracts are usually infiltrated with a mixture of inflammatory cells;** this infiltrate may spill over into the parenchyma, particularly where adjacent hepatocytes have undergone necrosis. The bile duct epithelia may proliferate, particularly in cases of HCV hepatitis, forming poorly defined ductular structures (cholangioles).[47]

In the recovery phase of acute hepatitis, the lobule remains somewhat disorganized because hepatocytes can proliferate faster than normal cord-sinusoid-cord relationships can be established. Regenerating hepatocytes lack uniformity in size and are pale, the result of diminished numbers of cytoplasmic organelles. Double and triple nuclei in regenerating cells are commonly observed. Residual clumps of inflammatory cells may persist for some time.

Chronic Viral Hepatitis

Symptomatic, biochemical, or serologic evidence of continuing or relapsing hepatic disease for more than 6 months, optimally with histologically documented inflammation and necrosis, is taken to mean chronic hepatitis. Although the hepatitis viruses are responsible for most cases of chronic hepatitis, there are many other etiologies (each described later): Wilson's disease, alpha₁-antitrypsin deficiency, chronic alcoholism, drugs (isoniazid, alphamethyldopa, methotrexate), and autoimmunity.

Since 1968, chronic hepatitis has been classified according to the extent of inflammation:[48]

1. *Chronic persistent hepatitis,* in which inflammation is confined to the portal tracts.
2. *Chronic active hepatitis,* in which portal tract inflammation spills into the parenchyma and surrounds regions of necrotic hepatocytes.
3. *Chronic lobular hepatitis,* in which persistent inflammation is confined to the lobule.[49]

It is now apparent that the primary determinant of disease progression, and therefore prognosis, is the etiologic form of hepatitis. Therefore, although histologic information may provide information helpful for patient management, *classification of chronic hepatitis strictly by histologic criteria is obsolete and should not be used.*[50] This is particularly important because therapy that is effective for one cause of chronic hepatitis may be ineffective, or potentially detrimental, in other forms of the disease.[51]

The likelihood of chronic hepatitis following acute viral infection, discussed earlier, can be summarized:

HAV: Extremely rare.

HBV: Develops in more than 90% of infected neonates and 5% of infected adults, of whom one-fourth progress to cirrhosis.

HCV: *Develops in more than 50% of infected patients, of whom half progress to cirrhosis.*

HDV: Rare in acute HDV/HBV coinfection; a more severe chronic hepatitis is the most frequent outcome of HDV superinfection.

HEV: Does not produce chronic hepatitis.

Chronic hepatitis with HBV, and apparently with HCV, contributes significantly to the development of primary hepatocellular carcinoma (see later). The clinical features of chronic hepatitis are extremely variable and are not predictive of outcome. In some patients, the only signs of chronic disease are persistent elevations of serum transaminases, hence the facetious designation "transaminitis." The most common symptom is fatigue; less common symptoms are malaise, loss of appetite, and occasional bouts of mild jaundice. Physical findings are few, if any, the most common being spider angiomas, palmar erythema, mild hepatomegaly, hepatic tenderness, and mild splenomegaly. Laboratory studies may reveal prolongation of the prothrombin time and, in some instances, hyperglobulinemia, hyperbilirubinemia, and mild elevations in alkaline phosphatase. Occasionally in cases of HBV, and rarely in HCV, immune-complex diseases may develop secondary to the presence of circulating antibody-antigen complexes, in the form of vasculitis (subcutaneous or visceral, i.e., polyarteritis nodosa; see Chapter 11) or glomerulonephritis (see Chapter 20).

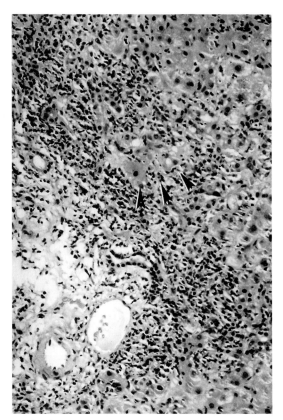

Figure 18-18. Piecemeal necrosis in hepatitis B virus infection. Chronic inflammatory cells are extending out from a portal tract *(left side)* to surround degenerating hepatocytes *(arrows)*. (Hematoxylin and eosin.)

MORPHOLOGY. The morphology of chronic hepatitis ranges from exceedingly mild to severe, to eventual cirrhosis. In the mildest form, an inflammatory infiltrate is limited to portal tracts, consisting of lymphocytes, macrophages, occasional plasma cells, and an occasional rare neutrophil or eosinophil. Liver architecture is usually well preserved but may exhibit vestiges of acute disease.

The histologic hallmark of progressive disease is **piecemeal necrosis,** whereby the chronic inflammatory infiltrate spills out from portal tracts into adjacent parenchyma, with associated necrosis of hepatocytes in the limiting plate (Fig. 18-18). There may be lobular inflammation with focal necrosis of hepatocytes. As with acute hepatitis, **bridging necrosis** may connect adjacent portal-portal, central-central, and portal-central zones. Although piecemeal and bridging necrosis do not imply inevitable progression of disease, **continued loss of hepatocytes results in fibrous septum formation, which, accompanied by hepatocyte re-** generation, results in cirrhosis. A schematic comparison of the morphologic changes in acute and chronic hepatitis is offered in Figure 18-19.

The aforementioned features are common to all forms of chronic hepatitis (viral or otherwise). In patients with chronic HCV hepatitis, lymphoid aggregates in portal tracts and mild fatty change are seen in about 50% of cases, and bile duct damage is seen in more than 90%.[52] Conversely, "ground-glass" hepatocytes are sometimes present in chronic HBV hepatitis.[53] Despite use of immunohistochemical techniques, it is frequently impossible to identify the etiology of chronic hepatitis on tissue samples, so great reliance must be placed on clinical, virologic, and serologic observations.

The clinical course is unpredictable. Patients may experience spontaneous remission or may have indolent disease without progression for many years. Conversely, some patients have rapidly progressive disease and develop cirrhosis within a few years. The major causes of death are cirrhosis, with liver failure and hepatic encephalopathy or massive hematemesis from esophageal varices and, in those with long-standing HBV (particularly neonatal) or HCV infection, hepatocellular carcinoma.

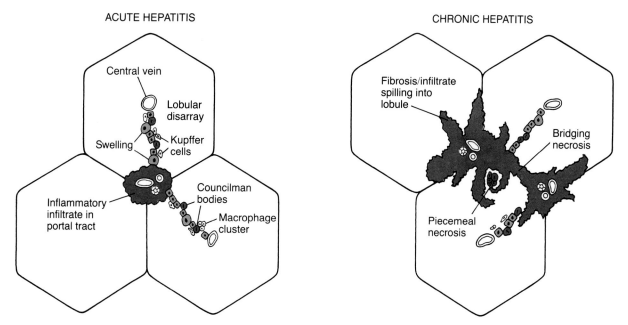

ACUTE HEPATITIS

Central vein
Lobular disarray
Swelling
Kupffer cells
Inflammatory infiltrate in portal tract
Councilman bodies
Macrophage cluster

CHRONIC HEPATITIS

Fibrosis/infiltrate spilling into lobule
Bridging necrosis
Piecemeal necrosis

Figure 18-19. A schematic comparison of the morphologic features of acute and chronic hepatitis.

AUTOIMMUNE HEPATITIS

Autoimmune hepatitis is a chronic hepatitis of unknown etiology, which has clinical and histologic features virtually indistinguishable from chronic viral hepatitis.[54] This disease may run an indolent or a severe and progressive course and typically responds dramatically to immunosuppressive therapy. Salient features include:

• Female predominance (70%), particularly young and perimenopausal women.
• The absence of viral serologic markers.
• Elevated serum IgG levels (> 2.5 gm/dl).
• High serum titers of autoantibodies in 80% of cases, including antinuclear (ANA), anti-smooth muscle (SMA), antimitochrondrial (AMA), and anti-liver and kidney microsome (LKM) antibodies. Because there is often a positive lupus erythematosus (LE) test, autoimmune hepatitis was formerly called "lupoid" hepatitis.
• An increased frequency of HLA B8 or DRw3.

The clinical diagnosis of autoimmune hepatitis is one of exclusion and circumstantial evidence[51] because uniform diagnostic criteria are lacking. Associated autoimmune diseases are present in up to 60% of patients, predominantly rheumatoid arthritis, rash, thyroiditis, Sjögren's syndrome, or ulcerative colitis. Clinical presentation is similar to other forms of chronic hepatitis; these tend to be the more severely affected patients, for whom immunosuppressive therapy is indicated. Autoimmune hepatitis, however, may present in an atypical fashion involving other organ systems, hampering diagnostic efforts.

Autoimmune hepatitis presents the entire spectrum of chronic hepatitis; symptomatic patients frequently exhibit aggressive disease,[52] with large areas of parenchymal collapse, severe piecemeal necrosis, and a prominent plasma cell infiltrate. Although patients usually respond to immunosuppression (in marked contrast to viral hepatitis), 5% of patients develop cirrhosis.

FULMINANT HEPATITIS

When hepatic insufficiency progresses from onset of symptoms to hepatic encephalopathy within 2 to 3 weeks, it is termed *fulminant hepatic failure*. A less rapid course, extending up to 3 months, is called *subfulminant failure*. Both patterns are fortunately uncommon and are caused mainly by rampant to fulminant viral hepatitis (50 to 65% of cases) and drug or chemical toxicity (25 to 30%). As Table 18-5 indicates, however, there are many other possible etiologies and ultimately some cases of unknown etiology. Drugs and chemicals act either as direct hepatotoxins or via idiosyncratic inflammatory reactions. Principally implicated are acetaminophen (in suicidal doses), isoniazid, antidepressants (particularly monoamine oxidase inhibitors), halothane, methyldopa, and the mycotoxins of the mushroom *Amanita phalloides*. The evolution of hepatic failure is extremely variable and is significantly influenced by the previous status of

Table 18-5. CAUSES OF FULMINANT OR
SUBFULMINANT LIVER FAILURE

Acute viral hepatitis
  Acute hepatitis A
  Acute hepatitis B
  Acute hepatitis C
  Acute hepatitis D (delta)
    Coinfection
    Superinfection
  Acute hepatitis E
  Acute hepatitis due to infection with herpesviruses
Acute drug-induced hepatitis
Acute hepatitis due to poisoning
Other causes
  Ischemic liver cell necrosis
  Obstruction of the hepatic veins
    Budd-Chiari syndrome
    Veno-occlusive disease
  Massive malignant infiltration of liver
  Wilson's disease
  Microvesicular steatosis
    Acute fatty liver of pregnancy
    Reye's syndrome
    Drug-induced microvesicular steatosis
  Autoimmune chronic active hepatitis
  Reactivation of chronic hepatitis B
  Hyperthermia (heat stroke)
  Liver transplantation
  Partial hepatectomy

With permission from Bernau, J., et al.: Fulminant and subfulminant liver failure: Definitions and causes. Semin. Liver Dis. 6(2):98, 1986. Thieme Medical Publishers, Inc.

the liver and patient age (younger patients fare better).

MORPHOLOGY. All causative agents produce essentially identical morphologic changes, and for all, the distribution of liver destruction is extremely capricious. **The entire liver may be involved or sometimes, for completely obscure reasons, only random areas.** An entire lobe may be spared, or patchy necrotic areas may be dispersed haphazardly throughout the liver. Progressive loss of liver substance leads to depression of affected areas; with massive involvement, the liver may shrink in the course of days to as little as 500 to 700 gm. In so doing, it is transformed into a red, limp organ covered by a wrinkled, too-large capsule (Fig. 18–20). Blotchy green bile staining may be present. On transection, necrotic areas have a muddy red, mushy appearance with patchy bile staining.

Histologically the necrosis may wipe out entire lobules or be less extreme, destroying the central and midzonal regions and sparing the periportal area of the lobule. Presumably, the most hypoxic zones are most vulnerable to severe insult. Complete destruction of contiguous lobules with liquefaction of hepatocytes leaves only a collapsed reticulin framework and preserved portal tracts (Fig. 18–21); portal tracts converge with shrinkage of the liver. There may be surprisingly little inflammatory reaction except possibly for an increase in lymphocytes, macrophages, and occasional neutrophils within the portal tracts.

Patient survival for more than a week permits secondary regenerative activity of surviving hepatocytes, which transiently take on the appearance of primitive ductules. With zonal necrosis, the parenchymal framework is preserved, and regeneration is orderly; native liver architecture may be completely restored in time. The Kupffer cells that survive the necrotizing process also proliferate and

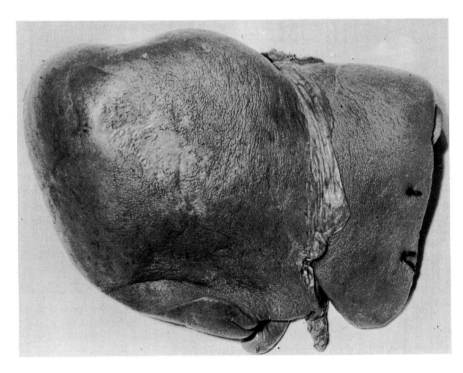

Figure 18–20. Massive necrosis. Liver is small (700 gm) and soft in consistency. Capsule is wrinkled.

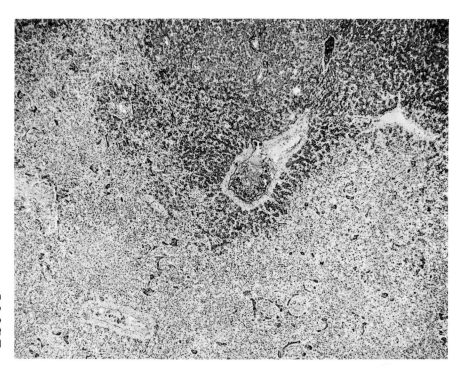

Figure 18-21. Massive necrosis. In the lower portion of field, complete necrosis is apparent, with absence of hepatocytes in many adjacent liver lobules. (Hematoxylin and eosin.)

become laden with lipofuscin and cellular debris. With more massive destruction of confluent lobules, regeneration is disorderly, yielding nodular masses of liver cells that may be separated by broad bands of scar tissue (**postnecrotic cirrhosis,** discussed next). Scarring is much more likely in those with a protracted course of submassive or patchy necrosis.

Fulminant hepatic failure may present with jaundice, encephalopathy, and fetor hepaticus, as described previously. Frequently, absent on physical examination are stigmata of chronic liver disease. Extrahepatic complications of the course of the illness include coagulopathy and bleeding, cardiovascular instability, renal failure, adult respiratory distress syndrome, electrolyte and acid-base disturbances, and sepsis. Depending on the magnitude of the insult and the sturdiness of the host, the mortality ranges from 25 to 90% in the absence of liver transplantation. One-year survival following liver transplantation approaches 60%.[55]

POSTNECROTIC CIRRHOSIS

This pattern of cirrhosis is characterized by irregularly sized nodules separated by variable but mostly broad scars. The most common known cause is previous viral infection; in about 20 to 25% of cases it evolves from chronic HBV infection; the contribution of chronic HCV may be even greater. In a small number of instances, there is a well-documented history of acute liver damage caused by some hepatotoxin, such as phosphorus;

carbon tetrachloride; mushroom poisoning; or a drug such as acetaminophen, oxyphenisatin, or alpha-methyldopa. Undoubtedly some cases represent end-stage alcoholic cirrhosis (see later), readily misinterpreted as postnecrotic cirrhosis in the absence of a history of chronic alcoholism. After all these possibilities have been excluded, there remains a large residual of uncertain origin. *A single attack of massive hepatic necrosis only infrequently gives rise to postnecrotic cirrhosis* because either it is fatal, or regeneration of the liver cells permits survival with little or no residual scarring.

MORPHOLOGY. Typically some time after an acute event or following years of chronic hepatitis, the liver exhibits nodules of varying size (some several centimeters in diameter) and broad bands or areas of depressed scarring (Fig. 18-22). Severe collapse may leave a shrunken liver less than 1 kg in size. Microscopically lobular architecture may be com-

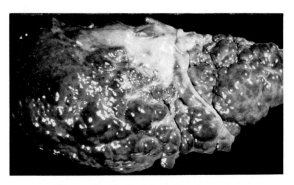

Figure 18-22. Postnecrotic cirrhosis.

pletely lost in the developing nodules and scar. Alternatively, **progressive chronic hepatitis of any etiology inexorably transforms a more normal-sized liver into a patchwork of variably sized nodules alternating with broad septal scars.** Eventually active liver cell necrosis becomes inconspicuous. Residua of portal tracts may be evident; bile stasis is variable. **Ultimately the diagnosis rests on excluding other bases for cirrhosis.**

The clinical course of postnecrotic cirrhosis is as varied as the origins of this form of cirrhosis. Death may ensue from the previously described complications of cirrhosis, including hepatocellular carcinoma.

LIVER ABSCESSES

In Developing Countries, liver abscesses are common; most represent parasitic infections, for example, amebic, echinococcal, and (less commonly) other protozoal and helminthic organisms. In developed countries, liver abscesses are uncommon. A low incidence of amebic abscesses (see Chapter 8) is encountered, usually in immigrants from endemic regions. Most abscesses are pyogenic, representing a complication of an infection elsewhere. The organisms reach the liver via (1) the portal vein, (2) arterial supply, (3) ascending infection in the biliary tract (*ascending cholangitis*), (4) direct invasion of the liver from a nearby source, or (5) a penetrating injury. The majority of hepatic abscesses used to result from portal spread of intra-abdominal infections (e.g., appendicitis, diverticulitis, colitis). With improved management of these conditions, spread now occurs primarily via the biliary tree or via the arterial supply in patients suffering from some form of immune deficiency, for example, old age with debilitating disease, immunosuppression, or cancer chemotherapy with marrow failure.[56] In these settings, abscesses may develop without a primary focus elsewhere.

MORPHOLOGY. Pyogenic hepatic abscesses may occur as solitary or multiple lesions, ranging in size from millimeters to massive lesions many centimeters in diameter. Bacteremic spread through the arterial or portal system tends to produce multiple small abscesses, whereas direct extension and trauma usually cause solitary large abscesses. Biliary abscesses, which are usually multiple, may be associated with purulent material in adjacent bile ducts. Gross and microscopic features are those to be seen in any abscess. Occasionally the causative organisms can be identified in the case of fungal or parasitic abscesses. On rare occasion, abscesses located in the subdiaphragmatic region, particularly amebic, may burrow into the thoracic cavity to produce empyema or a lung abscess. Rupture of subcapsular liver abscesses has also led to peritonitis or localized peritoneal abscesses.

Liver abscesses are associated with fever and in many instances right upper quadrant pain and tender hepatomegaly. Jaundice may result from extrahepatic biliary obstruction. Although antibiotic therapy may control smaller lesions, surgical drainage is often necessary for the larger lesions. Because diagnosis is frequently delayed and because patients are often elderly and have serious coexistent disease, the mortality rate with large liver abscesses ranges from 30 to 90%. With early recognition and appropriate management, up to 80% of patients may survive.[56]

DRUG-INDUCED AND TOXIN-INDUCED LIVER DISEASE

As the major drug-metabolizing and drug-detoxifying organ in the body, the liver is subject to potential damage from an enormous array of pharmaceutical and environmental chemicals. Injury may result from (1) direct toxicity; (2) hepatic conversion of a xenobiotic to an active toxin; or (3) via immune mechanisms, usually when the drug or a metabolite acts as a hapten to convert a cellular protein into an immunogen.[57] Principles of drug and toxic injury were discussed in Chapter 9. Here it suffices to recall that drug reactions may be classified as *predictable (intrinsic)* reactions or *unpredictable (idiosyncratic)* ones. Predictable drug reactions may occur in anyone who accumulates a sufficient dose. Unpredictable reactions depend on idiosyncrasies of the host, e.g., the host's propensity to mount an immune response to the antigenic stimulus and the rate at which the host metabolizes the agent. A broad classification of offending agents is offered in Table 18–6, with the following points of emphasis:

- The injury may be immediate or take weeks to months to develop, presenting only after severe liver damage has developed.
- The injury may take the form of *hepatocyte necrosis, cholestasis,* or *insidious onset of liver dysfunction.*
- *Drug-induced chronic hepatitis is clinically and histologically indistinguishable from chronic viral hepatitis.*

A diagnosis of drug-induced liver disease may be made based on a temporal association of liver damage with drug administration and, it is hoped, recovery on removal of the drug, combined with exclusion of other potential causes. *Exposure to a toxin or therapeutic agent should be included in the differential diagnosis of any form of liver disease.*

Table 18-6. DRUG-INDUCED AND TOXIN-INDUCED HEPATIC INJURY

TISSUE REACTION	EXAMPLES
Hepatocellular Damage	
Microvesicular fatty change	Tetracycline, salicylates, yellow phosphorus
Macrovesicular fatty change	Ethanol, methotrexate, amiodarone
Centrilobular necrosis	Bromobenzene, CCl_4, acetaminophen, halothane, rifampin
Diffuse or massive necrosis	Halothane, isoniazid, acetaminophen, α-methyldopa, trinitrotoluene, *Amanita phalloides* (mushroom) toxin
Hepatitis, acute and chronic	α-Methyldopa, isoniazid, nitrofurantoin, phenytoin, oxyphenisatin
Fibrosis-cirrhosis	Ethanol, methotrexate, amiodarone, most drugs that cause chronic hepatitis
Granuloma formation	Sulfonamides, α-methyldopa, quinidine, phenylbutazone, hydralazine, allopurinol
Cholestasis (with or without hepatocellular injury)	Chlorpromazine, anabolic steroids, erythromycin estolate, oral contraceptives, organic arsenicals
Vascular Disorders	
Veno-occlusive disease	Cytotoxic drugs, pyrrolizidine alkaloids (bush tea)
Hepatic or portal vein thrombosis	Estrogens, including oral contraceptives, cytotoxic drugs
Peliosis hepatis	Anabolic steroids, oral contraceptives, danazol
Hyperplasia and Neoplasia	
Adenoma	Oral contraceptives
Hepatocellular carcinoma	Vinyl chloride, aflatoxin, Thorotrast
Cholangiocarcinoma	Thorotrast
Angiosarcoma	Vinyl chloride, inorganic arsenicals, Thorotrast

ALCOHOLIC LIVER DISEASE

Alcohol abuse constitutes the major form of liver disease in most Western countries. These U.S. statistics attest to the magnitude of the problem:[58]

- More than 10 million Americans are alcoholics.
- Alcohol abuse causes 200,000 deaths annually, the fifth leading cause of death.
- Twenty-five per cent to 30% of hospitalized patients have problems related to alcohol abuse.

Chronic alcohol consumption has a variety of adverse effects, as pointed out in Chapter 9. Of greatest impact, however, are the three distinctive, albeit overlapping, forms of liver disease:[59] (1) hepatic steatosis, (2) alcoholic hepatitis, and (3) cirrhosis, collectively referred to as alcoholic liver disease. These conditions may exist independently of each other and do not necessarily represent a continuum of changes. Their morphology is presented first because this facilitates consideration of their pathogenesis.

HEPATIC STEATOSIS (FATTY LIVER)

MORPHOLOGY. Following even moderate intake of alcohol, small **(microvesicular)** lipid droplets accumulate in hepatocytes. With chronic intake of alcohol, lipid accumulates to the point of creating large clear **macrovesicular** spaces, compressing and displacing the nucleus to the periphery of the hepatocyte. This transformation is initially centrilobular, but in severe cases, it may involve the entire lobule (Fig. 18–23). The liver is often grossly enlarged, up to 4 to 6 kg, and is a soft, yellow, greasy organ. Although there is little or no fibrosis at the outset, with continued alcohol abuse, fibrous

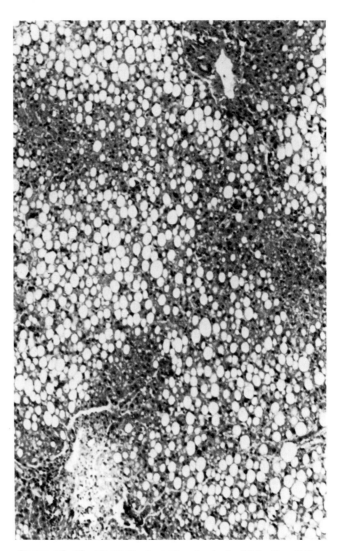

Figure 18–23. Alcoholic hepatic steatosis. Virtually all the hepatocytes contain large lipid vacuoles.

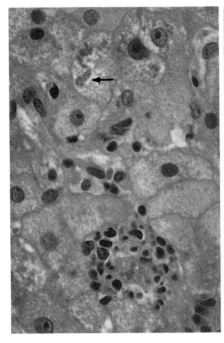
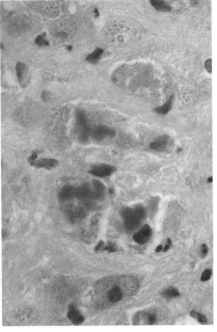

A

B

Figure 18–24. Alcoholic hepatitis. *A,* The cluster of neutrophils marks the site of a necrotic hepatocyte. A Mallory body is present in a second hepatocyte *(arrow). B,* Eosinophilic Mallory bodies are seen in hepatocytes, which are surrounded by fibrous tissue. (Hematoxylin and eosin.)

tissue develops around the central veins and extends into the adjacent sinusoids.[60] **Up to the time that fibrosis appears, the fatty change is completely reversible if there is further abstention from alcohol.**

ALCOHOLIC HEPATITIS

MORPHOLOGY. Alcoholic hepatitis exhibits the following: (1) **Liver cell necrosis**—Single or scattered foci of cells undergo swelling (ballooning) and necrosis, more frequently in the centrilobular regions of the lobule. (2) **Mallory bodies**—Scattered hepatocytes accumulate tangled skeins of cytokeratin intermediate filaments and other proteins, visible as eosinophilic cytoplasmic inclusions.[59] These may also be seen in primary biliary cirrhosis, Wilson's disease, chronic cholestatic syndromes, focal nodular hyperplasia, and hepatocellular carcinoma. (3) **Neutrophilic reaction**—Neutrophils permeate the lobule and accumulate around degenerating liver cells, particularly those having Mallory bodies. Lymphocytes and macrophages also enter portal tracts and spill into the lobule. (4) **Fibrosis**—Alcoholic hepatitis is almost always accompanied by a brisk sinusoidal and perivenular fibrosis; occasionally periportal fibrosis may predominate, particularly with repeated bouts of heavy alcohol intake. Typical features are illustrated in Figure 18–24. Fat may be present or entirely absent. Deranged iron processing in the alcoholic typically leads to a modest accumulation of hemosiderin in hepatocytes and Kupffer cells.[61]

ALCOHOLIC CIRRHOSIS

MORPHOLOGY. The final and irreversible form of alcoholic liver disease usually evolves slowly and insidiously. At first the cirrhotic liver is yellow-tan, fatty, and enlarged, usually weighing more than 2 kg. Over the span of years, it is transformed into a brown, shrunken, nonfatty organ, sometimes less than 1 kg in weight (Fig. 18–25). Cirrhosis may develop within 1 to 2 years in the setting of alcoholic hepatitis. Initially the developing fibrous septae are delicate and extend from central vein to portal regions as well as from portal tract to portal tract. Regenerative activity of the entrapped parenchymal acini generates fairly uniformly sized "micronodules." With time, the nodularity becomes more prominent; scattered nodules may become quite large, and occasionally nodules more than 2 cm in diameter may develop. As fibrous septae dissect and surround nodules, the liver becomes more fibrotic, loses fat, and shrinks progressively in size. Parenchymal islands are engulfed by ever wider bands of fibrous tissue, and the liver is converted into a mixed micronodular and macronodular pattern (Fig. 18–26). Further ischemic necrosis and fibrous obliteration of nodules eventually create broad expanses of tough, pale scar tissue, leaving residual parenchymal nodules that protrude like "hobnails" from the surface of the liver ("Laennec's cirrhosis"). By microscopy, the septae contain variable amounts of scattered lymphocytes and some reactive bile duct proliferation. Bile stasis often develops; Mallory bodies are only rarely evident at this stage. Thus, **end-stage alcoholic cirrhosis comes to resemble, both macroscopically and microscopically, postnecrotic cirrhosis.** The

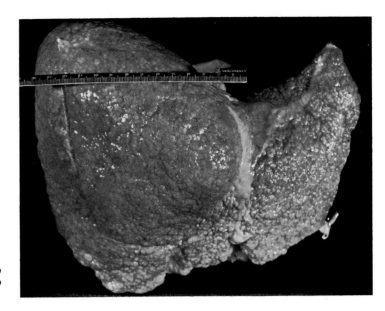

Figure 18-25. Alcoholic cirrhosis, showing the characteristic diffuse nodularity induced by the underlying fibrous scarring.

spectrum of morphologic changes associated with alcoholic liver is schematized in Figure 18-27.

PATHOGENESIS OF ALCOHOLIC LIVER DISEASE

The pharmacokinetics and metabolism of alcohol have been examined previously (see Chapter 9). Pertinent to our discussion is the hepatic disposition of alcohol and its by-products, which is associated with a myriad of detrimental events leading to hepatocellular dysfunction or outright necrosis, as follows:[62]

- Hepatocellular steatosis results from (1) the shunting of normal substrates away from catabolism and toward lipid biosynthesis owing to generation of excess nicotinamide-adenine dinucleotide (NADH) by alcohol dehydrogenase, (2) impaired assembly and secretion of lipoproteins, and (3) increased peripheral catabolism of fat.
- Induction of cytochromes P_{450} leads to augmented transformation of other drugs to toxic metabolites.
- Free radicals are generated during microsomal ethanol oxidizing system (MEOS) oxidation of alcohol, reacting with membranes and proteins.
- Alcohol directly affects microtubular and mitochondrial function and membrane fluidity.
- Acetaldehyde (the major metabolite of alcohol) induces lipid peroxidation and acetaldehyde-protein adduct formation, further disrupting microtubular function.
- Alcohol induces immunologic attack on hepatic neoantigens, possibly owing to alcohol-induced

or acetaldehyde-induced alteration in hepatic proteins.[63]

In addition, alcohol can become a major caloric source in the diet of an alcoholic, displacing other nutrients and leading to malnutrition and vitamin deficiencies. This is compounded by impaired digestive function, primarily related to chronic mucosal damage and pancreatitis. Alcohol-induced stimulation of fibrosis is multifactorial and remains

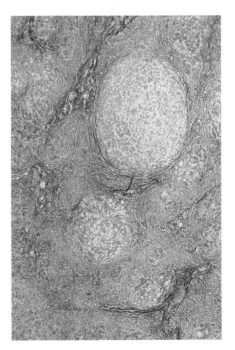

Figure 18-26. Alcoholic cirrhosis. Nodules of varying sizes are entrapped in fibrous tissue. Fatty change also is present (Masson trichrome).

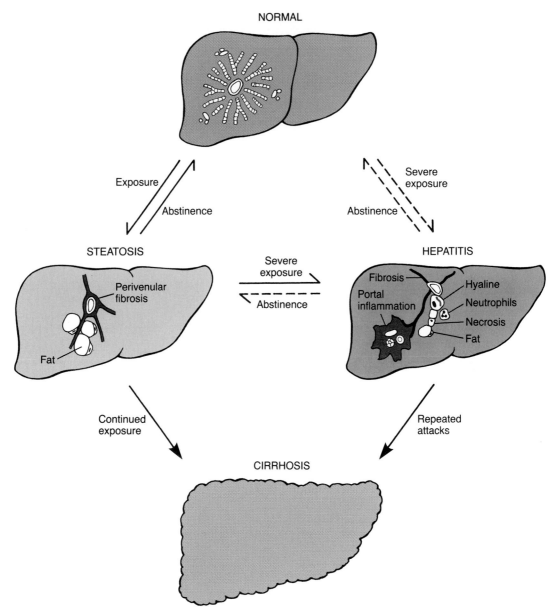

Figure 18-27. Alcoholic liver disease. The interrelationships among alcoholic steatosis, hepatitis, and cirrhosis are shown.

poorly understood; possible mechanisms were reviewed in Chapter 9.

CLINICAL COURSE

Short-term ingestion of up to 80 gm of ethanol per day (8 beers or 7 ounces of 80 proof liquor) generally produces mild, reversible hepatic changes, such as fatty liver. Daily ingestion of 160 gm or more of ethanol for 10 to 20 years is associated more consistently with severe injury; chronic intake of 80 to 160 gm/day is considered a borderline risk for severe injury. *Only 10 to 15% of alcoholics, however, develop cirrhosis.* For reasons that may relate to decreased gastric metabolism of ethanol[64] and differences in body composition, women

appear to be more susceptible to hepatic injury than men. Individual, possibly genetic, susceptibility must exist, but as yet no genetic markers of susceptibility have been identified. *In the absence of a clear understanding of the pathogenetic factors influencing the incidence of alcoholic liver disease, no "safe" upper limit for alcohol consumption can be proposed.* In addition, the relationship between hepatic steatosis and alcoholic hepatitis as precursors to cirrhosis, both causally and temporally, is not yet clear because cirrhosis may develop without antecedent evidence of steatosis or alcoholic hepatitis.

Clinically *hepatic steatosis* may become evident as mild elevation of serum bilirubin and alkaline phosphatase. Alternatively, there may be no clinical or biochemical evidence of liver disease. Severe hepatic compromise (e.g., malaise, anorexia, even hepatic failure and death)[65] is unusual. Alcohol withdrawal and the provision of an adequate diet are sufficient treatment.

In contrast, *alcoholic hepatitis* tends to appear relatively acutely, usually following a bout of heavy drinking. Symptoms and laboratory manifestations may range from none to fulminant hepatic failure. Between these two extremes are the nonspecific symptoms of malaise, anorexia, weight loss, upper abdominal discomfort, and tender hepatomegaly as well as hyperbilirubinemia and elevated alkaline phosphatase. Fever and a neutrophilic leukocytosis frequently occur. An acute cholestatic syndrome may appear, resembling large bile duct obstruction. The outlook is unpredictable; each bout of hepatitis incurs about a 10 to 20% risk of death. Cirrhosis is likely to appear in about one-third of patients within a few years if there are repeated bouts. With proper nutrition and total cessation of alcohol consumption, alcoholic hepatitis may slowly clear. In some patients, however, the hepatitis persists despite abstinence and progresses to cirrhosis.

The manifestations of *alcoholic cirrhosis* are similar to all forms of cirrhosis, presented earlier. In about 10% of patients, the alcoholic cirrhosis is discovered only at autopsy. Commonly the first signs of cirrhosis relate to complications of portal hypertension, sometimes as life-threatening variceal hemorrhage. Alternatively, malaise, weakness, weight loss, and loss of appetite precede the appearance of jaundice, ascites, and peripheral edema, the latter owing to impaired synthesis of albumin. The stigmata of cirrhosis (e.g., grossly distended abdomen, wasted extremities, caput medusae) may be dramatically evident. Laboratory findings reflect the developing hepatic compromise, with elevated serum transaminase levels, hyperbilirubinemia, variable elevation of serum alkaline phosphatase, hypoproteinemia, and anemia. In some instances, liver biopsy may be indicated because experience teaches that in about 10 to 20% of cases of presumed alcoholic cirrhosis, another disease process is found on biopsy.

In the end-stage alcoholic, the immediate causes of death are (1) hepatic coma; (2) a massive gastrointestinal variceal hemorrhage; (3) an intercurrent infection (to which these patients are predisposed); or (4) hepatorenal syndrome following a bout of alcoholic hepatitis. In about 3 to 6% of cases, death is related to the development of hepatocellular carcinoma.

INBORN ERRORS OF METABOLISM AND PEDIATRIC LIVER DISEASE

A distinct group of liver diseases is attributable to disorders of metabolism. Idiopathic hemochroma-

Table 18–7. CLASSIFICATION OF IRON OVERLOAD

Hereditary hemochromatosis
Secondary iron overload
  Anemia due to ineffective erythropoiesis
    β-Thalassemia
    Sideroblastic anemia
    Aplastic anemia
    Pyruvate kinase deficiency
  Liver disease
    Alcoholic cirrhosis
    Chronic viral hepatitis
    Following portocaval anastomosis
    Porphyria cutanea tarda
  Increased oral intake of iron
    African iron overload (Bantu siderosis)
  Congenital atransferrinemia
  Parenteral iron overload
    Red blood cell transfusions
    Iron-dextran injections
    Long-term hemodialysis

Adapted from Bacon, B.R.: Hemochromatosis. *In* Snape, W. (ed.): Consultations in Gastroenterology. Philadelphia, W.B. Saunders Co., in press.

tosis, Wilson's disease, and alpha$_1$-antitrypsin deficiency are well-characterized inherited disorders. Reye's syndrome is not an inherited disease but has metabolic features suggesting a predisposition to its development. We must also consider here neonatal hepatitis, a broad disease category encompassing rare inherited diseases and neonatal infections.

HEMOCHROMATOSIS

Hemochromatosis is defined as the excessive accumulation of body iron, most of which is deposited in the parenchymal cells of various organs, particularly liver and pancreas.[66] *Hereditary hemochromatosis* (HHC), also called *primary* or *idiopathic hemochromatosis*, is a homozygous recessive heritable disorder. Those disorders in which the source of excess iron can be defined are called *secondary hemochromatosis* (Table 18–7).

As discussed in Chapter 5, the total body iron pool ranges from 2 to 6 gm in normal adults; about 0.5 gm is stored in the liver, 98% of which is in hepatocytes. In HHC, total iron accumulation may exceed 50 gm. Clinically this disease exhibits the following features:

- Fully developed cases exhibit (1) *micronodular cirrhosis*—most patients; (2) *diabetes mellitus*—75 to 80%; and (3) *skin pigmentation*—75 to 80% of cases.
- Iron accumulation is lifelong; symptoms usually first appear in the fifth to sixth decades of life.
- The hemochromatosis gene is located on the short arm of chromosome 6, close to the HLA gene locus.[67] Associated HLA haplotypes include A3 in 70% of patients (versus 25% in the normal

population) and, to a lesser extent, B7, B14, or Bw35.
- Males predominate (5 to 7:1) with slightly earlier clinical presentation, partly because physiologic iron loss (menstruation, pregnancy) delays iron accumulation in women.

In white populations of northern European extraction, the gene frequency is estimated at approximately 6%.[68] The frequency of homozygosity is 0.45% (1 of every 220 people) and of heterozygosity 11% (1 of every 9 people), making HHC one of the most common inborn errors of metabolism.

PATHOGENESIS. For a general overview of iron physiology, the reader is referred to Chapter 5. In hemochromatotic patients, excessive intestinal iron absorption leads to net iron accumulation of 0.5 to 1.0 gm per year.[66] Mechanisms for regulation of intestinal iron absorption are obscure, and the functional defect of primary hemochromatosis is as yet unknown. Evidence suggests, however, that the liver and other parenchymal organs are innocent victims in this disease, acting only as iron-storage depots.

Symptoms typically develop after 20 gm of storage iron have accumulated. *The fundamental disease mechanism appears to be direct iron toxicity to host tissues,* mediated by the following proposed mechanisms:[66] (1) lipid peroxidation via iron-catalyzed free radical reactions; (2) iron stimulation of collagen formation; and (3) direct interactions of iron with DNA, leading to lethal alterations or predisposing to hepatocellular carcinoma. Whatever the actions of iron, it is reversible in cells not fatally injured, and removal of excess iron during therapy promotes recovery of tissue function.

The most common causes of *secondary hemochromatosis* are the severe anemias associated with ineffective erythropoiesis (see Chapter 13). In these disorders, the excess iron results not only from transfusions, but also from increased absorption of iron. Transfusions alone, as in aplastic anemias, usually lead to systemic hemosiderosis but little parenchymal cell injury except in extreme cases. *Alcoholic cirrhosis* may engender a modest increase in stainable iron within liver cells. This represents alcohol-induced redistribution of iron because total iron is not significantly increased.[69] A rather unusual form of iron overload resembling HHC was described in South African blacks ingesting large quantities of alcoholic beverage fermented in iron utensils ("Bantu siderosis"). Home-brewing in steel drums continues, and a genetic susceptibility to excess iron accumulation in this population has been implicated.[70]

MORPHOLOGY. Although iron overload occurs via excessive intestinal absorption, iron accumulates as ferritin and hemosiderin in the parenchymal tissues

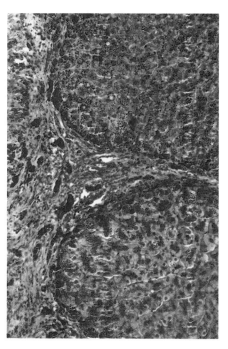

Figure 18–28. Hereditary hemochromatosis. The iron deposition in this cirrhotic liver is highlighted by the blue color imparted by Prussian blue stain.

of the body (liver, pancreas, myocardium, and endocrine glands) and in the linings of joints, without significant deposition in the bone marrow. In the **liver**, iron becomes evident first as golden-yellow hemosiderin granules in the cytoplasm of periportal hepatocytes, particularly in pericanalicular lysosomes. With increasing iron load, there is progressive involvement of the rest of the lobule; bile duct epithelium and Kupffer cell pigmentation are less marked. Because iron is a direct hepatotoxin, inflammation is characteristically absent. At this stage, the liver is typically slightly larger than normal, dense, and chocolate brown. Fibrous septa develop slowly, leading ultimately to a micronodular pattern of cirrhosis. The overall reduction in liver size is rarely marked.

The Prussian blue reaction (potassium ferrocyanide and hydrochloric acid) is used to stain the hemosiderin granules blue-black (Fig. 18–28). Because this stain does not stain ferritin-bound iron, **biochemical determination of hepatic iron concentration in unfixed tissue is the standard for quantitating iron content.** In normal individuals, it is less than 1000 μg/gm dry weight of liver. Adult patients with HHC exhibit over 10,000 μg iron/gm dry weight; hepatic iron concentrations in excess of 22,000 μg/gm dry weight are associated with the development of fibrosis and cirrhosis.[71]

The **pancreas** becomes intensely pigmented, has diffuse interstitial fibrosis, and may exhibit some parenchymal atrophy. Hemosiderin is found in both the acinar and the islet cells and sometimes in the interstitial fibrous stroma. The intensity of iron staining in the pancreatic islets correlates somewhat with the occurrence and severity of the diabetes. The **heart** is often enlarged and has hemosiderin granules within the myocardial fibers, inducing a striking brown coloration to the myocardium. A delicate interstitial fibrosis may appear. The **skin** usually has increased pigmentation, mainly owing to increased epithelial melanin (seen also with other forms of cirrhosis). A distinctive, metallic, slate-gray pigmentation is related to accumulation of hemosiderin in dermal macrophages and fibroblasts. With hemosiderin deposition in the **joint synovial linings,** an acute synovitis may develop. Excessive deposition of calcium pyrophosphate damages the articular cartilage, producing disabling arthritis referred to as pseudogout. The **testes** may be small and atrophic but are not usually significantly pigmented. It is thought that the atrophy is secondary to a derangement in the hypothalamic-pituitary axis. Other parenchymal organs, particularly endocrine (e.g., adrenals, thyroid), may also accumulate iron.

CLINICAL COURSE. Fully developed HHC features hepatomegaly, abdominal pain, skin pigmentation (particularly in sun-exposed areas), deranged glucose homeostasis or frank diabetes mellitus, cardiac dysfunction (arrhythmias, cardiomyopathy), and atypical arthritis. In some patients, the presenting complaint is hypogonadism, for example, amenorrhea in the female and loss of libido and impotence in the male. The classic triad of pigment cirrhosis with hepatomegaly, skin pigmentation, and diabetes mellitus may not develop. Death may result from cirrhosis or cardiac disease. The most common cause of death in established HHC is hepatocellular carcinoma, for which the risk is 200-fold greater than the general population.[72] Depletion of iron, and even reversal of cirrhosis, do not totally prevent the occurrence of this fatal neoplasm.

Fortunately hemochromatosis can be diagnosed long before irreversible tissue damage has occurred. Screening for HHC is accomplished by measuring serum iron, total iron binding capacity, and ferritin levels, followed by liver biopsy if indicated. Secondary causes of iron overload must be excluded, such as a history of numerous blood transfusions, grossly excessive iron ingestion, and dyserythropoietic syndromes. Most important for identification of patients with asymptomatic HHC is *screening of family members of probands,* which includes HLA typing. Heterozygotes for HHC also accumulate excessive iron, but not to the degree required to cause significant tissue damage. The natural course of the disease in homozygotes can be substantially altered by phlebotomy and the use of iron chelators. Patients with HHC diagnosed in the subclinical, precirrhotic stage and treated by regular phlebotomy have a normal life expectancy.[72]

WILSON'S DISEASE

This autosomal recessive disorder of copper metabolism is marked by the accumulation of toxic levels of copper in many tissues and organs, principally the liver, brain, and eye—hence the alternate designation *"hepatolenticular degeneration."* To understand Wilson's disease, we should briefly review normal copper absorption and transport.[73] Approximately 40 to 60% of daily ingested copper (2 to 5 mg) is absorbed in the stomach and duodenum and transported to the liver loosely complexed with albumin. Free copper dissociates and is transferred into hepatocytes, where it is incorporated into an alpha$_2$-globulin to form ceruloplasmin (a metallothionein) and resecreted into plasma. Ceruloplasmin accounts for 90 to 95% of plasma copper, although its biologic role is unknown because the contained six to seven atoms of copper per molecule are not readily exchangeable. Desialylated, senescent ceruloplasmin is endocytosed by the liver, where it is degraded within lysosomes. Delivery of copper to bile, presumably via lysosomes, constitutes the primary route for copper elimination;[74] urinary excretion of albumin-bound copper is miniscule. Estimated total body copper is only 50 to 150 mg.

Wilson's disease has a gene frequency of 1 : 200 to 400 and a disease incidence of approximately 1 : 200,000. The genetic defect is on chromosome 13, in linkage with the esterase D locus.[75] In this disease, the initial steps of copper absorption and transport to the liver are normal. The absorbed copper, however, fails to enter the circulation in the form of ceruloplasmin, and biliary excretion of copper is markedly diminished. Copper thus accumulates progressively in the liver, in excess of the metallothionein-binding capacity,[76] causing toxic liver injury. Usually by five years of age, nonceruloplasmin-bound copper spills over into the circulation, causing hemolysis and pathologic changes at other sites, such as brain, cornea, kidneys, bones, joints, and parathyroids. Concomitantly, urinary excretion of copper becomes markedly increased. The biochemical diagnosis of Wilson's disease is based on *a decrease in serum ceruloplasmin, increase in hepatic copper content, and increased urinary excretion of copper.* Serum copper levels are of no diagnostic value because they may be low, normal, or elevated, depending on the stage of evolution of the disease.

PATHOGENESIS. The nature of the metabolic error in Wilson's disease is unknown. The underlying defect may be *defective mobilization of copper from hepatocellular lysosomes for excretion into bile.* The resulting accumulation damages liver cells and suppresses apoceruloplasmin synthesis. Theories for the pathogenesis of copper-induced injury include (1) poisoning of hepatic enzymes, (2) copper binding to cytosolic proteins such as tubulin (perhaps accounting for the formation of Mallory bodies) or binding to sulfhydryl groups in proteins, and (3) the formation of free radicals.

MORPHOLOGY. In the mildest stages of Wilson's disease, the liver may exhibit only **fatty change** and focal hepatocyte necrosis. With more severe disease, **acute hepatitis** or **chronic hepatitis** develops, both of which are similar in histologic appearance to viral hepatitis (discussed earlier). Features that suggest Wilson's disease are the common occurrence of fatty change and nuclear vacuolization. With advancing disease, copper can be visualized with rhodanine or rubeanic acid stains in periportal hepatocytes, either as a reddish cytoplasmic blush or as distinct granules of varying size (lysosomal accumulations). Orcein stain highlights granules of intracellular copper-associated protein, possibly representing polymerized aggregates of copper-metallothionein.[77] Mallory bodies may be particularly prominent during the stage of acute hepatitis. With progression of chronic hepatitis, **cirrhosis** develops, often with ongoing necrosis of hepatocytes.

A rare manifestation that is indistinguishable from that caused by viruses or drugs is **massive hepatic necrosis.** Except for massive necrosis, the other patterns of hepatic damage appear to represent progressive stages in the evolution of full-blown cirrhosis. The histologic changes are not pathognomonic, both because copper accumulates in chronic obstructive cholestasis[78] and because histology cannot reliably distinguish Wilson's disease from viral-induced and drug-induced hepatitis (and vice versa). Most helpful is hepatic copper determination, which is characteristically in excess of 250 μg/gm dry weight.

The **neurologic changes** constitute toxic injury to neurons, most marked in the basal ganglia, particularly the putamen, sometimes leading to grossly visible cavitations. **Kayser-Fleischer rings** appear in the cornea in almost all patients with neurologic involvement. These green-to-brown deposits of copper in Desçemet's membrane (close to the limbus of the cornea) are characteristic but not pathognomonic of Wilson's disease because they may be found in other forms of chronic cholestasis.

CLINICAL COURSE. Most patients come to clinical attention in childhood or adolescence, usually with manifestations of liver disease, such as jaundice or hepatomegaly, in the absence of neurologic changes; the reverse is true in 40% of cases.[79] Thus, acute or chronic hepatitis may appear as early as the fourth or fifth year of life, only to clear and surface years later as fully developed cirrhosis. Alternatively, the disease may appear in younger adults insidiously as the result of fully evolved cirrhosis. When hepatic involvement remains subclinical, the condition comes to attention as a Parkinson-like movement disorder, as a psychiatric disturbance ranging from behavioral disorders to frank psychosis, or because of the ocular changes. Acute episodes of hepatic neuropsychiatric decompensation may complicate the clinical course. Early recognition permits the long-term use of copper chelators (e.g., penicillamine) to prevent the accumulation of copper and thus arrest the progression of organ damage. Fulminant hepatitis and unmanageable cirrhosis necessitate liver transplantation which appears to be curative.

ALPHA₁-ANTITRYPSIN DEFICIENCY

α_1-AT deficiency is an autosomal recessive disorder marked by abnormally low serum levels of this major protease inhibitor ("Pi"). The deficiency leads to the development of pulmonary disease (emphysema; see Chapter 15) and hepatic disease (cholestasis or cirrhosis).[80] α_1-AT is a small, 394 amino acid glycoprotein whose major function is the inhibition of proteases, particularly neutrophil elastase released at sites of cell injury and inflammation. The predominant site of α_1-AT synthesis is in hepatocytes, with some synthesis in macrophages.

You will recall from the emphysema section in Chapter 15 that the α_1-AT gene is located on human chromosome 14.[81] Among the 75 α_1-AT gene products that have been identified (denoted alphabetically by their relative migration on isoelectric gel migration), the most common phenotype is PiMM, occurring in 90% of individuals. Most allelic variants exhibit conservative substitutions in the polypeptide chain and produce normal functioning levels of α_1-AT. Some *deficiency variants*, including the S variant, result in a reduction in serum concentrations of α_1-AT without clinical manifestations. Homozygotes for the PiZZ protein, however, have circulating α_1-AT levels that are only 10% of normal levels and are at highest risk for developing clinical disease. *Expression of alleles is autosomal codominant*, and consequently PiMZ heterozygotes have intermediate plasma levels of α_1-AT. The gene frequency of PiZ is 0.0122 in the North American white population, yielding a PiZZ phenotype frequency of approximately 1:7000. Rare variants termed Pi-null have no detectable serum α_1-AT.

PATHOGENESIS. With most α_1-AT allelic genes, the mRNA is translated, and the protein is synthesized and secreted normally. Deficiency variants exhibit a selective defect in movement of this secretory protein from the endoplasmic reticulum (ER) to Golgi apparatus; this is most marked for the PiZ polypeptide, attributable to a single amino acid substitution of Glu_{342} to Lys_{342}.[81] The mechanism appears to be misfolding of the nascent polypeptide, resulting in (1) decreased ability for normal

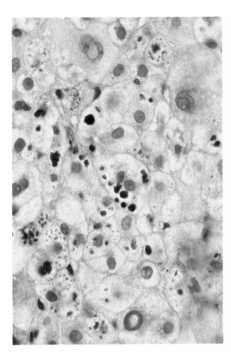

Figure 18-29. Alpha₁-antitrypsin deficiency. Periodic acid-Schiff diastase stain of liver, highlighting the characteristic red cytoplasmic granules. (Courtesy of Dr. I. Wanless, Toronto Hospital.)

folding, (2) accumulation of abnormally folded protein in the ER, and (3) enhanced lysosomal degradation of the aberrant protein.

As discussed in Chapter 15, pulmonary emphysema develops owing to a relative lack of antiprotease in the lungs, thus permitting tissue-destructive enzymes to run amok.[82] The mechanisms for development of liver disease, however, are not clear. All individuals with the PiZZ phenotype accumulate α_1-AT in the liver, yet only 8 to 20% develop clinical liver disease.[83] Familial factors may play a role, perhaps through genetic variability that increases the net balance of abnormally folded α_1-AT in the ER.

MORPHOLOGY. α_1-AT deficiency is characterized by the presence of round-to-oval cytoplasmic globular inclusions of impounded α_1-AT in hepatocytes, which in routine hematoxylin and eosin stains are acidophilic and indistinctly demarcated from the surrounding cytoplasm. They are strongly PAS positive and diastase resistant (Fig. 18-29). By electron microscopy, they lie within smooth, and sometimes rough, ER.[84] The globules also are present in diminished size and number in intermediate deficiency states.

The hepatic syndromes associated with PiZZ homozygosity are extremely varied, ranging from neonatal hepatitis without or with cholestasis and fibrosis (discussed shortly), to childhood cirrhosis, to cirrhosis that becomes apparent only late in life when liver scarring is well advanced.[85] The fibrous scarring of α_1-AT deficiency tends to be irregular, expanding and interconnecting portal tracts and encasing individual lobules or sometimes entrapping many adjacent lobules. Frequently piecemeal necrosis reminiscent of viral hepatitis can be identified in periportal regions, where the globules are most prominent. Infrequently fatty change and Mallory bodies are present. The diagnostic α_1-AT globules may be absent in the young infant.

CLINICAL COURSE. Neonatal hepatitis with cholestatic jaundice appears in 10 to 20% of newborns with the deficiency. In adolescence, presenting symptoms may be related to hepatitis or cirrhosis. Attacks of hepatitis may subside with apparent complete recovery, or they may become chronic and lead progressively to cirrhosis. Finally, the disease may remain silent until cirrhosis appears in middle to later life. Hepatocellular carcinoma develops in 2 to 3% of PiZZ adults, usually but not always in the setting of cirrhosis. The treatment, and cure, for severe hepatic disease is orthotopic liver transplantation, with restoration of normal α_1-AT synthesis and release.

REYE'S SYNDROME

Reye's syndrome is a rare disease characterized by fatty change in the liver and encephalopathy that in its most severe forms may be fatal. It primarily affects children younger than nine years (most younger than age four years), although older children and rarely adults are afflicted.[86] Typically, Reye's syndrome develops 3 to 5 days after a viral illness, heralded by pernicious vomiting and accompanied by irritability or lethargy and hepatomegaly. Except possibly for a brief period of obtundation or excitability, about three-quarters of the patients progress no further and recover with no residual effects.[87] The remaining 25% of patients have more serious illness, with progressively deeper levels of coma, accompanied by elevations in the serum levels of bilirubin, aminotransferases, and particularly ammonia. Survivors may be left with permanent neurologic impairments; death results from progressive deterioration of the mental state with delirium, convulsions, and coma. Rare patients die of liver failure. Therapy for Reye's syndrome is entirely symptomatic and supportive.

MORPHOLOGY. The major pathologic findings are in the liver and brain. **Liver** changes uniformly consist of microvesicular hepatic steatosis, seen during the first 3 to 7 days of the illness (Fig. 18-30). Hepatic mitochondrial injury is evidenced by pleomorphic enlargement and electron lucency of the matrices, with disruption of cristae. In the **brain,** cerebral edema is usually present; severity of the

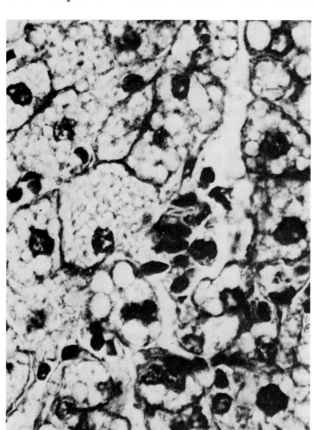

Figure 18–30. Reye's syndrome with microvesicular hepatic steatosis (fatty change). (Hematoxylin and eosin.)

edema corresponds to the severity of neurologic dysfunction. Astrocytes are swollen, and mitochondrial changes similar to those seen in the liver may develop. Inflammation is notably absent, as is any evidence of viral infection in the central nervous system. **Skeletal muscles, kidney,** and **heart** may also reveal microvesicular fatty change and mitochondrial alterations, although more subtle than those of the liver.

PATHOGENESIS. The pathogenesis of Reye's syndrome is generally believed to involve biochemical derangements alone or in combination with viral infection. Mitochondrial metabolism is profoundly affected, with reductions in activity of the citric acid cycle and urea cycle and defective beta-oxidation leading to accumulation of serum free fatty acids. An underlying inborn error of metabolism, particularly affecting fat metabolism (e.g., medium-chain acyl-CoA dehydrogenase deficiency),[88] has been identified in some patients exhibiting a Reye's-like syndrome. Accordingly *perhaps more subtle and yet to be identified metabolic disorders predispose a person to Reye's syndrome.* In the past, children who developed this condition had typi-

cally been given aspirin for the relief of viral-induced fever, but the role of salicylates in the pathogenesis of Reye's syndrome is not clear. Less than 0.1% of children receiving aspirin for a viral illness develop Reye's syndrome. Nevertheless, a national campaign condemning the use of aspirin in children with febrile illness may have served to break the Reye's syndrome epidemic. No specific virus has been identified.

NEONATAL HEPATITIS

Prolonged conjugated hyperbilirubinemia in the neonate, termed *neonatal cholestasis*, affects approximately 1 in 2500 live births. The major conditions causing it are (1) cholangiopathies, primarily *extrahepatic biliary atresia* (**EHBA**; see later) and (2) a variety of disorders causing conjugated hyperbilirubinemia in the neonate, collectively referred to as *neonatal hepatitis*.[89] *Neonatal cholestasis and hepatitis are not specific entities, nor are the disorders necessarily inflammatory.* Instead, the finding of "neonatal cholestasis" should evoke a diligent search for recognizable toxic, metabolic, and infectious liver diseases (Table 18–8). Once identifiable causes are excluded, one is left with the syndrome of "idiopathic" neonatal hepatitis, which shows considerable clinical overlap with EHBA.

The clinical presentation of infants with any form of neonatal cholestasis is fairly stereotypic, with few clinical clues regarding underlying etiology.[90] Affected infants have jaundice, dark urine, light or acholic stools, and hepatomegaly. Variable degrees of hepatic synthetic dysfunction may be identified, such as hypoprothrombinemia. Thus, liver biopsy is critical in distinguishing neonatal hepatitis from an identifiable cholangiopathy.

MORPHOLOGY. The morphologic features of neonatal hepatitis are as follows:

1. **Lobular disarray with focal liver cell necrosis**
2. **Panlobular giant cell transformation of hepatocytes**
3. **Prominent hepatocellular and canalicular cholestasis**
4. **Mild mononuclear infiltration of the portal areas**
5. **Reactive changes in the Kupffer cells**
6. **Extramedullary hematopoiesis**[91]

This predominantly parenchymal pattern of injury may blend imperceptibly into a ductal pattern of injury, with bile duct proliferation and fibrosis of portal tracts. Clear distinction from an obstructive cholangiopathy may thus be impossible. Specific features, which may permit diagnosis of a particular etiology, include the inclusions of α_1-AT or cytomegalovirus, and fatty change with cirrhosis, suggesting galactosemia or tyrosinemia. Electron

Table 18-8. CAUSES OF NEONATAL CHOLESTASIS

Neonatal hepatitis
  Idiopathic
  Viral
    Cytomegalovirus
    Rubella
    Reovirus 3
    Herpesviruses
    Enteroviruses
    Coxsackie virus
    ECHO virus
    Parvovirus
    Adenovirus
    Hepatitis B,C
  Bacterial and parasitic
    Bacterial sepsis
    Listeriosis
    Tuberculosis
    Syphilis
    Toxoplasmosis
Bile duct obstruction
  Extrahepatic biliary atresia
  Anomalies of the extrahepatic biliary tree
  Inspissated bile/mucous plug
  Cholelithiasis
  Tumors
Idiopathic syndromes of intrahepatic cholestasis
Toxic
  Drugs
  Parenteral nutrition
Metabollic diseases

Amino acid	Tyrosinemia
Lipid	Niemann-Pick disease
	Gaucher's disease
	Wolman's disease
Carbohydrate	Galactosemia
	Fructosemia
	Type IV glycogenosis
Bile acid metabolism	
Miscellaneous	α_1-Antitrypsin deficiency
	Cystic fibrosis
	Neonatal hemochromatosis
	Hypothyroidism
	Hypopituitarism

Miscellaneous
  Shock/hypoperfusion
  Intestinal obstruction
  Histiocytosis X
  Indian childhood cirrhosis
  Erythrophagocytic lymphohistiocytosis
  Autosomal trisomies
  Neonatal lupus erythematosus

Adapted from Suchy, F.J., and Shneider, B.L.: Neonatal jaundice and cholestasis. In Kaplowitz, N. (ed.): Liver and Biliary Diseases. Baltimore, Williams & Wilkins, 1992, p. 445.

microscopy may be helpful, e.g., by showing phospholipid whorls in Neimann-Pick disease.

Despite the long list of disorders associated with neonatal cholestasis, most are quite rare. "Idiopathic" neonatal hepatitis represents 50 to 60% of cases; about 20% are due to EHBA and 15% to α_1-AT deficiency. Differentiation of the two most common causes assumes great importance because definitive treatment of EHBA requires surgical intervention, whereas surgery may adversely affect the clinical course of a child with neonatal hepatitis. Fortunately discrimination can be made with clinical data in conjunction with liver biopsy in about 90% of cases.

INTRAHEPATIC BILIARY TRACT DISEASE

Biliary tract disorders cannot always be divided into those that affect only the intrahepatic or extrahepatic portions, particularly because extrahepatic biliary disorders incite secondary changes within the liver proper. Accordingly reference should be made to the subsequent section on the gallbladder and biliary tree, particularly biliary atresia, which affects both intrahepatic and extrahepatic bile ducts. In addition, hepatic bile ducts are frequently damaged as part of more general liver disease, as in drug toxicity, viral hepatitis, and transplantation. With these caveats, consideration is now given to the intrahepatic features of biliary tract disease, with salient features summarized in Table 18-9.

SECONDARY BILIARY CIRRHOSIS

Prolonged obstruction to the extrahepatic biliary tree results in profound alteration of the liver itself. The most common cause of obstruction is an impacted gallstone in the common bile duct (see later); other conditions include biliary atresia, malignancies of the biliary tree and head of the pancreas, and strictures resulting from previous surgical procedures. The initial morphologic features of *cholestasis* were described earlier and are entirely reversible with correction of the obstruction. Initiation of periportal fibrosis secondary to inflammation, however, eventually leads to *secondary biliary cirrhosis*. Secondary bacterial infection ("ascending cholangitis") may contribute to the damage; enteric organisms such as coliforms and enterococci are common culprits.

MORPHOLOGY. The end-stage obstructed liver exhibits extraordinary yellow-green pigmentation and is accompanied by marked icteric discoloration of body tissues and fluids. On cut surface, the liver is hard, with a finely granular appearance. Microscopically, large and small bile ducts are distended and frequently contain inspissated bile. Portal tracts are interconnected by inflamed fibrous septa and appear edematous; there is frequently a narrow zone of edema and ductular proliferation at the junction of parenchyma and septa. Cholestatic features may be severe, with cytoplasmic and canalicular accumulation of bile, extensive feathery degeneration of hepatocytes, and the for-

Table 18-9. DISTINGUISHING FEATURES OF DISORDERS ASSOCIATED WITH BILIARY CIRRHOSIS

	SECONDARY BILIARY CIRRHOSIS	PRIMARY BILIARY CIRRHOSIS	PRIMARY SCLEROSING CHOLANGITIS
Etiology	Extrahepatic bile duct obstruction: biliary atresia, gallstones, carcinoma of pancreatic head	Possibly autoimmune; associated with other autoimmune conditions	Unknown; possibly autoimmune; 50–70% of cases associated with inflammatory bowel disease
Sex Predilection	None	Female-to-male 6:1	Female-to-male 1:2
Symptoms and Signs	Pruritus, jaundice, malaise, dark urine, light stools, hepatosplenomegaly	Same as secondary biliary cirrhosis; insidious onset	Same as secondary biliary cirrhosis; insidious onset
Laboratory Findings	Conjugated hyperbilirubinemia, increased serum alkaline phosphatase, bile acids, cholesterol	Same as secondary biliary cirrhosis, plus elevated serum IgM, presence of autoantibodies, especially antimitochondrial antibody (AMA), hypercholesterolemia	Same as secondary biliary cirrhosis, plus hypergammaglobulinemia, elevated IgM
Distinctive Pathologic Findings of Bile Ducts	Prominent bile stasis in interlobular bile ducts, sometimes neutrophils in bile ducts; bile duct proliferation	Dense lymphocytic infiltrate around and in walls of interlobular bile ducts with granuloma formation and bile duct destruction	Periductal fibrosis and segmental stenosis of extrahepatic and intrahepatic biliary ducts

mation of bile lakes (see earlier discussion of cholestasis). Once the regenerative nodules of cirrhosis have formed, however, bile stasis may become less conspicuous. Ascending bacterial infection incites a supervening robust neutrophilic infiltration of bile ducts and cholangitic abscesses.

PRIMARY BILIARY CIRRHOSIS

Primary biliary cirrhosis (PBC) is a chronic, progressive, and often fatal cholestatic liver disease, characterized by the destruction of intrahepatic bile ducts, portal inflammation and scarring, and the eventual development of cirrhosis and liver failure.[92] The primary feature of this disease is a nonsuppurative, granulomatous destruction of medium-sized intrahepatic bile ducts; cirrhosis appears only late in the course.[93]

- This is primarily a disease of middle-aged women, with a female-to-male predominance in excess of 6:1. Age of onset is between 20 and 80 years, with the peak incidence between 40 and 50 years.
- The onset is insidious, usually presenting with pruritus. Jaundice develops late in the course.
- Hepatomegaly is typical. Xanthomas and xanthelasmas arise as a result of cholesterol retention. Stigmata of chronic liver disease are late features.
- The disease may be asymptomatic for years, running its course over two or more decades.

Serum alkaline phosphatase and cholesterol are almost always elevated; hyperbilirubinemia is a late development and usually signifies incipient hepatic decompensation. A striking feature of the disease is autoantibodies, especially antimitochondrial antibodies in more than 90% of patients. Particularly characteristic of primary biliary cirrhosis are "M2" antibodies to mitochondrial pyruvate dehydrogenase.[94] Extrahepatic manifestations associated with PBC include the sicca complex of dry eyes and mouth (Sjögren's syndrome), scleroderma, thyroiditis, rheumatoid arthritis, Raynaud's phenomenon, membranous glomerulonephritis, and celiac disease.

PATHOGENESIS. Many lines of evidence suggest an autoimmune etiology for PBC, including:[95]

- Abnormal expression of MHC class 1 and 2 antigens on biliary epithelium and accumulation of T cells around and within bile ducts.
- Expansion of B-lymphocyte clones producing antimitochondrial antibodies.
- Systemic abnormalities—polyclonal hypergammaglobulinemia, failure to convert IgM to IgG antibodies, and hypocomplementemia from complement activation and formation of immune complexes.

The underlying etiology, however, is not yet clear nor is the role of antimitochondrial antibodies.

MORPHOLOGY. PBC is the prototype of all conditions leading to small-duct biliary fibrosis and cirrhosis. Historically, four histologic stages have been described:[96]

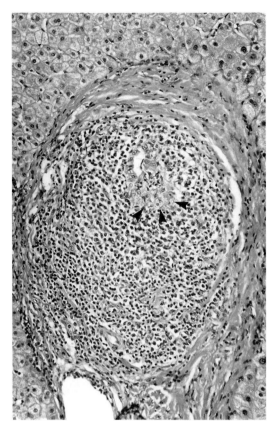

Figure 18–31. Primary biliary cirrhosis. A portal tract is markedly expanded by an infiltrate of lymphocytes and plasma cells. The granulomatous reaction to a bile duct undergoing destruction (florid duct lesion) is highlighted by the arrowheads. (Hematoxylin and eosin.)

1. The florid duct lesion (granulomatous destruction of interlobular bile ducts)
2. Ductular proliferation with periportal hepatitis
3. Scarring, with bridging necrosis and septal fibrosis
4. Cirrhosis

Although conceptually useful, these four stages cannot be reliably assessed histologically because **PBC is a focal and variable disease, and exhibits different degrees of severity in different portions of the liver.** Therefore it is more useful to regard PBC as being marked by damage **restricted to portal tracts,** followed by **progressive damage to the parenchyma.**[92]

Portal Tract Lesion. There is random, focal destruction of interlobular and septal bile ducts by granulomatous inflammation, entitled the **florid duct lesion** (Fig. 18–31). Affected portal tracts exhibit a dense infiltrate of lymphocytes (including lymphoid follicle formation), histiocytes, plasma cells, and a few eosinophils. Approximately 50% of biopsy specimens obtained early in the disease show ductal lesions. Granulomas and a lymphocytic infiltrate

may be present within the lobular parenchyma. Cholestasis is variably present.

Progressive Lesion. With more global hepatic involvement, normal interlobular bile ducts become infrequent, and secondary obstructive changes develop, similar to those seen in extrahepatic obstruction. Mallory bodies may be present in hepatocytes adjacent to portal tracts. Initially portal tract inflammation may be marked and spill over into the parenchyma, causing destruction of adjacent hepatocytes (piecemeal necrosis). With time, inflammation subsides, and granulomas and florid duct lesions become infrequent. Hepatocyte loss, fibrosis, and nodular regeneration lead to the gradual development of true cirrhosis. Macroscopically the liver does not at first appear abnormal, but as the disease progresses, bile stasis stains the liver green. The capsule remains smooth and glistening until a fine granularity appears, culminating in a well-developed, uniform micronodularity. Liver weight is at first normal to increased (owing to inflammation); ultimately liver weight is slightly decreased. **In most cases, the end-stage picture may be difficult to distinguish from secondary biliary cirrhosis or the cirrhosis that follows chronic active hepatitis.**

CLINICAL COURSE. Although PBC is basically a cholestatic disorder, it is extremely insidious in onset, and patients may be symptom free for many years. Eventually pruritus, fatigue, and abdominal discomfort develop, followed in time by secondary features: xanthomas and xanthelasmas; steatorrhea; and malabsorption-related osteomalacia, osteoporosis, or both. More general features of jaundice and hepatic decompensation, including portal hypertension and variceal bleeding, mark entry into the end stages of the disease. The major cause of death is liver failure, followed in order by massive variceal hemorrhage and intercurrent infection.

PRIMARY SCLEROSING CHOLANGITIS

Primary sclerosing cholangitis (PSC) is characterized by inflammation, obliterative fibrosis, and segmental dilatation of the intrahepatic and extrahepatic bile ducts.[97] *Characteristic "beading" of a barium column in radiographs of the intrahepatic and extrahepatic biliary tree is attributable to the irregular strictures and dilatations of affected bile ducts. PSC is commonly seen in association with inflammatory bowel disease (see Chapter 17), particularly chronic ulcerative colitis, which coexists in approximately 70% of patients.* Conversely, the prevalence of PSC in ulcerative colitis patients is about 4%. PSC tends to occur in the third through

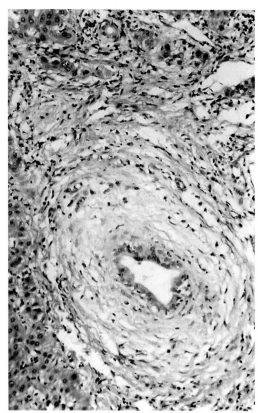

Figure 18–32. Primary sclerosing cholangitis. A bile duct undergoing degeneration is entrapped in a dense, "onion-skin" concentric scar.

fifth decades of life, and males predominate 2:1 (see Table 18–9).

PATHOGENESIS. The cause of PSC is unknown, despite its clear association with inflammatory bowel disease. Hypothesized mechanisms include toxin release by the inflamed gut and direct immunologic attack, although autoantibodies are usually absent.[98] Because hepatic artery infusions with 5-fluorodeoxyuridine and hepatic artery thrombosis after liver transplantation can generate a PSC-like picture, an ischemic contribution to bile duct loss in PSC patients has been postulated.[99]

MORPHOLOGY. PSC is a fibrosing cholangitis of bile ducts, with a lymphocytic infiltrate, progressive atrophy of the bile duct epithelium, and obliteration of the lumen (Fig. 18–32). The concentric periductal fibrosis around affected ducts ("onion-skin fibrosis") is followed by their disappearance, leaving behind a solid, cord-like fibrous scar. In between areas of progressive stricture, bile ducts become ectatic and inflamed, presumably the result of downstream obstruction. As the disease progresses, the liver becomes markedly cholestatic, culminating in biliary cirrhosis.

CLINICAL COURSE. Asymptomatic patients may come to attention based only on persistent elevation of serum alkaline phosphatase. Alternatively, progressive fatigue, pruritus, and jaundice may develop. Severely afflicted patients exhibit symptoms associated with chronic liver disease, including weight loss, ascites, variceal bleeding, and encephalopathy. Ten-year survival is on the order of 50 to 75%; progressive decline is arrested only by liver transplantation.

ANOMALIES OF THE BILIARY TREE

A heterogeneous group of lesions exists in which the primary abnormality is altered architecture of the intrahepatic biliary tree, presumably arising as a result of incomplete involution of embryonic bile duct remnants.[100] Lesions may be found incidentally during radiographic studies or at autopsy, or may become manifest as hepatosplenomegaly and portal hypertension in the absence of hepatic dysfunction, typically in late childhood, adolescence, or during adult years. Histologic abnormalities are diagrammed in Fig. 18–33; although one pattern usually predominates, it is not uncommon to find features of more than one pattern in the same liver.

MORPHOLOGY

Von Meyenburg Complexes. Close to or within portal tracts, these are small clusters of modestly dilated bile ducts embedded in a fibrous, sometimes hyalinized stroma. These "bile duct microhamartomas" contain inspissated bile concrements and may communicate with the biliary tree.

Polycystic Liver Disease. The liver contains multiple diffuse cystic lesions, numbering from a scattered few to hundreds. The cysts vary from 0.5 to 3–4 cm in diameter and are lined by cuboidal or flattened biliary epithelium and contain straw-colored fluid. They do not contain pigmented bile and appear to be detached from the biliary tree. Occasionally solitary liver cysts of biliary origin are identified, more commonly in women (4:1).

Congenital Hepatic Fibrosis. The portal tracts are enlarged by irregular and broad bands of collagenous tissue, forming septae and dividing the liver into irregular islands. Variable numbers of abnormally shaped bile ducts are embedded in the fibrous tissue, and bile duct remnants are distributed along the septal margins. Sometimes curved bile duct profiles are arranged in a concentric circle around portal tracts. These bile duct profiles are in continuity with the biliary tree.

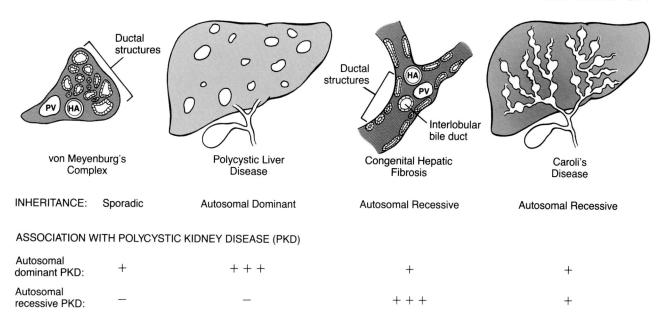

Figure 18-33. Bile duct anomalies. The morphologic features of the four major groups are diagrammed, along with apparent patterns of inheritance and associations with polycystic kidney disease.

Caroli's Disease. The larger ducts of the intrahepatic biliary tree are segmentally dilated and may contain inspissated bile. Pure forms are rare; this disease is usually associated with portal tract fibrosis of the congenital hepatic fibrosis type.[101]

CLINICAL COURSE. *Von Meyenburg complexes* are rather common and are usually without clinical significance except to avoid mistaking lesions radiographically for metastatic carcinoma. Patients with *polycystic liver disease* may develop abdominal tenderness or pain on stooping, occasionally requiring surgical intervention. There is a slight female predilection, with presentation common during pregnancy. Patients with *congenital hepatic fibrosis* may face complications of portal hypertension, particularly bleeding varices. *Caroli's disease* is frequently complicated by intrahepatic cholelithiasis (see later), cholangitis, and hepatic abscesses as well as by features of portal hypertension. There is an increased risk of cholangiocarcinoma (see later) with Caroli's disease and congenital hepatic fibrosis. A well-documented association exists for polycystic liver disease, and less often congenital hepatic fibrosis and Caroli's disease, with polycystic kidney disease (both infantile recessive and adult autosomal dominant; see Chapter 20). In such cases, renal impairment dominates the clinical picture and outlook.[102,103] It is presumed that a common pathogenesis underlies the renal and hepatic lesions, possibly relating to inadequate linking of parenchymal to tubuloductal anlage or deficient epithelial-mesenchymal interactions during embryogenesis. Choledochal cysts of the extrahepatic biliary tree (described later) also appear to fall into this broad category of diseases.

CIRCULATORY DISORDERS

Given the enormous flow of blood through the liver, it is not surprising that circulatory disturbances have considerable impact on liver status. In most instances, clinically significant liver compromise does not develop, but hepatic morphology may be strikingly affected. The general framework for discussing circulatory disturbances is offered in Figure 18–34.

LIVER INFARCTION

Liver infarcts are rare, thanks to the double blood supply to the liver. Nonetheless, thrombosis or compression of an intrahepatic branch of the hepatic artery by embolism, neoplasia, polyarteritis nodosa, or sepsis may result in a localized infarct that is usually anemic and pale tan. Hemorrhage may be present, owing to suffusion of portal blood. Occlusion of an intrahepatic branch of the portal vein does not cause ischemic infarction but instead results in a sharply demarcated area of red-blue discoloration inappropriately referred to as an *infarct of Zahn.* In this condition, there is no necrosis, only marked stasis in distended sinusoids, with secondary hepatocellular atrophy.

Interruption of the main hepatic artery does

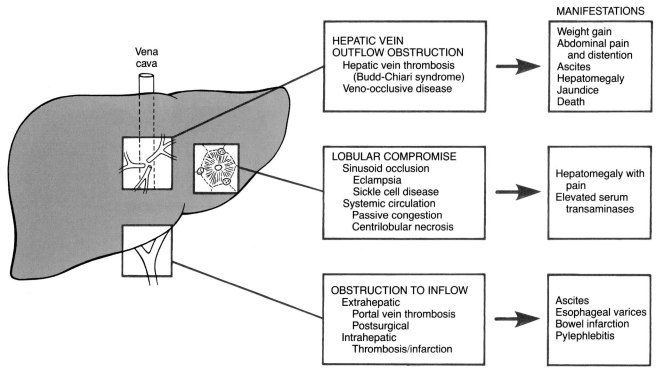

Figure 18-34. Hepatic circulatory disorders. The forms and clinical manifestations of compromised blood flow are contrasted.

not always produce ischemic necrosis of the organ, particularly if the liver is otherwise normal. Retrograde arterial flow through accessory vessels, when coupled with the portal venous supply, may be sufficient to sustain the liver parenchyma. The one exception is hepatic artery thrombosis (or transection) in the transplanted liver, which generally leads to loss of the organ.

PORTAL VEIN OBSTRUCTION AND THROMBOSIS

Blockage of the portal vein may be insidious and well tolerated or may be a catastrophic and potentially lethal event; most cases fall somewhere in between. *Extrahepatic causes of portal vein obstruction* include (1) massive enlargement of hilar lymph nodes owing to metastatic abdominal cancer; (2) *pylephlebitis* resulting from peritoneal sepsis (e.g., acute diverticulitis or appendicitis); (3) propagation of splenic vein thrombosis secondary to pancreatitis; and (4) postsurgical thrombosis following upper abdominal procedures. The most common *intrahepatic cause* is cirrhosis of the liver; intravascular invasion by primary or secondary cancer in the liver can occur. In all cases, retrograde propagation of thrombus or growth of tumor may completely occlude splanchnic inflow to the liver. Occlusive disease of the portal vein or its major radicles typically produces abdominal pain and in many cases massive ascites and esophageal

varices. Impairment of splanchnic blood flow often leads to profound bowel congestion and infarction. When the condition is secondary to pylephlebitis, anterograde spread of infection may yield multiple liver abscesses.

A condition deserving special mention is *Banti's syndrome,* characterized as splenomegaly, hypersplenism, and portal hypertension. More aptly termed *noncirrhotic* or *idiopathic portal hypertension,* this condition arises following subclinical occlusion of the portal vein, usually years after the occlusive event.[104] Postulated causes include neonatal omphalitis, dehydration, sepsis, or umbilical vein catheterization for exchange transfusion therapy; hypercoagulable myeloproliferative disorders; biliary tract surgery; peritonitis; and exposure to arsenicals. The prognosis is generally excellent, and clinical outcome relates primarily to the complications of chronic portal hypertension.

PASSIVE CONGESTION AND CENTRILOBULAR NECROSIS

These hepatic alterations were briefly characterized in Chapters 4 and 12 but are considered here in greater detail. They represent a morphologic continuum.[105]

MORPHOLOGY. Acute and chronic passive congestion of the liver usually reflects acute or slowly

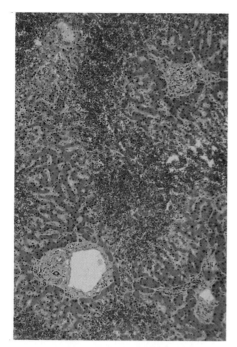

Figure 18–35. Centrilobular hemorrhagic necrosis. Centrilobular sinusoids are engorged with blood, and there is hemorrhage into the parenchymal space normally occupied by hepatocytes.

developing cardiac decompensation, most commonly right-sided failure. Because there is an element of preterminal circulatory failure with virtually every death, congestive hepatic changes are commonplace at autopsy. The liver is slightly enlarged, tense, and cyanotic, with rounded edges. On cut section, there is an excessive ooze of blood, and centrilobular areas are dusky and soft, surrounded by paler, fatty liver substance in the portal areas (the "nutmeg liver") shown in Figure 4–5). Microscopically there is congestion of centrilobular sinusoids. With time, centrilobular hepatocytes become atrophic, resulting in markedly attenuated liver cell cords.

Left-sided cardiac failure or shock may lead to hepatic hypoperfusion and hypoxia. In this instance, hepatocytes in the central region of the lobule undergo ischemic necrosis. **Centrilobular necrosis** is visible macroscopically as a slight depression of necrotic lobular centers. By microscopy, there is a sharp demarcation of viable and necrotic hepatocytes moving from portal tract to the centrilobular region. The necrosis is **coagulative,** in that the hepatocytes are pale staining and there is no inflammation. The combination of hypoperfusion and retrograde congestion act synergistically to generate **centrilobular hemorrhagic necrosis.** Necrotic centrilobular areas are suffused with blood, which both fills sinusoidal channels and occupies the parenchymal spaces where hepatocytes once existed (Fig. 18–35).

In most instances, the only clinical evidence of centrilobular necrosis is mild-to-moderate transient elevation of serum aminotransaminases. The parenchymal damage may be sufficient to induce mild-to-moderate jaundice. The elevated serum enzymes in these conditions have led to the designation "ischemic hepatitis," a regrettable term because there is no inflammation.

Cardiac Sclerosis

Chronic severe congestive heart failure may lead to fibrosis of the liver, an uncommon complication of sustained increased venous backpressure and centrilobular hypoxia. The pattern of liver fibrosis is distinctive, inasmuch as it is mostly centrilobular. The damage, however, rarely fulfills the accepted criteria for the diagnosis of cirrhosis (presented earlier), although the term *"cardiac cirrhosis"* has been applied to this condition. The clinical consequences of cardiac sclerosis are either negligible or identical to those of centrilobular hemorrhagic necrosis.

MORPHOLOGY. The scarring of cardiac sclerosis is delicate and subtle and easily missed on both gross and microscopic examination. Typically the liver is slightly reduced in size and has a fine pigskin grain on its external surface. Microscopically there is a subtle increase in fibrous tissue about the central veins, from which delicate strands fan out into the surrounding liver substance. Interconnection of the fibrous strands to produce bridging tracts of fibrous tissue is seen only in extreme examples, usually in association with tricuspid insufficiency.

PELIOSIS HEPATIS

Sinusoidal dilation occurs in any condition in which efflux of hepatic blood is impeded. *Peliosis hepatis* is a rare condition in which the dilatation is primary. It is most commonly associated with exposure to anabolic steroids and rarely oral contraceptives and danazol. Mottled and blotchy areas develop in the liver, consisting of irregular blood-filled lakes ranging from less than 0.1 to greater than 1 cm in diameter. Microscopically the lesions consist of irregular cystic spaces, either dilated sinusoids lined by an endothelium or dilated spaces of Disse. There are no intrinsic abnormalities in hepatocytes or hepatic venules. Although clinical signs are generally absent even in advanced peliosis, intra-abdominal hemorrhage or hepatic failure may rarely cause death. Peliotic lesions usually disappear after cessation of drug treatment.

HEPATIC VEIN THROMBOSIS (BUDD-CHIARI SYNDROME)

The Budd-Chiari syndrome was originally described for acute, usually fatal thrombotic occlusion of the hepatic veins. The definition has now been expanded to include subacute and chronic occlusive syndromes, characterized by hepatomegaly, weight gain, ascites, and abdominal pain. *Hepatic vein thrombosis is associated with (in order of frequency) polycythemia vera, pregnancy, the postpartum state, the use of oral contraceptives, paroxysmal nocturnal hemoglobinuria, and intra-abdominal cancers, particularly hepatocellular carcinoma.* All these conditions produce thrombotic tendencies or, in the case of liver cancers, sluggish blood flow. Membranous webs in the hepatic veins or in the inferior vena cava at the hepatic confluence also may give rise to obstruction. Such webs probably represent organized or recanalized thrombi of remote cause, although a congenital origin has been postulated. After all these potentiating conditions are excluded, about 30% of cases are idiopathic in origin. Untreated the mortality of acute Budd-Chiari syndrome is high. The chronic form of the syndrome is far less lethal, and about half the patients are alive after 5 years.

> **MORPHOLOGY.** With acutely developing thrombosis of the major hepatic veins or inferior vena cava, the liver is swollen and red-purple and has a tense capsule. Sometimes only the right or left hepatic vein is affected, producing subtotal involvement. On transection, the affected hepatic parenchyma reveals severe centrilobular congestion and necrosis. In instances in which the thrombosis is more slowly developing, the liver may show the centrilobular changes of cardiac sclerosis. The major veins may contain totally occlusive fresh thrombi, subtotal occlusion, or in chronic cases organized adherent thrombi. Membranous webs, if present, may be difficult to appreciate and should not be confused with the eustachian valve normally present in the inferior vena cava just below the right atrium.

VENO-OCCLUSIVE DISEASE

Originally described in Jamaican drinkers of pyrrolizidine alkaloid-containing bush tea, veno-occlusive disease now occurs primarily in the immediate weeks following bone marrow transplantation. The incidence is 5% in recipients of autologous marrow and up to 25% in allogeneic marrow recipients. Toxicity resulting from induction chemotherapy and radiotherapy appears to be the primary cause, enhanced by such factors as pre-existing hepatitis and older patient age. A diagnosis of veno-occlu-

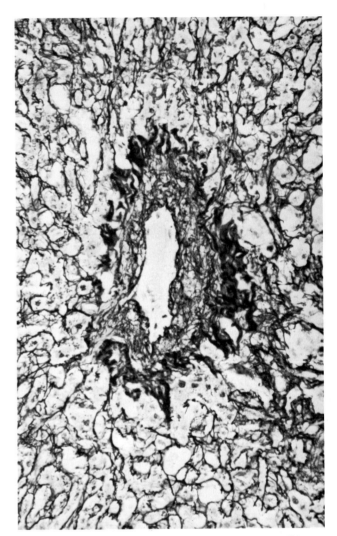

Figure 18–36. Veno-occlusive disease. A reticulin stain reveals the parenchymal framework of the lobule and the marked deposition of collagen within the lumen of the central vein.

sive disease is frequently made on clinical grounds only (tender hepatomegaly, ascites, weight gain, and jaundice), owing to the high risk of liver biopsy in these patients.

> **MORPHOLOGY.** Veno-occlusive disease is characterized by obliteration of hepatic vein radicles by varying amounts of subendothelial swelling and fine reticulated collagen. In acute disease, there is striking centrilobular congestion with hepatocellular necrosis and accumulation of hemosiderin-laden macrophages. As the disease progresses, obliteration of the lumen of the venule is easily identified using special stains for connective tissue (Fig. 18–36). With chronic or healed veno-occlusive disease, dense perivenular fibrosis radiating out into the parenchyma may be present, frequently with total obliteration of the venule; hemosiderin deposition is evident in the scar tissue, and congestion is mini-

mal. Because veno-occlusive disease affects the liver in an irregular fashion, acute or chronic features may be absent from liver biopsy samples.

The pathogenesis of veno-occlusive disease has been attributed (without rigorous proof) to toxic damage of the sinusoidal endothelium, allowing erythrocyte extravasation into the space of Disse, activation of the coagulation cascade, and downstream accumulation of debris in the central vein. Treatment of veno-occlusive disease has been largely supportive and has not significantly affected the mortality rates of 30 to 50%.

HEPATIC DISEASE ASSOCIATED WITH PREGNANCY

Although chronic liver disease can cause amenorrhea and infertility, patients with such conditions as alcoholic liver disease and viral or autoimmune chronic active hepatitis may become pregnant. Alternatively, such liver diseases can become manifest during pregnancy. Although these women require careful clinical management, there are no intrinsic differences in their liver disease from nonpregnant patients. A unique, very small subgroup of pregnant patients (0.1%),[106] however, develops hepatic complications directly attributable to pregnancy. For the unfortunate few, the outcome can be fatal.

PREECLAMPSIA AND ECLAMPSIA

Preeclampsia occurs in 7 to 10% of pregnancies and is characterized by maternal hypertension, proteinuria, peripheral edema, coagulation abnormalities, and varying degrees of disseminated intravascular coagulation. When hyperreflexia and convulsions occur, the condition is called *eclampsia*.[106] Hepatic disease is distressingly common in preeclampsia, usually as part of a syndrome of *he*molysis, *e*levated *l*iver enzymes, and *l*ow *p*latelets (HELLP syndrome).[107] Thus, monitoring of platelet count and serum liver enzyme levels in preeclamptic women has become standard practice.

MORPHOLOGY. The affected liver in preeclampsia is normal in size, firm and pale, with small red patches as a result of hemorrhage. Occasionally yellow or white patches of ischemic infarction can be seen. Microscopically **the periportal sinusoids contain fibrin deposits with hemorrhage into the space of Disse,** leading to periportal hepatocellular coagulative necrosis. In extreme cases, blood under pressure dissects through the portal connec-

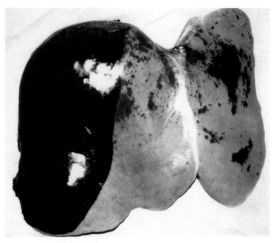

Figure 18–37. Eclampsia. Subcapsular hematoma dissecting under Glisson's capsule, in a fatal case of eclampsia. (Courtesy of Brian D. Blackbourne, M.D., Medical Examiner, San Diego, CA.)

tive tissue to form lakes of blood. Their coalescence and expansion can result in a **hepatic hematoma; dissection of blood under Glisson's capsule may lead to catastrophic hepatic rupture** (Fig. 18–37).

Patients with hepatic involvement in preeclampsia may exhibit modest-to-severe elevation of serum transaminases and mild elevation of serum bilirubin. Progressive hepatic involvement, leading to decreased synthesis of coagulation factors, signifies far-advanced, potentially lethal disease. There is considerable risk in performing a liver biopsy, despite the occasional need to distinguish this syndrome from acute fatty liver of pregnancy (discussed next). In mild cases, patients may be managed conservatively; *definitive treatment in severe cases requires termination of the pregnancy*. Patients who survive recover without sequelae.

ACUTE FATTY LIVER OF PREGNANCY

This disease exhibits a spectrum ranging from modest or even subclinical hepatic dysfunction to hepatic failure, coma, and death.[108] Affected women present in the latter half of pregnancy, usually in the third trimester. Symptoms may be directly attributable to incipient hepatic failure, including bleeding, nausea and vomiting, jaundice, or coma. In 20 to 40% of cases, the presenting symptoms may be those of coexistent preeclampsia. Alternatively, the patient may be free of symptoms and the suspicion raised by a progressive rise in serum transaminases.

MORPHOLOGY. The diagnosis of acute fatty liver of pregnancy cannot be made with certainty un-

less liver biopsy is performed, and the characteristic microvesicular fatty transformation of hepatocytes is demonstrated.[109] In severe cases, there may be lobular disarray with hepatocyte dropout, reticulin collapse, and portal tract inflammation, making distinction from viral hepatitis difficult. **Diagnosis depends on (1) a high index of suspicion and (2) confirmation of microvesicular steatosis using special stains (oil-red-O or Sudan black) on frozen tissue sections (routine processing of liver tissue for paraffin sections leaches the fat from hepatocytes).** Electron microscopy reveals fat accumulation in smooth and rough ER, distention of the Golgi apparatus by lipid, and mitochondrial enlargement with decreased cristae and crystalline inclusions.[106]

Although this condition most commonly runs a mild course, patients with acute fatty liver of pregnancy can progress within days to hepatic failure and death. There is thus considerable urgency in making a diagnosis early in the course, by performing a liver biopsy on an emergent basis before the onset of coagulopathy. *The primary treatment for acute fatty liver of pregnancy is termination of the pregnancy.* The hepatic failure and neurologic symptoms improve after delivery, but weeks of further intensive support and management of complications may be required. The pathogenesis of this condition is not known, although it does share features with Reye's syndrome (discussed earlier).

INTRAHEPATIC CHOLESTASIS OF PREGNANCY

The onset of pruritus in the third trimester, followed by darkening of the urine and occasionally light stools and jaundice, heralds the development of this enigmatic syndrome. Serum bilirubin (mostly conjugated) level rarely exceeds 5 mg/dl; alkaline phosphatase may be slightly elevated. Liver biopsy reveals mild cholestasis without necrosis. The pathophysiology is related to estrogenic hormones, in that intrahepatic cholestasis of pregnancy can be reproduced in susceptible individuals by estrogen administration, and the disease develops exclusively during pregnancy with a tendency to recur in subsequent gestations. Multiple factors appear to play a role, including (1) decreased inactivation of circulating estrogens, (2) alterations in hepatocellular secretory function, and (3) derangements in bile acid metabolism and enterohepatic circulation. Although intrahepatic cholestasis of pregnancy is generally a benign condition, the mother is at risk for gallstones and malabsorption, and the incidence of fetal distress, stillbirths, and prematurity is modestly increased.[106]

TRANSPLANTATION

The increasing use of transplantation for bone marrow, renal, hepatic, and other organ disorders has generated a challenging group of hepatic complications. For patients undergoing bone marrow transplantation, the liver may be damaged by toxic drugs or graft-versus-host disease, whereas patients receiving a liver transplant may encounter graft failure or graft rejection. Although the clinical settings are obviously different for each patient population, the common themes of toxic or immunologically mediated liver damage, infection of immunosuppressed hosts, and recurrent disease are readily apparent. The differential diagnoses for liver disease in transplantation are given in Table 18–10.

DRUG TOXICITY FOLLOWING BONE MARROW TRANSPLANTATION

"Liver toxicity" describes a general syndrome of hepatic dysfunction following administration of the drugs used to abrogate the bone marrow prior to bone marrow transplantation. It affects up to one-half of all such patients,[110] and is heralded by weight gain, tender hepatomegaly, edema, ascites, hyperbilirubinemia, and a fall in urinary sodium excretion. The onset is typically on the days immediately following donor marrow administration. The morphologic features are nonspecific and include hepatocyte necrosis and cholestasis; biopsy is not usually performed in these fragile patients. Clinical outcome is directly related to the severity of liver toxicity. Although persistent severe liver dysfunction is a harbinger of a fatal outcome, liver disease per se is not usually a direct cause of death, and most patients succumb to septicemia, pneumonia, bleeding, or multiorgan failure. Two specific forms of toxic liver damage evolving over weeks to several months are discussed elsewhere: veno-occlusive disease (see Fig. 18–36) and nodular regenerative hyperplasia (see below under section on tumors).

GRAFT-VERSUS-HOST DISEASE AND LIVER REJECTION

The liver has the unenviable position of being attacked by graft-versus-host and host-versus-graft mechanisms, in the respective settings of bone marrow transplantation and liver transplantation. Although these general processes are covered in detail in Chapter 6, morphologic features peculiar to the liver deserve comment.

MORPHOLOGY. Liver damage in acute graft-versus-host disease (10 to 50 days after bone marrow

Table 18-10. HEPATIC COMPLICATIONS IN BONE MARROW AND LIVER TRANSPLANTATION

TIMING	COMMON CAUSES	LESS COMMON CAUSES
Bone Marrow Transplantation		
Pretransplant	Viral hepatitis Malignant involvement	Drug toxicity Veno-occlusive disease Opportunistic infection Biliary tract disease
Day 0–25	Drug toxicity Veno-occlusive disease	Graft-versus-host disease Opportunistic infection Nodular regenerative hyperplasia Cholestasis of sepsis
Day 25–100	Acute graft-versus-host disease Veno-occlusive disease Opportunistic infections Drug toxicity	Veno-occlusive disease Toxicity from total parenteral nutrition Nodular regenerative hyperplasia
>Day 100	Chronic graft-versus-host disease Viral hepatitis (hepatotropic)	Opportunistic infections Drug toxicity Epstein-Barr virus–induced disorders
Liver Transplantation		
First week	Primary nonfunction/preservation injury Technical problems (e.g., vascular anastomoses) Acute rejection	Hyperacute rejection Drug toxicity
1 week–2 months	Acute rejection Opportunistic infections Nonspecific cholestasis Technical problems (e.g., biliary anastomosis)	Chronic vascular rejection Vanishing bile duct syndrome Hepatic artery thrombosis Drug toxicity
>2 months	Chronic vascular rejection Vanishing bile duct syndrome Recurrent disease Viral hepatitis (hepatotropic)	Opportunistic infections Portal vein thrombosis Drug toxicity Epstein-Barr virus–induced disorders

transplantation) is dominated by direct attack of donor lymphocytes on epithelial cells of the liver. This results in a hepatitic picture, with necrosis of hepatocytes and bile duct epithelial cells and inflammation of the parenchyma and portal tracts. In chronic hepatic graft-versus-host disease (usually greater than 100 days after transplantation), hepatic disease is generally limited to portal tracts, with variable inflammation, selective bile duct destruction, and eventual fibrosis.[111] Cholestasis may be observed in both acute and chronic graft-versus-host disease. Portal vein and hepatic vein radicles may exhibit lymphocytic inflammation and intimal proliferation, so-called **endothelialitis.** Differentiation of graft-versus-host disease from other potential causes of hepatic disease is assisted by identification of **bile duct destruction affecting most portal tracts, which is highly suggestive, and endothelialitis, which clinches the diagnosis.**

Acute cellular rejection of implanted livers exhibits features common to all solid organ transplants, including infiltration of a mixed population of inflammatory cells into portal tracts and bile duct and hepatocyte injury. Endothelialitis is a common feature; a regenerative response of both residual bile ducts and parenchymal hepatocytes is variably observed. Chronic rejection may affect both arteries and bile ducts. Severe obliterative arteritis of small and larger arterial vessels generates ischemic changes in the liver parenchyma. Alternatively or in combination with vascular rejection, progressive bile duct damage generates a "vanishing bile duct syndrome."[112] Both may lead to eventual loss of the graft.

NONIMMUNOLOGIC DAMAGE TO LIVER ALLOGRAFTS

Besides technical problems in the surgical procedure and the very rare *hyperacute rejection*, revascularization and perfusion of the donor liver may result in *preservation injury*, attributable to the generation of oxygen radicals in a hypoxic organ with insufficient reserves of oxygen scavengers to prevent damage. *The primary event appears to be necrosis and sloughing of the sinusoidal endothelium.*[113] Hepatocyte ballooning and cholestasis follow, with variable degrees of centrilobular necrosis.[114] With severe injury, the portal tracts also are damaged, resulting in inflammation, bile duct proliferation, and fibrosis. These histologic features may take weeks to months to resolve.

In the days to weeks following transplantation, several complications may threaten the ultimate viability of the graft. In contrast to the native liver, *hepatic artery thrombosis* is a sufficiently severe vascular insult to cause severe hepatic compromise.

Alternatively, *portal vein thrombosis* may be insidious and present only as variceal hemorrhage weeks to months later. *Bile duct obstruction* presents in the expected fashion.

TUMORS AND TUMOROUS CONDITIONS

Hepatic masses come to attention for a variety of reasons. They may generate epigastric fullness and discomfort or be detected by routine physical examination or radiographic studies for other indications. The most common benign lesions are *cavernous hemangiomas*, identical to those occurring elsewhere (see Chapter 11). They appear as discrete red-blue, soft nodules, usually less than 2 cm in diameter, and often directly beneath the capsule. The importance of recognizing these lesions is not to mistake them for metastatic tumors and not to perform blind percutaneous biopsies on them. *Cysts* of biliary origin have been addressed previously.

NODULAR HYPERPLASIAS

Solitary or multiple benign hepatocellular nodules may develop in the liver, in the absence of cirrhosis. *Focal nodular hyperplasia* appears as a well-demarcated but poorly encapsulated nodule, ranging up to many centimeters in diameter. Generally focal nodular hyperplasia is lighter than the surrounding liver and brown to tan (sometimes yellow). Typically there is a central gray-white depressed stellate scar from which radiate fibrous septa to the periphery. The central scar contains large vessels, usually arterial, which typically exhibit fibromuscular hyperplasia with eccentric or concentric narrowing of the lumen. The radiating septa contain foci of intense lymphocytic infiltrates and exuberant bile duct proliferation along septal margins. The parenchyma between the septa is composed largely of normal hepatocytes, although chronic cholestatic features (bile and copper retention) and marginal piecemeal necrosis may be present. Although this lesion is more common in women, the purported association with oral contraceptives is probably coincidental. Focal nodular hyperplasia occurs most frequently in young to middle-aged adults and does not appear to pose a risk for malignancy.

Arguably *nodular regenerative hyperplasia* is a diffuse, nonfibrosing version of focal nodular hyperplasia, affecting the entire liver with roughly spherical nodules of plump hepatocytes surrounded by rims of atrophic cells, *in the absence of fibrosis.*[115] *The variation in parenchymal architecture may be missed on a hematoxylin and eosin stain, and reticulin staining is required to appreciate the changes in hepatocellular architecture.* In contrast to focal nodular hyperplasia, the diffuse transformation of the liver into nodular regenerative hyperplasia is associated with the development of portal hypertension, with attendant symptoms. Nodular regenerative hyperplasia is a nonspecific transformation that may occur in association with such diverse conditions as bone marrow transplantation and primary biliary cirrhosis.[116]

Although the pathogenesis is not firmly established, the common factor in both conditions appears to be heterogeneity in hepatic blood supply, arising from focal obliteration of portal vein radicles with compensatory augmentation of arterial blood supply.[117]

ADENOMAS

Benign neoplasms may develop from hepatocytes ("liver cells") or bile duct epithelial cells. *Liver cell adenomas* tend to occur in young women who have used oral contraceptives and regress on discontinuance of use.[118] Liver cell adenomas have clinical significance for two reasons: (1) When they present as an intrahepatic mass, they may be mistaken for the more ominous hepatocellular carcinoma, and (2) subcapsular adenomas have a tendency to rupture, particularly during pregnancy (under estrogenic stimulation), causing severe intraperitoneal hemorrhage. Rarely they may harbor hepatocellular carcinoma. Bile duct adenomas, on the other hand, may not even be true neoplasms but instead may represent aggregates of reactive bile ducts.

MORPHOLOGY. Liver cell adenomas are pale, yellow-tan, and frequently bile-stained nodules, found anywhere in the hepatic substance but often beneath the capsule. They may reach 30 cm in diameter. Although they are usually well demarcated, encapsulation may not be grossly evident. Histologically liver cell adenomas are composed of sheets and cords of cells that may resemble normal hepatocytes or have some variation in cell and nuclear size. The cells may be well glycogenated, generating a cleared cytoplasm. Portal tracts are absent; instead prominent arterial vessels and draining veins are distributed through the substance of the tumor. A capsule that ranges from delicate collapsed reticulin to well-defined connective tissue usually separates the lesion from the surrounding parenchyma, but it may be deficient in places or entirely absent.

Bile duct adenomas are firm, pale, and usually single discrete nodules rarely more than 1 cm in diameter, frequently found in a subcapsular location. In contrast to the liver cell adenoma, they are almost never bile stained. Histologically they are composed of uniformly sized, epithelium-lined channels or ducts separated by a scant-to-abundant connective tissue stroma and sharply demarcated from the surrounding liver. Because the ducts are not cystically dilated, bile duct adenomas can be distinguished readily from von Meyenberg complexes (see earlier). Because of their small size, these adenomas are usually found incidentally.

MALIGNANT TUMORS

The liver and lungs share the dubious distinction of being the visceral organs most often involved in the metastatic spread of cancers. Primary carcinomas of the liver are relatively uncommon in North America and Western Europe (0.5 to 2% of all cancers) but represent 20 to 40% of cancers in countries endemic for viral hepatitis. Before embarking on a discussion of the major forms of malignancy affecting the liver, two rare forms of primary liver cancer deserve brief mention.

The *hepatoblastoma* is a tumor usually of young childhood, which exhibits two anatomic variants: (1) the *epithelial type,* composed of small, compact fetal or smaller embryonal cells, forming acini, tubules, or papillary structures vaguely recapitulating the development of the liver, and (2) the *mixed type,* containing an epithelial element interspersed with foci of mesenchymal differentiation that may consist of primitive mesenchyme, osteoid, cartilage, or striated muscle. Unless successfully resected, both variants are usually fatal within a few years. The *angiosarcoma* resembles those occurring elsewhere (see Chapter 11). The primary liver form is of interest because of its association with exposure to vinyl chloride, arsenic, or Thorotrast (once used in radiography as a hepatic contrast medium). The latent period between exposure to the putative carcinogen and the appearance of the neoplasm may be several decades. These highly aggressive neoplasms metastasize widely and generally kill within a year.

Primary Carcinoma of the Liver

There are basically two types of primary carcinoma of the liver: One is *hepatocellular carcinoma* (HCC); the other, composed of bile duct epithelium, is *cholangiocarcinoma.* HCC, grievously sometimes still called a "hepatoma," accounts for more than 90% of all primary liver cancers. Virtually all the remainder are cholangiocarcinomas; the mixed pattern is uncommon. There has been a major surge of interest in HCC because (1) epidemiologic and molecular biologic evidence has firmly established a causal relationship with hepatotropic virus infection, especially HBV, and (2)

interventions now available could dramatically reduce the incidence of this form of cancer.

EPIDEMIOLOGY. For HCC, annual incidence rates of 3 to 7 cases per 100,000 population in North and South America, northern and central Europe, and Australia compare with intermediate rates of up to 20 cases per 100,000 in countries bordering the Mediterranean. The greatest numbers of cases are found in Taiwan, Mozambique, and Southeast China, where annual incidence rates approach 150 per 100,000. Within each geographic area (low or high incidence), blacks have attack rates approximately fourfold higher than whites. Worldwide there is a clear predominance of males, ranging from 8:1 in countries with a high incidence of HCC to approximately 2:1 to 3:1 in populations with a low frequency.

The global distribution of HCC is strongly linked to the prevalence of HBV infection. In high-incidence regions, the HBV carrier state begins in infancy following vertical transmission of virus from infected mothers, conferring a 200-fold increased risk of HCC by adulthood.[119] In these regions, cirrhosis may be absent in up to half of HCC patients, and the cancer often occurs between 20 and 40 years of age. In the Western world, where HBV is not prevalent, cirrhosis is present in 85 to 90% of cases of HCC, frequently in the setting of other chronic liver diseases (including HCV infection); this cancer is seldom encountered before age 60.

From these statistics come two key points: (1) *On a global basis, primary liver cancer constitutes the most common visceral malignant tumor and in some populations is the most common cancer overall,* and (2) *attempts to elucidate the pathogenesis of primary liver cancer must take population differences into account.*

PATHOGENESIS. In Chapter 7, mechanisms of carcinogenesis are discussed in detail, including the role of HBV and aflatoxin in the pathogenesis of HCC. Several points deserve emphasis at this time:

- Three major etiologic associations for HCC have been established: HBV infection, aflatoxin exposure, and cirrhosis.
- Many other factors, including age, gender, chemicals, viruses, hormones, alcohol, nutrition, and cirrhosis *per se,* interact in the development of HCC. HCV also may be a major cause.
- The exact pathogenesis of HCC may vary between high-incidence populations in which HBV is the dominant cause, and low-incidence Western populations, in which other diseases are well represented, and where pathogenesis may be related to toxic damage or chronic inflammation.
- *The development of cirrhosis appears to be an important, but not requisite, contributor to the emergence of HCC.* Postulated direct causes and

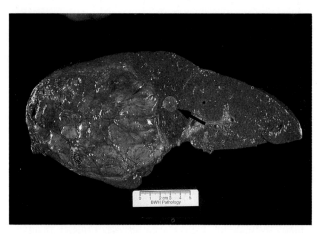

Figure 18–38. Hepatocellular carcinoma, massive type. A large neoplasm with extensive areas of necrosis replaces most of the right hepatic lobe in this noncirrhotic liver. A satellite tumor nodule is directly adjacent (arrow).

effects for injurious agents (e.g., alcohol, iron, and aflatoxin) have yet to be firmly established.

There is much to be learned about the pathogenesis of primary liver cancer in different disease conditions. For example, the disease most likely to give rise to HCC is in fact hereditary tyrosinemia, in which almost 40% of patients develop this tumor despite adequate dietary control.[120] *None of the influences related to HCC has any bearing on the development of cholangiocarcinoma:* The only recognized causal influences on this uncommon tumor are previous exposure to Thorotrast (formerly used in radiography of the liver) and invasion of the biliary tract by the liver fluke *Opisthorchis sinensis* and its close relatives. Most cholangiocarcinomas arise without evidence of antecedent risk conditions.

MORPHOLOGY. HCC, cholangiocarcinoma, or the mixed pattern may appear grossly as (1) a **unifocal** (usually large) mass; (2) **multifocal,** widely distributed nodules of variable size; or (3) a **diffusely infiltrative** cancer, permeating widely and sometimes involving the entire liver. All three patterns may cause liver enlargement (2000 to 3000 gm), particularly the unifocal massive and multinodular patterns. The diffusely infiltrative tumor may blend imperceptibly into a cirrhotic liver background. When discrete masses can be seen, they are basically yellow-white, punctuated sometimes by areas of hemorrhage or necrosis (Fig. 18–38). **HCCs sometimes take on a green hue when composed of well-differentiated hepatocytes capable of secreting bile. Cholangiocarcinomas are rarely bile stained** because differentiated bile duct epithelium does not synthesize pigmented bile. Infrequently with HCC, but often with cholangiocarcinoma, the tumor substance is extremely firm and gritty, related to dense desmoplasia. **All patterns**

of HCC have a strong propensity for invasion of vascular channels. Extensive intrahepatic metastases ensue, and occasionally long, snake-like masses of tumor invade the portal vein (with occlusion of the portal circulation) or inferior vena cava, extending even into the right side of the heart.

HCCs range from well-differentiated to highly anaplastic undifferentiated lesions. In well-differentiated and moderately well-differentiated tumors, cells recognizable as hepatocytic in origin are disposed either in a trabecular pattern (recapitulating liver cell plates; Fig. 18–39) or in an acinar, pseudoglandular pattern. Supporting connective tissue is minimal to absent, explaining the soft consistency of most HCCs. Bile may occasionally be seen in canalicular spaces or lumens between tumor cells, and bile canaliculi may be present ultrastructurally. Uncommonly the tumor may be made of "clear cells," containing abundant cytoplasmic glycogen and bearing a strong resemblance to clear-cell renal carcinomas. In poorly differentiated forms, tumor cells can take on a pleomorphic appearance with numerous anaplastic giant cells, or become small and completely undifferentiated cells, or may even resemble a spindle cell sarcoma.

A distinctive variant of HCC is the **fibrolamellar carcinoma.**[121] This tumor occurs in young men and women (20 to 40 years of age) with equal incidence, has no association with HBV or cirrhosis risk factors, and has a distinctly better prognosis. It usually constitutes a single large, hard "scirrhous" tumor with fibrous bands coursing through it. Histologically it is composed of well-differentiated polygonal cells growing in nests or cords and separated by parallel lamellae of dense collagen bundles (Fig. 18–40),[122] hence the name "fibrolamellar."

Cholangiocarcinomas resemble adenocarcinomas arising in other parts of the body and may exhibit the full range of morphologic variation. Most are well-differentiated sclerosing adenocarcinomas with clearly defined glandular and tubular structures lined by somewhat anaplastic cuboidal-to-low columnar epithelial cells. These neoplasms are often markedly desmoplastic, so dense collagenous stroma separates the glandular elements. Mucus is frequently present within cells and the lumina but not bile. There is no reliable histologic feature distinguishing intrahepatic cholangiocarcinoma from metastatic adenocarcinoma, and diagnosis depends on reasonable exclusion of an extrahepatic primary. Vascular invasion is less common with cholangiocarcinomas than with HCC.

HCC and cholangiocarcinoma differ somewhat in their patterns of spread. Hematogenous metastases to the lungs, bones (mainly vertebrae), adrenals, brain, or elsewhere are present at autopsy in about 50% of cases of cholangiocarcinoma. Disseminated hematogenous metastases are less frequent with HCC and may not be present, despite

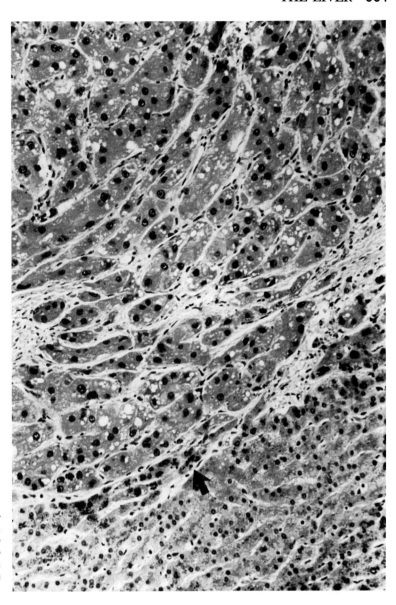

Figure 18-39. Hepatocellular carcinoma, trabecular type. Tumor occupies the upper left, and residual normal hepatic parenchyma the lower right of this image; the arrow marks the junction. Tumor cells have moderate variation in cell and nuclear size and shape but retain their resemblance to normal liver cells.

obvious venous invasion, until late in the course of the disease, when the lungs are frequently involved. Lymph node metastases to the perihilar, peripancreatic, and para-aortic nodes above and below the diaphragm are found in about half of all cholangiocarcinomas and less frequently with HCC.

CLINICAL COURSE. The clinical manifestations of primary liver cancer are seldom characteristic and in the Western population often are masked by those related to the background cirrhosis or chronic hepatitis. In areas of high incidence such as tropical Africa, patients usually have no clinical history of liver disease, although cirrhosis may be detected at autopsy. In both populations, most patients have ill-defined upper abdominal pain, malaise, fatigue, weight loss, and sometimes awareness of an abdominal mass or abdominal fullness. In many cases, the enlarged liver can be felt on pal-

pation, with sufficient irregularity or nodularity to permit differentiation from cirrhosis. Jaundice, fever, and gastrointestinal or esophageal variceal bleeding are inconstant findings.

Laboratory studies may be helpful but are rarely conclusive. Elevated levels of serum alpha-fetoprotein are found in 60 to 75% of patients with HCC. False-positive results, however, are encountered with yolk-sac tumors and many non-neoplastic conditions, including cirrhosis, massive liver necrosis, chronic hepatitis, normal pregnancy, fetal distress or death, and fetal neural tube defects such as anencephaly and spina bifida. The carcino-embryonic antigen levels are less often elevated and are even more nonspecific. Des-gamma-carboxyprothrombin, a prothrombin precursor resulting from failure to carboxylate glutamic acid residues, may be elaborated by liver cells and detected in the serum of 75 to 90% of patients with HCC.[123] All of these biochemical tests, however,

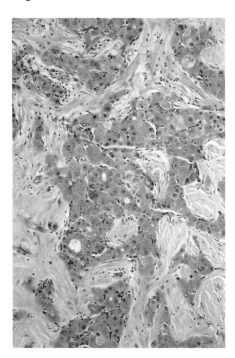

Figure 18-40. Fibrolamellar carcinoma. This hepatocellular neoplasm is composed of nests and cords of malignant-appearing hepatocytes separated by dense bundles of collagen. (Hematoxylin and eosin.)

often fail to detect small lesions, when curative resection might be possible. Most valuable for small tumors are ultrasonography, hepatic angiography, computed tomography, and magnetic resonance imaging scans.

The natural course of primary liver cancer is progressive enlargement of the primary mass until it encroaches on hepatic function or metastasizes, generally first to the lungs and then to other sites. Overall death usually occurs within 6 months of diagnosis from (1) cachexia, (2) gastrointestinal or esophageal variceal bleeding, (3) liver failure with hepatic coma, or, rarely, (4) rupture of the tumor with fatal hemorrhage.[124] The only ray of light in this otherwise dismal scene is *the possibility of significantly reducing the global mortality from HCC by immunization of high-risk populations against HBV, in whom infections are commonly acquired in early life.* Such public-health measures provide the extraordinary opportunity to eradicate a major cancer by a vaccination program.

The fibrolamellar variant of HCC is associated with a far more favorable outlook. It arises in otherwise healthy young adults and may be discovered while still amenable to surgical resection. About 60% of patients are alive at 5 years; the remainder succumb to progressive, unresectable disease. Cholangiocellular carcinoma is not usually detected until late in its course, and the clinical outlook is dismal, with death characteristically ensuing within 6 months.

Metastatic Tumors

Metastatic involvement of the liver is far more common than primary neoplasia. Although the most common primaries producing hepatic metastases are those of the breast, lung, and colon, any cancer in any site of the body may spread to the liver, including leukemias and lymphomas. Typically multiple nodular implants are found that often cause striking hepatomegaly and may replace more than 80% of existent hepatic parenchyma (Fig. 18-41). The liver weight can exceed several kilograms. There is a tendency for metastatic nodules to outgrow their blood supply, producing central necrosis and umbilication when viewed from the surface of the liver. Always surprising is the amount of metastatic involvement that may be present in the absence of clinical or laboratory evidence of hepatic functional insufficiency. Often the only clinical telltale sign is hepatomegaly, sometimes with nodularity of the free edge. With massive or strategic involvement (obstruction of major ducts), however, jaundice and abnormal elevations of liver enzymes may appear.

POSTMORTEM CHANGES

It is necessary to mention briefly the morphologic changes that occur after death, to avoid confusion with antemortem liver disease. Almost immediately, cytoplasmic glycogen is consumed, leading to a "leaner" appearance of hepatocytes in postmortem histologic sections. Depending on the adequacy and promptness of the methods used to preserve the body, including refrigeration, the liver may undergo postmortem autolysis. Usually it

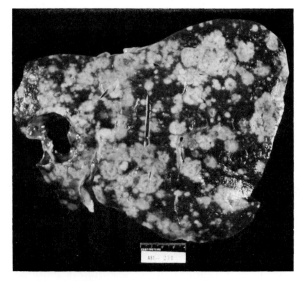

Figure 18-41. Multiple hepatic metastases from a primary gastric carcinoma.

begins to become evident about 24 hours after death and produces softening, discohesion, and enzymatic disintegration of cells in the complete absence of reactive inflammatory changes. The nuclei progressively fade, and the cells fall away from the reticular framework. With time, bacterial proliferation can be seen within the autolytic parenchyma. In some instances, gas-forming organisms such as *Clostridium welchii* are borne from the gastrointestinal tract to the liver through the portal system during the agonal stage of life. Growth of these organisms and the release of gas may produce visible or palpable gaseous bubbles *(foamy liver)*. Obviously no inflammatory response accompanies the bacterial invasion.

Appropriately, the description of postmortem changes brings to an end the consideration of the liver.

Biliary System

CONGENITAL ANOMALIES	DISORDERS OF THE	TUMORS	MISCELLANEOUS
DISORDERS OF THE	EXTRAHEPATIC BILE	CARCINOMA OF THE	DISORDERS OF THE
GALLBLADDER	DUCTS	GALLBLADDER	BILIARY TREE
CHOLELITHIASIS (GALLSTONES)	BILIARY ATRESIA	CARCINOMA OF THE	IATROGENIC INJURY TO THE
CHOLECYSTITIS	CHOLEDOCHOLITHIASIS AND	EXTRAHEPATIC BILE DUCTS	BILIARY TREE
Acute Calculous Cholecystitis	ASCENDING CHOLANGITIS		
Acute Acalculous	CHOLEDOCHAL CYSTS		
Cholecystitis			
Chronic Cholecystitis			

NORMAL

Disorders of the biliary tract affect a significant portion of the world's population. More than 95% of biliary tract disease is attributable to cholelithiasis (gallstones). In the United States, the annual cost of cholelithiasis and its complications is $6 to 8 billion, representing 1% of the national health care budget. Before further discussion, some comments about the normal structure and function of the biliary tree are in order.

Bile is the exocrine secretion of the liver, and humans secrete about 0.5 to 1.0 liter daily. Between meals, bile is stored in the gallbladder, which in the adult has a capacity of about 50 ml. Storage is facilitated by fivefold to tenfold concentration of bile through the coupled active absorption of electrolytes, with passive movement of water. In preparation for fat digestion, the gallbladder releases stored bile into the gut. This organ is not essential for biliary function because humans do not suffer from maldigestion or malabsorption of fat after cholecystectomy.

In contrast to the rest of the gastrointestinal tract, the gallbladder lacks a muscularis mucosa and submucosa and consists only of (1) a mucosal lining with a single layer of columnar cells; (2) a fibromuscular layer; (3) a layer of subserosal fat with arteries, veins, lymphatics, nerves, and paraganglia; and (4) a peritoneal covering except where the gallbladder lies adjacent to, or is even embedded, in the liver. The mucosal epithelium takes the form of numerous interlacing tiny folds, creating a honeycombed surface. In the neck of the gallbladder, these folds coalesce to form the *spiral valves of Heister*, which extend into the cystic duct. In combination with muscular action, these "valves" may assist in retaining bile between meals. The rapid taper of the gallbladder neck just proximal to the cystic duct is the site at which gallstones become impacted.

Sometimes small tubular channels *(ducts of Luschka)* are found buried within the gallbladder wall adjacent to the liver. The channels usually do not enter the gallbladder lumen but communicate with the intrahepatic biliary tree and rarely are patent accessory bile secretory ducts. Small outpouchings of the gallbladder mucosa may penetrate into and through the muscle wall *(Rokitansky-Aschoff sinuses)*; their prominence in the settings of inflammation and gallstone formation suggests that they are acquired herniations.

The confluence of the biliary tree is the common bile duct, which courses through the head of the pancreas for about 2 cm before disgorging its contents through the *ampulla of Vater* into the duodenal lumen. In approximately 60 to 70% of individuals, the main pancreatic duct joins the common bile duct to drain through a common

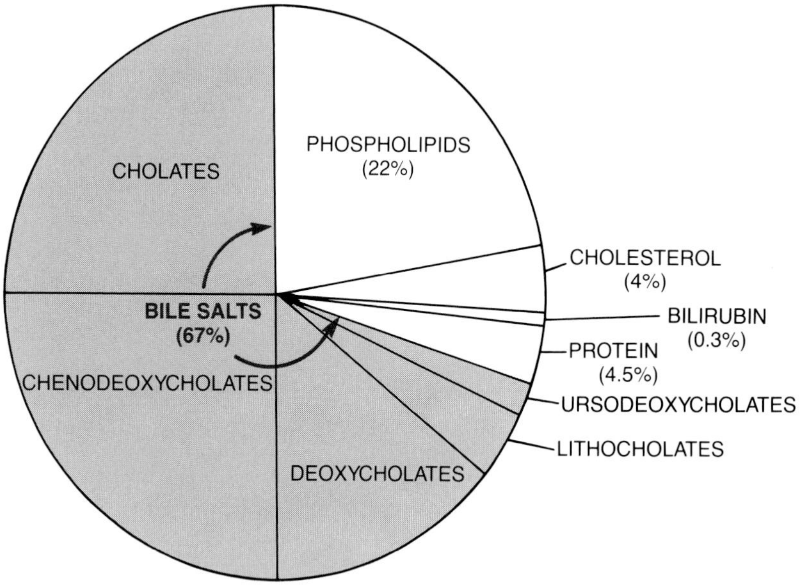

Figure 18-42. Typical solute composition of gallbladder and hepatic bile in health. (With permission from Carey, M.C.: Biliary lipids and gallstone formation. In Csomos, G., and Thaler, H. (eds.): Clinical Hepatology. Berlin, Springer-Verlag, 1983, pp. 52-69.)

channel; in the remainder, the two ducts run in parallel without joining. Scattered along the length of both the intrahepatic and the extrahepatic biliary tree are mucin-secreting submucosal glands. These become prominent near the terminus of the common bile duct, appearing as microscopic outpouchings that interdigitate with the spiraling smooth muscle of the ampullary sphincter. To the unwary, these buried glands may be mistaken for invasive cancer.

Newly secreted bile is a bicarbonate-rich fluid containing by weight about 3% organic solutes, of which two-thirds are bile salts (Fig. 18-42). Bile acids are the major catabolic products of cholesterol and are a family of water-soluble sterols with carboxylated side chains.[125] Bile salts act as highly effective detergents, solubilizing water-insoluble lipids secreted by the liver into the biliary tree and dietary lipids within the gut lumen. The principal secreted lipids (more than 95%) are *lecithins* (phosphatidylcholine), which are hydrophobic and have no appreciable aqueous solubility of their own. *These insoluble amphiphiles, however, enhance the cholesterol-solubilizing capacity of bile salts in bile.*[126] *Cholesterol* is a negligibly soluble steroid molecule with a single polar hydroxyl group, whose *solubility in bile is increased several millionfold by the presence of bile salts and lecithin.* About 95% of secreted bile salts are avidly reabsorbed in the intestines, primarily in the ileum, and returned to the liver via portal blood. *The enterohepatic circulation of bile salts constitutes a highly efficient mechanism for reuse of these essential physiologic molecules.*[127] Nevertheless, *the obligatory fecal loss of about half a gram of bile salts per day constitutes the major route for elimination of body cholesterol,* with a lesser contribution from cholesterol excreted directly into bile.

PATHOLOGY

CONGENITAL ANOMALIES

Although major developmental anomalies of the gallbladder and bile ducts are rare, anatomic variation is sufficiently common to present occasional surprises during surgery. The more distinctive variations, which also may be appreciated during ultrasonography, computed tomography, and magnetic resonance imaging scans, merit comment. The gallbladder may be *congenitally absent,* or there may be gallbladder *duplication* with conjoined or independent cystic ducts.[128] A longitudinal or transverse septum may create a *bilobed gallbladder.* *Aberrant locations* of the gallbladder occur in 5 to 10% of the population, most commonly partial or complete embedding in the liver substance. A *folded fundus* is the most common anomaly, creating the so-called *phrygian cap* (Fig. 18-43). *Agenesis* of all or any portion of the hepatic or common bile ducts and *hypoplastic* narrowing of biliary channels (true "biliary atresia") represent a spectrum of hepatobiliary malformations.

DISORDERS OF THE GALLBLADDER

CHOLELITHIASIS (GALLSTONES)

Gallstones afflict 10 to 20% of adult populations in developed countries. It is estimated that more than

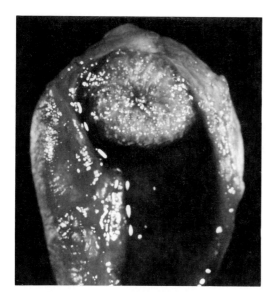

Figure 18–43. Phrygian cap of gallbladder. The fundus of the gallbladder is folded inward.

20 million persons in the United States have gallstones, totaling some 25 to 50 tons in weight.[129] About 1 million new patients annually are found to have gallstones, of whom approximately 600,000 undergo cholecystectomy. Nevertheless, the vast majority of gallstones (more than 80%) are "silent," and most individuals remain free of biliary pain or stone complications for decades. There are two main types of gallstones. In the West, *about 80% are cholesterol stones, containing more than 50% of crystalline cholesterol monohydrate. The remainder are composed predominantly of bilirubin calcium salts and are designated pigment stones.*

PREVALENCE AND RISK FACTORS. Certain populations are far more prone than others to develop gallstones. The major risk factors are cited in Table 18–11. The following applies to cholesterol gallstones.[130]

Ethnic-Geographic. The prevalence rates of cholesterol gallstones approach 75% in certain Native American populations: the Pima, Hopi, and Navajo[131]—whereas pigment stones are rare. Gallstones are more prevalent in industrialized societies and uncommon in underdeveloped or developing societies.

Age and Sex. The prevalence of gallstones increases throughout life. In the United States, less than 5 to 6% of the population under age 40 have stones, in contrast to 25 to 30% of those over age 80. The prevalence in white women is about twice as high as in men. With both aging and gender, hypersecretion of biliary cholesterol appears to play the major role.

Environmental Factors. Estrogenic influences, including oral contraceptives and pregnancy, increase the expression of hepatic lipoprotein recep-tors and stimulate hepatic hydroxymethylglutaryl co-enzyme A (HMG CoA) reductase activity. Thus, both cholesterol uptake and biosynthesis are increased. Clofibrate, used to lower blood cholesterol, increases hepatic HMG CoA reductase and decreases conversion of cholesterol to bile acids by reducing cholesterol 7α-hydroxylase activity. The net result of these influences is excess biliary secretion of cholesterol. Obesity and rapid weight loss also are strongly associated with increased biliary cholesterol secretion.

Acquired Disorders. Although gastrointestinal conditions may severely impair intestinal resorption of bile salts, there is compensatory enhanced hepatic conversion of cholesterol to bile salts, leading to less cholesterol excretion and no particular tendency to cholesterol stone formation. Gallbladder stasis, either neurogenic or hormonal, fosters a local environment favorable for both cholesterol and pigment gallstone formation.

Hereditary Factors. In addition to ethnicity, family history alone imparts increased risk, as do inborn errors of metabolism that (1) lead to impaired bile salt synthesis and secretion or (2) generate increased serum and biliary levels of cholesterol, such as defects in lipoprotein receptors (hyperlipidemia syndromes; see Chapter 11), which engender marked increases in cholesterol biosynthesis.

Certain risk factors are well established for the development of pigment stones. Disorders that are associated with elevated levels of unconjugated bilirubin in bile include hemolytic syndromes, severe ileal dysfunction (or bypass), and bacterial contamination of the biliary tree. The predominant type of gallstones in non-Western populations are pigment gallstones, primarily arising in the biliary

Table 18–11. RISK FACTORS FOR GALLSTONES

CHOLESTEROL STONES
Demography: Northern Europe, North and South America, Native Americans, Mexican Americans
Advancing age
Female sex hormones
  Female gender
  Oral contraceptives
  Pregnancy
Obesity
Rapid weight reduction
Gallbladder stasis
Inborn disorders of bile acid metabolism
Hyperlipidemia syndromes

PIGMENT STONES
Demography: Asian more than Western, rural more than urban
Chronic hemolytic syndromes
Biliary infection
Gastrointestinal disorders: ileal disease (e.g., Crohn's disease), ileal resection or bypass, cystic fibrosis with pancreatic insufficiency

tree in the setting of infections and parasitic infestations.

PATHOGENESIS. Cholesterol is rendered soluble in bile by aggregation with water-soluble bile salts and water-insoluble lecithins, both of which act as detergents.[126] *When cholesterol concentrations exceed the solubilizing capacity of bile (supersaturation), cholesterol can no longer remain dispersed and nucleates into solid cholesterol monohydrate crystals. Three conditions must be met to permit the formation of cholesterol gallstones: (1) Bile must be supersaturated with cholesterol; (2) nucleation must be kinetically favorable; and (3) cholesterol crystals must remain in the gallbladder long enough to agglomerate into stones* (Fig. 18–44). Nucleation is promoted by the presence of microprecipitates of inorganic or organic calcium salts, which may serve as nucleation sites for cholesterol stones. Approximately 4% of biliary solids are protein, and initiators or inhibitors of nucleation have been found in protein extracts of human bile.[130,132] Gallbladder stasis plays a key role in permitting stone formation. Defective or infrequent gallbladder emptying occurs in the settings of prolonged fasting, pregnancy, rapid weight loss, total parenteral nutrition, and spinal cord injury. Such stasis appears to result from intrinsic neuromuscular dysmotility and diminished responsiveness to CCK-octapeptide. By increasing the residence time of bile within the gallbladder, bile becomes more concentrated, thereby increasing cholesterol supersaturation as well.

In contrast to cholesterol gallstones, which are composed chiefly of cholesterol monohydrate, a normal constituent of bile, pigment gallstones are complex mixtures of abnormal insoluble calcium salts.[133] Precipitation of calcium salts of unconjugated bilirubin is critical.[134] In addition to the poorly understood contributions of bile pH and composition, the presence of unconjugated bilirubin in the biliary tree increases the likelihood of such precipitation. Infection of the biliary tract, as with *Escherichia coli, Ascaris lumbricoides,* or, in Asia, by the liver fluke *Opisthorchis sinensis,* induces deconjugation of excreted bilirubin glucuronides. Increased biliary excretion of conjugated bilirubin occurs during hemolysis. Because a low level (about 1%) of bilirubin glucuronides are deconjugated in the biliary tree even normally, under hemolytic conditions the aqueous solubility of free bilirubin may easily be exceeded. Eighty per cent of pigment and cholesterol stone patients, however, have no identifying risk factors.

MORPHOLOGY. Cholesterol stones arise exclusively in the gallbladder and consist of 100% down to around 50% cholesterol.[125] **Pure cholesterol stones** are pale yellow and round to ovoid and have a finely granular, hard external surface (Fig. 18–45), which on transection reveals a glistening radiating

crystalline palisade. With increasing proportions of calcium carbonate, phosphates, and bilirubin, the stones exhibit discoloration and may be lamellated and gray-white to black on transection. Most often, multiple stones are present that range up to several centimeters in diameter. Rarely there is a single, much larger stone that may virtually fill the fundus. Surfaces of multiple stones may be rounded or faceted, owing to tight apposition. **Stones composed largely of cholesterol are ra-**

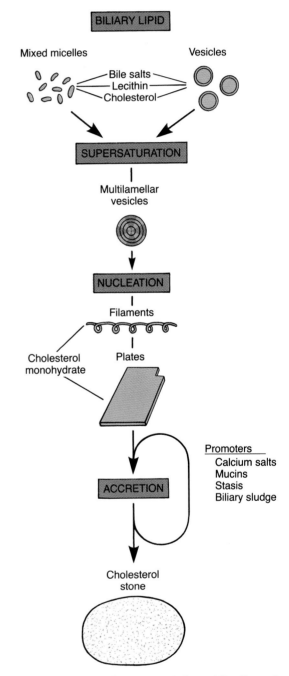

Figure 18–44. Schematic representation of the three stages of cholelithiasis: supersaturation, nucleation, and accretion.

diolucent; sufficient calcium carbonate is found in 10 to 20% of cholesterol stones to render them radiopaque.

Pigment gallstones are trivially classified as "black" and "brown."[133] In general, black pigment stones are found in sterile gallbladder bile, and brown stones are found in infected intrahepatic or extrahepatic ducts. "Black" pigment stones are composed of oxidized polymers of the calcium salts of unconjugated bilirubin, lesser amounts of calcium carbonate, calcium phosphate, and mucin glycoprotein and contain a modicum of cholesterol monohydrate crystals. "Brown" pigment stones contain pure calcium salts of unconjugated bilirubin, mucin glycoprotein, a substantial cholesterol fraction, and calcium salts of palmitate and stearate. The black stones are rarely greater than 1.5 cm in diameter, are almost invariably present in great number (with an inverse relationship between size and number; Fig. 18–46), and may crumble to the touch. Their contours are usually spiculated and molded. Brown stones tend to be laminated and soft and may have a soap-like or greasy consistency. Because of calcium carbonates and phosphates, **approximately 50 to 75% of black stones are radiopaque.** Brown stones, which contain only calcium soaps, are radiolucent. Mucin glycoproteins constitute the scaffolding and interparticle cement of all stones, whether pigment or cholesterol.

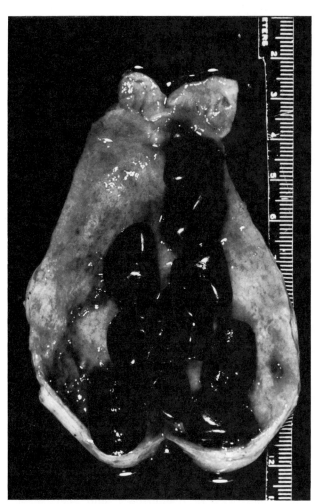

Figure 18–46. Pigment gallstones. They are jet black and are set against the background of a thickened fibrotic gallbladder with marked atrophy of the mucosa.

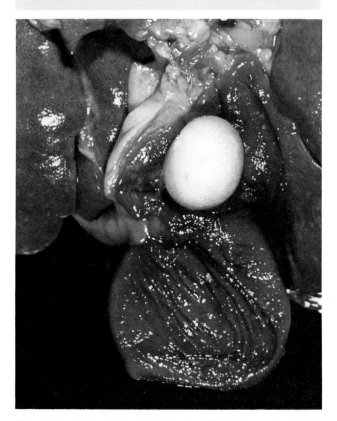

Figure 18–45. A pure cholesterol gallstone—pale yellow and semitransparent.

CLINICAL IMPLICATIONS. Gallstones may be present for decades before symptoms develop, and from 70 to 80% of patients remain asymptomatic throughout their lives. *It appears that asymptomatic patients convert to symptomatic ones at the rate of 1 to 3% per year, and the risk diminishes with time.*[135] Prominent among symptoms is biliary pain, which tends to be excruciating and constant or "colicky" (spasmodic), owing to the obstructive nature of gallstones in the biliary tree and perhaps in the gallbladder itself. Inflammation of the gallbladder (cholecystitis; see below), in association with obstructing and nonobstructing stones, also generates pain. More severe complications include empyema, perforation, fistulas, inflammation of the biliary tree (cholangitis), and obstructive cholestasis or pancreatitis with ensuant problems. The larger the calculi, the less likely they are to enter the cystic or common ducts to produce obstruction—the very small stones, or "gravel," are more dangerous. Occasionally a large stone may erode directly into an adjacent loop of small bowel, generating intestinal obstruction ("gallstone ileus"). Occasionally progressive mucosal removal of luminal lipids in obstructed, uninflamed gallbladders may leave clear mucinous secretions, so-called *hydrops* or *mucocele* of the gallbladder. More controversial is the increased risk for carcinoma of the gallbladder, discussed later.

CHOLECYSTITIS

Acute Calculous Cholecystitis

Inflammation of the gallbladder almost always develops in the setting of gallstones and on an acute or chronic basis. *Acute calculous cholecystitis is an acute inflammation of the gallbladder, precipitated 90% of the time by obstruction of the neck or cystic duct.* It is the primary complication of gallstones and the most common reason for emergency cholecystectomy. In general, patients have experienced previous episodes of biliary pain, but occasionally it is the first symptom of a previously unrecognized gallstone. *Acute calculous cholecystitis may appear with remarkable suddenness and constitute an acute surgical emergency or may present with mild symptoms that resolve without medical intervention.* Because this disease is the direct result of cholelithiasis, the patient populations tend to be the same as those with gallstones.

An attack of acute cholecystitis begins with progressive right upper quadrant or epigastric pain, frequently associated with mild fever, anorexia, tachycardia, diaphoresis, and nausea and vomiting. The upper abdomen is tender, but a distended tender gallbladder may be difficult to palpate. Most patients are free of jaundice; the presence of hyperbilirubinemia suggests obstruction of the common bile duct. Mild-to-moderate leukocytosis may be accompanied by mild elevations in serum alkaline phosphatase values. In the absence of medical attention, the attack usually subsides over 7 to 10 days and frequently within 24 hours. Up to 25% of patients, however, develop progressively more severe symptoms, requiring immediate medical intervention. In those patients that recover, recurrence is common.

PATHOGENESIS. Acute calculous cholecystitis is initially the result of chemical irritation and inflammation of the gallbladder wall in the setting of obstruction to bile outflow. With bile stasis phospholipases derived from the mucosa hydrolyze biliary lecithin to lysolecithin, which is toxic to the mucosa. The normally protective glycoprotein mucous layer is disrupted, exposing the mucosal epithelium to the direct detergent action of bile salts. Prostaglandins released within the wall of the distended gallbladder contribute to mucosal and mural inflammation. Distention and increased intraluminal pressure may also compromise blood flow to the mucosa. *These events occur in the ab-sence of bacterial infection;* only later in the course may bacterial contamination develop.

MORPHOLOGY. In **acute calculous cholecystitis,** the gallbladder is usually enlarged and tense and may assume a bright red or blotchy, violaceous to green-black discoloration, imparted by subserosal hemorrhages. The serosal covering is frequently layered by fibrin and, in severe cases, by a definite suppurative, coagulated exudate. In most cases, an obstructing stone is present in the neck of the gallbladder or the cystic duct. In addition to other possible stones, the gallbladder lumen is filled with a cloudy or turbid bile that may contain large amounts of fibrin and frank pus as well as hemorrhage. When the contained exudate is virtually pure pus, the condition is referred to as **empyema of the gallbladder.** In mild cases, the gallbladder wall is thickened and edematous and hyperemic. In more severe cases, it is transformed into a green-black necrotic organ, termed **gangrenous cholecystitis,** with small-to-large perforations. Histologically, the inflammatory reactions are not distinctive and consist of the usual patterns of acute inflammation, that is, edema, leukocytic infiltration, vascular congestion, frank abscess formation, or gangrenous necrosis.

The following complications may develop: (1) bacterial superinfection with ensuant cholangitis or sepsis; (2) gallbladder perforation with abscess formation; (3) gallbladder rupture with diffuse peritonitis; (4) biliary enteric (cholecystoenteric) fistula, allowing drainage of bile into adjacent organs, entry of air and bacteria into the biliary tree, and entry of gallstones into the intestine; and (5) aggravation of pre-existing medical illness, with cardiac, pulmonary, renal, or liver decompensation.

CLINICAL COURSE. Because many other conditions can present with right upper quadrant pain, even in patients with known gallstones, care must be taken to verify a diagnosis of acute cholecystitis, without subjecting the patient to undue delay.[135] *Surgical removal of the diseased gallbladder is the treatment of choice.* Although overall mortality from this disease is under 1%, several thousand deaths occur annually in the United States from this condition.

Acute Acalculous Cholecystitis

Between 5 and 12% of gallbladders removed for acute cholecystitis contain no gallstones. Most of these cases occur in the following circumstances: (1) the postoperative state after major, nonbiliary surgery; (2) severe trauma (e.g., car accidents, war injuries); (3) severe burns; (4) multisystem organ failure; (5) sepsis; (6) prolonged intravenous hyperalimentation; and (7) the postpartum state.[136]

Clinical symptoms are similar to those seen in acute calculus cholecystitis, but onset tends to be more insidious because symptoms are obscured by the generally grave clinical condition of the patient. A high proportion of patients, however, have no symptoms referable to the gallbladder; diagnosis therefore rests on a high index of suspicion. A more indolent form of acute acalculous cholecystitis may occur in the outpatient population in the setting of systemic vasculitis, severe atherosclerotic ischemic disease in the elderly, and acquired immunodeficiency syndrome (AIDS) (with a microbial complication).[137]

PATHOGENESIS. This disease is thought to develop ultimately as the result of ischemic compromise to the gallbladder. The cystic artery is an end-artery with essentially no collateral circulation. The interplay between contributing factors is unclear, but each of the following is thought to play some role:[138] (1) dehydration and multiple blood transfusions, leading to a pigment load; (2) gallbladder stasis, as may occur with hyperalimentation and assisted ventilation; (3) accumulation of biliary sludge, viscous bile, and gallbladder mucus, causing cystic duct obstruction in the absence of frank stone formation; (4) inflammation and edema of the wall, compromising blood flow; and (5) bacterial contamination of bile and generation of lysolecithins. Early recognition of this condition is critical because failure to do so almost ensures a fatal outcome. Overall mortality from acute acalculous cholecystitis is about 10%; this figure approaches 50% in the critically ill population.

MORPHOLOGY. There are no specific morphologic differences between acute calculous and acalculous cholecystitis except for the absence of macroscopic stones. Either as a result of the intrinsic nature of the disease or the frequent delay in diagnosis, the incidence of gangrene and perforation is much higher than in calculous cholecystitis.[135] In rare instances, primary bacterial infection can give rise to acute acalculous cholecystitis, including agents such as *Salmonella typhii* and staphylococci. Acute emphysematous cholecystitis results from gas-forming organisms, notably clostridia and coliforms, and typically in diabetics.

Chronic Cholecystitis

Chronic cholecystitis may be a sequel to repeated bouts of mild-to-severe acute cholecystitis, but in many instances, it develops in the apparent absence of antecedent acute attacks. Because it is associated with cholelithiasis in more than 90% of cases, the patient populations are the same as for the latter condition. The evolution of chronic cholecystitis is obscure, in that it is not clear that

gallstones play a direct role in the initiation of inflammation or the development of pain, particularly because chronic acalculous cholecystitis exhibits symptoms and histologic features similar to the calculous form. Rather, supersaturation of bile predisposes to both chronic inflammation and, in most instances, stone formation. Microorganisms, usually *E. coli* and enterococci, can be cultured from the bile in about one-third of cases. In contrast to acute calculous cholecystitis, obstruction of gallbladder outflow is not a requisite. Nevertheless, the symptoms for calculous chronic cholecystitis are similar to the acute form and range from biliary colic to indolent right upper quadrant pain and epigastric distress. Because most gallbladders removed at elective surgery for gallstones exhibit features of chronic cholecystitis, one must conclude that biliary symptoms often emerge after low-grade inflammation has become established.

MORPHOLOGY. The morphologic changes in chronic cholecystitis are extremely variable and sometimes minimal. The gallbladder may be contracted, normal in size, or enlarged, depending on the balance between the development of mural fibrosis and the contribution of obstruction to the inflammation. The serosa is usually smooth and glistening, but often it is dulled by subserosal fibrosis. Dense fibrous adhesions may remain as sequelae of pre-existent acute inflammation. On sectioning, the wall is variably thickened, rarely to more than three times normal. The wall has an opaque gray-white appearance and may be less flexible than normal. In the uncomplicated case, the lumen contains fairly clear, green-yellow, mucoid bile and usually stones (Fig. 18–47). The mucosa itself is generally preserved; when the lumen of the gallbladder is partially or totally obstructed, the gallbladder contents may be under sufficient pressure to cause mucosal thinning and atrophy.

Histologically the degree of inflammatory reaction is quite variable. In the mildest cases, only scattered lymphocytes, plasma cells, and macrophages are found in the mucosa and in the subserosal fibrous tissue. In more developed cases, there is marked subepithelial and subserosal fibrosis, accompanied by mononuclear cell infiltration. Inflammatory proliferation of the mucosa and fusion of the mucosal folds may give rise to buried crypts of epithelium within the gallbladder wall. Outpouchings of the mucosal epithelium through the wall **(Rokitansky-Aschoff sinuses)** may be quite prominent. Superimposition of acute inflammatory changes imply acute exacerbation of a previously chronically injured gallbladder.

In rare instances, extensive dystrophic calcification within the gallbladder wall may yield a **porcelain gallbladder,** notable for a markedly increased incidence of associated cancer. **Xanthogranulomatous cholecystitis** also is a rare condi-

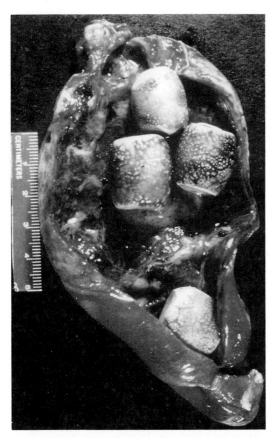

Figure 18–47. Chronic cholecystitis, demonstrating thickened gallbladder wall and luminal cholesterol stones.

tion in which the gallbladder is shrunken, nodular, and chronically inflamed with foci of necrosis and hemorrhage. This condition can be confused macroscopically for a malignancy. Finally, an atrophic, chronically obstructed gallbladder may contain only clear secretions, a condition known as **hydrops of the gallbladder**.

DISORDERS OF THE EXTRAHEPATIC BILE DUCTS

BILIARY ATRESIA

The infant presenting with neonatal cholestasis has been discussed previously in the context of intrahepatic disorders. A major contributor to neonatal cholestasis is *extrahepatic biliary atresia (EHBA)*, representing one-third of infants with neonatal cholestasis and occuring in approximately 1:10,000 live births. *EHBA is defined as a complete obstruction of bile flow owing to destruction or absence of all or part of the extrahepatic bile ducts.*[139] It is the single most frequent cause of death from liver disease in early childhood and accounts for 50 to 60% of children referred for liver transplantation, owing to the rapidly progressing secondary biliary cirrhosis.

PATHOGENESIS. *Most infants with EHBA are born with an intact biliary tree, which undergoes progressive inflammatory destruction in the weeks following birth.* In rare cases, there is evidence of bile duct destruction before birth. The cause of **EHBA** remains unknown, but various proposals ascribe the disease to (1) viral infection, particularly reovirus 3, cytomegalovirus, and rubella virus; (2) genetic inheritance, given reports of **EHBA** occurring in twins and **EHBA** occurring in families with anomalies of the intrahepatic biliary tree; and (3) anomalous embryologic development, given the 15 to 20% incidence of extrahepatic anomalies in **EHBA** patients, such as polysplenism, cardiovascular defects, malrotation, and bowel atresias.

MORPHOLOGY. The salient features of EHBA include inflammation and fibrosing stricture of the hepatic or common bile ducts, periductular inflammation of intrahepatic bile ducts, and progressive destruction of the intrahepatic biliary tree. On liver biopsy, florid features of extrahepatic biliary obstruction are evident, i.e., marked bile ductular proliferation, portal tract edema and fibrosis, and parenchymal cholestasis. When unrecognized or uncorrected, cirrhosis develops within 3 to 6 months of birth.

There is considerable variability in EHBA. When the disease is limited to the common duct (type I) or hepatic bile ducts (type II) with patent proximal branches, the disease is surgically correctable. Unfortunately, 90% of patients have type III biliary atresia, in which there also is obstruction of bile ducts at or above the porta hepatis. These cases are noncorrectable, because there are no patent extrahepatic ducts amenable to surgical anastomosis. Moreover, in most patients, bile ducts within the liver are initially patent but are progressively destroyed.

CLINICAL COURSE. Infants with EHBA present with neonatal cholestasis, discussed previously. These infants exhibit normal birth weight and postnatal weight gain, a slight female preponderance, and the progression of initially normal stools to acholic stools as the disease evolves. At the time of presentation, serum bilirubin values are usually in the 6 to 12 mg/dl range, with only moderately elevated transaminase and alkaline phosphatase levels. The success of surgical resection and bypass of the biliary tree is limited by subsequent bacterial contamination of the intrahepatic biliary tree and intrahepatic progression of the disease. Liver transplantation with accompanying donor bile ducts remains the primary hope for these young patients. Without surgical intervention, death usually occurs within 2 years of birth.

CHOLEDOCHOLITHIASIS AND ASCENDING CHOLANGITIS

These conditions are considered together because they so frequently go hand-in-hand. *Choledocholithiasis is the presence of stones within the biliary tree,* occurring in about 10% of patients with cholelithiasis. In Western nations, almost all stones are derived from the gallbladder, although both cholesterol and pigmented stones can form *de novo* anywhere in the biliary tree. In Asia, there is a much higher incidence of primary ductal and intrahepatic stone formation, usually pigmented. Choledocholithiasis may be asymptomatic or may cause symptoms from (1) obstruction, (2) pancreatitis, (3) cholangitis, (4) hepatic abscess, (5) secondary biliary cirrhosis, and (6) acute calculous cholecystitis.

Cholangitis is the term used for bacterial infection of the bile ducts. Cholangitis can result from any lesion creating obstruction to bile flow, most commonly choledocholithiasis. Uncommon causes include indwelling stents or catheters; tumors; acute pancreatitis; benign strictures; and rarely fungi, viruses, or parasites. Bacteria most likely enter the biliary tract through the sphincter of Oddi; infection of intrahepatic biliary radicles is termed *ascending cholangitis.* The bacteria are usually enteric gram-negative aerobes, such as *E. coli,* Klebsiella, Clostridium, Bacteroides, or Enterobacter, and group D streptococci. Cholangitis usually generates fever, chills, abdominal pain, and jaundice, accompanied by acute inflammation of the wall of the bile ducts with entry of neutrophils into the luminal space. Intermittence of symptoms suggests bouts of partial obstruction. The most severe form of cholangitis is suppurative cholangitis, in which purulent bile fills and distends bile ducts. These infections are prone to extending into the hepatic substance and causing liver abscesses. Because sepsis rather than cholestasis tends to dominate the picture, prompt diagnostic evaluation and intervention are imperative in these unstable patients.

CHOLEDOCHAL CYSTS

Choledochal cysts are congenital dilatations of the common bile duct, presenting most often in children before age 10 with the nonspecific symptoms of jaundice or recurrent abdominal pain typical of biliary colic, or both. Approximately 20% of patients become symptomatic only in adulthood; these sometimes occur in conjunction with cystic dilatation of the intrahepatic biliary tree (Caroli's disease; see earlier). The female-to-male ratio is 3 to 4:1.[140] These uncommon cysts may take the form of segmental or cylindrical dilatation of the common bile duct, diverticula of the extrahepatic ducts, or choledochoceles, which are cystic lesions that protrude into the duodenal lumen. Choledochal cysts predispose to stone formation, stenosis and stricture, pancreatitis, and obstructive biliary complications within the liver. In the older patient, the risk of bile duct carcinoma is elevated.

TUMORS

Although heterotopic tissues and carcinoids, fibromas, myomas, neuromas, hemangiomas, and their malignant counterparts have been described in the biliary tract, the neoplasms of primary clinical importance are those derived from the epithelium lining the biliary tree.[141] Adenomas are benign epithelial tumors, representing localized neoplastic growth of the lining epithelium. Adenomas are classified as tubular, papillary, and tubulopapillary and may be histologically indistinguishable from intestinal adenomas (see Chapter 17). In the gallbladder, they may be sessile or pedunculated and are generally under 1 cm in size and are visualized as immobile translucent lesions on imaging studies or found incidentally on cholecystectomy. Adenomas of the bile ducts are even less common and frequently present with obstructive symptoms. As with alimentary tract adenomas, a close relationship appears to exist with the development of carcinoma; some 10% of adenomas show evidence of carcinoma in situ.

CARCINOMA OF THE GALLBLADDER

Carcinoma of the gallbladder is the fifth most common cancer of the digestive tract, is slightly more common in women, and occurs most frequently in the seventh decade of life. Only rarely is it discovered at a resectable stage, and the mean 5-year survival has remained for many years at about 1%, despite surgical intervention.[142] Gallstones are present in 60 to 90% of patients but not 100%; in Asia, where pyogenic and parasitic disease of the biliary tree is common, the coexistence of gallstones is much lower. Whether gallbladders containing stones or infectious agents develop cancer as a result of irritative trauma and chronic inflammation remains uncertain.[135] Carcinogenic derivatives of bile acids also may play a role.

MORPHOLOGY. Carcinomas of the gallbladder exhibit two patterns of growth: **infiltrating** and **fungating.** The infiltrating pattern is more common

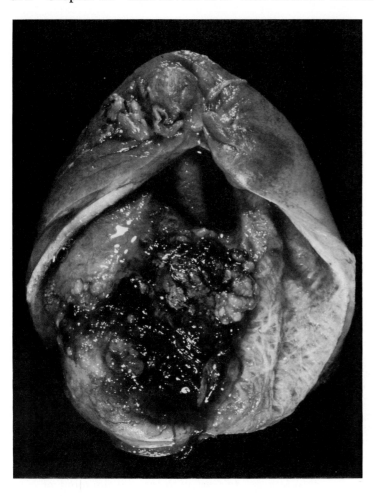

Figure 18-48. Carcinoma of the gallbladder as seen with the opened fundus. The neoplasm has fungated into the lumen and is partially hemorrhagic.

and usually appears as a poorly defined area of diffuse thickening and induration of the gallbladder wall that may cover several square centimeters or may involve the entire gallbladder. These tumors are scirrhous and have a firm consistency. The fungating pattern grows into the lumen as an irregular, cauliflower-like mass but at the same time invades the underlying wall. The luminal portion may be necrotic, hemorrhagic, and ulcerated (Fig. 18-48). The most common sites of involvement are the fundus and neck; about 20% involve the lateral walls. Direct penetration of the gallbladder wall into the liver bed or fistula formation to adjacent viscera may occur.

Most carcinomas of the gallbladder are adenocarcinomas. Some are papillary and others are infiltrative and poorly differentiated to undifferentiated (Fig. 18-49). About 5% are squamous cell carcinomas or have adenosquamous differentiation. A minority may exhibit carcinoid or a variety of mesenchymal features. By the time these neoplasms are discovered, **most have spread locally and invaded the liver,** and many have extended to the cystic duct and adjacent bile ducts and portahepatic lymph nodes. The peritoneum, gastrointestinal tract, and lungs are common sites of seeding; distant metastasis is uncommon.

CLINICAL COURSE. Preoperative diagnosis of carcinoma of the gallbladder is the exception rather than the rule, occurring in less than 20% of patients. Presenting symptoms are insidious and typically indistinguishable from those associated with cholelithiasis: abdominal pain, jaundice, anorexia, and nausea and vomiting. The fortunate patient develops a palpable, enlarged gallbladder and pain before extension of the tumor into adjacent structures, or has incidental carcinoma at the time of cholecystectomy for symptomatic gallstones. This cancer is sufficiently rare that prophylactic cholecystectomy for asymptomatic gallstones is not justified.

CARCINOMA OF THE EXTRAHEPATIC BILE DUCTS

This category refers to malignancies of the extrahepatic biliary tree, down to the level of the ampulla of Vater. Cancers arising in the immediate vicinity of the ampulla also include pancreatic carcinoma and adenomas of the ampullary orifice (see section on adenomas in Chapter 17); this particular group of tumors are referred to collectively as *periampullary carcinomas*.

Bile duct carcinoma is uncommon. The same age range is affected as in carcinoma of the gall-

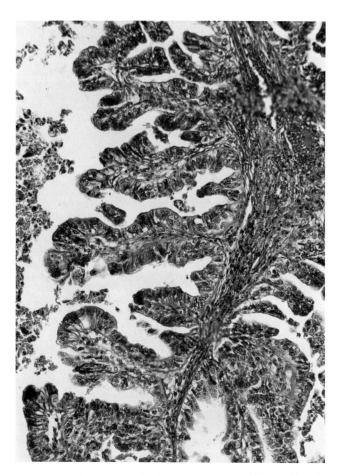

Figure 18–49. A detail of adenocarcinoma of the gallbladder, showing well-developed papillary formations.

bladder, but bile duct carcinoma is slightly more frequent in males. The role of gallstones is unconvincing because they are present in only 35 to 50% of cases. Choledochal cysts, ulcerative colitis, and chronic biliary infection with *Clonorchis sinensis* and *Giardia lamblia* impart an increased risk for bile duct carcinoma, but such cases represent a minority of patients.

MORPHOLOGY. These tumors are generally small lesions at the time of diagnosis. Most tumors appear as firm, gray nodules within the bile duct wall; some may be diffusely infiltrative lesions, and others are papillary, polypoid lesions. The vast majority of bile duct tumors are adenocarcinomas, which may or may not be mucin secreting. Uncommonly squamous features are present. For the most part, an abundant fibrous stroma accompanies the epithelial proliferation. Tumors arising from the part of the common bile duct between the cystic duct junction and the confluence of the right and left hepatic ducts at the liver hilus are called **Klatskin tumors.**[143] These tumors are notable for their slow-growing behavior, marked sclerosing characteristics, and the infrequent occurrence of distal metastases.

CLINICAL COURSE. Jaundice generally arises owing to obstruction, often preceded by decolorization of the stools, nausea and vomiting, and weight loss. Hepatomegaly is present in about 50% and a palpable gallbladder in about 25%.[142] Associated changes are elevated levels of serum alkaline phosphatase and transaminases and bile-stained urine. Differentiation of obstructive jaundice owing to calculous disease or other benign conditions from neoplasia is a major clinical problem because the presence of stones does not preclude the existence of concomitant malignancy. The majority of ductal cancers are not surgically resectable at the time of diagnosis, despite their small size. Mean survival times range from 6 to 18 months, regardless of whether aggressive resections or palliative surgery are performed.[144] Metastatic spread is uncommon because death comes so soon.

MISCELLANEOUS DISORDERS OF THE BILIARY TREE

Cholesterolosis of the gallbladder refers to focal accumulations of triglyceride and cholesterol-laden macrophages within the tips of mucosal folds directly beneath the columnar epithelium. The mucosal surface is studded with minute yellow flecks and polypoid projections producing the *"strawberry" gallbladder*. This condition causes no symptoms and does not predispose to cholecystitis. It has been attributed without proof to imbibition of cholesterol from supersaturated bile.

Inflammatory polyps constitute sessile mucosal projections, with a surface of columnar epithelial cells covering a fibrous stroma infiltrated with chronic inflammatory cells and lipid-laden macrophages. These lesions must be differentiated from neoplasms on imaging studies.

Adenomyosis of the gallbladder is characterized by hyperplasia of the muscularis, containing intramural hyperplastic diverticula or crypts. The localized form is sometimes termed an *adenomyoma*, but it is not a true neoplasm; it consists of a sessile mass in the fundus.[135] Segmental and diffuse forms can produce more generalized thickening of the gallbladder, hence the alternative name cholecystitis glandularis proliferans.

IATROGENIC INJURY TO THE BILIARY TREE

As a hollow viscus lying adjacent to the liver, the gallbladder is the occasional recipient of a needle thrust from percutaneous liver biopsy or transhepatic cholangiography. Needles are also intentionally introduced for diagnostic and therapeutic procedures. In both instances, subsequent leaks of irritant bile can give rise to chemically induced inflammation of the peritoneum, so-called *bile peritonitis*. Repeated infusion of chemotherapeutic agents into the hepatic artery for metastatic liver disease may cause iatrogenic *drug injury*. Because the intrahepatic and extrahepatic bile ducts and gallbladder are sustained by branches of this artery, chemically induced arterial obliteration can lead to a sclerosing cholangitis-like picture in the biliary tree with loss of intrahepatic bile ducts or an acute cholecystitis progressing to chronic fibrosis.[145] Finally, *biliary stricture* uncommonly follows operative trauma, involving iatrogenic injury to the biliary tree or the feeding vasculature. Less than 10% of strictures of the common bile duct are caused by pancreatitis, external trauma, and other rare causes. Strictures proximal to the cystic duct are usually malignant. With this melange of "goodies," we end the consideration of the liver and its appendages.

1. Rapaport, A.M.: The structural and functional units of the human liver (liver acinus). Microvasc. Res. 6:212, 1973.
2. Gumucio, J.J., and Chianale, J.: Liver cell heterogeneity and liver function. *In* Arias, I.M., et al. (eds.): The Liver: Biology and Pathobiology, 2nd. ed. New York, Raven Press, 1988, pp. 931–947.
3. Watanabe, N., et al.: Motility of bile canaliculi in the living animal: Implications for bile flow. J Cell Biol. 113:1069, 1991.
4. Riepe, S.P., and Galambos, J.T.: Cirrhosis. *In* Gitnick, G. (ed): Current Hepatology. Vol. IV. New York, John Wiley & Sons, 1984, p. 117.
5. Sherman, I.A., et al.: Hepatic microvascular changes associated with development of liver fibrosis and cirrhosis. Am. J. Physiol. 258:H460, 1990.
6. Anthony, P.P., et al.: The morphology of cirrhosis: Definition, nomenclature, and classification. Bull. W.H.O. 55:521, 1977.
7. Fauerholdt, L., et al.: Conversion of micronodular cirrhosis into macronodular cirrhosis. Hepatology 3:928, 1983.
8. Shah, M.C., and Barton, L.L.: Congenital syphilitic hepatitis. Pediatr. Infect. Dis. J. 8:891, 1989.
9. Scheig, R.: Defenestration of hepatic sinusoids in the pathogenesis of alcoholic hyperlipoproteinemia. Hepatology 11:148, 1990.
10. Maher, J.J., and McGuire, R.F.: Extracellular matrix gene expression increases preferentially in rat lipocytes and sinusoidal endothelial cells during hepatic fibrosis in vivo. J. Clin. Invest. 86:1641, 1990.
11. Friedman, S.L., et al: Isolated hepatic lipocytes and Kupffer cells from normal human liver: Morphological and functional characteristics in primary culture. Hepatology 15:234, 1992.
12. Maher, J.J.: Hepatic fibrosis caused by alcohol. Semin. Liver Dis. 10:66, 1990.
13. Groszman, R.J., and Atterbury, C.E.: The pathophysiology of portal hypertension: A basis for classification. Semin. Liver Dis. 2:177, 1982.
14. Korula, J.: Ascites: Pathogenesis, characteristics, complications, and treatment. *In* Kaplowitz, N. (ed): Liver and Biliary Diseases. Baltimore, Williams & Wilkins, 1992, pp. 529–541.
15. Slott, P.A., et al.: Origin, pattern, and mechanism of bile duct proliferation following biliary obstruction in the rat. Gastroenterology. 99:466, 1990.
16. Arias, I.M., et al.: Chronic nonhemolytic unconjugated hyperbilirubinemia with glucuronyl transferase deficiency. Am. J. Med. 47:395, 1969.
17. Watson, K.J.R., and Gollan, J.L.: Gilbert's syndrome. Bailliere's Clin. Gastroenterol. 3:337, 1989.
18. Kitamura, T., et al.: Defective biliary excretion of epinephrine metabolites in mutant (TR−) rats: Relation to the pathogenesis of black liver in the Dubin-Johnson syndrome and Corriedale sheep with an analogous excretory defect. Hepatology 15:1154, 1992.
19. Soltis, R.D.: New concepts in viral hepatitis. Geriatrics 36:62, 1981.
20. Lesnicar, G.: A prospective study of viral hepatitis A and the question of chronicity. Hepatogastroenterology 35:69, 1988.
21. Lemon, S.M.: Type A viral hepatitis. New developments in an old disease. N. Engl. J. Med. 313:1059, 1985.
22. Lemon, S.M.: Inactivated hepatitis A virus vaccines. Hepatology 15:1194, 1992.
23. Lau, J.Y.N., and Wright, T.L.: Molecular virology and pathogenesis of hepatitis B. Lancet 342:1335, 1993.
24. Miller, R.H.: Comparative molecular biology of the hepatitis viruses. Semin. Liver Dis. 11:113, 1991.
25. Katkov, W.N., and Dienstag, J.L.: Prevention and therapy of viral hepatitis. Semin. Liver Dis. 11:165, 1991.
26. Feitelson, M., and London, W.T.: Virus gene products as immunologic targets in acute hepatitis B. Lab. Invest. 62: 667, 1990.
27. Colombari, R., et al: Chronic hepatitis in multiple virus infection: Histopathological evaluation. Histopathology 22:319, 1993.
28. Milich, D.R.: Immune response to hepatitis B virus proteins: Relevance of the murine model. Semin. Liver Dis. 11:93, 1991.
29. Foster, G.R., et al.: Replication of hepatitis B and delta viruses: Appearance of viral mutants. Semin. Liver Dis. 11:121, 1991.
30. Carman, W.F., et al.: Vaccine-induced escape mutant of hepatitis B virus. Lancet 336:325, 1990.
31. Choo, Q., et al.: Isolation of a cDNA clone derived from a blood-borne non-A, non-B viral hepatitis genome. Science 224:359, 1989.
32. Weiland, O., and Schvarcz, R.: Hepatitis C: Virology, epidemiology, clinical course, and treatment. Scand. J. Gastroenterol. 27:337, 1992.
33. Plagemann, P.G.W.: Hepatitis C virus. Arch. Virol. 120: 165, 1991.
34. Puoti, M., et al.: Hepatitis C virus RNA and antibody response in the clinical course of acute hepatitis C virus infection. Hepatology 16:877, 1992.
35. Lok, A.S.F., et al.: Hepatitis C viremia in patients with hepatitis C virus infection. Hepatology 15:1007, 1992.
36. Farci, P., et al.: Lack of protective immunity against reinfection with hepatitic C virus. Science 258:135, 1992.
37. Hoofnagle, J.H.: Type D (delta) hepatitis. J.A.M.A. 261: 1321, 1989.
38. Caredda, F., et al.: Course and prognosis of acute HDV hepatitis. *In* Rizzetto, M., et al. (eds.): Hepatitis Delta Virus and Its Infection. New York; Alan R. Liss, 1987, pp. 267–276.
39. Goldsmith, R., et al.: Enzyme-linked immunosorbent assay for diagnosis of acute sporadic hepatitis E in Egyptian children. Lancet 339:328, 1992.
40. Bradley, D.W., et al.: Non-A, non-B hepatitis: Toward the discovery of hepatitis C and E viruses. Semin. Liver Dis. 11:128, 1991.
41. Huang, R.T. et al.: Isolation and identification of hepatitis E virus in Xinjiang, China. J. Gen. Virol. 73:1143, 1992.
42. Rosina, F., et al.: Risk of post-transfusion infection with the hepatitis delta virus: A multicenter study. N. Engl. J. Med. 312:1488, 1985.
43. Bianchi, L., and Gudat, F.: Sanded nuclei in hepatitis B: Eosinophilic inclusions in liver cell nuclei due to excess in hepatitis B core antigen formation. Lab. Invest. 35:1, 1976.

44. Gerber, M.A. and Thung, S.N.: The diagnostic value of immunohistochemical demonstration of hepatitis viral antigens in the liver. Hum. Pathol. 18:771, 1987.

45. Akyol, G., et al.: Detection of hepatitis C virus RNA sequences by polymerase chain reaction in fixed liver tissue. Modern Pathol. 5:501, 1992.

46. Dan, M., and Yaniv, R.: Cholestatic hepatitis, cutaneous vasculitis, and vascular deposits of immunoglobulin M and complement associated with hepatitis A virus infection. Am. J. Med. 89:103, 1990.

47. Scheuer, P.J., et al.: The pathology of hepatitis C. Hepatology 15:567, 1992.

48. De Groote, J., et al.: A classification of chronic hepatitis. Lancet 2:626, 1968.

49. Popper, H., and Schaffner, F.: The vocabulary of chronic hepatitis. N. Engl. J. Med. 284:1154, 1971.

50. Scheuer, P.J.: Classification of chronic viral hepatitis: A need for reassessment. J. Hepatol. 13:372, 1991.

51. Davis, F.L.: Chronic hepatitis. In Kaplowitz, N. (ed): Liver and Biliary Diseases. Baltimore, Williams & Wilkins, 1992; pp. 289–299.

52. Bach, N., et al: The histological features of chronic hepatitis C and autoimmune chronic hepatitis: A comparative analysis. Hepatology 15:572, 1992.

53. Deodhar, K.P., et al: Orcein staining of hepatitis B antigen in paraffin sections of liver biopsies. J. Clin. Pathol. 28:66, 1975.

54. Meyer zum Buschenfelde, K.-H.: Autoimmune hepatitis. Semin. Liver Dis. 11:183, 1991.

55. Douglas, D.D., and Rakela, J.: Fulminant hepatitis. In Kaplowitz, N. (ed.): Liver and Biliary Diseases. Baltimore, Williams & Wilkins, 1992; pp. 279–288.

56. Bertel, C.K., et al.: Treatment of pyogenic hepatic abscesses. Arch. Surg. 121:554, 1986.

57. Kaplowitz, N.: Drug metabolism and hepatotoxicity. In Kaplowitz, N. (ed.): Liver and Biliary Diseases. Baltimore, Williams & Wilkins, 1992, pp. 82–97.

58. Carithers, R.L., Jr.: Alcoholic hepatitis and cirrhosis. In Kaplowitz, N. (ed.): Liver and Biliary Diseases. Baltimore, Williams & Wilkins, 1992, pp. 334–346.

59. Ishak, K.G., et al.: Alcoholic liver disease: Pathologic, pathogenetic and clinical aspects. Alcoholism (N.Y.) 15:45, 1991.

60. Worner, T.M., and Lieber, C.S.: Perivenular fibrosis as precursor lesion of cirrhosis. J.A.M.A. 254:627, 1985.

61. Mihas, A.A., and Tavassoli, M.: The effect of ethanol on the uptake, binding, and desialylation of transferrin by rat liver endothelium: Implications in the pathogenesis of alcohol-associated hepatic siderosis. Am. J. Med. Sci. 301:299, 1991.

62. Lauterburg, B.H.: Pathogenesis of alcoholic liver disease. Schweiz Med. Wochenschr. 122: 609, 1992.

63. Paronetto, F.: Ethanol and the immune system. In Seitz, H.K., and Kommerell, H.B. (eds.): Alcohol-Related Diseases in Gastroenterology. Berlin, Springer-Verlag, 1985, pp. 269–281.

64. Frezza, M., et al.: High blood levels in women: The role of decreased gastric alcohol dehydrogenase activity and first-pass metabolism. N. Engl. J. Med. 322:95, 1990.

65. Randall, B.: Fatty liver and sudden death. Hum. Pathol. 11:147, 1980.

66. Nichols, G.M., and Bacon, B.: Hereditary hemochromatosis: Pathogenesis and clinical features of a common disease. Am. J. Gastroenterol. 84:851, 1989.

67. Lee, S.C., et al.: Localization of the haemochromatosis gene close to D6S105 (abstr). Hepatology 16:317, 1992.

68. Edwards, C.Q., et al.: Prevalence of hemochromatosis among 11,065 presumably healthy blood donors. N. Engl. J. Med. 318:1355, 1988.

69. LeSage, G.D., et al.: Hemochromatosis: Genetic or alcohol-induced? Gastroenterology 84:1471, 1983.

70. Gordeuk, V., et al.: Iron overload in Africa: Interaction between a gene and dietary iron content. N. Engl. J. Med. 326:95, 1992.

71. Bassett, M.L., et al.: Value of hepatic iron measurements in early hemochromatosis and determination of the critical iron level associated with fibrosis. Hepatology 6:24, 1986.

72. Niederau, C., et al.: Survival and causes of death in cirrhotic and in noncirrhotic patients with primary hemochromatosis. N. Engl. J. Med. 313:1256, 1985.

73. Gollan, J.L.: Copper metabolism, Wilson's disease, and hepatic copper toxicosis. In Zakim, D., and Boyer, T.D. (eds): Hepatology: A Textbook of Liver Disease. Philadelphia, W.B. Saunders Co., 1990; pp. 1249–1272.

74. Gross, J.B., et al.: Biliary copper excretion by hepatocyte lysosomes in the rat: Major excretory pathway in experimental copper overload. J. Clin. Invest. 83:30, 1989.

75. Frydman, M.: Genetic aspects of Wilson's disease. J. Gastroenterol. Hepatol. 5:483, 1990.

76. Nartey, N.O., et al.: Hepatic copper and metallothionein distribution in Wilson's disease (hepatolenticular degeneration). Lab. Invest. 57:397, 1987.

77. Elmes, M.E., et al.: Metallothionein and copper in liver disease with copper retention—a histopathological study. J. Pathol. 158:131, 1989.

78. Miyamura, H., et al.: Survey of copper granules in liver biopsy specimens from various liver abnormalities other than Wilson's disease and biliary diseases. Gastroenterol. Jap. 23:633, 1988.

79. Sternlieb, I.: Perspectives on Wilson's disease. Hepatology 12:1234, 1990.

80. Whitington, P.F.: Metabolic liver diseases of childhood. In Kaplowitz, N. (ed.): Liver and Biliary Diseases. Baltimore, Williams & Wilkins, 1992; pp. 456–478.

81. Perlmutter, D.H.: The cellular basis for liver injury in α_1-antitrypsin deficiency. Hepatology 13:172, 1991.

82. Gadek, J.E., et al.: Antielastases of the human alveolar structure: Implications for the protease-antiprotease theory of emphysema. J. Clin. Invest. 68:889, 1981.

83. Sveger, T.: The natural history of liver disease in alpha-1-antitrypsin deficient children. Acta Paediatr. Scand. 77:847, 1988.

84. Yunis, E.J., et al.: Fine structural observations of the liver in alpha-1-antitrypsin deficiency. Am. J. Pathol. 82:265, 1976.

85. Birrer, P., et al.: α_1-Antitrypsin deficiency and liver disease. J. Inherited Metab. Dis. 14:512, 1991.

86. Meythaler, J.N., and Varma, R.R.: Reye's syndrome in adults. Diagnostic considerations. Arch. Intern. Med. 147:61, 1987.

87. Holtzhauer, F.J., et al.: Reye's syndrome. An epidemiologic analysis of mild disease. Am. J. Dis. Child. 140:1231, 1986.

88. Kimura, S., and Amemiya, F.: Brain and liver pathology in a patient with carnitine deficiency. Brain Dev. 12:436, 1990.

89. Balistreri, W.F.: Neonatal cholestasis. Semin. Liver Dis. 7:67, 1987.

90. Balistreri, W.F.: Neonatal cholestasis: Medical progress. J. Pediatr. 106:171, 1985.

91. Craig, J.M., and Landing, B.H.: Form of hepatitis in neonatal period simulating biliary atresia. Arch. Pathol. Lab. Med. 54:321, 1952.

92. Scheuer, P.J.: Liver Biopsy Interpretation. London, Bailliere Tindall, 1988; pp. 53–62.

93. Rubin, E., et al.: Primary biliary cirrhosis. Chronic, non-suppurative, destructive cholangitis. Am. J. Pathol. 46:387, 1965.

94. Fussey, S.P.M., et al.: Clarification of the identity of the major M2 autoantigen in primary biliary cirrhosis. Clin. Sci. 80:451, 1991.

95. Mistry, P., and Seymour, C.A.: Primary biliary cirrhosis—from Thomas Addison to the 1990s. Q. J. Med. 82:185, 1992.

96. Scheuer, P.J.: Primary biliary cirrhosis. Proc. R. Soc. Med. 60:1257, 1967.

97. Lindor, K.D., et al.: Advances in primary sclerosing cholangitis. Am. J. Med. *89*:73, 1990.

98. Chapman, R.W.: Role of immune factors in the pathogenesis of primary sclerosing cholangitis. Semin. Liver Dis. *11*:1, 1991.

99. Ludwig, J., et al.: Floxuridine-induced sclerosing cholangitis: An ischemic cholangiopathy? Hepatology *9*:215, 1989.

100. Desmet, V.J.: Congenital diseases of intrahepatic bile ducts: Variations on the theme "ductal plate malformation." Hepatology *16*:1069, 1992.

101. Caroli, J.: Diseases of the intrahepatic biliary tree. Clin. Gastroenterol. *2*:147, 1973.

102. Cobben, J.M., et al.: Congenital hepatic fibrosis in autosomal-dominant polycystic kidney disease. Kidney Int. *38*:880, 1990.

103. Ramos, A., et al.: The liver in autosomal dominant polycystic kidney disease: Implications for pathogenesis. Arch. Pathol. Lab. Med. *114*:180, 1990.

104. Ohnishi, K., et al.: Portal hemodynamics in idiopathic portal hypertension (Banti's syndrome): Comparison with chronic persistent hepatitis and normal subjects. Gastroenterology *92*:751, 1987.

105. Arcidi, J.M., Jr., et al.: Hepatic morphology in cardiac dysfunction: A clinicopathologic study of 1000 subjects at autopsy. Am. J. Pathol. *104*:159, 1981.

106. Schorr-Lesnick, B., et al.: Liver diseases unique to pregnancy. Am. J. Gastroenterol. *86*:659, 1991.

107. Weinstein, L.: Syndrome of hemolysis, elevated liver enzymes, and low platelet count: A severe consequence of hypertension in pregnancy. Am. J. Obstet. Gynecol. *142*:159, 1982.

108. Riely, C.A.: Acute fatty liver of pregnancy. Semin. Liver Dis. *7*:47, 1987.

109. Rolfes, D.B., and Ishak, K.G.: Acute fatty liver of pregnancy: A clinicopathologic study of 35 cases. Hepatology *5*:1149, 1985.

110. McDonald, G.B., et al.: Liver disease after human marrow transplantation. Semin. Liver Dis. *7*:210, 1987.

111. Crawford, J.M., and Ferrell, L.D.: The liver in transplantation. In Rustgi, V.K., and Van Thiel, D.H. (eds.): The Liver in Systemic Diseases. New York, Raven Press, 1993, pp. 337–364.

112. Snover, D.C.: Problems in the interpretation of liver biopsies after liver transplantation. Am. J. Surg. Pathol. *13*(Suppl.1):31, 1989.

113. Caldwell-Kenkel, J.C., et al.: Kupffer cell activation and endothelial cell damage after storage of rat livers: Effects of reperfusion. Hepatology *13*:83, 1991.

114. Ng, I.O.L., et al.: Hepatocellular ballooning after liver transplantation: A light and electronmicroscopic study with clinicopathological correlation. Histopathology *18*:323, 1991.

115. Stromeyer, F.W., and Ishak, K.G.: Nodular transformation (nodular "regenerative" hyperplasia) of the liver: A clinicopathologic study of 30 cases. Hum. Pathol. *12*:60, 1981.

116. Nakanuma, Y.: Nodular regenerative hyperplasia of the liver: Retrospective survey in autopsy series. J. Clin. Gastroenterol. *12*:460, 1990.

117. Wanless, I.R.: Micronodular transformation (nodular regenerative hyperplasia) of the liver: A report of 64 cases among 2,500 autopsies and a new classification of benign hepatocellular nodules. Hepatology *11*:787, 1990.

118. Yager, J.D., et al.: Sex hormones and tumor promotion in liver. Proc. Soc. Exp. Biol. Med. *198*:667, 1991.

119. Beasley, R.P.: Hepatitis B virus, the major etiology of hepatocellular carcinoma. Cancer *61*:1942, 1988.

120. Etiology, Pathology and Treatment of Hepatocellular Carcinoma in North America. Houston, Gulf Publishing, 1991.

121. Craig, J.R., et al.: Fibrolamellar carcinoma of the liver. Cancer *46*:372, 1980.

122. Berman, M.A.: Fibrolamellar carcinoma of the liver: An immunohistochemical study of nineteen cases and a review of the literature. Hum. Pathol. *19*:784, 1988.

123. Soulier, J.-P., et al.: A new method to assay des-gamma-carboxyprothrombin. Results obtained in 75 cases of hepatocellular carcinoma. Gastroenterology *91*:1258, 1986.

124. Nagasue, N., et al.: The natural history of hepatocellular carcinoma. A study of 100 untreated cases. Cancer *54*:1461, 1984.

125. Hay, D.W., and Carey, M.C.: Pathophysiology and pathogenesis of cholesterol gallstone formation. Semin. Liver Dis. *10*:159, 1990.

126. Carey, M.C., and LaMont, J.T.: Cholesterol gallstone formation. 1. Physical-chemistry of bile and biliary lipid secretion. Prog. Liver Dis. *10*:139, 1992.

127. Carey, M.C., and Cahalane, M.J.: The enterohepatic circulation. In Arias, I., et al. (eds.): The Liver: Biology and Pathobiology. New York: Raven Press, 1988; pp. 573–616.

128. Janson, J.A., et al.: Choledocholithiasis and a double gallbladder. Gastrointest. Endosc. *38*:377, 1992.

129. Carey, M.C., and O'Donovan, M.A.: Gallstone disease: Current concepts on the epidemiology, pathogenesis and management. In Petersdorf, R.G., et al. (eds.): Harrison's Principles of Internal Medicine, Update V. New York, McGraw-Hill, 1984, pp. 139–168.

130. LaMont, J.T., and Carey, M.C.: Cholesterol gallstone formation. 2. Pathobiology and pathomechanics. Prog. Liver Dis. *10*:165, 1992.

131. Gibbons, A.: Geneticists trace the DNA trail of the first Americans. Science *259*:312, 1993.

132. Holzbach, R.T., et al.: Pathogenesis of cholesterol gallstone disease: The physico-chemical defect. In Northfield, T., et al. (eds.): Bile Acids in Health and Disease. Dordrecht, Kluwer Academic Publishers, 1988; pp. 117–133.

133. Cahalane, M.J., et al.: Physical-chemical pathogenesis of pigment gallstones. Semin. Liver Dis. *8*:317, 1988.

134. Carey, M.C.: Pathogenesis of gallstones. Rec. Prog. Med. *83*:379, 1992.

135. Malet, P.F.: Complications of cholelithiasis. In Kaplowitz, N. (ed.): Liver and Biliary Diseases. Baltimore, Williams & Wilkins, 1992, pp. 610–627.

136. Lin, K.Y.-K.: Acute acalculous cholecystitis: A limited review of the literature. Mt. Sinai J. Med. *53*:305, 1986.

137. Savoca, P.E., et al.: The increasing prevalence of acalculous cholecystitis in outpatients. Ann. Surg. *211*:433, 1990.

138. Williamson, R.C.N.: Acalculous disease of the gallbladder. Gut *29*:860, 1988.

139. Raweily, E.A., et al.: Abnormalities of intrahepatic bile ducts in extrahepatic biliary atresia. Histopathology *17*:521, 1990.

140. Oldham, K.T., et al.: Choledochal cysts presenting in late childhood and adulthood. Am. J. Surg. *141*:568, 1981.

141. Albores-Saavedra, J., et al.: The WHO Histological Classification of Tumors of the Gallbladder and Extrahepatic Bile Ducts: A commentary on the second edition. Cancer *70*:410, 1992.

142. Anderson, J.B., et al.: Adenocarcinoma of the extrahepatic biliary tree. Ann. R. Coll. Surg. *67*:139, 1985.

143. Klatskin G.: Adenocarcinoma of the hepatic duct at its bifurcation within the porta hepatis. Am. J. Med. *38*:241, 1965.

144. Lygidakis, N.J., and Van der Heyde, M.N.: Klatskin tumors. Semin. Liver Dis. *10*:85, 1992.

145. Andrews, J.C., et al.: Hepatobiliary toxicity of 5-fluoro-2'-deoxyuridine: Intra-arterial versus portal venous routes of infusion. Invest. Radiol. *26*:461, 1991.

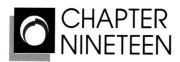

CHAPTER NINETEEN

The Pancreas

JAMES M. CRAWFORD, M.D., Ph.D., and RAMZI S. COTRAN, M.D.

The Exocrine Pancreas

NORMAL

In its posterior location in the upper abdomen, the pancreas is one of the "hidden" organs in the body. It is virtually impossible to palpate clinically. Diseases that impair its function evoke signs or symptoms only when far advanced, because there is such a large reserve of both exocrine and endocrine function. Some life-threatening lesions are manifested only by encroachment on neighboring structures, such as the gut and vertebral column. Thus, detection of pancreatic disease continues to be a source of frustration in modern medicine.

In the adult, the average pancreas is about 15 cm in length, weighs 60 to 140 gm, and consists of a head, a body, and a tail. The pancreas arises from the duodenum in the form of a dorsal bud and a shorter ventral bud.[1] Fusion of the two creates the composite head, with the dorsal bud being the primary source of the tapering body and tail. The ductal drainage systems anastomose, and the definitive pancreatic duct (the duct of Wirsung) is formed by fusion of the ventral duct with the distal portion of the dorsal duct. Occasionally, the proximal portion of the dorsal duct persists as the accessory duct of Santorini. Although there is much variability in the ductal system, in two-thirds of adults the major pancreatic duct does not empty directly into the duodenum but into the common bile duct just proximal to the ampulla of Vater, thus providing a common channel for pancreatic and biliary drainage.

The gross anatomic relationships of the pancreas include immediate proximity to the duodenum, ampulla of Vater, common bile duct, superior mesenteric artery, portal vein, spleen and its vascular supply, stomach, transverse colon, left lobe of the liver, and lower recesses of the lesser omental cavity (Fig. 19–1). The pancreas is a pinkish-tan organ with distinct coarse lobulations, the result of delicate collagen septa that subdivide the parenchyma into macroscopic lobules.

Histologically, the pancreas has two separate components, the exocrine and endocrine glands. The endocrine pancreas is described later in this chapter. The exocrine portion, constituting 80 to 85% of the organ, is made up of numerous small glands (acini) containing columnar to pyramidal epithelial cells radially oriented about the gland circumference. Small microvilli project from the apical surfaces of these secretory cells into the lumen. The acinar cells are deeply basophilic because of their abundant rough endoplasmic reticulum, located in the basal portion of the cell. The Golgi complex is well developed and is part of an apically oriented secretory complex that forms abundant membrane-bound zymogen granules containing digestive enzymes (Fig. 19–2). The ductal system of the pancreas is produced by progressive

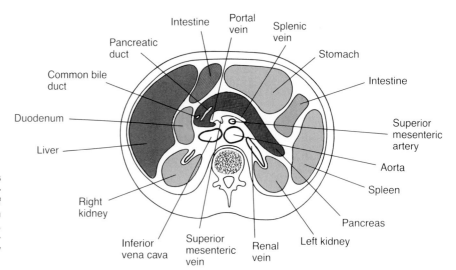

Figure 19-1. Anatomic relationships of the pancreas seen in a cross-section of the abdomen at the level of the upper lumbar vertebrae. (With permission from Go, V.W., et al. (eds): The Pancreas: Biology, Pathobiology, and Disease, 2nd ed. New York, Raven Press, 1993.)

anastomosis of the extremely fine radicles that drain each secretory acinus. The lining epithelium is at first cuboidal but becomes progressively higher to produce tall, columnar, mucus-secreting cells in the main ductal system. About the larger ducts, there are numerous accessory branching ducts and mucous glands.

It is hardly necessary here to reiterate the secretory functions of the pancreas and the regulatory mechanisms that control such activity. Several points, however, are directly pertinent to disease

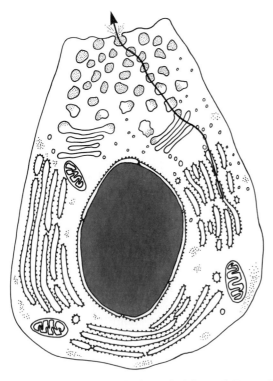

Figure 19-2. Ultrastructural characteristics of the acinar cell and the pathway (red line) for synthesis and secretion of zymogens.

processes and merit emphasis.[2] The pancreas secretes 1.5 to 3 liters per day of an alkaline fluid containing enzymes and proenzymes (zymogens). Secretion is adjusted to the workload that it is called on to handle, that is, the volume and character of the intestinal contents. The regulation of this secretion is a complex process that involves humoral and neural factors. The most important of these regulators are the hormones *secretin* and *cholecystokinin*, produced in the duodenum.[3] The former stimulates water and bicarbonate secretion by duct cells, and the latter enhances the discharge of zymogens by acinar cells. When the pancreas is stimulated to secretory activity, the zymogen granule-containing vesicles migrate to the apical plasma membrane, and rupture at the point of attachment to release their contents into the acinar lumen. Fats and alcohol are particularly active stimulators of secretin production and therefore, indirectly, of the pancreas.

A second point of interest relates to the elaboration of enzymes.[4] These include trypsin, chymotrypsin, aminopeptidases, elastase, amylases, lipases, and phospholipases. Trypsin itself is a key enzyme, as it catalyzes activation of the other enzymes. Self-digestion of the pancreas is prevented by several means: (1) these enzymes are synthesized as inactive proenzymes (with the exception of amylase and lipase); (2) they are sequestered in membrane-bound zymogen granules in the acinar cells; (3) activation of proenzymes requires conversion of inactive trypsinogen to active trypsin by duodenal enteropeptidase (enterokinase); (4) trypsin inhibitors are present within acini and pancreatic secretions; (5) intrapancreatic release of trypsin activates an enzyme(s) that degrades other zymogens to inert products; (6) lysosomal hydrolases are capable of degrading zymogen granules when normal acinar secretion is impaired or blocked; and (7) acinar cells are remarkably resistant to the action of trypsin, chymotrypsin, and phospholipase A_2.

PATHOLOGY

The most significant disorders of the exocrine pancreas are cystic fibrosis (see Chapter 10), acute and chronic pancreatitis, and tumors. It should be emphasized that, from the standpoints of both morbidity and mortality, diabetes mellitus (a disorder of endocrine metabolism) overshadows all other pancreatic disorders. However, a knowledgeable alertness to exocrine pancreatic disease is most necessary, since almost all these disorders are difficult to diagnose because of the hidden position and large reserve function of this organ, and because they appear under such diverse guises as a catastrophic "acute abdomen" or the silent growth of a carcinoma.

CONGENITAL ANOMALIES

Variations in pancreatic anatomy are usually of little clinical import, with some notable exceptions. The pancreas may be totally absent (agenesis), a condition that is regularly associated with widespread, severe malformations that are incompatible with life. The endocrine and exocrine elements may be hypoplastic. The gland may exist as two separate structures representing the persistence of the dorsal and ventral pancreas. The head of the pancreas may encircle the duodenum as a collar (annular pancreas), to sometimes cause subtotal duodenal obstruction and consequent clinical symptoms. Incomplete fusion of the two pancreatic anlagen creates pancreas divisum and predisposes to recurrent pancreatitis. Variable ductal anatomy of the pancreas may present particular problems to the endoscopist and surgeon. For example, the ducts of Wirsung and of Santorini may both persist as totally separate structures, with separate duodenal orifices. Failure to recognize aberrant ductal anatomy may lead to potential ligation or severance of ducts during surgery around the ampulla, causing serious sequelae.

ABERRANT PANCREAS

Aberrant, or ectopic, displaced pancreatic tissue is found in about 2% of careful routine postmortem examinations. The favored sites for ectopia are the stomach and duodenum, followed by the jejunum, Meckel's diverticulum, and the ileum. Usually, the rests are a few millimeters to centimeters in diameter, located in the submucosa. They are composed histologically of glands that appear completely normal, and not infrequently islets of Langerhans are present. Although usually incidental, such lesions may be visualized as sessile lesions, may cause pain from localized inflammation, or rarely may incite mucosal bleeding. About 2% of islet cell tumors arise in ectopic pancreatic tissue.

PANCREATITIS

Inflammation of the pancreas, almost always associated with acinar cell injury, is termed pancreatitis.[5] Clinically and histologically, pancreatitis presents as a spectrum, in both duration and severity. Acute pancreatitis includes a mild, self-limited form and a more serious type, acute hemorrhagic pancreatitis, which exhibits extensive hemorrhagic necrosis of the organ. Chronic pancreatitis is the process of continuous or relapsing inflammation of the pancreas, typically causing pain and leading to irreversible morphologic damage and permanent impairment of function.

ACUTE PANCREATITIS

Acute pancreatitis (also called "interstitial pancreatitis") is defined as an acute condition, typically presenting with abdominal pain and associated with raised levels of pancreatic enzymes (especially amylase and lipase) in the blood or urine.[5] Pancreatic inflammation is usually accompanied by edema and limited necrosis of pancreatic tissue. In its severe form, acute hemorrhagic pancreatitis, or "necrotizing pancreatitis," there is extensive fat necrosis in and about the pancreas and in other intra-abdominal fatty depots, and hemorrhage into the parenchyma of the pancreas.

EPIDEMIOLOGY AND PATHOGENESIS. Acute pancreatitis occurs most often in middle life. About 80% of cases are associated with two conditions: biliary tract disease and alcoholism (Table 19–1). Gallstones are present in 35 to 60% of cases of

Table 19–1. CONDITIONS AND ETIOLOGIC AGENTS ASSOCIATED WITH PANCREATITIS

CHOLELITHIASIS
ALCOHOLISM
IDIOPATHIC
OTHER CAUSES
  Abdominal operations
  Endoscopic procedures with injection into pancreatic duct
  Infection: bacterial, viral, and parasitic
  Ischemia or vasculitis
  Drugs
  Trauma
  Extension from adjacent inflamed tissues
  Mass lesions
  Endocrine/metabolic; hereditary hyperlipidemias, hypercalcemia, hemochromatosis, uremia, diabetic ketoacidosis, hypothermia

pancreatitis, and *about 5% of patients with gall-stones develop pancreatitis.* The percentage of cases of acute pancreatitis caused by alcoholism varies from 65% in the United States to 20% in Sweden and 5% or less in southern France and England.[6] The male-to-female ratio is 1:3 in the group with biliary tract disease, and 6:1 in those with alcoholism. Acute hemorrhagic pancreatitis represents about 5% of all cases of acute pancreatitis.

Among the less common causes of pancreatitis (see Table 19–1), several merit comment.[7]

- Rising antibody titers to the mumps and coxsackie viruses and to *Mycoplasma pneumoniae* in some patients suggest a role for these infectious agents.
- The helminth parasites *Ascaris lumbricoides* and *Clonorchis sinensis* are capable of occluding pancreatic ducts.
- Acute ischemia may be induced by vascular thrombosis, embolism, vasculitis (polyarteritis nodosa, systemic lupus erythematosus, Henoch-Schönlein purpura), and shock.
- Many drugs cause abdominal pain and elevated serum amylase levels. Those implicated in causing pancreatic injury are thiazide diuretics, azathioprine, estrogens, sulfonamides, furosemide, pentamidine, and procainamide.[8]
- Pancreatitis is occasionally associated with hyperlipoproteinemia (types I and V) and with hyperparathyroidism and other hypercalcemic states.

Of note, 10 to 20% of cases have no known associated processes and must be termed "idiopathic."

The ultimate pathogenetic process in acute pancreatitis is the proteolysis, lipolysis, and hemorrhage resulting from the destructive effect of pancreatic enzymes released from acinar cells. Thus, proteases (trypsin, chymotrypsin), lipases and phospholipases (which degrade lipids and membrane phospholipids), and elastase (which breaks down the elastic tissue of vessels) are the keys to pancreatic destruction. Trypsin, which is capable of activating all the other proenzymes, also converts prekallikrein to kallikrein, thereby activating the kinin system. The clotting and complement system is thus indirectly activated (see Chapter 3). These mediators further contribute to the local inflammation, thrombosis, tissue damage, and hemorrhage characteristic of acute hemorrhagic pancreatitis.

What remains to be clarified is how pancreatic enzymes are activated and released within the pancreas. Proposals about possible mechanisms of pancreatic injury (Fig. 19–3), based on animal studies, are as follows:[7]

1. *Duct obstruction* (see Fig. 19–3, *left*). Since the main pancreatic duct joins the common bile duct in two-thirds of normal individuals, gallstones impacted in the ampulla of Vater can, presumably, cause pancreatic obstruction. Continued pancreatic

secretion produces increased ductal pressure, which is thought to lead to rupture of small pancreatic ductules, extravasation of pancreatic secretions into the interstitium, digestive enzyme activation, and subsequent pancreatitis. How the enzymes become activated remains unclear. Reflux of bile *per se* is not felt to play a role.

The manner by which alcohol precipitates pancreatitis is unknown. It must be stated that *most cases of alcoholic pancreatitis now appear to be acute exacerbations of chronic pancreatitis, rather than acute pancreatitis* per se. Chronic alcohol ingestion causes secretion of a protein-rich pancreatic fluid, leading to deposition of inspissated protein plugs and their calcification. *These concretions also may cause obstruction of small pancreatic ducts,* followed by damage and degeneration of acini, and fibrosis.[9]

2. *Acinar cell injury* (see Fig. 19–3, *middle*) is an early event in the evolution of many forms of acute pancreatitis. Alcohol, in particular, may be directly toxic to acinar cells, leading to severe intercellular leak of digestive enzymes.

3. *Deranged intracellular transport of pancreatic enzymes* (see Fig. 19–3, *right*) is a more subtle alteration, in which apical secretion is inhibited in alcohol-induced pancreatitis. Instead, these enzymes are *missorted* to a vacuole containing lysosomal enzymes, leading to enzyme activation and rupture of these organelles.[10]

It is evident that much remains to be learned about the pathogenesis of pancreatitis.

MORPHOLOGY. The morphology of acute pancreatic necrosis stems directly from the action of activated pancreatic enzymes that are released into the pancreatic substance. The basic alterations are **(1) proteolytic destruction of pancreatic substance, (2) necrosis of blood vessels with subsequent hemorrhage, (3) necrosis of fat, and (4) an accompanying inflammatory reaction.** The extent and predominance of each of these features depend on the duration and severity of the process. In the very early stages, only interstitial edema is present. Soon after, focal and confluent areas of frank necrosis of endocrine and exocrine tissue are found. Neutrophilic infiltration and interstitial hemorrhage eventually ensue. The most characteristic histologic lesions of acute pancreatic necrosis are the focal areas of fat necrosis that occur in the pancreatic and peripancreatic fat (Fig. 19–4). Following enzymatic destruction, adipocytes are transformed into shadowy outlines of cell membranes filled with pink, granular, opaque precipitates. Amorphous basophilic calcium precipitates may be visible within the necrotic focus.

With severe pancreatic necrosis, a variegated pattern of blue-black hemorrhages and gray-white necrotic softening alternates with sprinkled foci of yellow-white, chalky fat necrosis

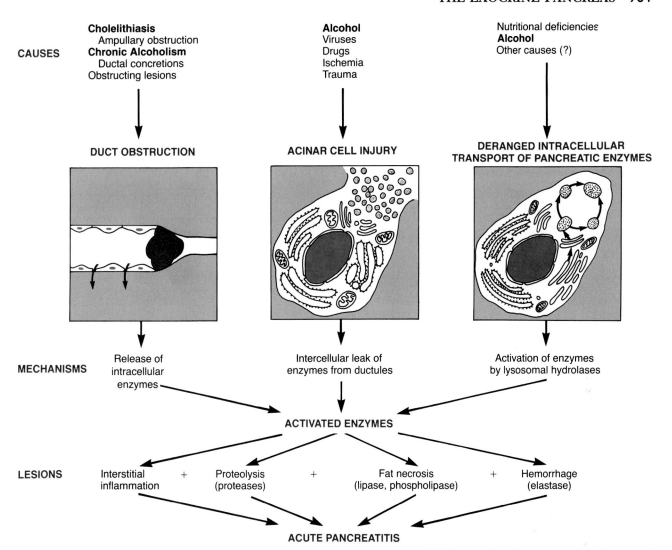

CAUSES

Cholelithiasis
   Ampullary obstruction
Chronic Alcoholism
   Ductal concretions
   Obstructing lesions

Alcohol
Viruses
Drugs
Ischemia
Trauma

Nutritional deficiencies
Alcohol
Other causes (?)

DUCT OBSTRUCTION

ACINAR CELL INJURY

**DERANGED INTRACELLULAR
TRANSPORT OF PANCREATIC ENZYMES**

MECHANISMS

Release of
intracellular
enzymes

Intercellular leak of
enzymes from ductules

Activation of enzymes
by lysosomal hydrolases

ACTIVATED ENZYMES

LESIONS

Interstitial   +   Proteolysis   +   Fat necrosis   +   Hemorrhage
inflammation   (proteases)   (lipase, phospholipase)   (elastase)

ACUTE PANCREATITIS

Figure 19-3. Pathogenesis of acute pancreatitis: duct obstruction, acinar cell injury, and a derangement in lysosomal traffic. See text. (Adapted and reproduced with permission from Longnecker, D.S.: Pathology and pathogenesis of diseases of the pancreas. Am. J. Pathol. *107:*103, 1982; and Steer, M.L., and Meldolesi, J.: Pathogenesis of acute pancreatitis. Annual Review of Medicine *39:*95, 1988; ©1988 by Annual Reviews Inc.)

(Fig. 19-5). The peritoneal cavity contains a serous and slightly turbid fluid in which globules of oil can be identified. Foci of fat necrosis may be found in any of the fat depots, such as in the omentum, mesentery of the bowel, abdominal wall, and even subcutaneous fat. Occasionally, liquefied areas are walled off by fibrous tissue to form small or large cystic spaces, known as **pancreatic abscesses.**

CLINICAL FEATURES. Abdominal pain is the cardinal manifestation of acute pancreatitis. Its severity varies from mild and tolerable, to severe and incapacitating. Localization in the epigastrium with radiation to the back is characteristic. Mild acute pancreatitis is diagnosed primarily by the presence of elevated plasma levels of amylase and lipase and exclusion of other causes of abdominal pain. *Full-blown, acute pancreatic necrosis is a medical emergency of the first magnitude.* These patients usually

have the sudden calamitous onset of an "acute abdomen" that must be differentiated from diseases such as ruptured acute appendicitis, perforated peptic ulcer, acute cholecystitis with rupture, and occlusion of mesenteric vessels with infarction of the bowel. Characteristically, the pain is constant and intense and is often referred to the upper back.

Many of the systemic features of severe acute pancreatitis can be attributed to release of toxic enzymes into the systemic circulation: *leukocytosis, hemolysis, disseminated intravascular coagulation, fluid sequestration (due to a leaky vasculature), adult respiratory distress syndrome, and diffuse fat necrosis. Peripheral vascular collapse, and shock with acute renal tubular necrosis may occur.* Explanations for the rapid development of shock include loss of blood volume, electrolyte disturbances, endotoxemia, and release of vasodilatory agents, such as bradykinin and prostaglandins.[11] Laboratory

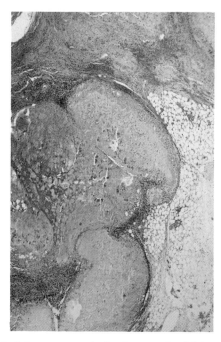

Figure 19-4. Low-power photomicrograph of fat necrosis in peripancreatic adipose tissue. Central focus of necrotic fat is surrounded by a rim of leukocytic infiltration (blue).

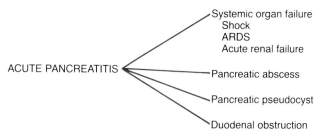

Figure 19-6. Complications and sequelae of acute pancreatitis.

findings include marked elevation of the serum amylase during the first 24 hours, followed within 72 to 96 hours by a rising serum lipase level. Glycosuria occurs in 10% of cases. Hypocalcemia may result from precipitation of calcium soaps in the fat necrosis; if persistent, it is a poor prognostic sign. Direct visualization of the enlarged inflamed pancreas by radiographic means is useful in the diagnosis of pancreatitis.

Despite palliative measures, about 5% of these patients die of shock during the first week of the clinical course. Acute adult respiratory distress syndrome and acute renal failure are ominous complications.[12] In surviving patients, sequelae

may include *pancreatic abscess, pseudocyst* (discussed later), and *duodenal obstruction* (Fig. 19–6).

CHRONIC PANCREATITIS

This entity might be more appropriately termed *chronic relapsing pancreatitis*, because it often represents progressive destruction of the pancreas by repeated flare-ups of silent or mildly symptomatic acute pancreatitis. The disease occurs in the same type of patient likely to develop acute pancreatitis —most commonly the middle-aged, male alcoholic, and less frequently the patient with biliary tract disease (Fig. 19–7). Hypercalcemia and hyperlipidemia also predispose to chronic pancreatitis. In as many as 12% of patients, recurrent pancreatitis is associated with *pancreas divisum*, presumably because of the combination of an anomalous ductal system and stenosis of the duodenal papilla. There are relatively rare special forms of chronic pancreatitis, such as *nonalcoholic tropical pancreatitis* and *familial hereditary pancreatitis*, of uncertain etiology. Familial pancreatitis begins in childhood and predisposes to the development of pancreatic carcinoma in later years. As many as 40% of patients with chronic pancreatitis have no recognizable predisposing factor.

The pathogenesis of chronic pancreatitis is as

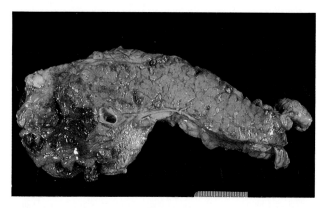

Figure 19-5. Acute hemorrhagic pancreatitis. Note the region of hemorrhagic necrosis in the head of the pancreas (left), and foci of chalky fat necrosis in pancreas and fat, best seen in tail of the pancreas (right).

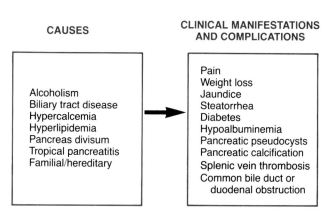

CAUSES	CLINICAL MANIFESTATIONS AND COMPLICATIONS
Alcoholism Biliary tract disease Hypercalcemia Hyperlipidemia Pancreas divisum Tropical pancreatitis Familial/hereditary	Pain Weight loss Jaundice Steatorrhea Diabetes Hypoalbuminemia Pancreatic pseudocysts Pancreatic calcification Splenic vein thrombosis Common bile duct or duodenal obstruction

Figure 19-7. Causes and consequences of chronic pancreatitis.

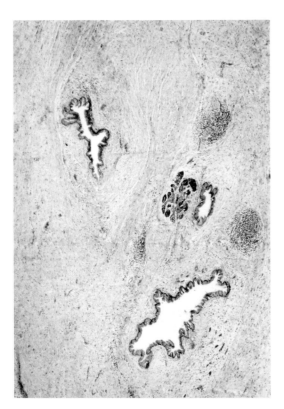

Figure 19–8. Chronic pancreatitis. Extensive fibrosis and atrophy has left only residual islets and ducts, with a sprinkling of chronic inflammatory cells and acinar tissue.

involve portions or all of the pancreas. A chronic inflammatory infiltrate around lobules and ducts is usually present. The interlobular and intralobular ducts are dilated and contain protein plugs in their lumina. The ductal epithelium may be atrophied or hyperplastic or may show squamous metaplasia (Fig. 19–9). Remaining islets become embedded in sclerosed tissue or severely damaged lobules, before they, too, disappear. **Grossly,** the gland is hard and exhibits foci of calcification and fully developed pancreatic calculi. These concretions vary from calculi invisible to the naked eye, to stones 1 cm to several centimeters in diameter, giving rise to the term "chronic calcifying pancreatitis." **Pseudocyst formation is common.**

With **chronic ductal obstruction,** the distribution of lesions is irregular, and the ductal epithelium generally is less severely damaged. Protein plugs and calcified stones are rare. The most common cause appears to be stenosis of the sphincter of Oddi associated with cholelithiasis. The lesions are more prominent in the head of the pancreas and regress after sphincterotomy. Any other obstructive lesion of the pancreatic ducts may result in this morphologic change, such as carcinoma or accidental surgical ligation of the duct.

varied as that of acute pancreatitis, and the distinction between acute and chronic pancreatitis remains blurred. The inciting events have been postulated as the following:[13]

1. *Ductal obstruction by concretions,* resulting from alcohol-induced alterations in acinar and ductal secretions, and in the biosynthesis of lithostathine (pancreatic stone protein); this protein normally inhibits intraluminal precipitation of calcium carbonates, yet is found in association with $CaCO_3$ as the main constituent of pancreatic stones.[14]

2. *Interstitial fat necrosis and hemorrhage,* which initiate a sequence of perilobular fibrosis, duct distortion, and altered pancreatic secretion and ductal flow — the "necrosis-fibrosis" hypothesis.[15]

Protein-calorie malnutrition probably plays a role in the tropical pancreatitis of Southeast Asia and parts of Africa, where alcohol consumption is extremely low.

MORPHOLOGY. Chronic pancreatitis is distinguished by **irregularly distributed fibrosis, reduced number and size of acini with relative sparing of the islets of Langerhans, and variable obstruction of pancreatic ducts of all sizes** (Fig. 19–8).[16] The lesions have a macroscopic lobular distribution and may

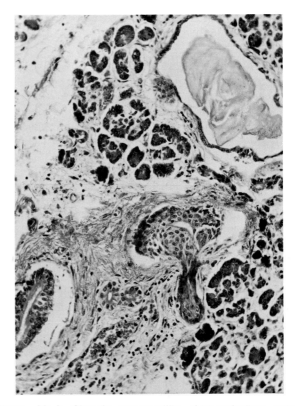

Figure 19–9. Chronic pancreatitis, demonstrating squamous metaplasia of one of the small ducts virtually obliterating its lumen. Note dilated duct above, filled with inspissated secretion.

CLINICAL FEATURES. Chronic pancreatitis can present as repeated attacks of mild to moderately severe abdominal pain, or persistent and intractable abdominal and back pain. Alternatively, the local disease may be entirely silent until pancreatic insufficiency and diabetes develop. In still other instances, the condition may present as recurrent episodes of mild jaundice or vague attacks of indigestion. The diagnosis of chronic pancreatitis thus requires a high index of suspicion. Attacks may be precipitated by alcohol abuse, overeating, or the use of opiates and other drugs. Abdominal imaging may show calcification in the region of the pancreas. Endocrine and exocrine insufficiency may lead to diabetes and steatorrhea, respectively. Pancreatic pseudocysts occur so frequently that they may perhaps be considered late features rather than complications of chronic pancreatitis. Profound weight loss and hypoalbuminemic edema are present in end-stage pancreatic insufficiency. Chronic pancreatitis appears to incur a modestly increased risk of pancreatic carcinoma.

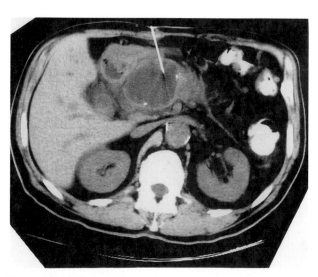

Figure 19–10. Pancreatic pseudocyst. In this CT scan of the upper abdomen, a percutaneous needle has been placed into a large cystic lesion in the body of the pancreas. (Courtesy of Peter A. Banks, M.D., Brigham and Women's Hospital, Boston.)

TUMORS

A variety of non-neoplastic and neoplastic masses involve this organ. The non-neoplastic masses almost invariably take the form of cysts, although neoplastic cystic masses also occur.

NON-NEOPLASTIC CYSTS

Cysts of the pancreas are infrequent, except when following chronic pancreatitis, in which case they are inflammatory *pseudocysts*. *Congenital cysts* are believed to result from anomalous development of the pancreatic ducts. Cysts in the kidney, liver, and pancreas frequently coexist in *congenital polycystic disease* (see Chapter 20). The pancreatic cysts range from microscopic lesions up to 3 to 5 cm in diameter. They are lined by a smooth, glistening membrane that may exhibit a ductal-type cuboidal epithelium or a completely atrophic, attenuated cell layer. The cysts are usually enclosed in a thin, fibrous capsule and are filled with a clear-to-turbid mucoid or serous fluid. In the rare entity *von Hippel–Lindau disease* angiomas are found in the retina and cerebellum or brain stem in association with cysts in the pancreas, liver, and kidneys.

Pseudocysts

Pseudocysts are localized collections of pancreatic secretions that develop following inflammation of the pancreas. They are to be distinguished from sterile *pancreatic abscesses*, which involve liquefac-

tive necrosis of severely damaged pancreatic parenchyma. Both entities lack a true epithelial lining, unlike congenital cysts. *Pseudocysts are by far the more common, and virtually all arise following acute or chronic pancreatitis.* Traumatic injury to the abdomen also may give rise to pseudocysts.

MORPHOLOGY. These cysts are usually solitary, and most measure 5 to 10 cm in diameter. They may be situated within the pancreatic substance, but more often they are found adjacent to the pancreas. The cyst walls may be thin, or thick and fibrous, and communication with pancreatic ducts may or may not be demonstrable. The fibrous capsule often exhibits a marked chronic inflammatory reaction, organizing blood clot, old blood pigment, precipitates of calcium, and cholesterol crystals.

Pseudocysts produce abdominal pain; hemorrhage and infection with generalized peritonitis are potential complications. However, their usual clinical significance lies in their being discovered as an abdominal mass in a location that strongly suggests a primary malignancy (Fig. 19–10). They are usually unilocular; this feature assists in distinguishing them from neoplastic cysts, which tend to be multiloculated.

NEOPLASMS

Cystic Tumors

Cystic tumors comprise 5% of all pancreatic neoplasms. They are usually located in the body or tail

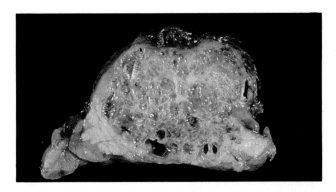

Figure 19-11. Pancreatic mucinous cystadenocarcinoma. Cross-section through a mucinous multiloculated cystic tumor in the body of the pancreas. The normal pancreatic tissue has been obliterated.

and present as painless, slow-growing masses. Some are multiloculated, cystic neoplasms filled with mucinous secretions (*mucinous cystic tumor*), resembling their histologic counterpart in the ovary (see Chapter 23). The only way of distinguishing the entirely benign form (*mucinous cystadenoma*) from its malignant counterpart (*cystadenocarcinoma*; Fig. 19-11) is by histologic assessment following complete surgical removal, usually by distal pancreatectomy. A rare cystic tumor with *serous* secretions (*microcystic adenoma*) is almost always benign.

An unusual *solid-cystic* (papillary-cystic) *tumor* is seen predominantly in adolescent girls and women younger than 35 years of age.[17] It is a large, rounded, well-circumscribed mass that has solid and cystic zones. Histologically, the tumor cells are small and uniform and have a finely granular eosinophilic cytoplasm. They grow in solid sheets or papillary projections. The tumors cause abdominal discomfort and pain and are usually cured with resection.

Carcinoma of the Pancreas

The term "carcinoma of the pancreas" is applied to carcinomas arising in the exocrine portion of the gland. *Virtually all these cancers begin in the ductal epithelium;* the acinar cells give origin to fewer than 1% of malignant tumors.[18] Tumors that arise from the islets of Langerhans are specifically designated as islet cell tumors and are considered in the section on the endocrine pancreas.

Pancreatic cancer continues to be a depressingly difficult problem. These highly fatal cancers have a deceptively silent growth habit, so that by the time they are diagnosed they are rarely curable: median survival time, regardless of therapy, is 2 to 3 months after diagnosis.[19] Pancreatic cancer accounts for 5% of all cancer deaths in the United States. There are 28,000 new cases and 26,000 deaths from the disease each year.[20] The incidence

rates are higher in blacks than in whites, in males than in females, in diabetics than in nondiabetics, and in the presence of hereditary chronic pancreatitis. These tumors occur most often in the sixth, seventh, and eighth decades of life, although about 10% of patients are much younger.

The incidence of pancreatic cancer is threefold that of 60 years ago, yet we remain ignorant of the causes of this disease. Smoking, diet, and chemical carcinogens have been implicated:[21] (1) The risk of pancreatic cancer among heavy smokers is at least 1.5 times that of nonsmokers; (2) there is a positive correlation between mortality from cancer of the pancreas and per capita consumption of fats and meat; and (3) there is a two- to fivefold long-term increased risk of pancreatic cancer following partial gastrectomy, possibly because of enhanced intestinal formation of N-nitroso compounds by bacteria.

These lesions may arise anywhere in the pancreas, but most studies show a fairly standard distribution: head of pancreas, 60%; body of pancreas, 15 to 20%; and tail of pancreas, 5%.[18] In 20% the tumor either is diffuse or has spread so widely as to preclude localization of its site of origin. Tumors of the head of the pancreas are in a strategic location to impinge on the ampulla of Vater, common bile duct, and duodenum and thus cause obstructive biliary symptoms relatively early in their life history. Some lesions, therefore, may be discovered before widespread metastasis has occurred. In contrast, cancers of the body and

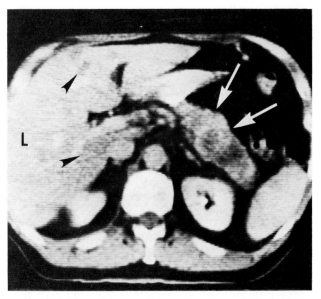

Figure 19-12. CT scan at midabdominal level demonstrating pancreatic carcinoma. Compare with Figure 19-1 to localize the other organs. Pancreatitic tail is enlarged and heterogeneous (arrows). Liver (L) contains multiple focal lucencies, corresponding to metastatic deposits (arrowheads). Stomach, spleen, and kidneys are also visible. (Courtesy of Dr. S. Seltzer, Brigham and Women's Hospital, Boston.)

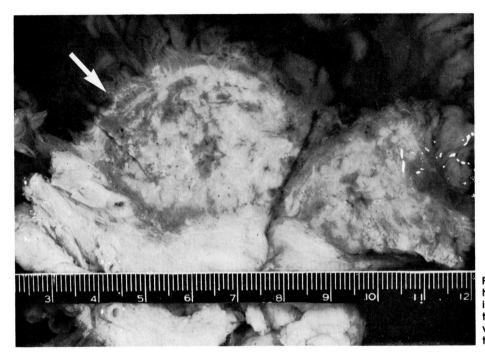

Figure 19–13. Carcinoma of the head of the pancreas. Mottled invasive tumor has grown into the wall of the duodenum, which appears at the upper extent of tumor *(arrow)*.

tail may grow silently until such time as extension to adjacent structures and metastatic dissemination preclude surgical intervention (Fig. 19–12).

MORPHOLOGY. Grossly, carcinomas of the **head of the pancreas** may be fairly small mass lesions that cause little or only moderate expansion of pancreatic tissue. They may be totally inapparent on external examination of the organ, creating only the impression of some increased consistency and irregular nodularity. Other lesions create masses up to 8 to 10 cm in diameter. The gray-white scirrhous, homogenous tumor infiltrates and replaces the lobular architecture of a normal pancreas. Such lesions have poorly defined, obviously infiltrative margins (Fig. 19–13). Larger tumors usually extend beyond the pancreas to invade the duodenum and common bile duct; biliary obstruction may occur by compression or outright growth of tumor into the biliary space. Extension to peripancreatic and portohepatic nodes, with metastasis to the liver, is not uncommon.

Carcinomas of the **body and tail** are usually large, hard, irregular masses that sometimes wipe out virtually the entire tail and body of the pancreas. Their consistency and appearance on cross-section is the same as that of carcinomas of the head of the gland, but **they frequently extend widely at the time of discovery.** They impinge on the adjacent vertebral column, extend through the retroperitoneal spaces inferiorly and superiorly, and occasionally invade the adjacent spleen or adrenal. They may extend into the transverse colon or stomach. Peripancreatic, gastric, mesenteric, omental, and portohepatic nodes are involved.

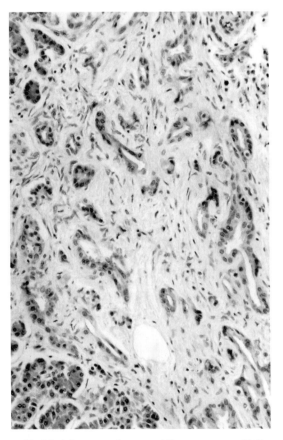

Figure 19–14. Adenocarcinoma of the pancreas. Malignant glands are invading pancreatic substance, seen at bottom left of photograph.

The liver may be strikingly seeded with tumor nodules to produce massive hepatomegaly.

The histologic appearance of pancreatic carcinoma is generally that of a **poorly differentiated adenocarcinoma forming abortive tubular structures or cell clusters and exhibiting an aggressive, deeply infiltrative growth pattern** (Fig. 19–14). Dense stromal fibrosis accompanies tumor invasion, and there is a proclivity for perineural invasion within and beyond the organ. The malignant glands are atypical, irregular, small, and bizarre and are usually lined by anaplastic cuboidal-to-columnar epithelial cells. Well to moderately differentiated tumors are the exception. Careful examination may reveal regions of ductal dysplasia and intraductal tumor growth, in keeping with the ductal origin of most of these tumors. About 10% of tumors assume either an **adenosquamous pattern** or the uncommon pattern of extreme anaplasia with **giant cell formation or sarcomatoid** histology. Rarely, carcinomas arise from acinar cells **(acinar cell carcinoma),** distinguished by the plump, polygonal eosinophilic appearance of the tumor cells.

CLINICAL FEATURES. Carcinomas of the pancreas, even those of its head, are insidious lesions that undoubtedly are present for months and possibly years before they produce symptoms referable to their expansive growth. The major symptoms include weight loss, abdominal pain, back pain, anorexia, nausea, vomiting and generalized malaise, and weakness. *Jaundice is present in about 90% of patients with carcinomas of the head and in 10 to 40% of those with cancer of the body or tail. Migratory thrombophlebitis,* known as *Trousseau's syndrome,* occurs in 10% of patients, attributed to the elaboration of platelet-aggregating factors and procoagulants from the tumor or its necrotic products (see Chapter 4). Ironically, Trousseau diagnosed his own fatal disease as cancer of the pancreas when he developed these spontaneously appearing and disappearing thromboses. This phenomenon is encountered in other forms of cancer as well.

The symptomatic course of pancreatic carcinoma is typically brief and progressive. Despite the tendency of lesions of the head of the pancreas to obstruct the biliary system at a relatively earlier date, fewer than 15% of pancreatic tumors overall are resectable at the time of diagnosis. One-year survival is less than 20%, and 5-year survival is only 3%.[21]

The Endocrine Pancreas

DIABETES MELLITUS
MORPHOLOGY OF DIABETES
  AND ITS LATE
  COMPLICATIONS

CLINICAL COURSE
ISLET CELL TUMORS
BETA-CELL TUMORS
  (INSULINOMA)

ZOLLINGER-ELLISON SYNDROME
  (GASTRINOMA)
OTHER RARE ISLET CELL TUMORS

NORMAL

The endocrine pancreas consists of about 1 million microscopic cellular units—the islets of Langerhans—and a few scattered cells within the small pancreatic ducts.[22] In the aggregate the islets in the adult human weigh only 1 to 1.5 gm. Embryologically, islet cells are of endodermal origin and form at many points along the pancreatic tubuloductal system. The first evidence of islet formation in the human fetus occurs at 9 to 11 weeks.

In the human adult, most islets measure 100 to 200 μm and consist of four major and two minor cell types. The four main types are *B (beta), A (alpha), D (delta),* and *PP (pancreatic polypeptide) cells.* These make up about 70, 20, 5 to 10, and 1 to 2%, respectively, of the islet cell population. They can be differentiated morphologically by their staining properties with certain dyes, by the ultrastructural morphology of their granules, and (most important) by their hormonal content in immunohistochemical studies that employ specific antibodies to individual hormones.

The *B cell (beta)* (Fig. 19–15) produces *insulin.* The description of insulin secretion by beta cells is detailed in the discussion of diabetes. The granules have rectangular profiles and a crystalline matrix and are surrounded by a halo (Fig. 19–16). Hyperplasia and neoplasia of these cells are responsible for the important clinical syndrome of hyperinsulinism. *A cells (alpha)* secrete *glucagon,*

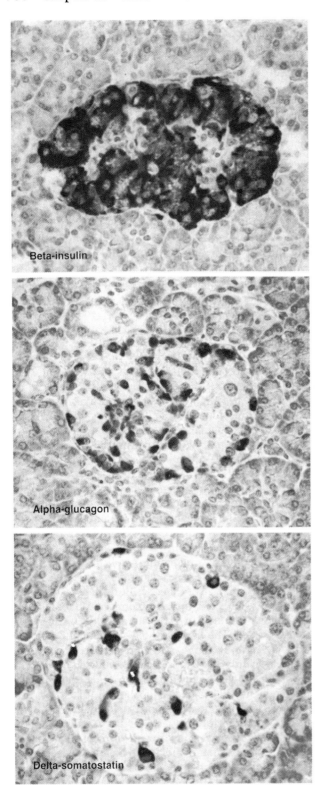

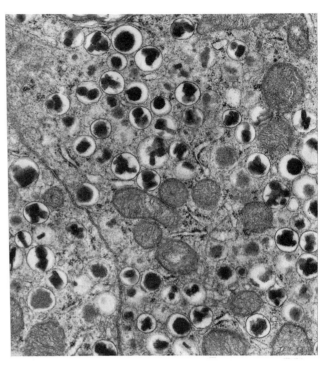

Figure 19-16. Electron micrograph of a portion of a beta cell with characteristic membrane-bound granules, each containing a dense, often rectangular core and a distinct halo. (Courtesy of Dr. A. Like, University of Massachusetts Medical School, Worcester.)

Figure 19-15. Islets stained by immunoperoxidase technique for insulin *(top)*, glucagon *(middle)*, and somatostatin *(bottom)*. The dark reaction product identifies beta, alpha, and delta cells, respectively. (Courtesy of Dr. A. Like, University of Massachusetts Medical School, Worcester.)

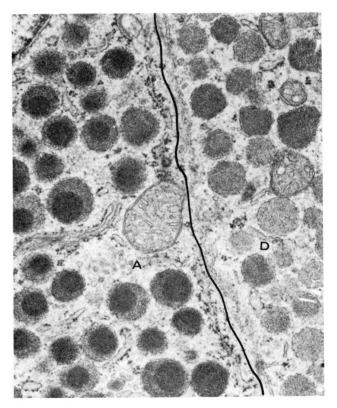

Figure 19-17. Portions of an alpha cell *(left,* A) and a delta cell *(right,* D). Granules in both cells have closely apposed membranes, but the alpha-cell granule exhibits a dense, round center. (Courtesy of Dr. A. Like, University of Massachusetts Medical School, Worcester.)

which induces hyperglycemia by its glycogenolytic activity in the liver. Alpha-cell granules are round, with closely applied membranes and a dense center (Fig. 19–17). *D cells* (delta) contain somatostatin, which suppresses both insulin and glucagon release. Delta cells have large, pale granules with closely applied membranes (see Fig. 19–17). *PP cells* have small, dark granules and are not only present in islets but also scattered in the exocrine pancreas. They contain a unique pancreatic polypeptide that exerts a number of gastrointestinal effects, such as stimulation of secretion of gastric and intestinal enzymes and inhibition of intestinal motility. The two rare cell types are *D1 cells* and *enterochromaffin cells.* D1 cells have distinctive granules by electron microscopy and elaborate *vasoactive intestinal polypeptide* (VIP), a hormone that induces glycogenolysis and hyperglycemia and also stimulates gastrointestinal fluid secretion and causes secretory diarrhea. *Enterochromaffin cells* synthesize serotonin and are the source of pancreatic tumors that induce the carcinoid syndrome.

We now turn to the two main disorders of islet cells: diabetes mellitus and islet cell tumors.

PATHOLOGY

Despite the minute size of the islets of Langerhans, even collectively, the endocrine pancreas is responsible for a disproportionate amount of morbidity and mortality. Diabetes mellitus alone ranks among the top ten causes of death in Western nations, and despite important improvements in its clinical management, to date it has not been possible to control significantly its lethal consequences. The various forms of neoplasia arising in the islets, although far less common, produce some fascinating, often difficult to diagnose endocrinopathies. The endocrine pancreas is therefore a source of significant clinical disease.

DIABETES MELLITUS

Diabetes mellitus represents a group of metabolic disorders in which there is impaired glucose utilization, inducing hyperglycemia. A defective or deficient insulin secretory response underlies the glucose underutilization. Fat and protein metabolism are also commonly affected.

CLASSIFICATION AND INCIDENCE. In this section, we deal principally with *primary or idiopathic diabetes mellitus,* which is by far the most common and important entity. Primary diabetes must be distinguished from *secondary diabetes,* which in-

Table 19–2. TYPES OF DIABETES

PRIMARY (IDIOPATHIC) DIABETES

IDDM (insulin-dependent diabetes mellitus (type I))
NIDDM (non–insulin-dependent diabetes mellitus (type II))
  Nonobese NIDDM
  Obese NIDDM
  Maturity-onset diabetes of the young (MODY)

SECONDARY DIABETES

Chronic pancreatitis
Postpancreatectomy
Hormonal tumors (e.g., pheochromocytoma, pituitary tumors)
Drugs (corticosteroids)
Hemochromatosis
Genetic disorders (e.g., lipodystrophy)

cludes forms of hyperglycemia associated with identifiable causes in which destruction of pancreatic islets is induced by inflammatory pancreatic disease, surgery, tumors, certain drugs, iron overload (hemochromatosis), and certain acquired or genetic endocrinopathies (Table 19–2).

Primary diabetes mellitus represents a heterogeneous group of disorders having hyperglycemia as a common feature. The National Diabetes Data Group of the National Institutes of Health developed a classification (Table 19–3), which basically divides primary diabetes into two variants that differ in their pattern of inheritance, insulin responses, and origins.[23]

- *Insulin-dependent diabetes mellitus (IDDM),* also called *type I diabetes,* and previously known as juvenile-onset and ketosis-prone diabetes. This

Table 19–3. TYPE I VS. TYPE II DIABETES

	IDDM (TYPE I)	NIDDM (TYPE II)
Clinical	Onset <20 years	Onset >30 years
	Normal weight	Obese
	Decreased blood insulin	Normal or increased blood insulin
	Islet cell antibodies	No islet cell antibodies
	Ketoacidosis common	Ketoacidosis rare
Genetics	50% concordance in twins	90–100% concordance in twins
	HLA-D linked	No HLA association
Pathogenesis	Autoimmunity	Insulin resistance
	Immunopathologic mechanisms	Relative insulin deficiency
	Severe insulin deficiency	
Islet cells	Insulitis early	No insulitis
	Marked atrophy and fibrosis	Focal atrophy and amyloid
	Beta-cell depletion	Mild beta-cell depletion

variant accounts for about 10 to 20% of all cases of idiopathic diabetes.

- *Non-insulin-dependent diabetes mellitus (NI-DDM)*, also called *type II diabetes* and previously referred to as adult-onset diabetes. This accounts for 80 to 90% of cases. Type II diabetes is further divided into obese and nonobese types and a third rare form, known as *maturity-onset diabetes of the young* (MODY). MODY is manifested by mild hyperglycemia and is transmitted as an autosomal dominant trait.

It should be stressed that while the two major types of diabetes have different pathogenetic mechanisms and metabolic characteristics, the *chronic, long-term complications in blood vessels, kidneys, eyes, and nerves occur in both types and are the major causes of morbidity and death in diabetes.*

With an annual toll of about 144,000 deaths, diabetes mellitus is the seventh leading cause of death in the United States.[24] It is estimated that 2 to 3% of the adult population have diabetes mellitus, and about as many have undiagnosed disease. The prevalence of type I diabetes varies widely around the world, as a reflection of some as yet obscure environmental factors in the pathogenesis of the disease and of genetic susceptibilities, as we shall see.

PATHOGENESIS

The pathogenesis of the two types will be discussed separately, but first we briefly discuss normal insulin metabolism, since some aspects of insulin release and action are important in the discussion of pathogenesis.

NORMAL INSULIN METABOLISM AND GLUCOSE HOMEOSTASIS. Normal glucose homeostasis is tightly regulated by three inter-related processes: *glucose production in the liver, uptake and utilization of glucose by peripheral tissues* (mostly muscle), and *insulin secretion*[25] (Table 19-4). Insulin secretion is modulated such that glucose production and utilization rise or fall to maintain normal blood glucose levels.

The human insulin gene is expressed in the beta cells of the pancreatic islets, where mature insulin mRNA is transcribed. Translation of the message occurs in the rough endoplasmic reticulum, yielding preproinsulin. There follows proteolytic cleavage of the prepeptide sequence to yield proinsulin and, in the Golgi apparatus, cleavage of the C-peptide to yield insulin sequences. Both insulin and C-peptide are then stored in secretory granules and secreted together after physiologic stimulation (Fig. 19-18). Release of insulin from beta cells is a biphasic process involving two pools of insulin. A rise in the blood glucose levels results in glucose uptake into beta cells, facilitated by an insulin-independent glucose-transporting protein, GLUT-2, and leading to an *immediate release of insulin*, presumably that stored in the beta-cell granules. If the secretory stimulus persists, a delayed and protracted response follows, which involves active synthesis of insulin. *The most important stimulus that triggers insulin release is glucose, which also initiates insulin synthesis.* Calcium influx, alpha-adrenergic agents, cAMP, and GLP (a glucagon-like peptide) are also involved in the process of insulin secretion. Other agents, including intestinal hormones, certain amino acids (leucine and arginine), and sulfonylureas, stimulate insulin release but not synthesis.

Insulin is a major anabolic hormone.[26] It is necessary for (1) transmembrane transport of glucose and amino acids, (2) glycogen formation in the liver and skeletal muscles, (3) glucose conver-

Table 19-4. THREE FACTORS IN REGULATION OF NORMAL GLUCOSE TOLERANCE

Hepatic glucose production
Glucose uptake and utilization
    Peripheral tissues (primarily muscle)
    Splanchnic (liver and GI tract)
Insulin secretion

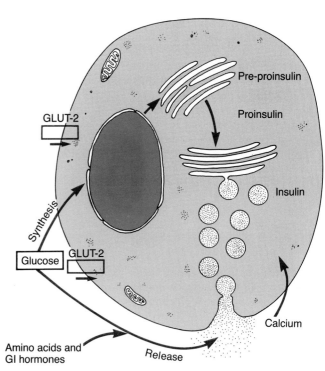

Figure 19-18. Insulin synthesis and secretion. Note that glucose stimulates both synthesis and secretion, while other agents—amino acids and certain gastrointestinal hormones—induce only secretion. GLUT-2 is an insulin-independent glucose transporter that facilitates diffusion of glucose into the cell.

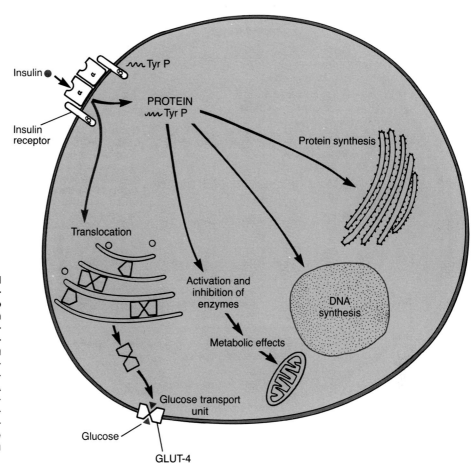

Figure 19-19. Schematic model of insulin action on an insulin-responsive cell. Insulin binds to the alpha subunit of the insulin receptor and activates tyrosine-specific protein kinase autophosphorylation (of the beta subunit) as well as phosphorylation of other intracellular proteins. This is followed by DNA synthesis, protein synthesis, altered mitochondrial metabolism, and translocation of glucose transport units from the Golgi apparatus to the plasma membrane.

sion to triglycerides, (4) nucleic acid synthesis, and (5) protein synthesis. *Its prime metabolic function is to increase the rate of glucose transport into certain cells in the body.* These are the striated muscle cells, including myocardial cells, fibroblasts, and fat cells, representing collectively about two-thirds of the entire body weight. In addition to these metabolic effects, *insulin and insulin-like growth factors initiate DNA synthesis in certain cells and stimulate their growth and differentiation.*

Insulin interacts with its target cells by first *binding to the insulin receptor,* composed of two glycoprotein subunits α and β (Fig. 19-19). Since the amount of insulin bound to the cells is affected by the availability of receptors, their number and function are important in regulating the action of insulin. Receptor-bound insulin triggers a number of intracellular responses, including activation or inhibition of insulin-sensitive enzymes in mitochondria, protein synthesis, and DNA synthesis. One of the important early effects of insulin involves translocation of *glucose transport protein units* (GLUTs) from the Golgi apparatus to the plasma membrane, thus facilitating cellular uptake of glucose. There are several forms of GLUTs, which differ in their tissue distribution, affinity for glucose, and sensitivity to insulin.[27] GLUT-4, present in muscle and adipose tissue, is the major insulin-regulatable transporter. GLUT-2, on the

other hand (as we have seen in Fig. 19-18), present in the liver and beta cells of the pancreas, is insulin independent and serves to facilitate rapid equilibration of glucose between extracellular and intracellular compartments.

Hepatic production of glucose by the liver is regulated by a number of hormones. Conversely, after glucose enters muscle cells, it is metabolized by oxidation to carbon dioxide and water or is stored by nonoxidative metabolism as *glycogen.* Glycogen synthesis is catalyzed by the rate-limiting *enzyme glycogen synthase.*[28] As we shall see, defects in all these regulatory steps in glucose homeostasis—insulin secretion, glucose transport, glucose production, and glucose utilization—are found in patients with type II non–insulin-dependent diabetes.[25]

PATHOGENESIS OF IDDM (TYPE I DIABETES). *This form of diabetes results from a severe, absolute lack of insulin caused by a reduction in the beta-cell mass.* IDDM usually develops in childhood, becoming manifest and severe at puberty. Patients *depend on insulin for survival.* Without insulin, they develop acute metabolic complications, such as ketoacidosis and coma.

A great deal has been learned about the pathogenesis of IDDM.[29] Three interlocking mechanisms are responsible for the islet cell destruction:

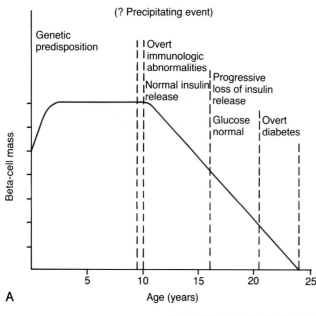

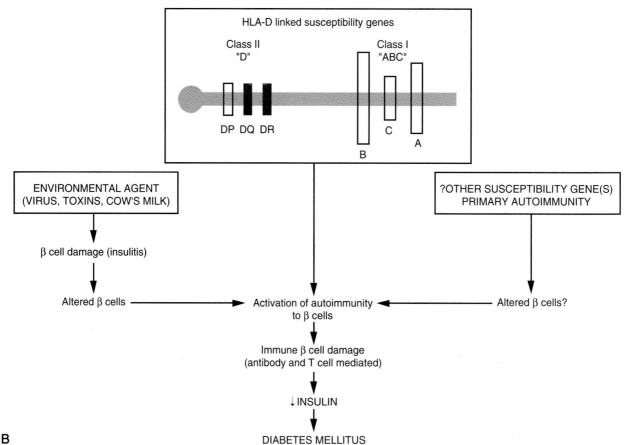

Figure 19-20. A, Stages in the development of type I diabetes mellitus (IDDM). The stages of diabetes are listed from left to right, and hypothetical beta-cell mass is plotted against age. B, Postulated mechanisms in the pathogenesis of type I diabetes. Susceptibility to the development of diabetes is enhanced by HLA-D–linked genes, which serve to activate or amplify autoimmune reactions to beta cells. Either environmental agents or other susceptibility genetic determinants are thought to alter beta cells and make them antigenic. Autoimmune reactions to beta cells result in antibody and T cell–mediated damage to cells, which in the absence of beta cells' regeneration, results in insulin depletion and diabetes. (A Reproduced with permission from Eisenbarth, G.E.: Type I diabetes—a chronic autoimmune disease. N. Engl. J. Med. *314:*1360, 1986.)

genetic susceptibility, autoimmunity, and an environmental insult. A postulated sequence of events involving these three mechanisms is shown in Figure 19–20A and B. It is thought that a *genetic susceptibility* to altered immune regulation, linked to specific alleles in the class II major histocompatibility complex (HLA-D), predisposes certain individuals to the development of *autoimmunity to islet beta-cell antigens.* The autoimmunity either develops spontaneously or, more likely, is triggered by an environmental agent (a virus, chemical, toxin, or dietary component), resulting in acute *insulitis* and damage to beta cells. An autoimmune reaction directed against beta-cell antigens then causes further beta-cell injury, and eventually when most of the beta cells are destroyed, overt diabetes mellitus appears (see Fig. 9–20A). Let us briefly review the three mechanisms in the sequence.

Genetic Susceptibility. It has long been known that diabetes mellitus can aggregate in families. However, the precise mode of inheritance of the susceptibility genes for type I diabetes remains unknown. Among identical twins, the concordance rate (i.e., both twins affected) is only approximately 50%. Only 5 to 10% of children of first-order relatives with IDDM develop the overt disease.

At least one of the susceptibility genes for IDDM resides in the genes encoding the class II antigens of the major histocompatibility region of chromosome 6 (HLA-D).[30] As should be known, the HLA-D region contains three subregions: DP, DQ, and DR (see Fig. 19–20B). The class II molecules are polymorphic, and each has numerous alleles. There seems to be an ordered hierarchy of susceptibility associated with the various class II genes.[31] By far the most common in whites is the *HLA-DQ3.2* (DQB1*0302) gene, which is present in 70% of patients. Individuals bearing this gene have an eightfold risk of developing IDDM compared with those not carrying the gene. (Because this gene is linked to HLA-DR4, earlier studies targeted DR4 as the most common variant.) Next in the hierarchy is HLA-DR3, and there is synergism between DQ3.2 and DR3 positive haplotypes, such that individuals bearing both types have an almost 20-fold increased risk of diabetes. Conversely, certain haplotypes, particularly HLA-DQ1.2, *decrease* the risk of IDDM. The precise mechanism by which these haplotypes influence the risk of IDDM is still unclear. Earlier explanations implicating differences in single amino acids in the antigen-binding cleft of the MHC class II molecule, presumably altering beta-cell antigen presentation, are insufficient.[32] It seems more likely that several clusters of distinct amino acid residues affect interactions between the DQ molecule and its bound peptide (antigen) or interactions with the T-cell receptor, or both, somehow facilitating the development of autoimmunity[31] (see Chapter 6).

Whether a second diabetogenic allele, not linked to the HLA region, is required for the development of diabetes (as is the case in a genetic model of diabetes [NOD] in mice) is under investigation.[33]

Autoimmunity. A role for autoimmunity in the pathogenesis of diabetes is supported by several morphologic, clinical, and experimental observations:[34]

• Lymphocytic infiltrates, often intense ("insulitis"), are frequently observed in the islets in cases of recent onset. Both CD4+ and CD8+ T cells are found within such infiltrates. Similar cells are found in animal models of type I dia-

betes. CD4+ T cells from diseased animals can transfer diabetes to normal animals, thus establishing the primacy of T-cell autoimmunity in type I diabetes.

• As many as 90% of patients with type I diabetes have circulating islet cell antibodies (ICA) when tested within a year of diagnosis. Asymptomatic relatives develop islet cell antibodies months to years before the clinical onset of diabetes. About half of first-degree relatives of diabetic children positive for islet cell antibodies eventually become insulin dependent, as opposed to 0.3% of ICA-negative subjects. Antibodies to a large variety of cytoplasmic and membrane islet cell antigens can be found, including a 64-kd glutamic acid decarboxylase (GAD), sialylglycolipids, and insulin.[35] The relative importance of such antigens in initiating the disease, and the role of antibodies to sequestered cytoplasmic cell antigens released by the initial injury, are under intense study. Currently, interest is in the role of the 64-kd GAD, because antibodies to GAD are the best predictors of impending IDDM, and T cell–mediated immunity to GAD is strongly associated with IDDM.[35]

• In experimental animals and humans the insulitis is associated with expression of class II molecules on beta cells as well as increased expression of class I antigens. Normal beta cells do not possess cell surface class II molecules. The aberrant expression of MHC molecules is induced by locally produced cytokines (e.g., interferon-gamma [IFN-γ]) derived from activated T cells. It is not known, however, whether the aberrant class II expression is a primary immune defect that leads to recognition of normal beta-cell antigens and a cascade of immune-mediated injury, or whether it is secondary to an inflammatory response initiated by some viral infection or toxin. In addition, it is not an absolute requisite for diabetes, since autoimmune diabetes can be induced in mice with MHC class II deficiency.[36]

• Approximately 10% of persons who have type I diabetes also have other organ-specific autoimmune disorders, such as Graves' disease, Addison's disease, thyroiditis, and pernicious anemia. In these patients there appears to be a broad derangement of immunoregulation.

To summarize, there is overwhelming evidence implicating autoimmunity and immune-mediated injury as causes of beta-cell loss in type I diabetes mellitus. Indeed, immunosuppressive therapy with cyclosporine prevents the development of, or ameliorates, type I diabetes in experimental animals and in children with this disease.[37]

Environmental Factors. Granted that a genetic susceptibility, leading to autoimmune destruction of islet cells, is the cause of insulin deficiency in type I diabetes, what triggers the autoimmune reaction? In the vast majority of cases the answer is unknown, leading to speculation that non–HLA-linked diabetogenic genes induce so-called *primary autoimmunity*, in which an immune response occurs against normal unaltered beta cells, causing the initial insulitis.

There is, however, a great deal of evidence that environmental factors are involved in triggering diabetes. The epidemiologic data are compelling. Finnish children have a 60- to 70-fold increased risk of type I diabetes compared with Korean children. In the northeastern United States, over the last 30 years there has been a tripling of type I diabetes in children younger than 15 years of age. In three studies in Japan, Israel, and Canada, emigrants assume a risk of type I diabetes closer to that of their destination country than to that of their country of origin.

Viruses are suspected as initiators of this disease.[38] There are seasonal trends in the diagnosis of new cases, often corresponding to the prevalence of common viral infections in the community. The viral infections implicated include mumps, measles, rubella, coxsackie B virus, and infectious mononucleosis.[39] Although many viruses are beta-cell tropic, direct virus-induced injury is rarely severe enough to cause diabetes mellitus. The most likely scenario is that viruses cause mild beta-cell injury, which is followed by an autoimmune reaction against altered beta cells in persons with HLA-linked susceptibility. One good example is the occurrence of type I diabetes in patients with congenital rubella. About 20% of those infected *in utero*, almost always those with HLA-DQ3.2 or DR3 genotype, go on to develop the disease in childhood or puberty. *Virus-associated IDDM thus appears to be a rare outcome of some relatively common viral infection, delayed by the long latency period necessary for progressive autoimmune loss of beta cells to occur and dependent on the modifying effects of MHC class II molecules.*[38]

A number of *chemical toxins*, including streptozotocin, alloxan, and pentamidine, also induce islet cell destruction in animals. In humans, pentamidine, a drug used for the treatment of parasitic infections, has been occasionally associated with the development of abrupt-onset diabetes, and cases of diabetes have also been reported after accidental or suicidal ingestion of Vacor, a pharmacologic agent used as a rat exterminator. These chemicals act either directly on islet cells or by triggering an immune mechanism.

Children who ingest *cow's milk* early in life have an incidence of IDDM higher than that of breast-fed children, and antibodies to bovine serum albumin (BSA) are present in patients with IDDM.[40] It has been suggested that BSA triggers autoimmunity by a process of *molecular mimicry*, since the described antibody is directed to a 17–amino acid peptide present both in BSA and in an islet beta-cell protein called *p69*.[41] The *p69* protein is induced on the surface of beta cells by cytokines (mainly IFN-γ). The following scenario is thus postulated. Absorption of peptides in cow's milk by the immature gut triggers a T- and B-cell response and the production of antibodies to the peptide. Infection (provoking cytokine production) subsequently induces surface expression of p69 on islet cells, causing destruction of beta cells by antibody and reactive T cells. Homologies between the antigenic peptide and the residues on the MHC II haplotypes may explain the varying risks of developing IDDM in children who ingest cow's milk.[40]

Figure 19–20B summarizes the postulated pathways in the pathogenesis of type I diabetes mellitus and the contribution of genetic, immunologic, and environmental factors.

PATHOGENESIS OF NON–INSULIN-DEPENDENT (NIDDM) DIABETES. Much less is known, unfortunately, about the pathogenesis of non–insulin-dependent diabetes, which is by far the most common type. About 10% of the population over 70 has NIDDM. The underlying causes are largely unidentified genetic factors and the effects of a Western lifestyle—obesity and overeating.[42] There is also an inverse relationship between the prevalence of NIDDM and a high level of physical activity.

Genetic factors are of even greater importance than in type I diabetes, and among identical twins the concordance rate is over 90%. Unlike type I, however, the disease is not linked to any HLA haplotype (except for weak HLA linkage in Pima Indians), and there is no evidence that autoimmune mechanisms are involved.

Except in a few subgroups, the mode of inheritance and the genetic defects are still unknown. In the maturity-onset type of diabetes (MODY), described earlier, inheritance is *autosomal dominant* and linked to chromosomes 7 and 20. The defect in chromosome 7 has been traced to mutations in the gene encoding the glucose-phosphorylating enzyme *glucokinase*, which serves as part of the glucose-sensing mechanism regulating insulin secretion in pancreatic beta cells.[43] There is also an association, in a subgroup of patients with NIDDM,[44] between polymorphic alleles of the gene for *glycogen synthase*, which as you recall, is the rate-limiting enzyme for glucose conversion to glycogen in muscle cells. Other rare mutations in insulin, insulin receptor, and mitochondrial genes have also been described.

Two metabolic defects that characterize NIDDM are (1) *a derangement in insulin secretion* that is insufficient relative to the glucose load, and (2) an inability of peripheral tissues to respond to insulin *(insulin resistance)*. The primacy of an insulin secretory defect versus insulin resistance is a matter of continuing debate. Most overtly diabetic patients exhibit both. In the following discussion each of these two factors is considered separately, beginning with the secretory defect (Fig. 19–21).

Insulin Deficiency. Early in the course of type II diabetes, *insulin secretion* appears to be normal and plasma insulin levels are not reduced. However, subtle defects in the function of beta cells can be demonstrated.[45] Perhaps the earliest detectable change is in the pattern of insulin secretion. In normal persons, insulin secretion occurs in a pulsatile or oscillatory pattern, whereas in patients with type II diabetes, the normal oscillations of insulin secretion are lost. At about the same time when fasting blood sugars reach 115 gm/ml, the rapid first phase of insulin secretion triggered by glucose is obtunded. This impaired insulin secretion caused by chronic hyperglycemia, referred to as *glucose toxicity*, is due in part to a reduction of GLUT-2 transporters, which, as you recall, facilitate glucose entry into B cells. In due course, most patients develop mild-to-moderate deficiency of insulin.

Assessment of insulin deficiency in type II diabetes is complicated by the frequent occurrence of obesity in these patients. *Obesity*, even in the absence of diabetes, is characterized by insulin resistance and hyperinsulinemia; however, when obese type II diabetics are compared with weight-matched nondiabetics, the insulin levels of obese diabetics are below those observed in obese nondiabetics, suggesting a relative insulin deficiency. Furthermore, in patients with moderately severe type II diabetes (fasting plasma glucose level of 200 to 300 gm/ml), it is possible to demonstrate an absolute deficiency of insulin. We can conclude, therefore, that *most patients with type II diabetes have a relative or absolute deficiency of insulin. However, this insulin deficiency is milder than that of type I diabetes and is not an early feature of this variant of diabetes.*

The cause of the insulin deficiency in type II diabetes is unknown. Unlike type I diabetes, there is no evidence for viral or immune-mediated injury to the islet cells. According to one view, all the somatic cells of diabetics, including pancreatic beta cells, are genetically vulnerable to injury, leading to accelerated cell turnover and premature aging and, ultimately, to a modest reduction in beta-cell mass.

Current interest is also focused on the role of *amylin* in type II diabetes.[46] This 37–amino acid peptide is normally produced by the beta cells, copackaged with insulin and cosecreted in the sinusoidal space. In patients with NIDDM, amylin tends to accumulate outside the beta cells, in close contact with their cell membranes. It eventually acquires the tinctorial characteristics of *amyloid*. Whether extracellular deposits of amylin contribute to the early disturbance in insulin secretion is controversial.

Insulin Resistance. Since in most patients with type II diabetes insulin deficiency is not of sufficient magnitude to explain the metabolic disturbances, it is logical to suspect impairment of the tissues' response to insulin. Indeed, *there is abundant evidence that insulin resistance is a major factor in the pathogenesis of type II diabetes.* Insulin resistance is a complex phenomenon, not restricted to the diabetes syndrome. In both obesity and pregnancy, insulin sensitivity of tissues decreases (even in the absence of diabetes). Hence either obesity or pregnancy may unmask subclinical type II diabetes by increasing the insulin resistance. *Obesity is an extremely important diabetogenic influence, and, not surprisingly, approximately 80% of type II diabetes patients are obese.* In many obese diabetics, especially early in the course of the disease, impaired glucose tolerance can be reversed by weight loss.

What is the cellular basis of insulin resistance? Although the answer is unclear, there is a decrease in the number of *insulin receptors*, and, more important, *postreceptor defects, including impaired postreceptor signaling, occur.* You may recall from our earlier discussion that binding of insulin to its receptors leads to translocation of GLUTs, particularly GLUT-4, to the cell membrane, which in turn facilitates transmembrane diffusion of glucose. Reduced synthesis and/or translocation of GLUT-4 in muscle and fat cells may account for insulin resistance in obesity as well as in NIDDM.

In addition to insulin resistance in peripheral tissues, there is increased glucose production in the liver, further aggravating the hyperglycemia.

To summarize, NIDDM is a complex, multifactorial disorder involving both impaired insulin release and end-organ insensitivity. Insulin resistance, frequently associated with obesity, produces excessive stress on beta cells, which may fail in the face of sustained need for a state of hyperinsulinism. Genetic factors are definitely involved, as is evident in patients with MODY, but in most cases of NIDDM how they fit into the puzzle remains unclear (see Fig. 19–21).

PATHOGENESIS OF THE COMPLICATIONS OF DIABETES. The morbidity associated with long-standing diabetes of either type results from complications such as *microangiopathy, retinopathy, nephropathy,* and *neuropathy.* Hence the basis of these chronic long-term complications is the subject of a great deal of research.[47] *Most of the available experimental and clinical evidence suggests that the complications of diabetes mellitus are a consequence of the metabolic derangements, mainly hyperglycemia.* The most telling evidence comes from the finding that kidneys, when transplanted into diabetics from nondiabetic donors, develop the lesions of diabetic nephropathy within 3 to 5 years after transplantation. Conversely, kidneys with lesions of diabetic

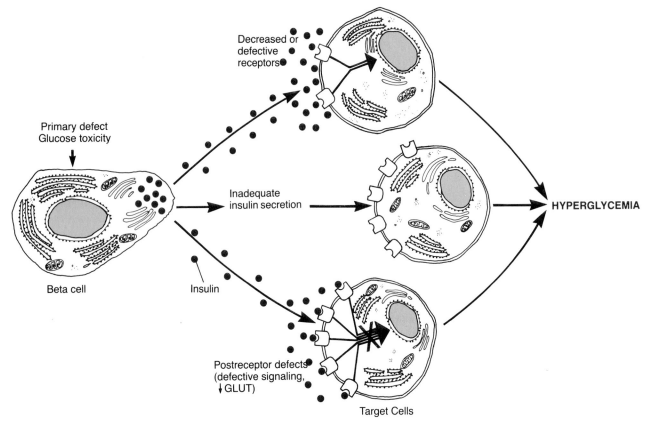

Figure 19–21. Postulated mechanisms in pathogenesis of type II diabetes: inadequate insulin secretion *(left)* and insulin resistance *(right)*. The causes of inadequate primary insulin secretion are unknown, but chronic hyperglycemia itself impairs beta-cell function (see text), owing to glucose toxicity. Insulin resistance can be due to decreased or abnormal insulin receptors or postreceptor defects.

nephropathy demonstrate a reversal of the lesion when transplanted into normal recipients. Recent multicenter studies clearly show delayed progression of diabetic complications by strict control of the hyperglycemia.[48]

Many mechanisms linking hyperglycemia to the complications of long-standing diabetes have been explored. Currently, two such mechanisms are considered important.

1. *Nonenzymatic glycosylation.* This refers to the process by which glucose chemically attaches to the amino group of proteins without the aid of enzymes.[48] Glucose forms chemically reversible glycosylation products with protein (named Schiff bases) that may rearrange to form more stable Amadori-type early glycosylation products, which are also chemically reversible (Fig. 19–22). The degree of enzymatic glycosylation is directly related to the level of blood glucose. Indeed, *the measurement of glycosylated hemoglobin (HbA$_{1c}$) levels in the blood is a useful adjunct in the management of diabetes mellitus.*

The early glycosylation products on collagen and other long-lived proteins in interstitial tissues and blood vessel walls, rather than dissociating, undergo a slow series of chemical rearrangements to form *irreversible advanced glycosylation end products (AGE),* which accumulate over the lifetime of the vessel wall. AGEs have a number of chemical and biologic properties which are potentially pathogenic (Table 19–5).[49,50]

- *AGE* formation occurs on proteins, lipids, and nucleic acids. On proteins, such as collagen, they cause cross-links *between* polypeptides of the collagen molecule and also *trap* nonglycosylated plasma or interstitial proteins. In large vessels, trapping low-density lipoprotein (LDL), for example, retards its efflux from the vessel wall and enhances the deposition of cholesterol in the intima, thus accelerating atherogenesis (see Chapter 11). In capillaries, including those of renal glomeruli, plasma proteins such as albumin bind to the glycosylated basement membrane, accounting in part for the increased basement membrane thickening characteristic of diabetic microangiopathy. *AGE cross-linked proteins are resistant to proteolytic digestion.* Thus, cross-linking decreases protein removal while enhancing protein deposition. AGE-induced cross-linking in collagen type IV in basement membrane may also impair the interaction of collagen with other ma-

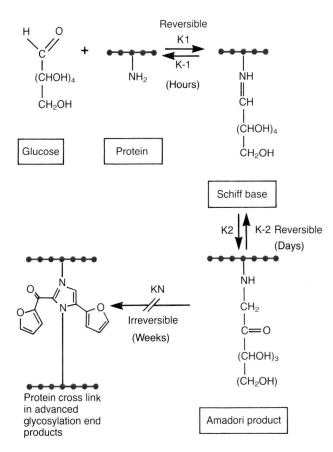

Figure 19–22. Nonenzymatic glycosylation of proteins. The advanced glycosylation product involves protein-protein cross-linking. Note that whereas the early glycosylation products are reversible, advanced end products are irreversible. (Modified from Brownlee, M., et al.: Advanced glycosylation end products in tissue and the biochemical basis of diabetic complications. N. Engl. J. Med. *318*:1315, 1988.)

trix components (laminin, proteoglycans), resulting in structural and functional defects in the basement membranes.
- AGEs bind to receptors on many cell types—endothelium, monocytes, macrophages, lymphocytes, and mesangial cells. Binding induces a variety of biologic activities, including monocyte emigration; release of cytokines and growth factors from macrophages; increased endothelial permeability; increased procoagulant activity on endothelial cells and macrophages; and enhanced proliferation of and synthesis of extracellular matrix by fibroblasts and smooth muscle cells. All these effects can potentially contribute to diabetic complications.
- Evidence that AGE products are pathogenic *in vivo* is derived from studies in experimental models of diabetes, in which neuropathy, retinopathy, and nephropathy are prevented or ameliorated by treatment with aminoguanidine, an agent that binds preferentially to precursors of AGE products and prevents their cross-linking to collagen. In humans it has been shown

Table 19–5. RELEVANT CHEMICAL AND BIOLOGIC PROPERTIES OF ADVANCED GLYCOSYLATION END PRODUCTS

CHEMICAL
Cross-link polypeptides of same protein (e.g., collagen)
Trap nonglycosylated proteins (e.g., LDL, Ig, complement)
Confer resistance to proteolytic digestion
Induce lipid oxidation
Inactivate nitric oxide
Bind nucleic acids
BIOLOGIC
Bind to AGE receptors on monocytes and mesenchymal cells
  Induce: Monocyte emigration
      Cytokines and growth factor secretion
      Increased vascular permeability
      Procoagulant activity
      Enhanced cellular proliferation
      Enhanced ECM production

ECM = extracellular matrix; LDL = low-density lipoprotein.
Adapted from Vlassara, H., Bucala, R., and Striker, L.: Pathogenic effects of advanced glycosylation: Biochemical, biological, and clinical implications. Lab. Invest. *70*:138, 1994; ©United States and Canadian Academy of Pathology, Inc. 1994.

that AGEs accumulate at a faster rate in arteries and plasma in diabetics than in control subjects, and AGE peptide serum levels correlate with the severity of nephropathy.

2. *Intracellular hyperglycemia with disturbances in polyol pathways.*[51] In some tissues (e.g., nerve, lens, kidney, and blood vessels) that do not require insulin for glucose transport, hyperglycemia leads to an increase in intracellular glucose. The excess glucose is metabolized to *sorbitol*, a polyol, by the enzyme aldose reductase and, eventually, to fructose (Fig. 19–23). The accumulated sorbitol and fructose lead to increased intracellular osmolarity and influx of water and, eventually, to osmotic cell injury. Sorbitol accumulation is asso-

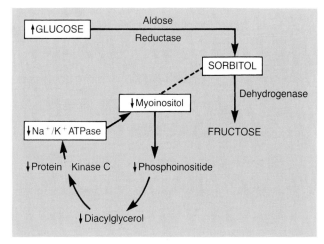

Figure 19–23. Intracellular hyperglycemia, the sorbitol pathway, and effects on *myo*-inositol. (Adapted from Greene, D.A., et al.: Sorbitol, phosphoinositides, and sodium potassium ATPase in the pathogenesis of diabetic complications. N. Engl. J. Med. *316*:599, 1987.)

ciated with a decrease in myo-*inositol content*, resulting in decreased phosphoinositide metabolism, diacylglycerol, protein kinase C, and Na+, K+-ATPase activity. This mechanism may be responsible for damage to Schwann cells and to pericytes of retinal capillaries, with resultant peripheral neuropathy and retinal microaneurysms, respectively. In the lens, osmotically imbibed water causes swelling and opacity. That this pathway may contribute to the ocular and neurologic complications of diabetes is supported by experimental studies in which pharmacologic inhibition of aldol reductase prevented the fall in *myo*-inositol content and the decrease in ATPase activity, as well as the development of cataracts and neuropathy.

METABOLIC DERANGEMENTS IN DIABETES. Insulin is a major anabolic hormone in the body, and therefore *derangement of insulin function affects not only glucose metabolism but also fat and protein metabolism.* Unopposed secretion of counter-regulatory hormones (glycogen, growth hormone, epinephrine) is now also thought to play a role in these metabolic derangements, which are most severe in type I diabetes. The assimilation of glucose into muscle and adipose tissue is sharply diminished or abolished. Not only does storage of glycogen in liver and muscle cease, but also reserves are depleted by glycogenolysis. Fasting hyperglycemia may reach levels many times greater than normal, and when the level of circulating glucose exceeds the renal threshold, glycosuria ensues. The excessive glycosuria induces an osmotic diuresis and thus *polyuria*, causing a profound loss of water and electrolytes (Na, K, Mg, P) (Fig. 19–24). This obligatory water loss combined with the hyperosmolarity resulting from the increased levels of glucose in the blood tends to deplete intracellular water, as, for example, in the osmoreceptors of the thirst centers of the brain. In this manner, intense thirst *(polydipsia)* appears. Increased appetite *(polyphagia)* develops, thus completing the classic triad of diabetic findings—*polyuria, polydipsia, and polyphagia.* With a deficiency of insulin, the scales swing from insulin-promoted anabolism to catabolism of proteins and fats. Proteolysis follows, and the glucogenic amino acids are removed by the liver and used as building blocks in gluconeogenesis.

Two important acute metabolic complications of diabetes mellitus follow, *diabetic ketoacidosis* and *nonketotic hyperosmolar coma.*

Diabetic ketoacidosis occurs exclusively in type I diabetes and is stimulated by *severe insulin deficiency coupled with absolute or relative increases of glucagon* (see Fig. 19–24). The insulin deficiency causes excessive breakdown of adipose stores, resulting in increased levels of free fatty acids. Oxidation of such free fatty acids within the liver through acetyl-CoA produces ketone bodies. *Glucagon* is the hormone that accelerates such fatty acid oxidation. The rate at which ketone bodies are formed may exceed the rate at which acetoacetic acid and beta-hydroxybutyric acid can be utilized by muscles and other tissues. Ketogenic amino acids aggravate the derangements in lipid metabolism. Ketogenesis thus increases, leading to ketonemia and ketonuria. If the urinary excretion of ketones is compromised by dehydration, the plasma hydrogen ion concentration increases, and *systemic metabolic ketoacidosis* results.

In type II diabetes, polyuria, polydipsia, and polyphagia may accompany the fasting hyperglycemia, but ketoacidosis is rare. Adults, particularly elderly diabetics, develop *nonketotic hyperosmolar coma,* a syndrome engendered by the severe dehydration resulting from sustained hyperglycemic diuresis, which is coupled with an inability of these patients to drink water. The absence of ketoacidosis and its symptoms (nausea, vomiting, respiratory difficulties) delays the seeking of medical attention in those patients until severe dehydration and coma have occurred.

MORPHOLOGY OF DIABETES AND ITS LATE COMPLICATIONS

The important morphologic changes in diabetes are related to its many late systemic complications, since they are the major causes of morbidity and mortality. There is extreme variability among patients in the time of onset, the severity of these complications, and the particular organ or organs involved. In most patients, regardless of the type

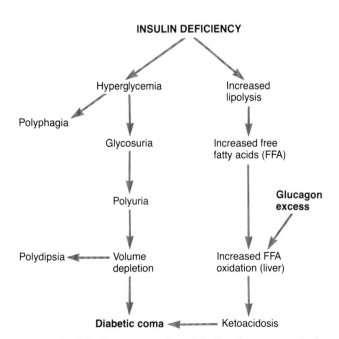

Figure 19–24. Sequence of metabolic derangements in diabetes mellitus.

of diabetes, when the disease has been present for 10 to 15 years, morphologic changes are likely to be found in the basement membranes of small vessels (*microangiopathy*), arteries (*atherosclerosis*), kidneys (*diabetic nephropathy*), retina (*retinopathy*), nerves (*neuropathy*), and other tissues, and clinical evidence of dysfunction in these organs is present.

ISLET CHANGES. Surprisingly, lesions in the pancreas are neither constant nor necessarily pathognomonic. They are more likely to be distinctive in type I than in type II. One or more of the following alterations may be present: (1) **Reduction in the size and number of islets.** This is most often seen in type I diabetes, particularly with rapidly advancing disease. Most of the islets are small, inconspicuous, and not easily detected in routinely stained sections. They are composed of thin cords of cells intermingled with fibrous stroma. Careful morphometric studies performed with special stains show reduction in beta cells even in type II disease, but this change is subtle and not easily detected. (2) **Increase in the size and number of islets.** This may be seen in diabetic or nondiabetic infants of diabetic mothers. Presumably, the maternal hyperglycemia leads to fetal hyperglycemia and compensatory hyperplasia of the fetal islets. (3) **Beta-cell degranulation.** This is most often encountered in the insulin-dependent variant and is thought to represent depletion of secretory stores of insulin in already damaged cells. (4) **Fibrosis of islets.** (5) **Amyloid replacement of islets** by an amorphous substance having the fibrillar substructure characteristic of amyloid (Fig. 19–25). As noted previously, amyloid deposits are composed of the polypeptide *amylin* (also called islet amyloid polypeptide (IAPP)). Both the collagenous and the amyloid deposits occur at first about the microcirculation within the islets and progressively extend to obliterate the surrounding cells. These changes may be found in type I but are more characteristic of the late chronic stages of type II. (6) **Leukocytic infiltrations** may take one of two forms. The most common pattern is a heavy lymphocytic infiltrate within and about the islets, referred to as **insulitis.** Insulitis is most frequent in young diabetics with a brief history of symptomatic diabetes. Eosinophilic infiltrates may also be found, particularly in diabetic infants who fail to survive the immediate postnatal period.

DIABETIC MICROANGIOPATHY. One of the most consistent morphologic features of diabetes is diffuse thickening of basement membranes.[52] The thickening is most evident in the capillaries of the skin, skeletal muscles, retina, renal glomeruli, and renal medulla, giving rise to the characteristic *diabetic microangiopathy* of these organs. However, it

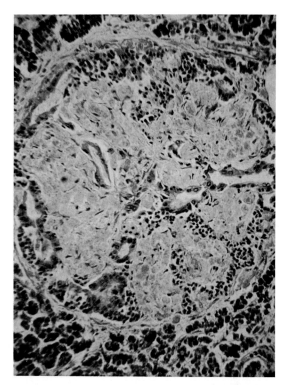

Figure 19–25. Amyloid deposition in an islet in the pancreas of a diabetic.

may also be seen in such nonvascular structures as renal tubules, Bowman's capsule, peripheral nerves, and placenta.

MORPHOLOGY. By light microscopy, the thickening appears as widening of the basement membrane by a homogeneous, sometimes multilayered hyaline substance, which is strongly positive with the periodic acid–Schiff (PAS) stain (Fig. 19–26). Under the electron microscope the thickening either may be homogeneous (Fig. 19–27) or, particularly in the skin, may consist of several laminated circumferential layers.[53] Despite the increased thickness of basement membranes, diabetic capillaries are more leaky than normal to plasma proteins. As will be seen, the microangiopathy has far-reaching implications, inducing serious lesions in the renal glomeruli and retina and possibly contributing to the increased vulnerability of the diabetic individual to neuropathy. It should be noted that similar microvascular lesions can be found in aged nondiabetic patients, but rarely to the extent seen in those with long-standing diabetes.[53]

The microangiopathy is clearly related to the hyperglycemia. A number of biochemical basement membrane alterations occur, including increased amounts and synthesis of collagen type IV and decreases in proteoglycans. The latter can account for the increased glomerular permeability characteristic of diabetic nephropathy. As explained earlier,

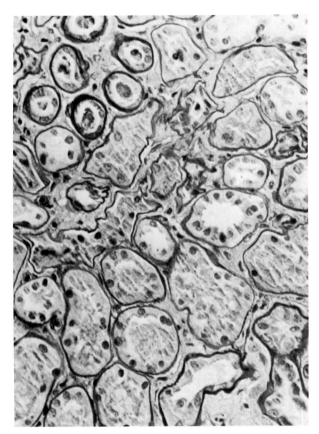

Figure 19–26. Periodic acid–Schiff stain of renal cortex showing thickening of basement membrane in a diabetic.

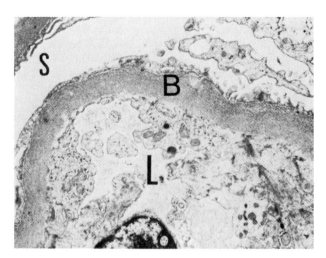

Figure 19–27. Markedly thickened glomerular basement membrane (B) in a diabetic. L = glomerular capillary lumen; S = urinary space.

there is evidence that *advanced glycosylation end products play a role in the pathogenesis of these changes.*

Hyaline arteriolosclerosis, the vascular lesion associated with hypertension, is both more prevalent and more severe in diabetics than in nondiabetics. However, it is not specific for diabetes and may be seen in elderly nondiabetics without hypertension. It takes the form of an amorphous, hyaline thickening on the wall of the arterioles, which causes narrowing of the lumen (see Chapter 11, Fig. 11–18). Not surprisingly, in the diabetic it is related not only to the duration of the disease but also to the level of the blood pressure.

ATHEROSCLEROSIS. Atherosclerosis begins to appear in most diabetics, whatever their age, within a few years of onset of both type I and type II diabetes. Fewer than 5% of nondiabetics as opposed to approximately 75% of diabetics younger than 40 years of age have moderate to severe atherosclerosis. Diabetic atherosclerotic lesions tend to be numerous and florid and to undergo the constellation of changes leading to complicated lesions, that is, ulceration, calcification, and superimposed thromboses. Thus, relatively early in the diabetic's life,

atherosclerosis may result in arterial narrowings or occlusions and attendant ischemic injury to organs; alternatively, it may induce aneurysmal dilatation, seen most often in the aorta, with the grave potential of rupture. *This large vessel disease accounts for the heavy toll exacted by myocardial infarction, cerebral stroke, and gangrene of the lower extremities in these patients.* Gangrene of the lower extremities is 100 times more common in diabetics than in nondiabetics.

The susceptibility of the diabetic to atherosclerosis is due to several factors (see Chapter 11). *Hyperlipidemia* occurs in one-third to one-half of patients, but even those with normal lipids have severe atherosclerosis. *High-density lipoprotein (HDL) levels are reduced* in type II diabetes, possibly enhancing susceptibility to atherogenesis. *Non-enzymatic glycosylation* of LDL renders it more recognizable by the LDL receptor, while glycosylated HDL is more readily degradable than normal HDL—both these effects enhance atherogenesis. LDL cross-linking to collagen increases with the degree of glycosylation of the collagen molecule, thus retarding cholesterol efflux from the arterial wall. Diabetics have *increased platelet adhesiveness* and response to aggregating agents. These changes are also likely to favor atherogenesis. Most patients with type II diabetes also tend to be *obese* and *hypertensive,* so that other contributing influences are present. Whatever the mechanism(s), all diabetics who have had the disease for at least 10 years, irrespective of the age of onset, are likely to have clinically significant atherosclerosis.

DIABETIC NEPHROPATHY. The kidneys are usually the most severely damaged organs in the diabetic. Renal failure, usually due to renal microvascular disease, accounts for many diabetic deaths in both juveniles and adults. Any one or any combination of the following major lesions may be found: (1)

glomerular involvement with three distinctive patterns: diffuse glomerulosclerosis, nodular glomerulosclerosis, and exudative lesions—these result in proteinuria, and in time progress to chronic renal failure; (2) *arteriolosclerosis,* including so-called benign nephrosclerosis and frequently associated with hypertension; (3) bacterial urinary tract infection, with *pyelonephritis* and sometimes *necrotizing papillitis.*

The glomerular and arteriolar lesions are the most important and are intimately linked to the overall diabetic microangiopathy. Since diabetic renal disease is one of the major causes of renal morbidity and mortality, the subject will be discussed in detail in Chapter 20.

DIABETIC OCULAR COMPLICATIONS. One of the most threatening aspects of diabetes mellitus is the development of visual impairment consequent to *retinopathy, cataract formation,* or *glaucoma.* Diabetic retinopathy is the fourth leading cause of all legal blindness (visual acuity of 20/200 or worse) in the United States today. In the development of diabetic retinopathy, the duration of disease appears to be a very important determinant. It has been estimated that if a patient is diagnosed as a diabetic at age 30, there is a 10% chance he will have some degree of diabetic retinopathy by age 37, a 50% chance by age 45, and a 90% chance by age 55. However, it should be appreciated that diabetic retinopathy does not always impose a visual handicap, depending on whether the macula is involved or not.

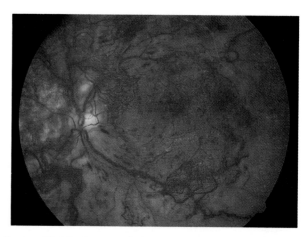

Figure 19-28. Severe diabetic retinopathy showing the optic nerve and macula. Note the large pale area of edema with numerous small new vessels (neovascularization) at periphery, and small hemorrhages. (Courtesy of Dr. Peggy Lindsey.)

MORPHOLOGY. Retinopathy consists of a constellation of changes that together are considered by many ophthalmologists to be virtually diagnostic of the disease. The lesion in the retina takes two forms—**nonproliferative,** or background, retinopathy and **proliferative retinopathy.** The former includes intraretinal or preretinal hemorrhages, retinal exudates, edema, venous dilatations, and, most important, thickening of the retinal capillaries (microangiopathy) and the development of microaneurysms. The retinal exudates can be either "soft" (microinfarcts) or "hard" (deposits of plasma proteins and lipids). The **microaneurysms** are discrete saccular dilatations of retinal choroidal capillaries that appear through the opthalmoscope as small red dots (Fig. 19–28). The pathogenesis of retinal microaneurysms is multifactorial. Selective **loss of retinal capillary pericytes** occurs early and is believed to be a consequence of changes in the basement membrane. Dilatations tend to occur at focal points of weakening, resulting from loss of pericytes. In addition, retinal edema resulting from excessive capillary permeability might cause focal collapse, making the vessels vulnerable to aneurysmal dilatation.

The so-called **proliferative retinopathy** is associated with neovascularization and fibrosis. This le-

sion can lead to serious consequences, including blindness, especially when it involves the macula. Vitreous hemorrhages can result from rupture of the newly formed capillaries. It is of interest that about half the patients with retinal microaneurysms also have nodular glomerulosclerosis. Conversely, **patients who have nodular glomerulosclerosis are almost certain to have retinal microaneurysms.**

DIABETIC NEUROPATHY. Peripheral nerves, brain, and spinal cord all may be damaged in long-standing diabetes. Most commonly encountered is *symmetric peripheral neuropathy* affecting both motor and sensory nerves of the lower extremities. It is characterized by Schwann cell injury, myelin degeneration, and also axonal damage. Damage to the Schwann cells or possibly axons is believed to be the primary event. The peripheral neuropathy is sometimes accompanied by disturbances in the neural innervation of the pelvic organs *(autonomic neuropathy),* leading to sexual impotence and bowel and bladder dysfunction.

The cause of the neuropathy is somewhat uncertain, and several explanations have been offered. It may be related to diffuse microangiopathy affecting the nutritional maintenance of the peripheral nerve. This mechanism seems to be the most likely explanation for *diabetic mononeuropathies* affecting, for example, obturator, femoral, or sciatic nerves. Disordered glucose metabolism, rather than vascular insufficiency, is believed to be the cause of polyneuropathies.

Accumulation of sorbitol, described earlier, appears to be responsible for the Schwann cell injury in this condition. Neuronal degeneration in the brain and spinal cord may also appear. In addition, the diabetic has some predisposition to cerebral infarctions and brain hemorrhages, the latter related to the hypertension seen so often in these patients. It is worth noting that neurons are vulnerable to the hypoglycemia encountered in insulin reactions and to the ketoacidosis of the uncontrolled diabetic state.

CLINICAL COURSE

It is difficult to sketch with brevity the diverse clinical presentations of diabetes mellitus, because the disease may appear as silently as a cat or storm in like an enraged bull. Only a few stereotypical responses can be presented.

Type I diabetes (IDDM), which begins by age 20 years in most patients, is dominated by signs and symptoms emanating from the disordered metabolism discussed earlier—polyuria, polydipsia, polyphagia, and ketoacidosis. The plasma insulin is low or absent, and glucagon levels are increased. Glucose intolerance is of the unstable or brittle type and is quite sensitive to administered exogenous insulin, deviations from normal dietary intake, unusual physical activity, infection, or other forms of stress. Inadequate fluid intake or vomiting may lead to disturbances in fluid and electrolyte balance. Thus, these patients are vulnerable, on the one hand, to *hypoglycemic episodes* and, on the other, to *ketoacidosis. Infection* may precipitate these conditions and, indeed, may precede the first manifestations of diabetes in some patients. Fortunately, these metabolic hazards are more avoidable with proper insulin therapy than the long-term sequelae.

Type II diabetes (NIDDM) may also present with polyuria and polydipsia, but unlike type I diabetes, the patients are often older (over 40 years) and frequently obese. In some cases medical attention is sought because of unexplained weakness or weight loss. Frequently, however, the diagnosis is made by routine blood or urine testing in asymptomatic individuals. Although patients with type II diabetes also have metabolic derangements, these are usually relatively mild and controllable, and so this form of the disease is not often complicated by ketoacidosis unless intercurrent infection or stress imposes new burdens. *In both forms of long-standing diabetes, atherosclerotic events such as myocardial infarction, cerebrovascular accidents, gangrene of the leg, and the microangiopathic complications, (nephropathy, retinopathy, neuropathy) are the most threatening and most frequent concomitants.*

Diabetics are also plagued by an enhanced susceptibility to infections, such as tuberculosis, pneumoconioses, pyelonephritis, and those affecting the skin. Collectively, such infections cause the deaths of about 5% of diabetic patients. The basis of this susceptibility is probably multifactorial; impaired leukocyte functions and poor blood supply secondary to vascular disease are involved. A trivial infection in a toe may be the first event in a long succession of complications (gangrene, bacteremia, and pneumonia) that ultimately lead to death.

As mentioned at the outset, this disease continues to be one of the top 10 "killers" in the United States. It is hoped that islet cell transplantation, which is still in the experimental stage, will lead to the cure of diabetes mellitus. Even then, the full benefit of islet cell replacement can be derived only early in the course of diabetes, before the myriad vascular complications have set in. Current studies show that good, early control of the hyperglycemia prevents or ameliorates some of the complications of diabetes.[48]

ISLET CELL TUMORS

Islet cell tumors[54] are rare in comparison with tumors of the exocrine pancreas. They are most common in adults and can occur anywhere along the length of the pancreas. They may be hormonally functional or entirely nonfunctional. The tumors may be single or multiple and benign or malignant, the latter metastasizing to lymph nodes and liver. When multiple, each tumor may be composed of a different cell type.

The three most common and distinctive clinical syndromes associated with hyperfunction of the islets of Langerhans are (1) *hyperinsulinism and hypoglycemia,* (2) *the Zollinger-Ellison syndrome (gastrinoma),* and (3) *multiple endocrine neoplasia.* Each of these may be caused by (1) diffuse hyperplasia of the islets of Langerhans, (2) benign adenomas that occur singly or multiply, and (3) malignant islet tumors. Multiple endocrine cell tumors are described in Chapter 25.

BETA-CELL TUMORS (INSULINOMA)

Beta-cell tumors (insulinomas) are the most common of islet cell tumors and may be responsible for the elaboration of sufficient insulin to induce clinically significant hypoglycemia. There is a characteristic clinical triad resulting from these pancreatic lesions: (1) Attacks of hypoglycemia occur with blood sugar levels below 50 mg/dl of serum; (2) the attacks consist principally of such central nervous system manifestations as confusion, stupor, and loss of consciousness and are clearly related to fasting or exercise; and (3) the attacks are promptly relieved by the feeding or parenteral administration of glucose. There are other causes of hypoglycemia when a patient manifests this classic triad, but the cause should first be sought in the pancreas.

MORPHOLOGY. Analysis of pancreatic islet lesions inducing hyperinsulinism indicates that about 70%

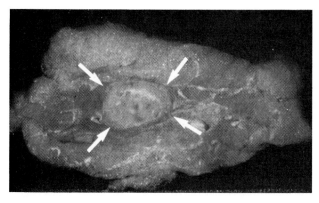

Figure 19–29. Islet cell adenoma of pancreas. Small, pale tumor is seen on transection of pancreas *(arrows)*.

are solitary adenomas, approximately 10% are multiple adenomas, 10% are metastasizing tumors that must be interpreted as carcinomas, and the remainder are a mixed group of diffuse hyperplasia of the islets and adenomas occurring in ectopic pancreatic tissue.[55] The **insulinomas** vary in size from minute lesions that are difficult to find even on the dissecting table to huge masses of over 1500 gm (Fig. 19–29). Most occur singly, but sometimes multiple adenomas are found scattered throughout the pancreas. They are usually encapsulated, firm, yellow-brown nodules, histologically composed of cords and nests of well-differentiated beta cells that do not differ from those of the normal islet (Fig. 19–30). On electron microscopy, the tumor cells exhibit the typical beta-cell granules, and by immunohistochemistry insulin can be visualized in tumor cells.

Five per cent of insulinomas are malignant. Histologically, these tumors display little evidence of anaplasia and may be impossible to differentiate from benign tumors. The diagnosis is made in the presence of metastasis or local invasion beyond the substance of the pancreas.

Hyperinsulinism may also be caused by **diffuse hyperplasia of the islets.** This change is found occasionally in adults but is characteristic of infants born of diabetic mothers. Long exposed to the hyperglycemia of the maternal blood, the infant responds by an increase in the size and number of its islets. In the postnatal period, these hyperactive islets may be responsible for serious episodes of hypoglycemia.[56]

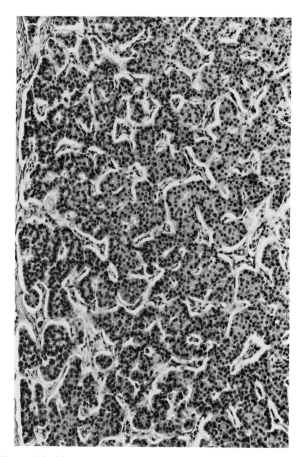

Figure 19–30. Islet cell adenoma of pancreas. The well-defined margin of an islet cell tumor. Note resemblance of tumor cells to normal islet cells.

A variety of functional and organic disorders, in addition to the beta-cell lesions, cause hypoglycemia. These include early diabetes mellitus, so-called insulin-sensitivity states, partial gastrectomy, starvation, diffuse liver disease, the glycogenoses, hypofunction of the anterior pituitary and adrenal cortex, a variety of extrapancreatic neoplasms, and idiopathic hypoglycemia.

ZOLLINGER-ELLISON SYNDROME (GASTRINOMA)

This syndrome is classically composed of the triad of recalcitrant peptic ulcer disease, gastric hypersecretion, and pancreatic islet cell tumor. Fundamental to the peptic ulcerations is gastric hypersecretion, induced by gastrin, so the tumor is also known as a *gastrinoma.* Although most common in the pancreas, 10 to 15% of gastrinomas occur in the duodenum. Serum gastrin levels are elevated, and indeed *hypergastrinemia can point to the pres-*

Although with newer evaluation procedures up to 80% of islet cell tumors may show excessive insulin secretion, the hypoglycemia is mild in all but 20%, and many cases never become clinically symptomatic. The critical laboratory findings in insulinomas are high circulating levels of insulin and a high insulin-to-glucose ratio. Surgical removal of the tumor is usually followed by prompt reversal of the hypoglycemia.

ence of early gastrinomas before the development of ulcer disease.

Approximately 60% of gastrinomas are malignant, and 40% are benign. Only spread to lymph nodes or metastasis marks the tumors as malignant. Some of the benign adenomas are multiple and occur in association with endocrine adenomas elsewhere, justifying their being classified as examples of multiple endocrine neoplasia. Seventy-five per cent of the ulcers occur in the usual sites within the stomach or, more often, in the first and second portions of the duodenum. Abnormally located peptic ulcers in the distal portions of the duodenum and jejunum occur in 25% of cases. In one of ten patients, there are multiple ulcerations. The stomach also shows hyperplasia of the acid-secreting parietal cells.

Patients with the Zollinger-Ellison syndrome present formidable problems in clinical management. They have striking gastric hypersecretion, which presumably produces the intractable ulcers. In addition, diarrhea is often sufficiently extreme to cause serious problems in fluid and electrolyte control, and many patients develop malabsorption syndromes. Moreover, the lesions in the pancreas not only may be malignant but also, even when benign, may be very small or multiple and difficult to discover at surgical exploration. It is not uncommon, therefore, for symptoms to be recurrent following removal of any apparent solitary lesion, with later discovery of additional lesions within the pancreas.

OTHER RARE ISLET CELL TUMORS

Alpha-cell tumors (glucagonomas) are associated with increased serum levels of glucagon and a syndrome consisting of mild diabetes mellitus, a characteristic migratory necrotizing skin erythema, and anemia. They occur most frequently in peri- and postmenopausal women and are characterized by extremely high plasma glucagon levels.

Delta-cell tumors (somatostatinomas) are associated with diabetes mellitus, cholelithiasis, steatorrhea, and hypochlorhydria. They are exceedingly difficult to detect preoperatively. High plasma somatostatin levels are required for diagnosis.

VIPoma (diarrheogenic islet cell tumor) is an islet cell tumor that induces a characteristic syndrome of *watery diarrhea, hypokalemia,* and *achlorhydria* (the WDHA syndrome) caused by release of *vasoactive intestinal polypeptide* (VIP) from the tumor. Some of these tumors are locally invasive and metastatic. Neural crest tumors, such as ganglioneuroma, neuroblastoma, neurofibroma, and

pheochromocytoma, can also be associated with the VIPoma syndrome.

Pancreatic *carcinoid tumors* producing serotonin and an atypical carcinoid syndrome are exceedingly rare. *Pancreatic polypeptide–secreting* islet cell tumors are endocrinologically asymptomatic, despite the presence of high levels of the hormone in plasma.

Some pancreatic and extrapancreatic tumors produce two or more hormones, usually simultaneously and occasionally in sequence. In addition to insulin, glucagon, and gastrin, islet cell tumors produce adrenocorticotropic hormone (ACTH), melanocyte-stimulating hormone (MSH), vasopressin, norepinephrine, and serotonin. These are called *multihormonal tumors* to distinguish them from the multiple endocrine neoplasias described before, in which a multiplicity of hormones are produced by several different glands.

1. Bockman, D.E.: Anatomy of the pancreas. *In* Go, V.L.W., et al. (eds.): The Pancreas: Biology, Pathobiology, and Disease. New York, Raven Press, 1993, pp. 1–8.
2. Meyer, J.G.: Pancreatic physiology. *In* Sleisenger, M.D., and Fordtran, J.S. (eds.): Gastrointestinal Disease: Pathophysiology, Diagnosis, Management. Philadelphia, W.B. Saunders Co., 1989, pp. 1777–1788.
3. Chey, W.Y.: Hormonal control of pancreatic exocrine secretion. *In* Go, V.L.W., et al. (eds.): The Pancreas: Biology, Pathobiology, and Disease. New York, Raven Press, 1993, pp. 403–424.
4. Rinderknecht, H.: Pancreatic secretory enzymes. *In* Go, V.L.W., et al. (eds.): The Pancreas: Biology, Pathobiology, and Disease. New York, Raven Press, 1993, pp. 219–252.
5. Singer, M.V., et al.: Revised classification of pancreatitis. Gastroenterology 89:683, 1985.
6. Ranson, J.H.C.: Risk factors in acute pancreatitis. Hosp. Pract. 20:69, 1985.
7. Steer, M.L.: Etiology and pathophysiology of acute pancreatitis. *In* Go, V.L.W., et al. (eds.): The Pancreas: Biology, Pathobiology, and Disease, 2nd ed. New York, Raven Press, 1993, pp. 581–591.
8. Scarpelli, D.G.: Toxicology of the pancreas. Toxicol. Appl. Pharmacol. 101:543, 1989.
9. Sarles, H.: Epidemiology and pathophysiology of chronic pancreatitis and the role of the pancreatic stone protein. Clin. Gastroenterol. 13:895, 1984.
10. Koike, H., et al.: Pancreatic effects of ethionine: Blockade of exocytosis and appearance of crinophagy and autophagy precede cellular necrosis. Am. J. Physiol. 242:G297, 1982.
11. Foulis, A.K., et al.: Endotoxemia and complement activation in pancreatitis. Gut 23:656, 1982.
12. Banks, P.A.: Predictors of severity in acute pancreatitis. Pancreas 6(Suppl. 1):S7, 1991.
13. Di Magno, E.P., et al.: Chronic pancreatitis. *In* Go, V.L.W., et al. (eds.): The Pancreas: Biology, Pathobiology, and Disease. New York, Raven Press, 1993, pp. 665–706.
14. Sarles, H., et al.: Pathogenesis and epidemiology of chronic pancreatitis. Annu. Rev. Med. 40:453, 1989.
15. Klöppel G., and Maillet, B.: The morphological basis for the evolution of acute pancreatitis into chronic pancreatitis. Virchows Arch. Pathol. Anat. Histopathol. 420:1, 1992.
16. Grendell, J.H., and Cello, J.P.: Chronic pancreatitis. *In* Sleisenger, M.H., and Fordtran, J.S. (eds.): Gastrointestinal Disease: Pathophysiology, Diagnosis, Management. Philadelphia, W.B. Saunders Co., 1989, pp. 1842–1871.
17. Nishihara, K., et al.: Papillary cystic tumors of the pan-

creas: Assessment of their malignant potential. Cancer 71:82, 1993.

18. Cubilla, A., and Fitzgerald, P.J.: Tumors of exocrine pancrease. In Atlas of Tumor Pathology, Tumor Fascicle Series. Washington, DC, Armed Forces Institute of Pathology, 1983, pp. 1–286.

19. Grodis, L., and Gold, E.B.: Epidemiology and etiology of pancreatic cancer. In Go, V.L.W., et al. (eds.): The Pancreas: Biology, Pathobiology, and Disease. New York, Raven Press, 1993, pp. 837–855.

20. Boring, C.C., et al.: Cancer Statistics, 1993. CA Cancer J. Clin. 43:7, 1993.

21. Warshaw, A.L., and Fernandez-del Castillo, C.: Medical progress: Pancreatic carcinoma. N. Engl. J. Med. 326:455, 1992.

22. Mendelsohn, G.: The endocrine pancreas and diabetes mellitus. In Mendelsohn, G. (ed.): Diagnosis and Pathology of Endocrine Diseases. Philadelphia, J.B. Lippincott Co., 1988, p. 273.

23. Bennett, P.H.: The diagnosis of diabetes: New internal classification and diagnostic crtieria. Annu. Rev. Med. 34:295, 1983.

24. Bennett, P.H.: Epidemiology of diabetes mellitus. In Rifkin, H., and Porte, D. (eds.): Diabetes Mellitus. New York, Elsevier, 1990, pp. 363–377.

25. DeFronzo, R.A., et al.: Pathogenesis of NIDDM: A balanced overview. Diabetes Care 15:319, 1992.

26. Kahn, R.: Molecular mechanisms of insulin action. Annu. Rev. Med. 36:429, 1985.

27. Garvey, W.T.: Glucose transport and NIDDM. Diabetes Care 15:397, 1992.

28. Thorburn, A.W., et al.: Multiple defects in muscle glycogen synthase activity contribute to reduced glycogen synthesis in non–insulin-dependent diabetes mellitus. J. Clin. Invest. 87:489, 1991.

29. Muir, A., et al.: The pathogenesis, prediction, and prevention of insulin-dependent diabetes mellitus. Endocrinol. Metab. Clin. North Am. 21:199, 1992.

30. Tait, B.D., and Harrison, L.C.: The major histocompatibility complex and IDDM. Baillieres Clin. Endocrinol. Metab. 5:211, 1991.

31. Nepom G.T.: Immunogenetics and IDDM. Diabetes Rev. 1:93, 1993.

32. Todd, J.A., et al.: A molecular basis for MHC Class II–associated autoimmunity. Science 240:1083, 1988.

33. Hatori, T., et al.: Thy-1–linked diabetogenetic gene but not MHC-linked gene causes the primary destruction of B-cells of the N.O.D. mouse. Diabetes 36(Suppl. 1):82A, 1987.

34. Rossini, A.A., et al.: Immunopathogenesis of diabetes mellitus. Diabetes Care 1:43, 1993.

35. Atkinson, M.A., and Maclaten, N.K.: Islet cell autoantigens in insulin-dependent diabetes. J. Clin. Invest. 92:1608, 1993.

36. Laufer, T.M., et al.: Autoimmune diabetes can be induced in transgenic major histocompatibility complex class II–deficient mice. J. Exp. Med. 178:589, 1993.

37. Herold, K.C., and Rubenstein, A.H.: Immunosuppression for insulin-dependent diabetes. N. Engl. J. Med. 318:701, 1988.

38. Yoon, J.W.: Role of viruses in the pathogenesis of IDDM. Ann. Intern. Med. 23:4327, 1991.

39. Craighead, J.E.: Viral diabetes. In Volk, B.W., and Arquilla, E.R. (eds.): The Diabetic Pancreas. New York, Plenum Medical Publishing, 1985, pp. 439–466.

40. Kostraba, J.N., et al.: Early exposure to cow's milk and solid foods in infancy, genetic predisposition, and risk of IDDM. Diabetes 42:288, 1993.

41. Karjalainen, J., et al.: A bovine albumin peptide as a possible trigger of insulin-dependent diabetes mellitus. N. Engl. J. Med. 327:302, 1992.

42. Weir, G.C.: A defective beta-cell glucose sensor as a cause of diabetes. N. Engl. J. Med. 328:729, 1993.

42a. Yki-Järvinen, H.: Pathogenesis of non–insulin-dependent diabetes mellitus. Lancet 343:91, 1994.

43. Froguel, P., et al.: Familial hyperglycemia due to mutations in glucokinase: Definition of a subtype of diabetes mellitus. N. Engl. J. Med. 328:697, 1993.

44. Groop, L.C., et al.: Association between polymorphism of the glycogen synthase gene and non–insulin-dependent diabetes mellitus. N. Engl. J. Med. 328:10, 1993.

45. Leahy, J.L., et al.: β-Cell dysfunction induced by chronic hyperglycemia. Diabetes Care 15:442, 1992.

46. Westermark, P., et al.: Islet cell amyloid polypeptide, a novel controversy in diabetes research. Diabetologia 35:297, 1992.

47. Nathan, D.M.: Long-term complications of diabetes mellitus. N. Engl. J. Med. 328:1676, 1993.

48. The Diabetes Control and Complications Trial Research Group: The effect of intensive treatment of diabetes on the development and progression of long-term complications in insulin-dependent diabetes mellitus. N. Engl. J. Med. 329:977, 1993.

49. Brownlee, M., et al.: Advanced glycosylation end products in tissue and the biochemical basis of diabetic complications. N. Engl. J. Med. 318:1314, 1988.

50. Vlassara, H., et al.: Pathogenic effects of advanced glycosylation: Biochemical, biological, and clinical implications. Lab. Invest. 70:135, 1994.

51. Greene, D.A., et al.: Sorbitol, phosphoinositides, and sodium potassium ATPase in the pathogenesis of diabetic complications. N. Engl. J. Med. 316:599, 1987.

52. Tisher, C.C., and Hostetter, T.: Diabetic nephropathy. In Tisher, C., and Brenner, B. (eds.): Renal Pathology, 2nd ed. Philadelphia, J.B. Lippincott, 1994, pp. 1387–1412.

53. Vracko, R.: A comparison of the microvascular lesions in diabetes mellitus with those of normal aging. J. Am. Geriatr. Soc. 30:201, 1982.

54. Bloodworth, J.M.B., and Creider, M.H.: The endocrine pancreas and diabetes mellitus. In Bloodworth, J.M.B., Jr. (ed.): Endocrine Pathology. Baltimore, Williams & Wilkins Co., 1982, pp. 556–720.

55. Freisen, S.R.: Tumors of the endocrine pancreas. N. Engl. J. Med. 306:580, 1982.

56. Eriksson, B., et al.: Neuroendocrine pancreatic tumors. J. Int. Med. 228:103, 1990.

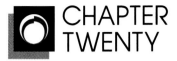
The Kidney

NORMAL

What is man but an ingenious machine designed to turn, with "infinite artfulness, the red wine of Shiraz into urine"? So said the story teller in Isak Dinesen's *Seven Gothic Tales*.[1] More accurately but less poetically, human kidneys serve to convert more than 1700 liters of blood per day into about 1 liter of a highly specialized concentrated fluid called urine. In so doing, the kidney excretes the waste products of metabolism, pre-

cisely regulates the body's concentration of water and salt, maintains the appropriate acid balance of plasma, and serves as an endocrine organ, secreting such hormones as erythropoietin, renin, and prostaglandins. The physiologic mechanisms that the kidney has evolved to carry out these functions require a high degree of structural complexity.

Each human adult kidney weighs about 150 gm. As the ureter enters the kidney at the hilus, it dilates into a funnel-shaped cavity, the *pelvis*, from which derive two to three main branches, the *major calyces;* the latter subdivide again into about three to four *minor calyces.* There are about 12 minor calyces in the human kidney. On cut sur-

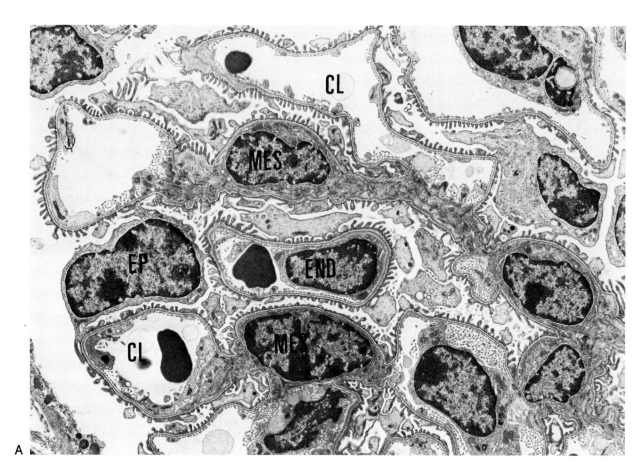

A

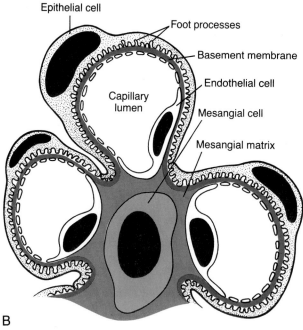

B

Figure 20–1. *A*, Low-power electron micrograph of renal glomerulus. CL = capillary lumen; MES = mesangium; END = endothelium; EP = visceral epithelial cells with foot processes. (Courtesy of Dr. Vicki Kelley, Brigham and Women's Hospital, Boston.) *B*, Schematic representation of a glomerular lobe.

face, the kidney is made up of a *cortex* and a *medulla*, the former 1.2 to 1.5 cm in thickness. The medulla consists of *renal pyramids*, the apices of which are called *papillae*, each related to a calyx. Cortical tissue extends into spaces between adjacent pyramids as the *renal columns of Bertin.* From the standpoint of its diseases, the kidney can be divided into four components: blood vessels, glomeruli, tubules, and interstitium.

BLOOD VESSELS. The kidney is richly supplied by blood vessels, and although both kidneys make up only 0.5% of the total body weight, they receive about 25% of the cardiac output. Of this, the cortex is by far the more richly vascularized, receiving 90% of the total renal circulation. The main renal artery divides into anterior and posterior sections at the hilus. From these, *interlobar arteries* emerge, course between lobes, give rise to the *arcuate arteries*, which arch between cortex and medulla, in turn giving rise to the *interlobular arteries.* From the interlobular arteries, *afferent arterioles* enter the glomerular tuft, where they progressively subdivide into 20 to 40 capillary loops arranged in several units or lobules. Capillary loops merge together to exit from the glomerulus as *efferent arterioles.* In general, efferent arterioles from superficial nephrons form a rich vascular network that encircles cortical tubules *(peritubular vascular network)*, while deeper juxtamedullary glomeruli give rise to the *vasa recta*, which descend as straight vessels to supply the outer and inner medulla. These descending arterial vasa recta then make several loops in the inner medulla and ascend as the *venous vasa recta.*

The anatomy of renal vessels has several important implications. First, because the arteries are largely end arteries, *occlusion of any branch results in infarction of the specific area it supplies.* Glomerular disease that interferes with blood flow through the glomerular capillaries has profound effects on the tubules, within both the cortex and the medulla, because *all tubular capillary beds are derived from the efferent arterioles.* The peculiarities of the blood supply to the renal medulla render them especially vulnerable to ischemia; *the medulla is relatively avascular*, and the blood in the capillary loops in the medulla has a remarkably low hematocrit value. Thus, minor interference with the blood supply of the medulla may result in medullary necrosis.

The glomerulus consists of an anastomosing network of capillaries invested by two layers of epithelium (Fig. 20–1). The visceral epithelium is incorporated into and becomes an intrinsic part of the capillary wall, whereas the parietal epithelium lines Bowman's space, the cavity in which plasma filtrate first collects. The glomerular capillary wall is the filtering membrane and consists of the following structures[2] (Fig. 20–2):

1. A thin layer of fenestrated *endothelial cells*, each fenestrum being about 70 to 100 nm in diameter.

2. A *glomerular basement membrane* (GBM) with a thick, electron-dense central layer, the *lamina densa*, and thinner, electron-lucent peripheral layers, the *lamina rara interna* and *lamina rara externa.*[3] The GBM consists of collagen, mostly type IV, laminin, polyanionic proteoglycans (mostly heparan sulfate), fibronectin, entactin, and several other glycoproteins.[3] Type IV collagen forms a network suprastructure to which the other glycoproteins attach (Fig. 20–3, *middle panel, top*).[4] The building block (monomer) of this network is a triple helical molecule made up of three α chains, composed of one or more of six types of α chains (α1 to α6 or COL4A1 to COL4A6), the most common consisting of α1, α2, α1 (see Fig. 20–3, *lower panel*). Each molecule consists of a 7S domain at the amino terminus; a triple helical domain in the middle; and a globular noncollagenous domain (NCI) at the carboxyl terminus. The NCI domain is important for helical formation and also for assembly of collagen monomers into dimers. The 7S domain, in turn, is involved in formation of tetramers, and thus a suprastructure evolves. The NCI domain, as we shall see, is critically involved in anti-GBM nephritis, and genetic defects in some of the α chains underlie hereditary nephritis.

3. The *visceral epithelial cells* (podocytes), structurally complex cells that possess interdigitating processes embedded in and adherent to the

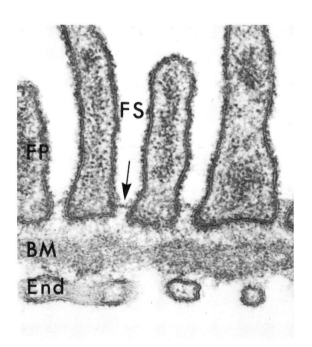

Figure 20–2. Glomerular filter consisting of fenestrated endothelium (End), basement membrane (BM), and foot processes (FP). FS = filtration slit. Arrow indicates the slit diaphragm. Note that the BM consists of a central lamina densa, labeled BM, sandwiched between two looser layers, the lamina rara interna and lamina rara externa.

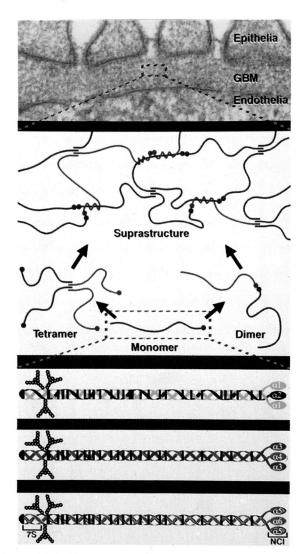

Figure 20–3. The structure of type IV collagen of the GBM. The *lower panel* shows the building block of the collagen network: collagen type IV monomers composed of three alpha chains (of possible six alpha chain types: $\alpha1-\alpha6$) arranged in a triple helix. The most common monomer is made up of $\alpha1/\alpha2$ chains, but in the kidney $\alpha3/\alpha4$ and $\alpha5/\alpha6$ chains are also present. Each monomer has an NC1 domain (carboxyl terminus), a triple helical domain, and a 7S amino acid terminus domain. The *middle panel* shows how monomers form dimers via their NC1 domains and tetramers at the 7S domain to develop a suprastructure to which other ECM components (proteoglycans, laminin, etc.) attach. (With permission from Hudson, B.G., and Reeders, S.T., and Tryggvason, K.: Structure, gene organization, and role in human diseases of type IV collagen. J. Biol. Chem. 268:1, 1993.)

contractile, phagocytic, and capable of proliferation, of laying down both matrix and collagen, and of secreting a number of biologically active mediators. They are, as we shall see, important players in many forms of human glomerulonephritis.

The major characteristics of glomerular filtration are an extraordinary high permeability to water and small solutes, accounted for by the highly fenestrated endothelium and impermeability to molecules of the size of albumin (+3.6-nm radius; 70,000 kd). The latter, called *glomerular barrier function*, discriminates among various protein molecules, depending on their size (the larger, the less permeable) and charge (the more cationic, the more permeable). This size- and charge-dependent barrier function is accounted for by the complex structure of the capillary wall, the integrity of the GBM, and the many anionic moieties present within the wall, including the acidic proteoglycans of the GBM and the sialoglycoproteins of epithelial and endothelial cell coats. The charge-dependent restriction is important in the virtually complete exclusion of albumin from the filtrate, because albumin is an anionic molecule of a pI ±4.5. The *visceral epithelial cell* is critical to the maintenance of glomerular barrier function: its slit diaphragm presents a distal diffusion barrier to the filtration of proteins, and it is the cell type that is largely responsible for synthesis of GBM components.

TUBULES. The structure of renal tubular epithelial cells varies considerably at different levels of the nephron and, to a certain extent, correlates with function. For example, the highly developed structure of the *proximal tubular cells*, with their abundant long microvilli, numerous mitochondria, apical canaliculi, and extensive intercellular interdigitations, is correlated with their major functions: reabsorption of two-thirds of filtered sodium and water as well as glucose, potassium, phosphate, amino acids, and proteins. The proximal tubule is particularly vulnerable to ischemic damage. Furthermore, toxins are frequently reabsorbed by the proximal tubule, rendering it also susceptible to chemical injury.

The juxtaglomerular (JG) apparatus snuggles closely against the glomerulus where the afferent arteriole enters it. The JG apparatus consists of (1) the *juxtaglomerular cells*, modified granulated smooth muscle cells in the media of the afferent arteriole that contain renin; (2) the *macula densa*, a specialized region of the distal tubule as the latter returns to the vascular pole of its parent glomerulus—here the tubular cells are more crowded and the cells are somewhat shorter and possess distinct patterns of interdigitation between adjacent membranes; and (3) the *lacis cells* or *nongranular cells*, which reside in the area bounded by the afferent arteriole, the macula densa, and the glomerulus. They resemble mesangial cells and

lamina rara externa of the basement membrane. Adjacent *foot processes* (pedicels) are separated by 20- to 30-nm-wide *filtration slits*, which are bridged by a thin diaphragm.

4. The entire glomerular tuft is supported by *mesangial cells* lying between the capillaries. Basement membrane–like *mesangial matrix* forms a meshwork through which the mesangial cells are scattered. These cells, of mesenchymal origin, are

appear to be continuous with them. The JG apparatus is a small endocrine organ, the JG cells being the principal sources of renin production in the kidney.

INTERSTITIUM. In the normal cortex, the interstitial space is compact, being occupied by the fenestrated peritubular capillaries and a small number of fibroblast-like cells. Any obvious expansion of the cortical interstitium is usually abnormal; this expansion can be due to edema or infiltration with acute inflammatory cells, as in acute interstitial diseases, or may be caused by accumulation of chronic inflammatory cells and fibrous tissue, as in chronic interstitial diseases. The amounts of proteoglycans in the interstitial tissue of the medulla increase with age and in the presence of ischemia.

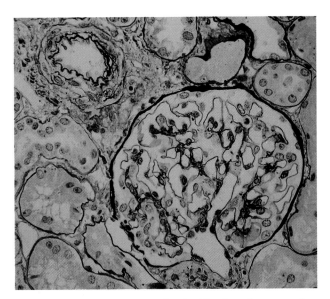

Figure 20–4. Glomerulus, stained with silver impregnation method. Note silver-positive *(black)* thin basement membranes of glomerulus and tubules.

PATHOLOGY

Renal diseases are responsible for a great deal of morbidity but, fortunately, are not major causes of mortality. To place the problem in some perspective, approximately 35,000 deaths are attributed yearly to renal disease in the United States, in contrast to about 750,000 to heart disease, 400,000 to cancer, and 200,000 to stroke. Morbidity, however, is by no means insignificant. Millions of persons are affected annually by nonfatal kidney diseases, most notably infections of the kidney or lower urinary tract, kidney stones, and urinary obstruction. Twenty per cent of all women suffer from infection of the urinary tract or kidney at some time in their lives, and at least 1% of the United States population develop renal stones. Similarly, dialysis and transplantation keep many patients alive who would formerly have died of renal failure, adding to the pool of renal morbidity. The cost of such programs now exceeds several billion dollars annually. Renal disease also has special importance to the clinician because so many of the deaths occur in young people.

Diseases of the kidney are as complex as its structure, but their study is facilitated by dividing them into those that affect the four basic morphologic components: glomeruli, tubules, interstitium, and blood vessels. This traditional approach is useful, since the early manifestations of disease affecting each of these components tend to be distinct. Further, some components appear to be more vulnerable to specific forms of renal injury; for example, *glomerular diseases are most often immunologically mediated, whereas tubular and interstitial disorders are more likely to be caused by toxic or infectious agents.* Nevertheless, some agents affect more than one structure. In addition the anatomic interdependence of structure in the kidney implies

that damage to one almost always secondarily affects the others. Disease primary in the blood vessels, for example, inevitably affects all the structures dependent on this blood supply. Severe glomerular damage impairs the flow through the peritubular vascular system; conversely, tubular destruction, by increasing intraglomerular pressure, may induce glomerular atrophy. Thus, whatever the origin, there is a tendency for all forms of chronic renal disease ultimately to destroy all four components of the kidney, culminating in chronic renal failure and what has been called *end-stage kidneys.* The functional reserve of the kidney is large, and much damage may occur before there is evident functional impairment. For these reasons, the early signs and symptoms are particularly important clinically.

The widespread use of renal biopsy has changed our concepts of renal disease, particularly of the various types of glomerulonephritis. A number of special stains and techniques are used to highlight morphologic and immunologic details in such biopsies. These include the following:

1. The **periodic acid–Schiff stain** (PAS), which outlines the basement membranes of glomeruli and tubules and highlights the mesangial matrix.
2. **Silver impregnation stains,** which also mark the glomerular and tubular basement membranes (Fig. 20–4).
3. **Immunofluorescence and immunoperoxidase studies,** which localize various types of immunoglobulins, antigens, complement, fibrin-related compounds, and cell surface markers.
4. **Electron microscopy,** which is frequently essen-

tial in resolving the fine details of glomerular lesions.
5. **Other special stains,** such as those for fibrin, amyloid, and lipids.

In this chapter we briefly review the clinical manifestations, pathogenesis, and pathology of the major renal diseases. These are dealt with in great detail in two recent comprehensive texts.[5,6]

CLINICAL MANIFESTATIONS OF RENAL DISEASES

The clinical manifestations of renal disease can be grouped into reasonably well-defined syndromes. Some are peculiar to glomerular diseases; others are present in diseases that affect any one of the components. Before we list the syndromes a few terms must be clarified.

Azotemia is a biochemical abnormality that refers to an elevation of the blood urea nitrogen (BUN) and creatinine levels and is related largely to a decreased glomerular filtration rate (GFR). Azotemia is produced by many renal disorders, but it also arises from extrarenal disorders. *Prerenal azotemia* is encountered when there is hypoperfusion of the kidneys (e.g., in hemorrhage, shock, volume depletion, and congestive heart failure) that impairs renal function *in the absence of parenchymal damage.* Similarly, *postrenal azotemia* is seen whenever urine flow is obstructed below the level of the kidney. Relief of the obstruction is followed by prompt correction of the azotemia.

When azotemia becomes associated with a constellation of clinical signs and symptoms and biochemical abnormalities, it is termed uremia. Uremia is characterized not only by failure of renal excretory function but also by a host of metabolic and endocrine alterations incident to renal damage. There is, in addition, secondary gastrointestinal (e.g., uremic gastroenteritis), neuromuscular (e.g., peripheral neuropathy), and cardiovascular (e.g., uremic fibrinous pericarditis) involvement, which are usually necessary for the diagnosis of uremia.

We can now turn to a brief description of the major renal syndromes:[7]

1. *Acute nephritic syndrome* is a glomerular syndrome dominated by the acute onset of usually grossly visible hematuria (red blood cells in urine), mild to moderate proteinuria, and hypertension; it is the classic presentation of acute poststreptococcal glomerulonephritis (GN).
2. The *nephrotic syndrome* is characterized by heavy proteinuria (over 3.5 gm per day), hypoalbuminemia, severe edema, hyperlipidemia, and lipiduria (lipid in the urine).
3. *Asymptomatic hematuria or proteinuria*, or a combination of these two, is usually a manifestation of subtle or mild glomerular abnormalities.
4. *Acute renal failure* is dominated by oliguria or anuria (no urine flow), with recent onset of azotemia. It can result from glomerular injury (e.g., crescentic glomerulonephritis), interstitial injury, or acute tubular necrosis.
5. *Chronic renal failure*, characterized by prolonged symptoms and signs of uremia, is the end result of all chronic renal diseases.
6. *Renal tubular defects* are dominated by polyuria (excessive urine formation), nocturia, and electrolyte disorders (e.g., metabolic acidosis). They are the result of either diseases directly affecting tubular structure (e.g., medullary cystic disease) or defects in specific tubular functions. The latter can be inherited (e.g., familial nephrogenic diabetes, cystinuria, renal tubular acidosis) or acquired (e.g., lead nephropathy).
7. *Urinary tract infection* is characterized by bacteriuria and pyuria (bacteria and leukocytes in the urine). The infection may be *symptomatic* or *asymptomatic*, and it may affect the kidney (*pyelonephritis*) or the bladder (*cystitis*) only.
8. *Nephrolithiasis* (renal stone) is manifested by renal colic, hematuria, and recurrent stone formation.

In addition to these renal syndromes, *urinary tract obstruction* and *renal tumors* represent specific anatomic lesions with often varied manifestations.

Renal Failure. Acute renal failure implies a rapid and frequently reversible deterioration of renal function. As a characteristic syndrome with a complex pathogenesis, it is discussed separately. Here the discussion is limited to *chronic renal failure*, which is the end result of a variety of renal diseases and is the major cause of death from renal disease.

Although exceptions abound, the evolution from normal renal function to symptomatic chronic renal failure progresses through four stages that merge into one another.

- *Diminished renal reserve.* In this situation the GFR is about 50% of normal. Serum BUN and creatinine values are normal, and the patients are asymptomatic. However, they are more susceptible to developing azotemia with an additional renal insult.
- *Renal insufficiency.* The GFR is 20 to 50% of normal. Azotemia appears, usually associated with anemia and hypertension. Polyuria and nocturia occur, as a result of decreased concentrating ability. Sudden stress (e.g., with nephrotoxins) may precipitate uremia.
- *Renal failure.* The GFR is less than 20 to 25% of normal. The kidneys cannot regulate volume and solute composition, and patients develop edema, metabolic acidosis, and hypocalcemia. Overt ure-

Table 20–1. PRINCIPAL SYSTEMIC MANIFESTATIONS OF CHRONIC RENAL FAILURE AND UREMIA

FLUID AND ELECTROLYTES
Dehydration
Edema
Hyperkalemia
Metabolic acidosis

CALCIUM PHOSPHATE AND BONE
Hyperphosphatemia
Hypocalcemia
Secondary hyperparathyroidism
Renal osteodystrophy

HEMATOLOGIC
Anemia
Bleeding diathesis

CARDIOPULMONARY
Hypertension
Congestive heart failure
Pulmonary edema
Uremic pericarditis

GASTROINTESTINAL
Nausea and vomiting
Bleeding
Esophagitis, gastritis, colitis

NEUROMUSCULAR
Myopathy
Peripheral neuropathy
Encephalopathy

DERMATOLOGIC
Sallow color
Pruritus
Dermatitis

mia may ensue, with neurologic, gastrointestinal, and cardiovascular complications.

- *End-stage renal disease.* The GFR is less than 5% of normal; this is the terminal stage of uremia.

The details of the pathophysiology of chronic renal failure are beyond the scope of this book and are well covered in various nephrology texts.[8,9] Table 20–1 lists the major systemic abnormalities in uremic renal failure.

CONGENITAL ANOMALIES

About 10% of all persons are born with potentially significant malformations of the urinary system. Renal dysplasias and hypoplasias account for 20% of chronic renal failure in children. Polycystic kidney disease (a congenital anomaly that becomes apparent in adults) is responsible for about 10% of chronic renal failure in humans.

Congenital renal disease can be hereditary but is most often the result of an acquired developmental defect that arises during gestation. As discussed in Chapter 10, defects in developmental genes, including the Wilms' tumor (WT-1)–associated genes, cause urogenital anomalies, and a "knockout" of the gene results in renal agenesis. As a rule, developmental abnormalities involve structural components of the kidney and urinary tract. However, enzymatic or metabolic defects in tubular transport, such as cystinuria and renal tubular acidosis, also occur. Here we shall restrict the discussion to structural anomalies involving primarily the kidney. Anomalies of the lower urinary tract are discussed in Chapter 21.

AGENESIS OF THE KIDNEY. Total bilateral agenesis, which is incompatible with life, is usually encountered in stillborn infants. It is often associated with many other congenital disorders (limb defects, hypoplastic lungs) and leads to early death. Unilateral agenesis is an uncommon anomaly that is compatible with normal life, if no other abnormalities exist. The opposite kidney is usually enlarged as a result of compensatory hypertrophy. Some patients eventually develop progressive glomerular sclerosis in the remaining kidney as a result of the adaptive changes in hypertrophied nephrons, discussed later in the chapter, and in time chronic renal failure.

HYPOPLASIA. Renal hypoplasia refers to failure of the kidneys to develop to a normal size. This anomaly may occur bilaterally, resulting in renal failure in early childhood, but it is more commonly encountered as a unilateral defect. True renal hypoplasia is extremely rare, most cases reported probably representing acquired scarring due to vascular, infectious, or other parenchymal diseases rather than an underlying developmental failure. Differentiation between congenital and acquired atrophic kidneys may be impossible, but *a truly hypoplastic kidney should show no scars and should possess a reduced number of renal lobes and pyramids:* six or fewer. In one form of hypoplastic kidney, *oligomeganephronia,* the kidney is small but the nephrons are markedly hypertrophied.

ECTOPIC KIDNEYS. The development of the definitive metanephros may occur in ectopic foci, usually at abnormally low levels. These kidneys lie either just above the pelvic brim or sometimes within the pelvis. They are usually normal or slightly smaller in size, but otherwise are not remarkable. Because of their abnormal position, kinking or tortuosity of the ureters may cause some obstruction to urinary flow, which predisposes to bacterial infections.

HORSESHOE KIDNEY. Fusion of the upper or lower poles of the kidneys produces a horseshoe-shaped structure continuous across the midline anterior to the great vessels. This anomaly is quite common and is found in about 1 in 500 to 1000 autopsies. Ninety per cent of such kidneys are fused at the lower pole, and 10% are fused at the upper pole.

CYSTIC DISEASES OF THE KIDNEY

Although not all cysts of the kidney are congenital, all types of cysts are discussed here for convenience.

Cystic diseases of the kidney are a heterogeneous group comprising hereditary, developmental but nonhereditary, and acquired disorders. As a group, they are important for several reasons: (1) they are reasonably common and often represent diagnostic problems for clinicians, radiologists, and pathologists; (2) some forms, such as adult polycystic disease, are major causes of chronic renal failure; (3) they can occasionally be confused with malignant tumors. A useful classification of renal cysts is as follows:[10]

1. Cystic renal dysplasia
2. Polycystic kidney disease
    a. Autosomal dominant (adult) polycystic disease
    b. Autosomal recessive (childhood) polycystic disease
3. Medullary cystic disease
    a. Medullary sponge kidney
    b. Nephronophthisis–uremic medullary cystic disease (UMCD) complex
4. Acquired (dialysis-associated) cystic disease
5. Localized (simple) renal cysts
6. Renal cysts in hereditary malformation syndromes (e.g., tuberous sclerosis)
7. Glomerulocystic disease
8. Extraparenchymal renal cysts (pyelocalyceal cysts, hilar lymphangitic cysts)

Only the more important of the cystic diseases will be discussed.

Pathogenesis of Cysts

Many theories have been suggested to explain the genesis of polycystic kidneys. Cysts are lined by tubular epithelium, and previous views invoked partial intratubular obstruction, causing dilatation proximal to obstructed sites; or defects of the extracellular matrix (ECM) of tubular basement membranes, causing loss of compliance of the tubular wall and cyst formation. Current studies, however, based on work on cystic disease in animals, as well as isolation and culture of cyst epithelium from humans, point to a *primary defect in tubular epithelial cell growth and differentiation.*[11] The epithelial cells lining cysts have a relatively high rate of proliferation, and this is correlated with high levels of proto-oncogene expression. Cysts are frequently detached from adjacent tubules and enlarge by active fluid *secretion* from the lining epithelial cells. In addition, the ECM produced by cyst-lining cells is abnormal. These findings have led to the hypothesis (Fig. 20–5) that

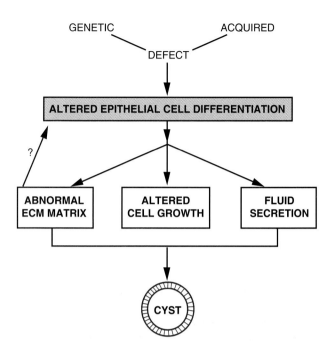

Figure 20–5. Possible mechanisms of cyst formation (see text).

cysts develop as a result of a genetic or acquired abnormality in cell differentiation, leading to sustained cellular proliferation, transepithelial fluid secretion, remodeling of the ECM, and cyst formation.[12] An alternative view is that the ECM defect is primary, the growth and secretion being secondary effects.[13] The gene for the most common hereditary form of cystic disease, adult autosomal dominant polycystic kidney disease, has been localized to the tip of the short arm of chromosome 16 and has been recently identified.

Cystic Renal Dysplasia

This disorder is due to an abnormality in metanephric differentiation *characterized histologically by the persistence in the kidney of abnormal structures—cartilage, undifferentiated mesenchyme, and immature collecting ductules—and by abnormal lobar organization.* Most cases are also associated with ureteropelvic obstruction, and ureteral agenesis or atresia, and other anomalies of the lower urinary tract. Renal dysplasia occurs as a sporadic disorder, without familial clustering.

MORPHOLOGY. Dysplasia can be unilateral or bilateral and is almost always cystic. Grossly, the kidney is usually enlarged, extremely irregular, and multicystic (Fig. 20–6A). The cysts vary in size from small microscopic structures to some that are several centimeters in diameter. They are lined by flattened epithelium. Histologically, although normal nephrons are present, many have immature ducts.

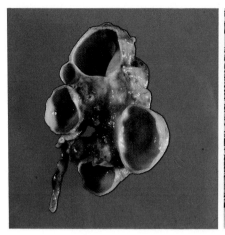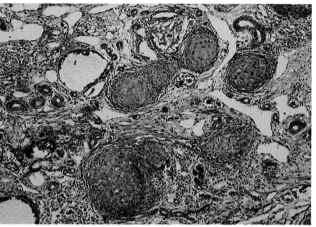

A   B

Figure 20-6. Renal dysplasia. *A,* Gross appearance. *B,* Histologic section showing disorganized architecture, dilated tubules, and islands of immature cartilage, PAS stain. (Courtesy of Dr. D. Schofield, Children's Hospital, Boston.)

The characteristic feature is the presence of islands of undifferentiated mesenchyme, often with cartilage, and immature collecting ducts (see Fig. 20-6B).

When unilateral, the dysplasia is discovered by the appearance of a flank mass that leads to surgical exploration and nephrectomy. Function in the opposite kidney is normal, and such patients have an excellent prognosis after surgical removal of the affected kidney. In bilateral renal dysplasia, renal failure may ultimately result.

Autosomal Dominant (Adult) Polycystic Kidney Disease

Adult polycystic kidney disease is a relatively common condition affecting roughly 1 of every 1000 persons and accounting for about 10% of cases requiring renal transplantation or chronic dialysis. The pattern of inheritance is *autosomal dominant,* with very high penetrance, approaching 100% in those surviving through their 70s or 80s. As noted earlier, the gene for an estimated 90% of cases is on chromosome 16 (APKD1). A second gene for some of the remaining 10% (termed APKD2 or non-APKD1) is on chromosome 4.[14] The disease is universally bilateral; unilateral cases reported probably represent multicystic dysplasia. The cysts initially involve only portions of the nephrons, so that renal function is retained until about the fourth or fifth decade of life. In some patients, however, the first symptoms may appear in early childhood, in the teens, or as late as 70 or 80 years of age. Patients with non-APKD1 genotype have an older age at onset and later development of renal insufficiency.[15] In time, most patients develop hypertension or progress to chronic renal failure.

The pathogenesis of cystic kidney disease in general has been discussed earlier (see Fig. 20-5). The mechanism of cyst formation in APKD awaits identification of the gene and the function of its protein product.

MORPHOLOGY. Grossly, the kidneys are usually bilaterally enlarged and may achieve enormous sizes, weights up to 4 kg for each kidney having been reported. The external surface appears to be composed solely of a mass of cysts, up to 3 to 4 cm in diameter, with no intervening parenchyma (Fig. 20-7A). However, microscopic examination reveals functioning nephrons dispersed between the cysts. The cysts may be filled with a clear serous fluid or, more usually, with turbid, red-to-brown, sometimes hemorrhagic fluid. As these cysts enlarge, they may encroach on the calyces and pelvis to produce pressure defects. The cysts arise from the tubules throughout the nephron and therefore have variable lining epithelia. Occasionally, papillary epithelial formations and polyps project into the lumen. Occasionally, Bowman's capsules are involved in cyst formation, and glomerular tufts may be seen within the cystic space.

Clinically, many of these patients remain asymptomatic until indications of renal insufficiency announce the presence of the underlying kidney disease. In others, hemorrhage or progressive dilation of cysts may produce pain. Excretion of blood clots causes renal colic. The larger masses usually apparent on abdominal palpation may induce a dragging sensation. Occasionally, the disease begins with the insidious onset of hematuria, followed by other features of progressive chronic renal disease, such as proteinuria (rarely more than 2 gm per day), polyuria, and hypertension.

Patients with polycystic kidney disease also tend to have other congenital anomalies: *about*

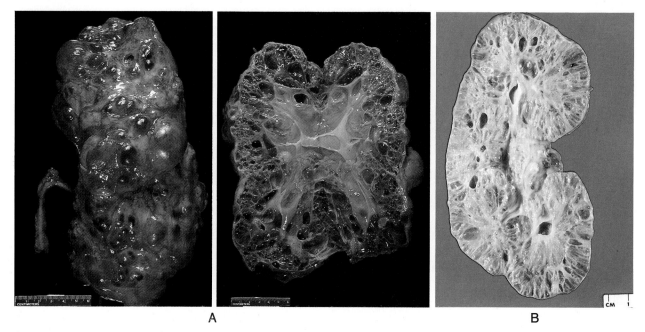

Figure 20–7. *A,* Autosomal dominant adult polycystic kidney, viewed from external surface A, and bisected. The kidney is markedly enlarged (note cm rule) with numerous dilated cysts. *B,* Autosomal recessive childhood polycystic kidney disease, showing smaller cysts and dilated channels at right angles to the cortical surface.

40% have one to several cysts in the liver (polycystic liver disease) that are usually asymptomatic. Cysts occur much less frequently in the spleen, pancreas, and lungs. *Intracranial berry aneurysms in the circle of Willis are present in 10 to 30% of patients,* and subarachnoid hemorrhages from these account for death in about 10% of patients. Mitral valve prolapse also occurs, consistent with a generalized defect in basement membranes in these patients. The clinical diagnosis is made by radiologic imaging techniques. CT scanning is highly sensitive and can detect cysts a few millimeters in diameter. Ultrasound is the least invasive and can confirm the diagnosis. This form of chronic renal failure is quite remarkable in that patients may survive for many years with azotemia slowly progressing to uremia. Ultimately, about one-third of adult patients die of renal failure; in another third, hypertension is responsible for death (cardiac disease, intracerebral hemorrhage, rupture of berry aneurysm). The remaining third die of unrelated causes.

Autosomal Recessive (Childhood) Polycystic Kidney Disease

This rare developmental anomaly is genetically distinct from adult polycystic kidney disease, having an *autosomal recessive* type of inheritance. *Perinatal, neonatal, infantile,* and *juvenile* subcategories have been defined, depending on time of presentation and presence of associated hepatic lesions. The first two are most common; serious manifestations are usually present at birth, and the young infant may succumb rapidly to renal failure.

MORPHOLOGY. Kidneys are enlarged and have a smooth external appearance. On cut section, numerous small cysts in the cortex and medulla give the kidney a sponge-like appearance. Dilated elongated channels are present at right angles to the cortical surface, completely replacing the medulla and cortex (see Fig. 20–7B). Microscopically, there is saccular or, more commonly, cylindrical dilatation of all collecting tubules. The cysts have a uniform lining of cuboidal cells, reflecting their origin from the collecting tubules. The disease is invariably bilateral. **In almost all cases, there are multiple epithelium-lined cysts in the liver as well as proliferation of portal bile ducts.**

Patients who survive infancy (infantile and juvenile form) may develop a peculiar type of hepatic fibrosis characterized by bland periportal fibrosis and proliferation of well-differentiated biliary ductules, a condition now termed *congenital hepatic fibrosis.* In older children, the hepatic picture in fact predominates. Such patients may develop portal hypertension with splenomegaly. Curiously, congenital hepatic fibrosis sometimes occurs in the absence of polycystic kidneys and has been reported occasionally in the presence of adult polycystic kidney disease.

Cystic Diseases of Renal Medulla

The two major types of medullary cystic disease are *medullary sponge kidney,* a relatively common and usually innocuous structural change, and *nephronophthisis–uremic medullary cystic disease complex,* almost always associated with renal dysfunction.

MEDULLARY SPONGE KIDNEY. *The term medullary sponge kidney should be restricted to lesions consisting of multiple cystic dilatations of the collecting ducts in the medulla.* The condition occurs in adults and is usually discovered radiographically, either as an incidental finding or sometimes in relation to secondary complications. The latter include calcifications within the dilated ducts, hematuria, infection, and urinary calculi. Renal function is usually normal. Grossly, the papillary ducts in the medulla are dilated, and small cysts may be present. The cysts are lined by cuboidal epithelium or occasionally by transitional epithelium. Unless there is superimposed pyelonephritis, cortical scarring is absent. The pathogenesis is unknown.

NEPHRONOPHTHISIS–UREMIC MEDULLARY CYSTIC DISEASE (UMCD) COMPLEX. This is a group of progressive renal disorders that usually have their onset in childhood. The common characteristic is the presence of a variable number of *cysts in the medulla associated with significant cortical tubular atrophy and interstitial fibrosis.* Although the presence of medullary cysts is important, the *cortical tubulointerstitial damage is the cause of the eventual renal insufficiency,* and some prefer the term *hereditary tubulointerstitial nephritis for this group.*[10] Four variants are recognized: (1) *sporadic, nonfamilial* (20%); (2) *familial juvenile nephronophthisis* (50%), inherited as a recessive disease; (3) *renal-retinal dysplasia* (15%), recessively inherited and associated with retinitis pigmentosa; and (4) *adult-onset medullary cystic disease,* dominantly inherited (15%). As a group this complex accounts for about 20% of cases of chronic renal failure in children and adolescents.

Affected children present first with polyuria and polydipsia, which reflect a marked tubular defect in concentrating ability. Sodium wasting and tubular acidosis are also prominent, findings consistent with initial injury to the distal tubules and collecting ducts. The expected course is progression to terminal renal failure over a period of 5 to 10 years.

MORPHOLOGY. Grossly, the kidneys are small, have contracted granular surfaces, and show cysts in the medulla, most prominently at the corticomedullary junction (Fig. 20–8). Small cysts are also seen in the cortices. The cysts are lined by flattened or cuboidal epithelium and are usually surrounded by either inflammatory cells or fibrous tissue. In the cortex there is widespread atrophy and thickening of the basement membranes of proximal and distal tubules together with interstitial fibrosis. Some glomeruli may be hyalinized, but, in general, glomerular structure is preserved.

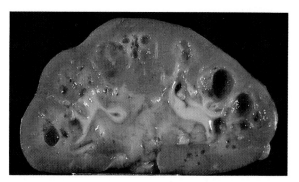

Figure 20–8. Uremic medullary cystic disease. Cut section of kidney showing cysts at corticomedullary junction and in medulla. (Courtesy of Dr. D. Schofield, Children's Hospital, Boston.)

There are few specific clues to diagnosis, because the medullary cysts may be too small to be visualized radiographically. The disease should be strongly considered in children or adolescents with otherwise unexplained chronic renal failure, a positive family history, and chronic tubulointerstitial nephritis on biopsy.

Acquired (Dialysis-Associated) Cystic Disease

The kidneys from patients with end-stage renal disease who have undergone prolonged dialysis sometimes exhibit numerous cortical and medullary cysts. The cysts measure 0.5 to 2 cm in diameter, contain clear fluid, are lined by either hyperplastic or flattened tubular epithelium, and often contain calcium oxalate crystals. They probably form as a result of obstruction of tubules by interstitial fibrosis or by oxalate crystals. Tumors, usually of the renal adenoma type but occasionally adenocarcinomas, may be present in the walls of these cysts, and sometimes the cysts bleed, causing hematuria. These complications are increasing in frequency with the growing population of patients with end-stage renal disease.

Simple Cysts

These occur as multiple or single usually cortical cystic spaces that vary in diameter over wide limits. Commonly, they are 1 to 5 cm but may reach 10 cm or more in size. They are translucent, lined by a gray, glistening, smooth membrane, and filled with clear fluid. Microscopically, these membranes are composed of a single layer of cuboidal or flattened cuboidal epithelium, which, in many instances, may be completely atrophic.

Simple cysts are common postmortem findings

Table 20-2. SUMMARY OF RENAL CYSTIC DISEASES

	INHERITANCE	PATHOLOGIC FEATURES	CLINICAL FEATURES OR COMPLICATIONS	TYPICAL OUTCOME	DIAGRAMMATIC REPRESENTATION
Adult polycystic kidney disease	Autosomal dominant	Large multicystic kidneys, liver cysts, berry aneurysms	Hematuria, flank pain, urinary tract infection, renal stones, hypertension	Chronic renal failure beginning at age 40–60 years	
Childhood polycystic kidney disease	Autosomal recessive	Enlarged, cystic kidneys at birth	Hepatic fibrosis	Variable, death in infancy or childhood	
Medullary sponge kidney	None	Medullary cysts on excretory urography	Hematuria, urinary tract infection, recurrent renal stones	Benign	
Familial juvenile nephronophthisis	Autosomal recessive	Corticomedullary cysts, shrunken kidneys	Salt wasting, polyuria, growth retardation, anemia	Progressive renal failure beginning in childhood	
Adult-onset medullary cystic disease	Autosomal dominant	Corticomedullary cysts, shrunken kidneys	Salt wasting, polyuria	Chronic renal failure beginning in adulthood	
Simple cysts	None	Single or multiple cysts in normal-sized kidneys	Microscopic hematuria	Benign	
Acquired renal cystic disease	None	Cystic degeneration in end-stage kidney disease	Hemorrhage, erythrocytosis, neoplasia	Dependence on dialysis	

without clinical significance. On occasion, hemorrhage into them may cause sudden distention and pain, and calcification of the hemorrhage may give rise to bizarre radiographic shadows. The main importance of cysts lies in their differentiation from kidney tumors, when they are discovered either incidentally or because of hemorrhage and pain during life. Radiologic studies show that, in contrast to renal tumors, renal cysts have smooth contours, are almost always avascular, and give fluid rather than solid signals on ultrasound.

Table 20–2 summarizes the characteristic features of the principal renal cystic diseases.

GLOMERULAR DISEASES

Glomerular diseases constitute some of the major problems in nephrology; indeed, chronic glomerulonephritis is one of the most common causes of chronic renal failure in humans. Glomeruli may be injured by a variety of factors and in the course of a number of systemic diseases. Immunologic diseases such as systemic lupus erythematosus (SLE), vascular disorders such as hypertension and polyarteritis nodosa, metabolic diseases such as diabetes mellitus, and some purely hereditary conditions such as Fabry's disease often affect the glomerulus. These are termed *secondary glomerular diseases* to differentiate them from those in which the kidney is the only or predominant organ involved. The latter constitute the various types of *primary glomerulonephritis* (GN) or, because some do not have a cellular inflammatory component, *glomerulopathy*. Here we shall discuss the various types of primary GN, and briefly review the secondary forms covered in other parts of this book.

Table 20–3 lists the most common forms of GN that have reasonably well-defined morphologic and clinical characteristics. In reviewing the specific types of GN, it is useful to consider each in terms of (1) clinical presentation, (2) the morphology of the glomerular lesion, and (3) the cause and pathogenesis.

CLINICAL MANIFESTATIONS

The clinical manifestations of glomerular disease are clustered into the five major glomerular syndromes described earlier and summarized in Table 20–4. Both the primary glomerulonephritides and the systemic diseases affecting the glomerulus can result in these syndromes. Thus, a critical point in the clinical differential diagnosis is first to exclude the major systemic disorders, of which the major

Table 20-3. GLOMERULAR DISEASES

PRIMARY GLOMERULOPATHIES
  Acute diffuse proliferative glomerulonephritis (GN)
    Poststreptococcal
    Nonpoststreptococcal
  Rapidly progressive (crescentic) glomerulonephritis
  Membranous glomerulopathy
  Lipoid nephrosis (minimal change disease)
  Focal segmental glomerulosclerosis
  Membranoproliferative glomerulonephritis
  IgA nephropathy
  Focal proliferative glomerulonephritis
  Chronic glomerulonephritis

SYSTEMIC DISEASES
  Systemic lupus erythematosus
  Diabetes mellitus
  Amyloidosis
  Goodpasture's syndrome
  Polyarteritis nodosa
  Wegener's granulomatosis
  Henoch-Schönlein purpura
  Bacterial endocarditis

HEREDITARY DISORDERS
  Alport's syndrome
  Fabry's disease

four are *diabetes mellitus, SLE, vasculitis,* and *amyloidosis.*

HISTOLOGIC ALTERATIONS

Various types of GN are characterized by one or more of four basic tissue reactions:

GLOMERULAR HYPERCELLULARITY. So-called *inflammatory diseases* of the glomerulus are associated with an increase in the number of cells in the glomerular tufts. This hypercellularity is caused by one or a combination of two of the following:

- *Cellular proliferation* of mesangial, endothelial, or, in certain cases, parietal epithelial cells
- *Leukocytic infiltration,* consisting of neutrophils, monocytes, and, in some diseases, lymphocytes

Table 20-4. THE GLOMERULAR SYNDROMES

Acute nephritic syndrome	Hematuria, azotemia, variable proteinuria, oliguria, edema, and hypertension
Rapidly progressive GN	Acute nephritis, proteinuria, and acute renal failure
Nephrotic syndrome	>3.5 gm proteinuria, hypoalbuminemia, hyperlipidemia, lipiduria
Chronic renal failure	Azotemia → uremia progressing over years
Asymptomatic hematuria or proteinuria	Glomerular hematuria; subnephrotic proteinuria

BASEMENT MEMBRANE THICKENING. By light microscopy, this change appears as thickening of the capillary walls, best seen in sections stained with PAS. On electron microscopy such thickening can be resolved as either (1) thickening of the basement membrane proper, as occurs in diabetic glomerulosclerosis; or, more commonly, (2) deposition of amorphous electron-dense material representing precipitated proteins, on the endothelial or epithelial side of the basement membrane, or within the GBM itself. *By far the most common type of thickening is due to extensive subepithelial deposition, as occurs in membranous GN,* discussed later. In most instances the deposits are thought to be immune complexes, although fibrin may also appear as an electron-dense material.

HYALINIZATION AND SCLEROSIS. Hyalinization or hyalinosis, as applied to the glomerulus, denotes the accumulation of material that is homogeneous and eosinophilic by light microscopy. By electron microscopy the material is extracellular and consists of amorphous substance (made up of precipitated plasma protein) as well as increased amounts of basement membrane or mesangial matrix. This change results in obliteration of structural detail of the glomerular tuft (sclerosis) and usually denotes the end result of various forms of glomerular damage.

Additional alterations include fibrin deposition, intraglomerular thrombosis, or deposition of abnormal materials (amyloid, "dense deposits," lipid). Because many of the primary glomerulonephritides are of unknown cause, they are often classified by their histology, as can be seen in Table 20-3. The histologic changes can be further subdivided into *diffuse,* involving all glomeruli; *global,* involving the entire glomerulus; *focal,* involving only a certain proportion of the glomeruli; *segmental,* affecting a part of each glomerulus; and *mesangial,* affecting predominantly the mesangial region. These terms are sometimes appended to the histologic classifications.

PATHOGENESIS OF GLOMERULAR INJURY

Although we know little of etiologic agents or triggering events, it is clear that immune mechanisms underlie most cases of primary GN and many of the secondary glomerular involvements[16-18] (Table 20-5). Experimentally, GN can be readily induced by antigen-antibody reactions, and glomerular deposits of immunoglobulins, often with various components of complement, are found in more than 70% of patients with GN. Thus, although cell-mediated and other immune mechanisms play roles, antibody-mediated injury has received the most attention.

Two forms of antibody-associated injury have

Table 20–5. IMMUNE MECHANISMS OF GLOMERULAR INJURY

I. Antibody-Mediated Injury
    A. *In situ* immune complex deposition
        1. Fixed intrinsic tissue antigens
            a. Goodpasture's antigen (Anti-GBM nephritis)
            b. Heymann's antigen (membranous GN)
            c. Mesangial antigens
            d. Others
        2. Planted antigens
            a. Exogenous (drugs, lectins, infectious agents)
            b. Endogenous (DNA, immunoglobulins, immune complexes, IgA)
    B. Circulating immune complex deposition
        1. Endogenous antigens (e.g., DNA, tumor antigens)
        2. Exogenous antigens (e.g., infectious products)
    C. Cytotoxic antibodies
II. Cell-Mediated Injury
III. Activation of Alternative Complement Pathway

been established: (1) injury by *antibodies reacting in situ within the glomerulus, either with insoluble fixed (intrinsic) glomerular antigens or with molecules planted within the glomerulus,* and (2) injury resulting from deposition of *soluble circulating antigen-antibody complexes* in the glomerulus. In addition, there is experimental evidence that *cytotoxic antibodies* directed against glomerular cell components may cause glomerular injury. These pathways are not mutually exclusive, and in humans all may contribute to injury.

In Situ Immune Complex Deposition

In this form of injury, antibodies react directly with intrinsic tissue or planted antigens. There are two well-established experimental models for anti–tissue-mediated glomerular injury, for which there are counterparts in human disease—antiglomerular basement membrane (anti-GBM) and Heymann's nephritis.

ANTI-GBM NEPHRITIS. In this type of injury, *antibodies are directed against intrinsic fixed antigens in the GBM, which induce a linear pattern of localization on immunofluorescence microscopy.* It has its experimental counterpart in so-called Masugi or nephrotoxic nephritis, produced in rats by injections of anti–rat kidney antibodies prepared in rabbits by immunization with rat kidney tissue. The injected antibodies bind along the entire length of the GBM, *resulting in a homogeneous, diffuse linear immunofluorescent pattern* (Figs. 20–9B and E). This is contrasted with the granular lumpy pattern seen in other *in situ* models or after deposition of circulating immune complexes. To come back to Masugi's model, it should be noted that the deposited immunoglobulin of the rabbit is foreign to the host and thus acts as an antigen

eliciting antibodies in the rat. This rat antibody then reacts with the rabbit immunoglobulin within the basement membrane, leading to further glomerular injury. This is referred to as the *autologous phase* of nephrotoxic nephritis, to distinguish it from the initial *heterologous phase* caused by the anti-GBM antibody. Often the anti-GBM antibodies cross-react with other basement membranes, especially those in the lung alveoli, resulting in simultaneous lung and kidney lesions *(Goodpasture's syndrome).* Anti-GBM nephritis accounts for fewer than 5% of cases of human GN. It is solidly established as the cause of injury in Goodpasture's syndrome, discussed later. Most instances of anti-GBM nephritis are characterized by very severe glomerular damage and the development of rapidly progressive renal failure. The basement membrane antigen responsible for classic anti-GBM nephritis of Goodpasture's syndrome is a component of the noncollagenous domain (NCI) of the $\alpha 3$ chain of collagen type IV, which, as was discussed earlier (see Fig. 20–3), is critical for GBM function.[3]

HEYMANN'S NEPHRITIS. The Heymann model of rat GN is induced by immunizing animals with preparations of proximal tubular brush border (see Fig. 20–9C). The rats develop antibodies to brush border antigens, and a membranous GN, closely resembling human membranous GN, develops (discussed later; see also Fig. 20–16). On electron microscopy, the nephritis is characterized by the presence of numerous electron-dense deposits (presumably immune reactants) along the *subepithelial aspect* of the basement membrane. The pattern of immune deposition by fluorescence microscopy is *granular* and *interrupted,* rather than linear (see Fig. 20–9D). It is now clear that the GN results largely from the reaction of antibody with the Heymann antigen, a 330-kd glycoprotein (GP330) located in coated pits on the basal surface of visceral epithelial cells and expressed on the brush border also.[19] Antibody binding to the cell membrane is followed by complement activation and then by patching, capping, and subsequent shedding of the immune aggregates from the cell surface to form the characteristic subepithelial deposits (see Fig. 20–9C).[20] Heymann's nephritis most resembles human membranous GN, in which the epithelial cell antigen appears to be a homologue of GP330.

It must be apparent that, in humans, anti-GBM disease and membranous GN (the counterpart of Heymann's nephritis) are autoimmune diseases, caused by antibodies to endogenous tissue components. What triggers these autoantibodies is unclear, but any one of the several mechanisms responsible for autoimmunity, discussed in Chapter 6, may be involved. Experimentally, several forms of autoimmune GN can be induced by drugs (e.g., mercuric chloride), infectious products (endotoxin), and the graft-versus-host reaction. In such models,

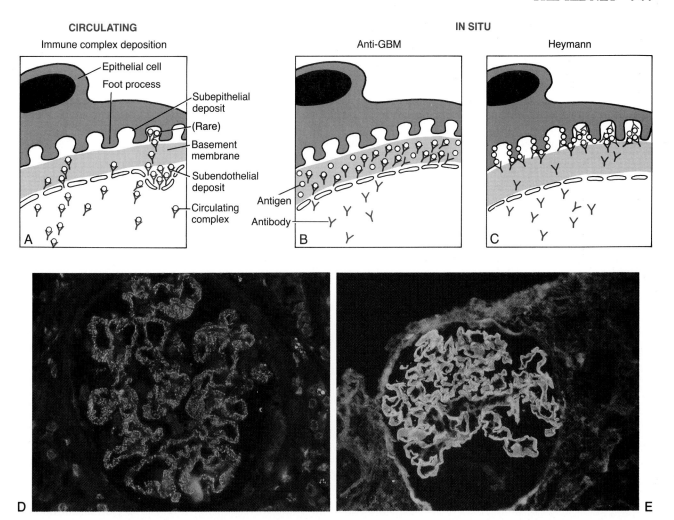

Figure 20-9. Antibody-mediated glomerular injury can result either from the deposition of circulating immune complexes (A) or from *in situ* formation of complexes exemplified by anti-GBM disease (B) or Heymann's nephritis (C). D and E, Two patterns of deposition of immune complexes as seen by immunofluorescence microscopy. D, *Granular*, characteristic of circulating and *in situ* immune complex nephritis. E, *Linear*, characteristic of classic anti-GBM disease.

there is an induced alteration of immune regulation associated with *polyclonal B-cell activation* and the induction of an array of autoantibodies that react with renal antigens.

ANTIBODIES AGAINST PLANTED ANTIGENS. Antibodies can react *in situ* with previously "planted" nonglomerular antigens. Such antigens may localize in the kidney by interacting with various intrinsic components of the glomerulus. There is increasing experimental support for such a mechanism. Planted antigens include cationic molecules that bind to glomerular capillary anionic sites; DNA, which has an affinity for GBM components; bacterial products, such as endostreptosin, a protein of group A streptococci; large aggregated proteins (e.g., aggregated IgG), which deposit in the mesangium because of their size; and immune complexes themselves, since they continue to have reactive sites for further interactions with free antibody, free antigen, or complement. There is no dearth of other possible planted antigens, including

viral, bacterial, and parasitic products and drugs. Most of these planted antigens induce a granular or heterogeneous pattern of immunoglobulin deposition by fluorescence microscopy, the pattern found also in circulating immune complex nephritis, discussed next.

Circulating Immune Complex Nephritis

In this type of nephritis, glomerular injury is caused by the trapping of circulating antigen-antibody complexes within glomeruli. The antibodies have no immunologic specificity for glomerular constituents, and the complexes localize within the glomeruli because of their physicochemical properties and the hemodynamic factors peculiar to the glomerulus (see Fig. 20-9A).

The pathogenesis of immune complex diseases (type III hypersensitivity reactions) was discussed in detail in Chapter 6. Here we shall briefly review the salient features that relate to glomerular injury.

The evocative antigens may be of endogenous origin, as in the case of the glomerulopathy associated with SLE, or they may be exogenous, as is likely in the glomerulonephritis that follows certain infections. Antigens implicated include bacterial products (streptococci), the surface antigen of hepatitis B virus (HBsAg), hepatitis C virus antigen or RNA, various tumor antigens, *Treponema pallidum*, *Plasmodium falciparum*, and several viruses. Frequently, the inciting antigen is unknown. Whatever the antigen may be, antigen-antibody complexes are formed in the circulation and then trapped in the glomeruli, where they produce injury, in large part through the binding of complement. The glomerular lesions usually consist of leukocytic infiltration in glomeruli and proliferation of mesangial and endothelial cells. Electron microscopy reveals the immune complexes as electron-dense deposits or clumps that lie *in the mesangium*, or between the endothelial cells and the GBM *(subendothelial deposits)*, or rarely between the outer surface of the GBM and the podocytes *(subepithelial deposits)*. Deposits may be located at more than one site in a given case. By immunofluorescence microscopy, *the immune complexes are seen as granular deposits either along the basement membrane or in the mesangium, or in both locations.* Once deposited in the kidney, immune complexes may eventually be degraded, mostly by phagocytic infiltrating monocytes and by mesangial cells, and the inflammatory changes may then subside. Such a course occurs when the exposure to the inciting antigen is short-lived and limited, as in most cases of poststreptococcal GN. However, if a continuous shower of antigens is provided, repeated cycles of immune complex formation, deposition, and injury may occur, leading to progressive GN.

Several factors affect glomerular localization of antigen, antibody, or complexes. The molecular charge and size of these reactants are clearly important. Highly cationic immunogens tend to cross the GBM, and the resultant complexes eventually achieve a subepithelial location. Highly anionic macromolecules are excluded from the GBM and either are trapped subendothelially or may, in fact, not be nephritogenic at all. Molecules with more neutral charge and their complexes tend to accumulate in the mesangium. Very large circulating complexes are not usually nephritogenic because they are cleared by the reticuloendothelial system and do not enter the GBM in sufficient quantities. The pattern of localization is also affected by changes in glomerular hemodynamics, mesangial function, and integrity of the charge-selective barrier in the glomerulus. These influences may underlie the variable pattern of immune reactant deposition and histologic change in various forms of GN (Fig. 20–10).

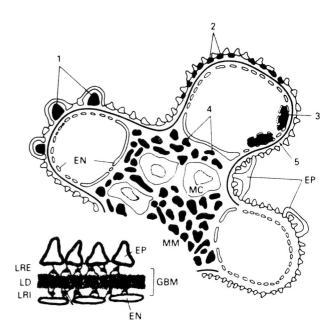

Figure 20–10. Localization of immune complexes in the glomerulus: (1) Subepithelial humps, as in acute GN; (2) epimembranous deposits, as in membranous and Heymann's GN; (3) subendothelial deposits, SLE and membranoproliferative GN; (4) mesangial deposits, as in IgA nephropathy; (5) basement membrane. LRE = lamina rara externa; LRI = lamina rara interna; LD = lamina densa. (Modified from Couser, W.G.: Mediation of immune glomerular injury. J. Am. Soc. Nephrol. *1:*13, 1990. © American Society of Nephrology.)

Cytotoxic Antibodies

In addition to causing immune deposits, antibodies directed to glomerular cell antigens may cause direct cell injury—often without deposits. Antibodies to mesangial cell antigens, for example, cause mesangiolysis followed by mesangial cell proliferation; antibodies to endothelial cell surface proteins cause endothelial injury; and antibodies to certain visceral epithelial cell glycoproteins cause proteinuria in experimental animals. This mechanism may well play a role in certain human immune disorders not associated with demonstrable immune deposits.

To conclude the discussion of antibody-mediated injury, it must be stated that in the largest proportion of cases of human GN, the pattern of immune deposition is granular and along the basement membrane or in the mesangium. However, it is not clear in human GN whether the deposition has occurred *in situ* or via circulating complexes, or by both mechanisms—because, as discussed earlier, immune complex trapping can either initiate or be superimposed on *in situ* formation. Single etiologic agents, such as hepatitis B and C, can cause either a membranous pattern of GN, suggesting *in situ* deposition, or a membranoproliferative pattern, more indicative of circulating complexes. It is best to consider that *antigen-antibody deposition in the glomerulus is a major pathway of glomerular injury; and that in situ immune reactions, trapping of circulating complexes, interactions between these two events, and local hemodynamic and structural determinants in the glomerulus all contribute to the diverse morphologic and functional alterations in GN.*

Cell-Mediated Immunity in Glomerulonephritis

There is increasing evidence that sensitized T cells, as a reflection of cell-mediated immune reactions, can cause glomerular injury. The idea is an attractive one, as it may account for the many instances of progressive GN in which either there are no immune deposits, or the deposits do not correlate with the severity of damage. Clues to its occurrence include the presence of macrophages and T lymphocytes in the glomerulus in some forms of human and experimental GN, *in vitro* evidence of lymphocyte reactivity on exposure to altered GBM antigen in progressive human GN, and a few successful attempts to transfer mild glomerular histologic alterations by lymphocytes in experimental GN.

Activation of Alternative Complement Pathway

Alternative complement pathway activation occurs in the clinicopathologic entity called *membranoproliferative glomerulonephritis (MPGN)*, sometimes independently of immune complex deposition, and also in some forms of proliferative GN. This mechanism is discussed later in the discussion of MPGN.

Mediators of Glomerular Injury

Once immune reactants or sensitized T cells have localized in the glomerulus, how does the glomerular damage ensue? The mediators—both cells and molecules—are largely similar to those involved in acute and chronic inflammation, described in Chapter 3, and only a few will be highlighted (Fig. 20–11A).[21]

Cells

Neutrophils infiltrate the glomerulus in certain types of GN, owing to activation of complement, resulting in generation of chemotactic agents (mainly C5a), and also via Fc-mediated immune adherence. Neutrophils release proteases, which cause GBM degradation; oxygen-derived free radicals, which cause cell damage; and arachidonic acid

metabolites, which contribute to the reductions in GFR.

Monocytes, macrophages, and *lymphocytes,* which infiltrate the glomerulus in antibody- and cell-mediated reactions, when activated release a vast number of biologically active molecules (described in Chapter 3).

Platelets aggregate in the glomerulus during immune-mediated injury. Their release of eicosanoids and growth factors may play a role in some of the manifestations of GN. Antiplatelet agents have beneficial effects in both human and experimental GN.

Resident glomerular cells, particularly mesangial cells, can be stimulated to produce several inflammatory mediators, including oxygen free radicals, cytokines, growth factors, eicosanoids, nitric oxide, and endothelin. In the absence of leukocytic infiltration they may initiate inflammatory responses in the glomerulus.

Soluble Mediators

Virtually all the inflammatory chemical mediators have been implicated in glomerular injury. The *chemotactic complement components* induce leukocyte influx and C5b-C9, the lytic component, causes cell lysis and also stimulates mesangial cells to produce other chemical mediators. *Eicosanoids, nitric oxide,* and *endothelin* are involved in the hemodynamic changes. *Cytokines,* particularly interleukin-1 (IL-1) and tumor necrosis factor (TNF), induce leukocyte adhesion and a variety of other effects. Of the *growth factors, platelet-derived growth factor (PDGF)* is involved in mesangial cell proliferation,[22] and transforming growth factor-beta (TGF-β) appears to be critical in the ECM deposition and hyalinization leading to glomerulosclerosis in chronic injury.[23]

The *coagulation system* may also be a mediator of glomerular damage. Fibrin is frequently present in the glomeruli in GN, and fibrinogen may leak into Bowman's space, serving as a stimulus to cell proliferation. Fibrin deposition is mediated largely by stimulation of macrophage procoagulant activity.

Other Mechanisms of Glomerular Injury

Other mechanisms may contribute to glomerular damage in certain primary renal disorders. Three that deserve special mention are epithelial cell injury, renal ablation glomerulopathy, and interstitial inflammation.

EPITHELIAL CELL INJURY. This can be induced experimentally by antibodies to visceral epithelial cell antigens; by toxins, such as puromycin aminonucleoside; conceivably by certain cytokines; or by unknown factors, as is the case in human lipoid

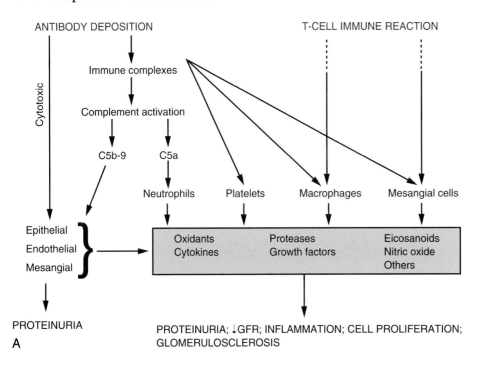

ANTIBODY DEPOSITION   T-CELL IMMUNE REACTION

Immune complexes

Complement activation

C5b-9   C5a

Neutrophils   Platelets   Macrophages   Mesangial cells

Epithelial
Endothelial
Mesangial

Oxidants   Proteases   Eicosanoids
Cytokines   Growth factors   Nitric oxide
                                 Others

PROTEINURIA
A

PROTEINURIA; ↓GFR; INFLAMMATION; CELL PROLIFERATION;
GLOMERULOSCLEROSIS

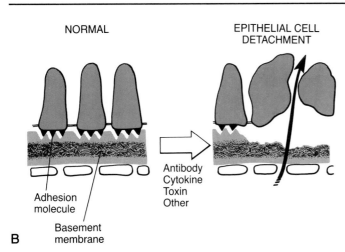

NORMAL   EPITHELIAL CELL
                              DETACHMENT

Antibody
Cytokine
Toxin
Other

Adhesion
molecule

Basement
membrane

B

Figure 20–11. *A,* Mediators of immune glomerular injury including cells and soluble mediators (see text). *B,* Epithelial cell injury. The postulated sequence is a consequence of antibodies against epithelial cell antigens, or toxins, or cytokines or other factors causing injury and detachment of epithelial cells, and protein leakage through defective GBM and filtration slits. (*A,* Redrawn and modified with permission from Couser, W.G.: Pathogenesis of glomerulonephritis. Kidney International. *44:*S19–S26, 1993. *B,* Adapted from Couser, W.G.: Mediation of immune glomerular injury. J. Am. Soc. Nephrol. *1:*13, 1990. © American Society of Nephrology.)

nephrosis, considered later. Such injury is reflected by morphologic changes in the visceral epithelial cells, which include loss of foot processes, vacuolization, retraction and *detachment* of cells from the GBM, and functionally by *proteinuria.* It is thought that the detachment of visceral epithelial cells is caused by loss of their adhesive interactions with the basement membrane, and that this detachment leads to protein leakage (see Fig. 20–11*B*).

RENAL ABLATION GLOMERULOPATHY (OR GLOMERULOSCLEROSIS). It has been documented that once any renal disease, glomerular or otherwise, destroys sufficient functioning nephrons to reduce the GFR to about 30 to 50% of normal, progression to end-stage renal failure proceeds inexorably. Such patients develop proteinuria, and their kidneys show widespread *glomerulosclerosis.* This progressive sclerosis appears to be initiated by the

adaptive changes that occur in the relatively unaffected glomeruli of diseased kidneys. Such a mechanism is suggested by experiments in rats subjected to ablation of renal mass by subtotal nephrectomy. *Compensatory hypertrophy* of the remaining glomeruli serves to maintain renal function in these animals, but proteinuria and glomerulosclerosis soon develop, leading eventually to total glomerular hyalinization and uremia. The glomerular hypertrophy is associated with hemodynamic changes, including increases in single-nephron GFR, blood flow, and transcapillary pressure (capillary hypertension), and often with systemic hypertension. The sequence of events (Fig. 20–12) leading to sclerosis entails endothelial and epithelial cell injury, increased glomerular permeability to proteins, accumulation of proteins in the mesangial matrix, and fibrin deposition. This is followed by proliferation of mesangial cells, increased depo-

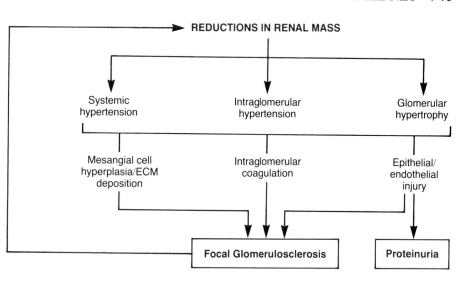

Figure 20-12. Renal ablation glomerulosclerosis. The adaptive changes in glomeruli (hypertrophy and glomerular capillary hypertension), as well as systemic hypertension, cause epithelial and endothelial injury and resultant proteinuria. The mesangial response, involving mesangial cell proliferation and extracellular matrix (ECM) production together with intraglomerular coagulation, causes the glomerulosclerosis. This results in further loss of functioning nephrons and a vicious circle of progressive glomerulosclerosis.

sition of mesangial matrix, and sclerosis of glomeruli. The latter results in further reductions in nephron mass and a vicious cycle of continuing glomerulosclerosis.[24] As we shall see, this so-called *renal ablation glomerulopathy* may play a role in a number of chronic renal diseases.

INTERSTITIAL INFLAMMATION IN GN. It has long been known that many human and experimental models of GN are associated with the presence of inflammatory cells—lymphocytes and macrophages—*in the interstitium.* In some instances, as in anti-GBM disease, the infiltrate may be related to cross-reacting antibodies with tubular basement membranes. In others, the nature of the infiltrate suggests an interstitial delayed hypersensitivity reaction. Recent evidence *suggests* that this interstitial reaction plays a role in both the acute and the progressive renal dysfunction in some forms of immune GN; however, the precise mechanisms of inflammatory cell accumulation and the manner by which such inflammation affects glomerular function are still unclear.

ACUTE GLOMERULONEPHRITIS

The first group of glomerular diseases we shall discuss are characterized anatomically by inflammatory alterations in the glomeruli and clinically by a complex of findings classically referred to as *the syndrome of acute nephritis.* The nephritic patient usually presents with hematuria, red cell casts in the urine, azotemia, oliguria, and mild to moderate hypertension. The patient also commonly has proteinuria and edema, but these are not as severe as those encountered in the nephrotic syndrome, discussed later. The acute nephritic syndrome may occur in such multisystem diseases as SLE and polyarteritis nodosa. Typically, however, it is characteristic of acute proliferative GN and is an im-

portant component of crescentic GN, which will be described later.

Acute Poststreptococcal (Proliferative) Glomerulonephritis

This glomerular disease is decreasing in frequency in the United States but continues to be a fairly common disorder worldwide.[25] It usually appears 1 to 4 weeks after a streptococcal infection of the pharynx or skin. It occurs most frequently in children six to ten years of age, but adults of any age can be affected.

ETIOLOGY AND PATHOGENESIS. Only certain strains of group A beta-hemolytic streptococci are nephritogenic, more than 90% of cases being traced to types 12, 4, and 1, which can be identified by typing of M protein of the cell wall. Skin infections are commonly associated with overcrowding and poor hygiene.

Poststreptococcal GN is an immunologically mediated disease. The latent period between infection and onset of nephritis is compatible with the time required for the building up of antibodies. Elevated titers to one or more of the streptococcal products are present in a great majority of patients. Serum complement levels are low, compatible with involvement of the complement system. The presence of granular immune deposits in the glomeruli suggests an immune complex–mediated mechanism, and so does the finding of electron-dense deposits. The streptococcal antigenic component(s) responsible for the immune reaction has eluded identification for years. A cytoplasmic antigen called *endostreptosin*, and several *cationic antigens*, including a proteinase related to the streptococcal erythrogenic toxin, are present in affected glomeruli, but whether these represent "planted

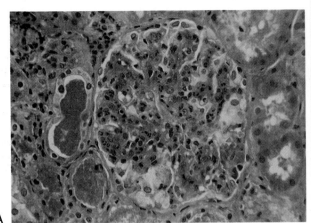
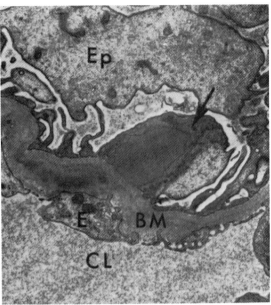

Figure 20–13. Poststreptococcal glomerulonephritis. *A,* Glomerular hypercellularity is due to intracapillary leukocytes and proliferation of intrinsic glomerular cells. Note red cell casts in tubules. *B,* Typical electron-dense subepithelial "hump" and intramembranous deposits.

antigens," or part of circulating immune complexes, or both, is unknown. GBM and immunoglobulins altered by streptococcal enzymes have also been implicated as antigens at one time or another.

MORPHOLOGY. The classic diagnostic picture is one of enlarged, hypercellular, relatively bloodless glomeruli (Fig. 20–13). The hypercellularity is caused by (1) proliferation of endothelial and mesangial cells and, in many cases, epithelial cells; and (2) infiltration by leukocytes, both neutrophils and monocytes. The proliferation and leukocyte infiltration are diffuse, that is, involving all lobules of all glomeruli. There is also swelling of endothelial cells, and the combination of proliferation, swelling, and leukocyte infiltration obliterates the capillary lumina. Small deposits of fibrin within capillary lumina and mesangium can be demonstrated by special stains. There may be interstitial edema and inflammation, and the tubules often contain red cell casts and may show evidence of degeneration.

By **immunofluorescence microscopy** there are granular deposits of IgG, IgM, and C3 in the mesangium and along the basement membrane. Although present, they are often focal and sparse. The characteristic **electron microscopic findings** are the discrete, amorphous, electron-dense deposits on the epithelial side of the membrane, often having the appearance of "humps" (see Fig. 20–13), presumably representing the antigen-antibody complexes at the epithelial cell surface. Subendothelial and intramembranous deposits are sometimes seen, and there is often swelling of endothelial and mesangial cells.

CLINICAL COURSE. In the classic case, a young child abruptly develops malaise, fever, nausea, oliguria, and hematuria (smoky or cocoa-colored urine) 1 to 2 weeks after recovery from a sore throat. The patients exhibit red cell casts in the urine, mild proteinuria (usually less than 1 gm/ day), periorbital edema, and mild to moderate hypertension. In adults, the onset is more apt to be atypical, with the sudden appearance of hypertension or edema, frequently with elevation of BUN. During epidemics caused by nephritogenic streptococcal infections, GN may be asymptomatic, discovered only when screening for microscopic hematuria. Important laboratory findings include elevations of antistreptococcal antibody titers (anticationic proteinase and anti-DNase B), a decline in the serum concentration of C3, and the presence of cryoglobulins in the serum.

More than 95% of children with poststreptococcal GN totally recover with conservative therapy aimed at maintaining sodium and water balance. Microscopic hematuria, mild proteinuria, and histologic changes confined to the mesangium may persist in some patients for several weeks or months, but even then complete long-term recovery is the rule. A small minority of children (perhaps less than 1%) do not improve, become severely oliguric, and develop a rapidly progressive form of GN (to be described later). Another 1 to 2% may undergo slow progression to chronic GN with or without recurrence of an active nephritic

Table 20-6. RAPIDLY PROGRESSIVE (CRESCENTIC)
GLOMERULONEPHRITIS (RPGN)

Postinfectious RPGN
Systemic diseases
    Systemic lupus erythematosus
    Goodpasture's syndrome
    Vasculitis (e.g., polyarteritis nodosa)
    Wegener's granulomatosis
    Henoch-Schönlein purpura
    Essential cryoglobulinemia
Idiopathic RPGN

picture. Prolonged and persistent heavy proteinuria and abnormal GFR mark patients with an unfavorable prognosis.

In adults, the disease is less benign. Although the overall prognosis in epidemics is good, in only about 60% of *sporadic cases* do the patients recover promptly. Some patients develop rapidly progressive GN. In the remainder the glomerular lesions fail to resolve quickly, as manifested by persistent proteinuria, hematuria, and hypertension. In some of these patients the lesions eventually clear totally, but others develop chronic GN.

NONSTREPTOCOCCAL ACUTE GN. A similar form of GN occurs sporadically in association with other bacterial infections (e.g., staphylococcal endocarditis, pneumococcal pneumonia, and meningococcemia), viral disease (e.g., hepatitis B, mumps, varicella, and infectious mononucleosis), and parasitic infections (malaria, toxoplasmosis). In all these, granular immunofluorescent deposits and subepithelial humps characteristic of immune complex nephritis are present.

RAPIDLY PROGRESSIVE (CRESCENTIC) GLOMERULONEPHRITIS (RPGN)

This represents a *clinicopathologic syndrome* in which glomerular damage is accompanied by rapid and progressive decline in renal function, frequently with severe oliguria or anuria, usually resulting in irreversible renal failure in weeks or months. *The syndrome is characterized histologically by the accumulation of cells in Bowman's space in the form of "crescents."*

CLASSIFICATION AND PATHOGENESIS. The conditions in which the syndrome of RPGN may occur can be grouped into three categories: (1) postinfectious (poststreptococcal) RPGN, (2) GN associated with systemic diseases, and (3) idiopathic RPGN (also called primary or isolated RPGN). As might be expected from the list of associated conditions (Table 20-6), no single pathogenic mechanism can explain all cases. There is little doubt, however, that in most cases the glomerular injury is immunologically mediated. In SLE, and in post-

streptococcal settings, RPGN is mediated by immune complexes.

RPGN associated with *Goodpasture's syndrome* is a classic example of anti-GBM nephritis. In this condition, described in Chapter 15, circulating anti-GBM antibodies can be detected in more than 95% of cases by radioimmunoassay. These antibodies cross-react with pulmonary alveolar basement membranes to produce the clinical picture of pulmonary hemorrhages associated with renal failure. Linear deposits of IgG, and in many cases C3, can be visualized by immunofluorescence along both the glomerular and the alveolar basement membranes.

The Goodpasture antigen, as noted, resides in the noncollagenous portion of the $\alpha 3$ chain of collagen type IV. What triggers the formation of these antibodies is unclear in most patients. Exposure to viruses or hydrocarbon solvents (found in paints and dyes) has been implicated in some patients, as have various drugs and cancers. Cigarette smoking appears to play a permissive role, since most patients who develop pulmonary hemorrhage are smokers. There is a high prevalence of DRW15/DQW6 haplotype in Goodpasture's syndrome, a finding consistent with the genetic predisposition to autoimmunity.

Idiopathic RPGN accounts for about half of all cases. In a fourth of these, linear glomerular deposits are found (as in Goodpasture's syndrome), but there is no pulmonary involvement. In another fourth, granular glomerular deposits are present, related to the deposition of immune complexes. But in about half the patients there are minimal immune deposits or none *(pauci-immune crescentic GN)*. Antineutrophil cytoplasmic antibodies (ANCA), which as we have seen (see Chapter 11) play a role in some forms of vasculitis, *are virtually always present in pauci-immune GN.* Both antimyeloperoxidase and anti–proteinase 3 variants can be present, and there is experimental evidence that such antibodies may be pathogenic.[27] Thus idiopathic *crescentic GN* can be caused by different pathogenic mechanisms: immune complexes, anti-GBM antibodies, and ANCA, all inducing severe glomerular injury.

MORPHOLOGY. The kidneys are enlarged and pale, often with petechial hemorrhages on the cortical surfaces. Depending on the underlying cause, the glomeruli may show focal necrosis, diffuse or focal endothelial proliferation, and mesangial proliferation. The histologic picture, however, is dominated by the formation of distinctive **crescents** (Fig. 20-14). Crescents are formed by proliferation of parietal cells and by migration of monocytes and macrophages into Bowman's space. Neutrophils and lymphocytes may be present. The crescents eventually obliterate Bowman's space and compress the glomerular tuft. Fibrin strands are promi-

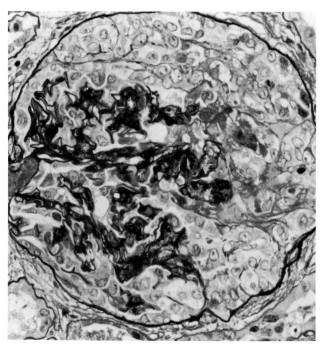

Figure 20-14. Rapidly progressive glomerulonephritis; PAS stain. Note the collapsed glomerular tuft and the mass of proliferating cells internal to Bowman's capsule. (Courtesy of Dr. Helmut Rennke, Brigham and Women's Hospital, Boston.)

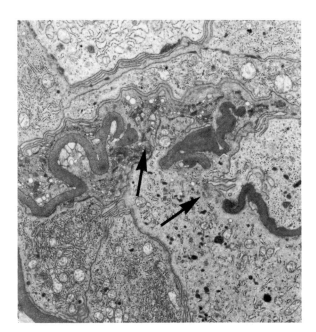

Figure 20-15. Rapidly progressive glomerulonephritis. Electron micrograph showing characteristic wrinkling of GBM with focal disruptions in its continuity (arrows).

nent between the cellular layers in the crescents, and some believe that it is the escape of fibrin into Bowman's space that incites crescent formation. Electron microscopy may, as expected, disclose subepithelial deposits in some cases, but in all cases shows distinct **ruptures in the GBM** (Fig 20-15). In time, most crescents undergo sclerosis.

As described in the section on pathogenesis, postinfectious cases exhibit granular immune deposits by fluorescence microscopy, Goodpasture's linear fluorescence, and idiopathic cases may have granular, linear, or little deposition.

CLINICAL COURSE. In Goodpasture's syndrome, the course may be dominated by recurrent hemoptysis or even life-threatening pulmonary hemorrhage. The renal manifestations of all forms include hematuria with red cell casts in the urine, moderate proteinuria occasionally reaching the nephrotic range, and variable hypertension and edema. Although milder forms of glomerular injury may subside, the renal involvement is usually progressive over a matter of weeks, culminating in severe oliguria. Assays for circulating anti-GBM antibodies are helpful in the diagnosis. Dramatic remission may follow early intensive plasmapheresis (plasma exchange) combined with steroids and cytotoxic agents in Goodpasture's syndrome. This therapy appears to reverse both pulmonary hemorrhage and renal failure. Plasma exchange presumably removes both the anti-GBM antibodies responsible

for initiating the damage and the secondary circulating mediators. The results are less dramatic in other forms of RPGN, particularly when therapy is instituted after oliguria develops. Despite therapy, patients may eventually require chronic dialysis or transplantation.

NEPHROTIC SYNDROME (NS)

Certain glomerular diseases (membranous GN, lipoid nephrosis, focal sclerosis) virtually always produce the nephrotic syndrome. In addition, many other forms of primary and secondary GN discussed in this chapter may evoke it. Before presenting the major diseases associated with NS, the pathophysiology of this clinical complex will be briefly discussed and the causes listed.

PATHOPHYSIOLOGY. The nephrotic syndrome includes massive proteinuria, with the daily loss of 3.5 gm or more of protein (less in children); hypoalbuminemia, with plasma albumin levels less than 3 gm per dl; generalized edema; and hyperlipidemia. The initial event is a derangement in glomerular capillary walls resulting in increased permeability to the plasma proteins. It will be remembered that the glomerular capillary wall, with its endothelium, GBM, and visceral epithelial cells, acts as a size and charge barrier through which the glomerular filtrate must pass. Any increased permeability resulting from either structural or physicochemical alterations allows protein to escape from the plasma into the glomerular filtrate. *Massive proteinuria results.*

The heavy proteinuria leads to depletion of serum albumin levels below the compensatory synthetic abilities of the liver, with consequent hypoalbuminemia and a reversed albumin-globulin ratio. Increased renal catabolism also contributes to the hypoalbuminemia. The generalized edema is, in turn, the consequence of the loss of colloid osmotic pressure of the blood and the accumulation of fluid in the interstitial tissues. There is also *sodium and water retention*, which aggravates the edema. This appears to be due to several factors, including compensatory secretion of aldosterone, mediated by the hypovolemia-enhanced antidiuretic hormone secretion; stimulation of the sympathetic system; and a reduction in the secretion of natriuretic factors, such as atrial peptides. Edema is characteristically soft and pitting, most marked in the periorbital regions and dependent portions of the body. It may be quite massive with pleural effusions and ascites.

The largest proportion of protein lost in the urine is albumin, but globulins are also excreted in some diseases. The ratio of low- to high-molecular-weight proteins in the urine in various cases of NS determines the so-called "selectivity" of proteinuria. A *highly selective proteinuria* consists mostly of low-molecular-weight proteins (albumin 66,000; transferrin 76,000), whereas a *poorly selective proteinuria* consists of higher-molecular-weight proteins in addition to albumin.

The genesis of the *hyperlipidemia* in the nephrotic syndrome is complex. Most patients have increased cholesterol, triglycerides, very low-density lipoprotein (VLDL), LDL, LP(a), and apoproteins, and, in some patients, there is a decrease in high-density lipoprotein (HDL). These defects seem to be due, in part, to *increased synthesis of lipoproteins in the liver, abnormal transport of circulating lipid particles, and decreased catabolism.* HDL, but not the larger lipoproteins, is also lost in the urine when severe proteinuria occurs. *Lipiduria* follows the hyperlipidemia, because not only albumin molecules but also lipoproteins leak across the glomerular capillary wall. The lipid appears in the urine either as free fat or as "oval fat bodies," representing lipoprotein resorbed by tubular epithelial cells and then shed along with the degenerated cells.

These patients are particularly vulnerable to *infection*, especially with staphylococci and pneumococci. The basis for this vulnerability could be related to loss of immunoglobulins or low-molecular-weight complement components (e.g., factor B) in the urine. *Thrombotic and thromboembolic complications* are also quite common in NS, owing in part to loss of anticoagulant factors (e.g., antithrombin III) and antiplasmin activity through the leaky glomerulus. *Renal vein thrombosis*, once thought to be a cause of NS, is most often a *consequence* of this hypercoagulable state.

Table 20–7. CAUSES OF NEPHROTIC SYNDROME

	PREVALENCE* (%)	
	Children	Adults
Primary Glomerular Disease		
Membranous GN	5	40
Lipoid nephrosis	65	15
Focal segmental glomerulosclerosis	10	15
Membranoproliferative GN	10	7
Other proliferative GN (focal, "pure mesangial," IgA nephropathy)	10	23
Systemic Diseases		
Diabetes mellitus		
Amyloidosis		
Systemic lupus erythematosus		
Drugs (gold, penicillamine, "street heroin")		
Infections (malaria, syphilis, hepatitis B, AIDS)		
Malignancy (carcinoma, melanoma)		
Miscellaneous (bee-sting allergy, hereditary nephritis)		

* Approximate prevalence of primary disease = 95% in children, 60% in adults. Approximate prevalence of systemic disease = 5% in children, 40% in adults.

CAUSES. The relative frequencies of the several causes of the nephrotic syndrome vary according to age. In children younger than age 15 years, for example, the nephrotic syndrome is almost always caused by a lesion primary to the kidney, whereas among adults it may often be associated with a systemic disease. Table 20–7 represents a composite derived from several studies of the causes of the nephrotic syndrome and is therefore only approximate. As the table indicates, the most frequent *systemic causes* of the nephrotic syndrome are SLE, diabetes, and amyloidosis. The renal lesions produced by these disorders are described elsewhere in this text. The most important of the *primary glomerular lesions* that characteristically lead to the nephrotic syndrome are *lipoid nephrosis (minimal change disease)* and *membranous GN.* The former is most important in children, the latter in adults. Two other primary lesions, *focal glomerulosclerosis* and *membranoproliferative GN*, also produce the nephrotic syndrome. These four lesions are discussed individually below.

MEMBRANOUS GLOMERULONEPHRITIS (MEMBRANOUS NEPHROPATHY)

Membranous glomerulonephritis (MGN) is a major cause of the nephrotic syndrome in adults. It is characterized by the presence of electron-dense, immunoglobulin-containing deposits along the epithelial (subepithelial) side of the basement membrane.[28] Early in the disease, the glomeruli may appear normal by light microscopy, but well-developed cases show *diffuse thickening of the capillary wall.*

MGN may occur in association with known

disorders or etiologic agents (secondary MGN). These include the following:

- Malignant epithelial tumors, particularly carcinoma of the lung and colon and melanoma
- Systemic lupus erythematosus
- Exposure to inorganic salts (gold, mercury)
- Drugs (penicillamine, captopril)
- Infections (chronic hepatitis B, syphilis, schistosomiasis, malaria)
- Metabolic disorders (diabetes mellitus, thyroiditis)

In about 85% of patients, the condition is truly "idiopathic."

ETIOLOGY AND PATHOGENESIS. Because of the uniform presence of immunoglobulins and complement in the subepithelial deposits, it is believed that MGN is a form of chronic antigen–antibody–mediated disease. In secondary MGN, specific antigens can sometimes be implicated. For example, MGN occurs in 10% of patients with SLE, presumably owing to deposition of autoantigen-antibody complexes. Exogenous (hepatitis B, Treponema antigens) or endogenous (thyroglobulin) antigens have been identified within deposits in some patients. In the vast majority of patients, however, including patients with idiopathic MGN, the antigens are unknown.

Genetic susceptibility is suggested by the increased prevalence of HLA-DR3 in European and HLA-DR2 in Japanese patients with MGN. This suggests possible defects in immune regulation.

Circulating immune complexes are found in only 15 to 25% of cases, and thus an *in situ* immune reaction involving glomerular or planted antigen is thought to account for the subepithelial immune deposits. The lesions bear a striking resemblance to those of experimental Heymann's nephritis, which, as you recall, is induced by antibodies to an intrinsic tissue antigen (GP330) present in the visceral epithelial cells. Susceptibility to Heymann's nephritis in rats is also linked to the HLA locus. Thus it is now postulated that idiopathic MGN, like Heymann's nephritis, is an autoimmune disease, linked to susceptibility genes, and caused by antibodies to an as yet unidentified renal antigen.

Begging the question of the nature of the immune deposits, how does the glomerular capillary wall become leaky? With the paucity of neutrophils, monocytes, or platelets in glomeruli and the virtually uniform presence of complement, current work points to a direct action of C5b-9, the membrane-attack complex of complement.

MORPHOLOGY. By light microscopy, the glomeruli either appear normal in the early stages of the disease or exhibit **uniform, diffuse thickening of the glomerular capillary wall** (Fig. 20–16A). By electron microscopy the apparent thickening is caused by irregular dense deposits between the basement membrane and the overlying epithelial cells, the latter having lost their foot processes (see Fig. 20–16B and D). Basement membrane material is laid down between these deposits, appearing as irregular spikes protruding from the GBM. These spikes are best seen by silver stains, which color the basement membrane black. In time, these spikes thicken to produce dome-like protrusions and eventually close over the immune deposits, burying them within a markedly thickened, irregular membrane. Immunofluorescence microscopy demonstrates that the granular deposits contain both immunoglobulins and complement (see Fig. 20–16C). As the disease advances, the membrane thickening progressively encroaches on the capillary lumina, and sclerosis of the mesangium may occur, and, in the course of time, glomeruli become totally hyalinized. The epithelial cells of the proximal tubules contain hyaline droplets, reflecting protein reabsorption, and there may be considerable mononuclear interstitial inflammation.

CLINICAL COURSE. In a previously healthy individual this disorder usually begins with the insidious onset of the nephrotic syndrome or, in 15% of patients, with non-nephrotic proteinuria. Hematuria and mild hypertension are present in 15 to 35% of cases. It is necessary in any patient with MGN to first rule out the secondary causes described earlier.

The course is irregular but generally indolent. Progression is associated with increasing sclerosis of glomeruli, rising BUN, relative reduction in the severity of proteinuria, and development of hypertension. Although proteinuria persists in more than 60% of patients, only about 10% die or go into renal failure within 10 years, and no more than 40% will eventually develop renal insufficiency. A relatively benign outcome occurs more commonly in women and in those with non-nephrotic range proteinuria and mild glomerular changes on electron microscopy. Because of the notoriously variable course of the disease, it has been difficult to evaluate the effectiveness of corticosteroids or immunosuppressive therapy in controlling the proteinuria or progression of chronic renal insufficiency.

MINIMAL CHANGE DISEASE (MCD) (LIPOID NEPHROSIS)

This relatively benign disorder is the most frequent cause of nephrotic syndrome in children. *It is characterized by diffuse loss of foot processes of epithelial cells in glomeruli that appear virtually normal by light microscopy* (see Table 20–7). The peak incidence is between two and six years of age. The disease sometimes follows a respiratory

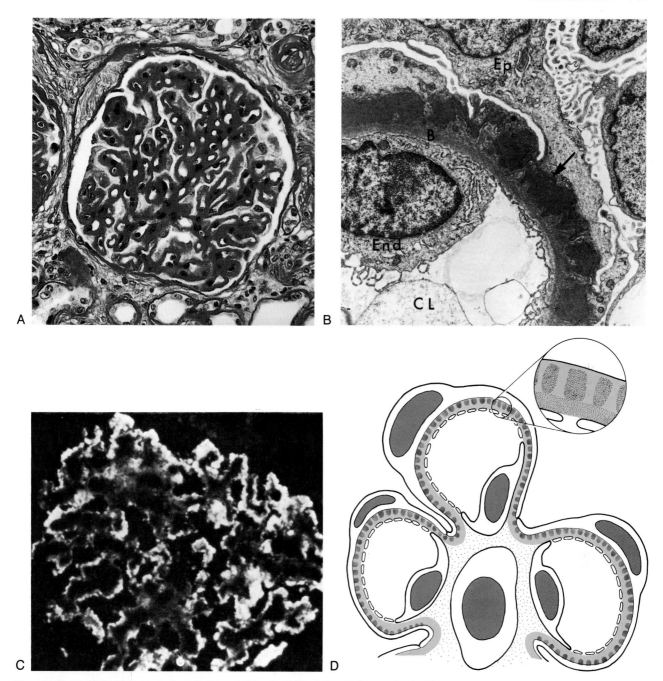

Figure 20–16. Membranous glomerulonephritis. *A*, PAS stain. Note marked diffuse thickening of capillary wall without increase in number of cells. *B*, Electron micrograph showing electron-dense deposits *(arrow)* along epithelial side of basement membrane (B). Note obliteration of foot process overlying deposits. CL = capillary lumen; End = endothelium; Ep = epithelium. *C*, Characteristic granular immunofluorescent deposits of IgG along GBM. *D*, Diagrammatic representation of membranous GN.

infection or routine prophylactic immunization. Its most characteristic feature is its usually dramatic response to corticosteroid therapy.

ETIOLOGY AND PATHOGENESIS. Although the absence of immune deposits in the glomerulus excludes classic immune complex mechanisms, several features of the disease point to an immunologic basis, including (1) the clinical associ-

ation with respiratory infections and prophylactic immunization; (2) the response to corticosteroid and immunosuppressive therapy; (3) the association with other atopic disorders (e.g., eczema, rhinitis); (4) the increased prevalence of certain HLA haplotypes in patients with minimal change disease associated with atopy (suggesting a possible genetic predisposition); (5) the increased incidence of MCD in patients with Hodgkin's disease, in

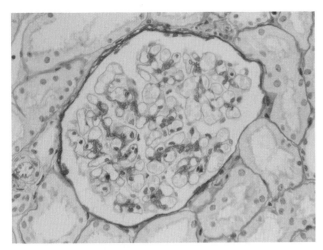

Figure 20–17. Minimal change disease. Thin section of glomerulus stained with PAS. Note thin basement membrane and absence of proliferation. Compare with membranous glomerulonephritis in Figure 20–16A.

made. The visceral epithelial changes are completely reversible after corticosteroid therapy and remission of the proteinuria. The cells of the proximal tubules are often laden with lipid, reflecting tubular reabsorption of lipoproteins passing through diseased glomeruli (thus, the term **lipoid nephrosis**). Immunofluorescence studies show no immunoglobulin or complement deposits.

CLINICAL COURSE. Despite massive proteinuria, renal function remains good, and there is commonly no hypertension or hematuria. The proteinuria usually is highly selective. The great majority (more than 90%) of children with MCD exhibit a rapid response to corticosteroid therapy. However, the nephrotic phase may recur, and some patients may become "steroid dependent." Nevertheless, the long-term prognosis for patients is excellent, and even steroid-dependent disease resolves when children reach puberty. Although adults are slower to respond to therapy, the long-term prognosis is also excellent. Because of its responsiveness to therapy, MCD must be differentiated from other causes of NS in children.

whom defects in T-cell–mediated immunity are well recognized; (6) the recurrence of proteinuria after transplantation in patients with the related disorder focal glomerulosclerosis, discussed later; and (7) reports of proteinuria-inducing factors in the plasma or lymphocyte supernatants of patients with lipoid nephrosis and focal glomerulosclerosis.[29] Such findings have led to a hypothesis that lipoid nephrosis involves some immune dysfunction, eventually resulting in the elaboration of a cytokine-like circulating substance that affects visceral epithelial cells and causes proteinuria. The ultrastructural changes clearly point to a primary visceral epithelial cell injury, and studies suggest that such injury results in loss of glomerular polyanions and the glomerular charge-barrier as the cause of proteinuria. Detachment of epithelial cells (see Fig. 20–11B), a consequence of diminished adhesion to GBM, may also contribute to protein loss.

FOCAL SEGMENTAL GLOMERULOSCLEROSIS (FSG)

As the name implies, *this lesion is characterized by sclerosis of some, but not all, glomeruli (thus, it is focal), and in the affected glomeruli only a portion of the capillary tuft is involved (thus, it is segmental).* Focal segmental glomerulosclerosis is frequently accompanied clinically by the nephrotic syndrome or heavy proteinuria.

FSG can be divided into (1) *idiopathic FSG;* (2) *FSG superimposed on another primary glomerular lesion* (e.g., IgA nephropathy); (3) *FSG associated with loss of renal mass (renal ablation FSG),* which occurs in advanced stages of other renal disorders, such as reflux nephropathy, analgesic abuse nephropathy, and unilateral renal agenesis; and (4) *secondary FSG,* associated with other known disorders or etiologic agents. Secondary FSG is a recognized manifestation of *heroin abuse* and *human immunodeficiency virus (HIV) infection.*

Idiopathic FSG accounts for 10 and 15% of cases of nephrotic syndrome seen among children and adults, respectively. About 80% of patients with this lesion have a nephrotic syndrome but differ from the usual patients with minimal change disease in the following respects: (1) they have a higher incidence of hematuria, reduced GFR, and hypertension; (2) their proteinuria is more often nonselective; (3) they respond poorly to corticosteroid therapy; (4) many progress to chronic GN, and at least 50% develop end-stage renal disease within 10 years; and (5) immunofluorescence mi-

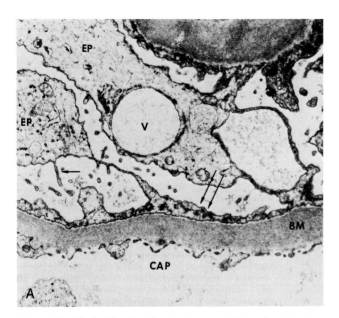

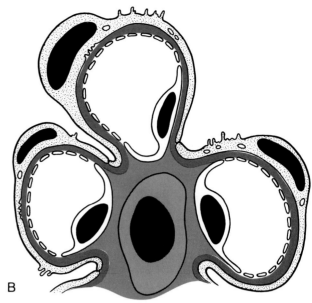

Figure 20–18. *A,* Ultrastructural characteristics of minimal change disease: loss of foot processes *(double arrows),* absence of deposits, vacuoles (V) and microvilli in visceral epithelial cells *(single arrow). B,* Schematic representation of minimal change disease, showing diffuse loss of foot processes.

croscopy shows deposition of IgM and C3 in the sclerotic segment.

MORPHOLOGY. By light microscopy, the segmental lesions may involve only a minority of the glomeruli and may be missed if insufficient glomeruli are present in the biopsy specimen (Fig. 20–19A). The lesions initially involve the juxtamedullary glomeruli, although they subsequently become more generalized. In the sclerotic segments there is collapse of basement membranes, increase in mesangial matrix, and deposition of hyaline masses **(hyalinosis),** often with lipoid droplets (Fig. 20–19B). Glomeruli

not exhibiting segmental lesions either appear normal on light microscopy or may show increased mesangial matrix and mesangial proliferation. On electron microscopy, nonsclerotic areas show the diffuse loss of foot processes characteristic of MCD, but in addition there is **pronounced, focal detachment of the epithelial cells with denudation of the underlying GBM.** By immunofluorescence microscopy, IgM and C3 are present within the hyaline masses in the sclerotic areas. In addition to the focal sclerosis, there is often rather pronounced hyaline thickening of afferent arterioles, and occasionally there are glomeruli that are completely sclerosed (global sclerosis). With the progression of

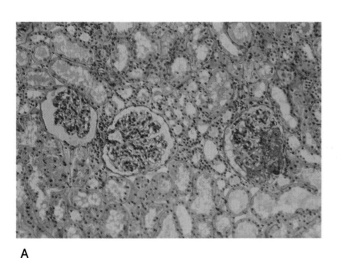

A

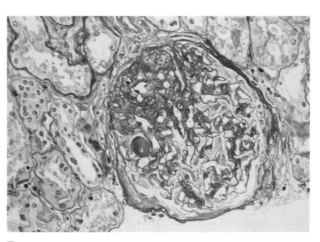

B

Figure 20–19. Focal segmental glomerulosclerosis. PAS stain. *A,* Low-power view showing segmental sclerosis in one of three glomeruli (at 3 o'clock). *B,* High-power view showing hyaline mass and lipid (small vacuoles) in sclerotic area.

the disease, increased numbers of glomeruli become involved, sclerosis spreads within each glomerulus, and there is an increase in mesangial matrix. In time this leads to total sclerosis of glomeruli, with pronounced tubular atrophy and interstitial fibrosis.

PATHOGENESIS. Whether idiopathic FSG represents a distinct disease or is simply a phase in the evolution of a subset of patients with MCD is a matter of conjecture, most workers favoring the latter explanation. The characteristic degeneration and focal disruption of visceral epithelial cells are thought to represent an accentuation of the diffuse epithelial cell change typical of MCD. *It is this epithelial damage that is the hallmark of FSG.* The hyalinosis and sclerosis represent entrapment of plasma proteins in extremely hyperpermeable foci and mesangial cell reaction to such proteins and to fibrin deposits. The recurrence of proteinuria in patients with focal sclerosis who receive renal allografts, sometimes within 24 hours of transplantation, suggests a systemic factor, such as a cytokine or a circulating toxin as the cause of the epithelial damage, and indeed a plasma factor causing proteinuria has recently been described in such patients.[30]

As was noted, *renal ablation FSG* occurs as a complication of other nonglomerular renal diseases causing reduction in functioning renal tissue, particularly reflux nephropathy and unilateral agenesis. These may lead to progressive glomerulosclerosis and renal failure. The pathogenesis of FSG in this setting is related to the adaptive glomerular hypertrophy and capillary hypertension occurring in remnant functioning nephrons of these kidneys, as detailed earlier in this chapter.

CLINICAL COURSE. As mentioned earlier, there is little tendency for spontaneous remission in idiopathic FSG, and responses to corticosteroid therapy are infrequent. In general, children have a better prognosis than adults. Progression of renal failure occurs at variable rates. About 20% of patients follow an unusually rapid course *(malignant focal sclerosis)*, with intractable massive proteinuria ending in renal failure within 2 years. Recurrences are seen in 25 to 50% of patients receiving allografts.

HIV-associated nephropathy occurs in 5 to 10% of HIV-infected patients, more frequently in blacks than whites, and the nephrotic syndrome may precede the development of acquired immunodeficiency syndrome (AIDS).[31] The glomerular lesions resemble those in idiopathic FSG, but in addition there is often a striking focal cystic dilatation of tubule segments, filled with proteinaceous material. Another characteristic finding is the presence of large numbers of tubuloreticular inclusions in endothelial cells. Such inclusions, also present in

SLE, have been shown to be induced by circulating interferon. They are not present in idiopathic FSG, and they may have diagnostic value in a biopsy specimen. The pathogenesis of HIV-related FSG is unclear, but viral DNA has been identified in renal biopsies in such patients.[32]

MEMBRANOPROLIFERATIVE GLOMERULONEPHRITIS (MPGN)

As the term implies, this group of disorders is characterized histologically by *alterations in the basement membrane and proliferation of glomerular cells.*[33] Because the proliferation is predominantly in the mesangium, a frequently used synonym is *mesangiocapillary GN.* MPGN accounts for 5 to 10% of cases of idiopathic NS in children and adults. Some patients present only with hematuria or proteinuria in the non-nephrotic range, and others have a combined nephrotic-nephritic picture. Like many other glomerulonephritides, histologic MPGN either can be associated with other systemic disorders and known etiologic agents (secondary MPGN) or may be primary, without known cause (idiopathic) in the kidney. Primary MPGN is divided into two major types on the basis of distinct ultrastructural, immunofluorescent, and probably pathogenic findings: type I and type II MPGN.

MORPHOLOGY. By light microscopy, both types are similar. The glomeruli are large and hypercellular. The hypercellularity is produced by proliferation of cells in the mesangium, although infiltrating leukocytes and parietal epithelial crescents are present in many cases. The glomeruli have a "lobular" appearance accentuated by the proliferating mesan-

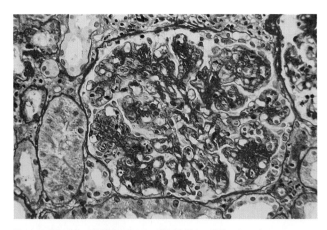

Figure 20–20. Membranoproliferative GN, showing mesangial cell proliferation, increased mesangial matrix, basement membrane thickening, leukocyte infiltration, and accentuation of lobular architecture. (Courtesy of Dr. H. Rennke.)

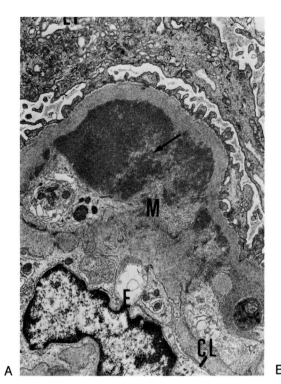

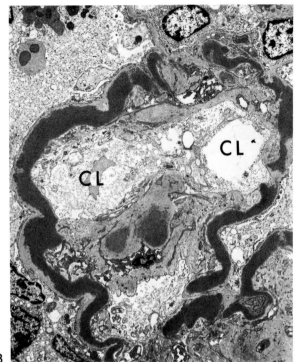

A

B

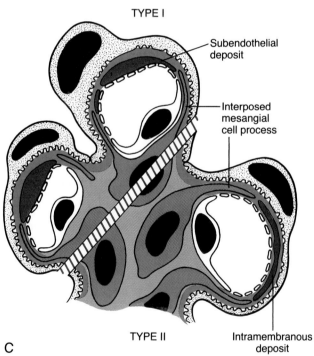

TYPE I

Subendothelial
deposit

Interposed
mesangial
cell process

TYPE II   Intramembranous
deposit

C

Figure 20–21. *A*, Membranoproliferative glomerulonephritis, type I. Note large subendothelial deposit *(arrow)* incorporated into mesangial matrix (M) through process of "mesangialization" (see text). E = endothelium; EP = epithelium; CL = capillary lumen. *B*, Type II MPGN, dense-deposit disease. There are markedly dense homogeneous deposits within basement membrane proper. CL = capillary lumen. *C*, Schematic representation of patterns in the two types of membranoproliferative glomerulonephritis, as seen by electron microscopy. In type I, there are *subendothelial deposits;* type II is characterized by *intramembranous dense deposits* (dense-deposit disease). In both, mesangial interposition gives the appearance of split basement membranes when viewed with the light microscope.

gial cells and increased mesangial matrix (Fig. 20–20). The GBM is clearly thickened, often focally, most evident in the peripheral capillary loops. The glomerular capillary wall often shows a "double-contour" or "tram-track" appearance, especially evident in silver or PAS stains. This is caused by "splitting" of the basement membrane because of the inclusion within it of processes of mesangial

cells extending into the peripheral capillary loops, so-called **mesangial interposition.**

Types I and II have altogether different ultrastructural and immunofluorescent features (Fig. 20–21A to C).

Type I MPGN (two-thirds of cases) is characterized by the presence of **subendothelial electron-dense deposits.** Mesangial and occasional subepithelial deposits may also be present (see Fig. 20–21). By immunofluorescence, C3 is deposited in a granular pattern, and IgG and early complement components (C1q and C4) are often also present, suggesting an immune complex pathogenesis.

In type II lesions, the lamina densa of the GBM is transformed into an irregular, ribbon-like, extremely electron-dense structure, due to the **deposition of dense material** of unknown composition in the GBM proper, giving rise to the term **dense-deposit disease.** In type II, C3 is present in irregular granular-linear foci in the basement membranes on either side, but not within the dense deposits. C3 is also present in the mesangium in characteristic circular aggregates (mesangial rings). **IgG is usually absent,** as are the early-acting complement components (C1q and C4).

Rare variants (type III) segregated because they exhibit both subendothelial and subepithelial deposits are associated with GBM disruption and reduplication.

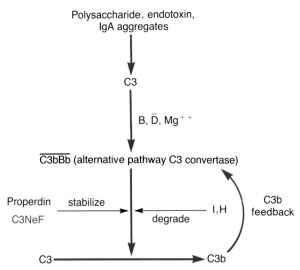

Figure 20–22. The alternative complement pathway. Note that C3NeF, present in the serum of patients with MPGN, acts at the same step as properdin, serving to stabilize the alternative pathway C3 convertase, thus enhancing C3 breakdown and causing hypocomplementemia.

PATHOGENESIS. *Although there are exceptions, most cases of type I MPGN present evidence of immune complexes in the glomerulus and activation of both classic and alternative complement pathways. The antigens involved are unknown.*

Conversely, most patients with dense-deposit disease (type II) have abnormalities that suggest activation of the alternative complement pathway. These patients have a consistently *decreased serum C3,* but normal C1 and C4, the immune complex–activated early components of complement. They also have diminished serum levels of factor B and properdin, components of the alternative complement pathway. In the glomeruli C3 and properdin are deposited, but not IgG. Recall that in the alternative complement pathway, C3 is directly cleaved to C3b (Fig. 20–22). The reaction depends on the initial interaction of C3 with such substances as bacterial polysaccharides, endotoxin, aggregates of IgA in the presence of factors B and $\bar{D}$, and magnesium. This leads to the generation of $\overline{C3bBb}$, the alternative pathway C3 convertase. The alternative C3 convertase is labile, being degraded by factors I and H, but it can be stabilized by properdin. More than 70% of patients with dense-deposit disease have in their sera a factor termed *C3 nephritic factor (C3NeF),* which acts at the same step as properdin, helping stabilize the alternative C3 convertase by binding to it (see Fig. 20–22). *C3NeF is indeed an immunoglobulin of the IgG class, an autoantibody to the alternative C3 convertase.* Dense-deposit disease may thus be considered an autoimmune disease. There is also decreased C3 synthesis by the liver, further contributing to the profound hypocomplementemia.

Precisely how C3NeF is related to glomerular injury, and the nature of the dense deposits are unknown. C3NeF activity also occurs in some patients with a genetically determined disease, *partial lipodystrophy,* some of whom develop type II MPGN.

CLINICAL COURSE. The principal mode of presentation is the nephrotic syndrome occurring in older children or young adults, although MPGN may begin as acute nephritis or, more insidiously, as mild proteinuria. Few remissions occur spontaneously in either type, and the disease follows a slowly progressive but unremitting course. Some patients develop numerous crescents and a clinical picture of rapidly progressive GN. About 50% develop chronic renal failure within 10 years. Treatments with steroids, immunosuppressive agents, and antiplatelet drugs have not been proved to be materially effective. There is a high incidence of recurrence in transplant recipients, particularly in type II disease. Dense deposits may recur in 90% of patients, although renal failure in the allograft is much less common.

Secondary MPGN[34] is usually of type I. It occurs in association with SLE, hepatitis B antigenemia, hepatitis C infection with cryoglobulinemia, infected ventriculoatrial shunts, schistosomiasis, alpha$_1$-antitrypsin deficiency, chronic liver diseases, and certain malignancies. As stated earlier, patients with partial lipodystrophy develop type II disease, associated with C3NeF.

IgA NEPHROPATHY (BERGER'S DISEASE)

This form of glomerulonephritis is characterized by the presence of prominent IgA deposits in the me-

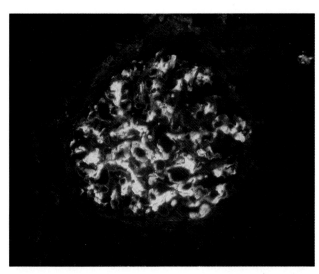

Figure 20-23. IgA nephropathy. Characteristic immunofluorescence deposition of IgA, principally in mesangial regions.

sangial regions detected by immunofluorescence microscopy.[35] The disease can be suspected by light microscopic examination, but diagnosis is made only by immunocytochemical techniques (Fig. 20-23). *IgA nephropathy is a very frequent cause of recurrent gross or microscopic hematuria* and is probably the most common type of glomerulonephritis worldwide. Mild proteinuria is usually present, and occasionally the nephrotic syndrome may develop. Rarely a patient may present with rapidly progressive crescentic GN.

While IgA nephropathy is an isolated renal disease, similar IgA deposits are present in a systemic disorder of children, *Henoch-Schönlein purpura,* to be discussed later, which has many overlapping features with IgA nephropathy. In addition, *secondary IgA nephropathy* occurs in patients with liver and intestinal diseases, as discussed later.

MORPHOLOGY. Histologically, the lesions vary considerably. The glomeruli may be normal or may show mesangial widening and segmental proliferation confined to some glomeruli (focal proliferative GN), diffuse mesangial proliferation (mesangioproliferative), or, rarely, overt crescentic GN. Healing of the focal proliferative lesion may lead to focal sclerosis. The characteristic immunofluorescent picture is of **mesangial deposition of IgA** (see Fig. 20-23), often with C3 and properdin and lesser amounts of IgG or IgM. Early complement components are usually absent. Electron microscopy confirms the presence of electron-dense deposits in the mesangium in the vast majority of cases. In some biopsies, prominent hyaline thickening of arterioles is present, a feature associated with a

greater likelihood of hypertension and progression to chronic renal failure.

PATHOGENESIS. IgA, the main immunoglobulin in mucosal secretions, is at low levels in normal serum, where it is present mostly in monomeric form, since the polymeric forms are catabolized in the liver. In patients with IgA nephropathy serum polymeric IgA1 (but not IgA2) is increased. In addition, circulating IgA1 immune complexes are present in some patients. A genetic influence is suggested by the occurrence of this condition in families and in HLA-identical brothers, and the increased frequency of certain HLA and complement phenotypes in some populations. The prominent mesangial deposition of IgA suggests entrapment of IgA immune complexes in the mesangium, and the absence of Clq and C4 in glomeruli points to activation of the alternative complement pathway. Taken together, these clues suggest a genetic or acquired abnormality of immune regulation leading to increased mucosal IgA synthesis in response to respiratory or gastrointestinal exposure to environmental agents (e.g., viruses, bacteria, food proteins). IgA1 and IgA1 complexes are then entrapped in the mesangium, where they activate the alternative complement pathway and initiate glomerular injury. In support of this scenario, IgA nephropathy occurs with increased frequency in patients with celiac disease and dermatitis herpetiformis (see Chapter 17), in whom intestinal mucosal defects are well defined, and in liver disease where there is defective hepatobiliary clearance of IgA complexes (*secondary IgA nephropathy*). The nature of the antigens is unknown. The deposited IgA1 appears to be polyclonal,[36] and it may be that a variety of antigens are involved in the course of the disease. Alternatively, qualitative alterations in the IgA1 molecule itself making it more likely to bind to mesangial antigens, and IgA antibodies reacting with mesangial cell autoantigens, have been invoked as mechanisms of glomerular IgA deposits.[37]

CLINICAL COURSE. The disease affects children and young adults and may occur within a day or two of mucosal infections of the respiratory, gastrointestinal, or urinary tract. Typically, the hematuria lasts for several days and then subsides, only to return every few months. IgA nephropathy is clinically a heterogeneous disease. Although most patients have an initially benign course, the disease appears to be slowly progressive: it is estimated that chronic renal failure develops in as many as 50% of cases over a period of 20 years. Onset in old age, heavy proteinuria, hypertension, and the presence of vascular sclerosis or crescents on biopsy are clues to an increased risk of progression. Recurrence of IgA deposits in transplanted kidneys occurs in 50% of cases, but with seemingly limited clinical consequence in most of these.

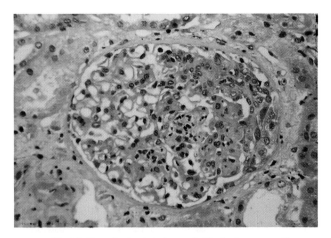

Figure 20–24. Focal glomerulonephritis in lupus erythematosus. There is segmental proliferation of cells and necrosis on the right. In the necrotic area there are neutrophils and fragmented nuclei (nuclear dust). The remainder of the glomerulus is not involved.

FOCAL PROLIFERATIVE AND NECROTIZING GLOMERULONEPHRITIS (FOCAL GN)

Focal glomerulonephritis represents a histologic entity in which glomerular proliferation is restricted to segments of individual glomeruli and commonly involves only a certain proportion of glomeruli. The lesions are predominantly proliferative and should be differentiated from those of focal sclerosis. Focal necrosis and fibrin deposition within the lesions often occur (Fig. 20–24).

Focal GN occurs under three circumstances:

1. It may be an early or mild manifestation of a systemic disease that sometimes involves entire glomeruli; among these are systemic lupus erythematosus, polyarteritis nodosa, Henoch-Schönlein purpura, Goodpasture's syndrome, subacute bacterial endocarditis, and Wegener's granulomatosis.

2. It may be a component of a known glomerular disease, such as a IgA nephropathy, as discussed earlier.

3. It can occur unrelated to any systemic or other renal disease and constitutes a form of *primary idiopathic focal GN.* It is necessary to exclude all other systemic disorders and IgA nephropathy by clinical and laboratory studies. The clinical manifestations may be mild, characterized by recurrent microscopic or gross hematuria or nonnephrotic proteinuria, but occasional cases present with a nephrotic syndrome.

CHRONIC GLOMERULONEPHRITIS

Chronic GN is best considered an end-stage pool of glomerular disease fed by a number of streams of specific types of glomerulonephritis, *most of which have been described earlier in this chapter (Fig. 20–25). Poststreptococcal GN is a rare antecedent of chronic GN, except in adults. Patients with rapidly progressive GN, if they survive the acute episode, usually progress to chronic GN. Membranous glomerulonephritis, membranoproliferative GN, and IgA nephropathy progress more slowly to chronic renal failure, whereas focal sclerosis often advances rather rapidly into chronic GN. Nevertheless, in any series of patients with chronic GN, a variable percentage of cases arise mysteriously with no antecedent history of any of the well-recognized forms of early GN.* These cases must represent the end result of relatively asymptomatic forms of GN, either known or still unrecognized, that progress to uremia. Clearly, the proportion of such unexplained cases depends on the availability of renal biopsy material from patients early in their disease.

MORPHOLOGY. The kidneys are symmetrically contracted and have diffusely granular, cortical surfaces. On section, the cortex is thinned, and there is an increase in peripelvic fat. The glomerular histology depends on the stage of the disease. In early cases, the glomeruli may still show evidence of the primary disease (e.g., membranous or membranoproliferative GN). However, there eventually ensues hyaline obliteration of glomeruli, transforming them into acellular eosinophilic PAS-positive masses (Fig. 20–26). The hyaline represents a combination of trapped plasma proteins, increased mesangial matrix, basement membrane–like material, and collagen. Because hypertension is an accompaniment of chronic GN, arterial and arteriolar sclerosis may be conspicuous. Marked atrophy of associated tubules, irregular interstitial fibrosis, and lymphocytic infiltration also occur.

Kidneys from patients with end-stage disease on long-term dialysis exhibit a variety of so-called "dialysis changes" that are unrelated to the primary disease. These include arterial intimal thickening caused by accumulation of smooth muscle–like cells and a loose, proteoglycan-rich stroma; calcification, most obvious in glomerular tufts and tubular basement membranes; extensive deposition of calcium oxalate crystals in tubules and interstitium; acquired cystic disease, discussed earlier; and increased numbers of renal adenomas and borderline adenocarcinomas.

Patients dying with chronic GN also exhibit pathologic changes **outside** the kidney that are related to the uremic state and are also present in other forms of chronic renal failure. Often clinically important, these include uremic pericarditis, uremic gastroenteritis, secondary hyperparathyroidism with nephrocalcinosis and renal osteodystrophy, left ventricular hypertrophy due to hypertension, and pulmonary changes of diffuse alveolar damage often ascribed to uremia (uremic pneumonitis).

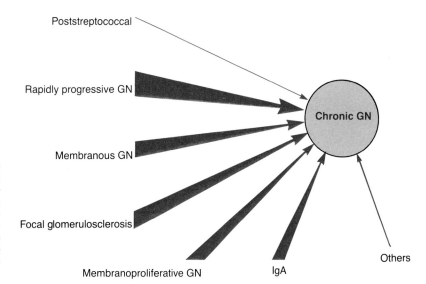

Poststreptococcal

Rapidly progressive GN

Membranous GN

Focal glomerulosclerosis

Membranoproliferative GN

IgA

Others

Chronic GN

Figure 20–25. Primary glomerular diseases leading to chronic glomerulonephritis. The thickness of the arrows reflects the approximate proportion of patients in each group who progress to chronic GN. Poststreptococcal (1 to 2%); rapidly progressive (crescentic) (90%); membranous (50%); focal glomerulosclerosis (50 to 80%); MPGN (50%); IgA nephropathy (30 to 50%).

CLINICAL COURSE. In most patients, chronic GN develops insidiously and slowly progresses to death in uremia over a span of years or possibly decades (see discussion of chronic renal failure). Not infrequently, patients present with such nonspecific complaints as loss of appetite, anemia, vomiting, or weakness. In some, the renal disease is suspected with the discovery of proteinuria, hypertension, or azotemia on routine medical examination. In others, the underlying renal disorder is discovered in the course of investigation of edema. *Most patients are hypertensive, and sometimes the dominant clinical manifestations are cerebral or cardiovascular.* In all, the disease is relentlessly progressive, although at widely varying rates. In nephrotic patients, as glomeruli become obliterated, the protein loss in the urine diminishes. If patients with chronic GN are not maintained on continued dialysis or if they do not receive a renal transplant, the outcome is invariably death.

Table 20–8 summarizes the main clinical and histologic features of the major forms of primary GN.

GLOMERULAR LESIONS ASSOCIATED WITH SYSTEMIC DISEASE

Many immunologically mediated, metabolic, or hereditary systemic disorders are associated with glomerular injury, and in some (e.g., SLE and diabetes mellitus) the glomerular involvement is a major clinical manifestation. Most of these diseases have been discussed elsewhere in this book. Here we shall briefly recall some of the lesions and discuss only those not considered in other sections.

Systemic Lupus Erythematosus

The various types of lupus nephritis are described and illustrated in detail in Chapter 6. As discussed, SLE gives rise to a heterogeneous group of lesions and clinical presentations. The clinical manifestations include recurrent microscopic or gross hematuria, acute nephritis, the nephrotic syndrome, chronic renal failure, and hypertension. Histologically, glomerular changes are classified into *mesan-*

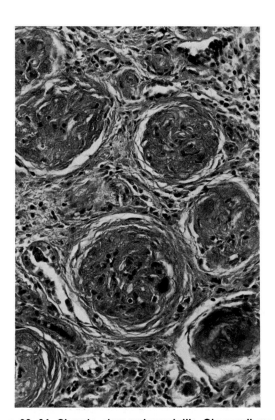

Figure 20–26. Chronic glomerulonephritis. Glomeruli are totally replaced by hyaline connective tissue.

Table 20–8. SUMMARY OF MAJOR PRIMARY GLOMERULONEPHRITIDES

DISEASE	MOST FREQUENT CLINICAL PRESENTATION	PATHOGENESIS	GLOMERULAR PATHOLOGY		
			Light Microscopy	*Fluorescence Microscopy*	*Electron Microscopy*
Poststreptococcal glomerulone-phritis	Acute nephritis	Antibody-mediated; circulating or planted antigen	Diffuse proliferation; leukocytic infiltration	Granular IgG and C3 in GBM and mesangium	Subepithelial humps
Goodpasture's syndrome	Rapidly progressive GN	Anti-GBM COL4A3 antigen	Proliferation; crescents	Linear IgG and C3; fibrin in crescents	No deposits; GBM disruptions; fibrin
Idiopathic RPGN	Rapidly progressive GN	Anti-GBM immune complex ANCA	Proliferation; focal necrosis; crescents	Linear IgG and C3 Granular

Negative or equivocal | No deposits Deposits may be present No deposits |
Membranous glomerulone-phritis	Nephrotic syndrome	Antibody-mediated; in situ Gp330 antigen	Diffuse capillary wall thickening	Granular IgG and C3; diffuse	Subepithelial deposits
Lipoid nephrosis	Nephrotic syndrome	Unknown, loss of glomerular polyanion	Normal; lipid in tubules	Negative	Loss of foot processes; no deposits
Focal segmental glomerulosclerosis	Nephrotic syndrome; non-nephrotic proteinuria	Unknown Ablation nephropathy ?Plasma factor	Focal and segmental sclerosis and hyalinosis	Focal; IgM and C3	Loss of foot processes; epithelial denudation
Membrano- Type I proliferative glomerulo-nephritis Type II	Nephrotic syndrome

Hematuria Chronic renal failure | (I) Immune complex

(II) Autoantibody: alternative complement pathway activation | Mesangial proliferation; basement membrane thickening; splitting | (I) IgG + C3; C1 + C4

(II) C3 ± IgG; no C1 or C4 | (I) Subendothelial deposits;

(II) Dense-deposit disease |
| IgA nephropathy | Recurrent hematuria and/or proteinuria | Unknown; see text | Focal proliferative GN; mesangial widening | IgA + IgG, M, and C3 in mesangium | Mesangial and paramesangial dense deposits |
| Chronic glomerulo-nephritis | Chronic renal failure | Variable | Hyalinized glomeruli | Granular or negative | — |

gial lupus nephritis, focal GN, diffuse proliferative GN, and diffuse membranous GN.[39]

Henoch-Schönlein Purpura

This syndrome consists of *purpuric skin lesions characteristically involving the extensor surfaces of arms and legs as well as buttocks; abdominal manifestations including pain, vomiting, and intestinal bleeding; nonmigratory arthralgia; and renal abnormalities.* The latter occur in one-third of patients and include gross or microscopic hematuria, proteinuria, and nephrotic syndrome. A small number of patients, mostly adults, develop a rapidly progressive form of GN with many crescents. Not all components of the syndrome need to be present, and individual patients may have purpura, abdomi-

nal pain, or urinary abnormalities as the dominant feature. The disease is most common in children three to eight years old, but it also occurs in adults, in whom the renal manifestations are usually more severe. There is a strong background of atopy in about one-third of patients, and onset often follows an upper respiratory infection.

MORPHOLOGY. Histologically, the renal lesions vary from mild focal mesangial proliferation to diffuse mesangial proliferation to relatively typical crescentic GN. Whatever the histologic lesions, the prominent feature by fluorescence microscopy is the **deposition of IgA, sometimes with IgG and C3 in the mesangial region** in a distribution similar to that described for IgA nephropathy. This has led to the belief that **IgA nephropathy and Henoch-**

Schönlein purpura are perhaps spectra of the same disease. The skin lesions consist of subepidermal hemorrhages and a necrotizing vasculitis involving the small vessels of the dermis. IgA is also present in such vessels. Vasculitis can also occur in other organs, such as the gastrointestinal tract, but is rare in the kidney.

The course of the disease is quite variable, but recurrences of hematuria may persist for many years after onset. Most children have an excellent prognosis. Patients with the more diffuse lesions or with the nephrotic syndrome have a somewhat poorer prognosis, and renal failure occurs in those with the crescentic lesions.

Bacterial Endocarditis

Glomerular lesions occurring in the course of bacterial endocarditis represent a type of immune complex nephritis initiated by bacterial antigen-antibody complexes. Clinically, hematuria and proteinuria of various degrees characterize this entity, but an acute nephritic presentation is not uncommon, and even rapidly progressive GN may occur in rare instances. The histologic lesions, when present, generally reflect these clinical manifestations. Milder forms have a focal and segmental necrotizing GN, whereas more severe ones exhibit a diffuse proliferative GN, and the rapidly progressive forms show large numbers of crescents.

Diabetic Glomerulosclerosis

Diabetes mellitus is a major cause of renal morbidity and mortality. End-stage kidney disease occurs in as many as 30% of insulin-dependent type I diabetics and accounts for 20% of deaths in patients younger than 40 years of age. By far the most common lesions involve the glomeruli and are associated clinically with three glomerular syndromes, including non-nephrotic proteinuria, nephrotic syndrome, and chronic renal failure.[40] However, diabetes also affects the arterioles, causing *arteriolar sclerosis;* increases susceptibility to the development of pyelonephritis, and particularly *papillary necrosis;* and causes a variety of tubular lesions. The term *diabetic nephropathy* is applied to the conglomerate of lesions that often occur concurrently in the diabetic kidney.

Proteinuria, sometimes in the nephrotic range, occurs in about 50% of both insulin-dependent and insulin-independent (type II) diabetics. It is usually discovered 12 to 22 years after the clinical appearance of diabetes, and (particularly in type I diabetics) often heralds the progressive development of chronic renal failure ending in death or end-stage disease within a period of 4 to 5 years. The

morphologic changes in the glomeruli include (1) capillary basement membrane thickening, (2) diffuse diabetic glomerulosclerosis, and (3) nodular glomerulosclerosis.

MORPHOLOGY

Capillary Basement Membrane Thickening. Widespread thickening of the glomerular capillary basement membrane (GBM) occurs in virtually all diabetics, irrespective of the presence of proteinuria, and is part and parcel of the diabetic microangiopathy. Pure capillary basement membrane thickening can be detected only by electron microscopy. Careful morphometric studies demonstrate that this thickening begins as early as 2 years after the onset of type I diabetes, and by 5 years amounts to about a 30% increase.[41] The thickening continues progressively, and usually concurrently with mesangial widening (Fig. 20–27). Simultaneously there is thickening of the tubular basement membranes.

Diffuse Glomerulosclerosis. This consists of diffuse increase in mesangial matrix, with mild proliferation of mesangial cells, and is always associated with the overall thickening of the GBM. The increase in mesangial volume appears to lag slightly behind basement membrane widening but becomes pronounced after 10 to 20 years of diabetes. The matrix depositions are PAS positive. The changes almost always begin in the vascular stalk and sometimes seem continuous with the invariably present hyaline thickening of arterioles (Fig. 20–28). As the disease progresses, the mesangial areas expand further and obliterate the mesangial cells, gradually filling the entire glomerulus **(obliterative diabetic glomerulosclerosis).**

Nodular Glomerulosclerosis. This is also known as **intercapillary glomerulosclerosis or Kimmelstiel-Wilson disease.** The glomerular lesions take the form of ovoid or spherical, often laminated, hyaline masses situated in the periphery of the glomerulus. They lie within the mesangial core of the glomerular lobules and often are surrounded by peripheral patent capillary loops (see Fig. 20–28). Usually, not all the lobules in the individual glomerulus are involved. **Uninvolved lobules and glomeruli all show striking diffuse glomerulosclerosis.** The nodules are PAS positive and contain lipids and fibrin. As the disease advances, the individual nodules enlarge and eventually compress and engulf capillaries, obliterating the glomerular tuft. As a consequence of the glomerular and arteriolar lesions, the kidney suffers from ischemia, develops tubular atrophy and interstitial fibrosis, and usually undergoes overall contraction in size.

Most workers believe that nodular glomerulosclerosis and the diffuse lesion are fundamentally similar lesions of the mesangium. The nodular lesion, however, is virtually pathognomonic of diabetes, so

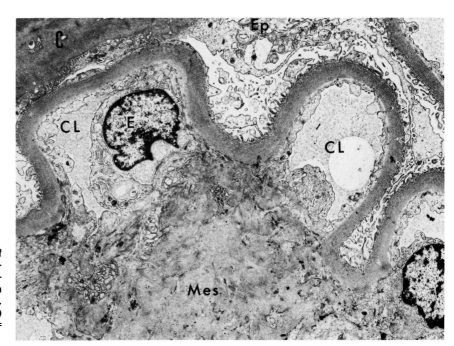

Figure 20–27. Electron micrograph of advanced diabetic glomerulosclerosis. Note massive increase in mesangial matrix (Mes) encroaching on glomerular capillary lumina (CL). GBM and Bowman's capsule (C) are markedly thickened. Ep = epithelium; E = endothelium.

long as care is taken to exclude membranoproliferative (lobular) GN, the GN associated with light-chain disease, and amyloidosis. Approximately 15 to 30% of long-term patients with diabetes develop nodular glomerulosclerosis, and in most instances it is associated with renal failure.

PATHOGENESIS. The pathogenesis of diabetic glomerulosclerosis is intimately linked with that of generalized diabetic microangiopathy, discussed in Chapter 19. The principal points are as follows:

1. The bulk of the evidence suggests that diabetic glomerulosclerosis *is caused by the metabolic defect*, that is, the insulin deficiency, or the result-

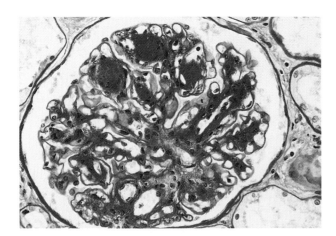

Figure 20–28. Diffuse and nodular diabetic glomerulosclerosis (PAS stain). Note diffuse increase in mesangial matrix and characteristic acellular PAS-positive nodules.

ant hyperglycemia, or some other aspects of glucose intolerance.

2. Biochemical alterations in diabetic GBM have been described, including increased amount and synthesis of collagen type IV and fibronectin, and decreased synthesis of proteoglycan heparan sulfate.

3. *Nonenzymatic glycosylation* of proteins, known to occur in diabetics and giving rise to advanced glycosylation end products (AGE), may contribute to the glomerulopathy. The mechanisms by which advanced glycosylation end products cause their effects were discussed in Chapter 19 (see Table 19–6).[42]

4. One hypothesis implicates *hemodynamic changes* in the initiation or modulation of diabetic glomerulosclerosis. It is well known that early-onset type I diabetics, particularly those with imperfectly controlled hyperglycemia, have an increased GFR, increased glomerular filtration area, increased glomerular capillary pressure, and *glomerular hypertrophy*.[43] Hemodynamic alterations and glomerular hypertrophy have been observed in experimental streptozotocin-induced diabetes in rats, where they are associated with proteinuria and can be reversed by diabetic control. It has been speculated that the subsequent morphologic alterations in the mesangium are somehow influenced by the glomerular hypertrophy and hemodynamic changes, akin to the adaptive responses to ablation of renal mass, discussed earlier.

To sum up, two processes seem to play a role in the fully developed diabetic lesions: a metabolic defect, possibly linked to advanced glycosylation end products, that accounts for the thickened GBM and increased mesangial matrix that occur in *all* patients; and hemodynamic effects, associated with glomerular hypertrophy, which leads to glomerulosclerosis in about 40% of patients.

CLINICAL COURSE. The clinical manifestations of diabetic glomerulosclerosis are linked to those of diabetes. The increased GFR typical of early-onset type I diabetics is associated with *microalbuminuria*, defined as urinary albumin excretion of 20 to 200 μg/minute of albumin. Microalbuminuria and increased GFR are important predictors of future overt diabetic nephropathy in these patients. Proteinuria then develops, which may be mild and asymptomatic initially, but gradually increases to nephrotic levels in some patients. This is followed by progressive loss of GFR, leading to end-stage renal failure within a period of 5 years. Systemic hypertension may precede the development of proteinuria and renal insufficiency. Indeed, recent evidence suggests that the risk of renal disease in type I diabetics is associated with a genetic predisposition to hypertension, and that hypertension increases the susceptibility to developing diabetic nephropathy in the presence of poor hyperglycemic control.

Although the prevalence of proteinuria and renal failure are comparable in type I and type II diabetics, the lesions are more heterogeneous and the cause less predictable in type II diabetics.[44] At present, the vast majority of patients with end-stage diabetic nephropathy are maintained on long-term dialysis, and a few receive renal transplantation. Diabetic lesions may recur in the renal allografts. Precise control of the blood sugar in diabetes has now been shown by several studies to delay or prevent the progression of glomerulopathy.[45] Similarly, inhibition of angiotensin by converting enzyme inhibitors (captopril) has a beneficial effect on progression, possibly by reversing the increased intraglomerular capillary pressure.[46]

Amyloidosis

Disseminated amyloidosis (see Chapter 6), whether it conforms to the so-called primary or secondary pattern of distribution, may be associated with deposits of amyloid within the glomeruli. The typical amyloid fibrils are present within the mesangium and subendothelium, and occasionally within the subepithelial space. Eventually, they obliterate the glomerulus completely. Recall that deposits of amyloid also appear in blood vessel walls and in the kidney interstitium. Amyloid can be detected on light microscopy by special stains, particularly by the characteristic birefringence after staining with Congo red. Patients with glomerular amyloid may present with heavy proteinuria or the nephrotic syndrome and later, owing to destruction

of the glomeruli, die in uremia. Characteristically, kidney size tends to be either normal or slightly enlarged.

Other Systemic Disorders

Goodpasture's syndrome, polyarteritis nodosa, and *Wegener's granulomatosis* are commonly associated with glomerular lesions and were discussed earlier. Suffice it to say here that the glomerular lesions in these three conditions can be very similar. In the early or mild forms of involvement there is focal and segmental, sometimes necrotizing, GN, and most of these patients will have hematuria with rather mild decline in GFR. In the more severe cases associated with rapidly progressive GN, there is also extensive necrosis, fibrin deposition, and the formation of epithelial crescents. It should be recalled, however, that these diseases have different pathogenetic mechanisms. Goodpasture's syndrome is mediated by anti-GBM antibodies and exhibits linear fluorescence of immunoglobulin and complement, polyarteritis nodosa is associated with immune complexes, and Wegener's granulomatosis with antineutrophil cytoplasmic antibodies (ANCA).

Essential mixed cryoglobulinemia is another rare systemic condition in which deposits of cryoglobulins composed principally of IgG-IgM complexes induce cutaneous vasculitis, synovitis, and focal or diffuse proliferative glomerulonephritis. Cryoglobulinemia secondary to infection (e.g., hepatitis C) may be associated with GN, usually of the MPGN type.

Plasma cell dyscrasias may also induce glomerular lesions. *Multiple myeloma* is associated with (1) amyloidosis, (2) deposition of monoclonal cryoglobulins in glomeruli, and (3) peculiar nodular lesions resembling those seen in nodular diabetic glomerulosclerosis and ascribed to the deposition of nonfibrillar light chains. This *light-chain nephropathy* also occurs in the absence of overt myeloma, usually associated with deposition of kappa chains in glomeruli. The glomeruli show PAS-positive mesangial nodules, lobular accentuation, and mild mesangial hypercellularity and need to be differentiated from diabetic nodules and membranoproliferative GN. These patients usually present with proteinuria or the nephrotic syndrome, hypertension, and progressive azotemia. Other renal manifestations of multiple myeloma are discussed later.

HEREDITARY NEPHRITIS

Hereditary nephritis refers to a group of heterogeneous hereditary-familial renal diseases associated primarily with glomerular injury.[47] The most well-

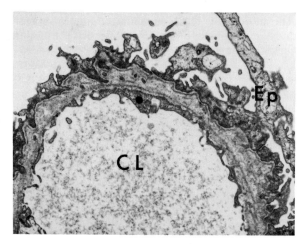

Figure 20–29. Hereditary nephritis. Electron micrograph of glomerulus with irregular thickening of basement membrane, lamination of lamina densa, and foci of rarefaction. Such changes may be present in other diseases but are most pronounced and widespread in hereditary nephritis. CL = capillary lumen; Ep = epithelium.

studied entity is so-called *Alport's syndrome, the name usually given to the disease in which nephritis is accompanied by nerve deafness and various eye disorders, including lens dislocation, posterior cataracts, and corneal dystrophy.* Males tend to be affected more frequently and more severely than females and are more likely to progress to renal failure. Females, however, are not completely spared. The most common presenting sign is gross or microscopic hematuria, frequently accompanied by erythrocyte casts. Proteinuria may occur and, rarely, the nephrotic syndrome develops. Symptoms appear at ages 5 to 20, and the onset of overt renal failure is between ages 20 and 50 in males. The auditory defects may be subtle, requiring extensive testing. The mode of inheritance is heterogeneous, being either X-linked or autosomal in most pedigrees.

MORPHOLOGY. Histologically, the glomeruli are always involved. The most common early lesion is segmental proliferation or sclerosis, or both. There is an increase in mesangial matrix, and in some patients the persistence of fetal-like glomeruli. In some kidneys, glomerular or tubular epithelial cells acquire a foamy appearance owing to accumulation of neutral fats and mucopolysaccharides **(foam cells)**. As the disease progresses, there is increasing glomerulosclerosis, vascular narrowing, tubular atrophy, and interstitial fibrosis. With the electron microscope, characteristic basement membrane lesions are found in some (but not all) patients with hereditary nephritis. The basement membrane shows irregular foci of thickening or attenuation, with pronounced splitting and lamination of the lamina densa (Fig. 20–29). Similar alterations are found in the tubular basement mem-

branes. Although such basement membrane changes may be seen focally in diseases other than hereditary nephritis, they are most widespread and pronounced in patients with this disorder.

PATHOGENESIS. Defective GBM synthesis underlies the renal lesions. In patients with X-linked disease, the defect has been traced to *mutations in the gene encoding the α5 chain (COL4A5) of collagen type IV,* a component of GBM.[48] The mutations are heterogeneous and affect all domains of α5 chain (see Fig. 20–3). This is thought to interfere with the structure and function of collagen type IV and thus the GBM network.[4] In addition, probably as a result of this defect, patients synthesize lesser amounts of other collagen components, including the α3 chain, which as you recall is the Goodpasture antigen. Indeed, glomeruli of some patients appear to lack the α3 chain and fail to react with anti-GBM antibodies from patients with Goodpasture's syndrome.[49] Certain patients with Alport's syndrome have additional mutations in the newly discovered α6 chain, associated with diffuse leiomyomatosis.[50]

DISEASES AFFECTING TUBULES AND INTERSTITIUM

Most forms of tubular injury also involve the interstitium, so the two are discussed together. Under this heading we present diseases characterized by (1) ischemic or toxic tubular injury, leading to *acute tubular necrosis* and acute renal failure, and (2) inflammatory involvement of the tubules and interstitium *(tubulointerstitial nephritis).*

ACUTE TUBULAR NECROSIS

Acute tubular necrosis (ATN) is a clinicopathologic entity characterized morphologically by destruction of tubular epithelial cells and clinically by acute suppression of renal function. It is the most common cause of acute renal failure (ARF). ARF signifies acute suppression of renal function and urine flow, falling within 24 hours to less than 400 ml. ARF can be caused by the following conditions:

1. *Organic vascular obstruction,* caused by diffuse involvement of the intrarenal vessels, such as in polyarteritis nodosa and malignant hypertension, and the hemolytic-uremic syndrome
2. *Severe glomerular disease,* such as rapidly progressive glomerulonephritis
3. *Acute tubulointerstitial nephritis,* most commonly occurring as a hypersensitivity to drugs

4. *Massive infection* (pyelonephritis), especially when accompanied by papillary necrosis

5. *Disseminated intravascular renal coagulation*

6. *Urinary obstruction* by tumors, prostatic hypertrophy, or blood clots (so-called postrenal ARF)

7. *Acute tubular necrosis* (ATN)

Here we discuss ATN; diffuse cortical necrosis follows in the next section. The other causes of ARF are discussed elsewhere in this chapter.

ATN is a reversible renal lesion that arises in a variety of clinical settings. Most of these, ranging from severe trauma to acute pancreatitis, have in common a period of inadequate blood flow to the peripheral organs, usually accompanied by marked hypotension and shock. The pattern of ATN associated with shock is called *ischemic ATN*. Mismatched blood transfusions and other hemolytic crises causing *hemoglobinuria* and several skeletal muscle injuries causing *myoglobinuria* also produce a picture resembling ischemic ATN, so-called *pigment-induced ATN*. The second pattern, called *nephrotoxic ATN*, is caused by a multitude of drugs, such as gentamicin, other antibiotics, and radiographic contrast agents, and poisons, including heavy metals (e.g., mercury), and organic solvents (e.g., carbon tetrachloride). Because of the many precipitating factors, ATN occurs quite frequently. Moreover, its reversibility adds to its clinical importance because proper management means the difference between full recovery and death.

PATHOGENESIS. The critical event in both ischemic and nephrotoxic ATN is believed to be *tubular damage* (Fig. 20–30).[51] Tubular epithelial cells are particularly sensitive to anoxia, and they are also vulnerable to toxins. Several factors predispose the tubules to toxic injury, including a vast electrically charged surface for tubular reabsorption, active transport systems for ions and organic acids, and the capability for effective concentration. Ischemia causes numerous structural and functional alterations in epithelial cells;[51] loss of cell polarity appears to be a functionally important early event. Because the medulla receives a small proportion of renal blood flow, it is particularly susceptible to ischemia. Thus, cortical and medullary tubules, including the functionally important *thick ascending limb*, are affected.[52] Once tubular injury has occurred, the progression to ARF may follow one of several hypothetic pathways (Fig. 20–31). (1) Tubular damage has been postulated to trigger vasoconstriction of preglomerular arterioles, resulting in reduced GFR due to *glomerulotubular feedback*. The *vasoconstriction* has been ascribed to activation of the renin-angiotensin system, but other vasoconstrictive agents, such as renin, adenosine, thromboxanes, and endothelin, have also been implicated. Alternatively or additionally, loss of vasodilator effects (prostaglandin, nitric oxide) may be involved. (2) Damage to the tubules can itself result in oliguria, because tubular debris could block urine outflow and eventually increase intratubular pressure, thereby decreasing the GFR. (3) Additionally, fluid from the damaged tubules could leak into the interstitium, resulting in increased interstitial pressure and collapse of the tubule. (4) Finally, there is some evidence of a direct effect of toxins on the ultrafiltration coefficient of the glomerular capillary wall. Which one of these mechanisms is most important in the onset of the oliguria is unclear, and it is likely that a combination of these effects is necessary. One or the other may predominate, depending on the inciting agents.

MORPHOLOGY. Ischemic ATN is characterized by focal tubular necrosis at multiple points along the nephron, with large skip areas in between, often accompanied by rupture of basement membranes (tubulorrhexis) and occlusion of tubular lumina by casts (see Fig. 20–30).[53] Tubular necrosis is often subtle but may be missed. The straight portion of the proximal tubule and the ascending thick limb in the renal medulla are especially vulnerable, but focal necrotic lesions may also occur in the distal tubule, often in conjunction with casts.

Eosinophilic hyaline casts, as well as pigmented granular casts, are extremely common, particularly in distal tubules and collecting ducts (Fig. 20–32). These casts consist principally of Tamm-Horsfall pro-

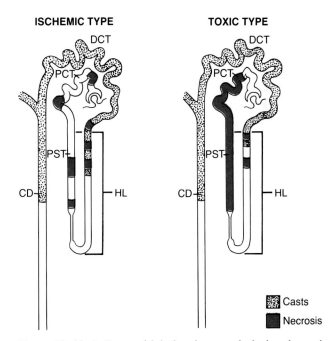

Figure 20–30. Patterns of tubular damage in ischemic and toxic ATN. In ischemic type, tubular necrosis is patchy, relatively short lengths of tubules are affected, and straight segments of proximal tubules (PST) and ascending limbs of Henle's loop (HL) are most vulnerable. In toxic ATN, extensive necrosis is present along proximal tubule segments (PCT) with many toxins (e.g., mercury), but necrosis of the distal tubule, particularly ascending Henle's loop, also occurs. In both types, lumina of distal convoluted tubules (DCT) and collecting ducts (CD) contain casts.

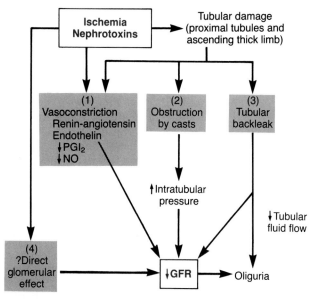

Figure 20-31. Possible pathogenetic mechanisms in acute renal failure. Sequence of events 1, 2, 3, and 4 is described in text.

tein (a specific urinary glycoprotein normally secreted by the cells of ascending thick limb and distal tubules) in conjunction with hemoglobin, myoglobin, and other plasma proteins. Other common findings in ischemic ATN are interstitial edema and accumulations of leukocytes within dilated vasa recta. There is also often evidence of **epithelial regeneration**: flattened epithelial cells with hyperchromatic nuclei and mitotic figures are often present. In the course of time, this regeneration repopulates the tubules so that if survival occurs no residual evidence of damage can be seen.

Toxic ATN is manifested by acute tubular injury, most obvious in the proximal convoluted tubules (see Fig. 20-30). Histologically, the tubular necrosis may be entirely nonspecific but is somewhat distinctive in poisoning with certain agents. With mercuric chloride, for example, severely injured cells not yet dead may contain large acidophilic inclusions. Later, these cells become totally necrotic, are desquamated into the lumen, and may undergo calcification. Carbon tetrachloride poisoning, in contrast, is characterized by the accumulation of neutral lipids in injured cells, but again, such fatty change is followed by necrosis. Ethylene glycol produces marked ballooning and hydropic or vacuolar degeneration of proximal convoluted tubules. Calcium oxalate crystals are often found in the tubular lumina in such poisoning.

CLINICAL COURSE. The clinical course of ATN may be divided into *initiating, maintenance,* and *recovery* stages. The *initiating phase,* lasting for about 36 hours, is dominated by the inciting medical, surgical, or obstetric event in the ischemic form of ATN. The only indication of renal involvement is a slight decline in urine output with a rise in BUN. At this point, oliguria could be explained on the basis of a transient decrease in blood flow to the kidneys.

The *maintenance stage* is characterized by sustained decreases in urine output to between 40 and 400 ml per day (oliguria), with salt and water overload, rising blood urea nitrogens, hyperkalemia, metabolic acidosis, and other manifestations of uremia dominating this phase. With appropriate attention to the balance of water and blood electrolytes, including dialysis, the patient can be carried over this oliguric crisis.

The *recovery phase* is ushered in by a steady increase in urine volume that may reach up to 3 liters per day. The tubules are still damaged, so that large amounts of water, sodium, and potassium are lost in the urinary flood. *Hypokalemia, rather than hyperkalemia, becomes a clinical problem.* There is a peculiar increased vulnerability to infection at this stage. Eventually, renal tubular function is restored, with improvement in concentrating ability. At the same time, BUN and creatinine levels begin to return to normal. Subtle tubular functional impairment may persist for months, but most patients who reach the recovery phase eventually recover completely.

The prognosis of ATN depends on the clinical setting surrounding its development. Recovery is expected with nephrotoxic ATN when the toxin

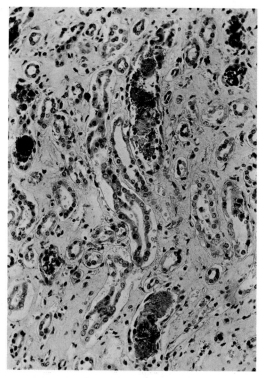

Figure 20-32. Ischemic ATN. Granular pigment casts are seen in collecting tubules. Some of the tubular epithelial cells in affected tubules are necrotic, whereas others are flattened, stretched out, and regenerating.

has not caused serious damage to other organs, such as the liver or heart. Conversely, in shock related to sepsis or extensive burns, the mortality rate may rise to over 50%.

Up to 50% of patients with ATN may not have oliguria, and may in fact have increased urine volumes. This so-called *nonoliguric ATN* occurs particularly often with nephrotoxins, and generally it tends to follow a more benign clinical course.

TUBULOINTERSTITIAL NEPHRITIS

This group of renal diseases is characterized by histologic and functional alterations that involve predominantly the tubules and interstitium.[54] Glomerular and vascular abnormalities may also be present but either are mild or occur only in advanced stages of these diseases. *The tubulointerstitial diseases have diverse causes and different pathogenetic mechanisms* (Table 20–9). Thus, the disorders are identified by cause or by associated disease (e.g., analgesic nephritis, irradiation nephritis).

Tubulointerstitial nephritis (TIN) can be acute or chronic. Acute TIN has an acute clinical onset and is characterized histologically by interstitial edema, often accompanied by leukocytic infiltra-

Table 20–9. TUBULOINTERSTITIAL DISEASES

INFECTIONS
Acute bacterial pyelonephritis
Chronic pyelonephritis (including reflux nephropathy)
Other infections (e.g., viruses, parasites)

TOXINS
Drugs
Acute hypersensitivity interstitial nephritis
Analgesic nephritis
Heavy metals
Lead, cadmium

METABOLIC DISEASES
Urate nephropathy
Nephrocalcinosis (hypercalcemic nephropathy)
Hypokalemic nephropathy
Oxalate nephropathy

PHYSICAL FACTORS
Chronic urinary tract obstruction
Radiation nephritis

NEOPLASMS
Multiple myeloma

IMMUNOLOGIC REACTIONS
Transplant rejection
Tubulointerstitial disease associated with glomerulonephritis
Sjögren's syndrome

VASCULAR DISEASES

MISCELLANEOUS
Balkan nephropathy
Nephronophthisis–medullary cystic disease complex
Other rare causes (sarcoidosis)
"Idiopathic" interstitial nephritis

tion and focal tubular necrosis. In *chronic interstitial nephritis* (CIN) there is infiltration with mononuclear cells, prominent interstitial fibrosis, and widespread tubular atrophy.

Clinically, these conditions are distinguished from the glomerular diseases by the absence, in early stages, of such hallmarks of glomerular injury as nephritic or nephrotic syndromes and by the presence of defects in tubular function. The latter may be quite subtle and include impaired ability to concentrate urine, evidenced clinically by polyuria or nocturia; salt wasting; diminished ability to excrete acids (metabolic acidosis); and isolated defects in tubular reabsorption or secretion. The advanced forms, however, may be difficult to distinguish clinically from other causes of renal insufficiency.

Some of the specific conditions listed in Table 20–9 are discussed elsewhere in this book. In this section we deal principally with pyelonephritis and interstitial diseases induced by drugs.

Pyelonephritis (PN) and Urinary Tract Infection

Pyelonephritis is a renal disorder affecting tubules, interstitium, and renal pelvis and is one of the most common diseases of the kidney. It occurs in two forms. *Acute PN* is caused by bacterial infection and is the renal lesion associated with urinary tract infection. *Chronic PN* is a more complex disorder: bacterial infection plays a dominant role, but other factors (vesicoureteral reflux, obstruction) are involved in its pathogenesis.

The term *urinary tract infection (UTI)* implies involvement of either the bladder (cystitis) or the kidneys and their collecting systems (pyelonephritis), or both. UTIs are extremely common disorders. It is important to realize, however, that bacterial infection of the urinary tract may be completely asymptomatic (asymptomatic bacteriuria) or may remain localized to the bladder without the development of renal infection. However, UTI always carries the potential of spread to the kidney.

ETIOLOGY AND PATHOGENESIS. The dominant etiologic agents, accounting for more than 85% of cases of UTI, are the gram-negative bacilli that are normal inhabitants of the intestinal tract.[55] By far the most common is *Escherichia coli,* followed by Proteus, Klebsiella, and Enterobacter. *Streptococcus faecalis,* also of enteric origin, staphylococci, and virtually every other bacterial and fungal agent can also cause lower urinary tract and renal infection.

In most patients with UTI, the infecting organisms are derived from the patient's own fecal flora. This is thus a form of *endogenous infection.* There are two routes by which bacteria can reach the

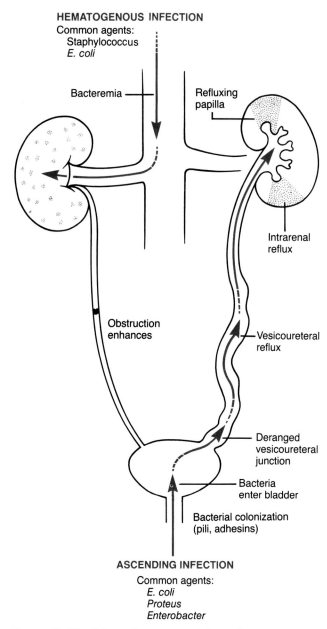

HEMATOGENOUS INFECTION
Common agents:
    Staphylococcus
    E. coli

Bacteremia

Refluxing papilla

Intrarenal reflux

Obstruction enhances

Vesicoureteral reflux

Deranged vesicoureteral junction

Bacteria enter bladder

Bacterial colonization (pili, adhesins)

ASCENDING INFECTION
Common agents:
    E. coli
    Proteus
    Enterobacter

Figure 20–33. Schematic representation of pathways of renal infection. *Hematogenous* infection results from bacteremic spread. More common is *ascending* infection, which results from a combination of urinary bladder infection, vesicoureteral reflux, and intrarenal reflux.

kidneys: (1) through the bloodstream (hematogenous infection), and (2) from the lower urinary tract (ascending infection) (Fig. 20–33). Although the hematogenous route is the less common of the two, acute pyelonephritis does result from seeding of the kidneys by bacteria from distant foci in the course of septicemia or infective endocarditis. Hematogenous infection is more likely to occur in the presence of ureteral obstruction, in debilitated patients, in patients on immunosuppressive therapy, and with nonenteric organisms, such as staphylococci and certain fungi.

Ascending infection is the most common cause of clinical pyelonephritis. Normal human bladder and bladder urine are sterile. The first step in the pathogenesis of ascending infection appears to be the *colonization of the distal urethra and introitus* (in the female) by coliform bacteria. This colonization is influenced by the ability of bacteria to adhere to vaginal or urethral mucosal cells. Such bacterial adherence, as was discussed in Chapter 8, involves the P-fimbriae (pili) of bacteria and other adhesive molecules that interact with receptors on the surface of uroepithelial cells.

From the urethra organisms may then gain entrance into the bladder during urethral catheterization or other instrumentation. Long-term catheterization, in particular, carries a high risk of infection. In the absence of instrumentation, *urinary infections are much more common in females*, and this has been variously ascribed to the shorter urethra in females, the absence of antibacterial properties such as are found in prostatic fluid, hormonal changes affecting adherence of bacteria to the mucosa, and urethral trauma during sexual intercourse, or a combination of these factors.

Ordinarily, organisms introduced into the bladder are cleared by the continual flushing of voiding and by antibacterial mechanisms. However, outflow obstruction or bladder dysfunction results in incomplete emptying and increased residual volume of urine. In the presence of stasis, bacteria introduced into the bladder can multiply unhindered without being unceremoniously flushed or destroyed by the bladder wall. Accordingly, UTI is particularly frequent among patients with lower urinary tract obstruction, such as may occur with benign prostatic hypertrophy, tumors, or calculi.

Although obstruction is an important predisposing factor in the pathogenesis of ascending infection, *it is incompetence of the vesicoureteral orifice* that allows bacteria to ascend the ureter into the pelvis. The normal ureteral insertion into the bladder is a competent one-way valve that prevents retrograde flow of urine, especially during micturition, when the intravesical pressure rises. An incompetent vesicoureteral orifice allows the reflux of bladder urine into the ureters (*vesicoureteral reflux, VUR*) (Fig. 20–34).[56] Reflux is most often due to a congenital, inherited absence or shortening of the intravesical portion of the ureter (Fig. 20–35), such that the ureter is not compressed during micturition. In addition, bladder infection itself, probably as a result of the action of bacterial or inflammatory products on ureteral contractility, can cause or accentuate VUR, particularly in children. The effect of VUR is similar to that of an obstruction in that after voiding there is residual urine in the urinary tract, which favors bacterial growth. Furthermore, VUR affords a ready mechanism by which the infected bladder urine can be propelled up to the renal pelves and deep into the renal parenchyma through open

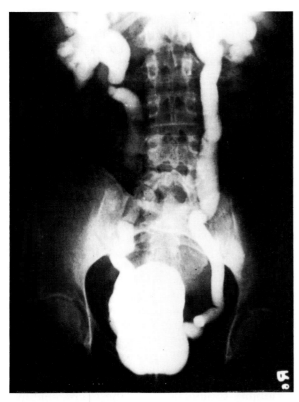

Figure 20-34. Vesicoureteral reflux demonstrated by a voiding cystourethrogram. Dye injected into bladder refluxes into both dilated ureters, filling pelvis and calyces.

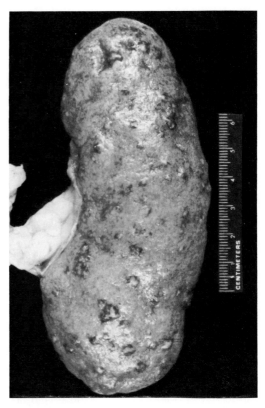

Figure 20-36. Acute pyelonephritis. Cortical surface is dotted with abscesses.

ducts at the tips of the papillae (intrarenal reflux). Intrarenal reflux is most common in the upper and lower poles of the kidney, where papillae tend to have flattened or concave tips rather than the convex pointed type present in the midzones of the kidney (and depicted in most text books). Reflux can be demonstrated radiographically by a voiding

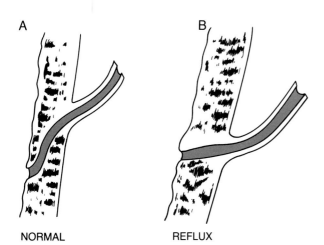

Figure 20-35. The vesicoureteric junction. In normal individuals (A), the intravesical portion of the ureter is oblique, such that the ureter is closed by muscle contraction during micturition. The most common cause of reflux is congenital complete or partial absence of intravesical ureter (B).

cystourethrogram: the bladder is filled with a radiopaque dye, and films are taken during micturition. VUR can be demonstrated in about 50% of infants and children with urinary tract infection (see Fig. 20-34).

Acute Pyelonephritis

Acute PN is an acute suppurative inflammation of the kidney caused by bacterial infection—whether hematogenous and induced by septicemic spread, or ascending and associated with VUR.

MORPHOLOGY. The hallmarks of acute PN are **patchy interstitial suppurative inflammation and tubular necrosis.** The suppuration may occur as discrete focal abscesses involving one or both kidneys, or as large, wedge-shaped areas of coalescent suppuration (Fig. 20-36). The distribution of these lesions is unpredictable and haphazard, but in PN associated with reflux, damage occurs most commonly in the lower and upper poles.

In the very early stages, the neutrophilic infiltration is limited to the interstitial tissue. Soon, however, the reaction involves tubules and produces a characteristic abscess with the destruction of the engulfed tubules (Fig. 20-37). Since the tubular lumina present a ready pathway for the extension of the infection, large masses of neutrophils frequently extend along the involved nephron into the col-

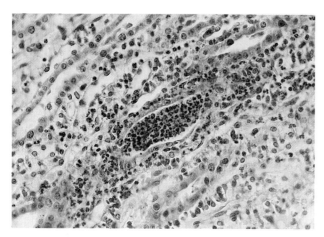

Figure 20–37. Acute pyelonephritis marked by an acute neutrophilic exudate within tubules and renal substance.

lecting tubules. Characteristically, the glomeruli appear to be resistant to the infection. Large areas of severe necrosis, however, eventually destroy the glomeruli, and fungal PN (e.g., Candida) often affects glomeruli.

Three complications of acute PN are encountered in special circumstances. **Papillary necrosis** is seen mainly in diabetics and in those with urinary tract obstruction. Papillary necrosis is usually bilateral but may be unilateral. One or all of the pyramids of the affected kidney may be involved. On cut section, the tips or distal two-thirds of the pyramids have gray-white to yellow necrosis that resembles infarction (Fig. 20–38). Microscopically, the necrotic tissue shows characteristic coagulative infarct necrosis, with preservation of outlines of tubules. The leukocytic response is limited to the junctions between preserved and destroyed tissue.

Pyonephrosis is seen when there is total or almost complete obstruction, particularly when it is high in the urinary tract. The suppurative exudate is unable to drain and thus fills the renal pelvis, calyces, and ureter, producing pyonephrosis.

Perinephric abscess implies extension of suppurative inflammation through the renal capsule into the perinephric tissue.

After the acute phase of PN, healing occurs. The neutrophilic infiltrate is replaced by one that is predominantly mononuclear with macrophages, plasma cells, and (later) lymphocytes. The inflammatory foci are eventually replaced by scars that can be seen on the cortical surface as fibrous depressions. Such scars are characterized microscopically by atrophy of tubules, interstitial fibrosis, and lymphocyte infiltrate and may resemble scars produced by ischemic or other types of injury to the kidney. **However, the pyelonephritic scar is almost always associated with inflammation, fibrosis, and deformation of the underlying calyx and pelvis,** reflecting the role of ascending infection and VUR in the pathogenesis of the disease.

CLINICAL COURSE. Acute PN is often associated with predisposing conditions, some of which were covered in the discussion of pathogenetic mechanisms. These include the following:

- *Urinary obstruction*, either congenital or acquired.
- *Instrumentation* of the urinary tract, most commonly catheterization.
- *Vesicoureteric reflux.*
- *Pregnancy.* Four to six per cent of pregnant women develop bacteriuria sometime during pregnancy, and 20 to 40% of these eventually develop symptomatic urinary infection if not treated.
- *Patient's sex and age.* After the first year of life (when congenital anomalies in males commonly become evident) and up to around age 40, infections are much more frequent in females. With increasing age, the incidence in males rises owing to the development of prostatic hypertrophy and frequent instrumentation.
- *Pre-existing renal lesions*, causing intrarenal scarring and obstruction.
- *Diabetes mellitus*, in which acute PN is caused by more frequent instrumentation, the general susceptibility to infection, and the neurogenic bladder dysfunction exhibited by patients.
- *Immunosuppression and immunodeficiency.*

When acute PN is clinically apparent, the onset is usually sudden, with pain at the costovertebral angle and systemic evidence of infection, such as fever and malaise. There are usually indications of bladder and urethral irritation, such as dysuria, frequency, and urgency. The urine contains many leukocytes (pyuria) derived from the inflammatory infiltrate, but pyuria does not differentiate upper from lower UTI. The finding of leukocyte casts (pus casts) indicates renal involvement, because casts are formed only in tubules.

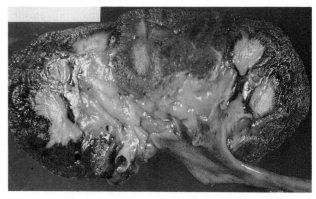

Figure 20–38. Papillary necrosis. Areas of pale gray necrosis are limited to papillae.

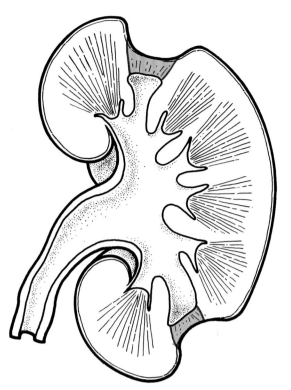

Figure 20–39. Coarse scars of chronic pyelonephritis associated with vesicoureteral reflux. The scars are usually polar and are associated with underlying blunted calyces.

The diagnosis of infection is established by quantitative urine culture.

Uncomplicated acute PN usually follows a benign course, and the symptoms disappear within a few days after the institution of appropriate antibiotic therapy. Bacteria, however, may persist in the urine, or there may be recurrence of infection with new serologic types of *E. coli* or other organisms. Such bacteriuria then either disappears or may persist sometimes for years. In the presence of unrelieved urinary obstruction, diabetes mellitus, and immunocompromise, acute PN may be more serious, leading to repeated septicemic episodes. The superimposition of papillary necrosis often leads to acute renal failure.

Chronic Pyelonephritis (CPN) and Reflux Nephropathy

CPN is a chronic tubulointerstitial renal disorder in which *chronic tubulointerstitial inflammation and renal scarring are associated with pathologic involvement of the calyces and pelvis* (Fig. 20–39). Pelvocalyceal damage is important in that virtually all the diseases listed in Table 20–9 produce chronic tubulointerstitial alterations, but except for CPN and analgesic nephropathy, none affects the calyces. CPN is an important cause of end-stage kidney disease, being found in 11 to 20% of patients in renal transplant or dialysis units.

CPN can be divided into two forms: chronic obstructive and chronic reflux–associated.

CHRONIC OBSTRUCTIVE PN. We have seen that obstruction predisposes the kidney to infection. Recurrent infections superimposed on diffuse or localized obstructive lesions lead to recurrent bouts of renal inflammation and scarring, resulting in a picture of CPN. In this condition, the effects of obstruction contribute to the parenchymal atrophy, and indeed it is sometimes difficult to differentiate the effects of bacterial infection from those of obstruction alone. The disease can be bilateral, as with obstructive anomalies of the urinary tract (e.g., posterior urethral valves), resulting in renal insufficiency unless the anomaly is corrected; or unilateral, such as occurs with calculi and unilateral obstructive anomalies of the ureter.

REFLUX NEPHROPATHY. This is by far the more common form of chronic pyelonephritic scarring. Renal involvement in reflux nephropathy occurs early in childhood, as a result of superimposition of a urinary infection on congenital VUR and intrarenal reflux, the latter conditioned by the number of potentially refluxing papillae. Reflux may be unilateral or bilateral; thus, the resultant renal damage either may cause scarring and atrophy of one kidney or may involve both and lead to chronic renal insufficiency. VUR occasionally causes renal damage in the absence of infection (sterile reflux), but only in the presence of severe obstruction.

MORPHOLOGY. The characteristic morphologic changes of CPN are seen on gross examination (see Fig. 20–39). The kidneys usually are irregularly scarred; if bilateral, the involvement is asymmetric. This contrasts with chronic glomerulonephritis, in which the kidneys are diffusely and symmetrically scarred. The hallmark of CPN is the coarse, discrete, corticomedullary scar overlying a dilated, blunted, or deformed calyx (Fig. 20–40). The scars can vary from one to several in number and may affect one or both kidneys. Most are in upper and lower poles, consistent with the frequency of reflux in these sites.

The microscopic changes involve predominantly tubules and interstitium. The tubules show atrophy in some areas and hypertrophy in others, or dilatation. Dilated tubules may be filled with colloid casts **(thyroidization).** There are varying degrees of chronic interstitial inflammation and fibrosis in the cortex and medulla. In the presence of active infection, there may be neutrophils in the interstitium and pus casts in the tubules. Arcuate and interlobular vessels disclose obliterative endarteritis in the scarred areas, and in the presence of hypertension hyaline arteriosclerosis is seen in the entire kidney. There is often fibrosis around the calyceal mucosa as well as marked chronic inflammatory infiltrate. Glomeruli may appear normal except for

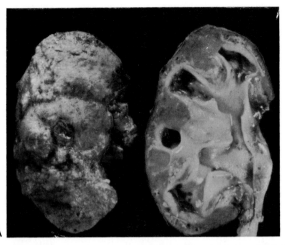
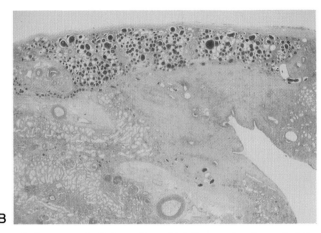

Figure 20–40. *A*, Chronic pyelonephritis. Surface *(left)* is irregularly scarred. Cut section *(right)* reveals characteristic dilatation and blunting of calyces. Ureter is dilated and thickened—a finding consistent with chronic vesicoureteral reflux. *B*, Low-power view showing corticomedullary renal scar with an underlying dilated deformed calyx. Note thyroidization of tubules in the cortex.

periglomerular fibrosis, but a variety of glomerular changes may be present, including ischemic fibrous obliteration as well as proliferation and necrosis ascribed to hypertension. Patients with CPN and reflux nephropathy who develop proteinuria in advanced stages exhibit secondary **focal segmental glomerulosclerosis,** as described later.

Xanthogranulomatous PN is an unusual and relatively rare form of CPN characterized by accumulation of foamy macrophages intermingled with plasma cells, lymphocytes, polymorphonuclear leukocytes, and occasional giant cells. Often associated with Proteus infections and obstruction, the lesions sometimes produce large, yellowish-orange nodules that may be confused with renal cell carcinoma.

CLINICAL COURSE. Chronic obstructive PN may be insidious in onset or may present the clinical manifestations of acute recurrent PN with back pain, fever, frequent pyuria, and bacteriuria. CPN associated with reflux may have a silent onset. These patients come to medical attention relatively late in the course of their disease because of the gradual onset of renal insufficiency and hypertension, or because of the discovery of pyuria or bacteriuria on routine examination. Reflux nephropathy is a common cause of hypertension in children. Loss of tubular function—in particular of concentrating ability—gives rise to polyuria and nocturia. Radiographic studies show asymmetrically contracted kidneys with characteristic coarse scars and blunting and deformity of the calyceal system. Significant bacteriuria may be present, but in the late stages it is often absent.

Although proteinuria is usually mild, some patients with pyelonephritic scars develop *focal segmental glomerulosclerosis* (FSG) with significant proteinuria, even in the nephrotic range, usually many years after the scarring has occurred and

often in the absence of continued infection or persistent VUR. The appearance of proteinuria and FSG is a poor prognostic sign, and many such patients proceed to chronic end-stage renal failure. The glomerulosclerosis is attributable to the adaptive glomerular alterations secondary to loss of renal mass caused by pyelonephritic scarring, described earlier in this chapter (renal ablation nephropathy).

Tubulointerstitial Nephritis (TIN) Induced by Drugs and Toxins

Toxins and drugs can produce renal injury in at least three ways: (1) they may trigger an interstitial immunologic reaction, exemplified by the acute hypersensitivity nephritis induced by such drugs as methicillin; (2) they may cause ARF, as described earlier; and (3) they may cause subtle but cumulative injury to tubules that takes years to become manifest, resulting in chronic renal insufficiency. The latter type of damage is especially treacherous, as it may be clinically unrecognized until significant renal damage has occurred. Such is the case with analgesic abuse nephropathy, which is usually detected only after the onset of chronic renal insufficiency.

Acute Drug-Induced Interstitial Nephritis

This is a well-recognized adverse reaction to a constantly increasing number of drugs. First reported after the use of sulfonamides, acute TIN most frequently occurs with synthetic penicillins (methicillin, ampicillin), other synthetic antibiotics (rifampin), diuretics (thiazides), nonsteroidal antiinflammatory agents (phenylbutazone), and miscellaneous drugs (phenindione, cimetidine).[57] The disease begins about 15 days (range, 2 to 40) after exposure to the drug and is characterized by *fever, eosinophilia* (which may be transient), *a skin rash*

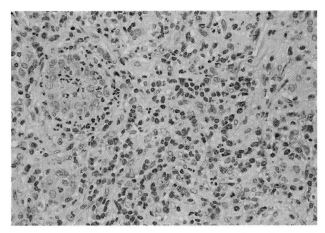

Figure 20–41. Drug-induced interstitial nephritis, with prominent eosinophilia and mononuclear infiltrate. (Courtesy of Dr. H. Rennke.)

in about 25% of patients, and *renal abnormalities.* The latter include hematuria, mild proteinuria, and leukocyturia (including eosinophils). A *rising serum creatinine level or ARF with oliguria develops in about 50% of cases,* particularly in older patients.

MORPHOLOGY. Grossly, the kidneys are usually slightly enlarged. Histologically, the abnormalities are in the interstitium, which shows pronounced edema and infiltration by mononuclear cells, principally lymphocytes and macrophages (Fig. 20–41). Eosinophils and neutrophils may be present, often in large numbers, and plasma cells and basophils are sometimes found in small numbers. With some drugs (e.g., methicillin, thiazides), interstitial granulomas with giant cells may be seen. Variable degrees of tubular necrosis and regeneration are present. The glomeruli are normal except in some cases caused by nonsteroidal anti-inflammatory agents when minimal change disease and the nephrotic syndrome develop concurrently.

PATHOGENESIS. Many features of the disease suggest an immune mechanism. Clinical evidence of hypersensitivity includes the latent period, the eosinophilia and skin rash, the fact that the onset of nephropathy is not dose related, and the recurrence of hypersensitivity following re-exposure to the same or a cross-reactive drug. IgE serum levels are increased in some patients, and IgE-containing plasma cells, and basophils, are sometimes present in the lesions, suggesting that a type I IgE-mediated late-phase response hypersensitivity may be involved in the pathogenesis (see Chapter 6). The mononuclear or granulomatous infiltrate, together with positive skin tests to drug haptens, suggests a delayed-hypersensitivity type reaction (type IV).

The most likely sequence of pathogenetic events is that the drugs act as haptens, which, during secretion by tubules, covalently bind to some cytoplasmic or extracellular component of tubular cells and become immunogenic. The resultant injury is then due to IgE and cell-mediated immune reactions to tubular cells or their basement membranes.

It is important to recognize drug-induced renal failure because withdrawal of the offending drug is followed by recovery, although it may take several months for renal function to return to normal and irreversible damage may occur occasionally in older subjects.

Analgesic Abuse Nephropathy

This is a form of chronic renal disease caused by excessive intake of analgesic mixtures and characterized morphologically by chronic tubulointerstitial nephritis with renal papillary necrosis.[58]

Analgesic nephropathy is of worldwide distribution. Its incidence reflects consumption of analgesics in various populations. In some parts of Australia and Western Europe it ranks as one of the most common causes of chronic renal insufficiency. Its incidence in the United States is relatively low but varies between states, being highest in the Southeast. The renal damage was first ascribed to phenacetin, but the analgesic mixtures consumed often contain, in addition, aspirin, caffeine, acetaminophen (a metabolite of phenacetin), and codeine. Patients who develop this disease usually ingest large quantities of analgesic mixtures (more than 2 kg of aspirin or phenacetin over 3 years). In most countries restrictions of over-the-counter sale of phenacetin or analgesic mixtures have significantly reduced the incidence of the disorder.[59]

PATHOGENESIS. Experimentally, papillary necrosis is readily induced by a mixture of aspirin and phenacetin, usually combined with water depletion. Most patients consume phenacetin-containing mixtures, and cases ascribed to ingestion of aspirin, phenacetin, or acetaminophen alone are uncommon. It is now clear that in the sequence of events leading to renal damage, *papillary necrosis occurs first, and cortical tubulointerstitial nephritis is a secondary phenomenon.* The phenacetin metabolite acetaminophen injures cells by both *covalent binding and oxidative damage.* Aspirin induces its potentiating effect by inhibiting the vasodilatory effects of prostaglandin, predisposing the papilla to ischemia. Thus, the papillary damage may be due to a combination of direct toxic effects of phenacetin metabolites as well as ischemic injury to both tubular cells and vessels.

MORPHOLOGY. Grossly, the kidneys are either normal or slightly reduced in size, and the cortex exhibits depressed and raised areas, the depressed areas representing cortical atrophy overlying necrotic papillae. The papillae show various stages of necrosis, calcification, fragmentation, and sloughing. **This gross appearance contrasts with the papillary necrosis seen in diabetic patients, in**

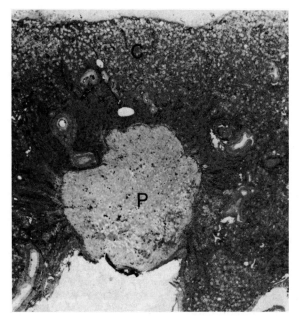

Figure 20–42. Analgesic nephropathy. Cortex (C) is scarred, and papilla (P) is transformed to a necrotic, structureless mass.

which all papillae are at the same stage of acute necrosis. Microscopically, the papillary changes may take one of several forms: in early cases there is patchy necrosis, but in the advanced form the entire papilla is necrotic, often remaining in place as a structureless mass with ghosts of tubules and foci of dystrophic calcification (Fig. 20–42). Segments of entire portions of the papilla may then be sloughed and excreted in the urine.

The cortical changes consist of loss and atrophy of these tubules, and interstitial fibrosis and inflammation. These changes are mainly due to obstructive atrophy caused by the tubular damage in the papilla, but superimposed pyelonephritic changes may be present. The cortical columns of Bertin are characteristically spared from this atrophy. The small vessels in the papilla and submucosa of the urinary tract exhibit characteristic PAS-positive basement membrane thickening (analgesic microangiopathy).

CLINICAL COURSE. Analgesic nephropathy is more common in women than in men and is particularly prevalent in individuals with recurrent headaches and muscular pain, in psychoneurotic patients, and in factory workers. Early renal findings include inability to concentrate the urine, as would be expected with lesions in the papilla. Acquired distal renal tubular acidosis contributes to the development of renal stones. Headache, anemia, gastrointestinal symptoms, and hypertension are common accompaniments of analgesic nephropathy. The anemia in particular is out of proportion to the renal insufficiency, owing to damage to red cells by the phenacetin metabolites. Urinary tract infection complicates about 50% of patients. Occasionally, entire tips of necrotic papillae are excreted, and these may cause gross hematuria or renal colic due to obstruction of the ureter by necrotic fragments. Progressive impairment of renal function may lead to chronic renal failure, but with *drug withdrawal and proper therapy for infection renal function may either stabilize or actually improve.*

Unfortunately, a serious complication sometimes occurs in patients who have survived because of their discontinuance of the offending drugs — namely, the development of *transitional papillary carcinoma of the renal pelvis.* Whether the carcinogenic effect is due to a metabolite of phenacetin or to some other component of the analgesic compounds is unsettled.

Other Tubulointerstitial Diseases

Urate Nephropathy

Three types of nephropathy can occur in patients with hyperuricemic disorders. *Acute uric acid nephropathy* is caused by the precipitation of uric acid crystals in the renal tubules, principally in collecting ducts, leading to obstruction of nephrons and the development of ARF. This type is particularly apt to occur in patients with leukemias and lymphomas who are undergoing chemotherapy; the drugs increase the destruction of neoplastic nuclei and the elaboration of uric acid. Precipitation of uric acid is favored by the acidic pH in collecting tubules.

Chronic urate nephropathy or gouty nephropathy occurs in patients with more protracted forms of hyperuricemia. The lesions are ascribed to the deposition of monosodium urate crystals in the acidic milieu of the distal tubules and collecting ducts, as well as in the interstitium. These deposits have a distinct histologic appearance, in the form of birefringent, needle-like crystals present either in the tubular lumina or in the interstitium (Fig. 20–43). The urates induce a *tophus* often surrounded by foreign body giant cells, other mononuclear cells, and a fibrotic reaction (see Chapter 27). Tubular obstruction by the urates causes cortical atrophy and scarring. Arterial and arteriolar thickening is common in these kidneys, owing to the relatively high frequency of hypertension in patients with gout. Clinically, urate nephropathy is a subtle disease associated with tubular defects that may progress slowly. Patients with gout who actually develop a chronic nephropathy commonly have evidence of increased exposure to lead, mostly by way of drinking "moonshine" whiskey contaminated with lead.

The third renal syndrome in hyperuricemia is *nephrolithiasis;* uric acid stones are present in 22%

of patients with gout and 42% of those with secondary hyperuricemia (see later discussion of renal stones).

Hypercalcemia and Nephrocalcinosis

Disorders characterized by hypercalcemia, such as hyperparathyroidism, multiple myeloma, vitamin D intoxication, metastatic bone disease, or excess calcium intake (milk-alkali syndrome), may induce the formation of calcium stones and deposition of calcium in the kidney (nephrocalcinosis). Extensive degrees of calcinosis, under certain conditions, may lead to a form of chronic tubulointerstitial disease and renal insufficiency. The first damage induced by the hypercalcemia is at the *intracellular level*, in the tubular epithelial cells, resulting in mitochondrial distortion and evidence of cell injury. Subsequently, calcium deposits can be demonstrated within the mitochondria, cytoplasm, and basement membrane. Calcified cellular debris then aids in obstruction of the tubular lumina and causes obstructive atrophy of nephrons with interstitial fibrosis and nonspecific chronic inflammation. Atrophy of entire cortical areas drained by calcified tubules may occur, and this accounts for the alternating areas of normal and scarred parenchyma seen in such kidneys.

The earliest functional defect is an inability to elaborate a concentrated urine. Other tubular defects, such as tubular acidosis and salt-losing nephritis, may also occur. With further damage, a slowly progressive renal insufficiency develops. This is usually due to nephrocalcinosis, but many of these patients also have calcium stones and secondary pyelonephritis.

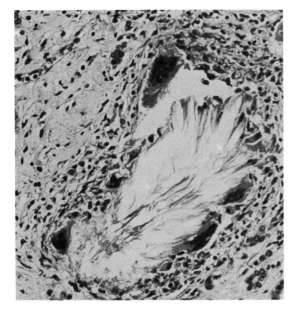

Figure 20–43. Urate crystals in renal medulla. Note inflammatory reaction with giant cells around needle-like crystals.

Table 20–10. RENAL INVOLVEMENT BY NONRENAL NEOPLASMS

1. Direct tumor invasion of renal parenchyma
   Ureters → obstruction
   Artery → renovascular hypertension
2. Hypercalcemia
3. Hyperuricemia
4. Amyloidosis
5. Excretion of abnormal proteins (multiple myeloma)
6. Radiotherapy
7. Chemotherapy
8. Infection
9. Glomerulopathy
   Immune complex GN (carcinomas)
   Lipoid nephrosis (Hodgkin's disease)

Multiple Myeloma

Nonrenal malignant tumors, particularly those of hematopoietic origin, affect the kidneys in a number of ways (Table 20–10). The most common involvements are tubulointerstitial, caused by complications of the tumor (hypercalcemia, hyperuricemia, obstruction of ureters) or therapy (irradiation, hyperuricemia, chemotherapy, infections in immunosuppressed patients). As the survival rate of patients with malignant neoplasms increases, so do these renal complications. We shall limit the discussion to the renal lesions in *multiple myeloma* that sometimes dominate the clinical picture in patients with this disease.

Renal involvement is a sometimes ominous manifestation of multiple myeloma, overt renal insufficiency occurring in half the patients with this disease.

The main cause of renal dysfunction is related to Bence Jones (light-chain) proteinuria, because renal failure correlates well with the presence and amount of such proteinuria and is extremely rare in its absence. Two mechanisms appear to account for the renal toxicity of Bence Jones proteins. First, some of these light chains appear to be directly toxic to epithelial cells; second, Bence Jones proteins combine with the urinary glycoprotein (Tamm-Horsfall protein) under acidic conditions to form large, histologically distinct tubular casts that obstruct the tubular lumina and also induce a peritubular inflammatory reaction.

Other factors that may contribute to renal failure include (1) vascular disease in the usually elderly population affected with myeloma; (2) hypercalcemia and hyperuricemia, which are often present in these patients; (3) amyloidosis, which occurs in 6 to 24% of patients with myeloma; and (4) urinary tract obstruction with secondary pyelonephritis.

MORPHOLOGY. Grossly, the kidneys usually are normal but sometimes are shrunken and pale because of extensive interstitial scarring. The most prominent changes are histologic. The tubular casts appear

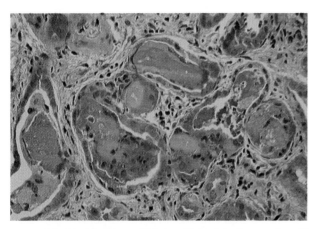

Figure 20–44. Myeloma kidney. Note tubular casts with multinucleate cells around them. (Courtesy of Dr. C. Alpers, University of Washington, Seattle.)

as pink-to-blue amorphous masses, sometimes concentrically laminated, filling and distending the tubular lumina. Some of the casts are surrounded by multinucleate giant cells, derived from either reactive tubular epithelium or mononuclear phagocytes (Fig. 20–44). The epithelium surrounding the cast is often necrotic, and the adjacent interstitial tissue usually shows a nonspecific inflammatory response. Occasionally, the casts erode their way from the tubules into the interstitium and here evoke a granulomatous inflammatory reaction.

Clinically, the renal manifestations are of several types. In the most common form, *chronic renal failure* develops insidiously and usually progresses slowly over a period of several months to years. Another form occurs suddenly and is manifested by *acute renal failure* with oliguria. Precipitating factors in these patients include dehydration, hypercalcemia, acute infection, and treatment with nephrotoxic antibiotics. *Proteinuria* occurs in 70% of patients with myeloma; the presence of significant non–light-chain proteinuria (e.g., albumin) suggests secondary amyloidosis or light-chain glomerulopathy, discussed earlier in the chapter.

DISEASES OF BLOOD VESSELS

Nearly all diseases of the kidney involve the renal blood vessels secondarily. Systemic vascular disease, such as various forms of vasculitis, also involves renal blood vessels, and often their effects on the kidney are clinically important. These were considered in Chapter 11. In this chapter, we shall discuss benign and malignant nephrosclerosis, lesions associated with hypertension, renal artery stenosis, and sundry lesions involving largely

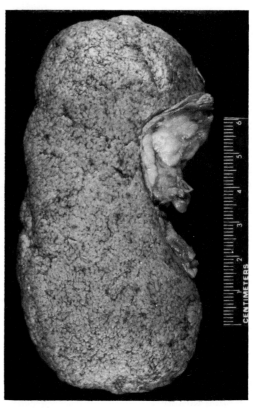

Figure 20–45. Benign nephrosclerosis illustrating fine leathery granularity of surface.

smaller vessels of the kidney. Hypertension was discussed in detail in Chapter 11.

BENIGN NEPHROSCLEROSIS

Benign nephrosclerosis (BNS), the term used for the kidney of benign hypertension, is associated with hyaline arteriolosclerosis, a lesion of arterioles described and illustrated in Chapter 11 (see Fig. 11–8). The resultant effect is focal ischemia of the renal parenchyma supplied by the thickened narrowed arteriole.

Some degree of BNS, albeit mild, is present at autopsy in many individuals over age 60. Hypertension and diabetes mellitus, however, increase the incidence and severity of the lesions in younger age groups.

MORPHOLOGY. Grossly, the kidneys are either normal in size or moderately reduced to average weights between 110 and 130 gm. The cortical surfaces have a fine, even granularity that resembles grain leather (Fig. 20–45). On section, the loss of mass is due mainly to cortical narrowing.

Histologically, there is narrowing of the lumina of arterioles and small arteries, caused by thickening and hyalinization of the walls (Fig.

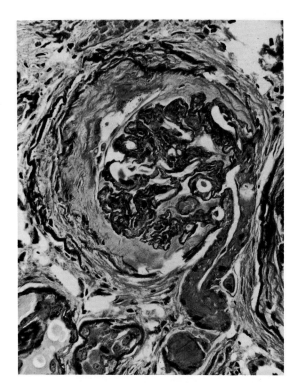

Figure 20–46. Benign nephrosclerosis—microscopic detail of a glomerulus and its afferent arteriole sectioned obliquely. The arteriole has hyaline, thickened walls, and a narrowed lumen. The glomerulus shows diffuse glomerulosclerosis and has marked fibrous thickening of the parietal layer of Bowman's capsule.

20–46). The hyaline material is composed of plasma proteins, lipids, and basement membrane material.

Consequent to the hyaline vascular narrowing, there is patchy ischemic atrophy, which consists of (1) foci of tubular atrophy and interstitial fibrosis and (2) a variety of glomerular alterations. The latter include collapse of glomerular basement membranes, deposition of collagen within Bowman's space, periglomerular fibrosis, and total sclerosis of glomeruli.

In addition to arteriolar hyalinization, the larger interlobular and arcuate arteries exhibit a characteristic lesion that consists of reduplication of the elastic lamina and increased fibrous tissue in the media, with consequent narrowing of the lumen. This change, called **fibroelastic hyperplasia,** often accompanies hyaline arteriolosclerosis and increases in severity with age and in the presence of hypertension.

Uncomplicated benign nephrosclerosis alone rarely causes renal insufficiency or uremia. There are usually moderate reductions in renal plasma flow, but the GFR is normal or slightly reduced. Occasionally, there is mild proteinuria. Patients with moderate degrees of benign nephrosclerosis appear to have lost an element of renal reserve and

Table 20–11. TYPES OF HYPERTENSION

PRIMARY OR ESSENTIAL HYPERTENSION

SECONDARY HYPERTENSION
 Renal
  Acute glomerulonephritis
  Chronic renal disease
  Renal artery stenosis
  Renal vasculitis
  Renin-producing tumors
 Endocrine
  Adrenocortical hyperfunction (Cushing's syndrome)
  Oral contraceptives
  Pheochromocytoma
  Acromegaly
  Myxedema
  Thyrotoxicosis (systolic)
 Vascular
  Coarctation of aorta
  Polyarteritis nodosa
  Aortic insufficiency (systolic)
 Neurogenic
  Psychogenic
  Increased intracranial pressure
  Polyneuritis, bulbar poliomyelitis, others

are thus more prone to developing azotemia in the face of volume depletion, surgical stress, or gastrointestinal hemorrhage. Renal failure may supervene in 5% of patients with prolonged benign hypertension, but in most patients it results from the development of the malignant or accelerated phase of hypertension, discussed next.

MALIGNANT PHASE OF HYPERTENSION (MALIGNANT NEPHROSCLEROSIS)

Malignant nephrosclerosis is the form of renal disease associated with the malignant or accelerated phase of hypertension.[60] This dramatic pattern of hypertension may occasionally develop in previously normotensive individuals but often is superimposed on pre-existing essential benign hypertension, or secondary forms of hypertension, or an underlying chronic renal disease, particularly glomerulonephritis or reflux nephropathy (Table 20–11). It is also a frequent cause of death from uremia in patients with scleroderma. Malignant hypertension is relatively uncommon, occurring in 1 to 5% of all patients with elevated blood pressure. In its pure form, it usually affects younger individuals, with a high preponderance in males and in blacks.

MORPHOLOGY. Grossly, the kidney size is dependent on the duration and severity of the hypertensive disease. Small, pinpoint petechial hemorrhages may appear on the cortical surface from rupture of arterioles or glomerular capillaries, giving the kidney a peculiar "flea-bitten" appearance.

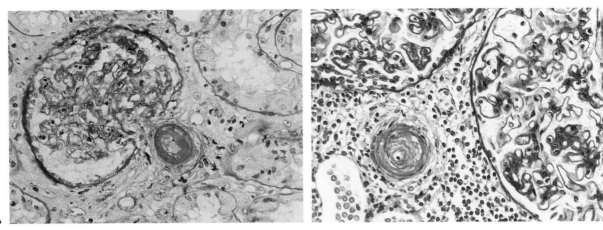

Figure 20–47. Malignant hypertension. A, Fibrinoid necrosis of afferent arteriole (PAS stain). B, Hyperplastic arteriolitis (onionskin lesion). Courtesy of Dr. Helmut Rennke, Brigham and Women's Hosptial, Boston.)

Two histologic alterations characterize blood vessels in malignant hypertension (Fig. 20–47).

1. **Fibrinoid necrosis of arterioles.** This appears as an eosinophilic granular change in the blood vessel wall, which stains positively for fibrin by histochemical or immunofluorescence techniques. In addition, there is often an inflammatory infiltrate within the wall, giving rise to the term **necrotizing arteriolitis.**

2. In the interlobular arteries and arterioles there is intimal thickening caused by a proliferation of elongated, concentrically arranged cells, smooth muscle cells, together with fine concentric layering of collagen. This alteration is known as **hyperplastic arteriolitis,** also referred to as "onionskinning." The lesion correlates well with renal failure in malignant hypertension. Sometimes the glomeruli become necrotic and infiltrated with neutrophils, and the glomerular capillaries may thrombose **(necrotizing glomerulitis).** The arteriolar and arterial lesions result in considerable narrowing of all vascular lumina, with ischemic atrophy and infarction distal to the abnormal vessels.

PATHOGENESIS. The triggers for the transition from benign to malignant hypertension are still unresolved. Malignant hypertension, however, is usually associated with remarkably high levels of renin, angiotensin, and aldosterone. Whatever the initial stimulus for the hyper-reninemia, experimental studies suggest that vasoconstriction and the severe increases in blood pressure accentuate the vascular necrosis that occurs in arterioles of the kidney and other organs. Such an increase in blood pressure causes endothelial injury, platelet thrombosis, fibroid necrosis, and intravascular coagulation; by producing ischemia, these perpetuate the vicious circle of hyper-reninemia in malignant hypertension. A variety of other vasoconstrictors (e.g., endothelin) or loss of vasodilators (e.g., nitric oxide) has also been implicated in causing the vasoconstriction and vascular damage.[60] Whatever the mechanism of malignant hypertension, the cause of the renal insufficiency is the profound ischemic change resulting from the arteriolar and arterial narrowing.

CLINICAL COURSE. The full-blown syndrome of malignant hypertension is characterized by diastolic pressures greater than 130 mm Hg, papilledema retinopathy, encephalopathy, cardiovascular abnormalities, and renal failure. Most often, the early symptoms are related to increased intracranial pressure and include headaches, nausea, vomiting, and visual impairments, particularly the development of scotomas or spots before the eyes. "Hypertensive crises" are sometimes encountered, characterized by episodes of loss of consciousness or even convulsions. At the onset of rapidly mounting blood pressure, there is marked proteinuria and microscopic or sometimes macroscopic hematuria, but no significant alteration in renal function. Soon, however, renal failure makes its appearance. The syndrome is a true medical emergency requiring the institution of aggressive and prompt antihypertensive therapy before the development of irreversible renal lesions. Before introduction of the new antihypertensive drugs, malignant hypertension was associated with a 50% mortality rate within 3 months of onset, progressing to 90% within a year. At present, however, about 75% of patients will survive 5 years, and 50% survive with precrisis renal function.

RENAL ARTERY STENOSIS

Unilateral renal artery stenosis is a relatively uncommon cause of hypertension, responsible for 2 to 5% of cases, but it is of importance because it is the most common curable form of hypertension, surgical treatment being successful in 70 to 80% of carefully selected cases in humans.[61] Furthermore, much of our knowledge of renal mechanisms in hypertension has come from studies of experimental and human renal artery stenosis.

The classic experiments of Goldblatt in 1934 showed that constriction of one renal artery in dogs results in hypertension, and that the magnitude of the effect is roughly proportional to the amount of constriction.[61a] Later experiments in rats confirmed these results, and in time it was shown that the hypertensive effect, at least initially, is due to stimulation of renin secretion by cells of the juxtaglomerular apparatus and the subsequent production of the vasoconstrictor angiotensin II. A large proportion of patients with renovascular hypertension have elevated plasma or renal vein renin levels, and almost all show a reduction of blood pressure when given competitive antagonists of angiotensin II. Further unilateral renal renin hypersecretion can be normalized after renal revascularization, in association with a decrease in blood pressure. Other factors, however, play a role in the maintenance of renovascular hypertension including *sodium retention* and, possibly, inhibition of medullary vasodepressor substances.

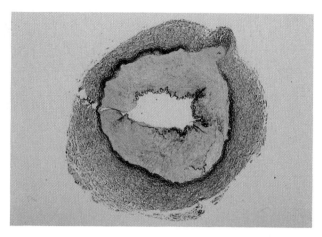

Figure 20–48. Fibromuscular dysplasia of renal artery, medial type (elastic tissue stain). Medium shows marked fibrous thickening, and lumen is stenotic. (Courtesy of Dr. Seymour Rosen, Beth Israel Hospital, Boston.)

MORPHOLOGY. The most common cause of renal artery stenosis (70% of cases) is occlusion by an atheromatous plaque at the origin of the renal artery. This lesion occurs more frequently in males, the incidence increasing with advancing age and diabetes mellitus. The plaque is usually concentrically placed, and superimposed thrombosis often occurs.

The second type of lesion leading to stenosis is so-called **fibromuscular dysplasia** of the renal artery. This is a heterogeneous group of lesions characterized by fibrous or fibromuscular thickening and may involve the initima, the media, or the adventitia of the artery. These lesions are thus subclassified into intimal, medial, and adventitial hyperplasia—the medial type being by far the most common (Fig. 20–48). The stenoses, as a whole, are more common in females and tend to occur in younger age groups (i.e., in the third and fourth decades). The lesions may consist of a single well-defined constriction or a series of narrowings, usually in the middle or distal portion of the renal artery. They may also involve the segmental branches and may be bilateral.

The ischemic kidney is usually reduced in size and shows signs of diffuse ischemic atrophy, with crowded glomeruli, atrophic tubules, interstitial fibrosis, and focal inflammatory infiltrate. The arterioles in the ischemic kidney are usually protected from the effects of high pressure, thus showing only mild arteriolosclerosis, in contrast to the contralateral nonischemic kidney, which may exhibit hyaline arteriolosclerosis, depending on the severity of the preceding hypertension.

CLINICAL COURSE. Few distinctive features suggest the presence of renal artery stenosis, and, in general, these patients resemble those presenting with essential hypertension. Occasionally, a bruit can be heard on auscultation of the kidneys. Elevated plasma or renal-vein renin, response to converting enzyme inhibitor (captopril), renal scans, and intravenous pyelography may aid with diagnosis but arteriography is required to localize the stenotic lesion. In properly selected patients, the cure rate after surgery is about 80% in fibromuscular dysplasias and 60 to 75% in atherosclerotic stenosis.

THROMBOTIC MICROANGIOPATHIES

A group of diseases with overlapping clinical manifestations are characterized morphologically by thrombosis in the interlobular arteries, afferent arterioles, and glomeruli together with necrosis and thickening of the vessel walls (Fig. 20–49), and clinically by *microangiopathic hemolytic anemia, thrombocytopenia, and renal failure.*[62] The morphologic changes are similar to those seen in malignant hypertension, but in these conditions they may precede development of hypertension or may be seen in its absence. The diseases include (1) childhood hemolytic-uremic syndrome, (2) various forms of adult hemolytic-uremic syndrome, and (3) thrombotic thrombocytopenic purpura.[63]

PATHOGENESIS. Although these disorders may have diverse causes, *endothelial injury and activation,* with intravascular thrombosis, appear to be the initiating mechanisms. The triggers for endo-

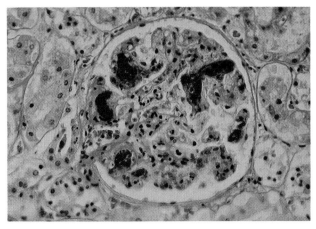

Figure 20–49. Fibrin stain showing platelet-fibrin thrombi (red) in glomerular capillaries characteristic of microangiopathic disorders.

thelial injury and activation can be bacterial endotoxins and cytotoxins, cytokines, viruses, or possibly antiendothelial antibodies, but in many cases they are unknown. Endothelial injury may mediate the microangiopathy in several ways. Endothelial denudation exposes a potentially thrombogenic subendothelial ECM. Reduced production of prostaglandin I_2 (PGI_2) and nitric oxide (both of which normally cause vasodilation and inhibit platelet aggregation) enhances platelet aggregation and vasoconstriction. Vasoconstriction can also be induced by endothelial-derived endothelin. Endothelial cells may also be *activated*, increasing their adhesivity to leukocytes, which themselves contribute to thrombosis, as described in Chapter 4. The glomerular lesions also bear a striking resemblance to those seen in the endotoxin-induced Shwartzman phenomenon.

Classic (Childhood) Hemolytic-Uremic Syndrome

This is the most well characterized of the hemolytic-uremic syndromes, since as many as 75% of cases occur in children with intestinal infection with *verocytotoxin*-producing *E. coli*. Verocytotoxins, so called because they cause damage to *vero* cells in culture, are similar to *Shiga* toxins produced by Shigella and described in detail in Chapter 8. Although relatively uncommon, epidemics traced to ingestion of infected ground meat (hamburgers) occur,[63] and the disease is one of the main causes of ARF in children. It is characterized by the *sudden onset, usually after a gastrointestinal or flu-like prodromal episode, of bleeding manifestations* (especially hematemesis and melena), *severe oliguria, hematuria, a microangiopathic hemolytic anemia, and (in some patients) prominent neurologic changes.* Hypertension is present in about half the patients.

The *pathogenesis* of this syndrome is clearly related to the Shiga-like toxin.[64] The toxin has a variety of effects on endothelium, causing increased adhesion of leukocytes, increased endothelin production and loss of endothelial nitric oxide (both favoring vasoconstriction), and in the presence of cytokines, such as TNF, it causes endothelial lysis. Indeed, Shiga toxin induces TNF synthesis in the kidney and potentiates the effects of both endotoxin and TNF. The resultant endothelial effects enhance both thrombosis and vasoconstriction, resulting in the characteristic microangiopathy. Verocytotoxin also binds to erythrocytes, activates monocytes, and affects platelet function.

MORPHOLOGY. The most important findings are in the kidney. Grossly, the kidneys may show patchy or widespread renal cortical necrosis (described later). Microscopically, the glomeruli show thickening of capillary walls, owing largely to endothelial and subendothelial swelling, and deposits of fibrin-related materials in the capillary lumina, subendothelially, and in the mesangium. Interlobular and afferent arterioles show fibrinoid necrosis and intimal hyperplasia and are often occluded by thrombi.

If the renal failure is managed properly with dialysis, most patients experience recovery in a matter of weeks. Recent studies, however, indicate that the long-term (15 to 25 years) prognosis is not uniformly favorable, as only 10 of 25 patients had normal renal function, and 7 had chronic renal failure.[65]

Adult Hemolytic-Uremic Syndrome (HUS)

A syndrome similar to that just described in children occurs in adults under a variety of settings:

1. *In association with infection,* such as typhoid fever, *E. coli* septicemia, viral infections, and shigellosis (postinfectious HUS). *Endotoxin,* or *Shiga toxin* (from Shigella species), plays a role in pathogenesis.

2. In women in relation to complications of pregnancy (placental hemorrhage) or the postpartum period. So-called *postpartum renal failure* usually occurs after an uneventful pregnancy, one day to several months following delivery, and is characterized by microangiopathic hemolytic anemia, oliguria, anuria, and initially mild hypertension. The condition has a grave prognosis, although in milder cases recovery may occur.

3. *Secondary hemolytic-uremic syndrome,* associated with vascular renal diseases such as scleroderma, SLE, and malignant hypertension or caused by chemotherapeutic and immunosuppressive drugs, such as mitomycin and cyclosporine.

4. *Hereditary hemolytic-uremic syndrome,* which also occurs in children and is characterized by recurrent attacks. The clinical and morphologic features are more or less similar to those in children.

Thrombotic Thrombocytopenic Purpura (TTP)

This entity, discussed earlier (see Chapter 12), is manifested by fever, neurologic symptoms, hemolytic anemia, thrombocytopenic purpura, and the presence of thrombi in glomerular capillaries and afferent arterioles. The disease is more common in females, and most patients are younger than 40 years of age. The entity overlaps considerably with hemolytic-uremic syndrome, and some consider both diseases part of the spectrum of the same entity. In classic TTP, however, central nervous system involvement is the dominant feature, whereas renal involvement occurs in only about 50% of patients. Histologically, eosinophilic granular thrombi are present predominantly in the terminal part of the interlobular arteries, afferent arterioles, and glomerular capillaries. The thrombi contain both platelets and fibrin and are found in arterioles of many organs throughout the body. Untreated, the disease was once highly fatal, but exchange transfusions and corticosteroid therapy have reduced mortality to less than 50%.

Other Vascular Disorders

ATHEROEMBOLIC RENAL DISEASE. Embolization of fragments of atheromatous plaques from the aorta or renal artery into intraparenchymal renal vessels occurs in elderly patients with severe atherosclerosis, especially after surgery on the abdominal aorta, aortography, or intra-aortic cannulization (Fig. 20–50). These emboli can be recognized in the walls of arcuate and interlobular arteries by their content of cholesterol crystals, which appear as rhomboid clefts. The clinical consequences of atheroemboli vary according to the number of emboli and the pre-existing state of renal function. Frequently, they have no functional significance. However, ARF may result in elderly patients in whom renal function is already compromised, principally after abdominal surgery on atherosclerotic aneurysms.

SICKLE CELL DISEASE NEPHROPATHY. Sickle cell disease in both the homozygous and the heterozygous forms may lead to a variety of alterations in renal morphology and function, some of which, fortunately uncommonly, produce clinically significant abnormalities. The various manifestations are termed "sickle cell nephropathy."

The most common clinical and functional ab-

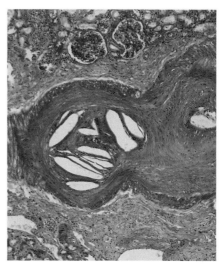

Figure 20–50. Atheroemboli with typical cholesterol clefts in interlobar artery.

normalities are *hematuria* and a *diminished concentrating ability.* These are thought to be largely due to accelerated sickling in the hypertonic hypoxic milieu of the renal medulla, which increases the viscosity of the blood during its passage through the vasa recta, leading to plugging of vessels and decreased flow. Patchy *papillary necrosis* may occur in both homozygotes and heterozygotes; this is sometimes associated with cortical scarring. *Proteinuria* is also common in sickle cell disease, occurring in about 30% of patients. It is usually mild to moderate, but on occasion the overt nephrotic syndrome arises, associated with a membranoproliferative glomerular lesion.

DIFFUSE CORTICAL NECROSIS. This is an uncommon condition that occurs most frequently following an obstetric emergency, such as abruptio placentae (premature separation of the placenta), septic shock, or extensive surgery. When bilateral and symmetric, it is uniformly fatal, but patchy cortical necrosis may permit survival. The cortical destruction has all the earmarks of ischemic necrosis. Glomerular and arteriolar microthrombi are found in some but by no means all cases; if present, they clearly contribute to the necrosis and renal damage. It is thought that the disorder results from disseminated intravascular coagulation (DIC, see Chapter 4) and vasoconstriction.

MORPHOLOGY. The gross alterations of the massive ischemic necrosis are sharply limited to the cortex (Fig. 20–51). The histologic appearance is that of acute ischemic infarction. The lesions may be patchy, with areas of apparently better preserved cortex. Intravascular and intraglomerular thromboses may be prominent but are usually focal, and occasionally acute necroses of small arterioles and capillaries may be present. Hemorrhages occur into

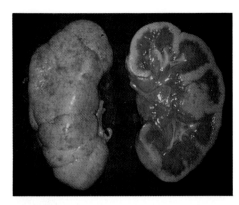

Figure 20–51. Diffuse cortical necrosis. Pale ischemic necrotic areas are confined to cortex and columns of Bertin.

the glomeruli, together with the precipitation of fibrin in the glomerular capillaries.

Massive acute cortical necrosis is of grave significance, since it gives rise to sudden anuria, terminating rapidly in uremic death. Instances of unilateral or patchy involvement are compatible with survival.

RENAL INFARCTS. The kidneys are favored sites for the development of infarcts, as one-fourth of the cardiac output passes through these organs. Although thrombosis in advanced atherosclerosis and the acute vasculitis of polyarteritis nodosa may occlude arteries, most infarcts are due to embolism. The major source of such emboli is mural thrombosis in the left atrium and ventricle as a result of myocardial infarction. Vegetative endocarditis, thrombosis in aortic aneurysms, and aortic atherosclerosis are less frequent sites for the origin of emboli.

MORPHOLOGY. Because the arterial supply to the kidney is of the "end-organ" type, most infarcts are of the "white" anemic type. They may occur as solitary lesions or may be multiple and bilateral. Within 24 hours infarcts become sharply demarcated, pale, yellow-white areas that may contain small irregular foci of hemorrhagic discoloration. They are usually ringed by a zone of intense hyperemia.

On section, they are wedge-shaped, with the base against the cortical surface and the apex pointing toward the medulla. There may be a very narrow rim of preserved subcortical tissue that has been spared by the collateral capsular circulation. In time, these acute areas of ischemic necrosis undergo progressive fibrous scarring, giving rise to depressed, **pale, gray-white scars** that assume a V shape on section. The histologic changes in renal infarction are those of ischemic coagulation necrosis, described in Chapters 1 and 4.

Many renal infarcts are clinically silent. Sometimes, pain and tenderness localized to the costovertebral angle occurs, and this is associated with showers of red cells in the urine. Large infarcts of one kidney are a well-known basis for hypertension.

URINARY TRACT OBSTRUCTION (OBSTRUCTIVE UROPATHY)

Recognition of urinary obstruction is important *because obstruction increases susceptibility to infection and to stone formation, and unrelieved obstruction almost always leads to permanent renal atrophy,* termed *hydronephrosis or obstructive uropathy.* Fortunately, many causes of obstruction are surgically correctable or medically treatable.

Obstruction may be sudden or insidious, partial or complete, unilateral or bilateral; it may occur at any level of the urinary tract from the urethra to the renal pelvis. It can be caused by lesions that are *intrinsic* to the urinary tract or *extrinsic* lesions that compress the ureter. The common causes are as follows (Fig. 20–52):

1. *Congenital anomalies.* Posterior urethral valves and urethral strictures, meatal stenosis, bladder neck obstruction; ureteropelvic junction narrowing or obstruction; severe vesicoureteral reflux

2. *Urinary calculi*

3. *Benign prostatic hypertrophy*

4. *Tumors.* Carcinoma of the prostate, bladder tumors, contiguous malignant disease (retroperitoneal lymphoma), carcinoma of the cervix or uterus

5. *Inflammation.* Prostatitis, ureteritis, urethritis, retroperitoneal fibrosis

6. *Sloughed papillae or blood clots*

7. *Normal pregnancy*

8. *Uterine prolapse and cystocele*

9. *Functional disorders.* Neurogenic (spinal cord damage) and other functional abnormalities of the ureter or bladder (often termed *dysfunctional obstruction*)

Hydronephrosis is the term used to describe dilatation of the renal pelvis and calyces associated with progressive atrophy of the kidney due to obstruction to the outflow of urine. Even with complete obstruction, glomerular filtration persists for some time because the filtrate subsequently diffuses back into the renal interstitium and perirenal spaces, where it ultimately returns to the lymphatic and venous systems. Because of this continued filtration, the affected calyces and pelvis become dilated, often markedly so. The high pressure in the pelvis is transmitted back through the collecting ducts into the cortex, causing renal atro-

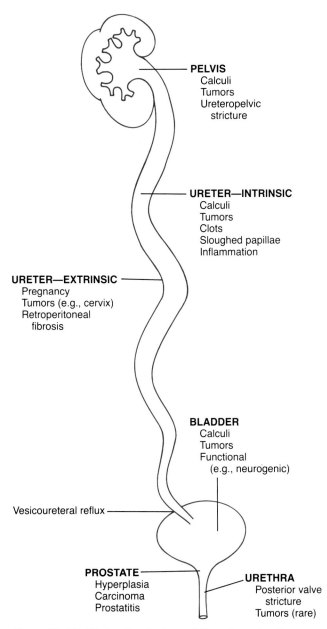

PELVIS
Calculi
Tumors
Ureteropelvic
   stricture

URETER—INTRINSIC
Calculi
Tumors
Clots
Sloughed papillae
Inflammation

URETER—EXTRINSIC
Pregnancy
Tumors (e.g., cervix)
Retroperitoneal
   fibrosis

BLADDER
Calculi
Tumors
Functional
   (e.g., neurogenic)

Vesicoureteral reflux

PROSTATE
Hyperplasia
Carcinoma
Prostatitis

URETHRA
Posterior valve
   stricture
Tumors (rare)

Figure 20–52. Obstructive lesions of the urinary tract.

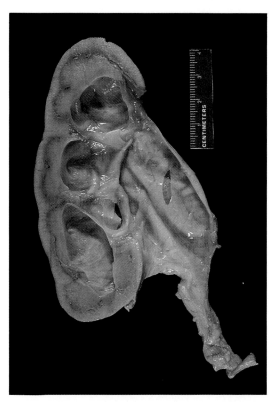

Figure 20–53. Hydronephrosis of kidney, with marked dilatation of pelvis and calyces and thinning of renal parenchyma.

phy, but it also compresses the renal vasculature of the medulla, causing a diminution in inner medullary plasma flow. The medullary vascular defects are reversible, but if protracted, obstruction will lead to medullary functional disturbances. Accordingly, the initial functional alterations are largely tubular, manifested primarily by impaired concentrating ability. Only later does the GFR begin to diminish.

MORPHOLOGY. When the obstruction is sudden and complete, the reduction of glomerular filtration usually leads to mild dilatation of the pelvis and calyces but sometimes to atrophy of the renal parenchyma. When the obstruction is subtotal or intermittent, glomerular filtration is not suppressed, and progressive dilatation ensues. Depending on the level of urinary block, the dilation may affect first the bladder or ureter and then the kidney.

Grossly, the kidney may have slight-to-massive enlargement. The earlier features are those of simple dilatation of the pelvis and calyces. Histologically, the picture is one of cortical tubular atrophy with interstitial fibrosis. Progressive blunting of the apices of the pyramids occurs, and eventually these become cupped. In far-advanced cases, the kidney may become transformed into a thin-walled cystic structure having a diameter of up to 15 to 20 cm (Fig. 20–53) with striking parenchymal atrophy, total obliteration of the pyramids, and thinning of the cortex.

CLINICAL COURSE. *Acute obstruction* may provoke pain attributed to distention of the collecting system or renal capsule. Most of the early symptoms are produced by the basic cause of the hydronephrosis. Thus, calculi lodged in the ureters may give rise to renal colic, and prostatic enlargements to bladder symptoms.

Unilateral, complete, or partial hydronephrosis may remain silent for long periods of time, since the unaffected kidney can maintain adequate renal function. Sometimes its existence first becomes apparent in the course of intravenous pyelography. It is regrettable that this disease tends to remain asymptomatic, because it has been shown that in its very early stages, perhaps the first few weeks, relief of such obstruction is compatible with reversion to normal function. *Ultrasound* is a useful noninvasive technique in the diagnosis of obstructive uropathy.

In *bilateral partial obstruction*, the earliest manifestation is that of inability to concentrate the urine, reflected by polyuria and nocturia. Some patients will have acquired distal tubular acidosis, renal salt wasting, and secondary renal calculi, *and a typical picture of tubulointerstitial nephritis* with scarring and atrophy of the papilla and medulla. Hypertension is common in such patients.

Complete bilateral obstruction results in oliguria or anuria and is incompatible with long survival unless the obstruction is relieved. Curiously, after relief of complete urinary tract obstruction, postobstructive *diuresis* occurs. This can often be massive, with the kidney excreting large amounts of urine rich in sodium chloride.

UROLITHIASIS (RENAL CALCULI, STONES)

Stones may form at any level in the urinary tract, but most arise in the kidney. Urolithiasis is a frequent clinical problem, affecting 5 to 10% of Americans in their lifetime.[67] Males are affected more often than females, and the peak age at onset is between 20 and 30 years. Familial and hereditary predisposition to stone formation has long been known. Many of the inborn errors of metabolism, such as gout, cystinuria, and primary hyperoxaluria, provide good examples of hereditary disease characterized by excessive production and excretion of stone-forming substances.

CAUSE AND PATHOGENESIS. There are four main types of calculi[67a] (Table 20–12): (1) *most stones (about 75%) are calcium-containing,* composed largely of calcium oxalate, or calcium oxalate mixed with calcium phosphate; (2) another 15% are so-called *"triple stones"* or *struvite stones,* composed of magnesium ammonium phosphate; (3) *6% are uric acid stones;* and (4) *1 to 2% are made up of cystine.* An organic matrix of mucoprotein, making up 1 to 5% of the stone by weight, is present in all calculi. Although there are many causes for the initiation and propagation of stones, *the most important determinant is an increased urinary concentration of the stones' constituents, such that it exceeds their solubility in urine (supersaturation).*[67] A *low urine volume* in some metabolically normal patients may also favor supersaturation.

Calcium oxalate stones (see Table 20–12) are associated in about 5% of patients with both *hypercalcemia* and *hypercalciuria,* occasioned by hy-

perparathyroidism, diffuse bone disease, sarcoidosis, and other hypercalcemic states. About 55% have *hypercalciuria without hypercalcemia.* This is caused by several factors, including hyperabsorption of calcium from the intestine *(absorptive hypercalciuria),* an intrinsic impairment in renal tubular reabsorption of calcium *(renal hypercalciuria),* or *idiopathic fasting hypercalciuria with normal parathyroid function.* As many as 20% are associated with increased uric acid secretion *(hyperuricosuric calcium nephrolithiasis),* with or without hypercalciuria. The mechanism of stone formation in this setting involves "nucleation" of calcium oxalate by uric acid crystals in the collecting ducts. Five per cent are associated with *hyperoxaluria,* either hereditary (primary oxaluria) or, more commonly, acquired by intestinal overabsorption in patients with enteric diseases. The latter, so-called *"enteric hyperoxaluria,"* also occurs in vegetarians, because much of their diet is rich in oxalates. *Hypocitraturia* associated with acidosis and chronic diarrhea of unknown cause may produce calcium stones. *In a variable proportion of patients with calcium stones* no cause can be found (idiopathic calcium stone disease).

Magnesium ammonium phosphate stones are formed largely following infections by urea-splitting bacteria (e.g., proteus and some staphylococci), which convert urea to ammonia. The resultant alkaline urine causes the precipitation of magnesium ammonium phosphate salts. These form some of the largest stones, as the amounts of urea excreted normally are huge. Indeed, so-called *staghorn calculi* are almost always associated with infection.

Table 20–12. TYPES OF RENAL STONES

	PERCENTAGE OF ALL STONES
Calcium Stones (Oxalate, Phosphate)	75
Hypercalcemia and hypercalciuria (5%)	
Hypercalciuria without hypercalcemia (55%)	
Absorptive	
Renal	
Idiopathic	
Hyperuricosuria (20%)	
Hyperoxaluria (5%)	
Enteric	
Primary	
Hypocitraturia	
No known metabolic abnormality	
Struvite (Mg++; NH₃; Ca++; PO₄)	10–15
Renal infection	
Uric Acid	6
Associated with hyperuricemia	
Associated with hyperuricosuria	
Idiopathic	
Cystine	1–2
Others or Unknown	±10

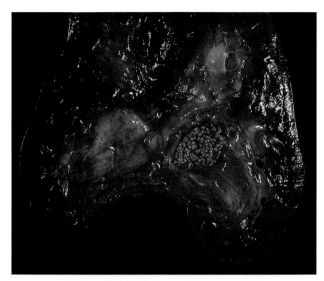

Figure 20-54. Nephrolithiasis. Large stone impacted in renal pelvis. (Courtesy of Dr. E. Mosher.)

Uric acid stones are common in patients with hyperuricemia, such as gout, and diseases involving rapid cell turnover, such as the leukemias. However, *more than half of all patients with urate calculi have neither hyperuricemia nor increased urinary excretion of uric acid.* In this group, it is thought that an unexplained tendency to excrete urine of pH below 5.5 may predispose to uric acid stones, as uric acid is insoluble in relatively acidic urine. In contrast to the radiopaque calcium stones, uric acid stones are radiolucent.

Cystine stones are associated with a genetically determined defect in the renal transport of certain amino acids, including cystine.

It can thus be appreciated that increased concentration of stone constituents, changes in urinary pH, decreased urine volume, and the presence of bacteria influence the formation of calculi. *However, many calculi occur in the absence of these factors, and conversely patients with hypercalciuria, hyperoxaluria, and hyperuricosuria often do not form stones.* It has, therefore, been postulated that stone formation is enhanced by a *deficiency in inhibitors of crystal formation in urine.* The list of such inhibitors is long, including pyrophosphate, diphosphonate, citrate, glycosaminoglycans, and a glycoprotein called *nephrocalcin.*

MORPHOLOGY. Stones are unilateral in about 80% of patients. The favored sites for their formation are within the renal calyces and pelves (Fig. 20-54) and in the bladder. If formed in the renal pelvis, they tend to remain small, having an average diameter of 2 to 3 mm. These may have smooth contours or may take the form of an irregular, jagged mass of spicules. Often, many stones are found within one kidney. Occasionally, progressive accretion of salts leads to the development of branching structures known as staghorn stones, which create a cast of the pelvic and calyceal system.

CLINICAL COURSE. Stones are of importance when they obstruct urinary flow or produce ulceration and bleeding. They may be present without producing any symptoms or significant renal damage. In general, smaller stones are most hazardous, as they may pass into the ureters, producing pain referred to as colic (one of the most intense forms of pain) as well as ureteral obstruction. Larger stones cannot enter the ureters and are more likely to remain silent within the renal pelvis. Commonly, these larger stones first manifest themselves by hematuria. Stones also predispose to superimposed infection, both by their obstructive nature and by the trauma they produce.

TUMORS OF THE KIDNEY

Both benign and malignant tumors occur in the kidney.[68] In general, the benign tumors are incidental findings at autopsy and rarely have clinical significance. Malignant tumors, on the other hand, are of great importance clinically and deserve considerable emphasis.[69] By far the most common of these malignant tumors is renal cell carcinoma, followed by Wilms' tumor, which is found in children and described in Chapter 10, and finally urothelial tumors of the calyces and pelves.

BENIGN TUMORS

CORTICAL ADENOMA. Small, discrete adenomas having origin in the renal tubules are found rather commonly (7 to 22%) at autopsy.

MORPHOLOGY. These are usually less than 2 cm in diameter. They are present invariably within the cortex and appear grossly as pale yellow-gray, discrete, seemingly encapsulated nodules. Microscopically, they are composed of complex, branching, papillomatous structures with numerous complex fronds that project into a cystic space. Cells may also grow as tubules, glands, cords, and totally undifferentiated masses of cells.

The cell type for all these growth patterns is quite regular and free of atypia. The cells are cuboidal to polygonal in shape, have regular small, central nuclei, and have a cytoplasm that may be filled with lipid vacuoles.

By histologic criteria, these tumors do not differ from renal cell adenocarcinoma. In this differential, the size of the tumor has been used as a diagnostic feature; tumors larger than 3 cm in diameter are likely to metastasize, whereas those smaller than 3 cm rarely do. This is obviously useful as a rule of thumb only, because adenocarcinomas may arise from adenomas. In addition, although most renal adenomas are incidental findings at autopsy, some of borderline size (2 to 3 cm) may be detected clinically during x-ray procedures or surgery. It seems appropriate to consider and treat those of borderline size as early cancers.

RENAL FIBROMA OR HAMARTOMA (Renomedullary Interstitial Cell Tumor). Occasionally, at autopsy, small foci of gray-white firm tissue, usually less than 1 cm in diameter, are found within the pyramids of the kidneys. Microscopic examination of these discloses fibroblast-like cells and collagenous tissue. Ultrastructurally, the cells have features of renal interstitial cells. The tumors have no malignant propensities.

ANGIOMYOLIPOMA. This is a benign tumor consisting of vessels, smooth muscle, and fat. *Angiomyolipomas are present in 25 to 50% of patients with tuberous sclerosis,* a disease characterized by lesions of the cerebral cortex that produce epilepsy and mental retardation, as well as a variety of skin abnormalities.

ONCOCYTOMA. This is an epithelial tumor composed of large, eosinophilic cells having small, rounded, benign-appearing nuclei. Ultrastructurally, the cells have numerous prominent mitochondria. Grossly the tumors are tan colored and relatively homogeneous. The tumors are usually well encapsulated. However, they may achieve a large size (up to 12 cm in diameter). The tumors have been divided histologically into three grades: grade 1 tumors, which represent the majority, are always benign and never metastasize. Higher grades can metastasize in a small percentage of cases.[70]

MALIGNANT TUMORS

Renal Cell Carcinoma (Hypernephroma, Adenocarcinoma of Kidney)

Renal cell carcinomas represent about 1 to 3% of all visceral cancers and account for 85 to 90% of all renal cancers in adults. They occur most often in older individuals, usually in the sixth and seventh decades of life, showing a male preponderance in the ratio of 3:1. Because of their gross yellow color and the resemblance of the tumor cells to clear cells of the adrenal cortex, they are also called *hypernephroma.* It is now clear that these tumors arise from tubular epithelium and are therefore renal adenocarcinomas.

Epidemiologic studies show a greater frequency of adenocarcinoma of the kidney in ciga-

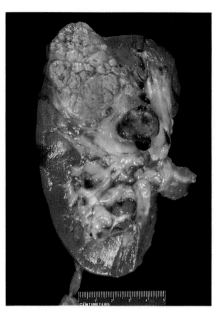

Figure 20–55. Renal cell carcinoma. Typical cross-section of yellowish, spherical neoplasm in one pole of kidney. Note tumor in dilated thrombosed renal vein.

rette, pipe, and cigar smokers. Genetic factors also play a role.[71] Nearly two-thirds of patients with the von Hippel-Lindau syndrome (VHL), characterized by hemangioblastomas of the central nervous system and retina (see Chapter 29), develop bilateral, often multiple renal cell carcinomas. The tumor suppressor gene for VHL is on the short arm of chromosome 3 (3p25-26) and encodes a protein that is involved in signal transduction or cell adhesion.[72] 3:8 and 3:11 translocations are also often found in familial cases of nonpapillary renal cell carcinoma, and mutations and deletions have been reported in sporadic cases. *Current studies thus implicate the VHL gene, or a gene related to VHL on chromosome 3, in renal carcinogenesis.* Other chromosomal abnormalities are seen in papillary cancers.

MORPHOLOGY. In its macroscopic appearance, the tumor is quite characteristic. It may arise in any portion of the kidney, but more commonly it affects the poles, particularly the upper one. Usually these neoplasms occur as solitary unilateral lesions. They are spherical masses, 3 to 15 cm in diameter, composed of bright yellow–gray-white tissue that distorts the renal outline. Commonly there are large areas of ischemic, opaque, gray-white necrosis, foci of hemorrhagic discoloration, and areas of softening. The margins are usually sharply defined and confined within the renal capsule (Fig. 20–55). However, small satellite nodules are often found in the surrounding substance, providing clear evidence of the aggressiveness of these lesions. As the tumor enlarges, it may bulge into the calyces and pelvis and eventually may fungate through

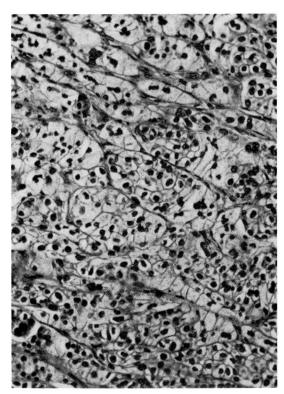

Figure 20-56. Renal cell carcinoma. Characteristic clear cell type.

the walls of the collecting system to extend even into the ureter. One of the striking characteristics of this tumor is its tendency to invade the renal vein (Fig. 20–56) and grow as a solid column of cells within this vessel. Further extension produces a continuous cord of tumor in the inferior vena cava and even in the right side of the heart.

Histologically, the growth pattern varies from papillary to solid, trabecular (cord-like), or tubular (resembling tubules). In any single tumor, all variations in patterns of growth may be present. The most common tumor cell type (70% of cases) is the **clear cell,** having a rounded or polygonal shape and abundant clear cytoplasm (see Fig. 20–56); the latter on special stains contains glycogen and lipids. Fifteen per cent are **papillary**, composed of either clear cells or **granular cells** (granular cell renal carcinoma). The latter have a moderately eosinophilic cytoplasm, grow in **sarcomatoid** pattern, and have a decidedly worse prognosis. Most tumors are well differentiated (grades I and II), but some (grade IV) show marked nuclear atypia with formation of bizarre nuclei and giant cells. The stroma is usually scanty but highly vascularized.

CLINICAL COURSE. The three classic diagnostic features of *costovertebral pain, palpable mass,* and *hematuria* unfortunately appear in only 10% of cases. The most reliable of the three is hematuria, which eventually appears in about 90% of cases. However, the hematuria is usually intermittent and may be microscopic; thus, the tumor may remain silent until it attains a large size. At this time, it gives rise to generalized constitutional symptoms, such as fever, malaise, weakness, and weight loss. This pattern of asymptomatic growth occurs in many patients, so that the tumor may have reached a diameter of more than 10 cm when it is discovered.

Renal cell carcinoma is classified as one of the great "mimics" in medicine, because it tends to produce a diversity of systemic symptoms not related to the kidney. In addition to the fever and constitutional symptoms mentioned earlier, renal cell carcinomas produce a number of paraneoplastic syndromes (see Chapter 7), ascribed to abnormal hormone production, including *polycythemia, hypercalcemia, hypertension, hepatic dysfunction, feminization or masculinization, Cushing's syndrome, eosinophilia, leukemoid reactions, and amyloidosis.*

One of the common characteristics of this tumor is its *tendency to metastasize widely before giving rise to any local symptoms or signs.* In 25% of new patients with renal cell carcinoma, there is radiologic evidence of metastases at presentation. The most common locations of metastasis are the lungs (over 50%) and bones (33%), followed in order by the regional lymph nodes, liver and adrenals, and brain. In 10 to 15% of cases, the primary tumor metastasizes across the midline to the opposite kidney.

It is essential that renal cell carcinomas be diagnosed at the earliest possible stage, which is usually accomplished during the investigation of hematuria in a middle-aged or an elderly patient. Renal ultrasonography, nephrotomography, computed tomography scanning, and intravenous pyelography aid in the differential diagnosis of a simple cyst from a tumor. Urinary cytology may also be helpful in identifying tumor cells.

The average 5-year survival of patients with renal cell carcinoma is about 45%, and up to 70% in the absence of distant metastases. With renal vein invasion or extension into the perinephric fat, the figure is reduced to approximately 15 to 20%. Nephrectomy is the treatment of choice.

Urothelial Carcinomas of Renal Pelvis

Approximately 5 to 10% of primary renal tumors occur in the renal pelvis (Fig. 20–57). These tumors span the range from apparently benign papillomas to frank papillary carcinomas, but, as with bladder tumors, the benign papillomas are difficult to differentiate from the low-grade papillary cancers.

Renal pelvic tumors usually become clinically

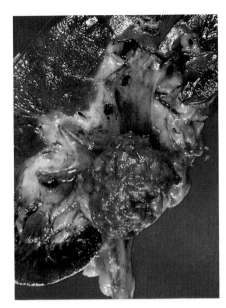

Figure 20–57. Urothelial carcinoma of renal pelvis. Pelvis has been opened to expose nodular irregular neoplasm, just proximal to the ureter.

apparent within a relatively short time because they lie within the pelvis and, by fragmentation, produce noticeable hematuria. They are almost invariably small when discovered. These tumors are almost never palpable clinically; however, they may block the urinary outflow and lead to palpable hydronephrosis and flank pain. Histologically, pelvic tumors are the exact counterpart of those found in the urinary bladder; for further details, reference should be made to that section.

Occasionally, urothelial tumors may be multiple, involving the pelvis, ureters, and bladder. In 50% of renal pelvic tumors there is a pre-existing or concomitant bladder urothelial tumor. Histologically, there are also foci of atypia or carcinoma in situ in grossly normal urothelium remote from the pelvic tumor. Although these facts point to a generalized "field" effect, caused by a carcinogenic influence on urothelium, recent evidence indicates that such multiple tumors have identical mutations in the p53 suppressor gene, suggesting seeding from a single progenitor focus.[73] There is a strikingly increased incidence of urothelial carcinomas of the renal pelvis and bladder in patients with analgesic nephropathy.

Infiltration of the wall of the pelvis and calyces is common, and renal vein involvement likewise occurs. For this reason, despite their apparently small, deceptively benign appearance, the prognosis for these tumors is not good. Five-year survival rates vary from 50 to 70% for low-grade superficial lesions to 10% with high-grade infiltrating tumors.

1. Dinesen, I.: Seven Gothic Tales. New York, Modern Library, 1939.
2. Kanwar, Y.S., and Venkatachalam, M.A.: Morphology of the glomerulus and juxtaglomerular apparatus. *In* Handbook of Physiology, Section of Renal Physiology, 2nd ed. Washington, DC, American Physiological Society, 1990.
3. Farquhar, M.G.: The glomerular basement membrane: A selective macromolecular filter. *In* Hay, E.D. (ed.): Cell Biology of the Extracellular Matrix, 2nd ed. New York, Plenum Press, 1991, pp. 365–412.
4. Hudson, B.G., Reeders, S.T., and Tryggvason, K., et al.: Structure, gene organization and role in human diseases of type IV collagen. J. Biol. Chem. *268*:1, 1993.
5. Heptinstall, R.H.: Pathology of the Kidney, 4th ed. Boston, Little, Brown & Co., 1992.
6. Tisher, C., and Brenner, B.M.: Renal Pathology, with Clinical and Pathological Correlations, 2nd ed. Philadelphia, J.B. Lippincott, 1994.
7. Brenner, B.M., et al. (eds.): Clinical Nephrology. Philadelphia, W.B. Saunders Co., 1987.
8. Schrier, R.W., and Gottschalk, C.W. (eds.): Diseases of the Kidney, 5th ed. Boston, Little, Brown & Co., 1993.
9. Brenner, B.M., and Rector, F. (eds.): The Kidney, 5th ed. Philadelphia, W.B. Saunders Co., 1994.
10. Gardner, K.D., Jr., and Bernstein, J.: The Cystic Kidney. Dordrecht, Kluwer Academic Publishers, 1990.
11. Gabow, P.A.: Autosomal dominant polycystic kidney disease. N. Engl. J. Med. *329*:332, 1993.
12. Grantham, J.J.: Fluid secretion, cellular proliferation, and the pathogenesis of renal epithelial cysts. J. Am. Soc. Nephrol. *3*:1843, 1993.
13. Calvet, J.P.: Polycystic kidney disease: Primary extracellular matrix abnormality or defective cellular differentiation. Kidney Int. *43*:101, 1993.
14. Reeders, S.T., et al.: Recent advances in the genetics of renal cystic disease. Mol. Biol. Med. *6*:81, 1989.
15. Parfrey, P.S., et al.: The diagnosis and prognosis of autosomal dominant polycystic kidney disease. N. Engl. J. Med. *323*:1085, 1990.
16. Atkins, R.C.: Pathogenesis of glomerulonephritis. *In* Nephrology, Vol. I. Proceedings of the Xth International Congress of Nephrology, Springer-Verlag, 1991.
17. Couser, W.G.: Pathogenesis of glomerulonephritis. Kidney Int. *44*:S19, 1993.
18. McCluskey, R.T.: Immunologic aspects of renal disease. *In* Heptinstall, R.H. (ed.): Pathology of the Kidney, 4th ed. Boston, Little, Brown & Co., 1992, pp. 169–260.
19. Kerjaschki, D.: Molecular pathogenesis of membranous nephropathy. Kidney Int. *41*:1090, 1992.
20. Andres, G., et al.: Formation of immune deposits and disease. Lab. Invest. *55*:550, 1989.
21. Couser, W.G.: Mediation of immune glomerular injury. J. Am. Soc. Nephrol. *1*:13, 1990.
21a. Schena, F.P., et al. (eds.): Molecular approaches to clinical nephrology. Kidney Int. *43*(Suppl. 39):S1, 1993.
22. Johnson, R.J., et al.: Role of platelet-derived growth factor in glomerular disease. J. Am. Soc. Nephrol. *4*:119, 1993.
23. Border, W.A., and Noble, N.A.: From serum sickness to cytokines: Advances in understanding the molecular pathogenesis of kidney disease. Lab. Invest. *68*:125, 1993.
23a. Yamamoto, T., et al.: Sustained expression of TGF-β1 underlies development of progressive kidney fibrosis. Kidney Int. *45*:916, 1994.
24. Rennke, H.G., et al.: The progression of renal disease: Structural and functional correlations. *In* Tisher, C.C., and Brenner, B. (eds.): Renal Pathology, 2nd ed. Philadelphia, J.B. Lippincott, 1994, pp. 116–139.
25. Rodriguez-Iturbe, J.: Acute post-streptococcal glomerulonephritis. *In* Schrier, R.W., and Gottschalk, C.W. (eds.): Diseases of the Kidney, 5th ed. Boston, Little, Brown & Co., 1993, pp. 1715–1730.
26. Couser, W.G.: Rapidly progressive glomerulonephritis. Am. J. Kidney Dis. *11*:449, 1988.
27. Jennette, J.C.: Pathogenic potential of anti-neutrophil cytoplasmic antibodies. Lab. Invest *70*:135, 1994.

27a. Wheeler, D.C., et al.: Lipid abnormalities in the nephrotic syndrome. Am. J. Kidney Dis. *23*:331, 1994.

28. Rosen, S., et al.: Membranous glomerulonephritis. *In* Tisher, C. and Brenner, B. (eds.): Renal Pathology, 2nd ed. Philadelphia, J.B. Lippincott, 1993, pp. 258–293.

29. Savin, V.: Mechanisms of proteinuria in noninflammatory glomerular diseases. Am. J. Kidney Dis. *21*:347, 1993.

30. Dantal, J., et al.: Effect of plasma protein absorption on protein excretion in kidney transplant recipients with recurrent nephrotic syndrome. N. Engl. J. Med. *330*:7, 1994.

30a. Ritz, E.: Pathogenesis of idiopathic nephrotic syndrome. N. Engl. J. Med. *330*:61, 1994.

31. Bourgoigne, E.T., et al.: The nephropathy related to acquired immune deficiency syndrome. Adv. Nephrol. *17*:113, 1988.

32. Kimmel, P.L., et al.: Viral DNA in renal biopsy tissue from HIV-infected patients with nephrotic syndrome. Kidney Int. *43*:1347, 1993.

33. White, R.H.: Mesangiocapillary glomerulonephritis. *In* Edelman, C.M., Jr. (ed.): Pediatric Kidney. Boston, Little, Brown & Co., 1992, pp. 1307–1324.

34. Johnson, R.J., et al.: Membranoproliferative glomerulonephritis associated with hepatitis C virus infection. N. Engl. J. Med. *328*:465, 1993.

35. Emancipator, S.N.: Primary and secondary forms of IgA nephritis. *In* Heptinstall, R.H. (ed.): Pathology of the Kidney, 4th ed. Boston, Little, Brown & Co., 1992, pp. 389–476.

36. van den Wall Bake, A.W.L., et al.: Shared idiotypes in mesangial deposits in IgA nephropathy are not disease-specific. Kidney Int. *44*:65, 1993.

37. van den Wall Bake, A.W.L.: Mechanisms of IgA deposition in the mesangium. Contrib. Nephrol. *104*:138, 1993.

38. Cameron, S.J.: The long-term outcome of glomerular diseases. *In* Schrier, R.W., and Gottschalk, C.W. (eds.): Diseases of the Kidney, 5th ed. Boston, Little, Brown & Co., 1993, pp. 1895–1958.

39. Schwartz, M.M.: The renal biopsy in lupus nephritis: Lessons from clinicopathological studies. Adv. Pathol. Lab. Med. *6*:423, 1993.

40. Mauer, M., et al.: Diabetic glomerulosclerosis. *In* Schrier, R.W., and Gottschalk, C.W. (eds.): Diseases of the Kidney, 5th ed. Boston, Little, Brown & Co., 1993, pp. 2153–2189.

41. Osterby, R., and Gundersen, H.G.: Glomerular size and structure in diabetes mellitus. Diabetologia *11*:225, 1975.

42. Vlassara, H., et al.: Pathogenic effects of advanced glycosylation: Biochemical, biological, and clinical implications for aging and diabetes. Lab. Invest. (in press).

43. Hostetter, T.H.: Mechanisms of diabetic nephropathy. Am. J. Kidney Dis. *23*:188, 1994.

44. Gambara, V., et al.: Heterogeneous nature of renal lesions in type II diabetes. J. Am. Soc. Nephrol. *3*:1458, 1993.

45. The Diabetes Control and Complications Trial Research Group: The effect of intensive treatment of diabetes on the development and progression of long-term complications in insulin-dependent diabetes mellitus. N. Engl. J. Med. *329*:977, 1993.

46. Lewis, E., et al.: The effect of angiotensin-converting-enzyme inhibition on diabetic nephropathy. N. Engl. J. Med. *329*:1456, 1993.

47. Grunfeld, J.P.: The clinical spectrum of hereditary nephritis. Kidney Int. *27*:83, 1985.

48. Tryggvason, K., et al.: Molecular genetics of Alport's syndrome. Kidney Int. *43*:38, 1993.

49. Savage, C.O.S., et al.: The Goodpasture's antigen in Alport's syndrome: Studies with monoclonal antibodies. Kidney Int. *30*:107, 1986.

50. Zhou, J., et al.: Deletion of the paired $\alpha5(IV)$ and $\alpha6(IV)$ collagen genes in inherited smooth muscle tumors. Science *261*:1167, 1993.

51. Bonventre, J.: Mechanisms of ischemic renal failure. Kidney Int. *43*:1160, 1993.

52. Brezis, M., and Epstein, F.H.: Cellular mechanisms of acute ischemic injury to the kidney. Annu. Rev. Med. *44*:27, 1993.

53. Oliver, J., et al.: The pathogenesis of acute renal failure associated with traumatic and toxic injury, renal ischemia, nephrotoxic damage, and the ischemic episode. J. Clin. Invest. *30*:1307, 1951.

54. Cotran, R.S., et al.: Tubulointerstitial diseases. *In* Brenner, B.M., and Rector, F. (eds.): The Kidney, 3rd ed. Philadelphia, W.B. Saunders Co., 1986, pp. 1143–1173.

55. Rubin, R.H., et al.: Urinary tract infection, pyelonephritis, and reflux nephropathy. *In* Brenner, B.M., and Rector, F.C. (eds.): The Kidney, 4th ed. Philadelphia, W.B. Saunders Co., 1991, pp. 1369–1429.

56. Bailey, R.R.: Vesicoureteric reflux and reflux nephropathy. Kidney Int. *44*:S80, 1993.

57. Buysen, J.G., et al.: Acute interstitial nephritis. Nephrol. Dial. Transplant. *5*:94, 1990.

58. Kincaid Smith, P., and Nanra, R.S.: Lithium-induced and analgesic-induced renal disease. *In* Schrier, R.W., and Gottschalk, C.W. (eds.): Diseases of the Kidney, 5th ed. Boston, Little, Brown & Co., 1993, pp. 1099–1130.

59. Nanra, R.S.: Analgesic nephropathy in the 1990's. Kidney Int. *44*:580, 1993.

60. Kincaid-Smith, P.: Malignant hypertension. J. Hypertension *9*:893, 1991.

61. Working Group on Renovascular Hypertension: Detection, evaluation, and treatment. Ann. Intern. Med. *147*:820, 1987.

61a. Goldblatt, H., et al.: Studies on experimental hypertension: I. Production of persistent elevation of systolic blood pressure by means of renal ischemia. J. Exp. Med. *59*:347, 1934.

62. Sommerfeld, D.L., et al.: Thrombotic microangiopathy. J. Am. Soc. Nephrol. *3*:35, 1992.

63. Ruggenenti, P., and Remuzzi, G.: Thrombotic microangiopathies. Crit. Rev. Oncol. Hematol. *11*:243, 1991.

64. Ashkenazi, S.: Role of bacterial cytotoxins in HUS and TTP. Annu. Rev. Med. *44*:11, 1993.

65. Gagnuandou, M.F., et al.: Long-term (15–25 years) prognosis of hemolytic-uremic syndrome. J. Am. Soc. Nephrol. *4*:275, 1993.

65a. Harel, Y., et al.: Renal specific induction of TNF by Shiga-like toxin. J. Clin. Invest. *92*:2110, 1993.

66. Falk, R., et al.: Prevalence and pathologic features of the sickle cell nephropathy and response to inhibition of angiotensin-converting enzyme. N. Engl. J. Med. *326*:910, 1992.

67. Pak, C.T.: Urolithiasis. *In* Schrier, R.W., and Gottschalk, C.W. (eds.): Diseases of the Kidney, 5th ed. Boston, Little, Brown & Co., 1993, pp. 729–743.

67a. Coe, F.L., et al.: The pathogenesis and treatment of kidney stones. N. Engl. J. Med. *327*:1141, 1993.

68. Brodsky, G.L., and Garnick, M.B.: Neoplasms in the adult kidney. *In* Tisher, C.C., and Brenner, B.M. (eds.): Renal Pathology, 2nd ed. Philadelphia, J.B. Lippincott Co. 1994, pp. 1540–1581.

69. Murphy, W.M., et al.: Tumors of the urinary bladder, urethra, ureters, renal pelves, and kidneys. *In* Armed Forces Institute of Pathology, Atlas of Tumor Pathology, 1994 (in press).

70. Morra, M.N., and Das, S.: Renal oncocytoma: A review of histogenesis, histopathology, diagnosis, and treatment. J. Urol. *150*:295, 1993.

71. Bane, B.C.: Renal cell carcinoma and other renal epithelial neoplasms: A cytogenetic and molecular update. Adv. Path. Lab. Med. *5*:419, 1992.

72. Latif, F.: Identification of the von Hippel–Lindau disease tumor suppressor gene. Science *260*:1317, 1993.

73. Habuchi, T., et al.: Metachronous multifocal development of urothelial cancers by intraluminal seeding. Lancet *342*:1087, 1993.

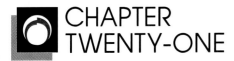
The Lower Urinary Tract

NORMAL STRUCTURE OF THE LOWER URINARY TRACT

Despite differing embryonic origins the various components of the lower urinary tract come to have many morphologic similarities. The renal pelves, ureters, bladder, and urethra (save for its terminal portion) are lined by a transitional epithelium (urothelium) that is two to three cells thick in the pelvis, three to five cells thick in the ureters, and five to seven cells thick in the bladder. These details come to have importance, since the number of layers increases when epithelial hyperplasia arises in inflammatory, preneoplastic, or neoplastic states. The surface layer consists of large, flattened "umbrella cells" that cover several underlying cells. Toward the basal layer the cells become smaller, or more cylindrical (particularly in contracted bladders), but are capable of some flattening when the underlying wall is stretched. This epithelium rests on a well-developed basement membrane, beneath which there is a lamina propria in the ureters, bladder, and urethra that sometimes contains a muscularis mucosae in the bladder. A well-developed musculature is present in the ureters and bladders that is capable, with obstruction to the flow of urine, of great thickening. The normal epithelial cells express surface blood group antigens (A, B, H) and epidermal growth factor receptors.

Several variants of the normal epithelial pattern may be encountered. Nests of urothelium or inbudding of the surface epithelium may be found occasionally in the mucosa lamina propria; these are sometimes referred to as *Brunn's nests*. Similarly, small cystic inclusions lined by cuboidal or columnar epithelium are sometimes found in the lamina propria.

Several points about the gross anatomy of these structures may come to have clinical significance. The ureters lie throughout their course in a retroperitoneal position. Retroperitoneal tumors or fibrosis may trap the ureters in neoplastic or dense, fibrous tissue, sometimes obstructing them. As ureters enter the pelvis, they pass anterior to either the common iliac or the external iliac artery. In the female pelvis, they lie close to the uterine arteries and are therefore vulnerable to injury in operations on the female genital tract. There are three points of slight narrowing: at the ureteropelvic junction, where they enter the bladder, and where they cross the iliac vessels, all providing loci where renal calculi may become impacted when they pass from the kidney to the bladder. As the ureters enter the bladder, they pursue an oblique course, terminating in a slit-like orifice. The obliquity of this intramural segment of the ureteral orifice permits the enclosing bladder musculature to act like a sphincteric valve, blocking the upward reflux of urine even in the presence of marked distention of the urinary bladder. As discussed in Chapter 20, a defect in the intravesical portion of the ureter leads to vesicoureteral reflux. The orifices of the ureters and urethra demarcate an area at the base of the bladder known as the trigone.

The bladder is almost entirely an extraperitoneal structure situated deep within the pelvis. It is in contact with the peritoneal cavity only in its most superior anterior aspect, where the peritoneum reflects from the anterior abdominal wall over the dome of the bladder. The close relationship of the female genital tract to the bladder is of considerable significance. It makes possible the spread of disease from one tract to the other. In middle-aged and elderly females, relaxation of pelvic support leads to prolapse (descent) of the uterus, pulling with it the floor of the bladder. In this fashion, the bladder is protruded into the vagina, creating a pouch—*cystocele*—that fails to empty readily with micturition. In the male, the seminal vesicles and prostate have similar close relationships, being situated just posterior and inferior to the neck of the bladder. Thus, enlargement of the prostate, so common in middle to later life, constitutes an important cause of urinary tract obstruction.

Ureters

As a generalization, the processes in which the ureters become involved are most commonly primary in the kidney or the bladder. Ureteral involvement, then, is usually overshadowed clinically and anatomically by the underlying disorders in these structures. Here we shall describe certain congenital anomalies, inflammations, and obstructive lesions.

CONGENITAL ANOMALIES

Congenital anomalies of the ureters occur in about 2 or 3% of all autopsies. They are, for the most part, of only incidental interest and have little clinical significance. Rarely, certain anomalies may contribute to obstruction to the flow of urine and thus cause clinical disease. Anomalies of the ureterovesical junction, potentiating reflux, are discussed with pyelonephritis in Chapter 20.

Double and bifid ureters. Double ureters (derived from a double or split ureteral bud) are almost invariably associated either with totally distinct double renal pelves or with the anomalous development of a very large kidney, having a partially bifid pelvis terminating in separate ureters. Double ureters may pursue separate courses to the bladder but commonly are joined within the bladder wall and drain through a single ureteral orifice.

Ureteropelvic junction obstruction (UPJ), a congenital disorder, results in hydronephrosis. It usually presents in male infants, more commonly in the left ureter, but it can be bilateral in 20% of cases and can affect female adults. It has been ascribed to abnormal organization of smooth muscle bundles at the UPJ, excess stromal deposition of collagen between smooth muscle bundles, or (very rarely) extrinsic compression by aberrant renal vessels. For unknown reasons, there is agenesis of the kidney on the opposite side in a significant number of cases.

Diverticula, saccular outpouchings of the ureteral wall, are uncommon lesions. They appear as congenital or acquired defects and are of importance as pockets of stasis and secondary infections. Dilatation, elongation, and tortuosity of the ureters *(hydroureter)* may occur as congenital anomalies or as acquired defects. Congenital hydroureter is thought to reflect some neurogenic defect in the innervation of the ureteral musculature. Massive enlargement of the ureter is known as *megaloureter* and is probably due to a functional defect of ureteral muscle. These anomalies are sometimes associated with some congenital defect of the kidney.

INFLAMMATION

Ureteritis may develop as one component of urinary tract infections. The morphologic changes are entirely nonspecific. Only infrequently does such ureteritis make a significant contribution to the clinical problem.

Persistence of infection or repeated acute exacerbations may give rise to chronic inflammatory changes within the ureters.

> **MORPHOLOGY.** In certain cases of long-standing chronic ureteritis, specialized reaction patterns are sometimes observed. The accumulation or aggregation of lymphocytes in the subepithelial region may cause slight elevations of the mucosa and produce a fine granular mucosal surface **(ureteritis follicularis).** At other times, the mucosa may become sprinkled with fine cysts varying in diameter from 1 to 5 mm **(ureteritis cystica).** These changes are also found in the bladder (they will receive fuller description later, in the section on urinary bladder). The cysts may aggregate to form small, grape-like clusters (Fig. 21–1). Histologic sections through such cysts demonstrate a lining of modified transitional epithelium with some flattening of the superficial layer of cells.

TUMORS AND TUMOR-LIKE LESIONS

Primary neoplasia of the ureter is very rare, metastatic seeding from other primary lesions occurring much more often than primary growths.

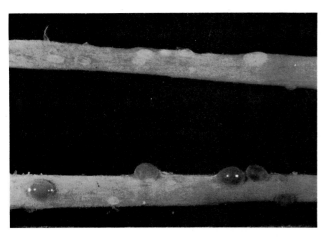

Figure 21–1. Opened ureters showing ureteritis cystica. Note smooth cysts projecting from the mucosa.

Small *benign tumors* of the ureter are generally of mesenchymal origin. They include the usual variety of neoplasms derived from fibrous tissue, blood vessels, lymphatics, and smooth muscle. These appear as well-encapsulated, submucosal nodules less than 1 cm in diameter, which are rarely of sufficient size to cause obstruction of the ureteral lumen. The *fibroepithelial polyp* is a curious tumor-like lesion that grossly presents as a small mass projecting into the lumen. The lesion occurs more commonly in the ureters (left more often than right) but may also appear in the bladder, renal pelves, and urethra. The polyp presents as a loose, vascularized connective tissue mass lying beneath the mucosa.

The primary *malignant tumors* of the ureter follow the identical patterns of those arising in the renal pelvis, calyces, and bladder, because all these structures are lined by the same transitional epithelium (urothelium). They may occlude the ureteral lumen (Fig. 21–2). They are found most frequently during the sixth and seventh decades of

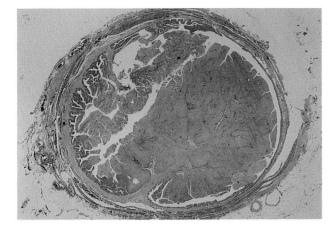

Figure 21–2. A papillary transitional cell carcinoma arising in the ureter and virtually filling the cross-section of the ureter.

life and are sometimes multiple and occasionally occur concurrently with similar neoplasms in the bladder or renal pelvis.

OBSTRUCTIVE LESIONS

A great variety of pathologic lesions may obstruct the ureters and give rise to hydroureter, hydronephrosis, and sometimes pyelonephritis (see Chapter 20). Obviously, it is not the ureteral dilatation that is of significance in these cases, but the consequent involvement of the kidneys. The more important causes, divided into those of intrinsic and those of extrinsic origin, are cited in Table 21–1 (see also Fig. 20–52). Only sclerosing retroperitoneal fibrosis will be further characterized.

SCLEROSING RETROPERITONEAL FIBROSIS. This entity of obscure origin is an uncommon cause of ureteral narrowing or obstruction and comes to medical attention by causing hydronephrosis.[1]

MORPHOLOGY. It is characterized by ill-defined fibrous masses that begin over the sacral promontory, encircle the lower abdominal aorta, and extend laterally through the retroperitoneum to enclose and encroach on the ureters. Microscopically, the inflammatory fibrosis is marked by a

Table 21–1. MAJOR CAUSES OF URETERAL OBSTRUCTION

INTRINSIC

Calculi	Of renal origin, rarely over 5 mm in diameter
	Larger renal stones cannot enter ureters
	Impact at loci of ureteral narrowing— ureteropelvic junction, where ureters cross iliac vessels, and where they enter bladder—and cause excruciating "renal colic"
Strictures	Congenital or acquired (inflammations, sclerosing retroperitoneal fibrosis)
Tumorous masses	Transitional cell carcinomas arising in ureters
	Rarely, benign tumors or fibroepithelial polyps
Blood clots	Massive hematuria from renal calculi, tumors, or papillary necrosis
Neurogenic causes	Interruption of the neural pathways to the bladder

EXTRINSIC

Pregnancy	Physiologic relaxation of smooth muscle or pressure on ureters at pelvic brim from enlarging fundus
Periureteral inflammation	Salpingitis, diverticulitis, peritonitis, sclerosing retroperitoneal fibrosis
Endometriosis	With pelvic lesions, followed by scarring
Tumors	Cancers of the rectum, bladder, prostate, ovaries, uterus, cervix, lymphomas, sarcomas. Ureteral obstruction is one of the major causes of death from cervical carcinoma

prominent inflammatory infiltrate of lymphocytes, often with germinal centers, plasma cells, and eosinophils. Sometimes, foci of fat necrosis and granulomatous inflammation are seen in and about the fibrosis.

The etiology of this condition is obscure. In some instances, there is a history of intake of the drug methysergide, an ergot derivative used for migraine. However, most cases have no obvious cause. Several cases have been reported with similar fibrotic changes in other sites (referred to as mediastinal fibrosis, sclerosing cholangitis, and Riedel's [fibrosing] thyroiditis), suggesting that the disorder is systemic in distribution but preferentially involves the retroperitoneum. Thus, a systemic autoimmune reaction, sometimes triggered by drugs, has been proposed.

Urinary Bladder

CONGENITAL ANOMALIES	METAPLASIAS	Inverted Papilloma	MESENCHYMAL TUMORS
INFLAMMATIONS	NEOPLASMS	Transitional Cell Carcinoma	SECONDARY TUMORS
ACUTE AND CHRONIC CYSTITIS	TRANSITIONAL CELL TUMORS	Other Types of Carcinoma	OBSTRUCTION
SPECIAL FORMS OF CYSTITIS	Exophytic (Benign) Papilloma		

Diseases of the bladder, particularly inflammation (cystitis), constitute an important source of clinical signs and symptoms. Usually, however, these disorders are more disabling than lethal. Cystitis is particularly common in young women of reproductive age and in older age groups of both sexes. Tumors of the bladder are an important source of both morbidity and mortality.

CONGENITAL ANOMALIES

DIVERTICULA. A bladder or vesical diverticulum consists of a pouch-like eversion or evagination of the bladder wall. Diverticula may arise as congenital defects but more commonly are acquired lesions from persistent urethral obstruction.

The *congenital form* may be due to a focal failure of development of the normal musculature or to some urinary tract obstruction during fetal development. *Acquired diverticula* are most often seen with prostatic enlargement (hyperplasia or neoplasia), producing obstruction to urine outflow and marked muscular thickening of the bladder wall. The increased intravesical pressure causes outpouching of the bladder wall and the formation of diverticula. They are frequently multiple and have narrow necks located between the interweaving hypertrophied muscle bundles (Fig. 21–3). In both the congenital and the acquired forms, the diverticulum usually consists of a round-to-ovoid, sac-like pouch that varies from less than 1 cm to 5 to 10 cm in diameter.

Diverticula are of clinical significance because they constitute sites of urinary stasis and predispose to infection and the formation of bladder calculi. They may also predispose to vesicoureteric reflux. Rarely, carcinomas may arise in bladder diverticuli.

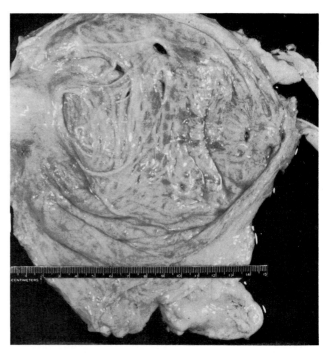

Figure 21–3. Acquired diverticula of the bladder. Note bladder distention as indicated by 15-cm rule and trabeculation of wall.

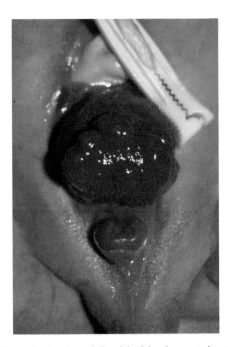

Figure 21–4. Exstrophy of the bladder in a male newborn. The clamped umbilical cord is seen above the hyperemic mucosa of the everted bladder. Below is an incompletely formed penis with marked epispadias. (Courtesy of Dr. Hardy Hendren, Surgeon-in-Chief, Children's Hospital, Boston.)

EXSTROPHY. Exstrophy of the bladder implies the presence of a developmental failure in the anterior wall of the abdomen and the bladder, so that the bladder either communicates directly through a large defect with the surface of the body or lies as an opened sac (Fig. 21–4). The exposed bladder mucosa may undergo colonic glandular metaplasia and is subject to the development of infections that often spread to upper levels of the urinary system. In the course of persistent chronic infections, the mucosa often becomes converted into an ulcerated surface of granulation tissue, and the preserved marginal epithelium becomes transformed into a stratified squamous type. There is an increased tendency toward the development later in life of carcinoma, mostly adenocarcinoma. These lesions are amenable to surgical correction, and long-term survival is possible.

MISCELLANEOUS ANOMALIES. *Vesicoureteral reflux* is the most common and serious anomaly. As a major contributor to renal infection and scarring, it was taken up earlier in Chapter 20 in the consideration of pyelonephritis. Abnormal connections between the bladder and the vagina, rectum, or uterus may create *congenital vesicouterine fistulas.*

Rarely, the *urachus* may remain patent in part or in whole (persistent urachus). When it is totally patent, a fistulous urinary tract is created that connects the bladder with the umbilicus. At times, the umbilical end or the bladder end remains patent, while the central region is obliterated. A seques-

tered umbilical epithelial rest or bladder diverticulum is formed that may provide a site for the development of infection. At other times, only the central region of the urachus persists, giving rise to *urachal cysts,* lined by either transitional or metaplastic epithelium. Carcinomas, mostly adenocarcinomas, have been reported to arise in such cysts.

INFLAMMATIONS

ACUTE AND CHRONIC CYSTITIS

The pathogenesis of cystitis and the common bacterial etiologic agents were discussed in the consideration of urinary tract infections. As emphasized earlier, bacterial pyelonephritis is frequently preceded by infection of the urinary bladder, with retrograde spread of microorganisms into the kidneys and their collecting systems. The common etiologic agents of cystitis are the coliforms— *Escherichia coli,* followed by Proteus, Klebsiella, and Enterobacter. *Tuberculous cystitis* is almost always a sequela to renal tuberculosis. *Candida albicans* (Monilia) and, much less often, cryptococcal agents cause cystitis, particularly in immunosuppressed patients or those receiving long-term antibiotics. Schistosomiasis *(S. hematobium)* is rare in the United States but is common in certain Middle Eastern countries, notably Egypt. Viruses (e.g., adenovirus), Chlamydia, and Mycoplasma may also be causes of cystitis. Patients receiving *cytotoxic antitumor drugs,* such as cyclophosphamide and busulfan, sometimes develop hemorrhagic cystitis.[2] Finally, radiation of the bladder region gives rise to *radiation cystitis.*

MORPHOLOGY. The great majority of cases of cystitis take the form of nonspecific acute or chronic inflammation of the bladder. Grossly, there is hyperemia of the mucosa, sometimes associated with exudate. When there is a hemorrhagic component, the cystitis is designated **hemorrhagic cystitis.** This form of cystitis sometimes follows radiation injury or antitumor chemotherapy and is often accompanied by epithelial atypia. Adenovirus infection also causes a hemorrhagic cystitis.

The accumulation of large amounts of suppurative exudate may merit the designation of **suppurative cystitis.** When there is ulceration of large areas of the mucosa, or sometimes the entire bladder mucosa, this is known as **ulcerative cystitis.**

Persistence of the infection leads to **chronic cystitis,** which differs from the acute form only in the character of the inflammatory infiltrate. There is more extreme heaping up of the epithelium with the formation of a red, friable, granular, sometimes ulcerated surface. Chronicity of the infection gives rise to fibrous thickening in the tunica propria and

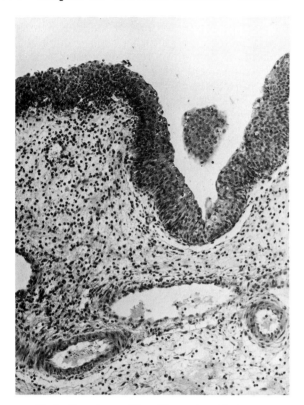

Figure 21-5. Chronic cystitis with a subepithelial mononuclear infiltrate and marked dilation of blood vessels.

consequent thickening and inelasticity of the bladder wall.

The histologic findings of most of these variants of acute and chronic nonspecific cystitis are exactly those that can be anticipated in any such nonspecific inflammation (Fig. 21-5). Mention might be made of special forms of chronic inflammatory reaction, the aggregation of lymphocytes into lymphoid follicles within the bladder mucosa and underlying wall, creating a variant of chronic cystitis known as **cystitis follicularis. Eosinophilic cystitis** is characterized by infiltration with submucosal eosinophils, together with fibrosis and occasionally giant cells.

All forms of cystitis are characterized by a triad of symptoms: (1) frequency, which in acute cases may necessitate urination every 15 to 20 minutes; (2) lower abdominal pain localized over the bladder region or in the suprapubic region; and (3) dysuria—pain or burning on urination. Associated with these localized changes, there may be systemic signs of inflammation such as elevation of temperature, chills, and general malaise. In the usual case, the bladder infection does not give rise to such a constitutional reaction.

The local symptoms of cystitis may be disturbing, but these infections are more important as antecedents to pyelonephritis. Cystitis is sometimes a secondary complication of some underlying dis-

order such as prostatic enlargement, cystocele of the bladder, calculi, or tumors. These primary diseases must be corrected before the cystitis can be relieved.

SPECIAL FORMS OF CYSTITIS

There is a multiplicity of so-called special variants of cystitis that are distinctive by either their morphologic appearance or their causation.

INTERSTITIAL CYSTITIS (HUNNER'S ULCER). This is a persistent chronic cystitis occurring most frequently in women and associated with inflammation and fibrosis of all layers of the bladder wall. Prominent in the inflammatory infiltrate are mast cells. A localized ulcer is often present. The condition is of unknown etiology but is thought by some to be of autoimmune origin, particularly because it is sometimes associated with lupus erythematosus and other autoimmune disorders. Alternatively, a chemical reaction to an excreted substance in urine, such as Tamm-Horsfall protein, is postulated.[3]

MALAKOPLAKIA. This designation refers to *a peculiar pattern of vesical inflammatory reaction characterized macroscopically by soft, yellow, slightly raised mucosal plaques 3 to 4 cm in diameter* (Fig. 21-6). Histologically, the plaques are made up of closely packed, large, foamy macrophages with occasional multinucleate giant cells and interspersed lymphocytes. The macrophages have an abundant

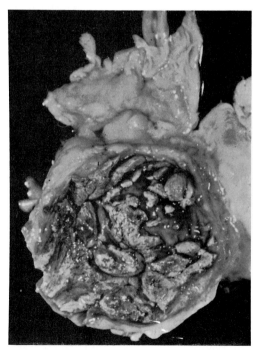

Figure 21-6. Malakoplakia of bladder showing classic broad, flat, inflammatory plaques.

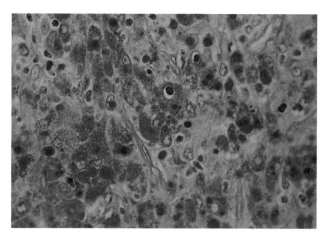

Figure 21-7. Malakoplakia, PAS stain. Note the large macrophages with granular PAS-positive cytoplasm and several dense, round Michaelis-Gutmann bodies surrounded by artefactual cleared holes in the upper middle field.

granular cytoplasm. The granularity is PAS positive and due to phagosomes stuffed with particulate and membranous debris of bacterial origin. In addition, laminated mineralized concretions known as Michaelis-Gutmann (MG) bodies are typically present, both within the macrophages and between cells (Fig. 21-7). Similar lesions have been described in the colon, lungs, bones, kidneys, prostate, and epididymis. Malakoplakia occurs with increased frequency in immunosuppressed transplant recipients.

The genesis of the malakoplakic lesion is still uncertain. Current opinion favors the hypothesis that the unusual-appearing macrophages and giant phagosomes result from defects in the phagocytic or degradative process. Thus, the phagosomes become overloaded with bacteria.

METAPLASIAS

The urothelium is subject to hyperplasia, dysplasia, and metaplasia under a variety of circumstances, including infections, nonspecific inflammation as may be caused by calculi, exposure to radiation, and a wide variety of excretory products of metabolized drugs. Whether these mucosal changes constitute preneoplastic alterations is speculative, but the factors leading to them may, if continued, contribute to cancer formation. Only the metaplasias are considered here; hyperplasia and dysplasia are further discussed in the section on bladder cancer.

Glandular metaplasia (intestinal metaplasia) of the bladder mucosa may appear with, or sometimes without, chronic cystitis. It is uncertain, therefore, whether the changes are related to chronic inflammation. Nests of transitional epithelium (Brunn's nests) grow downward into the lamina propria, with transformation of the central epithelial cells into columnar (colonic) forms lining slit-like or cystic spaces (sometimes referred to as *cystitis cystica*). These changes recapitulate those described earlier as ureteritis cystica. Large areas of glandular metaplasia are at increased risk for becoming cancerous.

Nephrogenic metaplasia is an uncommon lesion of the bladder, and rarely of the ureters or urethra, which takes the form of discrete, usually multiple, small (millimeters) mucosal projections. These are made up of clusters of benign-appearing tubular lumina within the lamina propria. It should be differentiated from adenocarcinoma.

Squamous metaplasia is a common reaction to long-standing chronic inflammation. It is often seen with exstrophy of the bladder, calculi, and schistosomal infections. The squamous changes may be limited to the trigonal area in cases with long-standing indwelling catheters. It is associated with an increased risk of squamous cell carcinoma.

NEOPLASMS

Neoplasms of the bladder pose biologic and clinical challenges. Despite significant inroads into their origins and improved methods of diagnosis and treatment they continue to exact a high toll in morbidity and mortality. About 95% are of urothelial origin, the remainder being mesenchymal tumors. The incidence of the epithelial tumors in the United States has been steadily increasing over the past years and is now more than 50,000 new cases annually. Despite improvements in detection and management of these neoplasms the death toll remains at about 10,000 annually, as the increased prevalence offsets such gains as have been made.

A simplified classification and frequency distribution of bladder epithelial tumors that is widely used (albeit not universally) is presented in Table 21-2. Some experts consider transitional cell papillomas to be transitional cell carcinomas (TCC) grade I on the grounds that differentiating one from the other both clinically and morphologically

Table 21-2. BLADDER EPITHELIAL TUMORS

BENIGN	
Transitional cell papilloma	2–3%
Inverted papilloma	rare
MALIGNANT	
Transitional cell carcinomas	90%
Grade I	20%
Grade II	} 60%
Grade III	
Carcinoma in situ	5–10%
(in the absence of other cancers)	
Squamous cell carcinomas	3–7%
Mixed	
Undifferentiated small cell carcinoma	rare
Adenocarcinoma	1%

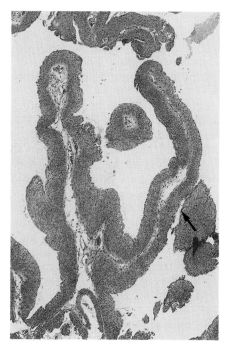

Figure 21-8. Low-power view of typical papillomatous growth of bladder. Note delicate axial stromal framework. (Courtesy of Dr. Christopher Corless.)

is very difficult and indeed imperfect.[4] Furthermore, TCC grades II and III are referred to as TCC "low grade" and "high grade," respectively. Here we shall continue to separate "papilloma" from TCC grade I because the former, when correctly identified, is a benign lesion, whereas the latter is malignant. Before considering what has been learned about their origins, the various lesions will be categorized morphologically.

TRANSITIONAL CELL TUMORS

Exophytic (Benign) Papilloma

These benign neoplasms, which may arise anywhere within the bladder, are difficult to distinguish from grade I papillary carcinomas, as pointed out. Pure papillomas are rare, representing about 2 to 3% of bladder tumors. Almost all are diploid.

> **MORPHOLOGY.** Papillomas usually arise singly, but multiple and sequential lesions may occur at varied and random locations. The individual tumor is usually a small (0.5 to 2.0 cm), delicate, soft, branching structure, superficially attached to the mucosa by a slender stalk. The individual finger-like papillae have a central core of loose fibrovascular tissue covered by normal-appearing transitional cells (Fig. 21-8) **seven or fewer layers in thickness.** The cells recapitulate the normal architecture of transitional urinary tract epithelium.

The usual papilloma is readily removed by transurethral resection, since it is attached only to the lamina propria. The frequency of recurrence varies among series. However, there are numerous reported instances in which new growths reappear. The regrowth may again be benign, but sometimes (about 3 to 5% of cases) it exhibits more marked irregularity of the epithelial cells sufficient to merit the diagnosis of transitional cell carcinoma. The line between the papilloma and its close relative the TCC grade I is finely drawn, but fortunately all well-differentiated papillary neoplasms, whether papilloma or TCC, seldom become invasive and provide a 95 to 98% 10-year survival rate.

Inverted Papilloma

These benign rarities merit only brief description. They appear as 1- to 3-cm solitary mucosal nodules that may be polypoid. The stalk-like structures of the exophytic papillomas just described grow into the lamina propria in the inverted papilloma. Anaplasia is seldom present as is invasion of the muscular wall.

Transitional Cell Carcinoma (TCC)

The great majority (90%) of bladder cancers are TCC, which includes grades I to III and carcinoma in situ. The remaining types cited in Table 21-2, save for squamous cell carcinomas, are on the whole uncommon.

> **MORPHOLOGY.** The gross appearance of all vesical cancers may be described as papillary or flat, and invasive or noninvasive (Fig. 21-9).

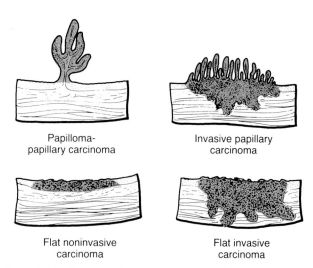

Papilloma-papillary carcinoma

Invasive papillary carcinoma

Flat noninvasive carcinoma

Flat invasive carcinoma

Figure 21-9. Four morphologic patterns of bladder tumors.

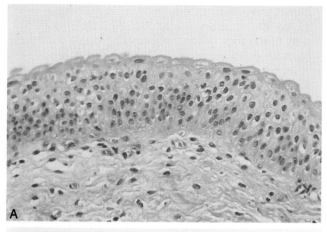

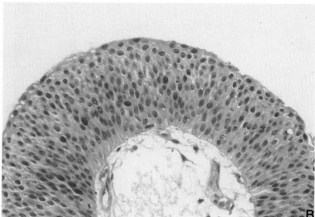

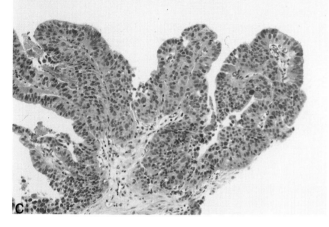

Figure 21–10. *A*, Normal bladder mucosa. *B*, TCC grade I. *C*, TCC grade III. (Courtesy of Dr. Christopher Corless.)

- **Papillary**—exophytic polypoid lesions attached by a stalk to the mucosa. Penetration of the basement membrane by the neoplastic cells may or may not be present.
- **Flat lesions**—growing as plaque-like thickenings of the mucosa without the formation of well-defined papillary structures. The neoplasm may be *in situ* or invasive (more often the latter), and these neoplasms generally tend to be more anaplastic than the papillary lesions.
- **Noninvasive**—thickening of the mucosa by proliferation of cancer cells, but without penetration of the basement membrane.
- **Invasive**—penetrating the mucosal basement membrane into the bladder wall, and possibly into contiguous structures.

Grading of the transitional cell neoplasms is based on the degree of atypia exhibited by the cancer cells (Fig. 21–10).

- **GRADE I**. The tumor cells display some atypia but are well differentiated and closely resemble normal transitional cells. Mitoses are rare. There is a significant increase in the number of layers of cells, that is, more than seven layers but only slight loss of polarity (see Fig. 21–10B).
- **GRADE II**. The tumor cells are still recognizable as of transitional origin. The number of layers of cells

is increased (often more than ten), as is the number of mitoses, and there is greater loss of polarity. Greater variability in cell size, shape, and chromaticity is present. In some tumors there may be areas of squamous differentiation.

- **GRADE III**. The tumor cells are barely recognizable as of transitional origin, and all the changes mentioned under grade II are more aggravated. In particular, there is evident disarray of cells with loosening and fragmentation of the superficial layers of cells. Occasional giant cells may be present. Sometimes the cells tend to flatten out, and the lesions come to resemble squamous cell carcinomas (see Fig. 21–10C). Alternatively, foci of glandular differentiation may be present.

Against this background we can now turn to the varying grades and patterns of TCC.

Transitional cell carcinomas range from noninvasive to invasive lesions, from flat to papillary, and from well-differentiated (grade I) to highly anaplastic, aggressive cancers (grades II and III). Overall, about half of all bladder cancers are high-grade anaplastic lesions. Most arise from the lateral or posterior walls, and many are multicentric.

Papillary neoplasms have a complicated fern-like structure composed of a delicate connective tissue stalk, covered by transitional epithelium that ranges from grade I to grade III. Most of these

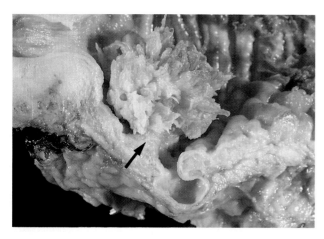

Figure 21-11. Sectioned bladder showing a grade I papillary transitional cell carcinoma projecting into the lumen *(arrow).* Note delicate arborizing structure and small stalk. Note also the small diverticulum adjacent to the attachment site of the stalk.

papillary lesions appear as small, red, elevated excrescences varying in size from less than 1 cm in diameter to large masses up to 5 cm in diameter. Multicentric origins may produce separate tumors. Some grade II and grade III papillary cancers spread over wide areas of the bladder wall.

Grade I lesions are almost always papillary (Fig. 21-11). Grade II neoplasms also are most often papillary but may be flat. Both the papillary and the flat patterns may be invasive or noninvasive. Noninvasive lesions are often referred to as "superficial" to differentiate them from carcinoma in situ, described later. The grade III transitional cell carcinomas represent the other end of the spectrum of anaplasia. Some of these lesions retain a papillary configuration, but many are flat or fungating, ne-

crotic, sometimes ulcerative, tumors that have unmistakably invaded deeply (Fig. 21-12). Frequently with the higher grade neoplasms, in areas of the bladder devoid of tumor, there may be areas of mucosal hyperplasia, dysplasia, or carcinoma in situ. In most analyses fewer than 10% of grade I but 80% of grade III TCC are invasive. Aggressive tumors may extend only into the bladder wall, but the more advanced stages invade the adjacent prostate, seminal vesicles, ureters, and retroperitoneum, and some produce fistulous communications to the vagina or rectum. About 40% of these deeply invasive tumors metastasize to regional lymph nodes. Hematogenous dissemination, principally to the liver, lungs, and bone marrow, generally occurs late, and only with highly anaplastic tumors.

Carcinoma in situ (CIS) is a high-grade abnormality of the full thickness of the bladder mucosa (Fig. 21-13). It usually occurs as a diffuse area of mucosal reddening, granularity, or thickening without producing an evident intraluminal mass. In some instances the in situ changes involve most of the bladder surface and may even extend into the ureters and urethra.[5] Although carcinoma in situ is most often found in bladders harboring well-defined TCC, about 5 to 10% of cases of carcinoma in situ occur in the absence of such tumors. In time, half of these lesions become invasive.

It is obvious that the extent of spread of cancer is the most important factor in determining the outlook for a patient. The staging system most commonly used is the Marshall modification of an earlier system (Table 21–3).[6]

Other Types of Carcinoma

Squamous cell carcinomas represent about 3 to 7% of bladder cancers. Presumably, they arise in areas of squamous metaplasia of the bladder mucosa. Mixed transitional cell carcinomas with areas of squamous carcinoma are more frequent than pure squamous cell carcinomas. Although the latter may be in situ, most are invasive, fungating tumors or infiltrative and ulcerative. True papillary patterns are almost never seen. The level of cytologic differentiation varies widely, from the highly differentiated lesions producing abundant keratohyaline pearls to very anaplastic giant cell tumors showing no evidence of squamous differentiation. They often cover large areas of the bladder and are deeply invasive by the time of discovery.

Adenocarcinomas of the bladder are rare. These tumors may arise from urachal remnants, from periurethral and periprostatic glands, or from cystitis cystica, or from metaplasia of transitional epithelium. Rare variants are the highly malignant **signet cell**

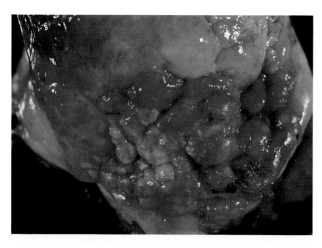

Figure 21-12. A grade III transitional cell carcinoma at an advanced stage. The aggressive multinodular neoplasm has fungated into the bladder lumen and spread over a wide area. Normal, somewhat edematous bladder mucosa is at the top of the illustration.

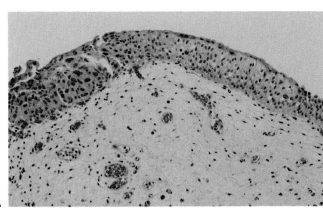

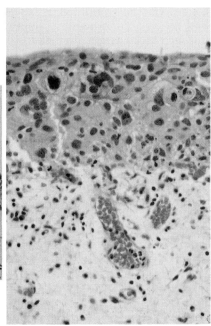

Figure 21–13. *A*, Low-power view of bladder with focus of carcinoma in situ *(left)*. *B*, High-power view of the focus of carcinoma in situ.

carcinoma and **mixed adenocarcinoma** and **transitional cell carcinomas.**

EPIDEMIOLOGY AND PATHOGENESIS. The incidence of carcinoma of the bladder resembles that of bronchogenic carcinoma, being more common in males than in females, in industrialized than in developing nations, and in urban than in rural dwellers. The male-to-female ratio for transitional cell tumors is approximately 3:1. About 80% of patients are between the ages of 50 and 80 years.

A number of factors have been implicated in the causation of TCC, some on substantial evidence, others are highly controversial. Some of the more important contributors will be cited.[7]

Table 21–3. BLADDER CANCER STAGING

DESCRIPTION	MARSHALL STAGE
Noninvasive	
Papillary	0
Carcinoma in situ	0
Invasive	
Lamina propria	A
Superficial muscle	B_1
Deep muscle	B_2
Perivesical tissue	C
Contiguous organs/tissues	D_1
Metastatic	
Regional lymph nodes	D_1
Distant sites	D_2

Modified from Grignon, D.J., and Srigley, J.R.: Superficially invasive transitional cell carcinoma. *In* Surgical Pathology of the Urothelial Tract: Conceptual and Diagnostic Problems: A Short Course of the U.S. and Canadian Academy of Pathology, New Orleans, March 1993, p. 8.

- *Industrial exposure to arylamines,* particularly 2-naphthylamine as well as related compounds, as was pointed out in the earlier discussion of chemical carcinogenesis (see Chapter 7). The cancers appear 15 to 40 years after the first exposure.
- *Cigarette smoking* is clearly the most important influence, increasing the risk three- to sevenfold, depending on the pack-years and smoking habits. It has been estimated that 50 to 80% of all bladder cancers among men can be attributed to the use of cigarettes. Cigars, pipes, and smokeless tobacco invoke a much smaller risk.
- *Schistosoma haematobium* infections are an established risk. The ova are deposited in the bladder wall and incite a brisk chronic inflammatory response that induces progressive mucosal squamous metaplasia and dysplasia and, in some instances, neoplasia. Approximately 70% of the cancers are squamous cell in type, the remainder being TCC.
- Long-term use of phenacetin, implicated also in analgesic nephropathy (see Chapter 20).
- Heavy long-term exposure to cyclophosphamide, an immunosuppressive agent, induces as noted hemorrhagic cystitis and increases the risk of bladder cancer almost tenfold after 12 years of exposure.
- Suggested but not established influences are excessive consumption of coffee or caffeine; long-term use of synthetic dietary sweeteners, for example, saccharin and cyclamates; and chronic alcohol consumption.

How the established influences induce tumor formation has not been unraveled, but a number of genetic alterations have been observed in TCC. It is speculated that carcinogenic influences cause cell injury followed by reparative activity. Continued exposure may lead to accumulation of mutations, some of which may be oncogenic. Particularly common (occurring in 30 to 60% of tumors studied) are chromosomal deletions of 9q, 11p, 13q, and 17p.[8] Other mutations have been observed, but less consistently. At least some of these deletions include sites of tumor suppressor genes (e.g., the p53 gene on chromosome 17p). Loss of DNA sequences from chromosome 9q is likely an important early event in bladder carcinogenesis. A significant percentage of superficial, noninvasive tumors show 9q deletions; others have lost one copy of chromosome 9 altogether. On the other hand, many invasive TCCs show deletions of 17p, including the region of the p53 gene, suggesting that, as in colonic carcinomas (see Chapter 7), alterations in p53 contribute to the progression of TCC. Increased expression of *ras*, c-*myc*, and epidermal growth factor receptors has also been observed in some bladder cancers, but the role of these factors in the progression of TCC is not yet defined. As more is learned of the genetic changes in bladder tumor development, there is the hope that noninvasive tests can be developed to detect tumor cells in the urine sediment of patients suspected of having cancer.

As has been pointed out, bladder tumors are often multifocal or are accompanied by areas of dysplasia and/or carcinoma in situ in contiguous or remote areas of the bladder mucosa. From these observations arose the concept that there is a "field change" affecting the entire bladder (a "restless epithelium"), out of which occasional cells "go over the line" to produce a tumor.[9] It is now proposed, on the basis of molecular analysis of X-chromosome inactivation[10] and p53 mutations[11] in individual tumors, however, that the multiple and recurrent tumors all are clonal in origin, deriving from a single transformed cell that "seeded" or permeated wide areas of mucosa, perhaps because of an acquired growth advantage. Progressive acquisition of additional mutations in cells derived from the original clone might lead to cancers of varying histology, occurring at various sites. It could also explain the tendency for subsequent recurrences over the span of years to become more anaplastic. So it is that most papillomas and grade I TCCs are diploid, whereas most grade II and III TCCs are aneuploid.

CLINICAL COURSE OF BLADDER CANCER. All bladder tumors classically produce painless hematuria. This is their dominant and sometimes only clinical manifestation. Occasionally, frequency, urgency, and dysuria accompany the hematuria. When the ureteral orifice is involved, pyelonephritis or hydronephrosis may follow. About 60% neoplasms, when first discovered, are single, and 70% localized to the bladder.

All transitional cell cancers, whatever their grade, have a tendency to recur following excision, and usually the recurrence exhibits greater anaplasia. Overall, about 60% of grade I papillary carcinomas recur, in contrast to 80 to 90% of grade III lesions. In many instances, the recurrence is seen at a different site, and the question of a new primary tumor must be entertained.

The prognosis depends on the histologic pattern, on the grade of the tumor, and principally on the stage when first diagnosed. Grade I TCCs yield a 98% 10-year survival rate regardless of the number of recurrences. Only a few patients with this grade of carcinoma have progression of their disease to a grade III lesion. In contrast, only about 30% of individuals with a grade III cancer survive 10 years; the tumor is progressive in 65%. Approximately 70% of patients with squamous cell carcinomas are dead within the year. Other factors may influence the prognosis. The expression of blood group antigens by tumor cells has proved to be a useful indicator of tumor behavior. Tumor cells that express A, B, and H antigens have a better prognosis than those that do not or lose this capacity. Analogously, the detection of a T antigen, increased c-*myc* expression, and multiple chromosomal mutations (cited earlier) all worsen the outlook. Almost half of all high-grade TCCs elaborate human chorionic gonadotropin even though the tumors show no chorionic differentiation. The finding of this hormone in the urine is thus a marker of an aggressive tumor.

The clinical challenge with these neoplasms is early detection. Although cytoscopy and biopsy are the mainstays of diagnosis, preneoplastic dysplasia, carcinoma in situ producing no or only subtle gross mucosal changes, and early small papillary lesions may be difficult to detect. Of value in these circumstances are *cytologic examinations and flow cytometric analyses of urinary sediment.* These diagnostic approaches are about 85% effective in detecting grade III TCC and squamous cell carcinomas and are almost as effective with carcinoma in situ. However, grade I TCC and some carcinoma in situ tumors are diploid and have only subtle anaplastic changes, reducing the effectiveness of cytologic and cytometric evaluations.[12] The perfect method of detecting all bladder cancers has yet to be discovered.

MESENCHYMAL TUMORS

BENIGN. A great variety of benign mesenchymal tumors may arise in the bladder. Collectively, they are rare. The most common is *leiomyoma.* They all tend to grow as isolated, intramural, encapsulated, oval-to-spherical masses, varying in diameter up to several centimeters. Occasionally, they assume submucosal pedunculated positions. They have the histologic features of their counterparts elsewhere.

SARCOMAS. True sarcomas are distinctly uncommon in the bladder. It is important to note that inflammatory pseudotumors, postoperative spindle cell nodules, and various carcinomas may assume sarcomatoid growth patterns, all sometimes mistaken histologically for sarcomas.[13] As a group, sarcomas tend to produce large masses (varying up to 10 to 15 cm in diameter) that protrude into the vesical lumen. Their soft, fleshy, gray-white gross appearance suggests their sarcomatous nature. *Rhabdomyosarcoma* takes one of two forms. The "adult" form occurs mostly in adults older than 40 years of age and shows a range of histology similar to rhabdomyosocarcomas of striated muscle (see Chapter 27). The other variant is the *embryonal rhabdomyosarcoma,* or *sarcoma botryoides,* encountered chiefly in infancy or childhood, and similar to those that occur in the female genital tract (see Chapter 23).

SECONDARY TUMORS

Secondary malignant involvement of the bladder is most often by direct extension from primary lesions in nearby organs, cervix, uterus, prostate, and rectum, in the order given. They may, on casual inspection of the bladder, appear as primary carcinomas of this organ. Hemorrhage, ureteral obstruction, and vesicovaginal fistulas are the common sequelae. Distinction between primary adenocarcinoma of the bladder (urethral or otherwise) from local extension of colorectal cancer can be difficult.

OBSTRUCTION

Obstruction to the bladder neck is of major clinical importance, not only for the changes induced in the bladder but also because of its eventual effect on the kidney. A great variety of intrinsic and extrinsic diseases of the bladder may narrow the urethral orifice and cause partial or complete vesical obstruction. In the male, the most important lesion is enlargement of the prostate gland due either to nodular hyperplasia or to carcinoma (Fig. 21–14). Vesical obstruction is somewhat less common in the female and is most often caused by cystocele of the bladder. The more infrequent causes can be listed as (1) congenital narrowings or strictures of the urethra; (2) inflammatory strictures of the urethra; (3) inflammatory fibrosis and contraction of the bladder following varying types of cystitis; (4)

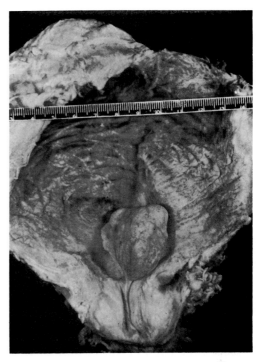

Figure 21–14. Hypertrophy and trabeculation of bladder wall secondary to polypoid hyperplasia of prostate.

bladder tumors — either benign or malignant — when strategically located; (5) secondary invasion of the bladder neck by growths arising in perivesical structures, such as the cervix, vagina, prostate, and rectum; (6) mechanical obstructions caused by foreign bodies and calculi; and (7) injury to the innervation of the bladder causing neurogenic or cord bladder.

> **MORPHOLOGY.** In the early stages, there is only some thickening of the bladder wall, presumably due to hypertrophy of the smooth muscle. The mucosal surface at this time may be entirely normal. With progressive hypertrophy of the muscular coat, the individual muscle bundles greatly enlarge and produce trabeculation of the bladder wall. In the course of time, crypts form and may then become converted into true acquired diverticula.

In some cases of acute obstruction or in terminal disease when the patient's normal reflex mechanisms are depressed, the bladder may become extremely dilated. The enlarged bladder may reach the brim of the pelvis or even the level of the umbilicus. In these cases, the bladder wall is markedly thinned, and the trabeculation becomes totally inapparent.

Urethra

INFLAMMATIONS

Urethritis is classically divided into gonococcal and nongonococcal urethritis. As noted earlier, gonococcal urethritis is one of the earliest manifestations of this venereal infection. Nongonococcal urethritis is very common and can be caused by a variety of bacteria, among which *E. coli* and other enteric organisms predominate. Urethritis is often accompanied by cystitis in females and by prostatitis in males. In many instances bacteria cannot be isolated. Various strains of Chlamydia (e.g., *C. trachomatis*) are the cause of 25 to 60% of nongonococcal urethritis in males and in about 20% in females. Mycoplasma *(Ureaplasma urealyticum)* also accounts for the symptoms of urethritis in many cases. Urethritis is also one component of *Reiter's syndrome,* which comprises the clinical triad of arthritis, conjunctivitis, and urethritis.

The morphologic changes are entirely typical of inflammation in other sites within the urinary tract. The urethral involvement is not itself a serious clinical problem but may cause considerable local pain, itching, and frequency, and may represent a forerunner of more serious disease in higher levels of the urogenital tract.

TUMORS

Urethral caruncle is an inflammatory lesion presenting a small, red, painful mass about the external urethral meatus in the female. Caruncles may be found at any age but are more common in later life. The lesion consists of a hemispheric, friable, 1- to 2-cm nodule that occurs singly, either just outside or just within the external urethral meatus. It may be covered by an intact mucosa but is extremely friable, and the slightest trauma may cause ulceration of the surface and bleeding. Histologically, it is composed of a *highly vascularized, young, fibroblastic connective tissue, more or less heavily infiltrated with leukocytes.* The overlying epithelium, where present, is either transitional or squamous cell in type. Surgical excision affords prompt relief and cure.

Papillomas of the urethra occur usually just within or on the external meatus. They may be of viral origin, analogous to those affecting the vulva.

Carcinoma of the urethra is an uncommon lesion. It tends to occur in advanced age in women and, in most instances, begins about the external meatus or on the immediately surrounding structures, such as the glans penis or the introitus in the female. Some apparently begin just inside the external meatus or even at a higher level within the urethra. Those that occur at or protrude from the external meatus appear as warty, papillary growths that at first resemble the sessile papillary carcinomas described in the bladder. As they progress, they tend to become ulcerated on their surfaces and to assume the characteristics of a fungating, ulcerating lesion (Fig. 21–15).

Most of these malignancies are squamous cell carcinomas. The papillary lesions that protrude

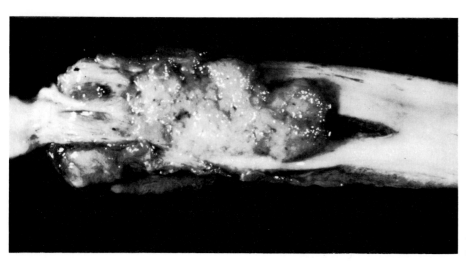

Figure 21–15. Carcinoma of urethra with typical fungating growth.

from the external meatus are apt to show a transitional cell growth that further heightens their similarity to bladder carcinoma. Uncommonly, an adenocarcinomatous growth pattern is found. Overall, they are more aggressive than bladder cancers, more often invasive, and more difficult to eradicate despite the fact that they seldom metastasize probably because most lead to death within a few years.

1. Mitchison, M.J.: Retroperitoneal fibrosis revisited. Arch. Pathol. Lab. Med. *110:*784, 1986.
2. deVries, C.R., and Freiha, F.S.: Hemorrhagic cystitis: A review. J. Urol. *143:*1, 1990.
3. Lynes, W.L., et al.: The histology of interstitial cystitis. Am. J. Surg. Pathol. *14:*969, 1990.
4. Murphy, W.M., et al.: Tumors of the urinary bladder, urethra, ureters, renal pelves, and kidneys. *In* Atlas of Tumor Pathology. Washington, DC, Armed Forces Institute of Pathology, 1994.
5. Lamm, D.L.: Carcinoma in situ. Urol. Clin. North Am. *19:*499, 1992.
6. Marshall, V.F.: The relation of the preoperative estimate to the pathologic demonstration of the extent of vesical neoplasms. J. Urol. *68:*714, 1952.
7. Rath, G.D.: Bladder Cancer, 1992. Postgrad. Med. *92:*105, 1992.
8. Dalbagni, G., et al.: Genetic alterations in bladder cancer. Lancet *342:*469, 1993.
9. Harris, A.L.: Bladder cancer—field origin versus clonal origin. N. Engl. J. Med. *326:*759, 1992.
10. Sidransky, D., et al.: Clonal origin of bladder cancer. N. Engl. J. Med. *326:*737, 1992.
11. Habuchi, T., et al.: Metachronous multifocal development of urothelial cancers by intraluminal seeding. Lancet *342:*1087, 1993.
12. Ro, J.Y., et al.: Cytologic and histologic features of superficial bladder cancer. Urol. Clin. North Am. *19:*435, 1992.
13. Jones, E.C., et al.: Inflammatory pseudotumor of the urinary bladder. Am. J. Surg. Pathol. *17:*264, 1993.

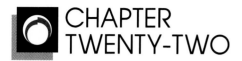

CHAPTER TWENTY-TWO

Male Genital System

PENIS

The penis can be affected by congenital anomalies, inflammations, and tumors, the most important of which are inflammations and tumors. The venereal infections (e.g., syphilis and gonorrhea) usually begin with penile lesions. Carcinoma of the penis, although not one of the more common neoplasms in North America, still accounts for about 1% of cancers in men.

CONGENITAL ANOMALIES

The penis is the site of many varied forms of congenital anomalies, only some of which have clinical significance. These range from congenital absence and hypoplasia to hyperplasia, duplication, and other aberrations in size and form. For the most part, these deviations in size and form are extremely uncommon and readily apparent on inspection. Certain other anomalies are more frequent and, therefore, have greater clinical significance.

HYPOSPADIAS AND EPISPADIAS. Malformation of the urethral groove and urethral canal may create abnormal openings either on the *ventral surface of the penis (hypospadias)* or on the *dorsal surface*

(epispadias). Such anomalies are commonly associated with failure of normal descent of the testes and with malformations of the urinary tract.[1] Even when isolated, these urethral defects may have clinical significance because often the abnormal opening is constricted, producing partial urinary obstruction and an attendant hazard of spread of bacterial contamination from the obstructed penile urethra into the bladder and remainder of the urinary tract. Moreover, these anomalies may have more serious consequences. When the orifices are situated near the base of the penis, normal ejaculation and insemination are hampered or totally blocked. These lesions, therefore, are possible causes of sterility in men.

PHIMOSIS. When the orifice of the prepuce is too small to permit its normal retraction, the condition is designated phimosis. Such an abnormally small orifice may result from anomalous development but may also be produced by inflammatory scarring of the prepuce. Phimosis is important because it interferes with cleanliness and permits the accumulation of secretions and detritus under the prepuce, favoring the development of secondary infections and possibly carcinoma. When a phimotic prepuce is forcibly retracted over the glans penis, marked constriction and subsequent swelling may block the replacement of the prepuce, creating

1007

what is known as *paraphimosis*. This condition not only is extremely painful, but also it may be a potential cause of urethral constriction and serious acute urinary retention.

INFLAMMATIONS

Inflammations of the penis almost invariably involve the glans and prepuce and include a wide variety of specific and nonspecific infections. The specific infections—syphilis, gonorrhea, chancroid, granuloma inguinale, lymphopathia venereum, genital herpes—are sexually transmitted and are discussed in Chapter 8. Only the nonspecific infections causing so-called balanoposthitis need description here.

Balanoposthitis is a nonspecific infection of the glans and prepuce caused by a wide variety of organisms, including pyogenic bacteria (staphylococci, coliforms), fungi *(Candida albicans)*, mycoplasmas, and chlamydia.[2] It is usually encountered in patients having phimosis or a large, redundant prepuce that interferes with cleanliness and predisposes to bacterial growth within the accumulated secretions and smegma. Such inflammations, if neglected, may lead to frank ulcerations of the mucosal covering of the glans. If they persist and become chronic, they lead to further inflammatory scarring of the phimosis, with aggravation of the underlying condition.

TUMORS

Tumors of the penis are, on the whole, uncommon. The most frequent neoplasms are carcinomas and a benign epithelial tumor—condyloma acuminatum. In addition to the clearly defined benign and malignant categories, however, there are some conditions that fall into an intermediate zone. These include the locally invasive giant condyloma (verrucous carcinoma) and Bowen's disease, which has the potential of developing into cancer.

Benign Tumors

Condyloma Acuminatum

This benign tumor is caused by human papillomavirus (HPV). It is related to the common wart (verruca vulgaris) and may occur on any moist mucocutaneous surface of the external genitals in either sex. There is ample evidence that HPV and associated diseases are sexually transmitted.[3] Of the various antigenically and genetically distinct types of HPV that have been identified, types 6 and 11 have been clearly associated with condylomata acuminata. The antigens and genome of these HPV types can be demonstrated in most lesions by

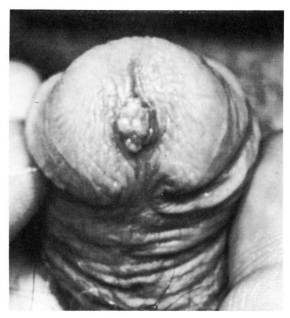

Figure 22–1. Condyloma acuminatum of the penis.

immunoperoxidase and DNA hybridization techniques, respectively.

MORPHOLOGY. As mentioned, condylomata acuminata may occur on the external genitalia or perineal areas. On the penis, these lesions occur most often about the coronal sulcus and inner surface of the prepuce. They consist of single or multiple sessile or pedunculated, red papillary excrescences that vary from 1 to several millimeters in diameter (Fig. 22–1). Histologically, a branching, villous, papillary connective tissue stroma is covered by a thickened hyperplastic epithelium that may have considerable superficial hyperkeratosis and thickening of the underlying epidermis (acanthosis) (Fig. 22–2). The normal orderly maturation of the epithelial cells is preserved. Clear vacuolization of the prickle cells (koilocytosis), characteristic of HPV infection, is noted in these lesions (Fig. 22–3). The basement membrane is usually intact, and there is no evidence of invasion of the underlying stroma. As far as we know, the vast majority of these lesions remain benign throughout their course.

Giant Condyloma (Buschké-Lowenstein Tumor, Verrucous Carcinoma)

Giant condyloma, as implied by its name, is much larger than condyloma acuminatum. It presents usually as a solitary exophytic lesion that may cover and destroy much of the penis. Like condyloma acuminatum, it is believed to be of viral origin because HPV 6 and 11 can be demonstrated within the tumor cells by DNA hybridization.[4] In

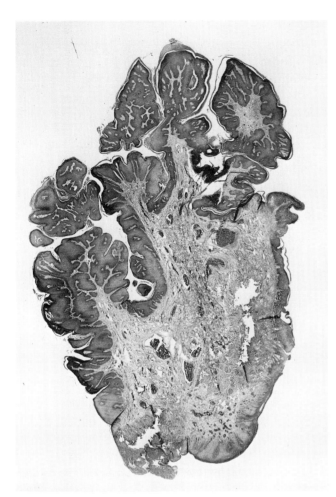

Figure 22–2. Condyloma acuminatum of the penis. Low magnification reveals the papillary (villous) architecture. (Courtesy of Dr. Jag Bhawan, Boston University School of Medicine, Boston.)

contrast to condyloma acuminatum, it is locally invasive and has a tendency for recurrence. Giant condylomata, however, differ from the unambiguously malignant squamous cell carcinomas in that they rarely, if ever, metastasize. Thus with respect to biologic behavior, giant condylomata occupy an intermediate position between the truly benign condyloma acuminatum and the squamous cell carcinoma.

MORPHOLOGY. Microscopically, the giant condyloma exhibits both upward and downward growth patterns. The exophytic part is almost indistinguishable from condyloma acuminatum, including the characteristic koilocytic change in the superficial layers. In its lower portion, the hyperplastic epithelium penetrates the underlying tissues along a broad front, in contrast to the finger-like invasion typical of squamous cell carcinoma. Cellular atypia is present along the superficially invasive margin.

Finally, a note about terminology. Giant condyloma is often referred to as Buschké-Lowenstein

tumor, after the names of the authors who first recognized it as an entity distinct from condyloma acuminatum. Subsequently, histologically identical lesions in the oral cavity were labeled *verrucous carcinomas*, and hence many authors prefer to apply this term to the genital lesions as well.

Carcinoma in situ

From the discussion in Chapter 7, it should be recalled that carcinoma in situ is a histologic term used to describe epithelial lesions having the cytologic changes of malignancy confined to the epithelium with no evidence of local invasion or distant metastases. It is considered a precancerous condition because of its potential to evolve into invasive cancer. In the external male genitalia, three lesions that display histologic features of carcinoma in situ have been described: *Bowen's disease, erythroplasia of Queyrat,* and *bowenoid papulosis.* Whether these are distinct clinical entities or instead are variants of a single underlying disorder is controversial, as will be evident from the following brief descriptions.

Bowen's disease occurs in the genital region of both males and females, usually in those over the

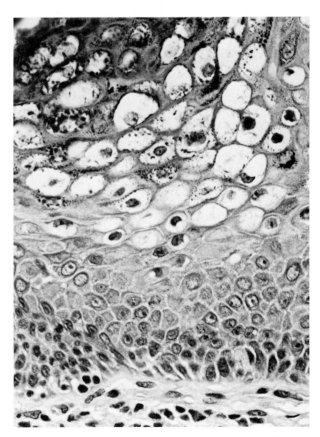

Figure 22–3. Condyloma acuminatum of the penis. The epithelium shows vacuolization (koilocytosis) characteristic of human papillomavirus (HPV) infection. (Courtesy of Dr. Jag Bhawan, Boston University School of Medicine, Boston.)

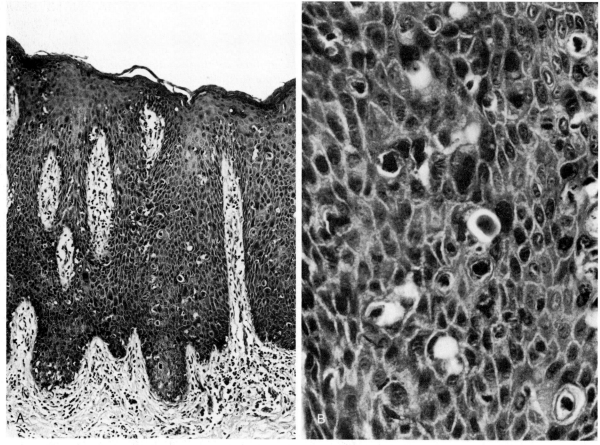

Figure 22-4. Bowen's disease (carcinoma in situ) of the penis. *A,* Low magnification shows an intact basement membrane. *B,* Higher magnification reveals dysplastic epithelial cells with several mitoses. (Courtesy of Dr. Jag Bhawan, Boston University School of Medicine, Boston.)

age of 35 years. In males it is prone to involve the shaft of the penis and the scrotum. Grossly it appears as a solitary, thickened, gray-white, opaque plaque with shallow ulceration and crusting. Histologically the epidermis shows proliferation with numerous mitoses, some atypical. The cells are markedly dysplastic with large hyperchromatic nuclei, and there is total lack of orderly maturation (Fig. 22-4). Nevertheless, *the dermal-epidermal border is sharply delineated by an intact basement membrane.* Over the span of years, Bowen's disease may become invasive and transform into typical squamous cell carcinoma in approximately 10 to 20% of patients. Another curious feature said to be associated with Bowen's disease is the occurrence of visceral cancer in approximately one-third of the patients. This view has been challenged, however, and hence this issue remains unresolved.[5]

Erythroplasia of Queyrat generally appears on the glans and prepuce as single or multiple shiny red, sometimes velvety plaques. Histologically, the dysplasia is of variable severity, ranging from mild disorientation of cells to a picture indistinguishable from that of Bowen's disease. Like Bowen's disease, it has the potential to develop into invasive carcinoma. In contrast to Bowen's disease, however, there is no reported association with visceral malignancy. Because the relationship between Bowen's disease and internal malignancy remains unresolved, it should be apparent that the distinction between erythroplasia of Queyrat and Bowen's disease is at best tenuous.

Bowenoid papulosis, the third member of the carcinoma in situ "family" of lesions affecting the external genitalia, occurs in sexually active adults. Clinically it differs from Bowen's disease by the younger age of patients and the presence of multiple (rather than solitary), pigmented (reddish brown) papular lesions. In some cases, the lesions may be verrucoid and readily mistaken for condyloma acuminatum. Histologically, however, bowenoid papulosis is indistinguishable from Bowen's disease.[6] Recent studies have revealed that the E6 and E7 portions of HPV type 16 DNA can be detected in virtually all cases by the polymerase chain reaction.[7]

Carcinoma

Squamous cell carcinoma of the penis represents about 1% of cancers in males in the United States.

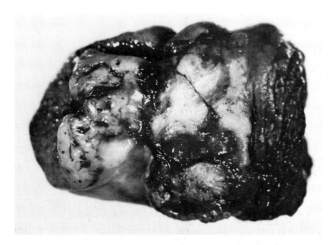

Figure 22–5. Squamous cell carcinoma of the penis with typical shaggy fungating ulcerations. (Courtesy of Dr. Fred Silva, Department of Pathology, University of Texas Health Science Center, Dallas.)

CLINICAL COURSE. Carcinoma of the penis is a slowly growing, locally metastasizing lesion[8] that often has been present for a year or more before it is brought to medical attention. Such delay is occasioned sometimes by the existence of a phimosis that completely hides the developing lesion but more often by unawareness of the significance of the developing papule. The lesions are nonpainful until they undergo secondary ulceration and infection. Frequently they bleed. Metastases to inguinal and iliac lymph nodes characterize the early stage, but widespread dissemination is extremely uncommon until the lesion is far advanced. The prognosis is related to the stage of advancement of the tumor. In persons with limited lesions without invasion of the inguinal lymph nodes, there is a 66% 5-year survival rate, whereas metastasis to the lymph nodes carries a grim 27% 5-year survival.

Because protection against this malignancy is apparently conferred by circumcision, carcinoma of the penis is extremely rare among Jews and Moslems and is correspondingly more common in regions of the world where circumcision is not routinely practiced.[8] The protection conferred by circumcision has traditionally been ascribed to its effectiveness in preventing accumulation of smegma, believed by some to be a source of as yet unidentified carcinogens. As with certain cancers of the female genital tract, however, there is evidence suggesting a possible causal association with HPV type 16 and, to a lesser extent, HPV type 18.[7,9] Carcinomas are usually found in patients between the ages of 40 and 70.

MORPHOLOGY. The lesion usually begins on the glans or inner surface of the prepuce near the coronal sulcus. The first observable changes are a small area of epithelial thickening accompanied by graying and fissuring of the mucosal surface. With progression, an elevated papule that often ulcerates develops. Despite the obviousness of such lesions, by the time most patients seek medical attention, large characteristic malignant ulcers are present, having necrotic, secondarily infected bases with ragged, irregular, heaped-up margins (Fig. 22–5). In far-advanced lesions, the ulceroinvasive disease may have destroyed virtually the entire tip of the penis or large areas of the shaft. A second pattern of macroscopic tumor growth is the papillary tumor that simulates the condyloma and progressively enlarges to form a cauliflower-like, ulcerated, fungating mass. Histologically both the papillary and ulceroinvasive lesions are squamous cell carcinomas similar to those that occur elsewhere on the skin surface.

TESTIS AND EPIDIDYMIS

The major pathologic involvements of the testis and epididymis are quite distinct. In the case of the epididymis, the most important and frequent involvements are inflammatory diseases, whereas in the testis the major lesions consist of tumors. Their close anatomic relationship, however, permits the extension of any of these processes from one organ to the other.

CONGENITAL ANOMALIES

With the exception of incomplete descent of the testes (cryptorchidism), congenital anomalies are extremely rare and include absence of one or both testes, fusion of the testes (so-called *synorchism*), and the formation of relatively insignificant cysts within the testis.

Cryptorchidism

Cryptorchidism is synonymous with undescended testes and is found in approximately 0.3 to 0.8% of the adult male population.[10] This anomaly represents a complete or incomplete failure of the intraabdominal testes to descend into the scrotal sac.

It will be recalled that in the fetus the testis arises within the celomic cavity, and then, by differential growth of the body as well as more rapid proliferation of the caudal end of the urogenital ridge, the testis comes to lie within the lower abdomen or brim of the pelvis, a process referred to as the internal descent. Following this, it descends through the inguinal canal into the scrotal sac — the external descent. On this basis, *malpositioned testes may be found at any point in this pathway of*

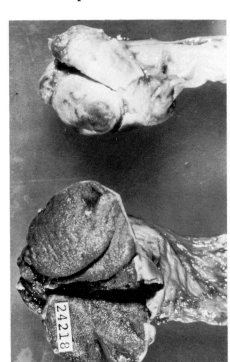

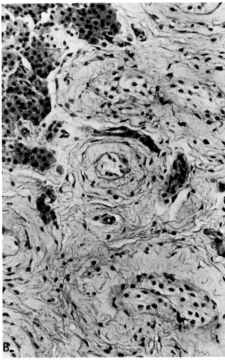

Figure 22-6. Testicular atrophy. A, The atrophic testis *(above)* is small and is replaced by white fibrous scars. Compare with cut surface of a normal testis *(below)*. B, Microscopically, the tubules are visible as shadowy structures with markedly thickened basement membranes. Note the prominence of Leydig cells in the upper left corner. (Courtesy of Dr. Fred Silva, Department of Pathology, University of Texas Health Science Center, Dallas.)

descent. The precise cause of cryptorchidism is still poorly understood. The vast majority of cases are idiopathic, but some cases are associated with specific genetic and hormonal factors. Cryptorchidism may be one of several congenital defects in chromosomal disorders such as trisomy 13. Because a normally functioning hypothalamic-pituitary axis is essential for testicular development and descent, cryptorchidism is associated with rare hormonal disorders that are characterized by a deficient secretion of luteinizing hormone–releasing hormone. In recent studies, testicular descent could be induced in some patients by administration of buserelin—an analogue of luteinizing hormone–releasing hormone.[11] The condition is completely asymptomatic, and it is found by the patient or the examining physician only when the scrotal sac is discovered not to contain the testis.

MORPHOLOGY. Cryptorchidism is unilateral in the majority of cases, but it may be bilateral in 25% of patients. Histologic changes in the malpositioned testis begin as early as two years of age. They are characterized by an arrest in the development of germ cells associated with marked hyalinization and thickening of the basement membrane of the spermatic tubules. Eventually the tubules appear as dense cords of hyaline connective tissue outlined by prominent basement membranes (Fig. 22-6). There is concomitant increase in interstitial stroma. Because Leydig cells are spared, they appear to be prominent. As might be expected with progressive tubular atrophy, the cryptorchid testis is small in size and is firm in consistency owing to fibrotic changes. Histologic deterioration, leading to a paucity of germ cells, has also been noted in the contralateral (descended) testis in patients with unilateral cryptorchidism, supporting a hormonal basis for the development of this condition.

Cryptorchidism is of more than academic interest for many reasons. When the testis lies in the inguinal canal, it is particularly exposed to trauma and crushing against the ligaments and bones. A concomitant inguinal hernia frequently accompanies such malposition of the testis. From the morphologic changes, it is apparent that bilateral cryptorchidism may result in sterility. Infertility, however, is also noted in a significant number of cases with uncorrected unilateral cryptorchidism because, as mentioned earlier, the contralateral descended testis may also be deficient in germ cells. In addition, the undescended testis is at a greater risk of developing testicular cancer than is the descended testis. It is generally accepted that cryptorchid patients have a 7- to 11-fold increase in the chance of developing a testicular tumor. The undescended testis requires surgical correction, preferably before histologic deterioration sets in at around two years of age.[12] Unfortunately, the placement of the testis within the scrotum does not preclude the possibility of a cancer developing at a later date, and fertility cannot be taken for granted. Indeed, malignant change may occur in the contralateral, normally descended testis. These observations suggest that cryptorchidism is associated with an intrinsic defect in testicular development and cellular differentiation that is unrelated to anatomic position.

REGRESSIVE CHANGES

Atrophy

Atrophy is the only important regressive change that affects the scrotal testis, and it may have a number of causes. These include (1) progressive atherosclerotic narrowing of the blood supply in old age; (2) the end stage of an inflammatory orchitis, whatever the etiologic agent; (3) cryptorchidism; (4) hypopituitarism; (5) generalized malnutrition, or cachexia; (6) obstruction to the outflow of semen; and (7) irradiation. In addition, (8) prolonged administration of female sex hormones, such as is used in treatment of patients with carcinoma of the prostate, may lead to atrophy, and (9) exhaustion atrophy may follow the persistent stimulation produced by high levels of follicle-stimulating pituitary hormone. The gross and microscopic alterations follow the pattern already described for cryptorchidism. When the process is bilateral, as it frequently is, sterility results. Atrophy or sometimes improper development of the testes occasionally occurs as a primary failure of genetic origin. The resulting condition, called Klinefelter syndrome, represents a sex chromosomal disorder that is discussed in detail in Chapter 5, along with other cytogenetic diseases.

INFLAMMATIONS

Inflammations are distinctly more common in the epididymis than in the testis. It is classically taught that, of the three major specific inflammatory states, *gonorrhea and tuberculosis almost invariably arise in the epididymis, whereas syphilis affects first the testis.*

Nonspecific Epididymitis and Orchitis

Epididymitis and possible subsequent orchitis are commonly related to infections in the urinary tract (cystitis, urethritis, genitoprostatitis), which presumably reach the epididymis and the testis through either the vas deferens or the lymphatics of the spermatic cord.

The cause of epididymitis varies with the age of the patient. Although uncommon in children, epididymitis in childhood is usually associated with a congenital genitourinary abnormality and infection with gram-negative rods. In sexually active men younger than age 35 years, the sexually transmitted pathogens *Chlamydia trachomatis* and *Neisseria gonorrhoeae* are the most frequent culprits. In men older than age 35, the common urinary tract pathogens, such as *Escherichia coli* and Pseudomonas, are responsible for most infections.[16]

MORPHOLOGY. The bacterial invasion sets up a nonspecific acute inflammation characterized by congestion, edema, and a white cell infiltration chiefly by neutrophils, macrophages, and lymphocytes. Although the infection, in the early stage, is more or less limited to the interstitial connective tissue, it rapidly extends to involve the tubules and may progress to frank abscess formation or complete suppurative necrosis of the entire epididymis. Usually, having involved the epididymis, the infection extends either by direct continuity or through tubular channels or lymphatics into the testis to evoke a similar inflammatory reaction within the testis. Such inflammatory involvement of the epididymis and testis is often followed by fibrous scarring, which, in many cases, leads to permanent sterility. Usually the interstitial cells of Leydig are not totally destroyed, so sexual activity is not disturbed. Any such nonspecific infection may become chronic.

Granulomatous (Autoimmune) Orchitis

Among middle-aged men, a rare cause of unilateral testicular enlargement is nontuberculous, granulomatous orchitis. It usually presents as a moderately tender testicular mass of sudden onset sometimes associated with fever. It may appear insidiously, however, as a painless testicular mass mimicking a testicular tumor, hence its importance.[13] Histologically the orchitis is distinguished by granulomas seen both within spermatic tubules and in the intertubular connective tissue. The lesions closely resemble tubercles but differ somewhat in having plasma cells and occasional neutrophils interspersed within the enclosing rim of fibroblasts and lymphocytes. Although an autoimmune basis is suspected, the cause of these lesions remains unknown.

Specific Inflammations

GONORRHEA. Extension of infection from the posterior urethra to the prostate, seminal vesicles, and thence to the epididymis is the usual course of a neglected gonococcal infection. Inflammatory changes similar to those described in the nonspecific infections occur, with the development of frank abscesses in the epididymis, resulting in extensive destruction of this organ. In the more ne-

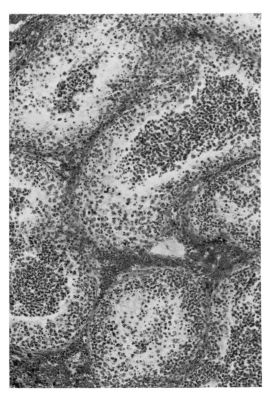

Figure 22–7. Acute severe mumps orchitis with extensive interstitial and intratubular exudation.

glected cases, the infection may thence spread to the testis and produce a suppurative orchitis.

MUMPS. Mumps is a systemic viral disease that most commonly affects school-aged children. Testicular involvement is extremely uncommon in this age group. In postpubertal males, however, orchitis may develop and has been reported in 20 to 30% of male patients. Most often, the acute interstitial orchitis develops about 1 week following onset of swelling of the parotid glands. Rarely cases of orchitis precede the parotitis or may be unaccompanied by parotid gland involvement.

The testicular involvement is unilateral in approximately 70% of the cases. In the acute stage, the inflammatory reaction is characterized by intense interstitial edema and mononuclear infiltration, consisting chiefly of lymphocytes, plasma cells, and macrophages. Neutrophils are usually not prominent, but in the more intense inflammatory responses frank suppuration may develop, and the tubular lumina may become filled with purulent exudate (Fig. 22–7). Because the process usually is unilateral, remains largely interstitial, and is characteristically patchy and haphazard, healing of the inflammatory reaction is usually not associated with infertility.

TUBERCULOSIS. *Tuberculosis almost invariably begins in the epididymis and may spread to the testis.* In many of these cases, there is associated tuberculous prostatitis and seminal vesiculitis, and it is believed that epididymitis usually represents a secondary spread from these other involvements of the genital tract.

The infection invokes the classic morphologic reactions of granulomatous inflammation characteristic of tuberculosis elsewhere.

SYPHILIS. The testis and epididymis are affected in both acquired and congenital syphilis, but *almost invariably the testis is involved first by the infection.* In many cases, the orchitis is not accompanied by epididymitis. The morphologic pattern of the reaction takes two forms: the production of gummas or a diffuse interstitial inflammation characterized by edema and lymphocytic and plasma cell infiltration with the characteristic hallmark of all syphilitic infections, i.e., obliterative endarteritis with perivascular cuffing of lymphocytes and plasma cells.

VASCULAR DISTURBANCES

TORSION. Twisting of the spermatic cord may cut off the venous drainage and the arterial supply to the testis. Usually, however, the thick-walled arteries remain patent so that intense vascular engorgement and venous infarction follow. The usual precipitating cause of such torsion is some violent movement or physical trauma. In most instances, however, there are predisposing causes, such as incomplete descent, absence of the scrotal ligaments or the gubernaculum testis, atrophy of the testis so it is abnormally mobile within the tunica vaginalis, abnormal attachment of the testis to the epididymis, or other abnormalities.

MORPHOLOGY. Depending on the duration of the process, the morphologic changes range from intense congestion to widespread extravasation of blood into the interstitial tissue of the testis and epididymis. Eventually hemorrhagic infarction of the entire testis occurs (Fig. 22–8). In these late stages, the testis is markedly enlarged and is con-

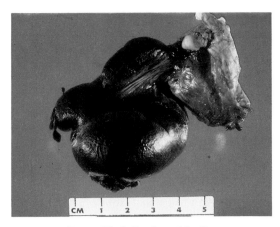

Figure 22–8. Torsion of testis.

verted virtually into a sac of soft, necrotic, hemorrhagic tissue.

TESTICULAR TUMORS

Testicular neoplasms span an amazing gamut of anatomic types. They are divided into two major categories: germ cell tumors and nongerminal tumors
derived from stroma or sex cord. Approximately
95% arise from germ cells. Most of these germinal
tumors are highly aggressive cancers capable of
rapid, wide dissemination, although with current
therapy the outlook for these patients has improved considerably. Many when limited to the
testis can be cured, and even with disseminated
tumors complete remissions can be achieved. Nongerminal tumors, in contrast, are generally benign,
but some elaborate steroids leading to interesting
endocrinologic syndromes.

Germ Cell Tumors

The incidence of testicular tumors in the United
States is approximately two per 100,000 males.
They cause about 0.15% of all male cancer deaths.
In the 15- to 34-year age group, when these neoplasms have a peak incidence, they constitute the
most common tumor of males and cause approximately 10% of all cancer deaths. Two smaller
peaks of incidence are encountered, in infancy and
in later life.

CLASSIFICATION AND HISTOGENESIS. Classifications of the testicular germ cell tumors abound
and, regrettably, vary widely. The major problems
are the differing concepts of the histogenesis of
these lesions and the endless variability in morphology among the various forms of neoplasms as
well as within a single tumor. As one might guess,
germ cells are multipotential, and once they become cancerous, they are not inhibited in their
lines of differentiation. Table 22–1 shows the
World Health Organization (WHO) classification,
most widely used in the United States. The proposed histogenesis of germ cell tumors of the testis
follows.

Testicular germ cell tumors may be divided
into two categories, based on whether they are
composed of a single histologic pattern or more
than one. Tumors with a *single* histologic pattern
constitute about 40% of all testicular neoplasms
and are listed in Table 22–1. In approximately
60% of the tumors, there is a *mixture of two or
more of the histologic patterns*. The most common
mixture is that of teratoma, embryonal carcinoma,
yolk sac tumor, and elements of choriocarcinoma.

The **WHO** classification is based on the view

Table 22–1. WHO PATHOLOGIC CLASSIFICATION OF
TESTICULAR TUMORS

GERM CELL TUMORS
  Tumors of one histologic pattern
    Seminoma
    Spermatocytic seminoma
    Embryonal carcinoma
    Yolk sac tumor (embryonal carcinoma, infantile type)
    Polyembryoma
    Choriocarcinoma
    Teratomas
      Mature
      Immature
      With malignant transformation
  Tumors showing more than one histologic pattern
    Embryonal carcinoma plus teratoma (teratocarcinoma)
    Choriocarcinoma and any other types (specify types)
    Other combinations (specify)
SEX CORD–STROMAL TUMORS
  Well-differentiated forms
    Leydig cell tumor
    Sertoli cell tumor
    Granulosa cell tumor
  Mixed forms (specify)
  Incompletely differentiated forms

that most tumors in this group originate from intratubular testicular germ cells. The precise relationship between the various histologic subtypes of
germ cell tumors is not clear. According to one
widely held view, the neoplastic germ cells may
give rise to seminoma, or they may transform into
totipotential tumor cells represented by embryonal
carcinoma. According to this view, embryonal carcinomas contain stem cells for all nonseminomatous
tumors. Depending on the line of differentiation of
embryonal carcinoma cells, tumors with different
histologic patterns result. The most undifferentiated state is represented by pure embryonal cell
carcinoma, whereas choriocarcinoma and yolk sac
tumor represent tumors in which the cells assume
the appearance of specific extraembryonic cell
types. Teratoma results from differentiation of the
embryonic carcinoma cells along the lines of all
three germ cell layers, and therefore teratomas
contain the greatest variety of neoplastic cells and
tissues. Some recent studies suggest that seminomas are not end-stage neoplasms. Like embryonal
carcinomas, seminomas may also act as precursors
from which other forms of testicular germ cell
tumors originate.[14] Although the precise histogenesis is of considerable interest in understanding the
histologic heterogeneity of testicular germ cell
tumors, the student will be relieved to note that
from a clinical standpoint there are only two important categories of germ cell tumors: seminomas
and nonseminomatous tumors. As will be discussed
later, this clinical distinction has important bear-
ings on treatment and prognosis.

PATHOGENESIS. As with all neoplasms, little is
known about the ultimate cause of germ cell
tumors. Several predisposing influences, however,

may be important: (1) cryptorchidism, (2) genetic factors, and (3) testicular dysgenesis, all of which may contribute to a common denominator—germ cell maldevelopment. Reference has already been made to the increased incidence of neoplasms in *undescended testes*. In most large series of testicular tumors, approximately 10% are associated with cryptorchidism.[15] The higher the location of the undescended testicle (intra-abdominal versus inguinal), the greater is the risk of developing cancer. The factors impinging on the cryptorchid testis that contribute to this increased risk of oncogenesis are not clear.

Genetic predisposition also seems to be important, although no well-defined pattern of inheritance has been identified. In support, striking racial differences in the incidence of testicular tumors can be cited. Blacks in Africa have an extremely low incidence of these neoplasms, which is unaffected by migration to the United States. Familial clustering has been reported, and according to one study, sibs of affected individuals have a tenfold higher risk of developing testicular cancer as compared with the general population.[16]

Patients with disorders of testicular development (testicular dysgenesis), including testicular feminization and Klinefelter syndrome, harbor an increased risk of developing germ cell tumors. The risk is highest in patients with testicular feminization.[17]

Regardless of the precise etiology, certain cytogenetic changes involving chromosomes 12 and 1 occur with regularity in all germ cell tumors. Much interest is focused on the isochromosome of the short arm of chromosome 12, i(12p), which is present in approximately 90% of these neoplasms, regardless of the histologic type. This abnormality is so rare in other tumor types that its presence is considered virtually diagnostic of a germ cell tumor.[18] It is of interest that i(12p) is also noted in ovarian germ cell neoplasms, suggesting that the events leading to this alteration may be critical to the molecular pathogenesis of germ cell neoplasms. The gene or genes on i(12p) that might be important in neoplastic transformation of germ cells have yet to be identified. In addition to the presence of i(12p), nonrandom gains of chromosomes 1, 7, 9, 12, 17, 21, 22, or X are seen in about 70% of the tumors.

With this background of pathogenesis, we can discuss the morphologic patterns of germ cell tumors, followed by the clinical features common to most germinal tumors.[19] The student can take comfort in the fact that some of the tumors listed in Table 22–1 are sufficiently rare to justify exclusion from the following discussion.

Seminoma

Seminomas are the most common type of germinal tumor (30%) and the type most likely to produce a uniform population of cells. They almost never

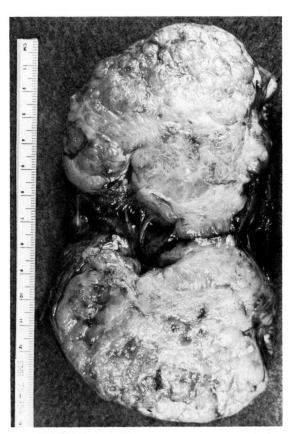

Figure 22–9. Seminoma. Testis is enlarged and virtually replaced by lobulated, homogeneous, gray-white tumor tissue. Hemorrhage and necrosis are not prominent. (Courtesy of Dr. Fred Silva, Department of Pathology, University of Texas Health Science Center, Dallas.)

occur in infants; they peak in the fourth decade, somewhat later than the collective peak. A nearly identical tumor arises in the ovary, where it is called dysgerminoma (see Chapter 23).

MORPHOLOGY. Three histologic variants of seminoma are described: typical (85%), anaplastic (5 to 10%), and spermatocytic (4 to 6%). The last-mentioned has been segregated into a separate category in the WHO classification and will be discussed later. All produce bulky masses, sometimes ten times the size of the normal testis.

The typical seminoma has a homogeneous, gray-white, lobulated cut surface, usually devoid of hemorrhage or necrosis (Fig. 22–9). In more than half the cases, the entire testis is replaced. Generally, the tunica albuginea is not penetrated, but occasionally extension to the epididymis, spermatic cord, or scrotal sac occurs.

Microscopically, the typical seminoma presents sheets of uniform, so-called seminoma cells divided into poorly demarcated lobules by delicate septa of fibrous tissue. **The classic seminoma cell is large and round-to-polyhedral and has a distinct cell membrane, a clear or watery-appearing cy-**

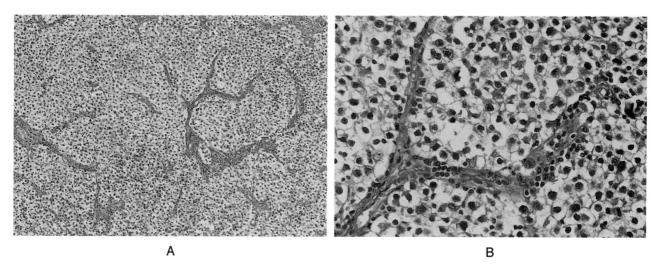

Figure 22-10. Seminoma. *A*, Low magnification shows clear seminoma cells divided into poorly demarcated lobules by delicate septa. *B*, High magnification shows clear cells with distinct cell membranes and lymphocytes infiltrating the septa. (Courtesy of Dr. Trace Worrell, Department of Pathology, University of Texas Southwestern Medical School, Dallas.)

toplasm, and a large, central hyperchromatic nucleus with one or two prominent nucleoli (Fig. 22–10). Mitoses are infrequent. The cytoplasm contains varying amounts of glycogen and, rarely, lipid vacuoles. Classic seminoma cells do not contain alpha-fetoprotein (AFP) or human chorionic gonadotropin (HCG). The tumor cells do stain positively for placental alkaline phosphatase.

Approximately 10% of seminomas contain syncytial giant cells that resemble the syncytiotrophoblast of the placenta both morphologically and in that they contain HCG. In this subset of patients, serum HCG levels are also elevated. The amount of stroma in typical seminomas varies greatly. Sometimes it is scant and at other times abundant. Usually, well-defined fibrous strands are present, creating lobules of neoplastic cells. The septa are usually infiltrated with T lymphocytes, and in some tumors they also bear prominent granulomas, that is, aggregates of histiocytes enclosed within a rim of fibroblasts and lymphocytes.

The anaplastic seminoma, as the name indicates, presents greater cellular and nuclear irregularity with more frequent tumor giant cells and many mitoses. Most critical to the identification of this pattern are the size of the cells and the presence of three or more mitoses per high-power field.

Spermatocytic Seminoma

Although related by name to seminoma, spermatocytic seminoma appears to be a distinctive tumor both clinically and histologically. It is an uncommon tumor, the reported incidence being approximately 4 to 6% of all seminomas. The age of involvement is much later than for most testicular tumors: Affected individuals are generally over the age of 65 years. In contrast to classic seminoma, it is a slow-growing tumor that rarely if ever produces metastases, and hence the prognosis is excellent.

MORPHOLOGY. Grossly, spermatocytic seminoma tends to be larger than classic seminoma and presents with a pale gray, soft, and friable cut surface. Spermatocytic seminomas have three cell populations, all intermixed: (1) medium-sized cells (15 to 18 μm), the most numerous, containing a round nucleus and eosinophilic cytoplasm; (2) smaller cells (6 to 8 μm), with a narrow rim of eosinophilic cytoplasm resembling secondary spermatocytes; and (3) scattered giant cells (50 to 100 μm), either uninucleate or multinucleate. With the electron microscope, tumor cells show nuclear and cytoplasmic features of spermatocytic maturation, thus justifying the term spermatocytic seminoma.

Embryonal Carcinoma

Embryonal carcinomas occur mostly in the 20- to 30-year age group. Although considerable progress has been made in treating these tumors, they are more aggressive than seminomas.

MORPHOLOGY. Grossly, the tumor is smaller than seminoma and usually does not replace the entire testis. On cut surfaces, the mass is often variegated, poorly demarcated at the margins, and punctuated by foci of hemorrhage or necrosis (Fig. 22–11). Extension through the tunica albuginea into the epididymis or cord is not infrequent. **Histologically, the cells grow in glandular, alveolar, or tubular patterns, sometimes with papillary convolutions** (Fig. 22–12). **More undifferentiated lesions may present sheets of cells.** The neoplastic cells

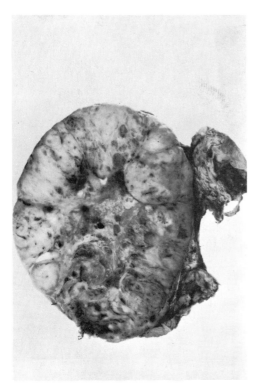

Figure 22-11. Embryonal carcinoma with extensive mottled necrosis and hemorrhage.

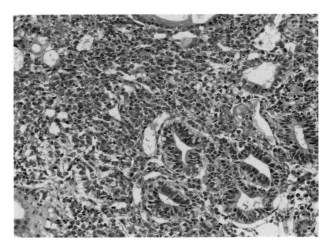

Figure 22-12. Embryonal carcinoma shows sheets of undifferentiated cells as well as glandular differentiation. The nuclei are large and hyperchromatic. (Courtesy of Dr. Trace Worrell, Department of Pathology, University of Texas Southwestern Medical School, Dallas.)

have an epithelial appearance and are large and anaplastic, with angry-looking hyperchromatic nuclei having prominent nucleoli. In contrast to seminoma, the cell borders are usually indistinct, and there is considerable variation in cell and nuclear size and shape. Mitotic figures and tumor giant cells are frequent. **Within this background, syncytial cells containing HCG or cells containing AFP, or both, may be detected by immunoperoxidase techniques. Because HCG and AFP are products of trophoblastic and yolk sac cells, respectively, their presence is indicative of a mixed tumor.**

If tumors containing HCG or AFP, or both, are excluded, it is estimated that pure embryonal cell carcinomas constitute about 3% of testicular germ cell tumors. If one includes mixed tumors, however, embryonal carcinoma cells are present in about 45% of tumors.

Yolk Sac Tumor

Also known as infantile embryonal carcinoma or endodermal sinus tumor, the yolk sac tumor is of interest because it is the most common testicular tumor in infants and children up to three years of age, and in this age group it has a very good prognosis. In adults the pure form of this tumor is rare; instead, yolk sac elements frequently occur in combination with embryonal carcinoma.

MORPHOLOGY. Grossly, the tumor is nonencapsulated, and on cross section it presents a homogeneous, yellow-white, mucinous appearance. Characteristic on microscopic examination is a lace-like (reticular) network of medium-sized cuboidal or elongated cells. In addition, papillary structures or solid cords of cells may be found. In approximately 50% of tumors, the so-called endodermal sinuses may be seen; these consist of a mesodermal core with a central capillary and a visceral and parietal layer of cells resembling primitive glomeruli. Present within and outside the cytoplasm are eosinophilic, hyalin-like globules in which AFP and alpha$_1$-antitrypsin can be demonstrated by immunocytochemical staining. The presence of AFP in the tumor cells is highly characteristic, and it underscores their differentiation into yolk sac cells.

Choriocarcinoma

This highly malignant form of testicular tumor is composed of both cytotrophoblast and syncytiotrophoblast. Identical tumors may arise in the placental tissue, ovary, or sequestered rests of totipotential cells, e.g., in the mediastinum or abdomen. Fortunately, in its "pure" form it is rare, constituting less than 1% of all germ cell tumors. As emphasized later, foci of choriocarcinoma are much more common in mixed patterns.

MORPHOLOGY. Despite their aggressive behavior, pure choriocarcinomas are usually small lesions. **Often they cause no testicular enlargement and are detected only as a small palpable nodule.** Because they are rapidly growing, they may out-

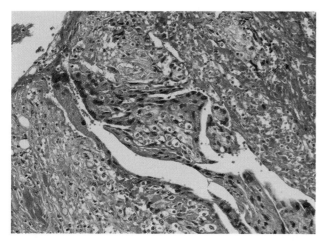

Figure 22–13. Choriocarcinoma shows clear cytotrophoblastic cells with central nuclei and syncytiotrophoblastic cells with multiple dark nuclei embedded in eosinophilic cytoplasm. Hemorrhage and necrosis are seen in the upper right field. (Courtesy of Dr. Trace Worrell, Department of Pathology, University of Texas Southwestern Medical School, Dallas.)

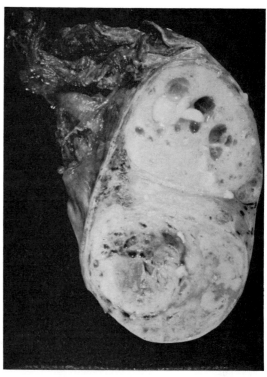

Figure 22–14. Teratoma of testis. The variegated cut surface reflects the multiplicity of tissue found histologically.

grow their blood supply, and sometimes the primary testicular focus is replaced by a small fibrous scar, leaving only widespread metastases. Typically, these tumors are small, rarely larger than 5 cm in diameter. Hemorrhage and necrosis are extremely common. Histologically, the tumors contain two cell types (Fig. 22–13). The syncytiotrophoblastic cell is large and has many irregular or lobular hyperchromatic nuclei and an abundant eosinophilic vacuolated cytoplasm. As might be expected, HCG can be readily demonstrated in the cytoplasm of syncytiotrophoblastic cells. The cytotrophoblastic cells are more regular and tend to be polygonal with distinct cell borders and clear cytoplasm; they grow in cords or masses and have a single, fairly uniform nucleus. Although most tumors contain both cellular elements, the presence of syncytiotrophoblast alone, documented by the presence of HCG in the cytoplasm, is considered adequate for diagnosis. More anatomic details are available in the discussion of these neoplasms in the female genital tract (see Chapter 23).

Teratoma

The designation teratoma refers to a group of complex tumors having various cellular or organoid components reminiscent of normal derivatives from more than one germ layer. They may occur at any age from infancy to adult life. Pure forms of teratoma are fairly common in infants and children, second only in frequency to yolk sac tumors. In adults, pure teratomas are rare, constituting 2 to 3% of germ cell tumors. As with embryonal carci-

nomas, their frequency in combination with other histologic types is about 45%.

MORPHOLOGY. Grossly, teratomas are usually large, ranging from 5 to 10 cm in diameter. Because they are composed of various tissues, the gross appearance is heterogeneous with solid, sometimes cartilaginous and cystic areas (Fig. 22–14). Hemorrhage and necrosis usually indicate admixture with embryonal carcinoma, choriocarcinoma, or both.

Histologically three variants are recognized, based on the degree of differentiation.

Mature teratomas are composed of a heterogeneous, helter-skelter collection of differentiated cells or organoid structures such as neural tissue, muscle bundles, islands of cartilage, clusters of squamous epithelium, structures reminiscent of thyroid gland, bronchial or bronchiolar epithelium, and bits of intestinal wall or brain substance, all embedded in a fibrous or myxoid stroma (Fig. 22–15). All the elements are differentiated. This mature variant occurs with relatively greater frequency in infancy and childhood. Similar tumors may occur in adults, but there is a far greater risk of small hidden foci of immature or malignant components that may escape detection despite rigorous sampling of the lesion. Thus, although teratomas may appear entirely mature and benign, such a diagnosis in an adult must be made with circumspection. Dermoid cysts, common in the ovary (see Chapter 23), are

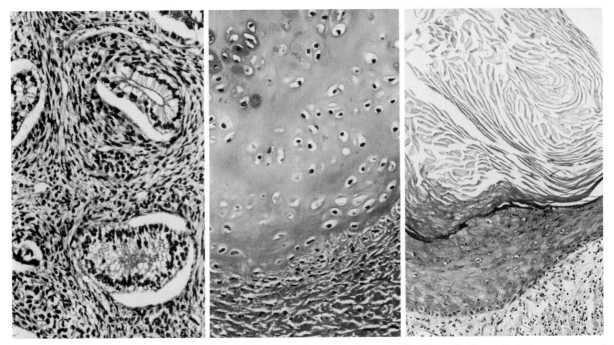

Figure 22–15. Mature teratoma. Three different fields from the same tumor with (1) well-differentiated mucus-secreting gland reminiscent of colonic (endodermal) mucosa on the left, (2) hyaline cartilage (mesodermal) in the middle, and (3) squamous stratified keratinizing epithelium (ectodermal) on the right. (Courtesy of Dr. Fred Silva, Department of Pathology, University of Texas Health Science Center, Dallas.)

rare in the testis. They represent a special form of mature teratoma.

Immature teratomas can be viewed as intermediate between mature teratoma and embryonal carcinoma. In contrast to the mature teratoma, elements of the three germ cell layers are incompletely differentiated and not arranged in organoid fashion. Even though the differentiation is incomplete, the nature of the embryonic tissue can be clearly identified; thus, poorly formed cartilage, neuroblasts, loose mesenchyme, and clusters of glandular structures may be seen lying helter-skelter. In some areas, more mature forms of these tissues may also be seen. Although these tumors are clearly malignant, they may not display clear-cut cytologic features of malignancy.

In contrast, the third variant—**teratoma with malignant transformation**—shows clear evidence of malignancy in derivatives of one or more germ cell layers. Thus, there may be a focus of squamous cell carcinoma, mucin-secreting adenocarcinoma, or a sarcoma. Immature and frankly malignant teratomas occur more commonly in adults.

In the child, differentiated mature teratomas may be expected to behave as benign tumors, and almost all these patients have a good prognosis. In the adult, it is difficult to be certain because, as pointed out, even apparently differentiated mature teratomas may harbor minute foci of cancer and should therefore be treated as malignant tumors.

Mixed Tumors

About 60% of testicular tumors are composed of more than one of the "pure" patterns. The most common mixture is that of teratoma, embryonal carcinoma, yolk sac tumor, and HCG-containing syncytiotrophoblast. Tumors with such a combination constitute 14% of testicular germ cell tumors. Other combinations include seminoma with embryonal carcinoma and embryonal carcinoma with teratoma. The latter has been called teratocarcinoma. In most instances, the prognosis is worsened by the inclusion of more aggressive elements: e.g., the teratoma with a focus of choriocarcinoma has a poorer outlook than that of pure teratoma. It is noteworthy that metastases of these mixed tumors may be composed of one or more of the various neoplastic components, and indeed a new line of differentiation sometimes appears.

CLINICAL FEATURES OF TESTICULAR TUMORS. From a clinical standpoint, tumors of the testis are segregated into two broad categories: *seminoma* and *nonseminomatous* germ cell tumors (NSGCT). The latter is an umbrella designation that includes tumors of one histologic type such as embryonal cell carcinoma as well as those with more than one histologic pattern. As is evident from the later discussion, seminomas and NSGCT not only present with somewhat distinctive clinical features, but also they differ with respect to therapy and prognosis. First we offer some general comments on the clinical manifestations of testicular tumors as a group.

Painless enlargement of the testis is the most common presenting feature of germ cell neoplasms. Indeed, any testicular mass should be considered neoplastic unless proved otherwise. Clinical differentiation between various types of germ cell tumors is at best imperfect because there are no distinctive clinical features to the testicular masses produced by these tumors.

Testicular tumors have a characteristic mode of spread, the knowledge of which is helpful in treatment. Lymphatic spread is common to all forms of testicular tumors, and in general retroperitoneal para-aortic nodes are the first to be involved. Subsequent spread may occur to mediastinal and supraclavicular nodes. Hematogenous spread is primarily to the lungs, but liver, brain, and bones may also be involved. Although most testicular tumors metastasize "true," the histology of metastases may sometimes be different from that of the testicular lesion. Thus an embryonal carcinoma may present a teratomatous picture in the secondary deposits. Conversely, a teratoma may show foci of choriocarcinoma in the lymph nodes. As discussed earlier, because all these tumors are derived from totipotential germ cells, the apparent "forward" and "backward" differentiation seen in different locations is not entirely surprising.

With this background, we can highlight the differences between seminoma and NSGCT. Seminomas tend to remain localized to the testis for a long time, and hence approximately 70% present in clinical stage I (see below). In contrast, approximately 60% of patients with NSGCT present with advanced clinical disease (stages II and III). Metastases from seminomas typically involve lymph nodes. Hematogenous spread occurs later in the course of dissemination. NSGCT not only metastasize earlier, but also use the hematogenous route more frequently. The rare choriocarcinoma is the most aggressive of NSGCT. It may not cause any testicular enlargement but instead spreads predominantly and rapidly by the bloodstream. Therefore, lungs and liver are involved early in virtually every case. From a therapeutic viewpoint, seminomas are extremely radiosensitive, whereas NSGCT are relatively radioresistant. To summarize, as compared with seminomas, NSGCT are biologically more aggressive and in general have a poorer prognosis.

Three clinical stages of testicular tumors are defined:

- Stage I: tumor confined to the testis
- Stage II: distant spread confined to retroperitoneal nodes below the diaphragm
- Stage III: metastases outside the retroperitoneal nodes or above the diaphragm

Stages II and III are further subdivided ("early" or "advanced") based on tumor burden in the secondary deposits.

Germ cell tumors of the testis often secrete polypeptide hormones and certain enzymes that can be detected in blood by sensitive assays. Such "biologic markers" include HCG, AFP, placental alkaline phosphatase, placental lactogen, and lactic dehydrogenase. HCG and AFP are widely used clinically and have proved to be valuable in the diagnosis and management of testicular cancer.[20]

AFP is the major serum protein of the early fetus and is synthesized by the fetal gut, liver cells, and yolk sac. One year after birth, the serum levels of AFP fall to less than 16 ng/ml, which is undetectable except by the most sensitive assays. HCG is a glycoprotein consisting of two dissimilar polypeptide units called alpha and beta. It is normally synthesized and secreted by the placental syncytiotrophoblast. The beta subunit of HCG has unique sequences not shared with other human glycoprotein hormones, and therefore the detection of HCG in the serum is based on a radioimmunoassay using antibodies to its beta chain. As might be expected from the histogenesis and morphology, elevated levels of these markers are most often associated with nonseminomatous tumors. Yolk sac tumors produce AFP exclusively, and choriocarcinomas elaborate only HCG. Either or both of these markers are elevated in more than 80% of patients with NSGCT at the time of diagnosis. In passing, it might be noted that elevated serum levels of AFP are also encountered with liver cell carcinomas. In the context of testicular tumors, the value of serum markers is threefold:

- In the evaluation of testicular masses.
- In the staging of testicular germ cell tumors. For example, following orchiectomy, persistent elevation of HCG or AFP indicates stage II disease even if the lymph nodes appear of normal size by computed tomography (CT) scanning.
- In monitoring the response to therapy. After eradication of tumors, there is a rapid fall in serum level of AFP and HCG. With serial measurements, it is often possible to predict recurrence before the patients become symptomatic or develop any other clinical signs of relapse.

The significance of elevated serum HCG levels in some patients with seminoma is not fully understood. The serum HCG is derived from the syncytial giant cells known to occur in some seminomas. According to current opinion, detection of HCG in the serum of patients with seminoma does not alter their prognosis.

The therapy and prognosis of testicular tumors depend largely on clinical stage and on the histologic type. Seminoma, which is extremely radiosensitive and tends to remain localized for long periods, has the best prognosis. More than 90% of patients with stage I and II disease can be cured. Among nonseminomatous tumors, the histologic subtype does not influence the prognosis significantly, and hence these are treated as a group.

Although they do not share the excellent prognosis of seminoma, 80 to 85% can achieve complete remission with aggressive chemotherapy, and most can be cured.

Tumors of Sex Cord– Gonadal Stroma

As indicated in Table 22–1, these tumors are subclassified based on their presumed histogenesis and differentiation. The two most important members of this group—Leydig cell tumors (derived from the stroma) and Sertoli cell tumors (derived from the sex cord)—are described here. Details of these tumors, and others not described, may be found in a recent review.[21]

Leydig (Interstitial) Cell Tumors

Tumors of Leydig cells are particularly interesting because they may elaborate androgens or androgens and estrogens, and, indeed, some have also elaborated corticosteroids. They arise at any age, although the majority of the reported cases have been noted between 20 and 60 years of age. As with other testicular tumors, the most common presenting feature is testicular swelling, but in some patients gynecomastia may be the first symptom. In children, hormonal effects, manifested primarily as sexual precocity, are the dominating features.

MORPHOLOGY. These neoplasms form circumscribed nodules, usually less than 5 cm in diameter. They have a distinctive golden-brown, homogeneous cut surface. Histologically, tumorous Leydig cells usually are remarkably similar to their normal forebears in that they are large and round or polygonal, and they have an abundant granular eosinophilic cytoplasm with a round central nucleus. Cell boundaries are often indistinct. The cytoplasm frequently contains lipid granules, vacuoles, or lipofuscin pigment, but, most characteristically, rod-shaped crystalloids of Reinke occur in about 25% of the tumors. Approximately 10% of the tumors in adults are invasive and produce metastases; most are benign.

Sertoli Cell Tumors (Androblastoma)

These tumors may be composed entirely of Sertoli cells or may have a component of granulosa cells. Some induce endocrinologic changes. Either estrogens or androgens may be elaborated but only infrequently in sufficient quantity to cause precocious masculinization or feminization. Occasionally, as with Leydig cell tumors gynecomastia appears.

MORPHOLOGY. These neoplasms appear as firm, small nodules with a homogeneous gray-white to yellow cut surface. Histologically, the tumor cells are arranged in distinctive trabeculae with a tendency to form cord-like structures resembling immature seminiferous tubules. The great majority of Sertoli cell tumors are benign, but occasional tumors (approximately 10%) are more anaplastic and pursue a malignant course.

Testicular Lymphoma

Although not primarily a tumor of the testis, testicular lymphoma is included here because affected patients present with only a testicular mass. *Lymphomas account for 5% of testicular neoplasms and constitute the most common form of testicular cancer in men over the age of 60.* In most cases, disseminated disease is already present at the time of detection of the testicular mass; only rarely does it remain confined to the testis. The histologic type in almost all cases is the diffuse large cell lymphoma (see non-Hodgkin's lymphomas, Chapter 14). The prognosis is extremely poor.

MISCELLANEOUS LESIONS OF TUNICA VAGINALIS

Brief mention should be made of the tunica vaginalis. As a serosa-lined sac immediately proximal to the testis and epididymis, it may become involved by any lesion arising in these two structures. Clear serous fluid may accumulate from neighboring infections or tumors, often spontaneously and without apparent cause *(hydrocele)*. Considerable enlargement of the scrotal sac is produced, which can be readily mistaken for testicular enlargement. By transillumination, however, it is usually possible to define the clear, translucent character of the contained substance, and many times the opaque testis can be outlined within this fluid-filled space.

Hematocele indicates the presence of blood in the tunica vaginalis. It is an uncommon condition usually encountered only when there has been either direct trauma to the testis or torsion of the testis with hemorrhagic suffusion into the surrounding tunica vaginalis or in hemorrhagic diseases associated with widespread bleeding diatheses.

Chylocele refers to the accumulation of lymph in the tunica and is almost always found in patients with elephantiasis who have widespread, severe lymphatic obstruction. For clarity's sake, mention should be made of the *spermatocele* and *varicocele*, which refer respectively to a small cystic accumulation of semen or to a dilated vein in the spermatic cord.

PROSTATE

Consideration of prostatic diseases will be facilitated by a brief introduction to the normal anatomy of the prostate. In the normal adult, the prostate weighs approximately 20 gm. It is a retroperitoneal organ encircling the neck of the bladder and urethra and is devoid of a distinct capsule. Classically, the prostate has been divided into five lobes, to which are attributed distinctive significance in the development of tumors and benign enlargements. These five lobes include a posterior, middle, and anterior lobe and two lateral lobes. These subdivisions, however, can be recognized only in the embryo. In the course of development, the five become fused into only three distinct lobes—two major lateral lobes and a small median lobe, which presumably includes the classic posterior lobe. Cross section of the gland, however, fails to disclose well-defined lobes, and only two lateral masses can be found on either side of the urethra as well as a much thinner median lobe, which forms the floor of the urethra.

Histologically, the prostate is a compound tubuloalveolar gland, which, in one plane of section, presents small to fairly large glandular spaces lined by epithelium. Characteristically, the glands are lined by two layers of cells: a basal layer of low cuboidal epithelium covered by a layer of columnar mucus-secreting cells. In many areas, there are small villous projections or papillary inbuddings of the epithelium. These glands all have a distinct basement membrane and are separated by an abundant fibromuscular stroma. Testicular androgens are clearly of prime importance in controlling prostatic growth because castration leads to atrophy of the prostate.

The only three pathologic processes that affect the prostate gland with sufficient frequency to merit discussion are inflammation, benign nodular enlargement, and tumors. Of these three, the benign nodular enlargements are by far the most common and occur so often in advanced age that they can almost be construed as a "normal" aging process. Prostatic carcinoma is also an extremely common lesion in men and therefore merits careful consideration. The inflammatory processes are, for the most part, of less clinical significance and can be treated briefly.

INFLAMMATIONS

Prostatitis may be divided into three categories: *acute* and *chronic bacterial prostatitis* and *chronic abacterial prostatitis.*[22] Differentiation among these

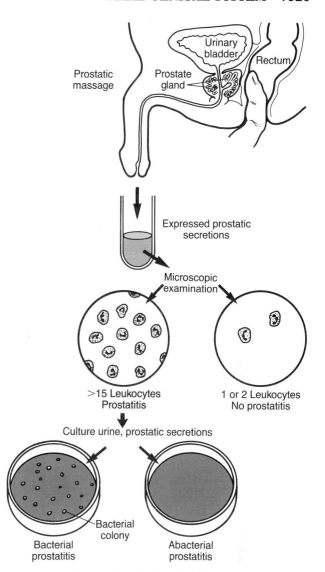

Figure 22-16. Prostatitis—bacterial and abacterial.

entities is based on quantitative bacterial cultures and microscopic examination of fractionated urine specimens and expressed prostatic secretions. If the first voided 10 ml of urine (urethral specimen) and the midstream urine (bladder specimen) do not show pyuria, the presence of more than 15 leukocytes per high-power field in prostatic secretions obtained by transrectal prostatic massage is considered diagnostic of prostatitis. Typically, the leukocytes are accompanied by fat-laden macrophages. In bacterial prostatitis (acute or chronic), cultures of expressed prostatic secretions are positive for bacterial growth, and the quantitative bacterial counts are significantly (>1 logarithm) higher than in cultures of urethral and bladder urine. In chronic abacterial prostatitis, however, the prostatic secretions are consistently negative for bacterial growth despite unambiguous evidence of prostatic inflammation (Fig. 22-16). Distinction between the three forms of prostatitis is important because treatment differs. In the ensuing discussion, the three conditions are characterized first, and then the morphologic features of all the forms are described together.

Acute bacterial prostatitis consists of an acute focal or diffuse suppurative inflammation in the prostatic substance. The bacteria responsible are similar in type and in incidence to those that cause urinary tract infections (UTI). Thus, most cases are caused by various strains of *E. coli*, other gram-negative rods, enterococci, and staphylococci. The organisms become implanted in the prostate usually by intraprostatic reflux of urine from the posterior urethra or from the urinary bladder, but occasionally they seed the prostate by the lympho-hematogenous routes from distant foci of infection. Prostatitis sometimes follows some surgical manipulation on the urethra or prostate gland itself, such as catheterization, cystoscopy, urethral dilatation, or resection procedures on the prostate. Clinically, acute bacterial prostatitis is associated with fever, chills, and dysuria. On rectal examination, the prostate is exquisitely tender and boggy. The diagnosis can be established by urine culture and clinical features.

Chronic bacterial prostatitis is difficult to diagnose and treat. It may present with low back pain, dysuria, and perineal and suprapubic discomfort. Alternatively, it may be virtually asymptomatic. *A very common historical characteristic is recurrent urinary tract infections (cystitis, urethritis) caused by the same organism.* Because most antibiotics penetrate the prostate poorly, bacteria find safe haven in the parenchyma and constantly seed the urinary tract. Diagnosis of chronic bacterial prostatitis depends on the documentation of leukocytosis in the expressed prostatic secretions along with positive bacterial cultures in the prostatic secretions. In the great majority of cases, there is no antecedent acute attack, and the disease appears insidiously and without obvious provocation. The implicated organisms are the same as those cited as causes of acute prostatitis.

Chronic abacterial prostatitis is the most common form of prostatitis seen today. *Clinically it is indistinguishable from chronic bacterial prostatitis. There is no history, however, of recurrent urinary tract infection.* Expressed prostatic secretions contain more than 15 leukocytes per high-power field, but bacterial cultures are uniformly negative. Because the affected patients are usually sexually active men, several sexually transmitted pathogens have been implicated. Both *Chlamydia trachomatis* and *Ureaplasma urealyticum* remain on trial as offending agents, but firm evidence incriminating them is lacking.[23]

MORPHOLOGY. Acute prostatitis may appear as minute, disseminated abscesses; as large, coalescent focal areas of necrosis; or as a diffuse

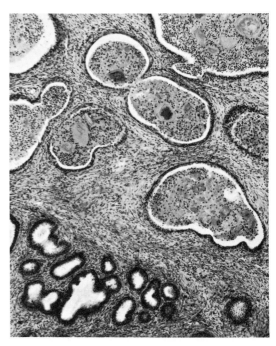

Figure 22–17. Acute prostatitis. Gland lumina are filled with neutrophils, and stroma contains a sprinkling of similar leukocytes.

edema, congestion, and boggy suppuration of the entire gland. When these reactions are fairly diffuse, they cause an overall soft, spongy enlargement of the gland.

Histologically, depending on the duration and severity of the inflammation, there may be minimal stromal leukocytic infiltrate accompanied by increased elaboration of prostatic secretion or leukocytic infiltration within gland spaces (Fig. 22–17). When abscess formation has occurred, focal or large areas of the prostatic substance may become necrotic. Such inflammatory reactions may totally subside and leave behind only some fibrous scarring and calcification. Alternatively, they may become chronic, particularly when the excretory ducts are plugged and the infection continues to smolder within walled-off minute abscesses in the prostatic substance.

Chronic prostatitis, both bacterial and abacterial, when correctly diagnosed, should be restricted to those cases of inflammatory reaction in the prostate characterized by the aggregation of numerous lymphocytes, plasma cells, and macrophages as well as neutrophils within the prostatic substance. It should be pointed out that, in the normal aging process, aggregations of lymphocytes are prone to appear in the fibromuscular stroma of this gland. All too often, such nonspecific aggregates are diagnosed as chronic prostatitis, even though the pathognomonic inflammatory cells, the macrophages and neutrophils, are not present.

BENIGN ENLARGEMENT

Nodular Hyperplasia (Benign Prostatic Hypertrophy or Hyperplasia)

Nodular hyperplasia, still referred to by the redundant term benign prostatic hyperplasia (all hyperplasias are benign), is an extremely common disorder in men over age 50. It is characterized by the formation of large, fairly discrete nodules in the periurethral region of the prostate. When sufficiently large, the nodules compress and narrow the urethral canal to cause partial, or sometimes virtually complete, obstruction of the urethra.

INCIDENCE. Although reports vary slightly, a careful examination of the prostate in an unselected series of autopsies disclosed nodular hyperplasia in approximately 20% of the men 40 years of age, a figure that increases to 70% by age 60 and to 90% by the eighth decade of life.[24] With this prevalence, it has been argued that nodular hyperplasia is not truly a disease but rather a normal aging process; this is a dilemma we can leave to the semanticists. Although clinically significant nodular hyperplasia is less prevalent, this is a problem of enormous magnitude. In 1990, more than 400,000 transurethral resections of the prostate were performed. In men older than 65 years of age, this surgical procedure is second only to cataract extraction.

ETIOLOGY. The cause of nodular hyperplasia is unknown, but there is little doubt that it is related to the action of androgens.[25] In both humans and dogs, hyperplasia of the prostate develops only with an intact testis. Dihydrotestosterone (DHT), which is derived from testosterone by the action of 5α-reductase, is believed to be the ultimate mediator of prostatic growth. In individuals with the autosomal recessive 5α-reductase deficiency, the development of the prostate is markedly impaired. For reasons not yet clear, with aging, DHT accumulates in the prostate, where it binds to nuclear receptors and causes prostatic hyperplasia.

The central role of DHT in causing nodular hyperplasia is supported by clinical observations in which an inhibitor of 5α-reductase was given to men with this condition. Therapy with 5α-reductase inhibitor markedly reduces the DHT content of the prostate.[26] Concomitantly there is a decrease in prostatic volume and urinary obstruction.[27] There is some experimental evidence that DHT-mediated prostatic hyperplasia is aided and abetted by estrogens. In castrated young dogs, prostatic hyperplasia can be induced by administration of androgens, an effect markedly enhanced by simultaneous administration of 17β-estradiol. In aging men, estradiol levels increase and possibly "sensitize" the prostate to the growth-promoting effects of DHT.

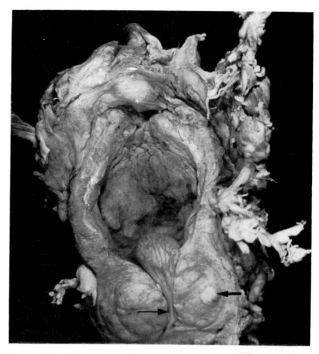

Figure 22–18. Nodular prostatic hyperplasia. Prostatic urethra and urinary bladder have been opened anteriorly to disclose enlarged prostatic gland that narrows urethral lumen to a slit *(small arrow)*. Note evident nodularity within prostatic gland *(large arrow)*. Urinary bladder is enlarged with hypertrophy of wall.

MORPHOLOGY. In the usual case of nodular enlargement, the prostatic nodules weigh between 60 and 100 gm. Not uncommonly, however, aggregate weights of up to 200 gm are encountered, and even larger masses have been recorded. Careful studies by McNeal have demonstrated that nodular hyperplasia of the prostate originates almost exclusively in the preprostatic region.[28] This area, which lies proximal to the verumontanum, corresponds to the "inner" periurethral portion of the classically defined middle and lateral lobes. This distribution is in striking contrast to that of prostatic carcinoma, which usually involves the posterior lobe.

From their origin in this strategic location, the nodular enlargements may encroach on the lateral walls of the urethra to compress it to a slit-like orifice, while at the same time nodular enlargement of the middle lobe may project up into the floor of the urethra as a hemispheric mass directly beneath the mucosa of the urethra (Fig. 22–18).

On cross-section of the affected prostate, the nodules usually are fairly readily identified (Fig. 22–19). They vary in color and consistency. In nodules with primarily glandular proliferation, the tissue is yellow-pink with a soft consistency, and a milky

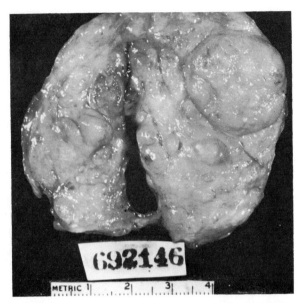

Figure 22-19. Nodular hyperplasia of prostate. Cut surface shows well-defined nodules of various sizes. (Courtesy of Dr. Fred Silva, Department of Pathology, University of Texas Health Science Center, Dallas.)

white prostatic fluid oozes out of these areas. In those primarily due to fibromuscular involvement, the nodule is pale gray, is tough, does not exude fluid, and is less clearly demarcated from the surrounding prostatic capsule. Although the nodules do not have true capsules, the compressed surrounding prostatic tissue creates a plane of cleavage about them, used by the surgeon in the enucleation of prostatic masses in so-called suprapubic prostatectomies.

Microscopically the nodularity may be due mainly to glandular proliferation or dilatation or to fibrous or muscular proliferation of the stroma. All three elements are involved in almost every case, although the epithelial element predominates in most cases. It takes the form of aggregations of small to large to cystically dilated glands, lined by two layers, an inner columnar and an outer cuboidal or flattened epithelium, based on an intact basement membrane (Fig. 22-20). The epithelium is characteristically thrown up into numerous papillary buds and infoldings, which are more prominent than in the normal prostate. Two other histologic changes are frequently found: (1) foci of squamous metaplasia and (2) small areas of infarction. The former tend to occur in the margins of the foci of infarction as nests of metaplastic, but orderly, squamous cells.

CLINICAL COURSE. Nodular hyperplasia of the prostate produces symptoms in approximately 50% of men who are 60 years or older. Symptoms, when produced, relate to two secondary effects:

(1) compression of the urethra with difficulty in urination and (2) retention of urine in the bladder with subsequent distention and hypertrophy of the bladder, infection of the urine, and the development of cystitis and renal infections.

These patients experience frequency, nocturia, difficulty in starting and stopping the stream of urine, overflow dribbling, and dysuria (painful micturition). In many cases, sudden, acute urinary retention appears for unknown reasons and persists until the patient receives emergency catheterization. In addition to these difficulties in urination, prostatic enlargement results in the inability to empty the bladder completely. Presumably this is due to the raised level of the urethral floor so that, at the conclusion of micturition, a considerable amount of residual urine is left. This residual urine provides a static fluid that is vulnerable to infection. On this basis, catheterization or surgical manipulation provides a real danger of the introduction of organisms and the development of pyelonephritis.

Many secondary changes occur in the bladder, such as hypertrophy, trabeculation, and diverticulum formation (see Chapter 21). Hydronephrosis or acute retention, with secondary UTI and even azotemia or uremia, may develop.

Finally, it should be noted that despite earlier claims that nodular hyperplasia predisposes to cancer of the prostate, most studies deny any association, and hence nodular hyperplasia is not considered to be a premalignant lesion.

TUMORS

Carcinoma

Carcinoma of the prostate is the most common form of cancer in males (followed closely by lung cancer) and the second leading cause of cancer death. It is currently estimated that approximately 200,000 new cases are detected every year, of which approximately one-fifth prove to be lethal.[29] In addition to these lethal neoplasms, there is an even more frequent anatomic form of prostatic cancer in which the cancer is discovered as an incidental finding, either at postmortem examination or in a surgical specimen removed for other reasons, e.g., nodular hyperplasia. In almost all these instances, the lesions are small and comprise only microscopic foci. Approximately 90% of these lesions do not cause trouble in the lifetime of the host; but which ones are the "bad apples"?[30]

INCIDENCE. Cancer of the prostate is a disease of men over age 50. The age-adjusted incidence in the United States is 69 per 100,000. Much more

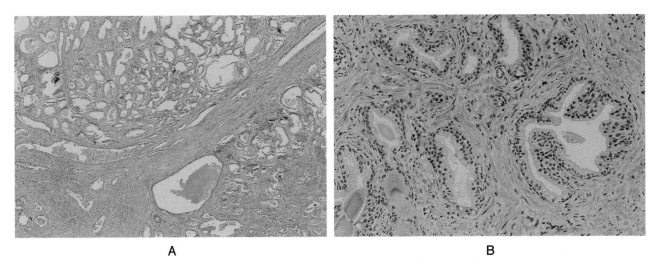

Figure 22-20. Nodular hyperplasia of prostate. *A*, Low-power view shows proliferation of glands, some cystically dilated within a well-defined nodule. *B*, High-power view shows hyperplastic glands with two layers of cells: an inner columnar and an outer cuboidal or flattened. (Courtesy of Dr. Trace Worrell, Department of Pathology, University of Texas Health Science Center, Dallas.)

revealing, however, are the age-specific rates, which are 4.8 in the 45- to 49-year age group but increase to a staggering 513 between the ages of 70 and 75 years.[31] The incidence of latent prostatic cancer is even higher. It increases from 10% in men in their fifth decade of life to approximately 60% in men in their eighties.[32] There are some remarkable and puzzling national and racial differences in the incidence of this disease. Prostatic cancer is extremely rare in Asians. The age-adjusted incidence (per 100,000) among Japanese is in the range of three to four and for the Chinese in Hong Kong only one, as compared with a rate of 50 to 60 among whites in the United States. The disease is even more prevalent among blacks, and indeed U.S. blacks not only have a markedly higher age-adjusted death rate from prostatic cancer than the white male population of the United States, but also the highest rate among 24 countries having reasonably accurate mortality data.[33] These differences are thought to be due to environmental influences because in Japanese migrants to the United States the incidence of the disease seems to have risen, but not nearly to the level of that of native-born Americans.

ETIOLOGY. Little is known about the causes of prostatic cancer. Several risk factors, such as age, race, family history, hormone levels, and environmental influences, are suspected of playing roles. The association of this form of cancer with advancing age and the enigmatic differences among races have already been mentioned. It is interesting to note that despite the striking geographic differences in the incidence of clinically evident prostate cancer, there is little variation in the incidence of latent carcinoma at autopsy. Could environmental factors be the key to progression from a histologic

to clinically evident tumor? The tendency for the incidence of this disease to rise among those enjoying a low-incidence rate when they migrate to a high-incidence locale is consistent with a role for environmental influences. Despite this suggestive evidence, it has not been possible to identify the critical environmental factors. As with many other cancers, increased consumption of fats has been implicated. It has been proposed that dietary fat intake influences the levels of hormones such as testosterone, which in turn affect the growth of prostate. This interesting hypothesis remains to be proved.

The role of the endocrine system in the induction of prostatic cancer is poorly understood. It is speculated that the endocrine changes of old age are related to its origin. Support for this general thesis lies in the inhibition of these tumors that can be achieved with orchiectomy. Neoplastic epithelial cells, like their normal counterparts, possess androgen receptors, which would suggest that they are responsive to these hormones. No significant or consistent alterations in the levels or metabolism of testosterone, however, have been disclosed in any studies. It seems more likely, therefore, that the role of hormones in this malignancy is essentially permissive. Androgens are required for the maintenance of the prostatic epithelium, which is then transformed by agents not yet characterized. There is no evidence for a role for HPV in the causation of prostate cancer.[34]

Several investigations have focused on a possible genetic basis of prostatic cancer. Although familial clustering has been observed, and in sporadic cases first-degree relatives have a higher risk, no specific chromosomal abnormalities have been detected. Some studies have suggested chromosomes 8, 10, and 16 as potential sites of gene(s)

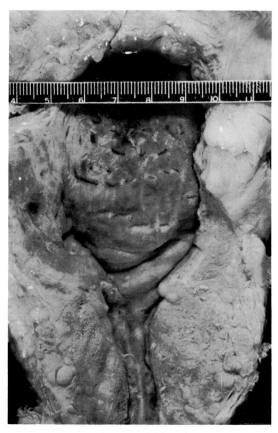

Figure 22–21. Carcinoma of the prostate. Carcinomatous tissue cannot be distinguished within prostate itself but has invaded floor of the urethra and infiltrated in the vesicle neck.

associated with neoplastic transformation of prostate cells,[35] but much remains to be learned.

MORPHOLOGY. In approximately 70% of cases, carcinoma of the prostate arises in the peripheral zone of the gland, classically in a posterior location, often rendering it palpable on rectal examination (Fig. 22–21). Characteristically on cross section of the prostate, **the neoplastic tissue is gritty and firm, but when embedded within the prostatic substance, it may be extremely difficult to visualize and be more readily apparent on palpation.** It should be noted, however, that uncommonly prostatic cancers are not hard, particularly those lesions that do not evoke a stromal proliferative reaction. Spread of prostate cancer occurs by direct local invasion and through the bloodstream and lymph. Local extension most commonly involves the seminal vesicles and the base of the urinary bladder, which may result in ureteral obstruction. Hematogenous spread occurs chiefly to the bones, particularly the axial skeleton, but some lesions spread widely to viscera. Massive visceral dissemination is an exception rather than the rule. The bony metastases may be osteolytic, but osteo-

are frequent and in men point strongly to prostatic cancer. The bones commonly involved, in descending order of frequency, are lumbar spine, proximal femur, pelvis, thoracic spine, and ribs. Lymphatic spread occurs initially to the obturator nodes followed by perivesical, hypogastric, iliac, presacral, and para-aortic nodes. Lymph node spread occurs frequently and often precedes spread to the bones. As we discuss later, metastases to the lymph nodes in apparently localized prostatic cancer have a significant impact on the prognosis.

Histologically most lesions are adenocarcinomas that produce well-defined, readily demonstrable gland patterns.[36] The glands are either small or medium-sized with a single uniform layer of cuboidal or low columnar epithelium. The outer basal layer of cells typical of normal and hyperplastic glands is often absent. Occasionally, the glands are somewhat larger, with a papillary or cribriform pattern. Typically, the neoplastic acini have an irregular shape and are distributed haphazardly in the stroma. The cytoplasm of the tumor cells is not distinctive: It may be pale or dark with marked eosinophilic staining. The appearance of nuclei is usually quite different from that in benign proliferations. They are large and vacuolated and contain one or more large nucleoli. There is some variation in nuclear size and shape, but in general pleomorphism is not marked. Mitotic figures are extremely uncommon. When well-differentiated tumors occur in sharply delimited rounded masses, they have to be distinguished from nodular hyperplasia. In general, malignant acini are smaller and closely spaced, "back-to-back" with little intervening stroma, and are lined by a single layer of cells (Fig. 22–22). Not all prostatic cancers, however, are well differentiated. In some poorly differentiated tumors, the glandular pattern is apparent only on careful examination; the tumor cells in such cases tend to grow in cords, nests, or sheets. Stromal production may be scant or quite extensive in certain lesions, producing a scirrhous-like consistency to the neoplasm.

The most reliable hallmarks of malignancy, especially in well-differentiated tumors, are clear evidence of invasion of the capsule with its lymphatic and vascular channels, perineurial invasion, or both (Fig. 22–23). The perineurial spaces, which are involved in most cases, are not lined by endothelium, and they do not represent lymphatics, as formerly believed.

In approximately 70% of cases, prostatic tissue removed for carcinoma also harbors presumptive precursor lesions referred to as duct-acinar dysplasia, or simply **prostatic intraepithelial neoplasia.** These lesions consist of large glands with intra-acinar proliferation of cells that demonstrate nuclear anaplasia. In contrast to frank cancer, however, there is no invasion, and the dysplastic cells

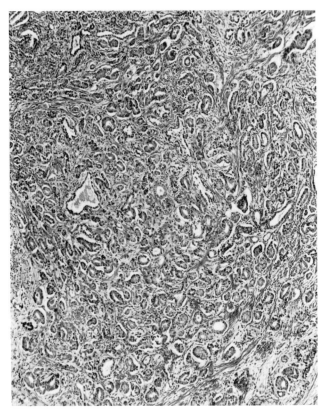

Figure 22–22. Well-differentiated adenocarcinoma of the prostate. Note numerous small acini lying "back to back."

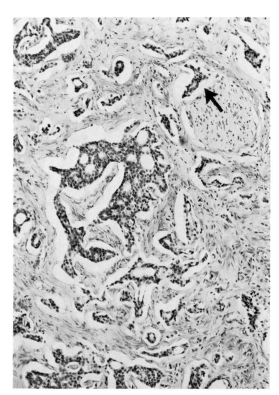

Figure 22–23. Carcinoma of the prostate. Cords of tumor cells permeate stroma. Perineurial invasion is present (arrow).

are surrounded by a layer of basal cells and an intact basement membrane. Direct transition between the dysplastic and the cancerous glands can be demonstrated only rarely.

GRADING AND STAGING. Carcinomas of the prostate, like most other forms of cancer, are graded and staged. Several grading systems have been described, of which the Gleason system is the best known.[32,36] A detailed discussion of grading is not presented here. Suffice it to say that all grading systems attempt to define histologic criteria (the arrangement and appearance of malignant glands and the degree of anaplasia of cancer cells) by which tumors of differing biologic behavior can be segregated. For example, the Gleason system is based on the degree of glandular differentiation and growth pattern of tumor in relation to the stroma. *Grading is of particular importance in prostatic cancer because there is in general fairly good correlation between the prognosis and the degree of differentiation.*

Staging of prostatic cancer is also important in the selection of the appropriate form of therapy and in establishing a prognosis. A staging system that is widely used in the United States is depicted in Figure 22–24.

DNA ploidy of tumor cells has emerged as a useful adjunct to staging and grading in the management of prostatic cancer. Patients with diploid tumors have a much better prognosis than those with aneuploid and tetraploid tumors.[37]

CLINICAL COURSE. As discussed earlier, the incidence of stage A cancers increases with age and approaches 60% or more in men past the age of 80 years. These microscopic cancers are asymptomatic and are discovered incidentally at autopsy or in tissue removed for nodular hyperplasia of the prostate. The long-term significance of these lesions is still not entirely clear.[30,38] It is generally accepted that the majority of patients with stage A1 cancer do not show evidence of progressive disease when followed for 10 or more years. Five per cent to 25% of patients, however, do develop local or distant spread. This is more likely in younger patients (<60 years) who have a longer life expectancy. For patients in this age group, some authorities recommend careful follow-up studies so if progression occurs, the cancer may be detected early, at a stage amenable to surgical cure.[39] Stage A2 lesions are more ominous. Approximately 30 to 50% can be expected to progress over a period of 5 years with a mortality of 20% if left untreated.

About 5 to 10% of patients with overt prostatic cancer are discovered in stage B. These patients do not have urinary symptoms, and the lesion is discovered by the finding of a suspicious

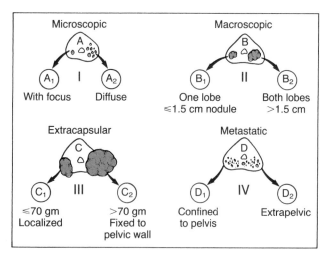

Figure 22–24. Staging of prostate cancer. Stage A: microscopic, not clinically palpable tumor (A₁, with focus in less than 5% of tissue examined, low grade; A₂, with multiple areas (more than 5%) or Gleason grade higher than 4). Stage B: palpable, macroscopic tumor (B₁, ≤1.5 cm in diameter, only in one lobe; B₂, >1.5 cm in diameter, or several nodules in both lobes). Stage C: tumor with extracapsular extension but still clinically localized (C₁, palpably extending into seminal vesicle but not fixed to pelvic wall; C₂, fixed to pelvic wall). Stage D: demonstrated metastatic tumor (D₁, metastases limited to three pelvic nodes or fewer; D₂, more extensive nodal or extrapelvic metastases, e.g., to bone). The tumor, node, and metastasis (TNM) staging for local tumors is indicated by Roman numerals I through IV. (Redrawn and adapted with permission from Gittes, R.F.: Carcinoma of the prostate. The New England Journal of Medicine 324:240, 1991.)

metastases may be missed by either of these two procedures, many centers use pelvic lymphadenectomy as a staging procedure. If pelvic lymph nodes are involved, curative surgery (radical prostatectomy) is not warranted. Osseous metastases may be detected by skeletal surveys or the much more sensitive radionuclide bone scanning.

Two biochemical markers, prostatic acid phosphatase and prostate-specific antigen (PSA), are of value in the diagnosis and management of prostate cancer. Both are produced by normal as well as neoplastic prostatic epithelium. Serum levels of prostatic acid phosphatase are elevated in patients whose tumor has extended beyond the capsule or metastasized, but it is not useful in the diagnosis of localized disease. PSA has largely supplanted prostatic acid phosphatase in the management of prostate cancer.[40] PSA is a product of prostatic epithelium and is normally secreted in the human semen. It is a serine protease whose function is to cleave and liquefy the seminal coagulum formed after ejaculation. In normal men, only minute amounts of PSA circulate in the serum. Elevated blood levels of PSA occur in association with localized as well as advanced cancer. Indeed, the PSA levels are proportional to the volume of the tumor. Serum levels of PSA are also raised in benign prostatic hyperplasia, although to a lesser extent. According to some investigators, for a given volume of the prostate, cancerous tissue yields higher level of serum PSA than does nodular hyperplasia.[40] This

nodule on rectal examination. You recall that most prostatic cancers arise in a subcapsular location removed from the urethra, and, therefore, urinary symptoms occur late. Most of these lesions are destined to progress unless eradicated by surgery or radiation.

More than 75% of patients with prostatic cancer present with stage C or D cancer. They come to clinical attention usually because of urinary symptoms, such as difficulty in starting or stopping the stream, dysuria, frequency, or hematuria. Pain is a late finding, reflecting involvement of capsular perineurial spaces. Some patients in stage D come to attention because of back pain caused by vertebral metastases. *The finding of osteoblastic metastases in bone is virtually diagnostic of this form of cancer in men* (Fig. 22–25). The outlook for these patients is poor.

Careful rectal digital examination is a useful, direct method for detection of early prostatic carcinoma because the posterior location of most tumors renders them easily palpable. Transrectal ultrasonography is an important adjunct for early detection as well as assessment of local spread. A transperineal or transrectal biopsy can confirm the diagnosis. Several procedures are used to determine the extent of disease. The involvement of lymph nodes may be detected by CT scans or magnetic resonance imaging. Because microscopic

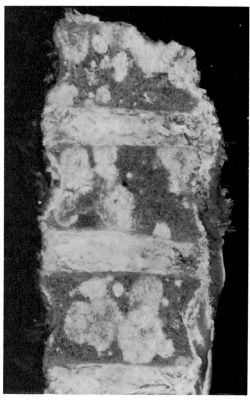

Figure 22–25. Metastatic osteoblastic prostatic carcinoma within vertebral bodies.

is not related to a greater production of PSA by cancer cells but perhaps results from greater diffusion of PSA from malignant acini to the stromal blood vessels. Thus, measurement of PSA density, that is, PSA levels per unit of prostate volume determined by transrectal ultrasonography, may increase the specificity of mild elevations of serum PSA levels. To summarize, because of the overlap in PSA values between patients with localized cancer and nodular hyperplasia, measurement of serum PSA alone cannot be used for the detection of early cancer. When combined with rectal examination and transrectal ultrasonography, however, measurement of PSA antigen levels is quite useful in detection of early stage cancers.[41,42] The monitoring of serum PSA levels is of even greater value in assessing the response to therapy. For example, an elevated PSA level after radical prostatectomy for localized disease is indicative of disseminated disease. Rising PSA levels after initial control of cancer herald recurrence or dissemination. Immunohistochemical localization of PSA is also helpful in determining whether a metastatic tumor originated in the prostate.

Cancer of the prostate is treated by surgery, radiotherapy, and hormonal manipulations. As might be expected, surgery and radiotherapy are most suited for treatment of patients with localized (stage A or B) disease. More than 90% of patients in this group can expect to live for 15 years. Endocrine therapy is the mainstay for treatment of advanced, metastatic carcinoma. Because prostatic cancer cells depend on androgens for their sustenance, the aim of endocrine manipulations is to deprive the tumor cells of testosterone. This can be achieved by orchiectomy or by administration of estrogens or synthetic agonists of luteinizing hormone–releasing hormone (LHRH). Although estrogens can inhibit testicular androgen synthesis directly, their principal effect appears to be suppression of pituitary luteinizing hormone (LH) secretion, which in turn leads to reduced testicular output of testosterone. Synthetic analogs of LHRH act similarly. Long-term administration of LHRH agonists (after an initial transient increase in LH secretion) suppresses LH release, achieving in effect a pharmacologic orchiectomy. Although antiandrogen therapy does induce remissions, tumor progression leads to emergence of testosterone-insensitive clones, and, hence, despite all forms of treatment, patients with disseminated cancers have a 10 to 40% likelihood of 10-year survival.

1. Opitz, J.M.: Editorial comment: Hypospadias. Am. J. Med. Genet. 21:57, 1985.
2. Vohra, S., and Badlani, G.: Balanitis and balanoposthitis. Urol. Clin. North Am. 19:143, 1992.
3. Grossman, H.B.: Premalignant and early carcinoma of the penis and scrotum. Urol. Clin. North Am. 19:221, 1992.
4. Boshart, M., and zur Hausen, V.: Human pappilomaviruses in Buschkè-Lowenstein tumors: Physical state of the DNA and identification of a tandem duplication in the non-coding region of a human papillomavirus 6 subtype. J. Virol. 58:963, 1986.
5. Kaye, V., et al.: Carcinoma in situ of penis: Is distinction between erythroplasia of Queyrat and Bowen's disease relevant? Urology 36:479, 1990.
6. Obalek, S., et al.: Bowenoid papulosis of the male and female genitalia: Risk of cervical neoplasia. J. Am. Acad. Dermatol. 14:433, 1986.
7. Sarkar, F.H., et al.: Detection of human papillomavirus in squamous neoplasms of the penis. J. Urol. 147:389, 1992.
8. Burgers, J.K., et al.: Penile cancer: Clinical presentation, diagnosis, and staging. Urol. Clin. North Am. 19:267, 1992.
9. Higgins, G.D., et al.: Differing prevalence of human papillomavirus RNA in penile dysplasias and carcinomas may reflect differing etiologies. Am. J. Clin. Pathol. 97:272, 1992.
10. Benson, R.C., et al.: Malignant potential of the cryptorchid testis. Mayo Clin. Proc. 66:372, 1991.
11. Bica, D.T.G., and Hadziselimovic, F.: Buserelin treatment of cryptorchidism: A randomized, double-blind, placebo-controlled study. J. Urol. 148:617, 1992.
12. Colodny, A.H.: Undescended testis—is surgery necessary? N. Engl. J. Med. 314:510, 1986.
13. Klein, F.A., et al.: Bilateral granulomatous orchitis: Manifestation of idiopathic systemic granulomatosis. J. Urol. 134:762, 1985.
14. Czaja, J.T., and Ulbright, T.M.: Evidence for the transformation of seminoma to yolk sac tumor, with histogenetic considerations. Am. J. Clin. Pathol. 97:468, 1992.
15. Sheldon, C.C.: Undescended testis and testicular torsion. Surg. Clin. North. Am. 65:1303, 1985.
16. Forman, D., et al.: Familial testicular cancer: A report of the U.K. family register, estimation of risk, and an HLA Class I sib-pair analysis. Br. J. Cancer 65:255, 1992.
17. Cassio, A., et al.: Incidence of intratubular germ cell neoplasia in androgen-insensitivity syndrome. Acta Endocrinol. (Copenh.) 123:416, 1990.
18. Ilson, D.H., et al.: Genetic analysis of germ cell tumors: Current progress and future prospects. Hem. Oncol. Clin. North Am. 5:1271, 1991.
19. Brodsky, G.L.: Pathology of testicular germ cell tumors. Hem. Oncol. Clin. North Am. 5:1095, 1991.
20. Bartlett, N.L., et al.: Serum markers in germ cell neoplasms. Hem. Oncol. Clin. North Am. 5:1245, 1991.
21. Dilworth, J.P., et al.: Non–germ cell tumors of testis. Urology 37:399, 1991.
22. Meares, E.M.: Prostatitis. Med. Clin. North Am. 75:405, 1991.
23. Shortliffe, L.M.D., et al.: The characterization of nonbacterial prostatitis: Search for an etiology. J. Urol. 148:1461, 1992.
24. Arrighi, H.M., et al.: Natural history of benign prostatic hyperplasia and risk of prostatectomy: The Baltimore Longitudunal Study of Aging. Urol. (Suppl.) 38:4, 1991.
25. Matzkin, H., and Braf, Z.: Endocrine treatment of benign prostatic hypertrophy: Current concepts. Urology 37:1, 1991.
26. McConnell, J.D., et al.: Finasteride, an inhibitor of 5α-reductase, suppresses prostatic dihydrotestosterone in men with benign prostatic hyperplasia. J. Clin. Endocrinol. Metab. 74:505, 1992.
27. Rittmaster, R.S.: Finasteride. N. Engl. J. Med. 330:120, 1994.
28. McNeal, J.: Pathology of benign prostatic hyperplasia. Urol. Clin. North Am. 17:477, 1990.
29. Boring, C.C., et al.: Cancer statistics, 1994. CA 44:7, 1994.
30. Smith, P.H.: The case for no initial treatment of localized prostate cancer. Urol. Clin. North Am. 17:827, 1990.
31. Hutchison, G.B.: Incidence and etiology of prostatic cancer. Urology 17 (Suppl. 3):4, 1981.
32. Gittes, R.F.: Carcinoma of the prostate. N. Engl. J. Med. 324(4):236, 1991.
33. Meilke, A.W., and Smith, J.A.: Epidemiology of prostate cancer. Urol. Clin. North Am. 17:709, 1990.

34. Effert, P.J., et al.: Human papillomavirus types 16 and 18 are not involved in human prostatic carcinogenesis: Analysis of archival human prostate cancer specimens by differential polymerase chain reaction. J. Urol. *147*:192, 1992.

35. Linehan, W.M.: Editorial. Molecular genetics of tumor suppressor genes in prostate carcinoma: The challenge and promise ahead. J. Urol. *147*:808, 1992.

36. Mostofi, F.K., et al.: Pathology of carcinoma of the prostate. Cancer (Suppl.) *70*:235, 1992.

37. Leiber, M.M.: DNA content/ploidy as prognostic factors in prostate cancer. Prostate (Suppl. 4):*119*, 1992.

38. Zhang, G., et al.: Long-term follow-up results after ex-

pectant management of stage A1 prostatic cancer. J. Urol. *146*:99, 1991.

39. Whitmore, W.: Stage A prostate cancer. J. Urol. *136*:883, 1986.

40. Cupp, M.R., and Oesterling, J.E.: Prostate specific antigen, digital rectal examination, and transrectal ultrasonography: Their roles in diagnosing early prostate cancer. Mayo Clin. Proc. *68*:297, 1993.

41. Stamey, T.A.: Editorial. Diagnosis of prostate cancer: A personal view. J. Urol. *147*:830, 1992.

42. Gustafsson, O., et al.: Diagnostic methods in the detection of prostate cancer: A study of a randomly selected population of 2,400 men. J. Urol. *148*:1827, 1992.

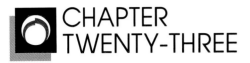

CHAPTER TWENTY-THREE

Female Genital Tract

CHRISTOPHER P. CRUM, M.D.

NORMAL

EMBRYOLOGY

The embryology of the female genital tract is relevant to both anomalies in this region and the histogenesis of various tumors.[1] The primordial germ cells arise in the wall of the yolk sac by the fourth week of gestation; by the fifth or sixth week, they migrate into the urogenital ridge. The mesodermal epithelium of the urogenital ridge then proliferates eventually to produce the epithelium and stroma of the gonad, and the dividing germ cells—of endodermal origin—are incorporated into these proliferating epithelial cells to form the ovary.[2] Failure of germ cells to develop may result in either absence of ovaries or premature ovarian failure.

Disruption of normal migration may account for extragonadal distribution of germ cells midline structures—retroperitoneum, mediastinum, and even pineal gland—and rarely may lead to tumors in these sites.

A second component of female genital development is the müllerian duct. At about the sixth week, invagination and subsequent fusion of the coelomic lining epithelium form the lateral müllerian (or paramesonephric) ducts. Müllerian ducts progressively grow caudally to enter the pelvis, where they swing medially to fuse. Further caudal growth brings these fused ducts into contact with the urogenital sinus, which eventually becomes the vestibule of the external genitalia. Normally, the unfused portions mature into the fallopian tubes, the fused caudal portion into the uterus and upper vagina and the urogenital sinus forming the lower vagina and vestibule. Consequently, the entire lining of the uterus and tubes as well as the ovarian surface is derived from coelomic epithelium (mesothelium). The fact that these various surfaces are derived from a similar origin explains the histologic similarities in both benign and malignant tumors at these sites.

In males, müllerian inhibiting substance[3] from the developing testis causes regression of the müllerian ducts, and the paired wolffian (or mesonephric) ducts form the epididymis and the vas deferens. Normally, the mesonephric duct regresses in the female, but remnants may persist into adult life as epithelial inclusions adjacent to the ovaries, tubes, and uterus. In the cervix and vagina, these rests may be cystic and are termed Gartner's duct cysts.

ANATOMY

During active reproductive life, the ovaries measure about $4 \times 2.5 \times 1.5$ cm in dimension. The ovary is divided into a cortex and a medulla. The cortex consists of a layer of closely packed spindle cells that resemble plump fibroblasts with scant intercellular ground substance and a thin outer layer of relatively acellular collagenous connective tissue. Follicles in varying stages of maturation are found within the outer cortex. With each menstrual cycle, one follicle develops into a graafian follicle enroute to ovulation and following ovulation is transformed into a corpus luteum. Corpora lutea of varying ages as well as corpora albicantia are also present in the cortex of the adult.

The medulla of the ovary is made up of a more loosely arranged mesenchymal tissue and may contain small clusters of round-to-polygonal, epithelial-appearing cells around vessels and nerves. These "hilus" cells, presumed to be vestigial remains of the gonad from its primitive "ambisexual" phase, are steroid producing and thus resemble the interstitial cells of the testis. Rarely, these cells give rise to masculinizing tumors (hilar cell tumors).

In the fallopian tube, the mucosa is thrown up into numerous delicate folds (plica) that on cross-

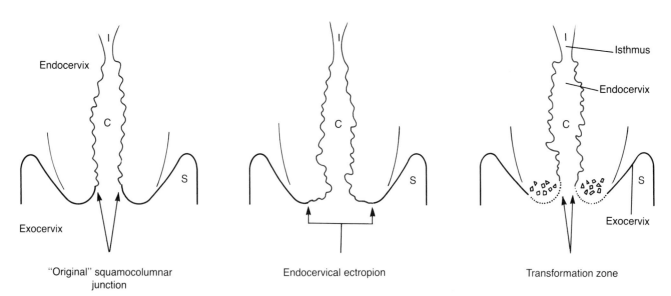

Figure 23-1. Schematic representation of normal cervix and transformation zone. *Left,* Diagram of a portio completely covered with native squamous epithelium. Squamocolumnar junction is at external os. *Middle,* Denotes an endocervical columnar ectropion with squamocolumnar junction located on exocervix below external os. *Right,* Indicates areas of ectropion now covered with squamous epithelium *(stippled line).* This area is the cervical transformation zone. (Modified with permission from Ferenczy, A., and Winkler, B.: Anatomy and histology of the cervix. *In* Kurman, R. (ed.): Blaustein's Pathology of the Female Genital Tract, 3rd ed. New York, Springer-Verlag, 1987. Reproduced with permission.)

section produce a papillary appearance. The lining epithelium consists of three cell types: ciliated columnar cell; nonciliated, columnar secretory cells; and so-called intercalated cells, which may simply represent inactive secretory cells.

The uterus varies in size, depending on the age and parity of the individual. During active reproductive life, it weighs about 50 gm and measures about $8.0 \times 6.0 \times 3.0$ cm in dimension. Pregnancies may leave small residual increases in these dimensions (up to 70 gm in weight) because the uterus rarely involutes completely to its original size. After menopause, the uterus undergoes atrophy, diminishing by up to one-half in dimension.

The uterus has three distinctive anatomic and functional regions: the cervix, the lower uterine segment, and the corpus. The cervix is further divided into the vaginal portion and the endocervix. The anatomic portion is visible to the eye on vaginal examination. It is covered by a stratified nonkeratinizing squamous epithelium continuous with the vaginal vault. The squamous epithelium converges centrally at a small opening termed the external os. In the normal cervix of nulliparous women, this os is virtually closed. Just cephalad to the os is the endocervix, which is lined by columnar, mucus-secreting epithelium that dips down into the underlying stroma to produce crypts (endocervical glands). The point at which the squamous and glandular epithelium meet is the squamocolumnar junction. The position of the junction is variable. Although its original position is at the cervical os (Fig. 23–1; *left*), in virtually all adult women who have borne children, the endocervix is everted, exposing the squamocolumnar junction to the naked eye (Fig. 23–1, *middle*). A combination of ingrowth of the squamous epithelium portion (epidermidalization) and intrinsic squamous differentiation of subcolumnar reserve cells (squamous metaplasia) transforms this area into squamous epithelium and produces the *transformation zone* (Fig. 23–1, *right*). During reproductive life, the squamocolumnar junction migrates cephalad on the leading edge of the transformation zone and may be invisible to the naked eye after menopause. As we shall see, it is in this transformation zone, including the squamocolumnar junction, where squamous carcinomas or precancerous lesions develop. The lower uterine segment, or isthmus, is the portion between the endocervix and the endometrial cavity.

ENDOMETRIAL HISTOLOGY AND MENSTRUAL CYCLE

The endometrial changes that occur during the menstrual cycle are keyed to the rise and fall in the levels of ovarian hormones, and the student should be familiar with the complex but fascinating interactions among hypothalamic, pituitary, and ovarian factors underlying maturation of ovarian follicles, ovulation, and the menstrual cycle. Suffice it to say that under the influence of the pituitary follicle-stimulating hormone (FSH) and luteinizing hormone (LH), development and ripening of a single ovum occur, and estrogen production by the enlarging ovarian follicle progressively rises during the first 2 weeks of the usual 28-day menstrual cycle. It reaches a peak, presumably just before ovulation, and then falls. Following ovulation, the estrogen levels again begin to rise to a plateau at about the end of the third week, but these levels are never as high as the preovulatory peak. The level of this hormone then progressively falls, beginning 3 to 4 days before the onset of menstruation. Progesterone, produced by the corpus luteum, rises throughout the last half of the menstrual cycle to fall to basal levels just before the onset of menstrual bleeding.

"Dating" the endometrium by its histologic appearance is helpful clinically to assess hormonal status, document ovulation, and determine causes of endometrial bleeding and infertility. We can begin with the shedding of the upper one-half to two-thirds of the endometrium during the menstrual period (Fig. 23–2). The basal third does not respond to the ovarian steroids and is retained at the conclusion of the menstrual flow. From the basal third of this preovulatory proliferative phase of the cycle, there is extremely rapid growth of both glands and stroma (proliferative phase). The glands are straight, tubular structures lined by quite regular, tall, pseudostratified columnar cells. Mitotic figures are numerous, and there is no evidence of mucus secretion or vacuolation (Fig. 23–3). The endometrial stroma is composed of thickly compacted spindle cells that have scant cytoplasm but abundant mitotic activity.

At the time of ovulation, the endometrium slows in its growth, and it ceases apparent mitotic activity within days immediately following ovulation. The postovulatory endometrium is initially marked by basal secretory vacuoles beneath the nuclei in the glandular epithelium (Fig. 23–4). This secretory activity is most prominent during the third week of the menstrual cycle, when the basal vacuoles progressively push past the nuclei. In the fourth week, the secretions are discharged into the gland lumina. When secretion is maximal, between 18 and 24 days, the glands are dilated. By the fourth week, the glands are tortuous, producing a serrated appearance when they are cut in their long axis (Fig. 23–5). This serrated or "sawtoothed" appearance is accentuated by secretory exhaustion and shrinking of the glands.

The stromal changes in late secretory phase are important for dating the endometrium and

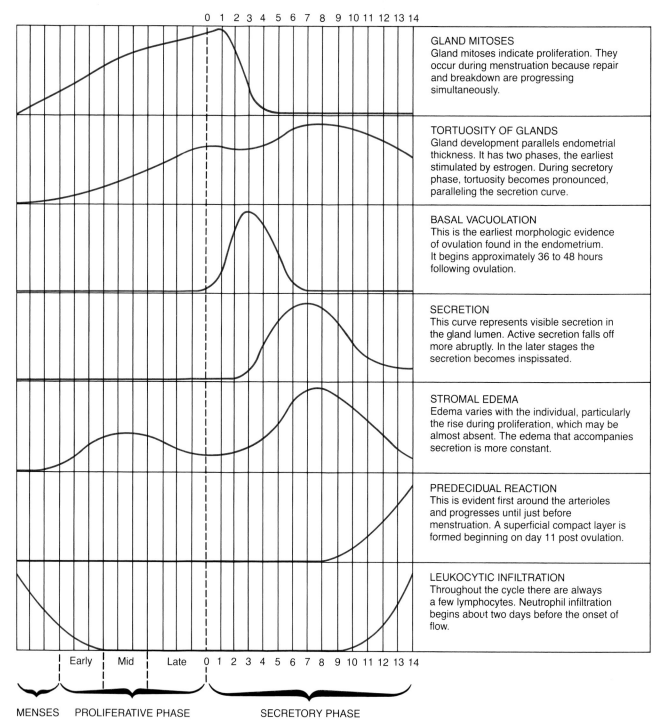

0 1 2 3 4 5 6 7 8 9 10 11 12 13 14

GLAND MITOSES
Gland mitoses indicate proliferation. They occur during menstruation because repair and breakdown are progressing simultaneously.

TORTUOSITY OF GLANDS
Gland development parallels endometrial thickness. It has two phases, the earliest stimulated by estrogen. During secretory phase, tortuosity becomes pronounced, paralleling the secretion curve.

BASAL VACUOLATION
This is the earliest morphologic evidence of ovulation found in the endometrium. It begins approximately 36 to 48 hours following ovulation.

SECRETION
This curve represents visible secretion in the gland lumen. Active secretion falls off more abruptly. In the later stages the secretion becomes inspissated.

STROMAL EDEMA
Edema varies with the individual, particularly the rise during proliferation, which may be almost absent. The edema that accompanies secretion is more constant.

PREDECIDUAL REACTION
This is evident first around the arterioles and progresses until just before menstruation. A superficial compact layer is formed beginning on day 11 post ovulation.

LEUKOCYTIC INFILTRATION
Throughout the cycle there are always a few lymphocytes. Neutrophil infiltration begins about two days before the onset of flow.

Early   Mid   Late   0 1 2 3 4 5 6 7 8 9 10 11 12 13 14

MENSES   PROLIFERATIVE PHASE   SECRETORY PHASE

Figure 23–2. Approximate quantitative changes in seven morphologic criteria found to be most useful in dating human endometrium. (Modified with permission from Noyes, R.W.: Normal phases of the endometrium. In Norris, H.J., et al. (eds.): The Uterus. Baltimore, Williams & Wilkins, 1973.)

consist of the development of prominent spiral arterioles by days 21 to 22. A considerable increase in ground substance and edema between the stromal cells occurs and is followed in days 23 to 24 by stromal cell hypertrophy with accumulation of cytoplasmic eosinophilia (predecidual change) and resurgence of stromal mitoses. Predecidual changes spread throughout the functionalis (the hormonally responsive upper zone) during days 24 to 28 and are accompanied by scattered neutrophils and occasional lymphocytes, which here do not imply inflammation. This is followed by disintegration of the functionalis and escape of blood into the stroma, which marks the beginning of menstrual shedding (Fig. 23–6).

The proliferative phase exhibits mitotic activ-

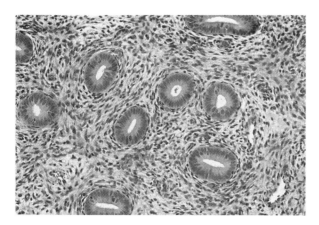

Figure 23-3. Normal proliferative endometrium, illustrating tube-like pattern of glands.

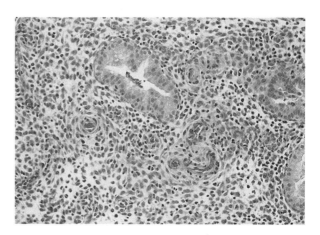

Figure 23-5. Late secretory endometrium with predecidual stromal changes.

ity in glandular and stromal cells; ovulation is confirmed by prominent basal vacuolation of glandular epithelial cells, secretory exhaustion, or predecidual changes. Obviously, ovulation cannot be confirmed during the proliferative phase or in the late stages of endometrial shedding when only the basalis is present.

PATHOLOGY

Diseases of the female genital tract are extremely common in clinical and pathologic practice and include complications of pregnancy, inflammations, tumors, and hormonally induced effects. The following discussion presents the pathology of the majority of clinical problems. Details can be found in current books of obstetric and gynecologic pathology and medicine.[4-9] The pathologic conditions

peculiar to each segment of female genital tract are discussed separately, but first we briefly review pelvic inflammatory disease (PID) and other infections because they can affect many of the segments concomitantly.

FEMALE GENITAL INFECTIONS

A large variety of organisms can infect the female genital tract and, in total, account for considerable suffering and morbidity. Some, such as Candida infections, trichomoniasis, and Gardnerella, are extremely common and may cause significant discomfort with no serious sequelae. Others, such as gonorrhea and Chlamydia, are major causes of female infertility, and others still, such as Mycoplasma infections, are implicated in spontaneous abortions. Viruses, principally the human papillomaviruses,

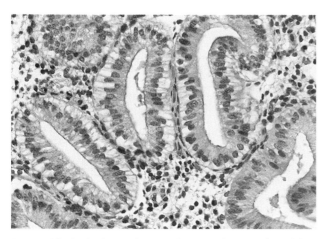

Figure 23-4. Postovulatory early secretory endometrium with prominent subnuclear vacuoles and alignment of nuclei.

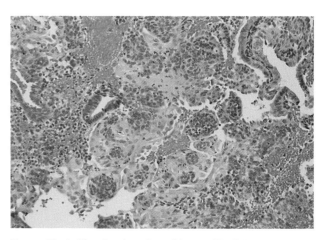

Figure 23-6. Menstrual endometrium, with disintegration of stroma and stromal hemorrhage.

appear to be involved in the pathogenesis of vulvar and cervical cancer.

Many of these infections are sexually transmitted, including trichomoniasis, gonorrhea, chancroid, granuloma inguinale, lymphogranuloma venereum, syphilis, Mycoplasma, Chlamydia, herpes, and human papillomavirus.[10] Most of these conditions have been adequately considered in Chapter 8. Here we touch only on selected aspects relevant to the female genital tract, including pathogens confined to the lower genital tract (vulva, vagina, and cervix) and those that involve the entire genital tract and are implicated in PID. Papillomaviruses are discussed subsequently under tumors.

INFECTIONS CONFINED TO LOWER GENITAL TRACT

In the lower genital tract, *herpes simplex* infection is common and usually involves the vulva, vagina, and cervix.[10] In sexually transmitted disease clinics, approximately one-half of patients have current or prior evidence of infection versus fewer than 10% of unselected women.[11] The frequency of genital herpes has increased dramatically in the past two decades, particularly in teenagers and young women, and herpes simplex virus type II (HSV II) infection is now one of the major sexually transmitted diseases. Of individuals infected, clinical symptoms are seen in about one-third.[11] The lesions begin 3 to 7 days after sexual relations and consist of painful red papules in the vulva that progress to vesicles and then coalescent ulcers. Cervical and vaginal involvement causes severe leukorrhea (genital discharge), and the initial infection produces systemic symptoms, such as fever, malaise, and tender inguinal lymph nodes. The vesicles and ulcers contain numerous virus particles, accounting for the high transmission rate during active infection. The lesions heal spontaneously in 1 to 3 weeks, but as with herpetic infections elsewhere, latent infection of regional nerve ganglia persists. About two-thirds of affected women suffer recurrences, which are less painful. Transmission may occur during active or inactive (latent) phases, although it is much less likely in asymptomatic carriers. The gravest consequence of HSV infection is transmission to the neonate during birth. This risk is highest if the infection is active during delivery and particularly if it is a *primary* (initial) infection in the mother.[12]

Mycotic and yeast (Candida) infections are common; about 10% of women are thought to be carriers of vulvovaginal fungi. Diabetes mellitus, oral contraceptives, and pregnancy may enhance the development of infection, which manifests as small white surface patches similar to monilial lesions elsewhere. It is accompanied by leukorrhea

and pruritus. The diagnosis is made by finding the organism in wet mounts of the lesions.

Acute or chronic vaginal infections are often caused by *Trichomonas vaginalis,* a large, flagellated ovoid protozoan that can be readily identified in wet mounts of vaginal discharge. Infections with this organism may occur at any age and are seen in about 15% of women in sexually transmitted disease clinics.[13] This infection is associated with a purulent vaginal discharge and discomfort; typically the underlying vaginal and cervical mucosa has a characteristic fiery red appearance, called "strawberry cervix." Histologically the inflammatory reaction is usually limited to the mucosa and immediately subjacent lamina propria.

Mycoplasma species account for some cases of vaginitis and cervicitis and have been implicated in spontaneous abortion and chorioamnionitis. *Gardnerella* is a gram-negative, small bacillus that is implicated in cases of vaginitis when other organisms (Trichomonas, fungi) cannot be found.

INFECTIONS INVOLVING LOWER AND UPPER GENITAL TRACT

Pelvic Inflammatory Disease (PID)

PID is a common disorder characterized by pelvic pain, adnexal tenderness, fever, and vaginal discharge; it results from infection by one or more of the following groups of organisms: gonococcus, chlamydia, and enteric bacteria. The gonococcus continues to be a common cause of PID, the most serious complication of gonorrhea in women (see Chapter 8). Chlamydia infection is now another well-recognized cause of PID. Besides these two, infections following spontaneous or induced abortions and normal or abnormal deliveries (called puerperal infections) are important in the production of PID. Such PID is polymicrobial and is caused by staphylococci, streptococci, coliform bacteria, and *Clostridium perfringens*.

Gonococcal inflammation begins usually in Bartholin's and other vestibular glands or periurethral glands; cervix involvement is common and frequently asymptomatic. From any of these loci, the organisms may spread upward to involve the tubes and tubo-ovarian region. The adult vagina is remarkably resistant to gonococcus, but in the child, presumably because of a more delicate lining mucosa, vulvovaginitis may develop. The nongonococcal bacterial infections that follow induced abortion, dilatation and curettage of the uterus, and other surgical procedures on the female genital tract are thought to spread from the uterus upward through the lymphatics or venous channels rather than on the mucosal surfaces. These infections therefore tend to produce less mucosal involvement but more reaction within the deeper layers.

> **MORPHOLOGY.** With the gonococcus, approximately 2 to 7 days after inoculation of the organism, inflammatory changes appear in the affected glands. Wherever it occurs, gonococcal disease is characterized by an acute suppurative reaction with inflammation largely confined to the superficial mucosa and underlying submucosa. Smears of the inflammatory exudate should disclose the intracellular gram-negative diplococcus, but absolute confirmation requires culture. If spread occurs, the endometrium is usually spared, for obscure reasons. Once within the tubes, an **acute suppurative salpingitis** ensues. The tubal serosa becomes hyperemic and layered with fibrin, the tubal fimbriae are similarly involved, and the lumen fills with purulent exudate that may leak out of the fimbriated end. Over days or weeks, the fimbriae may seal or become plastered against the ovary to create a **salpingo-oophoritis.** Collections of pus within the ovary and tube **(tubo-ovarian abscesses)** or tubal lumen **(pyosalpinx)** may occur. Adhesions of the tubal plica may produce gland-like spaces (follicular salpingitis). In the course of time, the infecting organisms may disappear, the pus undergoing proteolysis to a thin, serous fluid, to produce a **hydrosalpinx** or hydrosalpinx follicularis.
>
> PID caused by staphylococci, streptococci, and the other puerperal invaders tends to have less exudation within the lumina of the tube and less involvement of the mucosa, with a greater inflammatory response within the deeper layers. The infection tends to spread throughout the wall to involve the serosa and may often track into the broad ligaments, pelvic structures, and peritoneum. Bacteremia is a more frequent complication of streptococcal or staphylococcal PID than of gonococcal infections.

The complications of PID include (1) peritonitis; (2) intestinal obstruction owing to adhesions between the small bowel and the pelvic organs; (3) bacteremia, which may produce endocarditis, meningitis, and suppurative arthritis; and (4) infertility, one of the most commonly feared consequences of long-standing chronic PID. In the early stages, gonococcal infections are readily controlled with antibiotics, although regrettably penicillin-resistant strains have emerged. When the infection becomes walled off in suppurative tubes or tubo-ovarian abscesses, it is difficult to achieve a sufficient level of antibiotic within the centers of such suppuration to control these infections effectively. Postabortion and postpartum PIDs are also amenable to antibiotics but are far more difficult to control than the gonococcal infections. Sometimes it becomes necessary to remove the organs surgically.

VULVA

Diseases of the vulva in the aggregate constitute only a small fraction of gynecologic practice. Many inflammatory dermatologic diseases that affect hair-bearing skin elsewhere on the body may also occur on the vulva, so vulvitis may be encountered in psoriasis, eczema, and allergic dermatitis. The vulva is prone to skin infections because it is constantly exposed to secretions and moisture. Nonspecific vulvitis is particularly likely to occur in blood dyscrasias, uremia, diabetes mellitus, malnutrition, and avitaminoses. Most skin cysts (epidermal inclusion cysts) and tumors can also occur in the vulva. Here we discuss disorders peculiar to the vulva, including Bartholin's cyst, vestibular adenitis, vulvar dystrophies, and tumors of the vulva.

BARTHOLIN'S CYST

Acute infection of Bartholin's gland produces an acute inflammation of the gland (adenitis) and may result in a Bartholin's abscess. Bartholin's cysts are relatively common, occur at all ages, and result from obstruction of Bartholin's duct, usually by a preceding infection. These cysts may become quite large, up to 3 to 5 cm in diameter. The cyst is lined by either the transitional epithelium of the normal duct or squamous metaplasia. The cysts produce pain and local discomfort; the cysts are either excised or opened permanently (marsupialization).

VESTIBULAR ADENITIS

The vulvar vestibule is located in the posterior introitus at the entrance to the vagina and contains small glands in the submucosa (vestibular glands). Inflammation of these glands is associated with a chronic, recurrent, and exquisitely painful condition known as vestibular adenitis. The inflammatory condition, which involves the glands and mucosa, produces small ulcerations, which account for extreme point tenderness in the vestibule. The cause of the condition is unknown, and the condition is best relieved by surgical removal of the inflamed mucosa.[14]

VULVAR DYSTROPHY

A spectrum of inflammatory lesions of the vulva is characterized by opaque, white, scaly, plaque-like mucosal thickenings that produce vulvar discomfort and itching (pruritus). Because of their white appearance, these disorders traditionally have been termed "leukoplakia" by clinicians. This is a clinical descriptive term because *white plaques may indicate a variety of benign, premalignant, or malignant lesions.*[15] Hence a biopsy of "leukoplakia" may reveal one of several conditions: (1) vitiligo (loss of pigment); (2) inflammatory dermatoses (e.g., psoriasis, chronic dermatitis [see Chapter 26]); (3) carcinoma in situ, Paget's disease, or even invasive carcinoma; and (4) a variety of alterations of unknown etiology that elude proper classification. To eliminate the confusion generated by using multiple terms to characterize white vulvar lesions (e.g., kraurosis vulvae, leukoplakia, atrophic vulvitis), clinical descriptive terminology has been separated from histologic diagnosis. Excluding neoplasms and specific disease entities, nonspecific inflammatory alterations of the vulva have been placed under a single disease heading of *dystrophy* by the International Society for the Study of Vulvar Disease.[16] Under this heading, two entities are recognized: (1) *lichen sclerosus,* a characteristic disorder manifested by subepithelial fibrosis, and (2) *squamous hyperplasia,* characterized by epithelial hyperplasia and hyperkeratosis. The two forms may coexist in different areas of the same vulva, and the lesions are often multiple, making their clinical management particularly difficult.

Lichen Sclerosus

Lichen sclerosus can occur anywhere on the body. It leads to atrophy, fibrosis, and scarring and has been called "chronic atrophic vulvitis." The skin becomes pale gray and parchment-like, the labia are atrophied, and the introitus is narrowed. Histologically there is usually thinning of the epidermis, with disappearance of the rete pegs and replacement of the underlying dermis by dense collagenous fibrous tissue (Fig. 23–7). There is often marked hyperkeratosis and a mononuclear cell infiltrate about blood vessels. Clinically lichen sclerosus occurs in all age groups but is most common after menopause. Genetic as well as autoimmune and hormonal factors have been implicated in its pathogenesis.[17] At all ages, the disorder tends to be slowly developing, insidious, and progressive. It causes considerable discomfort and predisposes to acute infection but is usually of little systemic significance. Lichen sclerosus is not considered a premalignant lesion *per se,* but it increases the risk of subsequent carcinoma slightly. Only a small proportion of patients (about 1 to 4%) have actually been observed to develop carcinoma.[17]

Squamous Hyperplasia

Previously called "hyperplastic dystrophy," this lesion denotes hyperplasia of the vulvar squamous epithelium, frequently with hyperkeratosis. The

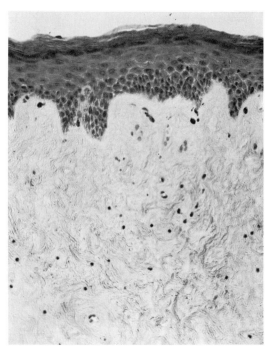

Figure 23–7. Lichen sclerosus illustrating atrophy of epidermis and dense sclerosis of dermis with total atrophy of dermal adnexal structures. (Courtesy of Dr. A. Hertig.)

epithelium is thickened and may show increased mitotic activity in both the basal and prickle cell layers (Fig. 23–8) with variable leukocytic infiltration of the dermis. Similar to lichen sclerosus, squamous hyperplasia is sometimes associated with carcinoma. It is not, however, considered a significant cancer precursor unless there is coexisting epithelial atypia, in which case it is classified as a pre-

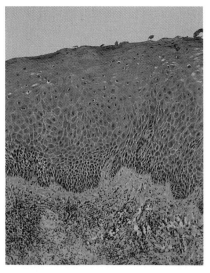

Figure 23–8. Squamous hyperplasia. Epithelial hyperplasia and dermal chronic inflammation.

cancerous lesion (vulvar intraepithelial neoplasia [VIN]).[18]

The pathogenesis of squamous hyperplasia is unknown. Because they may present as white vulvar plaques, they may be indistinguishable clinically from more serious disorders. Thus, biopsy is therefore indicated in all lesions, even those that are remotely suspicious.

TUMORS

Tumors of the vulva are the most important lesions to affect this region. Many types have been recorded, both benign and malignant, including fibromas, neurofibromas, angiomas, sweat gland tumors, carcinomas, malignant melanomas, and various types of sarcoma. All these forms are uncommon and moreover are histologically analogous to similar tumors occurring elsewhere in the body. Therefore attention is focused on the more common tumors and other proliferative lesions distinctive of the vulva.

Benign Tumors

Papillary Hidradenoma

Like the breast, the vulva contains modified apocrine sweat glands. In fact, the vulva may contain tissue closely resembling breast ("ectopic breast") and develops two tumors with counterparts in the breast. One of these, papillary hidradenoma, is identical in appearance to intraductal papillomas of the breast. The other, Paget's disease, is discussed later. Hidradenoma presents as a sharply circumscribed nodule, most commonly on the labia majora or interlabial folds, and may be confused clinically with carcinoma because of its tendency to ulcerate. Histologically hidradenomas consist of tubular ducts lined by a single or double layer of nonciliated columnar cells, with a layer of flattened "myoepithelial cells" underlying the epithelium. These myoepithelial elements are characteristic of sweat glands and sweat gland tumors.

Condyloma Acuminatum

Benign raised or wart-like (verrucous) conditions of the vulva occur in three forms. (1) By far the most common is the condyloma acuminatum, a papillomavirus-induced squamous lesion also called "venereal wart." (2) Another consists of mucosal polyps, which are benign stromal proliferations covered with squamous epithelium. (3) Another raised lesion, the syphilitic condyloma latum, is described in Chapter 8.

Condyloma acuminata are sexually transmitted, benign tumors that have a distinctly verrucous gross appearance (Fig. 23–9).[9] Although they may be solitary, they are more frequently multiple; often coalesce; and involve perineal, vulvar, and

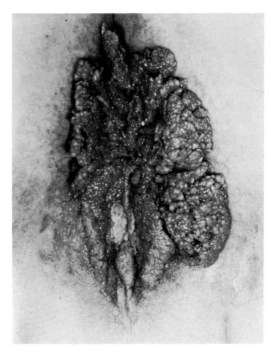

Figure 23–9. Numerous condylomas of vulva, almost obscuring labia minora. (Courtesy of Dr. A. Hertig.)

perianal regions as well as the vagina and, less commonly, the cervix. The lesions are identical to those found on the penis and around the anus in males (see Chapter 22). Histologically, they consist of branching, tree-like proliferation of stratified squamous epithelium supported by a fibrous stroma (Fig. 23–10A). Acanthosis, parakeratosis, hyperkeratosis, and, most specifically, nuclear atypia in the surface cells with perinuclear vacuolization (called koilocytosis) are present. Condylomata are caused by the human papillomavirus, specifically types 6 and 11,[20] which are associated with benign warts and replicate in the squamous epithelium. The virus life cycle is completed in the epithelium, specifically the mature superficial cells. This dependence of viral growth on squamous maturation is typical of human papillomavirus and produces a distinct cytologic change in the mature cells—koilocytotic atypia (nuclear atypia and perinuclear vacuolization)—which is considered a viral "cytopathic" effect. Except in immunosuppressed individuals, condyloma acuminata frequently regress spontaneously and are not considered to be precancerous lesions. They are, however, a marker for sexually transmitted disease.[20]

Malignant Tumors

Carcinoma and Vulvar Intraepithelial Neoplasia (VIN)

Carcinoma of the vulva is an uncommon malignancy (approximately one-eighth as frequent as

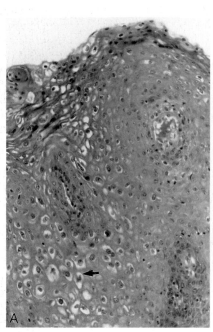
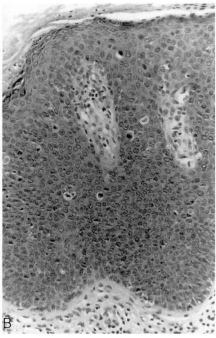

Figure 23-10. Histopathology of condyloma acuminatum and vulvar intraepithelial neoplasia (VIN). *A*, Cytoplasmic vacuolization (koilocytosis) and oval nuclei in superficial layers are characteristic of papillomavirus cytopathic effect and correlate with viral growth in these cells. *B*, VIN, with cellular atypia, nuclear crowding, and increased mitotic index.

cervical cancer) representing about 3% of all genital cancers in the female; approximately two-thirds occur in women over age 60 years.[21] Eight-five per cent of these malignant tumors are squamous cell carcinomas, the remainder being basal cell carcinomas, melanomas, or adenocarcinomas. In terms of etiology, pathogenesis, and clinical presentation, vulvar squamous cell carcinomas may be divided into two general groups.

The first group is associated with papillomaviruses, may be multicentric, and frequently coexists with or is preceded by a defined precancerous change, called vulvar intraepithelial neoplasia (VIN), also known as carcinoma in situ or Bowen's disease.[22] VIN is characterized by nuclear atypia in the epithelial cells, increased mitoses, and lack of surface differentiation (see Fig. 23–10B). Based on the severity of atypia, VIN may be graded as I (mild), II (moderate), or III (severe). These lesions usually present as white or pigmented plaques on the vulva; identical lesions are encountered in the male. VIN is appearing with increasing frequency in women under the age of 40. With or without associated invasive carcinoma, VIN is frequently multicentric, and from 10 to 30% are associated with another primary squamous neoplasm in the vagina or cervix. This association indicates a common etiologic agent. Indeed, 90% of cases of VIN and many associated cancers contain papillomavirus DNA, specifically types 16, 18, and other cancer-associated (high-risk) types.[22] Spontaneous regression of VIN lesions has been reported; the risk of progression to invasive cancer increases in older (over age 45) or immunosuppressed women.[22]

The second group of squamous cell carcinomas are associated with vulvar "dystrophies" (squamous cell hyperplasia or lichen sclerosus). The etiology of this group of carcinomas is unclear, and they are infrequently associated with papillomaviruses. In some cases, the associated dystrophies contain epithelial atypia (VIN), suggesting that precancerous changes can occur in these otherwise benign lesions and increase the risk of a subsequent cancer. Whether these cancers develop from exposure to specific carcinogens remains to be clarified.[23]

MORPHOLOGY. Vulvar squamous cell carcinomas begin as small areas of epithelial thickening that resemble leukoplakia but, in the course of time, progress to create firm, indurated, **exophytic** tumors or ulcerated, endophytic lesions. Although vulvar carcinomas are external tumors that are obviously apparent to the patient and the clinician, many are misinterpreted as dermatitis, eczema, or leukoplakia for long periods. The clinical manifestations evoked are chiefly those of pain, local discomfort, itching, and exudation because superficial secondary infection is common.

Histologically, tumors associated with human papillomavirus or VIN tend to be poorly differentiated, whereas others are usually well differentiated, with the formation of keratohyaline pearls and prickle cells (Fig. 23–11). Risk of metastatic spread is linked to the size of tumor, depth of invasion, and involvement of lymphatic vessels. The inguinal, pelvic, iliac, and periaortic lymph nodes are most commonly involved. Ultimately, lymphohematogenous dissemination involves the lungs, liver, and other internal organs. Patients with lesions less than 2 cm in diameter have a 60 to 80% 5-year

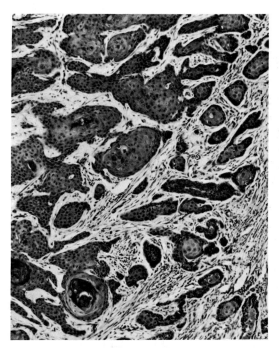

Figure 23-11. Carcinoma of vulva at medium power, illustrating typical invasive cords of squamous cell carcinoma.

survival rate after treatment with one-stage vulvectomy and lymphadenectomy; larger lesions with lymph node involvement yield a less than 10% 5-year survival rate.

Rare variants of squamous cell carcinoma include **verrucous carcinoma,** which may resemble condyloma acuminatum and presents as a large fungating tumor. Local invasion confirms the malignant nature of the lesion, but it rarely metastasizes and can be cured by wide excision.

Extramammary Paget's Disease

This curious and rare lesion of the vulva, and sometimes the perianal region, is similar in its skin manifestations to Paget's disease of the breast[24] (see Chapter 24). As a vulvar neoplasm, it manifests as a pruritic red, crusted, sharply demarcated, map-like area, occurring usually on the labia majora. It may be accompanied by a palpable submucosal thickening or tumor. The diagnostic microscopic feature of this lesion is the presence of large, anaplastic tumor cells lying singly or in small clusters within the epidermis and its appendages. These cells are distinguished by a clear separation ("halo") from the surrounding epithelial cells (Fig. 23-12) and a finely granular cytoplasm containing PAS, alcian blue, or mucicarmine-positive mucopolysaccharide. Ultrastructurally Paget's cells display apocrine, eccrine, and keratinocyte differentiation and presumably arise from primitive epithelial progenitor cells.[24]

In contrast to Paget's disease of the nipple, in which 100% of patients show an underlying ductal breast carcinoma, vulvar lesions are most frequently confined to the epidermis of the skin and adjacent hair follicles and sweat glands. The prognosis of Paget's disease is poor in uncommon cases with associated carcinoma, but intraepidermal Paget's disease may persist for many years, even decades, without the development of invasion. Because Paget's cells, however, often extend into skin appendages and may extend beyond the confines of the grossly visible lesion, they are prone to recurrence.

Malignant Melanoma

Melanomas of the vulva are rare, representing less than 5% of all vulvar cancers and 2% of all melanomas in women. Their peak incidence is in the sixth or seventh decade; they tend to have the same biologic and histologic characteristics as melanomas occurring elsewhere and are capable of widespread metastatic dissemination. The overall survival rate is less than 32%, presumably owing to delays in detection and a generally poor prognosis for mucosal melanomas. Prognosis is linked principally to depth of invasion, with greater than 60% mortality for lesions invading deeper than 1 mm.[25] Because it is initially confined to the epithelium, melanoma may resemble Paget's disease, both grossly and histologically. It can usually be differentiated by its uniform reactivity, using immunoperoxidase techniques, with antibodies to S100 protein, and by its lack of reactivity to content of carcinoembryonic antigen (CEA) and mucopolysaccharides.

VAGINA

The vagina is a portion of the female genital tract that is remarkably free from primary disease. In the adult, inflammations often affect the vulva and perivulvar structures and spread to the cervix without significant involvement of the vagina. The

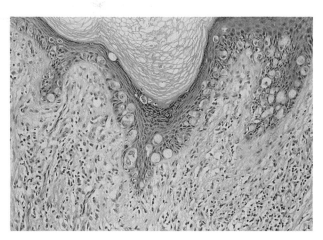

Figure 23-12. Paget's disease of vulva, with cluster of large clear tumor cells within squamous epithelium.

major serious primary lesion of this structure is the uncommon primary carcinoma. The remaining entities can therefore be cited quite briefly.

CONGENITAL ANOMALIES

Atresia and total absence of the vagina are both extremely uncommon. The latter usually occurs only when there are severe malformations of the entire genital tract. Septate, or double, vagina is also an uncommon anomaly that arises from failure of total fusion of the müllerian ducts and accompanies double uterus (uterus didelphis).

Gartner's duct cysts are relatively common lesions, found along the lateral walls of the vagina and derived from wolffian duct rests. They are 1- to 2-cm, fluid-filled cysts that occur submucosally. Other cysts include mucous cysts, which occur in the proximal vagina, are derived from müllerian epithelium, and often contain squamous metaplasia. Another müllerian-derived lesion—endometriosis, to be described later—may occur in the vagina and simulate a neoplasm.

PREMALIGNANT AND MALIGNANT NEOPLASMS

Most benign tumors of the vagina occur in reproductive-age women and consist of skeletal muscle (rhabdomyomas) or stromal (stromal polyps) tumors. The latter may contain cellular atypia but are benign, localized, and self-limited. Others include benign leiomyomas, hemangiomas, and rare mixed tumors. Clinically important malignant tumors in terms of frequency and biologic behavior are carcinoma and embryonal rhabdomyosarcoma (sarcoma botryoides).

Vaginal Intraepithelial Neoplasia and Squamous Cell Carcinoma

Primary carcinoma of the vagina is an extremely uncommon cancer (about 0.6 per 100,000 women yearly) accounting for about 1% of malignant neoplasms in the female genital tract, and of these, 95% are squamous cell carcinomas.[26] The greatest risk factor is a previous carcinoma of the cervix or vulva; from 1 to 2% of patients with an invasive cervical carcinoma eventually develop a vaginal squamous carcinoma. This has been attributed to the multicentric nature of squamous neoplasia in the lower genital tract (many are associated with papillomaviruses), inadequate removal of primary carcinomas, and the mutagenic effects of radiation therapy. The peak age incidence is between 60 and 70 years, and 90% of patients are over age 50. Vaginal carcinoma is frequently detected in association with a vaginal intraepithelial neoplasia (dys-

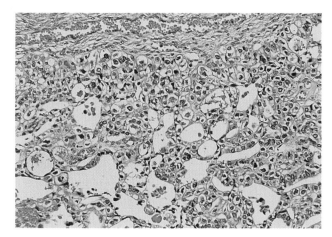

Figure 23-13. Clear cell adenocarcinoma showing vacuolated tumor cells forming glands.

plasia/carcinoma in situ). The latter occurs in slightly younger women and presumably precedes invasion.

MORPHOLOGY. Most often the tumor affects the upper posterior vagina, particularly along the posterior wall at the junction with the ectocervix. It begins as a focus of epithelial thickening, often in association with a vaginal intraepithelial neoplasm, progressing to a plaque-like mass that extends centrifugally and invades, by direct continuity, the cervix and perivaginal structures, such as the urethra, urinary bladder, and rectum. The lesions in the lower two-thirds metastasize to the inguinal nodes, whereas upper lesions tend to involve the regional iliac nodes and, in late advanced stages, distant organs via the blood. These lesions first come to the patient's attention by the appearance of irregular spotting or the development of a frank vaginal discharge (leukorrhea). At other times, they remain totally silent and become clinically manifest only with the onset of urinary or rectal fistulas.

Adenocarcinoma

Adenocarcinomas are rare but have received attention because of the increased frequency of clear cell adenocarcinomas in young women whose mothers had been treated with diethylstilbestrol (DES) during pregnancy (for a threatened abortion).[27] Fortunately, fewer than 0.14% of such DES-exposed young women develop adenocarcicoma. These tumors are usually discovered between the ages of 15 and 20 and are often composed of vacuolated, glycogen-containing cells, hence the term "clear cell" (Fig. 23-13).

MORPHOLOGY. The tumors are most often located on the anterior wall of the vagina, usually in the upper third, and vary in size from 0.2 to 10 cm in greatest diameter. These cancers can also arise in the cervix. A probable precursor of the tumor is vaginal adenosis, a condition in which glandular columnar epithelium of müllerian type either appears beneath the squamous epithelium or replaces it.[28] Adenosis presents clinically as red, granular foci contrasting with the normal pale pink, opaque vaginal mucosa. Microscopically the glandular epithelium may be either mucus-secreting, resembling endocervical mucosa, or so-called tuboendometrial, often containing cilia. Adenosis has been reported in 35 to 90% of the offspring of estrogen-treated mothers, but as mentioned earlier, malignant transformation is extremely rare.

Because of its insidious, invasive growth, vaginal cancer (squamous and adenocarcinoma) is difficult to cure. Thus early detection by careful follow-up is mandatory in DES-exposed women. Surgery and irradiation have successfully eradicated DES-related tumors in up to 80% of patients. Extension of cervical carcinoma to the vagina is much more common than primary malignancies of the vagina. Accordingly before a diagnosis of primary vaginal carcinoma can be made, a pre-existing cervical lesion must be ruled out.

Embryonal Rhabdomyosarcoma

Also called *sarcoma botryoides*, this is an interesting but very uncommon vaginal tumor most frequently found in infants and in children under the age of 5. The tumor consists predominantly of malignant embryonal rhabdomyoblasts and is thus a type of rhabdomyosarcoma.[33]

Grossly, these tumors tend to grow as polyploid, rounded, bulky masses that sometimes fill and project out of the vagina; they have the appearance and consistency of grape-like clusters (hence the designation "botryoides," grape-like) (Fig. 23–14). Histologically, the tumor cells are small and have oval nuclei, with small protrusions of cytoplasm from one end, so they resemble a tennis racket. Rarely striations can be seen within the cytoplasm. Beneath the vaginal epithelium, the tumor cells are crowded in a so-called cambium layer, but in the deep regions they lie within a loose fibromyxomatous stroma that is edematous and may contain many inflammatory cells. For this reason, the lesions can be mistaken for benign inflammatory polyps, leading to unfortunate delays in diagnosis and treatment. These tumors tend to invade locally and cause death by penetration into the peritoneal cavity or by obstruction of the urinary tract.

Conservative surgery, coupled with chemotherapy, appears to offer the best results in cases diagnosed sufficiently early.[30]

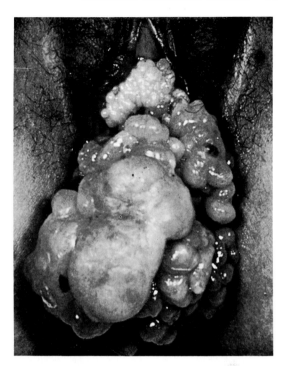

Figure 23–14. Sarcoma botryoides (embryonal rhabdomyosarcoma) of vagina appearing as a polypoid mass protruding from vagina. (Courtesy of Dr. A. Hertig.)

CERVIX

The cervix is both a sentinel for potentially serious upper genital tract infections and a target for viral or chemical carcinogens, which may lead to invasive carcinoma. The former constitutes one of the most common clinical complaints in gynecologic practice and frequently vexes both patient and clinician. The potential threat of cancer, however, is central to Papanicolaou smear screening programs and histologic interpretation of biopsies by the pathologist. Worldwide cervical carcinoma alone is responsible for about 5% of all cancer deaths in women.

INFLAMMATIONS

Acute and Chronic Cervicitis

At the onset of menarche, the production of estrogens by the ovary stimulates maturation (glycogen uptake) of cervical and vaginal squamous mucosa. As these cells are shed, the glycogen provides a substrate for endogenous vaginal aerobes and anaerobes, streptococci, enterococci, *Escherichia coli*, and staphylococci. The bacterial growth produces a drop in vaginal pH. The exposed endocervix is sensitive to these changes in chemical environment

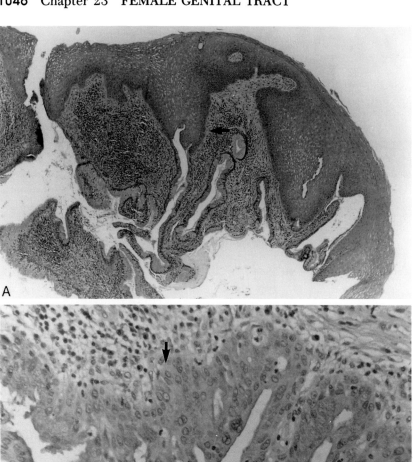

Figure 23–15. *A*, Low-power histology of chronic cervicitis and the cervical transformation zone. Mature squamous epithelium (epidermidalization) has replaced the columnar epithelium and covers the glands *(arrow)*. An inflammatory infiltrate is present in the submucosa. *B*, Immature squamous metaplasia developing in an endocervical gland. The arrows highlight layers of immature squamous cells displacing columnar cells toward the gland lumen.

and bacterial flora and responds by undergoing a transformation from columnar to squamous epithelium, as detailed previously.[31] The process and transformation is also hastened by trauma and other infections occurring in the reproductive years. As the squamous epithelium overgrows and obliterates the surface columnar papillae, it covers and obstructs crypt openings, with the accumulation of mucus in deeper crypts (glands) to form mucous (nabothian) cysts. This process is invariably associated with an inflammatory infiltrate composed of a mixture of polymorphonuclear leukocytes and mononuclear cells and, if the inflammation is severe, may be associated with loss of the epithelial lining (erosion or ulceration) and epithelial repair (reparative atypia or dysplasia of repair). All of these components characterize what is known as *chronic cervicitis* (Fig. 23–15).

Some degree of cervical inflammation may be found in virtually all multiparous and in many nulliparous adult women, and it is usually of little clinical consequence. Principal concerns include the potential presence of organisms, which may be clinically important. Specific infections by gonococci, chlamydia, mycoplasma, and herpes (mostly type II) may produce significant acute or chronic cervicitis and should be identified for their relevance to upper genital tract disease, pregnancy complications, or sexual transmission (Fig. 23–16).

MORPHOLOGY. The pathologic correlates of acute and chronic cervicitis include epithelial spongiosis (intercellular edema), submucosal edema, and a combination of epithelial and stromal changes. Acute cervicitis includes acute inflammatory cells, erosion, and reactive or reparative epithelial change. Chronic cervicitis includes inflammation, usually mononuclear, with lymphocytes, macrophages, and plasma cells. Necrosis and granulation tissue may also be present. Although the inflammation alone is not specific, some patterns are asso-

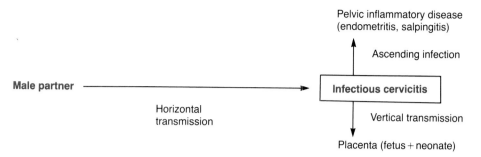

ciated with certain organisms. Herpesvirus is most strongly associated with epithelial ulcers (often with intranuclear inclusions in epithelial cells) and a lymphocytic infiltrate, and *C. trachomatis* with lymphoid germinal centers and a prominent plasmacytic infiltrate (Fig. 23–17). Epithelial spongiosis is associated with *T. vaginalis* infection.[32]

All the aforementioned changes are more pronounced in patients with clinical symptoms (mucopurulent cervicitis) or in whom specific organisms can be identified.[33] These changes, however, may be observed in culture-negative or asymptomatic women, underscoring the combined importance of culture, clinical evaluation, and Papanicolaou smear examination. Severe reparative changes may mimic precancerous lesions because cells undergoing repair are depleted of their normal content of glycogen and may contain nuclear atypia. They also may fail to stain brown with Schiller's solution (an iodine preparation), as detailed subsequently.

Endocervical Polyps

Endocervical polyps are relatively innocuous, inflammatory tumors that occur in 2 to 5% of adult women. Perhaps the major significance of polyps lies in their production of irregular vaginal "spotting" or bleeding that arouses suspicion of some more ominous lesion. Most polyps arise within the endocervical canal and vary from small and sessile to large, 5-cm masses that may protrude through the cervical os (Fig. 23–18). All are soft, almost mucoid, and are composed of a loose fibromyxomatous stroma harboring dilated, mucus-secreting endocervical glands and often accompanied by inflammation and squamous metaplasia. In almost all instances, simple curettage or surgical excision effects a cure.

INTRAEPITHELIAL AND INVASIVE SQUAMOUS NEOPLASIA

No form of cancer better documents the remarkable effects of prevention, early diagnosis, and curative therapy on the mortality rate than cancer of the cervix. Fifty years ago, carcinoma of the cervix was the leading cause of cancer deaths in women in the United States, but the death rate has dropped remarkably to its present rank as the eighth source of cancer mortality, causing about 4500 deaths annually (behind lung, breast, colon, pancreas, ovary, lymph nodes, and blood). In sharp

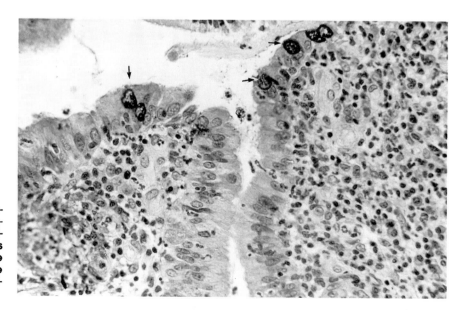

Figure 23–17. Severe chronic inflammation associated with chlamydia infection. An immunoperoxidase stain for chlamydia highlights distinct cytoplasmic vacuoles in the endocervical cells *(arrows)*. Note the intense inflammatory cell infiltrate.

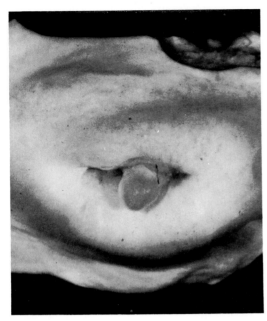

Figure 23-18. Endocervical polyp, protruding through external os.

contrast to this reduced mortality, the detection frequency of early cancers and precancerous conditions is very high. Annually there are an estimated 13,000 cases of new invasive cancer and 50,000 of advanced precancerous conditions.[34] Thus, it is evident that well over half of invasive cancers are cured by early detection and effective therapy, and even more important many more precancerous lesions that place the patients at risk for subsequent cancer are eradicated by timely, appropriate treatment. Much credit for these dramatic gains belongs to the effectiveness of the Papanicolaou cytologic test in detecting cervical precancers and to the accessibility of the cervix to colposcopy and biopsy.

PATHOGENESIS. To understand the pathogenesis of cervical cancer, it is important to understand the components involved in its development, which have been identified from a series of clinical, epidemiologic, pathologic, and molecular studies. Epidemiologic data have long implicated a sexually transmitted agent, based specifically on the risk factors for cervical cancer, which include (1) early age at first intercourse, (2) multiple sexual partners, and (3) a male partner with multiple previous sexual partners. All other risk factors are subordinate to these three influences, primarily multiple sexual partners. Potential risk factors that remain poorly understood include oral contraceptive use, cigarette smoking, parity, family history, associated genital infections, and lack of circumcision in the male sexual partner.[35,36] Concerning sexually transmitted agents, human papillomavirus is currently considered an important factor in cervical oncogenesis. As noted earlier, this virus is the known cause of the sexually transmitted vulvar condyloma acuminatum and has been isolated from vulvar and vaginal squamous cell carcinomas; it is also suspected to be an oncogenic agent in a variety of other squamous tumors or proliferative lesions of skin and mucous membranes, as detailed in Chapter 7.[37]

There is mounting evidence linking human papillomavirus to cancer in general and cervical cancer in particular: (1) Human papillomavirus DNA is detected by hybridization techniques in approximately 85% of cervical cancers and in approximately 90% of cervical condylomata and precancerous lesions.[37] (2) Specific human papillomavirus types are associated with cervical cancer (high risk) versus condylomata (low risk); low-risk types include types 6, 11, 42, and 44 and high-risk types 16, 18, 31, and 33.[38] (3) *In vitro* studies indicate that the high-risk human papillomavirus types have the capability to transform cells in culture (see Chapter 7), and this ability is linked to specific viral oncogenes (E6 and E7 genes), which differ in sequence between the high-risk and low-risk human papillomavirus types. Introduction of these nucleic acids into cultured keratinocytes produces morphologic changes nearly identical to precancerous changes, and under certain circumstances, these cells may form squamous tumors when injected into mice. (4) The physical state of the virus differs in cancers, being covalently linked (integrated) with the host genomic DNA. This is in contrast to free (episomal) viral DNA in condylomata and most precancerous lesions.[37,39] (5) The E6 oncoprotein of human papillomavirus type 16 and 18 (but not low-risk type 11) binds to the tumor suppressor gene p53 and accelerates its proteolytic degradation (see Chapter 7).

The evidence does not implicate human papillomavirus as the only factor. A high percentage of young women are infected with one or more human papillomavirus types during their reproductive years, and only a few develop cancer. Other cocarcinogens, the immune status of the individual, nutrition, and many other factors influence whether the human papillomavirus infection remains subclinical (latent), turns into a precancer, or eventually progresses to cancer. In addition, about 15% of cervical cancers are not associated with human papillomavirus, implying other modes of cancer development, including host gene mutations.[40] Figure 23-19 presents one attempt to explain the role of human papillomavirus in cervical carcinogenesis and its impact on the population in the United States.

Cervical Intraepithelial Neoplasia

The reason that Papanicolaou smear screening is so effective in preventing cervical cancer is that the

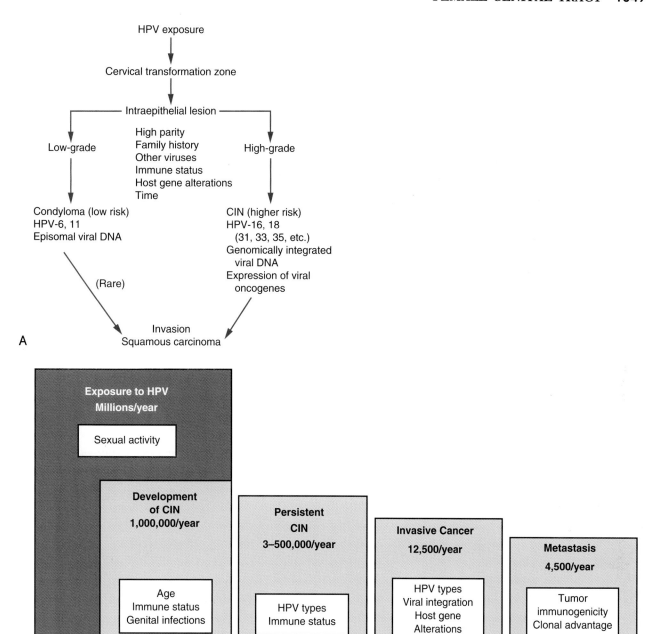

Figure 23–19. *A,* Postulated steps in the pathogenesis of cervical neoplasia. The conditions listed *(center)* are possible risk factors for cancer. *B,* Hypothetical schema for the role of human papillomavirus in cervical neoplasia, ranging from exposure to the virus to development of metastatic disease. The approximate number of individuals at each step yearly in the United States is enumerated; viral and host variables potentially involved in each step are enclosed within the smaller boxes.

majority of cancers are preceded by a precancerous lesion. This lesion may exist in the noninvasive stage for as long as 20 years and shed abnormal cells that can be detected on cytologic examination.[41] These precancerous changes should be viewed with the following in mind: (1) They represent a continuum of morphologic change with relatively indistinct boundaries; (2) they will not invariably progress to cancer and may spontaneously regress, with the risk of persisting or progressing to cancer increasing with the severity of the precancerous change; (3) they are associated with papillomaviruses, and "high-risk" human

papillomavirus types are found in increasing frequency in the higher grade precursors.[42,43]

Cervical precancers have been classified in a variety of ways. The oldest system is the dysplasia–carcinoma in situ system with mild dysplasia on one end and severe dysplasia/carcinoma in situ on the other. Another is the cervical intraepithelial neoplasia (CIN) classification, with mild dysplasias termed CIN grade I and carcinoma in situ lesions termed CIN III.[39] Still another reduces these entities to two, terming them low-grade and high-grade intraepithelial *lesions.*[53] Because these systems describe noninvasive lesions of indetermin-

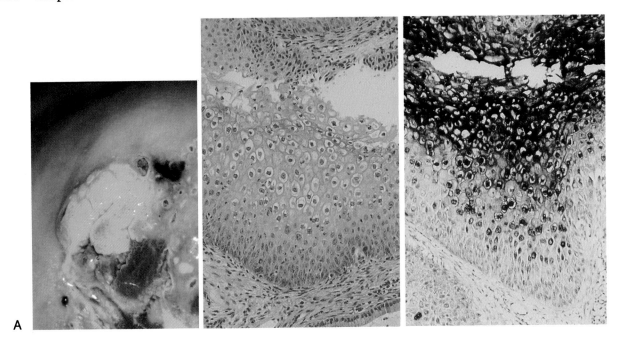

A

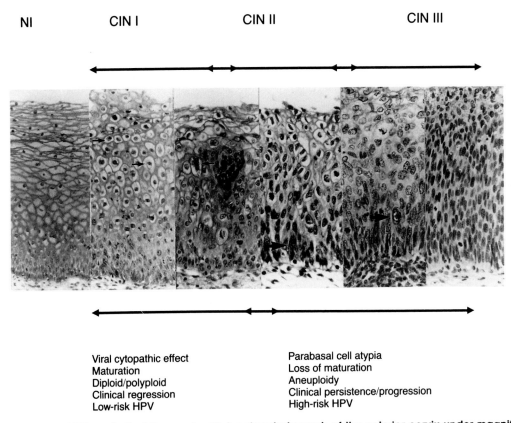

NI   CIN I   CIN II   CIN III

Viral cytopathic effect   Parabasal cell atypia
Maturation   Loss of maturation
Diploid/polyploid   Aneuploidy
Clinical regression   Clinical persistence/progression
Low-risk HPV   High-risk HPV

B

Figure 23–20. *A,* Condyloma (CIN grade I) of the cervix: (1) A colpophotograph of the anterior cervix under magnification depicts this as a discrete, raised, white lesion in the cervical transformation zone. The entrance to the endocervical canal is at the bottom of the picture. (2) Histology of a cervical condyloma, illustrating the prominent koilocytotic atypia in the upper epithelial cells, as evidenced by the prominent perinuclear halos. (3) Nucleic acid *in situ* hybridization of the same lesion for HPV nucleic acids. The blue staining denotes HPV DNA, which is typically most abundant in the koilocytes. *B,* The varied appearances of cervical intraepithelial neoplasia (CIN). This panel of epithelia range from normal (NI) to the highest grade (CIN III). Human papillomavirus (HPV) viral cytopathic effect (koilocytotic atypia; *small arrows*) is most prominent on the left (CIN I) and is joined by increasing nuclear atypia *(large arrows)* in the middle (CIN II) and accompanied by progressive loss of maturation on the right (CIN III) panels. Biologic (ploidy), clinical (regression/persistence), and viral (high-risk or low-risk HPV types) parameters are situated opposite their approximate histologic counterparts.

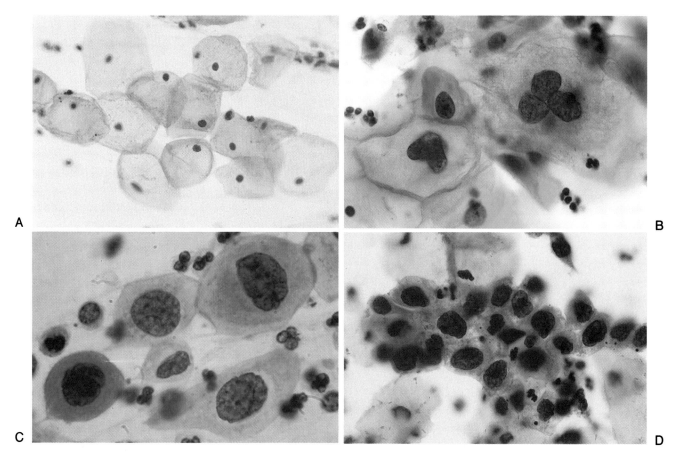

Figure 23–21. The cytology of cervical intraepithelial neoplasia, as seen on the Papanicolaou smear. A, Normal exfoliated superficial squamous epithelial cells. B, CIN I. C, CIN II. D, CIN III. Note the reduction in cytoplasm and increase in the nucleus-to-cytoplasm ratio, which occurs as the grade of the lesion increases. This reflects the progressive loss of cellular differentiation on the *surface* of the lesions from which these cells are exfoliated (see Fig. 23–20B).

ate biology that are usually easily treated, none of these classifications is indispensable to clinical management or immune to revision. In this chapter they are referred to using the CIN terminology.[42]

MORPHOLOGY. Figure 23–20 illustrates a spectrum of morphologic alterations that range from normal to the highest grade precancer. On the extreme low end of the spectrum of morphologic change are lesions that are indistinguishable histologically from condylomata acuminata and may be either raised (acuminatum) or macular (flat condyloma) in appearance. These lesions exhibit koilocytotic atypia (viral cytopathic effect) with few alterations in the other cells in the epithelium and fall within the range of CIN I (see Fig. 23–20A). These changes correlate strongly (but not invariably) with low-risk human papillomavirus types and genetically diploid or polyploid cell populations. The next change in the spectrum consists of the appearance of atypical cells in the lower layers of the squamous epithelium but nonetheless with persistent (but abnormal) differentiation toward the prickle and keratinizing cell layers. The atypical cells show changes in nucleocytoplasmic ratio; variation in nuclear size (anisokaryosis); loss of po-

larity; increased mitotic figures, including abnormal mitoses; and hyperchromasia —in other words, they take on some of the characteristics of malignant cells. These lesions fall within the range of CIN II. These features have been associated with aneuploid cell populations and correlate strongly with high-risk human papillomavirus types, probably reflecting early changes associated with the viral oncogenes of these viruses. As the spectrum evolves, there is progressive loss of differentiation with involvement of more and more layers of the epithelium, until it is totally replaced by immature atypical cells, exhibiting no surface differentiation (CIN III) (Fig. 23–20B).[42,43] The cellular changes on Papanicolaou smear that correspond to this histologic spectrum are illustrated in Figure 23–21.

CIN almost always begins at the squamocolumnar junction, in the transformation zone. The lowest grade CIN lesions, including condylomata, most likely do not progress, whereas lesions containing greater degrees of cellular atypia are at greater risk. Roughly one-third and two-thirds of CIN I and CIN II lesions, respectively, persist or progress to high grade. It is important to realize that not all lesions begin as condylomata or as CIN

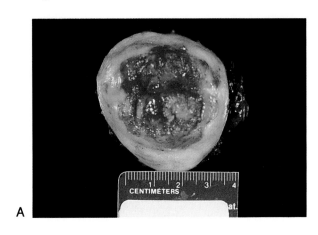

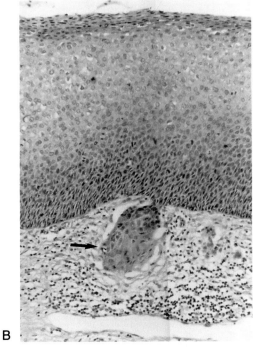

Figure 23–22. *A,* Carcinoma of cervix, well advanced. *B,* Early stromal invasion *(arrow)* occurring in a cervical intraepithelial neoplasm.

I and that they may enter at any point in the spectrum, depending on the associated human papillomavirus type and other host factors. The rates of progression are by no means uniform, and although HPV type is a potential predictor of lesion behavior, it is difficult to predict the outcome in an individual patient. These findings underscore that risk of cancer is conferred only in part by human papillomavirus type and depends on other carcinogens or genetic alterations that bring about the evolution of a precancer. Predictably lesions that have completely evolved (CIN III) constitute the greatest risk. CIN III is most frequently associated with invasive cancer when the latter is identified. Progression to invasive carcinoma, when it occurs, may develop in from a few months to over 20 years.[45]

Squamous Cell Carcinoma

Squamous cell carcinoma may occur at any age from the second decade of life to senility. The peak incidence is occurring at an increasingly younger age: 40 to 45 years for invasive cancer and about 30 years for high-grade precancers. This represents the combination of earlier onset of sexual activity (i.e., earlier acquisition of human papillomavirus infection) and active Papanicolaou smear screening programs in the United States, which detect either cancers or precancerous lesions at an earlier point in life.

MORPHOLOGY. Invasive cervical carcinoma manifests in three somewhat distinctive patterns: **fungating (or exophytic), ulcerating,** and **infiltrative cancer.** The most common variant is the fungating tumor, which produces an obviously neoplastic mass that projects above the surrounding mucosa (Fig. 23–22A). Advanced cervical carcinoma extends by direct continuity to involve every contiguous structure, including the peritoneum, urinary bladder, ureters, rectum, and vagina. Local and distant lymph nodes are also involved. Distant metastasis occurs to the liver, lungs, bone marrow, and other structures.

Histologically, about 95% of squamous carcinomas are composed of relatively **large cells,** either **keratinizing** (well-differentiated) or **nonkeratinizing** (moderately differentiated) patterns. A small subset of tumors (less than 5%) are poorly differentiated small cell squamous or more rarely small cell undifferentiated carcinomas **(neuroendocrine or oat cell carcinomas).** The latter closely resemble oat cell carcinomas of lung and have an unusually poor prognosis owing to early spread by lymphatics and systemic spread.[46,47]

Cervical cancer is staged as follows:

Stage 0. Carcinoma in situ (CIN III).
Stage I. Carcinoma confined to the cervix.
Ia. Preclinical carcinoma, i.e., diagnosed only by microscopy but showing:
Ia1. Minimal microscopic invasion of stroma (minimally invasive carcinoma) (Fig. 23–22B).
Ia2. Microscopic invasion of stroma of less than 5 mm in depth (microinvasive carcinoma).
Ib. Histologically invasive carcinoma of the cervix that is greater than stage Ia2.
Stage II. Carcinoma extends beyond the cervix but not onto the pelvic wall. Carcinoma involves the vagina but not the lower third.

Stage III. Carcinoma has extended onto pelvic wall. On rectal examination, there is no cancer-free space between the tumor and the pelvic wall. The tumor involves the lower third of the vagina.

Stage IV. Carcinoma has extended beyond the true pelvis or has involved the mucosa of the bladder or rectum. This stage obviously includes those with metastatic dissemination.

Ten to twenty-five per cent of cervical carcinomas constitute **adenocarcinomas, adenosquamous carcinomas, undifferentiated carcinomas,** or other rare histologic types. The **adenocarcinomas** presumably arise in the endocervical glands. They look grossly and behave like the squamous cell lesions and may be associated with papillomaviruses but arise in a slightly older age group.[47,48] The **adenosquamous carcinomas** have mixed glandular and squamous patterns and are thought to arise from the reserve cells in the basal layers of the endocervical epithelium. They tend to have a less favorable prognosis than squamous cell carcinoma of similar stage. **Clear cell adenocarcinomas** of the cervix in DES-exposed women are similar to those occurring in the vagina, described earlier.

CLINICAL COURSE. It is apparent from the preceding discussion that cancer of the cervix and its precursors evolve slowly over the course of many years. During this interval, the only sign of disease may be the shedding of abnormal cells from the cervix. For these reasons, it is generally acknowledged that periodic Papanicolaou smears should be performed on all women after they become sexually active. Cytologic examination merely detects the possible presence of a cervical precancer or cancer; it does not make an absolute diagnosis, which requires histologic evaluation of appropriate biopsy specimens. Identification of abnormalities is facilitated by colposcopic examination of the cervix, in which CIN lesions are characterized by white patches on the cervix following the application of acetic acid.[41] In addition, distinct vascular mosaic or punctuation patterns can be appreciated. Highly abnormal vascular patterns regularly accompany invasive cervical cancer. Ultimately when these cancers become clinically overt, they usually produce irregular vaginal bleeding, leukorrhea, bleeding or pain on coitus, and dysuria.

Modes of treatment of squamous neoplasia of the cervix depend on the stage of the neoplasm; treatment of precursors includes Papanicolaou smear follow-up (for mild lesions), cryotherapy, laser, wire loop excision, and cone biopsy. Invasive cancers usually result in hysterectomy and for advanced lesions radiation. Approximately 1 in 500 patients with a treated CIN III eventually develops an invasive cancer. The prognosis and survival for invasive carcinomas depend largely on the stage at which cancer is first discovered.[46]

With current methods of treatment, there is a 5-year survival rate of about 80 to 90% with stage I, 75% with stage II, 35% with stage III, and 10 to 15% with stage IV disease. Most patients with stage IV cancer die as a consequence of local extension of the tumor—e.g., into and about the urinary bladder and ureters, leading to ureteral obstruction, pyelonephritis, and uremia—rather than distant metastases.[46]

BODY OF UTERUS AND ENDOMETRIUM

The uterus, stimulated continually by hormones, denuded monthly of its endometrial mucosa, and inhabited periodically by fetuses, is subject to a variety of disorders, the most common of which result from endocrine imbalances, complications of pregnancy, and neoplastic proliferation. Together with the lesions that affect the cervix, the lesions of the corpus of the uterus and the endometrium account for the great preponderance of gynecologic practices.

INFLAMMATIONS

The endometrium and myometrium are relatively resistant to infections, primarily because the endocervix normally forms a barrier to ascending infection. Thus, although chronic inflammation in the cervix is an expected and frequently insignificant finding, it is a concern when present in the endometrium, excluding the menstrual phase. Acute endometritis is uncommon and limited to bacterial infections that arise after delivery or miscarriage. Retained products of conception are the usual predisposing influence, causative agents including group A hemolytic streptococci, staphylococci, and other bacteria. The inflammatory response is chiefly limited to the interstitium and is entirely nonspecific. Removal of the retained gestational fragments by curettage is promptly followed by remission of the infection.

Chronic Endometritis

Chronic inflammation of the endometrium occurs in the following settings:[49] (1) in patients suffering from chronic PID; (2) in postpartal or postabortal endometrial cavities, usually due to retained gestational tissue; (3) in patients with intrauterine contraceptive devices (IUDs); and (4) in tuberculosis, either from miliary spread or more commonly from drainage of tuberculous salpingitis (Fig. 23–23). The latter is distinctly rare in Western countries. The chronic endometritis in all these cases represents a secondary disease, and under these circumstances there is a plausible cause.

In about 15% of cases, no such primary cause is obvious, yet plasma cells (which are not present

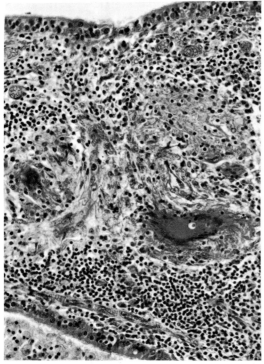

Figure 23–23. Tuberculous endometritis. Note granuloma with giant cells.

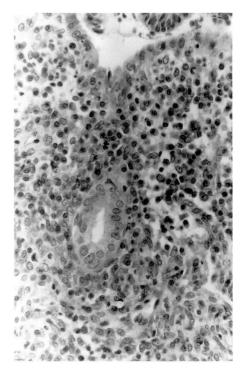

Figure 23–24. Chronic endometritis. Note the abundant plasma cells surrounding this endometrial gland.

in normal endometrium) are seen together with macrophages and lymphocytes (Fig. 23–24). Some women with this so-called nonspecific chronic endometritis have such gynecologic complaints as abnormal bleeding, pain, discharge, and infertility. Chlamydia may be involved and is commonly associated with both acute (polymorphonuclear leukocytes) and chronic (e.g., lymphocytes, plasma cells) inflammatory cell infiltrates. The organisms may or may not be successfully cultured.[32,50] Importantly antibiotic therapy is indicated because it may prevent other sequelae (e.g., salpingitis).

ADENOMYOSIS

The endomyometrial interface is usually sharply demarcated. Some endometrial glands, however, may extend beneath this interface to form nests deep within the myometrium, producing a condition known as adenomyosis. The cause is unknown; it occurs in approximately 15 to 20% of uteri. Adenomyosis causes expansion (enlargement) of the uterine wall and may be visible on gross examination as numerous small cysts. Microscopically irregular nests of endometrial stroma, with or without glands, are arranged within the myometrium, separated from the basalis by at least 2 to 3 mm. In some patients, the most important consequence of adenomyosis relates to shedding of the endometrium during the menstrual cycle (Fig. 23–25). Hemorrhage within these small adenomyotic nests

results in menorrhagia, colicky dysmenorrhea, dyspareunia, and pelvic pain, particularly during the premenstrual period.

ENDOMETRIOSIS

Endometriosis is the term used to describe the presence of endometrial glands or stroma in abnormal locations outside the uterus. It occurs in the following sites, in descending order of frequency: (1) ovaries; (2) uterine ligaments; (3) rectovaginal septum; (4) pelvic peritoneum; (5) laparotomy scars; and (6) rarely in the umbilicus, vagina, vulva, or appendix.

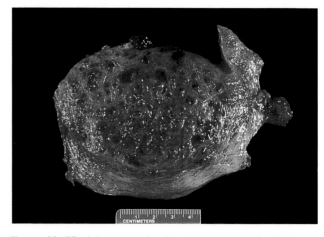

Figure 23–25. Adenomyosis. An unusual variant with functional endometrial nests producing foci of hemorrhagic cysts within uterine wall.

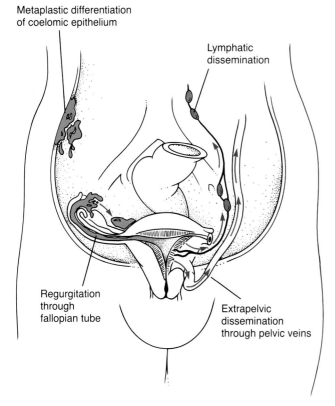

Figure 23-26. Depiction of the potential origins of endometrial implants.

Endometriosis is an important clinical condition; it often causes infertility, dysmenorrhea, pelvic pain, and other problems. The disorder is principally a disease of women in active reproductive life, most often in the third and fourth decades.

Three potential explanations exist to explain the origin of these dispersed lesions; they are not mutually exclusive (Fig. 23–26).[51]

1. The regurgitation theory. Retrograde menstruation through the fallopian tubes occurs regularly even in normal women and could mediate spread of endometrial tissue to the peritoneal cavity.
2. The metaplastic theory. Endometrium could arise directly from coelomic epithelium, which in the last analysis is the origin of the endometrium itself.
3. The vascular or lymphatic dissemination theory. This theory would explain the presence of endometriotic lesions in the lungs or lymph nodes, a phenomenon not explainable by the first two theories.

Genetic, hormonal, and immune factors have also been postulated to increase susceptibility of some women to endometriosis.

MORPHOLOGY. The foci of endometrium are almost invariably under the influence of the ovarian hormones and therefore undergo the cyclic menstrual changes with periodic bleeding. This produces nodules with a red-blue to yellow-brown appearance on or just beneath the serosal surfaces in the site of involvement. When the disease is extensive, organizing hemorrhage causes extensive fibrous adhesions between tubes, ovaries, and other structures and obliteration of the pouch of Douglas. The ovaries may become markedly distorted by large cystic spaces (3 to 5 cm in diameter) filled with brown blood debris to form so-called "chocolate cysts" (Fig. 23–27A).

The histologic diagnosis of endometriosis is usually straightforward but may be difficult in long-standing cases in which the endometrial tissue is obscured by the fibro-obliterative response. A histologic diagnosis of endometriosis is satisfied if two of the three following features are identified: endometrial glands, stroma, and hemosiderin pigment (see Fig. 23–27B).

CLINICAL COURSE. Clinical signs and symptoms usually consist of severe dysmenorrhea, dyspareunia, and pelvic pain owing to the intrapelvic bleeding and periuterine adhesions. Pain on defecation reflects rectal wall involvement, and dysuria reflects involvement of the serosa of the bladder. Intestinal disturbances may appear when the small intestine is affected. Menstrual irregularities are common, and infertility is the presenting complaint in 30 to 40% of women.

FUNCTIONAL ENDOMETRIAL DISORDERS (DYSFUNCTIONAL UTERINE BLEEDING)

During active reproductive life, the endometrium is constantly engaged in the dynamics of shedding and regrowth. It is controlled by the rise and fall of pituitary and ovarian hormones, and this control is executed by proper timing of hormonal release and both absolute and relative amounts. Alterations in this fine-tuning mechanism may result in a spectrum of disturbances, including atrophy, abnormal proliferative or secretory patterns, and hyperplasia.[52]

By far the most common problem is the occurrence of excessive bleeding during or between menstrual periods. The causes of abnormal bleeding from the uterus are many and vary among women of different age groups (Table 23–1). In some instances, bleeding is the result of a well-defined organic lesion, such as submucosal leiomyoma, endometrial polyp, or adenocarcinoma; however, the largest single group is so-called dysfunctional uterine bleeding. This is defined as abnormal bleeding in the presence of a functional disturbance rather than an organic lesion of the endometrium or uterus.[52]

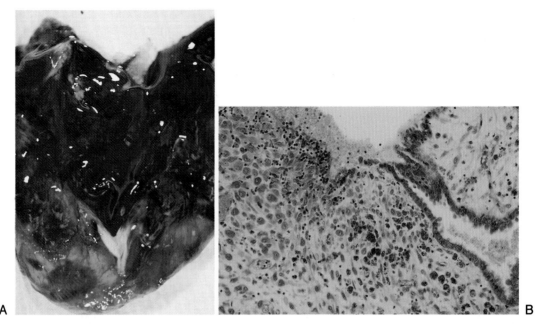

Figure 23–27. *A*, Endometriosis. This ovary has been sectioned to reveal a large endometriotic cyst containing necrotic brown material consisting of degenerated blood (chocolate cyst). *B*, Lining of endometriotic cyst from a pregnant patient. On the right is an endometrial gland; on the left is endometrial stroma with plump stromal cells characteristic of decidual changes. In the center are numerous macrophages containing hemosiderin.

Anovulatory Cycle

In most instances, dysfunctional bleeding is due to the occurrence of an anovulatory cycle, which results in excessive and prolonged estrogenic stimulation without the development of the progestational phase that regularly follows ovulation. Less commonly, lack of ovulation is the result of (1) an endocrine disorder, such as thyroid disease, adrenal disease, or pituitary tumors; (2) a primary lesion of the ovary, such as a functioning ovarian tumor (granulosa–theca cell tumors) or polycystic ovaries (see section on ovaries); or (3) a generalized metabolic disturbance, such as marked obesity, severe malnutrition, or any chronic systemic disease. In most patients, however, anovulatory cycles are unexplainable, probably occurring because of subtle hormonal imbalances. Anovulatory cycles are most common at menarche and the perimenopausal period.

Failure of ovulation results in prolonged, excessive endometrial stimulation by estrogens. Under these circumstances, the endometrial glands undergo mild architectural changes, including cystic dilatation (persistent proliferative endometrium). Unscheduled breakdown of the stroma may also occur ("anovulatory menstrual"), with no evidence of the endometrial secretory activity. More severe consequences of anovulation are discussed under Endometrial Hyperplasia.

Table 23–1. CAUSES OF ABNORMAL UTERINE BLEEDING BY AGE GROUP

AGE GROUP	CAUSE(S)
Prepuberty	Precocious puberty (hypothalamic, pituitary, or ovarian origin)
Adolescence	Anovulatory cycle
Reproductive age	Complications of pregnancy (abortion, trophoblastic disease, ectopic pregnancy)
	Organic lesions (leiomyoma, adenomyosis, polyps, endometrial hyperplasia, carcinoma)
	Anovulatory cycle
	Ovulatory dysfunctional bleeding (e.g., inadequate luteal phase)
Perimenopause	Anovulatory cycle
	Irregular shedding
	Organic lesions (carcinoma, hyperplasia, polyps)
Postmenopause	Organic lesions (carcinoma, hyperplasia, polyps)
	Endometrial atrophy

Inadequate Luteal Phase

This term refers to the occurrence of inadequate corpus luteum function and low progesterone output, with an irregular ovulatory cycle. Clinically the condition often manifests as infertility and either increased bleeding or amenorrhea. Endometrial biopsy performed at an estimated postovulatory date shows secretory endometrium, which, however, lags in its secretory characteristics with respect to the expected date.

Oral Contraceptives and Induced Endometrial Changes

As might be suspected, the use of oral contraceptives containing synthetic or derivative ovarian steroids induces a wide variety of endometrial changes, depending on the steroid used and the dose. A common response pattern is a discordant appearance between glands and stroma,[53] usually with inactive glands amidst a stroma showing large cells with abundant cytoplasm reminiscent of the decidua of pregnancy. When such therapy is discontinued, the endometrium reverts to normal. All these changes have been minimized with the newer low-dose contraceptives.

Menopausal and Postmenopausal Changes

Because the menopause is characterized by anovulatory cycles, architectural alterations in the endometrial glands may be present transiently, followed by ovarian failure and atrophy of the endometrium. As discussed next, a component of anovulatory cycles and uninterrupted estrogen production includes mild hyperplasias with cystic dilatation of glands. If this is followed by complete ovarian atrophy and loss of stimulus, the cystic dilatation may remain, while the ovarian stroma and gland epithelium undergo atrophy. In this case, so-called cystic atrophy results.[61] Such cystic changes should not be confused with more active cystic hyperplasia, which exhibits evidence of glandular and stromal proliferation.

ENDOMETRIAL HYPERPLASIA

Endometrial hyperplasia is another cause of abnormal bleeding that differs from typical anovulation by the degree of glandular epithelial alterations in the endometrium. Endometrial hyperplasia deserves special attention because of its relationship to endometrial carcinoma. More than 40 years ago, Hertig and Sommers[54] proposed a progression of endometrial changes from hyperplasia through a spectrum of atypical changes leading eventually, in some cases, to endometrial carcinoma. Numerous studies have since largely confirmed the malignant potential of certain endometrial hyperplasias and the concept of a continuum of glandular atypia culminating, in some cases, in carcinoma.[55]

As mentioned previously, endometrial hyperplasia is related to an abnormally high, prolonged level of estrogenic stimulation with diminution or absence of progestational activity. Thus hyperplasia occurs most commonly around menopause or in association with persistent anovulation in younger women. Conditions leading to hyperplasia include polycystic ovarian disease—including Stein-

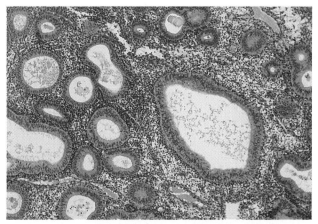

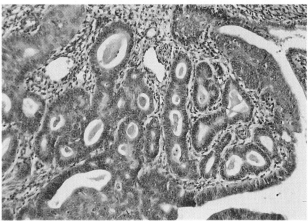

Figure 23–28. A, Simple (cystic, mild) hyperplasia with dilatation of glands. B, Complex hyperplasia of a nest of closely packed glands.

Leventhal syndrome—functioning granulosa cell tumors of the ovary, excessive cortical function (cortical stroma hyperplasia), and prolonged administration of estrogenic substances (estrogen replacement therapy). These are the same influences postulated to be of pathogenetic significance in a portion of endometrial carcinomas, discussed later.

MORPHOLOGY. Endometrial hyperplasia exhibits a continuum of alterations in gland architecture, epithelial growth pattern and cytology, and the grade increases as a function of the severity of these changes.

Lower grade hyperplasias include simple hyperplasia and complex hyperplasia. **Simple hyperplasia,** also known as cystic or mild hyperplasia, is characterized by the presence of architectural alterations in glands of various sizes, producing irregularity in gland shape with cystic alterations. The epithelial growth pattern and cytology are similar to proliferative endometrium, although mitoses are not as prominent (Fig. 23–28A). The stroma between glands also is frequently increased. These lesions uncommonly progress to adenocarcinoma; cystic hyperplasia frequently evolves into cystic at-

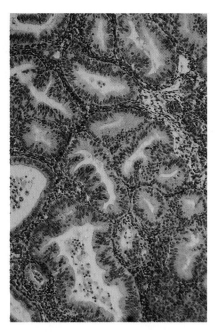

Figure 23-29. Severe atypical hyperplasia. Note both marked crowding of glands and piling up of glandular epithelium. Compare with Figure 23-28.

rophy in which the epithelium and stroma become atrophic. **Complex hyperplasia,** also known as adenomatous hyperplasia without atypia, exhibits an increase in the number and size of endometrial glands, with gland crowding and a disparity in their size and irregularity in their shape. The glands undergo "budding" with finger-like outpouchings into the adjacent endometrial stroma. The lining epithelium may appear more stratified than simple hyperplasia but is regular in contour and devoid of conspicuous cytologic atypia (see Fig. 23-28B). In the absence of cytologic atypia, less than 5% of these lesions evolve into carcinoma.

Higher grade hyperplasias are usually termed **atypical hyperplasia,** or adenomatous hyperplasia with atypia. In addition to glandular crowding and complexity, epithelial lining is irregular, characterized by stratification, scalloping, and tufting. Importantly, there is cellular atypia with cytomegaly, loss of polarity, hyperchromatism, prominence of nucleoli, and altered nuclear cytoplasmic ratio (Fig. 23-29). Mitotic figures are common. Predictably, in the most severe forms, cytologic and architectural atypia may resemble frank adenocarcinoma, and an accurate distinction between atypical hyperplasia and cancer may not be made without hysterectomy (Fig. 23-30). In one study, 23% of patients with atypical hyperplasias eventually developed adenocarcinoma.[55] In another study in which atypical hyperplasias were treated with progestin therapy alone, 50% persisted despite therapy, 25% recurred, and 25% progressed to carcinoma.[56]

It should be emphasized that interpretation of endometrial hyperplasia may be extremely subjective and precise classification elusive.[57] It is important therefore in any assessment of an endometrial hyperplastic lesion for the pathologist to indicate the degree of atypia in a manner clearly understandable by the clinician. The selection of diagnostic terminology may mean the difference between cyclic progestin therapy on one hand and continuous high-dose progestin therapy or hysterectomy (or both) on the other.

TUMORS

The uterine corpus, including its endometrium and myometrium, is affected by a great variety of neoplastic growths. These can be benign or malignant and arise from (1) the endometrial glands (endometrial polyp, endometrial carcinoma), (2) the endometrial stroma (stromal nodule and stromal sarcoma), (3) the müllerian mesoderm differentiating into both glandular and stromal elements (mixed mesodermal tumors), or (4) the smooth muscle of the myometrium (leiomyoma, leiomyosarcoma). The most common of these tumors are the endometrial polyps, leiomyomas, and endometrial carcinomas.

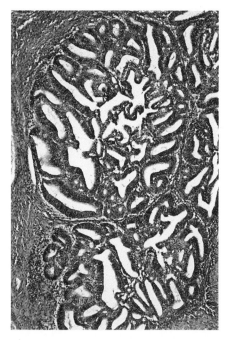

Figure 23-30. Well-differentiated endometrial adenocarcinoma. Discrete glands are less easily identified because the epithelium is arranged in a confluent pattern without intervening stroma. Compare with Figure 23-29.

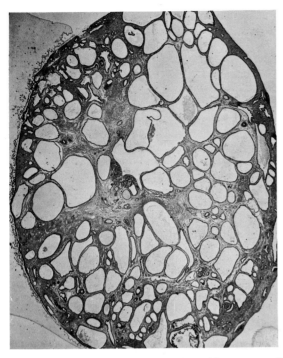

Figure 23-31. Cystic endometrial polyp at low power, illustrating cystic dilatation of glands. (Courtesy of Dr. A. Hertig.)

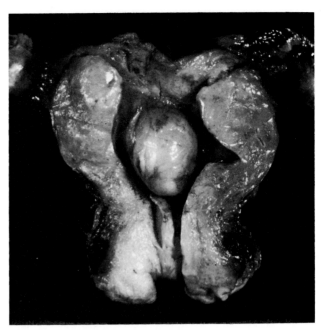

Figure 23-32. Submucosal leiomyoma appearing as a bulbous polyp, protruding into endometrial cavity.

Benign Tumors

Endometrial Polyps

Endometrial polyps are sessile masses of variable size that project into the endometrial cavity. They may be single or multiple and are usually 0.5 to 3.0 cm in diameter but occasionally large and pedunculated. Polyps may be asymptomatic or may cause abnormal bleeding if they ulcerate or undergo necrosis. Histologically, they are generally of two types, made up of (1) functional endometrium, paralleling the adjacent cycling endometrium, or (2) more commonly hyperplastic endometrium, mostly of the cystic variety. Such polyps may develop in association with generalized endometrial hyperplasia and are responsive to the growth effect of estrogen but exhibit no progesterone response (Fig. 23–31). Rarely, adenocarcinomas may arise within endometrial polyps. Endometrial polyps have been observed in association with the administration of tamoxifen, an antiestrogen frequently used in the therapy of breast cancer.[58] Cytogenetic studies indicate that the stromal cells in endometrial polyps are clonal with chromosomal (6p21) rearrangements, indicating that genetic alterations may play a role in their development.[59]

Leiomyomas

Leiomyomas are the most common tumors in women and are referred to in colloquial usage as "fibroids." The tumors are found in at least 25% of women in active reproductive life and are more common in blacks. These tumors are estrogen responsive; they regress or even calcify following castration or menopause and may undergo rapid increase in size during pregnancy. Their cause is unknown, although similar to endometrial polyps, chromosomal aberrations may play a role in their pathogenesis.[60]

MORPHOLOGY. Leiomyomas are sharply circumscribed, discrete, round, firm, gray-white tumors varying in size from small, barely visible nodules to massive tumors that fill the pelvis. Except in rare instances, they are found within the myometrium of the corpus. Only infrequently do they involve the uterine ligaments, lower uterine segment, or cervix. They can occur within the myometrium (**intramural**), just beneath the endometrium (**submucosal**) (Fig. 23–32), or beneath the serosa (**subserosal**) (Fig. 23–33).

Whatever their size, the characteristic whorled pattern of smooth muscle bundles on cut section usually makes these lesions readily identifiable on gross inspection. Large tumors may develop areas of yellow-brown to red softening (red degeneration).

Histologically, the leiomyoma is composed of whorled bundles of smooth muscle cells that resemble the architecture of the uninvolved myometrium (Fig. 23–34). Usually, the individual muscle cells are uniform in size and shape and have the characteristic oval nucleus and long, slender bipolar cytoplasmic processes. Mitotic figures are

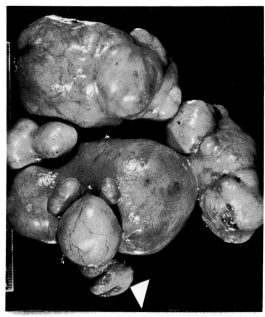

Figure 23-33. Multiple subserosal leiomyomas of the uterus. The uterine body is "lost" in irregular mass, but the cervix is visible as the most pendant portion of the specimen (arrow).

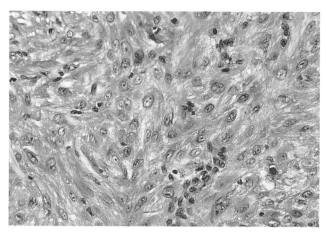

Figure 23-34. Leiomyoma showing well-differentiated, regular, spindle-shaped smooth muscle cells.

scarce. Benign variants of leiomyoma include atypical or bizarre (symplastic) tumors with nuclear atypia and giant cells and cellular leiomyomas. Importantly, both contain a very low mitotic index. An extremely rare variant, called **benign metastasizing leiomyoma,** consists of a uterine tumor that extends into vessels and migrates to other sites, most commonly the lung.

Leiomyomas of the uterus, even when extensive, may be asymptomatic. The most important symptoms are produced by submucosal leiomyomas (abnormal bleeding), compression of the bladder (urinary frequency), sudden pain if disruption of blood supply occurs, and impaired fertility. Myomas in pregnant women increase the frequency of spontaneous abortion, fetal malpresentation, uterine inertia, and postpartum hemorrhage. Malignant transformation (leiomyosarcoma) within a leiomyoma is extremely rare.

Malignant Tumors

Carcinoma of the Endometrium

Endometrial carcinoma is the most common invasive cancer of the female genital tract and accounts for 7% of all invasive cancer in women, excluding skin cancer. At one time, it was far less common than cancer of the cervix, but earlier detection and eradication of CIN and an increase in endometrial carcinomas in younger age groups have reversed this ratio. There are now 34,000 new endometrial cancers per year, compared with 13,000 new invasive cervical cancers.[34] Despite their high frequency, endometrial cancers usually arise in postmenopausal women and cause abnormal (postmenopausal) bleeding. This permits early detection and cure at an early stage.

INCIDENCE AND PATHOGENESIS. Carcinoma of the endometrium is uncommon in women younger than 40 years of age. The peak incidence is in the 55- to 65-year-old woman. A higher frequency of this form of neoplasia is seen with (1) obesity, (2) diabetes (abnormal glucose tolerance is found in more than 60%), (3) hypertension, and (4) infertility — women who develop cancer of the endometrium tend to be single and nulliparous and to give a history of functional menstrual irregularities consistent with anovulatory cycles. Infrequently both endometrial and breast carcinomas arise in the same patient.[61]

In terms of potential pathogenesis, two general groups of endometrial cancer can be identified. The first and the most well studied develops on a background of prolonged estrogen stimulation and *endometrial hyperplasia.*[73] Both conditions — hyperplasia and cancer — appear related to obesity and anovulatory cycles. Additional support includes the following: (1) Women with ovarian estrogen-secreting tumors have a higher risk of endometrial cancer. (2) Endometrial cancer is extremely rare in women with ovarian agenesis and in those castrated early in life. (3) Estrogen replacement therapy is associated with increased risk in women, and prolonged administration of DES to laboratory animals may produce endometrial polyps, hyperplasia, and carcinoma. (4) In postmenopausal women, there is greater synthesis of estrogens in body fats from adrenal and ovarian androgen precursors, a finding that may partly explain why there is increased risk of endometrial cancer with age and obesity.

Endometrial carcinomas that are associated

with the aforementioned risk factors tend to be well differentiated and mimic normal endometrial glands ("*endometrioid*") in histologic appearance. This group of tumors is generally associated with a more favorable prognosis, as described subsequently.[62]

A second and not insignificant subset of patients with endometrial cancer less commonly exhibits the stigmata of hyperestrinism or pre-existing hyperplasia and acquires the disease at a somewhat older age on average. In this group, tumors are generally more poorly differentiated, including tumors that resemble subtypes of ovarian carcinomas *(serous carcinomas)*. Overall these tumors have a poorer prognosis than endometrioid tumors, and the factors predisposing to their development are obscure.

MORPHOLOGY. Grossly, endometrial carcinoma presents either as a localized polypoid tumor or as a diffuse tumor involving the entire endometrial surface (Fig. 23–35).[74] Generally, spread occurs via direct myometrial invasion with eventual spread to the periuterine structures by direct continuity. Spread into the broad ligaments may create a clinically palpable mass. Eventually dissemination to the regional lymph nodes occurs, and in the late stages, the tumor may be hematogenously borne to the lungs, liver, bones, and other organs. In certain types, specifically papillary serous carcinoma, relatively superficial endometrial involvement may be associated with extensive peritoneal disease, suggesting spread via routes—that is, tubal or lymphatic transmission—other than direct invasion.

Histologically, most endometrial carcinomas (about 85%) are **adenocarcinomas** characterized by more or less well-defined gland patterns lined by malignant stratified columnar epithelial cells (Fig. 23–36). They are classically defined as well-

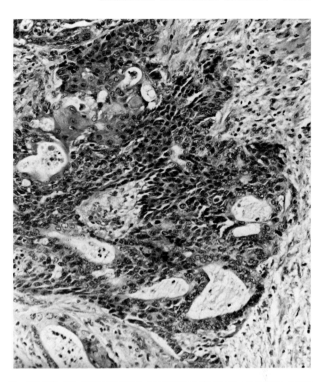

Figure 23–36. Endometrial adenocarcinoma, showing solid and gland components, focal squamous change *(upper left)*, and myometrial invasion. (Courtesy of Dr. William Welch, Brigham and Women's Hospital, Boston.)

differentiated (grade 1), with easily recognizable glandular patterns; moderately differentiated (grade 2), showing well-formed glands mixed with solid sheets of malignant cells; or poorly differentiated (grade 3), characterized by solid sheets of cells with barely recognizable glands and a greater degree of nuclear atypia and mitotic activity.

The more well-differentiated tumors tend to be those of endometrioid differentiation. Two to twenty per cent of endometrioid carcinomas contain foci of squamous differentiation. Squamous elements most commonly are histologically benign in appearance (called **adenocarcinoma with squamous metaplasia** or, more traditionally, **adenoacanthoma**) when associated with well-differentiated adenocarcinomas. Less commonly, moderate or poorly differentiated endometrioid carcinomas contain squamous elements that appear frankly malignant. Such tumors have also been termed **"adenosquamous carcinomas"** if more than 10% of the tumor is squamous.[63,64]

Although classification as a poorly differentiated adenocarcinoma typically requires a loss of glandular differentiation and the presence of solid growth, two histologic patterns behave as poorly differentiated regardless of their degree of differentiation and include **papillary serous carcinomas** and **clear cell carcinomas.** Serous carcinomas in particular are a highly aggressive form of uterine cancer.[64]

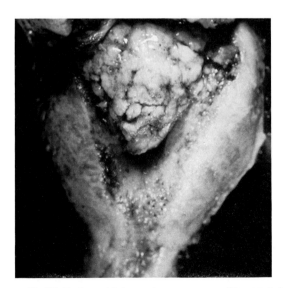

Figure 23–35. Endometrial carcinoma, presenting as a fungating mass in the fundus of the uterus.

Staging of endometrial adenocarcinoma is as follows:[65]

Stage I. Carcinoma is confined to the corpus uteri itself.

Stage II. Carcinoma has involved the corpus and the cervix.

Stage III. Carcinoma has extended outside the uterus but not outside the true pelvis.

Stage IV. Carcinoma has extended outside the true pelvis or has obviously involved the mucosa of the bladder or the rectum.

Cases in various stages can also be subgrouped with reference to histologic type of adenocarcinoma as follows:

G1. Well-differentiated adenocarcinoma.

G2. Differentiated adenocarcinoma with partly solid areas.

G3. Predominantly solid or entirely undifferentiated carcinoma, including all serous and clear cell carcinomas.

CLINICAL COURSE. Carcinoma of the endometrium may be asymptomatic for periods but usually produces irregular vaginal bleeding with excessive leukorrhea. Uterine enlargement in the early stages may be deceptively absent. Cytologic detection on Papanicolaou smears is variable and most likely with serous carcinomas, which shed discohesive clusters of cells. Ultimately the diagnosis must be established by curettage and histologic examination of the tissue.

As would be anticipated, the prognosis heavily depends on the clinical stage of the disease when discovered and its histologic grade and type. In the United States, most women (about 80%) have stage I disease clinically and have well-differentiated or moderately well-differentiated lesions histologically. Surgery, alone or in combination with irradiation, yields close to 90% 5-year survival in stage I disease. This rate drops to 30 to 50% in stage II and to less than 20% in any of the other, more advanced stages of the disease.

Mixed Müllerian and Mesenchymal Tumors

Collectively sarcomas make up 5% or less of uterine tumors; mixed mesodermal tumors, leiomyosarcomas, and endometrial stromal sarcomas are the most common variants.[66]

MALIGNANT MIXED MESODERMAL TUMORS (MIXED MÜLLERIAN TUMORS). Malignant mixed müllerian tumors (MMMTs) consist of endometrial adenocarcinomas in which malignant mesenchymal (stromal) differentiation takes place.[67] They are called mixed tumors because they consist of malignant glandular and stromal (sarcomatous) elements, and the latter tend to differentiate into a variety of malignant mesodermal components, including muscle, cartilage, and even osteoid.[68] Presumably both components are originally derived from the same cell, a concept supported by the fact that the stromal cells often stain positive with epithelial cell markers. MMMTs occur in postmenopausal women and manifest similar to adenocarcinoma, with postmenopausal bleeding. Many affected patients give a history of previous radiation therapy.

MORPHOLOGY. Grossly, such tumors are somewhat more fleshy in appearance than adenocarcinomas, may be bulky and polypoid, and sometimes protrude through the cervical os. On histology, the tumors consist of adenocarcinoma admixed with the stromal (sarcoma) elements; alternatively the tumor may comprise two distinct and separate epithelial and mesenchymal components. If sarcoma components mimic extrauterine tissues (i.e., striated muscle cells, cartilage, adipose tissue, and bone), the tumors are termed **heterologous MMMTs.** If the mesenchymal component consists of malignant endometrial or smooth muscle differentiation, the term **carcinosarcoma** or **homologous MMMT** is used.

Prognosis is determined primarily by depth of invasion and stage. Similar to endometrial carcinoma, the prognosis may be influenced in addition by the grade and type of the adenocarcinoma, being poorest with serous differentiation. It is noteworthy that mixed müllerian tumors usually metastasize as adenocarcinomas. The tumors are highly malignant and have a 5-year survival rate of 25 to 30%.[69]

Leiomyosarcomas

These uncommon malignancies arise *de novo* directly from the myometrium or endometrial stroma, which undergoes smooth muscle differentiation. Their origin from a pre-existing leiomyoma is a controversial issue, and most believe that such occurrences are extremely rare.

MORPHOLOGY. Leiomyosarcomas grow within the uterus in two somewhat distinctive patterns: bulky, fleshy masses that invade the uterine wall, or polypoid masses that project into the uterine lumen. Histologically, they contain a wide range of atypia, from those that are extremely well differentiated to anaplastic lesions that have the cytologic abnormalities of wildly growing sarcomas (Fig. 23–37). The distinction of leiomyosarcomas from leiomyomas is based on the combination of degree of nuclear atypia and mitotic index. With few exceptions, the presence of ten or more mitoses per 10 high-power (400×) fields indicates malignancy, with or without cellular atypism. If the tumor contains nuclear atypia or large (epithelioid) cells, five mitoses per 10 high-power fields are sufficient to justify a diagnosis of malignancy.[62,70] Rare exceptions include mitotically active leiomyomas in very

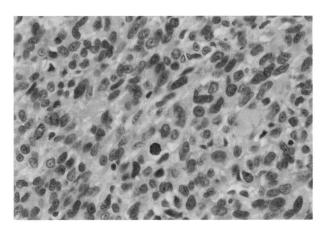

Figure 23-37. Leiomyosarcoma. Cells are irregular in size and have hyperchromatic nuclei. A mitotic figure is in the center (compare with Figure 23-34).

young or pregnant women, and caution should be exercised in interpreting such neoplasms as malignant.

Leiomyosarcomas are equally common before and after menopause, with a peak incidence at 40 to 60 years of age. These tumors have a striking tendency to recur after removal, and more than half the cases eventually metastasize via the bloodstream to distant organs, such as lungs, bone, and brain. Dissemination throughout the abdominal cavity is also encountered. The 5-year survival rate averages about 40%. The well-differentiated lesions have a better prognosis than the anaplastic lesions, which have a very low 5-year survival rate of about 10 to 15%.

Endometrial Stromal Tumors

The endometrial stroma occasionally gives rise to neoplasms, which may closely or remotely resemble normal stromal cells. Similar to most neoplasms, they may be well or poorly differentiated. Stromal neoplasms are divided into three categories: (1) benign stromal nodules; (2) low-grade stromal sarcoma, or endolymphatic stromal myosis; and (3) endometrial stromal sarcoma. *Stromal nodule* is a well-circumscribed aggregate of endometrial stromal cells in the myometrium and is of little consequence. *Low-grade stromal sarcoma* consists of well-differentiated endometrial stroma lying between muscle bundles of the myometrium and is distinguished from stromal nodules by the penetration of lymphatic channels, hence the term *endolymphatic stromal myosis*. About half of these tumors recur sometimes after 10 to 15 years; distant metastases and death from metastatic tumor occur in about 15% of cases. *Endometrial stromal sarcoma* is the overtly malignant subset of stromal tumors. These tumors infiltrate the stroma with indistinct margins and contain cells

with a wide range of atypia, including highly undifferentiated lesions with wild pleomorphic tumor giant cells and numerous mitoses. As with all sarcomas, these cancers invade vessels and are capable of widespread metastasis. Five-year survival rates average 50%.[62]

FALLOPIAN TUBES

The most common disorders in these structures are inflammations, followed in frequency by ectopic (tubal) pregnancy (see discussion later in this chapter) and endometriosis.

INFLAMMATIONS

Suppurative salpingitis may be caused by any of the pyogenic organisms, and often more than one is involved. The gonococcus still accounts for more than 60% of cases of suppurative salpingitis, with chlamydia less often a factor. These tubal infections are a part of PID described earlier in this chapter (Fig. 23-38).

Tuberculous salpingitis is extremely uncommon in the United States and accounts for probably not more than 1 to 2% of all forms of salpingitis. It is more common, however, in parts of the world where tuberculosis is prevalent and is an important cause of infertility in these areas.

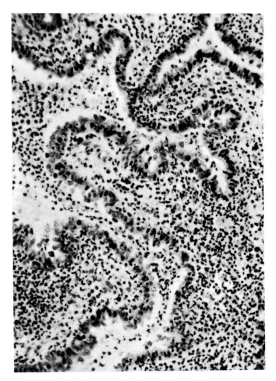

Figure 23-38. Acute salpingitis with a diffuse neutrophilic exudate within both the mucosal folds and the lumen.

TUMORS AND CYSTS

The most common primary lesions of the fallopian tube (excluding endometriosis) are minute, 0.1- to 2-cm, translucent cysts filled with clear serous fluid, called paratubal cysts. Larger varieties are found near the fimbriated end of the tube or in the broad ligaments and are referred to as *hydatids of Morgagni*. These cysts are presumed to arise in remnants of the müllerian duct and are of little more than academic significance.

Tumors of the fallopian tube are uncommon. Benign tumors include *adenomatoid tumors* (mesotheliomas), which occur subserosally on the tube or sometimes in the mesosalpinx. These small nodules are the exact counterparts of those already described in relation to the testes or epididymides (see Chapter 22) and are benign. *Adenocarcinoma* of the fallopian tubes is rare and has a papillary architecture with tubal (papillary serous) differentiation. Because these tumors are uncommonly diagnosed when confined to the tube, they have a poor prognosis. To be distinguished as a primary tubal cancer versus a metastasis of ovarian or endometrial origin, the bulk of the tumor must be in the tube, involve the lumen, and arise from the mucosa.

OVARIES

The most common types of lesions encountered in the ovary include functional or benign cysts and tumors. Intrinsic inflammations of the ovary (oophoritis) are uncommon, usually accompanying tubal inflammation. Rarely, a primary inflammatory disorder involving ovarian follicles (autoimmune oophoritis) occurs and is associated with infertility.

NON-NEOPLASTIC AND FUNCTIONAL CYSTS

Follicular and Luteal Cysts

Cystic follicles in the ovary are so common as to be virtually physiologic. They originate in unruptured graafian follicles or in follicles that have ruptured and immediately sealed.

MORPHOLOGY. These cysts are usually multiple. They range in size up to 2 cm in diameter; are filled with a clear serous fluid; and are lined by a gray, glistening membrane. Occasionally, larger cysts exceeding 2 cm—follicular cysts—may be diagnosed by palpation or ultrasonography and cause pelvic pain (Fig. 23–39). Histologically granulosa

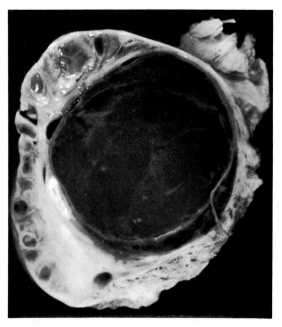

Figure 23–39. Follicular-luteal cysts of the ovary, showing one large cyst and multiple subcortical smaller cavities.

lining cells can be identified if the intraluminal pressure has not been too great. The outer theca cells may be conspicuous with increased cytoplasm and a pale appearance (luteinized). As discussed subsequently, when this alteration is pronounced (hyperthecosis), it may ultimately result in increased estrogen production and endometrial abnormalities. An impressive physiologic condition accompanying pregnancy is theca-lutein hyperplasia of pregnancy, in which the theca interna proliferate and may form small nodules in the ovarian cortex.

Granulosa **luteal cysts** (cystic corpora lutea) are normally present in the ovary. These cysts are lined by a rim of bright yellow luteal tissue containing luteinized granulosa cells. Occasionally they rupture and cause a peritoneal reaction. When advanced, the combination of old hemorrhage and fibrosis may make their distinction from endometriotic cysts difficult.

Polycystic Ovaries and Stromal Hyperthecosis

In polycystic ovarian disease (PCOD), the central pathologic abnormality is numerous cystic follicles or follicle cysts. When associated with oligomenorrhea, the clinical term *Stein-Leventhal syndrome* has been applied. These patients have persistent anovulation, obesity (40%), hirsutism (50%), and rarely virilism.[71]

MORPHOLOGY. The ovaries are usually twice normal size, are gray-white with a smooth outer cortex, and are studded with subcortical cysts 0.5 to 1.5 cm in diameter. Histologically, there is a thickened superficial cortex beneath which are innumerable follicle cysts with hyperplasia of the theca interna (follicular hyperthecosis). Corpora lutea are frequently but not invariably absent.

The initiating event in PCOD is not clear, but theoretically increased secretion of LH stimulates the theca lutein cells of the follicles, with excessive production of androgen (androstenedione), which is converted to estrone. For years, these endocrine abnormalities were attributed to primary ovarian dysfunction because large wedge resections of the ovaries sometimes restored fertility. It is now believed that the ovarian and hormonal changes are the result of unbalanced or asynchronous release of LH by the pituitary owing to disruption of hypothalamic control of pituitary secretion.[72] Other mechanisms, including hyperprolactinemia, may be involved in up to 25% of cases.[71] PCOD is currently managed by administering drugs that either regulate the menstrual cycle or induce ovulation.

Stromal hyperthecosis, also called cortical stromal hyperplasia, is a disorder of ovarian stroma most commonly seen in postmenopausal women but may blend with PCOD in younger women. The disorder is characterized by uniform enlargement of the ovary (up to 7 cm) with a white to tan appearance on sectioning. The involvement is usually bilateral and microscopically consists of hypercellular stroma with luteinization of the stromal cells, which are visible as discrete nests with vacuolated cytoplasm. The clinical presentation and effects on the endometrium are similar to PCOD, although virilization may be striking.[71]

OVARIAN TUMORS

Tumors of the ovary are common forms of neoplasia in women.[73,74] Among cancers of the female genital tract, the incidence of ovarian cancer ranks below only carcinoma of the cervix and the endometrium. Ovarian cancer accounts for 6% of all cancers in the female and is the fifth most common form of cancer in women in the United States (excluding skin cancer). In addition, because many of these ovarian neoplasms cannot be detected early in their development, they account for a disproportionate number of fatal cancers, being responsible for almost half of the deaths from cancer of the female genital tract. There are numerous types of ovarian tumors, both benign and malignant. About 80% are benign, and these occur mostly in young women between the ages of 20 and 45 years. The malignant tumors are more common in older women, between the ages of 40 and 65 years.

Risk factors for ovarian cancer are much less clear than for other genital tumors[75] with general agreement on two risk factors: nulliparity and family history. There is a higher frequency of carcinoma in unmarried women and in married women with low parity. Gonadal dysgenesis in children is associated with a higher risk of ovarian cancer. The risk of developing ovarian cancer in women 40 to 59 years of age who have taken oral contraceptives is reduced.[76] The most intriguing risk factor is genetic and candidate host genes, which may be altered in susceptible families (i.e., ovarian cancer genes). Several are being considered, and at least one (BRCA1) increases susceptibility to breast

Table 23–2. OVARIAN NEOPLASMS (1993 WHO CLASSIFICATION)*

1. Surface epithelial-stromal tumors
   Serous tumors
     Benign (cystadenoma)
     Of borderline malignancy
     Malignant (serous cystadenocarcinoma)
   Mucinous tumors, endocervical-like and intestinal-type
     Benign
     Of borderline malignancy
     Malignant
   Endometrioid tumors
     Benign
     Of borderline malignancy
     Malignant
     Epithelial—stromal
       Adenosarcoma
       Mesodermal (müllerian) mixed tumor
   Clear cell tumors
     Benign
     Of borderline malignancy
     Malignant
   Transitional cell tumors
     Brenner tumor
     Brenner tumor of borderline malignancy
     Malignant Brenner tumor
     Transitional cell carcinoma (non–Brenner-type)
2. Sex cord–stromal tumors
   Granulosa-stromal cell tumors
     Granulosa cell tumors
     Tumors of the thecoma-fibroma group
   Sertoli-stromal cell tumors; androblastomas
   Sex-cord tumor with annular tubules
   Gynandroblastoma
   Steroid (lipid) cell tumors
3. Germ cell tumors
   Teratoma
     Immature
     Mature (adult)
       Solid
       Cystic (dermoid cyst)
     Monodermal (e.g., struma ovarii, carcinoid)
   Dysgerminoma
   Yolk sac tumor (endodermal sinus tumor)
   Mixed germ cell tumors
4. Malignant, NOS
5. Metastatic nonovarian cancer (from nonovarian primary)

NOS = Not otherwise specified.
*Modified.

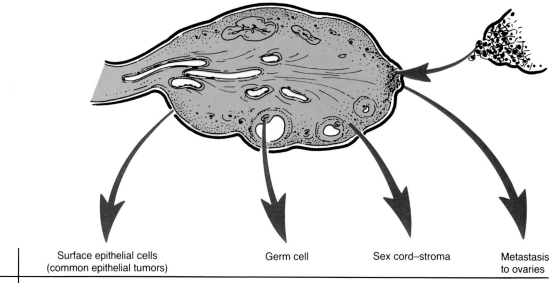

Origin	Surface epithelial cells (common epithelial tumors)	Germ cell	Sex cord–stroma	Metastasis to ovaries
Frequency	65–70%	15–20%	5–10%	5%
Age group affected	20 + years	0–25 + years	All ages	Variable
Types	• Serous tumor • Mucinous tumor • Endometrioid tumor • Clear cell tumor • Brenner tumor • Unclassifiable	• Teratoma • Dysgerminoma • Endodermal sinus tumor • Choriocarcinoma	• Fibroma • Granulosa–theca cell tumor • Sertoli-Leydig cell tumor	

Figure 23–40. Derivation of various ovarian neoplasms and some data on their frequency and age distribution.

cancer and resides on chromosome 17q21. Approximately 30% of ovarian adenocarcinomas express high levels of HER-2/*neu* oncogene, which correlates with a poor prognosis. Mutations in a host tumor suppressor gene p53 are found in 50% of ovarian carcinomas.[77]

The classification of ovarian tumors given in Table 23–2 and Figure 23–40 is a simplified version of the World Health Organization (WHO) Histological Classification, which separates ovarian neoplasms according to the most probable tissue of origin. It is now believed that tumors of the ovary arise ultimately from one of three ovarian components: (1) the surface coelomic epithelium, which embryologically gives rise to the müllerian epithelium, i.e., the fallopian tubes (ciliated columnar [serous] cells), the endometrial lining (nonciliated, columnar cells), or the endocervical glands (mucinous nonciliated cells); (2) the germ cells, which migrate to the ovary from the yolk sac and are totipotential; and (3) the stroma of the ovary, which includes the sex cords, forerunners of the endocrine apparatus of the postnatal ovary. There is, as usual, a group of tumors that defy classification, and finally there are secondary or metastatic tumors, the ovary being a common site of metastases from a variety of other cancers.

Table 23–3. CERTAIN FREQUENCY DATA FOR MAJOR OVARIAN TUMORS

TYPE	PERCENTAGE OF MALIGNANT OVARIAN TUMORS	PERCENTAGE THAT ARE BILATERAL
Serous	40	
Benign (60%)		25
Borderline (15%)		30
Malignant (25%)		65
Mucinous	10	
Benign (80%)		5
Borderline (10%)		10
Malignant (10%)		20
Endometrioid carcinoma	20	40
Undifferentiated carcinoma	10	—
Clear cell carcinoma	6	40
Granulosa cell tumor	5	5
Teratoma		15
Benign (96%)		
Malignant (4%)	1	Rare
Metastatic	5	>50
Others	3	—

Although some of the specific tumors have distinctive features and are hormonally active, the vast majority are nonfunctional and tend to produce relatively mild symptoms until they have reached a large size. Malignant tumors have usually spread outside the ovary by the time a definitive diagnosis is made. Some of these tumors, principally epithelial tumors, tend to be bilateral. Table 23–3 lists these tumors and their subtypes and shows the frequency of bilateral occurrence. Abdominal pain and distention, urinary and gastrointestinal tract symptoms owing to compression by tumor or cancer invasion, and abdominal and vaginal bleeding are the most common symptoms. The benign forms may be entirely asymptomatic and occasionally are unexpected findings on abdominal or pelvic examination or during surgery.

Tumors of Surface (Coelomic) Epithelium

The great majority of primary neoplasms in the ovary fall within this category. There are three major types of such tumors: serous, mucinous, and endometrioid. Mixtures of these epithelia frequently occur in the same tumor. Neoplasms composed of these three cell types range from clearly benign, to tumors of borderline malignancy, to malignant tumors.[74] These neoplasms range in size and composition. Tumors may be small and grossly imperceptible or massive, filling the pelvis and even the abdominal cavity. Components of the tumors may include cystic areas (cystadenomas), cystic and fibrous areas (cystadenofibromas), and predominantly fibrous areas (adenofibromas). On gross examination, the risk of malignancy increases as a function of the amount of discernible solid epithelial growth, including papillary projections of soft tumor, thickened tumor lining the cyst spaces, or solid necrotic friable tissue depicting necrosis.

Although termed epithelial in differentiation, these tumors are derived from coelomic mesothelium and are graphic reminders of this tissue's ability to evolve into serous (tubal), endometrioid (endometrium), and mucinous (cervix) epithelia present in the normal female genital tract. Why these tumors predominate in the ovary is a mystery but appears linked to the incorporation of coelomic epithelium into the ovarian cortex to form mesothelial inclusion cysts. This incorporation occurs via the formation of surface adhesions, atrophy with epithelial infolding, and repair of ovulation sites. The close association of ovarian carcinomas with either the ovarian surface mesothelium or inclusion cysts may explain the development of extraovarian carcinomas of similar histology from similar coelomic epithelial rests (so-called endosalpingiosis) in the mesentery.

Serous Tumors

These common cystic neoplasms are lined by tall, columnar, ciliated epithelial cells and are filled with clear serous fluid. Although the term serous appropriately describes the cyst fluid, it has become synonymous with the tubal-like epithelium in these tumors. Together the benign, borderline, and malignant types account for about 30% of all ovarian tumors. About 75% are benign or of borderline malignancy and 25% malignant. Serous cystadenocarcinomas account for approximately 40% of all cancers of the ovary and are the most common malignant ovarian tumors. Benign and borderline tumors are most common between the ages of 20 and 50. Cystadenocarcinomas occur later in life on average, although somewhat earlier in familial cases.

MORPHOLOGY. Grossly, the characteristic serous tumor has one or a few fibrous walled cysts averaging 10 to 15 cm in diameter and occasionally up to 40 cm. Benign tumors contain a smooth glistening cyst wall with no epithelial thickening or small papillary projections (i.e., papillary cystadenoma). Borderline tumors contain an increasing amount of papillary projections. Larger amounts of solid or papillary tumor mass, irregularity in the tumor mass, and fixation or nodularity of the capsule are all important indicators of probable malignancy (Fig. 23–41). Bilaterality is common, occurring in 20% of benign cystadenomas, 30% of borderline tumors, and approximately 66% of cystadenocarcinomas. Histologically, the lining epithelium is composed of columnar epithelium with abundant cilia in benign tumors (Fig. 23–42). Microscopic papillae may be found. Tumors of borderline malignancy contain increased complexity of the stromal papillae with stratification of the epithelium and nuclear atypia, but destructive infiltrative growth into the stroma is not seen. Cystadenocarcinomas exhibit even more complex growth with infiltration or frank effacement of the underlying stroma by solid growth (Fig. 23–43). The individual tumor cells in the carcinomatous lesions display the usual features of all malignancy, and with the more extreme degrees of atypia, the cells may become quite undifferentiated. The presence of concentric calcifications (psammoma bodies) characterizes serous tumors, although they are not specific for neoplasia when found alone.

The biologic behavior of serous tumors depends on both degree of differentiation and distribution. Importantly, serous tumors may occur on the surface of the ovaries and, rarely, as primary tumors of the peritoneal surface. Predictably, unencapsulated serous tumors of the ovarian surface are more likely to extend to the peritoneal surfaces, and prognosis is closely related to the histo-

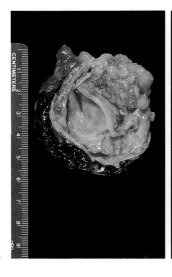

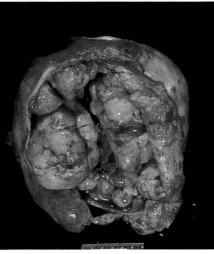

A

B

Figure 23–41. *A,* Borderline serous cystadenoma opened to display a cyst cavity lined by delicate papillary tumor growths. *B,* Cystadenocarcinoma. The cyst is opened to reveal a large, bulky tumor mass.

logic appearance of the tumor and its growth pattern on the peritoneum. Borderline tumors can also originate from or extend to the peritoneal surfaces and may remain localized, causing no symptoms, or slowly spread, producing intestinal obstruction or other complications after many years. Frank carcinomas infiltrate the soft tissue and form large intra-abdominal masses and rapid deterioration. For this reason, careful pathologic classification of the tumor, even if it has extended to the peritoneum, is relevant to both prognosis and selection of therapy.[78] The 5-year survival for borderline and malignant tumors confined within the ovarian mass is 100% and 70%, whereas the 5-year survival for the same tumors involving the peritoneum

is about 90% and 25%, respectively. Because of their protracted course, borderline tumors may recur after many years, and 5-year survival is not synonymous with cure.

Mucinous Tumors

These tumors closely resemble their serous counterparts. They are somewhat less common, accounting for about 25% of all ovarian neoplasms. They occur principally in middle adult life and are rare before puberty and after menopause. Eighty per cent are benign or borderline, and about 15% are malignant. Mucinous cystadenocarcinomas are relatively uncommon and account for only 10% of all ovarian cancers.

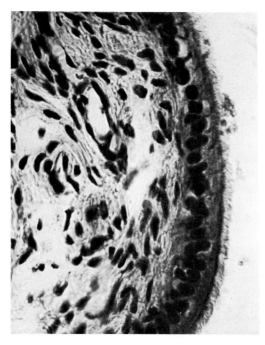

Figure 23–42. Histologic detail of classic ciliated, columnar lining epithelial cells of serous cystadenoma.

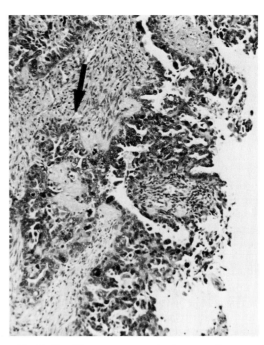

Figure 23–43. Papillary serous cystadenocarcinoma of the ovary with loss of orientation and piling up of atypical epithelium.

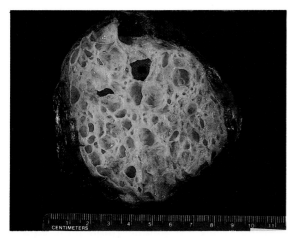

Figure 23-44. A mucinous cystadenoma with its multicystic appearance and delicate septa. Note the presence of glistening mucin within the cysts.

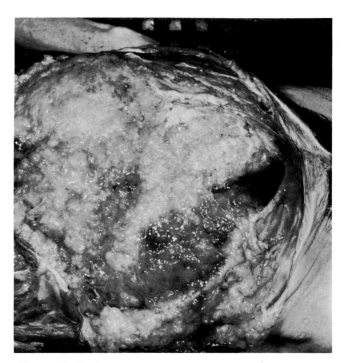

Figure 23-45. Pseudomyxoma peritonei (ovarian), viewed at autopsy with abdominal wall laid back to expose massive overgrowth of gelatinous metastatic tumor.

MORPHOLOGY. Grossly, the mucinous tumors differ from the serous variety in several ways. They are characterized by more cysts of variable size and a rarity of surface involvement and are less frequently bilateral. Approximately 5% of mucinous cystadenomas and 20% of mucinous cystadenocarcinomas are bilateral. Mucinous tumors tend to produce larger cystic masses, and some have been recorded with weights of more than 25 kg. Grossly they appear as multiloculated tumors filled with sticky, gelatinous fluid rich in glycoproteins (Fig. 23-44). Like serous tumors, ovarian mucinous tumors may be complicated by involvement of the peritoneal surfaces by tumor and the collection of extensive mucinous material resembling cystic contents within the peritoneal cavity. This rare condition is termed **pseudomyxoma peritonei,** and complicates primarily borderline or malignant neoplasms. The major complication of this condition relates to extensive interadherence and adhesion of the viscera, which produce a matting together of the abdominal contents (Fig. 23-45) and intestinal obstruction, not unlike that seen in serous tumors with similar involvement.

Histologically, benign mucinous tumors are characterized by a lining of tall columnar epithelial cells with apical mucin and the absence of cilia, akin to benign cervical or intestinal epithelia (Fig. 23-46). Borderline tumors exhibit abundant gland-like or papillary growth with nuclear atypia and stratification and are strikingly similar to tubular adenomas or villous adenomas of the intestine. Cystadenocarcinomas contain more solid growth with conspicuous epithelial cell atypia and stratification, loss of gland architecture and necrosis, and are similar to colonic cancer in appearance. Because both borderline and malignant mucinous cyst-

adenomas form complex glands in the stroma, the documentation of clear-cut stromal invasion, which is uncomplicated in serous tumors, is subjective, and some authors describe a category of

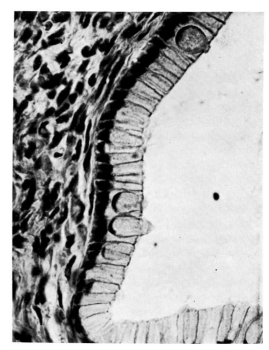

Figure 23-46. Histologic detail of classic nonciliated, mucin-secreting, columnar lining epithelium of a mucinous cystadenoma of the ovary. (Courtesy of Dr. A. Hertig.)

"noninvasive" mucinous carcinomas for those tumors with marked epithelial atypia without obvious stromal alterations. Approximate 10-year survivals for stage I borderline, noninvasive malignant, and frankly invasive malignant tumors are greater than 95%, 90%, and 66%, respectively.[79]

Endometrioid Tumors

These neoplasms account for approximately 20% of all ovarian cancers, excluding endometriosis, which is considered non-neoplastic. Most endometrioid tumors are carcinomas. Less commonly, benign forms — usually cystadenofibromas — are encountered.[80] They are distinguished from serous and mucinous tumors by the presence of tubular glands bearing a close resemblance to benign or malignant endometrium. For obscure reasons, 15 to 30% of endometrioid carcinomas are accompanied by a carcinoma of the endometrium, and the relatively good prognosis in such cases suggests that the two may arise independently rather than by metastatic spread from one another.[81] About 15% of cases with endometrioid carcinoma coexist with endometriosis, although an origin directly from ovarian coelomic epithelium is also possible.[82]

MORPHOLOGY. Grossly, endometrioid carcinomas present as a combination of solid and cystic areas, similar to other cystadenocarcinomas. Forty per cent involve both ovaries, and such bilaterality usually, although not always, implies extension of the neoplasm beyond the female genital tract. Histologically, glandular patterns bearing a strong resemblance to those of endometrial origin are seen. The overall 5-year survival rate is 40 to 50%.

Clear Cell Adenocarcinoma

This uncommon pattern of surface epithelial tumor of the ovary is characterized by large epithelial cells with abundant clear cytoplasm. Because these tumors sometimes occur in association with endometriosis or endometrioid carcinoma of the ovary and resemble clear cell carcinoma of the endometrium, they are now thought to be of müllerian duct origin and variants of endometrioid adenocarcinoma.[74] The clear cell tumors of the ovary can be predominantly solid or cystic. In the solid neoplasm, the clear cells are arranged in sheets or tubules. In the cystic variety, the neoplastic cells line the spaces. The 5-year survival rate is approximately 50% when the tumors are confined to the ovaries; however, these tumors tend to be aggressive, and with spread beyond the ovary, a survival of 5 years is exceptional.

Cystadenofibroma

Cystadenofibromas are variants in which there is more pronounced proliferation of the fibrous stroma that underlies the columnar lining epithelium. These benign tumors are usually small and multilocular and have rather simple papillary processes that do not become so complicated and branching as those found in the ordinary cystadenoma. They may be composed of mucinous, serous, endometrioid, and transitional (Brenner tumors) epithelium. Borderline lesions with cellular atypia and rarely tumors with focal carcinoma occur, but metastatic spread of either is extremely uncommon.

Brenner Tumor

Brenner tumors are uncommon adenofibromas in which the epithelial component consists of nests of transitional cells resembling those lining the urinary bladder. Less frequently, the nests contain microcysts or glandular spaces lined by columnar, mucin-secreting cells. For reasons not clear, Brenner tumors are occasionally encountered in mucinous cystadenomas.[83]

MORPHOLOGY. These neoplasms may be solid or cystic, are usually unilateral (approximately 90%), and vary in size from small lesions less than 1 cm in diameter to massive tumors up to 20 and 30 cm. The fibrous stroma, resembling that of the normal ovary, is marked by sharply demarcated nests of epithelial cells (Fig. 23–47) resembling the epithelium of the urinary tract, often with mucinous glands in their center. Infrequently, the stroma is composed of somewhat plump fibroblasts resembling theca cells, and such neoplasms may have hormonal activity. The vast majority of Brenner tumors are benign, but borderline (proliferative Brenner tumor) and malignant counterparts have been reported.

Several reports have emphasized the occurrence of ovarian tumors, which are composed in part or all of neoplastic epithelium similar to transitional carcinoma of the bladder but without a coexisting Brenner component. Referred to as *transitional cell carcinoma*, these tumors arise from coelomic epithelium or from selective differentiation of existing carcinomas. This form of differentiation is of interest because of speculation that transitional cell tumors are uniquely susceptible to chemotherapy, with correspondingly more favorable prognosis.[84]

Clinical Course of Surface Epithelial Tumors

All ovarian epithelial carcinomas produce similar clinical manifestations, most commonly lower abdominal pain and abdominal enlargement. Gastrointestinal complaints, urinary frequency, dysuria, pelvic pressure, and many other symptoms may appear. Benign lesions are easily resected with cure. The malignant forms, however, tend to cause the progressive weakness, weight loss, and cachexia characteristic of all malignancies. If the car-

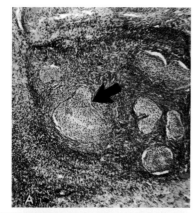

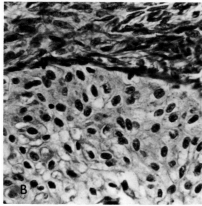

Figure 23–47. Brenner tumor. *A,* Low-power micrograph showing spindle cell component and nests of epithelial cells *(arrow). B,* High-power detail of characteristic epithelial nests.

cinomas extend through the capsule of the tumor to seed the peritoneal cavity, massive ascites is common. Characteristically, the ascitic fluid is filled with diagnostic exfoliated tumor cells. The peritoneal seeding that these malignancies produce

is quite distinctive: They tend to seed all serosal surfaces diffusely with 0.1- to 0.5-cm nodules of tumor. These surface implants rarely invade deeply into the underlying parenchyma of the organ. The regional nodes are often involved, and metastases may be found in the liver, lungs, gastrointestinal tract, and elsewhere. Metastasis across the midline to the opposite ovary is discovered in about half the cases by the time of laparotomy and heralds a progressive downhill course to death within a few months or years.

Because ovarian carcinomas often remain undiagnosed until very large, many patients are first seen with lesions that are no longer confined to the ovary. This is perhaps the primary reason for the relatively poor 5- and 10-year survival rates for these patients, compared with rates in cervical and endometrial carcinoma. For these reasons, specific biochemical markers for tumor antigens or tumor products in the plasma of these patients are being sought vigorously. One such marker is a high-molecular-weight glycoprotein present in more than 80% of serous and endometrioid carcinomas, known as CA-25, but whether its use will influence outcome is unproven.

Germ Cell Tumors

Germ cell tumors constitute 15 to 20% of all ovarian tumors.[74] The vast majority are benign cystic teratomas, but the remainder, which are found principally in children and young adults, have a higher incidence of malignant behavior and pose problems in histologic diagnosis and in therapy. They bear a remarkable homology to germ tumors in the male testis (see Chapter 22) and arise from germ cell differentiation in a similar manner (Fig. 23–48).

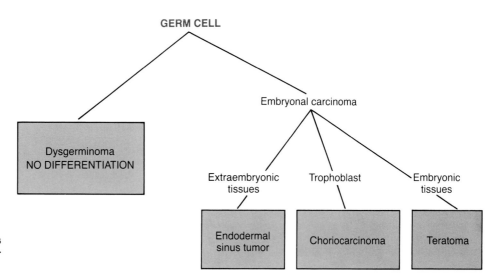

Figure 23–48. Histogenesis and interrelationships of tumors of germ cell origin.

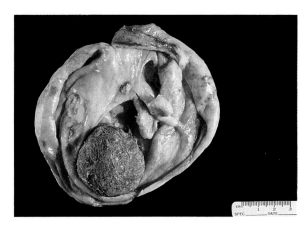

Figure 23-49. Opened mature cystic teratoma (dermoid cyst) of the ovary. Hair *(bottom)* and a mixture of tissues are evident.

Teratomas

Teratomas are divided into three categories: (1) mature (benign), (2) immature (malignant), and (3) monodermal or highly specialized.

MATURE (BENIGN) TERATOMAS. The vast majority of benign teratomas are cystic and are better known in clinical parlance as dermoid cysts. These neoplasms are invariably benign and are presumably derived from the ectodermal differentiation of totipotential cells. Cystic teratomas are usually found in young women during the active reproductive years.[74]

MORPHOLOGY. Benign teratomas are bilateral in 10 to 15% of cases. Characteristically, they are unilocular cysts containing hair and cheesy sebaceous material (Fig. 23-49). On section they reveal a thin wall lined by an opaque, gray-white, wrinkled, apparent epidermis. From this epidermis, hair shafts frequently protrude. Within the wall, it is common to find tooth structures and areas of calcification.

Histologically, the cyst wall is composed of stratified squamous epithelium with underlying sebaceous glands, hair shafts, and other skin adnexal structures (Fig. 23-50). In most cases, structures from other germ layers can be identified, such as cartilage, bone, thyroid tissue, and other organoid formations (Fig. 23-51). Dermoid cysts are sometimes incorporated within the wall of a mucinous cystadenoma. **About 1% of the dermoids undergo malignant transformation of any one of the component elements—e.g., thyroid carcinoma, melanoma, but most commonly squamous cell carcinoma.**

In rare instances, a teratoma is solid but is composed entirely of benign-looking heterogeneous collections of tissues and organized structures derived from all three germ layers. These tumors presumably have the same histogenetic ori-

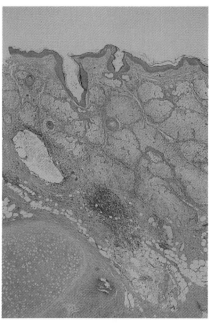

Figure 23-50. Dermoid cyst. Low-power view of skin, underlying sebaceous glands, and cartilage *(lower left).*

gin as dermoid cysts but lack preponderant differentiation into ectodermal derivatives. **These neoplasms may be initially difficult to differentiate from the malignant, immature teratomas, which almost always are largely solid.**

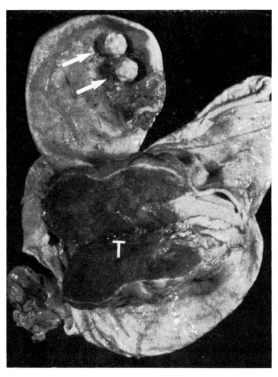

Figure 23-51. Mature cystic teratoma of the ovary, opened to illustrate several abortive tooth structures *(arrows)* and a darker area of thyroid substance (T).

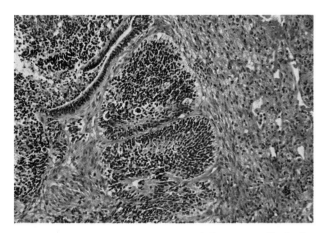

Figure 23–52. Immature teratoma of the ovary, illustrating primitive neuroepithelium.

The origin of teratomas has been a matter of fascination for centuries. Some common beliefs blamed witches, nightmares, or adultery with the devil. The current parthenogenetic theory suggests origin from a meiotic germ cell. The karyotype of all benign ovarian teratomas is 46,XX. From the results of chromosome-banding techniques and the distribution of electrophoretic variants of enzymes in the normal and teratoma cells, Linder and co-workers[86] suggested that tumors arise from an ovum after the first meiotic division. Other derivations have been proposed.[87]

IMMATURE MALIGNANT TERATOMAS. These are rare tumors that differ from benign teratomas in that the component tissue resembles that observed in the fetus or embryo rather than adult. The tumor is found chiefly in prepubertal adolescents and young women, the mean age being 18.[88]

> **MORPHOLOGY.** The tumors are bulky and have a smooth external surface. On section they have a solid or predominantly solid structure. There are areas of necrosis and hemorrhage. Hair, grumous material, cartilage, bone, and calcification may be present. Microscopically, there are varying amounts of immature tissue differentiating toward cartilage, glands, bone, muscle, nerve, and others. An important risk for subsequent extraovarian spread is the histologic grade of tumor (I through III), which is based on the proportion of tissue (in histologic sections) containing immature neuroepithelium (Fig. 23–52).

Immature teratomas grow rapidly and frequently penetrate the capsule with spread or metastases. Stage I tumors, however, particularly those with low-grade (grade I) histology, have an excellent prognosis. Higher grade tumors confined to the ovary are generally treated with prophylactic chemotherapy. Most recurrences develop in the first 2 years, and absence of disease beyond this period carries an excellent chance of cure.

MONODERMAL OR SPECIALIZED TERATOMAS. The specialized teratomas are a remarkable, rare group of tumors, the most common of which are struma ovarii and carcinoid. They are always unilateral, although a contralateral teratoma may be present. Struma ovarii is composed entirely of mature thyroid tissue. Interestingly these thyroidal neoplasms may hyperfunction, producing hyperthyroidism. The ovarian carcinoid, which presumably rises from intestinal epithelium in a teratoma, might in fact be functioning, particularly in large (greater than 7 cm) tumors, producing 5-hydroxytryptamine and the carcinoid syndrome. Primary ovarian carcinoid can be distinguished from metastatic intestinal carcinoid, the latter virtually always bilateral. Even more rare is the strumal carcinoid, a combination of struma ovarii and carcinoid in the same ovary. Primary carcinoids are uncommonly (less than 2%) malignant.

Dysgerminoma

The dysgerminoma[89] is best remembered as the ovarian counterpart of the seminoma of the testis. Similar to the latter, it is composed of large vesicular cells having a cleared cytoplasm, well-defined cell boundaries, and centrally placed regular nuclei. Relatively uncommon tumors, the dysgerminomas account for about 2% of all ovarian cancers yet form about half of malignant germ cell tumors. They may occur in childhood, but 75% occur in the second and third decades. Some occur in patients with gonadal dysgenesis, including pseudohermaphroditism. Most of these tumors have no endocrine function. A few produce elevated levels of chorionic gonadotropin and may have syncytiotrophoblastic giant cells on histologic examination.

> **MORPHOLOGY.** Usually unilateral (80 to 90%), they most frequently are solid tumors ranging in size from barely visible nodules to masses that virtually fill the entire abdomen. On cut surface, they have a yellow-white to gray-pink appearance and are often soft and fleshy. Histologically, the dysgerminoma cells are dispersed in sheets or cords separated by scant fibrous stroma. As in the seminoma, the fibrous stroma is infiltrated with mature lymphocytes and occasional granulomas. Occasionally, small nodules of dysgerminoma are encountered in the wall of an otherwise benign cystic teratoma; conversely, a predominantly dysgerminomatous tumor may contain a small cystic teratoma.

All dysgerminomas are malignant, but the degree of histologic atypia is variable, and only about one-third are aggressive. Thus a unilateral tumor that has not broken through the capsule and has not spread has an excellent prognosis (up to 96% cure rate) after simple salpingo-oophorectomy. These neoplasms are extremely radiosensitive, and even those that have extended beyond the ovary can generally be controlled by radiotherapy. Overall survival exceeds 80%.

Endodermal Sinus (Yolk Sac) Tumor

This tumor is rare but is the second most common malignant tumor of germ cell origin. It is thought to be derived from a multipotential embryonal carcinoma by selection and differentiation toward yolk sac structure[82] (see Fig. 23–48). Similar to the yolk sac, the tumor is rich in alpha-fetoprotein and alpha-antitrypsin. Its characteristic histologic feature is a glomerulus-like structure composed of a central blood vessel enveloped by germ cells within a space similarly lined by germ cells (Schiller-Duval body). Similar structures are observed in the yolk sac of the rat placenta. Conspicuous intracellular and extracellular hyaline droplets are present in all tumors, and some of these can be stained for alpha-fetoprotein by immunoperoxidase techniques.

Most patients are children or young women presenting with abdominal pain and a rapidly developing pelvic mass. The tumors usually appear to involve a single ovary but grow rapidly and aggressively. These tumors were once almost uniformly fatal within 2 years of diagnosis, but combination chemotherapy has measurably improved the outcome.

Choriocarcinoma

More commonly of placental origin, the choriocarcinoma, similar to the endodermal sinus tumor, is an example of extraembryonic differentiation of malignant germ cells. It is generally held that a germ cell origin can be certified only in the prepubertal girl because after this age, an origin from an ovarian ectopic pregnancy cannot be excluded.

Most ovarian choriocarcinomas exist in combination with other germ cell tumors, and pure choriocarcinomas are extremely rare. Histologically they are identical with the more common placental lesions, described later. These ovarian primaries are ugly tumors that generally have metastasized widely through the bloodstream to the lungs, liver, bone, and other viscera by the time of diagnosis. As with all choriocarcinomas, they elaborate high levels of chorionic gonadotropins that are sometimes helpful in establishing the diagnosis or highlighting recurrences. In contrast to choriocarcinomas arising in placental tissue, those arising in the ovary are generally unresponsive to chemotherapy and are highly fatal.

Other Germ Cell Tumors

These include (1) embryonal carcinoma, another highly malignant tumor of primitive embryonal elements, histologically similar to tumors arising in the testes (see Chapter 22); (2) polyembryoma, a malignant tumor containing so-called embryoid bodies; and (3) mixed germ cell tumors containing various combinations of dysgerminoma, teratoma, endodermal sinus tumor, and choriocarcinoma.

Sex Cord–Stromal Tumors

These ovarian neoplasms are derived from the ovarian stroma, which in turn is derived from the sex cords of the embryonic gonad. Because the undifferentiated gonadal mesenchyme eventually produces structures of specific cell type in both male (Sertoli and Leydig) and female (granulosa and theca) gonads, tumors emulating all of these cell types can be identified in the ovary.[90] Moreover, because some of these cells normally secrete estrogens (theca cells) or androgens (Leydig cells), their corresponding tumors may be either feminizing (granulosa–theca cell tumors) or masculinizing (Leydig cell tumors).

Granulosa-Theca Cell Tumors

This designation embraces ovarian neoplasms composed of varying proportions of granulosa and theca cell differentiation. These tumors are composed almost entirely of granulosa cells or a mixture of granulosa and theca cells. Collectively these neoplasms account for about 5% of all ovarian tumors. Although they may be discovered at any age, approximately two-thirds occur in postmenopausal women.

MORPHOLOGY. Granulosa cell tumors are usually unilateral and vary from microscopic foci to large, solid, and cystic encapsulated masses. Tumors that are endocrinologically active have a yellow coloration to their cut surfaces, produced by contained lipids. The pure thecomas are solid, firm tumors.

The granulosa cell component of these tumors takes one of many histologic patterns. The small, cuboidal-to-polygonal cells may grow in anastomosing cords, sheets, or strands (Fig. 23–53). In occasional cases, small, distinctive, gland-like structures filled with an acidophilic material recall immature follicles (Call-Exner bodies). When these structures are evident, the diagnosis is rendered considerably more simple. The thecoma component consists of clusters or sheets of cuboidal-to-polygonal cells. In some tumors, the granulosa or theca cells may appear more plump with ample cytoplasm characteristic of luteinization (i.e., luteinized granulosa–theca cell tumors).

Granulosa–theca cell tumors have clinical importance for two reasons: (1) their potential elaboration of large amounts of estrogen and (2) the small but distinct hazard of malignancy in the

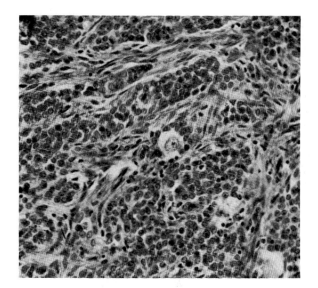

Figure 23–53. Granulosa cell tumor.

granulosa cell forms. Functionally active tumors in young girls (juvenile granulosa cell tumors) may produce precocious sexual development in prepubertal girls. In adult women, they may be associated with endometrial hyperplasia, cystic disease of the breast, and endometrial carcinoma. About 10 to 15% of patients with steroid-producing tumors eventually develop an endometrial carcinoma. Occasional granulosa cell tumors produce androgens, masculinizing the patient.

The additional clinical significance of these

tumors lies in the fact that all are potentially malignant. It is difficult, from the histologic evaluation of granulosa cell tumors, to predict their biologic behavior.[74] The estimates of clinical malignancy (recurrence, extension) range from 5 to 25%. In general, malignant tumors pursue an indolent course in which local recurrences may be amenable to surgical therapy. Recurrences within the pelvis and abdomen may appear many years (10 to 20) after removal of the original tumor. The 10-year survival rate is approximately 85%. Tumors composed predominantly of theca cells are almost never malignant.

Thecoma-Fibromas

Tumors arising in the ovarian stroma that are composed of either fibroblasts (fibromas) or more plump spindle cells with lipid droplets (thecomas) are relatively common and account for about 4% of all ovarian tumor types (Fig. 23–54A). Because many tumors contain a mixture of these cells, they are termed fibroma-thecomas. Pure thecomas are very rare, but tumors in which these cells predominate may be hormonally active. Most are composed principally of fibroblasts and are for practical purposes hormonally inactive.

Fibroma-thecomas of the ovary are unilateral in about 90% of cases and usually are solid, spherical or slightly lobulated, encapsulated, hard, gray-white masses covered by glistening, intact ovarian serosa (Fig. 23–54B). Histologically, they are com-

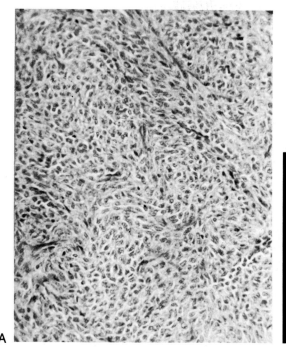

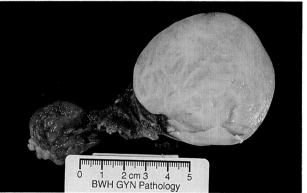

Figure 23–54. *A,* Thecoma-fibroma composed of plump, differentiated stromal cells with thecal appearance. (Courtesy of Dr. A. Hertig and the Armed Forces Institute of Pathology.) *B,* Large bisected fibroma of ovary apparent as a white, firm mass *(right).* The fallopian tube is attached.

posed of well-differentiated fibroblasts with a more or less scant collagenous connective tissue interspersed between the cells. Areas of thecal differentiation may be identified and can be confirmed by fat stains. This exercise, however, is considered unnecessary on clinical grounds.

In addition to the relatively nonspecific findings of pain and pelvic mass, the tumors may be accompanied by two curious associations. The first is ascites, found in about 40% of cases, in which the tumors measure more than 6 cm in diameter. Uncommonly, there is also hydrothorax, usually only of the right side. This combination of findings, i.e., ovarian tumor, hydrothorax, and ascites, is designated Meigs' syndrome. The genesis is unknown. The second association is with the basal cell nevus syndrome, described in Chapter 26. Rarely, cellular tumors with mitotic activity and increased nuclear cytoplasmic ratio are identified; because they may pursue a malignant course, they are termed fibrosarcomas.[91]

Sertoli-Leydig Cell Tumors (Androblastoma)

These tumors recapitulate, to a certain extent, the cells of the testis at various stages of develop-

ment.[92] They commonly produce masculinization or at least defeminization, but a few have estrogenic effects. They occur in women of all ages, although the peak incidence is in the second and third decades. The embryogenesis of such male-directed stromal cells remains a puzzle. These tumors are unilateral and resemble granulosa–theca cell neoplasms.

The cut surface is usually solid and varies from gray to golden brown in appearance (Fig. 23–55A). Histologically the well-differentiated tumors exhibit tubules composed of Sertoli cells or Leydig cells interspersed with stroma (see Fig. 23–55B). The intermediate forms show only outlines of immature tubules and large eosinophilic Leydig cells. The poorly differentiated tumors have a sarcomatous pattern with a disorderly disposition of epithelial cell cords. Leydig cells may be absent. Heterologous elements, such as mucinous glands, bone, and cartilage, may be present in some tumors.

The incidence of recurrence or metastasis by Sertoli-Leydig cell tumors is less than 5%. These neoplasms may block normal female sexual development in children and may cause defeminization

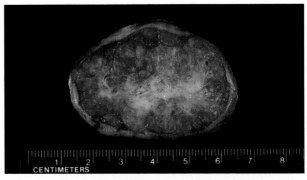

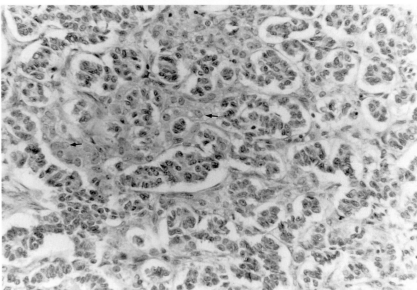

Figure 23–55. Sertoli cell tumor. A, Gross photograph illustrating characteristic golden-yellow appearance of tumor; B, photomicrograph showing well-differentiated Sertoli cell tubules. A few larger cells (Leydig cells) are noted between the tubular structures (arrows). (Courtesy of Dr. William Welch, Brigham and Women's Hospital, Boston.)

of women, manifested by atrophy of the breasts, amenorrhea, sterility, and loss of hair. The syndrome may progress to striking virilization, that is, hirsutism, male distribution of hair, hypertrophy of the clitoris, and voice changes.

Other Sex Cord-Stromal Tumors

Normally, the ovarian hilus contains clusters of polygonal cells arranged around vessels (hilar cells). *Hilus cell tumors (pure Leydig cell tumor)* are derived from these cells, are rare, are unilateral, and are characterized histologically by large, lipid-laden cells with distinct borders. A typical cytoplasmic structure characteristic of Leydig cells— Reinke crystalloids—is usually present. Typically, the patients present clinically with evidence of masculinization, hirsutism, voice changes, and clitoral enlargement. The tumors are unilateral. The most consistent laboratory finding is an elevated 17-ketosteroid excretion level unresponsive to cortisone suppression. Treatment is surgical excision. True hilus cell tumors are almost always benign. Occasionally histologically identical tumors occur in the cortical stroma *(nonhilar Leydig cell tumors).*

In addition to Leydig cell tumors, the stroma rarely may give rise to tumors composed of pure luteinized cells, producing small benign tumors rarely more than 3 cm in diameter. The tumor may produce the clinical effects of androgen, estrogen, or progestogen stimulation.

As mentioned previously, the ovary in pregnancy may exhibit microscopic nodular proliferations of theca cells in response to gonadotropins. Rarely a frank tumor may develop—termed *pregnancy luteoma*—which closely resembles a corpus luteum of pregnancy. These tumors have been associated with virilization in the pregnant patient and in their respective female infants.

Gonadoblastoma is an uncommon tumor thought to be composed of germ cells and sex cord–stroma derivatives. It occurs in individuals with abnormal sexual development and in gonads of indeterminate nature. Eighty per cent are phenotypic females, and 20% are phenotypic males with undescended testicles and female internal secondary organs. Microscopically, the tumor consists of nests of a mixture of germ cells and sex cord derivatives resembling immature Sertoli and granulosa cells. A coexistent dysgerminoma occurs in 50% of the cases. The prognosis is excellent if the tumor is completely excised.[93]

Metastatic Tumors

The most common "metastatic" tumors of the ovary are probably derived from tumors of müllerian origin: the uterus, fallopian tube, contralateral ovary, or pelvic peritoneum. Although technically metastases, they are accepted as part of the "field

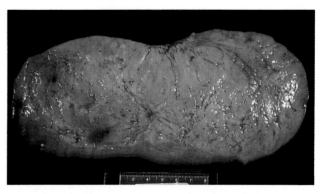

Figure 23-56. Krukenberg's tumor (metastatic gastric carcinoma) of the ovary.

effect" of müllerian neoplasia. The most common extramüllerian primaries are the breast and gastrointestinal tract, including stomach, biliary tract, and pancreas. A classic example of metastatic gastrointestinal neoplasia to the ovaries is termed Krukenberg's tumor, which are bilateral metastases composed of mucin-producing, signet-ring cancer cells, most often of gastric origin (Fig. 23–56).[94]

GESTATIONAL AND PLACENTAL DISORDERS

Diseases of pregnancy and pathologic conditions of the placenta are important causes of intrauterine or perinatal death, congenital malformations, intrauterine growth retardation, maternal death, and a great deal of morbidity for both mother and child.[6,95] Here we discuss only a limited number of disorders in which knowledge of the morphologic lesions contributes to an understanding of the clinical problem.

PLACENTAL INFLAMMATIONS AND INFECTIONS

Infections may occur in the placenta (placentitis, villitis),[96] in the fetal membranes (chorioamnionitis), and in the umbilical cord (funisitis).[97] They reach the placenta by two pathways: (1) ascending infection through the birth canal and (2) hematogenous (transplacental) infection. Ascending infections are by far the most common and are most often bacterial; in many such instances, localized infection of the membranes by an organism produces premature rupture of membranes and entry for the organisms. Sexual intercourse has been implicated in enhancing ascending infections.[95] The amniotic fluid may be cloudy with purulent exudate, and the chorion-amnion histologically contains a leukocytic polymorphonuclear infiltration with accompanying edema and congestion of the vessels. The infection frequently elicits a fetal response with umbilical cord vasculitis. Extension into the villous space may produce a septic intervillous thrombus.

Uncommonly, bacterial infections of the placenta and fetal membranes may arise by the hematogenous spread of bacteria directly to the placenta. Histologically, the villi are most often affected (villitis). Classically, TORCH (toxoplasma and others [syphilis, tuberculosis, listeriosis], rubella, cytomegalovirus, herpes simplex) should be considered, although the cause is usually obscure and may involve immunologic phenomena.[7] (See also Chapter 10.)

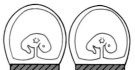

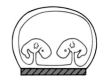

Dichorionic diamnionic   Dichorionic diamnionic (fused)

Monochorionic diamnionic   Monochorionic monoamnionic

— Chorion —— Amnion ▨▨▨ Placenta

Figure 23–57. Diagrammatic representation of the various types of twin placentation and their membrane relationships. (Adapted with permission from Gersell, D., et al.: In Kurman, R. (ed): Blaustein's Pathology of the Female Genital Tract. New York, Springer-Verlag, 1987.)

PLACENTAL ABNORMALITIES AND TWIN PLACENTAS

Abnormalities in placental shape, structure, and implantation are not uncommon. Accessory placental lobes, bipartite placenta (placenta made up of two equal segments), and circumvallate placenta (having an extrachorial part) are examples of abnormalities that have limited clinical significance.

Placenta accreta[97] is caused by partial or complete absence of the decidua with adherence of the placenta directly to the myometrium. It is important for two reasons: (1) Postpartum bleeding, often life-threatening, occurs because of failure of placental separation; (2) in up to 60% of cases, it is associated with placenta previa, a condition in which the placenta implants in the lower uterine segment or cervix, often with serious antepartum bleeding and premature labor. Many cases of placenta previa–associated accreta occur in cesarean section scars.

Twins arise from fertilization of two ova (dizygotic) or from division of one fertilized ovum (monozygotic). There are three basic types of twin placentas (Fig. 23–57):[98] dichorionic diamnionic (which may be fused); monochorionic diamnionic; and monochorionic monoamnionic. Monochorionic placentas imply monozygotic (identical) twins, and the time at which splitting occurs determines whether one or two amnions are present. Dichorionic gestation may occur with either monozygotic or dizygotic twins and is not specific.

SPONTANEOUS ABORTION

Ten to 15% of recognized pregnancies terminate in spontaneous abortion. Studies, however, using highly sensitive immunoassay of chorionic gonado-

tropin to detect pregnancy identified an additional 22% loss of presumably fertilized and implanted ova in otherwise healthy women.[99] The causes for this early loss of pregnancy are still mysterious, but as one good writer said, "There's many a slip 'twixt implantation and the crib."[100]

The causes of recognized spontaneous abortion are both fetal and maternal. Defective implantation inadequate to support fetal development and death of the ovum or fetus in uteri because of some genetic or acquired abnormality constitute the major origins of spontaneous abortion. Numerous studies have indicated chromosomal abnormalities in more than one-half of spontaneous abortuses.[101]

Maternal influences, which are less well understood, include inflammatory diseases, both localized to the placenta and systemic; uterine abnormalities; and possibly trauma. The role of trauma is generally overemphasized and must be considered a rare-to-exceptional trigger of spontaneous abortion. Toxoplasma, mycoplasma, listeria, and viral infections have also been implicated as causes of abortion.

The morphologic changes usually seen in endometrial curettage specimens depend, of course, on the interval between fetal death and passage of the products of conception.[102] Generally there are focal areas of decidual necrosis with intense neutrophilic infiltrations, thrombi within decidual blood vessels, and considerable amounts of hemorrhage, both recent and old, within the necrotic decidua. Placental villi may be markedly edematous and devoid of blood vessels. The changes encountered in the ovum or fetus are highly variable. In many spontaneous abortions, no fetal products can be identified, but when they are present, they should be carefully examined for anomalies that would suggest specific genetic or karyotypic defects. Chromosomal studies are recommended in

(1) habitual or recurrent abortion and (2) when there is a malformed fetus.

ECTOPIC PREGNANCY

Ectopic pregnancy is the term applied to implantation of the fetus in any site other than normal uterine location. The most common site is within the tubes (approximately 90%).[103] The other sites are the ovary, the abdominal cavity, and the intrauterine portion of the fallopian tube (cornual pregnancy). Ectopic pregnancies occur about once in every 150 pregnancies. The most important predisposing condition in 35 to 50% of patients is PID with chronic salpingitis. Other factors are peritubal adhesions owing to appendicitis or endometriosis, leiomyomas, and previous surgery. Fifty per cent, however, occur in tubes that are apparently normal. Intrauterine devices (IUDs) may also increase risk.

Ovarian pregnancy is presumed to result from the rare fertilization and trapping of the ovum within the follicle just at the time of its rupture. Abdominal pregnancies may develop when the fertilized ovum drops out of the fimbriated end of the tube. In all these abnormal locations, the fertilized ovum undergoes its usual development with the formation of placental tissue, amniotic sac, and fetus, and the host implantation site develops decidual changes.

> **MORPHOLOGY.** In tubal pregnancy, the placenta is poorly attached to the wall of the tube. Intratubal hemorrhage may thus occur from partial placental separation without tubal rupture (Fig. 23–58). Tubal pregnancy is the most common cause of hematosalpinx and should always be suspected when a tubal hematoma is present. More often, the placental tissue invades the tubal wall and causes tubal rupture and intraperitoneal hemorrhage. Less commonly, the tubal pregnancy may undergo spontaneous regression and resorption of the entire gestation. Still less commonly, the tubal pregnancy is extruded through the fimbriated end into the abdominal cavity (tubal abortion).

The clinical course of ectopic pregnancy is punctuated by the onset of severe abdominal pain about 6 weeks following a previous normal menstrual period, when rupture of the tube leads to a pelvic hemorrhage. In such cases, the patient may rapidly develop a shock-like state with signs of an acute abdomen, and early diagnosis becomes critical. Chorionic gonadotropin assays, ultrasound studies, and laparoscopy may be helpful. Endometrial biopsy specimens may or may not disclose decidual changes but, excluding the extremely rare dual pregnancy, do not exhibit chorionic villi. It

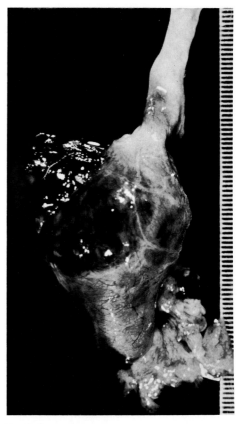

Figure 23–58. Tubal pregnancy with marked dilatation and rupture of distal end of tube by the contained pregnancy and subsequent hemorrhage.

must be remembered that rupture of a tubal pregnancy constitutes a medical emergency.

TOXEMIA OF PREGNANCY (PRE-ECLAMPSIA AND ECLAMPSIA)

Toxemia of pregnancy refers to a symptom complex characterized by hypertension, proteinuria, and edema (pre-eclampsia). It occurs in about 6% of pregnant women, usually in the last trimester and more commonly in primiparas than in multiparas. Certain of these patients become more seriously ill, developing convulsions; this more severe form is termed eclampsia. Patients with eclampsia develop disseminated intravascular coagulation (DIC) with lesions in the liver, kidneys, heart, placenta, and sometimes the brain. There is no absolute correlation between the severity of eclampsia and the magnitude of the anatomic changes.

PATHOGENESIS. The many theories on the nature of toxemia of pregnancy[104] are beyond our scope, but three events that seem to be of prime importance in this disorder are addressed: placental ischemia, hypertension, and DIC (Fig. 23–59). The causes of the initial events of toxemia are unknown, but evidence points to an abnormality of

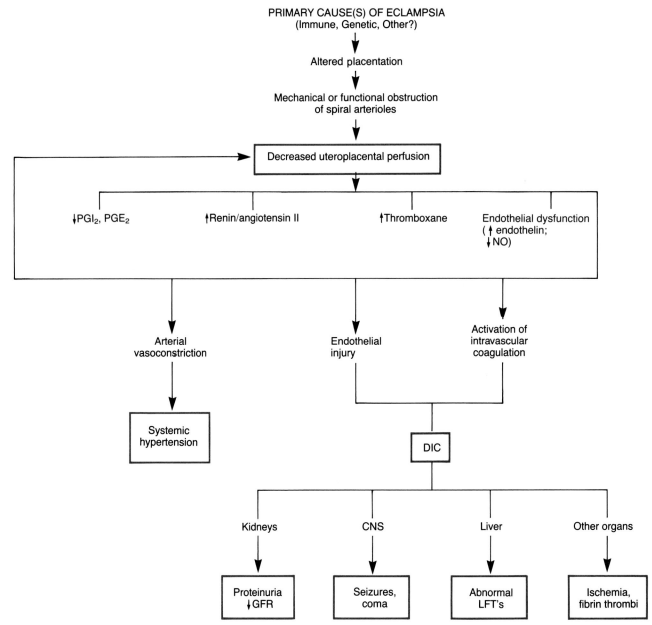

Figure 23-59. Proposed sequence of events in the pathogenesis of toxemia of pregnancy. The main features are (1) decreased uteroplacental perfusion; (2) increased vasoconstrictors and decreased vasodilators, resulting in local and systemic vasoconstriction; and (3) disseminated intravascular coagulation (DIC). (Adapted from Friedman, S.A.: Obstet. Gynecol. 71:122, 1988 (reprinted by permission of the American College of Obstetricians and Gynecologists); and Khong, T.Y., et al.: Br. Med. J. 93:1049, 1986.)

placentation.[105] This may involve an abnormality in both trophoblast invasion and the development of the physiologic alterations in the placental vessels required to perfuse the placental bed adequately. Immunologic, genetic, and other acquired factors have been postulated as the cause of such abnormality. The net effect is a shallow implantation with incomplete conversion of decidual vessels to vessels adequate for the pregnancy state.[105] The resultant perfusion abnormality produces placental ischemia, the basis for the toxemic placenta. It is thought that this decreased uteroplacental perfusion induces the stimulation of vasoconstrictor sub-

stances (thromboxane, angiotensin, endothelin) and the inhibition of vasodilator influences (PGI_2, PGE_2, nitric oxide) from the ischemic placenta. The resultant DIC, hypertension, and organ damage ensue (see Fig. 23–59).

As to the pathogenesis of DIC in toxemia, endothelial damage, abnormalities in the level and activities of coagulation factors, and primary platelet alteration may play a role.[106] For example, during toxemia, the placental ischemia leads to a higher output of thromboplastic substances, and antithrombin III levels are reduced. The characteristic lesions in eclampsia are in large part due to thrombosis of arterioles and capillaries throughout the body, particularly in the liver, kidneys, brain, pituitary, and placenta.

The mechanism of toxemic hypertension appears to involve the renin-angiotensin mechanism and prostaglandins.[107] Normal pregnant women develop a resistance to the vasoconstrictive and hypertensive effects of angiotensin, but women with toxemia lose such resistance, developing a tendency to hypertension. Prostaglandins of the E series, produced in the uteroplacental vascular bed during pregnancy, are thought to mediate the normal resistance of pregnant women to angiotensin, and prostaglandin production is indeed decreased in the placenta of toxemic women. Thus the increase in angiotensin hypersensitivity, characteristic of toxemia, may be due to decreased synthesis of prostaglandin by the toxemic placenta. There is also evidence that renin production by the toxemic placenta is increased, another potentially vasoconstrictive event. Figure 23–59 presents a hypothetical schema for the pathogenesis of eclampsia.

MORPHOLOGY. The liver lesions, when present, take the form of irregular, focal, subcapsular, and intraparenchymal hemorrhages. On histologic examination, there are fibrin thrombi in the portal capillaries with foci of characteristic peripheral hemorrhagic necrosis.

The **kidney** lesions are variable. Glomerular lesions are diffuse, at least when assessed by electron microscopy. They consist of striking swelling of endothelial cells, the deposition of fibrinogen-derived amorphous dense deposits on the endothelial side of the basement membrane, and mesangial cell hyperplasia. Immunofluorescent studies confirm the abundance of fibrin in glomeruli. In the more well-defined cases, fibrin thrombi are present in the glomeruli and capillaries of the cortex. When the lesion is far advanced, it may produce complete destruction of the cortex in the pattern referred to as bilateral renal cortical necrosis (see Chapter 20).

The **brain** may have gross or microscopic foci of hemorrhage along with small-vessel thromboses. Similar changes are often found in the **heart** and the **anterior pituitary**. The **placenta** is the site of variable changes, most of which reflect ischemia and vessel injury. (1) Placental infarcts, which occur in normal full-term placentas, are larger and more numerous. (2) There is increased frequency of retroplacental hematomas. (3) There is evidence of increased villous ischemia: formation of prominent syncytial knots, thickening of trophoblastic basement membrane, and villous hypovascularity. (4) A characteristic finding in the walls of uterine vessels is striking fibrinoid necrosis and intramural lipid deposition (acute atherosis) (Fig. 23–60).

CLINICAL COURSE. Pre-eclampsia usually starts after the 32nd week of pregnancy but begins earlier in patients with hydatidiform mole or pre-ex-

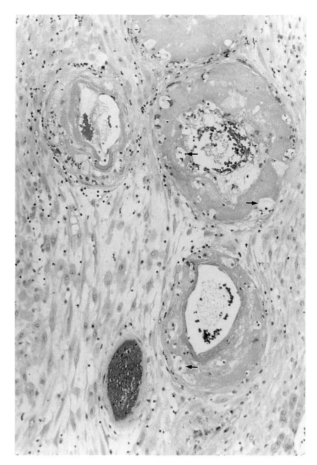

Figure 23–60. Acute atherosis of uterine vessels in eclampsia. Note fibrinoid necrosis of the vessel walls, subendothelial macrophages *(arrows)*, and perivascular lymphocytic infiltrate. (Courtesy of Dr. Drucilla J. Roberts.)

isting kidney disease or hypertension. The onset is usually insidious, characterized by hypertension and edema, with proteinuria following within several days. Headaches and visual disturbances are common. Eclampsia is heralded by central nervous system involvement, including convulsions and eventual coma. Mild and moderate forms of toxemia can be controlled by bed rest, a balanced diet, and antihypertensive agents, but induction of delivery is the only definitive treatment of established pre-eclampsia and eclampsia. Proteinuria and hypertension usually disappear within 1 or 2 weeks after delivery except in patients in whom these findings predated the pregnancy.

GESTATIONAL TROPHOBLASTIC DISEASE

Gestational trophoblastic disease constitutes a spectrum of tumors and tumor-like conditions characterized by proliferation of pregnancy-associated trophoblastic tissue of progressive malignant potential. The lesions include the hydatidiform mole (complete and partial), the invasive mole, and the frankly malignant choriocarcinoma.[62,108] Gestational trophoblastic disease is important for the following reasons:

- The hydatidiform mole is a common complication of gestation, occurring about once in every 1000 to 2000 pregnancies in the United States and curiously far more commonly in the Far East.
- It has become possible, by monitoring the circulating levels of human chorionic gonadotropin, to determine the early development of persistent trophoblastic disease.
- Choriocarcinoma, once a dreaded and uniformly fatal complication, is now highly responsive to chemotherapy in most cases.[109]

Hydatidiform Mole (Complete and Partial)

Hydatidiform mole is characterized by cystic swelling of the chorionic villi, accompanied by variable trophoblastic proliferation. The most important reason for the correct recognition of true moles is that they are the most common precursors of choriocarcinoma.[108] Most patients present in the fourth or fifth month of pregnancy with vaginal bleeding and with a uterus that is usually, but not always, larger than expected for the duration of pregnancy. These moles can occur at any age during active reproductive life, but the risk is higher in pregnant women in their teens or between the ages of 40 and 50 years. For poorly explained reasons, the incidence varies considerably in different regions of the world: 1 in 1000 pregnancies in the United States but 10 in 1000 in Indonesia.[110]

TYPES AND PATHOGENESIS. Two types of benign, noninvasive moles—complete and partial—can be differentiated by histologic, cytogenetic, and flow cytometric studies (Table 23–4).[111] In complete (or classic mole), all or most of the villi are edema-

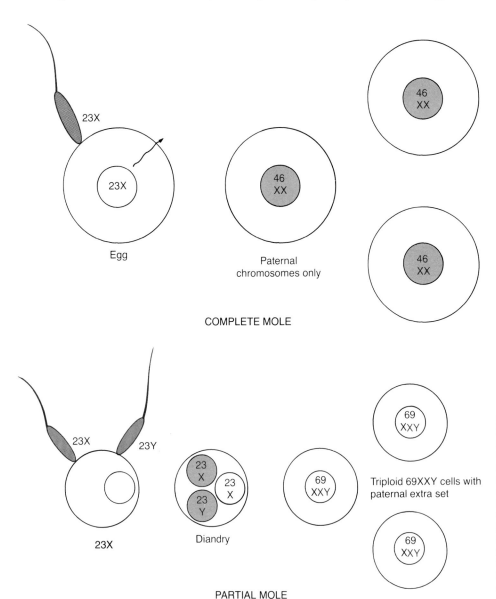

COMPLETE MOLE

PARTIAL MOLE

Figure 23–61. Patterns of fertilization to account for chromosomal origin of complete (46XX) and triploid partial moles (XXY). In a complete mole, a single sperm fertilizes an egg that has lost its chromosomes. Partial moles are due to fertilization of an egg by two sperm—one 23X and one 23Y. (Adapted with permission from Szulman, A.E.: Syndromes of hydatidiform moles: Partial vs. complete. J. Reprod. Med. 29:788, 1984.)

Table 23–4. FEATURES OF COMPLETE VERSUS PARTIAL HYDATIDIFORM MOLE

FEATURE	COMPLETE MOLE	PARTIAL MOLE
Karyotype	46,XX (46,XY)	Triploid
Villous edema	All villi	Some villi
Trophoblast proliferation	Diffuse; circumferential	Focal; slight
Atypia	Often present	Absent
Serum HCG	Elevated	Less elevated
HCG in tissue	++++	+
Behavior	2% choriocarcinoma	Rare choriocarcinoma

HCG = Human chorionic gonadotropin.

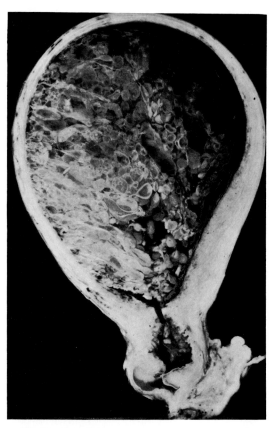

Figure 23–62. Hydatidiform mole. The uterus is filled with the classic mass of grape-like clusters. (Courtesy of Dr. A. Hertig. With permission from Anderson, W.A.D.: Textbook of Pathology. St. Louis, C.V. Mosby Co., 1971.)

tous, and there is diffuse trophoblast hyperplasia. Cytogenetic studies of these moles show that more than 90% have a 46,XX diploid pattern, all derived from the sperm (a phenomenon called androgenesis). They are presumed to be derived from fertilization, by a single sperm of an egg that has lost its chromosomes (Fig. 23–61). The remaining 10% are from the fertilization of such an empty egg by two sperm (46,XX and 46,XY). In both circumstances, embryonic development does not occur, and thus complete moles show no fetal parts.

In partial moles, some of the villi are edematous, and other villi show only minor changes; the trophoblastic proliferation is focal. In these moles, the karyotype is triploid (e.g., 69,XXY) or even occasionally tetraploid (92,XXXY). The moles result from fertilization of an egg with two sperm, one bearing 23,X and the other 23,Y (see Fig. 23–61). The embryo is viable for weeks, and thus fetal parts may be present when the resultant mole is aborted. In contrast to complete moles, partial moles are rarely followed by choriocarcinoma.

MORPHOLOGY. In most instances, moles develop within the uterus, but they may occur in any ectopic site of pregnancy. When discovered, usually in the fourth or fifth month of gestation, the uterus is usually larger (but may be normal sized, or even smaller) than anticipated for the duration of the pregnancy. The uterine cavity is filled with a delicate, friable mass of thin-walled, translucent, cystic, grape-like structures (Fig. 23–62). Careful dissection may disclose a small, usually collapsed amniotic sac. Fetal parts are frequently seen in partial moles but are never found in complete moles (unless a twin pregnancy).

In **partial moles** (Fig. 23–63A), the villous edema involves only a proportion of villi, and the trophoblastic proliferation is focal and slight.

Microscopically, the **complete mole** shows hydropic swelling of most chorionic villi and virtual absence or inadequate development of vascularization of villi. The central substance of the villi is a loose, myxomatous, edematous stroma, and they may be covered by a layer of chorionic epithelium, both cytotrophoblast and syncytial trophoblast (see Fig. 23–63B). At the opposite end of the spectrum are moles having similar cystic dilation of villi, accompanied, however, by circumferential and striking proliferation of the chorionic epithelium to produce sheets and masses of both cytotrophoblast and syncytial trophoblast. Histologic grading does not predict the outcome;[112] therefore all moles should be carefully followed by monitoring of the human chorionic gonadotropin levels.

CLINICAL COURSE. Most patients have abnormal uterine bleeding that usually begins early in the course of the pregnancy and is accompanied by the passage of a thin, watery fluid and bits of tissue seen as small, grape-like masses. The uterine enlargement is more rapid than anticipated. Ultrasound examination permits a definitive diagnosis in most cases.

In the classic case, quantitative analysis of human chorionic gonadotropin shows levels of hormone greatly exceeding those produced by a normal pregnancy of similar age. Serial hormone de-

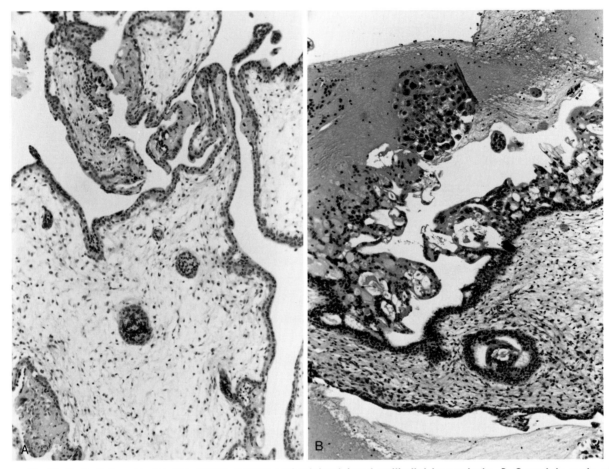

Figure 23–63. *A,* Partial mole showing villous edema and minimal focal epithelial hyperplasia. *B,* Complete mole with widespread trophoblast hyperplasia. (Courtesy of Dr. J. Lage.)

termination indicates a rapidly mounting level that climbs faster than the usual normal single or even multiple pregnancy.

Once the diagnosis is made, the mole must be removed by thorough curettage. In patients not desirous of further childbearing, hysterectomy may be performed. The course following curettage alone depends on the malignant potential of the removed uterine contents. From many studies, it is clear that 80 to 90% of these moles remain benign and give no further difficulty. Ten per cent develop into invasive moles and 2.5% into choriocarcinoma.[113]

blood vessels. Hydropic villi may embolize to distant sites, such as lungs and brain, but do not grow in these organs as true metastases, and even before the advent of chemotherapy, they eventually regressed unless fatal hemorrhage occurred. Clinically the tumor is manifested by vaginal bleeding and irregular uterine enlargement. It is always associated with a persistent elevated human chorionic gonadotropin level and varying degrees of luteinization of the ovaries. The tumor responds well to chemotherapy. Although invasive mole is biologically benign, rupture of the uterus may lead to hemorrhage.

Invasive Mole

This is defined as a mole that penetrates and may even perforate the uterine wall. There is invasion of the myometrium by hydropic chorionic villi, accompanied by proliferation of both cytotrophoblast and syncytiotrophoblast. The tumor is locally destructive and may invade parametrial tissue and

Choriocarcinoma

Gestational choriocarcinoma is an epithelial malignancy of trophoblastic cells derived from any form of previously normal or abnormal pregnancy.[108] Although most cases arise in the uterus, ectopic pregnancies provide extrauterine sites of origin. Choriocarcinoma is a rapidly invasive, widely me-

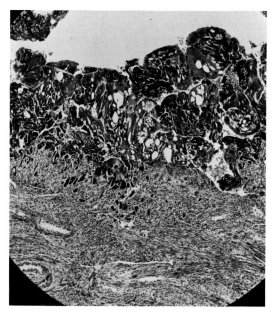

Figure 23–64. Low-power view of choriocarcinoma of uterine wall showing invasion of underlying myometrium.

tastasizing malignancy, but once identified, it responds well to chemotherapy.

INCIDENCE. This is an uncommon condition that arises in 1 in 20,000 to 30,000 pregnancies in the United States. It is much more common in some Asian countries, for example, 1 in 2500 pregnancies in Ibadan. It is preceded by several conditions: 50% arise in hydatidiform moles, 25% in previous abortions, approximately 22% in normal pregnancies, and the rest in ectopic pregnancies and genital and extragenital teratomas. About 1 in 40 hydatidiform moles may be expected to give rise to a choriocarcinoma, in contrast to 1 in approximately 150,000 normal pregnancies.

MORPHOLOGY. Classically, the choriocarcinoma is a soft, fleshy, yellow-white tumor, with a marked tendency to form large pale areas of ischemic necrosis, foci of cystic softening, and extensive hemorrhage. Histologically, it is a purely epithelial cellular malignancy that does not produce chorionic villi and that grows, as do other cancers, by the abnormal proliferation of both cytotrophoblast and syncytiotrophoblast (Figs. 23–64 and 23–65).

It is sometimes possible to identify anaplasia within such abnormal proliferation replete with abnormal mitoses. The tumor invades the underlying myometrium, frequently penetrates blood vessels and lymphatics, and in some cases extends out onto the uterine serosa and adjacent structures. In its rapid growth, it is subject to hemorrhage, ischemic necrosis, and secondary inflammatory infiltration.

In fatal cases, metastases are found in the lungs, brain, bone marrow, liver, and other organs.

Occasionally, metastatic choriocarcinoma is discovered without a detectable primary in the uterus (or ovary), presumably because the primary has undergone total necrosis.

CLINICAL COURSE. Classically, the uterine choriocarcinoma does not produce a large, bulky mass. It becomes manifest only by irregular spotting of a bloody, brown, sometimes foul-smelling fluid. This discharge may appear in the course of an apparently normal pregnancy, after a miscarriage, or after a curettage.

Sometimes the tumor does not appear until months later. Usually, by the time the tumor is discovered locally, radiographs of the chest and bones already disclose the presence of metastatic lesions. The human chorionic gonadotropin titers are elevated to levels above those encountered in hydatidiform moles. Occasional tumors, however, produce little hormone, and some tumors have become so necrotic as to become functionally inactive.

Widespread metastases are characteristic of these tumors. Favored sites of involvement are the lungs (50%) and vagina (30 to 40%), followed in descending order of frequency by the brain, liver, and kidney.

The treatment of trophoblastic neoplasms depends on the type and stage of tumor and includes evacuation of the contents of the uterus, surgery, and chemotherapy. The results of chemotherapy for gestational choriocarcinoma are spectacular and have resulted in up to 100% cure or remission in

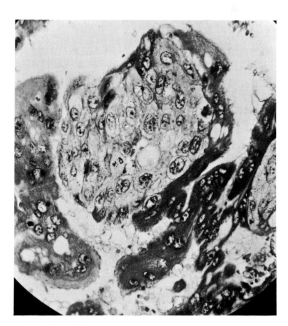

Figure 23–65. High-power detail of choriocarcinoma illustrating the two types of epithelial cells—cytotrophoblast and syncytiotrophoblast.

all patients except some who had high-risk metastatic trophoblastic disease. Many of the cured patients have had normal subsequent pregnancies and deliveries. By contrast, nongestational choriocarcinomas are much more resistant to therapy.

Placental Site Trophoblastic Tumor

This rare tumor is characterized by the presence of proliferating trophoblastic tissue deeply invading the myometrium and is composed largely of an *intermediate trophoblast*. These cells are usually mononuclear, rather than syncytial, but are larger and have more abundant cytoplasm than the regular cytotrophoblast; in contrast to syncytiotrophoblast (which produces human chorionic gonadotropin), intermediate trophoblast cells are immunoreactive for human placental lactogen. This lesion differs from choriocarcinoma in the absence of cytotrophoblastic elements and in the low level of human chorionic gonadotropin production. The tumors are locally invasive, but many are self-limited and subject to cure by curettage. Malignant variants, however, have been reported; they are distinguished by a high mitotic index, extreme cellularity, extensive necrosis, local spread, or even widespread metastases. About 10% result in disseminated metastases and death.[108,114]

1. McLean, J.M.: Embryology and anatomy of the female genital tract and ovary. *In* Fox, H. (ed.): Haines and Taylor's Obstetrical and Gynaecologic Pathology, 4th ed. Edinburgh, Churchill Livingstone, 1987, pp. 1–50.
2. Parmley, T.: Embryology of the female genital tract. *In* Kurman, R. (ed.): Blaustein's Pathology of the Female Genital Tract, 4th ed. New York, Springer-Verlag, 1994 (in press).
3. Donahoe, P.K.: The diagnosis and treatment of infants with intersex abnormalities. Pediatr. Clin. North Am. 34:1333, 1987.
4. Kurman, R. (ed.): Blaustein's Pathology of the Female Genital Tract, 4th ed. New York, Springer-Verlag, 1994 (in press).
5. Fox, H. (ed.): Haines and Taylor's Obstetrical and Gynaecologic Pathology, 4th ed. Edinburgh, Churchill Livingstone, 1987.
6. Benirschke, K., and Kaufmann, P.: Pathology of the Human Placenta, 2nd ed. New York, Springer-Verlag, 1990.
7. Danforth, D.N. (ed.): Obstetrics and Gynecology, 5th ed. Philadelphia, Harper & Row, 1988.
8. Buchsbaum, H. (ed.): Gynecology and Obstetrics. Hagerstown, MD, Harper & Row, 1988.
9. Knapp, R.C., and Berkowitz, R.S. (eds.): Gynecologic Oncology, 2nd ed. New York, McGraw-Hill, 1993.
10. Holmes, K.K., et al. (eds.): Sexually Transmitted Diseases. New York, McGraw-Hill, 1984.
11. Koutsky, L.A. et al.: The frequency of unrecognized type 2 herpes simplex virus infection among women. Implications for the control of genital herpes. Sex. Transm. Dis. 17:2, 1990.
12. Prober, C.G.: Herpetic vaginitis in 1993. Clin. Obstet. Gynecol. 36:177–187, 1993.
13. Wolner-Hanssen, P., et al.: Clinical manifestations of vaginal trichomoniasis. J.A.M.A. 261:4, 1989.
14. Mann, M.S., et al.: Vulvar vestibulitis: Significant clinical variables and treatment outcome. Obstet. Gynecol. 79:1, 1992.
15. Wilkinson, E.J.: Normal histology, and nomenclature of the vulva and malignant neoplasms, including VIN. Dermatol. Clin. 10:283–296, 1992.
16. Report of the ISSVD Terminology Committee. Proceedings of the VIII World Congress (1986), Stockholm, Sweden. J. Reprod. Med. 31:973, 1986.
17. Wilkinson, E.J.: Premalignant and malignant diseases of the vulva. *In* Kurman, R. (ed.): Blaustein's Pathology of the Female Genital Tract, 4th ed. New York, Springer-Verlag, 1994 (in press).
18. Crum, C.P.: Vulvar intraepithelial neoplasia: Histology and associated viral changes. Contemp. Issues Surg. Pathol. 9:119, 1987.
19. Lynch, P.J.: Condyloma acuminata. Clin. Obstet. Gynaecol. 28:142, 1985.
20. Gissman, L., et al.: Human papilloma virus type 6 and 11 DNA sequences in genital and laryngeal papillomas. Proc. Natl. Acad. Sci. (U.S.A.) 80:560, 1983.
21. Zaino, R.J.: Carcinoma of the vulva, urethra, and Bartholin's glands. Contemp. Issues Surg. Pathol. 9:119, 1987.
22. Crum, C.P.: Carcinoma of the vulva: Epidemiology and pathogenesis. Obstet. Gynecol. 79:3, 1992.
23. Leibowitch, M., et al.: The epithelial changes associated with squamous cell carcinoma of the vulva: A review of the clinical, histological and viral findings in 78 women. Br. J. Obstet. Gynaecol. 97:1135, 1990.
24. Michael, H., and Roth, L.M.: Paget's disease, skin appendage tumors, and cysts of the vulva. Contemp. Issues Surg. Pathol. 9:25, 1987.
25. Chung, A. F., et al.: Malignant melanoma of the vulva: A report of 44 cases. Obstet. Gynecol. 45:6, 1975.
26. Hilborne, L.H., and Fu, Y.S.: Intraepithelial, invasive and metastatic neoplasms of the vagina. Contemp. Issues Surg. Pathol. 9:181–208, 1987.
27. Herbst, A.L.: Clear cell adenocarcinoma and the current status of DES-exposed females. Cancer 48:484, 1981.
28. Scully, R.E., and Welch, W.R.: Pathology of the female genital tract after prenatal exposure to diethylstilbestrol. *In* Herbst, A.L., and Bern, H.A. (eds.): Developmental Effects of Diethylstilbestrol in Pregnancy. New York, Thieme-Stratton, 1981, pp. 26–45.
29. Copeland, L.J., et al.: Sarcoma botryoides of the female genital tract. Obstet. Gynecol. 66:262, 1985.
30. Cancer Manual, 8th ed. Boston, American Cancer Society, 1990, p. 390.
31. Coppleson, M., and Reid, B.: Preclinical Carcinoma of the Cervix Uteri. Oxford, Pergamon, 1967.
32. Winkler, B., and Crum, C.P.: *Chlamydia trachomatis* infection of the female genital tract. Pathogenetic and clinicopathologic correlations. Pathol. Annu. 5:193–221, 1984.
33. Kiviat, N.B., et al.: Histopathology of endocervical infection by Chlamydia trachomatis, herpes simplex virus, Trichomonas vaginalis, and Neisseria gonorrheae. Hum. Pathol. 21:831–837, 1990.
34. Silverberg, E., and Lubera, J.: Cancer statistics. Cancer 39:1, 1989.
35. Koutsky, L.A., et al.: A cohort study of the risk of cervical intraepithelial neoplasia grade 2 or 3 in relation to papillomavirus infection. N. Engl. J. Med. 327:1272–1278, 1992.
36. Herrero, R., et al.: Sexual behavior, venereal diseases, hygiene practices and invasive cervical cancer in a high-risk population. Cancer 65:380–386, 1990.
37. zur Hausen, H., and Schneider, A.: The role of human papilloma viruses in human urogenital cancer. *In* Salzman, N., and Howley, P. (eds.): The Papovaviridae. New York, Plenum Press, 1987, pp. 245–263.
38. Lorincz, A.T., et al.: Human papillomavirus infection of

the cervix: Relative risk associations of 15 common an-ogenital types. Obstet. Gynecol. *79*:328–337, 1992.

39. Crum, C.P., and Nuovo, G.J.: Genital Papillomaviruses and Related Neoplasms. New York, Raven Press, 1991.

40. Crook, T., and Vousden, K.H.: Properties of p53 mutations detected in primary and secondary cervical cancers suggest mechanisms of metastasis and involvement of environmental carcinogens. Embo J. *11*:3935–3940, 1992.

41. Wright, T., et al.: Precursors of cervical carcinoma. *In* Kurman, R. (ed.): Blaustein's Pathology of the Female Genital Tract, 4th ed. New York, Springer-Verlag, 1994 (in press).

42. Richart, R.M.: Cervical intraepithelial neoplasia. *In* Sommers, S.C.: Pathology Annual. New York, Appleton-Century-Crofts, 1973, pp. 301–328.

43. Crum, C.P., et al.: Cervical papillomaviruses segregate within morphologically distinct precancerous lesions. J. Virol. *54*:675–681, 1985.

44. The Bethesda System for reporting cervical/vaginal cytologic diagnoses. Report of the 1991 Bethesda Workshop. Am. J. Surg. Pathol. *16*:914–916, 1992.

45. Ostor, A.G.: Natural history of cervical intraepithelial neoplasia: A critical review. Int. J. Gynecol. Pathol. *12*:186–192, 1993.

46. Van Nagell, J.R., et al.: Small cell cancer of the uterine cervix. Cancer *40*:2243–2249, 1977.

47. Rotman, M., et al.: Prognostic factors in cervical carcinoma: Implications in staging and management. Cancer *48*:560, 1981.

48. Smotkin, D., et al.: Human papillomavirus DNA in adenocarcinoma and adenosquamous carcinoma of the uterine cervix. Obstet. Gynecol. *68*:241–244, 1986.

49. Rotterdam, H.: Chronic endometritis. A clinicopathologic study. Pathol. Annu. *13*(Part 2):209, 1978.

50. Kiviat, N.B., et al.: Endometrial histopathology in patients with culture-proved upper genital tract infection and laparoscopically diagnosed acute salpingitis. Am. J. Surg. Pathol. *14*:167–175, 1990.

51. Fox, H., and Buckley, C.H.: Current concepts of endometriosis. Clin. Obstet. Gynecol. *11*:279, 1984.

52. Dahlenbach-Hellweg, G.: Histopathology of the Endometrium, 4th ed. New York, Springer-Verlag, 1993.

53. Ober, W.B.: Effects of oral and intrauterine administration of contraceptives on the uterus. Hum. Pathol. *8*:513, 1977.

54. Hertig, A.T., and Sommers, S.C.: Genesis of endometrial carcinoma. 1. Study of prior biopsies. Cancer *2*:964, 1949.

55. Kurman, R.J., et al.: The behavior of endometrial hyperplasia. A long-term study of untreated hyperplasia in 170 patients. Cancer *56*:403, 1985.

56. renczy, A., and Gelfand, M.: The biologic significance of cytologic atypia in progestogen-treated endometrial hyperplasia. Am. J. Obstet. Gynecol. *160*:126–131, 1989.

57. Winkler, B., et al.: Pitfalls in the diagnosis of endometrial neoplasia. Obstet. Gynecol. *64*:185–194, 1984.

58. Corley, D., et al.: Postmenopausal bleeding from unusual endometrial polyps in women on chronic tomoxifen therapy. Obstet. Gynecol. *79*:111–116, 1992.

59. Fletcher, J.A., et al.: Clonal 6p21 rearrangement is restricted to the mesenchymal component of an endometrial polyp. Genes Chromosom. Cancer *5*:260–263, 1992.

60. Fletcher, J.A., et al.: Chromosome aberrations in uterine smooth muscle tumors: Potential diagnostic relevance and cytogenetic instability. Cancer Res. *50*:4092–4097, 1990.

61. Brinton, L.A., et al.: Reproductive, menstrual, and medical risk factors for endometrial cancer: Results from a case-control study. Am. J. Obstet. Gynecol. *167*:1317–1325, 1992.

62. Silverberg, S.G., and Kurman, R.J.: Atlas of Tumor Pathology. Tumors of the Uterine Corpus and Gestational Trophoblastic Disease. Washington, DC, Armed Forces Institute of Pathology, 1991, pp. 219–287.

63. Connelly, P.J., et al.: Carcinoma of the endometrium. III. Analysis of 865 cases of adenocarcinoma and adenoacanthoma. Obstet. Gynecol. *59*:569, 1982.

64. Hendrickson, M.R., et al.: Adenocarcinoma of the endometrium: Analysis of 256 cases with disease limited to uterine corpus. Analysis of prognostic variables. Gynecol. Oncol. *12*:373, 1982.

65. Cowles, T.A., et al.: Comparison of clinical and surgical staging in patients with endometrial carcinoma. Obstet. Gynecol. *66*:413, 1985.

66. Christopherson, W.M., and Richardson, M.: Uterine mesenchymal tumors. Pathol. Annu. *16*:215, 1981.

67. Geisinger, K.R., et al.: Malignant mixed müllerian tumors. Cancer *54*:1281, 1987.

68. Chu, M.T., et al.: Expression of various antigens by different components of uterine mixed Müllerian tumors. Acta Pathol. *38*:35, 1988.

69. Silverberg, S.G., et al.: Carcinosarcoma (malignant mixed mesodermal tumor of the uterus). Int. J. Gynecol. Pathol. *9*:1, 1990.

70. Buscema, J., et al.: Epithelioid leiomyosarcoma. Cancer *47*:1192, 1986.

71. Young, R.H., and Scully, R.E.: Ovarian pathology in infertility. *In* Kraus, F.T. (ed.): Pathology of Reproductive Failure. Baltimore, Williams & Wilkins, 1991, pp. 104–139.

72. McKenna, T.J.: Pathogenesis and treatment of polycystic ovary syndrome. N. Engl. J. Med. *318*:558, 1988.

73. Russel, P., and Bannatyne, P.: Surgical Pathology of the Ovaries. Edinburgh, Churchill Livingstone, 1989.

74. Young, R.H., et al.: The ovary. *In* Sternberg S., et al. (eds.): Diagnostic Surgical Pathology. New York, Raven Press, 1994.

75. Piver, M.S., et al.: Epidemiology and etiology of ovarian cancer. Semin. Oncol. *18*:177–184, 1991.

76. Cramer, D.W., et al.: Factors affecting the association of contraceptives and ovarian cancer. N. Engl. J. Med. *307*:1047, 1982.

77. Bast, R.C., et al.: Malignant transformation of ovarian epithelium. J. Natl. Cancer Inst. *84*:557–558, 1992.

78. Bell, D.A., et al.: Peritoneal implants of ovarian serous borderline tumors. Cancer *62*:2212–2222, 1988.

79. Watkin, W., et al.: Mucinous carcinoma of the ovary. Cancer *69*:208–212, 1992.

80. Snyder, R.R., et al.: Endometrial proliferative and low malignant potential tumors of the ovary. Am. J. Surg. Pathol. *12*:661, 1988.

81. Eifel, P., et al.: Simultaneous presentation of carcinoma involving the ovary and uterine corpus. Cancer *50*:163–170, 1982.

82. Teilum, G.: Special Tumors of Ovary and Testis and Related Extragonadal Lesions. Philadelphia, W.B. Saunders Co., 1976.

83. Shevchuk, M.M., et al.: Histogenesis of Brenner tumors. I. Histology and ultrastructure. II. Histochemistry and CEA. Cancer *46*:2607, 1980.

84. Silva, E.G., et al.: Ovarian carcinomas with transitional cell carcinoma pattern. Cancer *93*:457–465, 1990.

85. Altaras, M.M., et al.: The role of cancer antigen CA 125 in the management of various epithelial carcinomas. Gynecol. Oncol. *30*:26, 1988.

86. Linder, D., et al.: Pathogenetic origin of benign ovarian teratomas. N. Engl. J. Med. *292*:63, 1975.

87. Mutter, G.L.: Teratoma genetics and stem cells: A review. Obstet. Gynecol. Surv. *42*:661, 1987.

88. Norris, H.J., et al.: Immature (malignant) teratoma of the ovary. A clinical and pathological study of 58 cases. Cancer *37*:2359, 1976.

89. Gordon, T., et al.: Dysgerminoma. A review of 158 cases from the Emil Novak ovarian tumor registry. Obstet. Gynecol. *58*:497, 1981.

90. Young, R.H., and Scully, R.: Ovarian sex cord-stromal tumors. Recent progress. Int. J. Gynecol. Pathol. *1*:101, 1982.

91. Prat, J., and Scully, R.E.: Cellular fibromas and fibrosarcomas of the ovary. Cancer *47*:2663, 1981.

92. Roth, L.M., et al.: Sertoli-Leydig cell tumors: A clinicopathologic study of 34 cases. Cancer *48*:187, 1981.

93. Scully R.E.: The ovary. *In* Wolfe, H. (ed.): Endometrial Pathology. New York, Springer-Verlag, 1986.

94. Young, R.H., and Scully, R.E.: Metastatic tumors of the ovary. *In* Kurman, R.J. (ed.): Blaustein's Pathology of the Female Genital Tract, 4th ed. New York, Springer-Verlag, 1994 (in press).

95. Naeye, R.L.: Disorders of the Placenta Fetus and Neonate: Diagnosis and Clinical Significance. St. Louis, Mosby-Year Book, 1992, pp. 113–114.

96. Grossman, J.H.: Infections affecting the placenta. *In* Lavery, J.P. (ed.): The Placenta. Rockville, MD, Aspen Publishing, 1987, pp. 131–134.

97. Morrison, J.E.: Placenta accreta: A clinicopathologic review of 67 cases. Obstet. Gynecol. Annu. *7*:107, 1978.

98. Lage, J.M., et al.: The twin placenta. *In* Lavery, J.P. (ed.): The Placenta. Rockville, MD, Aspen Publishing, 1987, p. 67.

99. Wilcox, A.J.: Incidence of early loss of pregnancy. N. Engl. J. Med. *319*:189, 1988.

100. Little, A.B.: There's many a slip 'twixt implantation and the crib. N. Engl. J. Med. *319*:241, 1988.

101. Kalousek, D.K., and Lau, A.E.: Pathology of spontaneous abortion. *In* Dimmick, J.E., and Kalousek, D.K. (eds.): Developmental Pathology of the Embryo and Fetus. Philadelphia, J.B. Lippincott Co., 1992, p. 62.

102. Rushton, D.I.: Examination of products of conception from previable human pregnancies. J. Clin. Pathol. *34*:819, 1981.

103. Hockberger, R.S.: Ectopic pregnancy. Obstet. Gynecol. Emerg. *5*:481, 1987.

104. Weiner, G.P.: The clinical spectrum of pre-clampsia. Am. J. Kidney Dis. *9*:312, 1987.

105. Khong, T.Y., et al.: Inadequate maternal vascular response to placentation in pregnancies complicated by pre-eclampsia and by small for gestational age infants. B.M.J. *93*:1049, 1986.

106. Ferris, T.F.: Pregnancy, preeclampsia and the endothelial cell. N. Engl. J. Med. *325*:1439–1440, 1991.

107. Friedman, S.A.: Pre-clampsia: A review of the role of prostaglandins. Obstet. Gynecol. *71*:122, 1988.

108. Lage, J.M., and Young, R.H.: Pathology of trophoblastic disease. *In* Clement, P.B., and Young, R.H. (eds.): Tumors and Tumor-like Conditions of the Uterine Corpus and Cervix, New York, Churchill Livingstone, 1993, pp. 419–475.

109. Berkowitz, R.S., and Goldstein, D.P.: Management of molar pregnancy and gestational trophoblastic tumors. *In* Knapp, R.C., and Berkowitz, R.S. (eds.): Gynecologic Oncology. New York, McGraw-Hill, 1993, pp. 328–340.

110. Bracken, M.B., et al.: Epidemiology of hydatidiform mole and choriocarcinoma. Epidemiol. Rev. *6*:52, 1984.

111. Lage, J.M., et al.: Hydatidiform moles. Application of flow cytometry to diagnosis. Am. J. Clin. Pathol. *89*:596, 1988.

112. Genest, D.R., et al.: A clinico-pathologic study of 153 cases of complete hydatidiform mole (1980–1990): Histologic grade lacks prognostic significance. Obstet. Gynecol. *78*:402–409, 1991.

113. Lurain, J.R., et al.: Natural history of hydatidiform mole after primary evacuation. Am. J. Obstet. Gynecol. *145*:591, 1983.

114. Finkler, N.J., et al.: Clinical experience with placental site trophoblastic tumors at the New England Trophoblastic Disease Center. Obstet. Gynecol. *71*:854, 1988.

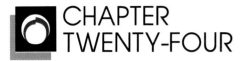
The Breast

The Female Breast

NORMAL

ANATOMY AND HISTOLOGY. The resting mammary gland consists of six to ten major duct systems, each of which is subdivided into lobules, the functional units of the mammary parenchyma (Fig. 24–1).[1] Each ductal system drains through a separate main excretory or *lactiferous sinus.* Successive branching of the lactiferous ducts distally eventually leads to the terminal ducts. Before puberty, the complex system of branching ducts ends blindly, but at the beginning of menarche, it proliferates distally, giving rise to some 30 epithelium-lined *ductules* or *acini.* Each terminal duct and its ductules compose the *terminal duct lobular units* (see Fig. 24–1).

The areola, nipple, and mouths of the main lactiferous ducts are covered by stratified squamous epithelium. The lining of the major breast ducts changes to a pseudostratified columnar and then double-layered cuboidal epithelium. A low, flattened layer of cells *(myoepithelial cells)* can be identified beneath the more prominent lining epithelium. Myoepithelial cells contain myofilaments oriented parallel to the long axis of the duct. A basement membrane follows faithfully the contour of ducts and ductules.[1] The lobules are enclosed in a loose, delicate, myxomatous stroma that contains a scattering of lymphocytes *(intralobular connective tissue),* and the individual lobules are enclosed within a denser, collagenous, fibrous *interlobular stroma.*

Just as the endometrium rises and ebbs with each menstrual cycle, so does the breast.[2] Following the menstrual period, with the progressive rise in estrogen, the ductal and ductular cells begin to proliferate and continue to develop throughout the menstrual cycle. During the secretory phase of the menstrual cycle, under the influence of progesterone, proliferation of the terminal duct structure increases, and there is vacuolization and increased mitotic activity of basal epithelial cells. The stromal cells proliferate, and there is, in addition, stromal edema. This combined stimulatory effect of estrogen and progesterone on the intralobular breast elements accounts for the sense of fullness commonly experienced by women during the premenstrual phase of the cycle. When menstruation occurs, the fall in estrogen and progesterone levels is followed by desquamation of epithelial cells, atrophy of the intralobular connective tissue, disappearance of the stromal edema, and overall shrinkage in the size of the ducts and gland buds.

It is only with the onset of pregnancy that the breast assumes its complete morphologic maturation

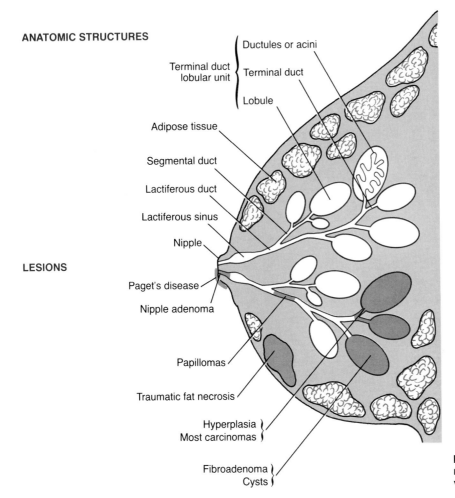

ANATOMIC STRUCTURES

Ductules or acini

Terminal duct lobular unit { Terminal duct

Lobule

Adipose tissue

Segmental duct

Lactiferous duct

Lactiferous sinus

Nipple

LESIONS

Paget's disease

Nipple adenoma

Papillomas

Traumatic fat necrosis

Hyperplasia }
Most carcinomas }

Fibroadenoma }
Cysts }

Figure 24–1. Anatomy of the breast and major lesions at each site within the various units.

and functional activity. From each gland bud, numerous true secretory glands pouch out to form grape-like clusters. As a consequence, there is a reversal of the usual stromal-glandular relationship so that, by the end of the pregnancy, the breast is composed almost entirely of glands separated by a relatively scant amount of stroma. The secretory glands are lined by cuboidal cells, and in the third trimester, secretory vacuoles of lipid material are found within the cells. Immediately following birth the secretion of milk begins (Fig. 24–2). Breast lesions arising during pregnancy may exhibit similar secretory changes (lactating adenoma or fibroadenoma).

Following lactation, the glands once again regress and atrophy, the ducts shrink, and the total breast size diminishes remarkably. However, complete regression to the stage of the normal virginal breast usually does not occur, and some increase of glandular parenchyma remains as a permanent residual.

After the third decade, the ducts and lobules further atrophy with more shrinkage of the intra- and interlobular stroma. The lobules may almost totally disappear in the very aged, leaving only ducts to create a morphologic pattern that comes close to that of the male. However, in most women there is sufficient persistent estrogenic stimulation, possibly of adrenal origin, to maintain the vestigial remnants of lobules that differentiate even the very aged female breast from the male breast.

PATHOLOGY

Lesions of the breast are preponderantly confined to the female. In the male, the breast is a rudimentary structure relatively insensitive to endocrine influences and apparently resistant to neoplastic growth. In the female, on the other hand, the more complex breast structure, the greater breast volume, and the extreme sensitivity to endocrine influences all predispose this organ to a number of pathologic conditions.

Most diseases of the breast present as palpable masses, inflammatory lesions, nipple secretion, or mammographic abnormalities. Although fortunately

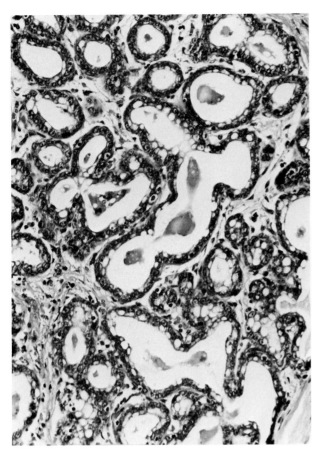

Figure 24-2. Lactating breast. Note the hyperplasia of glands, vacuolization of cells, and secretion in lumina.

most are benign, cancer of the breast is the second most common cause of cancer deaths and one of the most dreaded diseases of women. In this chapter, therefore, the conditions to be described should be considered in terms of their possible confusion clinically with cancer.[3-5]

An overall perspective of the frequency of various breast problems can be gained from an analysis of a large series of patients with breast complaints who were seen in a surgical outpatient

department.[6] About 30% of the women were considered, after careful evaluation, to have no breast disease. Almost 40% were diagnosed as having fibrocystic changes. Slightly more than 10% had biopsy-proven cancer, and about 7% had a benign tumor (fibroadenoma). The remainder were suffering from a miscellany of benign lesions (Fig. 24-3). Three features of this study deserve particular note: (1) *A significant proportion of women having no recognizable breast disease have sufficient irregularity of the "normal" breast tissue to cause concern and to necessitate clinical evaluation;* (2) *fibrocystic changes are the dominant breast problem;* and (3) *cancer, unhappily, is all too frequent.*

CONGENITAL ANOMALIES

These anomalies run the gamut from congenital absence to abnormal numbers of breasts, but as a group these entities are of limited clinical significance.

SUPERNUMERARY NIPPLES OR BREASTS. These result from the persistence of epidermal thickenings along the milk line, extending from the axilla to the perineum, both below the adult breast and above it in the anterior axillary fold. Rarely, the disorders that affect the normally situated breast may arise in these heterotopic foci, and occasionally the cyclic changes of the menstrual cycle cause painful premenstrual enlargements.

ACCESSORY AXILLARY BREAST TISSUE. The normal ductal systems sometimes extend over the entire anterolateral chest wall and into the axillary fossa. Simple mastectomies commonly do not remove all this epithelial tissue. Such tissue may also give rise to tumors that appear to be outside the breast and, therefore, are commonly misidentified as lesions of the axillary lymph nodes or even metastases from an occult breast cancer.

CONGENITAL INVERSION OF NIPPLES. This occurs in many women, particularly those who have large or pendulous breasts. Commonly, this inversion is corrected during the growth activity of pregnancy, or it may sometimes be corrected by simple traction on the nipples. Nipple inversion is of clinical significance, since it may frustrate attempts at nursing and may also be confused with acquired retraction of the nipple, sometimes observed in mammary cancer and in inflammation of the breasts.

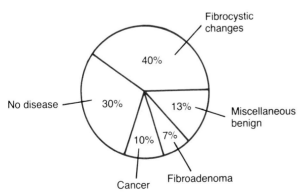

Figure 24-3. Representation of the findings in a series of women seeking evaluation of apparent breast "lumps."

INFLAMMATIONS

Inflammations of the breast are, on the whole, uncommon and consist of only a relatively few forms of acute and chronic disease. Of these, the most important is nonspecific acute mastitis, virtually confined to the lactating period. Breast abscesses are included under the heading of acute mastitis. The other forms of mastitis consist of plasma cell mastitis or mammary duct ectasia (an entity of obscure etiology), granulomatous mastitis, and post-traumatic lesions.

ACUTE MASTITIS AND BREAST ABSCESS

During the early weeks of nursing, the breast is rendered vulnerable to bacterial infection by the development of cracks and fissures in the nipples. The disease is not confined to the postpartum state, however, and eczema and other dermatologic conditions of the nipples may be predisposing factors. From this portal of entry, *Staphylococcus aureus* usually, or streptococci less commonly, invade the breast substance.

MORPHOLOGY. Usually the disease is unilateral. The staphylococcus tends to produce a localized area of acute inflammation that may progress to the formation of single or multiple abscesses. The streptococcus tends to cause, as it does in all tissues, a diffuse spreading infection that eventually involves the entire organ. Surgical drainage and antibiotic therapy may limit the spread of the infection, but when extensive necrosis occurs, the destroyed breast substance is replaced by fibrous scar as a permanent residual of the inflammatory process. Such scarring may create a localized area of increased consistency sometimes accompanied by retraction of the skin or the nipple, changes that may later be mistaken for a neoplasm.

MAMMARY DUCT ECTASIA

This condition is characterized chiefly by dilatation of ducts, inspissation of breast secretions, and a marked periductal and interstitial chronic granulomatous inflammatory reaction, sometimes associated with large numbers of plasma cells *(plasma cell mastitis).*[5] This disorder tends to occur in the fifth or sixth decade of life, usually in multiparous women, and is thought to result from obstruction of ducts due to inspissation of secretions. The etiology is unknown, but the association with pituitary adenomas or elevated prolactin levels suggests a role for prolactin secretion in the pathogenesis.[7]

MORPHOLOGY. The condition usually affects a single area of the breast substance drained through one of the major excretory ducts. A poorly defined

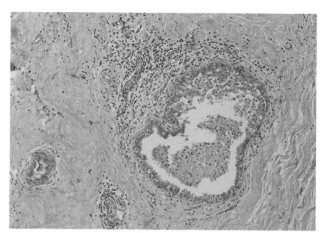

Figure 24–4. Duct ectasia. Duct is partially filled with lipid-laden macrophages. Ductal epithelium is destroyed, and periductal tissue is infiltrated with leukocytes.

area of induration, thickening, or ropiness results. On section, thick, cheesy material can be extruded from the ducts by slight pressure.

The dilated ducts are filled by granular, necrotic, acidophilic debris that contains principally lipid-laden macrophages (Fig. 24–4). The lining epithelial cells of the ducts may persist in small foci but for the most part are necrotic and atrophic. There is sometimes **squamous metaplasia** of lactiferous ducts. The periductal and interductal inflammation is manifested by heavy infiltrates of neutrophils, lymphocytes, and histiocytes, with in some cases a striking predominance of plasma cells. Occasionally, there is a granulomatous inflammation around cholesterol deposits. Fibrosis may eventually produce skin retraction that can be confused with carcinoma.

This lesion is of clinical significance because it can be mistaken for a carcinoma clinically, grossly, and by mammography.

FAT NECROSIS

Focal necrosis of fat tissues in the breast, followed by an inflammatory reaction, is an uncommon lesion that tends to occur as an isolated, sharply localized process in one breast. If strict criteria are used to differentiate this entity from mammary duct ectasia, almost all patients give a history of trauma, prior surgical intervention, or radiation therapy.[5]

MORPHOLOGY. In the early stages, the focus may consist of hemorrhage and, later, central liquefactive necrosis of fat. Still later, it may be an ill-defined nodule of gray-white, firm tissue containing small foci of chalky white or hemorrhagic debris.

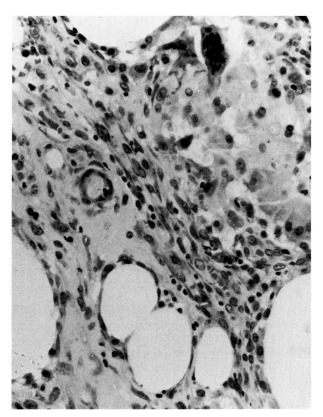

Figure 24–5. Fat necrosis. Note foamy macrophages and giant cell (top right), inflammation, and beginning fibrosis.

Histologically, the central focus of necrotic fat cells is surrounded by lipid-filled macrophages and an intense neutrophilic infiltration. Then, over the next few days, progressive fibroblastic proliferation, increased vascularization, and lyphocytic and histiocytic infiltration wall off the focus. By this time, the central necrotic fat cells have disappeared and may be represented only by foamy, lipid-laden macrophages and spicules of crystalline lipids. Still later, foreign body giant cells, calcium salts, and blood pigments make their appearance, and eventually the focus is replaced by scar tissue or is encysted and walled off by collagenous tissue (Fig. 24–5).

The major clinical significance of the condition is its possible confusion with a tumor, when fibrosis has created a clinically palpable mass, and focal calcification is seen on mammography.

FIBROCYSTIC CHANGES (FIBROCYSTIC DISEASE)

These designations are applied to a miscellany of morphologic changes in the female breast ranging from those that are entirely innocuous to those that are associated with an increased risk of carcinoma. One feature of all these changes is that they often produce palpable lumps—although some are so mild as to be clinically silent and so common as to be present in some 60 to 90% of breasts in routine autopsies.[7] Despite the many "good-byes to fibrocystic disease,"[8] the term, though unsatisfactory, seems to be ingrained in clinical usage. "Fibrocystic change" is more appropriate, since the alterations are often of no clinical significance.[9]

The morphologic features run the gamut from lesions that consist principally of cysts, to those characterized by an overgrowth of fibrous stroma, to lesions in which both stromal and epithelial proliferation occurs, to other types in which epithelial proliferation predominates.[5] Despite this marked variability, it is possible to distinguish three dominant patterns of morphologic change: (1) *cyst formation and fibrosis* (simple fibrocystic change and gross cysts), (2) *epithelial hyperplasia* (ductal and lobular), and (3) *sclerosing adenosis*. Of these, epithelial hyperplasia—particularly when atypical—is particularly associated with the increased risk of carcinoma.[3,10,11]

INCIDENCE AND PATHOGENESIS. Together these variants compose the single most common disorder of the breast and account for more than one-half of all surgical operations on the female breast. In a study of the so-called normal breast, that is, in unselected postmortem cases, significant changes were found in 29% and minimal disease was found in an additional 24%.[12] At least 10% of women develop clinically apparent cystic disease.[13] The condition is unusual before adolescence, is diagnosed frequently between the ages of 20 and 40, peaks at or just before the menopause, and rarely develops after the menopause. However, premenopausal lesions may persist into the more advanced years.

Hormonal imbalances are considered to be basic to the development of this multipatterned disorder. The excess of estrogens may represent an absolute increase, as in the rarely associated functioning ovarian tumors, or may be related to a deficiency of progesterone, as seen in anovulatory women. There is also some evidence of abnormal end-organ metabolism of hormones in the pathogenesis of cystic disease. Oral contraceptive use decreases the risk of fibrocystic disease, presumably because it supplies a balanced source of progesterone and estrogen.

CYSTS AND FIBROSIS (SIMPLE FIBROCYSTIC CHANGE)

This is the most common type of alteration, characterized by an increase in fibrous stroma associated with dilatation of ducts and the formation of cysts of various sizes. Gross cysts, over 3 mm in diame-

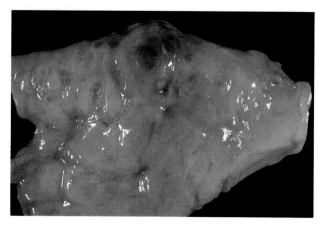

Figure 24-6. Cystic change of breast, showing a "blue-dome cyst."

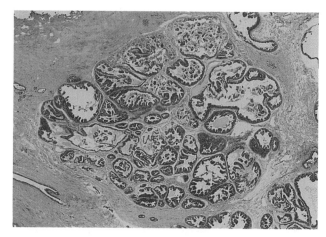

Figure 24-7. Cystic change of breast. Multiple cystic spaces, some filled with precipitated fluid with stromal fibrosis. Most of the cysts exhibit apocrine metaplasia (see Fig. 24-8).

ter, should be differentiated from *microcysts*,[13] since the latter are found so commonly in all women in the middle years of life that they cannot be construed as disease or as justification for surgery.

MORPHOLOGY. Grossly, a large cyst may be formed within one breast, but the disorder is usually multifocal and often bilateral. As a result of the dense stroma and cystic dilatation of the ducts, the involved areas both on palpation and by gross examination have an ill-defined diffuse increase in consistency and discrete nodularities. Closely aggregated, small cysts produce a shotty texture. Larger, particularly solitary, cysts evoke the greatest alarm as isolated firm masses that are deceptively unyielding. Secretory products within cysts of the breast calcify, resulting in microcalcifications detected by mammography. Unopened, these cysts are brown to blue **(blue-dome cysts)**, owing to the contained semitranslucent, turbid fluid (Fig. 24-6). Histologically, in smaller cysts, the epithelium is more cuboidal to columnar and is sometimes multilayered in focal areas (Fig. 24-7). In larger cysts, it may be flattened or may even be totally atrophic. Occasionally, epithelial proliferation leads to piled-up masses or small papillary excrescences. Frequently, cysts are lined by large polygonal cells having an abundant granular, eosinophilic cytoplasm, with small, round, deeply chromatic nuclei, so-called **apocrine metaplasia** (Fig. 24-8); such apocrine epithelium is found not uncommonly in the normal breast and is **virtually always benign.** Epithelial overgrowth and papillary projections are common in cysts lined by apocrine epithelium (see Fig. 24-7).

The stroma about all forms of cysts is usually compressed fibrous tissue, having lost its normal, delicate, myxomatous appearance. Stromal lymphocytic infiltration is common in this and all other variants of fibrocystic disease.

EPITHELIAL HYPERPLASIA

The fibrocystic changes can be accompanied by epithelial hyperplasia, and as mentioned earlier, this histologic variant increases the risk of the subsequent development of carcinoma. This is not to say that all foci of epithelial hyperplasia (termed *epitheliosis* by British pathologists) are premalignant, leading inevitably to carcinoma; indeed, only a small proportion apparently are. But it is this pattern of alteration that should concern the pathologist, who is called to differentiate among benign hyperplasia, atypical but still noncancerous hyperplasia, and carcinoma. The more severe and atypical the hyperplasia, the greater the risk of developing cancer. These hyperplasias may sometimes coexist with other fibrocystic changes, but on occasion they form the predominant pattern.

MORPHOLOGY. The gross appearance is usually that of the accompanying fibrosis, cysts, or adenosis. Microscopically, proliferation causes an increase

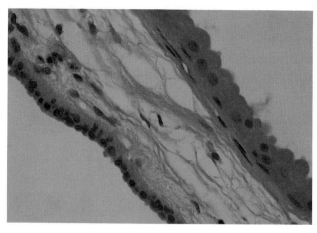

Figure 24-8. Normal lining (left) and apocrine metaplasia (right).

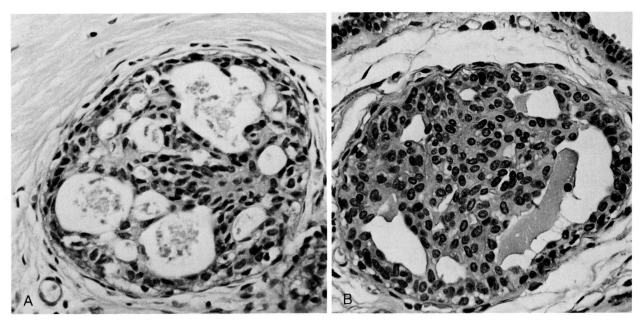

Figure 24–9. *A,* Moderate duct epithelial hyperplasia. Note that cells fill part of the duct lumen. *B,* More florid duct epithelial hyperplasia, with irregular lumina at the periphery—so-called fenestrations. (Courtesy of Dr. Noel Weidner, University of California at San Francisco.)

in the layers of the duct-lining epithelium beyond the usual double layer. Sometimes the proliferating epithelium takes the form of solid masses extending and encroaching into the duct lumen, partially obliterating it, but usually irregular lumina **(so-called fenestrations)** can be discerned at the periphery of the cellular masses (Fig. 24–9). Alternatively, papillary epithelial projections may grow into the lumen **(ductal papillomatosis).** (Fig. 24–10). If extensive, this is termed **florid papillomatosis.** Both papillary and solid proliferations may sometimes show various degrees of cellular and architectural atypia **(atypical hyperplasia).** The differentiation of the latter from intraductal carcinoma, discussed later, may be difficult. In general, greater cellular uniformity, more regular sharply defined gland lumina (so-called **cribriform pattern**), and nuclear hyperchromasia favor intraductal carcinoma.

Atypical lobular hyperplasia is the term used to describe hyperplasias of the terminal duct and ductules (acini) that have some—but not all—the features of lobular carcinoma in situ, described later in this chapter. Cytologically, the atypical cells of atypical lobular hyperplasia resemble those of lobular carcinoma in situ but do not fill or distend more than 50% of the terminal duct units.[3] Atypical lobular hyperplasia, particularly when it affects ducts (rather than only acini), is associated with an increased risk of invasive carcinoma.[14]

or *acini.* It is less common than cysts or epithelial hyperplasia. Although long thought to be a completely innocuous lesion, recent studies have shown a slightly increased risk of subsequent cancer.

MORPHOLOGY. Grossly, areas of sclerosing adenosis can be masked by the cystic changes, but sometimes they have a **hard cartilaginous consistency that begins to approximate that found in breast cancer.** On section, the involved area is not well localized and does not have the chalky yellow-white foci and streaks that identify breast carcinoma, an important gross differential feature.

Proliferation of small ducts, canaliculi, and gland buds may yield masses of small gland patterns, or nests and cords of cells within a fibrous stroma. The lobular arrangement is maintained. Usually, in such an area, many or at least some well-defined glands can be identified, but frequently they are closely aggregated so that glands lined by single or multiple layers of cells are backed up to each other **(adenosis).** At other times, the stromal overgrowth distorts and compresses the glands. Occasionally, the fibrous growth may totally compress the lumina to create the appearance of solid cords or double strands of cells lying within the dense stroma, a histologic pattern that at times verges on the appearance of carcinoma (Fig. 24–11).

SCLEROSING ADENOSIS

This variant is characterized histologically by *intralobular fibrosis and proliferation of small ductules*

OTHER LESIONS

Pure *fibrosis* is an infrequent variant in which a relatively well-delineated mass is associated with

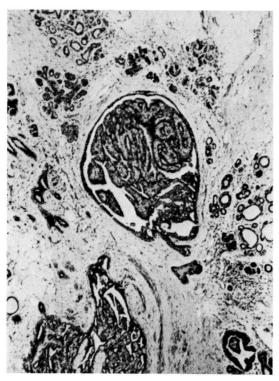

Figure 24-10. Papillary epithelial hyperplasia in fibrocystic disease. Two ducts show hyperplastic epithelium thrown into papillary projections. Note also fibrosis and small cysts. (Courtesy of Dr. Noel Weidner, University of California at San Francisco.)

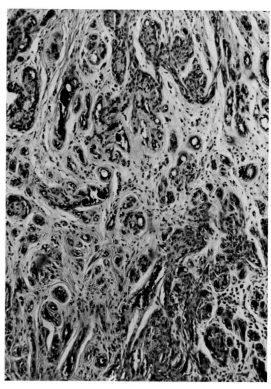

Figure 24-11. Sclerosing adenosis of the breast. The epithelial hyperplasia has produced the nests of cells, which appear quite disorderly. The overgrowth of fibrous tissue enmeshes and partially obliterates many of the epithelial nests, creating a pattern to be differentiated from the infiltrative growth of a cancer.

dense stromal fibrous tissue unaccompanied by cysts or epithelial hyperplasia. It may be a variant of fibroadenoma or complex sclerosing lesion. It does not predispose to carcinoma.

Radial scar (benign sclerosing ductal proliferation) is characterized histologically by ductal proliferation with an abundant central fibrosis and elastosis, giving it the gross microscopic appearance of a scar.[15] It is often associated with other features of a cystic disease. It may be difficult to differentiate from a special type of cancer called tubular carcinoma, described later.

CLINICAL SIGNIFICANCE OF FIBROCYSTIC CHANGES

The many patterns of breast pathology included under the designation fibrocystic change have clinical importance for three reasons: (1) Clinically, they produce masses in the breast that require differentiation from carcinoma, (2) microcalcifications are frequently detected on mammography, and (3) *some* may predispose to the subsequent development of carcinoma.[16] Certain clinical features of fibrocystic disease tend to differentiate it from cancer, but the only certain way of making the distinction is pathologic examination.

What is the relationship between the morpho-

logic variants of fibrocystic change and carcinoma? *Current evidence is that patients with some morphologic variants of fibrocystic disease have a higher than expected attack rate of cancer of the breast.* The increased risk of different subtypes is as follows (Fig. 24-12):

- No *increased risk of breast carcinoma:* fibrosis, cystic changes, apocrine metaplasia, mild hyperplasia
- *Slightly increased risk—1.5 to 2 times:* sclerosing adenosis, hyperplasia (moderate to florid), ductal papillomatosis (marked)
- *Significantly increased risk—5 times:* atypical hyperplasia, ductal or lobular
- *A family history of breast cancer increases the risk in all categories,* for example, to about tenfold with atypical hyperplasia

Fortunately, a minority of biopsies reveal atypical epithelial hyperplasia. Thus, the majority of women having "lumps" related to fibrocystic change can be reassured that there is little or no increased predisposition to cancer.

In summary, *the association between fibrocystic change and cancer is proportional to the degree of epithelial hyperplasia and atypia seen.* In a study of 301 patients in whom a histologic diagnosis of

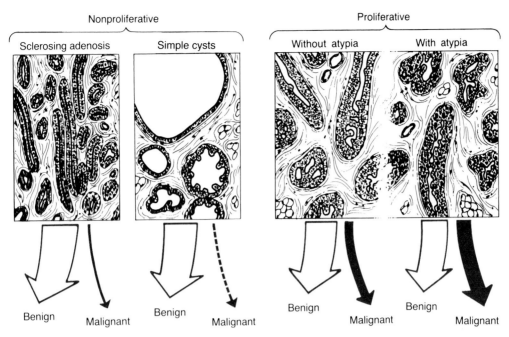

Figure 24-12. Depiction, by the sizes of the arrows, the risk of malignant transformation of the various patterns of fibrocystic change.

atypical hyperplasia was made on biopsy but in whom the breast was not removed, the cumulative risk of breast cancer (both in situ and infiltrating) was 10% at 55 months.[17]

TUMORS

Neoplasms constitute the most important, albeit not the most common, lesions of the female breast. A great variety of tumors may occur in the female breast, made up as it is of a covering integument, adult fat, mesenchymal connective tissue, and epithelial structures. These tumors run the gamut of the neoplasms that may arise from stratified squamous epithelium, glandular structures, and mesenchymal connective tissue. Some are skin papillomas, squamous cell carcinomas of the skin, adenomas, papillomas of ducts, carcinomas of glandular duct origin, and virtually every variety of benign and malignant mesenchymal tumor, such as fibroma and fibrosarcoma, granular cell tumor, chondrosarcoma, lipoma and liposarcoma, osteogenic sarcoma, and angioma and angiosarcoma. Only the more common tumors specialized to the breast, however, will be discussed.

FIBROADENOMA

The most common benign tumor of the female breast is the fibroadenoma. As the name implies, it is *a new growth composed of both fibrous and glan-*

dular tissue. Cytogenetic studies have shown that only the fibrous (stromal) component is clonal.[18] The tumor appears to arise from the specialized intralobular stroma, perhaps explaining why these lesions do not arise in other soft tissue sites. Occurring at any age within the reproductive period of life, they are somewhat more common before age 30. Multiple small areas closely resembling a fibroadenoma are sometimes found in cases of cystic disease, termed *fibroadenomatosis.*

MORPHOLOGY. The fibroadenoma grows as **a spherical nodule that is usually sharply circumscribed and freely movable from the surrounding breast substance.** These tumors frequently occur in the upper outer quadrant of the breast. They vary in size from under 1 cm to giant forms 10 to 15 cm in diameter **(giant fibroadenoma),** but most are surgically removed when 2 to 4 cm in diameter (Fig. 24-13). On section they are grayish white, and often contain slit-like spaces. They are well circumscribed and can often be shelled out.[5]

The histologic pattern is essentially one of delicate, cellular, fibroblastic stroma resembling intralobular stroma, enclosing glandular and cystic spaces lined by epithelium. Intact, round-to-oval gland spaces may be present, lined by single or multiple layers of cells (pericanalicular fibroadenoma) (Fig. 24-14A). In other areas, the connective tissue stroma appears to have undergone more active proliferation with compression of the gland spaces. In consequence, glandular lumina are collapsed or compressed into slit-like, irregular clefts, and the epithelial elements then appear as

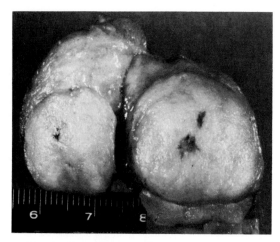

Figure 24–13. Fibroadenoma. Discrete mass bulges above level of surrounding breast tissue.

narrow strands or cords of epithelium lying with the fibrous stroma (intracanalicular fibroadenoma) (see Fig. 24–14B). Both pericanalicular and intracanalicular patterns often coexist in the same tumor.

The epithelium of the fibroadenoma is normally responsive and can undergo lactational change during pregnancy. An increase in size, or

not uncommonly infarction and inflammation, may lead to a fibroadenoma mimicking carcinoma in a pregnant woman.

Fibroadenoma usually appears as a solitary, discrete, freely movable nodule within the breast. Slight increase in size may occur during the late phases of each menstrual cycle, and pregnancy may stimulate growth. Postmenopausally, regression or calcification may result.

PHYLLODES TUMOR

Phyllodes tumors, like fibroadenomas, arise from intralobular stroma but may recur or be frankly malignant. These tumors are much less common than fibroadenomas and are distinguished from them on the basis of cellularity, mitotic rate, nuclear pleomorphism, loss of the usual biphasic pattern of stroma and associated benign epithelium, and infiltrative borders. The low-grade tumors are seen most commonly and may recur locally but only rarely metastasize. Rare high-grade lesions behave aggressively with local recurrences common, as well as distant hematogenous metastases.[19] As is true of other sarcomas, lymph node metastases are rare. The term *cystosarcoma phyllodes* is sometimes used for these lesions; however, the

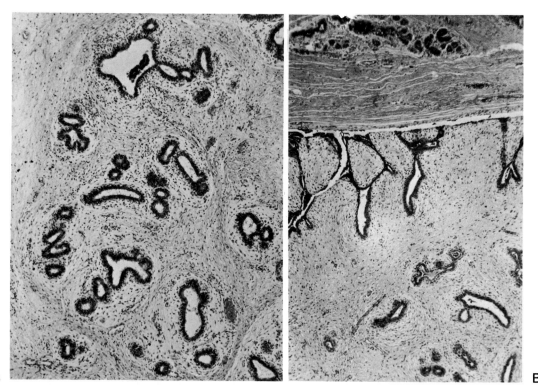

A   B

Figure 24–14. A, Fibroadenoma showing morphology referred to as pericanalicular variant. B, Fibroadenoma. Margin of nodule, with capsule and separation from compressed breast substance above. Growth is in part intracanalicular, particularly near capsule, with compression of gland spaces. Toward bottom, pattern is pericanalicular.

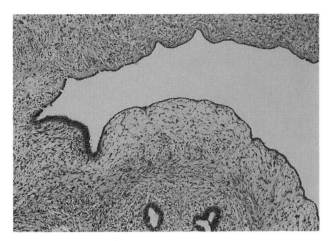

Figure 24–15. Phyllodes tumor. Note the typical stromal nodule projecting into a cyst, giving the gross phyllode (leaf-like) pattern.

majority of the tumors behave in a relatively benign fashion.

MORPHOLOGY. The tumors vary in size, from a few centimeters to massive lesions involving the entire breast. The larger lesions often are lobulated owing to the presence of nodules of proliferating stroma lined by epithelium (phyllodes is Greek for leaf-like) (Fig. 24–15). This growth pattern can also occasionally be seen in larger fibroadenomas and is not in and of itself an indicator of malignancy. Histologically, lower grade lesions resemble fibroadenomas but with increased cellularity and mitotic figures. High-grade lesions may be difficult to distinguish from other types of soft tissue sarcomas and may have foci of mesenchymal differentiation (e.g., rhabdomyosarcomatous differentiation).

INTRADUCTAL PAPILLOMA

As the name implies, this is a neoplastic papillary growth within a duct. Most of these lesions are solitary and are found within the principal lactiferous ducts or sinuses. They present clinically as (1) serous or bloody nipple discharge; (2) a small subareolar tumor, a few millimeters in diameter; and (3) rarely, nipple retraction.

MORPHOLOGY. The tumors are rarely more than 1 cm in diameter. As mentioned, they are usually located in the major ducts, close to the nipple. Histologically, the tumor is composed of multiple papillae, each having a connective tissue axis covered by cuboidal or cylindrical epithelial cells

(Fig. 24–16). In the truly benign papilloma, two cell types are seen in the luminal mass—epithelial and myoepithelial.[5]

The distinction between a benign but atypical intraductal papilloma and an intraductal papillary carcinoma may be difficult. In general, severe cytologic atypia, the absence of myoepithelial cells, abnormal mitotic figures, pseudostratification, the absence of a vascular connective tissue core, the presence of cell strands bridging the duct lumen (forming a so-called **cribriform pattern**), and the absence of hyalinization or apocrine metaplasia favor a malignant rather than benign papillary tumor.

Complete excision of the duct system should be performed in order to avoid local recurrences. The present consensus is that most solitary intraductal papillomas are benign and are *not* the precursors of papillary carcinoma. However, *multiple intraductal papillomas* should be distinguished from the group, since they are more likely to recur and are associated with an increased risk of development of carcinoma. They form poorly delineated, palpable tumors in which multiple papillary lesions in ducts occupy peripheral sectors of the breast.

Nipple adenoma and *florid papillomatosis of the nipple* are terms used to describe tumors of the nipple exhibiting papillary hyperplasia of the duct epithelium, intermixed with fibrosis. They should be differentiated from intraductal papilloma, as they are associated with concomitant or subsequent carcinoma in 16% of cases.[5]

CARCINOMA

Breast cancer causes some 20% of cancer deaths among females and has been called the "foremost cancer" in women.[20-22] The incidence has been increasing steadily over the past 80 years such that currently one of every nine women in the United States will develop cancer in their lifetime. Understandably, then, breast cancer has received a great deal of appropriate publicity and has been the focus of intensive study relative to its origins, diagnostic methods, and treatment. Although much has been gained, particularly in early diagnosis, the age-adjusted death rate from breast cancer in females in the United States has virtually remained stable over the past 30 years, now being about 27 per 100,000. Each year, 43,000 women die of the disease. It is both ironic and tragic that a neoplasm arising in an exposed organ, readily accessible to self-examination and clinical diagnosis, continues to exact such a heavy toll.

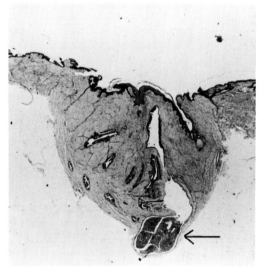

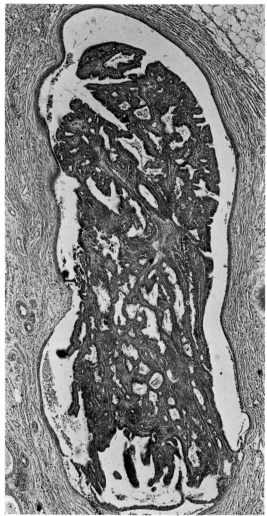

Figure 24-16. Intraductal papilloma. A, Low-power view of nipple showing tumor in lactiferous duct (arrow). B, High-power view showing well-differentiated papillary tumor.

INCIDENCE AND EPIDEMIOLOGY. Cancer of the female breast is rarely found before the age of 25 except in certain familial cases. It may occur at any age thereafter, with a peak incidence at or after the menopause.

Few cancers have been subjected to more intensive epidemiologic study. Observations bearing on the incidence of this disease can be summarized as follows:[23,24]

- *Geographic influences:* Five times more common in the United States than in Japan and Taiwan.
- *Genetic predisposition:* Well defined. The magnitude of risk is in proportion to the number of close relatives with breast cancer and the age when cancer occurred in relatives. The younger the relatives at the time of development of cancer and the more bilateral cancers, the greater the genetic predisposition. Thus, the risk is 1.5 to 2 times for women with one first-degree relative with breast cancer, 4 to 6 times for those with two affected relatives. There are uncommon high-risk families with apparent autosomal dominant transmission and familial association of

breast and ovarian carcinomas. Breast cancer affects 25% of patients with the Li-Fraumeni syndrome (multiple sarcomas and carcinomas), which, as described in Chapter 7, is associated with germ-line mutations of the tumor suppressor gene p53.

- *Increasing age:* Uncommon before age 25, but then a steady rise to the time of menopause, followed by a slower rise throughout life.
- *Length of reproductive life:* Risk increases with early menarche and late menopause.
- *Parity:* More frequent in nulliparous than in multiparous women.
- *Age at first child:* Increased risk when older than 30 years of age at time of first child.
- *Obesity:* Increased risk attributed to synthesis of estrogens in fat depots.
- *Exogenous estrogens:* Moderately increased risk with high-dosage therapy for menopausal symptoms.
- *Oral contraceptives:* No clear-cut increased risk; attributed to balanced content of estrogens and progestins in currently used oral contraceptives.
- *Fibrocystic changes with atypical epithelial hyper-*

plasia: Increased risk, as noted in earlier discussion of this condition.

• *Carcinoma of the contralateral breast or endometrium:* Increased risk.

ETIOLOGY AND PATHOGENESIS. The epidemiologic data cited above and studies of mammary tumors *in vitro* and in experimental animals point to three sets of influences that may be important in breast cancer: (1) genetic factors, (2) hormonal imbalances, and (3) environmental factors. In animals, viruses can clearly interact with these influences to cause cancer, but no such viral etiology has yet been documented in humans.

Genetic predisposition undoubtedly exists, as evidenced by the markedly increased risk in first-degree relatives of cancer patients. In mice, high cancer strains can be achieved by genetic inbreeding. As noted, germ-line mutations in the tumor suppressor gene p53 (the Li-Fraumeni syndrome) account for rare cases of familial cancer.[26] The genetic basis of the majority of familial breast cancer is now being vigorously sought, and a breast cancer susceptibility gene has recently been traced to a small locus in chromosome 17q21 in a large number of families in whom breast cancer develops at an early age.[25] Named *BRCA1* (breast carcinoma 1) gene, it is also linked to ovarian cancer.[26]

Endogenous estrogen excess, or more accurately, hormonal imbalance, clearly plays a significant role. Many of the risk factors mentioned — long duration of reproductive life, nulliparity, and late age at first child — imply increased exposure to estrogen peaks during the menstrual cycle. Functioning ovarian tumors that elaborate estrogens are associated with breast cancer in postmenopausal women. Recent studies have confirmed associations among excess urinary estrogens, frequency of ovulation, age at menarche, and increased breast cancer risk.[27] There are also hints of how the estrogens may act. Normal breast epithelium possesses estrogen and progesterone receptors. These have been identified in some but not all breast cancers. A variety of growth promoters (transforming growth factor-alpha/epithelial growth factor [TGF-α/EGF], platelet-derived growth factor [PDGF], and fibroblast growth factor [FGF]) and growth inhibitors (TGF-β) are secreted by human breast cancer cells, and many studies suggest that they are involved in an autocrine mechanism of tumor progression. Production of these growth factors is dependent on estrogen, and it is thought that interactions between circulating hormones, hormone receptors on cancer cells, and autocrine growth factors induced by tumor cells are involved in breast cancer progression.[28]

Environmental influences are suggested by the variable incidence of breast cancer in genetically homogeneous groups and the geographic differences in incidence. Various items in diets have been implicated, but the role of high-fat diet, previously well accepted, is now questioned.[29] Coffee addicts will be pleased to know that there is no substantial evidence that caffeine consumption increases the risk, but studies suggest that moderate alcohol consumption is associated with a 1.5 increased risk of breast cancer. The role of *viruses* has been pursued since Bittner's brilliant discovery in 1936 that a filterable agent, transmitted through the mother's milk, causes breast cancer in suckling mice.[30] The virus, called mouse mammary tumor virus (MMTV), was later identified as a retrovirus. Subsequently, there were many hints of the existence of an analogous virus in breast cancer of humans, but the findings have not been conclusive.

More has been learned of the possible contributions of *oncogenes* and *tumor suppressor genes* to breast cancer.[31,32] In particular, amplification of the *erb* B2/*neu* gene (which is similar to the gene for the receptor to EGF) is found in from 5% to as many as 30% of cancers, associated with overexpression of the protein product of the gene in carcinoma cells (p185$^{\text{erb 2}}$). Overexpression of the gene product is associated with poor prognosis in patients with lymph node–positive breast cancer. Insertion of an activated *erb* B2/*neu* oncogene in transgenic mice results in the formation of breast adenocarcinomas. Amplification of the *int-2* (homologous to FGF), c-*ras*, and c-*myc* genes has also been described in human breast cancer. Finally, somatic mutations of p53 and Rb suppressor genes occur in 50% and 20% of breast cancers, respectively.[32]

CLASSIFICATION AND DISTRIBUTION. Curiously, carcinoma is more common in the left breast than in the right, in a ratio of 110:100. The cancers are bilateral or sequential in the same breast in 4% or more of cases.

Among breast carcinomas small enough for their general areas of origin to be identified, approximately 50% arise in the upper outer quadrant; 10% in each of the remaining quadrants; and about 20% in the central or subareolar region. As will be seen, the site of origin influences the pattern of nodal metastasis to a considerable degree.

An overview of the range in tumor histologic types based on a World Health Organization (WHO) classification is as follows:[33]

A. Noninvasive
  1a. Intraductal carcinoma
  1b. Intraductal carcinoma with Paget's disease
  2. Lobular carcinoma in situ
B. Invasive (infiltrating)
  1a. Invasive ductal carcinoma — not otherwise specified (NOS)
  1b. Invasive ductal carcinoma with Paget's disease
  2. Invasive lobular carcinoma
  3. Medullary carcinoma
  4. Colloid carcinoma (mucinous carcinoma)
  5. Tubular carcinoma

Table 24-1. INCIDENCE OF HISTOLOGIC TYPES OF INVASIVE BREAST CANCER

	%
Invasive duct carcinoma	
Pure	52.6
Combined with other types	22.0
Medullary carcinoma	6.2*
Colloid carcinoma	2.4
Paget's disease	2.3
Other pure types	2.0
Other combined types	1.6
Infiltrating lobular carcinoma	4.9
Combined lobular and ductal	6.0

* With strict histologic criteria, medullary carcinoma incidence is 1 to 5%.

Modified from Fisher, E., et al.: The pathology of invasive breast cancer: A syllabus derived from the findings of the National Surgical Adjuvant Breast Project. Cancer 36:1, 1975.

6. Adenoid cystic carcinoma
7. Apocrine carcinoma
8. Invasive papillary carcinoma

Only the more common types will be discussed. The incidence of the various types of infiltrating carcinomas collected from a national study is shown in Table 24-1.

Noninvasive (In Situ) Carcinoma

INTRADUCTAL CARCINOMA. Intraductal carcinoma was once considered a rare lesion, but with the increased use of mammography, which detects early and small lesions, it now constitutes approximately 20 to 30% of carcinomas. It is defined as a malignant population of cells that lack the capacity to invade through the basement membrane and, therefore, are incapable of distant metastasis. However, these cells can spread throughout a duc-

tal system and produce extensive lesions involving an entire sector of a breast. Movement of these cells up the main duct and into the nipple skin results in the clinical appearance of **Paget's disease of the nipple**, described later.

Histologically, these tumors are divided into five subtypes: comedocarcinoma, solid, cribriform, papillary, and micropapillary. Except for comedocarcinoma, these lesions are usually clinically occult and are detected as incidental findings in breast biopsies or by mammography. **Comedocarcinoma** is characterized by rapidly proliferating, high-grade malignant cells (Fig. 24–17B). The cells in the center of the ducts are often necrotic and commonly calcify. These necrotic cells are detected grossly on cut section by punctate areas of cheesy necrotic material ("comedone" like) (see Fig. 24–17A) or on mammography as linear and branching microcalcifications. The growth pattern can also be *solid* or **cribriform,** the latter indicating the presence of duct-like structures within the primary dilated ducts (Fig. 24–18). Rarely, these intraductal carcinomas have a predominantly papillary pattern and are called **intraductal papillary carcinomas.**

Comedocarcinoma, and probably all other subtypes, are thought to be precursors or predictors of invasive cancer. In women with intraductal carcinoma treated with lumpectomy alone, recurrences or invasion occurs in from 0 to 10% of low-grade or intermediate nonpalpable tumors to 40% of high-grade comedocarcinomas.

LOBULAR CARCINOMA IN SITU. This is a histologically unique lesion manifested by proliferation, in one or more terminal ducts and/or ductules (acini), of cells that are loosely cohesive, are somewhat larger than normal, and have rare mitoses and oval or round nuclei with small nucleoli (Fig. 24–19). These lesions can be seen in breasts removed

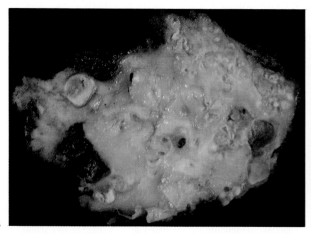
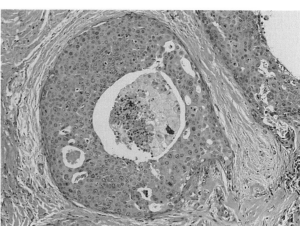

Figure 24-17. *A*, Gross appearance of comedocarcinoma, showing typical white necrotic centers. *B*, Comedocarcinoma. Intraductal proliferation of malignant cells. Note central necrosis.

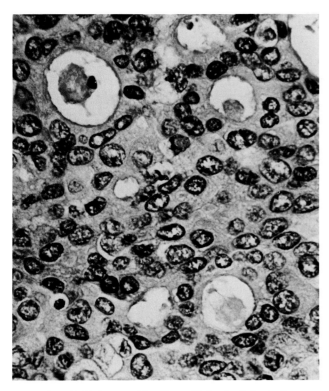

Figure 24-18. High magnification of intraductal carcinoma, showing cribriform pattern, and large cells with hyperchromatic nuclei. Compare with Figure 24-9, which shows hyperplastic lesions.

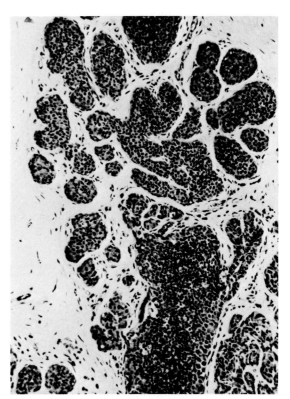

Figure 24-19. Lobular carcinoma in situ. Note proliferation of well-differentiated tumor cells in terminal ducts and ductules.

for fibrocystic disease, in the vicinity of invasive carcinoma, or admixed with the foci of intraductal carcinoma. They are frequently multifocal and bilateral. The frequency in which such change may develop into invasive carcinoma varies. In patients **not** treated with mastectomy and followed for 24 years,[35] the frequency of subsequent carcinoma developing in the same or **contralateral** breast was 30%, nine times greater than that expected for the general population. The infiltrating carcinomas that developed were either ductal or lobular.[34] **The lesion is thus a marker for invasive carcinoma.**

Invasive (Infiltrating) Carcinoma

INVASIVE DUCTAL CARCINOMA NOS (NOT OTHERWISE SPECIFIED). As mentioned, this is the most common type, accounting for 65 to 80% of all mammary cancers. Most exhibit a marked increase in dense, fibrous tissue stroma, giving the tumor a hard consistency **(scirrhous carcinoma).** These growths occur as fairly sharply delimited nodules of **stony-hard** consistency that average 1 to 2 cm in diameter and rarely exceed 4 to 5 cm. On palpation, they may have an infiltrative attachment to the surrounding structures with fixation to the underlying chest wall, dimpling of the skin, and re-

traction of the nipple (Fig. 24-20). The mass is quite characteristic on cut section. **It is retracted below the cut surface, has a hard cartilaginous consistency, and produces a grating sound when scraped.** Within the central focus, there are small pinpoint foci or streaks of chalky-white necrotic tumor and small foci of calcification.

Histologically, the **tumor consists of malignant duct lining cells diposed in cords, solid cell nests, tubules, glands, anastomosing masses, and mixtures of all these.** In many cases, clear-cut intraductal components can also be seen. The cells clearly invade the connective tissue stroma (Fig. 24-21). The cytologic detail of tumor cells varies from small cells with moderately hyperchromatic regular nuclei to huge cells with large irregular and hyperchromatic nuclei. Frequently, invasion of perivascular and perineural spaces as well as blood and lymphatic vessels is readily evident. Tumors are graded according to (1) the degree of nuclear atypia and (2) histologic differentiation (tubule formation) into well differentiated, moderately differentiated, and poorly differentiated (Fig. 24-22).

MEDULLARY CARCINOMA. This variant accounts for 1 to 5% of all mammary carcinomas. The average size is 2 to 3 cm, but some produce large, fleshy tumor masses up to 5 cm in diameter or greater.[36] These tumors do not have the striking desmoplasia (formation of fibrous tissue) of the usual carcinoma

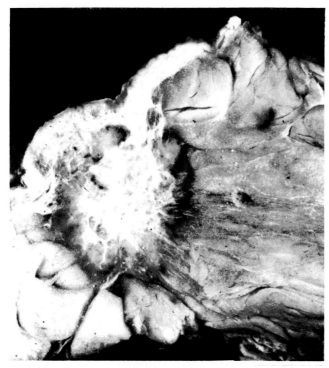

Figure 24-20. Carcinoma of the breast, infiltrating. The cut surface illustrates the lack of demarcation, the fixation to the skin, and the chalky foci of necrosis within the mass.

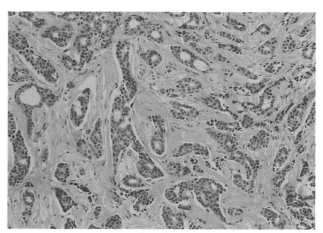

Figure 24-22. Infiltrating duct carcinoma (low-power view). Note tumor cells in cords and tubules infiltrating stroma (see Fig. 24-21 for high-power view).

24-23). It is the lymphoid infiltrate that gives these tumors their special significance, since such tumors have a distinctly better prognosis than the usual infiltrating duct carcinomas, even in the presence of axillary lymph node metastases. The ten-year survival rate is more than 70%.

COLLOID OR MUCINOUS CARCINOMA. This unusual variant tends to occur in older women and grows slowly over the course of many years. The tumor is extremely soft and has the consistency and appearance of pale gray-blue gelatin. It may occur in **pure form,** in which at least 75% of the tumor is mucinous or **mixed,** in association with other types of infiltrating duct carcinoma.

Histologically, in "pure" mucinous carcinomas there are large lakes of lightly staining, amorphous mucin that dissect and extend into contiguous tissue spaces and planes of cleavage. Floating within this mucin are small islands and isolated neoplastic cells, sometimes forming glands (Fig. 24-24). Vacuolation of at least some of the cells is characteristic. In "mixed" mucinous tumors, the tumor exhibits

and, therefore, are distinctly more yielding on external palpation and on cut section. On section, the tumor has a soft, fleshy consistency and tends to be discrete. Foci of necrosis and hemorrhage are large and numerous. Histologically, the carcinoma is characterized by (1) solid, syncytium-like sheets of large cells with vesicular, often pleomorphic nuclei, containing prominent nucleoli and frequent mitoses (the syncytial cells occupy more than 75% of the tumor), and (2) a moderate-to-marked lymphocytic infiltrate between these sheets, with a scant fibrous component (Fig.

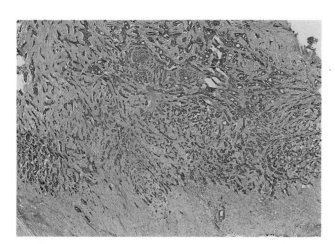

Figure 24-21. Infiltrating duct carcinoma, well differentiated.

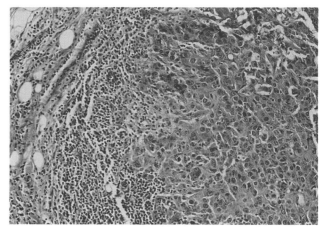

Figure 24-23. Medullary carcinoma with lymphoid infiltrate. Note lymphocytes infiltrating syncytial epithelial tumor.

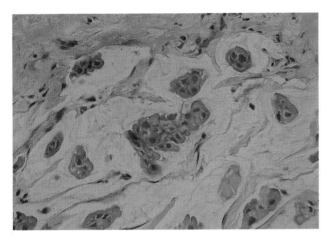

Figure 24-24. Colloid carcinoma. Note lakes of lightly staining mucin with small islands of tumor cells.

large areas with mucin as well as areas of typical nonmucinous invasive duct carcinoma.

The survival rate is appreciably greater in pure colloid carcinoma than in the mixed type or the usual infiltrating duct carcinoma, and lymph node metastases are infrequent.

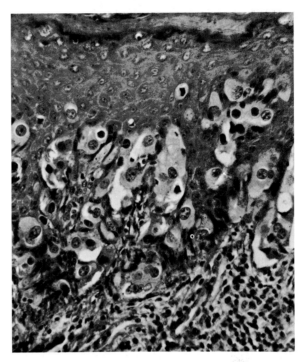

Figure 24-25. Paget's disease of the breast. Paget's cells dot the epithelium.

PAGET'S DISEASE. Paget's disease of the nipple is a form of ductal carcinoma that arises in the main excretory ducts of the breast and extends **intraepithelially** to involve the skin of the nipple and areola. Careful morphologic study has demonstrated that **the skin lesions are invariably associated with an underlying ductal carcinoma in situ, or less commonly invasive duct carcinoma, arising deeper within the breast.**

The most striking gross characteristics of this lesion involve the skin. The skin of the nipple and areola is frequently fissured, ulcerated, and oozing. There is surrounding inflammatory hyperemia and edema and, occasionally, total nipple ulceration. An underlying lump or mass is present in 50 to 60% of cases.

The histologic hallmark of this entity is the involvement of the epidermis by malignant cells, referred to as Paget's cells. These cells are large, have abundant clear or lightly staining cytoplasm, and nuclei with prominent nucleoli (Fig. 24–25). The cells usually stain positively for mucin, epithelial membrane antigens, and low-molecular-weight keratins. In addition to the Paget's cells, the other histologic criteria of ductal carcinoma are present. The prognosis is dependent on the extent of the underlying carcinoma.

INVASIVE LOBULAR CARCINOMA. This is a distinct morphologic form of mammary cancer that probably arises from the terminal ductules of the breast lobule. Although making up only 5 to 10% of breast carcinomas, **invasive lobular carcinomas** are of

particular interest for at least two reasons: (1) They tend to be bilateral far more frequently than those arising in ducts (the likelihood of cancer in the contralateral breast being on the order of 20%), and (2) they tend to be multicentric within the same breast.

Grossly, the tumor is rubbery and poorly circumscribed but sometimes appears as a typical scirrhous type. Histologically, it consists of strands of infiltrating tumor cells, often only one cell in width (in the form of a single file), loosely dispersed throughout the fibrous matrix (Fig. 24–26). The cells are small and uniform-staining with relatively little

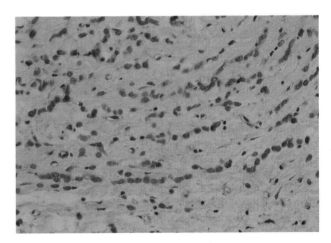

Figure 24-26. Carcinoma of the breast, infiltrating lobular type. A single file of tumor cells are embedded within a dense fibrous stroma.

cytologic pleomorphism. Irregularly shaped, solid nests and sheets may also occur in continuity with the single-file pattern. The tumor cells are frequently arranged in concentric rings about normal ducts. However, differentiation between ductal and lobular infiltrating carcinoma may very often be quite difficult, and in some tumors mixed ductal and lobular patterns, as well as intermediate cancers, exist.

FEATURES COMMON TO ALL INVASIVE CANCERS. There are additional morphologic features common to all infiltrative breast carcinomas, whatever the histologic types. As focal lesions, they extend progressively in all directions. In the course of time, they may become adherent to the deep fascia of the chest wall and thus become **fixed in position.** Extension to the skin may cause not only fixation but also **retraction and dimpling of the skin,** an important characteristic of malignant growth. At the same time, the lymphatics may become so involved as to block the local area of skin drainage and cause lymphedema and thickening of the skin, a change that has for years been referred to as **peau d'orange** (orange peel). When the tumor involves the main excretory ducts, particularly in the intraduct variety, **retraction of the nipple** may develop. Certain carcinomas tend to infiltrate widely through the breast substance, involve the majority of the lymphatics, and produce acute swelling, redness, and tenderness of the breast, referred to clinically as **inflammatory carcinoma.** This is not a special morphologic pattern but merely implies widespread involvement of dermal lymphatic channels. It has a high incidence of systemic metastases.

The utilization of **mammography** has allowed the detection of malignant tumors before they reach palpable size (Fig. 24–27). Tumors may be detected because of their increased density relative to surrounding adipose tissue (most marked in postmenopausal women) or because of microcalcifications. However, some tumors remain occult by radiography. Microcalcifications associated with malignancies tend to be smaller, more numerous, and more tightly clustered than microcalcifications associated with benign processes. Histologically, they are seen in association with necrotic cells or in abnormal secretory vacuoles in malignant cells.

Spread of the tumor eventually occurs through the lymphohematogenous routes. The pathways of lymphatic dissection are in all possible directions: **lateral** to the axilla, **superior** to the nodes above the clavicle and the neck, **medial** to the other breast, **inferior** to the abdominal viscera and lymph nodes, and **deep** to the nodes within the chest, particularly along the internal mammary arteries. The two most favored directions of drainage are the axillary nodes and the nodes along the internal mammary artery.

Overall, about half of all patients have metas-tases to lymph nodes at the time of initial diagnosis of breast cancer. **The pattern of nodal spread is heavily influenced by the location of the cancer in the breast.** Tumors arising in the outer quadrants involve the axillary nodes alone in about 50% of cases and have both internal mammary and axillary involvement in an additional 15% of cases. In contrast, cancers arising in the inner quadrants and center of the breast affect the axilla alone in about 25% of cases. In an additional 40%, internal mammary nodes are affected, along with axillary involvement. The supraclavicular nodes are the third most favored site of nodal spread. **Distant metastases via the bloodstream may affect virtually any organ of the body.** Favored sites for dissemination are the lungs, bones, liver, adrenals, brain, and meninges. In these locations human cells can be detected in pleural fluid, peritoneal cavity, or cerebrospinal fluid by cytologic examination (Fig. 24–28).

GRADING AND STAGING OF BREAST CANCER. The many histologic grades and stages of breast cancer have been subdivided into smaller homogeneous

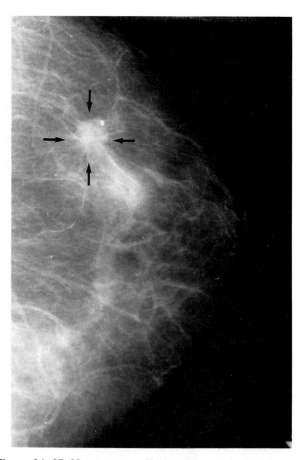

Figure 24–27. Mammogram. Horizontal section (nipple at 3 o'clock), showing a small, stellate-shaped carcinoma *(arrows).* There is a small, superimposed, incidental calcification. (Courtesy of Dr. Jack E. Meyer, Brigham and Women's Hospital, Boston.)

groups to standardize comparisons of results of various therapeutic modalities among clinics. From the histologic classification described earlier, cancers may be roughly divided as follows:

Nonmetastasizing: intraductal or in situ lobular carcinoma

Uncommonly metastasizing: pure mucinous or colloid cancer; medullary cancer; tubular adenocarcinoma; adenoid cystic carcinoma

Moderately to highly metastasizing: all other types

The American Joint Committee on Cancer Staging divides the clinical stages as follows:

STAGE I. A tumor less than 2 cm in diameter without nodal involvement and no metastases

STAGE II. A tumor less than 5 cm in diameter with involved but movable axillary nodes and no distant metastases or a tumor greater than 5 cm without nodal involvement or distant metastases

STAGE III. All breast cancers of any size with possible skin involvement, pectoral and chest wall fixation, and nodal involvement including axillary nodes and internal mammary lymph nodes, fixed but without disseminated metastases

STAGE IV. Any form of breast cancer with or without nodal involvement, pectoral fixation, skin ulceration, or chest wall fixation, but having disseminated metastases

CLINICAL COURSE. Cancers of the breast are usually first discovered by the patient or physician as a solitary, painless mass in the breast or owing to mammographic abnormalities during screening. The older the patient with a single breast lesion, the more likely is it to be cancer. On the average, these palpable lesions are 4 cm in diameter when first found, and approximately two-thirds have already

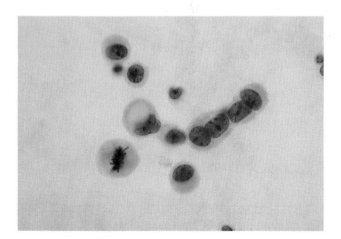

Figure 24–28. Cerebrospinal fluid showing metastatic breast cancer cells: Note duct-like structure, a signet-ring mucus-containing cell, and a mitotic figure. (Courtesy of Dr. Edmund Cibas, Brigham and Women's Hospital, Boston.)

spread to axillary or other nodes. Intraductal cancers, which rarely produce palpable masses, come to attention by the appearance of a discharge (sometimes hemorrhagic) from the nipple but most commonly after mammographic study.

Because early treatment of localized disease is the best hope of total eradication, an enormous effort is being made to identify breast cancers at an early stage. Currently, emphasis is being placed on more frequent, regular medical examinations and mammography as screening techniques. Mammography has uncovered a great number of carcinomas in situ or cases of "minimal cancer." The current consensus is to recommend mammography at age 40 and every 1 or 2 years thereafter, except in high-risk groups, in whom screening could begin earlier.

A number of factors influence the prognosis of breast cancer.[38]

1. *The size of the primary tumor,* tumors of less than 2 cm being associated with favorable prognosis.

2. *Lymph node involvement and the number of lymph nodes exhibiting metastases.* For example, with no histologic involvement of axillary lymph nodes the 5-year survival rate is close to 80%; those with one to three positive nodes have a 50% 5-year survival rate. The disease-free survival rate falls off to 21% in the presence of four or more positive nodes.

3. *The histologic type and grade of tumor.* This has been discussed earlier but can be appreciated from an older study of 30-year follow-up of 1458 consecutive operable cancers treated by radical mastectomy. The survival rate for intraductal carcinoma was 74%; for papillary carcinoma, 65%; for medullary carcinoma, 58%; for colloid, 58%; for infiltrating lobular, 34%; and for infiltrating ductal, 29%.[39]

4. *The presence or absence of estrogen and progesterone receptors.* The number of estrogen receptors in breast cancer cells can be high, intermediate, or absent and is proportional to the degree of cell differentiation and of the potential responsiveness of the tumor to the antiestrogen therapy, oophorectomy, or tamoxifen. Seventy per cent of tumors with estrogen receptors regress after hormonal manipulation, whereas only 5% of those that are negative respond to these procedures. The highest response rates are in patients with tumors containing both estrogen and progesterone receptors. On the whole, cancers with high levels of estrogen receptors have a better prognosis than those with intermediate levels or no receptors.

5. *The proliferative rate of the tumor and aneuploidy,* increased and scattered DNA values as measured by flow cytometry, are indicators of poor outcome in some studies—in particular, the fraction of cells scattered outside the modal peaks of DNA histograms (Fig. 24–29).[40]

6. *The presence of amplified or activated onco-*

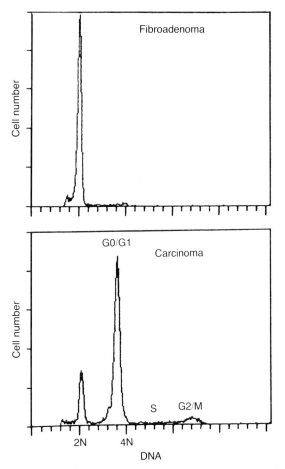

Figure 24-29. Flow cytometric histograms of a benign breast tumor *(top)* and ductal carcinoma *(bottom)*. The histogram of the benign lesion contains a single peak, representing G_0/G_1 phase euploid nuclei having 2N DNA content. The histogram of the malignant lesion shows, in addition, an aneuploid population having near-tetraploid G_0/G_1 phase DNA content. (Courtesy of Dr. David Weinberg, Department of Pathology, Brigham and Women's Hospital, Boston.)

genes, particularly c-*erbB2* in tumor tissue, as discussed earlier.

7. *The degree of angiogenesis in the tumor.* Indeed recent studies show a higher correlation between vessel density (reflecting angiogenesis; see Chapter 7) and the subsequent development of metastases than many other predictors of prognosis.[41] This increased vascularization is demonstrated by staining VIII tissues for endothelial antigens, such as Factor VIII (Fig. 24-30).

Other obvious poor prognostic signs include extensive edema or multiple nodules in the skin of the breast, fixation to the chest wall, spread to internal mammary lymph nodes, supraclavicular metastases, inflammatory carcinoma, and of course, distant metastases.

Overall, *axillary node status is the single most important prognostic factor for patients with early breast cancer.* However, 20 to 30% of patients with histologically negative lymph nodes will suffer recurrences and die of their disease within 10 years. For these reasons, there are continued searches for better biologic markers of prognosis and more effective treatment modalities. Current therapeutic approaches include combinations of simple mastectomy or segmental resection of the mass (lumpectomy) with or without lymph node dissection, postoperative irradiation, and chemotherapy — with ardent proponents for each of the many combinations.

The overall 5-year survival rate for stage I cancer is 80%; for stage II, 65%; for stage III, 40%; and for stage IV, 10%. It should be noted that recurrence may appear late, even after 10 years, but with each passing year free from disease, the prognosis improves. In the overall view of breast cancers, the 10-year survival is still no more than 50%.

Thus, this discussion of breast cancer ends virtually where it began. The clinical problem is monumental despite great efforts to solve it, and there is much yet to be learned.

MISCELLANEOUS MALIGNANCIES. Malignant neoplasia may arise from the skin of the breast, sweat glands, sebaceous glands, and hair shafts, or from the connective tissues and fatty stroma. These tumors are identical to their counterparts found in other sites of the body. Those arising from skin grow as basal or squamous cell carcinoma. Cancers arising in the skin adnexa grow as carcinomas of sweat gland or sebaceous gland origin. Malignancies of the interlobar stroma are, of course, sarcomas and include fibrosarcomas, myxosarcomas, liposarcomas, angiosarcomas, chondrosarcomas, and osteogenic sarcomas, the last-named primarily derived from metaplastic differentiation of the fibro-

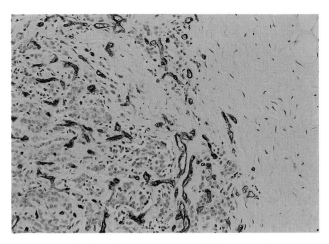

Figure 24-30. Infiltrating carcinoma *(left)* reacted by immunoperoxidase for factor VIII, which stains endothelium brown. Note markedly increased density of blood vessels (angiogenesis) in tumor compared to surrounding stroma *(right)*. (Courtesy of Dr. Noel Weidner, University of California at San Francisco.)

blasts. As a general rule, sarcomas occur in the same age range as carcinomas and differ chiefly in their rate of growth. They tend to produce large, bulky, fleshy masses that cause rapid increase in breast size with considerable distortion of breast contour. Attachment to the skin surface and ulcer-ation are, perhaps, more common with this rapid growth than with carcinomas. Sarcomas as a group frequently metastasize via the blood to distant organs, particularly the lungs. The clinical outlook in these cases is poor. *Angiosarcomas*, in particular, are the most rapidly fatal of breast tumors.

The Male Breast

GYNECOMASTIA
CARCINOMA

PATHOLOGY

The rudimentary male breast is relatively free from pathologic involvement. Only two processes occur with sufficient frequency to merit considera-tion.

GYNECOMASTIA

Lobules are not found in the normal male breast. As in the female, the male breast is subject to hor-monal influences, and gynecomastia (enlargement of the male breast) may occur as a result of an imbalance between estrogens, which stimulate breast tissue, and androgens, which counteract these effects. It is encountered under a variety of normal and abnormal circumstances. It may be found at the time of puberty or in the very aged, in the latter presumably owing to a relative in-crease in adrenal estrogens as the androgenic func-tion of the testis fails. It is one of the manifesta-tions of Klinefelter's syndrome and may occur in those with functioning testicular neoplasma, such as Leydig's cell and, rarely, Sertoli's cell tumors. It may occur at any time during adult life when there is cause for hyperestrinism. The most important cause of hyperestrinism in the male is cirrhosis of the liver, since the liver is responsible for metabo-lizing estrogen. Drugs such as alcohol, marijuana, heroin, and some of the psychoactive agents have also been associated with gynecomastia.[42]

MORPHOLOGY. Grossly, the lesion may be unilat-eral or bilateral. A button-like, subareolar enlarge-ment develops. In farther advanced cases, the swelling may simulate the adolescent female breast.

Microscopically, there is proliferation of a dense, periductal hyaline, collagenous connective tissue, but more striking are the changes in the epi-thelium of the ducts. There is marked hyperplasia of the ductal linings with the piling up of mul-tilayered epithelium (Fig. 24–31). The individual cells are fairly regular, columnar to cuboidal with regular nuclei. Occasionally there may be some variation in cell size and considerable disorientation of the heaped-up lining cells. Anaplasia is absent.

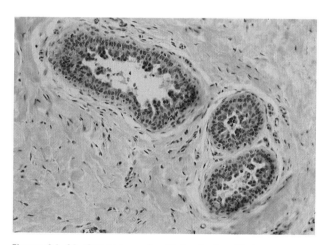

Figure 24–31. Gynecomastia. Note ducts with hyperplastic multilayered epithelium and periductal hyalinization and fibrosis.

The lesion is readily apparent on clinical examination and must be differentiated only from the seldom-occurring carcinoma of the male breast. Gynecomastia is chiefly of importance as an indicator of hyperestrinism, suggesting the possible existence of a functioning testicular tumor, or the possible presence of cirrhosis of the liver.

CARCINOMA

Carcinoma arising in the male breast is a very rare occurrence, with a frequency ratio to breast cancer in the female of 1:100. It occurs in advanced age. Because of the scant amount of breast substance in the male, the malignancy rapidly infiltrates to become attached to the overlying skin and underlying thoracic wall.[43] Ulceration through the skin is perhaps more common than in the female. These tumors behave exactly as do the invasive ductal carcinomas in the female but, on the whole, tend to have less striking desmoplasia and, hence, less of the hard, scirrhous quality. Dissemination follows the same pattern as in women, and axillary lymph node involvement is present in about one-half of cases at the time of discovery of the lesion. Distant metastases to the lungs, brain, bone, and liver are common.

Acknowledgment. We wish to thank Dr. Susan Lester for invaluable help with this chapter and for contributing the color illustrations.

1. Stirling, J.W., and Chandler, J.A.: The fine structure of the normal, resting terminal ductal–lobular unit of the female breast. Virchows Arch. (Pathol. Anat.) *372*:205, 1976.
2. Longacre, T.A., and Bartow, S.A.: A correlative morphologic study of human breast and endometrium in the menstrual cycle. Am. J. Surg. Pathol. *10*:382, 1986.
3. Page, D.L., and Anderson, T.J.: Diagnostic Histopathology of the Breast. New York, Churchill-Livingstone, 1988.
4. Carter, D.: Interpretation of Breast Biopsies, 2nd ed. New York, Raven Press, 1991.
5. Rosen, P.P., and Oberman, H.A.: Tumors of the mammary gland. *In* Atlas of Tumor Pathology, 3rd series, (series ed., J. Rosai), Fascicle 7. Washington, DC, Armed Forces Institute of Pathology, 1993.
6. Ellis, H., and Cox, P.J.: Breast problems in 1,000 consecutive referrals to surgical out-patients. Postgrad. Med. J. *60*:653, 1984.
7. Shousha, S., et al.: Mammary duct ectasia and pituitary adenoma. Am. J. Surg. Pathol. *12*:180, 1988.
8. Hutter, R.V.P.: Goodby to "fibrocystic disease." N. Engl. J. Med. *312*:179, 1985.
9. Consensus Statement by the Cancer Committee of the College of American Pathologists: Is "fibrocystic disease" of the breast precancerous? Arch. Pathol. Lab. Med. *110*:171, 1986.
10. Bodian, C.A., et al.: Prognostic significance of proliferative breast disease. Cancer *71*:3896, 1993.
11. Rosen, P.: Editorial. Cancer *71*:3894, 1993.
12. Frantz, V.K., et al.: Incidence of chronic cystic disease in so-called "normal breast": A study on 225 postmortem examinations. Cancer *4*:762, 1951.
13. Haagensen, C.D., et al. (eds): Breast Carcinoma: Risk and Detection. Philadelphia, W.B. Saunders Co., 1981.
14. Page, D.L., et al.: Ductal involvement by cells of atypical lobular hyperplasia in the breast. Hum. Pathol. *19*:201, 1988.
15. Andersen, J.A., et al: A symposium of sclerosing duct lesions of the breast. Pathol. Annu. *21*(Part II):145, 1986.
16. Harris, J.R., et al.: Breast Disease, 2nd ed. Philadelphia, J.B. Lippincott Co., 1991.
17. Ashikari, R., et al.: A clinicopathologic study of atypical lesions of the breast. Cancer *33*:310, 1974.
18. Fletcher, J.A., et al.: Lineage-restricted clonality in biphasic solid tumors. Am. J. Pathol. *138*:1199, 1991.
19. Cohn-Cedermark, G., et al.: Prognostic factors in cystosarcoma phyllodes. Cancer *68*:2017, 1991.
20. Holford, T.R., et al.: Trends in female breast cancer in Connecticut and the United States. J. Clin. Epidemiol. *44*:29, 1991.
21. Harris, J.R., et al.: Breast cancer. N. Engl. J. Med. *327*:319, 390, 473, 1992.
22. Marshall, E.: Search for a killer: Focus shifts from fats to hormones. Science *259*:618, 1993.
23. Willet, W.C.: Recent findings regarding lifestyle risk factors in the epidemiology of breast and colon cancer. *In* Fortner, J.G., and Rhoads, J.E. (eds.): Accomplishments in Cancer Research. Philadelphia, J.B. Lippincott Co., 1993, pp. 164–177.
24. Malkin, D., et al.: Germ line p53 mutations in a familial syndrome of breast cancer, sarcomas, and other neoplasms. Science *250*:1233, 1990.
25. Hall, J.M., et al.: Linkage of early-onset familial breast cancer to chromosome 17q21. Science *250*:1684, 1990.
26. Roberts, L.: Zeroing in on a breast cancer susceptibility gene. Science *259*:622, 1993.
27. McMahon, B. et al.: Urine estrogens, frequency of ovulation, and breast cancer risk. Int. J. Cancer *40*(6):721, 1987.
28. Dickson, R.B., and Lippman, M.E.: Molecular determinants of growth, angiogenesis, and metastases in breast cancer. Semin. Oncol. *19*:286, 1992.
29. Willett, W., et al.: Dietary fat and fiber in relation to the risk of breast cancer: An eight-year study. J.A.M.A. *268*:2037, 1992.
30. Bittner, J.J.: Some possible effects of nursing on mammary gland tumor incidence in mice. Science *84*:162, 1936.
31. Shay, J.W., et al.: Toward a molecular understanding of human breast cancer: A hypothesis. Breast Cancer Res. Treat. *25*:83, 1993.
32. Leslie, K.O., and Howard, P.: Oncogenes and antioncogenes in human breast carcinoma. Pathol. Annu. *27*(Pt. 1):321, 1992.
33. The World Health Organization Histologic Typing of Breast Tumors, 2nd ed. Am. J. Clin. Pathol. *78*:806, 1982.
34. Fechner, R.E.: One century of mammary carcinoma in situ. What have we learned? Am. J. Clin. Pathol. *100*:654, 1993.
35. Rosen, P.P.: Lobular carcinoma in situ of the breast. Am. J. Surg. Pathol. *2*:225, 1978.
36. Rapier, V., et al.: Medullary breast carcinoma: A reevaluation of 95 cases of breast cancer with inflammatory stroma. Cancer *61*:2503, 1988.
37. Figueroa, J.A., et al.: Prognostic factors in early breast cancer. Am. J. Med. Sci. *305*:176, 1993.
38. Visscher, D.W., et al.: Clinical significance of pathologic, cytometric, and molecular parameters in carcinoma of the breast. Adv. Pathol. Lab. Med. *5*:123, 1992.
39. Adair, F.E., et al.: Long-term follow-up of breast cancer patients: The 30-year report. Cancer *33*:1145, 1974.
40. Weinberg, D.S.: Proliferation indices in solid tumors. Adv. Pathol. Lab. Med. *5*:163, 1992.
41. Weidner, N., et al.: Tumor angiogenesis: A new signifi-

cant and independent prognostic indicator in early-stage breast carcinoma. J. Natl. Cancer Inst. *84*:1875, 1992.

42. Braunstein, G.D.: Gynecomastia. N. Engl. J. Med. *328*:490, 1993.

43. Hultborn, R., et al.: Male breast carcinoma: A study of the total material reported to the Swedish Cancer Registry, 1958–1967, with respect to clinical and histological parameters. Acta Oncol. *26*:241, 1987.

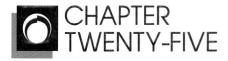

CHAPTER TWENTY-FIVE

The Endocrine System

Cellular homeostasis throughout the body is regulated by the nervous system and the endocrine system. These two systems are closely integrated, particularly in the hypothalamus, which modulates pituitary activity, and in the widely dispersed neuroendocrine cells, which compose the formerly called APUD (Amine Precursor Uptake and Decarboxylation) system.

In this chapter, our attention is directed to the endocrine system. The hormones elaborated by the endocrine glands interact with their target organs via cell receptors, for the most part, specific for particular hormones. According to changing concepts, they are of three basic types: (1) surface membrane receptors, (2) cytoplasmic receptors, and (3) ill-defined intranuclear receptors. A few words on each type of receptor follow.

- *Polypeptide (e.g., pituitary) and amine (e.g., cate-cholamine) hormones interact with receptors on the surfaces of cells.* Binding of the hormone (the ligand) to its receptor induces an apparent conformational or biochemical change in the receptor, which, usually through the mediation of a protein kinase and signal transducer–G protein pathway, activates one or more second messengers that ultimately modify the cell's function. The second messengers are not always known, as, for example, for pituitary growth hormone, but a large number of candidate messengers have been described, in addition to cyclic AMP, including tyrosine kinase, membrane phospholipids (e.g., inositol triphosphate), and shifts in the intracellular level of ionized calcium. The latter often leads to some interaction with a calcium-binding protein, such as calmodulin, or a calcium-binding kinase.
- *Steroid hormones appear to penetrate the lipid-*

rich membranes of cells readily and interact with receptors, mostly within the cytoplasm, but in some instances within the nucleus. In either event, the hormone-receptor complex, after translocation into the nucleus (in the case of cytoplasmic receptors), binds to DNA and activates specific genes, resulting in transcription and translation of new proteins, which mediate the hormone's effects.

- *Thyroid hormone receptors are located mainly within the nucleus, directly associated with the DNA, but some may be cytoplasmic.* First the hormones bind to sites on the cell surface, and then the protein-hormone complexes are internalized to the nuclei or cytoplasm. Thereafter, the hormone-receptor complex activates in some way the transcription of specific genes in the manner described for steroid hormones.

The function of the endocrine glands is subject to control, either by the interaction of stimulatory and inhibitory hormones produced in the hypothalamus, as is the case with the pituitary gland, or by feedback mechanisms, as occurs with the peripheral endocrine glands under pituitary control. For example, when cortisol levels are insufficient to maintain homeostasis, the inhibitory effects of cortisol on the hypothalamic secretion of corticotropin-releasing hormone (CRH) and, in turn, adrenocorticotropin (ACTH) are reduced, leading to increased ACTH release and increased synthesis of cortisol. When the cortisol levels are normalized, CRH and ACTH synthesis is suppressed. This hormonal feedback mechanism may be modified by factors other than hormones, such as is seen with cortisol biosynthesis, which is also regulated by cation levels in the serum, serum osmolarity, and extracellular fluid volume.

Diseases of the endocrine system (endocrinopathies) are best understood in the context of the broad categories of "too much" or "too little" hormone production.

Thanks are owed to Dr. Ronald A. DeLellis, New England Medical Center, Boston, for permission to draw on his comparable chapter in the previous edition of this book.

1113

Pituitary Gland

NORMAL

Few organs in the body are smaller or more important than the pituitary gland. In the adult, it weighs about 0.5 gm and measures 10 to 15 mm in greatest diameter. As is well known, it is composed of two functionally separate components: an anterior lobe (adenohypophysis) made up of secretory epithelial cells and a neurosecretory posterior lobe (neurohypophysis). The anterior lobe is derived embryologically from an extension of the oral canal, called Rathke's pouch, which grows upward toward the base of the brain. It is eventually cut off from its origins by the growth of the sphenoid bone, which creates a saddle-like depression, the sella turcica, in which the definitive pituitary nestles. Rests of epithelial cells may deposit along the course of growth, and these anlagen may persist to give rise later to a pharyngeal pituitary or to an extrasellar craniopharyngioma (see section on hypothalamic tumors, later in this chapter). The posterior lobe, by contrast, is derived from an outpouching of the floor of the third ventricle, which grows downward alongside the anterior lobe. The neural connection of the posterior lobe persists as the pituitary stalk, thus to maintain anatomic continuity between the hypothalamus and the neurohypophysis. An extension of the dura called the diaphragma sellae roofs over the sella. Separating the anterior and posterior lobes is a vestigial intermediate lobe.

Histologically, the posterior and anterior lobes are entirely dissimilar. The posterior lobe is composed of tangled, unmyelinated nerve fibers containing secretory granules of stored posterior pituitary hormones—vasopressin (antidiuretic hormone [ADH]) and oxytocin. These hormones are produced in the hypothalamus and transported through neural connections to the posterior lobe. Glia-like pituicytes are dispersed between the nerve fibers. The vestigial pars intermedia may be totally absent or marked by only small cystic or cleft-like spaces.

The anterior lobe (adenohypophysis) is the major secretory portion of the pituitary. Traditionally, it was said to be composed of three cell types as seen with aniline dye stains: acidophils and basophils (composing the chromophils) and chromophobes. Five cell types, producing the six major tropic hormones, however, can be differentiated immunocytochemically using specific monoclonal antibodies against the various hormones (Fig. 25–1):

- *Somatotrophs*, producing growth hormone (GH) —acidophilic
- *Mammotrophs*, producing prolactin (Prl)—acidophilic
- *Corticotrophs*, producing proopiomelanocortin, from which ACTH, melanocyte-stimulating hormone (MSH), endorphins, and lipotropin are derived—basophilic
- *Thyrotrophs*, producing thyroid-stimulating hormone (TSH)—basophilic
- *Gonadotrophs*, producing both follicle-stimulating hormone (FSH) and luteinizing hormone (LH)—basophilic

TSH, FSH, and LH all are glycoproteins composed of an alpha subunit, common to all three, and different beta subunits specific to each hormone. Sometimes these subunits are found in the blood. All the secretory cells contain, under the electron microscope, membrane-bound granules, varying in size from 50 to 1000 nm, containing stored tropic hormone, somewhat distinctive for each particular hormone. There are, in addition in the anterior pituitary, about 15 to 20% of cells that fail to react with antibodies to any of the known hormones. These are the so-called *chromophobes*, which can be divided into three groups: (1) cells that are secretorily inactive, are sparsely granulated, and contain minute amounts of hormone below the threshold of clinical manifestations and immunohistochemical demonstration; (2) nonsecretory (null) cells; and (3) uncommon oncocytes derived from the previous cell types.

The functional activity of the secretory cells is regulated by the hypothalamus through its release of stimulatory and inhibitory factors (hormones),

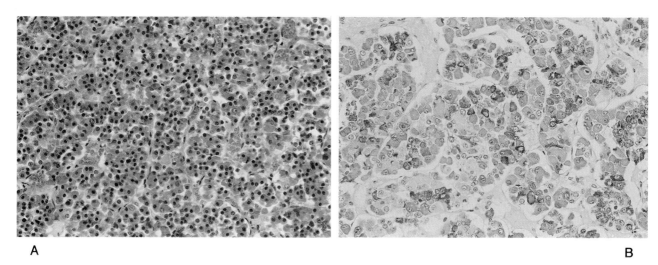

A
B

Figure 25-1. Photomicrograph of normal pituitary and immunostain of human growth hormone.

PATHOLOGY

and by feedback control mechanisms (described earlier).

Disorders of the pituitary may be divided into those involving primarily the anterior lobe and those involving the posterior lobe. Uncommonly, certain lesions, such as tumors, damage both.

Diseases affecting predominantly the adenohypophysis come to attention as a consequence of either of the following:

- *Increased or decreased tropic hormone production.* The former is referred to as hyperpituitarism and, until proved otherwise, relates to a functioning anterior lobe tumor, but rarely it is hypothalamic in origin or due to loss of feedback inhibition. Hypopituitarism has more varied origins and appears whenever there is destruction of at least 75% of the anterior lobe by a nonfunctioning tumor, infection, or other process. Rarely it is hypothalamic in origin.
- *Local effects.* Less commonly, anterior lobe disorders come to attention because of local consequences, which can be divided into three patterns:

1. Demonstration of enlargement of the sella turcica by x-ray film, computed tomography (CT) scan, or magnetic resonance imaging (MRI), related to some expansile lesion, such as a neoplasm of the pituitary (Fig. 25-2).
2. A visual field defect from encroachment of the expanding diseased pituitary on the immediately adjacent optic chiasm or optic nerves.

Classically this takes the form of a bitemporal hemianopsia, or less commonly, some other pattern of visual impairment.

3. Very infrequently, manifestations of increased intracranial pressure, such as headache, nausea, and vomiting, owing to a particularly large pituitary neoplasm.

Obviously, the individual patient may have any or none of these features, and the pituitary disease is discovered only at postmortem. The major disorders of the anterior pituitary will be considered

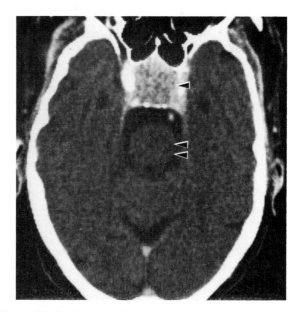

Figure 25-2. Computed tomography scan of transverse plane of skull at level of pituitary fossa, revealing enlargement of sella caused by an expansile pituitary adenoma *(arrowhead)*. Compare its size with transverse dimension of brain stem *(double arrowhead)*. (Courtesy of Dr. Calvin Rumbaugh, Department of Radiology, Brigham and Women's Hospital, Harvard Medical School, Boston.)

Table 25–1. FREQUENCY OF ADENOMA TYPES IN UNSELECTED SURGICAL MATERIAL OF 1043 BIOPSIES

GH cell adenoma	
Densely granulated	6.71
Sparsely granulated	7.28
Prl cell adenoma	
Densely granulated	0.58
Sparsely granulated	26.65
Mixed GH cell–Prl cell adenoma	4.80
Acidophil stem cell adenoma	2.20
Mammosomatotroph adenoma	1.44
Corticotroph cell adenoma	8.05
Silent ("corticotroph") adenoma	5.95
TSH cell adenoma	0.96
Gonadotroph cell adenoma	6.42
Null cell adenoma	
Non-oncocytic	16.30
Oncocytic	8.92
Plurihormonal adenoma	3.74

With permission from Horvath, E., and Kovacs, K.: Pituitary gland. Pathol. Res. Pract. *183*:129, 1988.

under the headings of (1) hyperpituitarism—anterior lobe tumors, and (2) disorders associated with hypopituitarism.

HYPERPITUITARISM— ANTERIOR LOBE TUMORS

Until proved otherwise, hyperfunction of the anterior pituitary means an adenoma; carcinomas, particularly functioning carcinomas, are rare. Equally rarely, the hyperfunction is attributable to a hypothalamic disorder with excessive stimulation of the pituitary. The frequency of the various adenomas is presented in Table 25–1.

To be noted: Some adenomas produce more than one hormone (e.g., GH and Prl). In some of these instances, two cell populations are present—somatotrophs and mammotrophs. In other instances, the cells appear to be somewhat less differentiated and are presumed to be the progenitors of both cell types and both hormones, or the adenomas are monomorphous and composed of bihormonal somatomammotrophs. Clinically, a small number of other adenomas are also plurihormonal, but in the great majority of instances, clinical manifestations relate only to a single hormone, that is, such additional functional activity as may be demonstrable on immunostaining is at too low a level to be clinically significant.[1] At the other extreme are nonfunctional adenomas that, by their expansile growth, destroy the surrounding normal anterior lobe and so lead to hypopituitarism, as will be pointed out subsequently.

The great majority of adenomas are monoclonal in origin, even those that are plurihormonal, suggesting that most arise from a single somatic cell. Indeed, some plurihormonal tumors may arise from clonal expansion of primitive, pluripotential cells, which then differentiate in several directions simultaneously. To date, efforts to identify genetic alterations associated with adenoma production have not yielded definitive findings, but of interest several studies point to a somatic mutation in a subset of GH-secreting adenomas that converts the alpha subunit of a G protein into a possible oncogene, referred to as *gsp*.[2] You may recall that G proteins are involved in the signal transduction pathways of hormone secretion and, putatively, in growth-regulatory pathways.

GENERAL MORPHOLOGY. Hypophyseal adenomas can be divided into microadenomas (less than 10 mm in diameter) or macroadenomas (greater than 10 mm and ranging up to several centimeters in diameter). Microadenomas are surprisingly common and have been reported in 40% of unselected autopsies; in most cases, they were incidental findings and hence would not be represented in surgical series. Although microadenomas tend to occur singly, multiple lesions may be present in the same gland, but the possibility of multiple foci of hyperplasia cannot always be excluded. They are virtually always located within the hypophysis itself. Macroadenomas may be entirely intrasellar and restricted to a portion of the anterior lobe, may totally obliterate the anterior lobe and possibly the posterior lobe in their expansile outgrowth, or may erode the bony enclosure and extend into adjacent structures to become seemingly invasive. Adenomas confined to the sella are usually delicately or poorly encapsulated and surrounded only by condensed reticulin. Large, rapidly growing lesions may break through their capsules to extend along broad fronts, into neighboring structures, such as the optic chiasm and adjacent cranial nerves, the base of the brain, cavernous sinuses, and sphenoid bone (Fig. 25–3).

Microscopically, all adenomas have a fairly uniform appearance. The more or less uniform polygonal cells are arranged in sheets, cords, or nests, having only a delicate, vascularized stroma. Sometimes, pseudoglandular or papillary formations are present. Small or large foci of ischemic necrosis may be present, and psammoma bodies may be found, accompanied by hemorrhage. When this involves most of the adenoma, it is sometimes referred to as **pituitary apoplexy.** Some adenomas, usually those that are more rapidly growing, have some variation in cell and nuclear size and shape. This appearance, however, is not a reliable indicator of malignancy, which can be diagnosed only on the basis of metastases. Ultrastructurally, in most adenomas associated with well-defined hormonal syndromes, abundant or sparse secretory granules can be identified in the cytoplasm of the tumor cells, as will be pointed out subsequently.

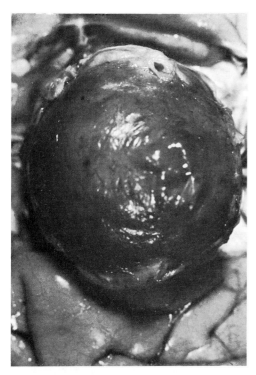

Figure 25-3. Close-up detail of a pituitary adenoma still attached to the brain. Compressed vessels and nerves are apparent about periphery.

SOMATOTROPIC ADENOMAS. *Almost all patients with excess GH, leading usually to acromegaly or gigantism, have an underlying somatotropic acidophilic macroadenoma.* Only rarely is hyperplasia of somatotrophs, or hypothalamic disease, responsible. Acromegaly appears when the GH excess occurs in adults. It is characterized by "megaly" of the acral parts, with enlargement of the head, hands, and feet; jutting jaw; large tongue; and soft tissue enlargement. These changes have generally been developing for decades before being recognized, hence the opportunity for the adenomas to reach substantial size. When somatotropic adenomas appear in children before the epiphyses have closed, gigantism results, as seen in the circus giants of old. Today, gigantism has become vanishingly rare. About half of somatotropic adenomas are composed of densely granulated uniform mature cells that yield strong immunostaining for GH. The other half are sparsely granulated adenomas, more often composed of somewhat more pleomorphic acidophils, that yield a weak reaction for GH. Indeed, the manifestations of acromegaly may be poorly developed in these cases, and only local manifestations of a pituitary tumor are present.

About one-third of GH-producing adenomas are bihormonal and also elaborate Prl. Most of these adenomas have recognizable populations of somatotrophs and mammotrophs, that is, they are bimorphous. Rarely these tumors are monomorphous and composed of apparent precursors of the two differentiated cell types. Clinically, in these cases, features of acromegaly may be present but are usually not marked, along with hyperprolactinemia, which is clinically silent. In some instances, despite the presence of sparse Prl granules in the neoplastic cells, Prl cannot be detected in the circulating blood.

PROLACTINOMAS. Prl-secreting adenomas are the most common form of pituitary tumor, and most are sparsely granulated (see Table 25-1). Prl cell hyperplasia is rare. It should be cautioned, however, that hyperprolactinemia may also result from other causes, for example, hypothalamic lesions, drugs that impair dopaminergic transmission (methyldopa, reserpine), and estrogen therapy. Whatever its basis, hyperprolactinemia may induce hypogonadism in both the male and the female and galactorrhea in the female. This tumor underlies almost a quarter of cases of amenorrhea. Men may manifest impotence and infertility.

Anatomically, about two-thirds of Prl-secreting tumors are macroadenomas, usually composed of sparsely granulated acidophilic cells (Fig. 25-4). The remainder are microadenomas. Indeed, most unsuspected pituitary tumors found at autopsy are composed of Prl cells, but with usual hematoxylin and eosin stains, these neoplasms may appear chromophobic or, at the most, weakly acidophilic. Immunohistochemical methods are required to identify the tropic hormone present in the sparse granules. Foci of calcification can be seen in about 10 to 15% of these adenomas. The cells are usually quite uniform in size and shape and sometimes may expand the sella turcica to produce local changes.

CORTICOTROPH TUMORS. Most of these are small, basophilic microadenomas. The excess production of ACTH leads to adrenal hypersecretion of cortisol and the production of Cushing's disease (see section on adrenal, later in this chapter). A less common variant of corticotroph adenoma is referred to as *chromophobic;* it is responsible for less well-defined symptoms of cortisol excess. These more or less silent tumors tend to be large and sometimes induce local changes. The classic, basophilic corticotropic adenoma yields strong reactions on immunostaining for ACTH and other proopiomelanocortin-related peptides. A distinctive alteration, referred to as Crooke's hyaline change, is sometimes seen in the corticotrophs, largely in the nontumorous surrounding anterior lobe, and will be discussed in the consideration of Cushing's syndrome discussed later.

Infrequently the excess elaboration of ACTH is attributable to foci of hyperplasia of corticotrophs or multiple microadenomas. The differentiation of these two morphologic patterns is almost impossible.

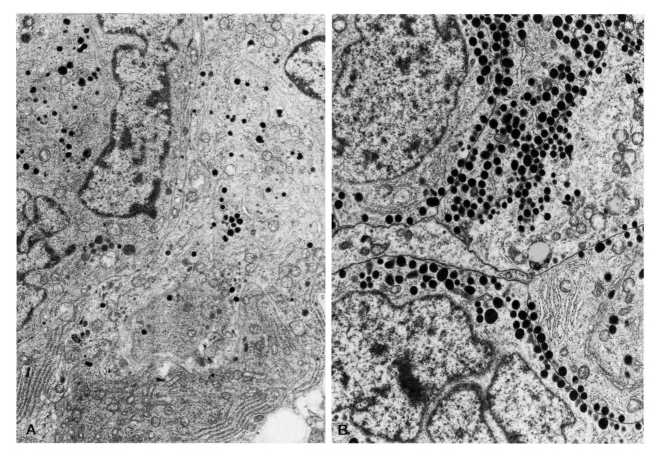

Figure 25–4. *A,* Electron micrograph of a sparsely granulated prolactinoma. The tumor cells contain abundant granular endoplasmic reticulum (indicative of active protein synthesis) and small numbers of secretory granules (6000 ×). *B,* Electron micrograph of densely granulated growth hormone–secreting adenoma. The tumor cells are filled with large membrane-bound secretory granules (6000 ×). (Courtesy of Dr. Eva Horvath, St. Michael's Hospital, Toronto, Ontario.)

OTHER FUNCTIONING ADENOMAS. Gonadotrophs account for about 6% of pituitary tumors. In men, they are usually associated with increased serum levels of FSH, with little evidence of increased LH secretion. The presenting manifestation is usually hypogonadism. In the majority of instances, overproduction of the beta subunit of FSH can also be identified. In women, there is often no evidence of increased gonadotropin secretion, although levels of LH may be detectable in the serum. In both men and women, the tumors tend to be large and sometimes accompanied by local manifestations. Histologically, immunoreactivity for gonadotropins may be weak and is also somewhat patchy throughout the lesion. Tumors in men frequently exhibit some variation in cell size and shape, whereas those in women tend to be composed of relatively uniform small cells. The number of secretory granules within these cells correlates with their basophilia.

Thyrotroph adenomas are too uncommon for further comment, but because they elaborate the glycoprotein thyrotropin releasing hormone (TRH), they are basophilic with aniline dye.

CARCINOMA. Adenohypophyseal adenocarcinomas are quite rare, and most are not functional. Although these malignant tumors range from well differentiated, resembling somewhat atypical adenomas, to poorly differentiated, with variable degrees of pleomorphism and the features characteristic of carcinomas in other locations, the diagnosis of carcinoma of the adenohypophysis requires the demonstration of metastases, usually to lymph nodes, bone, liver, and sometimes elsewhere.

DISORDERS ASSOCIATED WITH HYPOPITUITARISM

Hypofunction of the adenohypophysis may result from lesions in the hypothalamus or in the anterior lobe of the pituitary. Hypothalamic lesions are on the whole extremely rare: Only the suprasellar craniopharyngioma, glioma, and germ cell tumor occur with frequency sufficient to merit description (see later). Such tumors may produce a variety of clinical syndromes, including diabetes insipidus, growth acceleration, stunting of growth, and delayed puberty.[3] *About 90% of cases of hypopituitarism arise from destructive processes directly involving the adenohypophysis, the three most common being nonsecretory adenomas, Sheehan's pituitary necrosis, and the empty sella syndrome.* The remaining causes of pituitary insufficiency include metastatic neoplasms, pituitary apoplexy (hemorrhage), disruption of blood supply by systemic arteritis or thrombosis of cavernous venous sinuses, inflammatory destruction of the anterior lobe by sarcoidosis or infections, surgical or radiation ablation of the pituitary, and a variety of metabolic disorders. Whatever the underlying disorder, pituitary hypofunction is unlikely to be manifested until at least 75% of the anterior lobe is destroyed.

The clinical manifestations of destructive lesions of the adenohypophysis are extremely variable, and many will be mentioned later along with the various causative conditions. Only a few comments are offered here.

Lack of GH *per se* in the adult is virtually undetectable except by radioimmunoassay of the hormone level. In the prepubertal child, it causes symmetric retardation of growth, so-called *pituitary dwarfism.* Frequently, sexual development is also retarded. Hypogonadotropism in women induces amenorrhea, loss of axillary and pubic hair, sterility, and atrophy of the ovaries and external genitalia. In men, hypogonadotropism is manifested by testicular atrophy, sterility, and loss of axillary and pubic hair. Often there is a notable absence of hair or recession of the hairline. All these manifestations are related to loss of gonadal function. Other deficits may induce hypothyroidism related to a lack of TSH or hypoadrenalism related to a deficiency of ACTH, followed in time by atrophy of the thyroid and adrenals. Thus, thyroid, adrenal, or gonadal insufficiency related to lacks of pituitary tropic hormones must be differentiated from primary disorders of these organs. The destructive process, whatever its nature, may also affect the posterior pituitary and add to the symptom complex. It should be noted that panhypopituitarism rarely, if ever, induces weight loss, and so the older designation of "Simmonds' cachexia" is clearly inappropriate.

Remarks here will be confined to the three most common causes of hypopituitarism, followed by brief comments on hypothalamic tumors, which sometimes also cause pituitary insufficiency.

NONSECRETORY CHROMOPHOBE PITUITARY ADENOMAS

About 25 to 30% of diagnosed pituitary tumors are nonfunctioning clinically; that is, there are no recognizable manifestations of excess anterior lobe hormones. Instead these patients come to clinical attention because of so-called local effects, including abnormalities in the visual fields, headaches, or hypofunction of one of the target endocrine organs under pituitary control (e.g., hypothyroidism or hypogonadism). Generally, these adenomas are large when first discovered because they remain clinically silent for many years. On gross inspection, they cannot be differentiated from secretory adenomas. Histologically, the majority can be classified as null cell adenomas, or oncocytomas. The former are composed of cells either totally lacking secretory granules or having only a scant number of them. Immunocytochemical reactions in these sparsely granulated lesions reveal that many have demonstrable FSH, free alpha-hormone and beta-hormone subunits, or, less frequently, LH. Oncocytomas are composed of cells having an abundant eosinophilic granular cytoplasm that is literally packed with mitochondria. These oncocytic cells are thought to derive from sparsely granulated cells or null cells.[4]

SHEEHAN'S SYNDROME

Also known as postpartum pituitary necrosis, this syndrome results from sudden infarction of the anterior lobe precipitated by obstetric hemorrhage or shock.[5] During pregnancy, the pituitary enlarges to almost twice its normal size, compressing the blood supply. Sudden systemic hypotension precipitates vasospasm of the vessels and thus ischemic necrosis of much or all of the anterior lobe, sparing the posterior lobe, which is less vulnerable to anoxia.

Other pathogenetic mechanisms, however, may be involved, such as disseminated intravascular coagulation (DIC) or (more rarely) sickle cell anemia, cavernous sinus thrombosis, temporal arteritis, or traumatic injury of vessels. The incidence appears to be increased in individuals with long-standing diabetes mellitus. With these varied origins, *Sheehan's syndrome may be encountered in nonpregnant women as well as in men.* In most instances, there is destruction of 95 to 99% of the anterior lobe, most evident as a gonadotropic deficiency having the features described but possibly accompanied by failure of lactation in the puerperium. Concomitantly the deficiency of TSH and ACTH may induce hypothyroidism and adrenocortical insufficiency. Less extensive destruction of the anterior lobe may be asymptomatic or may present as loss of only one of the tropic hormones. Strangely, the loss of pituitary function may not become evident for years after the initiating event, attributed to continued destruction of marginal viable cells as they become trapped in the postinfarction scarring.

Whatever the pathogenesis, the infarcted

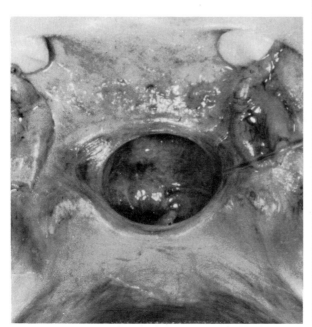
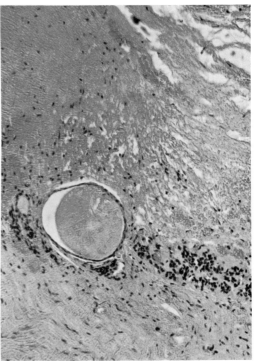

Figure 25–5. *A, In situ* view of sella turcica in a patient dying of far-advanced pituitary insufficiency. Residual gland substance remains *in situ* and can be seen as a minute nubbin of tissue protruding from midline of posterior wall of sella *(below). B,* Microscopic view of anterior lobe of pituitary illustrated in *A.* Complete fibrous atrophy of anterior lobe is evident above pars intermedia, indicated in photograph by cystic space. Posterior lobe is below and appears normal.

adenohypophysis at the outset appears soft, pale, and ischemic or hemorrhagic. Over time, the ischemic area is resorbed and replaced by fibrous tissue. In some long-standing cases, the gland scars down to a fibrous nubbin weighing less than 0.1 gm, attached to the wall of an empty sella.

EMPTY SELLA SYNDROME

This uncommon condition has a number of origins. Most often it is related to herniation of the arachnoid through some defect in the diaphragma sellae —either an abnormally large aperture through which the hypophyseal stalk passes or a defect elsewhere. The cerebrospinal fluid (CSF) pressure eventually causes atrophy of the pituitary, creating the appearance of an empty sella (Fig. 25–5). Other possible causes are Sheehan's syndrome, total infarction of an adenoma followed by fibrous scarring, and ablation of the gland by either surgery or radiation.[6] In most individuals with this condition, sufficient parenchyma is preserved to prevent pituitary insufficiency, but occasionally there is either panhypopituitarism or inadequate secretion of one or more of the tropic hormones. In some cases, the sella is not only empty but also enlarged, and so on radiography or CT scan it is easily mistaken for an expansile pituitary neoplasm.

HYPOTHALAMIC SUPRASELLAR TUMORS

Neoplasms in this location are extremely uncommon but may induce hypofunction or hyperfunction of the anterior pituitary, diabetes insipidus (discussed below), or combinations of these manifestations. The most commonly implicated lesions are gliomas (sometimes arising in the chiasm) and craniopharyngiomas. The craniopharyngioma is derived from vestigial remnants of Rathke's pouch; some arise within the sella, but most are suprasellar. Most commonly seen in children and young adults, they are usually benign.

MORPHOLOGY. Craniopharyngiomas average 3 to 4 cm in diameter; they may be encapsulated and solid but more commonly are cystic and sometimes multiloculated. More than three-fourths of these tumors contain sufficient calcification to be visualized radiographically. In their strategic location, they often encroach on the optic chiasm or nerves and not infrequently bulge into the floor of the third ventricle and base of the brain.

The histologic pattern is quite variable and recapitulates the enamel organ of the tooth. Thus, these tumors are also known as **adamantinomas** or **ameloblastomas.** Nests or cords of stratified squamous or columnar epithelium are embedded in a loose fibrous stroma. Often the nests of squamous cells gradually merge into a peripheral layer of columnar cells. In the cystic variants, the lining stratified squamous or columnar epithelium may be flat and regular or thrown up into papillary projections. Calcification and metaplastic bone formation occur in the necrotic centers of the solid tumors as well as in the cystic variety. Infrequently, anaplastic changes are encountered in the epithelial cells, but cancerous behavior is rare.

POSTERIOR PITUITARY SYNDROMES

Disorders arising out of posterior pituitary dysfunction are rare. Most relate to primary suprasellar hypothalamic lesions that were detailed above. The consequences of dysfunction of the posterior pituitary take the form of ADH (or arginine vasopressin) deficiency or inappropriate release. The only known functions of oxytocin are potentiation of uterine contraction during labor and stimulation of contraction of lactating glands in the breast to force milk into the excretory ducts during suckling.

ADH deficiency induces diabetes insipidus, characterized by polyuria, excessive thirst, and polydipsia. The origins of this syndrome include (1) neoplastic or inflammatory involvement of the hypothalamohypophyseal axis (e.g., suprasellar tumors, metastatic cancer, abscesses, meningitis, tuberculosis, and sarcoidosis), (2) surgical or radiation injury to the hypothalamohypophyseal axis (e.g., surgical or irradiation hypophysectomy), (3) severe head injuries, and (4) idiopathic causes. Occasionally, patients with idiopathic diabetes insipidus have regressive alterations of obscure etiology of ganglion cells in the hypothalamus. Rarely, the idiopathic form of this syndrome is familial and apparently inherited as a Mendelian dominant.

Inappropriate ADH secretion implies persistent release of ADH unrelated to the plasma osmolarity. Thus, there is excessive reabsorption of water from the glomerular filtrate, abnormal retention of water with expansion of the extracellular fluid volume, consequent hyponatremia and hemodilution, and inability to excrete a dilute urine. The most common cause of inappropriate secretion is paraneoplastic elaboration of ADH by a variety of tumors, particularly small cell bronchogenic carcinoma, accounting for more than four-fifths of all cases. Other neoplasms associated with ectopic production of ADH include thymoma, carcinoma of the pancreas, and lymphoma. Infrequently disorders of the central nervous system (CNS) underlie this syndrome, such as intracerebral hemorrhages or thromboses, subarachnoid hemorrhage, subdural hematoma, and infections in and about the CNS. Pulmonary disorders, including pneumonia and tuberculosis, and drugs have also been associated with this disorder.

Thyroid Gland

THYROTOXICOSIS (HYPERTHYROIDISM)	SUBACUTE GRANULOMATOUS (DE QUERVAIN'S) THYROIDITIS	DIFFUSE NONTOXIC (SIMPLE) GOITER	Papillary Carcinoma
HYPOTHYROIDISM	SUBACUTE LYMPHOCYTIC (PAINLESS) THYROIDITIS	MULTINODULAR GOITER	Follicular Carcinoma
CRETINISM		TUMORS	Anaplastic Carcinoma
MYXEDEMA	GRAVES' DISEASE	ADENOMAS	Medullary Thyroid Carcinoma
THYROIDITIS	DIFFUSE AND	OTHER BENIGN TUMORS	MISCELLANEOUS LESIONS
HASHIMOTO'S THYROIDITIS	MULTINODULAR GOITER	MALIGNANT TUMORS	Congenital Anomalies
			Systemic Thyroidal Changes

NORMAL

The thyroid gland develops as a tubular evagination from the root of the tongue, called the foramen caecum. It grows downward anterior to the trachea and thyroid cartilage to reach its adult site. The distal end proliferates to form the adult gland, whereas the remainder degenerates and disappears, usually by the fifth to sixth week of development. Incomplete descent may lead to the formation of the thyroid at loci abnormally high in the neck, producing a lingual or aberrant subhyoid thyroid. Excessive descent leads to substernal thyroid glands. Malformations of branchial pouch differentiation may result in intrathyroidal sites of the thymus or parathyroid glands. The implication of these deviations from the norm may become all too evident in the patient who has a total thyroidectomy and subsequently develops hypoparathyroidism.

In the adult, the normal thyroid weighs 20 to 25 gm. Two large lateral lobes are connected in the midline by a broad isthmus from which, on occasion, a pyramidal lobe may protrude superiorly. Occasionally in a very thin person, this normal pyramidal structure may be mistaken for a thyroid nodule. The gland is made up of acini or follicles lined by regular cuboidal cells and separated by a scant fibrovascular stroma. Small collections of lymphocytes are dispersed in the stroma. Scattered in the follicular epithelium and interstitium are the neuroectodermal calcitonin-secreting C cells, recognizable only by immunocytochemical techniques.

The biosynthesis of the hormones of the thyroid triiodothyronine (T_3) and thyroxine (T_4) is widely available elsewhere.

Once released into the blood, T_4 and T_3 are bound to an alpha globulin: thyroxine-thyronine-binding globulin (TBG). Other plasma proteins, including prealbumin and albumin, participate to a lesser extent in this binding. T_3 is bound less firmly by TBG and very little by other plasma proteins. Because the metabolic state of cells is regulated by the unbound fractions, unbound or free T_3 is more available to the cells of the body than is the small fraction of free T_4.[7]

The thyroid gland is one of the most responsive organs in the body. T_3 and T_4, or more accurately, free T_3 and T_4, act through specific nuclear receptors to modulate cell growth and functional activity of all kinds. The gland responds to many stimuli and is in a constant state of adaptation. During puberty, pregnancy, and physiologic stress from any source, the gland increases in size and becomes more active. This functional lability is reflected in transient hyperplasia of the thyroidal epithelium. At this time, thyroglobulin is resorbed, and the follicular cells become tall and columnar, sometimes forming small infolded buds or papillae. When the stress abates, involution occurs, that is, the height of the epithelium falls, colloid accumulates, and the follicular cells resume their normal size and architecture. Failure of this normal balance between hyperplasia and involution may produce major or minor deviations from the usual histologic pattern.

The function of the thyroid gland can be inhibited by a variety of chemical agents, collectively referred to as goitrogens. Because they suppress T_3 and T_4 synthesis, the level of TSH increases, and subsequent hyperplastic enlargement of the gland (goiter) follows (Fig. 25–6). Most important among these compounds are certain drugs used in the treatment of hyperthyroidism. The antithyroid agents, thiourea and mercaptoimidazole, inhibit the oxidation of iodide and block production of the thyroid hormones. There follows diminished negative feedback on the pituitary and hypothalamus, leading to increased levels of TSH and TRH, resulting in thyroid hyperplasia and enlargement. Iodide, when given to patients with thyroid hyperfunction, also blocks the release of thyroid hormones but through different mechanisms. Iodides in large doses inhibit proteolysis of thyroglobulin. Thus, thyroid hormone is synthesized and incorporated within increasing amounts of colloid, but it is not released into the blood. Following thiourea therapy, the gland lacks thyroglobulin colloid and is extremely cellular, but with iodine treatment, the follicles become distended with thyroglobulin and the stromal vascularization compressed, creating the appearance of an inactive gland.

PATHOLOGY

Diseases of the thyroid are of great importance because most are amenable to medical or surgical management. *They present principally as thyrotoxicosis (hyperthyroidism), hypothyroidism, and diffuse or focal enlargement of the gland (goiter).*

There is no simple correlation between morphologic lesions and resultant clinical manifestations. A multinodular goiter, for example, in one instance may be associated with normal thyroid function, in another with hyperfunction, and in yet another with hypofunction. It is best, therefore, at the outset to present the clinical syndromes of hyperthyroidism and hypothyroidism and then discuss the various thyroid lesions, relating each to its possible clinical significance.

THYROTOXICOSIS (HYPERTHYROIDISM)

Thyrotoxicosis is a hypermetabolic state encountered much more often in women, caused by elevated levels of free T_3 and T_4 in the blood. When these elevated levels arise from hyperfunction of the thyroid, as occurs in Graves' disease, the thyrotoxicosis may correctly be called hyperthyroidism. When the increased hormone levels reflect excessive leakage of hormone out of a nonhyperactive gland, however, it is properly referred to as thyrotoxicosis. Long usage often equates these terms. By either name, the syndrome is manifested by nervousness, palpitations, rapid pulse, fatigability, muscular weakness, weight loss with good appetite, diarrhea, heat intolerance, warm skin, ex-

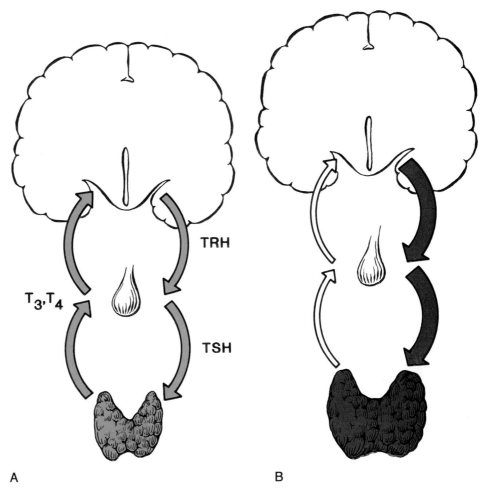

Figure 25–6. *A,* Thyroid hormone synthesis is controlled by both hypothalamic thyrotropin-releasing hormone (TRH) and pituitary thyroid-stimulating hormone (TSH) secretion in classic negative-feedback loop. Low levels of triiodothyronine (T₃) and thyroxine (T₄) stimulate the release of TSH and TRH. TSH stimulates the thyroid to synthesize T₃ and T₄; when levels rise sufficiently, the release of TRH and TSH is suppressed. *B,* In individuals with suppressed T₃ and T₄ synthesis, TRH and TSH are increased. The persistent stimulation of the thyroid by TSH results in thyroid enlargement (goiter). (Courtesy of Dr. Ronald A. DeLellis, New England Medical Center, Boston.)

A

B

cessive perspiration, emotional lability, menstrual changes, a fine tremor of the hand (particularly when outstretched), eye changes, and variable enlargement of the thyroid gland.

MORPHOLOGY. The skin is warm, moist, and flushed, related both to peripheral vasodilation to increase the heat loss and to the general hyperdynamic circulatory state. **Eye changes often call attention to the hyperthyroidism.** Typically, patients have a wide-eyed stare produced by retraction of the upper eyelid accompanied often by upper lid lag as it falls behind the globe on slow downward gaze. In Graves' disease, there is also protrusion of the globe (proptosis) secondary to immunoinflammatory changes in the retro-orbital tissues (Fig. 25–7). **Cardiac manifestations are among the earliest and most consistent features of hyperthyroidism.** Tachycardia, palpitations, and cardiomegaly are common. Arrhythmias, particularly fibrillation, occasionally appear and are often supraventricular. The basis for these arrhythmias is not clear. Myocardial changes, such as foci of lymphocytic and eosinophilic infiltration, mild fibrosis in the interstitium, fatty changes in myofibers, and an increase in size and

number of mitochondria, have been described.[8] These changes are not frequent, and other possible concomitant pathogeneses have not been rigorously ruled out, so debate continues about so-called **thyrotoxic cardiomyopathy.** The cardiomegaly is equally obscure and is usually attributed to increased workload. Only uncommonly does cardiac failure occur in these patients, usually in the elderly in whom an episode of myocardial infarction may have occurred.

Other findings throughout the body include atrophy and fatty infiltration of skeletal muscle, sometimes with focal interstitial lymphocytic infiltrates; minimal fatty changes in the liver, sometimes accompanied by mild periportal fibrosis and a mild lymphocytic infiltrate; osteoporosis; and generalized lymphoid hyperplasia with lymphadenopathy.

Thyrotoxicosis may be caused by a variety of disorders (Table 25–2). The three common causes collectively account for virtually 99% of cases. Among these, Graves' disease is the most frequent, particularly in patients younger than 40 years of age; alone it accounts for 85% of cases. This dis-

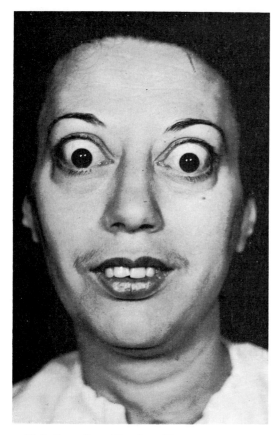

Figure 25-7. Hyperthyroidism in a 27-year-old woman.

ease, which is truly "hyperthyroidism," is also known as diffuse toxic hyperplasia to differentiate it from the thyrotoxicosis related to toxic nodular goiter, whether it is a solitary nodule (presumably an adenoma) or multinodular.[9] Only a few brief comments are merited on the rare causes of hyperthyroidism. Metastatic, well-differentiated thyroid carcinoma may sometimes elaborate sufficient thyroid hormones to cause hyperthyroidism. Similarly, acute or subacute thyroiditis during the stage of active cell injury may be associated with sufficient release of stored hormones to induce transient

Table 25-2. DISORDERS ASSOCIATED WITH HYPERTHYROIDISM

COMMON
Diffuse toxic hyperplasia (Graves' disease)
Toxic multinodular goiter
Toxic adenoma

UNCOMMON
Acute or subacute thyroiditis
Hyperfunctioning thyroid carcinoma
Choriocarcinoma or hydatidiform mole
TSH-secreting pituitary adenoma
Neonatal thyrotoxicosis associated with maternal Graves' disease
Struma ovarii (ovarian teratomatous thyroid)
Iodide-induced hyperthyroidism
Iatrogenic (exogenous) hyperthyroidism

manifestations of hyperthyroidism. Choriocarcinomas and hydatidiform moles may produce not only chorionic gonadotropin but also sometimes a TSH-like material.[10] Increased levels of thyroid hormones may rarely be caused by TSH-secreting pituitary tumors or pituitary stimulation by excessive hypothalamic release of TRH. Thyroid hyperfunction can be also induced by excess iodine ingestion in patients with various thyroid disorders. This pattern is sometimes referred to as *jodbasedow disease.* The iodine ingestion permits T_3, T_4 synthesis and precipitates the thyrotoxicosis. Equally rarely, patients receiving thyroid hormone medication for hypothyroidism or for other reasons (misguided attempts at weight control) may develop iatrogenic or factitious hyperthyroidism. In all, the same hypermetabolic syndrome results.

HYPOTHYROIDISM

Any structural or functional derangement of the thyroid that impairs its output of hormone leads to the hypometabolic state of hypothyroidism. The clinical manifestations depend on the age when it first appears. When present during development and infancy, it results in *cretinism* with its associated physical and mental retardation. The term *cretin* was derived from the French *chrétien,* meaning Christian or Christ-like, and was applied to these unfortunates because they were considered to be so mentally retarded as to be incapable of sinning. When hypothyroidism first appears in older children or adults, it is termed *myxedema.* This designation calls attention to the accumulation of hydrophilic mucopolysaccharides in connective tissue throughout the body, leading to a distinctive, edematous, doughy thickening of the skin that is resistant to pitting.

The causes of hypothyroidism in both infants and adults can be divided into several categories (Table 25-3). Among these various disorders, the most frequent in the United States is primary idiopathic hypothyroidism, also known as atrophic autoimmune thyroiditis. This condition is variously reported to cause 15 to 60% of cases of hypothyroidism. Patients are frequently HLA-DR3 or B8. There is substantial evidence that this condition is caused by blocking autoantibodies to the TSH receptor. Significantly, these thyrotropin-blocking autoantibodies may disappear spontaneously or with therapy with recovery from the hypothyroidism.[11] A large resection of the gland for the treatment of hyperthyroidism or excision of a primary neoplasm is probably the second most common cause of hypothyroidism. The gland may also be ablated by radiation, whether in the form of radioiodine administered for the treatment of hyperthyroidism or exogenous irradiation. Together, surgical-induced and radiation-induced thyroidal

Table 25-3. CAUSES OF HYPOTHYROIDISM

INSUFFICIENT THYROID PARENCHYMA
Developmental
Radiation injury (radioiodine, external radiation)
Surgical ablation
Hashimoto's thyroiditis

INTERFERENCE WITH THYROID HORMONE SYNTHESIS
Idiopathic primary hypothyroidism (possible immune blockade of TSH receptors)
Heritable biosynthetic defects
Iodine deficiency
Drugs (lithium, iodides, p-aminosalicylic acid, others)
Hashimoto's thyroiditis

SUPRATHYROIDAL
Pituitary lesions reducing TSH secretion
Hypothalamic lesions that reduce thyrotropin-releasing hormone delivery

ablation account for most of the remaining cases of hypothyroidism. Infrequently, hypothyroidism arises because of a disorder in the hypothalamus or adenohypophysis that reduces serum TSH levels.

CRETINISM

This uncommon condition is marked by retardation of both physical and intellectual growth. It is seldom apparent at birth but, depending on the severity of hormone lack, becomes evident over ensuing weeks to months. By the time the changes become unmistakably evident, they are largely irreversible, and so a strong case can be made for laboratory screening of neonates who fail to thrive. Its relative rarity justifies considerable brevity.

The fully developed syndrome is characterized by dry, rough skin; widely set eyes; periorbital puffiness; a flattened, broad nose; and an overly large protuberant tongue. When the thyroidal deficit is present during early fetal development, as may occur with severe iodine lack, agenesis of the thyroid, or a congenital biosynthetic defect, there is impaired skeletal growth and retarded development of the brain. *Endemic cretinism* occurs wherever endemic goiter (see the section on diffuse nontoxic goiter, later in this chapter) is prevalent, generally related to a dietary lack of iodine. *Sporadic cretinism*, in contrast, is usually caused by some congenital developmental failure in thyroid gland formation (sporadic athyrotic cretinism) or by some biosynthetic defect in thyroid hormone formation.[12]

MYXEDEMA

The term *myxedema* is applied to hypothyroidism in the older child or adult. The clinical manifestations vary with the age at onset of the deficiency. The older child shows signs and symptoms inter-mediate between those of the cretin and those of the adult with hypothyroidism. In the adult, the condition appears insidiously and may take years to reach the level of clinical suspicion. Basically, it is characterized by slowing of physical and mental activity. The initial symptoms are fatigue, lethargy, cold intolerance, and general listlessness and apathy. Speech and intellectual functions become slowed. With the passage of time, periorbital edema develops along with a thickened, dry, coarse skin. Eventually the facial features become thickened and the tongue enlarged, and the distinctive peripheral edema described earlier worsens. At this time, there is extreme physical and mental torpor. Other systems share in the general lethargy with decreased sweating, constipation, and slowness of motor function. In well-advanced myxedema, the heart is flabby and enlarged, with dilated chambers. Histologically, there is sometimes swelling of the myofibers with some loss of striations, accompanied by an increase of interstitial mucopolysaccharide-rich edema fluid. A similar fluid sometimes accumulates within the pericardial sac. To these changes the term *myxedema heart* or *hypothyroid cardiomyopathy* has been applied. There may also be some retardation in skeletal growth and in CNS development; the latter, however, is more characteristic of cretinism.

With this overview of the clinical consequences of disturbed thyroid function, we can turn to the disorders causing it.

THYROIDITIS

There are many forms of thyroiditis. Some are ill defined (e.g., interstitial thyroiditis), and some are quite rare (e.g., palpation thyroiditis). One slightly less uncommon form is suppurative or infectious thyroiditis produced by microbial seeding of the thyroid. Almost always the infection is primary elsewhere, and the agents blood-borne; rarely there is direct traumatic seeding of the gland. Sometimes, immunologic incompetence potentiates these infections. The most frequent causes are Staphylococcus, Streptococcus, Salmonella, Enterobacter, *Mycobacterium tuberculosis*, and fungi (Candida, Aspergillus, Mucor). Viral thyroiditis is a special case, discussed later (see the section on subacute granulomatous thyroiditis, later in this chapter). The thyroid may also be involved in sarcoidosis. Whatever the cause, the inflammatory involvement may cause painful enlargement of the gland, but almost always the condition is self-limited or controllable with appropriate therapy. Thyroid function usually is not significantly affected, and there are few residual effects except for possible small foci of scarring.

Another uncommon form is *Riedel's fibrous thyroiditis*, which is also known as Riedel's struma.

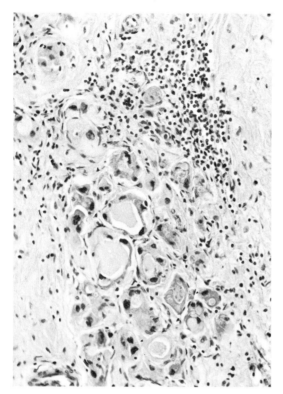

Figure 25-8. High-power view of Riedel's thyroiditis illustrating extensive fibrosis, scant lymphocytic infiltration, and a few residual distorted thyroid follicles.

This obscure condition of unknown cause is marked by glandular atrophy, hypothyroidism, and replacement of the thyroid by fibrous tissue, with adhesion to surrounding structures (Fig. 25–8). Because of this dense adherence and replacement of the glandular substance by firm, gray tissue, Riedel's thyroiditis may be misconstrued as a neoplasm. Sometimes this condition is associated with mysterious fibrosis of other sites, particularly retroperitoneal fibrosis (*multifocal fibrosclerosis*). Much more common and clinically significant are the following more or less well-defined forms of thyroiditis: (1) Hashimoto's thyroiditis, (2) subacute granulomatous thyroiditis, and (3) subacute lymphocytic thyroiditis.

HASHIMOTO'S THYROIDITIS

Also referred to as *struma lymphomatosa* or *lymphadenoid goiter*, Hashimoto's thyroiditis is marked by an intense infiltrate of lymphocytes admixed with plasma cells that virtually replace the thyroid parenchyma. These terms apply to the classic goitrous variant of Hashimoto's thyroiditis, but it should be noted there is a less common atrophic variant marked largely by fibrosis with a scant lymphoid infiltrate. Whatever the morphologic variety, Hashimoto's thyroiditis is of importance for several reasons:

1. It is the most common cause of goitrous hypothyroidism in regions that have a sufficiency of iodine.

2. It is a major cause of nonendemic goiter in children.

3. It is the first described and the archetype of organ-specific, autoimmune diseases.

Most patients with long-standing Hashimoto's thyroiditis become hypothyroid, but a few, in midcourse, develop hyperthyroidism, sometimes called *hashitoxicosis*. This concurrence is more than fortuitous because both Hashimoto's thyroiditis and Graves' disease are thought to be autoimmune in origin and share some features of their autoimmune reactions. Predominantly a disease of women with a female-to-male ratio of 5:1, the incidence of this condition increases with age.

ETIOLOGY AND PATHOGENESIS. There is considerable evidence that Hashimoto's thyroiditis is an autoimmune disease resulting perhaps from a defect in the function of thyroid-specific suppressor T cells. Whether this immunologic deficit is genetic in origin or is acquired remains uncertain, although there are suggestions of autosomal dominant inheritance.[13] Also supporting a genetic basis is the association of Hashimoto's disease with major histocompatibility complex (MHC) class II genes HLA-DR5 in patients with the goitrous form of Hashimoto's thyroiditis and HLA-DR3 in those with the atrophic variant. A defect in thyroid-specific suppressor cell function is then postulated to permit the emergence of CD4+ helper T cells, targeted on thyroid cell antigens, which cooperate with B cells in the thyroid to produce a constellation of autoantibodies. Probably most important are antibodies to thyroid peroxidases (formerly called antimicrosomal antibodies). Other autoantibodies are specific for thyroglobulin, an additional colloid antigen distinct from thyroglobulin, the TSH receptor, and still others. Despite all these autoantibodies, there is no clear understanding of whether damage to the thyroid gland results from cell-mediated immunity or humoral immunity or both. On the one hand, autoimmune thyroiditis can be transferred in various animal species by immune serum. On the other hand, the majority of lymphocytes in experimental models of Hashimoto's thyroiditis have been shown to be CD8+ cytolytic T cells, suggesting a causal role for cell-mediated immunity.[14] Significantly patients with this condition frequently suffer from a variety of other presumed autoimmune diseases, for example, systemic lupus erythematosus, Sjögren's syndrome, rheumatoid arthritis, pernicious anemia, type II diabetes, and Graves' disease.

MORPHOLOGY. As noted before, there is a goitrous and an atrophic variant of Hashimoto's thyroiditis.

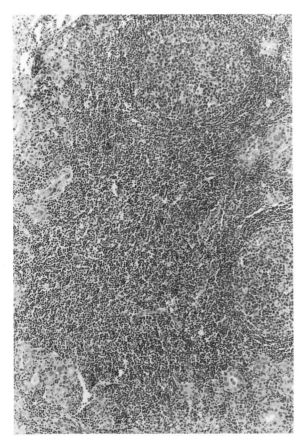

Figure 25–9. Hashimoto's thyroiditis. The thyroid parenchyma is largely replaced by a heavy lymphocytic infiltrate containing two evident lymphoid follicles. Only some marginal thyroid follicles are present in the field.

The goitrous form is characterized by diffuse, possibly asymmetric, moderate enlargement of the gland; the capsule is intact and only rarely adherent. The cut surface reveals replacement of the normally brown, meaty thyroid substance by a somewhat nodular, pale gray, rubbery tissue. However much these changes may resemble a tumor, the diffuseness of the involvement and the integrity of the capsule argue against such a diagnosis. **Microscopically in the goitrous form, there is extensive replacement of the underlying parenchyma by lymphocytes, plasma cells, immunoblasts, and macrophages, sometimes with the formation of lymphoid germinal centers** (Fig. 25–9). Isolated follicles containing deeply stained colloid or clusters of so-called **Hürthle cells** or *oncocytes* having an abundant, brightly eosinophilic granular cytoplasm persist. The Hürthle cells are thought to represent a degenerated state of the follicular epithelium. In the goitrous variant of Hashimoto's thyroiditis, the fibrosis is usually delicate and confined largely to the interlobular septa.

The less common atrophic variant reveals much more abundant fibrosis with a commensurate decrease in the lymphoid infiltrate. As a conse-

quence, there is little or no glandular enlargement, and in some instances, the fibrosis produces a reduction in thyroid size. This fibrosing reaction does not extend beyond the capsule, differentiating this pattern of Hashimoto's disease from the previously described Riedel's struma.

CLINICAL COURSE. The classic clinical presentation of this disease is goitrous enlargement of the thyroid in a middle-aged woman associated with hypothyroidism. Sometimes, particularly in the patient with the atrophic variant of Hashimoto's thyroiditis, there is no goitrous enlargement, only hypothyroidism. In most patients, antithyroid peroxidase antibodies can be identified in the serum, but they may also be found in the absence of clinical disease. Early the patient is metabolically normal, but with the passage of time, thyroid function decreases with a rise in the serum TSH and a fall in T_3 and T_4 levels. Although damage to the thyroid gland is the obvious cause of the failing thyroid function, a contributing influence may be TSH receptor–blocking antibodies.

Occasionally, patients with Hashimoto's thyroiditis present with hyperthyroidism, attributed to anti-TSH receptor–stimulating antibodies, such as are seen in Graves' disease. In time, however, hypothyroidism supervenes. Although the clinical and laboratory features alone may be sufficient for a diagnosis, needle biopsy may be required to confirm it and to rule out the possibility of neoplastic involvement. Generally, the prognosis is excellent in these patients with appropriate hormonal replacement therapy. There is, however, a small increased risk of lymphoma (on the order of 1 patient in 200) and arguably an increased risk of carcinoma.

SUBACUTE GRANULOMATOUS (DE QUERVAIN'S) THYROIDITIS

The term *de Quervain's thyroiditis* is restricted to a distinctive form of self-limited granulomatous inflammation of the thyroid gland, which is also referred to as *giant cell* or *granulomatous thyroiditis*. The peak incidence is in the second to fifth decades of life, with a female-to-male ratio of $3:1$.[15] There is a fairly strong association with HLA-B35.

Although the cause is still uncertain, considerable circumstantial evidence suggests a viral etiology. For example, there is a more than chance association between onset of the thyroiditis and a previous viral infection (mumps, measles, influenza, adenovirus, coxsackievirus, echovirus). Antibodies to these infections can be identified in about half the cases. Clinically, the condition is reminiscent of an infection, with fever, painful tender enlargement of the thyroid gland, and a self-limited course measured in months.

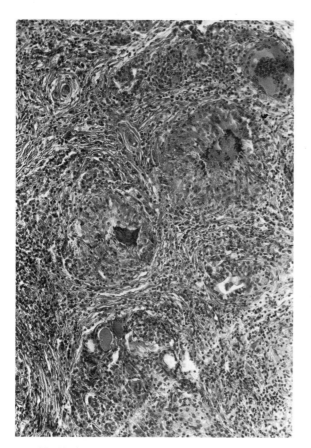

Figure 25–10. Subacute thyroiditis. Two granulomatous foci enclosing remnants of colloid are evident in midfield. Note large giant cell *(above right)*. (Courtesy of Dr. Merle Legg, New England Deaconess Hospital, Boston.)

MORPHOLOGY. The gland may be subtly or markedly enlarged. Usually the enlargement appears asymmetric or focal on palpation, but sometimes the whole gland is irregularly involved. It may be slightly adherent to surrounding structures. On cut section, the involved areas are firm and yellow-white and stand out from the more rubbery, normal brown thyroid substance. Histologically, the changes are patchy and depend on the stage of the disease. Early in the active inflammatory phase, scattered follicles may be entirely disrupted and replaced by neutrophils forming microabscesses. **Later the more characteristic features appear in the form of aggregations of cells about damaged follicles. It is not certain whether these cells are follicular in origin or instead are plump macrophages. Possibly both types are present admixed with multinucleate giant cells enclosing naked pools or fragments of colloid** (Fig. 25–10), hence the designation "granulomatous thyroiditis." In later stages of the disease, a chronic inflammatory infiltrate and fibrosis may replace the foci of injury. Different histologic stages are sometimes found in

the same gland, suggesting waves of destruction over a period of time.[16]

CLINICAL COURSE. The presentation of this condition is extremely variable. Three patterns can be identified: (1) an acute systemic febrile reaction with elevation of the sedimentation rate; (2) sudden painful enlargement of the gland, sometimes mimicking "sore throat" or "earache"; or (3) less painful enlargement accompanied by transient manifestations of hyperthyroidism. Obviously, more than one may coexist in the same patient. Whatever form the disease takes at onset, the condition is self-limited, and over the span of weeks to months, the tenderness usually abates along with the fever and manifestations of hyperthyroidism. Indeed, with extensive destruction of the gland, transient hypothyroidism may supervene.

Characteristically, the T_3 and T_4 levels are increased as a result of damage to the follicles, and the radioactive iodine uptake is low because of suppression of TSH. After recovery, generally within 6 to 8 weeks, normal thyroid function returns.

SUBACUTE LYMPHOCYTIC (PAINLESS) THYROIDITIS

This poorly understood condition is an uncommon cause of goitrous hyperthyroidism. The only changes in the gland are foci of lymphocytic infiltration, sometimes accompanied by an increase in interstitial fibrous tissue. There is no tendency to formation of lymphoid germinal centers and few, if any, plasma cells. This form of thyroiditis usually comes to attention because of goitrous enlargement of the gland or hyperthyroidism, or both. One survey indicated that subacute lymphocytic thyroiditis was responsible for about 15% of all cases of hyperthyroidism in North America. There are, however, none of the other stigmata of Graves' disease (see below). In the absence of hyperthyroidism and with only modest goitrous enlargement, the condition may well pass unrecognized, particularly because it is self-limited and without sequelae. Sometimes it is followed by a period of hypothyroidism.

The origin of this form of thyroiditis and its place in the spectrum of thyroiditis are obscure. There is no association with previous viral infections, and autoimmune reactions are inconstant and evanescent. Generally, the T_3 and T_4 levels are increased. Antithyroid antibodies may be identified in relatively low titers. Although this form of thyroiditis may occur at any age in either sex, it is most common in women and during the postpartum period. There is no evidence that it constitutes a precursor of Hashimoto's disease or so-called primary idiopathic myxedema.

GRAVES' DISEASE

The term Graves' disease is restricted to a syndrome marked by hyperthyroidism caused by a hyperfunctioning diffuse hyperplastic goiter, sometimes accompanied by infiltrative ophthalmopathy and infiltrative dermopathy. The most striking features of the ophthalmopathy, when present, are lid lag, upper lid retraction, stare, weakness of eye muscles, diplopia, periorbital edema, and notably proptosis to the point at which the lids cannot close. The dermopathy takes the form of localized areas of edematous skin over the dorsa of the legs or feet, having plaque-like or nodular conformations. Perplexingly, it has been referred to as localized myxedema. *Although Graves' disease is said to consist of a triad of features, the dermopathy is present in only 10 to 15% of cases, and there may be no ophthalmopathy or it may not be readily evident, so the diagnosis rests largely on the documentation of thyrotoxicosis related to a diffuse toxic goiter.* You recall from the earlier discussion that there are many other possible causes of thyrotoxicosis (e.g., toxic multinodular goiter and toxic adenoma), but none of them is associated with the eye and skin changes sometimes found in Graves' disease.

Graves' disease is said to present in 1.5 to 2% of women in the United States but is only one-tenth as common among men. There is an increased frequency of haplotypes HLA-B8 and DR3 among whites with the disease but, interestingly, different haplotypes among Asians. Familial predisposition has been noted frequently. There is also a well-defined relationship between Graves' disease and other autoimmune thyroid disorders, notably Hashimoto's thyroiditis, perhaps because both conditions have somewhat similar immunologic origins. Sometimes the hyperthyroidism supervenes on pre-existing Hashimoto's thyroiditis, referred to as hashitoxicosis. As might be expected, other autoimmune diseases, such as pernicious anemia and rheumatoid arthritis, occur with greater-than-chance frequency in patients with Graves' disease.

ETIOLOGY AND PATHOGENESIS. The evidence is quite compelling that the thyroid changes in Graves' disease are autoimmune in origin and initiated by IgG antibodies against specific domains of the TSH receptor. Central to the pathogenesis are the following:

One class of TSH receptor autoantibodies is known as thyroid-stimulating antibodies (TSAb) or thyroid-stimulating immunoglobulin (TSI). *In vitro,* they stimulate the function of thyroid cells as evidenced by increased generation of cAMP, reflecting increased adenylate cyclase activity. Another distinctive autoantibody binds to the TSH receptor and inhibits TSH binding, referred to as thyrotropin-binding inhibitor immunoglobulin (TBII). By binding to the TSH receptor, it mimics the action of TSH, and, therefore, both TSI and TBII are responsible for the hyperfunction of the thyroid gland in Graves' disease, but in certain instances, by blocking TSH, TBII may also inhibit thyroid cell activity. This capacity to stimulate but sometimes to inhibit has been ascribed to distinct epitopes on the large TSH receptor molecule, producing distinctive subsets of TBII with differing impact on thyroid cell function. Whether the TSI are also responsible for the proliferation of follicular epithelial cells and growth of the thyroid remains controversial because certain groups have identified distinctive thyroid growth immunoglobulins (TGI).[17] Other investigators, however, contend that the TSI antibodies subsume this role. The various other autoantibodies that have been identified can be reserved for the "thyromaniacs."

The trigger for the initiation of the autoimmune reaction in Graves' disease remains uncertain. Because no environmental agent has been implicated, a scenario much like that of Hashimoto's thyroiditis is proposed. It is theorized that in association with a certain genotype, perhaps related to the DR genes, there is an organ-specific defect in suppressor T-cell function, permitting the emergence and proliferation of CD4+ helper T cells targeted on TSH-receptor epitopes. These cells may then cooperate with B cells, leading to the formation of a range of thyroid-specific autoantibodies.

The ophthalmopathy of Graves' disease is also thought to be autoimmune in origin. Often there is a marked lymphocytic infiltrate in the extraocular eye muscles as well as in the retro-orbital fibrofatty tissues. The lymphocytes are T cells (CD4+ or CD8+). There is also an increase of glycosaminoglycans in the orbital fat and fibrous tissue and extraocular muscles. Together these changes account for the protrusion (extrusion) of the eyes.[18] The basis for these changes is uncertain, but a T cell–mediated reaction with the local release of cytokines and growth factors is proposed.

MORPHOLOGY. In most cases of diffuse hyperplasia, the gland is uniformly but not markedly enlarged. Increases in weight to over 80 to 90 gm are uncommon. The capsule is intact and not adherent. On cut section, the parenchyma has a soft, yielding, meaty appearance closely resembling normal muscle. Preoperative iodine administration causes the accumulation of colloid and alters this gross appearance.

The dominant histologic feature is "too many cells." This appearance is imparted by an increase in height of the lining epithelium to form tall columnar cells and an increase in the number of cells, causing them to pile up in pseudopapillary buds (without fibrovascular cores) and encroach on the colloid. For the most part, these papillae represent simple, nonbranching projections. Occasionally, the

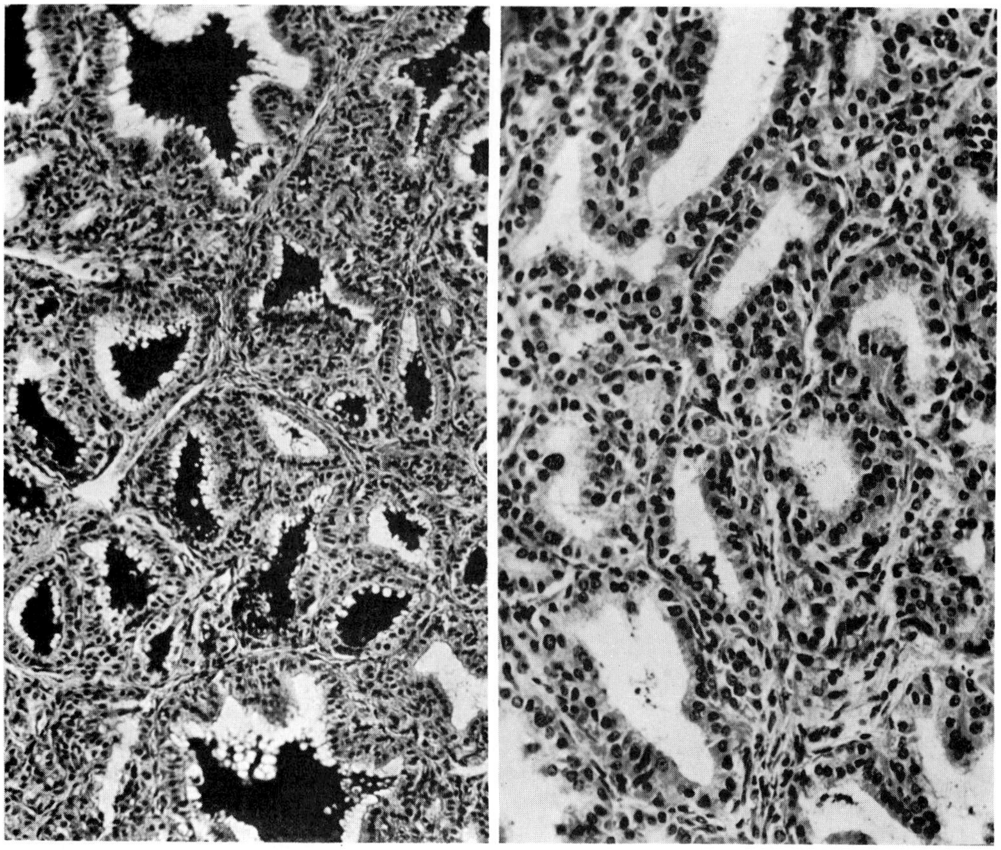

Figure 25–11. *A,* Microscopic view of diffuse thyroid hyperplasia. Cellularity of follicles and resorption of colloid are evident. High columnar epithelium and small projections into follicular spaces are visible. *B,* High-power view of diffuse thyroid hyperplasia, illustrating total absence of colloid, increase in height of epithelium, and buckling of lining cells into follicular spaces.

papillae are sufficiently large to mushroom out and virtually fill the follicles. The cells may show slight variation in size and shape, but no striking atypicality is present. The Golgi apparatus is hypertrophied, the mitrochondria increased in number, and the microvilli more abundant. Colloid is markedly diminished and, when present, has a thin, pale pink, watery appearance (Fig. 25–11). There is a striking increase in the amount of lymphoid tissue in the interfollicular stroma and, in some areas, large lymphoid follicles. The accumulation of lymphoid tissue in the thyroid is only one aspect of the generalized lymphoid hypertrophy found throughout the body, with enlargement of lymph nodes and thymus and hyperplasia of the lymphoid tissue of the spleen. There is inevitably a markedly increased vascularization of the thyroid gland.

This classic histologic pattern may be significantly altered by preoperative medication. Iodine promotes colloid storage, devascularization, and involution of the gland, whereas thiourea derivatives tend to produce marked hyperplasia. Thus, it is impossible, from histologic examination, to evaluate the functional activity of pretreated surgical specimens.

When present, the exophthalmos is related to an increase in the volume of the extraocular muscles and orbital tissues secondary to edema, increased deposits of hydrophilic mucopolysaccharides, fibrosis, and lymphocytic infiltrates (infiltrative ophthalmopathy). Later, fibrosis and contractures of the extraocular muscles occur and lead to the incoordination of eye movements, diplopia, and sometimes ophthalmoplegia.

CLINICAL COURSE. Graves' disease presents, principally in young women, as thyrotoxicosis associated with modest symmetric enlargement of the thyroid gland. When ophthalmopathy and dermopathy are also present, the diagnosis is almost certain. Confirmation usually requires one or more of the following findings: increased radioactive iodine uptake, decreased TSH levels, and above-normal serum levels of total and free T_3 and T_4.

In most cases of Graves' disease, the thyrotoxicosis is persistent, but it may wax and wane. There are many ways of controlling it, but these forms of treatment are without effect on the ophthalmopathy. In most cases, the eye changes run a benign course and spontaneously remit. They can, however, become progressively worse when the proptosis precludes closure of the lids, with corneal injuries and ulcerations and, ultimately, loss of the eye(s). On a happier note, there is little evidence to suggest an increased frequency of thyroidal cancer in patients with Graves' disease.

DIFFUSE AND MULTINODULAR GOITER

Diffuse goiter and multinodular goiter are the consequences of hypertrophy and hyperplasia of follicular epithelium secondary to some derangement that hampers thyroid hormone output with compensatory elevation of the TSH level. The degree of thyroid enlargement is proportional to the level and duration of thyroid hormone lack, but optimally, in most cases, the increased thyroid mass eventually achieves a euthyroid state, although hypothyroidism or hyperthyroidism may result in some cases. At the outset, the goitrous enlargement is diffuse, but for poorly understood reasons and in the course of time, it is likely to become nodular, as described subsequently.

DIFFUSE NONTOXIC (SIMPLE) GOITER

This designation specifies a form of goiter that (1) diffusely involves the entire gland without producing nodularity and (2) is not associated usually with either hyperfunction or hypofunction. Because the enlarged follicles are filled with colloid, the term *colloid goiter* has been applied to this condition. It occurs in both an endemic and a sporadic distribution.

The term *endemic goiter* refers to the high incidence of simple goiter in particular geographic locales in more than 10% of the population. It is extremely common throughout the world and is thought to affect more than 200 million individuals. It is most prevalent in mountainous areas, such as the Alps, Andes, and Himalayas, but also may occur in nonmountainous regions remote from the sea, such as central Africa where iodized salt is not used. *A deficient intake of iodine is the dominant cause of the disease.* The lack of iodine leads to decreased synthesis of thyroid hormone and a compensatory increase in TSH, leading to follicular cell hypertrophy and hyperplasia and goitrous enlargement. The enlarged mass of follicular cells increases hormone output until a euthyroid state is achieved.

Variations in the prevalence of endemic goiter in locales with similar levels of iodine deficiency point to the existence of other causative influences, particularly dietary substances referred to as goitrogens. Calcium and fluorides in the water supply promote goiter formation. A number of foods, including cabbage, cassava, cauliflower, Brussels sprouts, turnips, and others belonging to the Brassica and Crucifera plants, have been documented to be goitrogenic in animals and humans. Native populations subsisting largely on cassava root are at particular risk. Cassava contains a thiocyanate that inhibits iodide transport within the thyroid, worsening any possible concurrent iodine deficiency. Pollution of water supplies may also in some way be goitrogenic. Depending on the severity of iodine lack and goitrogenic influences, the thyroid enlargement may appear in early childhood, but usually it peaks at about puberty or soon thereafter, affecting females more often than males. Severe iodine deficiency during fetal development may produce cretinism.

Nonendemic or sporadic simple goiter is much less common than the endemic variety. There is a striking female preponderance with a ratio of 8:1 and a peak incidence at puberty or in young adult life. The cause of this condition is rarely evident. Although it is natural to assume that increased levels of TSH stimulate the glandular enlargement, it has not been possible to document elevated levels in all patients. Conceivably, a number of influences act in concert. A minimal iodine lack, for example, when coupled with increased demand for thyroid hormones or a partial biosynthetic block might lead to goiter formation. First appearance at puberty in girls underscores the role of increased physiologic demand. During pregnancy, estrogen-induced increased levels of the thyroid-binding globulins (TBG) may lower the levels of free T_3 and T_4 and reduce feedback inhibition of TSH. Dietary goitrogens may be superimposed on these causal influences. It is evident that much is speculative.

Uncommon causes of sporadic goiter are hereditary biosynthetic defects in thyroid hormone synthesis, all transmitted as autosomal recessive conditions.[19] The four major ones are (1) iodide transport defect, (2) organification defect, (3) dehalogenase defect, and (4) iodotyrosine coupling defect.

MORPHOLOGY. Two stages can be identified in the evolution of the diffuse nontoxic goiter, the hyperplastic stage and colloid involution. In the stage of hyperplasia, the gland is modestly enlarged and rarely exceeds 100 to 150 gm. It is diffusely, symmetrically involved and markedly hyperemic. Histologically, the follicular epithelium is columnar, and the newly generated follicles are small with only scanty colloid. The duration of the hyperplastic stage is extremely variable. With the increased mass of cells, a euthyroid state is achieved, and follicular cell growth ceases and is

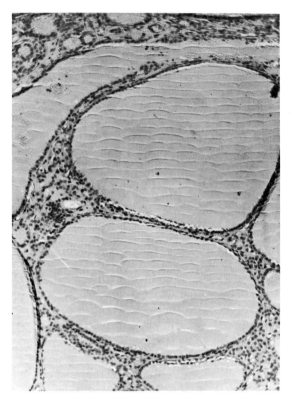

Figure 25–12. Diffuse nontoxic goiter. Follicles are distended with colloid, and epithelial lining is flattened.

followed by colloid accumulation.[20] Now the thyroid becomes markedly enlarged, sometimes to 500 gm or more. At this stage, follicles enlarge as they become filled with colloid, and the epithelium undergoes progressive flattening (Fig. 25–12). For reasons that are unclear, **the accumulation of colloid is not uniform throughout the gland, and some follicles are hugely distended, whereas others remain small and may even retain small papillary infoldings of hyperplastic cells.** The accumulated colloid produces a marked increase in consistency and a gelatinous, glistening cut surface, hence the designation **colloid goiter.**

CLINICAL COURSE. In children, sporadic goiter due to a congenital biosynthetic defect may induce cretinism (see section on hypothyroidism and cretinism). By contrast, the clinical significance of nontoxic diffuse goiter in adults depends largely on its ability to achieve a state of euthyroidism, which is generally the rule. Rare patients are hypothyroid, and the TSH level is almost invariably elevated, as it may be to a lesser extent in marginally euthyroid individuals. The goitrous enlargement may be nonvisible, even with the head raised, or plainly evident. During the early stages of endemic goiter, administration of iodine brings about regression, but later it is without effect. An important aspect of the diffuse goiter is that it may become transformed into a nodular goiter.

MULTINODULAR GOITER

Nearly all long-standing simple goiters become transformed into multinodular goiters. They may be nontoxic or may induce thyrotoxicosis (toxic multinodular goiter), also called *Plummer's disease.* This condition differs from Graves' disease insofar as there is no associated ophthalmopathy or dermopathy, and the hypermetabolism is usually less severe. Rarely, multinodular goiters are associated with hypothyroidism. Whatever their functional state, *multinodular goiters produce the most extreme thyroid enlargements and are more frequently mistaken for neoplastic involvement than any other form of thyroid disease.* Because they derive from simple goiter, they occur in both sporadic and endemic forms, having the same female-to-male distribution and presumably the same origins but affecting older individuals because they are late complications. There is no understanding, however, of the basis of the transformation into the nodular pattern. Because normal thyroid cells are heterogeneous with respect to response to TSH and ability to replicate, the development of nodules may reflect clonal proliferation of cells having differing proliferative potentials.[21] It is further speculated that with such uneven follicular hyperplasia, generation of new follicles and uneven accumulation of colloid, tensions and stresses are produced that lead to rupture of follicles and vessels followed by hemorrhages, scarring, and sometimes calcifications. The scarring adds to the tensions, and in this cyclical manner nodularity appears. Moreover, the pre-existent stromal framework of the gland may more or less enclose areas of expanded parenchyma, contributing to the nodularity.[22]

MORPHOLOGY. The multinodular goiter is marked by its heterogeneity. **Typical features include (1) nodularity created by islands of colloid-filled or hyperplastic follicles, (2) random irregular scarring, (3) focal hemorrhages and hemosiderin deposition, (4) focal calcifications in areas of scarring, and (5) microcyst formations (Fig. 25–13).**

The goitrous enlargement may be monstrous and achieve a weight of more than 2000 gm. The pattern of enlargement is quite unpredictable and may involve one lobe far more than the other, producing lateral pressure on midline structures, such as the trachea and esophagus (Fig. 25–14). In other instances, the goiter grows behind the sternum and clavicles to produce the so-called **intrathoracic** or **plunging goiter.** Occasionally, most of it is hidden behind the trachea and esophagus, yet in other instances, one nodule may so stand out as to impart the clinical appearance of a solitary nodule. On cut section, there is an overall hetero-

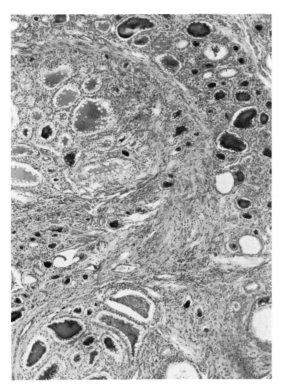

Figure 25–13. Multinodular goiter illustrating scarring and variation in size of follicles.

geneous multinodularity; some of the nodules are poorly circumscribed, but others appear to accumulate scarring and condensation of the thyroid stroma about themselves to create the appearance of complete encapsulation similar to that found in the true adenoma. Thus have arisen the misnomers **adenomatous goiter** and **multiple colloid adenomatous goiter** for this condition.

CLINICAL COURSE. From the clinical standpoint, multinodular goiters are of importance because of (1) size and location of the goitrous mass; (2) possible abnormal function, usually thyrotoxicosis; and (3) their differentiation from neoplasms. When sufficiently enlarged, the goiter may cause not only cosmetic disfigurement but also dysphagia, a choking sensation, and (with compression of the trachea) an inspiratory stridor. These manifestations are particularly prominent when the goiter enlarges into the thoracic inlet behind the sternum, sometimes inducing a superior vena caval syndrome, that is, distention of the veins of the neck and upper extremities, edema of the eyelids and conjunctiva, and syncope on coughing. Hemorrhages into the goiter may induce sudden painful enlargement, worsening the obstructive symptoms.

In fewer than half the patients, hyperfunction appears—toxic multinodular goiter. The thyrotoxicosis, when present, is in general moderate,

and cardiovascular manifestations tend to predominate, possibly because these goiters usually appear in older patients who are likely to have underlying heart disease. Thus, atrial fibrillation, tachycardia, and sometimes heart failure may be encountered. The radioactive iodine uptake and serum levels of T_3 and T_4 may be only slightly elevated. Scintiscans of the gland reveal one of two patterns: The radioiodine may accumulate in patchy foci throughout the gland or, less commonly, in only one or a few hyperfunctioning ("hot") nodules.

The differentiation of a multinodular goiter with a dominant nodule from a thyroid tumor may be difficult, both clinically and anatomically. Scintiscan, ultrasonography, CT, and MRI may be helpful in ruling out neoplasia by revealing hidden diffuse multinodularity, but often fine-needle aspiration is necessary. There is some evidence that these goiters increase the risk of developing cancer, but the data are not unequivocal.

TUMORS

Nodules in the thyroid have always commanded a great deal of attention because of the fear of their being cancerous. The estimated incidence of solitary palpable nodules in the adult population of the United States is about 2 to 4%; it is significantly higher in endemic goitrous regions. The female-to-male ratio is about 3 to 4:1. Most of these solitary masses prove to be dominant nodules within a multinodular goiter, cysts, or asymmetric enlargements of various non-neoplastic conditions, such as Hashimoto's thyroiditis. When such nodules prove to be neoplastic, in well over 90% of instances, they are adenomas. Thyroid cancer is rare, with an annual incidence in the United States of approximately 25 to 35 cases per million population. Moreover, as will be seen subsequently, most are indolent, permitting a 90% survival at 20 years. It is apparent then that thyroid carcinomas are uncommon clinical problems.

Despite all the epidemiologic data, a patient is not a statistic, and so every nodule demands careful appraisal. It is well beyond our scope to delve into the details of the clinical differential diagnosis, but a few points are noteworthy:

- A solitary nodule is more likely to be neoplastic than multiple nodules, for reasons that must be obvious.
- Functioning nodules that take up radioactive iodine and therefore appear "warm" or "hot" on scintiscans are more likely to be benign than malignant.
- The younger the patient (under the age of 40),

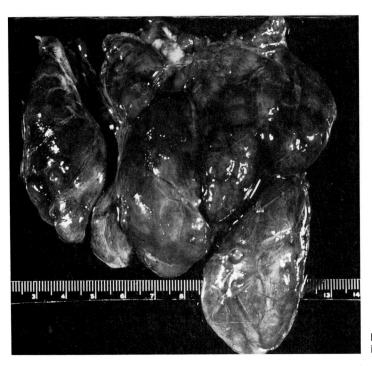

Figure 25-14. Completely distorted thyroid comprising a multinodular goiter.

the greater the likelihood of neoplasia because non-neoplastic nodularity, such as may be produced by Hashimoto's thyroiditis or multinodular goiter, tends to appear in older individuals.

• A nodule in a male is more ominous than one in a female because most non-neoplastic disorders are much more frequent in females.

Despite these generalizations and a rigorous clinical evaluation, it is frequently necessary to resort to morphologic diagnosis often based on fine-needle aspiration.[23] Using this diagnostic modality, false-positive errors are very uncommon in experienced hands. Two per cent to 15% of aspirates, however, are unsatisfactory for evaluation, and about 35% are indeterminate or read as "suspicious"; among these, 20% prove to be malignant on surgical excision.

ADENOMAS

Virtually all adenomas of the thyroid present as solitary, discrete masses. With rare exception, they all are derived from follicular epithelium and so might all be called *follicular adenomas*. Microscopically, a variety of patterns can be identified that recapitulate stages in the embryogenesis of the normal thyroid, and so they have been divided into fetal, embryonal, simple, and colloid subtypes or, more simply, into microfollicular and macrofollicular patterns. There is little virtue in these classifications because mixed patterns are common, and ultimately all have the same clinical and biologic

significance. Numerous studies have made it clear that adenomas are not forerunners of cancer except in the exceptional instance.

MORPHOLOGY. It is difficult, even morphologically, to differentiate an adenoma from a nodule in a multinodular goiter. In theory, the adenoma is completely encapsulated, has a homogeneous architecture within the capsule that differs from that outside of the capsule, and by its expansile growth compresses the surrounding non-neoplastic thyroid substance (Fig. 25–15). Non-neoplastic nodules, however, may fulfill these criteria.

Follicular adenomas average about 3 cm in diameter, but some are much larger (up to 10 cm in diameter) or smaller. Infrequently, two or even more are present. On cross-section, they range in color from tan to gray, are soft and fleshy, and appear to be discretely encapsulated. Sometimes there are foci of softening, hemorrhage, or central fibrosis, particularly in the larger adenomas. Even more rarely, there may be extensive central necrosis, virtually transforming the adenoma into a cyst.

Microscopically, the follicular architecture is well developed in many and poorly developed in some but is more or less uniform throughout the lesion. The various patterns tend to recapitulate the embryologic development of the thyroid gland (Fig. 25–16). Thus, **trabecular adenomas** are composed of closely packed cells forming cords or trabeculae of cells with only here and there small abortive follicles. Some have numerous small, well-developed follicles lined by flattened epithelial

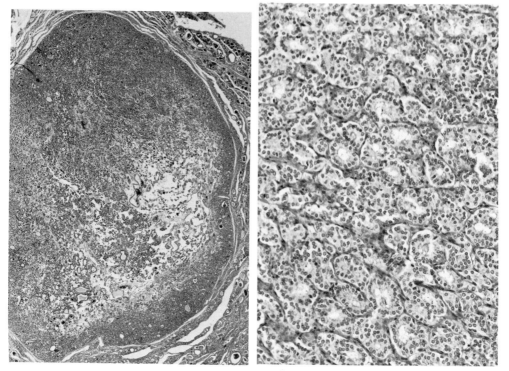

Figure 25-15.   Figure 25-16A.

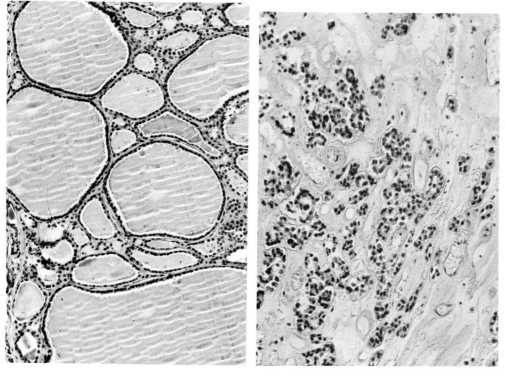

Figure 25-16B.   Figure 25-16C.

Figure 25-15. Low-power view of follicular adenoma of thyroid, illustrating discrete encapsulation and demarcation from surrounding thyroid substance.

Figure 25-16. A to C, Three types of follicular adenoma, illustrating variability in acinar size, colloid content, and amount of interstitial connective tissue. C represents the type formerly referred to as a fetal adenoma.

cells widely separated by an abundant loose myxoid stroma **(fetal adenomas)**. Others have follicles of normal size lined by cuboidal cells with scant interfollicular connective tissue. At the other extreme are lesions with large colloid-filled follicles lined by flattened epithelial cells **(colloid adenomas)**. Cytologically, the epithelial cells in all reveal little variation in cell and nuclear morphology. Occasionally, as noted, there are foci of hemorrhage, fibrosis, or calcification.

Several variations may appear. Infrequently, adenomas are composed of tightly packed spindle cells with some significant variation in cellular size and nuclear morphology. These have been variously called spindle cell adenomas or "atypical adenomas." The term "atypical," however, is generally reserved for follicular adenomas revealing some pleomorphism and variability in cell and nuclear size. This pleomorphism can be so marked that it verges on that seen in follicular carcinoma, to be described, and in all likelihood many atypical lesions represent well-differentiated follicular carcinomas.

Another rare variant is the Hürthle cell adenoma, composed of large, eosinophilic, granular cells identical to those encountered in various nonneoplastic thyroidal lesions (e.g., Hashimoto's thyroiditis). A final variation is the so-called papillary adenoma distinguished by papillary excrescences within large follicular or cystic spaces. The papillae may be large and branched and show some variation in cytologic morphology. According to most experts, such lesions are better considered as papillary carcinomas because identical tumors have invaded and metastasized.

CLINICAL SIGNIFICANCE. The principal importance of adenomas is their clinical differentiation from cancers, as has already been emphasized. In addition, they may (1) slowly increase in size to cause pressure symptoms in the neck, (2) achieve a certain size and then plateau, (3) suddenly enlarge and become painful owing to intralesional hemorrhages, and (4) rarely synthesize T_3 or T_4 and cause hyperthyroidism that is usually mild and unassociated with ophthalmopathy.

Most adenomas are "cold," but some, particularly those associated with hyperfunction, accumulate sufficient radioiodine to appear "warm" or "hot" on scintiscans. It is the "cold" nodules that evoke the most clinical concern because cancers are very infrequently functional. Although theoretically autonomous, an adenoma occasionally has some dependence on TSH and so can be induced to regress by the administration of thyroid hormones, which suppress TSH secretion. Finally, as has already been emphasized, the risk of malignant transformation is small to negligible.

OTHER BENIGN TUMORS

Solitary nodules of the thyroid gland may also prove to be cysts.[24] The great preponderance of these lesions represent cystic degeneration of a follicular adenoma; the remainder probably arise in multinodular goiters. They are often filled with a brown, turbid fluid containing blood, hemosiderin pigment, and cell debris. Additional benign rarities include dermoid cysts, lipomas, hemangiomas, and teratomas (seen mainly in infants).

MALIGNANT TUMORS

Thyroid cancers, as noted earlier, are uncommon in the United States; in 1991 they caused 1000 deaths, two-thirds among females, representing fewer than 1% of all cancer deaths. Almost all are carcinomas. Lymphomas and mesenchymal sarcomas are rarities. In middle age, thyroid carcinoma is two to three times more common in women than in men. Before puberty, there is no sex difference, and the female preponderance disappears in postmenopausal life. Possibly relevant is the fact that most well-differentiated thyroid carcinomas have estrogen receptors. The morphologic variants of thyroid carcinoma with their approximate frequencies are as follows:

- Papillary carcinoma—75 to 85%
- Follicular carcinoma—10 to 20%
- Medullary thyroid carcinoma—5%
- Anaplastic carcinoma—rare

Papillary carcinoma includes several major variants. These together with the well-differentiated forms of follicular carcinoma are referred to as well-differentiated tumors to distinguish them from all the other thyroid carcinomas, collectively referred to as poorly differentiated tumors. This subdivision is significant for two reasons: (1) Well-differentiated tumors represent 90 to 95% of all thyroid cancers, and (2) only about 9% of patients with these forms of thyroid cancer die of their disease, in contrast to poorly differentiated tumors, which include some of the most aggressive forms of malignancy in the body.

PATHOGENESIS. The incidence of thyroid cancer, particularly papillary carcinomas, has been steadily increasing for decades. Although part of the increasing incidence may be related to better case finding and improved reporting, some significant part is thought to represent the consequence of past practices of irradiation of the head and neck areas for many benign conditions, such as tonsillar or thymic enlargement, acne, and other skin disorders. *Irradiation during the first two decades of life is particularly carcinogenic to the thyroid.*[25] From 4 to 9% of irradiated infants have developed thyroid carcinoma after a mean latent period of 20 years. Almost 7% of Japanese survivors of the atomic bombs developed thyroid cancers. Fortunately, the doses of radiation employed in diagnostic x-ray films of the head and neck or with the use of radioisotopes in scintiscans, or even the larger doses used in the treatment of thyroid disease, have not proved tumorigenic. The only other known predisposition to thyroid cancer is certain (and only certain) forms of thyroid disease. Most clearly implicated is Hashimoto's thyroiditis with its increased risk of lymphoma and slightly increased risk of carcinoma, and possibly (but controversial) nontoxic nodular goiter.[26] Diffuse hyperplastic goiter is not implicated, and only rarely is an adenoma, as pointed out earlier.

Some insights have been gained into the possible genetic origins of papillary thyroid carcinoma. It is clear that all are monoclonal, and activation of a new oncogene named *PTC* (papillary thyroid carcinoma) has been identified in 20 to 30% of these tumors. *PTC* appears to be the product of the recombination of a tyrosine-kinase domain of the *RET* proto-oncogene on chromosome 10[27] with an uncharacterized gene to create the hybrid sequence *RET/PTC*. The *RET* proto-oncogene is also implicated in the genesis of medullary thyroid carcinoma and pheochromocytoma occurring in the familial MEN (multiple endocrine neoplasia) syndrome IIa, described later. Against this background we can turn to the various patterns.

Papillary Carcinoma

As noted earlier, this is the predominant form of thyroid cancer. These tumors may occur at any age but are found most often in the third to fifth decades, with a 2 to 3 : 1 female preponderance.

MORPHOLOGY. Because papillary carcinomas have a propensity for invading lymphatics, including those within the thyroid gland, they often appear as multifocal tumors, and regional lymph node metastases are present at the time of diagnosis in 50% of cases but only rarely (approximately 5%) more distant spread. When unifocal, they range in size from minute lesions, discovered incidentally in thyroid tissue removed for other reasons, to 7 to 10 cm in diameter. Indeed, tiny tumors less than 1 cm in diameter have been reported in up to one-third of routine postmortems.[28] Whether these "occult" lesions might have progressed or possibly regressed is unknown; but many must remain silent throughout life, or else clinically significant thyroid neoplasms would be much more common. Whatever their size, this form of thyroid carcinoma is rarely encapsulated but instead infiltrates surrounding thyroid parenchyma and rarely the perithyroidal soft tissues. On cross-section, these lesions are

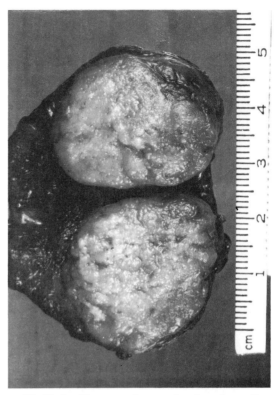

Figure 25–17. Papillary carcinoma showing deceptive apparent encapsulation. (Courtesy of Dr. Merle Legg, New England Deaconess Hospital, Boston.)

gray-white and firm and sometimes have foci of calcification or areas of cystic change (Fig. 25–17). Histologically, these neoplasms range from those that are predominantly papillary (about a third) to those that are in some part follicular in appearance (about 30%) to lesions having equal parts of papillary and follicular architecture. Whatever the distribution, all behave the same. Only the pure follicular carcinoma has a different behavior. All papillary carcinomas reveal some branching papillae having a fibrovascular stalk covered by a single to multiple layers of cuboidal epithelial cells (Fig. 25–18). In most neoplasms, the epithelium covering the papillae comprises very well-differentiated, uniform, orderly, cuboidal cells, but at the other extreme are those with fairly anaplastic epithelium showing considerable variation in cell and nuclear morphology. Nonetheless, the characteristic hallmarks of papillary neoplasms can be found in all:

• Hypochromatic "empty" nuclei devoid of nucleoli ("Orphan Annie eyes") (Fig. 25–19).
• Nuclear grooves.
• Eosinophilic intranuclear inclusions representing invaginations of cytoplasm.
• Psammoma bodies, usually within the cores of papillae, sometimes surrounded by calcific lamellations. These structures are almost never found in follicular and medullary carcinomas and so, when

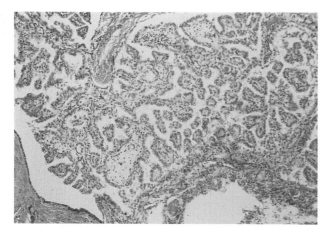

Figure 25–18. Papillary carcinoma. A low-power view showing the elaborately branching papillae.

present, are diagnostic of a papillary carcinoma. Indeed, it is said that whenever a psammoma body is found within a lymph node or perithyroidal tissues, a "hidden" papillary carcinoma must be suspected.

Other features sometimes present are areas of follicular architecture (described next); foci of squamous metaplasia; a prominent lymphocytic infiltrate, occasionally with germinal follicles; and areas of apparent ischemic necrosis leading sometimes to gross cystic change.

There are variant forms of papillary carcinoma that are important to recognize because despite their differences, they behave like the more usual lesions.

The **encapsulated variant** constitutes about 10% of all papillary neoplasms. It is usually confined to the thyroid gland, is well encapsulated, rarely presents with vascular or lymph node dissemination, and so in most cases has an excellent prognosis. Such lesions in the past have been called **papillary adenoma.**

The **follicular variant** has the characteristic nuclei of the papillary carcinoma but has an almost totally follicular architecture. Like most papillary cancers, they are unencapsulated and infiltrative. The true follicular carcinoma is usually encapsulated, frequently shows vascular and/or focal capsular invasion, and has a less favorable prognosis.

A **tall cell variant** is marked by tall columnar cells with intensely eosinophilic cytoplam covering the papillary structures and lining the follicular patterns. These tumors tend to be large with prominent vascular invasion and often are associated with local and distant metastases. They tend to occur in older individuals and have the poorest prognosis of all forms of papillary carcinoma. Because of their eosinophilic cytoplasm, they may be misdiagnosed as Hürthle cell tumors.

The additional variants of papillary carcinoma

are too uncommon to merit comment. Whatever the pattern of the papillary neoplasm, the great preponderance reveal thyroglobulin and sometimes T_3 and T_4 on immunostaining. Low-molecular-weight keratin is also frequently present.

Papillary carcinomas are the most frequent form of thyroid cancer, particularly in young individuals.[29] Uncommonly they produce mild or moderate degrees of thyrotoxicosis. These tumors would appear "warm" to "hot" on scintiscans. Most papillary lesions, however, are "cold" palpable masses. As noted frequently, there are cervical lymph node metastases at the time of diagnosis but rarely remote spread. The prognosis with these tumors is on the whole excellent, providing a 90% survival at 20 years. Favorable factors include (1) female sex, (2) under 20 years of age (providing an almost 100% curability, even with lymph node metastases), (3) confinement to the thyroid gland (especially important in older individuals), and (4) well-differentiated cytologic morphology. Larger, poorly differentiated lesions in older individuals, particularly in men, with extension beyond the thyroid yield only a 20% 10-year survival.

Follicular Carcinoma

These tumors account for about 10 to 20% of all thyroid cancers. They have a peak incidence in the fifth and sixth decades with a threefold female preponderance. The prevalence of these tumors has been increasing, particularly in areas of iodine deficiency, suggesting that goiters, particularly multinodular goiters, provide a soil for their origin.

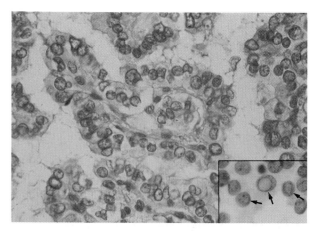

Figure 25–19. Papillary carcinoma. The cross-sections of several papillae covered by cuboidal epithelium having the characteristic "empty," "Orphan Annie eyes" nuclei. *Inset* shows a few cells with scant cytoplasm obtained on fine-needle aspiration having characteristic intranuclear inclusions. (Courtesy of Dr. Edmund Cibas, Brigham and Women's Hospital, Boston.)

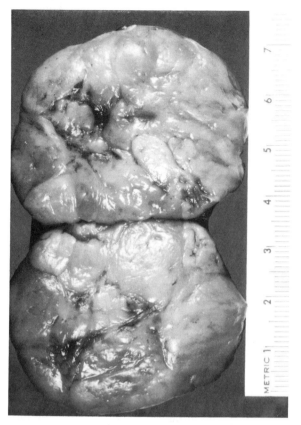

Figure 25-20. Cut surface of a follicular carcinoma with complete replacement of thyroid lobe. (Courtesy of Dr. Merle Legg, New England Deaconess Hospital, Boston.)

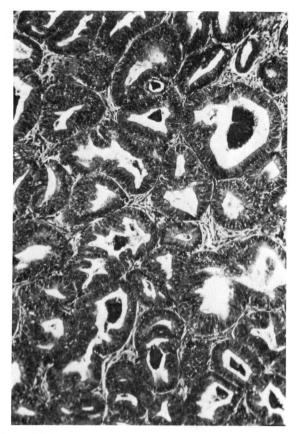

Figure 25-21. Follicular carcinoma of the thyroid. A few of the glandular lumina contain recognizable colloid.

MORPHOLOGY. Typically, follicular carcinomas are encapsulated tumors that are sometimes exceedingly difficult to differentiate from follicular adenomas. In some, penetration of the capsule is evident with moderate to massive infiltration of the thyroid (Fig. 25-20). They are gray to tan to pink on transection and, on occasion, are somewhat translucent when large, colloid-filled follicles are present. Central fibrosis and foci of calcification are often found.

Microscopically, follicular carcinomas vary considerably in their architecture, but whatever the pattern, the nuclei lack the features typical of papillary carcinoma, and psammoma bodies are not present. It is important to note the absence of these details because, as you recall, some papillary carcinomas, with their much better prognoses, may appear almost entirely follicular. Most often follicular carcinomas present a microfollicular architecture with relatively uniform, orderly, cuboidal cells lining the sometimes colloid-filled follicles (Fig. 25-21), creating more than a passing resemblance to thyroid architecture. Such lesions, when encapsulated, are easily misinterpreted as follicular adenomas or "atypical" adenomas, giving rise to the belief that adenomas sometimes become cancerous. These encapsulated tumors often reveal mi-croscopic invasion into the capsule and vascular invasion. Although they were at one time referred to as "angioinvasive" adenomas, it is now clear that they represent cancers (Fig. 25-22). Indeed, when both capsule and blood vessels are invaded, distant metastases are present in about half of the cases. With more evident extension through and beyond the capsule as well as vascular invasion, the metastatic rate approaches 75%.[30] Immunostaining sometimes reveals thyroglobulin and thyroid hormones in this pattern of carcinoma.

Less commonly, follicular carcinomas present trabecular architecture or solid sheets of polygonal to spindled cells, but abortive follicles can generally be found. The cells in these variants may be somewhat more variable in size and shape, but marked anaplasia is unusual. An additional variant is composed mostly or entirely of eosinophilic oxyphilic cells, which have abundant cytoplasm and relatively uniform, round to oval nuclei, closely simulating Hürthle cells. Despite the cytologic variability, all patterns of follicular carcinoma have the same biologic behavior. They have little propensity for invading lymphatics, and therefore regional lymph nodes are rarely involved, but vascular invasion is common, with spread to bone, lungs, liver, and elsewhere.

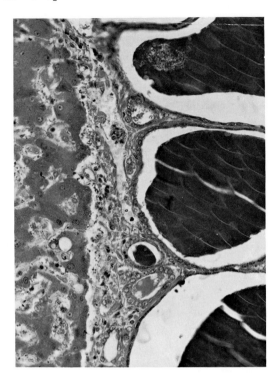

Figure 25-22. High-power detail of follicular carcinoma of thyroid that has metastasized to liver. Normal liver cells (left) can be seen in approximation to extremely well-differentiated cancer.

CLINICAL COURSE. Most follicular carcinomas present as slowly enlarging, painless thyroid nodules requiring differentiation from adenomas. At a later stage, the mass may appear somewhat irregular and multilobate. Metastases may or may not be evident at the time of diagnosis. The better differentiated lesions take up radioactive iodine and therefore may appear "warm" on scintiscan. The prognosis depends entirely on the size of the primary, the presence or absence of capsular and vascular invasion, and so some extent the level of anaplasia in the lesion. Encapsulated lesions without capsular or vascular invasion are amenable to total excision and cure, but sometimes metastases appear years after excision of the primary. Larger invasive cancers yield only a 30% survival at 5 years, which drops to 20% at 10 years. Because many of the well-differentiated lesions synthesize thyroglobulin, some palliation has been achieved by the administration of TSH followed by radioiodine.

Anaplastic Carcinoma

Fortunately, fewer than 5% of thyroid carcinomas fall into this category. They tend to occur in elderly individuals, particularly in endemic goitrous regions. There are basically three histologic patterns: (1) spindle cell carcinomas, (2) giant cell lesions, and (3) rarest of all the small cell carci-

noma. All grow quite rapidly and are usually large, bulky masses by the time they come to clinical attention. The spindle cell tumors often take on a sarcomatoid appearance. The giant cell lesions are the most anaplastic of malignant tumors afflicting humans. They are characterized by bizarre-shaped, giant, often multinucleated forms with numerous mitoses. The small cell variant may be difficult to distinguish from lymphomas or from metastases arising in the small cell bronchogenic carcinoma.

Infrequently, admixtures of papillary and follicular carcinoma are found in these anaplastic tumors, suggesting transformation of a better differentiated carcinoma into an anaplastic one. All tend to increase in size rapidly (over the span of months), metastasize widely, and prove fatal within a year unless controlled by some form of therapy. The cause of death is more often the consequence of local invasion of a major structure (e.g., the trachea) than the dissemination of the neoplasm.

Medullary Thyroid Carcinoma

Differing from all the previously described thyroid carcinomas, medullary thyroid carcinomas (MTCs) are neuroendocrine neoplasms of parafollicular (C) cell origin. As pointed out earlier, neuroendocrine cells are widely dispersed in the body and are capable of elaborating a variety of amine and polypeptide bioactive products. In the thyroid, neoplasms of these cells—MTC—have three distinctive features: (1) Most secrete calcitonin, which indeed constitutes a biochemical marker of these neoplasms; (2) many of these tumors have a distinctive amyloid stroma; and (3) about 20 to 25% occur in association with the MEN syndromes IIa and IIb. Uncommonly, these tumors may also occur in other familial patterns: familial MTC unassociated with other endocrine lesions, von Hippel–Lindau disease, and neurofibromatosis. In addition to calcitonin, MTC may elaborate a large variety of products, including somatostatin, prostaglandins, serotonin, ACTH, carcinoembryonic antigen, neuron-specific enolase, histaminase, and others. The amyloid stroma is believed to represent the deposition of modified calcitonin molecules.

Although the peak incidence of these sporadic tumors is in the fifth or sixth decade of life, in the MEN syndromes the MTC occurs in the third or fourth decade, and in the familial MTC pattern it occurs in elderly individuals.[31] The MEN IIa syndrome has now been ascribed to a germ line mutation in the RET proto-oncogene on the long arm of chromosome 10. You may recall that this oncogene is also involved in the origin of papillary thyroid carcinoma.

MORPHOLOGY. Grossly, two patterns can be discerned: (1) discrete tumors in one lobe or (2) nu-

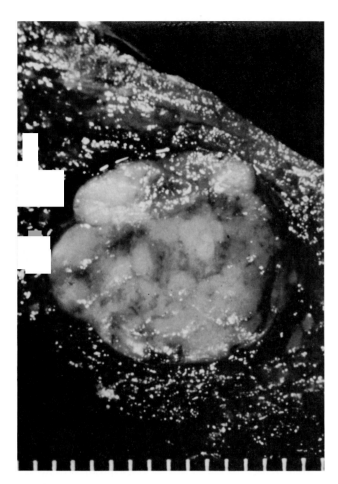

Figure 25-23. Medullary carcinoma of thyroid. These tumors typically show a solid pattern of growth and do not have connective tissue capsules.

merous nodules that usually involve both lobes. The sporadic neoplasms tend to originate in one lobe, and usually the other lobe of the thyroid gland is unaffected, although rarely it also harbors a similar tumor interpreted as a metastasis across the midline. The familial tumors, on the other hand, are commonly bilateral and multicentric early in their course. In both, the tumor tissue is usually firm, pale gray to tan, and infiltrative (Fig. 25-23). Frequently, there is spotty calcification and minimal to extensive fibrosis. There may also be foci of hemorrhage and necrosis in larger lesions. Histologically, whatever the setting, the tumor cells are usually polygonal or spindled and disposed in organoid nests separated by a scant to abundant fibrovascular stroma. In somewhat fewer than half of the cases, the stroma contains broad bands of amyloid that has the same histochemical and refractile properties as that of the amyloid found in other settings (Fig. 25-24). In some tumors, the neoplastic epithelial cells are disposed in trabecular or ribbon patterns, and in others there is apparent follicle formation. Infrequently, MTC reveals masses of cells

closely resembling those of intestinal carcinoids. A range of other histologic variations have also been described. Ultrastructural studies usually disclose, in all cytologic patterns, membrane-bound secretory granules that represent sites of storage of calcitonin and other elaborated products (Fig. 25-25). Multiple foci of C-cell hyperplasia occasionally accompany the neoplasm in familial cases but are rare in the sporadic tumors. It is hypothesized that the genetic abnormality underlying the familial syndromes leads to the hyperplasia of the C cells, and some subsequent event, involving one or more cells, leads to tumor formation.

CLINICAL COURSE. Sporadic MTC usually comes to the physician's attention as a thyroid mass, but occasionally the investigation of dysphagia, hoarseness, cough, or other local signs leads to its discovery. Uncommonly, some paraneoplastic syndrome associated with its secretory activity calls attention to the existence of the tumor (e.g., diarrhea attributable to calcitonin or possibly vasoactive intestinal

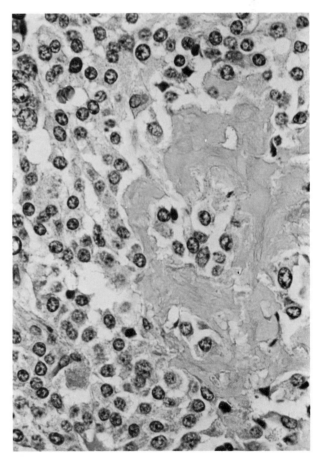

Figure 25-24. Medullary carcinoma with amyloid stroma. High-power detail revealing round-to-polygonal tumor cells with an abundant intercellular amyloidic stroma. (Courtesy of Drs. M. Warhol and L. Weiss, Department of Pathology, Brigham and Women's Hospital, Harvard Medical School, Boston.)

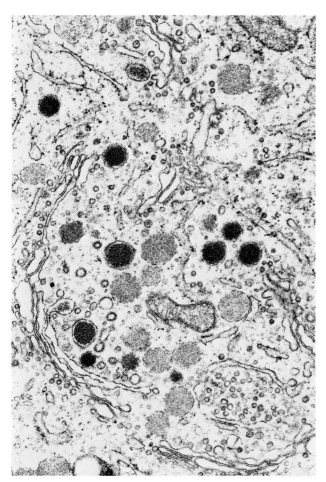

Figure 25–25. Electron micrograph of medullary thyroid carcinoma. These cells contain membrane-bound secretory granules that are the sites of storage of calcitonin and other peptides (30,000 ×).

polypeptide). By contrast, in the familial settings, MTC is usually asymptomatic when discovered and the diagnosis is established by screening family members of an affected patient for elevated levels of calcitonin, in some instances after the administration of provocative agents. The diagnostic problem is significantly increased when other secretory tumors are present in the polyendocrine syndromes (e.g., pheochromocytomas).

The aggressiveness of medullary carcinomas varies widely. In the familial medullary carcinoma syndrome, the tumors tend to be indolent, with a 10-year survival approaching 90%. On the other hand, those associated with MEN IIb are aggressive (as are the neoplasms that arise sporadically), with a 30 to 50% 10-year survival. Death is usually the consequence of lymphatic and hematogenous dissemination commonly to regional nodes, lung, liver, and bone.

MISCELLANEOUS LESIONS

This noncommittal heading is adopted to cover some congenital anomalies of the thyroid gland and sundry other involvements, some encountered in systemic diseases.

CONGENITAL ANOMALIES

Thyroglossal duct or *cyst* is the most common clinically significant congenital anomaly. A persistent sinus tract may remain as a vestigial remnant of the tubular development of the thyroid gland. Parts of this tube may be obliterated, leaving small segments to form cysts. These occur at any age and may not become evident until adult life. Mucinous, clear secretion may collect within these cysts to form either spherical masses or fusiform swellings, rarely over 2 to 3 cm in diameter. These are present in the midline of the neck anterior to the trachea. Segments of the duct and cysts that occur high in the neck are lined by stratified squamous epithelium, which is essentially identical with that covering the posterior portion of the tongue in the region of the foramen caecum. Those anomalies that occur in the lower neck more proximal to the thyroid gland are lined by epithelium resembling the thyroidal acinar epithelium. Characteristically, subjacent to the lining epithelium, there is an intense lymphocytic infiltrate. Superimposed infection may convert these lesions into abscess cavities, and rarely they give rise to cancers.

SYSTEMIC THYROIDAL CHANGES

Notable in this category are systemic amyloidosis, with deposits in the stromal connective tissue chiefly about vessels, and hemochromatosis, with the accumulation of hemosiderin pigment within thyroidal epithelium and within fibroblasts in the stroma. These involvements rarely produce functional abnormalities. The thyroid may be seeded by any blood-borne infection or disseminated disease, as pointed out in the consideration of thyroiditis. It is sometimes seeded by metastatic cancers, including lymphomas and leukemias. Necropsy studies have identified thyroid involvement in 4 to 24% of patients dying of disseminated cancer.[41]

Parathyroid Glands

PRIMARY
HYPERPARATHYROIDISM

SECONDARY
HYPERPARATHYROIDISM

HYPOPARATHYROIDISM

PSEUDOHYPOPARA-
THYROIDISM AND
PSEUDOPSEUDOHYPO-
PARATHYROIDISM

NORMAL

The four parathyroid glands, upper and lower pairs, are derived from the pharyngeal pouches, which also give rise to the thymus and other structures. Of surgical importance, about 10% of individuals have only two or three glands. In the adult, the parathyroid is a yellow-brown, ovoid, encapsulated nodule weighing approximately 35 to 40 mg. The superior glands are almost always located close to the upper posterior aspect of the thyroid, but the inferior glands are more footloose and may be found anywhere down to the deep recesses of the mediastinum.

In early infancy and childhood, the parathyroids are composed almost entirely of solid sheets of chief cells. The amount of stromal fat increases up to age 25, to reach a maximum of approximately 30% of the gland, and then it plateaus. The precise proportion of fat is determined largely by constitutional factors; fat individuals have fat glands and vice versa.

In adults, most of the glands are composed of *chief cells*, but these give rise to several transitional forms as will be evident subsequently. The chief cells vary from light to dark pink with hematoxylin and eosin stains, depending on their glycogen content. They are polygonal, 12 to 20 μm in diameter, and have central, round, uniform nuclei. In addition, they contain lipofuscin pigment and secretory granules of parathyroid hormone (PTH). Sometimes these cells have a *"water clear"* appearance owing to lakes of glycogen. *Oxyphil cells* and transitional oxyphils are found throughout the normal parathyroid either singly or in small clusters. They are slightly larger than the chief cells, have acidophilic cytoplasm, and are tightly packed with mitochondria. Glycogen granules are also present in these cells, but secretory granules are sparse or absent. The chief cell is the major source of PTH.

PTH, encoded by a gene mapped at chromosome 11p15, is rapidly released from chief cells whenever there is a fall in the serum ionic calcium level. Circulating PTH is an 84 amino acid linear polypeptide derived by sequential cleavage in the chief cell of a larger "pre-pro" form. Its biologic activity resides within the 34 residues at the amino terminus. Smaller nonfunctional fragments of the hormone, apparently lacking the critical amino-terminal domain, also circulate. These assume importance because, although they are biologically inert, they contain epitopes that react in certain radioimmunoassays for PTH.

The metabolic function of PTH in supporting the serum calcium level is complex but can be briefly summarized as follows:

1. PTH mobilizes calcium from bone.
2. It increases renal tubular reabsorption of calcium, thereby conserving it.
3. It promotes renal production of 1,25-$(OH)_2D_3$, active in intestinal absorption of calcium (see discussion of vitamin D in Chapter 9).
4. It lowers the serum phosphate level by enhancing phosphaturia.

PTH increases the resorption of bone, releasing calcium and phosphorus into the blood. At first it binds to specific receptors on osteoblasts, which in turn transmit some signal to osteoclasts, which lack receptors but are responsible for resorption of bone and mobilization of calcium.[32] The PTH membrane-receptor complex interacts with a membrane-bound G protein, leading to activation of adenylate cyclase and a "second" messenger. cAMP is the favored second messenger, but alternatively, calcium either alone or in concert with cAMP may serve as a second messenger, and there are also other possible candidates. Ultimately, the many actions of PTH on the cells and organs of the body all serve to support the serum calcium level whenever it falls below normal. In turn, PTH secretion is regulated by the plasma calcium level in a classic feedback loop. Understandably, then, any disorder leading to an excess of PTH induces hypercalcemia.

PATHOLOGY

The anatomic disorders of the parathyroid gland are best considered in relation to their effects on function, that is, hyperparathyroidism and hypoparathyroidism. The former can be further divided into primary hyperparathyroidism, which results from disorders intrinsic to the glands that produce autonomous hypersecretion of PTH leading to hypercalcemia and hypophosphatemia, and secondary hyperparathyroidism, also associated with excessive production of PTH but only as a response to some basic disease causing hypocalcemia or whenever there is some apparent insensitivity of the parathyroids to the serum calcium levels. The following discussion covers primary hyperparathyroidism, secondary hyperparathyroidism, hypoparathyroidism, and the uncommon pseudohypoparathyroidism.

PRIMARY HYPERPARATHYROIDISM

Primary hyperparathyroidism (PHPT) is characterized by some parathyroid lesion responsible for excessive secretion of PTH. The excess PTH has three major effects:

1. It increases bone resorption and calcium mobilization from the skeleton.

2. It increases renal tubular reabsorption and retention of calcium.

3. It increases renal synthesis of 1,25-$(OH)_2D_3$, thereby enhancing gastrointestinal calcium absorption.

The net effect is hypercalcemia. Although there are many other clinical causes of hypercalcemia, in more than 90% of cases, it either is related to hyperparathyroidism or is cancer-related. The frequency of the various parathyroid lesions underlying the hyperfunction is somewhat controversial, but the weight of opinion favors the following:

- Adenoma—75 to 80%
- Primary hyperplasia (diffuse or nodular)—10 to 15%
- Parathyroid carcinoma—less than 5%

The elevated serum calcium level has no effect on the autonomously functioning tumors, adenomas, and carcinomas, and with the primary hyperplasias, the glands continue to hyperfunction because of some apparent defect in the calcium receptor mechanism of chief cells normally involved in sensing the serum calcium levels.

The basis of hypercalcemia in association with a wide variety of nonendocrine cancers was discussed in Chapter 7, in the section on paraneoplastic syndromes. It will suffice here that two mechanisms appear to be involved. In one, there is

some paracrine effect of metastatic tumor cells by cytokines or other factors, producing local osteolysis. Principally implicated in this mechanism are breast carcinomas, multiple myeloma, and other hematologic cancers. The other mechanism of hypercalcemia involves apparent elaboration by cancers, not necessarily in contact with bone, of a humoral factor mobilizing calcium from the skeleton. Principally implicated in this mechanism are squamous cell carcinoma of the lung and renal, bladder, and ovarian carcinomas. The putative humoral factor has not been unequivocally identified, but currently most evidence points to a PTH-related peptide (PTHrP) having close homology with the normal hormone and capable of interacting with PTH receptors in vitro.[33] PTHrP is not simply a fragment of PTH because the gene for it is located on chromosome 12p12-11, whereas the gene encoding the normal hormone is, you recall, at chromosome 11. Whether such other humoral factors as prostaglandins, transforming growth factor-beta (TGF-β), and osteoclast-activating factor may also be involved has not yet been excluded.

With the widespread use of multiphasic testing, which includes determination of the serum calcium level, the diagnosis of hypercalcemia attributable to hyperparathyroidism has become much more common than it was 2 or 3 decades ago. The annual incidence is now estimated to be about 25 cases per 100,000 population in the United States and Europe with a 3:1 female preponderance. Most cases occur in the sixth to later decades of life. With current methods of detection, the great majority of cases of PHPT are asymptomatic when diagnosed or have only vague complaints of weakness, easy fatigability, and a wide variety of affective dysfunctions. In years past, PHPT came to attention because of "bone and stone" disease. The majority of patients had a variety of urinary complaints, mostly attributable to hypercalciuria and renal stone formation. Analogously, about one-third to one-half of patients had skeletal disease (osteitis fibrosa cystica) caused by prolonged osteoclastic hyperactivity. Renal stones and bone disease are now encountered in fewer than 10% of patients with PHPT.

Although the great majority of cases occur sporadically, uncommonly, you recall, the condition may appear in the familial MEN syndrome I or IIa. In these settings, the parathyroid disorder usually takes the form of diffuse or nodular hyperplasia, but rarely it appears to be an adenoma in MEN I. Homozygous loss of a putative suppressor gene on chromosome 11q11-13 can be demonstrated in most familial cases.[34] Significantly the same mutation has been found in about 25% of sporadic adenomas. There is evidence that loss of these genes permits expression of a novel cyclin possibly involved in cell replication. Against this background, we can turn to the parathyroid lesions underlying PHPT.

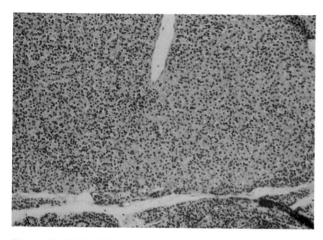

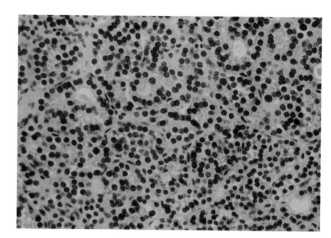

Figure 25–26. Solidly chief cell parathyroid adenoma (low-power view) revealing clear delineation from the residual gland below.

Figure 25–27. High-power detail of a chief cell parathyroid adenoma. There is some slight variation in nuclear size but no anaplasia and some slight tendency to follicular formation.

MORPHOLOGY. Adenomas. Almost always solitary, adenomas average 0.5 to 5.0 gm in weight but may be much larger. Although two may be present concomitantly in the same or different glands, nodular hyperplasia must always be ruled out when more than one adenoma is present; in fact, the morphologic differentiation is at best difficult and sometimes impossible. Theoretically in the adenoma, as contrasted with nodular hyperplasia, there is a distinct capsule about which a rim of residual normal parathyroid may be found possibly compressed by the expansile growth. Typically, there is little or no stromal fat within the adenoma, in contrast to the admixture of parathyroid cells and fat in the normal gland and scant fat cells in the hyperplastic gland. Finally, when a functional adenoma is present, the unaffected glands should be unenlarged and possibly suppressed and smaller than normal. Moreover, adenomas can be shown to be monoclonal, whereas hyperplasia is polyclonal.

For obscure reasons, most adenomas are located in the inferior glands. Perversely, they may also be found in such ectopic sites as within the thymus or thyroid, attached to the pericardium or behind the esophagus, and so may be exceedingly difficult to find surgically. They are well-encapsulated, soft, tan to red lesions. Most are composed predominantly of chief cells, but often they contain foci of oxyphil and transitional cells usually present as islands within a background of the chief cells (Fig. 25–26). Although characteristically the chief cells look quite normal, they may be slightly larger than usual with some variation in cell and nuclear size. Occasionally, binucleate forms can be found. The cells are disposed usually in sheets but, occasionally, in trabeculae or even in follicular patterns (Fig. 25–27). Although oxyphil cells are

traditionally thought to be nonfunctional, rarely a hyperfunctioning adenoma is composed of these cells. In larger lesions, there may be areas of infarct necrosis or hemorrhage.

Primary Hyperplasia. Primary hyperplasia may occur sporadically or in the MEN syndromes I and IIa. In all these settings, the anatomic changes are identical. Although classically all four glands are involved, frequently there is asymmetry, sometimes very marked, with apparent sparing of one or two of the glands. Glands that appear macroscopically normal, however, may reveal some evidence of hyperplasia on microscopic evaluation. The combined weight of all glands rarely exceeds 1.0 gm and often is less than 0.5 gm. The hyperplasia may be either diffuse or nodular and most often is composed predominantly of chief cells (Fig. 25–28) but sometimes water clear cells and, in almost all instances, islands or nodules of oxyphils. Poorly developed, delicate, fibrous strands may envelop the nodules. The cells in the diffuse hyperplasia or within the nodules are arranged in a wide variety of patterns—solid sheets, nests, trabeculae, or sometimes follicular structures. There is generally little variability in cell and nuclear size, but occasionally binucleate cells are encountered. One of the more distinctive features of primary hyperplasia is the dispersal of occasional fat cells throughout the hyperplastic areas, but overall the total amount of fat is reduced. The uneven involvement of the glands sometimes causes clinical difficulties because one or two dominantly enlarged glands may be removed in the mistaken belief that they harbor adenomas, only to have recurrence of the hyperfunction when the remaining hyperplastic glands become more active. Indeed, in a survey of a large number of cases of hyperplasia, only 7% of

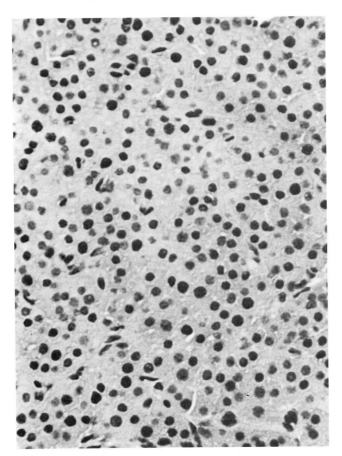

Figure 25–28. Marked chief cell hyperplasia of the parathyroid.

the patients had enlargement of all glands, and in almost half, only two glands were enlarged. This asymmetry is more typical of the nodular pattern than of the diffuse variety.[35]

Carcinoma. Fewer than 5% of cases of PHPT are caused by carcinomas. These tumors present as gray-white, irregular masses that sometimes exceed 10 gm in weight and enlarge usually one parathyroid gland. Many are small, however, and readily mistaken for an adenoma. Histologically, the neoplastic cells may be of variable size and shape but are usually remarkably uniform and not too dissimilar from normal parathyroid cells. They are disposed in nodular or trabecular patterns, although occasionally solid sheets are seen. Typically, there is a dense fibrous capsule enclosing most of the mass. **There is general agreement that a diagnosis of carcinoma based on cytologic detail is unreliable, and local invasion and metastasis constitute the only reliable criteria of malignancy.** Local recurrence occurs in about one-third of the cases, and more distant dissemination in another third. Survival for many years is the rule, however, and death results more often from the complications of hyperparathyroidism than from the spread of the disease.

CLINICAL COURSE. Classically, full-blown **PHPT** presents a diversity of clinical manifestations:

- *Renal*—recurrent nephrolithiasis, nephrocalcinosis
- *Skeletal*—osteitis fibrosa cystica or at least loss of bone mineral with osteoporosis
- *Gastrointestinal*—nausea, vomiting, peptic ulceration, pancreatitis
- *Cardiovascular*—headaches, lethargy, depression, loss of memory, seizures
- *Muscular*—generalized weakness
- *Other*—skin and eye changes

Recurrent nephrolithiasis (see Chapter 20) and osteitis fibrosa cystica (see Chapter 27) are now unusual, as was mentioned before. Indeed, about half of the cases are virtually asymptomatic when first seen except for vague complaints of lethargy, fatigability, and muscular weakness. The diagnosis is established by the demonstration of hypercalcemia and hypophosphatemia, often accompanied by increased urinary excretion of nephrogenous cAMP. PHPT is definitively diagnosed by an elevated immunoassay for PTH. Sometimes the astute clinician discovers PHPT in trying to understand intractable peptic ulceration or recurrent pancreatitis or in the investigation of hypertension. It should be cautioned, however, that there is still some uncertainty as to whether PHPT is causally associated with the hypertension because the elevated blood pressure improves in only about half of the patients after control of the parathyroid hyperfunction. Uncommonly, in long-standing PHPT, foci of metastatic calcification (see Chapter 1) are found, usually only at postmortem examination.

SECONDARY HYPERPARATHYROIDISM

This syndrome most often appears in patients with renal failure ("uremic hyperparathyroidism") but also with marked vitamin D deficiency or osteomalacia (see Chapter 9). The rare condition pseudohypoparathyroidism, characterized by a deficient response to PTH at the level of the end organ receptors, may also produce secondary hyperparathyroidism. The origin of hyperparathyroidism in renal failure is attributed to phosphate retention and hypocalcemia leading to compensatory parathyroid hyperfunction. In addition, the renal disease may contribute to the hypocalcemia by (1) a reduction in the synthesis of $1,25\text{-}(OH)_2D_3$ with impaired intestinal absorption of calcium and (2) some poorly understood state of skeletal resistance to the calcemic action of vitamin D and PTH. It should be noted, however, that uremic hyperparathyroidism may be observed in the absence of hypocalcemia. Similarly, vitamin D deficiency may

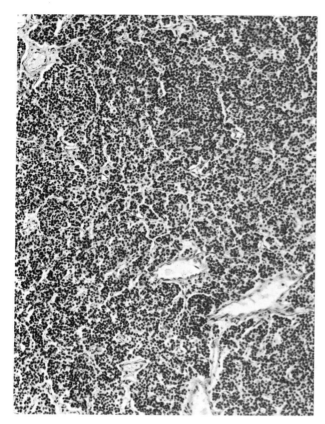

Figure 25–29. Diffuse secondary hyperplasia of parathyroid, illustrating extensive replacement of the normally contained fat.

directly stimulate PTH secretion. Whatever the precise mechanism, it is clear that patients with renal failure and rarely the other conditions mentioned develop secondary parathyroid hyperfunction with hyperplasia principally of the chief cells and most notably skeletal changes comprising a mixture of osteitis fibrosa cystica and osteomalacia, referred to as *renal osteodystrophy* (see Chapter 27). The other manifestations of parathyroid hyperfunction are less prominent than with PHPT.

MORPHOLOGY. The anatomic changes in secondary hyperparathyroidism mimic those of primary hyperplasia. Usually all glands are affected, but infrequently one, two, or even three may be spared. As with the primary disease, the hyperplasia may be diffuse or nodular and consist mainly of chief cells admixed with areas of water clear cells or oxyphil cells. The fat is usually reduced in amount or largely replaced by the hyperplastic cells (Fig. 25–29). As with the primary disease, metastatic calcifications may develop (see Chapter 1).

In many instances, the glands revert to normal if the basic clinical derangement is brought under control by, for example, renal transplantation. With long-standing secondary hyperplasia, however, reversion to normal may not occur, contributing to the possibility that *secondary hyperplasia may in time convert into autonomous adenoma formation, sometimes referred to as tertiary hyperparathyroidism.* Evidence suggests that this transition may involve an allelic loss on chromosome 11 similar to the genomic changes found in some sporadic primary adenomas.[36]

HYPOPARATHYROIDISM

Because hypoparathyroidism is largely a functional clinical disorder with few distinctive anatomic changes, the reader will be pleased to learn that relatively little will be said about it here. There are a large number of possible causes of deficient PTH secretion resulting in hypocalcemia. The major ones are as follows:

- *Surgically induced*—inadvertent removal of all glands during thyroidectomy; excision of the parathyroids in the mistaken belief that they are lymph nodes during radical neck dissection for some form of malignant disease; or removal of too large a proportion of parathyroid tissue in the treatment of PHPT, for example, removal of three glands in a patient lacking the normal complement of four glands
- *Congenital absence of all glands* as in DiGeorge's syndrome, described earlier.
- *Autoimmune disease* as occurs in the polyglandular-autoimmune syndrome with accompanying adrenal and ovarian failure, mucocutaneous candidiasis, and pernicious anemia
- *Sundry rare familial autosomal (dominant, recessive, and X-linked) and metabolic (hypomagnesemia) syndromes*

The clinical manifestations of hypoparathyroidism in these various settings may be exceedingly subtle and almost undecipherable without the documentation of hypocalcemia, but with more overt deficiency, the manifestations include the following:

- *Increased neuromuscular excitability* related to the decreased serum ionized calcium concentration. Classically, this is elicited with subclinical disease by tapping along the course of the facial nerve, which induces contractions of the muscles of the eye, mouth, or nose (Chvostek's sign). Alternatively, occluding the circulation to the forearm and hand by inflating a blood pressure cuff about the arm for several minutes induces carpal spasm within seconds, which disappears as soon as the cuff is deflated (Trousseau's sign). When the PTH deficiency becomes overt, tetany appears with muscle cramps, carpopedal spasms, laryngeal stridor, and convulsions.

- *Mental changes* ranging from irritability to depression to frank psychosis.
- *Intracranial changes*—calcifications in the basal ganglia and a parkinsonian-like syndrome. There may also be elevation of the CSF pressure and papilledema.
- *Calcification of the lens* leading to cataract formation.
- *Abnormalities in cardiac conduction*, mainly prolongation of the QT interval and T-wave changes and, rarely, heart block.

The diagnosis can be suspected by the finding of hypocalcemia but requires for confirmation markedly depressed or undetectable serum levels of PTH.

PSEUDOHYPOPARATHYROIDISM AND PSEUDOPSEUDOHYPO-PARATHYROIDISM

These rare conditions are mentioned only because, although poorly understood, they appear to involve some abnormality in the PTH-receptor complex interaction resulting in failure of responsiveness to the PTH. Hypocalcemia results, leading to secondary parathyroid hyperfunction, unanticipated elevated serum PTH levels, and a constellation of skeletal and other developmental abnormalities.

Adrenal Cortex

HYPERFUNCTION OF ADRENAL CORTEX (HYPERADRENALISM) CUSHING'S SYNDROME PRIMARY HYPERALDOSTERONISM	CONGENITAL ADRENAL HYPERPLASIA; ADRENOGENITAL SYNDROMES 21-Hydroxylase Deficiency HYPOFUNCTION OF ADRENAL CORTEX (HYPOADRENALISM)	PRIMARY ACUTE ADRENOCORTICAL INSUFFICIENCY WATERHOUSE-FRIDERICHSEN SYNDROME PRIMARY CHRONIC ADRENOCORTICAL INSUFFICIENCY (ADDISON'S DISEASE)	SECONDARY ADRENOCORTICAL INSUFFICIENCY NONFUNCTIONAL CORTICAL NEOPLASMS OTHER LESIONS OF THE ADRENAL

NORMAL

The adrenals, as you know, are composed of two totally separate functional units—a central compartment of catecholamine-producing medulla about which is wrapped the steroid-secreting cortex. This section deals only with disorders of the adrenal cortex. Later, those of the medulla will be considered. In the adult, the normal adrenal weighs about 4 gm, but with acute stress, lipid depletion may reduce the weight, or prolonged stress, such as dying after a long chronic illness, may induce hypertrophy and hyperplasia of the cortical cells and more than double the weight of the normal gland. Before birth, the cortex is composed largely of a wide fetal zone that, after birth, involutes and is replaced by the well-known three functional zones. Beneath the capsule is the narrow zona glomerulosa consisting of closely packed groups and clusters of cuboidal to columnar cells with darkly staining nuclei and scanty cytoplasm containing only scant lipid. An equally narrow zona reticularis abuts the medulla composed of aggregates of deeply acidophilic nonvacuolated ("compact" or "dark") cells devoid of apparent lipid but containing large accumulations of lipochrome pigment. Intervening is the broad zona fasciculata, which makes up about 75% of the total cortex. It is composed of radial cords or columns of polyhedral cells somewhat larger than those of the glomerulosa appearing somewhat paler ("clear cells") in routine tissue stain because of the microvacuolation of the cytoplasm. The fine vacuoles contain lipids, mostly cholesterol and cholesterol esters, but only small amounts of corticosteroids. When stimulated to elaborate steroids, the clear cells are transformed into compact cells as the stored cholesterol is depleted.

As you know, three major classes of steroids are elaborated in the cortex: the mineralocorticoids in the zona glomerulosa and the glucocorticoids and sex steroids in the inner two zones, which serve as a functional unit. Aldosterone accounts for

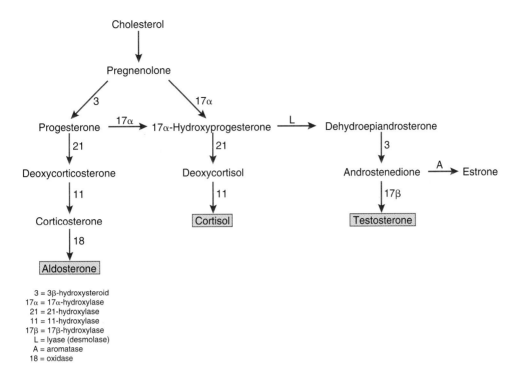

Figure 25-30. Normal adrenal steroid biosynthesis.

95% of the mineralocorticoid activity; its production is largely under the control of the serum renin-angiotensin and potassium levels and to a minor degree is modulated by ACTH. The major glucocorticoid is cortisol (commonly used synthetic analogues are cortisone, prednisone, and dexamethasone, the last two more potent than cortisol). The biosynthesis of cortisol is largely regulated by ACTH, itself regulated by hypothalamic CRH (see section on normal pituitary). In a classic feedback loop, the levels of ACTH released by the anterior pituitary are regulated by the circulating cortisol levels. It is hardly necessary here to review in detail the biosynthesis of the various steroids; a schema of the pathways and the enzymes involved is provided in Figure 25-30. A few details, however, merit emphasis because they are helpful in understanding the disorders of the adrenal cortex. It is evident that the biosynthesis of each of the three major classes of steroids begins with cholesterol and involves sequential transformations catalyzed by specific cortical enzymes. A functional deficiency of one of these enzymes may block a pathway and the synthesis of the end product, while channeling steroidogenesis into alternative pathways, as is exemplified by the adrenogenital syndrome (see later).

The clinical manifestations of most adrenal disorders can be interpreted in terms of their impact on the production of specific corticosteroids. *Corti-sol,* the principal glucocorticoid, as well as testosterone circulates in the blood largely bound to plasma proteins (a high-affinity, low-capacity globulin called cortisol-binding globulin or transcortin and low-affinity, high-capacity albumin). The small fraction of free unbound cortisol is physiologically active; freely enters target cells by diffusion; binds to a cytoplasmic, specific, high-affinity receptor protein; and is then translocated into the nucleus, where it binds to specific regulatory sequences in DNA (binding sites) to enhance transcription of specific glucocorticoid-responsive genes. As an ultimate consequence of these molecular actions, certain enzymes are activated, others inhibited, and nucleic acid synthesis in most cells inhibited, the totality of which has far-reaching implications on intermediary metabolism. Among the major effects are inhibition of glucose uptake in most tissues, predisposing to glucose intolerance, hyperglycemia, and diabetes mellitus.

Protein catabolism occurs in many tissues, not only affecting muscle mass and strength but also providing glycogenic amino acids for gluconeogenesis. Cortisol also reduces the reabsorption of calcium and phosphorus in the kidney; the wastage of these two minerals leads in time to osteoporosis. It causes selective lysis of T cells both in the peripheral blood and in peripheral lymphoid organs, impairing both cellular and humoral immunity. It also blocks transcription of cytokine genes and the elaboration of many macrophage factors involved in the inflammatory response, such as interleukin-1 (IL-1), IL-6, and tumor necrosis factor (TNF). Studies indicate that glucocorticoids also diminish endothelial cell expression of adhesion molecules ELAM-1 and ICAM-1, critical for neutrophil adhesion and emigration.[37] Thus, individuals on long-term cortisone or prednisone therapy are particularly vulnerable to microbiologic infections, such as tuberculosis, and have poor wound healing. Many of these actions are exemplified by some of the hyperadrenal disorders to be considered.

The major activity of *aldosterone* is restricted to the kidney. It is a major regulator of extracellular fluid volume and of potassium metabolism. In the kidney, aldosterone promotes reabsorption of sodium and excretion of potassium. Thus, excess aldosterone leads to sodium retention, an increase in the extracellular fluid volume, and a predisposition to hypertension. Simultaneously, hypokalemia appears. With a deficiency of aldosterone, the opposite changes are seen.

Testosterone, the major androgenic steroid, accentuates male characteristics and inhibits female characteristics. Thus, excesses of androgens lead to virilization in the female, manifested principally by hirsutism, acne, amenorrhea, clitoral enlargement, atrophy of the breasts and uterus, deepening of the voice, and receding hairline. Masculinization is difficult to detect in the man but can lead to precocious puberty in boys. Trace amounts of estrogens are also produced by cortical cells insufficient to have much physiologic effect, but in rare instances, neoplasms may elaborate sufficient quantities to induce feminization.

PATHOLOGY

Diseases of the adrenal cortex can be conveniently divided into those associated with cortical hyperfunction and steroid excess and those characterized by cortical hypofunction.[38] Two rare or incidental conditions that do not fit into either category merit only mention here. Developmental failures may lead to several subtypes of congenital adrenal hypoplasia producing hyperpigmentation and manifestations of adrenal failure in the newborn. One is autosomal recessive and the other X-linked recessive, the latter sometimes accompanied by Duchenne muscular dystrophy. Unless recognized promptly and treated with replacement steroid therapy, these syndromes can be rapidly fatal. The other slightly more common, but more trivial, developmental anomaly is the occurrence of ectopic nests or nodules of cortical cells (rarely with medullary cells) located in the great majority of instances in the kidney, testis, or ovary. These ectopic nodules rarely have clinical significance except when they cause a surface protrusion and are misinterpreted at surgical exploration or on a CT scan as a tumor or, once every million years, give rise to a neoplasm.

HYPERFUNCTION OF ADRENAL CORTEX (HYPERADRENALISM)

Just as there are three basic types of corticosteroids elaborated by the adrenal cortex—glucocorticoids, mineralocorticoids, and sex steroids—so there are three distinctive hyperadrenal clinical syndromes: (1) Cushing's syndrome, characterized by an excess of cortisol; (2) hyperaldosteronism; and (3) adrenogenital syndromes with an excess of androgens. Rarely a neoplasm is associated, predominantly with female sex steroids, and equally rarely mixed syndromes are encountered, for example, when both cortisol and androgens are produced in excess.

CUSHING'S SYNDROME

Cushing's syndrome is caused by a chronic excess of cortisol. The condition is then in essence "hypercortisolism." The major distinctive clinical and laboratory features are presented in Table 25–4. Most of these manifestations can be directly attributed to the excess cortisol, but some (e.g., hirsutism, acne, and menstrual abnormalities) probably reflect concomitant hypersecretion of androgens.

Table 25–4. MAJOR FEATURES OF CUSHING'S SYNDROME WITH APPROXIMATE FREQUENCY

CLINICAL FEATURES	PERCENTAGES
Central obesity (about trunk and upper back)	85–90
Moon facies	85
Weakness and fatigability	85
Hirsutism	75
Hypertension	75
Plethora	75
Glucose intolerance/diabetes	75/20
Osteoporosis	75
Neuropsychiatric abnormalities	75–80
Menstrual abnormalities	70
Skin striae (sides of lower abdomen)	50

PATHOGENESIS. There are four possible sources of excess cortisol. The most obvious and most common is prolonged administration of a glucocorticoid for therapeutic reasons, such as for immunosuppression following transplantation. The development of Cushing's syndrome under these circumstances is a calculated risk and is usually recognized early and aborted by modification of the therapy. The other three spontaneous sources of the hypercortisolism can be categorized as endogenous Cushing's syndrome:

- Pituitary hypersecretion of ACTH
- Ectopic production of ACTH or CRH by a nonendocrine neoplasm
- Hypersecretion of cortisol by an adrenal adenoma, carcinoma, or nodular hyperplasia—ACTH independent (Fig. 25–31)

Pituitary hypersecretion of ACTH accounts for 65 to 70% of cases of endogenous hypercortisolism. Usually there is a basophilic microadenoma, but sometimes a macroadenoma, and rarely a sparsely granulated chromophobic adenoma (see previous discussion of pituitary adenomas). Out of deference to the neurosurgeon who first published the full description of this syndrome and related it to a pituitary lesion, this pituitary form of Cushing's *syndrome* is referred to as Cushing's *disease.* In about 15% of the cases of Cushing's disease, no pituitary adenoma can be found but instead only corticotroph hyperplasia. Was an undiscovered microadenoma present in such cases? When the pituitary is hyperplastic in some cases of Cushing's disease, controversy persists as to whether the basic abnormality is hypothalamic "overdrive" with excess production of CRH. It may well be that this pathway may obtain in particular cases.[39] Whatever the primary condition, in Cushing's disease, *the adrenals are bilaterally hyperplastic, and in most cases, there are readily measurable elevated serum levels of ACTH.* This pattern of the condition is more common in females, 8:1, usually in young adult life.

"Ectopic" ACTH secretion by nonpituitary tumors accounts for about 10 to 15% of cases of endogenous Cushing's syndrome. Differentiation of this form of the disease from that of pituitary origin is difficult but usually can be accomplished by imaging and laboratory studies. Although theoretically any tumor might secrete ACTH, those most commonly associated are small cell carcinoma of the lung, carcinoids of the bronchus or pancreas, malignant thymoma, pheochromocytoma, medullary carcinoma of the thyroid, and gastrinomas. In addition, there are rare reports of ectopic secretion of corticotropin-releasing factor, which in turn leads to overproduction of ACTH.[40] As in the pituitary variant, the adrenal glands undergo bilateral cortical hyperplasia, but often the rapid downhill course of the patients with these cancers cuts short the adrenal enlargement. This variant of Cushing's syndrome is more common in men and usually occurs in the fifth and sixth decades of life.

Adrenal adenoma, carcinoma, and cortical hyperplasia are responsible for about 20 to 25% of cases of Cushing's syndrome. This pattern is ACTH independent because the adrenal lesion is directly responsible for autonomous hypersecretion of cortisol. Adenomas and carcinomas are about equally common in adults; in children, carcinomas predominate. Autonomous hyperplasia is uncommon, as will be detailed later. The cortical carcinomas tend to produce more marked hypercortisolism than the adenomas or hyperplastic processes. In those instances with a unilateral neoplasm, the uninvolved adrenal cortex and that in the opposite gland undergo atrophy because of suppression of ACTH secretion. Thus, *adrenal Cushing's syndrome is marked by elevated levels of cortisol but low serum levels of ACTH.*

MORPHOLOGY. The basic lesions of Cushing's syndrome are found in the pituitary and adrenal glands.

In the **pituitary,** regardless of the cause of Cushing's syndrome, increased levels of cortisol produce feedback effects on the nontumorous (and sometimes tumorous) corticotrophs, referred to as Crooke's **hyaline degeneration of the basophils.** Perinuclear or patchy foci of cytoplasm take on a basophilic hyalinization that obscures underlying details. Electron microscopy reveals that the hyaline is made up of aggregates of intermediate cytokeratin filaments (normally present in small numbers). In addition, in the pituitary variant of Cushing's syndrome, most often there is a basophilic microadenoma. Less often a basophilic macroadenoma, a sparsely granulated chromophobic adenoma, or diffuse hyperplasia of the corticotrophs is found. The last-mentioned variant—diffuse hyperplasia—is rare.

The **adrenals** have one of the following abnormalities: (1) diffuse hyperplasia; (2) nodular hyperplasia; (3) an adenoma, rarely a carcinoma, of the adrenal cortex; or (4) cortical atrophy, bilateral in cases of exogenous glucocorticoid administration, or in the uninvolved and contralateral gland when there is a functioning cortical neoplasm. **Diffuse hyperplasia** is found in 60 to 70% of cases of Cushing's syndrome. Both glands are enlarged, either subtly or markedly, and have rounded edges weighing up to 25 to 40 gm. The cortex is widened and composed predominantly of lipid-poor reticularis and inner fasciculata cells that are normal in size and appearance. **Nodular hyperplasia** accounts for about 15 to 20% of cases of Cushing's syndrome. The nodular hyperplasia takes the form of bilateral, 0.5- to 2.0-cm, yellow nodules scattered throughout the cortex, separated by intervening areas of widened cortex (Fig. 25–32). The

EXOGENOUS CUSHING'S SYNDROME (CS)

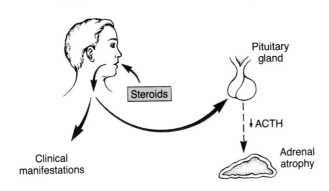

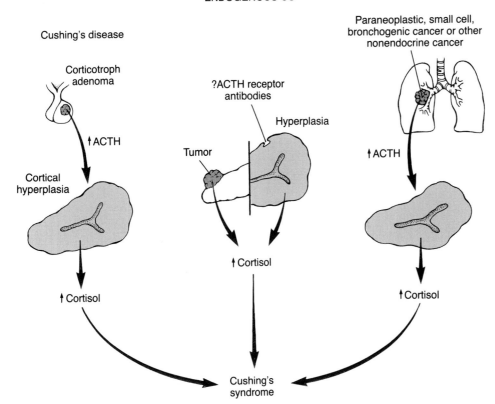

Figure 25–31. The exogenous and three endogenous pathogenetic pathways of Cushing's syndrome.

uninvolved cortex and nodules are composed of a mixture of lipid-laden and lipid-poor compact cells showing some variability in cell and nuclear size with occasional binucleate forms. The combined adrenals may weigh up to 30 to 50 gm. This macronodularity appears to be an extension of the diffuse hyperplasia because the cortex between the nodules exactly resembles that found in the diffuse form of this condition. Most cases of hyperplasia are associated with elevated serum levels of ACTH whether of adrenal or ectopic origin. Rarely when no increased level of ACTH can be found, autoantibodies to the ACTH receptors are suspected as the basis for the hyperplasia (as with Graves' disease). Uncommonly, more often in children but sometimes in adults, a **diffuse micronodular** hyperplasia is seen. This pattern is quite distinctive inasmuch as it may be unilateral, and the glands are not enlarged but are studded with multiple, small, dark brown to black pigmented nodules, hence the synonym "pigmented micronodular adrenal disease."[41] The cells within and between the nodules are small and compact and have little pleomorphism. Within the nodules, they contain a finely divided cytoplasmic pigment having some of the characteristics of lipofuscin and others of neuro-

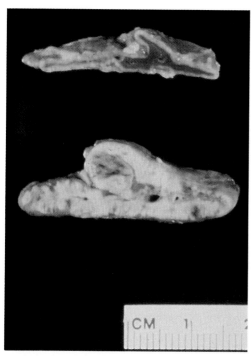

Figure 25-32. Cross-section of nodular hyperplasia contrasted with normal adrenal.

melanin. This form of micronodular hyperplasia is ACTH independent, in contrast to the macronodular variant. At least in some instances, the micronodular disease is familial and autosomal dominant.

Adenomas or carcinomas of the adrenal cortex as the source of cortisol secretion are not macroscopically distinctive from nonfunctioning adrenal neoplasms to be described. Both the benign and malignant lesions are more common in women in the fourth to sixth decades of life. The adenomas are surrounded by thin or well-developed capsules, and most weigh less than 30 gm (Fig. 25-33). Microscopically, they are composed of mixtures of lipid-rich and lipid-poor cortical cells with little variation in cell and nuclear size. Whether all of these lesions are true neoplasms or simply localized nodular proliferations remains uncertain. The carcinomas, by contrast, tend to be large, unencapsulated masses frequently exceeding 200 to 300 gm in weight, having all of the anaplastic characteristics of cancer, as will be detailed later. With both functioning benign and malignant tumors, such unaffected cortex as remains in the ipsilateral and contralateral glands reveals atrophic changes with shrinkage in width and shrinkage of the zona reticularis and fasciculata but sparing of the zona glomerulosa, which makes up most of the residual cortex.

CLINICAL COURSE. The classic clinical features of Cushing's syndrome, mentioned in Table 25-4, whatever the genesis, are fairly easily recognized. In addition, there is often increased bruisability and poor wound healing. The diagnosis is confirmed by the demonstration of increased cortisol production, elevated plasma levels of cortisol metabolites such as 17-hydroxycorticoid, or both. A major question, however, remains: Which variant of Cushing's syndrome is it, if effective therapy is to be instituted? It is beyond our scope to delve into the intriguing differential algorithm generally applied, except to point out that fundamental observations include the circulating level of ACTH and the ability of high doses of dexamethasone to suppress the levels of ACTH, as well as CT scans of the pituitary and adrenal regions for possible demonstrable neoplasms and ultrasonography of the adrenals. Sometimes sampling of the adrenal venous effluent on one or both sides is necessary. When the cause of the hypercortisolism can be corrected, as with an adrenal or pituitary adenoma, the prognosis is excellent. It is less favorable in many of the other variants.

Brief mention should be made of *Nelson's syndrome*, which represents enlargement of a pituitary adenoma in a patient with Cushing's disease whose adrenals have been removed. Sometimes there is also pituitary enlargement owing to corticotroph hypertrophy. The loss of the feedback inhibition of cortisol in the adrenalectomized patient underlies Nelson's syndrome. It is often accompanied by intense skin pigmentation presumably related to excess production of ACTH and closely related melanocyte-stimulating hormone peptides.

PRIMARY HYPERALDOSTERONISM

Primary hyperaldosteronism (PHA) is the generic term for a small group of closely related, uncommon syndromes, all characterized by chronic excess aldosterone secretion independent or virtually independent of the renin-angiotensin system. As you know, whenever there is some reason for increased production of renin-angiotensin, as may occur with renal ischemia or any chronic edematous state, there is a secondary rise in the aldosterone secretion, referred to as "secondary hyperaldosteronism" to differentiate it from the condition under consideration here. *PHA is characterized by suppression of plasma renin activity, hypokalemia, sodium retention, and hypertension.* The causes of PHA are as follows:

COMMON CAUSES

- A solitary aldosterone-secreting adenoma, also referred to as *Conn's syndrome*—approximately 65% of cases

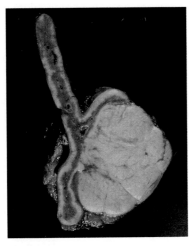

Figure 25–33. Gross view of adrenal adenoma in a case of Cushing's syndrome. The residual cortex is atrophic.

- Bilateral idiopathic hyperplasia of adrenals— approximately 30% of cases

UNCOMMON CAUSES

- Glucocorticoid-suppressible hyperaldosteronism
- Adrenal cortical carcinoma
- Familial nonglucocorticoid-suppressible variant
- Others

Collectively, all these causes of **PHA** can be found in only about 0.05 to 0.2% of all hypertensive patients.[42] The following discussion will be restricted to the two common causes and the glucocorticoid-suppressible variant, which is the most frequent of the uncommon causes (Fig. 25–34).

MORPHOLOGY. Aldosterone-producing adenomas are almost always solitary, small (less than 2 cm in diameter), encapsulated lesions, more often found on the left than on the right. They tend to occur in women more often than men in the fourth to fifth decades of life. They are often sufficiently buried within the gland not to produce visible enlargement, a point to be remembered when interpreting sonographic or scanning images. They are bright-yellow on cut section and, surprisingly, are composed of lipid-laden cortical cells more closely resembling fasciculata cells than glomerulosa cells (the normal source of aldosterone). Sometimes there are admixed smaller zona glomerulosa cells. In general, the cells tend to be uniform in size and shape and resemble mature cortical cells, but occasionally there is some nuclear and cellular pleomorphism but no evidence of anaplasia.

Bilateral idiopathic hyperplasia is marked by diffuse and focal hyperplasia of cells resembling those of the normal zona glomerulosa interspersed with small adrenocortical nodules composed of lipid-laden cells having the electron microscopic

features of normal zona fasciculata. These changes are highly reminiscent of those found in the nodular hyperplasia of Cushing's syndrome, suggesting prolonged exposure to an abnormal secretagogue of as yet unknown nature. Several potential candidates have been described, most of the evidence favoring a non-ACTH pituitary glycoprotein.[43]

Glucocorticoid-suppressible hyperaldosteronism is an uncommon cause of PHA that runs in families and appears to be the result of a mutation leading to some developmental derangement in the zonation of the adrenal cortex (which normally progresses from the capsule inward). As a result, hybrid cells appear in the interface between the zona glomerulosa and the zona fasciculata, which elaborate hybrid steroids in addition to both cortisol and aldosterone. The prolonged activation of aldosterone secretion appears to be under the continuous influence of ACTH and hence is suppressible by exogenous administration of dexamethasone.

CLINICAL COURSE. What makes the hypertension of **PHA** distinctive is the accompanying hypokalemia, which results from renal potassium wasting. In addition, there are a variety of neuromuscular manifestations, including weakness, paresthesias, visual disturbances, and occasionally frank tetany. Sodium retention increases the total body sodium and expands the extracellular fluid volume, leading to elevation of the serum sodium concentration and an increase in intracellular sodium with increased vascular reactivity. The hypertension is in some part a result of the sodium retention. The expanded extracellular fluid volume and hypokalemia both impose a burden on the heart, sometimes causing electrocardiographic changes and cardiac decompensation. The diagnosis of PHA is confirmed by the elevated levels of aldosterone and depressed levels of renin in the circulation. Even when the diagnosis of PHA is made (and sometimes the presentation is subtle), it is necessary to distinguish among the various causes, particularly the differentiation of an adenoma, which is amenable to surgical excision, and bilateral idiopathic hyperplasia, calling for medical therapy. Uncommon as PHA may be, it should not be overlooked clinically because it provides an opportunity to cure a form of hypertension.

CONGENITAL ADRENAL HYPERPLASIA; ADRENOGENITAL SYNDROMES

Disorders of sexual differentiation are uncommon and often difficult diagnostic problems. They take a variety of forms, some of which are her-

PRIMARY HYPERALDOSTERONISM

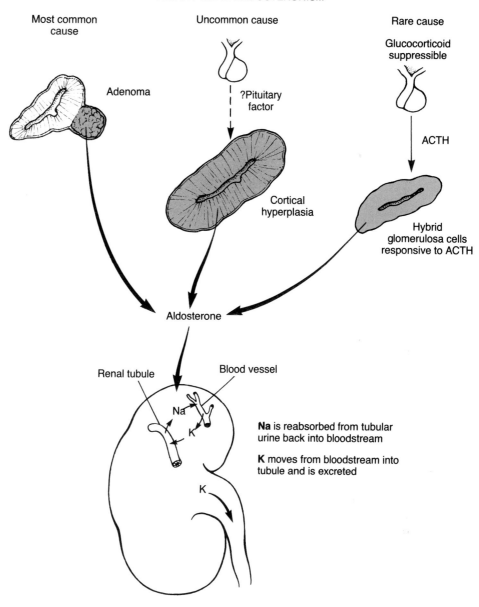

Most common
cause

Uncommon cause

Rare cause

Adenoma

?Pituitary
factor

Glucocorticoid
suppressible

ACTH

Cortical
hyperplasia

Hybrid
glomerulosa cells
responsive to ACTH

Aldosterone

Renal tubule   Blood vessel

Na

K

Na is reabsorbed from tubular
urine back into bloodstream

K moves from bloodstream into
tubule and is excreted

K

Figure 25–34. The major causes of primary hyperaldosteronism and its principal effects on the kidney.

maphroditism, pseudohermaphroditism, virilization in the female, and precocity in the male (see also Chapter 5). Gonadal disorders underlie some, but some are of adrenal origin.[44]

Adrenogenital syndrome, also called *adrenal virilism,* is quite uncommon and may be caused by an androgen-secreting adrenal carcinoma but may also be caused by a small group of congenital metabolic errors, each characterized by a deficiency or total lack of a particular enzyme involved in the biosynthesis of cortical steroids, particularly cortisol. Steroidogenesis is then channeled into other pathways leading to increased production of androgens, which accounts for the virilization.

Simultaneously, the deficiency of cortisol permits increased secretion of ACTH, resulting in adrenal hyperplasia. Certain enzyme defects may also impair aldosterone secretion, adding "salt wasting" to the virilizing syndrome. Other particular enzyme lacks may be incompatible with life or, in a rare instance, may involve only the aldosterone pathway without involving cortisol synthesis. Thus, there is a spectrum of these syndromes, and with each one there may be a total lack of a particular enzyme or a mutation that only mildly impairs the effectiveness of the enzyme. Figure 25–35 illustrates the consequence of a 21-hydroxylase deficiency, which alone accounts for about 85 to 90%

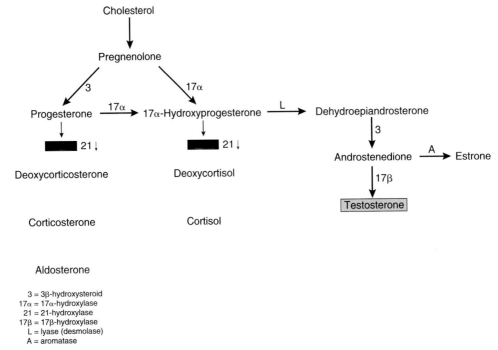

3 = 3β-hydroxysteroid
17α = 17α-hydroxylase
21 = 21-hydroxylase
17β = 17β-hydroxylase
L = lyase (desmolase)
A = aromatase

Figure 25-35. Diagram of steroid biosynthesis in adrenogenital syndrome with blocks induced by a lack of 21-hydroxylase.

of all cases of adrenal virilism. The following remarks are therefore confined to this disorder.

21-Hydroxylase Deficiency

21-Hydroxylase deficiency may range from a total lack to a mild loss, depending on the nature of the mutation.[45] Three distinctive syndromes have been segregated: (1) salt-wasting adrenogenitalism, (2) simple virilizing adrenogenitalism, and (3) nonclassic adrenogenitalism, which implies mild disease that may be entirely asymptomatic or associated only with symptoms of androgen excess during childhood or puberty.

The *salt-wasting syndrome* results from an inability to convert progesterone into deoxycorticosterone because of a total lack of the hydroxylase. Thus, there is virtually no synthesis of mineralocorticoids and concomitantly a block in the conversion of hydroxyprogesterone into deoxycortisol with deficient cortisol synthesis. This pattern usually comes to light because *in utero* the electrolytes and fluids can be maintained by the maternal kidneys, but soon after birth the salt wasting, hyponatremia, and hyperkalemia induce acidosis, hypotension, cardiovascular collapse, and possibly death. The concomitant block in cortisol synthesis and excess production of androgens, however, lead to virilization, which is easily recognized in the female at birth or indeed *in utero* but is difficult to recognize in the male. Various degrees of virilization are encountered, ranging from mild clitoral

enlargement to complete labioscrotal fusion to marked clitoral enlargement enclosing the urethra, thus producing a phalloid organ. Males with this disorder are generally unrecognized at birth but come to clinical attention 5 to 15 days later because of some salt-losing crisis.

Simple virilizing adrenogenital syndrome without salt wasting may appear with a less than total 21-hydroxylase defect because with less severe deficiencies the level of mineralocorticoid, although reduced, is sufficient for salt reabsorption, but the lowered glucocorticoid level fails to cause feedback inhibition of ACTH secretion. Thus, the level of aldosterone is mildly reduced, testosterone increased, and ACTH elevated, with resultant adrenal hyperplasia.

Nonclassic adrenal virilism is much more common than the "classic" patterns already described. These patients may be virtually asymptomatic or have mild manifestations. The diagnosis can be made only by demonstration of biosynthetic defects in steroidogenesis and by genetic studies, as will become evident subsequently.

All the adrenogenital syndromes are autosomal recessive disorders transmitted by a single gene located on chromosome 6p21.3 within the HLA (major histocompatibility) complex.[45] The various forms of deficiency are associated with specific haplotypes, and it appears, therefore, that there are multiple alleles at 6p21.3, with a range of mutations, accounting for the different phenotypes. Thus, HLA-A3;BW47;DR7 is associated with some of the cases of the classic salt-wasting or simple

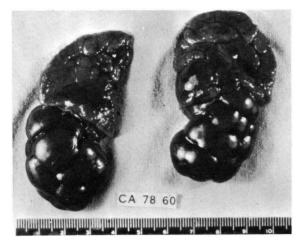

Figure 25–36. Adrenogenital syndrome in an infant with massive nodular enlargement of adrenals to the point at which they approximate the size of kidneys.

virilizing syndromes, but HLA-B14;DR1 is related to the nonclassic disease. Particular mutations affecting both the maternal and the paternal alleles account for various degrees of enzymatic compromise. The classic forms of 21-hydroxylase deficiency appear with homozygous inheritance of mutations that either prevent synthesis of the hydroxylase or code for a completely inactive enzyme. By contrast, the nonclassic disease might represent inheritance of one severe and one mild mutation or conceivably two mild mutations. Because a range of mutations may account for some compromise in the activity of the 21-hydroxylase, the nonclassic disease is much more common than the classic.

MORPHOLOGY. The defect in cortisol synthesis with consequent elevation of ACTH levels leads to bilateral adrenal hyperplasia, sometimes up to 10 to 15 times their normal weights (Fig. 25–36). On cut section, the widened cortex appears brown owing to total depletion of all lipid with widening of all zones, in particular the zona reticularis and the zona glomerulosa in the salt-wasting disorder. Small nodular formations may appear within the widened cortex. Despite the striking hyperplasia, cells appear relatively normal in size and shape. There is no evidence of significant pleomorphism.

HYPOFUNCTION OF ADRENAL CORTEX (HYPOADRENALISM)

Adrenocortical hypofunction may be caused by any anatomic or metabolic lesion of the cortex that impairs the output of cortical steroids, or it may be secondary to a deficiency of ACTH (Table 25–5). The clinicoanatomic patterns of adrenocortical insufficiency can be considered under the following headings: (1) primary acute adrenocortical insufficiency (adrenal crisis), (2) primary chronic adrenocortical insufficiency (Addison's disease), and (3) secondary adrenocortical insufficiency.

PRIMARY ACUTE ADRENOCORTICAL INSUFFICIENCY

Acute adrenocortical insufficiency is an uncommon clinical problem that may appear in a variety of settings, as follows:

• As a "crisis" in patients with chronic adrenocortical insufficiency precipitated by any form of stress that requires an immediate increase in steroid output from glands incapable of responding.
• From too rapid withdrawal of steroids from patients whose adrenals have been suppressed by long-term steroid administration, or from failure to increase the level of administered steroids during stress in a bilaterally adrenalectomized patient.
• As a result of some massive destruction of the adrenals.

  • In neonates, following prolonged and difficult delivery, with considerable trauma and hypoxia, leading to extensive adrenal hemorrhages beginning in the medulla and extending into the cortex. Newborns are particularly vulnerable because they are often deficient in prothrombin for at least several days after birth.
  • In postsurgical patients who develop disseminated intravascular coagulation (DIC) with consequent hemorrhagic infarction of the adrenals, potentiated by anticoagulation therapy.
  • When massive adrenal hemorrhage complicates a bacteremic infection, in this setting called the Waterhouse-Friderichsen (W-F) syndrome.

WATERHOUSE-FRIDERICHSEN SYNDROME

This uncommon but catastrophic syndrome is characterized by the following:

1. An overwhelming septicemic infection most often caused by meningococci but occasionally other highly virulent organisms, such as gonococci, pneumococci, or staphylococci
2. Rapidly progressive hypotension leading to shock

Table 25-5. ADRENOCORTICAL INSUFFICIENCY

PRIMARY INSUFFICIENCY	SECONDARY INSUFFICIENCY

Loss of cortex
  Idiopathic (autoimmune)
  Infection (mycobacteria, fungi)
  AIDS, opportunistic microbes
  Acute hemorrhagic necrosis (Waterhouse-Friderichsen
    syndrome)
  Amyloidosis
  Sarcoidosis, hemochromatosis
  Metastatic carcinoma
Metabolic failure in hormone production
  Congenital adrenal hypoplasia
  Drug- and steroid-induced inhibition of ACTH or cortical
    cell function
	Hypothalamic pituitary disease
	  Neoplasm, inflammation (sarcoidosis, tuberculosis, pyo-
	    gens, fungi)
	Hypothalamic pituitary suppression
	  Long-term steroid administration
	  Steroid-producing neoplasms

3. DIC with widespread purpura, particularly of the skin

4. Rapidly developing adrenocortical insufficiency associated with massive bilateral adrenal hemorrhage

The W-F syndrome may occur at any age but is somewhat more common in children. The basis for the adrenal hemorrhage is uncertain but could be attributable to direct bacterial seeding of small vessels in the adrenal, the development of DIC, endotoxin-induced vasculitis, or some form of hypersensitivity vasculitis. *Whatever the basis, the adrenals are converted to sacs of clotted blood virtually obscuring all underlying detail* (Fig. 25-37). Histologic examination reveals that the hemorrhage starts within the medulla in relationship to thin-walled venous sinusoids and then suffuses peripherally into the cortex, often leaving islands of recognizable cortical cells. Thus, there is continuing uncertainty as to whether the shock is related to adrenocortical insufficiency or to massive overwhelming infection. When recognized promptly and treated effectively with antibiotics, recovery is possible, but the clinical course is usually devastatingly abrupt, and short and prompt recognition and appropriate therapy must be instituted immediately or death follows within hours to a few days. The fact that administered steroids appear to be beneficial suggests that at least in some instances there is some element of adrenocortical insufficiency.

PRIMARY CHRONIC ADRENOCORTICAL INSUFFICIENCY (ADDISON'S DISEASE)

Addison's disease is a rare condition caused by any chronic destructive process in the adrenal cortex. Clinical manifestations appear insidiously at any age, more often in adults but not until at least 90% of the functioning cortical cells have been de-

stroyed. Although all races and both sexes may be affected, certain causes of Addison's disease (autoimmune adrenalitis) are much more common in whites, particularly in women.

ETIOLOGY AND PATHOGENESIS. A large number of diseases may attack the adrenal cortex, including

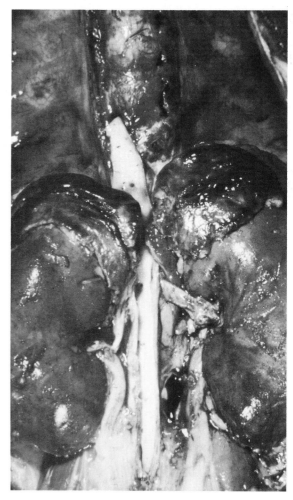

Figure 25-37. Waterhouse-Friderichsen syndrome in a child. The dark, hemorrhagic adrenal glands are distended with blood.

lymphomas, amyloidosis, sarcoidosis, hemochromatosis, fungal infections, and adrenal hemorrhages, but more than 90% of all cases are attributable to autoimmune adrenalitis, tuberculosis, or metastatic cancers.

Autoimmune adrenalitis alone is responsible for 60 to 70% of cases. In about half of these instances, the adrenal is the sole target of the autoimmune reaction, but in the remainder, other endocrine glands are concomitantly affected. These polyglandular syndromes have been subdivided into three types: Type I represents the combination of candidiasis, hypoparathyroidism, and adrenal insufficiency; type II is marked by coexistent adrenal and thyroid disease (Schmidt's syndrome) sometimes accompanied by insulin-dependent diabetes; and type III is a polyglandular disease but not with adrenal involvement. Type I affects males and females equally, but type II is three times more common in females than in males and usually in adult life.[46] Circulating antiadrenal antibodies are present in about half of the cases of autoimmune adrenalitis as well as other types of antibodies related to involvement of other organs or tissues. The basis for this autoimmune attack is obscure, just as in the case of Graves' disease, but there is a well-defined increased incidence of certain histocompatibility antigens in these patients, particularly HLA types B8 and DR3, suggesting some genetic predisposition.

Tuberculous adrenalitis was once the most common cause of Addison's disease. Now it accounts for 10 to 15% of cases in the United States but is much more frequent in other parts of the world. The adrenal involvement is almost always a dissemination from a primary disease elsewhere, most often the lungs but sometimes the genitourinary tract. With tuberculous adrenalitis, not only is the cortex involved, but also the medulla, resulting in loss not only of glucocorticoids but also mineralocorticoids and catecholamines. In passing, we should note that fungi may also rarely produce similar disease (e.g., histoplasmosis, coccidioidomycosis, and blastomycosis).

Metastatic cancer is a relatively uncommon cause of adrenocortical insufficiency because the tumorous infiltration of the glands, however massive, usually spares sufficient islands of tissue to permit marginal adrenal function. When metastases are responsible for Addison's disease, the glands are usually massively involved and may each weigh more than 100 to 200 gm. Common primaries spreading to the adrenal are bronchogenic, gastric, and breast carcinomas as well as malignant melanomas and lymphomas.

MORPHOLOGY. The anatomic changes in the adrenal glands of course depend on the underlying disease, but because nothing need be said about tuberculosis and metastatic tumors, further remarks

will be limited to the autoimmune adrenalitis. Typically, the glands are smaller than normal and may be reduced to leaf-like structures difficult to find at postmortem. Histologically, there is diffuse atrophy of all zones with small, shrunken, lipid-sparse cells having abundant cytoplasmic lipofuscin. Around and between the cells there is a diffuse, extensive infiltration of lymphocytes admixed with plasma cells and macrophages (Fig. 25–38). The adrenal medulla is unaffected. The lymphocytic infiltration differentiates this form of atrophy from that seen in other conditions.

CLINICAL COURSE. Addison's disease begins insidiously and does not come to attention until at least 90% of the cortex of both glands is destroyed, and the levels of circulating glucocorticoids and mineralocorticoids are significantly lowered. Major manifestations, when they appear, are weakness, fatigability, anorexia, nausea and vomiting, weight loss, hypotension, and hyperpigmentation of the skin,

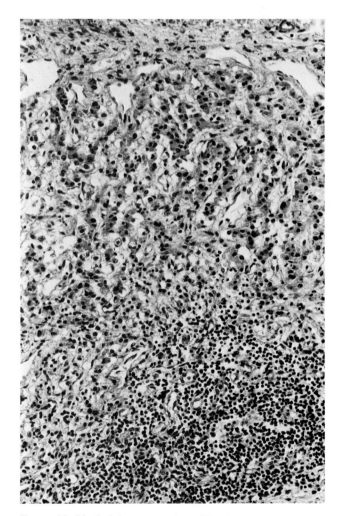

Figure 25–38. Autoimmune adrenalitis. In addition to loss of all but a subcapsular rim of cortical cells, there is an extensive mononuclear cell infiltrate.

particularly of sun-exposed areas and at pressure points, such as the neck, elbows, knees, and knuckles. Less consistently present are diarrhea, constipation, salt craving, and ill-defined abdominal pain that sometimes mimics an "acute abdomen." Blood pressure is generally subnormal and may be associated with postural dizziness. Classically, the serum levels of sodium, chloride, bicarbonate, and glucose are below normal as well as the plasma cortisol and urinary steroid excretory products, such as 17-ketosteroids and 17-hydroxycorticoids. The serum potassium level is elevated largely because of aldosterone deficiency, and there is salt wasting, lowered circulating blood volume, and hypotension. In primary adrenocortical insufficiency, the circulating ACTH levels are elevated. Often, however, especially with milder disease, the laboratory values may be within the normal range. Confirmation of the diagnosis can be achieved by stimulating ACTH secretion and determining whether the adrenals are capable of responding. With Addison's disease, there is little or no cortex to respond.

Although this condition is readily managed by steroids, death may occur in the untreated patient because of acute adrenal insufficiency superimposed on the chronic condition, hyperkalemic cardiac arrhythmias, or a hypoglycemic cerebral crisis (Addisonian crisis). Any of these complications may be precipitated, in the already fragile metabolic state, by stress, such as an intercurrent illness.

SECONDARY ADRENOCORTICAL INSUFFICIENCY

Any disorder of the hypothalamus and pituitary, such as metastatic cancer, infection, infarction, or irradiation, that reduces the output of ACTH leads to a syndrome of hypoadrenalism having many similarities to Addison's disease. Analogously, prolonged administration of exogenous glucocorticoids suppresses the output of ACTH and adrenal function. *With secondary disease, the hyperpigmentation of primary Addison's disease is lacking because melanotropic hormone levels are low.* The manifestations also differ inasmuch as secondary hypoadrenalism is characterized by deficient cortisol and androgen output but normal or near-normal aldosterone synthesis. Thus, in adrenal insufficiency secondary to pituitary malfunction, there is no marked hyponatremia and hyperkalemia, although a liberal intake of water may induce dilutional lowering of the serum sodium level.

ACTH deficiency may occur alone, but in some instances, it is only one part of panhypopituitarism, associated with multiple primary tropic hormone deficiencies. The differentiation of secondary disease from Addison's disease can be confirmed with demonstration of low levels of plasma ACTH in the former. In patients with primary disease, the destruction of the adrenal cortex does not permit a response to exogenously administered ACTH in the form of increased plasma levels of cortisol, whereas in those with secondary hypofunction, there is a prompt rise in plasma cortisol levels.

Depending on the extent of ACTH lack, the adrenals may be moderately to markedly reduced in size. They may come to have a leaf-like appearance and, indeed, be extremely difficult to find in the periadrenal fat. The cortex may be reduced to a thin ribbon having an unusually heavy fibrous capsule and scattered subcapsular cortical cells composed largely of zona glomerulosa. The medulla is unaffected.

NONFUNCTIONAL CORTICAL NEOPLASMS

It is evident from preceding sections that the proliferative lesions of the adrenal cortex range from diffuse hyperplasia to nodular hyperplasia to benign and malignant tumors and that all these proliferative processes may be associated with steroidogenesis. In addition, there are nonfunctional benign and malignant tumors of the adrenal cortex.[47]

Usually, nonfunctional **adenomas** are poorly encapsulated masses of yellow-orange adrenocortical tissue ranging up to 2.5 cm in diameter. Some nestle within the adrenal cortex, others appear to be within the medulla, and still others protrude under the capsule. Some may achieve a larger size and exhibit areas of hemorrhage, cystic degeneration, and calcification. The encapsulation may be poorly defined and may appear at places to be deficient. In contrast to functional adenomas, which are associated with atrophy of the adjacent cortex, the cortex adjacent to nonfunctional adenomas is of normal thickness.

Some **cortical carcinomas** may not be associated with the biosynthesis of steroid hormones. These tumors are highly malignant and usually large when discovered, many exceeding 20 cm in diameter. On cut section, they are predominantly yellow but frequently have hemorrhagic, cystic, and necrotic areas (Fig. 25–39). Many appear to be more or less encapsulated. Histologically, they range from lesions showing mild degrees of atypia to wildly anaplastic neoplasms composed of monstrous giant cells (Fig. 25–40). Between these extremes are found cancers with moderate degrees of anaplasia, some predominantly composed of spindle cells. Carcinomas, particularly those of bronchogenic origin, may metastasize to the adre-

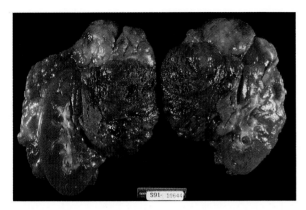

Figure 25-39. Adrenal carcinoma. The bright yellow tumor dwarfs the kidney and compresses the upper pole. It is largely hemorrhagic and necrotic.

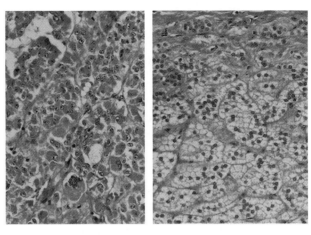

Figure 25-40. Adrenal carcinoma *(left)* revealing marked anaplasia, contrasted with normal cortical cells *(right)*.

nals, and they may be extremely difficult to differentiate from primary cortical carcinomas.

Adrenal cancers have a strong tendency to invade the adrenal vein, vena cava, and lymphatics. Metastases to regional and periaortic nodes are common as well as distant hematogenous spread to the lungs and other viscera. Bone metastases are unusual.

OTHER LESIONS OF THE ADRENAL

Adrenal cysts are relatively uncommon lesions; however, with the use of sophisticated abdominal imaging techniques, the frequency of these lesions appears to be increasing. The larger cysts may produce an abdominal mass and flank pain. It should be remembered that both cortical and medullary neoplasms may undergo necrosis and cystic degeneration and may present as "nonfunctional" cysts.

The adrenal myelolipoma is an unusual lesion composed of mature fat and hematopoietic cells. Although most of these lesions represent incidental findings, occasional myelolipomas may reach massive proportions. Foci of myelolipomatous change may be seen in cortical tumors and in adrenals with cortical hyperplasia.

Adrenal Medulla

PHEOCHROMOCYTOMA
TUMORS OF EXTRA-
  ADRENAL
  PARAGANGLIA

NORMAL

The adrenal medulla is composed of specialized neural crest (neuroendocrine) cells; it is, as you know, enveloped by the adrenal cortex. It is the major source of catecholamines—epinephrine, norepinephrine, dopamine—in the body. The neurosecretory cells are round to oval, have prominent cytoplasmic membrane–bound granules of stored catecholamines, and are supported by a richly vascularized scant stroma of spindled and sustentacular cells. Because the secretary cells are a part of the neuroendocrine system, they are also capable of synthesizing a wide variety of bioactive amines and peptides, such as histamine, serotonin, renin, chromogranin A, and neuropeptide hormones. When fixed in dichromate solutions (e.g., Zenker's), the cytoplasmic granules appear brown as a result of oxidation and polymerization of the stored catecholamines (the chromaffin reaction). It should be cautioned, however, that although neuroendocrine cells, in a tumor for example, may yield a positive chromaffin reaction, it does not necessarily indicate that the stored catecholamines are being released, and so a positive reaction does not necessarily imply a secretory function.

There is also a widely dispersed extra-adrenal system of clusters and nodules of similar neuroendocrine cells, which together with the adrenal medulla make up the paraganglion system. These extra-adrenal paraganglia are closely associated with the autonomic nervous system and can be divided into three groups based on their anatomic distribution: (1) branchiomeric, (2) intravagal, and (3) aorticosympathetic (Fig. 25–41). The branchiomeric and intravagal paraganglia associated with the parasympathetic system are located close to the major arteries and cranial nerves of the head and neck and include the carotid bodies (see Chapter 16). The intravagal paraganglia, as the term implies, are distributed along the vagus nerve. The aorticosympathetic chain is found in association with segmental ganglia of the sympathetic system and therefore is distributed mainly alongside of the abdominal aorta. The notorious organs of Zuckerkandl, close to the aortic bifurcation, belong to this group. The visceral paraganglia, as the term implies, are located within organs such as the urinary bladder. Histologically, all of the paraganglia are composed of cells closely resembling those of the adrenal medulla. Although many are functional, some are nonfunctional, and there is poor correspondence between the chromaffin reaction and the level of catecholamine release. Certain of the branchiomeric paraganglia, the carotid bodies in particular, are chemoreceptors capable of monitoring the oxygen and carbon dioxide levels in the blood.

Norepinephrine functions as a local neurotransmitter, chiefly of sympathetic postganglionic neurons. Only small amounts reach the circulation. Epinephrine (adrenaline) is secreted into the vascular system. It interacts with alpha-adrenergic and beta-adrenergic effector cells, membrane-bound specific receptors, which then activate second messengers and a cascade of enzymatic reactions mediating the systemic actions of epinephrine, for example, increasing the force and rate of myocardial contractions and causing vasoconstriction of most vascular beds. The principal metabolites of the catecholamines are metanephrine, normetanephrine, vanillylmandelic acid (VMA), and homovanillic acid (HVA).

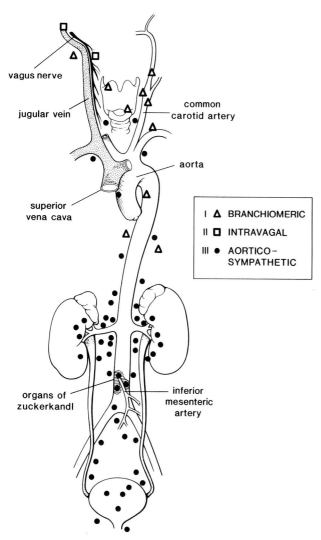

Figure 25–41. Schematic representation of paraganglion system demonstrates sites of paraganglion cell nests, in which neoplasms may form. Extra-adrenal portion of paraganglion system is grouped into three families based on anatomic distribution, innervation, and microscopic structure: (1) branchiomeric, (2) intravagal, and (3) aorticosympathetic. (With permission from Whalen, R.K., et al.: Extra-adrenal pheochromocytoma. J. Urol. 147:1–10, 1992; © Williams & Wilkins, 1992.)

In the figure, labeled: vagus nerve, jugular vein, superior vena cava, organs of zuckerkandl, common carotid artery, aorta, inferior mesenteric artery. Legend: I △ BRANCHIOMERIC, II □ INTRAVAGAL, III ● AORTICO-SYMPATHETIC

PATHOLOGY

Most significant disorders arising in the medulla are neoplasms. As might be expected from the cell types indigenous to the paraganglion system, the tumors include pheochromocytomas, neuroblastomas, ganglioneuromas, and variants of these neoplasms. Only the first requires description here (neuroblastomas and ganglioneuromas; Chapter 10).

PHEOCHROMOCYTOMA

This uncommon neoplasm is of great interest because despite its rarity, it is associated with cate-

Table 25-6. FAMILIAL SYNDROMES WITH PHEOCHROMOCYTOMA

SYNDROME	COMPONENTS
MEN, type II or IIA	Medullary thyroid carcinomas and C cell hyperplasia
	Pheochromocytomas and adrenal medullary hyperplasia
	Parathyroid hyperplasia
MEN, type III or IIB	Medullary thyroid carcinomas and C cell hyperplasia
	Pheochromocytomas and adrenal medullary hyperplasia
	Mucosal neuromas
	Marfanoid features
von Hippel-Lindau	Renal, hepatic, pancreatic, and epididymal cysts
	Renal cell carcinomas
	Pheochromocytomas
	Angiomatosis
	Cerebellar hemangioblastomas
von Recklinghausen	Neurofibromatosis
	Café au lait skin spots
	Schwannomas, meningiomas, gliomas
	Pheochromocytomas
Sturge-Weber	Cavernous hemangiomas of fifth cranial nerve distribution
	Pheochromocytomas

Modified with permission from Silverman, M.L., and Lee, A.K.: Anatomy and pathology of the adrenal glands. Urol. Clin. North Am. 16:417, 1989.

cholamine-induced hypertension that can be cured by excision of the neoplasm. Although only about 0.1 to 0.3% of hypertensive patients have an underlying pheochromocytoma, the hypertension can be fatal when the pheochromocytoma goes unrecognized. Occasionally, one of these tumors produces other biogenic steroids or peptides and so may be associated with Cushing's syndrome or some other endocrinopathy.

About 85% of pheochromocytomas arise in the medulla of the adrenals, the remainder in any of the extra-adrenal paraganglia, more often below the diaphragm. Extra-adrenal tumors that are chromaffin-negative are sometimes called paragangliomas to differentiate them from functioning pheochromocytomas. Although 90% of pheochromocytomas occur sporadically, about 10% occur in one of the several, mostly autosomal dominant, familial syndromes listed in Table 25-6. About 14% of individuals with von Hippel–Lindau disease develop pheochromocytomas.[48] The familial MEN syndrome IIa (described more fully later) is characterized by mutations of the *RET* proto-oncogene on chromosome 10, and this mutant gene can be found in the pheochromocytomas and medullary thyroid carcinomas occurring in this syndrome.

Although the nonfamilial pheochromocytomas most often occur in adults between 40 and 60 years of age, with a slight female preponderance, in the familial syndromes many arise in childhood, with a strong male preponderance. Most tumors in the familial syndromes are bilateral (70%), but in the nonfamilial setting only 10 to 15% are bilateral. Another highly significant difference is that 2 to 10% of adrenal pheochromocytomas—but 20 to 40% of extra-adrenal tumors—are malignant.

MORPHOLOGY. In the MEN syndromes, the adrenal medullary involvement may take the form of diffuse or nodular hyperplasia, sometimes accompanied by one or more discrete neoplasms. There is the suggestion, then, that the pheochromocytomas arise through a sequence of diffuse hyperplasia, nodular hyperplasia, and, finally, an overt neoplasm in this setting. Significantly, occasional intramedullary tumors are associated with diffuse hyperplasia in the opposite medulla.

The average weight of a pheochromocytoma is 100 gm, but variations from just over 1 gm to almost 4000 gm have been recorded.[49] The larger tumors are well demarcated by either connective tissue or compressed cortical or medullary tissue. Fibrous trabeculae, richly vascularized, pass into the tumor and produce a lobular pattern. In many tumors, remnants of the adrenal gland can be seen, stretched over the surface or attached at one pole. On section, the cut surface has a pale gray or brown color, and areas of hemorrhage, necrosis, or cyst formation can be observed, particularly in the larger lesions (Fig. 25-42). When a suitable dichromate fixative (Zenker's or Helly's solution) is used, the tumor turns brown-black owing to oxidation of stored catecholamines, hence, the term chromaffin.

The cytologic patterns in pheochromocytomas are quite variable.[49] The tumors are composed of mature-appearing medullary cells that possess an

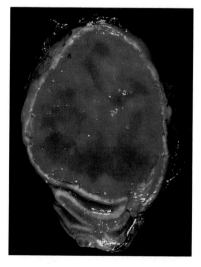

Figure 25-42. The gray-pink pheochromocytoma with areas of hemorrhage is enclosed within an attenuated cortex. The comma-shaped residual adrenal is seen below.

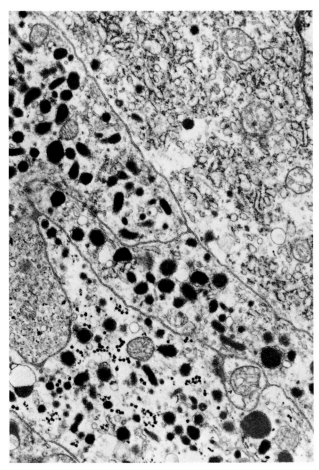

Figure 25–43. Electron micrograph of pheochromocytoma. This tumor contains membrane-bound secretory granules in which catecholamines are stored (30,000 ×).

cytomas may have an identical histologic appearance, the only absolute criterion of malignancy is metastasis. Local invasion is unreliable. Metastases occur most frequently to the related lymph nodes, liver, lungs, and bones, and survival after such spread rarely exceeds 3 years.

CLINICAL COURSE. *The dominant clinical feature in patients with pheochromocytoma is hypertension.* About one-third of patients have sustained hypertension rendered distinctive by paroxysmal attacks. In another third, the hypertension is intermittent; in the remaining third, it is sustained without paroxysms. The paroxysms may be precipitated by emotional stress, exercise, changes in posture, and palpation in the region of the tumor. The elevations of pressure are induced by the sudden release of catecholamines that may acutely precipitate congestive heart failure, pulmonary edema, myocardial infarction, ventricular fibrillation, cerebral hemorrhage, and even death. The cardiac complications are attributable, at least in some instances, to what has been called *catecholamine cardiomyopathy* or *catecholamine heart muscle disease.* The myocardial changes have been attributed to ischemic damage secondary to the catecholamine-induced vasomotor constriction of the myocardial circulation or to direct toxicity. Histologically, there are focal areas of myocytolysis and occasionally myofiber necrosis and interstitial fibrosis, sometimes with mononuclear inflammatory infiltrates. These cardiac lesions are often superimposed on hypertensive changes or alterations incident to coronary artery disease, and so, not surprisingly, patients may have anginal chest pain.

abundant basophilic cytoplasm bearing secretory granules, best seen in dichromate-fixed tissue or with the electron microscope (Fig. 25–43). Uncommonly, the dominant cell type is spindle cell or small cell. The functional activity of a neoplasm cannot be judged by the abundance of granules, as noted earlier. The cells are arranged either in large trabeculae, punctuated by thin-walled sinusoids often lined by the tumor cells themselves, or in small alveoli enclosed within a fibrovascular stroma derived from the tumor capsule (Fig. 25–44). Various patterns may be found in any one tumor. Cellular and nuclear pleomorphism is often present, especially in the alveolar group of lesions, and giant and bizarre cells are commonly seen. Mitotic figures are rare; moreover, they do not imply malignancy. Occasionally, tumor cells can be found lying in the capillaries or sinusoids. This is not indicative of malignancy because it has been observed in tumors that are benign in their behavior. **Because malignant and benign pheochromo-**

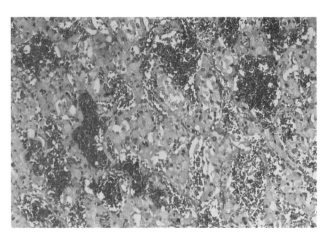

Figure 25–44. A highly vascularized field. The tumor cells have abundant cytoplasm and small central nuclei and are separated into clusters by slender fibrovascular septa.

The sudden release of catecholamines may provoke a number of other symptoms during or following the paroxysm, including headache, sweating, anxiety or fear of impending death, tremor, fatigue, nausea and vomiting, abdominal pain, and visual disturbances. These findings in combination with the hypertension, particularly if paroxysmal, point strongly to the appropriate diagnosis.[50] Measurement of urinary catecholamines and their metabolites, principally metanephrine and VMA, is necessary to confirm it. Once the diagnosis is made, localization can usually be reliably accomplished by CT or MRI scan or ultrasonography because most tumors are larger than 2 cm.

TUMORS OF EXTRA-ADRENAL PARAGANGLIA

There is considerable confusion in the literature regarding the terminology of these tumors. Some experts refer to them simply as paragangliomas. Others refer to the functioning neoplasms as extra-adrenal pheochromocytomas and restrict the term paraganglioma to the nonfunctioning tumors.[51] To add to the confusion, those arising in the carotid (carotid body tumors; see Chapter 16) and jugulotympanic bodies are sometimes referred to as "chemodectomas" because these paraganglia sense the oxygen and carbon dioxide levels of the blood. Despite the infrequency and small size of paragan-

gliomas, they are of great clinical importance because from 10 to 40% are malignant and recur after resection, and overall about 10% metastasize widely, causing death.

They are very uncommon and occur about one-tenth as frequently as adrenal pheochromocytomas. Most are discovered in the second and third decades of life, with no significant sex predisposition. They are, however, much more often multicentric (15 to 25% of cases) than adrenal tumors.

MORPHOLOGY. Typically, they range from 1 to 6 cm in diameter and are firm and tan-red. Despite encapsulation, well developed or scant, they are often densely adherent to adjacent vessels and difficult to excise. Histologically, they are composed of well-differentiated neuroendocrine cells with indistinct outlines, so they may give the appearance of syncytia. The cells are disposed typically in small clusters (*zellballen*) or cords separated by prominent fibrovascular stroma. Some tumors completely mimic the appearance of adrenal pheochromocytomas. Distinctive within the cells in most tumors are dark neurosecretory granules that contain catecholamines. Sometimes the cells are spindle shaped. Mitoses are usually infrequent, but occasional tumors are overtly anaplastic and pleomorphic and contain numerous mitoses. The malignancy rates (up to 40%) for paraganglion tumors are significantly higher than those for adrenal pheochromocytomas. The more anaplastic lesions may disseminate widely and cause death.

Thymus

DEVELOPMENTAL
  DISORDERS
THYMIC HYPERPLASIA
THYMOMAS

NORMAL

Once an organ buried in obscurity within the mediastinum, the thymus has risen to a star role in cell-mediated immunity, as detailed in Chapter 6. Here our interest centers on the disorders of the gland itself.

The thymus is embryologically derived from the third and, inconstantly, the fourth pair of pharyngeal pouches along with the lower pair of parathyroid glands. Not surprisingly, one or two parathyroids occasionally become enclosed within the thymic capsule, an aberrance that may plague the parathyroid surgeon. At birth, the thymus weighs 10 to 35 gm and continues to grow in size until puberty, when it achieves a maximum weight of 20 to 50 gm. Thereafter, it undergoes progressive atrophy to little more than 5 to 15 gm in the elderly. This age-related involution is accompanied by replacement of the thymic parenchyma by fibrofatty tissue. The rate of thymic growth in the child and involution in the adult is extremely variable, and so it is difficult to determine weight appropriate for age.

The fully developed thymus is pyramid shaped, well encapsulated, and composed of two fused lobes. Fibrous extensions of the capsule divide each lobe into numerous lobules, each of which has an outer cortical layer enclosing the central medulla. A diversity of cell types populate the thymus, but thymic epithelial cells and lymphocytes of T-cell lineage predominate. Directly beneath the capsule, the epithelial cells are closely packed, but deeper in the cortex and medulla, they create a structural lattice containing lymphocytes. In the cortex, they have an abundant cytoplasm and pale vesicular nuclei with finely divided chromatin and only small nucleoli; cytoplasmic extensions interconnect with adjacent cells. In contrast, the epithelial cells in the medulla have only scant cytoplasm devoid of interconnecting processes; are more oval in shape; and may be "spindled" with oval, darkly staining nuclei. Whorls of these cells create the well-known *Hassall's corpuscles* having keratinized cores.

As you know from the earlier consideration of the thymus in relation to immunity (see Chapter 6), stem cells of marrow origin migrate to the thymus and there give rise to T cells. Peripherally, in the lobules there is a fairly narrowly defined layer of prothymocyte lymphoblasts that give rise to the more mature thymocytes (T cells) found in the cortex and medulla. Most of the thymocytes in the cortex are small, compact lymphocytes bearing CD1, CD2, and CD3 markers as well as CD4 and CD8. The medulla harbors relatively fewer lymphocytes, but they resemble those found in the peripheral circulation and so are slightly larger than the cortical lymphocytes and by surface markers can be divided mainly into CD4+ (T4) and CD8+ (T8) lymphocytes as well as some precursors. In addition, macrophages, dendritic cells, and rare neutrophils, eosinophils, B lymphocytes, and scattered myoid (muscle-like) cells may be found within the thymus. The myoid cells are of particular interest because, as will be seen subsequently, the thymus in some obscure manner is related to myasthenia gravis, a musculoskeletal disorder of apparent immune origin.

PATHOLOGY

Morphologic lesions in the thymus are associated with a variety of systemic conditions ranging from immunologic to hematologic to neoplastic.

Fortunately, the changes within the thymus itself are of relatively limited nature and can be adequately considered under the following headings: (1) developmental disorders, (2) thymic hyperplasia, and (3) thymomas. The changes associated with myasthenia gravis are considered in Chapter 28.

DEVELOPMENTAL DISORDERS

Thymic hypoplasia or *aplasia* is seen in DiGeorge syndrome accompanied by parathyroid developmental failures. As detailed in Chapter 6, this condition is marked by a total absence or severe lack of cell-mediated immunity and often hypoparathyroidism. Developmental defects may also involve the heart and great vessels as well as other sites.

Thymic cysts are uncommon lesions that are usually discovered incidentally at postmortem or at surgery. They are probably developmental in origin, rarely exceed 4 cm in diameter, may be spherical or arborizing, and are lined by stratified to columnar epithelium. The fluid contents may be serous to mucinous and are often modified by hemorrhage, recent or old. Cysts rarely distort the contour of the thymus itself and are without clinical significance.

THYMIC HYPERPLASIA

The term thymic hyperplasia in reality applies to the appearance of lymphoid follicles within the thymus, creating what is referred to as *thymic follicular hyperplasia*. The gland may not appear enlarged, but admittedly it is nearly impossible to judge normal size and weight of the thymus because of the vagaries of aging atrophy and fatty involution. The lymphoid follicles are not different from those encountered in lymph nodes, have germinal centers, and contain both dendritic reticular cells and B lymphocytes, which, you recall, are present in scant numbers in the normal thymus (Fig. 25–45). Although follicular hyperplasia may occur in chronic inflammatory and immunologic states, it is most frequently encountered in myasthenia gravis and is present in about 65 to 75% of these cases. In this neuromuscular disorder, autoantibodies to acetylcholine receptors impair transmission of impulses across the myoneural junctions. Conceivably, follicular hyperplasia involving B cells participates in the formation of these autoantibodies. Similar thymic changes are sometimes encountered in Graves' disease, systemic lupus erythematosus, systemic sclerosis, and rheumatoid arthritis as well as other autoimmune disorders. A few scattered follicles, however, are sometimes discovered in the thymus of patients dying of completely unrelated conditions, and so the diagnosis

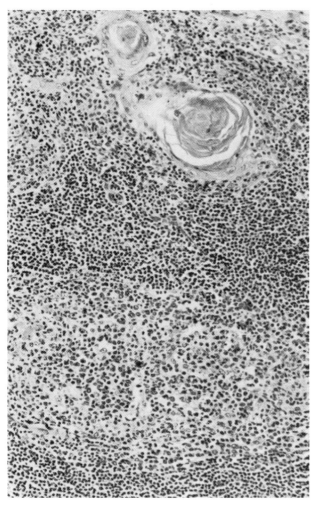

Figure 25-45. Thymic lymphoid hyperplasia in a patient with myasthenia gravis. A Hassall's corpuscle is seen in the upper portion of the illustration. A lymphoid follicle is present in the lower portion.

of follicular hyperplasia requires that the involvement be diffuse.

THYMOMAS

A diversity of neoplasms may arise in the thymus —germ cell tumors, lymphomas, Hodgkin's disease, and carcinoids as well as others—but *the designation "thymoma" should be restricted to tumors of thymic epithelial cells.* Such tumors typically have in addition a scant or rich background of lymphocytes (thymocytes), but this population of cells is secondary, not monoclonal, not tumorous, and therefore does not contribute to the biology or clinical behavior of these neoplasms.

Thymomas have been classified and reclassified in an effort to create subsets of clinical and prognostic usefulness. No effort will be made here to present these varied classifications; we shall re-

sort to one that has the virtues of simplicity and clinical usefulness. According to this approach, thymomas can be divided into the following categories:

- Benign thymoma—cytologically and biologically benign
- Malignant thymoma

  - Type I—cytologically benign but biologically aggressive and capable of local invasion and, rarely, distant spread
  - Type II, also called "thymic carcinoma"—cytologically malignant with all of the features of cancer and comparable behavior

All categories, benign and malignant, are tumors of adults, usually older than 40 years of age, and are rare in children. Males and females are affected equally. Most arise in the anterior, superior mediastinum but sometimes in the neck, thyroid, pulmonary hilus, or elsewhere. They are uncommon in the posterior mediastinum. They account for only 20 to 30% of tumors in the antero-superior mediastinum because this is also a common location for nodular sclerosing Hodgkin's disease as well as lymphomas.

MORPHOLOGY. Macroscopically, thymomas are lobulated, firm, gray-white masses up to 15 to 20 cm in longest dimension. They sometimes have areas of cystic necrosis and calcification even in tumors that later prove to be biologically benign. The majority appear encapsulated, but in about 20 to 25%, there is apparent penetration of the capsule and infiltration of perithymic tissues and structures.

Microscopically, virtually all thymomas are made up of a mixture of epithelial cells and a variable infiltrate of non-neoplastic lymphocytes.[52] The relative proportions of the epithelial and lymphocytic components are of little significance. In **benign thymomas,** the epithelial cells tend to resemble those of the medulla and are often elongated or spindle shaped, producing what is called a "medullary thymoma." Tumors that have a significant proportion of medullary-type epithelial cells are almost always completely benign. Frequently there is an admixture of the plumper, rounder, cortical-type epithelial cells, and some are composed largely of such cells. This pattern of thymoma often has few lymphocytes. Hassall's corpuscles are rarely present and, when found, often appear as poorly formed suggestive whorls. They are of no diagnostic significance because they may represent residual normal thymic tissue. Some experts would call this pattern a "mixed thymoma." The medullary and mixed patterns account for well over 50% of all thymomas.

The designation **malignant thymoma type I** as used here implies a cytologically benign tumor, which is locally invasive and sometimes has the capacity for widespread metastasis. These tumors account for about 20 to 25% of all thymomas. They are composed of varying proportions of epithelial cells and lymphocytes; the epithelial cells, however, tend to be of the cortical variety with abundant cytoplasm and rounded vesicular nuclei. Palisading of these cells about blood vessels is sometimes seen. Some spindled epithelial cells may be present as well. Nothing in the cytoarchitecture of these lesions permits recognition of their aggressive nature other than the fact that so-called cortical thymomas are thought to be frequently invasive and tend to occur in younger patients. **The critical distinguishing feature of these neoplasms is penetration of the capsule with invasion into surrounding structures.** The extent of invasion has been subdivided into various stages, which are somewhat beyond our scope, but it suffices that with minimal invasion, complete excision yields a greater than 90% 5-year survival. Extensive invasion is often accompanied by metastasis and is associated with a less than 50% 5-year survival.

Malignant thymoma type II is better designated **"thymic carcinoma."** They represent about 5% of thymomas. In contrast to the type I malignant thymomas, these are cytologically malignant, having all of the features of anaplasia seen in most forms of cancer. Macroscopically, they are usually fleshy, obviously invasive masses sometimes accompanied by metastases to such sites as the lungs. The majority are **squamous cell carcinomas, either well or poorly differentiated.** The next most common malignant pattern is the so-called **lymphoepithelioma** composed of cytologically anaplastic cortical-type epithelial cells scattered against a dense background of benign-appearing lymphocytes. Some of these tumors have revealed traces of Epstein-Barr virus genome. A variety of other histologic patterns of thymic carcinoma have been described, including sarcomatoid variants, basaloid carcinoma, and clear cell carcinoma.

CLINICAL COURSE. Many thymomas are discovered incidentally during the course of some form of cardiac surgery. Of those that come to clinical attention, about 40% present as thymic masses either on imaging studies or because of local pressure symptoms and 50% because of their association with myasthenia gravis. Only about 10% of thymomas are associated with so-called systemic paraneoplastic syndromes, such as Graves' disease, pernicious anemia, dermatomyositis-polymyositis, and Cushing's syndrome. The basis for these associations is still obscure but cannot be attributed simply to the generation in the thymus of autoreactive T cells.

Pineal Gland

PINEALOMAS

NORMAL

The rarity of clinically significant lesions (virtually only tumors) justifies brevity in the consideration of the pineal gland. It is a minute, pine cone–shaped organ (hence its name), weighing 100 to 180 mg and lying between the superior colliculi at the base of the brain. It is composed of a loose, neuroglial stroma enclosing nests of epithelial-appearing pineocytes containing well-defined neurosecretory granules (melatonin). Silver impregnations reveal that these cells have long, slender processes reminiscent of primitive neuronal precursors intermixed with the processes of astrocytic cells.

PATHOLOGY

All tumors involving the pineal are rare; most (50 to 70%) arise from sequestered embryonic germ cells. They most commonly take the form of so-called *germinomas* replicating testicular seminoma (see Chapter 22) or ovarian dysgerminoma (see Chapter 23). Other lines of germ cell differentiation include embryonal carcinomas; choriocarcinomas; mixtures of germinoma, embryonal carcinoma, and choriocarcinoma; and, uncommonly, typical teratomas (usually benign). Whether to characterize these germ cell neoplasms as pinealomas is still a subject of debate, but most "pinealophiles" favor restricting the term "pinealoma" to neoplasms arising from the pineocytes.

PINEALOMAS

These neoplasms are divided into two categories, pineoblastomas and pineocytomas, based on their level of differentiation, which in turn correlates with their neoplastic aggressiveness.[53]

MORPHOLOGY. Pineoblastomas are encountered mostly in young people and appear as soft, friable, gray masses punctuated with areas of hemorrhage and necrosis. They typically invade surrounding structures, that is, hypothalamus, midbrain, and lumen of the third ventricle. Histologically, they are composed of masses of pleomorphic cells two to four times the diameter of an erythrocyte. Large hyperchromatic nuclei appear to occupy almost the entire cell, and mitoses are frequent. The cytology is that of medulloblastoma-neuroblastoma of the brain. Large, poorly formed rosettes are sometimes present in the pineoblastoma, reminiscent of those seen in their "first cousins" in the brain. A further similarity is the tendency of pineoblastomas to spread via the CSF. As might be expected, the enlarging mass may compress the aqueduct of Sylvius, giving rise to internal hydrocephalus and all its consequences. Survival beyond 1 or 2 years is rare.

In contrast, **pineocytomas** occur mostly in adults and are much slower growing than pineoblastomas. They tend to be well-circumscribed, gray or hemorrhagic masses that compress but do not infiltrate surrounding structures. **Histologically, they exhibit divergent glial and neuronal differentiation.** On the one hand, the neoplasm may be largely astrocytomatous. These areas stain positively for glial fibrillary acidic protein. On the other hand, it may be composed largely of pineocytes having darkly staining, round to oval, fairly regular nuclei that stain for neuron-specific enolase. Particularly distinctive of the pineocytoma are the pseudorosettes rimmed by rows of pineocytes. The centers of these rosettes are filled with eosinophilic cytoplasmic material representing tumor cell processes. These cells are set against a background of thin, fibrovascular, anastomosing septa that divide the tumor into lobular masses.

In addition to the monomorphic pineocytomas, there are many instances in which mixed patterns are encountered, in part astrocytic, in part pineocytomatous, sometimes having neuronal-type cells.

The clinical course of patients with pineocytomas is prolonged, averaging 7 years. The manifestations are the consequence of their pressure effects and consist of visual disturbances, headache, mental deterioration, and sometimes dementia-like behavior. The lesions being located where they are, it is understandable that successful excision is at best difficult.

Multiple Endocrine Neoplasia

Having completed a consideration of the disorders of the various endocrine glands, it is appropriate to turn to three autosomal dominant MEN syndromes (some cases of MEN I may be recessive) characterized by hyperplasia or tumors in several endocrine glands simultaneously. The essential features of these syndromes are presented in Table 25–7.

MEN I (Wermer's) syndrome is basically characterized by parathyroid, pancreatic, and pituitary involvements. The parathyroids reveal either hyperplasia or multiple adenomas in 90 to 95% of cases, and the resultant hypercalcemia with its attendant changes (e.g., kidney stones) most often brings these patients to clinical attention. Pancreatic islet cell lesions, most often adenomas but sometimes carcinomas, and rarely hyperplasia are present in about a third of the patients and are responsible for most of the fatalities resulting from this syndrome. These islet cell lesions elaborate one or more of the following products in descending order of frequency: gastrin, insulin, serotonin, vasoactive intestinal polypeptide, and sometimes other products. The hypergastrinemia may lead to Zollinger-Ellison syndrome (see Chapter 17) with its peptic ulcerations, or hyperinsulinism may produce serious hypoglycemia. The pituitary involvement takes the form of adenomas, found in about 10 to 15% of these patients. For the most part, these tumors are nonfunctioning, and the pituitary changes are incidental only, but occasionally the adenomas become sufficiently large to produce local "mass effects." Uncommonly, there is also adrenocortical hyperfunction owing to hyperplasia or an adenoma and hyperfunction of the thyroid gland. These changes, however, are not prominent in most patients with MEN I.

The basis for the concurrent dispersed lesions remains largely mysterious. A mutation in chromosome 11q11-q13, however, has been identified in

Table 25–7. MULTIPLE ENDOCRINE NEOPLASIA SYNDROMES

	MEN I (WERMER'S SYNDROME)	MEN II OR IIa (SIPPLE'S SYNDROME)	MEN IIb OR III
Pituitary	Adenomas		
Parathyroid	Hyperplasia+++ Adenomas+	Hyperplasia+ Adenomas	Hyperplasia
Pancreatic islets	Hyperplasia+ Adenomas+++ Carcinoma++		
Adrenal	Cortical hyperplasia++	Pheochromocytoma++	Pheochromocytoma+++
Thyroid	C-cell hyperplasia±	Medullary carcinoma+++	Medullary carcinoma++
Extraendocrine changes			Mucocutaneous ganglioneuromas Marfanoid habitus
Mutant gene locus	11q11-13	10 (near centromere)	Unknown

Relative frequency; +, uncommon; +++, common.

the majority of cases, but this alteration is firmly linked only to the parathyroid lesions and indeed is also present in sporadic parathyroid adenomas but has not been clearly linked to the pancreatic and pituitary lesions. The mutation is thought to be responsible for loss of a tumor suppressor gene on chromosome 11. This syndrome often remains silent and is not discovered until late in life.

MEN II (Sipple's) syndrome, sometimes referred to as MEN IIa, is clinically and genetically distinct from MEN I and is best remembered as the "medullary thyroid carcinoma–pheochromocytoma" syndrome. Parathyroid hyperplasia or adenoma is inconsistently present, and so only about 10% of patients with MEN II have clinical evidence of hypercalcemia or renal stones. The MTC, which is frequently multifocal, dominates this syndrome, producing almost always elevated serum levels of calcitonin. In some instances, only C-cell hyperplasia is found as a possible precursor to tumor development. The medullary carcinoma may also elaborate prolactin, ACTH, serotonin, and vasoactive intestinal polypeptide as well as other bioactive products. Pheochromocytomas, frequently bilateral and often extra-adrenal, are present in about one-half of the patients. Although the pheochromocytomas are generally benign, the medullary thyroid tumors pursue a typical malignant course, as described earlier.

MEN II has been linked to germ line mutations of the *RET* proto-oncogene on chromosome 10q11.2, underscoring the separation of this syndrome from MEN I. The *RET* proto-oncogene can be identified in the MTC and pheochromocytomas of MEN II (but not in the parathyroid tumors) and is also involved in the genesis of papillary thyroid carcinomas. The age at diagnosis of this syndrome ranges from childhood to the advanced years.

MEN IIb or III is best remembered as the "mucosal neuroma" syndrome; otherwise it is very similar to MEN IIa. In MEN III, typically there is MTC and pheochromocytoma, but these neoplasms are accompanied by striking and often disfiguring neuromas or ganglioneuromas of the lips, oral cavity, eyes, respiratory tract, gastrointestinal tract, bladder, and elsewhere. Other additional inconstant features are a marfanoid bodily habitus and parathyroid hyperplasia. As in MEN IIa, the medullary carcinomas of the thyroid may elaborate a variety of bioactive products, producing confusing clinical manifestations. The neuromas bring this syndrome to the physician's attention usually in the early decades of life and are responsible for a mean duration of survival of about three or four decades, in contrast to the six or seven decades with MEN II or IIa.

Of recent date, familial cases have been linked to a mutation in the RET proto-oncogene differing from that involved in MEN IIA.[54] To be noted, about half of the cases are apparently sporadic.

1. Giannattasio, G., and Bassetti, M.: Human pituitary adenomas: Recent advances in morphologic studies. J. Endocrinol. Invest. 13:435, 1990.
2. Lyons, J., et al.: Two G protein oncogenes in human endocrine tumors. Science 249:655, 1990.
3. Sung, D.I.: Suprasellar tumors in children: A review of clinical manifestations and managements. Cancer 50:1420, 1982.
4. Kovacs, K.: The pathology of clinically nonfunctioning pituitary adenomas. Pathol. Res. Pract. 187:571, 1991.
5. Sheehan, H.L.: Postpartum necrosis of the anterior pituitary. J. Pathol. Bacteriol. 45:189, 1987.
6. Spaziante, R.: The empty sella. Surg. Neurol. 16:418, 1981.
7. DeGroot, L.J.: Mechanism of thyroid hormone action. Adv. Exp. Med. Biol. 299:1, 1991.
8. Skelton, C.L.: The heart and hyperthyroidism. N. Engl. J. Med. 307:1206, 1982.
9. Werner, S.C.: Toxic goiter. In Werner, S.C., and Ingbar, S.H. (eds.): The Thyroid, 4th ed. Hagerstown, MD, Harper & Row, 1978, p. 591.
10. Amir, S.M., et al.: In vitro responses to crude and purified hCG in human thyroid membranes. J. Clin. Endocrinol. Metab. 51:51, 1980.
11. Takasu, N., et al.: Disappearance of thyrotropin-blocking antibodies and spontaneous recovery from hypothyroidism in autoimmune thyroiditis. N. Engl. J. Med. 326:513, 1992.
12. Hamilton, W.: Sporadic cretinism. Dev. Med. Child. Neurol. 18:384, 1976.
13. Rapoport, B.: Pathophysiology of Hashimoto's thyroiditis and hypothyroidism. Annu. Rev. Med. 42:91, 1991.
14. Mariotti, S., et al.: Recent advances in the understanding

of humoral and cellular mechanisms implicated in thyroid autoimmune disorders. Clin. Immunol. Immunopathol. 50:S73, 1989.

15. Volpe, R.: Subacute thyroiditis. In Soto, R.J., et al. (eds.): Progress in Clinical and Biological Research. New York, Alan R. Liss, 1981, p. 115.

16. Harach, H.R., and Williams, E.D.: The pathology of granulomatous diseases of the thyroid. Sarcoidosis 7:19, 1990.

17. Smyth, P.P., et al.: Thyroid growth-stimulating immunoglobulins in goitrous disease: Relationship to thyroid-stimulating immunoglobulins. Acta Endocrinol. (Copenh.) 111:321, 1986.

18. Bahn, R.S., and Heufelder, A.E.: Pathogenesis of Graves' ophthalmopathy. N. Engl. J. Med. 329:1468, 1993.

19. Zonana, J., and Rimoin, D.L.: Genetic disorders of the thyroid gland. Med. Clin. North Am. 59:1263, 1975.

20. Studer, H., and Ramelli, F.: Simple goiter and its variants: Euthyroid and hyperthyroid multinodular goiters. Endocr. Rev. 3:40, 1982.

21. Peter, H.J., et al.: The pathogenesis of "hot" and "cold" follicles in multinodular goiters. J. Clin. Endocrinol. Metab. 55:941, 1982.

22. Ramelli, F., et al.: Pathogenesis of thyroid nodules in multinodular goiter. Am. J. Pathol. 109:215, 1982.

23. Miller, J.M.: Evaluation of thyroid nodules; accent on needle biopsy. Med. Clin. North Am. 69:1063, 1985.

24. Mazzaforri, E.L.: Management of a solitary thyroid nodule. N. Engl. J. Med. 328:553, 1993.

25. Robbins, J., et al.: Thyroid cancer: A lethal endocrine neoplasm. Ann. Intern. Med. 115:133, 1991.

26. Cole, W.H.: Incidence of carcinoma of the thyroid in nodular goiter. Semin. Surg. Oncol. 7:61, 1991.

27. Santoro, M., et al.: Ret oncogene activation in human thyroid neoplasms is restricted to the papillary cancer subtype. J. Clin. Invest. 89:1517, 1992.

28. LiVolsi, V.A.: Papillary neoplasms of the thyroid: Pathologic and prognostic features. Am. J. Clin. Pathol. 97:426, 1992.

29. Carcangiu, M.L., et al.: Papillary thyroid carcinoma: A study of its many morphologic expressions and clinical correlates. Pathol. Annu. 20:1, 1985.

30. Watne, A.L., et al.: Follicular carcinoma of the thyroid. Semin. Surg. Oncol. 7:87, 1991.

31. Lairmore, T.C., and Wells, S.A., Jr.: Medullary carcinoma of the thyroid: Current diagnosis and management. Semin. Surg. Oncol. 7:92, 1991.

32. Fukayama, S., et al.: Human parathyroid hormone (PTH)–related protein and human PTH: Comparative biological activities on human bone cells and bone resorption. Endocrinology 123:2841, 1988.

33. Mallette, L.E.: The parathyroid polyhormones: New concepts in the spectrum of peptide hormone action. Endocr. Rev. 12:110, 1991.

34. Friedman, E., et al.: Allelic loss from chromosome 11 in parathyroid tumors. Cancer Res. 52:6804, 1992.

35. Tominaga, Y., et al.: Histological and clinical features of nonfamilial primary parathyroid hyperplasia. Pathol. Res. Pract. 188:115, 1992.

36. Falchetti, A., et al.: Progression of uremic hyperparathyroidism involves allelic loss on chromosome 11. J. Clin. Endocrinol. Metab. 76:139, 1993.

37. Cronstein, B.N.: A mechanism for the antiinflammatory effects of corticosteroids: The glucocorticoid receptor regulates leukocyte adhesion to endothelial cells and expression of endothelial-leukocyte adhesion molecule 1 and intercellular adhesion molecule 1. Proc. Natl. Acad. Sci. U.S.A. 89:9991, 1992.

38. Kannan, C.R.: Diseases of the adrenal cortex. Disease-a-Month 34:601, 1988.

39. Schteingart, D.E.: Cushing's syndrome. Endocrinol. Metab. Clin. North Am. 18:311, 1989.

40. Belsky, J., et al.: Cushing's syndrome due to ectopic production of corticotropin-releasing factor. J. Clin. Endocrinol. Metab. 60:496, 1985.

41. Travis, W.D., et al.: Primary pigmented nodular adrenal cortical disease: A light and electron microscopic study of 8 cases. Am. J. Surg. Pathol. 13:921, 1989.

42. Young, W.F., et al.: Primary aldosteronism: Diagnosis and treatment. Mayo Clin. Proc. 65:96, 1990.

43. Melby, J.C.: Clinical review 1: Endocrine hypertension. J. Clin. Endocrinol. Metab. 69:697, 1989.

44. Miller, W.L.: Congenital adrenal hyperplasias. Endocrinol. Metab. Clin. North Am. 20:721, 1991.

45. White, P.C., and Noe, M.I.: Genetic basis of endocrine disease: II. Congenital adrenal hyperplasia due to 21-hydroxylase deficiency. J. Clin. Endocrinol. Metab. 74:6, 1992.

46. Meyerson, J., et al.: Polyglandular autoimmune syndrome: Current concepts. Can. Med. Assoc. J. 138:605, 1988.

47. Page, D.L., et al.: Tumors of the Adrenal (Fascicle 23). Washington, DC, Armed Forces Institute of Pathology, 1986.

48. Hartmut, P.H., et al.: Pheochromocytomas, multiple endocrine neoplasia type 2, and von Hippel–Lindau disease. N. Engl. J. Med. 329:1531, 1993.

49. Goldfien, A.: Phaeochromocytoma. Clin. Endocrinol. Metab. 10:607, 1981.

50. Stein, P.P., and Black, H.R.: A simplified diagnostic approach to pheochromocytoma: A review of the literature and report of one institution's experience. Medicine 70:46, 1991.

51. Whalen, R.K., et al.: Extra-adrenal pheochromocytoma. J. Urol. 147:1, 1992.

52. Hammond, E.H., and Flinner, R.L.: The diagnosis of thymoma: A review. Ultrastruc. Pathol. 15:419, 1991.

53. Disclafani, A., et al.: Pineocytomas. Cancer 63:302, 1989.

54. Romeo, G. et al.: A mutation in the RET proto-oncogene associated with multiple endocrine neoplasia type 2B and sporadic medullary thyroid carcinoma. Nature 367:375, 1994.

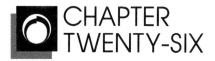

CHAPTER
TWENTY-SIX

The Skin

GEORGE F. MURPHY, M.D., and MARTIN C. MIHM, Jr., M.D.

THE SKIN AS A PROTECTIVE ORGAN

More than 100 years ago, the noted pathologist Rudolph Virchow portrayed the skin as a protective covering for more delicate and functionally sophisticated internal viscera.[1] At that time, the skin was appreciated primarily as a passive barrier to fluid loss and mechanical injury. By routine light microscopy, early investigators could visualize only the tough epidermal layer composed of stratified squamous epithelial cells, the leathery underlying dermis, and the cushion of subcutaneous fat that lay beneath. This level of understanding changed little over the century that followed. During the past three decades, however, enormously productive avenues of scientific inquiry have demonstrated skin to be a complex organ in which precisely regulated cellular and molecular interactions govern many crucial responses to our environment.

We now know that skin is composed of a num-ber of interdependent cell types (Fig. 26–1). *Melanocytes* within the epidermis are cells responsible for the production of a brown pigment (melanin) that represents an important endogenous screen against harmful ultraviolet rays in sunlight. *Langerhans cells*[2] are dendritic histiocytic cells that take up and process antigenic signals and communicate this information to lymphoid cells. *Squamous epithelial cells (keratinocytes)* are major sites for the biosynthesis of soluble molecules (cytokines) important in the functional regulation of adjacent epidermal cells and cells forming the nearby dermal microenvironment[3] (Fig. 26–2).

Factors affecting the delicate homeostasis that exists among skin cells may result in conditions as diverse as wrinkles and hair loss, blisters and rashes, and even life-threatening cancers and disorders of immune regulation. For example, chronic exposure to sunlight fosters premature cutaneous aging, blunting of immunologic responses to environmental antigens, and the development of a variety of premalignant and malignant cutaneous neo-

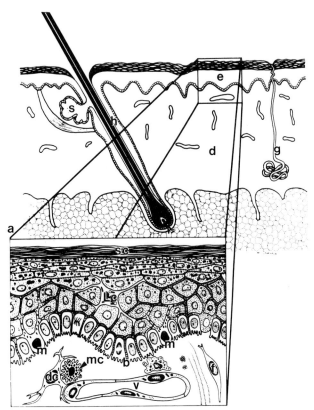

Figure 26–1. A, The skin is composed of an epidermal layer (e) from which specialized adnexae (hair follicles (h), sweat glands (g), and sebaceous glands (s)) descend into the underlying dermis (d). **B,** This projection of the epidermal layer (e) and underlying superficial dermis demonstrates the progressive upward maturation of basal cells (b) into cornified squamous epithelial cells of the stratum corneum (sc). Melanin-containing dendritic melanocytes (m) and midepidermal dendritic Langerhans cells (Lc) are also present. The underlying dermis contains small vessels (v), fibroblasts (f), perivascular mast cells (mc), and dendrocytes (dc), potentially important in dermal immunity and repair.

plasms. Ingested agents, such as therapeutic drugs, can cause an enormous number of skin rashes, or exanthems. And internal disorders, such as diabetes mellitus, amyloidosis, and lupus erythematosus, also may have important manifestations in the skin.

Definition of Terms

Before describing the clinical features and characteristic histology of skin disorders, we will define some descriptive terms used in dermatopathology.

Macroscopic Terms

Macule   Circumscribed area of any size characterized by its flatness and usually distinguished from surrounding skin by its coloration.

Papule   Elevated solid area 5 mm or less across.

Nodule   Elevated solid area greater than 5 mm across.

Plaque   Elevated flat-topped area, usually greater than 5 mm across.

Vesicle   Fluid-filled raised area 5 mm or less across.

Bulla   Fluid-filled raised area greater than 5 mm across; a large blister.

Blister   Common term used for vesicle or bulla.

Pustule   Discrete, pus-filled, raised area.

Wheal   Itchy, transient, elevated area with variable blanching and erythema formed as the result of dermal edema.

Scale   Dry, horny, platelike excrescence; usually the result of imperfect cornification.

Lichenification   Thickened and rough skin characterized by prominent skin markings; usually the result of repeated rubbing in susceptible persons.

Excoriation   A traumatic lesion characterized by breakage of the epidermis, causing a raw linear area, i.e., a deep scratch. Such lesions are often self induced.

Onycholysis   Loss of integrity of the nail substance.

Microscopic Terms

Hyperkeratosis   Hyperplasia of the stratum corneum often associated with a qualitative abnormality of the keratin.

Parakeratosis   Mode(s) of keratinization characterized by the retention of the nuclei in the stratum corneum. On mucous membranes, parakeratosis is normal.

Acanthosis   Epidermal hyperplasia.

Dyskeratosis   Abnormal keratinization occurring prematurely within individual cells or groups of cells below the stratum granulosum.

Acantholysis   Loss of intercellular connections resulting in loss of cohesion between keratinocytes.

Papillomatosis   Hyperplasia of the papillary dermis with elongation and/or widening of the dermal papillae.

Lentiginous   Referring to a linear pattern of melanocyte proliferation within the epidermal basal cell layer; lentiginous melanocytic hyperplasia can occur as a reactive change or as part of a neoplasm of melanocytes.

Spongiosis   Intercellular edema of the epidermis.

Exocytosis   Infiltration of the epidermis by inflammatory or circulating blood cells.

Erosion   Discontinuity of the skin, exhibiting incomplete loss of the epidermis.

Ulceration   Discontinuity, often excavative, of skin exhibiting complete loss of the epidermis and portions of the dermis and even subcutaneous fat.

Vacuolization   Formation of vacuoles within or adjacent to cells; often refers to basal cell–basement membrane zone area.

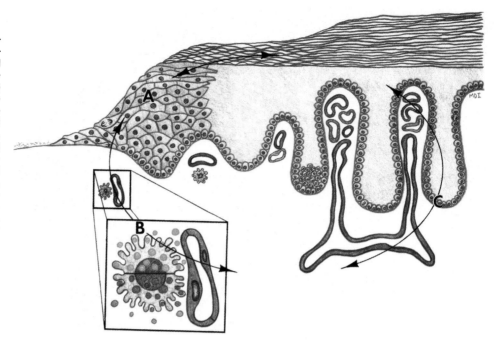

Figure 26-2. Schematic representation of dynamic interaction between epidermal layer and dermal layer. Keratinocytes at edge of ulcer (A) produce cytokines and factors that influence both keratinization and the function of underlying dermal cells (B). Dermal cells (B), such as mast cells, also release cytokines (green granules) and proteases (red granules), which may regulate both endothelial cells and overlying keratinocytes. Perturbations in these complex regulatory interactions between epidermal cells and dermal cells may contribute to the formation of pathologic processes, such as psoriasis (C), in which both compartments become morphologically abnormal.

DISORDERS OF PIGMENTATION AND MELANOCYTES

Skin pigmentation historically has had major societal implications. Cosmetic desire for increased pigmentation (tanning) has resulted in many deleterious alterations that will be described in the pages that follow. Focal or widespread loss of pigmentation not only renders individuals extraordinarily vulnerable to the harmful effects of sunlight (as in albinism) but also has resulted in severe emotional stresses and, in some cultures, profound social and economic discrimination (as in vitiligo). Change in pre-existing pigmentation may signify important primary events in the skin (e.g., malignant transformation of a mole) or disorders of internal viscera (e.g., in Addison's disease).

VITILIGO

Vitiligo is a common disorder characterized by partial or complete loss of pigment-producing melanocytes within the epidermis. All races are affected, but lesions are most noticeable in darkly pigmented individuals. Lesions may be entirely inapparent in lightly pigmented skin until tanning occurs in the surrounding normal skin.

Clinically, lesions are asymptomatic, flat, well-demarcated zones (macules) of pigment loss (Fig. 26-3). Their size varies from few to many centimeters, and their distribution often involves the

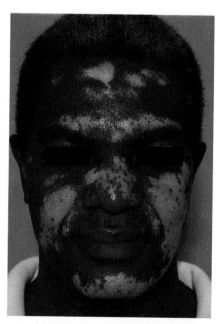

Figure 26-3. Vitiligo. Well-demarcated zones of pigment loss result from depletion of melanocytes that produce small melanin granules.

wrists, axillae, and perioral, periorbital, and anogenital skin.

MORPHOLOGY. Histologically, vitiligo is characterized by loss of melanocytes, as defined by electron microscopy. This is in contrast to some forms of **albinism,** in which melanocytes are present but no melanin pigment is produced because of a lack of or defect in the tyrosinase enzyme. Both conditions may be differentiated from other forms of hypopigmentation (unrelated to the absence of melanocytes or tyrosinase enzyme) by demonstrating diminished or absent activity of melanocyte tyrosinase on the melanin pigment precursor dopa (dihydroxyphenylalanine). This histochemical stain is useful because melanocytes or their melanogenic potential cannot be reliably quantified in routine H and E sections.

Why are melanocytes progressively lost or destroyed in vitiligo? Theories of pathogenesis include (1) autoimmunity, (2) neurohumoral factors, and (3) self-destruction of melanocytes by toxic intermediates of melanin synthesis. Most evidence supports autoimmune causation, focusing on the presence of circulating antibodies against melanocytes[4] and the association of vitiligo with disorders possibly involving autoimmune mechanisms, such as pernicious anemia, Addison's disease, and autoimmune thyroiditis. Recently, abnormalities in Langerhans cells[5] and T lymphocytes in the peripheral blood[6] have also been described, suggesting that aberrations in cell-mediated immunity may also be operative in the pathogenesis of vitiligo.

FRECKLE (EPHELIS)

Freckles are the most common pigmented lesions of childhood in light-skinned whites. They are small (1 to 10 mm in diameter), tan-red or light brown macules that first appear in early childhood after sun exposure. Once present, freckles will fade and reappear in a cyclic fashion with winter and summer, respectively.

MORPHOLOGY. The observed hyperpigmentation of the freckle is the result of increased amounts of melanin pigment within basal keratinocytes; melanocytes are relatively normal in number, although they may be slightly enlarged. It is unclear as to whether the freckle represents a focal abnormality in pigment production by a discrete field of melanocytes, enhanced pigment donation to adjacent basal keratinocytes, or both.

MELASMA

Melasma is a masklike zone of facial hyperpigmentation commonly seen in pregnancy—hence its designation as the "mask of pregnancy." It presents as poorly defined, blotchy macules involving the cheeks, temples, and forehead bilaterally. Sunlight may accentuate this pigmentation, which often resolves spontaneously, particularly after the end of pregnancy.

MORPHOLOGY. Histologically, two patterns have been recognized:[10] an **epidermal type,** in which there is increased melanin deposition in the basal layers, and a **dermal type,** characterized by macrophages in the superficial (papillary) dermis that have phagocytized melanin from the adjacent epidermal layer (a process referred to as **melanin pigment incontinence**). These two types may be distinguished by the use of a Wood's light. This is important because melasma of the epidermal type may respond to the topical bleaching agent hydroquinone.

The pathogenesis of melasma appears to relate to functional alterations in melanocytes resulting in enhanced pigment transfer to basal keratinocytes or to dermal macrophages. Apart from its association with pregnancy, melasma may occur during the administration of oral contraceptives or hydantoins, or it may be idiopathic.

LENTIGO

Until now, we have been addressing disorders of pigmentation that do not involve proliferation of melanocytes. The term "lentigo" (plural "lentigines") refers to a common benign hyperplasia of melanocytes occurring at all ages, but often in infancy and childhood. There is no sex or racial predilection, and the cause and pathogenesis are unknown. These lesions may involve mucous membranes as well as the skin, and they appear as small (5 to 10 mm across), oval, tan-brown macules. Unlike freckles, lentigines do not darken when exposed to sunlight.

MORPHOLOGY. The essential histologic feature of the lentigo is linear melanocytic hyperplasia that produces a hyperpigmented basal cell layer. So characteristic is this linear melanocytic hyperplasia that the term **"lentiginous"** is often used to describe similar patterns of growth in unrelated melanocytic tumors, such as in lentiginous nevi and acral lentiginous melanomas. Elongation and thinning of the rete ridges are also commonly seen in a lentigo.

NEVOCELLULAR NEVUS (PIGMENTED NEVUS, MOLE)

Most of us have at least a few moles and probably regard them as mundane and uninteresting. It may be surprising to learn, then, that moles or nevi represent one of the most diverse, dynamic, and biologically instructive tumors of the skin! Strictly

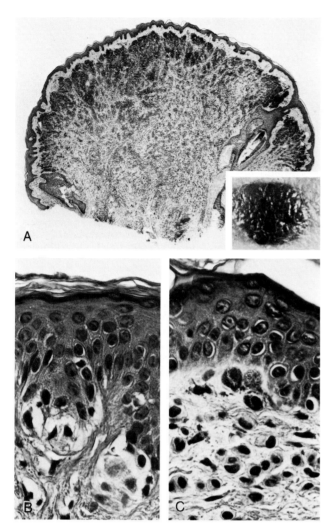

highly dendritic single cells that normally are interspersed among basal keratinocytes, to round-to-oval cells that grow in aggregates, or "nests," along the dermal-epidermal junction (see Fig. 26-4B). Nuclei of nevus cells are uniform and rounded in contour, contain inconspicuous nucleoli, and show little or no mitotic activity. Such lesions are believed to represent an early developmental stage in nevocellular nevi, and are called **junctional nevi.** Eventually, most junctional nevi grow into the underlying dermis as nests or cords of cells **(compound nevi),** and in older lesions, the epidermal nests may be lost entirely to form pure **dermal nevi** (see Fig. 26-4C). Clinically, compound and dermal nevi are often more elevated than junctional nevi.

Progressive growth of nevus cells from the dermoepidermal junction into the underlying dermis is accompanied by a process termed "maturation." Whereas less mature, more superficial nevus cells are larger, tend to produce melanin pigment, and grow in nests, more mature, deeper nevus cells are smaller, produce little or no pigment, and grow in cords. The most mature nevus cells may be found at the deepest extent of lesions, where they often acquire fusiform contours and grow in fascicles resembling neural tissue.[12,13] This striking metamorphosis correlates with enzymatic changes (progressive loss of tyrosinase activity and acquisition of cholinesterase activity in deeper, nonpigmented, nerve-like nevus cells). **This sequence of maturation of individual nevus cells is of diagnostic importance in distinguishing some benign nevi from melanomas, which usually show little or no maturation.**

Figure 26-4. Nevocellular nevus. Lesions are symmetrical and uniform in clinical *(A, inset)* and histologic *(A)* appearance. Junctional nevi *(B)*, characterized by rounded nests of nevus cells at the dermoepidermal junction, may progress in time to become compound and pure dermal nevi *(C)*, exhibiting migration of nevus cells into the underlying dermis.

speaking, the term "nevus" denotes any congenital lesion of the skin. "Nevocellular" nevus, however, refers to any congenital or acquired neoplasm of melanocytes.

Clinically, common acquired nevocellular nevi are tan-to-brown, uniformly pigmented, small (usually less than 6 mm across), solid regions of elevated skin (papules) with well-defined, rounded borders (Fig. 26-4A). There are numerous clinical and histologic types of nevocellular nevi, and the clinical appearance may be quite variable. Table 26-1 provides a comparative summary of salient clinical and histologic features of the more commonly encountered forms of melanocytic nevi.

MORPHOLOGY. Nevocellular nevi are formed by melanocytes that have been transformed from

Although nevocellular nevi are common, their clinical and histologic diversity necessitates thorough knowledge of their appearance and natural evolution, lest they become confused with other skin conditions, notably malignant melanoma. The biologic importance of some nevi, however, resides in their recent recognition as an important model of tumor progression (dysplastic nevi and the heritable melanoma syndrome).

DYSPLASTIC NEVI

The association of nevocellular nevi with malignant melanoma was made over 160 years ago,[8] although it was not until 1978 that a true precursor of malignant melanoma was described in detail. In 1978, Clark and colleagues detailed the characteristics of lesions they termed "BK" moles[9] (a name derived from the first letters of the last names of the initial two families studied).

Clinically, BK moles—or dysplastic nevi, as they are frequently called—are larger than most acquired nevi (often greater than 5 mm across) and

Table 26–1. VARIANT FORMS OF NEVOCELLULAR NEVI

NEVUS VARIANT	DIAGNOSTIC ARCHITECTURAL FEATURES	DIAGNOSTIC CYTOLOGIC FEATURES	CLINICAL SIGNIFICANCE
Congenital nevus	Deep dermal and sometimes subcutaneous growth around adnexae, neurovascular bundles, and blood vessel walls	Identical to ordinary acquired nevi	Present at birth; large variants have increased melanoma risk
Blue nevus	Non-nested dermal infiltration, often with associated fibrosis	Highly dendritic, heavily pigmented nevus cells	Black-blue nodule; often confused with melanoma clinically
Spindle and epithelioid cell nevus (Spitz's nevus)	Fascicular growth	Large, plump cells with pink-blue cytoplasm; fusiform cells	Common in children; red-pink nodule; often confused with hemangioma clinically
Halo nevus	Lymphocytic infiltration surrounding nevus cells	Identical to ordinary acquired nevi	Host immune response against nevus cells and surrounding normal melanocytes
Dysplastic nevus	Large, coalescent intraepidermal nests	Cytologic atypia	Potential precursor of malignant melanoma

may occur as hundreds of lesions on the body surface (Fig. 26–5A). They are flat macules to slightly raised plaques with a "pebbly" surface. They usually show variability in pigmentation (variegation) and borders that are irregular in contour. Unlike ordinary moles, dysplastic nevi have a tendency to occur on non–sun-exposed as well as on sun-exposed body surfaces. Dysplastic nevi have been documented in multiple members of families prone to the development of malignant melanoma (the heritable melanoma syndrome).[10] In these cases, genetic analyses have demonstrated the trait to be inherited as an autosomal dominant, possibly involving a susceptibility gene located on the short arm of chromosome 1, near the Rh locus.[11] Dysplastic nevi also may occur as isolated lesions not associated with the heritable melanoma syndrome, in which case the risk of malignant change appears to be low. Transitions from these lesions to early melanoma have actually been documented clinically and histologically within a period as short as several weeks. However, most dysplastic nevi are clinically stable lesions.

MORPHOLOGY. Histologically (see Fig. 26–5B), dysplastic nevi consist of compound nevi with both architectural and cytologic evidence of abnormal growth. **Nevus cell nests within the epidermis may be enlarged and exhibit abnormal fusion or coalescence with adjacent nests. As part of this process, single nevus cells begin to replace the normal basal cell layer along the dermoepidermal junction, producing so-called lentiginous hyperplasia** (recall the definition of this term earlier). Cytologic atypia consisting of irregular, often angulated, nuclear contours and hyperchromasia is frequently observed. Associated alterations also occur in the superficial dermis. These consist of a usually sparse lymphocytic infiltrate, loss of melanin pigment from presumably destroyed nevus cells,

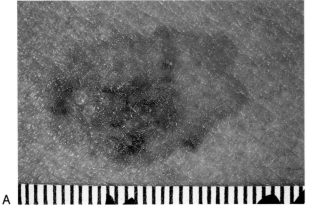

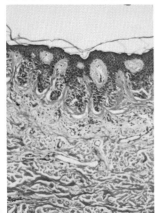
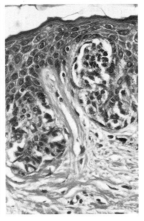

Figure 26–5. Dysplastic nevus. A, The nevus has an irregular contour, variegated color, and a typical center of darker pigment with a "pebbly" surface. B, Low (left) and high (right) magnification of the histology of a dysplastic nevus, showing poorly formed and coalescent nests of nevus cells associated with eosinophilic linear fibrosis forming concentric lamellae within the underlying papillary dermis.

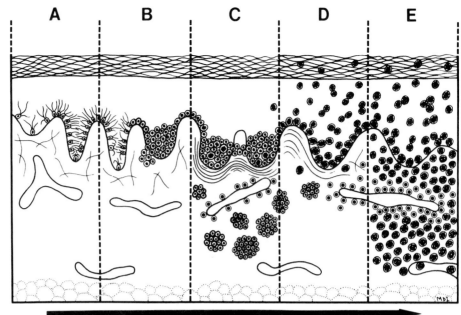

Figure 26-6. Steps of tumor progression in dysplastic nevi: *A*, Lentiginous melanocytic hyperplasia; *B*, lentiginous junctional nevus; *C*, lentiginous compound nevus with abnormal architectural and cytologic features (dysplastic nevus); *D*, early melanoma, or radial growth phase melanoma (large dark cells in epidermis); *E*, advanced melanoma (vertical growth phase) with malignant spread into the dermis and vessels.

Time

phagocytosis of this pigment by dermal macrophages (melanin pigment incontinence), and a peculiar linear fibrosis surrounding the epidermal rete ridges that are involved by the nevus. All of these features assist in the histologic recognition of a dysplastic nevus.

Several lines of evidence support the concept that some *dysplastic nevi are precursors of malignant melanoma.* In one study[12] it was shown that in a large number of families prone to the development of melanoma, over 5% of family members developed melanoma over an 8-year follow-up period, and new melanomas occurred only in individuals with dysplastic nevi. From this database, it was concluded that the actuarial probability of persons with the dysplastic nevus syndrome developing melanoma is 56% at age 59! Dysplastic nevi also demonstrate expression of some abnormal cell surface antigens,[13] karyotypic abnormalities,[14] and *in vitro* vulnerability to mutagenic effects of ultraviolet light.[15]

Clark and associates[16] have proposed steps whereby benign nevi may undergo aberrant differentiation to become dysplastic and eventually metastasizing malignant tumors (Fig. 26-6). Parallels may be found in neoplasia involving other organ systems, and thus dysplastic nevi are regarded by some as a general model of tumor progression.

MALIGNANT MELANOMA

Malignant melanoma is a relatively common neoplasm that not long ago was considered almost uniformly deadly. Although the great preponderance arise in the skin, other sites of origin include the oral and anogenital mucosal surfaces, esophagus, meninges, and notably the eye. The following comments apply to cutaneous melanomas, but later a few words will be directed to intraocular melanomas.

Today as a result of increased public awareness of the earliest signs of skin melanomas, most are cured surgically.[17] Nonetheless, the incidence of these lesions is on the rise, necessitating vigorous surveillance for their development.

As with epithelial malignancies of the skin (see later), sunlight appears to play an important role in the development of skin malignant melanoma. For example, men commonly develop this tumor on the upper back, whereas women have a relatively high incidence on both the back and the legs. Lightly pigmented individuals are at higher risk for the development of melanoma than darkly pigmented individuals. Sunlight, however, does not seem to be the only predisposing factor, and the presence of a pre-existing nevus (e.g., a dysplastic nevus), hereditary factors, or even exposure to certain carcinogens (as in the case of experimental melanomas in rodent models) may play a role in lesion development and evolution.[18]

Clinically, malignant melanoma of the skin is usually asymptomatic, although itching may be an early manifestation. *The most important clinical sign of the disease is change in color in a pigmented lesion.* Unlike benign (nondysplastic) nevi, melanomas exhibit striking variations in pigmentation, appearing in shades of black, brown, red, dark blue, and gray (Fig. 26-7A). Occasionally, zones of white or flesh-colored hypopigmentation are also

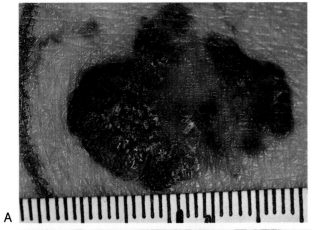

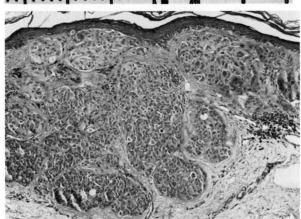

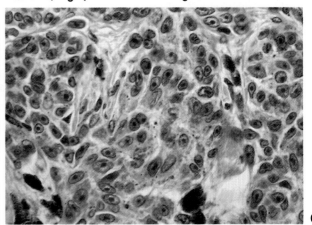

Figure 26-7. Malignant melanoma. *A*, Clinically, lesions are irregular in contour and pigmentation. Macular areas correlate with the radial growth phase, while raised areas usually correspond to nodular aggregates of malignant cells in the vertical phase of growth. *B*, Photomicrograph of lesion in the vertical phase of growth, demonstrating nodular aggregates of infiltrating cells. *C*, High-power view of malignant melanoma cells.

present. The borders of melanomas are not smooth, round, and uniform, as in nevocellular nevi, but irregular and often "notched." In summary, the clinical warning signs of melanoma are (1) enlargement of a pre-existing mole; (2) itching or pain in a pre-existing mole; (3) development of a new pigmented lesion during adult life; (4) irregularity of the borders of a pigmented lesion; and (5) variegation of color within a pigmented lesion.

Central to understanding the complicated histology of malignant melanoma is the concept of radial and vertical growth.[19] *Simply stated, radial growth indicates the tendency of a melanoma to grow horizontally within the epidermal and superficial dermal layers, often for a prolonged period of time. During this stage of growth, melanoma cells do not have the capacity to metastasize. Specific types of radial growth phase melanoma include lentigo maligna, superficial spreading, and acral/mucosal lentiginous. These are defined on the basis of architectural and cytologic features of growth within the epidermal layer as well as biologic behavior (e.g., lentigo maligna type of radial growth typically occurs on sun-damaged facial skin of the elderly and may continue for as long as several decades before the tumor develops the capacity to metastasize). With time, the pattern of growth as-*sumes a vertical component, and the melanoma now grows downward into the deeper dermal layers as an expansile mass lacking cellular maturation, with a tendency for the cells to become smaller as they descend into the reticular dermis (stage V, Fig. 26-7B). This event is heralded clinically by the development of a nodule in the relatively flat radial growth phase, and correlates with the emergence of a clone of cells with true metastatic potential.*[20] Interestingly, the probability of metastasis in such as lesion may be predicted by simply measuring in millimeters the depth of invasion of this vertical growth phase nodule below the granular cell layer of the overlying epidermis.[21] Recently, prediction of clinical outcome has been refined by taking into account factors such as number of mitoses and degree of infiltrative lymphocytic response within the tumor nodule.[22]

MORPHOLOGY. Individual melanoma cells usually are considerably larger than nevus cells. They contain large nuclei with irregular contours having chromatin characteristically clumped at the periphery of the nuclear membrane and prominent red (eosinophilic) nucleoli. These cells grow as poorly formed nests or as individual cells at all levels of the epidermis and, in the dermis, as expansile, balloon-like nodules (Fig. 26–7B). **The nature and extent of the vertical growth phase determine the biologic behavior of malignant melanoma,** and thus it is important to observe and record vertical growth phase parameters in a pathology report.[23]

Melanoma of the eye is about one-twentieth as common as melanoma of the skin. Most intraocular melanomas arise in the melanocytes of the uvea (i.e., iris, ciliary body, and choroid), but they can also originate in the pigmented epithelium of the retina.

Most of these tumors occur in the posterior choroid and may either spread laterally, lifting the retina, or bulge into and penetrate the vitreous chamber. Unlike the cutaneous type, they are composed of two distinctive cell types—spindle and epithelioid—having differing clinical implications. *Spindle cell melanomas* have cohesive cells, which may be arranged in interlocking bundles. The nuclei are spindle shaped and surrounded by scant to abundant cytoplasm, which sometimes contains melanin granules. *Epithelioid melanomas* are not distinct from other lesions grossly, but are composed of poorly cohesive large cells with abundant, sometimes pigmented, cytoplasm. *Mixed* patterns are in fact the most common.

Although many factors (e.g., tumor size) are important, cell type is of major prognostic significance. Lesions composed completely or predominantly of spindle cells are of low aggressiveness, do not tend to metastasize, and permit about a 75% survival at 15 years. Thus, many eye surgeons recommend careful surveillance and enucleation only if and when there is obvious progressive increase in size. In contrast, epithelioid melanomas provide only about a 35% survival at 15 years despite early enucleation, owing to late metastasis.

BENIGN EPITHELIAL TUMORS

Benign epithelial neoplasms are common and usually biologically inconsequential, although they may represent significant sources of psychologic discomfort for the patient. These tumors, derived from the keratinizing stratified squamous epithelium of the epidermis and hair follicles (keratinocytes) and the ductular epithelium of cutaneous glands, may recapitulate the cell layers from which they arise. Clinically, they are often confused with malignancy, particularly when they are pigmented or inflamed, and histologic examination of a biopsy specimen is frequently required to establish a definitive diagnosis.

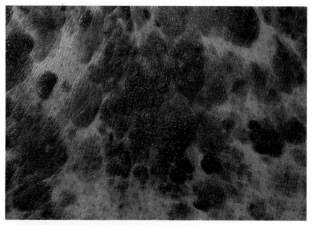

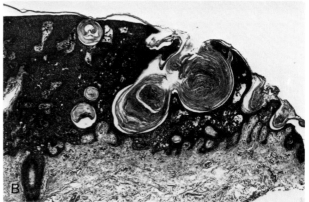

Figure 26–8. Seborrheic keratoses. Multiple coalescent, coin-like pigmented lesions on the back *(A)* are composed of well-demarcated, orderly proliferations of basaloid cells forming small, keratin-filled cysts *(B)*.

SEBORRHEIC KERATOSES

These common epidermal tumors occur most frequently in middle-aged or older individuals. They arise spontaneously and may become particularly numerous on the trunk, although the extremities, head, and neck may also be involved. In people of color, multiple small lesions on the face are termed *dermatosis papulosa nigra.*

Clinically, seborrheic keratoses (also called senile keratoses) have characteristic features. They appear as round, flat, coinlike plaques that vary in diameter from millimeters to several centimeters (Fig. 26–8A). They are uniformly tan to dark brown in color and usually show a velvety to granular surface. Lesions may give the impression that they are "stuck on" and may be easily peeled off. Inspection with a hand lens will usually reveal small, round, porelike ostia impacted with keratin (a feature helpful in differentiating these pigmented lesions from melanomas).

MORPHOLOGY. Histologically, these neoplasms are exophytic and demarcated sharply from the adjacent epidermis (see Fig. 26–8B). They are composed of sheets of small cells that most resemble basal cells of the normal epidermis. Variable melanin pigmentation is present within these basaloid cells, accounting for the brown coloration clinically. Exuberant keratin production (hyperkeratosis) occurs at the surface of seborrheic keratoses, and small keratin-filled cysts (horn cysts) and downgrowths of keratin into the main tumor mass (pseudo–horn cysts) are characteristic features. Interestingly, when seborrheic keratoses become irritated and inflamed, they undergo squamous differentiation[24] and are characterized by foci of "whirling" squamous cells resembling eddy currents in a stream. A biologic explanation for this intriguing phenomenon awaits discovery. When seborrheic keratoses involve the epithelium of hair follicles, they may grow in an endophytic fashion, and they generally also show the effects of inflammation; such lesions are termed **inverted follicular keratoses.**

The occurrence of seborrheic keratoses explosively in large numbers, as part of a paraneoplastic syndrome (sign of Leser-Trelat), raises important pathogenetic issues. In one report, for example, a patient was noted to have developed the sign of Leser-Trelat in association with a malignant melanoma.[25] The melanoma was shown to produce an alpha-transforming growth factor (a growth factor closely related to epidermal growth factor). Because this factor exerts its effects by interaction with receptors on basal keratinocytes, it was hypothesized that the seborrheic keratoses were related to its abnormal production by the melanoma. Interestingly, when the melanoma was excised surgically, the number of seborrheic keratoses decreased.

ACANTHOSIS NIGRICANS

"Acanthosis nigricans" is used to describe thickened (acanthosis = hyperplasia of the stratum spinosum of the epidermis), hyperpigmented zones of skin involving most commonly the flexural areas (axillae, skin folds of the neck, groin, and anogenital regions). It is an important cutaneous marker for associated benign and malignant conditions, and, accordingly, is divided into two types.[26] The benign type, which constitutes about 80% of all cases, develops gradually and usually occurs in childhood or during puberty. It may occur (1) as an autosomal dominant trait with variable penetrance; (2) in association with obesity or endocrine abnormalities (particularly with pituitary and pineal tumors and with diabetes); and (3) as part of a number of rare congenital syndromes. As with seborrheic keratoses, acanthosis nigricans may result from abnormal production of epidermal growth-

promoting factors by a variety of tumors.[25] This latter occurrence may account for many instances of the malignant type, in which lesions arise in middle-aged and older individuals, often in association with an underlying adenocarcinoma. Because the occurrence of acanthosis nigricans may precede the overt clinical symptoms and signs of the underlying process, knowledge and recognition of this entity is of great diagnostic importance.

> **MORPHOLOGY.** All forms of acanthosis nigricans have similar histologic features. The epidermis undulates sharply to form numerous repeating peaks and valleys. Variable hyperplasia may be seen, along with hyperkeratosis and slight basal cell layer hyperpigmentation (but no melanocytic hyperplasia).

FIBROEPITHELIAL POLYP

The fibroepithelial polyp has many names (acrochordon, squamous papilloma, skin tag) and is one of the most common cutaneous lesions. It is generally detected as an incidental finding in middle-aged and older individuals on the neck, trunk, face, and intertriginous areas as a soft, flesh-colored, baglike tumor attached to the skin surface by a small, often slender stalk.

> **MORPHOLOGY.** Histologically, these tumors are merely fibrovascular cores covered by benign squamous epithelium. It is not uncommon to discover ischemic necrosis in histologic sections (the result of torsion that produced the pain and swelling that precipitated their removal).

Fibroepithelial polyps are usually biologically inconsequential, although they have been associated with diabetes and intestinal polyposis. It is of interest that along with nevocellular nevi (discussed earlier) and hemangiomas (see later), they often become more numerous or prominent during pregnancy.

EPITHELIAL CYST (WEN)

Epithelial cysts are common lesions formed by the downgrowth and cystic expansion of the epidermis or of the epithelium forming the hair follicle. The lay term "wen" derives from the Anglo-Saxon wenn, meaning a lump or tumor. These cysts are filled with keratin and variable amounts of admixed, lipid-containing debris derived from sebaceous secretions. Clinically, they are dermal or subcutaneous, well-circumscribed, firm, and often moveable nodules. When large, they may be dome-shaped and flesh-colored and often become painful upon traumatic rupture.

> **MORPHOLOGY.** Histologically, epithelial cysts are divided into several types according to the structural components of their walls. The **epidermal inclusion cyst** has a wall nearly identical to the epidermis and is filled with laminated strands of keratin. **Pilar** and **trichilemmal cysts** have a wall that resembles follicular epithelium, without a granular cell layer and filled by a more homogeneous mixture of keratin and lipid. The **dermoid cyst** is similar to the epidermal inclusion cyst, but it also shows multiple appendages (such as small hair follicles) budding outward from its wall. Finally, **steatocystoma multiplex** constitutes a curious cyst with a wall resembling the sebaceous gland duct from which numerous compressed sebaceous lobules originate. The importance of recognition of this cyst derives from the often dominantly heritable nature of the lesion.

KERATOACANTHOMA

Keratoacanthoma is a rapidly developing neoplasm that clinically and histologically may mimic well-differentiated squamous cell carcinoma (see later discussion), but it heals spontaneously, without treatment! Men are more often affected than women, and lesions most frequently affect sun-exposed skin of whites over 50 years of age.[27]

Clinically, keratoacanthomas appear as flesh-colored, dome-shaped nodules with a central, keratin-filled plug, imparting a crater-like topography. Lesions range in size from 1 cm to several centimeters across and have a predilection for the cheeks, nose, ears, and dorsa of the hands.

> **MORPHOLOGY.** Histologically, keratoacanthomas are characterized by a central, keratin-filled crater, surrounded by proliferating epithelial cells that extend upward in a lip-like fashion over the sides of the crater and downward into the dermis as irregular tongues (Fig. 26–9A). This epithelium is composed of enlarged cells showing evidence of reactive cytologic atypia. These cells have a characteristically "glassy" eosinophilic cytoplasm (see Fig. 26–9B) and produce keratin abruptly (without the development of an intervening granular cell layer). This mode of keratinization is analogous to that of the normal hair follicle and similar to that seen in the pilar cyst described earlier, giving rise to speculation that the keratoacanthoma is a neoplasm of follicular epithelium. The early tumor infiltrates into the collagen and elastic fibers and entraps them.

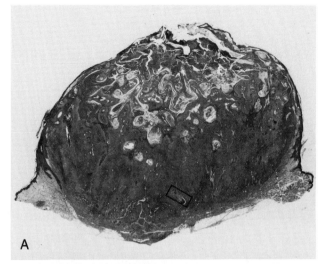
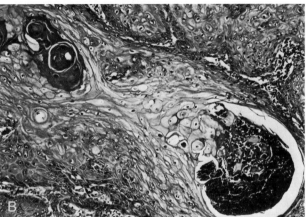

Figure 26–9. Keratoacanthoma. A, At low power, the crater-like architecture may be appreciated. **B,** Higher power view of the small rectangle in A. These tumors are composed of large, glassy squamous cells that form islands of keratin *(upper left).* The dark mass in the lower right corner is a characteristic aggregate of neutrophils within the tumor.

> Little, if any, host inflammatory response is present during this rapidly proliferative phase, but as the lesion evolves, there is some stromal response that is fibrotic and contains numerous inflammatory cells.

ADNEXAL (APPENDAGE) TUMORS

There are literally hundreds of benign neoplasms arising from cutaneous appendages.[28] Although some show no aggressive behavior and remain localized, they may be confused with certain types of cutaneous cancers (e.g., basal cell carcinoma; see later discussion). Certain appendage tumors are associated with Mendelian patterns of inheritance and occur as multiple disfiguring lesions. In some

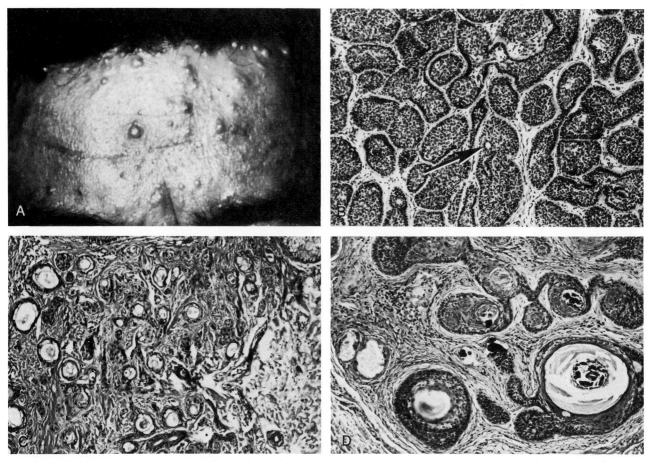

Figure 26-10. Adnexal tumors. Although the clinical appearance is often nondescript (*A* shows multiple cylindromas), the histologic features of each are characteristic. *B*, Cylindroma; *C*, syringoma; *D*, trichoepithelioma. Note the rare ducts in the cylindroma (*arrow*) and the numerous ducts in the syringoma. The trichoepithelioma resembles primitive hair follicle differentiation.

instances, these lesions serve as markers for internal malignancy, as in the case of multiple trichilemmomas and breast carcinoma of Cowden's syndrome.[29] Selected examples are provided here to illustrate neoplasms of hair follicles, eccrine glands, and apocrine glands.

Clinically, appendage tumors are often nondescript, solitary or multiple papules and nodules. Some have a predisposition for occurrence on specific body surfaces. For example, the *eccrine poroma* occurs predominantly on the palms and soles. The *cylindroma*, an appendage tumor with apocrine differentiation, usually occurs on the forehead and scalp (Fig. 26–10*A*), where coalescence of nodules with time may produce a hatlike growth, hence the name *"turban tumor."* These lesions may be dominantly inherited and first appear early in life. *Syringomas*, lesions of eccrine differentiation, on the other hand, usually occur as multiple, small, tan papules in the vicinity of the lower eyelids. *Trichoepitheliomas*, showing follicular differentiation, are dominantly inherited when they are seen as multiple, semitransparent, dome-

shaped papules that involve the face, scalp, neck and upper trunk.

MORPHOLOGY. The **cylindroma** is composed of islands of basaloid cells that seem to fit together like pieces of a jigsaw puzzle within a fibrous dermal matrix (see Fig. 26–10*B*). The **syringoma** shows some eccrine ductular differentiation within small, tadpole-like islands and strands of basaloid epithelium (see Fig. 26–10*C*). The **trichoepithelioma** is a proliferation of basaloid cells that forms hair follicle–like structures (see Fig. 26–10*D*). The **trichilemmoma** is a localized proliferation of pale pink, glassy cells that resembles the uppermost portion of the hair follicle (infundibulum). Table 26–2 summarizes common adnexal tumors according to histologic features that recapitulate mature adnexal counterparts.

Although most appendage tumors are benign, malignant variants do exist. *Sebaceous carcinoma*, for example, arises from the meibomian glands of

Table 26-2. COMMON ADNEXAL TUMORS AND MATURE COUNTERPARTS

ADNEXAL TUMORS	MATURE COUNTERPART	COMMON FEATURES	CLINICAL SIGNIFICANCE
Trichoepithelioma Trichofolliculoma	Hair follicle	Hair matrix, outer root sheath differentiation	Multiple trichoepitheliomas —dominant inheritance
Sebaceous adenoma Sebaceous epithelioma	Sebaceous gland	Cytoplasmic lipid vacuoles	Association with internal malignancy
Syringocystadenoma papilliferum	Apocrine gland	Apocrine-type ("decapitation") secretion	May develop in mixed epidermal-adnexal hamartomas of face and scalp termed "nevus sebaceus"
Syringoma	Eccrine gland	Eccrine ducts lined by membranous eosinophilic cuticles; tadpole-like epithelial structures	May be confused with basal cell carcinoma clinically

the eyelid and may follow an aggressive biologic course with systemic metastases. *Eccrine* and *apocrine carcinomas* are often confused with metastatic adenocarcinomas to the skin because of their tendency for abortive gland formation.

PREMALIGNANT AND MALIGNANT EPIDERMAL TUMORS

ACTINIC KERATOSIS

Prior to the development of overt malignancy of the epidermis, a series of progressively dysplastic changes occurs, a phenomenon analogous to the atypia that precedes carcinoma of the squamous mucosa of the uterine cervix (see Chapter 23). Because this dysplasia is usually the result of chronic exposure to sunlight and is associated with build-up of excess keratin, these lesions are called actinic keratoses. As would be expected, they occur in a particularly high incidence in lightly pigmented individuals. Exposure to ionizing radiation, hydrocarbons, and arsenicals may induce similar lesions.

Lesions are usually less than 1 cm in diameter; are tan-brown, red, or skin-colored; and have a rough, sandpaperlike consistency. Some lesions may produce so much keratin that a "cutaneous horn" develops (Fig. 26–11A). Such horns may become so developed that they actually resemble the horns of animals! Skin sites commonly involved by sun exposure (face, arms dorsum of hands) are most frequently affected. The lips may also develop similar lesions (actinic cheilitis).

MORPHOLOGY. Cytologic atypia is seen in the lowermost layers of the epidermis and may be asso-

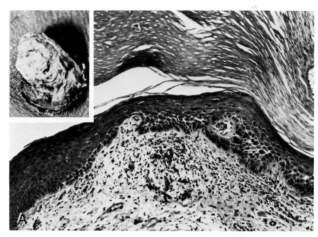
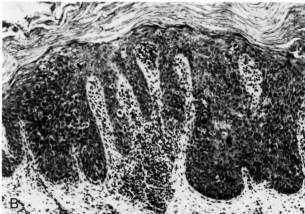

Figure 26–11. *A*, Actinic keratosis. Basal cell layer atypia (normal epidermis, *on left*) is associated with marked hyperkeratosis and parakeratosis that may result in the clinical appearance of a horn *(inset)*. *B*, Progression to full-thickness atypia heralds the development of squamous cell carcinoma in situ.

ciated with hyperplasia of basal cells (see Fig. 26–11A), or, alternatively, with early atrophy that results in diffuse thinning of the epidermal surface of the lesion. The atypical basal cells usually have evidence of dyskeratosis with pink or reddish cytoplasm. Also, intercellular bridges are present, in contrast to basal cell carcinoma (see later discussion), in which the cytoplasm is usually basophilic and the cells lack intercellular bridges identifiable by light microscopy. The dermis contains thickened, blue-gray elastic fibers (elastosis), a probable result of abnormal dermal elastic fiber synthesis by sun-damaged fibroblasts[30] within the superficial dermis. The stratum corneum is thickened and, unlike in normal skin, nuclei in the cells in this layer are often retained (a pattern termed "parakeratosis").

Whether all actinic keratoses would eventuate in skin cancer (usually squamous cell carcinoma), if given enough time, is conjectural. Indeed, it is likely that many lesions regress or remain stable during a normal lifespan. However, enough do become malignant to warrant local eradication of these potential precursor lesions. This can usually be accomplished by gentle curettage, freezing, or topical application of chemotherapeutic agents.

SQUAMOUS CELL CARCINOMA

Squamous cell carcinoma is the most common tumor arising on sun-exposed sites in older people. Except for lesions on the lower legs, these tumors have a higher incidence in men than in women. Implicated as predisposing factors, in addition to sunlight, are industrial carcinogens (tars and oils), chronic ulcers and draining osteomyelitis, old burn scars, ingestion of arsenicals, ionizing radiation, and in the oral cavity tobacco and betel nut chewing. Patients with xeroderma pigmentosum (see Chapter 7), and immunosuppressed individuals also have a high incidence of this neoplasm.

Squamous cell carcinomas that have not invaded through the basement membrane of the dermoepidermal junction (in situ carcinoma) appear as sharply defined, red scaling plaques. More advanced, invasive lesions are nodular, show variable

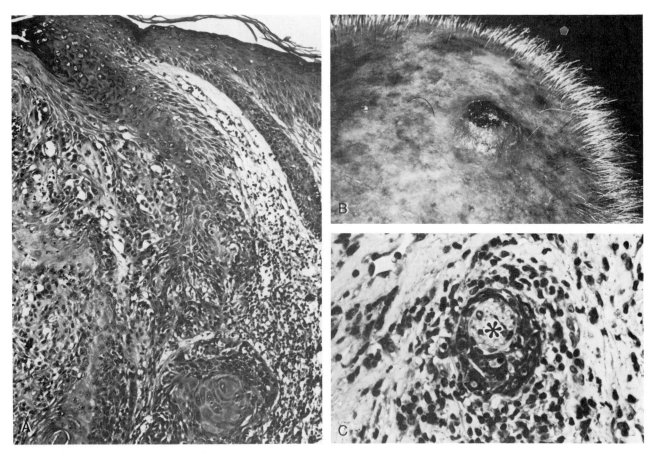

Figure 26–12. Invasive squamous cell carcinoma. *A,* Tongues of atypical squamous epithelium have transgressed the basement membrane, invading deeply into the dermis. *B,* Such lesions are often nodular and ulcerated clinically. *C,* Tumor cells highlighted by staining with labeled antibodies to keratin surround a dermal nerve twig (*), indicative of the locally aggressive nature of this neoplasm.

keratin production appreciated clinically as hyperkeratosis, and may ulcerate (Fig. 26–12). Well-differentiated lesions may be indistinguishable from keratoacanthoma (see previous section). When the mucosa is involved, a zone of white thickening is seen, an appearance caused by a variety of disorders and referred to clinically as *leukoplakia*.

> **MORPHOLOGY.** Unlike actinic keratoses, squamous cell carcinoma in situ is characterized by highly atypical cells at **all levels** of the epidermis (see Fig. 26–11B). When these cells break through the basement membrane, the process has become invasive. Invasive squamous cell carcinoma (see Fig. 26–12) exhibits variable differentiation, ranging from tumors formed by polygonal squamous cells arranged in orderly lobules and exhibiting numerous large zones of keratinization, to neoplasms formed by highly anaplastic, rounded cells with foci of necrosis and only abortive, single-cell keratinization (dyskeratosis). These latter tumors may be so poorly differentiated that electron microscopy for the detection of keratinocyte intercellular attachment sites (desmosomes) or reaction of tissue with antibodies to keratin or epithelial membrane-associated antigens may be necessary to definitively establish cell lineage.
>
> Invasive squamous cell carcinomas are usually discovered while small and resectable; fewer than 5% have metastases to regional nodes.

The most commonly accepted exogenous cause of squamous cell carcinoma is exposure to ultraviolet light with subsequent DNA damage and associated mutagenicity. Individuals who are immunosuppressed as a result of chemotherapy or organ transplantation, or who have xeroderma pigmentosum, are at increased risk for developing neoplasms.[31] A considerable proportion of these are squamous cell carcinomas, implicating aberrations in local immune networks in the skin in the production of an atmosphere permissive to neoplasia. Sunlight, in addition to its effect on DNA, also seems to have a direct and at least a transient immunosuppressive effect on skin by affecting the normal surveillance function of antigen-presenting Langerhans cells in the epidermis.[32] In experimental animals, it now appears that although Langerhans cells responsible for T-lymphocyte activation are injured by ultraviolet light, similar cells responsible for the selective induction of suppressor lymphocyte pathways are resistant to UV damage.[33,34] Such a phenomenon could result in local imbalances in T-cell function that would favor tumorigenesis and progression. DNA sequences of certain viruses (e.g., human papillomavirus HPV36) have been detected recently in DNA extracted from potential precursors of squamous cell carcinoma,[35] suggesting a role for these agents in the evolution of certain cutaneous epithelial neoplasms. Finally, certain chemical agents appear to have direct mutagenic effects by producing DNA adducts with subsequent oncogene activation.[36]

BASAL CELL CARCINOMA

Basal cell carcinomas are common, slow-growing tumors that rarely metastasize. They have a tendency to occur at sites subject to chronic sun exposure and in lightly pigmented people. As with squamous cell carcinoma, the incidence of basal cell carcinoma rises sharply with immunosuppression and in patients with inherited defects in DNA replication or repair (xeroderm pigmentosum; see Chapter 7). The rare, dominantly inherited basal cell nevus syndrome[37] is associated with the development of numerous basal cell carcinomas in early life and with abnormalities of bone, nervous system, eyes, and reproductive organs.

Clinically, these tumors present as pearly papules often containing prominent, dilated subepidermal blood vessels (telangiectasias) (Fig. 26–13A). Some tumors contain melanin pigment and, thus, appear similar to nevocellular nevi or melanomas. Advanced lesions may ulcerate, and extensive local invasion of bone or facial sinuses may occur after many years of neglect or in unusually aggressive tumors, justifying the past designation "rodent ulcers."

> **MORPHOLOGY.** Histologically, tumor cells resemble those in the normal basal cell layer of the epidermis. They arise from the epidermis or follicular epithelium and do not occur on mucosal surfaces. Two patterns are seen, either **multifocal growths** originating from the epidermis and extending over several square centimeters or more of skin surface (multifocal superficial type), or **nodular lesions** growing downward deeply into the dermis as cords and islands of variably basophilic cells with hyperchromatic nuclei, embedded in a mucinous matrix, and often surrounded by many fibroblasts and lymphocytes (see Fig. 26–13B). The cells forming the periphery of the tumor cell islands tend to be arranged radially with their long axes in approximately parallel alignment (palisading). The stroma shrinks away from the epithelial tumor nests, creating clefts or separation artifacts that assist in differentiating basal cell carcinomas from certain appendage tumors also characterized by proliferation of basaloid cells.

MERKEL CELL CARCINOMA

This rare neoplasm is derived from the infrequent and functionally obscure *Merkel cell* of the epidermis, a neural crest–derived cell putatively impor-

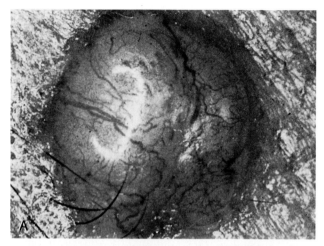

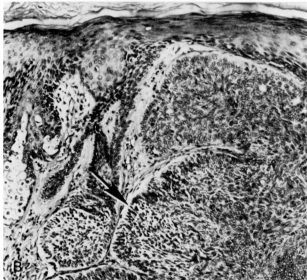

Figure 26-13. Basal cell carcinoma. Pearly, telangiectatic nodules (A) are composed of nests of basaloid cells within the dermis (B) that are often separated from the adjacent stroma by thin clefts (arrow).

tant for tactile sensation in lower animals.[38] These potentially lethal tumors are composed of small, round malignant cells containing neurosecretory-type cytoplasmic granules. Pathologists must be aware of this rare primary skin tumor since it may closely resemble metastatic small cell carcinoma from lung or certain lymphomas that spread to the dermis.

TUMORS OF THE DERMIS

The dermis is composed of a variety of different elements, including smooth muscle, pericytes, fibroblasts, neural tissue, and endothelium. All of these components can give rise to neoplasia within the skin, but many of these tumors also arise in soft tissue and viscera unrelated to skin (e.g., leiomyo-

sarcoma) or occur as part of a syndrome primarily affecting another organ system (e.g., as with cutaneous neurofibromas in neurofibromatosis). In this section, therefore, only representative dermal neoplasms that arise primary in the skin, that have unique characteristics in the skin, or that have not been detailed in other chapters are considered.

BENIGN FIBROUS HISTIOCYTOMA

Benign fibrous histiocytoma refers to a heterogeneous family of morphologically and histogenetically related benign dermal neoplasms of fibroblasts and histiocytes. (They are also discussed with the soft tissue tumors in Chapter 27.) These tumors are usually seen in adults, and often occur on the legs of young to middle-aged women. Their biologic behavior is indolent, and they should not be confused with malignant fibrous histiocytoma, which arises *de novo* in skin and in extracutaneous sites and often has an aggressive clinical course.

On gross inspection, these neoplasms are tan to brown, firm papules (Fig. 26–14A). Lesions are asymptomatic to slightly tender, and their size may increase and decrease slightly over time. Actively growing lesions may reach several centimeters in diameter, and, with time, they often become flattened. The tendency for fibrous histiocytomas to dimple inward upon lateral compression is helpful in distinguishing them from nodular melanomas, which protrude when similarly manipulated.

MORPHOLOGY. The most common form of fibrous histiocytoma is referred to as a **dermatofibroma.** These tumors are formed by benign, spindle-shaped fibroblasts arranged in a well-defined, non-encapsulated mass within the mid-dermis (see Fig. 26–14B). Extension of these cells into the subcutaneous fat is frequently observed. The majority of cases demonstrate a peculiar form of overlying epidermal hyperplasia, characterized by downward elongation of hyperpigmented rete ridges ("dirty fingers" pattern). Although foamy histiocytes may be seen in dermatofibromas, they are generally not conspicuous. Other tumors are composed predominantly of these foamy histiocytes admixed with a paucity of fibroblasts. Finally, variants containing numerous blood vessels and deposits of hemosiderin may be encountered **(sclerosing hemangiomas).**

The histogenesis of fibrous histiocytomas remains a mystery. Many cases have a history of antecedent trauma, suggesting an abnormal response to injury, perhaps analogous to the deposition of increased amounts of altered collagen in a hypertrophic scar or keloid.

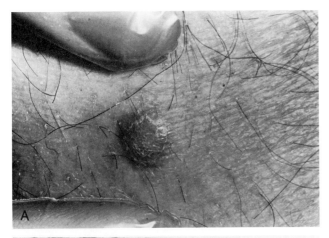

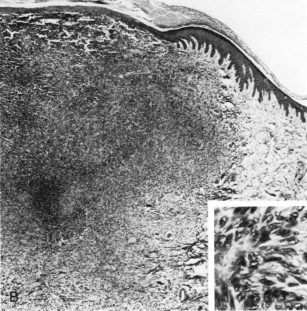

Figure 26–14. Benign fibrous histiocytoma (dermatofibroma). On excision, this firm, tan papule on the leg *(A)* shows a localized nodular proliferation of benign-appearing fibroblasts within the dermis *(B, inset)*. Note the characteristic overlying epidermal hyperplasia near the edge of the lesion.

DERMATOFIBROSARCOMA PROTUBERANS

Dermatofibrosarcoma protuberans is best regarded as a well-differentiated, primary fibrosarcoma of the skin. These tumors are slow growing, and although they are locally aggressive, they rarely metastasize.

Clinically, they are firm, solid nodules that arise most frequently on the trunk. They often develop as aggregated "protuberant" tumors within a firm (indurated) plaque and may ulcerate.

MORPHOLOGY. Microscopically, these neoplasms are very cellular, composed of fibroblasts arranged radially, reminiscent of blades of a pinwheel, a pattern referred to as "storiform." Mitoses are usually present but are not as numerous as in a moderately or poorly differentiated fibrosarcoma (see section on soft tissue tumors in Chapter 27). In contrast to that in dermatofibroma, the overlying epidermis is generally thinned. Deep extension from the dermis into subcutaneous fat is frequently present, hindering attempts at complete surgical removal.

XANTHOMAS

Xanthomas are tumor-like collections of foamy histiocytes within the dermis. They may be associated with familial (see Chapter 5) or acquired disorders resulting in hyperlipidemia, with lymphoproliferative malignancies, or without any underlying disorder.

On the basis of clinical appearance, xanthomas are divided into five types. Because identification of these types may provide important clinical markers of the underlying hyperlipoproteinemia, the classes of lipid abnormality (types I to V) are specified for each kind of clinical lesion.[39] *Eruptive xanthomas* (types I, IIB, III, IV, V) occur as sudden showers of yellow papules that wax and wane according to variations in plasma triglyceride and lipid content. They occur on the buttocks, posterior thighs, knees, and elbows. *Tuberous* (types IIA, III; rarely IIB, IV) and *tendinous* (types IIA, III; rarely IIIB) *xanthomas* occur as yellow nodules; the latter frequently are found on the Achilles tendon and the extensor tendons of the fingers. *Plane xanthomas* (type III; IIA associated with primary biliary cirrhosis) are linear yellow lesions in the skin folds, especially the palmar creases. *Xanthelasma* (types IIA, III; also without lipid abnormality) refers to soft yellow plaques on the eyelids.

MORPHOLOGY. Histologically, all types are characterized by dermal accumulation of benign-appearing histiocytes with abundant, finely vacuolated (foamy) cytoplasm. Cholesterol (free and esterified), phospholipids, and triglycerides are present within cells. The cellularity of the infiltrate is variable, and with the exception of xanthelasma, lesions may also be surrounded by inflammatory cells and fibrosis about the central zone of lipid-laden cells.

DERMAL VASCULAR TUMORS

Benign vascular neoplasms (capillary and cavernous hemangiomas), malformations (nevus flammeus or "port-wine stain"), multifocal angioproliferative lesions (Kaposi's sarcoma, bacillary angiomatosis), and malignant vascular tumors (angiosarcomas) are not infrequently encountered in the skin, and are discussed in depth in Chapter 11.

TUMORS OF CELLULAR IMMIGRANTS TO THE SKIN

Aside from tumors that arise directly from epidermal and dermal cells, several proliferative disorders of the skin involve primarily cells whose progenitors have arisen elsewhere, but which exhibit a peculiar homing to the cutaneous microenvironment. Examples of such cells are epidermal Langerhans cells, which arise from precursors in the bone marrow and which, in their mature form, traffic freely from skin to regional lymph nodes by way of dermal lymphatics; T lymphocytes that are normally in residence in low numbers in the dermis and epidermis; and dermal mast cells derived from marrow precursors The proliferative lesions to be discussed in this section—namely, histiocytosis X, cutaneous T-cell lymphoma, and mastocytosis—are primary cutaneous disorders that arise from these three cell types, respectively.

HISTIOCYTOSIS X

Histiocytosis X has been described in detail in a previous chapter (see Chapter 14). In the skin, this condition presents in multiple forms, including solitary or multiple lesions ranging from papules to nodules to scaling erythematous plaques that in infants may resemble seborrheic dermatitis (see previous discussion).

MORPHOLOGY. Histologically, histiocytosis X involving the skin has several patterns, all of which may show marked infiltration of the skin. The first is that of a diffuse dermal infiltrate of large, round-to-ovoid cells with pale pink cytoplasms containing indented, often bland nuclei (Fig. 26–15A). A second pattern consists of a clustering of similar cells into small aggregates that resemble granulomas. The third is characterized by a dermal infiltrate of cells with foamy, xanthoma-like cytoplasm. Variable numbers of eosinophils may also be observed, particularly with their first pattern. Because these patterns are not specific, ultrastructural identification of specific organelles (Birbeck granules) characteristic of the Langerhans cells from which histiocytosis X cells are believed to originate is helpful. Likewise, special immunohistochemical methods to identify cell surface markers common to Langerhans cells and histiocytosis X cells (CD1 antigen)[41] may be necessary to establish a definitive histologic diagnosis (see Fig. 26–15B).

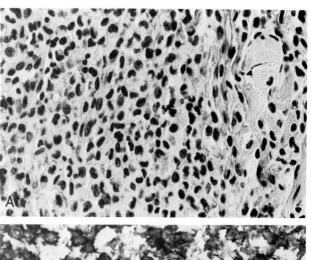

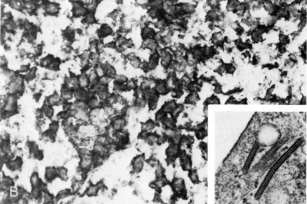

Figure 26–15. Histiocytosis X. *A*, Dermal infiltration by bland mononuclear cells with infolded nuclei presents a nonspecific histologic pattern. *B*, However, immunohistochemical demonstration of Langerhans cell CD1 antigen or ultrastructural detection of Birbeck granules *(inset)* permitted accurate diagnosis in this case.

MYCOSIS FUNGOIDES (CUTANEOUS T-CELL LYMPHOMA)

Cutaneous T-cell lymphoma (CTCL) represents a spectrum of lymphoproliferative disorders affecting the skin (see also Chapter 14). Two types of malignant T-cell disorders were originally recognized; mycosis fungoides (MF), a chronic proliferative process, and a nodular eruptive variant, *mycosis fungoides d'emblée*. It is now known that a variety of presentations of T-cell lymphoma occur, including MF, the eruptive nodular type, and an adult T-cell leukemia or lymphoma type.[42] The latter disorder may have a rapid progressive downhill course.

Mycosis fungoides is the T-cell lymphoproliferative disorder that arises primarily in the skin and that may evolve into generalized lymphoma.[43] Most affected individuals have disease that remains localized to the skin for many years; a minority have rapid systemic dissemination. This condition may occur at any age, but most commonly it afflicts persons over 40 years of age.

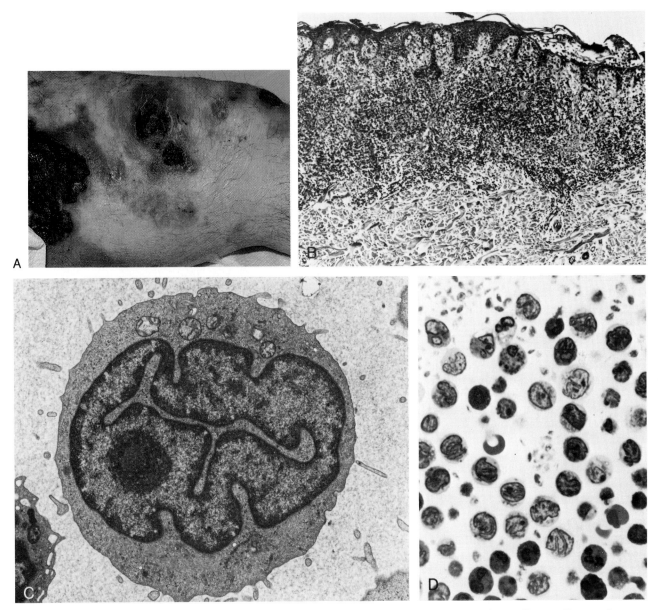

Figure 26–16. Cutaneous T-cell lymphoma. The histologic correlate of ill-defined, erythematous, often scaling, and occasionally ulcerated plaques (A) is an infiltrate of atypical lymphocytes that show a tendency to accumulate beneath the epidermal layer (B) and to invade the epidermis as small microabscesses. C, Unlike most benign lymphocytes, these cells have markedly irregular nuclear contours. D, With advanced disease, they may be detected in white cell fractions (buffy coat) of the peripheral blood.

Clinically, lesions of the MF type of CTCL include scaly, red-brown patches; raised, scaling plaques that may even be confused with psoriasis; and fungating nodules. Eczema-like lesions typify early stages of disease when obvious visceral or nodal spread has not occurred. Raised, indurated, irregularly outlined, erythematous plaques may then supervene. Development of multiple, large (up to 10 cm or more in diameter), red-brown nodules correlates with systemic spreading. Sometimes plaques and nodules ulcerate, as depicted in Figure 26–16A. Lesions may affect numerous body surfaces, including the trunk, extremities, face, and scalp. In some individuals, seeding of the blood by malignant T cells is accompanied by diffuse erythema and scaling of the entire body surface (erythroderma), a condition known as *Sézary syndrome* (see Chapter 14).

MORPHOLOGY. The hallmark of CTCL of the mycosis fungoides type histologically is the identification of the **Sézary-Lutzner** cells. These are T-helper cells (CD4 antigen–positive) that characteristically form band-like aggregates within the superficial dermis (see Fig. 26–16B) and invade the epidermis as single cells and small clusters **(Pautrier's microabscesses).** These cells have markedly infolded nuclear membranes, imparting a "hyperconvoluted" or "cerebriform" contour (see Fig. 26–16C). Although patches and plaques show pronounced epidermal infiltration by Sézary-Lutzner cells (epidermotropism), in more advanced nodular lesions the malignant T cells often lose this epidermotropic tendency, grow deeply into the dermis, and eventually seed lymphatics and the peripheral circulation (see Fig. 26–16D).

The cause of CTCL is under active investigation. The discovery that a highly aggressive form of T-cell lymphoma or leukemia in adults is caused by infection of helper T cells by a specific retrovirus (human T-cell leukemia virus, or HTLV-I)[43] (see section on RNA oncogenic viruses in Chapter 7) raises the possibility that conventional CTCL may also have an infectious causation.

Topical therapy with steroids or ultraviolet light is often employed for early lesions of CTCL, whereas more aggressive systemic chemotherapy is indicated for advanced disease. In patients with circulating malignant cells, exposure of blood cells removed from the body to photosensitizing agents and ultraviolet A irradiation, followed by reinfusion into the patient (extracorporeal photopheresis[44]), has shown promise as a novel therapeutic approach to disseminated CTCL.

MASTOCYTOSIS

The term "mastocytosis" refers to a spectrum of rare disorders characterized by increased numbers of mast cells in the skin and, in some instances, in other organs. A localized cutaneous form of the disease that affects predominantly children and accounts for more than 50% of all cases is termed *urticaria pigmentosa*. These lesions are multiple, although solitary mastocytomas may also occur, usually shortly after birth. About 10% of patients with mast cell disease have overt systemic mastocytosis, with mast cell infiltration of many organs. These individuals are often adults, and unlike the case with localized cutaneous disease, the prognosis may be poor.

The clinical picture of mastocytosis is highly variable. In urticaria pigmentosa, lesions are multiple and widely distributed, consisting of round-to-oval, red-brown, nonscaling papules and small plaques. Solitary mastocytomas present as one or several tan-brown nodules that may be pruritic or exhibit blister formation. In systemic mastocytosis, skin lesions similar to those of urticaria pigmentosa are accompanied by mast cell infiltration of bone marrow, liver, spleen, and lymph nodes. Many of the signs and symptoms of mastocytosis are due to the effects of histamine, heparin, and other substances released as a result of degranulation. *Darier's sign* refers to a localized area of dermal edema

and erythema (wheal) that occurs when lesional skin is rubbed. *Dermatographism* refers to an area of dermal edema resembling a hive that occurs in normal skin as a result of localized stroking with a pointed instrument. Pruritus and flushing triggered by certain foods, temperature changes, alcohol, and certain drugs (morphine, codeine, aspirin); watery nasal discharge (rhinorrhea); rarely gastrointestinal or nasal bleeding, possibly due to the anticoagulant effects of heparin; and bone pain as a result of osteoblastic and osteoclastic involvement may all be seen in systemic disease.

MORPHOLOGY. The histologic picture varies from a subtle increase in the numbers of spindle-shaped and stellate mast cells about superficial dermal blood vessels to large numbers of tightly packed, round-to-oval mast cells in the upper to mid-dermis (Fig. 26–17A) in urticaria pigmentosa or solitary mastocytoma. Variable fibrosis, edema, and small numbers of eosinophils may also be present. Mast cells may be difficult to differentiate from lymphocytes in routine, H and E-stained sections, and special "metachromatic" stains (toluidine blue or Giemsa) must be used to visualize their granules. Even with these stains, extensive degranulation may result in failure to detect these cells by light microscopy, and ultrastructural analysis must then be performed (see Fig. 26–17B).

ACUTE INFLAMMATORY DERMATOSES

Inflammatory dermatoses are usually mediated by local or systemic immunologic factors, although the causes for most remain a mystery. Literally thousands of specific inflammatory dermatoses exist. In general, acute lesions last from days to weeks and are characterized by inflammation (often marked by mononuclear cells, not neutrophils), edema, and, in some, epidermal, vascular, or subcutaneous injury. Chronic lesions, on the other hand, persist for months to years and often show significant components of altered epidermal growth (atrophy or hyperplasia) or dermal fibrosis. The lesions discussed here are selected as examples of the more commonly encountered dermatoses within the acute category.

URTICARIA

Urticaria (hives) is a common disorder of the skin characterized by localized mast cell degranulation and resultant dermal microvascular hyperpermea-

edematous plaques. Individual lesions may coalesce to form annular, linear, or arciform configurations. Sites of predilection for urticarial eruptions include any area exposed to pressure, such as the trunk, distal extremities, and ears. Persistent urticaria may simply be the result of inability to eliminate the causative antigen, or may herald underlying disease (e.g., collagen-vascular disorders, Hodgkin's disease).

MORPHOLOGY. The histologic features of urticaria may be so subtle that many biopsy specimens at first resemble normal skin. Usually there is a very sparse superficial perivenular infiltrate consisting of mononuclear cells and rare neutrophils. Eosinophils may be present, often in the mid-reticular dermis. Collagen bundles are more widely spaced than in normal skin, a result of superficial dermal edema fluid that does not stain in routinely prepared tissue. Superficial lymphatic channels are dilated in an attempt to accommodate this transudated edema fluid.

In most cases urticaria results from antigen-induced release of vasoactive mediators from mast cell granules via sensitization with specific IgE antibodies.[45] This *IgE-dependent* degranulation can follow exposure to a number of antigens (pollens, foods, drugs, insect venom) and specifically results from bridging of cell-bound IgE molecules by multivalent ligand, as discussed in Chapter 6. *IgE-independent* urticaria may result from substances that in certain individuals incite directly the degranulation of mast cells, such as opiates, certain antibiotics, curare, and radiographic contrast media. Another cause of IgE-independent urticaria is exposure to chemicals, such as aspirin, that suppress prostaglandin synthesis from arachidonic acid. Hereditary angioneurotic edema is the result of an inherited deficiency of C1 activator (C1 esterase inhibitor) that results in uncontrolled activation of the early components of the complement system (so-called complement-mediated urticaria).[46]

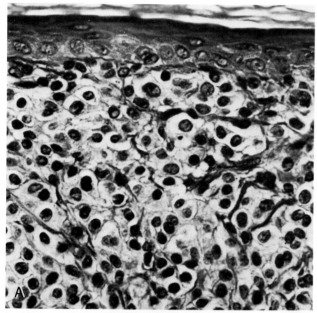

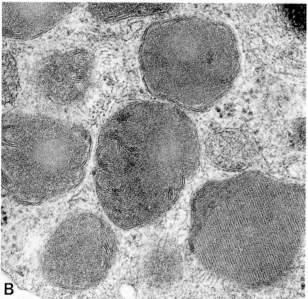

Figure 26–17. Mastocytosis. *A,* Numerous ovoid cells with uniform, centrally located nuclei are observed in the dermis. *B,* By electron microscopy, most of these cells are found to contain cytoplasmic granules typical of mast cells. These are membrane-bound and contain scroll- and lattice-like material.

bility, culminating in pruritic edematous plaques called wheals. Angioedema is closely related to urticaria and is characterized by deeper edema of both the dermis and the subcutaneous fat.

Clinically, urticaria most often occurs between the ages of 20 and 40, although all age groups are susceptible. Individual lesions develop and fade within hours (usually less than 24 hours), and episodes may last for days or persist for months. Lesions vary from small, pruritic papules to large

ACUTE ECZEMATOUS DERMATITIS

Eczema is a clinical term that embraces a number of pathogenetically different conditions. All are characterized by red, papulovesicular, oozing, and crusted lesions early on that with persistence eventuate into raised, scaling plaques. Clinical differences permit classification of eczematous dermatitis into the following categories: (1) allergic contact dermatitis; (2) atopic dermatitis; (3) drug-related eczematous dermatitis; (4) photoeczema-

Table 26–3. CLASSIFICATION OF ECZEMATOUS DERMATITIS

TYPE	CAUSE OR PATHOGENESIS	HISTOLOGY*	CLINICAL FEATURES
Contact dermatitis	Topically applied chemicals Pathogenesis: delayed hypersensitivity	Spongiotic dermatitis	Marked itching or burning or both; requires antecedent exposure
Atopic dermatitis	Unknown, may be heritable	Spongiotic dermatitis	Erythematous plaques in flexural areas; family history of eczema, hay fever, or asthma
Drug-related eczematous dermatitis	Systemically administered antigens or haptens (e.g., penicillin)	Spongiotic dermatitis; eosinophils often present in infiltrate; deeper infiltrate	Eruption occurs with administration of drug; remits when drug is discontinued
Photoeczematous eruption	Ultraviolet light	Spongiotic dermatitis; deeper infiltrate	Occurs on sun-exposed skin; phototesting may help in diagnosis
Primary irritant dermatitis	Repeated trauma (rubbing)	Spongiotic dermatitis in early stages; epidermal hyperplasia in late stages	Localized to site of trauma

* All types, with time, may develop chronic changes.

tous dermatitis; and (5) primary irritant dermatitis (Table 26–3).

The Greek word "eczema," meaning "to boil over," vividly describes the clinical appearance of acute eczematous dermatitis. The most obvious example is an acute contact reaction to poison ivy, characterized by pruritic, edematous, oozing plaques, often containing small and large blisters (vesicles and bullae) (Fig. 26–18A). Such lesions are prone to bacterial superinfection, which produces a yellow crust (impetiginization). With time, persistent lesions become less "wet" (fail to ooze or form vesicles) and become progressively scaly (hyperkeratotic) as the epidermis thickens (acanthosis).

MORPHOLOGY. Spongiosis—the accumulation of edema fluid within the epidermis—characterizes acute eczematous dermatitis, hence the synonym "spongiotic dermatitis." Whereas in urticaria, edema is localized to the perivascular spaces of the superficial dermis, in spongiotic dermatitis edema seeps into the intercellular spaces of the epidermis, splaying apart keratinocytes located primarily in the stratum spinosum. Intercellular bridges become prominent, giving a "spongy" appearance to the epidermis (see Fig. 26–18B). Mechanical shearing of intercellular attachment sites (desmosomes) and cell membranes by progressive accumulation of intercellular fluid may result in the formation of intraepidermal vesicles.

During the earliest stages of the evolution of spongiotic dermatitis, there is a superficial, perivascular, lymphocytic infiltrate associated with papillary dermal edema and mast cell degranulation. The pattern and composition of this infiltrate may provide clues to the underlying cause.[47] For example, spongiotic dermatitis resulting from certain drugs will show a lymphocytic infiltrate, **often con-**

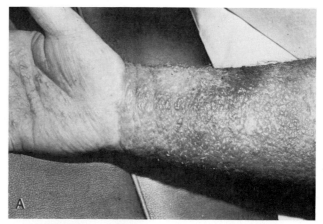

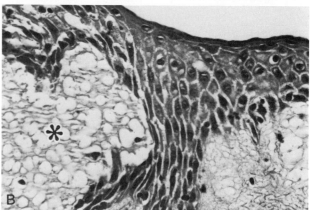

Figure 26–18. Eczematous dermatitis. *A*, In an acute allergic contact dermatitis, numerous vesicles appear at the site of antigen exposure (in this case, laundry detergent). *B*, Histologically, intercellular edema produces widened intercellular spaces within the epidermis, eventually resulting in small, fluid-filled intraepidermal vesicles (•).

taining eosinophils, and extending around deep as well as superficial dermal vessels.

Spongiotic dermatitis due to contact hypersensitivity (e.g., poison ivy dermatitis) has been studied extensively with regard to pathogenesis. It appears that an early event in the genesis of these lesions is local cytokine release in the vicinity of dermal postcapillary venules.[48,49]

This results in "endothelial activation" whereby endothelial cells express molecules on their plasma membranes that promote adhesion of circulating T lymphocytes with immunologic memory for the sensitizing antigen or hapten. Once these memory T cells enter the site of antigen challenge via activated microvessels, they elaborate a potent array of lymphokines that signal recruitment of large numbers of inflammatory cells to the site of antigen contact. This process occurs within 24 hours and accounts for the initial erythema and pruritus that characterize cutaneous delayed hypersensitivity in the acute, spongiotic phase.

ERYTHEMA MULTIFORME

Erythema multiforme is an uncommon, self-limited disorder that appears to be a hypersensitivity response to certain infections and drugs. Erythema multiforme is a prototype of a cytotoxic reaction pattern (one typified by extensive epithelial cell degeneration and death). This disorder affects individuals of any age and is associated with the following conditions: (1) infections such as herpes simplex, mycoplasma infections, histoplasmosis, coccidioidomycosis, typhoid, and leprosy, among others; (2) administration of certain drugs (sulfonamides, penicillin, barbiturates, salicylates, hydantoins, and antimalarials); (3) malignancy (carcinomas and lymphomas); and (4) collagen-vascular diseases (lupus erythematosus, dermatomyositis, and periarteritis nodosa).

Clinically, patients present with an array of "multiform" lesions including macules, papules, vesicles, and bullae, as well as the characteristic target lesion consisting of a red macule or papule with a pale, vesicular or eroded center (Fig. 26–19A). Although lesions may be widely distributed, symmetric involvement of the extremities frequently occurs. An extensive and symptomatic febrile form of the disease, which is more common in children, is called the *Stevens-Johnson syndrome.* Typically, erosions and hemorrhagic crusts involve the lips and oral mucosa, although the conjunctiva, urethra, and genital and perianal areas may also be affected. Infection of involved areas may result in life-threatening sepsis. Another variant, termed *toxic epidermal necrolysis,* results in diffuse necrosis and sloughing of cutaneous and mucosal epithelial surfaces, producing a clinical situation analogous to an extensive burn.

> **MORPHOLOGY.** Histologically, early lesions show a superficial perivascular, lymphocytic infiltrate associated with dermal edema and margination of lymphocytes along the dermoepidermal junction, where they are intimately associated with degenerating and necrotic keratinocytes. With time, there is upward migration of lymphocytes into the epidermis. Discrete and confluent zones of epidermal necrosis occur with concomitant blister formation (see Fig. 26–19B). Epidermal sloughing leads to shallow erosions. Histologically the **"target lesion"** exhibits central necrosis surrounded by a rim of perivenular inflammation.

Erythema multiforme has potential immunologic similarities to other conditions characterized by cytotoxic epidermal cell injury (e.g., acute graft-versus-host disease,[50] skin allograft rejection,[51] and fixed drug eruptions[52]). Many of the lymphocytes responsible for the cytotoxic response

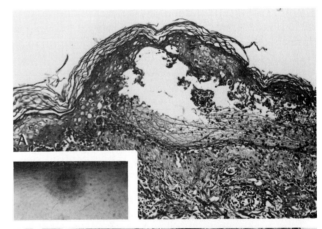

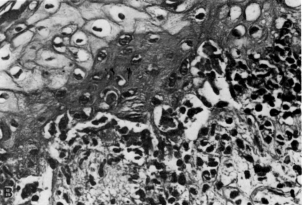

Figure 26–19. Erythema multiforme. *A,* The target-like clinical lesion *(inset)* is a central blister or zone of epidermal necrosis surrounded by macular erythema. *B,* Higher magnification of a biopsy specimen from the erythematous edge shows numerous lymphocytes in intimate contact with degenerating basal epidermal cells.

are of the supressor-cytotoxic phenotype, expressing CD8 molecules on their surfaces.

ERYTHEMA NODOSUM AND ERYTHEMA INDURATUM

Panniculitis is an inflammatory reaction in the subcutaneous fat that may affect (1) principally the connective tissue septa separating lobules of fat, or (2) predominantly the lobules of fat themselves. *Erythema nodosum* is the most common form of panniculitis and usually has an acute presentation. Its occurrence is often associated with infections (beta-hemolytic streptococcal infection, tuberculosis, and, less commonly, coccidioidomycosis, histoplasmosis, and leprosy), drug administration (sulfonamides, oral contraceptives), sarcoidosis, inflammatory bowel disease, and certain malignancies, but many times a cause cannot be elicited. Many types of panniculitis have a subacute to chronic course.

Panniculitis often involves the lower legs. Erythema nodosum presents acutely as poorly defined, exquisitely tender, erythematous nodules that may be better felt than seen. Fever and malaise may accompany the cutaneous signs. Over the course of weeks, lesions usually flatten and become bruise-like, leaving no residual clinical scars, while new lesions develop. Biopsy of a deep wedge of tissue is usually required to establish a definitive diagnosis.

Erythema induratum is an uncommon type of panniculitis that affects primarily adolescents and menopausal women. Although the cause is not known, most observers today regard this disorder as the result of a primary vasculitis affecting deep vessels supplying lobules of the subcutis, with subsequent necrosis and inflammation within the fat. Erythema induratum presents as an erythematous, slightly tender nodule that usually goes on to ulcerate. Originally considered a hypersensitivity response to tuberculosis, erythema induratum today most commonly occurs without an associated underlying disease.

> **MORPHOLOGY.** The histopathology of erythema nodosum is distinctive. In early lesions, there is widening of the connective tissue **septa** owing to edema, fibrin exudation, and neutrophilic infiltration (Fig. 26–20). Later, infiltration by lymphocytes, histiocytes, multinucleated giant cells, and occasional eosinophils is associated with septal fibrosis. Vasculitis is not present. In erythema induratum, on the other hand, the fat **lobule** is involved by granulomatous inflammation and zones of caseous necrosis. Early lesions show necrotizing vasculitis affecting small to medium-sized arteries and veins in the deep dermis and subcutis.

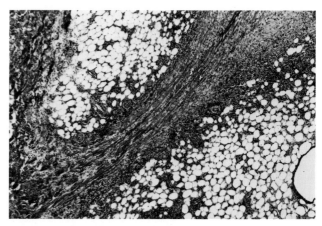

Figure 26–20. Erythema nodosum. A septum of the subcutaneous fat is preferentially infiltrated and widened by inflammatory cells.

Erythema nodosum and erythema induratum are but two examples of many types of panniculitis. *Weber-Christian disease (relapsing febrile nodular panniculitis)* is a rare form of lobular, nonvasculitic panniculitis seen in children and adults. It is marked by crops of erythematous plaques or nodules, predominantly on the lower extremities, created by deep-seated foci of inflammation with aggregates of foamy histiocytes admixed with lymphocytes, neutrophils, and giant cells. *Factitial panniculitis*, as a result of self-inflicted trauma or injection of foreign or toxic substances, is a form of secondary panniculitis that often poses profound problems in definitive clinical and pathologic diagnosis and may present a distinct set of therapeutic challenges. Deep mycotic infections in immunocompromised individuals may produce histologic changes that mimic primary panniculitis. Finally, disorders such as lupus erythematosus (see later) may occasionally have deep inflammatory components with associated panniculitis.

CHRONIC INFLAMMATORY DERMATOSES

This category focuses on those persistent inflammatory dermatoses that exhibit their most characteristic clinical and histologic features over many months to years. Unlike the normal cutaneous surface, the skin surface in some chronic inflammatory dermatoses is roughened as a result of excessive or abnormal scale formation and shedding (desquamation) (Fig. 26–21). However, not all scaling lesions are inflammatory. Witness the hereditary ichthyoses with fish-like scales as the result of some de-

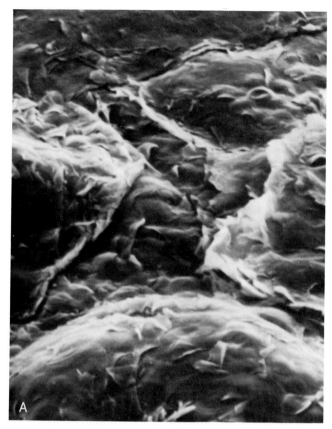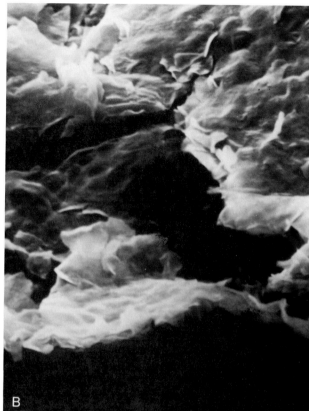

Figure 26–21. The surface morphology of hyperkeratosis assessed by scanning electron microscopy. Unlike the normal cutaneous surface *(A)* that is covered by relatively smooth and contiguous squamous cells of the stratum corneum, chronic dermatoses often exhibit excessive stratum corneum production *(B)*, producing an irregular and roughened surface. (Courtesy of Dr. Robert Lavker, University of Pennsylvania.)

fect in the adhesive properties of cells in the stratum corneum.

PSORIASIS

Psoriasis is a common chronic inflammatory dermatosis affecting as many as 1 to 2% of people in the United States. Persons of all ages may develop the disease. Psoriasis is sometimes associated with arthritis, myopathy, enteropathy, spondylitic heart disease, and AIDS. Psoriatic arthritis may be mild or produce severe deformities resembling the joint changes seen in rheumatoid arthritis.

Clinically, psoriasis most frequently affects the skin of the elbows, knees, scalp, lumbosacral areas, intergluteal cleft, and glans penis. The most typical lesion is a well-demarcated, pink to salmon-colored plaque covered by loosely adherent scales that are characteristically silver-white in color (Fig. 26–22). Variations exist, with some lesions occurring in annular, linear, gyrate, or serpiginous configurations. Psoriasis can be one cause of total-body erythema and scaling known as *erythroderma*. Nail changes[53] occur in 30% of cases of psoriasis and

consist of yellow-brown discoloration (often likened to an oil slick), with pitting, dimpling, separation of the nail plate from the underlying bed (onycholysis), thickening, and crumbling. In the rare variant called *pustular psoriasis*, multiple small pustules form on erythematous plaques. This type of psoriasis is either benign and localized (hands and feet) or generalized and life-threatening, with associated fever, leukocytosis, arthralgias, diffuse cutaneous and mucosal pustules, secondary infection, and electrolyte disturbances.

MORPHOLOGY. Established lesions of psoriasis have a characteristic histologic picture. Increased epidermal cell turnover results in marked epidermal thickening (acanthosis), with regular downward elongation of the rete ridges. Mitotic figures are easily identified well above the basal cell layer, where, in normal skin, mitotic activity is confined (Fig. 26–23). **The stratum granulosum is thinned or absent, and extensive overlying parakeratotic scale is seen.** Typical of psoriatic plaques is thinning of the portion of the epidermal cell layer that overlies the tips of dermal papillae (suprapapillary plates) and dilated, tortuous blood vessels within

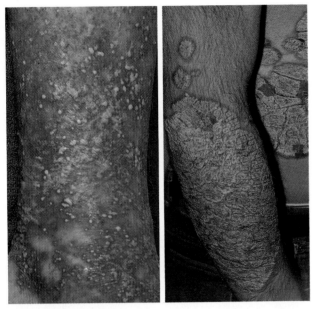

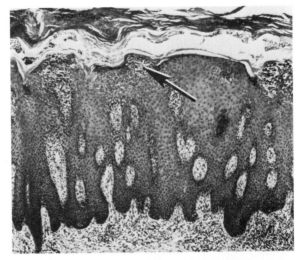

Figure 26–23. Psoriasis. Histologically, established lesions demonstrate marked epidermal hyperplasia, parakeratotic scale, and, importantly, minute microabscesses of neutrophils *(arrow)* within the superficial epidermal layers.

Figure 26–22. Clinical evolution of psoriasis. Early and eruptive lesions may be dominated by signs of inflammation and erythema *(left panel)*. Established, chronic lesions demonstrate erythema surmounted by characteristic silver-white scale *(right panel)*. Rarely, the early inflammatory phase predominates throughout the course of the disease (pustular psoriasis).

these papillae. This constellation of changes results in abnormal proximity of dermal vessels within the dermal papillae to the overlying parakeratotic scale, and it accounts for the characteristic clinical phenomenon of multiple, minute, bleeding points when the scale is lifted from the plaque **(Auspitz sign)**. Neutrophils form small aggregates within slightly spongiotic foci of the superficial epidermis **(spongiform pustules)** and within the parakeratotic stratum corneum **(Munro's microabscesses)**. In pustular psoriasis, larger abscess-like accumulations of neutrophils are present directly beneath the stratum corneum.

Determination of the pathogenesis of psoriasis is one of the most important challenges in dermatopathologic research. An increased incidence of disease in association with certain HLA types suggests that genetic factors participate in the predisposition for disease development. The genesis of new lesions at sites of trauma (the *Koebner phenomenon*) is undoubtedly providing some basic yet elusive pathogenetic clue. Evidence has recently been accumulated that psoriasis may be a type of complement-mediated reaction localized to the stratum corneum.[54] According to this hypothesis, exogenous or endogenous damage to the stratum corneum of certain individuals results in the unmasking of stratum corneum antigens. These antigens elicit the formation of specific autoantibodies that bind to the stratum corneum, fix complement,

and activate the complement cascade. Release locally of C3a, C5a, and C567 then leads to neutrophil activation and accumulation, a phenomenon likely aided by arachidonic acid metabolites, including leukotrienes. Neutrophils within the stratum corneum then release neutral serine proteases, which unmask more antigen and perpetuate the process. Proliferative factors for underlying keratinocytes are released as a consequence of these events and result in increased epidermal turnover and the hyperplasia and scale formation so characteristic of psoriasis.

Another possibility, however, is that the primary defect in psoriasis resides in the enhanced ability of superficial dermal microvessels to recruit neutrophils. It is possible that psoriatic endothelial cells are unusually sensitive to cytokine stimuli that regulate display of endothelial-leukocyte adhesion molecules, possibly as a result of genetically determined enhancement of cytokine receptor expression. Such hypotheses are the subject of active investigation.

LICHEN PLANUS

"Pruritic, purple, polygonal papules" are the presenting signs of this disorder of skin and mucous membranes. Lichen planus is self-limiting and generally resolves spontaneously one to two years after onset, often leaving zones of postinflammatory hyperpigmentation (see later). Oral lesions may persist for years. Malignant degeneration has been noted to occur in chronic mucosal and paramucosal lesions of lichen planus, although the

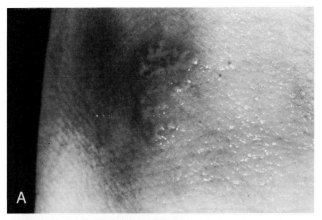

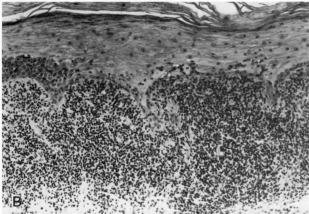

Figure 26–24. Lichen planus. *A,* A small erythematous plaque, covered with oil to render the stratum corneum translucent, shows characteristic Wickham's striae. *B,* Biopsy of this lesion demonstrates the band-like infiltrate of lymphocytes at the dermoepidermal junction and pointed rete ridges ("saw-toothing"; compare with Figure 26–1).

destructive infiltration of lymphocytes is a redefinition of the normal, smoothly undulating configuration of the dermoepidermal interface to a more angulated zig-zag contour ("saw-toothing"). Anucleate, necrotic basal cells may become incorporated into the inflamed papillary dermis, where they are referred to as **colloid** or **Civatte bodies.** Although this destructive relationship between lymphocytes and epidermal cells bears some similarities to that in erythema multiforme (discussed previously), lichen planus shows changes of chronicity —namely, epidermal hyperplasia (or rarely atrophy) and thickening of the granular cell layer and stratum corneum (hypergranulosis and hyperkeratosis, respectively). Lichen planus preferentially affecting the epithelium of hair follicles is referred to as **lichen planopilaris.**

The precise pathogenesis of lichen planus is not known. It is plausible that release of antigens at the levels of the basal cell layer and the dermoepidermal junction may elicit a cell-mediated immune response in lichen planus. Supporting this notion are data indicating that infiltrates of primarily T lymphocytes associated with hyperplasia of Langerhans cells are fundamental to lesion formation and evolution.[56]

LUPUS ERYTHEMATOSUS (LE)

The manifestations of systemic lupus erythematosus (SLE) are described in detail in Chapter 6. However, a localized, cutaneous form of LE, with no associated systemic manifestations, occurs and is called *discoid lupus erythematosus (DLE).* Patients who present with DLE usually do not go on to develop systemic disease. However, over one-third of patients with SLE may exhibit, during their course, lesions that are clinically and histologically indistinguishable from those of the discoid type. Thus, it is often impossible to distinguish patients with SLE from those with DLE on the basis of clinical and histologic inspection of skin lesions alone.

Cutaneous lesions usually consist of either poorly defined malar erythema (usually seen in systemic disease) or large, sharply demarcated erythematous scaling plaques (Fig. 26–25A). These "discoid" plaques may occur in either pure cutaneous LE or SLE. Cutaneous manifestations of LE may occur or worsen with sun exposure. The epidermal surface of lesions is shiny or scaly, and lateral compression often produces wrinkling, a sign of epidermal atrophy. Through this thinned epidermis, dilated and tortuous blood vessels (telangiectasia) and small zones of hypo- and hyperpigmentation may be seen. Small, keratotic plugs in

direct pathogenetic relationship has not been shown.[55]

Cutaneous lesions consist of itchy, violaceous, flat-topped papules that may coalesce focally to form plaques. These papules are often highlighted by white dots or lines called *Wickham's striae* (Fig. 26–24A). Multiple lesions are characteristic and are symmetrically distributed, particularly on the extremities, often about the wrists and elbows, and on the glans penis. In 70% of cases, oral lesions are present as white, reticulated, or netlike areas involving the mucosa. As in psoriasis, the Koebner phenomenon (see above) may be seen in lichen planus.

MORPHOLOGY. Lichen planus is characterized histologically by a dense, continuous infiltrate of lymphocytes along the dermoepidermal junction (see Fig. 26–24B). The lymphocytes are intimately associated with basal keratinocytes, which show degeneration, necrosis, and a resemblance in size and contour to more mature cells of the stratum spinosum (squamatization). A consequence of this

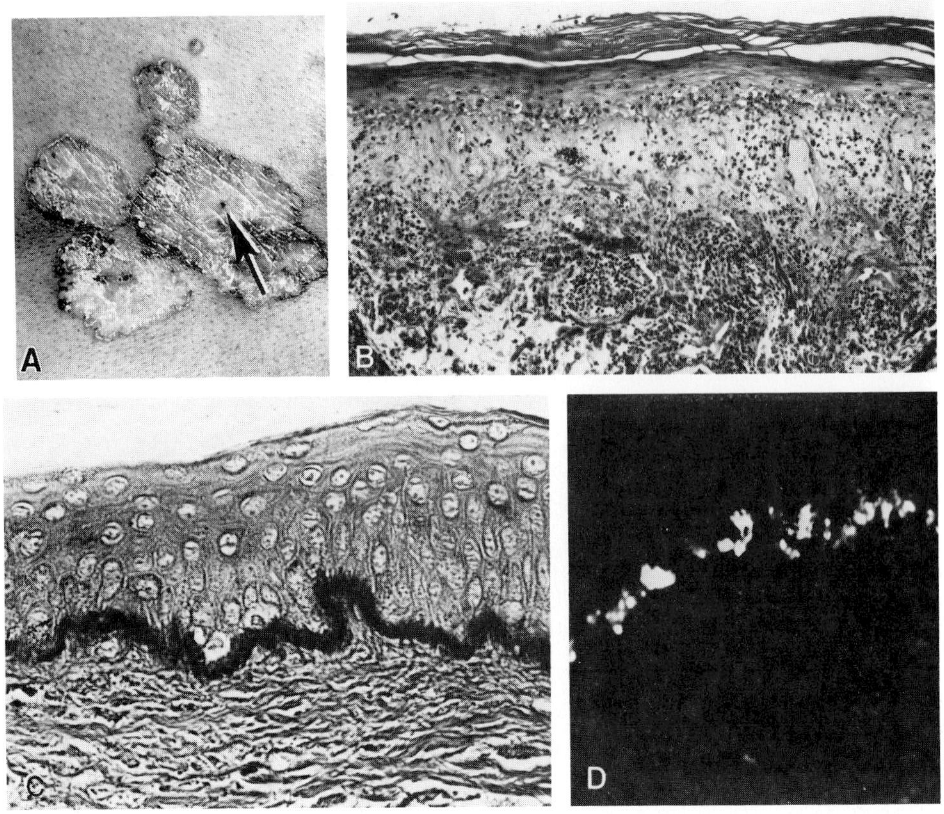

Figure 26-25. Lupus erythematosus. *A,* Discoid plaques show erythema and excessive scale. The histology of a biopsy taken from the center of such a plaque *(arrow)* is depicted in *B. B,* There is an infiltrate of lymphocytes within the superficial (and often deep) dermis, marked thinning of the epidermis, and hyperkeratosis. *C* and *D,* Chronic damage to the basal cell layer is characteristically associated with thickening of the basement membrane zone *(C)* and granular deposits of immunoglobulin and complement at the dermoepidermal junction *(D).*

follicular ostia may be appreciated with a hand lens.

MORPHOLOGY. Histologically, lesions of DLE are characterized by an infiltrate of lymphocytes along the dermoepidermal or the dermal-follicular epithelial junction, or both (see Fig. 26–25*B*). Deep perivascular and periappendageal (e.g., around sweat glands) infiltrates are also observed, and preferential infiltration of subcutaneous fat is called **lupus profundus.** The basal cell layer generally shows diffuse vacuolization. The epidermal layer is markedly thinned or atrophied, with loss of the normal rete ridge pattern. Variable hyperkeratosis is present on the epidermal surface. Involved hair follicles also may show epithelial atrophy and their infundibula are frequently dilated and plugged with keratin. Periodic acid–Schiff (PAS) stain of established lesions reveals marked thickening of the epidermal basement membrane zone (see Fig. 26–25*C*), and **direct immunofluorescence shows a characteristic granular band of immunoglobulin and complement along the dermoepidermal and dermal-follicular junctions (so-called lupus band test[57])** (see Fig. 26–25*D*).

The immunopathogenesis of lupus erythematosus is discussed extensively elsewhere in this text (see Chapter 6). In the skin, it is believed that both humoral and cell-mediated mechanisms collaborate to result in destruction of pigment-containing basal cells.[58] Humoral mechanisms of injury may involve both formation and deposition of immune complexes and components C5b to C9 ("membrane attack complex")[59] (see Chapter 3) in dermoepithelial junction.

ACNE VULGARIS

Acne vulgaris is a chronic inflammatory dermatosis affecting the hair follicle. It is virtually universal in the middle-to-late teenage years, affecting both males and females, although males tend to have more severe disease. Acne is seen in all races, but it is said to be milder in people of Asian descent. Acne vulgaris in adolescents is believed to occur as a result of physiologic hormonal variations and alterations in hair follicle maturation. The clinical features of acne may be induced or exacerbated by drugs (corticosteroids, ACTH, testosterone, gonadotropins, contraceptives, trimethadone, iodides, and bromides), occupational contactants (cutting oils, chlorinated hydrocarbons, and coal tars), and occlusive conditions such as heavy clothing and tropical climates. Some families seem to be particularly affected by acne, suggesting a heritable factor.

Acne is divided into noninflammatory and inflammatory types, although both may coexist. The former consists of open and closed comedones (singular, comedo). *Open comedones* consist of small follicular papules containing a central black keratin plug. This color is the result of oxidation of melanin pigment (not dirt). *Closed comedones* are follicular papules without a visible central plug. Because the keratin plug is trapped beneath the epidermal surface, these lesions are potential sources of follicular rupture and inflammation. Inflammatory acne is characterized by erythematous papules, nodules, and pustules. Severe variants (e.g., acne conglobata) result in profound scarring and sinus tract formation.

> **MORPHOLOGY.** Histologically, comedones form as an expanding mass of lipid and keratin within the midportion of the hair follicle. With gradual expansion, the follicle becomes dilated and the follicular epithelium and sebaceous glands atrophy. Resultant open comedones have large, patulous orifices, whereas those of closed comedones are identifiable only microscopically. Variable lymphohistiocytic infiltrates are present in and around affected follicles, and extensive acute and chronic inflammation accompanies follicular rupture. Dermal abscesses may form in association with rupture, and gradual resolution, often with scarring, ensues.

The pathogenesis of acne is incompletely understood. Endocrine factors have been implicated (especially androgens) because castrated persons never develop the condition. However, these do not appear to be the sole or primary cause.[60] It has been postulated that bacterial lipases of *Propionibacterium acnes* break down sebaceous oils, liberating highly irritating fatty acids resulting in the earliest inflammatory phases of acne.[61] Inhibition of lipase production is a rationale for administration of antibiotics to patients with inflammatory acne.[62] The synthetic vitamin A derivative 13-*cis*-retinoic acid (isotretinoin) has brought about remarkable clinical improvement in some cases of severe acne.[63]

BLISTERING (BULLOUS) DISEASES

Although vesicles and bullae (blisters) occur as a secondary phenomenon in a number of unrelated conditions (e.g., herpesvirus infection, spongiotic dermatitis, erythema multiforme, and thermal burns), there exists a group of disorders in which blisters are the primary and most distinctive features. These bullous diseases, as they are called,

produce visually dramatic clinical lesions, and in some instances (e.g., pemphigus vulgaris) are uniformly fatal if untreated. Blisters can occur at multiple levels within the skin (Fig. 26–26), and assessment of these levels is essential to formulating an accurate histologic diagnosis.

PEMPHIGUS

Pemphigus is a rare autoimmune blistering disorder resulting from loss of the integrity of normal intercellular attachments within the epidermis and mucosal epithelium.[64] The majority of individuals who develop pemphigus are in the fourth to sixth decades of life, and men and women are affected equally. There are four clinical and pathologic variants: (1) pemphigus vulgaris; (2) pemphigus vegetans; (3) pemphigus foliaceus; and (4) pemphigus erythematosus.

Pemphigus vulgaris, by far the most common type (accounting for over 80% of cases worldwide), involves mucosa and skin, especially on the scalp, face, axilla, groin, trunk, and points of pressure. It may present as oral ulcers that persist sometimes for months before skin involvement appears. Primary lesions are very superficial vesicles and bullae that rupture easily, leaving shallow erosions covered with dried serum and crust. *Pemphigus vegetans* is a rare form that usually presents not with blisters but with large, moist, verrucous (wartlike), vegetating plaques studded with pustules on the groin, axilla, and flexural surfaces. *Pemphigus foliaceus* is a more benign form of pemphigus that occurs in an epidemic form in South America, as well as in isolated cases in other countries. Sites of predilection are the scalp, face, chest, and back, and the mucous membranes are only rarely affected. Bullae are so superficial that only zones of erythema and crusting, sites of previous blister rupture, are usually present on physical examination. *Pemphigus erythematosus* is considered to be a localized, less severe form of pemphigus foliaceus that may selectively involve the malar area of the face in a lupus erythematosus–like fashion.

> **MORPHOLOGY.** The common denominator, histologically, in all forms of pemphigus is **acantholysis.** This term implies dissolution, or lysis, of the intercellular adhesion sites within a squamous epithelial surface. Acantholytic cells that are no longer attached to other epithelial cells lose their polyhedral shape and characteristically become rounded. In pemphigus vulgaris and pemphigus vegetans, acantholysis selectively involves the layer of cells immediately above the basal cell layer. (The vegetans variant has considerable overlying epidermal

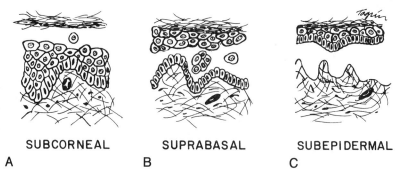

Figure 26-26. Schematic representation of sites of blister formation. *A*, In subcorneal blister, stratum corneum forms roof of bulla (as in impetigo or pemphigus foliaceus). *B*, In suprabasal blister, a portion of epidermis including stratum corneum forms the roof (as in pemphigus vulgaris). *C*, In subepidermal blister, entire epidermis separates from dermis (as in bullous pemphigoid and dermatitis herpetiformis).

SUBCORNEAL   SUPRABASAL   SUBEPIDERMAL

A   B   C

hyperplasia.) The **suprabasal acantholytic blister** that forms is characteristic of pemphigus vulgaris (Fig. 26–27). In pemphigus foliaceus, a blister forms by similar mechanisms but, unlike the case with pemphigus vulgaris, selectively involves the superficial epidermis at the level of the stratum granulosum. Variable superficial dermal infiltration by lymphocytes, histiocytes, and eosinophils accompanies all forms of pemphigus.

Sera from patients with pemphigus contain antibodies (IgG) to intercellular cement substance of skin and mucous membranes.[65] This phenomenon is the basis for direct and indirect diagnostic immunofluorescence testing of skin and serum, respectively. Lesional sites show a characteristic net-like pattern of intercellular IgG deposits localized to sites of developed or incipient acantholysis (Fig. 26–28). Although cultured skin exposed to pemphigus antiserum develops acantholysis, it now appears that at least some of the acantholytic process is not the direct result of antibody-induced damage, but rather is the consequence of synthesis and liberation of a serine protease, plasminogen activa-

tor, by epidermal cells, an event that is triggered by the pemphigus antibody.[66,67]

BULLOUS PEMPHIGOID

Originally considered to be a form of pemphigus, bullous pemphigoid has been recognized for almost the last four decades as a distinct and relatively common autoimmune, vesiculobullous disease. Generally affecting elderly individuals, bullous pemphigoid shows a wide range of clinical presentations, with localized-to-generalized cutaneous lesions and involvement of mucosal surfaces.

Clinically, lesions are tense bullae, filled with clear fluid, on normal or erythematous skin (Fig. 26–29A). The size may reach 4 to 8 cm in diameter. The bullae do not rupture as easily as the blisters seen in pemphigus, and, if uncomplicated by infection, heal without scarring. Sites of occurrence include the inner aspects of the thighs, flexor surfaces of the forearms, axillae, groin, and

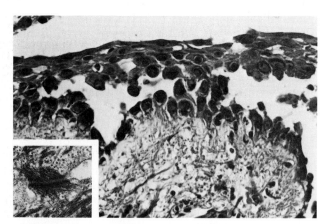

Figure 26-27. Pemphigus vulgaris. Suprabasal acantholysis results in an intraepidermal blister in which rounded (acantholytic) epidermal cells are identified. Dissolution of intercellular cement substance of keratinocyte attachment plaques (desmosomes *(inset)*) results in acantholysis in this disorder.

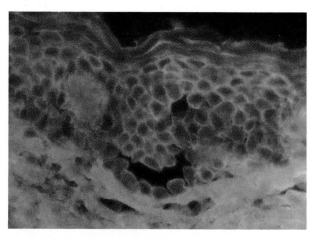

Figure 26-28. Direct immunofluorescence of pemphigus vulgaris. There is deposition of immunoglobulin along the plasma membranes of epidermal keratinocytes in a fish-net-like pattern. Also note the early suprabasal separation due to loss of cell-cell adhesion (acantholysis).

lower abdomen. Oral involvement is present in up to one-third of patients, usually following the development of cutaneous lesions. Some patients may present with urticarial plaques, with extreme associated pruritus.

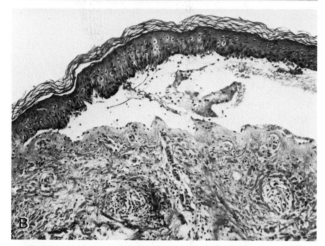

MORPHOLOGY. The separation of bullous pemphigoid from pemphigus, establishing the former as a distinctive entity, was based on the seminal observation of Lever that pemphigoid resulted from a **subepidermal, nonacantholytic** blister.[68] Early lesions show a superficial and sometimes deep perivascular infiltrate of lymphocytes and variable numbers of eosinophils, occasional neutrophils, superficial dermal edema, and associated basal cell layer vacuolization. The vacuolated basal cell layer eventually gives rise to a fluid-filled blister (see Fig. 26–29B).

The immunopathology of bullous pemphigoid[69] features *linear* basement membrane zone deposition of immunoglobulin and complement (recall that the pattern for lupus erythematosus was similar, but granular in character). Ultrastructural studies have shown that circulating antibody reacts with antigen present in the narrow clear zone (lamina lucida) of the epidermal basement membrane that separates the underlying lamina densa from the plasma membrane of the basal cells (see Fig. 26–29C). Some reactivity also occurs in the basal cell–basement membrane attachment plaques (hemidesmosomes). The antigen present at these sites has been named "bullous pemphigoid antigen" and is now recognized as a normal constituent of the dermoepidermal junction. In bullous pemphigoid, it is likely that the generation of autoantibodies to this basement membrane component results in the fixation of complement and subsequent tissue injury at this site via locally recruited neutrophils and eosinophils. In some individuals, pemphigus may herald the presence of underlying lymphoreticular neoplasms, and the term "paraneoplastic pemphigus" recently has been proposed for this association.[70]

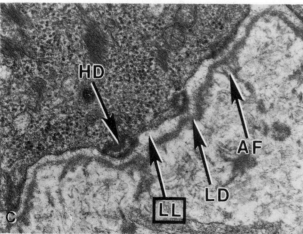

Figure 26–29. Bullous pemphigoid. Clinical bullae (A) result from basal cell layer vacuolization, producing a subepidermal blister (B). C, Bullous pemphigoid antigen is located in the lamina lucida (LL) of the basement membrane zone and in the lowermost portion of the basal cell cytoplasm. HD = hemidesmosome; LD = lamina densa; AF = anchoring fibrils.

DERMATITIS HERPETIFORMIS

Dermatitis herpetiformis, first described by Duhring[71] in 1884, is a rare and fascinating entity characterized by urticaria and vesicles. Males tend to be affected more frequently than females, and the age of onset is often in the third and fourth decades, although disease has been known to develop at any age after weaning. A major association is with celiac disease (see Chapter 17); both the vesicular dermatosis and the enteropathy respond to a diet free of gluten (see later).

The urticarial plaques and vesicles of dermati-

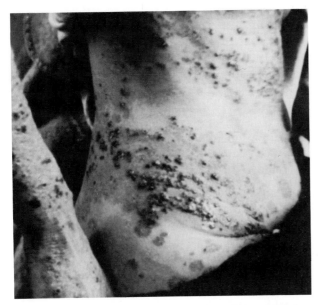

Figure 26–30. One of the original cases of dermatitis herpetiformis described by Duhring. (From the Duhring Collection of the Department of Dermatology of the University of Pennsylvania.)

tis herpetiformis are extremely pruritic. They characteristically occur bilaterally and symmetrically, involving preferentially the extensor surfaces, elbows, knees, upper back, and buttocks. Figure 26–30 illustrates one of the original Duhring cases. Vesicles are frequently grouped, as are those of true herpesvirus, and hence the name "herpetiform."

MORPHOLOGY. Histologically, the early lesions of dermatitis herpetiformis are characteristic. Fibrin and neutrophils accumulate selectively at the **tips of dermal papillae,** forming small "microabscesses" (Fig. 26–31A). The basal cells overlying these microabscesses show vacuolization, and minute zones of dermoepidermal separation (microscopic blisters) may occur at the tips of involved papillae. In time, these zones coalesce to form a true subepidermal blister. Eosinophils may occur in the infiltrates of older lesions, creating confusion with the histologic picture of bullous pemphigoid. Attention to the early alterations at the blister edge, however, usually allows for separation of these two disorders. By direct immunofluorescence, dermatitis herpetiformis shows granular deposits of **IgA** selectively localized in the tips of dermal papillae, where they are deposited on anchoring fibrils (see Fig. 26–31B).

Gluten is the protein moiety that persists subsequent to the removal of water and starch from defatted flour. Gliadin is a class of protein found in the gluten fraction of flour. Patients with dermatitis herpetiformis may develop antibodies of the IgA and IgG classes to gliadin and reticulin, a component of the anchoring fibrils that tether the epidermal basement membrane to the superficial dermis. In addition, individuals with certain histocompatibility types (HLA-B8 and HLA-DRw3) are particularly prone to this disease. It is tempting to speculate that genetically predisposed persons may develop IgA antibodies in the gut to components of dietary gluten, and that these antibodies (or immune complexes) then cross react or are deposited in the skin, resulting in clinical disease. Although it is clear that some individuals with dermatitis herpetiformis and enteropathy respond to a gluten-free diet (as with celiac disease), the immunopathogenesis of the disease remains to be fully clarified.[72]

Figure 26–31. Dermatitis herpetiformis. *A,* Neutrophilic microabscess selectively involving the dermal papilla. *B,* Direct immunofluorescence demonstrates granular IgA deposits within four adjacent dermal papillae. These deposits are specifically localized to the anchoring fibrils.

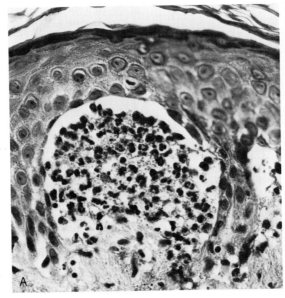
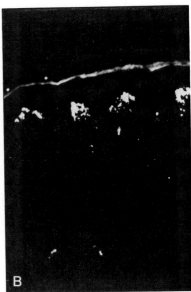

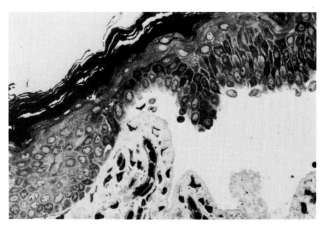

Figure 26–32. Epidermolysis bullosa. A noninflammatory subepidermal blister in this case has formed at the level of the lamina lucida.

NONINFLAMMATORY BLISTERING DISEASES — PORPHYRIA, EPIDERMOLYSIS BULLOSA

To this point, we have discussed inflammatory blistering diseases. However, some primary disorders characterized by vesicles and bullae are not mediated by inflammatory mechanisms. Two such diseases are *porphyria* and *epidermolysis bullosa.*

Porphyria refers to a group of uncommon inborn or acquired disturbances of porphyrin metabolism. Porphyrins are pigments normally present in hemoglobin, myoglobin, and cytochromes. The classification of porphyrias is based on both clinical and biochemical features. The five major types are (1) congenital erythropoietic porphyria; (2) erythrohepatic protoporphyria; (3) acute intermittent porphyria; (4) porphyria cutanea tarda; and (5) mixed porphyria. Cutaneous manifestations consist of urticaria and vesicles that heal with scarring and that are exacerbated by exposure to sunlight. The primary alterations by light microscopy are a *subepidermal vesicle with associated marked thickening of superficial dermal vessels.* The pathogenesis of these alterations is not well understood.

Epidermolysis bullosa constitutes a group of disorders unified by the common link of blisters that develop at sites of pressure, rubbing, or trauma, at or soon after birth. The different types of epidermolysis bullosa, however, are likely to be unrelated with regard to pathogenesis. In the *junctional type,* for example, blisters occur in otherwise histologically normal skin at precisely the level of the lamina lucida (Fig. 26–32). In the scarring *dystrophic types,* blisters develop beneath the lamina densa, presumably in association with rudimentary or defective anchoring fibrils. In the *simplex type,* degeneration of the basal cell layer of the epidermis results in clinical bullae. The histologic changes are so subtle that electron microscopy may

be required to differentiate among these types in clinically ambiguous settings!

INFECTION AND INFESTATION

Although the skin is a protective organ, it frequently succumbs to the attack of microorganisms, parasites, and insects. We have already discussed the possible role of bacteria in the pathogenesis of common acne, and the dermatoses resulting from viruses are too numerous to list. In the setting of the immunocompromised patient, ordinarily trivial cutaneous infections may be life-threatening.

Many disorders, such as herpes simplex and herpes zoster, the viral exanthems, and deep fungal infections, are discussed in Chapter 8. In addition, immune reactions in skin provoked by infectious agents, such as the annular erythema termed "erythema chronica migrans," a harbinger of Lyme disease, are also discussed in Chapter 8. Here we address a representative sampling of common infections and infestations whose primary clinical manifestations are in the skin.

VERRUCAE (WARTS)

Verrucae are common lesions of children and adolescents, although they may be encountered at any age. They are caused by papillomaviruses that belong to the DNA-containing papovavirus group. Transmission of disease usually involves direct contact between individuals or autoinoculation. Verrucae are generally self-limiting, regressing spontaneously within six months to two years.

The classification of verrucae is based largely on clinical morphology and location. *Verruca vulgaris* is the most common type of wart. These lesions occur anywhere, but most frequently on the hands, particularly on the dorsal surfaces and periungual areas, where they appear as gray-white to tan, flat to convex, 0.1- to 1-cm papules with a rough, pebble-like surface (Fig. 26–33A). *Verruca plana,* or *flat wart,* is common on the face or the dorsal surfaces of the hands. These warts are slightly elevated, flat, smooth, tan papules that are generally smaller than verruca vulgaris. *Verruca plantaris* and *verruca palmaris* occur on the soles and palms, respectively. Rough, scaly lesions may reach 1 to 2 cm in diameter, coalesce, and be confused with ordinary calluses. *Condyloma acuminatum (venereal wart)* occurs on the penis, female genitalia, urethra, perianal areas, and rectum. These lesions appear as soft, tan, cauliflower-like masses that in occasional cases reach many centimeters in diameter.

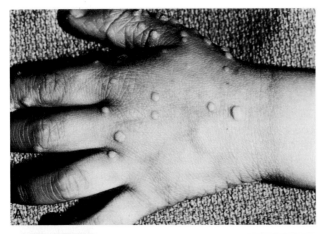

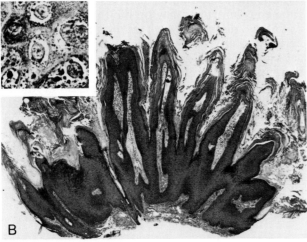

Figure 26-33. Verrucae. *A*, Multiple papules with rough, pebble-like surfaces are present. *B*, Histologically, such lesions show papillomatous epidermal hyperplasia and cytopathic alterations that include nuclear pallor and prominent keratohyaline granules *(inset)*.

MORPHOLOGY. Histologic features common to verrucae include epidermal hyperplasia that is often undulant in character (so-called verrucous or papillomatous epidermal hyperplasia—see Fig. 26–33B) and cytoplasmic vacuolization (koilocytosis) that preferentially involves the more superficial epidermal layers, producing halos of pallor surrounding infected nuclei. Electron microscopy of these zones reveals numerous viral particles within nuclei. Infected cells may also demonstrate prominent and apparently condensed keratohyaline granules and jagged eosinophilic intracytoplasmic keratin aggregates as a result of viral cytopathic effects. These cellular alterations are not as prominent in condylomas; hence their diagnosis is based primarily on hyperplastic papillary architecture containing wedge-shaped zones of koilocytosis.

It is now recognized that the clinically different types of warts just described result not solely because of the anatomically different sites in which

they arise but also as a consequence of distinct types of human papillomavirus. Over 49 types of papillomavirus that can produce warts in humans have been identified in studies utilizing molecular hybridization and restriction enzyme analyses. For example, anogenital warts are caused predominantly by papillomavirus types 6 and 11. In contrast, there is a tendency for lesions induced by type 16 to show some degree of associated dysplasia.[73] Moreover, type 16 has also been associated with *in situ* squamous cell carcinoma of the genitalia and with *bowenoid papulosis* (genital lesions of young adults with the histology of *in situ* carcinoma but with a biologic course of spontaneous regression).[74] These findings are consonant with previous observations of the association of types 16 and 18 with carcinomas of the uterine cervix (see Chapter 23).[75] The potential relationship of papillomavirus to carcinoma is reinforced by the rare heritable condition termed *epidermodysplasia verruciformis*. In this disorder, patients develop multiple flat warts, some of which evolve to become invasive squamous cell carcinoma. The genomes of papillomavirus types 5 and 8 have been detected in some of these cutaneous tumors.[76] Thus, the types of papillomavirus differ not only in the morphology of the lesions they produce but also in their oncogenic potential.

MOLLUSCUM CONTAGIOSUM

Molluscum contagiosum is a common, self-limiting, viral disease of the skin caused by a poxvirus. The virus is characteristically brick-shaped, has a dumbbell-shaped DNA core, and measures 300 nm in maximum dimension. Infection is usually spread by direct contact, particularly among children and young adults.

Clinically, multiple lesions may occur on the skin and mucous membranes, with a predilection for the trunk and anogenital areas. Individual lesions are firm, often pruritic, pink to skin-colored umbilicated papules generally ranging in diameter from 0.2 to 0.4 cm. Rarely, "giant" forms occur measuring up to 2.0 cm in diameter. A curdlike material can be expressed from the central umbilication. Smearing this material onto a glass slide and staining with Giemsa reagent often shows diagnostic "molluscum bodies."

MORPHOLOGY. Microscopically, lesions show cup-like verrucous epidermal hyperplasia (Fig. 26–34A). The pathognomonic structure is the **molluscum body,** which occurs as a large (up to 35 μm), ellipsoid, homogeneous, cytoplasmic inclusion in cells of the stratum granulosum and the stratum corneum (see Fig. 26–34B). These inclusions are eosinophilic in the blue-purple (on H and E stain) stratum granulosum and acquire a red to pale blue hue in

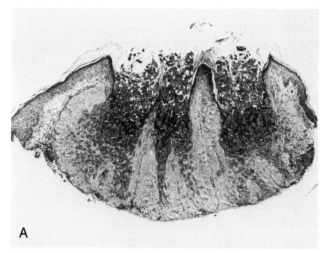

A

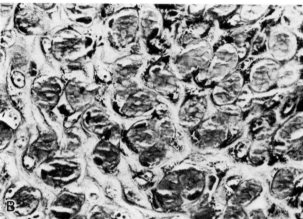

B

Figure 26–34. Molluscum contagiosum. A focus of cup-like verrucous epidermal hyperplasia (A) contains numerous cells with ellipsoid cytoplasmic inclusions (molluscum bodies) (B).

the red stratum corneum. Numerous virions are present within molluscum bodies.

IMPETIGO

This common superficial infection of the skin usually caused by staphylococci or streptococci is discussed in Chapter 8. Impetigo is frequently seen in normal children as well as in adults in poor health. Cultures most frequently grow coagulase-positive staphylococci or group A beta-hemolytic streptococci, or both. Nephritogenic strains of Streptococcus cause impetigo, particularly in tropical areas and in the southern United States.[77]

The condition usually involves exposed skin, particularly that of the face and hands. Initially it is an erythematous macule, but multiple small pustules rapidly supervene. As pustules break, shallow erosions form, covered with drying serum, giving the characteristic clinical appearance of *honey-colored crust*. If the crust is not removed, new lesions form about the periphery and extensive epidermal damage may ensue. A bullous form of impetigo occurs in children.

MORPHOLOGY. The characteristic microscopic feature of impetigo is accumulation of neutrophils beneath the stratum corneum, often with the formation of a subcorneal pustule. Special stains reveal the presence of bacteria in these foci. Nonspecific, reactive epidermal alterations and superficial dermal inflammation accompany these findings. Rupture of pustules results in superficial layering of serum, neutrophils, and cellular debris to form the characteristic crust.

SUPERFICIAL FUNGAL INFECTIONS

As opposed to deep fungal infections, superficial fungal infections of the skin are confined to the stratum corneum, where they are caused primarily by dermatophytes. These organisms grow in the soil and on animals and produce a number of diverse and characteristic clinical lesions.

Tinea capitus usually occurs in children and is only rarely seen in infants and adults. It is a dermatophytosis of the scalp characterized by asymptomatic, often hairless patches of skin associated with mild erythema, crust formation, and scale. *Tinea barbae* is a dermatophyte infection of the beard area that affects adult men; it is a relatively uncommon disorder. *Tinea corporis*, on the other hand, is a common superficial fungal infection of the body surface that affects persons of all ages, but particularly children. Predisposing factors include excessive heat and humidity, exposure to infected animals, and chronic dermatophytosis of the feet or nails. The most common type of tinea corporis is an expanding, round, slightly erythematous plaque with an elevated scaling border (Fig. 26–35A). *Tinea cruris* occurs most frequently in the inguinal areas of obese men during warm weather. Heat, friction, and maceration all predispose to its development. The infection usually first appears on the upper inner thighs, with gradual extension of moist, red patches that have raised, scaling borders. *Tinea pedis (athlete's foot)* affects 30 to 40% of the population at some time in their lives. There is diffuse erythema and scaling, often initially localized to the web spaces. Most of the inflammatory tissue reaction, however, has recently been shown to be the result of bacterial superinfection and not directly related to the primary dermatophytosis.[78] Spread to, or primary infection of, the nails is referred to as *onychomycosis*. This produces discoloration, thickening, and deformity of

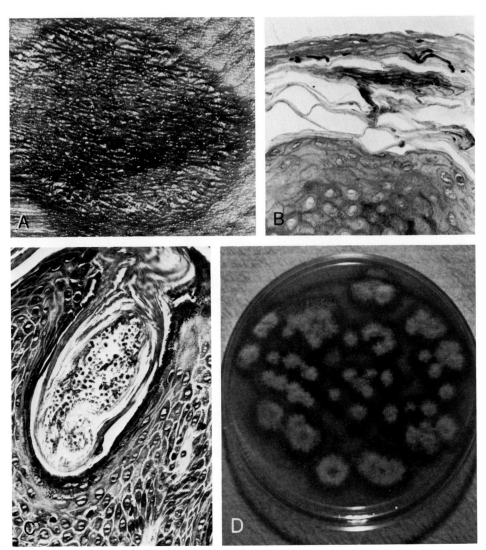

Figure 26–35. Tinea. *A,* Characteristic plaque of tinea corporis. PAS stain reveals hyphae *(B)* and yeast forms *(C)* within the stratum corneum and hair shaft in tinea corporis and tinea capitis, respectively. *D,* Scraping and culture of infected sites will often permit growth of offending organisms, facilitating their definitive classification.

the nail plate. *Tinea versicolor* usually occurs on the upper trunk and is highly distinctive in appearance. Caused by *Malassezia furfur,* the lesions consist of groups of macules of all sizes, lighter or darker than surrounding skin, with a fine peripheral scale.

MORPHOLOGY. The histologic features of all dermatophytoses are variable, depending on the antigenic properties of the organism, the corresponding host response, and the degree of bacterial superinfection that occurs.[78] Fungal cell walls, rich in mucopolysaccharides, stain bright pink to red with PAS stain. They are present in the anucleate cornified layer of lesional skin, hair, or nails (see Fig. 26–35B and C), and scraping of these areas and subsequent culture of organisms will usually produce colonial growth that permits definitive classification of the offending species (see Fig. 26–35D). Reactive epidermal changes may produce a pattern that mimics a mild eczematous dermatitis.

ARTHROPOD BITES, STINGS, AND INFESTATIONS

Arthropods are ubiquitous, and we all are prone to the bites, stings, and other discomforts they cause. The arthropods include Arachnida (spiders, scorpions, ticks, and mites); Insecta (lice, bedbugs, bees, wasps, fleas, flies, and mosquitos); and Chilopoda (centipedes). All can cause skin lesions, but there is a wide variability in clinical patterns of reaction. Some persons suffer minimal symptoms, others considerable discomfort, and some may die as a consequence of a bite or sting. Arthropods can produce lesions in several ways: (1) by direct irritant effects of insect parts or secretions; (2) by immediate or delayed hypersensitivity responses (including an anaphylactic reaction) to retained or injected body parts or secretions; (3) by specific effects of venoms (e.g., the black widow spider venom produces severe cramps and excruciating pain; the brown recluse spider venom contains po-

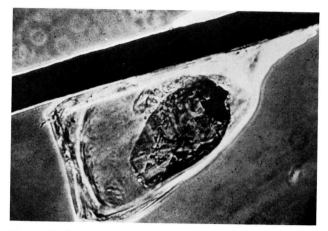

Figure 26-36. Pediculosis. Egg case (nit) of head louse attached to hair shaft.

tent enzymes that produce tissue necrosis); and (4) by serving as vectors for secondary invaders, such as bacteria, rickettsiae, and parasites.

Macroscopically, arthropod bites may be urticarial or inflamed papules and nodules, sometimes with ulceration. Individual lesions may last for several weeks. With the tick bite caused by *Ixodes scapularis (dammini)*, the vector for the spirochete that causes Lyme disease (see Chapter 8), a characteristic expanding, erythematous plaque (erythema migrans) develops. Such extensive necrosis may result from the bite of the brown recluse spider that radical surgical excision of the involved area is often necessary. *Scabies* is a contagious, pruritic dermatosis caused by the mite *Sarcoptes scabiei*. The female mite burrows under the stratum corneum, producing burrows (linear, poorly defined streaks, 0.2 to 0.6 cm in length) on the interdigital skin, palms, wrists, periareolar skin of women, and genital skin of men. *Pediculosis* is caused by the head louse, crab louse, and body louse. The disease is pruritic, and the louse, or its eggs, attached to hair shafts can usually be seen with the unaided eye (Fig. 26–36). In pediculosis of the scalp, impetigo and enlarged cervical lymph nodes may be frequent complications, especially in children. The pubic louse · may be transmitted through sexual contact. Infection with the body louse ("vagabond's disease") is usually characterized by areas of hyperpigmentation and scratch marks (excoriations).

MORPHOLOGY. The histologic picture of arthropod bites is highly varied. The classic lesion shows a wedge-shaped perivascular infiltrate of lymphocytes, histiocytes, and eosinophils within the dermis. There may be a central zone of exceedingly focal epidermal necrosis, directly under which birefringent insect mouthparts may be found (the site of the bite is called the punctum). In some bites, a primarily urticarial reaction is seen histologically, whereas in others the inflammatory infiltrate is so florid and dense that it may superficially resemble a cutaneous lymphoma. Spongiosis, resulting in intraepidermal blisters, is present in some biopsy specimens, and, in certain settings, insect bites even resemble bullous pemphigoid.

Careful correlation with a clinical history of exposure to insects and the clinical finding of clustered or linear lesions facilitate the clinicopathologic diagnosis.

Acknowledgments. Dr. Gerald Lazarus graciously provided the clinical photographs. Clinical panels of Figures 26–4, 26–18, 26–29B and C, and 26–35 were reproduced with permission from F.A. Davis Co., Philadelphia. Dr. Michael Ioffreda provided the excellent medical illustrations. Ms. Diana Whitaker gave expert technical assistance in the preparation of illustrations. Finally, we thank the histotechnologists of the Dermatopathology Laboratory of the Hospital of the University of Pennsylvania for the superb slides, upon which the photomicrography was performed.

1. Virchow, R.: Cellular Pathology. London, John Churchill, 1860, p. 33.
2. Murphy, G.F.: Cell membrane glycoproteins and Langerhans cells. Hum. Pathol. *16*:103, 1985.
3. Kupper, T.: Epidermal cytokines. *In* Shevach, E., and Oppenheim, J. (eds.): The Immunophysiology of Cells and Cytokines. Oxford, Oxford University Press, 1988.
4. Hertz, K.C., et al.: Autoimmune vitiligo, detection of antibodies to melanin-producing cells. N. Engl. J. Med. *297*:634, 1977.
5. Palkowski, M.R., et al.: Langerhans cells in hair follicles of the depigmenting C57B1/Ler-vit.vit mouse. A model for human vitiligo. Arch. Dermatol. *123*:1022, 1987.
6. Grimes, P.E., et al.: T cell profiles in vitiligo. J. Am. Acad. Dermatol. *14*:196, 1986.
7. Sanchez, N.P., et al.: A clinical, light microscopic, ultrastructural, and immunofluorescence study. J. Am. Acad. Dermatol. *4*:698, 1981.
8. Norris, W.: A case of fungoid disease. Edinburgh Med. Surg. J. *16*:562, 1820.
9. Clark, W.H., Jr., et al.: Origin of familial malignant melanomas from heritable melanotic lesions: The BK mole syndrome. Arch. Dermatol. *114*:732, 1978.
10. Reimer, R.R., et al.: Precursor lesions in familial melanoma: A new genetic preneoplastic syndrome. J.A.M.A. *239*:744, 1978.
11. Greene, M.H., et al.: Familial cutaneous malignant melanoma: Autosomal dominant trait possibly linked to the Rh locus. Proc. Natl. Acad. Sci. U.S.A. *80*:6071, 1983.
12. Greene, M.H., et al.: The high risk of melanoma in melanoma prone families with dysplastic nevi. Ann. Intern. Med. *102*:458, 1985.
13. Ruiter, D.J., et al.: Major histocompatibility antigens and mononuclear inflammatory infiltrate in benign nevomelanocytic proliferations and malignant melanoma. J. Immunol. *129*:2808, 1982.
14. Caporaso, N., et al.: Cytogenetics in hereditary malignant melanoma and dysplastic nevus syndrome: Is dysplastic nevus syndrome a chromosome instability disorder? Cancer Genet. Cytogenet. *24*:299, 1987.
15. Smith, P.J., et al.: Abnormal sensitivity to UV-radiation in cultured skin fibroblasts from patients with hereditary cutaneous malignant melanoma and dysplastic nevus syndrome. Int. J. Cancer *30*:39, 1987.

16. Clark, W.H., et al.: A study of tumor progression: The precursor lesions of superficial spreading and nodular melanoma. Hum. Pathol. *15*:1147, 1985.
17. Mihm, M.C.: The clinical diagnosis, classification and histogenetic concepts of the early stages of cutaneous malignant melanomas. N. Engl. J. Med. *284*:1078, 1971.
18. Mihm, M.C.: Malignant melanoma. *In* Demis, D.J. (ed.): Clinical Dermatology. Baltimore, Harper & Row, 1984, p. 104.
19. Murphy, G.F., et al.: Clinicopathologic types of malignant melanoma: Relevance to biologic behavior and diagnostic surgical approach. J. Dermatol. Surg. Oncol. *11*:673, 1985.
20. Imber, M.J., and Mihm, M.C.: Biological and prognostic significance of vertical growth phase characteristics in malignant melanoma. *In* Mihm, M.C., and Murphy, G.F. (eds.): Pathobiology and Recognition of Malignant Melanoma. Baltimore, Williams & Wilkins, 1988, p. 19.
21. Breslow, A.: Thickness, cross-sectional areas and depth of invasion in the prognosis of cutaneous melanoma. Ann. Surg. *182*:572, 1970.
22. Clark, W.H., Jr., et al.: Model predicting survival in stage I melanoma based on tumor progression. J. Natl. Cancer Inst. *81*:1893, 1989.
23. Murphy, G.F., and Mihm, M.C.: Histologic reporting of malignant melanoma. *In* Mihm, M.C., and Murphy, G.F. (eds.): Pathobiology and Recognition of Malignant Melanoma. Baltimore, Williams & Wilkins, 1988, p. 79.
24. Mevorah, B., and Mishima, Y.: Cellular response of seborrheic keratosis following croton oil irritation and surgical trauma. Dermatologica *131*:452, 1965.
25. Ellis, D.L., et al.: Melanoma, growth factors, acanthosis nigricans, the sign of Leser-Trelat, and multiple acrochordons. A possible role for alpha-transforming growth factor in cutaneous paraneoplastic syndromes. N. Engl. J. Med. *317*:1582, 1987.
26. Curth, H.O.: Classification of acanthosis nigricans. Int. J. Dermatol. *15*:592, 1976.
27. Fitzpatrick, T.B., et al.: Color Atlas and Synopsis of Clinical Dermatology. New York, McGraw-Hill Book Company, 1983, p. 284.
28. Murphy, G.F., and Elder, D.: Atlas of Tumor Pathology: Non-melanocytic Tumors of the Skin. Washington, DC, Armed Forces Institute of Pathology, 1991, pp. 61–154.
29. Starink, T.M., et al.: The cutaneous pathology of cutaneous lesions of Cowden's disease: New findings. J. Cutan. Pathol. *11*:331, 1984.
30. Thielmann, H.W., et al.: DNA repair synthesis in fibroblast strains from patients with actinic keratosis, squamous cell carcinoma, basal cell carcinoma, or malignant melanoma after treatment with ultraviolet light, *N*-acetoxy-2-acetyl-aminofluorene methyl methanesulfonate, and *N*-methyl-*N*-nitrosourea. J. Cancer Res. Clin. Oncol. *113*:171, 1987.
31. Penn, I.: Neoplastic consequences of transplantation and chemotherapy. Cancer Detect. Prev. *1*(Suppl):149, 1987.
32. Cooper, K.D., et al.: Effects of ultraviolet radiation on human epidermal cell alloantigen presentation: Initial depression of Langerhans cell–dependent function is followed by the appearance of T6⁻ Dr⁺ cells that enhance epidermal alloantigen presentation. J. Immunol. *134*:129, 1985.
33. Granstein, R.D.: Epidermal I-J-bearing cells are responsible for transferable suppressor cell generation after immunization of mice with ultraviolet radiation–treated epidermal cells. J. Invest. Dermatol. *84*:206, 1985.
34. Granstein, R.D., et al.: Epidermal cells in activation of suppressor lymphocytes: Further characterization. J. Immunol. *138*:4055, 1987.
35. Kawashima, M., et al.: Characterization of a new type of human papillomavirus (HPV) related to HPV5 from a case of actinic keratosis. Virology *154*:389, 1986.
36. Hochwalt, A.E., et al.: Mechanism of H-ras oncogene activation in mouse squamous carcinoma induced by an alkylating agent. Cancer Res. *48*:556, 1988.
37. Gorlin, R.J., et al.: The multiple basal cell nevi syndrome. Cancer *18*:89, 1965.
38. Wick, M.R., et al.: Primary neuroendocrine carcinomas of the skin (Merkel cell tumors). A clinical, histologic, and ultrastructural study of thirteen cases. Am. J. Clin. Pathol. *79*:6, 1983.
39. Lever, W.F., and Schaumburg-Lever, G.: Histopathology of the Skin. Philadelphia, J.B. Lippincott, 1983, p. 385.
40. Gottlieb, G., and Ackerman, A.B.: Kaposi's Sarcoma: A Text and Atlas. Philadelphia, Lea & Febiger, 1988.
41. Murphy, G.F., et al.: Distribution of T cell antigens in histiocytosis X cells. Quantitative immunoelectron microscopy using monoclonal antibodies. Lab. Invest. *48*:90, 1983.
42. Knobler, R.M., and Edelson, R.L.: Lymphoma cutis: T cell type. *In* Murphy, G.F., and Mihm, M.C., Jr. (eds.): Lymphoproliferative Disorders of the Skin. Boston, Butterworths, 1980, p. 176.
43. Murphy, G.F.: Cutaneous T cell lymphoma. *In* Fenoglio-Preiser, C.M. (ed.): Advances in Pathology. Chicago, Year Book Medical Publishers, 1988.
44. Rook, A.H., et al.: Combined therapy of the Sézary syndrome with extra-corporeal photochemotherapy and low dose interferon alpha: Clinical, molecular, and immunologic observations. Arch. Dermatol. *127*:1535, 1991.
45. Roitt, I.M., et al.: Immunology. St. Louis, C.V. Mosby Company, 1985, p. 199.
46. Frank, M., et al.: Hereditary angioedema. The clinical syndrome and its management. Ann. Intern. Med. *84*:580, 1976.
47. Murphy, G.F., et al.: Reaction patterns in the skin and special dermatologic techniques. *In* Moschella, S. (ed.): Dermatology. Philadelphia, W.B. Saunders Company, 1984, p. 104.
48. Waldorf, H.A., et al.: Early cellular events in evolving cutaneous delayed hypersensitivity in humans. Am. J. Pathol. *131*:477, 1991.
49. Walsh, L.J., et al.: Human dermal mast cells contain and release tumor necrosis factor alpha, which induces leukocyte adhesion molecule 1. Proc. Natl. Acad. Sci. U.S.A. *88*:4220, 1991.
50. Guillén, F.J., et al.: Acute cutaneous graft-versus-host disease to minor histocompatibility antigens in a murine model: Evidence that large granular lymphocytes are the effector cells in the immune response. Lab. Invest. *137*:1874, 1986.
51. Guillén, F.J., et al.: Inhibition of rat skin allograft rejection by cyclosporin. In situ characterization of the impaired local immune response. Transplantation *41*:734, 1986.
52. Murphy, G.F., et al.: Cytotoxic T lymphocytes and phenotypically abnormal epidermal dendritic cells in fixed cutaneous eruptions. Hum. Pathol. *16*:1264, 1985.
53. Zaias, N.: Psoriasis of the nail. A clinical-pathologic study. Arch Dermatol. *99*:567, 1969.
54. Beutner, E.H., et al.: Autoimmunity in psoriasis. *In* Beutner, E.H., et al. (eds.): Immunopathology of the Skin. New York, John Wiley and Sons, 1987, p. 703.
55. Kronenberg, K., et al.: Malignant degeneration of lichen planus. Arch. Dermatol. *104*:304, 1971.
56. Bhan, A.K., et al.: T cell subset populations in lichen planus: In situ characterization using monoclonal anti-T cell antibodies. Br. J. Dermatol. *105*:617, 1981.
57. Harrist, T.J., and Mihm, M.C.: The specificity and usefulness of the lupus band test. Arthritis Rheum. *23*:479, 1980.
58. Rubenstein, M.H., et al.: Lichen planus and lupus erythematosus: Two disorders with pigment incontinence of possible immunologically mediated origin. *In* Fitzpatrick, T.B., et al. (eds.): Biology of Diseases of Dermal Pigmentation. Tokyo, University of Tokyo Press, 1981, p. 151.
59. Biesecker, G., et al.: Cutaneous localization of membrane attack complex in discoid and systemic lupus erythematosus. N. Engl. J. Med. *306*:264, 1982.
60. Strauss, J.S., and Pochi, P.E.: Recent advances in androgen metabolism and their relation to the skin. Arch. Dermatol. *100*:621, 1969.

61. Voss, J.G.: Acne vulgaris and free fatty acids. Arch. Dermatol. *109*:849, 1974.

62. Webster, G.F., et al.: Inhibition of lipase production in *Propioni bacterium acnes* by sub-minimal inhibitory concentrations of tetracycline and erythromycin. Br. J. Dermatol. *104*:453, 1981.

63. Mills, O.H., and Kligman, A.M.: Treatment of acne by vitamin A (retinol). Semin. Dermatol. *1*:245, 1985.

64. Ahmed, A.R.: Clinical features of pemphigus. *In* Ahmed, A.R. (ed.): Clinics in Dermatology — Pemphigus. Philadelphia, J.B. Lippincott Company, 1983, p. 13.

65. Beutner, E.H., and Jordan, R.E.: Demonstration of skin antibodies in sera of pemphigus vulgaris patients by indirect immunofluorescent staining. Proc. Soc. Exp. Biol. Med. *117*:505, 1964.

66. Hashimoto, K., et al.: Anti-cell surface pemphigus autoantibody stimulates plasminogen activator activity of human epidermal cells. J. Exp. Med. *157*:259, 1983.

67. Morioka, S., et al.: Involvement of urokinase-type plasminogen activator in acanthosis induced by pemphigus. J. Invest. Dermatol. *189*:474, 1987.

68. Lever, W.F.: Pemphigus. Medicine *32*:1, 1953.

69. Imber, M.J., et al.: The immunopathology of bullous pemphigoid. *In* Ahmed, A.R. (ed.): Clinics in Dermatology — Bullous Pemphigoid. Philadelphia, J.B. Lippincott Company, 1987, p. 81.

70. Anhalt, G.J., et al.: Paraneoplastic pemphigus: An autoimmune mucocutaneous disease associated with neoplasia. N. Engl. J. Med. *323*:1729, 1990.

71. Duhring, L.: Dermatitis herpetiformis. J.A.M.A. *3*:225, 1984.

72. Hall, R.P.: The pathogenesis of dermatitis herpetiformis: Recent advances. J. Am. Acad. Dermatol. *16*:1129, 1987.

73. von Krogh, et al.: Advantage of human papillomavirus typing in the clinical evaluation of genitoanal warts. J. Am. Acad. Dermatol. *18*:495, 1988.

74. Ikenberg, H., et al.: Human papillomavirus type-16–related DNA in genital Bowen's disease and bowenoid papulosis. Int. J. Cancer *32*:563, 1983.

75. Zachow, K.R., et al.: Detection of human papillomavirus DNA in anogenital neoplasia. Nature *300*:771, 1982.

76. Ostrow, R., et al.: Human papillomavirus DNA in cutaneous primary and metastasized squamous cell carcinoma from patients with epidermodysplasia verruciformis. Proc. Natl. Acad. Sci. U.S.A. *79*:1634, 1982.

77. Dillon, H.C.: Streptococcal skin infection and glomerulonephritis. *In* Hoeprick, P.D. (ed.): Infectious Diseases. 2nd ed. New York, Harper & Row, 1977.

78. Leyden, J.J., and Kligman, A.M.: Interdigital athlete's foot. The interaction of dermatophytes and resident bacteria. Arch. Dermatol. *114*:1466, 1978.

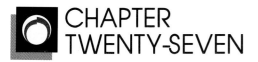
Skeletal System and Soft Tissue Tumors

ANDREW E. ROSENBERG, M.D.

Bones

NORMAL

The skeletal system is composed of 206 bones, which are diverse in size and shape (tubular, flat, cuboid) and exemplify how form reflects function. Bones play a vital role in mineral homeostasis, house the hematopoietic elements, provide mechanical support for movement and protection, and determine the attributes of body size and shape. The bones are interconnected by a variety of joints, which allow for a range of movement and stability (discussed later).

Bone is a type of connective tissue. It is unique because it is one of the few tissues that normally mineralize. Biochemically it is defined by its special blend of organic matrix (35%) and inor-

ganic elements (65%). The inorganic component, calcium hydroxyapatite $(Ca_{10}(PO_4)_6(OH)_2)$, is the mineral that gives bone strength and hardness and is the storehouse for 99% of the body's calcium, 80% of the body's phosphorus, and 65% of the body's sodium and magnesium. The formation of hydroxyapatite crystal in bone is a phase transformation from liquid to solid analogous to the conversion of water to ice. The process involves the initiation and induction of mineralization by the organic matrix and is tightly regulated by numerous factors, many of which are still unknown.[1] The rate of mineralization can vary, but normally there is a 12- to 15-day lag time between the formation of the matrix and its mineralization. Bone that is unmineralized is known as *osteoid*.

The organic component includes the cells of bone and the proteins of the matrix. Although bone cells constitute only 2% of bone weight, they are responsible for its formation and maintenance throughout life. The bone-forming cells include the osteoprogenitor cells, osteoblasts, and osteocytes.

- *Osteoprogenitor* cells are pluripotential mesenchymal stem cells that are located in the vicinity of all bony surfaces; when appropriately stimulated, they have the capacity to undergo cell division and produce offspring that differentiate into osteoblasts. This phenomenon is vital to growth and repair of bone.
- *Osteoblasts* are located on the surface of bone and synthesize, transport, and arrange the many proteins of matrix, detailed later (Fig. 27–1). They also initiate the process of mineralization. Osteoblasts are formed in groups of up to 400 cells at a time whose activity is coordinated because bone is made in structural units that are greater than the capacity of single cells. Osteoblasts have receptors for hormones (parathyroid hormone, vitamin D, and estrogen), cytokines, and growth factors (which regulate differentiation, growth, and metabolism of bone cells). Once osteoblasts become surrounded by matrix, they are known as osteocytes.
- *Osteocytes* are not as metabolically active as osteoblasts, but they play an important role in the control of the daily fluctuations in serum calcium and phosphorus levels. Although encased by bone, osteocytes communicate with surface cells and other osteocytes via an intricate network of tunnels through the matrix known as canaliculi.

The osteocyte cell processes traverse the canaliculi, and their contacts along gap junctions allow the transfer of surface membrane potentials and substrates.

The *osteoclast* is the cell responsible for bone resorption. It is derived from a granulocyte-monocyte precursor cell located in the hematopoietic marrow. The osteoclast is multinucleated (6 to 12 nuclei) and is intimately related to the bone surface (Fig. 27–2). The scalloped *resorption pits* they produce and frequently reside in are known as *Howship's lacunae.* The portion of the osteoclast cell membrane overlying the resorption surface is modified by numerous villous extensions, known as the ruffled border, which serve to increase the membrane surface area. The plasmalemma bordering this region is specialized and forms a seal with the underlying bone, preventing leakage of digestion products. This self-contained extracellular space is analogous to a secondary lysosome, and the osteoclast acidifies it with a hydrogen pump system, which solubilizes the mineral.[2] The osteoclast also releases into this space a multitude of enzymes that help disassemble the matrix proteins into amino acids and liberate and activate growth factors and other enzymes, such as collagenase, which have been previously deposited and bound to the matrix by osteoblasts. Thus as bone is broken down to its elemental units, substances are released that initiate its renewal.

The *proteins of bone* include type I collagen

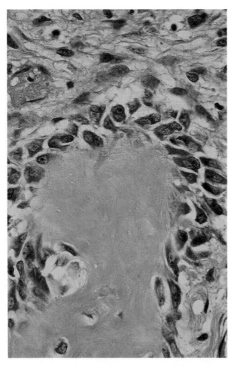

Figure 27–1. Active osteoblasts synthesizing bone matrix. The surrounding spindle cells represent osteoprogenitor cells.

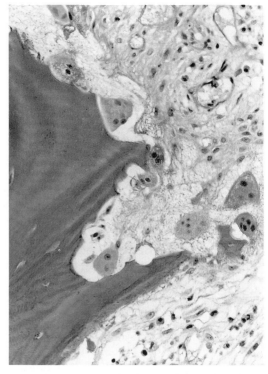

Figure 27–2. A group of osteoclasts resorbing bone.

and a family of noncollagenous proteins that are derived mainly from osteoblasts. Type I collagen forms the backbone of matrix and accounts for 90% of the organic component. Osteoblasts deposit collagen either in a random weave known as *"woven bone"* or in an orderly, layered manner designated *"lamellar bone"* (Fig. 27–3). Normally, woven bone is seen in the fetal skeleton and is formed at growth plates. Its advantages are that it is produced quickly and it resists forces equally from all directions. The presence of woven bone in the adult is always indicative of a pathologic state; however, it is not diagnostic of a particular disease. For instance, in circumstances requiring rapid reparative stability, such as a fracture, woven bone is produced. It is also formed around sites of infection and composes the matrix of bone-forming tumors. *Lamellar bone, which gradually replaces woven bone during growth, is deposited much more slowly and is stronger than woven bone.* There are four different types of lamellar bone, three being present only in the cortex—circumferential, concentric, and interstitial (Fig. 27–4). The fourth type, *trabecular lamellae,* composes the bone trabeculae, in which the lamellae are oriented parallel to the long axis of the trabeculum.

The noncollagenous proteins of bone are bound to the matrix and grouped according to

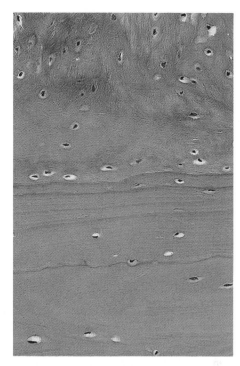

Figure 27–3. Woven bone *(top)* deposited on the surface of pre-existing lamellar bone *(bottom).*

Normal bone

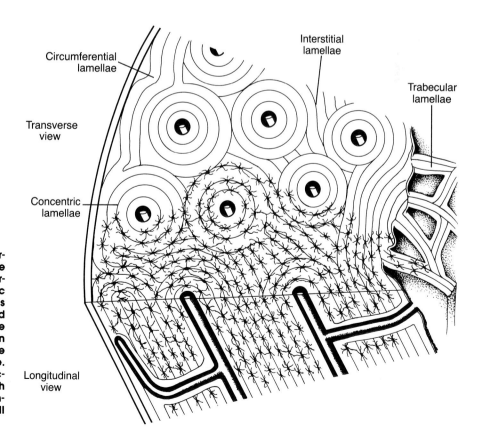

Figure 27–4. The schematic of normal bone structure reveals the subperiosteal and endosteal circumferential lamellae, concentric lamellae about vascular cores creating Haversian systems, and the interstitial lamellae that fill the spaces in between the Haversian systems. The trabecular lamellae extend from the endosteal surface. The individual lamellae are punctuated by osteocytic lacunae with their finely ramifying and interconnecting canals, which contain cell processes.

Table 27–1. PROTEINS OF BONE MATRIX

OSTEOBLAST-DERIVED PROTEINS
  Collagen
    Type I
  Cell adhesion proteins
    Osteopontin, fibronectin, thrombospondin
  Calcium-binding proteins
    Osteonectin, bone sialoprotein
  Proteins involved in mineralization
    Osteocalcin
  Enzymes
    Collagenase, alkaline phosphatase
  Growth factors
    IGF-1, TGF-β, PDGF
  Cytokines
    Prostaglandins, IL-1, IL-6

PROTEINS CONCENTRATED FROM SERUM
  Beta HS microglobulin
  Albumin

IGF-1 = Insulin-like growth factor-1; TGF-β = transforming growth factor-beta; PDGF = platelet-derived growth factor; IL-1, IL-6 = interleukin-1, interleukin-6.

their function as adhesion proteins, calcium-binding proteins, mineralization proteins, enzymes, cytokines, and growth factors[3] (Table 27–1). Of these, only osteocalcin is unique to bone. It is measurable in the serum and used as a sensitive, specific marker for osteoblast activity. The cytokines and growth factors control bone cell proliferation, maturation, and metabolism.[4] They are important in translating mechanical and metabolic signals into local bone cell activity and eventual skeletal adaptation. The skeleton is uniquely able to adapt to new physical forces; witness the repositioning of teeth by the forces of braces.

MODELING AND REMODELING

Osteoblasts and osteoclasts act in coordination and are considered the functional unit of bone known as the "basic multicellular unit." The processes of bone formation and resorption are tightly coupled, and their balance determines skeletal mass at any point in time.[5] As the skeleton grows and enlarges (modeling), bone formation predominates. Once the skeleton has reached maturity, the breakdown and renewal of bone that constitutes skeletal maintenance is called remodeling. Peak bone mass is achieved in early adulthood, and at this stage approximately 5 to 10% of the skeleton is turned over or remodeled yearly and the amount of bone formed and resorbed by the basic multicellular units is in equilibrium. Beginning in the third decade of life, however, the amount of bone resorbed exceeds that which has been formed, so there is a steady decrement in skeletal mass.

In the formation and maintenance of the skeletal system, the osteoblast provides much of the local control because it not only produces bone matrix, but also plays an important role in mediating osteoclast activity. Many of the primary stimulators of bone resorption, such as parathyroid hormone, parathyroid hormone–related protein, interleukin-1, interleukin-6, and tumor necrosis factor-beta (TNF-β), have minimal or no direct effect on osteoclasts. Indeed the osteoblast has receptors for these substances, and evidence suggests that once the osteoblast receives the appropriate signal, it releases a soluble mediator that induces osteoclast bone resorption. The cytokines and growth factors, especially transforming growth factor-beta (TGF-β), released from the matrix during digestion act as a feedback loop and trigger the formation and activation of osteoblasts to synthesize and deposit an equivalent amount of new bone in the resorption pit (Fig. 27–5). In this fashion, bone formation and resorption are temporally and spatially related and can be controlled by systemic and local factors.

GROWTH AND DEVELOPMENT

Bone tissue is made only by osteoblasts. After its formation, further increase in size is achieved only by the deposition of new bone on a pre-existing surface. This mechanism of appositional growth is key to understanding the facets of skeletal development.

Primitive mesenchyme is the precursor of the earliest skeleton. Bones derived from intramembranous formation, such as the cranium and portions of the clavicles, are formed by osteoblasts directly from the mesenchyme. In contrast, in the process of enchondral bone formation, the mesenchyme first creates a cartilaginous model, or anlage of the future bone. Subsequently around the eighth week of gestation, the cartilage in the center of the bone undergoes degradative changes, mineralizes, and is removed by osteoclast-type cells. This process, which progresses up and down the length of the bone, allows for the ingrowth of blood vessels and osteoprogenitor cells, which provide the bone-forming cells. A similar sequence of events occurs separately in the epiphyses. A plate of the cartilage model becomes entrapped between the expanding centers of ossification and is known as the physis or growth plate. The chondrocytes within the growth plate undergo a series of events, including proliferation, growth, degradation, and mineralization (Fig. 27–6). Cartilage mineralization is a signal for its resorption. Remnant struts act as scaffolding for the deposition of bone on its surfaces, and these structures form the primary spongiosa. The process of enchondral ossification also occurs at the base of articular cartilage, and by these mechanisms bones increase in length and articular surfaces increase in diameter.

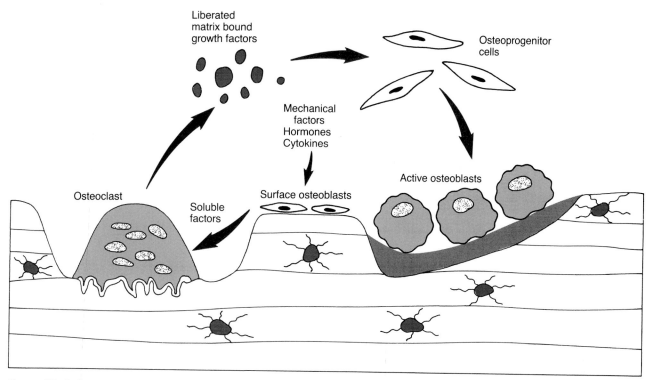

Figure 27-5. Bone resorption and formation are coupled processes that are controlled by systemic factors and local cytokines, some of which are deposited in the bone matrix. Cytokines are key in the communication between osteoblasts and osteoclasts.

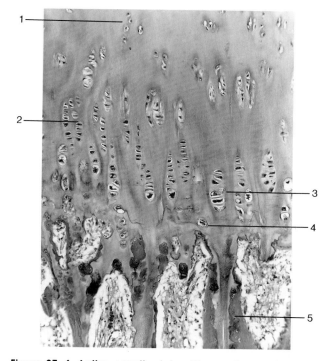

Figure 27-6. Active growth plate with ongoing enchondral ossification. 1, Reserve zone; 2, zone of proliferation; 3, zone of hypertrophy; 4, zone of mineralization; 5, primary spongiosa.

PATHOLOGY

The skeletal system is as subject to circulatory, inflammatory, neoplastic, metabolic, and congenital disorders as the other organ systems of the body. Indeed the complexity of its growth, development, maintenance, and relationships with other organ systems makes it unusually vulnerable to adverse influences. Not surprisingly then primary and secondary diseases of bone are varied and numerous. The spectrum of bone disorders is broad and the classification system not standardized, and so we prefer here to categorize the various disorders according to their perceived biologic defect.

DEVELOPMENTAL ABNORMALITIES

MALFORMATIONS

Congenital malformations of bone are generally uncommon. Simple anomalies include the failure of development of a bone (e.g., congenital absence of a phalanx, rib, or clavicle), the formation of extra bones (supernumerary ribs), the fusion of two adjacent digits (syndactylism), or the development of long spider-like digits (arachnodactylism). The association of the last anomaly with Marfan's syndrome is discussed in Chapter 5. Anomalies that affect the skull and vertebral column, such as craniorachischisis (failure of closure of the spinal column and skull), are frequently of great clinical importance. This defect produces a persistent opening through which the meninges and central nervous system herniate to produce a meningomyelocele or meningoencephalocele (see Chapter 29).

ACHONDROPLASIA

Achondroplasia is the most common disease of the growth plate and is a major cause of dwarfism. It can occur in heterozygous and homozygous forms, but approximately 80% of the cases represent new mutations. *Heterozygous achondroplasia* is autosomal dominant. The affected infant has shortened proximal extremities, a trunk of relatively normal length, and an enlarged head with bulging forehead and conspicuous depression of the root of the nose. The skeletal abnormalities are usually not associated with changes in longevity, intelligence, or reproductive status. *Homozygous achondroplasia* occurs in the rare situation when both parents are heterozygous achondroplastic dwarfs. The infants suffer respiratory insufficiency secondary to a small chest cavity and frequently die at birth or soon after. The skeletal changes are similar but more severe than in the heterozygote variant, and platyspondyly is prominent.

MORPHOLOGY. The histologic abnormalities in achondroplasia can be found in the growth plates. The zones of proliferation and hypertrophy are narrowed and disorganized and contain clusters of large chondrocytes instead of well-formed columns.[6] At the base of the growth plate, there is premature deposition of horizontal struts of bone that seals the plate and prevents further growth. Appositional intramembranous bone formation is not disrupted; therefore the cortices form normally and appear thickened in relation to the short length of the bone. The actual defect causing achondroplasia has not been identified.

DISEASES ASSOCIATED WITH ABNORMAL MATRIX

Many of the bone matrix components have been only recently identified, and their interactions are far more complex than originally imagined. Therefore this field of skeletal pathology is still in its early stages of discovery. Examples of the potential importance of abnormalities in bone matrix are the diseases associated with deranged metabolism of type I collagen and decreased bone mass, and the various mucopolysaccharidoses.

OSTEOGENESIS IMPERFECTA

Osteogenesis imperfecta (OI) is a group of phenotypically related disorders that are caused by deficiencies in the synthesis of type I collagen. Although OI, or "brittle bone" disease, has prominent skeletal manifestations, other anatomic structures rich in type I collagen, such as joints, eyes, ears, skin, and teeth, are affected as well. The genetic defects in OI reside in mutations in the genes that code for the alpha-1 and alpha-2 chains of the collagen molecule.[7] The mutations are usually point substitutions or deletions, with the more common ones inherited in an autosomal dominant fashion. Mutations resulting in the production of qualitatively normal collagen that is synthesized in decreased amounts are associated with mild skeletal abnormalities. More severe or lethal phenotypes result from genetic defects producing abnormal collagen molecules that cannot form the triple helix of collagen. The clinical expression of OI constitutes a spectrum of disorders all marked by extreme skeletal fragility; therefore classification into distinct variants is somewhat arbitrary and artificial. Nonetheless, four major subtypes have been segregated (Table 27–2). New and less well characterized variants are still being identified.

MORPHOLOGY. The type II variant of OI is at one end of the spectrum and is uniformly fatal *in utero* or during the perinatal period. It is characterized by extraordinary bone fragility with multiple fractures occurring when the fetus is still within the womb (Fig. 27–7). In contrast, the type I form, which is usually transmitted as an autosomal dominant disorder but is rarely due to a new mutation, permits a normal life span but with an increased number of fractures during childhood, which decrease in frequency after puberty. Other findings include blue sclerae caused by a decreased collagen content, making the sclera translucent and allowing partial visualization of the underlying choroid; hearing loss related to both a sensorineural deficit and impeded conduction owing to abnormalities in the bones of the middle and inner ear; and dental imperfections (small, misshapen, and blue-yellow teeth) secondary to a deficiency in dentin. Morphologically, **the basic abnormality in all forms of OI is "too little bone,"** thus constituting a type of osteoporosis with marked cortical thinning and attenuation of trabeculae. In some variants, the skeleton fails to model properly, and there are persistent foci of hypercellular woven bone.[8]

Table 27–2. OSTEOGENESIS IMPERFECTA

SUBTYPE	INHERITANCE	COLLAGEN DEFECT	MAJOR CLINICAL FEATURES
OI I Postnatal fractures, blue sclerae	Autosomal dominant	Decreased synthesis pro-α1(1) chain Abnormal pro-α1(1) or pro-α2(1) chains	Compatible with survival Normal stature Skeletal fragility Dentinogenesis imperfecta Hearing impairment Joint laxity Blue sclerae
OI II Perinatal lethal	Most autosomal recessive Some autosomal dominant ?New mutations	Abnormally short pro-α1(1) chain Unstable triple helix Abnormal or insufficient pro-α2(1)	Death in utero or within days of birth Skeletal deformity with excessive fragility and multiple fractures Blue sclerae
OI III Progressive deforming	Autosomal dominant (75%) Autosomal recessive (25%)	Altered structure of pro-peptides of pro-α2(1) Impaired formation triple helix	Compatible with survival Growth retardation Multiple fractures Progressive kyphoscoliosis Blue sclerae at birth that become white Hearing impairment Dentinogenesis imperfecta
OI IV Postnatal fractures, normal sclerae	Autosomal dominant	Short pro-α2(1) chain Unstable triple helix	Compatible with survival Moderate skeletal fragility Short stature Sometimes dentinogenesis imperfecta

The recognition of particular variants and their modes of inheritance is important in genetic counseling.

MUCOPOLYSACCHARIDOSES

The mucopolysaccharidoses, as discussed in Chapter 5, are a group of lysosomal storage diseases that are caused by deficiencies in the enzymes that degrade dermatan sulfate, heparan sulfate, chondroitin sulfate, and keratan sulfate. The implicated enzymes are mainly acid hydrolases. Mesenchymal cells, especially chondrocytes, play an important role in the metabolism of extracellular matrix mucopolysaccharides and therefore are most severely affected. Consequently, many of the skeletal manifestations of the mucopolysaccharidoses result from abnormalities in hyaline cartilage, including the cartilage anlage, growth plates, costal cartilages, and articular surfaces. It is not surprising therefore that these patients are frequently of short stature, have chest wall abnormalities, and have malformed bones.

OSTEOPOROSIS

Osteoporosis is a general term denoting increased porosity of the skeleton resulting from a reduction in bone mass. It may be localized to a certain bone or region, as in disuse osteoporosis of a limb, or may involve the entire skeleton, as a manifestation of a metabolic bone disease. Generalized osteoporosis may be primary or secondary (Table 27–3).[9] Secondary osteoporosis is associated with conditions other than age or menopause. *When the term osteoporosis is used in an unqualified manner, it usually refers to the common primary forms, senile and postmenopausal osteoporosis, in which the critical loss of bone mass makes the skeleton vulnerable to fractures.* About 15 million individuals suffer from primary osteoporosis in the United States, and their medical care costs close to $1 billion annually. Effective treatment and prevention are imperative. The following discussion relates to senile and postmenopausal osteoporosis, the dominant forms.

Peak bone mass is achieved during young adulthood. Its magnitude is determined largely by hereditary factors; however, physical activity, muscle strength, diet, and hormonal state all contribute.[10] A major genetic factor involves the vitamin D receptor gene.[11] Once maximal skeletal mass is attained, a small deficit accrues with every resorption and formation cycle because the remodeling sequence is not completely effective. Accordingly age-related bone loss, which may average 0.7% per year, is a normal and predictable biologic phenomenon, similar to the graying of hair. Both sexes are affected equally and whites more so than blacks. Differences in the peak skeletal mass in males

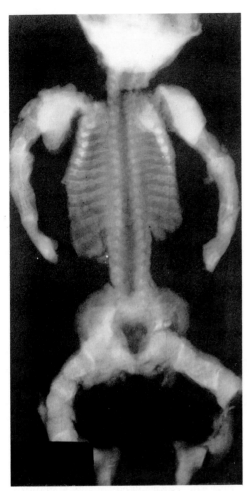

Figure 27-7. Skeletal radiograph of fetus with lethal type II osteogenesis imperfecta. Note the numerous fractures of virtually all bones, resulting in accordion-like shortening of the limbs.

Table 27-3. CATEGORIES OF GENERALIZED OSTEOPOROSIS

PRIMARY
Postmenopausal
Senile
Idiopathic juvenile
Idiopathic middle adulthood

SECONDARY
Endocrine Disorders
  Hyperparathyroidism
  Hyperthyroidism
  Hypothyroidism
  Hypogonadism
  Acromegaly
  Cushing's syndrome
  Prolactinoma
  Diabetes, type 1
  Addison's disease

Neoplasia
  Multiple myeloma
  Carcinomatosis
  Mast cell disease

Gastrointestinal
  Malnutrition
  Malabsorption
  Subtotal gastrectomy
  Hepatic insufficiency
  Vitamin C, D deficiencies

Rheumatologic Disease

Drugs
  Anticoagulants
  Chemotherapy
  Corticosteroids
  Anticonvulsants
  Lithium
  Alcohol

Miscellaneous
  Osteogenesis imperfecta
  Immobilization
  Pulmonary disease
  Chronic obstructive pulmonary disease
  Homocystinuria
  Gaucher's disease
  Anemia

versus females and in blacks versus whites may partially explain why certain populations are prone to develop this disorder.

PATHOGENESIS. The law of perversity states that the more common a condition, the less known about its cause—witness baldness, atherosclerosis, and cancer. Not surprisingly then some of the origins of primary osteoporosis are unknown; however, there is little doubt but that it is the result of an imbalance between bone resorption and formation. Although much remains unknown, discoveries in the molecular biology of bone have put forth some new intriguing hypotheses (Fig. 27–8).

Age-related changes in bone cells and matrix have a strong impact on bone metabolism. Osteoblasts from elderly individuals have reduced reproductive and biosynthetic potential when compared with osteoblasts from younger individuals. Also, proteins deposited in the matrix (such as growth factors, which both are mitogenic to osteoprogenitor cells and stimulate osteoblastic synthetic activity) lose their biologic punch over time. The end

result is a skeleton populated by bone-forming cells that have a diminished capacity to make bone. This form of osteoporosis, also known as senile osteoporosis, is categorized as a *"low turnover variant."*

Reduced physical activity increases the rate of bone loss in experimental animals and humans. The bone loss seen in an immobilized or paralyzed extremity, the reduction of skeletal mass observed in astronauts subjected to a gravity-free environment for prolonged periods, and the higher bone density in athletes as compared with nonathletes all support a role for physical activity in preventing bone loss. Studies have shown that the type of exercise is important because load magnitude influences bone density more than the number of load cycles. Because muscle contraction is the dominant source of skeletal loading, it is logical that resistance exercises, such as weight training, are a more effective

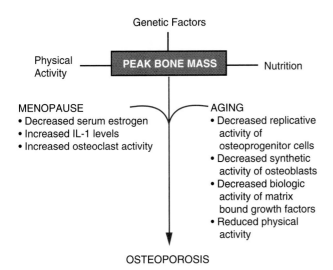

Figure 27–8. Pathophysiology of postmenopausal and senile osteoporosis.

does not keep pace, leading to what is classified as a "high turnover" form of osteoporosis.

MORPHOLOGY. The entire skeleton is affected in postmenopausal and senile osteoporosis (Fig. 27–9), but certain regions tend to be more severely involved than others. In postmenopausal osteoporosis, the subtle increase in osteoclast activity mainly affects bones or portions of bones that have increased surface area, such as the cancellous compartment of vertebral bodies. The osteoporotic trabeculae are thinned and lose their interconnections, leading to progressive microfractures and eventual collapse. In senile osteoporosis, the osteoporotic cortex is thinned by subperiosteal and endosteal resorption, and the Haversian systems are widened. In severe cases, the Haversian systems are so enlarged that the cortex mimics cancellous bone. Such bone as remains is of normal composition.

stimulus for increasing bone mass than repetitive endurance activities, such as jogging. Certainly the decreased physical activity that is associated with aging contributes to senile osteoporosis.

Increased parathyroid hormone levels or function or marginal-to-insufficient intake of vitamin D, despite wishful thinking, cannot be ascribed significant roles in the development of senile and postmenopausal osteoporosis. The body's calcium nutritional state, however, has been recognized as a factor in the development of osteoporosis. The data have shown that adolescent girls (but not boys) have calcium intake levels that are less than those that are recommended. This calcium deficiency occurs during a period of rapid bone growth, stunting the peak bone mass ultimately achieved; thus these individuals are at greater risk of developing osteoporosis.

Postmenopausal osteoporosis is characterized by a hormone-dependent acceleration of bone loss. In the decade following menopause, the yearly reduction in bone mass may reach up to 2% of cortical bone and 9% of cancellous bone. Women may lose as much as 35% of their cortical bone and 50% of their trabecular bone within the 30 to 40 years after menopause; no surprise that 1 out of every 2 women suffers an osteoporotic fracture in contrast to 1 in 40 men. *Estrogen deficiency is believed to play the major role in this phenomenon as evidenced by the increased incidence of osteoporosis in women and by the fact that estrogen replacement beginning at the menopause reduces the rate of bone loss.* The relationship between estrogen and bone mass is mediated by cytokines. It has been demonstrated that decreased estrogen levels result in increased secretion of interleukin-1 by blood monocytes.[12] Interleukin-1 is the most potent known stimulator of osteoclast recruitment and activity. Compensatory osteoblastic activity occurs, but it

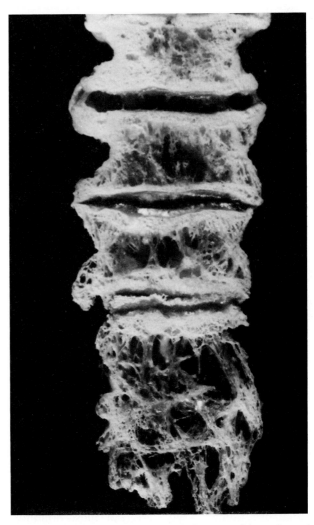

Figure 27–9. Vertebral osteoporosis in a specimen cleared of soft tissue, leaving only the residual bone structure. There is striking cortical thinning and loss of trabeculae with compression fracture of the upper three bodies (compare vertical dimensions with the lowest vertebra shown).

CLINICAL COURSE. The clinical manifestations of structural failure of the skeleton depend on which bones are involved. Vertebral fractures, which frequently occur in the thoracic and lumbar regions, are potentially very painful. Multiple level fractures can cause significant loss of height and various deformities, including lumbar lordosis and kyphoscoliosis. Femoral neck and wrist fractures are common. Complications of overt fractures of the femoral neck, pelvis, or spine, such as pulmonary embolism and pneumonia, are frequent and result in 40,000 to 50,000 deaths per year, which is more than the combined mortality from carcinomas of the breast and endometrium.

Osteoporosis cannot be reliably detected in plain radiographs until 30 to 40% of the bone mass is lost. Moreover, blood levels of calcium, phosphorus, and alkaline phosphatase are not revealing in uncomplicated cases. Osteoporosis therefore can be a difficult condition to diagnose accurately because (1) it remains asymptomatic until skeletal fragility is well advanced; (2) it is only one of a group of osteopenic skeletal disorders characterized by "too little" bone, which can be difficult to differentiate; and (3) there is no easy, sensitive, and specific method to determine the degree of bone loss. Currently the best procedures that accurately estimate the amount of bone loss, aside from biopsy, are various radiographic imaging techniques, such as single-energy photon absorptiometry, dual-energy absorptiometry, and quantitative computed tomography (CT). In essence, these techniques measure bone density. Once the diagnosis of osteoporosis is established, an attempt to identify its etiology should be made and the various secondary causes ruled out.

DISEASES CAUSED BY OSTEOCLAST DYSFUNCTION

OSTEOPETROSIS

Osteopetrosis refers to a group of rare hereditary diseases that are characterized by osteoclast dysfunction, which results in diffuse symmetric skeletal sclerosis (Fig. 27–10). The term osteopetrosis was coined because of the stone-like quality of the bones; however, the bones are abnormally brittle and fracture "like a piece of chalk." Osteopetrosis, which is also known as *marble bone disease* and *Albers-Schönberg disease*, has been classified into at least four variants based on both the mode of inheritance and the clinical findings. The autosomal recessive "malignant" type and the autosomal dominant "benign" type are the most common variants.

The precise nature of the osteoclast dysfunction in these disorders is unknown.[13] An exception

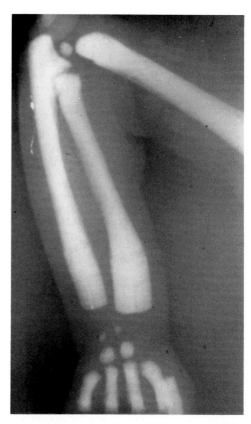

Figure 27–10. Radiograph of upper extremity in patient with osteopetrosis. The bones are diffusely sclerotic, and the distal metaphyses of the ulna and radius are poorly formed (Erlenmeyer's flask deformity).

is the variant associated with carbonic anhydrase II deficiency. Carbonic anhydrase II is an enzyme required by osteoclasts and renal tubular cells to excrete hydrogen ions and acidify their environment. The absence of this enzyme prevents osteoclasts from solubilizing and resorbing matrix and blocks the acidification of urine by the renal tubular cells. Experimental models have shown that in animals osteopetrosis can also be caused by a retrovirus infection, a mutation in the gene coding for macrophage colony-stimulating factor, and mutations in the C-src gene. It is likely that some of these mechanisms will be linked to the human disorders.

MORPHOLOGY. The morphologic changes of osteopetrosis are explained by deficient osteoclast activity. Grossly the bones lack a medullary canal, and the ends of long bones are bulbous (Erlenmeyer's flask deformity) and misshapen. The neural foramina are small and compress exiting nerves. The primary spongiosa, which is normally removed during growth, persists and fills the medullary cavity, leaving no room for the hematopoietic marrow, and prevents the formation of mature trabeculae (Fig. 27–11).[14] Bone that forms is not remodeled and tends to be woven in architecture. In the end, these intrinsic abnormalities cause the bone to be brittle. Histologically there are no consistent changes in osteoclast number; they have been reported to be increased, normal, or decreased in number.

The malignant autosomal recessive pattern usually becomes evident *in utero* or soon after birth. Fractures, anemia, and hydrocephaly are often seen resulting in postpartum mortality. Patients who survive into their infancy have cranial nerve problems (optic atrophy, deafness, facial paralysis) and repeated, often fatal infections because of the inadequacies of the marrow produced in extramedullary sites. The extramedullary hematopoiesis also causes prominent hepatosplenomegaly. The manifestations of the autosomal dominant benign form may not be detected until adolescence or adulthood, when it is discovered on x-ray films performed because of numerous fractures. These patients may also have milder cranial nerve deficits and anemia.

Because osteoclasts are derived from marrow monocyte stem cells, bone marrow transplants provide affected patients with progenitor cells that can produce normal functioning osteoclasts.

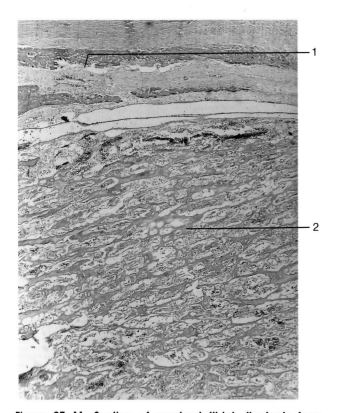

Figure 27–11. Section of proximal tibial diaphysis from fetus with osteopetrosis. The cortex (1) is being formed, and the medullary cavity (2) is abnormally filled with primary spongiosa replacing the hematopoietic elements.

PAGET'S DISEASE (OSTEITIS DEFORMANS)

This unique skeletal disease can be characterized as a "collage of matrix madness." At the outset, Paget's disease is marked by regions of furious osteoclastic bone resorption that is followed by a period of hectic bone formation. The net effect, as the bone cell activity quiets down, is a gain in bone mass; however, the newly formed bone is disordered and architecturally unsound. *This repetitive, overlapping sequence forms the basis of dividing Paget's disease into (1) an initial osteolytic stage, followed by (2) a mixed osteoclastic-osteoblastic stage, which ends with a predominance of osteoblastic activity and evolves ultimately into (3) a burnt-out quiescent osteosclerotic stage.*

Paget's disease usually begins in the fifth decade of life, becomes progressively more common thereafter, and has a slight male predominance. An intriguing aspect is the striking variation in prevalence both within certain countries and throughout the world. Paget's disease is relatively common in whites in England, France, Austria, regions of Germany, Australia, New Zealand, and the United States. The exact incidence is difficult to determine because most affected individuals are asymptomatic, but it is estimated to affect 5 to 11% of the populations in these countries. In contrast, Paget's disease is rare in the native populations of Scandinavia, China, Japan, and Africa.

PATHOGENESIS. When Sir James Paget first described this condition in 1876, he attributed the skeletal changes to an inflammatory process, hence the term "osteitis deformans." It is ironic that after numerous alternative causes have been explored, Sir James Paget may be finally proved correct. Current evidence strongly suggests that Paget's disease is a slow virus infection caused by a paramyxovirus. This likens it to other slow virus diseases, such as subacute sclerosing leukoencephalitis and kuru, produced by the same family of viruses.[15] Viral particles resembling the nucleocapsids of paramyxovirus have been seen in the cytoplasm and nuclei of osteoclasts, and immunologic analyses have identified antigens associated with both the measles and respiratory syncytial viruses (both paramyxoviruses) in osteoclasts from affected sites. More recently *in situ* hybridization studies have localized canine distemper virus (a type of paramyxovirus) in Pagetic osteoclasts, osteoblasts, and osteocytes.[16] It is now hypothesized that the target of the virus is the osteoblast with permissive transmission to the osteoclast; however, the cell-associated viral particles have been identified only in the osteoclasts. Retroviruses such as the paramyxovirus can also induce the secretion of interleukin-6 from infected cells, such as fibroblasts and macrophages; this cytokine is produced in large amounts by osteoblasts and is a potent stimulator of osteoclast recruitment and resorptive activity.[17] Intriguing as these observations may be, to date no virus can be isolated from affected tissue.

MORPHOLOGY. Paget's disease is a focal process with remarkable variation in its stage of development in separate sites. The histologic hallmark is the **mosaic pattern** of lamellar bone. This pattern, which is likened to a jigsaw puzzle, is produced by prominent cement lines that anneal haphazardly oriented units of lamellar bone (Fig. 27-12). In the initial lytic phase, there are the waves of osteoclastic activity and numerous resorptive pits. The osteoclasts are abnormally large and have many more than the normal 10 to 12 nuclei; sometimes 100 nuclei are present. Osteoclasts persist in the mixed phase, but now many of the bone surfaces are lined by prominent osteoblasts. The marrow adjacent to the bone-forming surface is replaced by loose connective tissue that contains osteoprogenitor cells and numerous blood vessels, which transport nutrients and catabolites to and from these metabolically active sites. The newly formed bone may be woven or lamellar, but eventually all of it is remodeled into lamellar bone. As the mosaic pattern unfolds and the cell activity decreases, the fibrovascular lining tissue recedes and is replaced by normal marrow. In the end, the bone becomes a caricature of itself: larger than normal and composed of coarsely thickened trabeculae and cortices that are soft and porous and lack structural stability (Fig. 27-13). These aspects make the bone vulnerable to deformation under stress and to fracture.

CLINICAL COURSE. Paget's disease occurs in one or more bones and is monostotic (tibia, ilium, femur, skull, vertebra, humerus) in about 15% of cases and polyostotic (pelvis, spine, skull) in the re-

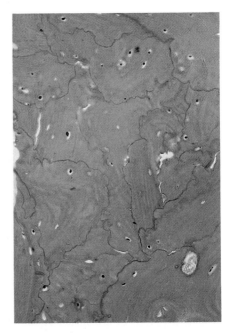

Figure 27-12. Mosaic pattern of lamellar bone pathognomonic of Paget's disease.

mainder.[18] The axial skeleton or proximal femur is involved in up to 80% of cases. Even though no bone is immune, involvement of the ribs, fibula, and small bones of the hands and feet is unusual. The diagnosis can frequently be made from its characteristic radiographic findings. Pagetic bone is typically enlarged with thick coarsened cortices and cancellous bone (Fig. 27-14). The laboratory findings are not diagnostic but usually include an elevated serum level of alkaline phosphatase and increased urinary excretion of hydroxyproline. Clinical findings are extremely variable and depend on the extent and site of the disease. Most cases are mild, do not cause symptoms, and are discovered as an incidental radiographic finding;

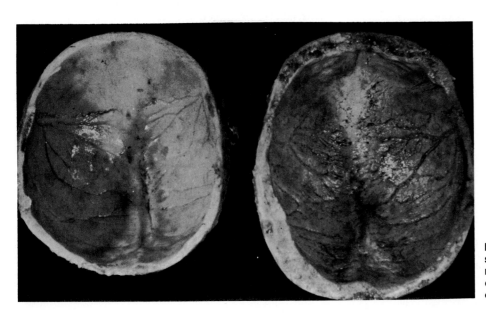

Figure 27-13. Paget's disease of skull. Irregular thickening of right calvarium is obvious by comparison with normal control on left.

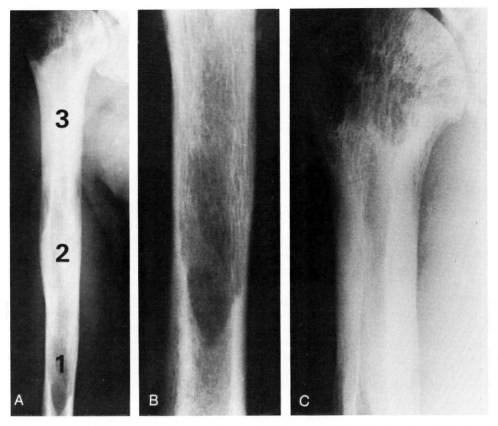

Figure 27–14. Paget's disease of the humerus. The three sequential stages, (1) lytic, (2) mixed, and (3) sclerotic, are shown in *A*. Area 1, the lytic stage, is seen in close-up in *B*. Area 2, the mixed stage (upper portion of *B*) reveals central and endosteal cortical resorption and replacement by less compact new bone. Area 3, the sclerotic stage, with irregular thickening of both cortical and trabecular bone, is seen in *C*. (From Maldague, B., and Malghem, J.: Dynamic radiologic pattern of Paget's disease of bone. Clin. Orthop. *217*:127, 1987.)

Paget's disease, however, can produce a variety of skeletal, neuromuscular, and cardiovascular complications. Pain is the most common problem and is localized to the affected bone. It is caused by a combination of microfractures and bone overgrowth that compresses spinal and cranial nerve roots. Bone overgrowth in the craniofacial skeleton may produce a leonine facies and a cranium so heavy that it becomes difficult for the patient to hold the head erect. The weakened Pagetic bone may lead to invagination of the base of the skull (platybasia) and compression of the posterior fossa structures. Weight bearing causes anterior bowing of the femora and tibiae and distorts the femoral heads, resulting in the development of severe secondary osteoarthritis. Chalkstick-type fractures are the next most common complication and usually occur in the long bones of the lower extremities. Compression fractures of the spine result in spinal cord injury and the development of kyphoses. The hypervascularity of Pagetic bone warms the overlying skin, and in severe polyostotic disease, the increased blood flow behaves as an arteriovenous shunt leading to high output heart failure or exacerbation of underlying cardiac disease. A variety of tumors and tumor-like conditions develop in Pagetic bone. The benign lesions include giant

cell tumor, giant cell reparative granuloma, and extraosseous masses of hematopoiesis. The most dreaded complication is the development of sarcoma, which occurs in 5 to 10% of patients with severe polyostotic disease. The sarcomas are usually osteosarcoma, malignant fibrous histiocytoma or chondrosarcoma,[19] and they arise in the long bones, pelvis, skull, and spine.

Paget's disease is usually not a serious or life-threatening disease in the absence of malignant transformation. Most patients have mild symptoms that are readily suppressed by medical therapy, including calcitonin and diphosphonates.

DISEASES ASSOCIATED WITH ABNORMAL MINERAL HOMEOSTASIS

RICKETS AND OSTEOMALACIA

Rickets and osteomalacia represent a group of diseases of divergent causes that are characterized by a defect in matrix mineralization, most often related to a lack of vitamin D or some disturbance in its metabolism. The term rickets refers to the disorder in children in which deranged bone growth produces distinctive skeletal deformities. In the adult, the disorder is called osteomalacia because the bone that forms during the remodeling process is undermineralized. This results in osteopenia and predisposition to insufficiency fractures. Both rickets and osteomalacia have already been considered in the discussion of vitamin D in Chapter 9.

HYPERPARATHYROIDISM

Hyperparathyroidism is classified into primary and secondary types, as discussed in Chapter 25. Primary hyperparathyroidism results from autonomous hyperplasia or a tumor, usually an adenoma, of the parathyroid gland, whereas secondary hyperparathyroidism is commonly caused by prolonged states of hypocalcemia resulting in compensatory hypersecretion of parathyroid hormone. Whatever the basis, the increased parathyroid hormone levels are detected by receptors on osteoblasts, which then initiate the release of mediators that stimulate osteoclast activity. Thus, through a chain of signals, the skeletal manifestations of hyperparathyroidism are caused by unabated osteoclastic bone resorption. The following points should be noted:

- As in all metabolic bone disease, the entire skeleton is affected in hyperparathyroidism, even though some sites are more severely affected than others.
- The anatomic changes of severe hyperparathyroidism known as *osteitis fibrosa cystica* are now rarely encountered because hyperparathyroidism is currently being diagnosed and treated at an early stage for reasons previously discussed (see Chapter 25, section on hyperparathyroidism).
- Secondary hyperparathyroidism is usually not as severe or as prolonged as primary hyperparathyroidism; hence the skeletal abnormalities tend to be more mild.

MORPHOLOGY. For reasons unknown, the increased osteoclast activity in hyperparathyroidism affects cortical bone (subperiosteal, osteonal, and endosteal surfaces) more severely than cancellous bone. Subperiosteal resorption produces thinned cortices and loss of the lamina dura around the teeth. The resultant x-ray pattern is virtually diagnostic of hyperparathyroidism and is often visible along the radial aspect of the middle phalanges of the index and middle fingers. Intracortical bone resorption is caused by a spearhead arrangement of osteoclasts that bore along and enlarge Haversian and Volkmann's canals. These "cortical cutting cones" are characteristic of hyperparathyroidism.

In cancellous bone, osteoclasts tunnel into and "dissect" centrally along the length of the trabeculae, creating the appearance of railroad tracks and producing what is known as dissecting osteitis (Fig. 27-15). The correlative radiographic finding is a decrease in bone density or osteopenia. Because bone resorption and formation are coupled processes, it is not surprising that osteoblast activity is also increased in hyperparathyroidism. In the regions of bone cell activity, the marrow spaces around the affected surfaces are replaced by fibrovascular tissue.

Microfractures and secondary hemorrhages occur that elicit an influx of multinucleated macrophages and an ingrowth of reactive fibrous tissue to create an apparent mass known as "brown tumor" (Fig. 27-16). The brown color of this reactive lesion is the result of the vascularity, hemorrhage, and hemosiderin deposition. Frequently these lesions undergo cystic degeneration. The combined picture of increased bone cell activity, peritrabecular fibrosis, and cystic brown tumors is the hallmark of severe hyperparathyroidism and is known as **generalized osteitis fibrosa cystica (von Recklinghausen's disease of bone).**

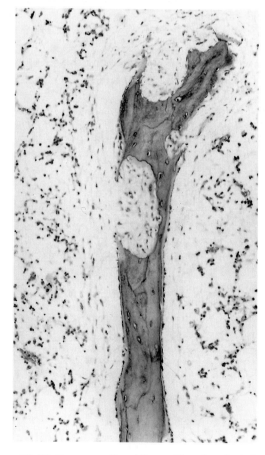

Figure 27-15. Hyperparathyroidism with osteoclasts boring into the center of a trabeculum (dissecting osteitis).

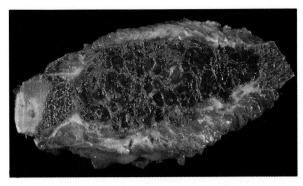

Figure 27-16. Resected rib, harboring expansile brown tumor adjacent to costal cartilage.

The decrease in bone mass predisposes to fractures, deformities caused by the stress of weight bearing, and joint pain and dysfunction as the lines of normal weight bearing are altered. Control of hyperparathyroidism allows the bony changes to regress significantly or disappear completely.

RENAL OSTEODYSTROPHY

Renal osteodystrophy is the term used to describe collectively all of the skeletal changes of chronic renal disease, including (1) increased osteoclastic bone resorption mimicking osteitis fibrosa cystica, (2) delayed matrix mineralization (osteomalacia), (3) osteosclerosis, (4) growth retardation, and (5) osteoporosis. The interrelation between renal failure, secondary hyperparathyroidism, and altered vitamin D metabolism is well recognized, and as advances in medical technology have prolonged the lives of patients with renal diseases, their impact on skeletal homeostasis has assumed greater clinical importance.[20]

The pathophysiology underlying the melange of skeletal lesions is complex and is simplified here:

- Chronic renal failure results in phosphate retention and hyperphosphatemia.
- Hyperphosphatemia can produce secondary hyperparathyroidism by causing hypocalcemia.
- Contributing to the hypocalcemia are (1) decreased conversion of the vitamin D metabolite $25\text{-}(OH)\text{-}D_3$ to $1,25\text{-}(OH)_2\text{-}D_3$ by damaged and shrunken kidneys; (2) inhibition by the high levels of phosphorus of the renal hydroxylase involved in the conversion of $25\text{-}(OH)\text{-}D_3$ to the more active metabolite; and (3) reduced intestinal absorption of calcium because of low levels of $1,25\text{-}(OH)_2\text{-}D_3$.
- Renal failure and low levels of $1,25\text{-}(OH)_2\text{-}D_3$ render bone more unresponsive to parathyroid hormone, and thus the parathyroids are stimu-

lated to increased activity to maintain serum calcium levels.
- The resultant secondary hyperparathyroidism produces increased osteoclast activity.
- A shift in the set point for calcium-regulated parathyroid hormone secretion results in the parathyroid glands being more sensitive to the depressed serum ionized calcium levels.
- Decreased degradation and excretion of parathyroid hormone occur because of compromised renal function.
- The lowered levels of $1,25\text{-}(OH)_2\text{-}D_3$ and serum calcium contribute to osteomalacia.

Other factors that are important in the genesis of osteodystrophy in chronic renal failure include hyperphosphatemia, metabolic acidosis, iron accumulation in bone, and aluminum deposition at the site of mineralization. Aluminum deposition is considered to be *a major cause* and has received a lot of attention because of its iatrogenic origin.[20] The sources of the aluminum include dialysate solutions prepared from water with a high aluminum content and oral aluminum-containing phosphate binders. The aluminum, which has an affinity for the mineralization front, interferes with the deposition of calcium hydroxyapatite and hence results in osteomalacia. Aluminum not only is toxic to bone but also has been implicated as the cause of dialysis encephalopathy and microcytic anemia in patients with chronic renal failure.

FRACTURES

Fractures are classified as *complete* or *incomplete (greenstick); closed (simple)* when the overlying tissue is intact, or *compound* when the fracture site *communicates* with the skin surface; and *comminuted* when the bone is splintered, or *displaced* when the ends of the bone at the fractures site are not aligned. If the break occurs in bone already altered by a disease process, it is a *pathologic fracture*. A *stress fracture* develops slowly and follows a period of increased physical activity in which the bone is subjected to new repetitive loads, as in sports training or marching in military boot camp.

Bone is unique in its ability to repair itself; it can completely reconstitute itself by reactivating processes that normally occur during embryogenesis. This process is a highly regulated cascade that can be artificially separated into overlapping histologic, biochemical, and biomechanical stages. The completion of each stage initiates its successor, which is accomplished by continuous communication among the various constituents.

MORPHOLOGY. Immediately following fracture, rupture of blood vessels results in a hematoma, which fills the fracture gap and surrounds the area of bone injury. This also provides a fibrin mesh, which helps seal off the fracture site and at the same time serves as a framework for the influx of inflammatory cells and ingrowth of fibroblasts and capillary buds. Simultaneously degranulated platelets and migrating inflammatory cells release platelet-derived growth factor (PDGF), TGF-β, and fibroblast growth factor (FGF), which activate the osteoprogenitor cells in the periosteum, medullary cavity, and surrounding soft tissues.[21] Thus by the end of the first week, the hematoma is organizing, and the adjacent tissue is being modulated for future matrix production. This fusiform and predominantly **soft tissue callus (procallus)** provides some anchorage between the ends of the fractured bones but offers no structural rigidity for weight bearing.

Subsequently, the activated periosteal osteoblasts deposit trabeculae of woven bone that are oriented perpendicular to the cortical axis and also within the medullary cavity. The activated mesenchymal cells in the soft tissues surrounding the fracture line differentiate into chondroblasts that make fibrocartilage and hyaline cartilage enveloping the fracture site. In an uncomplicated fracture, the repair tissue reaches its maximal girth at the end of the second or third week, which helps stabilize the fracture site, but it is not yet strong enough for weight bearing. As the intramedullary and subperiosteal reactive woven bone approaches the newly formed cartilage along the fracture line, the cartilage undergoes enchondral ossification such as normally occurs at the growth plate. In this fashion, the fractured ends are bridged by a **bony callus,** and as the callus mineralizes, its stiffness and strength increase to the point that controlled weight bearing can be tolerated (Fig. 27–17).

In the early stages of callus formation, an excess of fibrous tissue, cartilage, and bone is produced. If the bones are not perfectly aligned, the volume of callus is greatest in the concave portion of the fracture site. As the callus matures and transmits weight-bearing forces, the portions that are not physically stressed are resorbed, and in this manner the callus is reduced in size until the shape and outline of the fractured bone have been reestablished. The medullary cavity is also restored, and after this has been completed, it may be impossible to demonstrate the site of previous injury.

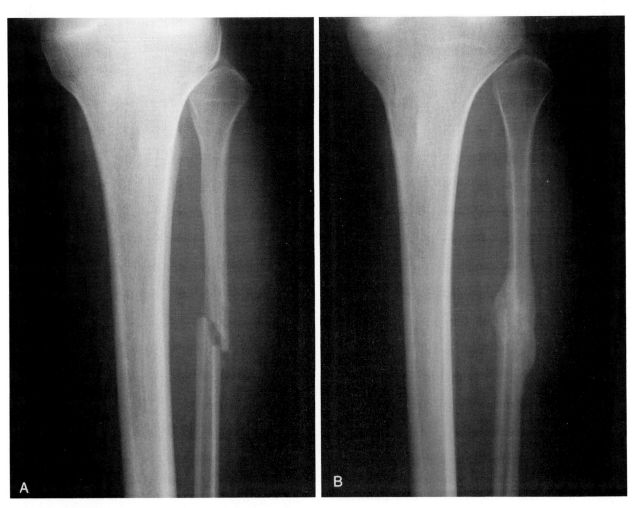

Figure 27–17. *A,* A recent fracture of the fibula. *B,* The marked callus formation 6 weeks later. (Courtesy of Dr. Barbara Weissman, Brigham and Women's Hospital, Boston.)

Unfortunately, the sequence of events in the healing of a fracture can be easily impeded or even blocked. Displaced and comminuted fractures all too frequently result in some deformity. The devitalized fragments of splintered bone require resorption, and this delays healing, enlarges the callus, and requires extremely long periods of remodeling, so in essence there is a permanent abnormality. Inadequate immobilization permits constant movement at the fracture site so the normal constituents of callus do not form. Consequently, the callus may be composed mainly of fibrous tissue and cartilage, which perpetuates the instability and can result in delayed union and non-union. If a non-union allows for too much motion along the fracture gap, the central portion of the callus undergoes cystic degeneration, and the luminal surface can actually become lined by synovial-like cells creating a false joint or *pseudoarthrosis.* In the setting of a non-union or pseudoarthrosis, the normal healing process can be reinstituted if the interposed soft tissues are removed and the fracture site stabilized. A very serious obstacle to healing is infection of the fracture site, which is a real risk in comminuted and open fractures. The infection must be eradicated before bony union can also be achieved. Bone repair cannot be viewed in isolation; this complex process can be derailed by inadequate levels of calcium or phosphorus, vitamin deficiencies, systemic infection, diabetes, and vascular insufficiency. Generally, with children and young adults, in whom most uncomplicated fractures are found, practically perfect reconstitution can be anticipated. In older age groups in whom fractures tend to occur on a background of some other disease (osteoporosis, osteomalacia), repair is less optimal and often requires mechanical methods of immobilization to facilitate healing.

OSTEONECROSIS (AVASCULAR NECROSIS)

Infarction of bone and marrow is a relatively common event and can occur in the medullary cavity of the metaphysis or diaphysis and the subchondral region of the epiphysis.

All instances of bone necrosis result from ischemia; however, the mechanisms that produce it are varied and include (1) mechanical vascular interruption (fracture), (2) thrombosis and embolism (nitrogen bubbles in dysbarism) (see section on changes in atmospheric pressure in Chapter 9), (3) vessel injury (vasculitis, radiation therapy, Gaucher's disease), (4) increased intraosseous pressure with vascular compression (possibly steroid-induced necrosis), and (5) venous hypertension.[22] The disease states associated with bone infarcts are diverse (Table 27–4), and in many the cause of the necrosis is uncertain. Indeed, aside from fracture,

Table 27–4. DISORDERS ASSOCIATED WITH OSTEONECROSIS

Idiopathic
Trauma
Corticosteroid administration
Infection
Dysbarism
Radiation therapy
Connective tissue disorders (rheumatoid arthritis, systemic lupus erythematosus, CREST)
Pregnancy
Gaucher's disease
Sickle cell and other anemias
Clotting disorders
Alcohol abuse
Chronic pancreatitis
Tumors
Epiphyseal disorders

the most common causes of bone necrosis are idiopathic and prior steroid administration. The pathophysiology underlying steroid-induced bone infarcts is obscure; however, it has followed short-term high doses, long-term smaller doses, and even intra-articular injections.

MORPHOLOGY. The pathologic features of bone necrosis are the same regardless of the etiology. In medullary infarcts, the necrosis is geographic and involves the cancellous bone and marrow. The cortex is usually not affected because of its collateral blood flow. In subchondral infarcts, a triangular or wedge-shaped segment of tissue that has the subchondral bone plate as its base and the center of the epiphysis as its apex undergoes necrosis. The overlying articular cartilage remains viable because it receives nutrition from the synovial fluid. The dead bone, recognized by its empty lacunae, is surrounded by necrotic adipocytes that frequently rupture, releasing their fatty acids that bind calcium and form insoluble calcium soaps, which may remain for life. In the healing response, osteoclasts resorb the necrotic trabeculae; however, those that remain act as scaffolding for the deposition of new living bone in a process known as "creeping substitution." In subchondral infarcts, the pace of "creeping substitution" is too slow to be effective, so there is eventual collapse of the necrotic cancellous bone and distortion of the articular cartilage (Fig. 27–18).

CLINICAL COURSE. The symptoms associated with bone necrosis are varied and depend on the location and extent of infarction. Typically, subchondral infarcts cause chronic pain that is initially associated only with activity but then becomes progressively more constant until finally it is present at rest. In contrast, medullary infarcts are clinically silent except for larger ones occurring in Gaucher's disease, dysbarism, and hemoglobinopathies. Medullary infarcts usually remain stable over time and rarely are the site of malignant transfor-

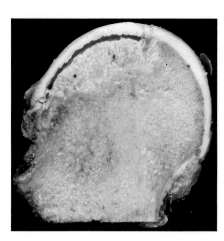

Figure 27-18. Femoral head with subchondral wedge-shaped pale area of osteonecrosis. The space between the overlying articular cartilage and the bone is caused by trabecular compression fractures without repair.

mation. Subchondral infarcts, however, often collapse and may predispose to severe, secondary osteoarthritis. More than 10% of the 500,000 joint replacements performed annually in the United States are for treatment of the complications of osteonecrosis.

INFECTIONS — OSTEOMYELITIS

Osteomyelitis, by definition, means inflammation of bone and marrow, and the common use of the term virtually always implies infection. Osteomyelitis may be a complication of any systemic infection; it frequently manifests, however, in the skeleton as a primary solitary focus of disease. All types of organisms, including viruses, parasites, fungi, and bacteria, can produce osteomyelitis, but infections caused by certain pyogenic bacteria and mycobacteria are the most common. Currently in the United States, Third World immigrants and immunosuppressed patients have made infections by rare exotic organisms more common; thus the diagnosis and treatment of osteomyelitis have become more challenging.

PYOGENIC OSTEOMYELITIS

Pyogenic osteomyelitis is almost always caused by bacteria, and virtually every known organism has been involved at one time or another. The organisms may reach the bone by (1) hematogenous spread, (2) extension from a contiguous site, and (3) direct implantation. Most cases of osteomyelitis are hematogenous in origin and develop in the long bones or vertebral bodies in otherwise healthy individuals.[23] The initiating bacteremia may follow trivial occurrences, such as occult injury to the intestinal mucosa during defecation, vigorous chewing of hard foods, or minor infections of the skin.

Staphylococcus aureus is responsible for 80 to 90% of the cases of pyogenic osteomyelitis in which an organism is recovered. *Escherichia coli*, Pseudomonas, and Klebsiella are more frequently isolated from patients having genitourinary tract infections or who are intravenous drug abusers. Mixed bacterial infections, including anaerobes, are seen in the setting of direct spread or inoculation of organisms during surgery or open fractures. In the neonatal period, *Haemophilus influenzae* and group B streptococci are frequent pathogens, and patients with sickle cell disease, for unknown reasons, are predisposed to Salmonella infection. Unfortunately in almost 50% of cases of typical pyogenic osteomyelitis, no organisms can be isolated because the bacteria are eradicated by prior antibiotic therapy, sampling for culture is inadequate, or culture methods are suboptimal.

The location of the lesions within specific bones is influenced by the vascular circulation, which changes with age. In the neonate, the metaphyseal vessels penetrate the growth plate, resulting in frequent infection of the metaphysis, epiphysis, or both. In children, localization of microorganisms in the metaphysis is typical. After growth plate closure, the metaphyseal vessels reunite with their epiphyseal counterparts and provide a route for the bacteria to seed the epiphyses and subchondral regions in the adult.

MORPHOLOGY. The morphology of osteomyelitis depends on the stage (acute, subacute, or chronic) and location of the infection. Once localized in bone, the bacteria proliferate and induce an acute inflammatory reaction. The released toxins and destructive enzymes reduce the local pH and oxygen tension, increase the intraosseous pressure, and cause cell death. The entrapped bone undergoes necrosis within the first 48 hours, and the bacteria and inflammation spread within the shaft of the bone and may percolate throughout the Haversian systems to reach the periosteum. In children, the periosteum is loosely attached to the cortex; therefore sizeable **subperiosteal** abscesses may form, which can trek for long distances along the bone surface. Lifting of the periosteum further impairs the blood supply to the affected region, and both the suppurative and the ischemic injury may cause segmental bone necrosis; the dead piece of bone is known as the **"sequestrum."** Rupture of the periosteum leads to a soft tissue abscess and the eventual formation of a **draining sinus.** Sometimes the sequestrum crumbles and forms free foreign bodies that pass through the sinus tract.

In infants, but uncommonly in adults, epiphyseal infection spreads through the articular surface or along capsular and tendoligamentous insertions into a joint to produce septic or suppurative arthritis, sometimes causing extensive destruction of the articular cartilage and permanent disability. An analogous process involves the vertebrae, in which the infection destroys the hyaline cartilage end plate and intervertebral discs and spreads into adjacent vertebrae.

Over time, the host response evolves, and after the first week of infection, chronic inflammatory cells become more numerous and stimulate osteoclastic bone resorption, ingrowth of fibrous tissue, and deposition of reactive bone in the periphery. In the presence of a sequestrum, the reactive woven or lamellar bone may be deposited as a sleeve of living tissue known as the **"involucrum,"** around the segment of devitalized bone (Fig. 27–19). Several morphologic variants of osteomyelitis have been given eponyms because of their distinguishing features: **Brodie's abscess** is a small intraosseous abscess that frequently involves the cortex and is walled off by reactive bone; **sclerosing osteomyelitis of Garré** typically develops in the jaw and is associated with extensive new bone formation that obscures much of the underlying osseous structure.

Clinically hematogenous osteomyelitis may manifest as an acute systemic illness with malaise, fever, chills, leukocytosis, and marked-to-intense throbbing pain over the affected region. The presentation may be more subtle, however, with only unexplained fever, particularly in infants, or conversely only localized pain in the absence of fever

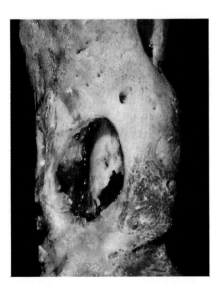

Figure 27–19. Resected femur in patient with draining osteomyelitis. The drainage tract in the subperiosteal shell of viable new bone (involucrum) reveals the inner native necrotic cortex (sequestrum).

in adults. The diagnosis can be strongly suggested by the characteristic x-ray findings of a lytic focus of bone destruction surrounded by a zone of sclerosis. In many untreated patients, blood cultures are positive; in the remainder, however, biopsy and culture are required to identify the pathogen. The combination of antibiotics and surgical drainage when necessary is usually curative; in 5 to 25% of cases, however, acute osteomyelitis fails to resolve and persists as chronic infection. Chronicity may develop when there is delay in diagnosis, extensive bone necrosis, abbreviated antibiotic therapy, inadequate surgical débridement, and weakened host defenses. Acute flare-ups may mark the clinical course of chronic infection; they can occur after years of dormancy, are usually spontaneous, and have no obvious cause. Other complications of chronic osteomyelitis include pathologic fracture, secondary amyloidosis, endocarditis, sepsis, the development of squamous cell carcinoma in the sinus tract, and rarely sarcoma in the infected bone.

TUBERCULOUS OSTEOMYELITIS

A resurgence of tuberculous osteomyelitis is occurring in industrialized nations, attributed to the influx of immigrants from underdeveloped countries and the greater numbers of immunosuppressed people. In developing countries, the affected individuals are usually adolescents or young adults, whereas in the indigenous population of the United States, the victims tend to be older except for those who are immunosuppressed. It is estimated that 1 to 3% of patients with pulmonary or extrapulmonary tuberculosis have osseous infection.

The organisms are usually blood borne and originate from a focus of active visceral disease. Direct extension (e.g., from a pulmonary focus into a rib or from tracheobronchial nodes into adjacent vertebrae) or spread via draining lymphatics may also be involved. The bony infection is usually solitary and in some cases may be the only manifestation of tuberculosis. Similar to the more common pulmonary form, it may fester for years before being recognized. In AIDS patients, the bone infection is frequently multifocal. The spine (especially the thoracic and lumbar vertebrae) is the most common site of skeletal involvement, followed by the knees and hips. Tuberculous osteomyelitis tends to be more destructive and resistant to control than pyogenic osteomyelitis. The infection spreads through large areas of the medullary cavity and causes extensive necrosis. In the spine *(Pott's disease)*, the infection breaks through intervertebral discs to involve multiple vertebrae and extends into the soft tissues forming abscesses. Typically, the patients present with pain on motion, localized tenderness, low-grade fevers, chills, and weight loss. In some cases, the patients may complain of an inguinal mass that represents a cold fluctuant psoas abscess originating in a vertebral infection. Severe destruction of vertebrae frequently results in permanent compression fractures that produce significant scoliotic or kyphotic deformities and neurologic deficits secondary to spinal cord and nerve compression. Other complications of tuberculous osteomyelitis include tuberculous arthritis, sinus tract formation, and amyloidosis.

SKELETAL SYPHILIS

Syphilis *(Treponema pallidum)* and yaws *(Treponema pertenue)* both can involve bone. Currently, syphilis is experiencing a resurgence; however, bone involvement remains infrequent because the disease is readily diagnosed and treated before this stage develops.

Skeletal syphilis may be congenital or acquired. In congenital syphilis, the bone lesions begin to appear about the fifth month of gestation and are fully developed at birth. The spirochetes tend to localize in areas of active enchondral ossification (osteochondritis) and in the periosteum (periostitis). In acquired syphilis, bone disease may begin early in the tertiary stage, which is usually 2 to 5 years after the initial infection. The bones most frequently involved are those of the nose, palate, skull, and extremities, especially the long tubular bones such as the tibia. The syphilitic "saber shin" is produced by massive reactive periosteal bone deposition on the medial and anterior surfaces of the tibia. The "saddle nose" is the result of inflammatory destruction and collapse of the nasal and palatal bones.

MORPHOLOGY. The histology of congenital syphilitic periostitis is characterized by edematous granulation tissue containing numerous plasma cells and necrotic bone. This type of response is also seen in acquired syphilis; the morphology of acquired disease, however, is distinguished by gummata. A gumma is composed of tissue that has undergone central necrosis surrounded by layers of granulomatous and nonspecific chronic inflammation. The spirochetes can be demonstrated in the inflammatory tissue with special silver stains. The gumma is a smoldering inflammatory process that can cause massive destruction if not treated.

BONE TUMORS AND TUMOR-LIKE LESIONS

Bone tumors come in all sizes and appearances and range in their biologic potential from the innocuous to the rapidly fatal. This diversity makes it critical to accurately diagnose, stage, and appropriately treat tumors so the patients not only survive but also maintain optimal function of the affected body parts.

Bone tumors are generally classified according to the normal cell or tissue type they recapitulate. Those lesions that do not have normal tissue counterparts are grouped according to their distinct clinicopathologic features. All cell and tissue types indigenous to bone are represented in the classification scheme, and an indicator of their wide variety and incidence is provided in Table 27–5. Overall, matrix-producing (chondrogenic, osteogenic) and fibrous tumors are the most common, and among the benign tumors, osteochondroma and fibrous cortical defect are the most numerous. Excluding malignant neoplasms of marrow origin (myeloma, lymphoma, and leukemia), osteosarcoma is the most common primary cancer of bone, followed by chondrosarcoma and Ewing's sarcoma.

The precise incidence of specific bone tumors is not known because biopsy is not performed on many benign lesions. It is safe to estimate, however, that benign tumors outnumber their malignant counterparts by at least several hundredfold. Benign tumors have their greatest frequency within the first three decades of life, whereas in the elderly a bone tumor is likely to be malignant. In the United States, about 2100 bone sarcomas are diagnosed per year, and they are responsible annually for the death of approximately 1300 people.

Although these neoplasms as a group affect all ages, arise in virtually every bone of the body, and occur in males slightly more frequently than in females, specific types of tumors target certain age groups[24] and anatomic sites. For instance, most osteosarcomas occur during adolescence, and about half arise around the knee either in the distal femoral or proximal tibial metaphysis. Interestingly, these are the sites of greatest skeletal growth activity. In contrast, chondrosarcomas tend to develop in mid to late adulthood and to involve the trunk, limb girdles, and proximal long bones. Chondroblastomas and giant cell tumors almost always arise in the epiphysis of long bones, and in comparison Ewing's sarcoma, osteofibrous dysplasia, and adamantinoma most often arise in the diaphysis. Thus the location of a tumor provides important diagnostic information.

Although the etiology of most bone tumors is unknown, current evidence strongly suggests that genetic alterations underlie their development. For instance, in the Li-Fraumeni and hereditary retinoblastoma cancer syndromes, the development of bone sarcomas has been linked to mutations affecting specific tumor suppressor genes (discussed later). Bone infarcts, chronic osteomyelitis, Paget's disease, radiation, and metal prostheses are also associated with an increased incidence of bone neoplasia. To date, however, no consistent mutation has been identified in these settings, and such

Table 27-5. CLASSIFICATION OF 8542 PRIMARY TUMORS OF BONE IN MAYO CLINIC PATIENTS

HISTOLOGIC TYPE	TOTAL CASES	BENIGN	CASES	MALIGNANT	CASES
Hematopoietic	3401 (39.8%)			Myeloma	2932
				Malignant lymphoma	469
Chondrogenic	1822 (21.3%)	Osteochondroma	727	Primary chondrosarcoma	545
		Chondroma	245	Secondary chondrosarcoma	89
		Chondroblastoma	79	Dedifferentiated chondrosarcoma	79
		Chondromyxoid fibroma	39	Mesenchymal chondrosarcoma	19
Osteogenic	1638 (19.2%)	Osteoid osteoma	245	Osteosarcoma	1274
		Osteoblastoma	63	Parosteal osteosarcoma	56
Unknown origin	878 (10.3%)	Giant cell tumor	425	Ewing's tumor	402
				Malignant giant cell tumor	28
				Adamantinoma	23
Histiocytic origin	62 (0.7%)	Fibrous histiocytoma	10	Malignant (fibrous) histiocytoma	52
Fibrogenic	315 (3.7%)	Metaphyseal fibrous defect (fibroma)	99	Desmoplastic fibroma	9
				Fibrosarcoma	207
Notochordal	262 (3.1%)			Chordoma	262
Vascular	147 (1.7%)	Hemangioma	80	Hemangioendothelioma	60
				Hemangiopericytoma	7
Lipogenic	7 (0.1%)	Lipoma	6	Liposarcoma	1
Neurogenic	10 (0.1%)	Neurilemmoma	10		
Total	8542 (100%)		2028		6514

From Dahlin, D.C., and Unni, K.K.: Bone Tumors, 4th ed. Springfield, IL, Charles C Thomas, 1986, p.8, by permission of Mayo Foundation.

secondary neoplasms account for only a small fraction of all skeletal tumors.

Clinically, bone tumors have a variety of presentations. The more common benign lesions are frequently asymptomatic and are detected as an incidental finding. Many tumors, however, produce pain or are noticed as a slow-growing mass. In some circumstances, the first hint of a tumor's presence is a sudden pathologic fracture. Radiographic analysis plays an important role in diagnosing these lesions. In addition to providing the exact location and extent of tumor, imaging studies can detect features that help limit diagnostic possibilities and give clues to the aggressiveness of the tumor. Ultimately in most instances, histologic examination is necessary. Although light microscopy is usually sufficient, special techniques, such as electron microscopy, immunohistochemistry, and cytogenetic analysis, may be required to help distinguish between certain types of tumors, especially small round cell neoplasms. In addition to classifying the tumor, when dealing with a sarcoma, its histologic grade also needs to be determined. This has been shown to be the most important prognostic feature of a bone sarcoma and has been incorporated into the major staging systems of bone neoplasms (Table 27–6).

BONE-FORMING TUMORS

Common to all these neoplasms is the production of bone by the neoplastic cells. Except in osteoma,

the tumor bone is usually deposited as woven trabeculae and is variably mineralized.

Osteoma

Osteomas are generally slow-growing tumors of little clinical significance except when they cause obstruction of a sinus cavity, impinge on the brain or eye, interfere with function of the oral cavity, or produce cosmetic problems. Osteomas do not transform into osteosarcoma.

MORPHOLOGY. Osteomas are bosselated, round-to-oval sessile tumors that project from the subperiosteal or endosteal surfaces of the cortex. Subperiosteal osteomas most often arise on or inside the

Table 27-6. ENNEKING STAGING SYSTEM FOR SARCOMAS OF BONE AND SOFT TISSUE

STAGE	HISTOLOGIC GRADE	SITE	METASTASES
IA	Low	Intracompartmental	Absent
IB	Low	Extracompartmental	Absent
IIA	High	Intracompartmental	Absent
IIB	High	Extracompartmental	Absent
III	Low or high	Intracompartmental or extracompartmental	Present

The compartment of a bone is bounded by its periosteum, even if lifted.

skull and facial bones. They are usually solitary and detected in middle adult life, with a slight male predominance. Multiple osteomas are seen in the setting of Gardner's syndrome (see Chapter 17, section on intestinal familial polyposis). They are composed of a composite of woven and lamellar bone that is frequently deposited in a cortical pattern with Haversian-like systems. Some variants contain a component of trabecular bone in which the intertrabecular spaces are filled with hematopoietic marrow. Histologically the reactive bone induced by infection, trauma, or hemangiomas may simulate an osteoma and should be considered in the differential diagnosis.

Osteoid Osteoma and Osteoblastoma

Osteoid osteoma and osteoblastoma have identical histologic features but differ in size, sites of origin, and symptoms. By definition, osteoid osteomas are less than 2 cm in greatest dimension and osteoblastomas are larger.

Osteoid osteoma usually occurs in the second and third decades of life (75% of patients are less than 25 years old), and males outnumber females 2:1. They can arise in any bone but have a predilection for the appendicular skeleton (50% of cases involve femur or tibia), where they commonly arise in the cortex and less frequently within the medullary cavity. Osteoid osteomas are painful. The pain, which is caused by excess prostaglandin E_2 production, is severe in relation to the small size of the lesion and is characteristically nocturnal and dramatically relieved by aspirin.[25]

Osteoblastoma occurs in the same age group and has the same gender distribution as osteoid osteoma. Osteoblastoma differs from osteoid osteoma in that it involves the spine more frequently; it may not be painful, or if pain is present, it is dull, achy, and not very responsive to salicylates; and it is not associated with a marked bony reaction.

MORPHOLOGY. Grossly, both osteoid osteoma and osteoblastoma are round-to-oval masses of hemorrhagic, gritty, tan tissue. Histologically, they are well circumscribed and composed of a morass of randomly interconnecting trabeculae of woven bone that are prominently rimmed by osteoblasts (Fig. 27–20). The stroma surrounding the tumor bone is loose connective tissue that contains many dilated and congested capillaries. Importantly, the relatively small size and well-defined margins of these tumors in combination with the benign cytologic features of the neoplastic osteoblasts help distinguish them from osteosarcoma. Osteoid osteomas,

especially those that arise beneath the periosteum, usually elicit a tremendous amount of reactive bone formation that encircles the lesion. The actual tumor, known as the **nidus**, manifests radiographically as a small round lucency that is variably mineralized (Fig. 27–21).[26] Although larger, osteoblastomas also appear on x-ray film as a partially mineralized lytic mass that has sharp margins.

Osteoid osteoma and osteoblastoma are readily treated by conservative surgery; if not entirely excised, they can recur. The possibility of malignant transformation is remote except when tumors are treated with radiation, which promotes this dreaded complication.

Osteosarcoma

Osteosarcoma is defined as a malignant mesenchymal tumor in which the cancerous cells produce bone matrix. It is the most common primary malig-

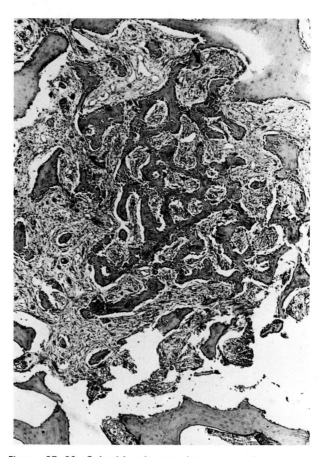

Figure 27–20. Osteoid osteoma. Low-power view reveals entire lesion enclosed within peripheral sclerotic wide bone spicules. The lesion is composed of anastomosing trabeculae of woven bone rimmed by prominent osteoblasts. The intertrabecular spaces are filled with vascular loose connective tissue.

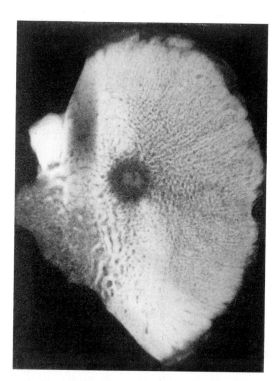

Figure 27-21. Specimen radiograph of intracortical osteoid osteoma. The round radiolucency with central mineralization represents the lesion and is surrounded by abundant reactive bone that has massively thickened the cortex.

nant tumor of bone exclusive of myeloma and lymphoma and accounts for approximately 20% of primary bone cancers. About 1000 cases are newly diagnosed each year in the United States. Osteosarcoma occurs in all age groups but has a bimodal age distribution. Approximately 75% occur in patients younger than 20 years of age.[27] The smaller second peak (secondary osteosarcoma) occurs in the elderly, who frequently suffer from conditions known to be associated with the development of osteosarcoma (Paget's disease, bone infarcts, and prior irradiation). Hereditary osteochondromas, enchondromas, and fibrous dysplasia are also sometimes complicated by osteosarcomas. Overall, males are more commonly affected than females (1.6:1). The tumors usually arise in the metaphyseal region of the long bones of the extremities, and almost 60% occur about the knee. Their locations in descending order of frequency are the distal femur, proximal tibia, proximal humerus, and proximal femur (Fig. 27-22). Any bone may be involved, however, and in persons beyond the age of 25, the incidence in flat bones and long bones is almost equal.

PATHOGENESIS. Mutations are fundamental to the development of osteosarcoma. As pointed out earlier (see Chapter 7), patients with hereditary retinoblastomas have a several hundredfold greater risk of subsequently developing osteosarcoma. These patients inherit a mutant allele of the retinoblastoma gene, a well-known tumor suppressor

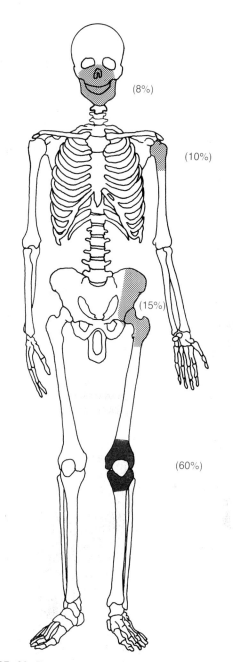

DISTRIBUTION OF OSTEOSARCOMA

Figure 27-22. The major sites of origin of osteosarcomas. Numbers in parentheses are approximate percentages.

gene, described in detail in Chapter 7. When the remaining allele is somatically inactivated, uncontrolled proliferation follows. Mutations in the retinoblastoma gene are uncommon in sporadic osteosarcoma; however, mutations in another suppressor gene, p53, are frequently present. Located on the short arm of chromosome 17, germline mutations of the p53 gene (Li-Fraumeni syndrome) have been implicated in the development of most nonhereditary osteosarcomas as well as many other types of cancer, as has already been discussed (see

Chapter 7).[28] It is also interesting that many osteosarcomas develop at sites of greatest bone growth where bone cell mitotic activity is at its peak — e.g., the base of the femoral growth plate where primary spongiosa is being formed and in Pagetic bone with its frenzy of bone formation and resorption. It is not surprising then that the large dog breeds such as St. Bernards and Great Danes have a high incidence of this type of tumor (data are not available on the frequency in professional basketball players).

The classification scheme of osteosarcoma is complex but important because particular variants frequently require specific modes of therapy. More than 12 different subtypes of osteosarcoma have been described, and they are grouped according to (1) the anatomic portion of the bone from which they arise (intramedullary, intracortical, or surface), (2) degree of differentiation, (3) multicentricity (synchronous, metachronous), (4) secondary osteosarcoma associated with pre-existing disorders (6 to 10%) (benign tumors, Paget's disease, bone infarcts, previous radiation), and (5) histologic variants (osteoblastic, chondroblastic, fibroblastic, telangiectatic, small cell, and giant cell).[29] The most common subtype is conventional osteosarcoma, which arises in the metaphysis of long bones and is primary, solitary, intramedullary, and poorly differentiated and produces a predominantly bony matrix.

CLINICAL COURSE. Osteosarcomas typically present as painful, progressively enlarging masses. Sometimes a sudden fracture of the bone is the first symptom. These aggressive neoplasms spread through the bloodstream, and at the time of diagnosis, approximately 20% of patients have demonstrable pulmonary metastases. In those who die of the neoplasm, 90% have metastases to the lungs, bones, brain, and elsewhere. Radiographs of the primary tumor usually show a large destructive, mixed lytic and blastic mass that has permeative margins (Fig. 27–25). The tumors frequently break through the cortex and lift the periosteum, resulting in reactive periosteal bone formation. The triangular shadow between the cortex and raised ends of periosteum is known radiographically as *Codman's triangle* and is characteristic but not diagnostic of this tumor. Laboratory studies are usually normal except for possibly an elevated serum alkaline phosphatase, which is nonspecific.

Advances in treatment have substantially improved the prognosis of osteosarcoma. Currently the long-term survival rate has been increased to approximately 60% from the historic controls of 25%.[30]

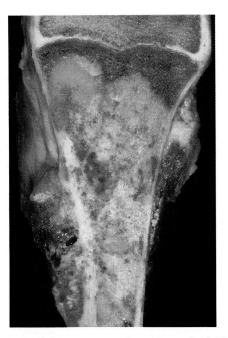

Figure 27–23. Osteosarcoma of upper end of tibia. The tan-white tumor fills most of the medullary cavity of the metaphysis and proximal diaphysis. It has infiltrated through the cortex, lifted the periosteum, and formed soft tissue masses on both sides of the bone.

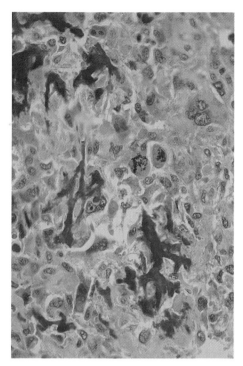

Figure 27–24. Coarse pattern of dark-appearing neoplastic bone produced by the anaplastic malignant tumor cells. Note the mitotic figures.

CARTILAGE-FORMING TUMORS

Cartilage tumors are characterized by the formation of hyaline or myxoid cartilage; fibrocartilage and elastic cartilage are rare components. As in most types of bone tumors, benign cartilage tumors are much more common than malignant ones.

Osteochondroma

Osteochondroma, also known as an *exostosis,* is a benign, cartilage-capped outgrowth that is attached to the underlying skeleton by a bony stalk. It is a relatively common lesion and can be solitary or multiple. Multiple osteochondromas occur in *mul-*

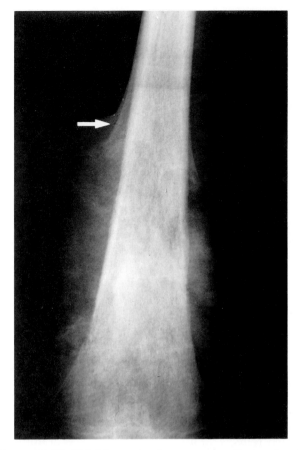

Figure 27–25. Distal femoral osteosarcoma with prominent bone formation extending into the soft tissues. The periosteum that has been lifted has laid down a proximal triangular shell of reactive bone, known as Codman's triangle *(arrow).*

tiple hereditary exostosis, which is an autosomal dominant hereditary disease. Osteochondromas are believed to result from displacement of the lateral portion of the growth plate, which then proliferates in a direction diagonal to the long axis of the bone and away from the nearby joint (Fig. 27–26). Solitary osteochondromas are usually first diagnosed in late adolescence and early adulthood, but multiple osteochondromas become apparent during childhood. For unknown reasons, males are af-

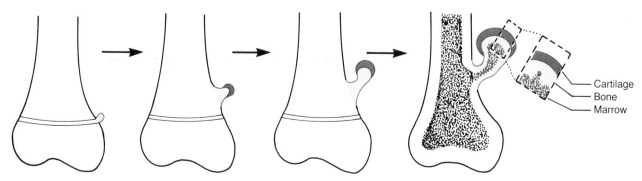

Cartilage
Bone
Marrow

Figure 27–26. A schematic of the development over time of an osteochondroma, beginning with an outgrowth from the epiphyseal cartilage.

fected three times more often than females. They usually arise from the metaphysis near the growth plate of long tubular bones. Occasionally they develop from bones of the pelvis, scapula, and ribs, and in these sites they are frequently sessile and have short stalks. Rarely do these benign lesions involve the short tubular bones of the hands and feet.

> **MORPHOLOGY.** Osteochondromas are mushroom shaped and range in size from 1 to 20 cm. The outer layer of the head of the osteochondroma is composed of benign hyaline cartilage varying in thickness and is delineated peripherally by perichondrium. The cartilage has the appearance of disorganized growth plate and undergoes enchondral ossification, with the newly made bone forming the inner portion of the head and stalk. The cortex of the stalk merges with the cortex of the host bone so the medullary cavity of the osteochondroma and bone are in continuity.

Clinically, osteochondromas present as slow-growing masses, which can be painful if they impinge on a nerve or if the stalk is fractured. In many cases, they are detected as an incidental finding. In multiple hereditary exostosis, the underlying bones may be bowed and shortened, which reflects an associated disturbance in epiphyseal growth. Osteochondromas usually stop growing at the time of growth plate closure; however, some may continue to enlarge during adulthood. Most behave in an innocent fashion. In less than 1% of cases, however, they give rise to a chondrosarcoma or some other type of sarcoma. The risk of this complication is substantially higher in patients with the hereditary syndrome.

Chondroma

Chondromas are benign tumors of hyaline cartilage. They may arise within the medullary cavity, where they are known as *enchondromas,* or on the surface of bone, where they are called *subperiosteal* or *juxtacortical chondromas.* Enchondromas are the most common of the intraosseous cartilage tumors. They occur equally in both sexes and are most frequent in the third to fifth decades of life.

Enchondromas are usually solitary, located in the metaphyseal region of tubular bones, and the favored sites are the short tubular bones of the hands and feet.[31] *The syndrome of multiple enchondromas or enchondromatosis is known as Ollier's disease, and if the enchondromatosis is associated with soft tissue hemangiomas, the disorder is called Maffucci's syndrome.* Chondromas are hypothesized to develop from rests of growth plate cartilage that subsequently proliferate and slowly enlarge. Based on this theory, it is not surprising that these tumors arise mainly in bones that develop from enchondral ossification.

> **MORPHOLOGY.** They usually do not get bigger than 3 cm and grossly are gray-blue and translucent and have a nodular configuration. Microscopically, the nodules of cartilage are well circumscribed, have a hyaline matrix, and are hypocellular, and the neoplastic chondrocytes that reside in lacunae are cytologically benign (Fig. 27–27). At the periphery of the nodules, the cartilage undergoes enchondral ossification, and the center frequently calcifies and dies. The chondromas in Ollier's disease and Maffucci's syndrome may demonstrate a greater degree of cellularity and cytologic atypia and can be difficult to distinguish from chondrosarcoma.

Most enchondromas are asymptomatic and are detected as an incidental finding. Occasionally they are painful and cause pathologic fracture. The cartilage tumors in enchondromatosis may be so numerous and large that they produce severe deformities. The radiographic features are characteristic because the unmineralized nodules of cartilage produce well-circumscribed oval lucencies that are surrounded by a thin rim of radiodense bone ("o ring sign").[31] If the matrix calcifies, it is detected as irregular opacities, and although the nodules scallop the endosteum, they do not result in complete cortical destruction (Fig. 27–28). The growth potential of chondromas is limited, and most remain stable. If operated on, they may recur if nodules of tumor are left behind. It is uncommon for a solitary chondroma to undergo sarcomatous transformation. This phenomenon occurs much more frequently in enchondromatoses. In addition, patients with Maffucci's syndrome are at risk for developing other types of malignancies, including ovarian carcinomas and brain gliomas.

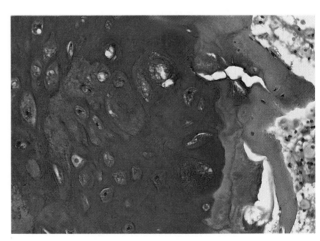

Figure 27–27. Enchondroma with nodule of hyaline cartilage on left rimmed by a thin layer of reactive bone.

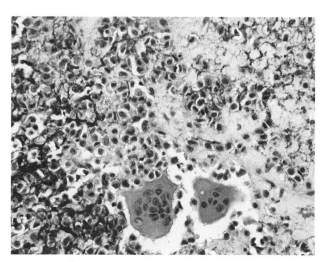

Figure 27-29. Chondroblastoma with scant mineralized matrix surrounding chondroblasts in a chicken wire-like fashion most evident on left.

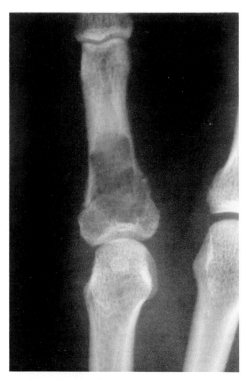

Figure 27-28. Enchondroma of phalanx with pathologic fracture. The radiolucent nodules of hyaline cartilage scallop the endosteal surface.

Chondroblastoma

Chondroblastoma is a rare benign tumor that accounts for less than 1% of primary bone tumors. It usually occurs in young patients (second decade) with a male-to-female ratio of 2:1. Most arise about the knee, and less common sites, such as the pelvis and ribs, are affected in older patients. Its pathogenesis is unknown; however, chondroblastoma has a striking predilection for epiphyses and apophyses (epiphyseal equivalents, i.e., iliac crest).[32]

MORPHOLOGY. The tumor is very cellular and is composed of sheets of compact polyhedral chondroblasts that have well-defined cytoplasmic borders, moderate amounts of pink cytoplasm, and nuclei that are hyperlobulated with longitudinal grooves (Fig. 27-29). Mitotic activity and necrosis are frequently present. The tumor cells make primitive-appearing hyaline matrix that surrounds cells in a lace-like fashion; nodules of well-formed hyaline cartilage are distinctly uncommon. When the matrix calcifies, it produces the characteristic "chicken-wire" pattern of mineralization. Scattered through the lesion are non-neoplastic osteoclast-type giant cells. Occasionally the tumors undergo prominent hemorrhagic cystic degeneration. The morphologic differential diagnosis includes chondrosarcoma, giant cell tumor, and pigmented villonodular synovitis that has invaded into bone.

Chondroblastomas are usually painful, and because of their location near a joint, they also cause effusions and restrict joint mobility. Radiographically they produce a well-defined geographic lucency that commonly has spotty calcifications. Surgical treatment is usually thorough curettage; however, recurrences are not uncommon. Pulmonary metastasis is a rare complication and usually occurs in a lesion that has undergone prior pathologic fracture or repeated curettage. Apparently, in these circumstances the tumor cells are pushed into ruptured vessels giving them access to the systemic circulation.

Chondromyxoid Fibroma

Chondromyxoid fibroma is the rarest of cartilage tumors and because of its varied morphology can be mistaken for sarcoma. It affects patients in their second and third decades of life with a definite male preponderance. The tumors most frequently arise in the metaphysis of long tubular bones; however, they may involve virtually any bone of the body.

MORPHOLOGY. The tumors range from 3 to 8 cm in greatest dimension and are well circumscribed, solid, and glistening tan-gray. Microscopically, there are nodules of poorly formed hyaline cartilage and myxoid tissue delineated by fibrous septae. The cellularity varies; however, the areas of greatest cellularity are at the periphery of the nodules. In the cartilaginous regions, the tumor cells are situated in lacunae; in the myxoid areas, however, the cells are stellate, and their delicate cell processes extend through the mucinous ground substance and approach or contact neighboring cells (Fig. 27-30). In contrast to other benign cartilage tumors, the neoplastic cells in chondromyxoid fibroma show varying degrees of cytologic atypia, including the presence of large hyperchromatic nuclei. Other findings include small foci of calcification of the cartilaginous matrix and scattered non-neoplastic, osteoclast-type giant cells.[33]

Patients with chondromyxoid fibroma usually complain of localized dull, achy pain. In most instances, x-ray films demonstrate an eccentric geographic lucency that is well delineated from the adjacent bone by a rim of sclerosis. Occasionally the tumor expands the overlying cortex. The treatment of choice is simple curettage, and even though they may recur, they do not pose a threat for malignant transformation or metastasizing.

Chondrosarcoma

Chondrosarcomas comprise a group of tumors that have a broad spectrum of clinical and pathologic findings. The feature common to all is the production of neoplastic cartilage. Chondrosarcoma is morphologically subclassified into conventional intramedullary and juxtacortical, clear cell, dedifferentiated,[34] and mesenchymal variants.

Chondrosarcoma of the skeleton is about half as frequent as osteosarcoma and is the second most common malignant matrix-producing tumor of bone. Patients with chondrosarcoma are usually in their fourth decade of life or are older. The clear cell and especially the mesenchymal variants occur in younger patients (second or third decade). The tumor affects men twice as frequently as women and has no predilection for any particular race. Although a significant number of chondrosarcomas arise in association with a pre-existing enchondroma, only a few develop within an osteochondroma, chondroblastoma, fibrous dysplasia, or in the setting of Paget's disease.

MORPHOLOGY. Conventional chondrosarcoma is composed of malignant hyaline and myxoid cartilage. The large bulky tumors are composed of nodules of gray-white, somewhat translucent glistening tissue (Fig. 27–31). In predominantly myxoid variants, the tumors are viscous and gelatinous and ooze from the cut surface. Spotty calcifications are typically present, and central necrosis may create cystic spaces. The adjacent cortex is thickened or eroded, and the tumor grows with broad "pushing fronts" into the surrounding soft tissue. The malignant cartilage infiltrates the marrow space and encompasses pre-existing bony trabeculae. Depending on the grade, the tumor varies in degree of cellularity, cytologic atypia, and mitotic activity (Fig. 27–32).[35] Low-grade or grade 1 lesions demonstrate mild hypercellularity, and the chondrocytes have plump vesicular nuclei with small nucleoli. Binucleate cells are sparse, and mitotic figures are very difficult to find. Portions of the matrix frequently mineralize, and the cartilage may undergo enchondral ossification. By contrast, grade 3 chondrosarcomas are characterized by marked hypercellularity and extreme pleomorphism with bizarre tumor giant cells; mitoses are easily identified. Pure grade 3 chondrosarcomas are uncommon; cartilage this atypical is more frequently a component of chondroblastic osteosarcoma.

Approximately 10% of conventional low-grade chondrosarcomas have a second high-grade component that has the morphology of a poorly differentiated sarcoma, such as malignant fibrous histiocytoma, fibrosarcoma, or osteosarcoma. It is hypothesized that in these "dedifferentiated chondrosarcomas" the well-differentiated component evolves into the more aggressive element. The hallmark of clear cell chondrosarcoma is sheets of large malignant chondrocytes that have abundant clear cytoplasm, numerous osteoclast-type giant cells, and intralesional reactive bone formation. The latter often causes confusion with osteosarcoma. Mesenchymal chondrosarcoma is composed of islands of well-differentiated hyaline cartilage surrounded by sheets of small round cells that resemble either hemangiopericytoma or Ewing's sarcoma.

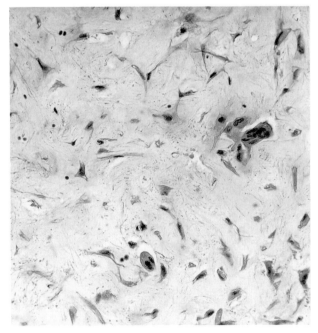

Figure 27–30. Chondromyxoid fibroma with prominent stellate and spindle cells surrounded by myxoid matrix. Occasional osteoclast-type giant cells are also present.

Chondrosarcomas commonly arise in the central portions of the skeleton, including the pelvis, shoulder, and ribs. The clear cell variant is unique

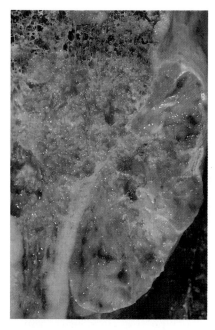

Figure 27-31. Chondrosarcoma with lobules of hyaline and myxoid cartilage permeating throughout the medullary cavity, growing through the cortex, and forming a relatively well-circumscribed soft tissue mass.

in that it originates in the epiphyses of long tubular bones. In contrast to enchondroma, chondrosarcoma rarely involves the distal extremities. These tumors usually present as painful, progressively enlarging masses. The nodular growth pattern of the cartilage produces prominent endosteal scalloping radiographically. A slow-growing, low-grade tumor causes reactive thickening of the cortex, whereas a more aggressive high-grade neoplasm destroys the cortex and forms a soft tissue mass.[35] On x-ray film, the calcified matrix appears as flocculent densities; the more radiolucent the tumor, the greater the likelihood it is high grade. There is a direct correlation between the grade and the biologic behavior of the tumor. Fortunately, most conventional chondrosarcomas are relatively indolent and fall into the range of grade 1 and grade 2. In one analysis, the 5-year survival rate of patients with grades 1, 2, and 3 were 90%, 81%, and 43%. None of the grade 1 tumors metastasized, whereas 70% of the grade 3 tumors disseminated. Another prognostic feature is size; tumors greater than 10 cm behave significantly more aggressively than smaller tumors. When chondrosarcomas metastasize, they preferentially spread to the lungs and skeleton.

FIBROUS AND FIBRO-OSSEOUS TUMORS

Tumors composed solely or predominantly of fibrous elements are diverse and include some of the most common lesions of the skeleton.

Fibrous Cortical Defect and Nonossifying Fibroma

Fibrous cortical defects are extremely common, being found in 30 to 50% of all children older than 2 years. They are believed to be developmental defects rather than neoplasms. The vast majority arise eccentrically in the metaphysis of the distal femur and proximal tibia, and almost one-half are bilateral or multiple. Often they are small, about 0.5 cm in diameter. Those that grow to 5 or 6 cm in size, however, develop into nonossifying fibromas and are usually not detected until adolescence.

MORPHOLOGY. Both fibrous cortical defects and nonossifying fibromas produce elongated, sharply demarcated radiolucencies that are surrounded by a thin zone of sclerosis (Fig. 27-33). They consist of gray and yellow-brown tissue and are cellular lesions composed of fibroblasts and histiocytes. The cytologically benign fibroblasts are frequently arranged in a storiform (pinwheel) pattern, and the histiocytes are either multinucleated giant cells or clusters of foamy macrophages (Fig. 27-34).

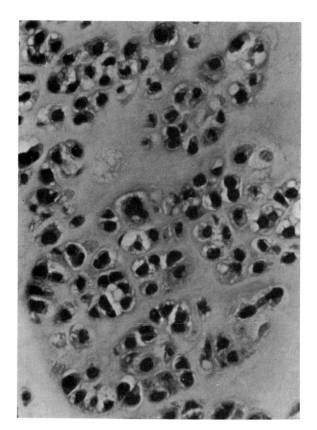

Figure 27-32. Anaplastic chondrocytes within a chondrosarcoma.

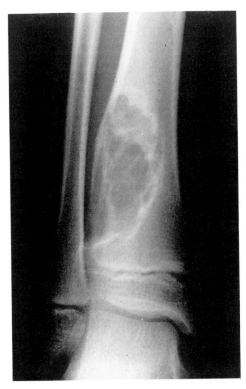

Figure 27–33. Nonossifying fibroma of the distal tibial metaphysis producing an eccentric lobulated radiolucency that is surrounded by a sclerotic margin.

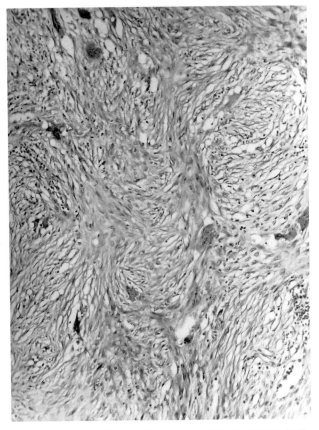

Figure 27–34. Storiform pattern created by benign spindle cells with scattered osteoclast-type giant cells characteristic of fibrous cortical defect and nonossifying fibroma.

Fibrous cortical defects are asymptomatic and are usually detected on x-ray film as an incidental finding. The vast majority have limited growth potential and undergo spontaneous resolution within several years, being replaced by normal cortical bone. The few that progressively enlarge into nonossifying fibromas may present with pathologic fracture or require biopsy and curettage to exclude other types of tumors.

Fibrous Dysplasia

This benign tumor-like lesion of bone is best characterized as a localized developmental arrest; all of the components of normal bone are present, but they do not differentiate into their mature structures. The lesions appear in three distinctive but sometimes overlapping clinical patterns: (1) involvement of a single bone (monostotic); (2) involvement of multiple, but never all, bones (polyostotic); and (3) polyostotic disease associated with café-au-lait skin pigmentations and endocrine abnormalities, especially precocious puberty.[36]

Monostotic fibrous dysplasia accounts for 70% of all cases. It occurs equally in males and females, usually in early adolescence, and often stops growing at the time of growth plate closure. The ribs, femur, tibia, jaw bones, calvarium, and humerus are most commonly affected in descending order of frequency. The lesion is usually asymptomatic and discovered incidentally. Fibrous dysplasia can cause marked enlargement and distortion of bone, so if the craniofacial skeleton is involved, disfigurement occurs. Monostotic disease does not evolve into the polyostotic form.

Polyostotic fibrous dysplasia without endocrine dysfunction accounts for 27% of all cases. It appears at a slightly earlier age than the monostotic type and may continue to cause problems into adulthood. The bones affected in descending order of frequency are the femur, skull, tibia, humerus, ribs, fibula, radius, ulna, mandible, and vertebrae. Craniofacial involvement is present in 50% of patients who have a moderate number of bones affected and in 100% of patients with extensive skeletal disease. All forms of polyostotic disease have a propensity to involve the shoulder and pelvic girdles, resulting in severe sometimes crippling deformities (e.g., shepherd-crook deformity of the proximal femur) and spontaneous, often recurrent fractures.

Polyostotic fibrous dysplasia associated with café-au-lait skin pigmentation and endocrinopathies is known as the McCune-Albright syndrome and accounts for 3% of all cases. The endocrinopathies result from a somatic (not hereditary) mutation occurring during embryogenesis and include sexual precocity, hyperthyroidism, pituitary adenomas that secrete growth hormone, and primary adrenal hyperplasia with Cushing's syndrome. The mutation involves the gene that codes for a stimulatory guanine nucleotide-binding protein, and it results in the excess production of cyclic adenosine monophosphate leading to endocrine gland hyperfunction.[37] The most common clinical presentation is precocious sexual development, and in this setting, females are affected more often than males. The bone lesions are often unilateral, and the skin pigmentation is usually limited to the same side of the body. The cutaneous macules are classically large; are dark to "café-au-lait;" have irregular serpiginous borders (coastline of Maine), and are found primarily on the neck, chest, back, shoulder, and pelvic region.

MORPHOLOGY. Grossly, the lesions of fibrous dysplasia are well circumscribed and intramedullary and vary greatly in size. Larger lesions expand and distort the bone. The lesional tissue is tan-white and gritty and is composed of curvilinear trabeculae of woven bone surrounded by a moderately cellular fibroblastic proliferation. The shapes of the trabeculae mimic "Chinese letters," and the bone lacks osteoblastic rimming (Fig. 27–35). Nodules of hyaline cartilage with the appearance of disorganized growth plate are also present in approximately 20% of cases. Cystic degeneration, hemorrhage, and foamy macrophages are other common findings.

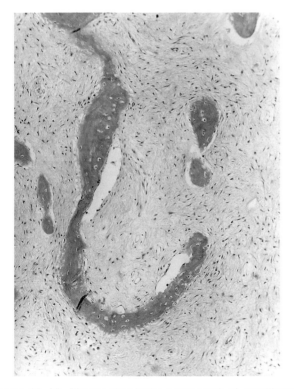

Figure 27–35. Fibrous dysplasia composed of curvilinear trabeculae of woven bone that lack conspicuous osteoblastic rimming and arise in a background of fibrous tissue.

CLINICAL COURSE. The natural history of fibrous dysplasia is variable and depends on the extent of skeletal involvement. Patients with monostotic disease usually have minimal symptoms. The lesion is readily diagnosed by radiograph because of its typical "ground-glass" appearance and well-defined margination. Lesions that fracture or cause significant symptoms are cured by conservative surgery. Polyostotic involvement is frequently associated with progressive disease, and often skeletal complications, such as recurring fractures, long bone deformities, and distorting involvement of the craniofacial bones, calling attention to the disorder at an early age. A rare complication, usually in the polyostotic involvement, is malignant transformation of a lesion into a sarcoma, such as osteosarcoma, or malignant fibrous histiocytoma. The risk of this occurrence is increased if the lesion has been irradiated.

Fibrosarcoma and Malignant Fibrous Histiocytoma

Fibrosarcoma and malignant fibrous histiocytoma are fibroblastic collagen-producing sarcomas of bone. They have overlapping clinical, radiographic, and pathologic features, and their distinction is based on somewhat arbitrary morphologic criteria. They occur at any age, but most affect the middle-aged and elderly. Fibrosarcoma has a nearly equal sex distribution, whereas malignant fibrous histiocytoma occurs more frequently in men. Both sarcomas usually arise *de novo;* a minority, however, are secondary tumors and develop in pre-existing benign tumors, bone infarcts, Pagetic bone, and fields of previous radiation.

MORPHOLOGY. Grossly, these tumors are large, hemorrhagic, tan-white masses that destroy the underlying bone and frequently extend into the soft tissues. Fibrosarcoma is composed of malignant fibroblasts arranged in a "herringbone pattern." The level of differentiation determines the amount of collagen produced and degree of cytologic atypia. Bizarre multinucleated cells are not common, and most fibrosarcomas have the appearance of a low-to-intermediate grade malignancy. Malignant fibrous histiocytoma consists of a background of spindled fibroblasts in a storiform pattern admixed with large, ovoid, bizarre, multinucleated tumor giant cells. Morphologically some tumor cells resemble neoplastic histiocytes; however, the evidence shows they are actually fibroblasts. Malignant fibrous histiocytoma is generally a high-grade pleomorphic tumor.[38]

Fibrosarcoma and malignant fibrous histiocytoma present as enlarging painful masses that usually arise in the metaphyses of long bones and pelvic flat bones. Pathologic fracture is a frequent complication. Radiographically they are permeative and lytic and often extend into the adjacent soft tissue. The prognosis of these two sarcomas depends on their grade; high-grade tumors have a poor prognosis with about a 20% 5-year survival.

MISCELLANEOUS TUMORS

Ewing's Sarcoma and Primitive Neuroectodermal Tumor

Ewing's sarcoma is a primary malignant small round cell tumor of bone. It has long posed a difficult diagnostic problem because by light microscopy Ewing's cells resemble those of lymphoma, rhabdomyosarcoma, neuroblastoma, and small cell carcinoma of the lung. Originally classified as an endothelial neoplasm, current evidence indicates that many Ewing's sarcomas exhibit a primitive neural phenotype. The identification of an 11;22 chromosomal translocation in both Ewing's sarcoma and primitive neuroectodermal tumors of soft tissue further supports this contention.[39] The translocation results in the production of a fusion protein in which the carboxy-terminus of the protein EWS (for Ewing's sarcoma), which normally contains an RNA binding domain, is replaced by a DNA binding transcription factor termed FLI-1. The functions of both the native EWS protein and the EWS–FLI-1 fusion protein are as yet undetermined. It is now believed that Ewing's sarcoma and primitive neuroectodermal tumor of bone are closely related tumors that differ in their degree of differentiation.[40] Diagnostically, tumors that demonstrate neural differentiation by light microscopy, immunohistochemistry, or electron microscopy are labeled primitive neuroectodermal tumors, and those that are undifferentiated by these analyses are diagnosed as Ewing's sarcoma.[41] Ewing's sarcoma is the term used to represent these two tumors in this discussion.

Ewing's sarcoma accounts for approximately 6 to 10% of primary malignant bone tumors and follows osteosarcoma as the second most common bone sarcoma in children. Of all bone sarcomas, Ewing's sarcoma has the youngest average age at presentation: most patients are 10 to 15 years old, and approximately 80% are younger than 20 years. Males are affected slightly more frequently than females, and there is a striking predilection for whites; blacks are rarely afflicted.

MORPHOLOGY. Arising in the medullary cavity, Ewing's sarcoma usually invades the cortex and periosteum, producing a soft tissue mass. The tumor is tan-white and frequently contains areas of hemorrhage and necrosis. It is composed of sheets of uniform small, round cells that are slightly larger than lymphocytes (Fig. 27–36). They have scant cytoplasm, which may appear clear because it is rich in glycogen. The presence of Homer-Wright pseudorosettes (in which the tumor cells are arranged in a circle about a central fibrillary space) is indicative of neural differentiation. Although the tumor contains fibrous septae, there is generally little stroma. Necrosis may be prominent, and there are relatively few mitotic figures despite the dense cellularity of the tumor.

Ewing's sarcoma usually arises in the diaphysis of long tubular bones, especially the femur and the flat bones of the pelvis. It presents as a painful enlarging mass, and the affected site is frequently tender, warm, and swollen. Interestingly some patients have systemic findings, including fever, elevated sedimentation rate, anemia, and leukocytosis, which mimic infection. Plain x-ray films show a destructive lytic tumor that has permeative margins. The characteristic periosteal reaction produces layers of reactive bone deposited in an "onionskin" fashion. The diagnosis often depends on the characteristic 11;22 translocation and a specific MIC2 antigenic marker on the tumor cells.

The treatment of Ewing's sarcoma includes chemotherapy and surgery with or without radiation. The advent of effective chemotherapy has dramatically improved the prognosis from a dismal 5 to 15% to a 75% 5-year survival rate; 50% are long-term cures.

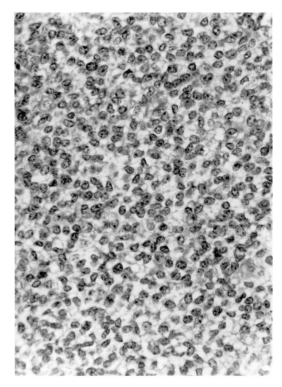

Figure 27–36. Ewing's sarcoma composed of sheets of small, round cells with small amounts of clear cytoplasm.

Giant Cell Tumor

Giant cell tumor is so named because it contains a profusion of multinucleated, osteoclast-type giant cells, giving rise to the synonym "osteoclastoma." Giant cell tumor is a relatively uncommon benign but locally aggressive neoplasm. It usually arises during the third to fifth decades, and there is a slight female predominance. Giant cell tumors are postulated to have a monocyte-macrophage lineage,[42] and the giant cells are believed to form via fusion of mononuclear cells.

> **MORPHOLOGY.** These tumors are large and redbrown and frequently undergo cystic degeneration. They are composed of uniform oval mononuclear cells that have indistinct cell membranes and appear to grow in a syncytium. The mononuclear cells are the proliferating component of the tumor, and mitoses are frequent. Scattered within this background are numerous osteoclast-type giant cells having 100 or more nuclei that are identical to those of the mononuclear cells (Fig. 27-37). Necrosis, hemorrhage, hemosiderin deposition, and reactive bone formation are common secondary features. The histologic differential diagnosis includes other giant cell lesions, such as the brown tumor seen in hyperparathyroidism, giant cell reparative granuloma, chondroblastoma, and pigmented villonodular synovitis. The morphologic identity between the nuclei of the stromal cells and those of the giant cells helps distinguish giant cell tumor from these other lesions.

Giant cell tumors in adults involve both the epiphyses and the metaphyses, but in adolescents they are confined proximally by the growth plate and are limited to the metaphysis. The majority of giant cell tumors arise around the knee (distal femur and proximal tibia), but virtually any bone may be involved, including the sacrum, pelvis, and small bones of the hands and feet. The location of these tumors in the ends of bones near joints frequently causes patients to complain of arthritic symptoms. Occasionally they present as pathologic fractures. Most are solitary; however, multiple or multicentric tumors do occur, especially in the distal extremities. Radiographically, giant cell tumors are large, purely lytic, and eccentric and erode into the subchondral bone plate (Fig. 27-38). The overlying cortex is frequently destroyed, producing a bulging soft tissue mass delineated by a thin shell of reactive bone. The margins with the adjacent bone are fairly circumscribed but seldom sclerotic. The biologic unpredictability of these neoplasms complicates their management. Conservative surgery such as curettage is associated with a 40 to 60% recurrence rate. Giant cell tumors are histologically benign; up to 4%, however, metastasize to the lungs usually after prior surgery, suggesting

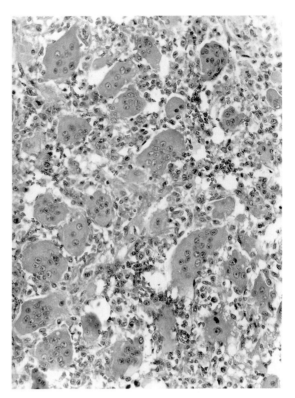

Figure 27-37. Benign giant cell tumor illustrating abundance of multinucleated giant cells with background mononuclear stromal cells.

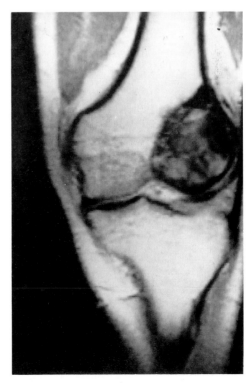

Figure 27-38. MRI of giant cell tumor that replaces most of femoral condyle and extends to the subchondral bone plate.

dislodgement of tumor emboli. The metastatic deposits have the same morphology as the primary tumor. Sarcomatous transformation of a giant cell tumor, either *de novo* or following previous treatment, is a rare event.

METASTATIC TUMORS TO THE SKELETON

Metastatic tumors are the most common form of skeletal malignancy. The pathways of spread include (1) direct extension, (2) lymphatic or vascular dissemination, (Batson's venous plexus) and (3) intraspinal seeding. Carcinomas of the breast, prostate, lung, kidney, and thyroid are the most common sources, and they usually reach the skeleton via the vascular system. In adults, more than 75% of skeletal metastases originate from cancers of the prostate, breast, kidney, and lung. Tumors that spread to bone in children include neuroblastoma, Wilms' tumor, osteosarcoma, Ewing's sarcoma, and rhabdomyosarcoma.

The radiographic manifestations of metastases may be purely lytic, purely blastic, or mixed lytic and blastic. In lytic lesions, the metastatic cells secrete substances, such as prostaglandins, interleukins, and parathyroid hormone–related protein, that stimulate osteoclastic bone resorption; the tumor cells themselves do not directly resorb bone.

Carcinomas of the kidney, lung, and gastrointestinal tract and malignant melanoma produce this type of bone destruction. Similarly, metastases that elicit a sclerotic response, especially prostate adenocarcinoma, do so by stimulating osteoblastic bone formation. Most metastases induce a mixed lytic and blastic reaction.

HYPERTROPHIC OSTEOARTHROPATHY

In association with some underlying disease, three changes may appear: (1) periosteal new bone formation primarily at the distal ends of long bones, metacarpals, and proximal phalanges (visible only radiographically); (2) nonspecific arthritis of the adjacent joints; and (3) clubbing of the fingertips, rendering them swollen, dusky, and cyanotic with "watch-glass" deformity of the nails. Most often involved is bronchogenic carcinoma, but sometimes other intrathoracic tumors, including lung metastases, chronic lung infections, or chronic liver disease is seen.

Clubbing alone may occur secondary to the same conditions but also with cyanotic heart disease, infective endocarditis, inflammatory bowel disease, and cancer of the esophagus. Rarely the periosteal or finger changes are apparently primary and familial.

The relationships of these reactions to each other and to the underlying diseases are obscure, but, significantly, resection of the cancer (e.g., bronchogenic) often reverses them.

Joints

OSTEOARTHRITIS
RHEUMATOID ARTHRITIS
JUVENILE RHEUMATOID
   ARTHRITIS

SERONEGATIVE SPON-
   DYLOARTHROPATHIES
INFECTIOUS ARTHRITIS
CRYSTAL ARTHROPATHIES

GOUT AND GOUTY ARTHRITIS
CALCIUM PYROPHOSPHATE
   CRYSTAL DEPOSITION
   DISEASE
TUMORS OF JOINTS AND
   RELATED STRUCTURES

GANGLION AND SYNOVIAL
   CYST
VILLONODULAR SYNOVITIS

NORMAL

Synovial joints of primary interest have a joint space that allows for a wide range of motion. Situated between the ends of bones formed via enchondral ossification, they are strengthened by a dense fibrous capsule and reinforced by ligaments

and muscles. The boundary of the joint space is formed by the synovial membrane, which is firmly anchored to the underlying capsule. Its contour is smooth except near the osseous insertion, where it is thrown into numerous villous folds. The surface lining of cuboidal cells or synoviocytes are arranged one to four cell layers deep. They are not present over the cartilage surfaces. Traditionally they are segregated into type A cells (macrophage-like), which are phagocytic and synthesize hyaluronic acid, and type B cells (fibroblast-like), which produce various proteins. The type A and B cells are now best considered one cell population that alters its phenotype according to the functional demands. The synovial lining lacks a basement membrane and merges with the underlying loose connective tissue stroma that is generally vascular. The absence of a basement membrane allows for quick exchange between blood and synovial fluid. The clear, viscous synovial fluid is a filtrate of plasma containing hyaluronic acid that acts as a lubricant and provides nutrition for the articular hyaline cartilage.

Articular cartilage is a unique connective tissue ideally suited to serve as an elastic shock absorber and wear-resistant surface. It lacks a blood supply and does not have lymphatic drainage nor innervation. Adult articular cartilage varies in thickness from 2 to 4 mm and is thickest both at the periphery of concave surfaces and in the central portions of convex surfaces. The hyaline cartilage is composed of type II collagen, water, proteoglycans, and chondrocytes, each of which has specific functions. The collagen fibers are arranged in arches so near the surface they are horizontal in orientation—this allows the cartilage to resist tensile stresses and transmit vertical loads. The water and proteoglycans give hyaline cartilage its turgor and elasticity and play an important role in limiting friction. The chondrocytes synthesize the matrix as well as enzymatically digest it. These processes are normally in equilibrium. The half-life of the different components ranges from weeks (proteoglycans) to years (type II collagen). Matrix turnover is carefully controlled as chondrocytes secrete the degradative enzymes in an inactive form and enrich the matrix with enzyme inhibitors (Table 27–7). Diseases that destroy articular cartilage do so by activating the catabolic enzymes and decreasing the production of inhibitors, thereby accelerating the rate of matrix breakdown. The chondrocytes react by increasing matrix production; however, the response is usually inadequate. Cytokines such as interleukin-1 and tumor necrosis factor (TNF) trigger the degradative process, and their sources include chondrocytes, synoviocytes, fibroblasts, and inflammatory cells. Destruction of articular cartilage by indigenous cells is an important mechanism in many joint diseases.

Table 27–7. CARTILAGE MATRIX DEGRADATIVE ENZYMES AND THEIR INHIBITORS

ENZYME	INHIBITOR
Collagenase	Tissue inhibitor of metalloproteinases
Stromelysin	Tissue inhibitor of metalloproteinases
Gelatinase	Tissue inhibitor of metalloproteinases
Tissue plasminogen activator	Plasminogen activator inhibitor

PATHOLOGY

OSTEOARTHRITIS

Osteoarthritis (OA), also called *degenerative joint disease (DJD)*, is the most common type of joint disease. Billions of dollars are spent annually for its treatment and for lost days of work. *It is characterized by the progressive erosion of articular cartilage.* The term OA implies a role for inflammation in its pathogenesis; however, inflammatory cells are usually not prominent and are a secondary phenomenon. OA is now considered to be a disease of cartilage, in which intrinsic biochemical and metabolic alterations result in its breakdown.[43]

In the great majority of instances, OA appears insidiously, without apparent initiating cause as an aging phenomenon (idiopathic or primary OA). In these cases, the disease is usually oligoarticular but may be generalized. In about 5% of cases, OA may appear in younger individuals having some predisposing condition, such as previous macrotraumatic or repeated microtraumatic injuries to a joint; a congenital developmental deformity of a joint(s); or some underlying systemic disease, such as diabetes, ochronosis, hemochromatosis, or marked obesity. In these settings, the disease is called secondary OA and often involves one or several predisposed joints—witness the shoulder or elbow involvements in baseball players and knees in basketball players. Gender has some influence on distribution. The knees and hands are more commonly affected in women and the hips in men.

PATHOGENESIS. The association between OA and aging is nonlinear; the prevalence increases exponentially beyond the age of 50. About 80 to 90% of individuals, of both sexes, have evidence of OA by the time they reach 65 years of age; thus OA joins heart disease and cancer as one of the dividends of the "golden years."[44] The age-related changes in cartilage include alterations in the proteoglycans and collagen, which decrease tensile strength and shorten "fatigue life." Despite this relationship, it is an oversimplification to consider OA as merely a disease of cartilage "wear and tear." Chondrocytes play a primary role in the process and constitute the cellular basis of the disease. For example, chondrocytes in osteoarthritic cartilage produce interleukin-1 which is known to initiate matrix breakdown. Secondary mediators come into play, such as prostaglandin derivatives, TNF-α, and TGF-β, which induce the release of lytic enzymes from chondrocytes while inhibiting matrix synthesis.[45] The precise biologic events leading to the secretion of cytokines, however, have not been clearly defined.

MORPHOLOGY. In the early stages of OA, the chondrocytes proliferate forming "clones." This is accompanied by biochemical changes as the water content of the matrix increases and the concentration of proteoglycans decreases. Subsequently vertical and horizontal fibrillation and cracking of the matrix occur as the superficial layers of the cartilage are degraded. Gross examination at this stage reveals a granular articular surface that is softer than normal. Eventually full-thickness portions of the cartilage are sloughed, and the exposed subchondral bone plate becomes the new articular surface. Friction smooths and burnishes the exposed bone, giving it the appearance of polished ivory (bone eburnation). Concurrently there is thickening of the subchondral bone plate and rebuttressing and sclerosis of the underlying cancellous bone. Small fractures through the articulating bone are common, and the dislodged pieces of cartilage and subchondral bone tumble into the joint forming loose bodies (joint mice). The fracture gaps allow synovial fluid to be forced into the subchondral regions in a one-way, ball-valve–like mechanism. The loculated fluid collection increases in size, forming fibrous walled cysts (Fig. 27–39). Mushroom-shaped osteophytes (bony outgrowths) develop at the margins of the articular surface and are capped by fibrocartilage and hyaline cartilage that gradually ossifies. The synovium shows minor alterations in comparison to the destruction of the articular surface and is congested and fibrotic and may have scattered chronic inflammatory cells. In severe disease, a fibrous synovial pannus covers the peripheral portions of the articular surface.

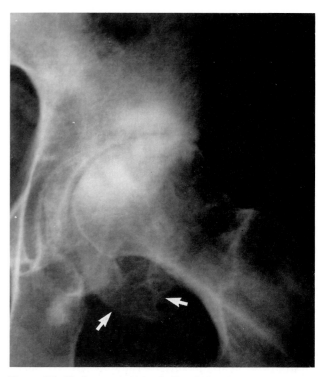

Figure 27–40. Severe osteoarthritis of hip. The joint space is narrowed, there is subchondral sclerosis and peripheral osteophyte lipping (arrows).

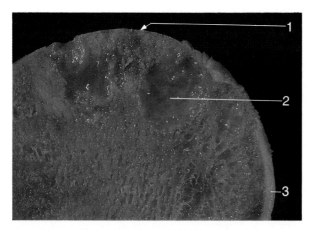

Figure 27–39. Transection of the femoral head with severe osteoarthritis. Thickened subchondral bone plate now acting as the articular surface (1). Large subchondral cysts (2). Residual articular cartilage at periphery (3).

CLINICAL COURSE. OA is an insidious disease. Patients with primary disease are usually asymptomatic until they are in their fifties. If a young patient has significant manifestations of OA, a search for some underlying cause should be made. Characteristic symptoms include deep, achy pain that worsens with use; morning stiffness; crepitus; and limitation of range of movement. Impingement on spinal foramina by osteophytes results in cervical and lumbar nerve root compression with radicular pain, muscle spasms, muscle atrophy, and neurologic deficits. Typically only one or a few joints are involved except in the uncommon generalized variant. The joints commonly involved include the hips, knees, lower lumbar and cervical vertebrae, proximal and distal interphalangeal joints of the fingers, first carpometacarpal joints, and first tarsometatarsal joints of the feet (Fig. 27–40). Characteristic in women but not in men are "Heberden's nodes" in the fingers representing prominent osteophytes at the distal interphalangeal joints. The wrists, elbows, and shoulders are usually spared. There are still no satisfactory means of preventing primary OA nor are there any methods of halting its progression. The disease may stabilize for years at any stage but more often is slowly progressive over the remaining years of life and is second only to cardiovascular diseases in causing long-term disability.

RHEUMATOID ARTHRITIS

Rheumatoid arthritis (RA) is a chronic systemic inflammatory disorder that may affect many tissues and organs — skin, blood vessels, heart, lungs, and muscles — but principally attacks the joints, producing a nonsuppurative proliferative synovitis that often progresses to destruction of the articular cartilage and ankylosis of the joints. Although the cause of RA remains unknown, there is convincing evidence (discussed later) that autoimmunity plays a pivotal role in its chronicity and progression, likening this condition to other so-called connective tissue diseases.

About 1% of the world's population is afflicted by RA, women three to five times more often than men. The peak incidence is in the third and fifth decades of life, but no age is immune. The genesis of the condition is best considered after the morphology.

MORPHOLOGY

Musculoskeletal System. RA causes a broad spectrum of morphologic alterations; the most severe are manifested in the joints. Initially the synovium becomes edematous, thickened, and hyperplastic transforming its smooth contour to one covered by delicate and bulbous fronds (Fig. 27–41). A dense perivascular inflammatory infiltrate composed of lymphoid follicles (mostly CD4+ helper T cells), plasma cells, and macrophages fills the synovial stroma. The vascularity is increased with superficial hemosiderin deposits and scattered giant cells. Aggregates of organizing fibrin cover portions of the synovium and float in the joint space as "rice bodies." Neutrophils accumulate in the synovial fluid and cluster along the surface but usually do not penetrate deep to the synoviocytes. The fluid, although turbid and increased in volume, forms a poor mucin clot on exposure to acetic acid. The inflamed and hyperemic synovium creeps over the articular surface forming a **pannus** and causes erosion of the underlying cartilage (Fig. 27–42). The mediators released by the inflammatory cells and synoviocytes result in osteoclastic activity, allowing the synovium to penetrate into the bone forming juxta-articular erosions, subchondral cysts, and osteoporosis. In time, after the cartilage has been destroyed, the fibrocellular pannus bridges the apposing bones, forming a fibrous ankylosis that eventually ossifies ultimately resulting in bony ankylosis.

Tendinoligamentous involvement frequently accompanies the arthritis. The inflamed synovial sheaths cause irreversible damage or even rupture of the tendons and ligaments. Occasionally the inflammation extends into the adjacent muscles.

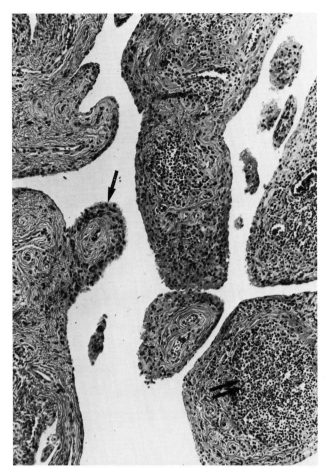

Figure 27–41. Rheumatoid arthritis. The villous hypertrophy of the synovium is shown with proliferation of the synoviocytes *(arrow)* and aggregates of inflammatory cells *(double arrows)* within the villi.

Skin. Rheumatoid nodules are the most common cutaneous manifestation. They occur in approximately 25% of patients, usually those with severe disease, and arise in regions that are subjected to pressure, including the ulnar aspect of the forearm, elbows, occiput, and lumbosacral area. Less commonly they form in the lungs, spleen, pericardium, myocardium, heart valves, aorta, and other viscera. Rheumatoid nodules are firm, nontender, and round to oval and in the skin arise in the subcutaneous tissue. Microscopically they have a central zone of fibrinoid necrosis surrounded by a prominent rim of epithelioid histiocytes and numerous lymphocytes and plasma cells (Fig. 27–43).

Blood Vessels. Patients with severe erosive disease, rheumatoid nodules, and high titers of rheumatoid factor are at risk of developing vasculitic syndromes (see Chapter 11). Rheumatoid vasculitis is potentially catastrophic, and the different types vary according to the size and nature of the affected vessels. Frequently segments of small ar-

PROGRESSION OF RHEUMATOID ARTHRITIS

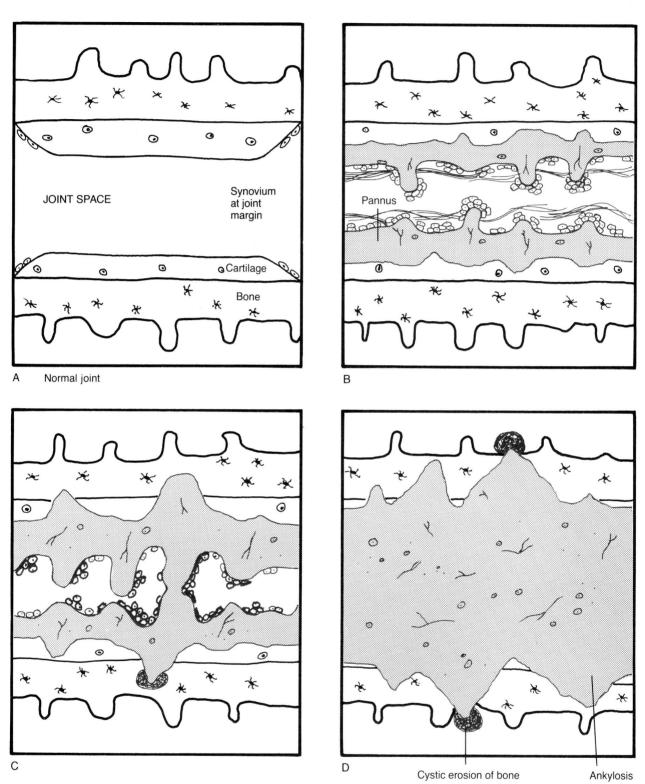

Figure 27–42. Rheumatoid arthritis—its progressive development. *A*, The normal joint with thin synovium. *B*, Polypoid fibrovascular thickening of the synovium with synoviocyte hyperplasia, producing a pannus that is eroding into articular cartilage. *C*, Continued growth of the pannus and erosion of cartilage with penetration into the subchondral bone and cyst formation. *D*, Complete filling of joint space with pannus producing ankylosis of the joint.

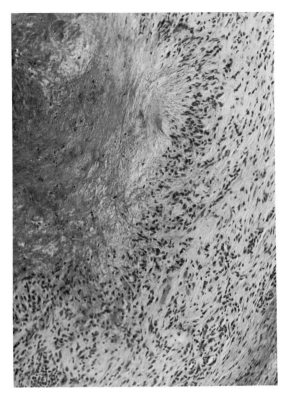

Figure 27-43. Subcutaneous rheumatoid nodule with an area of necrosis *(upper left)* surrounded by a palisade of macrophages and scattered chronic inflammatory cells.

teries, such as vasa nervorum and digital arteries, are obstructed by endarteritis obliterans and medial necrosis resulting in peripheral neuropathy, ulcers, and gangrene. The involvement is similar to that in polyarteritis nodosa except that in RA the kidneys are not involved. Leukocytoclastic venulitis produces purpura, cutaneous ulcers, and nail bed infarcts.

Other Organs. Nonspecific inflammation, rheumatoid nodules, and vasculitis can affect virtually all organ systems, especially the eyes, lungs, and heart (see rheumatoid heart in Chapter 12). The combined features of RA, splenomegaly, and neutropenia are known as **Felty's syndrome.**

PATHOGENESIS. Although much remains uncertain, it is currently believed that *RA is triggered by exposure of an immunogenetically susceptible host to an arthritogenic microbial antigen.* In this manner, an acute arthritis is initiated, but it is a continuing autoimmune reaction in which T cells play a central role with the local release of inflammatory mediators and lytic cytokines that ultimately destroy the joint. Therefore involved in the causation are (1) genetic susceptibility, (2) a primary exogenous arthritogen, (3) an autoimmune reaction within synovial membranes, and (4) mediators of the joint damage.

Genetic predisposition is clearly a major determinant of susceptibility to RA. There is a high rate of concordance between monozygotic twins and a well-defined familial predisposition. More important, the majority (65 to 80%) of individuals who develop RA are HLA-DR4 or DR1 or both.[46] The importance of these haplotypes rests on the concept of "shared epitopes." All the DR alleles associated with susceptibility to RA share a common region of four amino acids located in the antigen-binding cleft of the DR molecule adjacent to the T-cell receptor. Presumably, this is the specific binding site of the arthritogen(s) that initiates the inflammatory synovitis.

It is generally believed that the initiator of the disease is a microbial agent, but its identity continues to be elusive.[47] Epstein-Barr virus (EBV) is a prime suspect,[48] but closely following are retroviruses, parvoviruses, mycobacteria, Borrelia, and Mycoplasma as well as numerous others. For each, tentative support is offered, but the evidence implicating EBV is particularly intriguing. Autoimmunity to type II collagen can be demonstrated in most patients with RA. Perhaps the EBV and type II collagen share some cross-reactive epitopes, and conceivably an immunologic reaction against EBV might therefore affect joint cartilage rich in type II collagen.

An autoimmune reaction in which T cells play the pivotal role is widely held to be responsible for the chronic destructive nature of RA, once an inflammatory synovitis has been initiated by an exogenous agent. T cells, mainly CD4+ memory cells, appear within the affected joints early in the development of RA. Soon the endothelial cells of synovial capillaries are activated with the expression of ICAM-1 (intercellular adhesion molecule-1), leading to further attachment and transmigration of other inflammatory cells. This sequence is further enhanced by release of IL-1, TNF-α, and IFN-γ. The activated CD4+ cells simultaneously activate monocytes-macrophages and promote the release of monokines and at the same time activate B cells with antibody production in affected joints. About 80% of individuals with RA have autoantibodies to the Fc portion of autologous IgG (rheumatoid factors). These are mostly IgM antibodies, perhaps generated within joints, but they may be of other classes. These self-associate (RA-IgG) to form immune complexes in the sera, synovial fluid, and synovial membranes. These circulating immune complexes underlie many of the extra-articular manifestations of RA. Rheumatoid factor, however, is not present in some patients with the disease (seronegative). It is sometimes found in other disease states and even in otherwise healthy people; thus these immune complexes are probably not critical to the causation of RA. Nonetheless, substantial quantities of immune complexes are localized within the inflamed cartilage, activating complement and augmenting the synovial inflammatory reaction, and contributing to the degradation of cartilage.

What *mediators* then bring about the destructive-proliferative synovitis? Sensitized CD4+ lymphocytes, activated B cells, and particularly macrophages elaborate within the inflammatory synovium a diversity of cytokines, including IL-1, IL-2, IL-3, IL-4, IL-6, IFN-γ, GM-CSF, TGF-β, TNF-α, and TNF-β. Simultaneously neutrophils and synoviocytes contribute proteases and elastases. How all these interact is not completely clear, but some seminal observations have been made. TNF-α produced locally by macrophages appears to play a central role, but many of its actions are matched by IL-1.[49] *TNF-α or IL-1 induces resorption of cartilage and bone by stimulating release of collagenases from synovial cells; up-regulates expression of adhesion molecules such as ICAM-1, ELAM-1, and V-CAM by endothelial cells favoring the accumulation of white cells in the inflamed synovium; inhibits synthesis of proteoglycans in cartilage; and stimulates proliferation of fibroblasts via platelet-derived growth factor.* Collectively, these actions might well lead to destruction of articular cartilage and subsequent pannus formation. Significantly, anti–TNF-α and/or IL-1 antibodies have a protective effect on a collagen-induced arthritis in mice. Tantalizing as all these observations may be, the genesis of RA is still a puzzle.

CLINICAL COURSE. The clinical course of RA is extremely variable. The disease begins slowly and insidiously in more than half of the patients. Initially, there is malaise, fatigue, and generalized musculoskeletal pain, and only after several weeks to months do the joints become involved, sometimes monoarticular, at other times oligoarticular, and in some instances polyarticular (usually symmetrically). The involved joints are swollen, warm, painful, and particularly stiff on arising or following inactivity. Approximately 10% of patients have an acute onset, with severe symptoms and polyarticular involvement developing within a few days. In the typical patient, the onset is insidious with progressive joint involvement over a period of months to years, with initial minimal limitation of motion that, in time, becomes more severe. The disease course may be slow or rapid and fluctuate over a period of years, with the greatest damage occurring during the first 4 to 5 years. Approximately 20% of patients enjoy periods of partial or complete remission, but the symptoms inevitably return and involve previously unaffected joints. The pattern of joint involvement varies, but generally the small joints are affected before the larger ones. Symptoms usually develop in the small joints of the hands (metacarpophalangeal and proximal interphalangeal joints) and feet, followed by the wrists, ankles, elbows, and knees. Uncommonly the upper spine is involved, but the lumbosacral region and hips are usually spared. The radiographic hallmarks are joint effusions, juxta-articular osteopenia with erosions, and narrowing of the joint space with loss of articular cartilage (Fig. 27–44). Destruction of tendons, ligaments, and joint capsules produces characteristic deformities, including radial deviation of the wrist, ulnar deviation of the fingers, and flexion-hyperextension abnormalities of the fingers (swan-neck, boutonnière). The end result is deformed joints that have no stability and

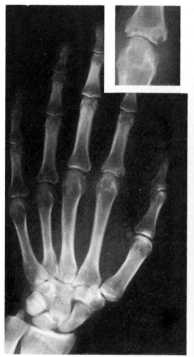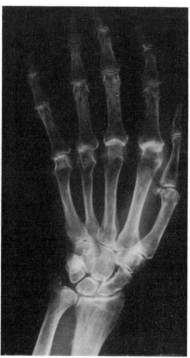

A B

Figure 27–44. Rheumatoid arthritis. *A,* Early disease, most marked in second metacarpophalangeal joint, where there is narrowing of joint space and marginal erosions on both radial and ulnar aspects of proximal phalanx *(see inset). B,* More advanced disease with loss of articular cartilage, narrowing of joint spaces of virtually all the small joints, and ulnar deviation of fingers. There is dislocation of second, third, and fourth proximal phalanges produced by advanced articular disease. (Courtesy of Dr. John O'Connor, Boston University Medical Center.)

minimal or no range of motion. Large synovial cysts, such as Baker's cyst in the posterior knee, may develop as the increased intra-articular pressure causes outpouchings of the synovium.

There are no specific laboratory tests diagnostic of RA. As pointed out, rheumatoid factor is present in most but not all patients with rheumatoid arthritis and also appears in many other conditions. Analysis of synovial fluid confirms an inflammatory arthritis with its attendant changes but is nonspecific. The diagnosis is made primarily on the clinical features and requires the presence of four of the following criteria:[50] (1) morning stiffness, (2) arthritis in three or more joint areas, (3) arthritis of hand joints, (4) symmetric arthritis, (5) rheumatoid nodules, (6) serum rheumatoid factor, and (7) typical radiographic changes.

It is difficult to predict the natural history of the disease for individuals. The fortunate patients have a mild onset and relatively short-term symptoms with no sequelae. Most, however, have progressive disease for life. Overall, life expectancy is reduced by a mean of 3 to 7 years. The fatalities are usually due to complications of RA, such as systemic amyloidosis, and to iatrogenic effects of therapy, e.g., gastrointestinal bleeding related to long-term use of aspirin and infections associated with long-term steroid use.

JUVENILE RHEUMATOID ARTHRITIS

Juvenile rheumatoid arthritis (JRA) is one of the more common connective tissue diseases of children and is a major cause of functional disability in this age group.[51] By definition, it begins before the age of 16, and most patients are diagnosed during early childhood. There is a 2:1 female predominance except in the subgroup that has a systemic onset, in which the sexes are equally affected. JRA differs from RA in adults in that (1) oligoarthritis is more common, (2) systemic onset is more frequent, (3) large joints are affected more than small joints, (4) rheumatoid nodules and rheumatoid factor are usually absent, and (5) antinuclear antibody seropositivity is common. Genetic susceptibility, abnormal immunoregulation, cytokine production, and viral infection may all play a role in the pathogenesis.[52] The morphology of the joint pathology, including the marked synovitis, is similar to the alterations in adult RA. The development of symptoms, such as fatigue, joint stiffness, and limited range of motion, is generally slow and gradual. Commonly targeted joints in all forms of the disease are the knees, wrists, elbows, and ankles. They become warm and swollen and are often involved symmetrically. Pericarditis, myocarditis, pulmonary fibrosis, glomerulonephritis, uveitis, and growth retardation are potential extra-articular manifestations. A systemic onset may begin rather abruptly, associated with high spiking fevers, migratory and transient skin rash, hepatosplenomegaly, and serositis. Satisfactory recovery occurs in 70 to 90% of patients, and in only 10% severe joint deformities persist.

SERONEGATIVE SPONDYLOARTHROPATHIES

The seronegative spondyloarthropathies lacking rheumatoid factor include ankylosing spondylitis, Reiter's syndrome, psoriatic arthritis, and enteropathic arthritis. They all share overlapping clinical features, and many are associated with HLA-B27.

Ankylosing spondyloarthritis, also known as *rheumatoid spondylitis* and *Marie-Stumpell disease,* is a chronic inflammatory joint disease of axial joints, especially the sacroiliac joints. It usually occurs in males and begins in adolescence. Approximately 90% of affected individuals are HLA-B27 positive. Analogous to RA, this immunogenetic phenotype may predispose to the development of autoantibodies directed at joint elements following infection.[53] Histologically a chronic synovitis causes destruction of articular cartilage and bony ankylosis, especially in the sacroiliac and apophyseal joints (between tuberosities and processes). Inflammation of tendinoligamentous insertion sites eventuates in bony outgrowths and ossification of the annulus fibrosus, which compound the fibrous and bony ankylosis producing severe spinal immobility. The patients characteristically present with low back pain, which frequently follows a chronic progressive course. Involvement of peripheral joints, such as the hips, knees, and shoulders, occurs in at least one-third of patients. Uveitis, aortitis, and amyloidosis are other recognized complications.

Reiter's syndrome is classically defined as the triad of arthritis, nongonococcal urethritis or cervicitis, and conjunctivitis. Most affected individuals are male and in the third to fourth decades of life, and more than 80% are positive for HLA-B27. The evidence suggests that the disease is caused by an autoimmune reaction initiated by prior infection. The implicated infections are gastrointestinal (Shigella, Salmonella, Yersinia, Campylobacter) and genitourinary (Chlamydia). Arthritic symptoms usually develop within several weeks of the inciting bout of urethritis or diarrhea. Joint stiffness and low back pain are common early symptoms. The ankles, knees, and feet are affected most often, frequently in an asymmetric pattern. Synovitis of digital tendon sheaths produces the "sausage" finger or toe and leads to calcaneal spurs and bony outgrowths from tendinous insertions. Patients with severe chronic disease have involvement of the spine that is indistinguishable from ankylosing spondylitis. Extra-articular involvement manifests as keratoderma blennorrhagicum, balanitis circinata, conjunctivitis, cardiac conduction abnormalities, and aortic regurgitation. The natural behavior of Reiter's syndrome is extremely variable. The episodes of arthritis usually wax and wane over a period of several weeks to half a year. Almost 50% of patients have recurrent arthritis, tendinitis, fasciitis, and lumbosacral back pain that can cause significant functional disability.

Psoriatic arthritis is uncommon and affects 5% of the psoriatic population. There is no sex predilection, and the disease manifests between the age of 35 and 45. The etiology is not clearly defined, but there is evidence of genetic predisposition; HLA typing has not correlated specific phenotypes with the distribution or severity of disease. Involved synovium shows papillary hyperplasia with dense chronic inflammation, similar to that seen in RA. Synovial vessels commonly show prominent endothelial cells, thickened walls, and transmural inflammation. The joint symptoms develop slowly but are acute in onset in one-third of patients. The patterns of joint involvement are diverse. The distal interphalangeal joints of the hands and feet are first affected in an asymmetric distribution in more than 50% of patients. The large joints, such as the ankles, knees, hips, and wrists, may be involved as well.[54] Inflammation of the digit tendon sheaths produces the "sausage" finger. Sacroiliac and spinal disease occurs in 20 to 40% of patients. Aside from conjunctivitis and iritis, extra-articular manifestations are uncommon and are similar in scope to those in the other seronegative spondyloarthropathies. Psoriatic arthritis is not as severe as RA because remissions are more frequent, and the joint destruction less marked.

Enteropathic arthritis is associated with or induced by various inflammatory disorders of the bowel. It usually appears in patients who are HLA-B27 positive. *About 10 to 20% of patients with ulcerative colitis or Crohn's disease experience a migratory oligoarthritis* of the large joints and spine that lasts for several months to years. Although the arthritis is not associated with permanent joint damage, it is sometimes complicated by ankylosing spondylitis with all its sequelae. Any type of bacterial infection may also be followed by a postenteric arthritis,[55] which appears abruptly and usually involves the knees and ankles but sometimes the wrists, fingers, and toes. The arthritis lasts for about a year and then generally clears and only rarely is accompanied by ankylosing spondylitis.

INFECTIOUS ARTHRITIS

Microorganisms of all types can seed joints during hematogenous dissemination. Articular structures can also become infected by direct inoculation or by contiguous spread from a soft tissue abscess or focus of osteomyelitis. Infectious arthritis is potentially serious because it can cause rapid destruction of the joint and produce permanent deformities.

Bacterial infections almost always cause an acute suppurative arthritis. The bacteria usually seed the joint during an episode of bacteremia; in neonates, however, there is an increased incidence of contiguous spread from underlying epiphyseal osteomyelitis. The most common organisms are gonococcus, Staphylococcus, Streptococcus, *Haemophilus influenzae* and gram-negative bacilli (*E. coli*, Salmonella, Pseudomonas, and others). *H. influenzae* arthritis predominates in children under 2 years of age, *S. aureus* is the main causative agent in older children and adults, and the gonococcus is encountered during late adolescence and young adulthood. Individuals with sickle cell disease are prone to infection with Salmonella at any age. These joint infections affect the sexes equally except for gonococcal arthritis, which is seen mainly in sexually active women. Predisposing conditions include immune deficiencies (congenital and acquired), debilitating illness, joint trauma, chronic arthritis of any etiology, and intravenous drug abuse.

The classic presentation is the sudden development of an acutely painful and swollen infected joint that has a restricted range of motion. Systemic findings of fever, leukocytosis, and elevated sedimentation rate are common. In disseminated gonococcal infection, the symptoms are more subacute. In 90% of nongonococcal cases, the arthritis involves only a single joint, usually the knee followed in frequency by the hip, shoulder, elbow, wrist, and sternoclavicular joints. Axial articulations are more commonly involved in drug addicts. Gonococcal arthritis tends to be oligoarticular and is often associated with a skin rash and with a genetic deficiency of C5, C6, or C7. Prompt recognition and effective therapy prevent rapid joint destruction whatever the etiology.

Tuberculous arthritis, a chronic progressive monoarticular disease, occurs in all age groups, especially adults. It usually develops as a complication of adjoining osteomyelitis or following hematogenous dissemination from a visceral (usually pulmonary) site of infection.

Tuberculous arthritis has an insidious onset and causes gradual progressive pain. Systemic symptoms may or may not be present. Mycobacterial seeding of the joint induces the formation of confluent granulomas with central caseous necrosis. The affected synovium may grow as a pannus over the articular cartilage and erode into bone along the joint margins. Chronic disease results in severe destruction with fibrous ankylosis and obliteration of the joint space. The weight-bearing joints are usually affected, especially the hips, knees, and ankles in descending order of frequency. Prompt, effective therapy is necessary to prevent extensive damage.

Lyme arthritis, as previously discussed in Chapter 8, is caused by infection with the spirochete *Borrelia burgdorferi*. The initial infection of the skin is followed within several days or weeks by dissemination of the organism to other sites, especially the joints.

Approximately 80% of patients with Lyme disease develop joint symptoms within a few weeks to 2 years following the onset of the disease.[56] The arthritis tends to be remitting and migratory and primarily involves large joints, especially the knees, shoulders, elbows, and ankles in descending order of frequency. Usually one or two joints are affected at a time, and the attacks last for a few weeks to months with periods of remission. Infected synovium takes the form of a chronic papillary synovitis with synoviocyte hyperplasia, fibrin deposition, mononuclear cell infiltrates (especially helper/inducer T cells), and onionskin thickening of arterial walls. The morphology in severe cases can closely resemble that of RA. Silver stains may reveal small numbers of organisms in the vicinity of blood vessels in approximately 25% of cases. Chronic arthritis with pannus formation develops in approximately 10% of patients, resulting in permanent deformities.

CRYSTAL ARTHROPATHIES

Articular crystal deposits are associated with a variety of acute and chronic joint disorders. Endogenous crystals shown to be pathogenic include monosodium urate, calcium pyrophosphate dihydrate, and basic calcium phosphate (hydroxyapatite). Exogenous crystals, such as corticosteroid ester crystals, talcum, polyethylene, and methylmethacrylate, may also induce joint disease. Silicone, polyethylene, and methylmethacrylate are used in prosthetic joints, and their debris, which accumulates with long use and wear, may result in local arthritis and failure of the prosthesis. Endogenous and exogenous crystals produce disease by triggering a cascade that results in cytokine-mediated cartilage destruction.[57]

GOUT AND GOUTY ARTHRITIS

Gout is the common end point of a group of disorders that produce hyperuricemia. It is marked by transient attacks of *acute arthritis* initiated by crystallization of urates within and about joints, leading eventually to *chronic gouty arthritis* and the deposition of masses of urates in joints and other sites creating *tophi*. Most but not all patients with chronic gout also develop urate nephropathy. Although hyperuricemia is a sine qua non for the development of gout, it is not the sole determinant

as the following data indicate. More than 10% of the population of the Western Hemisphere have hyperuricemia, but gout develops in fewer than 0.5% of the population. A plasma urate level above 7 mg/dl is considered elevated because it exceeds the saturation value for urate at normal body temperature and blood pH.

The various conditions producing hyperuricemia and gout are shown in Table 27–8, which divides them into "primary gout," in which the basic metabolic defect is unknown or gout is the main manifestation of a known defect, and "secondary gout," in which the cause of the hyperuricemia is known or gout is not the main clinical dysfunction.

It is beyond our scope to review uric acid metabolism completely, but a few words are indicated. As you know, uric acid is the end product of purine metabolism. Two pathways are involved in purine synthesis:[58] (1) a *"de novo"* pathway, in which purines are synthesized from nonpurine precursors, and (2) a *"salvage"* pathway, in which free purine bases derived from the breakdown of nucleic acids of endogenous or exogenous origin are recaptured (salvaged) (Fig. 27–45). Hypoxanthine guanine phosphoribosyl transferase (HGPRT) is involved in the salvage pathway. A deficiency of this enzyme leads to increased synthesis of purine nucleotides through the *de novo* pathway and hence increased production of uric acid. A complete lack of HGPRT occurs in the uncommon X-linked Lesch-Nyhan syndrome, seen only in males and characterized by hyperuricemia, severe neurologic deficits with mental retardation and self-mutilation, and in some cases gouty arthritis.[59] Less severe deficiencies of the enzyme may also induce hyperuricemia and gouty arthritis with only mild

Table 27–8. CLASSIFICATION OF GOUT

CLINICAL CATEGORY	METABOLIC DEFECT
Primary Gout (90% of Cases)	
Enzyme defects unknown (85 to 90% of primary gout)	Overproduction of uric acid Normal excretion (majority) Increased excretion (minority) Underexcretion of uric acid with normal production
Known enzyme defects— e.g., partial HGPRT deficiency (rare)	Overproduction of uric acid
Secondary Gout (10% of Cases)	
Associated with increased nucleic acid turnover— e.g., leukemias	Overproduction of uric acid with increased urinary excretion
Chronic renal disease	Reduced excretion of uric acid with normal production
Inborn errors of metabolism—e.g., complete HGPRT deficiency	Overproduction of uric acid with increased urinary excretion (Lesch-Nyhan syndrome)

HGPRT = Hypoxanthine guanine phosphoribosyl transferase.

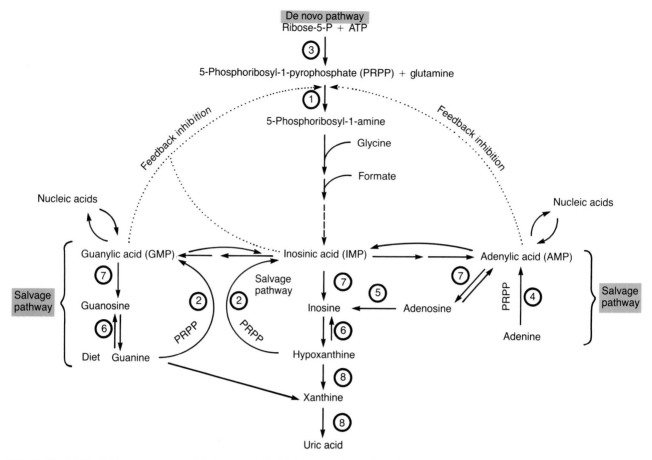

Figure 27–45. Outline of purine metabolism. (1) Amidophosphoribosyltransferase; (2) hypoxanthineguanine phosphoribo-syltransferase; (3) PP-ribose-P synthetase; (4) adenine phosphoribosyltransferase; (5) adenosine deaminase; (6) purine nucleoside phosphorylase; (7) 5′-nucleotidase; (8) xanthine oxidase. (Modified from Kelley, W.N., and Wyngaarden, J.B.: Clinical syndromes associated with hypoxanthine-guanine phosphoribosyl transferase deficiency. *In* Stanbury, J.B., et al. (eds.): Metabolic Basis of Inherited Disease. New York, McGraw-Hill Book Co., 1982, p. 1115. Copyright © 1982 by McGraw-Hill, Inc. Used by permission.)

neurologic deficits, but together these causes of gout are uncommon. The great majority of cases of gout are "primary," in which, frustratingly, the metabolic defect underlying the increased levels of uric acid is unknown.

PATHOGENESIS. Many factors play a role in the conversion of asymptomatic hyperuricemia into primary gout. Some of these are:

- Age of the individual and duration of the hyperuricemia—gout rarely appears before 20 to 30 years of hyperuricemia.
- Genetic predisposition—in addition to the well-defined X-linked abnormalities of HGPRT, primary gout follows multifactorial inheritance and therefore runs in families.
- Heavy alcohol consumption predisposes.
- Obesity predisposes.
- Certain drugs predispose—e.g., thiazides.
- Lead toxicity predisposes to saturnine gout (see Chapter 9).

Central to the pathogenesis of the arthritis is precipitation of monosodium urate (MSU) crystals into the joints. Synovial fluid is a poorer solvent

for MSU than plasma, and so with hyperuricemia the urates in the joint fluid become supersaturated, particularly in the peripheral joints, which may have temperatures as low as 20°C in the ankle. With prolonged hyperuricemia, microtophi of urates develop in the synovial lining cells and in the joint cartilage. Some unknown event, possibly trauma, then initiates release of crystals into the synovial fluid followed by a cascade of events. The released crystals are chemotactic and also activate complement, with the generation of C3a and C5a leading to the accumulation of neutrophils and macrophages in the joints and synovial membranes. Phagocytosis of crystals induces release of toxic free radicals and leukotrienes (LTB$_4$). Death of the neutrophils releases destructive lysosomal enzymes, and the macrophages and synoviocytes secrete a variety of mediators, including IL-1, IL-6, and IL-8, and TNF-α which further intensify the inflammatory reaction and augment the injury to the articular structures.[60] Activation of Hageman factor pours fuel onto the fire. Thus comes about an acute arthritis, which typically remits (days to weeks) even untreated. A schematic of some of these events is shown in Figure 27–46.

Repeated attacks of acute arthritis lead eventually to chronic arthritis and the formation of tophi in the inflamed synovial membranes and periarticular tissue as well as elsewhere. In time, severe damage to the cartilage and the function of the joints develops. It is not known why the chronic arthritis is asymptomatic for intervals of days to months even though synovial crystals are undoubtedly present in abundance in the joints.

MORPHOLOGY. The distinctive morphologic changes in gout are (1) acute arthritis, (2) chronic tophaceous arthritis, (3) tophi in various sites, and sometimes (4) gouty nephropathy.

Acute arthritis is characterized by a dense neutrophilic infiltrate that permeates the synovium and synovial fluid. The MSU crystals are frequently found in the cytoplasm of the neutrophils and are arranged in small clusters in the synovium. They are long, slender, and needle shaped and are negatively birefringent. The synovium is edematous and congested and contains scattered lymphocytes, plasma cells, and macrophages. When the episode of crystallization abates and many of the crystals are resolubilized, the acute attack remits.

Chronic tophaceous arthritis evolves from the repetitive precipitation of urate crystals during acute attacks. The urates may heavily encrust the articular surfaces and form visible deposits in the synovium (Fig. 27–47). The synovium becomes hyperplastic, fibrotic, and thickened by inflammatory cells and forms a pannus that destroys the underlying cartilage, leading to juxta-articular bone erosions. In severe cases, fibrous or bony anklyosis ensues, resulting in partial-to-complete loss of joint function.

Tophi are the pathognomonic hallmark of gout. They are formed by large aggregations of urate crystals surrounded by an intense inflammatory reaction of macrophages, lymphocytes, and large foreign body giant cells, which may have completely or partially engulfed masses of crystals (Fig. 27–48). Tophi may appear in the articular cartilage of joints and also in the periarticular ligaments, tendons, and soft tissues, including the olecranon and patellar bursae, Achilles tendons, and ear lobes. Less frequently they may appear in the kidneys, nasal cartilages, skin of the fingertips, palms, or soles as well as elsewhere. Superficial tophi can lead to large ulcerations of the overlying skin.

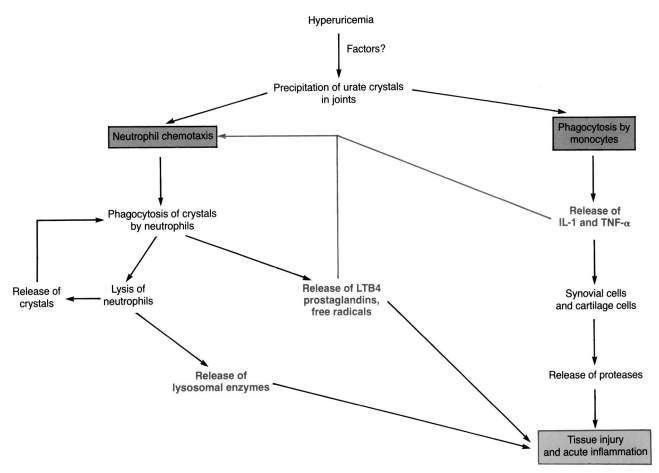

Figure 27–46. Pathogenesis of acute gouty arthritis.

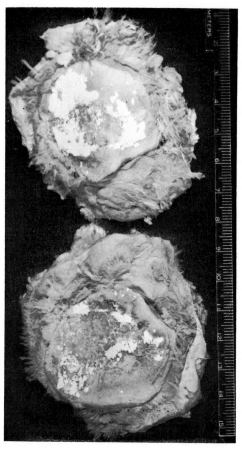

Figure 27–47. Gouty deposits of patella. Articular surfaces of patellas are encrusted with white deposits of urates.

(in descending order of frequency): insteps, ankles, heels, knees, wrists, fingers, and elbows. Untreated, acute gouty arthritis may last for hours to weeks, but gradually there is complete resolution, and the patient enters an asymptomatic intercritical period. Although some patients never have another attack, most experience a second acute episode within months to a few years. In the absence of appropriate therapy, the attacks recur at shorter intervals and frequently become polyarticular. Eventually over the span of years, symptoms fail to resolve completely with the development of disabling chronic tophaceous gout. On average, it takes about 12 years between the initial acute attack and the development of chronic tophaceous arthritis. At this stage, x-ray films show characteristic juxta-articular bone erosion caused by the crystal deposits and loss of the joint space. Progression leads to severe crippling disease. Often in the background there is hypertension. Renal manifestations sometimes appear in the form of renal colic associated with the passage of gravel and stones. Indeed about 20% of those with chronic gout die of renal failure. The diagnosis of gout should not be missed because numerous drugs are available to abort or prevent acute attacks of arthritis and mobilize tophaceous deposits. Their use is important because many aspects of the disease are related to the duration and severity of the hyperuricemia. Generally gout does not materially shorten one's life span, but it may impair its quality.

Gouty nephropathy (see Chapter 20) embraces (1) the deposition of MSU crystals in the medullary interstitium sometimes forming tophi, (2) intratubular precipitations or free uric acid crystals, and (3) the production of uric acid renal stones, particularly in patients with marked hyperexcretion of uric acid. Secondary complications may ensue, such as pyelonephritis, particularly when the urates induce some urinary obstruction.[61]

CLINICAL CORRELATION. The natural history of gout passes through four stages: (1) asymptomatic hyperuricemia, (2) acute gouty arthritis, (3) intercritical gout, and (4) chronic tophaceous gout. Asymptomatic hyperuricemia appears around puberty in males and after the menopause in females. After a long interval of years, acute arthritis appears in the form of the sudden onset of excruciating joint pain associated with localized hyperemia, warmth, and exquisite tenderness. Yet constitutional symptoms are uncommon except possibly mild fever. The vast majority of first attacks are monoarticular; 50% occur in the first metatarsophalangeal joint. Eventually about 90% of patients experience acute attacks in the following locations

CALCIUM PYROPHOSPHATE CRYSTAL DEPOSITION DISEASE

Calcium pyrophosphate crystal deposition disease (CPPD), also known as *pseudogout* and *chondrocalcinosis*, is one of the most common disorders associated with intra-articular crystal formation.[62] It usually occurs in individuals over 50 years of age and becomes more common with increasing age, rising to a prevalence of 30 to 60% in those 85 years or older. The sexes and races are equally affected. CPPD can be divided into sporadic (idiopathic), hereditary, and secondary types. The secondary form is linked with various disorders, including previous joint damage, hyperparathyroidism, hemochromatosis, hypomagnesemia, hypothyroidism, ochronosis, and diabetes. The conditions leading to crystal formation are not entirely known but include altered activity of the cartilage matrix enzymes that produce and degrade pyrophosphate resulting in its accumulation and eventual crystallization with calcium.

The crystals first develop in the articular matrix, menisci, and intervertebral discs, and as the deposits enlarge, they may rupture and seed the joint. They form chalky white friable deposits,

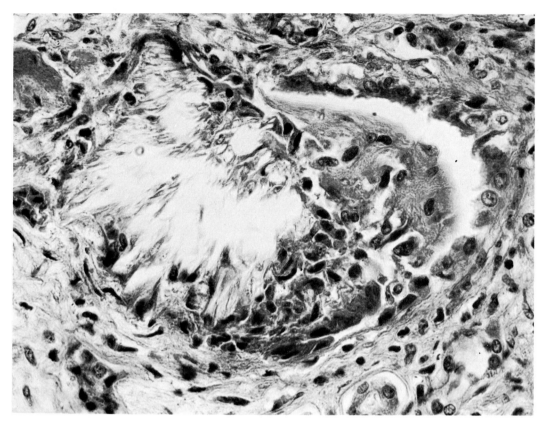

Figure 27–48. A tophus of gout. The group of slender urate crystals is surrounded by a reaction of fibroblasts, occasional lymphocytes, and giant cells.

which are seen histologically in stained preparations as oval blue-purple aggregates. Individual crystals are generally 0.5 to 5 μm in greatest dimension and weakly birefringent (Fig. 27–49).

CPPD is frequently asymptomatic; however, it is a great "simulator" because it produces acute, subacute, or chronic arthritis that may mimic other disorders, such as OA or RA. The joint involvement may last from several days to weeks and may be monoarticular or polyarticular; the knees, followed by the wrists, elbows, shoulders, and ankles, are most commonly affected. Ultimately, approximately 50% of patients experience significant joint damage. There is no therapy that prevents or retards the crystal formation.

TUMORS OF JOINTS AND RELATED STRUCTURES

Reactive tumor-like lesions, such as ganglions, synovial cysts, and osteochondral loose bodies, commonly involve joints and tendon sheaths. They usually result from trauma or degenerative processes and are much more common than neoplasms. Primary neoplasms are unusual and tend to reca-

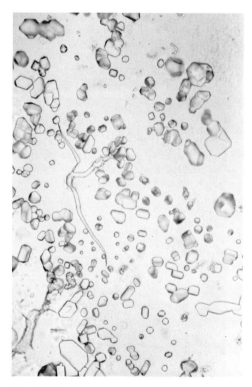

Figure 27–49. Smear preparation of calcium pyrophosphate crystals.

pitulate the cells and tissue types (synovial membrane, fat, blood vessels, fibrous tissue, and cartilage) native to joints and related structures. Benign tumors are much more frequent than their malignant counterparts, which are rare and discussed with the soft tissue tumors.

GANGLION AND SYNOVIAL CYST

A *ganglion* is a small (1 to 1.5 cm) cyst that is almost always located near a joint capsule or tendon sheath. A common location is around the joints of the wrist, where it appears as a firm, fluctuant, pea-sized translucent nodule. It arises from cystic or myxoid degeneration of connective tissue; hence the cyst wall lacks a true cell lining. The lesion may be multilocular and enlarges through coalescence of adjacent areas of myxoid change. The fluid that fills the cyst is similar to synovial fluid; however, there is no communication with the joint space.

Herniation of synovium through a joint capsule or massive enlargement of a bursa may produce a *synovial cyst.* A well-recognized example is the synovial cyst that forms in the popliteal space in the setting of rheumatoid arthritis (Baker's cyst). The synovial lining may be hyperplastic and contain inflammatory cells and fibrin but is otherwise unremarkable.

VILLONODULAR SYNOVITIS

Villonodular synovitis is the term for several closely related benign neoplasms that develop in the synovial linings of joints, tendon sheaths, and

bursae. They were previously considered reactive synovial proliferations (hence the designation "synovitis"); however, cytogenetic studies have demonstrated consistent chromosomal aberrations in these lesions, indicating that they arise from a clonal proliferation of cells and are neoplastic.[63] The prototypes of these tumors are pigmented villonodular synovitis (PVNS) and giant cell tumor of tendon sheath (GCT), which is also known as *localized nodular tenosynovitis.* Although PVNS tends to involve one or more joints diffusely, GCT usually occurs as a discrete nodule on a tendon sheath. Both PVNS and GCT usually arise in the third to fifth decades of life and affect the sexes equally.

MORPHOLOGY. Grossly, the lesions of PVNS and GCT are both red-brown to mottled orange-yellow. In PVNS, much or all of the smooth synovium in a joint, most often the knee, is converted into a tangled mat by red-brown folds and finger-like projections (Fig. 27–50). In contrast, GCT is localized, is well circumscribed, and resembles a small walnut. The tumor cells in both lesions are polyhedral, are moderately sized, and resemble synoviocytes (Fig. 27–51). In PVNS, they spread along the surface and infiltrate the subsynovial compartment. In GCT, the cells grow in a solid nodular aggregate that may be attached to the synovium by a pedicle. Other frequent findings in both lesions include hemosiderin deposits, foamy macrophages, multinucleated giant cells, and zones of sclerosis.

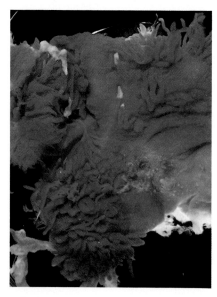

Figure 27–50. Excised synovium with fronds and nodules typical of PVNS.

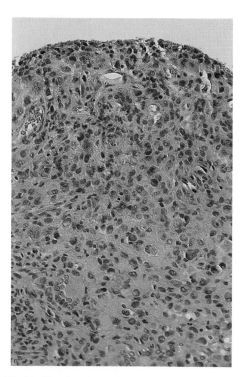

Figure 27–51. Sheets of proliferating cells in PVNS bulging into the synovial lining.

PVNS usually presents as a monoarticular arthritis that affects the knee in 80% of cases, followed in frequency by the hip, ankle, and calcaneocuboid joints.[64] Patients typically complain of pain, locking, and recurrent swelling. Tumor progression limits the range of movement of the joint and causes it to become stiff and firm. Sometimes a palpable mass can be appreciated. Aggressive tumors erode into adjacent bones and soft tissues, causing confusion with other types of neoplasia.

In contrast, GCT manifests as a solitary, slow-growing, painless mass that frequently involves the tendon sheaths along the wrists and fingers; it is the most common mesenchymal neoplasm of the hand and so is often labeled "fingeroma." Cortical erosion of adjacent bone occurs in approximately 15% of cases. Surgery is the recommended treatment for both lesions; PVNS has a significant recurrence rate because it is difficult to excise.

Soft Tissue Tumors and Tumor-Like Lesions

FATTY TUMORS
LIPOMA
LIPOSARCOMA
FIBROUS TUMORS AND TUMOR-LIKE LESIONS
REACTIVE PSEUDOSARCOMATOUS PROLIFERATIONS

Nodular Fasciitis
Myositis Ossificans
Palmar, Plantar, and Penile Fibromatosis
Desmoid (Aggressive Fibromatosis)
FIBROMA

FIBROSARCOMA
FIBROHISTIOCYTIC TUMORS
Benign Fibrous Histiocytoma
Malignant Fibrous Histiocytoma
TUMORS OF SKELETAL MUSCLE

RHABDOMYOSARCOMA
TUMORS OF SMOOTH MUSCLE
LEIOMYOMA
LEIOMYOSARCOMA
SYNOVIAL SARCOMA

Traditionally, soft tissue tumors (STTs) are defined as "mesenchymal proliferations that arise in the extraskeletal, nonepithelial tissue of the body exclusive of the viscera, coverings of the brain, and lymphoreticular system." They are classified according to the tissue they recapitulate (muscle, fat, fibrous tissue, vessels, and nerves). Some have no normal tissue counterpart but have constant clinicopathologic features warranting their designation as distinct entities. The true frequency of STTs is difficult to estimate because most benign lesions are not removed. A conservative estimate is that benign tumors outnumber their malignant counterparts by a ratio of at least 100:1. In the United States, only 5700 sarcomas are diagnosed annually (0.8% of invasive malignancies), yet they are responsible for 2% of all cancer deaths, reflecting their lethal nature.

The etiology of most STTs is unknown; however, there are documented associations between radiation therapy and rare instances of chemical burns, heat burns, or trauma with the subsequent development of a sarcoma. Exposure to phenoxyherbicides and chlorophenols has also been implicated in some cases.[65] The increased incidence of Kaposi's sarcoma in acquired immunodeficiency syndrome (AIDS) and in immunosuppressed patients has also suggested that viruses and defective immunocompetence may be causative factors. Most

STTs occur sporadically, but a small minority are associated with genetic syndromes, the most notable of which are neurofibromatosis type I or von Recklinghausen's disease (malignant schwannoma), Gardner's syndrome (fibromatosis), and Osler-Weber-Rendu syndrome (telangiectasia). Derangements in certain tumor suppressor genes, such as p53 and retinoblastoma gene, have been identified in some STTs; however, the molecular basis of most of these neoplasms remains unknown.

They may arise in any location, although approximately 40% occur in the lower extremity, especially the thigh; 20% in the upper extremities; 10% in the head and neck; and 30% in the trunk and retroperitoneum. Regarding sarcomas, males are affected more frequently than females (1.4:1), and approximately 40% develop in the middle-aged and elderly. The 15% that arise in children constitute the fourth most common malignancy in this age group and follow brain tumors, hematopoietic cancers, and Wilms' tumor in frequency. Specific sarcomas tend to appear in certain age groups, for example, rhabdomyosarcoma in childhood, synovial sarcoma in young adulthood, and liposarcoma and malignant fibrous histiocytoma in middle to late adult life.

Before discussion of individual entities, some generalizations are in order that influence the prognosis of a patient with a soft tissue sarcoma:

- Size has an important bearing on prognosis—the larger the mass, the poorer the outlook.
- Accurate histologic classification contributes significantly to establishing the prognosis of a sarcoma. Important diagnostic features are cell morphology and architectural arrangement (Tables 27–9 and 27–10). Unfortunately, often these features are not sufficient to distinguish one from another, particularly with poorly differentiated aggressive tumors. Great reliance must often be placed on immunohistochemistry, electron microscopy, cytogenetics, and molecular genetics. Whatever the type, the grade of a soft tissue sarcoma is of great importance. Grading, usually I to III, is based largely on the degree of differentiation, the average number of mitoses per high power field, cellularity, pleomorphism, and an estimate of the extent of necrosis (presumably a reflection of rate of growth).[66] No agreement has been reached on the relative importance of each of these variables, but extent of necrosis is thought to be particularly significant.[67]
- Staging determines the prognosis and chances of successful excision of a tumor. Several staging systems have been proposed for these sarcomas; the one most widely used is presented in Table 27–6 (in introduction to bone tumors).
- In general, tumors arising in superficial locations, for example, skin and subcutis, have a better prognosis than deep-seated lesions. Metastatic disease develops in 80% of patients with deep-seated, high-grade sarcomas larger than 20 cm. Overall the 10-year survival rate for sarcomas is approximately 40%.

With this brief background, we can turn to the individual tumors and tumor-like lesions. Fortunately, many of the STTs have already been presented elsewhere—tumors of peripheral nerve (see Chapter 28); tumors of vascular origin, including Kaposi's sarcoma (see Chapter 11); and those of smooth muscle origin (see the section on the uterus, Chapter 23).

Table 27–9. MORPHOLOGY OF CELLS IN SOFT TISSUE TUMORS

CELL TYPE	FEATURES	TUMOR TYPE
Spindle cell	Rod-shaped, long axis twice as great as short axis	Fibrous, fibrohistiocytic, smooth muscle, Schwann cell
Small round cell	Size of a lymphocyte with little cytoplasm	Rhabdomyosarcoma, primitive neuroectodermal tumor
Epithelioid	Polyhedral with abundant cytoplasm; nucleus is centrally located	Smooth muscle, Schwann cell, endothelial, epithelioid sarcoma

Table 27–10. ARCHITECTURAL PATTERNS IN SOFT TISSUE TUMORS

PATTERN	TUMOR TYPE
Fascicles of spindle cells intersecting at right angles	Smooth muscle
Short fascicles of spindle cells radiating from a central point (like spokes on a wheel)—storiform	Fibrohistiocytic
Nuclei arranged in columns—palisading Herringbone	Schwann cell Fibrosarcoma
Mixture of fascicles of spindle cells and groups of epithelioid cells—biphasic	Synovial sarcoma

FATTY TUMORS

LIPOMA

Benign tumors of fat, that is, lipomas, are the most common STT of adulthood. They are subclassified according to particular morphologic features as conventional lipoma, fibrolipoma, angiolipoma, spindle cell lipoma, myelolipoma, and pleomorphic lipoma.

MORPHOLOGY. The conventional lipoma, the most common subtype, is a thinly encapsulated aggregate of mature adipocytes that is several centimeters in greatest dimension. It arises in the subcutis of the proximal extremities and trunk during mid adult life when individuals become sedentary. Infrequently they are large, intramuscular, and poorly circumscribed.

Lipomas are soft, mobile, and painless (except angiolipoma) and are usually cured by simple excision.

LIPOSARCOMA

Liposarcomas tend to appear in the fifth to seventh decade but uncommonly occur in children. They usually arise in the deep soft tissues of the proximal extremities and retroperitoneum and are notorious for developing into large tumors.

MORPHOLOGY. Histologically, liposarcomas can be divided into well-differentiated, myxoid, round cell, and pleomorphic variants. The cells in well-differentiated liposarcomas are readily recognized as lipocytes, and the tumor is easily mistaken for a lipoma. In the other variants, the cells indicative of fatty differentiation are known as lipoblasts, which mimic fetal fat cells. They contain round cytoplas-

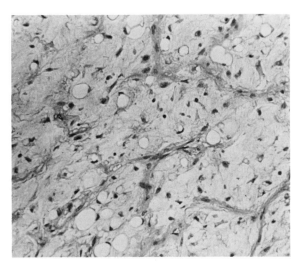

Figure 27–52. Myxoid liposarcoma with abundant ground substance in which are scattered adult-appearing fat cells and more primitive cells, some containing small lipid vacuoles (lipoblasts).

mic vacuoles of lipid that scallop the nucleus. The myxoid variant is most common and is composed of a myxoid background containing stellate mesenchymal cells with only scattered lipoblasts. The vascularization is prominent and disposed in a "chicken-wire" pattern (Fig. 27–52).

Studies reveal that the myxoid variant (but not the other variants) contains a characteristic, balanced chromosomal translocation t(12;16). This translocation moves the CHOP (C/EBP homologous protein) transcription factor coding sequence of chromosome 12 to the 3′ end of a gene with unknown function on chromosome 16, termed TLS (translocated in liposarcoma). The result is the production of a fusion protein with the amino-terminus encoded by TLS and the carboxy-terminus encoded by CHOP.[68] The TLS-CHOP fusion protein has an as yet undetermined role in the pathogenesis of myxoid liposarcoma. The well-differentiated and myxoid variants are relatively indolent; the round cell and pleomorphic variants, however, usually behave aggressively, tend stubbornly to recur, and have the worst prognosis.

FIBROUS TUMORS AND TUMOR-LIKE LESIONS

REACTIVE PSEUDOSARCOMATOUS PROLIFERATIONS

Reactive pseudosarcomatous proliferations are nonneoplastic lesions that develop in response to some form of local injury (physical or ischemic) and are composed of metabolically active fibroblasts or related mesenchymal cells. Clinically they are alarming because they develop suddenly and grow rapidly, and histologically they cause concern because they mimic sarcomas with hypercellularity, mitotic activity, and a primitive appearance. Representative of this family of lesions are nodular fasciitis and myositis ossificans.

Nodular Fasciitis

Nodular fasciitis, also known as *infiltrative* or *pseudosarcomatous fasciitis*, is the most common reactive pseudosarcoma. It most often occurs in adults on the volar aspect of the forearm, followed in order of frequency by the chest and back. Patients typically present with a several week history of a solitary, rapidly growing, and sometimes painful mass. Preceding trauma is noted in only 10 to 15% of cases.

MORPHOLOGY. The lesion arises in the deep dermis, subcutis, or muscle. Grossly, it is several centimeters in greatest dimension, is nodular in configuration, and has poorly defined margins. By light microscopy, nodular fasciitis is richly cellular and consists of plump immature-appearing fibroblasts arranged randomly or in irregular short fascicles simulating cells growing in tissue culture (Fig. 27–53). The cells vary in size and shape (spindle to stellate) and have conspicuous nucleoli and abundant mitotic figures. Frequently the stroma is myxoid and contains extravasated red blood cells. The histologic differential is extensive, but important lesions that should be excluded are fibromatosis and spindle cell sarcomas. Because nodular fasciitis is reactive, the lesion rarely recurs following excision.

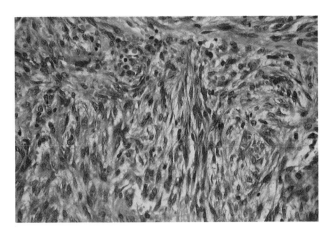

Figure 27–53. Nodular fasciitis. The rich cellularity and the resemblance to a spindle cell sarcoma are evident. (Courtesy of Dr. J. Corson, Brigham and Women's Hospital, Boston.)

Other pseudosarcomas related to nodular fasciitis are proliferative fasciitis and proliferative myositis. These lesions occur in slightly older patients and develop in the proximal extremities; the proliferating fibroblasts are large and round, have prominent nucleoli, and resemble ganglion cells.

Myositis Ossificans

Myositis ossificans is distinguished from the other fibroblastic proliferations by the presence of metaplastic bone.[69] It usually develops in athletic adolescents and young adults after an episode of trauma. The lesion arises in the subcutis and musculature of the proximal extremities. The clinical findings are related to its stage of development; in the early phase, the involved area is swollen and painful, and within the subsequent several weeks, it becomes more circumscribed and firm. Eventually it evolves into a painless, hard, well-demarcated mass.

> **MORPHOLOGY.** Grossly the usual lesion is 3 to 6 cm in greatest dimension. Most are well delineated and have soft glistening centers and a firm gritty periphery. The microscopic findings vary according to the age of the lesion; in the earliest phase, the lesion is the most cellular and consists of plump, elongated fibroblast-like cells arranged in poorly formed fascicles. Morphologic zonation begins within 3 weeks; the center retains its population of fibroblasts; however, it merges with an adjacent intermediate zone that contains osteoblasts depositing ill-defined trabeculae of woven bone. The most peripheral zone contains well-formed and mineralized trabeculae that closely resemble cancellous bone. Frequently skeletal muscle fibers and regenerating muscle giant cells are trapped within the margins. Eventually, the entire lesion ossifies, and the intertrabecular spaces become filled with marrow. The mature lesion is completely ossified.

The radiographic findings parallel the morphologic progression. Initially the x-ray films may show only soft tissue fullness, but at about 3 weeks, patchy flocculent radiodensities form in the periphery. The radiodensities become more extensive with time and slowly encroach on the radiolucent center (Fig. 27-54). Myositis ossificans must be distinguished from extraskeletal osteosarcoma. The latter occurs in elderly patients, the proliferating cells are cytologically malignant, and the tumor lacks the zonation of myositis ossificans. The most peripheral regions of osteosarcoma are the most cellular and primitive, which is the reverse of myositis ossificans. Myositis ossificans is usually cured with simple excision, and rarely does it undergo malignant transformation.

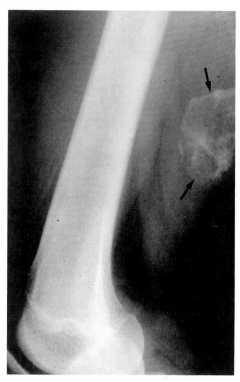

Figure 27-54. A focus of peripherally mineralized myositis ossificans involving posterior thigh (arrows).

Palmar, Plantar, and Penile Fibromatosis

These more bothersome than serious lesions constitute a small group of superficial fibromatoses. They are characterized by nodular or poorly defined fascicles of mature-appearing fibroblasts surrounded by abundant dense collagen. Ultrastructural studies indicate that many of these cells are myofibroblasts and therefore presumably contractile.

> **MORPHOLOGY.** In the palmar variant **(Dupuytren's contracture),** there is irregular or nodular thickening of the palmar fascia either unilaterally or bilaterally (50%). Over a span of years, attachment to the overlying skin causes puckering and dimpling. At the same time, a slowly progressive flexion contracture develops, mainly of the fourth and fifth fingers of the hand. Essentially similar changes are seen with **plantar fibromatosis** except that flexion contractures are uncommon and bilateral involvement is infrequent. In **penile fibromatosis (Peyronie's disease),** a palpable induration or mass appears usually on the dorsolateral aspect of the penis. It may cause eventually abnormal curvature of the shaft or constriction of the urethra, or both.

Although not surprisingly males are affected more frequently than females in Peyronie's disease, male predominance is true of the other patterns as well. In about 20 to 25% of cases, the palmar and plantar fibromatoses after a period of time stabilize and do not progress, and in some instances, they resolve spontaneously. Some recur after excision, particularly the plantar lesion.

Desmoid (Aggressive Fibromatosis)

Biologically desmoids lie in the interface between exuberant fibroproliferations and low-grade fibrosarcomas. On the one hand, they present frequently as large, infiltrative masses that may recur after incomplete excision but, on the other hand, may be small masses composed of banal well-differentiated fibroblasts that do not metastasize. They may occur at any age but are most frequent in the second to fourth decades. Desmoids are divided into extra-abdominal, abdominal, and intra-abdominal, but all have essentially similar gross and microscopic features. Extra-abdominal desmoids occur in men and women with equal frequency and arise principally in the musculature of the shoulder, chest wall, back, and thigh.[70] Abdominal desmoids generally arise in the musculoaponeurotic structures of the anterior abdominal wall in women during or after pregnancy. Intra-

abdominal desmoids tend to occur in the mesentery or pelvic walls, often in patients having Gardner's syndrome (see section on familial polyposis, Chapter 17).

MORPHOLOGY. These lesions occur as unicentric, gray-white, firm, poorly demarcated masses varying from 1 to 15 cm in greatest diameter. They are rubbery and tough and infiltrate surrounding structures. Histologically, they are composed of plump fibroblasts having minimal variation in cell and nuclear size interspersed within a densely collagenous background (Fig. 27–55). Mitoses are infrequent. Regenerative muscle cells when trapped within these lesions may take on the appearance of multinucleated giant cells.

In addition to their possibly being disfiguring or disabling, desmoids are occasionally painful. Although curable by adequate excision, they stubbornly recur in the local site when incompletely removed. The rare reports of metastasis of a desmoid must be interpreted as misidentification of a low-grade fibrosarcoma.

FIBROMA

Despite the widespread distribution of connective tissue throughout the body, fibromas are surprisingly limited in their origin, and fibrosarcomas are one of the less common STTs. Many lesions previously called fibromas have been reclassified as "fibromatosis."

Fibromas most often arise in ovaries or along nerve trunks (neurofibroma). Circumscribed nodules referred to as "fibromas" occur about the teeth, but these may be reactive.

MORPHOLOGY. Fibromas are usually small tumors that are firm, encapsulated, and pearly gray on cross-section. Wherever they arise, they are composed of typical spindled fibroblasts either closely packed with scant intervening collagen or separated by abundant collagen. In most, mitoses are rare, but in so-called "cellular fibromas" of the ovary, scattered mitoses may be present; thus the differentiation between these cellular lesions and fibrosarcomas may be difficult.

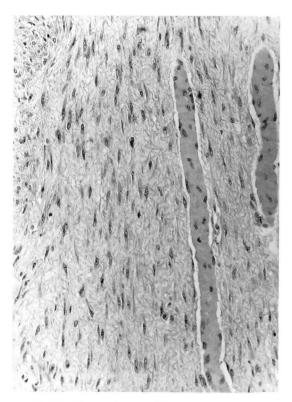

Figure 27–55. Fibromatosis infiltrating between skeletal muscle cells.

FIBROSARCOMA

Fibrosarcomas may occur anywhere in the body but are most common in the retroperitoneum, in the thigh, about the knee, and in the distal extremities. Many tumors previously considered fibrosarcoma have been reclassified as aggressive fibromatosis (desmoid) or malignant fibrous histiocytoma.

> **MORPHOLOGY.** Typically, these neoplasms are unencapsulated, infiltrative, soft, "fish-flesh" masses often having areas of hemorrhage and necrosis. Better differentiated lesions may appear deceptively encapsulated. Histologic examination discloses all degrees of differentiation, from slowly growing tumors that closely resemble "cellular fibromas" sometimes having spindled cells growing in a "herringbone" fashion (Fig. 27–56) to highly cellular neoplasms dominated by architectural disarray, pleomorphism, frequent mitoses, and areas of necrosis.

Recurrence occurs in more than half of the cases, and in about 25%, metastases are present at the time of diagnosis. Overall 60 to 80% of patients survive 5 years with present methods of treatment.

FIBROHISTIOCYTIC TUMORS

Fibrohistiocytic tumors contain both fibroblastic and histiocytic elements. Originally they were believed to be neoplasms of histiocytes that had the capacity to express certain properties of fibroblasts. Studies suggest, however, that the fundamental phenotype of the neoplastic cells most closely resembles fibroblasts. Therefore the term fibrohistiocytic should be viewed as descriptive in nature and not one that connotes histogenetic origin.

Benign Fibrous Histiocytoma

Benign fibrous histiocytoma is a relatively common lesion that usually occurs in the dermis and subcutis. It is painless and slow-growing, and most often presents in middle adult life as a firm, small (up to 1 cm), mobile nodule. Multiple nodules are present in as many as one-third of cases.

Most benign fibrous histiocytomas consist of a proliferation of bland spindle cells arranged in a storiform pattern.[71] These are often referred to as "dermatofibromas." Other variants, however, may contain numerous blood vessels and hemosiderin deposition, giving rise to the designation "sclerosing hemangioma." Still others may be richly punctuated with foamy histiocytes and are called "histiocytomas." All are variations on a common theme, and in all the margins are infiltrative, but the tumor does not invade the overlying epidermis, which is frequently hyperplastic. Adequate treatment is simple excision.

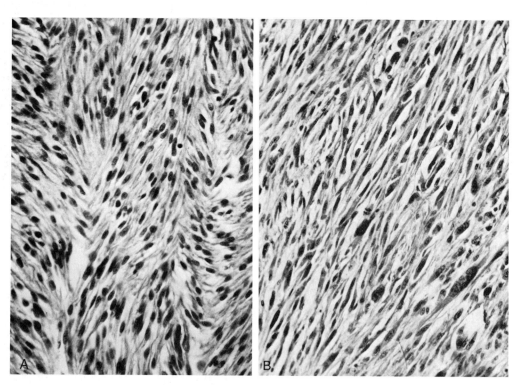

Figure 27–56. Fibrosarcoma. *A,* A better differentiated tumor with spindle cells forming a classic herringbone pattern. *B,* There is considerable anaplasia of cells with marked variation in size and shape. Scattered giant cells are readily evident.

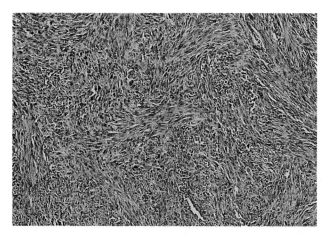

Figure 27–57. Malignant fibrous histiocytoma revealing fascicles of plump spindled cells in a swirling (storiform) pattern, typical but not pathognomonic of this neoplasm. (Courtesy of Dr. J. Corson, Brigham and Women's Hospital, Boston.)

Malignant Fibrous Histiocytoma

Malignant fibrous histiocytoma is a controversial sarcoma of adults. Some believe all MFHs are misinterpretations of other types of sarcoma. They usually arise in the musculature of the proximal extremities and the retroperitoneum.[72]

MORPHOLOGY. They are usually gray-white unencapsulated masses but often appear deceptively circumscribed. They are frequently large (5 to 20 cm). Malignant fibrous histiocytomas have been categorized into storiform-pleomorphic, myxoid, inflammatory, giant cell, and angiomatoid variants based on their histologic features. The storiform-pleomorphic type is the most common (about two-thirds) and as the name indicates is composed of malignant spindle cells oriented in a storiform pattern with scattered large, round pleomorphic cells (Fig. 27–57). The other patterns can be deduced by their names.

Most variants of malignant fibrous histiocytoma are aggressive, recur unless widely excised, and have a metastatic rate of 30 to 50% except for the cutaneous tumors, which rarely disseminate.[73] The angiomatoid variant is also indolent and in contrast to the other types occurs in adolescents and young adults.[74]

TUMORS OF SKELETAL MUSCLE

Skeletal muscle neoplasms, in contrast to other groups of tumors, are almost all malignant. The benign variant, rhabdomyoma, is distinctly rare. The so-called cardiac rhabdomyoma is probably hamartomatous in origin.

RHABDOMYOSARCOMA

Rhabdomyosarcomas, the most common soft tissue sarcomas of childhood and adolescence, usually appear within the first two decades of life. They may arise in any anatomic location, but, surprisingly, most develop in the head and neck, genitourinary tract, and retroperitoneum, where there is little if any skeletal muscle as a normal constituent.[75] Only in the extremities do they appear in relation to skeletal muscle.

MORPHOLOGY. Rhabdomyosarcoma is histologically subclassified into the embryonal, alveolar, and pleomorphic variants. The rhabdomyoblast is the diagnostic cell in all types and contains eccentric, eosinophilic, granular cytoplasm rich in thick and thin filaments. The rhabdomyoblasts may be round or elongate; the latter are known as "tadpole" or "strap" cells (Fig. 27–58). Ultrastructurally, rhabdomyoblasts contain sarcomeres, and immunohistochemically they stain with antibodies to vimentin, actin, desmin, and myoglobin.[76]

Embryonal rhabdomyosarcoma includes the variant known as "*sarcoma botryoides.*" This is the most common variant accounting for 66% of rhabdomyosarcomas. It occurs in children under the age of 10 years and typically arises in the nasal cavity, orbit, middle ear, prostate, and paratesticular region. The sarcoma botryoides subtype develops in the walls of hollow mucosal lined structures, such as the nasopharynx, common bile duct, bladder, and vagina.[77]

MORPHOLOGY. Embryonal rhabdomyosarcoma appears as a soft gray infiltrative mass. Most when first seen are many centimeters in size. The tumor

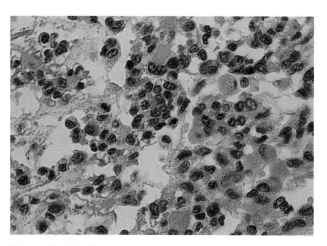

Figure 27–58. Rhabdomyosarcoma. The rhabdomyoblasts vary in size and some have abundant cytoplasm, but no cross-striations are evident.

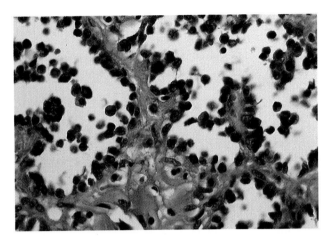

Figure 27–59. Alveolar rhabdomyosarcoma with numerous spaces lined with tumor cells.

cells mimic skeletal muscle in its various stages of embryogenesis and consist of sheets of both malignant round and spindled cells in a variably myxoid stroma. Sarcoma botryoides grows in a polypoid fashion, producing the appearance of a cluster of grapes protruding into a hollow structure, such as the bladder or vagina. Where the tumor abuts the mucosa of an organ, the tumor cells form a submucosal zone of hypercellularity known as the cambium layer. Rhabdomyoblasts with visible cross striations are present in most cases.

Alveolar rhabdomyosarcoma occurs in early to middle adolescence and commonly arises in the deep musculature of the extremities.[78] The tumor is traversed by a network of fibrous septae that divide the cells into clusters or aggregates; as the central cells become necrotic and drop out, a crude resemblance to pulmonary alveoli is created (Fig. 27–59). The tumor cells are discohesive and moderate in size, and many have little cytoplasm. Cells with cross striations are identified in only about 30% of cases. Cytogenetic studies have shown a translocation between chromosomes 2 and 13 (q35-37; q14) in this type of rhabdomyosarcoma.[79]

Pleomorphic rhabdomyosarcoma is characterized by numerous large, sometimes multinucleated, bizarre tumor cells. This variant is uncommon, has a tendency to arise in the deep soft tissue of adults, and can be confused histologically with malignant fibrous histiocytoma.

Rhabdomyosarcomas are aggressive neoplasms and are usually treated with a combination of surgery, radiation, and chemotherapy. The histologic variant influences survival.[80] The botryoid subtype has the best prognosis followed by the embryonal, pleomorphic, and alveolar variants. Overall, approximately 65% of patients are cured of their disease.

TUMORS OF SMOOTH MUSCLE

LEIOMYOMA

Leiomyomas, benign smooth muscle tumors, often arise in the uterus, where they represent the most common neoplasm in the female. These are described in detail in the uterine section of Chapter 23. Leiomyomas may also arise in the walls of blood vessels, in deep soft tissue, and in the skin and subcutis from the arrector pili muscles found in the skin, nipples, scrotum, and labia (genital leiomyomas). Those arising in the arrector muscles (pilar leiomyomas) are frequently multiple and painful. The tendency to multiple lesions is thought to be hereditary and transmitted as an autosomal dominant trait. In whatever setting, these lesions tend to occur in adolescence and early adult life.

MORPHOLOGY. They are usually not larger than 1 to 2 cm in greatest dimension and are composed of fascicles of spindle cells that tend to intersect each other at right angles. The tumor cells have blunt-ended, elongated nuclei and show minimal atypia and few mitotic figures.

Solitary lesions are easily cured; however, they may be so numerous that complete surgical removal is impractical.

LEIOMYOSARCOMA

Leiomyosarcomas are relatively uncommon and account for 7% of soft tissue sarcomas. They occur in adults and afflict women more frequently than men. Most develop in the skin and deep soft tissues of the extremities and retroperitoneum. Only rarely do they arise in pre-existing leiomyomas.

MORPHOLOGY. Leiomyosarcomas present as painless firm masses. Retroperitoneal tumors may be large and bulky and cause abdominal symptoms. Histologically they are characterized by malignant spindle cells that have "cigar-shaped" nuclei arranged in interweaving fascicles. Morphologic variants include tumors with a prominent myxoid stroma and others with epithelioid cells. Ultrastructurally, malignant smooth muscle cells contain bundles of thin filaments with dense bodies and pinocytotic vesicles, and individual cells are surrounded by basal lamina. Immunohistochemically they stain with antibodies to vimentin, actin, and desmin.

The treatment depends on the size, location, and grade of the tumor. Superficial or cutaneous leiomyosarcomas are usually small and have a good prognosis, whereas those of retroperitoneum are large, cannot be entirely excised, and cause death by both local extension and metastatic spread.

SYNOVIAL SARCOMA

Synovial sarcoma is so named because its morphology resembles developing synovium. It accounts for approximately 10% of all soft tissue sarcomas and ranks as the fourth most common sarcoma. They usually occur in the third to fifth decades of life. Although the term synovial sarcoma implies an origin from the joint linings, less than 10% are intra-articular. Most develop in the vicinity of the large joints of the extremities, and about 60 to 70% involve the lower extremity, especially around the knee.[81] Patients usually present with a deep-seated mass that has been noted for several years. Uncommonly these tumors occur in the parapharyngeal region or in the abdominal wall.

MORPHOLOGY. The histologic hallmark of synovial sarcoma is the biphasic morphology of the tumor cells, that is, epithelial-like and spindle cells. Despite the mimicry, the tumor cells do not have the features of synoviocytes. The epithelial-like cells are cuboidal to columnar and form glands or grow in solid cords. The spindle cells are arranged in densely cellular fascicles that surround the epithe-lial-like cells (Fig. 27–60). Some synovial sarcomas are monophasic in that they are composed of only spindled or epithelial-like cells. Lesions composed solely of spindled cells are easily mistaken for fibrosarcomas. A characteristic feature, when present, are round calcified concretions that can be detected radiographically. Immunohistochemistry can be helpful in identifying these tumors because the epithelial-like and sometimes spindle cell portions yield positive reactions for keratin and epithelial membrane antigen, differentiating these tumors from most other sarcomas.[82] In addition, synovial sarcomas can almost always be shown to have a reciprocal translocation between chromosomes X and 18, referred to as t(x; 18) (p. 11.2; q11.2).[83]

Synovial sarcomas are treated aggressively with limb-sparing therapy.[84] The 5-year survival rate varies from 25 to 62%, and only 11 to 30% of patients live for 10 years or longer. Common sites of metastases are the regional lymph nodes, lungs, and skeleton.

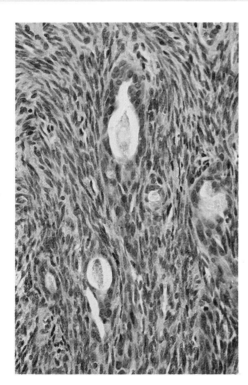

Figure 27–60. Synovial sarcoma revealing the classic biphasic spindle cell and glandular-like histology.

1. Glimcher, M.J.: The nature of the mineral component of bone and the mechanism of calcification. In Avioli, L.V., and Krane, S.M. (eds.): Metabolic Bone Disease and Clinically Related Disorders, 2nd ed. Philadelphia, W.B. Saunders Co., 1990, pp. 42–68.
2. Barron, R.: Molecular mechanisms of bone resorption by the osteoclast. Anat. Rec. 224:317, 1989.
3. Young, M.F., et al.: Structure, expression, and regulation of the major noncollagenous matrix proteins of bone. Clin. Orthop. Rel. Res. 281:275, 1992.
4. MacDonald, B.R., and Gowen, M.: Cytokines and bone. Br. J. Rheumatol. 31:149, 1992.
5. Marcus, R.: Normal and abnormal bone remodeling in man. Annu. Rev. Med. 38:129, 1987.
6. Gilbert, E.F., et al.: Pathologic changes of osteochondrodysplasia in infancy. Pathol. Ann. 22(part 2):282, 1987.
7. Byers, P.H., and Steiner, R.D.: Osteogenesis imperfecta. Annu. Rev. Med. 43:269, 1992.
8. Bullough, P.G., et al.: The morbid anatomy of the skeleton in osteogenesis imperfecta. Clin. Orthop. Rel. Res. 159:42, 1981.
9. Gallager, J.C.: Pathophysiology of osteoporosis. Semin. Nephrol. 12:109, 1992.
10. Chestnut, C.H.: Theoretical overview: Bone development, peak bone mass, bone loss, and fracture risk. Am. J. Med. 91(Suppl. 5B):25, 1991.
11. Mundy, G. R.: Boning up on genes. Nature 367:216, 1994.
12. Pacifici, R.: Is there a causal role for IL-1 in postmenopausal bone loss? Calcif. Tiss. Int. 50:295, 1992.
13. Marks, S.C.: Osteopetrosis—multiple pathways for the interception of osteoclast function. Appl. Pathol. 5:172, 1987.
14. Shapiro, F., et al.: Human osteopetrosis: Histologic, ultrastructural, and biochemical study. J. Bone Joint Surg. 62A:384, 1980.
15. Mirra, J.M.: Pathogenesis of Paget's disease based on viral etiology. Clin. Orthop. 217:162, 1987.
16. Gordon, M.T., et al.: Canine distemper virus localized in bone cells of patients with Paget's disease. Bone 12:195, 1992.
17. Bataille, R.: Etiology of Paget's disease of bone: A new perspective. Calcif. Tiss. Int. 50:293, 1992.

18. Meunier, P.J. et al.: Skeletal distribution and biochemical parameters of Paget's disease. Clin. Orthop. *217*:37, 1987.

19. Hadjipavlou, A., et al.: Malignant transformation in Paget's disease of bone. Cancer *70*:2802, 1992.

20. Sutton, R.A.L., and Cameron, E.C.: Renal osteodystrophy: Pathophysiology. Semin. Nephrol. *12*:91, 1992.

21. Bolander, M.: Regulation of fracture repair by growth factors. Proc. Soc. Exp. Biol. Med. *200*:165, 1992.

22. Mankin, H.: Nontraumatic necrosis of bone (osteonecrosis). N. Engl. J. Med. *326*:1473, 1992.

23. Ray, M.J., and Bassett, R.L.: Pyogenic vertebral osteomyelitis. Orthopaedics *8*:506, 1985.

24. Senac, M.O., et al.: Primary lesions of bone in the first decade of life: Retrospective survey of biopsy results. Radiology *160*:491, 1986.

25. Klein, M.H., and Shankman, S.: Osteoid osteoma: Radiologic and pathologic correlation. Skel. Radiol. *21*:23, 1992.

26. Nemoto, O., et al.: Osteoblastoma of the spine: A review of 75 cases. Spine *15*:1272, 1990.

27. Klein, M.J., et al.: Osteosarcoma: Clinical and pathological considerations. Orthop. Clin. North Am. *20*:327, 1989.

28. Lane, D.P.: p53, guardian of the genome. Nature *358*:15, 1992.

29. Unni, K.K., and Dahlin, D.C.: Osteosarcoma: Pathology and classification. Semin. Roentgenol. *24*:143, 1989.

30. Glasser, D.B. et al.: Survival, prognosis, and therapeutic response in osteogenic sarcoma. Cancer *69*:698, 1992.

31. Ragsdale, B.D., et al.: Radiology as gross pathology in evaluating chondroid lesions. Hum. Pathol. *20*:930, 1989.

32. Kurt, A.-M., et al.: Chondroblastoma of bone. Hum. Pathol. *20*:965, 1989.

33. Zillmer, D.A., and Dorfman, H.D.: Chondromyxoid fibroma of bone: Thirty-six cases with clinicopathologic correlation. Hum. Pathol. *20*:952, 1989.

34. Daly, P.J., et al.: Dedifferentiated chondrosarcoma of bone. Orthopaedics *12*:763, 1989.

35. Rosenthal, D.I., et al.: Chondrosarcoma: Correlation of radiological and histological grade. Radiology *150*:21, 1984.

36. Lee, P.A., et al.: McCune-Albright syndrome: Long-term follow-up. J.A.M.A. *256*:2980, 1986.

37. Weinstein, L.S., et al.: Activating mutations of the stimulatory G protein in the McCune-Albright syndrome. N. Engl. J. Med. *325*:1688, 1991.

38. Huvos, A.G., et al.: The pathology of malignant fibrous histiocytoma of bone. Am. J. Surg. Pathol. *9*:853, 1985.

39. May, W.A., et al.: Ewing's Sarcoma 11; 22 translocation produces a chimeric transcription factor that requires the DNA-binding domain encoded by FLI-1 for transformation. Proc. Natl. Acad. Sci. U.S.A. *90*:5752, 1993.

40. Dehner, L.P.: Primitive neuroectodermal tumor of bone. Am. J. Surg. Pathol. *17*:1, 1993.

41. Schmidt, D., et al.: Malignant peripheral neuroectodermal tumor and its necessary distinction from Ewing's sarcoma. Cancer *68*:2251, 1991.

42. Meideiros, L.J., et al.: Giant cells and mononuclear cells of giant cell tumor of bone resemble histiocytes. Appl. Immunohistochem. *1*:115, 1993.

43. Hamerman, D.: The biology of osteoarthritis. N. Engl. J. Med. *320*:1322, 1989.

44. Moskowitz, R.W.: Primary osteoarthritis: Epidemiology, clinical aspects, and general management. Am. J. Med. *83*(Suppl. 5A):5, 1987.

45. Howell, D.S.: Etiopathogenesis of osteoarthritis. *In* Moskowitz, R.W., et al. (eds.): Osteoarthritis: Diagnosis and Medical/Surgical Management, 2nd ed. Philadelphia, W.B. Saunders Co., 1992, p. 233.

46. Sewell, K.T., and Trentham, D.E.: Pathogenesis of rheumatoid arthritis. Lancet *341*:283, 1993.

47. Harris, E.D., Jr.: Rheumatoid arthritis: Pathophysiology and implications for therapy. N. Engl. J. Med. *322*:1277, 1990.

48. Roudier, J., et al.: Susceptibility to rheumatoid arthritis maps to a T-cell epitope shared by HLA-Dw4DR beta-1 chain and the Epstein-Barr virus glycoprotein gp110. Proc. Natl. Acad. Sci. U.S.A. *86*:5140, 1989.

49. Brennan, F.M., et al.: Tumor necrosis factor-alpha—a pivotal role in rheumatoid arthritis. Br. J. Rheumatol. *31*:293, 1992.

50. Arnett, F.C., and Committee: The American Rheumatism Association 1987 revised criteria for the classification of rheumatoid arthritis. Arthritis Rheum. *31*:315, 1988.

51. Cassidy, J.T., et al.: The development of classification criteria for children with juvenile rheumatoid arthritis. Bull. Rheumat. Dis. *38*:1, 1989.

52. Fernandez-Vina, M.A., et al.: HLA antigens in juvenile arthritis: Pauciarticular and polyarticular juvenile arthritis are immunogenetically distinct. Arthritis Rheum. *33*:1787, 1990.

53. Williams, R.C., Jr., et al.: Molecular mimicry, ankylosing spondylitis, and reactive arthritis—something missing? Scand. J. Rheumatol. *21*:105, 1992.

54. Helliwell, P., et al.: A re-evaluation of the osteoarticular manifestations of psoriasis. Br. J. Rheumatol. *30*:339, 1991.

55. Lahesmaa, R., et al.: Molecular mimicry between HLA-B27 and Yersinia, Salmonella, Shigella, and Klebsiella with the same region of HLA alpha-1 helix. Clin. Exp. Immunol. *86*:399, 1991.

56. Steere, A.C., et al.: The clinical evolution of Lyme arthritis. Ann. Intern. Med. *107*:725, 1987.

57. Terkeltaub, R.A., and Ginsberg, M.H.: The inflammatory reaction to crystals. Rheum. Dis. Clin. North Am. *14*:353, 1988.

58. German, D.C., and Holmes, E.W.: Hyperuricemia and gout. Med. Clin. North Am. *70*:419, 1986.

59. Agudelo, C.A., and Wise, C.M.: Gout and hyperuricemia. Curr. Opin. Rheumatol. *3*:684, 1991.

60. DiGiovine, F.S., et al.: Interleukin 1 (IL-1) as a mediator of crystal arthritis: Stimulation of T cell and synovial fibroblast mitogenesis by urate crystal–induced IL-1. J. Immunol. *138*:3213, 1987.

61. Dykman, D., et al.: Hyperuricemia and uric acid nephropathy. Arch. Intern. Med. *147*:1341, 1987.

62. Fam, A.G.: Calcium pyrophosphate crystal deposition disease and other crystal deposition disease. Curr. Opin. Rheumatol. *4*:574, 1992.

63. Fletcher, J.A., et al.: Trisomy 5 and trisomy 7 are nonrandom aberrations in pigmented villonodular synovitis: Confirmation of trisomy 7 in uncultured cells. Genes Chrom. Cancer *4*:264, 1992.

64. Flandry, F., and Hughston, J.C.: Pigmented villonodular synovitis. J. Bone Joint Surg. *69A*:942, 1987.

65. Wingren, G., et al.: Soft tissue sarcoma and occupational exposures. Cancer *66*:806, 1990.

66. Leyvraz, S., et al.: Histological diagnosis and grading of soft-tissue sarcomas. Semin. Surg. Oncol. *4*:3, 1988.

67. Kulander, B.G., et al.: Grading of soft tissue sarcomas: Necrosis is a determinant of survival. Mod. Pathol. *2*:205, 1989.

68. Crozat, A., et al.: Fusion of CHOP to a novel RNA-binding protein in human myxoid liposarcoma. Nature *363*:640, 1993.

69. Nuova, M.A., et al.: Myositis ossificans with atypical clinical, radiographic, or pathologic findings: A review of 23 cases. Skel. Radiol. *21*:87, 1992.

70. Markhede, G., et al.: Extra-abdominal desmoid tumors. Acta Orthop. Scand. *57*:1, 1986.

71. Vilanova, J.R., and Flint, A.: The morphological variations of fibrous histiocytomas. J. Cutan. Pathol. *1*:155, 1974.

72. Rooser, B., et al.: Malignant fibrous histiocytoma of soft tissue. Cancer *67*:499, 1991.

73. Pezzi, C.M., et al.: Prognostic factors in 227 patients with malignant fibrous histiocytoma. Cancer *69*:2098, 1992.

74. Costa, M.J., and Weiss, S.W.: Angiomatoid malignant fibrous histiocytoma: A follow-up study of 108 cases with evaluation of possible histologic predictors of outcome. Am. J. Surg. Pathol. *14*:1126, 1990.

75. Malogolowkin, M., and Ortega, J.A.: Rhabdomyosarcoma of childhood. Pediatr. Ann. *17*:253, 1992.
76. Parham, D.M., et al.: Immunohistochemical study of childhood rhabdomyosarcomas and related neoplasms. Cancer *67*:3072, 1991.
77. Brand, E., et al.: Rhabdomyosarcoma of the uterine cervix: Sarcoma botryoides. Cancer *60*:1552, 1987.
78. Reboul-Marty, J., et al.: Prognostic factors of alveolar rhabdomyosarcoma in childhood. Cancer *68*:493, 1991.
79. Barr, F.G., et al.: Molecular and cytogenetic analysis of chromosomal arms 2q and 13q in alveolar rhabdomyosarcoma. Gene Chrom. Cancer *3*:153, 1991.
80. Maurer, H.M., et al.: The Intergroup Rhabdomyosarcoma Study—II. Cancer *71*:1904, 1993.
81. Soule, E.H.: Synovial sarcoma. Am. J. Surg. Pathol. *10*(Suppl. 1):78, 1986.
82. Ordonez, N.G.: Synovial sarcoma: An immunohistochemical and ultrastructural study. Hum. Pathol. *21*:733, 1990.
83. Limon, J., et al.: Cytogenetics of synovial sarcoma: Presentation of 10 new cases and review of the literature. Gene Chrom. Cancer *3*:338, 1991.
84. Oda, Y., et al.: Survival in synovial sarcoma: A multivariate study of prognostic factors with special emphasis on the comparison between early death and long-term survival. Am. J. Surg. Pathol. *17*:35, 1993.

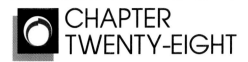

CHAPTER
TWENTY-EIGHT

Peripheral Nerve and Skeletal Muscle

UMBERTO DE GIROLAMI, M.D., DOUGLAS C. ANTHONY, M.D., Ph.D.,
and MATTHEW P. FROSCH, M.D., Ph.D.

NORMAL STRUCTURE AND GENERAL REACTIONS OF THE MOTOR UNIT

The functional unit of the neuromuscular system is the *motor unit,* which consists of (1) a *lower motor neuron* in the anterior horn of the spinal cord, (2) the *axon* of that neuron, and (3) the multiple *muscle fibers* it innervates (Fig. 28–1).

Lower motor neurons are distributed in the anterior horns in columns or groups arranged somatotopically so that cells lying medially innervate proximal muscles, and those lying laterally supply the distal musculature. The number of muscle fibers within the unit varies considerably. Muscles with highly refined movements, like the extrinsic muscles of the eye, have a high neuron-to-muscle fiber ratio (1:10); those with relatively coarse and

stereotyped movements, like calf muscles, have a much lower ratio (1:2000).[1]

PERIPHERAL NERVE

The principal structural component of peripheral nerve is the *nerve fiber*—an axon with its Schwann cells and myelin sheath. A nerve consists of numerous fibers that are grouped into fascicles by connective tissue sheaths. *Myelinated* and *unmyelinated* nerve fibers are intermingled across the fascicle (Fig. 28–2). In the sural nerve, the one most commonly biopsied and a relatively pure sensory nerve, myelinated fibers range between 2 and 15 μm in diameter and have a bimodal distribution; small axons, which average 4 μm, are about twice as numerous as the larger axons, which average

1273

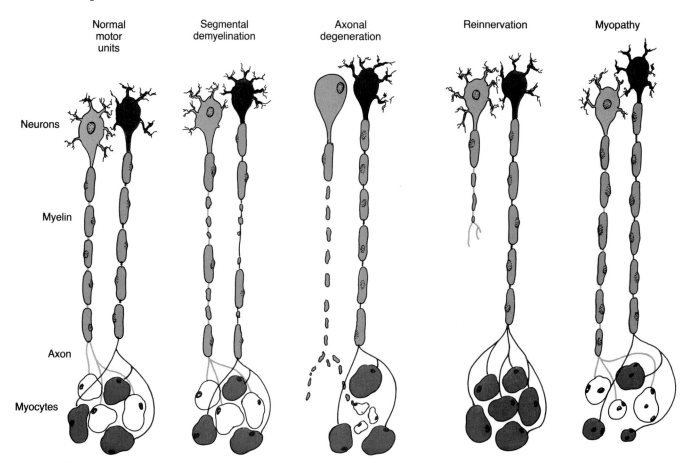

Figure 28-1. Normal and abnormal motor units. *Segmental demyelination:* Random internodes of myelin are injured and are remyelinated by multiple Schwann cells, while the axon and myocytes remain intact. *Axonal degeneration:* The axon and its myelin sheath undergo anterograde degeneration, with resulting denervation atrophy of the myocytes within its motor unit. *Reinnervation:* Sprouting of adjacent uninjured motor axons leads to fiber type grouping of myocytes, while the injured axon attempts axonal sprouting. *Myopathy:* Scattered myocytes of adjacent motor units are small (degenerated or regenerated), whereas the neurons and nerve fibers are normal.

11 μm.[2] Axons are myelinated in segments *(internodes)* separated by *nodes of Ranvier.* A single Schwann cell supplies the myelin sheath for each internode. The thickness of the myelin sheath is directly proportional to the diameter of the axon,[3] and the larger the axon diameter, the longer the internodal distance. Unmyelinated axons, more numerous than myelinated axons, range in size from 0.2 to 3 μm. They occur in groups of 5 to 20 and are enveloped and isolated from each other by the cytoplasm of one Schwann cell. Regardless of their association with myelinated or unmyelinated fibers, Schwann cells have pale oval nuclei with an even chromatin distribution and an elongated bipolar cell body. By electron microscopy, Schwann cells, unlike fibroblasts, have a basement membrane.

Peripheral axons contain organelles and cytoskeletal structures, including microfilaments, neurofilaments, microtubules, mitochondria, vesicles, smooth endoplasmic reticulum, and lysosomes. Dense-cored and coated vesicles are located in the nerve terminals. Protein synthesis does not occur in the axon, and axoplasmic flow delivers proteins

and other substances synthesized in the perikaryon down the axon.[4] A retrograde transport system serves as a feedback system for the cell body.

The connective tissue sheaths of peripheral nerve include the *epineurium,* which encloses the entire nerve; the *perineurium,* a multilayered concentric connective tissue sheath that encloses each fascicle; and the *endoneurium,* which surrounds individual nerve fibers. The nerve microenvironment is regulated by the *perineurial barrier* (formed by the tight junctions between perineurial cells), the *blood-nerve barrier,* and the *nerve–cerebrospinal fluid* (CSF) barrier.[5] Endoneurial capillaries derive from the vasa nervorum, and their endothelial cells form tight junctions to establish the blood-nerve barrier. This barrier has been found to be relatively less competent within nerve roots, dorsal root ganglia, and autonomic ganglia than along the rest of the nerve. The nerve-CSF barrier is formed by the tight junctions between the cells that form the outer layer of the arachnoid membrane. These cells fuse with the perineurium of the roots and cranial nerves as they leave the subarachnoid

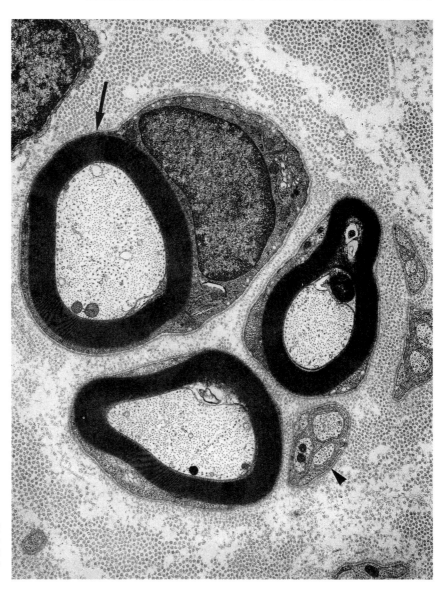

Figure 28–2. Electron micrograph of myelinated *(large arrow)* and unmyelinated *(arrowhead)* fibers in human sural nerve. One Schwann cell nucleus is present.

space, and the motor and sensory fibers, which are separated within anterior and posterior roots, intermingle within the mixed sensorimotor nerves that exit the spinal canal.

SKELETAL MUSCLE

Skeletal muscles are composed of syncytia *(muscle fibers, myocytes)* derived from numerous cells. The multiple nuclei are normally located just beneath the plasma membrane *(sarcolemma)*; they are slender, oval, and oriented parallel to the length of the fiber with evenly distributed chromatin and inconspicuous nucleoli. Internal nuclei, best seen in transverse section as nuclei within the center of the fiber, are estimated to be found in no more than about 3% of normal adult fibers;[6] they occur

in higher frequency in some pathologic conditions. *Satellite cells*, a reserve cell population, are located adjacent to the sarcolemma and are covered by basement membrane, which encircles the entire muscle fiber.

The entire cytoplasm of the muscle fiber is filled with *myofilaments*, which form the contractile apparatus of *myofibrils* (Fig. 28–3). A myofibril is composed of identical repeating units *(sarcomeres)*, which consist of interlaced, longitudinally directed thin filaments (actin) and thick filaments (myosin) and perpendicularly disposed Z *bands* (primarily α-actinin). The T system, involved in calcium release during excitation, is an invagination of the sarcolemmal membrane into the interior of the cell. The T system runs parallel to the Z bands, accompanied on each side by sarcoplasmic around endoplasmic reticulum. Between the myofibrils is cytoplasm (sarcoplasm), which accounts for 40% of the volume of the fiber and contains myo-

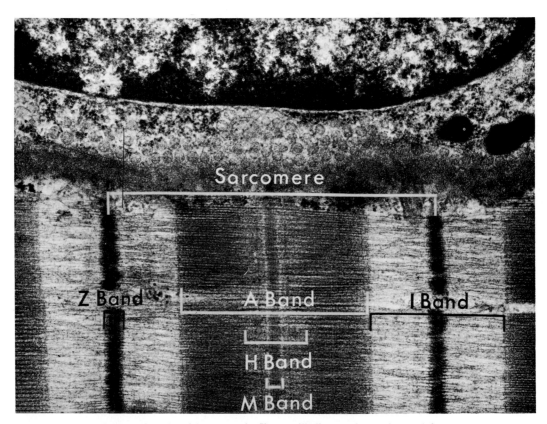

Figure 28–3. Electron micrograph of parts of two muscle fibers with the nucleus of one *(above)* and the most superficial myofibrils of the other *(below)*. Principal features of pattern of cross striations are identified on figure (34,000 ✕). (Courtesy of Bloom, W., and Fawcett, D.W.: A Textbook of Histology, 9th ed. Philadelphia, W.B. Saunders Co., 1968, p. 277.)

globin, glycogen, mitochondria, lysosomes, and lipid vacuoles.

The adult muscle fiber on transverse section is polygonal; in infancy, fibers tend to be round, as are those of the extrinsic eye muscles and some facial muscles in adults. The cross-sectional diameter of individual fibers varies, depending on the specific muscle and its functional status. In humans, two major types of fibers, *type 1* and *type 2*, have been defined on the basis of histochemistry and physiology (Table 28–1). Type 1 fibers are high in myoglobin and oxidative enzymes and have many mitochondria, in keeping with their ability to perform tonic contraction; operationally, they are most often defined by their dark staining for ATPase at pH 4.2 but light staining at pH 9.4. Type 2 fibers are rich in glycolytic enzymes and are involved in rapid phasic contractions; they stain dark with ATPase at pH 9.4 but light at pH 4.2. *Since the motor neuron determines fiber types, all fibers of a single unit are of the same type.* These fibers are distributed randomly across the muscle, giving rise to the *checkerboard* pattern of alternating light and dark fibers as demonstrated with ATPase or other forms of histochemical staining (Fig. 28–4A). There is variability in the relative abundance of fiber types between muscles.[6]

Muscle spindles are fusiform structures that re-spond to stretch in muscles and thus have a role in maintaining tone. They consist of specialized muscle and nerve fibers, delimited by a connective tissue capsule.

The connective tissue sheath of muscles in-

Table 28–1. MUSCLE FIBER TYPES

	TYPE 1	TYPE 2
Action	Sustained force Weight-bearing	Sudden movements Purposeful motion
Enzyme content	NADH dark staining ATPase pH 4.2 dark staining ATPase pH 9.4 light staining	NADH light staining ATPase pH 4.2 light staining ATPase pH 9.4 dark staining
Lipids	Abundant	Scant
Glycogen	Scant	Abundant
Ultrastructure	Many mitochondria Wide Z band	Few mitochondria Narrow Z band
Physiology	Slow-twitch	Fast-twitch
Color	Red	White
Prototype	Soleus (pigeon)	Pectoral (pigeon)

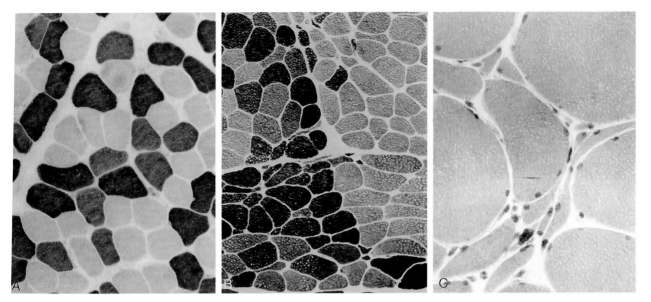

Figure 28-4. *A*, ATPase histochemical staining, at pH 9.4, of normal muscle showing random (checkerboard) distribution of type I (light) and type II (dark) fibers. *B*, In contrast, with reinnervation, fibers of a single histochemical type are grouped together. *C*, A cluster of atrophic fibers (group atrophy).

cludes the *endomysium*, which surrounds individual muscle fibers; the *perimysium*, which groups muscle fibers into primary and secondary bundles (fasciculi); and the *epimysium*, which envelops single muscles or large groups of fibers.

The two main responses of peripheral nerve to injury are based on the target of the insult: the Schwann cell or the axon. Diseases that attack the Schwann cell lead to a loss of myelin *(segmental demyelination)*. In contrast, primary involvement of the neuron and its axon leads to *axonal degeneration*. The two principal pathologic processes seen in skeletal muscle are those consequent to interruption of innervation *(denervation)* and those due to a primary abnormality of the muscle fiber itself *(myopathy)*.

SEGMENTAL DEMYELINATION

Segmental demyelination occurs when there is dysfunction of the Schwann cell and/or damage to the myelin sheath; there is no primary abnormality of the axon. The process affects some Schwann cells, and their corresponding internodes, while sparing others (see Fig. 28-1). The disintegrating myelin is engulfed initially by Schwann cells and later by macrophages. The denuded axon provides a stimulus for remyelination. A population of cells within the endoneurium has the capacity to replace injured Schwann cells. These cells proliferate and encircle the axon and, in time, remyelinate the denuded portion.[7] Newly formed myelinated internodes, however, are shorter than normal, and several are required to bridge the demyelinated re-

gion (see Fig. 28-1). The new myelin sheath is also thin in proportion to the diameter of the axon.

With sequential episodes of demyelination and remyelination, there is an accumulation of tiers of Schwann cell processes that, on transverse section, appear as concentric skeins of cell cytoplasm surrounding the axon *(onion bulbs*, Fig. 28-5). In time, most chronic demyelinating neuropathies are also associated with axonal injury.

AXONAL DEGENERATION AND MUSCLE FIBER ATROPHY

Axonal degeneration is characterized by primary destruction of the axon, with secondary disintegration of its myelin sheath. The damage to the axon may be due either to a discrete, localized event (e.g., trauma, ischemia) or to an underlying abnormality of the neuron *(neuronopathy)* or its axon *(axonopathy)*. When axonal degeneration occurs as the result of transection, the distal portion of the fiber undergoes *Wallerian degeneration* (Fig. 28-6). Within a day, the axon breaks down, and the affected Schwann cells begin to catabolize myelin and later engulf axon fragments, forming small oval compartments *(myelin ovoids)*. Macrophages are recruited into the area and participate in the phagocytosis of axonal and myelin-derived debris.[8] The stump of the proximal portion of the severed nerve shows degenerative changes involving only the most distal two or three internodes and then undergoes regenerative activity. In the slowly evolving neuronopathies or axonopathies, evidence of myelin breakdown is scant because

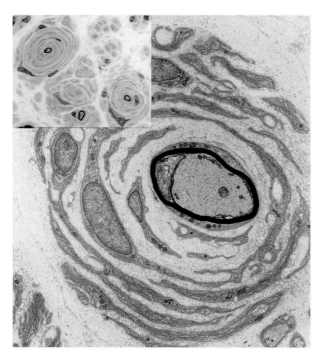

Figure 28–5. Electron micrograph of a single, thinly myelinated axon surrounded by concentrically arranged proliferating Schwann cells, forming an onion bulb. (Courtesy of G. Richard Dickersin, M.D., from the book Diagnostic Electron Microscopy: A Text-Atlas. Igaku-Shoin Medical Publishers, New York, New York; 1988, p. 600.) *Inset*, Light microscopic appearance of an onion bulb neuropathy.

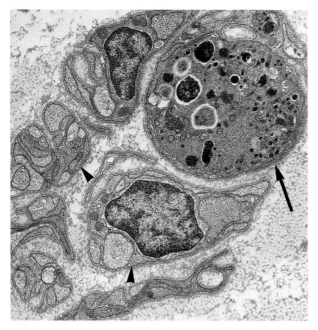

Figure 28–6. Electron micrograph of a degenerating axon *(large arrow)* adjacent to several intact unmyelinated fibers *(arrowheads)*. The axon is markedly distended and contains numerous degenerating organelles and dense bodies.

only a few fibers are degenerating at any given time.

When axonal degeneration occurs, the muscle fibers within that motor unit lose their neural input and undergo *denervation atrophy*. Denervation of muscle leads to down-regulation of myosin and actin synthesis, with a decrease in cell size and resorption of myofibrils, but cells remain viable.[9] In cross-section, the atrophic fibers are smaller than normal and have a roughly triangular shape ("angulated"). There is also cytoskeletal reorganization of some muscle cells, which results in a rounded zone of disorganized filaments *(target fiber)*.

Type 2 fiber atrophy can occur in association with inactivity or disuse in a variety of clinical settings. One of the best examples is the inactivity of a limb that occurs when a plaster cast is applied. The affected muscles may show severe atrophy, especially of the type 2 fibers. A similar picture occurs with disuse, regardless of the cause, in pyramidal tract disorders, neurodegenerative diseases, and mental retardation. As a result, type 2 atrophy is a common finding in muscle biopsies.

NERVE REGENERATION AND REINNERVATION

The proximal stumps of degenerated axons can develop new growth cones that extend along the course of the degenerated axon. The presence of multiple, closely aggregated, thinly myelinated, small-caliber axons is evidence of regeneration *(regenerating cluster)*. This regrowth of axons is a slow process, apparently limited by the rate of the slow component of axonal transport, the movement of tubulin, actin, and intermediate filaments, on the order of 2 mm/day.[10] In spite of its slow pace, axonal regeneration accounts for some of the potential for functional recovery following peripheral axonal injury.

Before the regeneration of axons, however, reinnervation of muscle occurs when surviving axons in the vicinity of denervated myocytes extend sprouts that reinnervate the denervated muscle and incorporate these fibers into their motor unit. Since these orphaned fibers assume the fiber type of their neighbors, a localized group of fibers with the same histochemical properties develops *(type grouping)* (see Fig. 28–4B). *Group atrophy* occurs when a type group becomes denervated (see Fig. 28–4C).

PRIMARY REACTIONS OF THE MUSCLE FIBER

Segmental necrosis, destruction of only a portion of a myocyte, may be followed by *myophagocytosis* as macrophages infiltrate the region. *Regeneration* occurs when peripherally located satellite cells proliferate and reconstitute the destroyed portion of the fiber. The regenerating cell has large internalized nuclei and prominent nucleoli, and the cytoplasm, laden with RNA, becomes basophilic. Other characteristics of myopathic injury include vacuolation, alterations in structural proteins or organelles, and accumulation of intracytoplasmic deposits. Whatever the cause, the loss of fibers is associated with extensive deposition of collagen and fatty infiltration. Fiber *hypertrophy* occurs in response to increased load, either in the setting of exercise or in pathologic conditions in which muscle fibers are injured. Large fibers may divide along a segment (*muscle fiber splitting*) so that, in cross-section, a single large fiber contains a cell membrane traversing its diameter, often with adjacent nuclei.

DISEASES OF PERIPHERAL NERVE

INFLAMMATORY NEUROPATHIES

Acute Inflammatory Demyelinating Polyradiculoneuropathy (Guillain-Barré Syndrome)

Guillain-Barré syndrome (GBS) is one of the most common life-threatening diseases of the peripheral nervous system. The annual incidence is 1 to 2 cases per 100,000 persons in the United States,[11,12] and many patients spend weeks in hospital intensive care units before recovering normal function. With improved respiratory care and support, the mortality rate has fallen from 25% in the past but is still considerable, with some 2 to 5% dying of respiratory paralysis, autonomic instability, and the complications of tracheostomy.[12]

The disease is characterized by an ascending paralysis, with weakness beginning in the distal limbs, but rapidly advancing to affect more proximal muscle functions. Deep tendon reflexes disappear early in the process; although sensory involvement can often be detected, it is less troublesome than the weakness. The nerve conduction velocity is slowed, and there is an elevation of the CSF protein level in the absence of increased cells.

MORPHOLOGY. The dominant histopathologic finding is **inflammation of peripheral nerve**, manifested as perivenular and endoneurial infiltration by lymphocytes, macrophages, and a few plasma cells. The invading cells vary in number, from a sparse seeding of the perivenous spaces to large collections of mononuclear cells disseminated throughout the entire nerve. Although immune-mediated segmental demyelination is considered the primary lesion in GBS,[13] damage to axons characteristically is also present, particularly at autopsy. Electron microscopy has identified an early effect on myelin sheaths. The cytoplasmic processes of macrophages penetrate the basement membrane of Schwann cells, particularly in the vicinity of the nodes of Ranvier, and extend between the myelin lamellae, stripping away the myelin sheath from the axon. Ultimately, the remnants of the myelin sheath are engulfed by the macrophages. Remyelination follows the demyelination and appears to be the same as that following segmental demyelination from other causes.

Inflammatory foci and demyelination are widely distributed throughout the peripheral nervous system, although their intensity is so variable that they may be difficult to identify in an individual case. The most intense inflammatory reaction is often localized in spinal and cranial motor roots and the adjacent parts of the spinal and cranial nerves. The posterior roots, the dorsal root ganglia, the autonomic ganglia, and the more distal parts of nerves are also involved to a lesser extent.

Approximately two-thirds of cases are preceded by an acute, influenza-like illness, usually viral, from which the patient usually has recovered by the time the neuropathy becomes symptomatic. There has been no consistent demonstration of any infectious agent in peripheral nerves in these patients, and the possibility of an immunologically mediated disorder of obscure origin is now generally favored.[13] A similar inflammatory disease of peripheral nerves can be induced in experimental animals by sensitization to peripheral nerve myelin or its components. A T-cell–mediated immune response ensues, accompanied by segmental demyelination, effected by macrophages. Transfer of these T cells to a naive animal results in comparable lesions.[14] Moreover, lymphocytes from patients with GBS have been shown to produce demyelination in tissue cultures of myelinated nerve fibers. Circulating antibodies may also play a part,[15] and plasmapheresis has been reported to be beneficial.

Chronic Inflammatory Demyelinating Polyradiculoneuropathy (CIDP)

In some patients, inflammatory demyelinating polyradiculopathy, instead of occurring as an acute illness as in GBS, follows a subacute or chronic course usually with relapses and remissions, in some instances over several years. There is often a symmetric, mixed sensorimotor polyneuropathy, although some patients have predominantly sensory or motor impairment. Clinical response has been reported with steroid treatment and plasmapheresis. The histologic appearance is similar to that in GBS. Some peripheral nerves show evidence of recurrent demyelination and remyelination with well-developed onion-bulb structures.

INFECTIOUS POLYNEUROPATHIES

Leprosy

Leprosy is the result of infection with *Myocobacterium leprae,* an acid-fast, rod-like organism of relatively low virulence that is found within the cells of the host (see Chapter 8). There is a spectrum of clinical manifestations extending from *lepromatous leprosy,* in which there is active growth of *M. leprae* and spread of organisms through the affected tissues, to *tuberculoid leprosy,* which is characterized by a vigorous immune response and very sparse evidence of the microorganisms.[16]

MORPHOLOGY. In lepromatous leprosy, Schwann cells are often invaded by *M. leprae,* which proliferate and eventually infect other cells. There is evidence of segmental demyelination and remyelination, and loss of both myelinated and unmyelinated axons. As the infection advances, endoneurial fibrosis and multilayered thickening of the perineurial sheaths occurs. Tuberculoid leprosy shows evidence of active cell-mediated immune response to *M. leprae,* with nodular granulomatous inflammation situated in the dermis. The inflammation injures cutaneous nerves in the vicinity; axons, Schwann cells, and myelin are lost, and there is fibrosis of the perineurium and endoneurium.

Diphtheric Neuropathy

This disorder results from the effects of the diphtheria exotoxin on peripheral nerves and begins with paresthesias and weakness; early loss of proprioception and vibratory sensation is common.

MORPHOLOGY. The earliest changes are seen in the sensory ganglia, where the incomplete blood-nerve barrier allows entry of the toxin.[17] There is selective demyelination of axons that extends into adjacent anterior and posterior roots as well as into the mixed sensorimotor nerve.

Varicella-Zoster Virus (VZV)

This virus is one of the few that produce lesions in the peripheral nervous system. Latent infection of neurons in the sensory ganglia of the spinal cord and brain stem follows chickenpox, and reactivation leads to a painful, vesicular skin eruption in the distribution of sensory dermatomes *(shingles),* most frequently thoracic or trigeminal. The virus may be transported along the sensory nerves to the skin, where it establishes an active infection of epidermal cells. In a small proportion of patients, weakness is also apparent in the same distribution. Although the factors giving rise to reactivation are not fully understood, decreased cell-mediated immunity is of major importance in many cases.[18]

MORPHOLOGY. Affected ganglia show neuronal destruction and loss, usually accompanied by abundant mononuclear inflammatory infiltrates. Regional necrosis with hemorrhage may also be found. Peripheral nerve shows axonal degeneration following the death of the sensory neurons. Focal destruction of the large motor neurons of the anterior horns or cranial nerve motor nuclei may be seen at the corresponding levels. Intranuclear inclusions generally are not found in the nervous system.

HEREDITARY NEUROPATHIES

The genetic and pathophysiologic basis of many of the hereditary peripheral neuropathies remains unknown; in the absence of such understanding, these disorders have been classified on the basis of the mode of inheritance, the functional modalities affected, and the cellular and molecular pathology. *As the molecular basis of hereditary neuropathy is further defined, adjustments in the classification scheme can be anticipated.*

Most hereditary neuropathies affect both strength and sensation and have been termed *hereditary motor and sensory neuropathies (HMSN).*[19] In others, symptoms are usually limited to numbness, pain, and/or autonomic dysfunction such as orthostatic hypotension; these diseases have been termed *hereditary sensory and autonomic neuropathies (HSAN)* (Table 28–2). In addition, some hereditary neuropathies are notable for the deposition of amyloid within the nerve; these *familial amyloid polyneuropathies* have a clinical presentation similar to that of the HSAN. The pathologic findings of many of the hereditary neuropathies are those of an axonal neuropathy, with fiber loss being the most prominent finding, although other neuropathologic features are useful in distinguishing between different diseases. The characteristics

Table 28–2. HEREDITARY SENSORY AND AUTONOMIC NEUROPATHIES

DISEASE	INHERITANCE	CLINICAL FINDINGS	PATHOLOGIC FINDINGS
HSAN I	Autosomal dominant	Predominantly sensory neuropathy, often presenting in young adults with secondary consequences such as foot ulcers	Axonal degeneration (myelinated fibers affected more than unmyelinated)
HSAN II	Autosomal recessive (some cases are sporadic)	Predominantly sensory neuropathy, presenting in infancy or early childhood	Axonal degeneration (myelinated fibers affected more than unmyelinated); nerve biopsy may reveal complete absence of myelinated fibers
HSAN III (Riley-Day syndrome; familial dysautonomia)	Autosomal recessive (most often in Jewish children)	Predominantly autonomic neuropathy, often presenting in infancy with symptoms such as postural hypotension, absence of tears, and excessive sweating	Axonal degeneration (unmyelinated fibers affected more than myelinated); atrophy and loss of sensory and autonomic ganglion cells

of neuropathies associated with known biochemical abnormalities are presented in Table 28–3.

Hereditary Motor and Sensory Neuropathy I (HMSN I)

There are three common forms of HMSN. The most common hereditary peripheral neuropathy, *Charcot-Marie-Tooth disease, hypertrophic form* *(HMSN I)*, usually presents in childhood or early adulthood. The progressive muscular atrophy of the calf seen in these patients gave rise to the common clinical term *peroneal muscular atrophy.* Patients may be asymptomatic, but when they present, it is often with symptoms such as distal muscle weakness, atrophy of the calf, or secondary orthopedic problems of the foot (e.g., *pes cavus*). In some patients, there is palpable nerve enlargement, which gives rise to the term "hypertrophic

Table 28–3. HEREDITARY NEUROPATHIES WITH KNOWN METABOLIC CAUSE

DISEASE	METABOLIC DEFECT	INHERITANCE	CLINICAL FINDINGS	PATHOLOGIC FINDINGS
Adrenoleukodystrophy	Fatty acyl-CoA ligase activity (peroxisomal transporter enzyme)	X-linked; 4% of female carriers are symptomatic	Mixed motor and sensory neuropathy, adrenal insufficiency, spastic paraplegia; onset between 10 and 20 for males (leukodystrophy); between 20 and 40 for females (myeloneuropathy)	Axonal degeneration (myelinated and unmyelinated); segmental demyelination, with onion bulbs; electron microscopy: linear inclusions in Schwann cells
Familial amyloid polyneuropathies	Point mutations in transthyretin; rare pedigrees involve other molecules	Autosomal dominant	Sensory and autonomic dysfunction; age at onset varies with site of mutation	Amyloid deposits in vessel walls and connective tissue with axonal degeneration
Porphyria (acute intermittent, coproporphyria, variegate)	Enzymes involved in heme synthesis	Autosomal dominant	Acute episodes of neurologic dysfunction, psychiatric disturbances, abdominal pain, seizures, proximal weakness, autonomic dysfunction; attacks may be precipitated by drugs	Acute and chronic axonal degeneration; regenerating clusters
Refsum's disease	Phytanic acid α-hydroxylase (peroxisomal enzyme)	Autosomal recessive	Mixed motor and sensory neuropathy with palpable nerves; ataxia, night blindness, retinitis pigmentosa, ichthyosis; age at onset before 20 years (a genetically distinct infantile form also exists)	Severe onion-bulb formation

neuropathy." The disorder is usually autosomal dominant, and although it is slowly progressive, the disability is usually limited in severity and a normal life span is typical. It is now apparent that this disease is genetically heterogeneous. In most pedigrees, the altered gene on chromosome 17 has been identified as encoding a myelin-specific protein, PMP-22 (type 1A).[20] A separate locus has been identified on chromosome 1 (myelin protein P$_o$; type 1B[21]), and some pedigrees show no linkage to either of these sites (type 1C). In addition some pedigrees have a genetic locus on the X chromosome, with mutations in the gene for the gap junction protein connexin.[22]

MORPHOLOGY. Histologic examination shows multiple onion bulbs, more pronounced in distal than in proximal nerves (see Fig. 28–5). The axon is often present in the center of the onion bulbs. The myelin sheath may be thin or absent. In the longitudinal plane, individual segments of the axon may show evidence of segmental demyelination. There is also degeneration of the posterior columns of the spinal cord in these patients.

The relationship between the molecular abnormalities and the observed peripheral nerve pathology is not well understood. The presence of onion bulbs and segmental demyelination suggest that Schwann cell abnormalities form the basis of the neuropathy. Alternatively, there are other features that suggest an axonal disturbance, including the distal predominance of onion bulbs, nonrandom distribution of segmental demyelination, and reports of motor neuron loss.

HMSN II

There is also a neuronal form of Charcot-Marie-Tooth disease, HMSN II, that presents with signs and symptoms similar to those of HMSN I, although nerve enlargement is not seen and the disease presents at a slightly later age. This form is less common than HMSN I, and the autosomal dominant genetic locus has not been identified, although it appears to be distinct from those identified for HMSN I.[23]

MORPHOLOGY. Nerve biopsies in this disorder show loss of myelinated axons as the predominant finding, although occasional onion bulbs may be present. In addition, segmental demyelination of internodes is infrequent. These findings suggest that the primary cellular dysfunction is the axon or neuron.

HMSN III

Patients with *Dejerine-Sottas disease (HMSN III)* often present in infancy with a delay in the acquisition of motor skills, such as walking. Distal weakness is accompanied by truncal weakness, and the weakness and atrophy are usually not limited to the legs as in HMSN I or II. Areflexia may also be present, and the velocity of nerve conduction is markedly reduced. A dramatic finding on physical examination is the presence of *enlarged peripheral nerves that can be detected by palpation*. The disorder is slowly progressive, often resulting in severe neurologic impairment; it is inherited in an autosomal recessive pattern, and the gene locus has not been identified.

MORPHOLOGY. The size of individual peripheral nerve fascicles is increased, often dramatically, with abundant onion bulb formation as well as segmental demyelination. There is usually evidence of axonal loss, and those axons that remain are often of diminished caliber. All of these findings are usually most severe in the distal portions of the peripheral nervous system; however, autopsy studies have shown that similar findings may be present in spinal roots.

ACQUIRED METABOLIC AND TOXIC NEUROPATHIES

Peripheral Neuropathy in Adult-Onset Diabetes Mellitus

Several distinct patterns of diabetes-related peripheral nerve abnormalities have been recognized and can be broadly categorized as *distal symmetric sensory or sensory-motor neuropathy, autonomic neuropathy,* and *focal or multifocal asymmetric neuropathy*. Individuals may develop any combination of these lesions, and in fact the first two are often found together.

The most common of these patterns of injury is the symmetric neuropathy that involves distal sensory and motor nerves. These patients develop decreased sensation in the distal extremities with comparably less evident motor abnormalities. The loss of pain sensation can result in the development of ulcers that, because of the diffuse microvascular injury in diabetes, heal poorly and are a major cause of morbidity.

MORPHOLOGY. The predominant pathologic finding is an axonal neuropathy; as with other chronic axonal neuropathies, there also is some segmental demyelination. There is a relative loss of small mye-

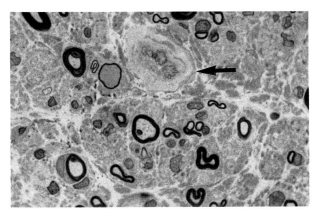

Figure 28–7. Diabetic neuropathy with marked loss of myelinated fibers, a thinly myelinated fiber, and thickening of endoneurial vessel wall *(arrow).*

linated fibers and of unmyelinated fibers, but large fibers are also affected. Endoneurial arterioles show thickening, hyalinization, and intense PAS-positivity in their walls and extensive reduplication of the basement membrane (Fig. 28–7).[24,25] The microvascular changes seen in nerves from diabetics suggest that the lesions may be due to ischemia, although the pattern of a symmetric and distal process is more commonly seen in association with intoxication or metabolic dysfunction.

Another manifestation of peripheral neuropathy in diabetic patients is *dysfunction of the autonomic nervous system;* this affects 20 to 40% of diabetics, nearly always in association with a distal sensorimotor neuropathy.[26] The basis of these abnormalities remains ambiguous, but pathologic findings suggest some differences from the symmetric sensorimotor neuropathy.

In some patients, especially elderly adults with a long history of diabetes, neuropathy manifests itself as a disorder of single individual nerves *(mononeuropathy)* or of several individual nerves in an asymmetric distribution *(multiple mononeuropathy or mononeuropathy multiplex).* Unilateral ocular nerve palsy, with sparing of reflexes, is a recognized clinical syndrome.

Metabolic and Nutritional Causes of Peripheral Neuropathy

As many as 65% of patients with renal failure have clinical evidence of peripheral neuropathy *(uremic neuropathy)* prior to dialysis.[27] This is typically a distal, symmetric neuropathy that may be asymptomatic or may be associated with muscle cramps,

distal dysesthesias, and diminished deep tendon reflexes.

MORPHOLOGY. In these patients, it appears that axonal degeneration is the primary event, with degenerating fibers and fiber loss. In addition, some fibers have thin myelin sheaths indicative of previous demyelination; however, these changes have been interpreted as a secondary event **(secondary demyelination).** Regeneration and recovery are common following dialysis, although they are usually complete only in mild cases.

Peripheral neuropathy can also develop in patients with chronic liver disease, chronic respiratory insufficiency,[27] and thyroid dysfunction. *Thiamine deficiency* is characterized by axonal neuropathy, a clinical condition termed neuropathic *beriberi.* Axonal neuropathies also occur with deficiencies of vitamins B_{12} (cobalamin), B_6 (pyridoxine), and E (α-tocopherol).

Neuropathies Associated with Malignancy

Direct infiltration or compression of peripheral nerves by tumor is a common cause of mononeuropathy and may be the presenting symptom of cancer. These neuropathies include brachial plexopathy from neoplasms of the apex of the lung, obturator palsy from pelvic malignancies, and cranial nerve palsies from intracranial tumors and tumors of the base of the skull. A polyradiculopathy involving the lower extremity may develop when the cauda equina is involved by meningeal carcinomatosis.

In distinction to these phenomena, which all involve direct interaction between neoplastic cells and nerve, a diffuse, symmetric peripheral neuropathy may occur in patients with a distant carcinoma, and is considered a remote, or *paraneoplastic,* effect (see Chapter 7). The most common paraneoplastic neuropathy is a sensorimotor lesion, characterized by weakness and sensory deficits that are often more pronounced in the lower extremities and that progress over months to years. The neuropathy is most often associated with carcinoma of the lung, especially small cell carcinoma; as many as 2 to 5% of patients with lung cancer may have clinical evidence of peripheral neuropathy. Patients with the less frequent pure sensory neuropathy present with numbness and paresthesias, symptoms that may precede the identification of the malignancy by 6 to 15 months. Paraneoplastic sensory neuropathy, although less common than the sensorimotor form, is even more strongly associated with small cell carcinoma of the lung.[28]

MORPHOLOGY. The sensory manifestations are due to degeneration of dorsal root ganglion cells, with a proliferative response by the surrounding satellite cells. Inflammatory infiltrates, composed of plasma cells and lymphocytes with a predominance of CD8+ T cells, are found in the ganglia and may extend into the adjacent nerves. Axonal degeneration is seen in both the peripheral nervous system and in the dorsal columns of the spinal cord.

Although the pathogenetic mechanism of paraneoplastic sensory neuropathy is not established, an immunologic mechanism has been suggested based on the presence of inflammatory infiltrates within the dorsal root ganglia and the identification of a circulating polyclonal IgG antibody. This antibody (anti-Hu), which has been identified in patients with small cell carcinoma of the lung and a subacute sensory neuropathy, binds to a 35 to 38 kd RNA-binding protein expressed by neurons and the tumor.[29]

Patients with plasma cell dyscrasias may develop a peripheral neuropathy in one of two recognized ways. The first is through the deposition of light chain amyloid in peripheral nerves. While it is uncommon to have peripheral nerve involvement in reactive systemic amyloidosis (AA type), 20% of patients with amyloid derived from immunoglobulin (AL type) have a peripheral neuropathy. The initial symptoms include weakness, and amyloid is deposited in the peripheral nervous system.

Patients with plasma cell dyscrasias may develop a peripheral neuropathy independent of the presence or deposition of amyloid. They often present with a symmetric sensorimotor neuropathy that progresses over months to years. Although the pathogenesis of this neuropathy is not established, in a subset of these patients with IgM monoclonal gammopathy the protein is deposited within peripheral nerve. In addition, in 50% of patients with IgM monoclonal gammopathy and peripheral neuropathy, the IgM binds to myelin-associated glycoprotein (MAG), a 100-kd glycoprotein with a 30% carbohydrate content, present in myelin.[30] Patients with osteosclerotic myeloma have a higher frequency of neuropathy than those with osteolytic tumors.

Toxic Neuropathies

Peripheral neuropathies can occur following exposure to industrial or environmental chemicals, biologic toxins, or therapeutic drugs.[31] Prominent among the environmental chemicals causing neuropathy are heavy metals, including lead and arsenic (see Chapter 9). In addition, many organic compounds are known to be neurotoxic; some examples are listed in Table 28–4.

Table 28–4. TOXIC NEUROPATHIES DUE TO ORGANIC COMPOUNDS

TOXIC AGENT	SOURCE OF EXPOSURE	MOLECULAR BASIS	CLINICAL FINDINGS	PATHOLOGIC FINDINGS
Ethanol	Alcoholic beverages	Probable superimposed nutritional deficiencies	Slowly progressive distal sensorimotor neuropathy	Axonal degeneration (myelinated and unmyelinated fibers)
Acrylamide	Industry (polymerizing agent used as flocculant and for grouting)	Unknown	Numbness and sweating of hands and feet, progressing to distal sensorimotor neuropathy	Axonal degeneration, most pronounced in distal nerve (large-caliber fibers most affected)
Hexane	Industry (solvent), and inhalant abuse ("glue sniffing")	Protein alkylation; impaired intermediate filament transport	Distal symmetric sensorimotor polyneuropathy	Enlarged axons filled with neurofilaments; axonal degeneration predominantly affecting large-caliber axons
Organophosphorus esters	Industry (pesticides, petroleum additives, plasticizers) and contaminated food products	Induction of esterase activity ("neurotoxic esterase"); altered protein phosphorylation	Rapidly progressive distal sensorimotor polyneuropathy after latent phase (7–21 days)	Axonal degeneration affecting long axons of the peripheral and central nervous systems
Vinca alkaloids	Medicine (vincristine used in cancer chemotherapy)	Impaired assembly of microtubules	Diminished ankle jerk earliest sign; subsequent progression to sensorimotor neuropathy	Axonal degeneration; large intravenous doses may cause accumulation of filaments in cell bodies

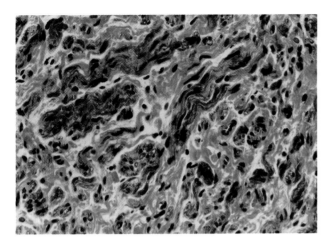

Figure 28-8. Traumatic neuroma showing disordered orientation of nerve fiber bundles (purple), intermixed with connective tissue (blue).

TRAUMATIC NEUROPATHIES

Peripheral nerves are commonly injured in the course of trauma. *Lacerations* result from cutting injuries and can complicate fractures when a sharp fragment of bone lacerates the nerve. *Avulsions* occur when tension is applied to a peripheral nerve, often as the result of a force applied to one of the limbs.

> **MORPHOLOGY.** Following laceration and avulsion injuries, axons degenerate along the entire distal extent of the involved nerve. Distal to the site of injury, the changes are very similar to other forms of axonal degeneration, with the entire axonal cylinder fragmenting into oval structures. The direct mechanical interruption of nerve integrity is associated with hemorrhage, and there is transection of the connective tissue planes. Regeneration of peripheral nerve axons does occur, albeit slowly, and is dependent on axonal growth cones tracking along Schwann cells and their basal lamina. Regrowth may be complicated by discontinuity between the proximal and distal portions of the nerve sheath as well as the misalignment of individual fascicles.
>
> Axons, even in the absence of correctly positioned distal segments, may continue to grow, resulting in a mass of tangled axonal processes known as a **traumatic neuroma (pseudoneuroma or amputation neuroma)**. Within this mass, small bundles of axons appear randomly oriented; each, however, is surrounded by organized layers containing Schwann cells, fibroblasts, and perineurial cells (Fig. 28–8).

Compression neuropathy (entrapment neuropathy) occurs when a peripheral nerve is compressed, often within an anatomic compartment.

Carpal tunnel syndrome is the most common entrapment neuropathy and results from compression of the median nerve at the level of the wrist within the compartment delimited by the transverse carpal ligament. Females are more commonly affected than males, and the problem is frequently bilateral. The disorder may be observed with any condition that can cause decreased available space within the carpal tunnel, such as tissue edema, but predisposing factors include pregnancy, degenerative joint disease, hypothyroidism, amyloidosis (especially that related to β_2-microglobulin deposition in renal dialysis patients), and excessive usage of the wrist.[32,33] Symptoms are limited to dysfunction of the median nerve, including numbness and paresthesias of the tips of the thumb and first two digits.

Additional entrapment neuropathies include involvement of the ulnar nerve at the level of the elbow, the peroneal nerve at the level of the knee, and the radial nerve in the upper arm, as seen after sleeping with the arm improperly positioned ("Saturday night palsy"). Another form of compression neuropathy is found in the foot, affecting the interdigital nerve at intermetatarsal sites. This problem, which occurs nearly exclusively in women, leads to foot pain (metatarsalgia). The histologic findings of the lesion *(Morton's neuroma)* include evidence of chronic compressive injury.

TUMORS OF PERIPHERAL NERVE

Both benign and malignant tumors can be derived from elements of the nerve sheath. These are discussed in association with tumors of the central nervous system (CNS) (see Chapter 29).

DISEASES OF SKELETAL MUSCLE

MUSCULAR DYSTROPHIES

The muscular dystrophies are a heterogeneous group of inherited disorders characterized clinically by progressively severe muscular weakness and wasting, often beginning in childhood.

X-Linked Muscular Dystrophy

The two most common forms of muscular dystrophy are X-linked: *Duchenne's muscular dystrophy* (DMD) and *Becker's muscular dystrophy (BMD)*. *Duchenne's muscular dystrophy*, the most severe of the dystrophies, with an incidence of about

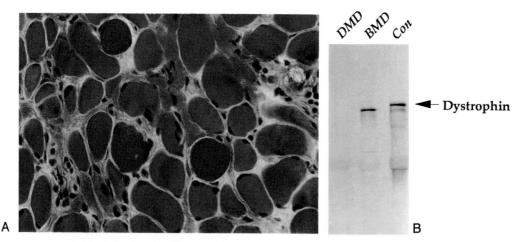

Figure 28-9. *A,* Duchenne's muscular dystrophy showing variation in muscle fiber size, increased endomysial connective tissue, and regenerating fibers (blue hue). *B,* Western blot showing absence of dystrophin in DMD and altered dystrophin size in BMD compared to control (CON). (Courtesy of Dr. L. Kunkel, Children's Hospital, Boston.)

1 per 10,000 males,[34] becomes clinically manifest by the age of five years with weakness leading to wheelchair dependence by 10 to 12 years of age, and progresses relentlessly until death by the early 20s. Boys with DMD are normal at birth, and early motor milestones are met on time. Walking, however, is often delayed, and the first indications of muscle weakness are clumsiness and inability to keep up with peers. Weakness begins in the pelvic girdle muscles and then extends to the shoulder girdle. The use of *Gower's maneuver,* requiring the assistance of the upper extremities to stand up, is a characteristic sign. Enlargement of the calf muscles associated with weakness, a phenomenon termed *pseudohypertrophy,* is an important clinical finding. The increased muscle bulk is caused initially by an increase in the size of the muscle fibers and then, as the muscle atrophies, by an increase in fat and connective tissue. Pathologic changes are also found in the heart, and patients may develop heart failure or arrhythmias. Although there are no well-established structural abnormalities of the CNS, cognitive impairment appears to be a component of the disease and is severe enough in some patients to be considered mental retardation.[35] Serum creatine kinase is elevated during the first decade of life but returns to normal in the later stages of the disease. Death results from respiratory insufficiency, pulmonary infection, and cardiac decompensation.

Approximately one-third of cases of DMD represent new mutations;[34] in the remaining families, obligate female carriers are usually clinically asymptomatic but often have elevated serum creatine kinase and show minimal myopathic histologic abnormalities on muscle biopsy.

Although *Becker's muscular dystrophy (BMD)* involves the same genetic locus, it is less common and much less severe than Duchenne's muscular dystrophy. The onset occurs later in childhood or in adolescence, and is accompanied by a slower and more variable rate of progression, although there is considerable variation between pedigrees. Many patients have a nearly normal life span. Cardiac disease is much rarer in these patients. Although the clinical features originally suggested a relationship between BMD and DMD, the allelic nature of the two diseases is now clear.

MORPHOLOGY. Histopathologic abnormalities common to DMD and BMD include (1) **variation in fiber size** (diameter) (due to the presence of both small and giant fibers, sometimes with fiber splitting); (2) **increased numbers of internalized nuclei** (beyond the normal range of 3%); (3) **degeneration, necrosis, and phagocytosis of muscle fibers;** (4) **regeneration of muscle fibers;** and (5) **proliferation of endomysial connective tissue** (Fig. 28-9A). DMD cases also often show enlarged, rounded, hyaline fibers that have lost their normal cross-striations, believed to be hypercontracted fibers; this finding is rare in BMD. Both type 1 and type 2 fibers are involved, and no alterations in the proportion or distribution of fiber types are evident. Histochemical reactions sometimes fail to identify distinct fiber types in DMD. In later stages, the muscles eventually become almost totally replaced by fat and connective tissue, an appearance indistinguishable from the end-stage of other severe muscle diseases. Cardiac involvement, when present, consists of nonspecific interstitial fibrosis, more prominent in the subendocardial layers. Despite the clinical evidence of CNS dysfunction in DMD, no consistent neuropathologic abnormalities have been described.

The molecular genetic and biochemical investigations of DMD represent a major recent achievement in the understanding and diagnosis of this disease. The gene is enormous $(2.5 \times 10^6$ base

Table 28–5. MISCELLANEOUS MUSCULAR DYSTROPHIES

DISEASE	INHERITANCE	CLINICAL FINDINGS	PATHOLOGIC FINDINGS
Fascioscapulohu-meral (FSH) mus-cular dystrophy	Autosomal domi-nant	Variable age at onset (most com-monly 10–30 years); weakness of muscles of face, neck, and shoulder girdle (gene localized to 4q35)	Dystrophic myopathy, but also often including inflammatory in-filtrate of muscle
Oculopharyngeal muscular dys-trophy	Autosomal domi-nant	Onset in midadult life; ptosis and weakness of extraocular mus-cles; difficulty in swallowing	Dystrophic myopathy, but often in-cluding rimmed vacuoles in type 1 fibers
Limb-girdle dys-trophy (hetero-geneous group)	Autosomal reces-sive and spo-radic cases are common	Onset often 10–30 years; weak-ness of proximal muscles of upper and lower extremities; usually slowly progressive but prognosis extremely variable	Variable findings of dystrophic my-opathy
Emery-Dreifuss muscular dys-trophy	X-linked	Variable onset (most common 10–20 years); prominent contrac-tures, especially of elbows and ankles	Mild myopathic changes

pairs with more than 80 exons) and is located in the Xp21 region, encoding a 427-kd protein, termed *dystrophin*.[36] The size of the gene has made genetic analysis extremely complicated; dele-tions appear to represent a large proportion of mu-tations, with frameshift and point mutations ac-counting for the rest. Antisera raised against dystrophin have shown that it is normally located adjacent to the sarcolemmal membrane in myo-cytes. Muscle biopsies from patients with DMD show minimal evidence of dystrophin by both staining and direct measurements (Western blot).[37] BMD patients, who also have mutations in the dys-trophin gene, have identifiable protein, usually of an abnormal molecular weight, reflecting mutations that allow synthesis of some dystrophin (see Fig. 28–9B). The molecule has been further localized to sites of I and M bands and has been suggested to play a role in maintaining the integrity of the myocyte membrane during the shape changes asso-ciated with contraction. The recent advances in the molecular understanding of DMD point to possibil-ities for genetic therapy.

Other forms of muscular dystrophy share many of the histologic features of DMD and BMD but have distinct clinical and pathologic features (Table 28–5).

Myotonic Dystrophy

Myotonia, the sustained involuntary contraction of a group of muscles, is the cardinal neuromuscular symptom in this disease.[38] Patients often complain of "stiffness" and have difficulty in releasing their grip, as following a handshake. Myotonia can often be elicited by percussion of the thenar eminence. The disease begins in late childhood with gait dif-ficulty secondary to weakness of foot dorsiflexors, then progresses to weakness of the hand intrinsic

muscles and wrist extensors. Atrophy of muscles of the face and ptosis ensue, leading to the typical facial appearance. Cataracts, which are present in virtually every patient, may be detected early in the course of the disease with slit-lamp examina-tion. Other associated abnormalities include frontal balding, gonadal atrophy, cardiomyopathy, smooth muscle involvement, decreased plasma IgG, and an abnormal glucose tolerance test. Dementia has been reported in some cases. Inherited as an auto-somal dominant trait, the disease tends to increase in severity and come on at a younger age in suc-ceeding generations, a phenomenon termed *antici-pation*. The disease may present as congenital weakness and is then associated with maternal in-heritance. In these cases, symptoms are severe, with facial diplegia, feeding difficulties, and respi-ratory insufficiency.

MORPHOLOGY. Pathologically, skeletal muscle may show features of a dystrophy similar to Duchenne's muscular dystrophy. In addition, there is a striking increase in the number of internal nuclei, which on longitudinal section may form conspicuous chains. Another well-recognized abnormality is the **ring fiber**, with a subsarcolemmal band of cytoplasm that appears distinct from the center of the fiber. The rim contains myofibrils that are oriented cir-cumferentially in relation to the longitudinally ori-ented fibrils in the rest of the fiber. The ring fiber may be associated with an irregular mass of sarco-plasm **(sarcoplasmic mass)** extending outward from the ring. These stain blue with H&E, red with Gomori trichrome, and intensely blue with the nico-tinamide-adenine dinucleotide (NADH) histochemi-cal reaction. The relation of the ring fiber to clinical myotonia is not understood. Histochemical tech-niques have demonstrated a relative atrophy of type 1 fibers early in the course of the disease in

Table 28-6. CONGENITAL MYOPATHIES

DISEASE	INHERITANCE	CLINICAL FINDINGS	PATHOLOGIC FINDINGS
Central core disease	Autosomal dominant (or sporadic)	Early-onset hypotonia and non-progressive weakness; associated skeletal deformities; may develop malignant hyperthermia	Cytoplasmic cores are lightly eosinophilic and distinct from surrounding sarcoplasm; only found in type 1 fibers, which usually predominate
Nemaline myopathy	Variable	Weakness, hypotonia, and delayed motor development in childhood; may also be seen in adults; usually nonprogressive; involves proximal limb muscles most severely; skeletal abnormalities may be present	Aggregates of subsarcolemmal spindle-shaped particles (nemaline rods); occur predominantly in type 1 fibers; derived from Z-band material (α-actinin)
Centronuclear myopathy	Autosomal recessive; rarer severe X-linked recessive; later onset autosomal dominant; sporadic	Presents in infancy or early childhood with prominent involvement of extraocular and facial muscles, hypotonia, and slowly progressive limb muscle weakness	Abundance of centrally located nuclei involving the majority of muscle fibers; central nuclei are usually confined to type 1 fibers, which are small in diameter, but can occur in both fiber types

some cases. Of all the dystrophies, only myotonic dystrophy shows pathologic changes in the intrafusal fibers of muscle spindles, with fiber splitting, necrosis, and regeneration.

The gene for myotonic dystrophy has been localized to 19q13.2–13.3; cloning by several groups[39] demonstrated that the gene codes for a protein kinase, termed *myotonin-protein kinase.* Located in the 3' untranslated region of the gene, it is a trinucleotide repeat, consisting of $(CTG)_n$. The disease phenotype is associated with expansion of this region; in normal subjects fewer than 30 repeats are present, whereas in severely affected individuals several thousand may be present.[40] The mutation is not stable within a pedigree; with each generation, more repeats accumulate, and this appears to correspond to the phenomenon of anticipation. Expansion of the trinucleotide repeat influences the eventual level of protein product.

CONGENITAL MYOPATHIES

The congenital myopathies are a group of disorders defined largely on the basis of the pathologic findings within muscle. Most of these conditions share common clinical features, including onset in early life, nonprogressive or slowly progressive course, proximal or generalized muscle weakness, and hypotonia. Those affected at birth or in early infancy may present as "floppy babies" because of hypotonia or may have severe joint contractures *(arthrogryposis)*; however, both hypotonia and arthrogryposis may also be caused by other neuromuscular dysfunction.

The best-characterized myopathies are listed in Table 28–6, and Figure 28–10 shows the structural characteristics of nemaline myopathy, one of the most distinctive types.

MYOPATHIES ASSOCIATED WITH INBORN ERRORS OF METABOLISM

Many of the myopathies associated with metabolic disease are found in the setting of disorders of glycogen synthesis and degradation (see Chapter 5). Myopathies can also result from disorders of mitochondrial metabolism.

Lipid Myopathies

In order to undergo beta-oxidation, cytoplasmic fatty acyl-CoA esters are conjugated with carnitine through the action of carnitine palmitoyl transferase (CPT), transported across the inner mitochondrial membrane, and then re-esterified to acyl-CoA esters. Deficiencies affecting the carnitine system can lead to the accumulation of lipid droplets within muscle *(lipid myopathies)* and can result from a deficiency of either carnitine or carnitine palmitoyl transferase.

Carnitine deficiency may be limited to muscle (myopathic carnitine deficiency) or may be secondary to diminished systemic levels (systemic carnitine deficiency). The cardinal symptom of the so-called myopathic form of disease is weakness; the age at onset is variable. Since it has recently been recognized that systemic carnitine deficiency can occur as a result of several disorders of beta-oxidation of fatty acids, including medium chain acyl-CoA dehydrogenase (MCAD) deficiency,[41] it has been suggested that systemic carnitine deficiency is not a single disease entity.

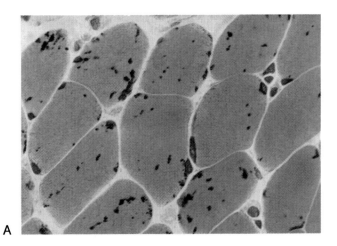

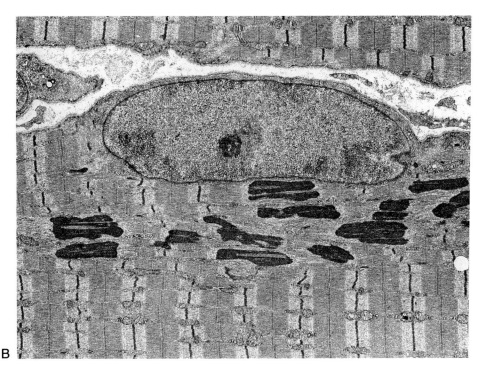

Figure 28-10. *A,* Nemaline myopathy with numerous rod-shaped, intracytoplasmic inclusions (dark purple structures). *B,* Electron micrograph of subsarcolemmal nemaline bodies, showing material of Z-band density.

In contrast, CPT deficiency often presents as recurrent myoglobinuria.[42] Episodic acute myonecrosis *(rhabdomyolysis)* follows prolonged exercise and leads to the release of myoglobin into plasma, which when excreted gives the urine an alarmingly dark color (myoglobinuria). Renal failure can occur following massive episodes of rhabdomyolysis and is a serious complication of CPT deficiency.

MORPHOLOGY. In all of the lipid myopathies the principal morphologic characteristic is accumulation of lipid within myocytes. The myofibrils are separated by vacuoles which stain with oil red O or Sudan black and have the typical appearance of lipid by electron microscopy. The vacuoles occur predominantly in type 1 fibers and they are dispersed diffusely throughout the fiber.

Mitochondrial Myopathies

Approximately one-fifth of the proteins involved in mitochondrial oxidative phosphorylation are encoded by the mitochondrial genome (mtDNA); additionally, this 16.6-kb circular genome codes for mitochondrial specific tRNA and rRNA species.[43] The remainder of the mitochondrial enzyme complexes are encoded in the nuclear genome. Diseases that involve the mtDNA show maternal inheritance, since the oocyte contributes the mitochondria to the embryo. Potential understanding of the tissue specificity of these diseases comes from the observation that the proportion of normal to abnormal mitochondria can vary from cell to cell and tissue to tissue *(heteroplasmy)*, although some of the mitochondrial diseases do not show this phenomenon. Mitochondrial metabolic defects

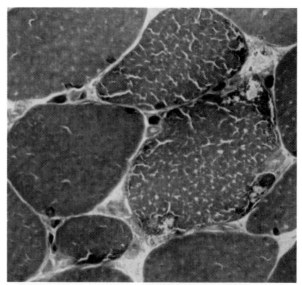

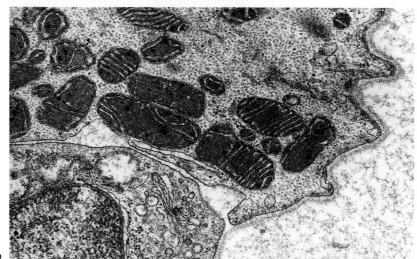

Figure 28–11. *A,* Mitochondrial myopathy showing an irregular fiber with subsarcolemmal collections of mitochondria that stain red on trichrome staining *(ragged red fiber). B,* Electron micrograph of mitochondria from biopsy in *A,* showing "parking lot" inclusions.

identified so far include defects in respiratory chain protein complexes I, III, and IV.[44] The diseases typically present in young adulthood (less often in infancy) and manifest with proximal muscle weakness, sometimes with severe external ophthalmoplegia. The weakness may be accompanied by other neurologic symptoms, lactic acidosis, and cardiomyopathy, so that this group may also be classified as mitochondrial encephalomyopathies (see Chapter 29).

MORPHOLOGY. The most consistent pathologic finding is aggregates of abnormal mitochondria that are demonstrable only by special techniques. These occur subsarcolemmally in type 1 muscle cells; with severe involvement they may extend throughout the fiber. The abnormal mitochondria impart a blotchy red appearance to the muscle fiber on Gomori trichrome stain. Since they are also associated with distortion of the myofibrils, the muscle fiber contour becomes irregular on cross-section, and the descriptive term **"ragged red fibers"** has been applied to them (Fig. 28–11A).[45] The electron microscopic appearance is often distinctive: there are increased numbers of, and abnormalities in the shape and size of, mitochondria, some of which contain paracrystalline **parking-lot inclusions** or alterations in the structure of cristae (Fig. 28–11B).[46]

There is variability in presentation and progression of the disorders in this category, and the precise classification is undergoing change as their biochemical basis is being clarified; however, several clinical syndromes have been identified that are consistently associated with abnormalities in mitochondrial DNA (mtDNA). *Chronic progressive external ophthalmoplegia* is characterized by a myopathy with prominent weakness of external ocular movements. *Kearns-Sayre syndrome* ("ophthalmoplegia plus") is characterized by ophthalmoplegia, pigmentary degeneration of the retina, and complete heart block. Other findings include short stature and cerebellar ataxia. A large deletion of mtDNA has been identified in Kearns-Sayre syndrome,[45,47] in contrast to the mitochondrial encephalomyopathies, which are associated with point mutations.[48,49]

INFLAMMATORY MYOPATHIES

There are a variety of inflammatory diseases involving muscle, including infectious myositis (see Chapter 8), noninfectious inflammatory muscle disease (polymyositis, dermatomyositis, and inclusion body myositis [see Chapter 6]), and inflammatory processes associated with diffuse systemic inflammatory disease (see Chapter 6).

TOXIC MYOPATHIES

Thyroid Dysfunction

Thyrotoxic myopathy presents most commonly as an acute or a chronic proximal muscle weakness that may precede the onset of other signs of thyroid dysfunction. Exophthalmic ophthalmoplegia is characterized by swelling of the eyelids, edema of the conjunctiva, and diplopia.

Another muscle disease associated with thyroid dysfunction is thyrotoxic periodic paralysis, which is characterized by episodic weakness that is often accompanied by hypokalemia. Males are affected four times more often than females, with a high incidence in individuals of Japanese descent. Periodic paralysis may also be seen as a familial disease independent of thyroid dysfunction. Variants associated with elevated, depressed, or normal serum potassium levels are well known. Hyperkalemic periodic paralysis has recently been shown to be caused by specific mutations in the sodium channel of muscle.

> **MORPHOLOGY.** In thyrotoxic myopathy, there is fiber necrosis, regeneration, and interstitial lymphocytes. In chronic thyrotoxic myopathy, there may be only slight variability of fiber size, mitochondrial hypertrophy, and focal myofibril degeneration; fatty infiltration of muscle is seen in very severe cases. In thyrotoxic periodic paralysis, as in the other periodic paralyses, there is dilatation of the sarcoplasmic reticulum and intermyofibril vacuoles during episodes of weakness. Exophthalmic ophthalmoplegia is limited to the extraocular muscles, which may be edematous and enlarged.

In hypothyroidism, there may be cramping or aching of muscles, and movements and reflexes are slowed. Findings include fiber atrophy, an increased number of internal nuclei, glycogen aggregates, and, occasionally, deposition of mucopolysaccharides in the connective tissue.

Ethanol (Alcoholic) Myopathy

"Binge" drinking of alcohol is known to produce an acute toxic syndrome of rhabdomyolysis with accompanying myoglobinuria, which may lead to renal failure. Clinically, the patient may acutely develop pain that is either generalized or confined to a single muscle group. Some patients have a complicated clinicopathologic syndrome consisting of proximal muscle weakness with electrophysiologic evidence of myopathy superimposed on alcoholic neuropathy.

> **MORPHOLOGY.** Histopathologic studies of acute alcoholic myopathy have shown swelling of myocytes, with fiber necrosis, myophagocytosis, and regeneration. There may also be evidence of denervation.

Drug-Induced Myopathies

Proximal muscle weakness and atrophy can occur as a result of the deleterious effects of steroids on muscle, whether in Cushing syndrome or during therapeutic administration of steroids. The severity of clinical disability is variable and not directly related to the steroid level or the therapeutic regimen.

> **MORPHOLOGY. Steroid myopathy** is characterized by muscle fiber atrophy, predominantly affecting type 2 fibers.[6] When the myopathy is severe, there may be a bimodal distribution of fiber sizes, with type 1 fibers of nearly normal caliber and markedly atrophic type 2 fibers. Electron microscopy has shown dilatation of the sarcoplasmic reticulum and thickening of the basal laminae.

Chloroquine, originally used in treatment of malaria but subsequently utilized in other clinical settings, can produce a proximal myopathy in humans.

> **MORPHOLOGY.** The most prominent finding in chloroquine myopathy is the presence of vacuoles within myocytes.[50] Two types of vacuoles have been described: autophagic membrane-bound vacuoles containing membranous debris and curvilinear bodies with short curved membranous structures with

alternating light and dark zones. Vacuoles can be seen in as many as 50% of the myocytes, most commonly type 1 fibers, and with progression, myocyte necrosis may develop.

DISEASES OF THE NEUROMUSCULAR JUNCTION

MYASTHENIA GRAVIS

Now recognized as one of the most well-defined forms of autoimmune disease, myasthenia gravis is a muscle disease with characteristic temporal and anatomic patterns as well as drug responses. The weakness fluctuates, with alterations occurring over days, hours, or even minutes, and intercurrent medical conditions can lead to exacerbations of the weakness. When there is compromised respiratory function, the patient has a *crisis*, which may occur spontaneously. Extraocular muscles are involved in the vast majority of cases and are often the site of first disability, with ptosis and diplopia causing the patient to seek medical attention. Involvement of the limbs is also found but is only rarely seen in isolation. It was noted early on that patients had a transient improvement in strength in response to administration of anticholinesterase agents; this remains the most diagnostic feature of the clinical examination (Tensilon test).[51] Electrophysiologic studies are notable for decrement in motor responses with repeated stimulation; nerve conduction studies are normal. Sensory as well as autonomic functions are not affected. The analysis of neuromuscular transmission in myasthenia gravis is consistent with a decrease in the number of muscle acetylcholine receptors (AChRs). Circulating antibodies to the AChR have been demonstrated in nearly all patients with myasthenia gravis,[51] and the disease can be passively transferred to animals.

The disease has an incidence of about 3 in 100,000 persons.[52] When arising before age 40, it is most commonly seen in women, but in older patients there is equal occurrence between the sexes. Interestingly, in light of the immune-mediated etiology of the disease, thymic abnormalities are common in these patients. The most common finding is thymic hyperplasia, seen in about 65 to 75% of patients; the more dramatic finding of a thymoma is found in approximately 15%. Regardless of the pattern of thymic pathology, most patients have a clinical response to thymectomy.

MORPHOLOGY. By light microscopic examination, muscle biopsies from patients with myasthenia are usually unrevealing. In severe cases, disuse changes with type 2 fiber atrophy may be found. The postsynaptic membrane is simplified, with loss of AChRs from the region of the synapse. Immune complexes as well as the membrane attack complex of the later components of the complement cascade can be found along the postsynaptic membrane as well.

The circulating anti-AChR antibodies apparently increase the degradation rate of the AChR,[53] leading to a decreased receptor number, and also appear to fix complement and lead to direct injury to the postsynaptic membrane. Despite the evidence that these antibodies play a critical pathogenic role in the disease, there is not always a correlation between antibody levels and neurologic deficit.

Other Diseases of the Neuromuscular Junction

Lambert-Eaton myasthenic syndrome (LEMS) usually develops as a paraneoplastic process, most commonly with small cell carcinoma of the lung (60% of cases), although it can be found in the absence of underlying malignancy.[54] Patients develop proximal muscle weakness along with evidence of autonomic dysfunction. No clinical improvement is found with the Tensilon test, and electrophysiologic studies show evidence of enhanced neurotransmission with repetitive stimulation. These clinical features allow this disorder to be distinguished from myasthenia gravis.

Detailed electrophysiologic studies performed on muscle biopsies from patients with LEMS have shown that the single vesicle content of ACh is normal and that the postsynaptic membrane is normally responsive to ACh, but that fewer vesicles are released in response to each presynaptic action potential. Although antibodies directed against the AChR are not present in these patients, their sera contain IgG species that allow passive transfer of LEMS-type electrophysiologic findings to animals.[55]

Disruption of presynaptic neurotransmitter release occurs in the infrequently observed condition *botulism*, caused by a toxin derived from *Clostridium botulinum*. The toxin is inactivated by proper processing of prepared foods but can be generated *in situ* with anaerobic wound infections or with intestinal overgrowth in patients with constipation. It interrupts neuromuscular transmission, leading to paralysis; the ability to produce a long-lasting block of muscular activity has led to its use in the treatment of various dystonic movement disorders, including blepharospasm, spasmodic torticollis, and laryngeal dystonia.[56]

TUMORS OF SKELETAL MUSCLE

These are discussed with other soft tissue tumors (see Chapter 27).

1. Adams, R.D., and Victor, M.: Principles of Neurology, 5th ed. New York, McGraw-Hill, 1993.
2. Dyck, P.J., et al.: The morphometric composition of myelinated fibers by nerve, level, and species related to nerve micro-environment and ischaemia. Electroencephalogr. Clin. Neurophysiol. (Suppl.) 36:39, 1982.
3. Smith, K.J., et al.: Internodal myelin volume and axon surface area. A relationship determining myelin thickness? J. Neurol. Sci. 55:231, 1982.
4. Grafstein, B., and Forman, D.S.: Intracellular transport in neurons. Physiol. Rev. 60:1167, 1980.
5. Rechthand, E., and Rapoport, S.I.: Regulation of the microenvironment of peripheral nerve: Role of the blood-nerve barrier. Prog. Neurobiol. 28:303, 1987.
6. Dubowitz, V.: Muscle Biopsy: A Practical Approach, 2nd ed. London, Baillière Tindal, 1985.
7. DeVries, G.H.: Schwann cell proliferation. In Dyck, P.J., et al. (eds.): Peripheral Neuropathy, Vol. 1. Philadelphia, W.B. Saunders Co., 1993, pp. 290–298.
8. Stoll, G., et al.: Wallerian degeneration in the peripheral nervous system: Participation of both Schwann cells and macrophages in myelin degradation. J. Neurocytol. 18:671, 1989.
9. Tischler, M.E., et al.: Different mechanisms of increased proteolysis in atrophy induced by denervation or unweighting of rat soleus muscle. Metabolism 39:756, 1990.
10. Wujek, J.R., and Lasek, R.J.: Correlation of axonal regeneration and slow component B in two branches of a single axon. J. Neurosci. 3:243, 1983.
11. Koobatian, T.J., et al.: The use of hospital discharge data for public health surveillance of Guillain-Barré syndrome. Ann. Neurol. 30:618, 1991.
12. Farkkila, M., et al.: Survey of Guillain-Barré syndrome in southern Finland. Neuroepidemiology 10:236, 1991.
13. Hartung, H.P., and Toyka, K.V.: T-cell and macrophage activation in experimental autoimmune neuritis and Guillain-Barré syndrome. Ann. Neurol. (Suppl.) 27:S57, 1990.
14. Linington, C., et al.: Cell adhesion molecules of the immunoglobulin supergene family as tissue-specific autoantigens: Induction of experimental allergic neuritis (EAN) by P0 protein-specific T cell lines. Eur. J. Immunol. 22:1813, 1992.
15. Ilyas, A.A., et al.: Anti-GM$_1$ IgA antibodies in Guillain-Barré syndrome. J. Neuroimmunol. 36:69, 1992.
16. Kaur, G., et al.: A clinical, immunological, and histological study of neuritic leprosy patients. Int. J. Lepr. Other Mycobact. Dis. 59:385, 1991.
17. Waksman, B.H.: Experimental study of diphtheritic polyneuritis in the rabbit and guinea pig. III. The blood-nerve barrier in the rabbit. J. Neuropathol. Exp. Neurol. 20:35, 1961.
18. Wilson, A., et al.: Subclinical varicella-zoster virus viremia, herpes zoster, and T lymphocyte immunity to varicella-zoster viral antigens after bone marrow transplantation. J. Infect. Dis. 165:119, 1992.
19. Dyck, P.J., et al.: Hereditary motor and sensory neuropathies. In Dyck, P.J., et al. (eds.): Peripheral Neuropathy, Vol. 2. Philadelphia, W.B. Saunders Co., 1993, pp. 1094–1136.
20. Takahashi, E., et al.: Localization of PMP-22 gene (candidate gene for the Charcot-Marie-Tooth disease 1A) to band 17p11.2 by direct R-banding fluorescence in situ hybridization. Jpn. J. Hum. Genet. 37:303, 1992.
21. Hayasaka, K., et al.: Charcot-Marie-Tooth neuropathy type 1B is associated with mutations of the myelin P$_o$ gene. Nature Genetics 5:31, 1993.
22. Bergoffen, J., et al.: Connexin mutations in X-linked Charcot-Marie-Tooth disease. Science 262:2039, 1993.
23. Loprest, L.J., et al.: Linkage studies in Charcot-Marie-Tooth disease type 2: Evidence that CMT types 1 and 2 are distinct genetic entities. Neurology 42:597, 1992.
24. Beggs, J., et al.: Innervation of the vasa nervorum: Changes in human diabetics. J. Neuropathol. Exp. Neurol. 51:612, 1992.
25. Behse, F., et al.: Nerve biopsy and conduction studies in diabetic neuropathy. J. Neurol. Neurosurg. Psychiatry 40:1072, 1977.
26. Llewelyn, J.G., et al.: Sural nerve morphometry in diabetic autonomic and painful sensory neuropathy: A clinicopathological study. Brain 114:867, 1991.
27. Asbury, A.K.: Neuropathies with renal failure, hepatic disorders, chronic respiratory insufficiency, and critical illness. In Dyck, P.J., et al. (eds.): Peripheral Neuropathy, Vol. 2. Philadelphia, W.B. Saunders Co., 1993, pp. 1251–1265.
28. Dayan, A.D., et al.: Association of carcinomatous neuromyopathy with different histological types of carcinoma of the lung. Brain 88:435, 1965.
29. Graus, F., et al.: Sensory neuronopathy and small cell lung cancer: Antineuronal antibody that also reacts with the tumor. Am. J. Med. 80:45, 1986.
30. Latov, N., et al.: Plasma neuropathy and anti-MAG antibodies. Crit. Rev. Neurobiol. 3:301, 1988.
31. Spencer, P.S., and Schaumburg, H.H.: Experimental and Clinical Neurotoxicology. Baltimore, Williams & Wilkins, 1980.
32. Fuchs, P.C., et al.: Synovial histology in carpal tunnel syndrome. J. Hand Surg. (St. Louis) 16:753, 1991.
33. Ullian, M.E., et al.: Beta$_2$-microglobulin–associated amyloidosis in chronic hemodialysis patients with carpal tunnel syndrome. Medicine 68:107, 1989.
34. Van Essen, A.J., et al.: Birth and population prevalence of Duchenne muscular dystrophy in The Netherlands. Hum. Genet. 88:258, 1992.
35. Hodgson, S.V., et al.: Correlation of clinical and deletion data in Duchenne and Becker muscular dystrophy, with special reference to mental ability. Neuromusc. Dis. 2:269, 1992.
36. Hoffman, E.P., et al.: Dystrophin: The protein product of the Duchenne muscular dystrophy locus. Cell 51:919, 1987.
37. Gold, R., et al.: The use of monoclonal antibodies in diagnostic tests for Becker and Duchenne muscular dystrophy. J. Neurol. 240:21, 1993.
38. Ptacek, L.J., et al.: Genetics and physiology of the myotonic muscle diseases. N. Engl. J. Med. 328:482, 1993.
39. Shelbourne, P., et al.: Direct diagnosis of myotonic dystrophy with a disease-specific DNA marker. N. Engl. J. Med. 328:471, 1993.
40. Brook, J.D., et al.: Molecular basis of myotonic dystrophy: Expansion of a trinucleotide (CTG) repeat at the 3' end of a transcript encoding a protein kinase family member. Cell 68:799, 1992.
41. Roe, C.R., and Coates, P.M.: Acyl-CoA dehydrogenase deficiencies. In Scriver, C.R., et al. (eds.): The Metabolic Basis of Inherited Disease, Vol. 1. New York, McGraw-Hill, 1989, pp. 889–914.
42. Tonin, P., et al.: Metabolic causes of myoglobinuria. Ann. Neurol. 27:181, 1990.
43. Clayton, D.A.: Structure and function of the mitochondrial genome. J. Inherit. Metab. Dis. 15:439, 1992.
44. Hammans, S.R., et al.: A molecular genetic study of focal histochemical defects in mitochondrial encephalomyopathies. Brain 115:343, 1992.
45. Rowland, L.P., et al.: Clinical syndromes associated with ragged red fibers. Rev. Neurol. 147:467, 1991.
46. Lindal, S., et al.: Mitochondrial diseases and myopathies: A series of muscle biopsy specimens with ultrastructural changes in the mitochondria. Ultrastruct. Pathol. 16:263, 1992.

47. Sparaco, M., et al.: Neuropathology of mitochondrial encephalomyopathies due to mitochondrial DNA defects. J. Neuropathol. Exp. Neurol. *52*:1, 1993.

48. Moraes, C.T., et al.: The mitochondrial tRNA(Leu(UUR)) mutation in mitochondrial encephalomyopathy, lactic acidosis, and strokelike episodes (MELAS): Genetic, biochemical, and morphological correlations in skeletal muscle. Am. J. Hum. Genet. *50*:934, 1992.

49. Ciafaloni, E., et al.: MELAS: Clinical features, biochemistry, and molecular genetics. Ann. Neurol. *31*:391, 1992.

50. Kumamoto, T., et al.: Experimental chloroquine myopathy: Morphological and biochemical studies. Eur. Neurol. *29*:202, 1989.

51. Phillips, L.H., Jr., and Melnick, P.A.: Diagnosis of myasthenia gravis in the 1990s. Semin. Neurol. *10*:62, 1990.

52. Phillips, L.H., Jr., et al.: The epidemiology of myasthenia gravis in central and western Virginia. Neurology *42*:1888, 1992.

53. Tzartos, S.J., et al.: The main immunogenic region (MIR) of the nicotinic acetylcholine receptor and the anti-MIR antibodies. Molec. Neurobiol. *5*:1, 1991.

54. Gutmann, L., et al.: Trends in the association of Lambert-Eaton myasthenic syndrome with carcinoma. Neurology *42*:848, 1992.

55. Kim, Y.I., and Neher, E.: IgG from patients with Lambert-Eaton syndrome blocks voltage-dependent calcium channels. Science *239*:405, 1988.

56. Cohen, S.R., et al.: Botulinum toxin for relief of bilateral abductor paralysis of the larynx: Histologic study in an animal model. Ann. Otol. Rhinol. Laryngol. *98*:213, 1989.

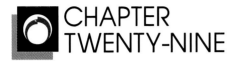

CHAPTER TWENTY-NINE

The Central Nervous System

UMBERTO DE GIROLAMI, M.D., MATTHEW P. FROSCH, M.D., Ph.D., and DOUGLAS C. ANTHONY, M.D., Ph.D.

The brain is an enormously heterogeneous organ, subdivided into many sets of structurally disparate but functionally inter-related sets of neurons, not necessarily contiguous in space. Neurons, the most important cellular constituents of the nervous system, are incapable of cell division in adults. Consequently, destruction of a small number of neurons, with a specific function, can have far-reaching clinical implications. Neurons differ greatly from one another—in the pattern of their interconnections, the architecture of their dendritic arborization, the neurotransmitters they use for synaptic transmission, their regional blood flow and glucose requirements, and their state of functional activity at a given moment. A pool of neurons, not necessarily contiguous in space, may thus show *selective vulnerability* to a disease because of some shared features, such as metabolic properties. The nervous system has unique physiologic properties, including the regulation of blood circulation, metabolic substrate requirements, the absence of a lymphatic system, a special cerebrospinal fluid (CSF) circulation, limited immunologic surveillance, and unique responses to injury and wound healing. It is, in a sense, a prisoner of the skeleton within the body it controls—more specifically, within the skull and spinal canal. As a result, it is vulnerable to disastrous consequences ensuing from what may be trivial pathologic processes in other organs (see reference texts[1,2]).

NORMAL CELLS AND THEIR REACTIONS TO INJURY

The principal cellular components of the central nervous system (CNS) are neurons, glia, and the cells that make up the meninges and blood vessels.

NEURONS

Neurons vary considerably in structure and function.[3] They are located in the gray matter and are organized either as aggregates (nuclei) or as elongated columns and layers, such as the six-layered cerebral cortex. Cortical and some subcortical neurons are arranged somatotopically within a given region, thus imparting another order of topographic-functional specificity. There are but a few well-characterized basic histopathologic *neuronal reactions to injury.*

- *Axonal reaction* is the response visible in the neuronal cell body (perikaryon) after the axon is cut or damaged. It is a reparative process associated with upregulation of protein synthesis.

Morphologically, it consists of enlargement and rounding of the cell body, with peripheral displacement of the nucleus, enlargement of the nucleolus, and dispersion of Nissl substance, particularly in the center of the cell (chromatolysis).

- *Acute cell injury (red neuron)* refers to changes that accompany acute CNS anoxia or other related injuries that result in death of the cell. The change is histologically visible at 12 hours and consists of shrinkage of the cell body, pyknosis of the nucleus, disappearance of the nucleolus, and loss of Nissl substance with intense eosinophilia of the cytoplasm. Often, the nucleus assumes the angulated shape of the shrunken perikaryon.

- *Atrophy and neuronal degeneration* occur in many slowly progressive neurologic diseases and are characterized by a loss of neurons, often selectively involving functionally related systems. The characteristic histologic feature is cell loss and reactive gliosis. When the process is at an early stage, this cell loss is difficult to detect; the associated glial changes are often the best indicator of the pathologic process at this stage. A similar sequence is seen following destruction of innervating axons, a process termed trans-synaptic degeneration.

- *Intraneuronal deposits* can occur as part of the aging process, with storage of complex lipids *(lipofuscin)*. They may also be seen in genetically determined disorders of metabolism in which substrate or other intermediates may accumulate. These generally give rise to a swollen cell body where the "stored" abnormal metabolite results in death of the cell. Viral diseases can also lead to abnormal intranuclear or intracytoplasmic deposits (inclusions), as seen in herpetic infection (Cowdry body) and in rabies (Negri body) (described later). Some degenerative diseases of the CNS are associated with neuronal intracytoplasmic deposits (e.g., neurofibrillary tangles of Alzheimer's disease, and Lewy bodies of Parkinson's disease).

GLIA

Glia are derived from neuroectoderm (astrocytes, oligodendrocytes, ependyma) or from bone marrow (microglia). Glial cells act as a supporting system for the neurons and their cellular processes, and also have a primary role in repair, fluid balance, and energy metabolism. Their nuclear size and shape generally serve to distinguish them, as their cytoplasm is not visible with ordinary H&E preparations. Astrocytes have round to oval nuclei (10 μm wide) with evenly dispersed, pale chromatin; oligodendrocytes have denser, more homogeneous chromatin in a rounder and smaller nucleus (8 μm); and microglia have elongated, irregular

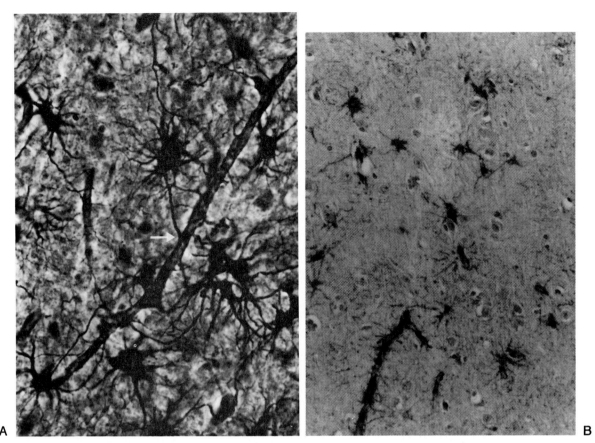

Figure 29-1. *A,* Astrocytes and their processes. Some processes extend toward blood vessels *(white arrow)* (Cajal gold sublimate). *B,* Immunoperoxidase staining for GFAP shows astrocytic cytoplasm and well-developed processes (red).

nuclei (5 to 10 μm) with clumped chromatin. Ependyma, on the other hand, do have visible cytoplasm; they are columnar epithelial–like cells with a ciliated border facing the ventricular surface and with a pale, vesiculated nucleus, about 8 μm, at the abluminal end of the cell.

Astrocytes

This cell is found in both gray and white matter and derives its name from the star-shaped appearance imparted by its multiple, branching cytoplasmic processes visible with metallic impregnation techniques or immunoperoxidase preparations for glial fibrillary acidic protein (GFAP) (Fig. 29–1). Their characteristic ultrastructural feature is the presence of intracytoplasmic intermediate filaments. Some astrocytic processes are directed toward neurons, where they are believed to act as metabolic buffers or detoxifiers, suppliers of nutrients, and electrical insulators. Astrocytes are the principal cells responsible for repair and scar formation in the brain, a process referred to as *gliosis;* fibroblasts, located mainly around large blood ves-

sels in the subarachnoid space, participate only to a limited extent.

- *Gliosis* is the most important histopathologic indicator of CNS injury, regardless of etiology. Astrocytes respond to injury by hypertrophy and hyperplasia. The nucleus enlarges and becomes vesicular, and the nucleolus is prominent. The previously scant cytoplasm expands to a bright pink, somewhat irregular swath around an eccentric nucleus, from which emerge numerous stout, ramifying processes *(gemistocytic astrocytes).* Immunohistochemistry for GFAP splendidly demonstrates the extraordinary metamorphosis. In long-standing lesions, the nuclei become small and dark and lie in a dense net of processes (glial fibrils). The factors that initiate astrocytic proliferation and gliosis are poorly understood; growth factors have been suggested to play a role.
- *Rosenthal fibers* are thick, elongated, brightly eosinophilic structures, somewhat irregular in contour, located within astrocytic processes. They consist, in large part, of αB-crystallin, a lens protein that is normally synthesized in trace amounts by astrocytes. They are typically found in long-standing gliosis, as around vascular malformations, or in certain tumors (cerebellar pilo-

cytic astrocytomas). In *Alexander's disease*, a leukodystrophy, they are present in abundance in periventricular, perivascular, and subpial locations.

- *Corpora amylacea,* or polyglucosan bodies, are round, basophilic, periodic acid–Schiff (PAS)–positive, concentrically lamellated structures ranging between 5 and 50 μm and located wherever there are astrocytic end processes, especially in the subpial zones. They represent a degenerative change in the astrocyte, and they occur in increasing numbers with advancing age; little is known of their pathogenesis or pathophysiologic significance. The *Lafora bodies* seen in the cytoplasm of neurons (as well as hepatocytes, myocytes, and other cells) in myoclonic epilepsy (Unverricht's disease, Lafora's disease) are of similar structure and biochemical composition.
- The *Alzheimer type II astrocyte* is a gray matter astrocyte having a two- to three-fold nuclear enlargement, loss of central chromatin with an intranuclear glycogen droplet, and a prominent nuclear membrane and nucleolus. Despite the name, such cells occur especially in patients with hyperammonemia due to chronic liver disease or hereditary metabolic disorders of the urea cycle.

Oligodendrocytes

Oligodendrocytes are a main cellular constituent of the white matter, where they line up beside myelinated fibers; they are also present along the myelinated fibers within the gray matter. Special techniques bring out radially arranged cytoplasmic processes, shorter and sparser and more delicate than those of astrocytes. The principal function of oligodendrocytes is the production and maintenance of CNS myelin; Schwann cells have an equivalent role in the peripheral nervous system (PNS). The potential for oligodendrocytes to proliferate or regenerate myelin after injury is under investigation.

Ependyma

Ependyma line the ventricular system and extend into the central canal of the spinal cord. They form a single layer of cuboidal-to-columnar cells (variably ciliated) with a row of nuclei on the basal surface resting on a dense feltwork of specialized astrocytes (subependymal glia). After cytotoxic injury or with the expansion of the ventricular system, as occurs in hydrocephalus, the ensuing gaps in the ventricular lining are filled by proliferating subependymal glia, *ependymal granulations.*

Microglia

Microglia are mesoderm-derived cells whose primary function is to serve as a fixed macrophage system; they are CD4+. They respond to injury by (1) proliferation; (2) developing elongated nuclei *(rod cells)*, as in neurosyphilis; (3) forming aggregates about small foci of tissue necrosis *(microglial nodules);* or (4) congregating around portions of dying neurons *(neuronophagia).* In addition to microglia, blood-derived macrophages are the principal phagocytic cells present in inflammatory foci.[4–6]

COMMON PATHOPHYSIOLOGIC COMPLICATIONS

The brain is suspended in CSF, enclosed in a fixed, rigidly confined space, the skull, and its closely applied, tough, inelastic connective tissue, the dura mater. There are two extensions of dura that are not intimately applied to the bone: the *falx*, running above the corpus callosum, separates the two cerebral hemispheres, and the *tentorium*, extending over the superior surface of the cerebellum, separates the contents of the anterior and middle fossae from those of the posterior fossa. The configuration of the cranial vault and its contents, together with the blood-brain barrier (BBB) and the CSF circulation, render the brain susceptible to three common and inter-related pathophysiologic phenomena: herniation, brain edema, and hydrocephalus.[7]

HERNIATIONS

The volume available to the intracranial contents (brain, CSF, and blood) is fixed by the skull. As a result, the introduction of additional tissue or fluid leads to an *increase in pressure.* Increased intracranial pressure can result from any space-occupying mass lesion within the brain parenchyma or meningeal spaces (e.g., tumor, abscess, hematoma), a diffuse process (e.g., cerebral edema, encephalitis, subarachnoid hemorrhage), or increased volume of CSF (hydrocephalus). An important manifestation of increased intracranial pressure, often preceeding overt clinical symptoms, is *papilledema*, a swelling of the nerve head (optic disc) that bulges into the vitreous of the eye. An increase in intracranial pressure, if unchecked, may lead to extremely serious brain damage due to brain *herniation* (Fig. 29–2).

MORPHOLOGY. On gross examination, when the increased intracranial pressure is due to a diffuse expansile process within the brain, as in cerebral edema, there is flattening of the cortical gyri over

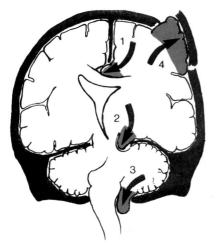

Figure 29-2. Herniations of the brain: (1) subfalcine, (2) transtentorial, (3) tonsillar, and (4) transcalvarial. (From Fishman, R.A.: Brain edema. N. Engl. J. Med. 293:706, 1975. Reprinted, by permission, from the New England Journal of Medicine.)

the convexities and compression of the lateral ventricles to slit-like cavities (well seen on radiologic studies). When the pathologic process is focal, the local expansion may cause the brain to be displaced or herniated past the free edge of one of the dural partitions or down the foramen magnum. Herniations are classified by the part that is herniated or the structure under or through which it has been pushed. Expansion of a cerebral hemisphere may lead to displacement of the medial aspect of the hemisphere (cingulate gyrus) under the falx, producing **subfalcine herniation.** This can sometimes cause compression of the anterior cerebral artery and give rise to infarction of the brain in that vascular territory.

A space-occupying lesion in the temporal lobe or more lateral portions of the cerebral hemisphere is likely to lead to **transtentorial (uncal or uncinate) herniation.** The medial part of the temporal lobe (uncus) slips over the free edge of the opening of the tentorium, beside the cerebral peduncles and the posterior cerebral artery as it wraps around the midbrain. This can result in several clinically important consequences: (1) alterations in consciousness to the point of coma, secondary to compression of the midbrain by the impinging uncus; (2) stretching or compression of the oculomotor nerve (ipsilateral, contralateral, or both), with partial ophthalmoplegia and pupillary dilatation; (3) compression of the contralateral cerebral peduncle against the free edge of the tentorium **(Kernohan notch),** with resulting hemiparesis ipsilateral to the initiating lesion (both cerebral peduncles may be compressed in the setting of severe swelling); (4) aqueductal compression and hydrocephalus, further raising the intracranial pressure; and (5) intermittent compression of the posterior

cerebral artery (ipsilateral, contralateral, or both), with hemorrhagic infarction of the occipital lobes.

Persistent downward displacement of brain stem structures leads to tearing of the penetrating arteries off the basilar artery which supply the brainstem (veins are torn as well), with irreversible hemorrhagic destruction of the midbrain and pons, often in the midline (**Duret hemorrhages;** Fig. 29-3). Downward movement of the contents of the posterior fossa, as occurs with mass lesions in the cerebellar hemispheres, results in **tonsillar herniation** (or coning). One or both cerebellar tonsils are displaced into the foramen magnum, with compression of the medulla and its vital respiratory centers, causing death. Other forms of herniation include upward extension of the cerebellum past the tentorium, as occasionally seen in patients with posterior fossa lesions, and herniation of brain tissue through surgical or traumatic skull defects.

CEREBRAL EDEMA

Edema within the brain is of great clinical significance and may be life-threatening, since the brain has little room to expand within the rigid skull. Furthermore, effective lymphatic drainage is essentially absent in humans (although experimental studies suggest that some lymphatic drainage is possible). Removal of excess fluid is dependent largely on CSF transport. The *blood-brain barrier* (BBB) closely regulates the movement of fluids and all other substances into and out of the brain; *tight junctions between brain capillary endothelial cells*

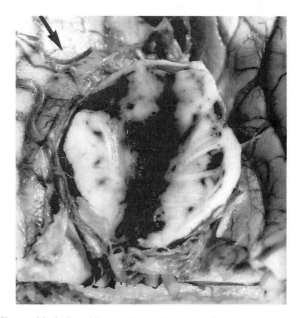

Figure 29-3. Duret hemorrhage involving the midline of the upper pons. Note the transtentorial herniation of the temporal lobe *(arrow).*

constitute the cellular barrier. Capillary basement membranes and pericapillary astrocytic processes also have important barrier functions. In addition to its physiologic role, the BBB is a major factor influencing drug and toxin access to the CNS.

Accumulation of fluid outside the vascular compartment can occur secondary to increased vascular permeability *(vasogenic edema)*, as a result of altered cell regulation of fluid *(cytotoxic edema)*, or via transudation of fluid from the ventricular system across the ependymal lining *(interstitial edema)*. Combinations of these three patterns commonly occur in a given disease state.

MORPHOLOGY

Vasogenic Edema. On macroscopic examination, the edematous region of the brain is soft and swollen; the gyri are flattened, and the ventricles compressed. The process is especially pronounced in the white matter, where microscopically there are multiple small vacuoles in the tissue, poor staining, separation of the myelinated fibers, and hyperchromasia of cell nuclei. Ultrastructural studies in experimental animals show widening of the extracellular spaces between the normally closely apposed myelinated fibers, distention of endothelial cells and pericapillary astrocytic foot processes (sometimes with obliteration of the capillary lumen), and eventually breakdown of myelin.

Cytotoxic Edema. This process is most evident in gray matter. Microscopically, the cells are swollen and vacuolated. In experimental animals, ultrastructural examination demonstrates fluid accumulation within the processes of neurons and glia or within myelin lamellae.

HYDROCEPHALUS

Hydrocephalus is defined as enlargement of the ventricles with an associated increase in the volume of CSF. In the normal adult, CSF is produced at a rate of 500 ml/day; since the total CSF volume is about 140 to 150 ml, it is renewed every 6 to 8 hours.[8] The fluid is secreted by the epithelial cells of the choroid plexus tufts located in the floor of the lateral ventricles and the roof of the third and fourth ventricles. Cells of the arachnoid villi provide unidirectional transport of CSF from the subarachnoid space to the venous sinuses. Hydrocephalus usually results from blockage of CSF flow anywhere along this pathway; only rarely does overproduction of CSF by choroid plexus papillomas account for hydrocephalus. *Noncommunicating hydrocephalus* is the result of blockage anywhere along the ventricular system, most often involving blockage of the aqueduct or occlusion of one of the foramina of Monro, leading to disproportionate enlargement of a segment of the ventricular system, with the isolated portion not communicating with the subarachnoid space. In *communicating hydrocephalus*, the obstruction is along the subarachnoid path of CSF flow, including the sites of its absorption.

In infants and children when fusion of the cranial bones has not yet occurred, hydrocephalus produces enlargement of the head. Hydrocephalus requires prompt surgical intervention, with the placement of drainage shunts or elimination of the cause, if possible. In this age group, the most common causes are congenital malformations, intrauterine or perinatal infections, vascular diseases, and neoplasms.

In adults, hydrocephalus can occur with any obstruction of CSF flow, as mentioned previously, be it sudden or gradual, and leads to increased intracranial pressure. *Normal pressure hydrocephalus* refers to a clinical syndrome typically found in the elderly, and characterized by mental slowness, incontinence, and gait disturbances associated with a slowly evolving hydrocephalus. The basis for the functional disturbances is not understood, but the symptoms are sometimes ameliorated by surgical insertion of a shunt. In processes leading to brain atrophy (e.g., Alzheimer's disease) or when there is extensive tissue loss, compensatory expansion of the ventricular system and of the entire CSF compartment results in *hydrocephalus ex vacuo*.

MORPHOLOGY. The extent and distribution of the ventricular enlargement depend on the duration and site of the obstruction; for example, a tumor blocking one of the foramina of Monro will result in unilateral enlargement of the lateral ventricle, while a diffuse leptomeningitis of long-standing, with blockage of the foramina of Luschka and Magendie, will widen the entire ventricular system (Fig. 29–4A and B). The white matter is compressed, and microscopically there is interruption of the ependymal lining with ependymal granulations, interstitial periventricular edema with thinning out of myelinated fibers, and comparatively good preservation of the cortical gray matter.

MALFORMATIONS AND DEVELOPMENTAL DISEASES

Background knowledge of neuroembryology is essential to understand CNS malformations. The anatomic pattern of the malformation reflects the stage of formation of the brain at the time of injury. The pathogenesis and etiology of CNS malformations are largely unknown. Etiologic agents can either lead to the failure of normal develop-

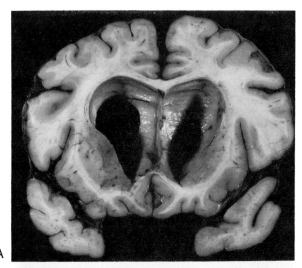

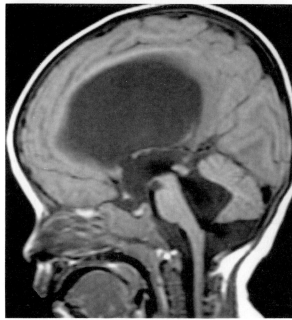

Figure 29-4. *A,* Hydrocephalus. Dilated lateral ventricles seen in a coronal section through frontal lobes. *B,* Mid-sagittal plane T1-weighted magnetic resonance image of a child with communicating hydrocephalus, involving all ventricles. (*B,* Courtesy of Dr. P. Barnes, Children's Hospital, Boston.)

ment or result in tissue destruction.[9] There is recent evidence that homeotic and other genes are expressed in a regulated fashion during the segmental development of the brain; understanding these genes and their function may help explain some brain malformations.[10]

NEURAL TUBE DEFECTS (NTD)

Failure to close a portion of the neural tube, or reopening of a region of the tube after successful closure, may lead to one of several malformations. All are characterized by abnormalities involving both neural tissue and overlying bone and/or soft tissues. *Anencephaly* is a malformation of the anterior end of the neural tube, with absence of the brain and calvarium. It occurs in 1 to 5 per 1000 live births, more commonly in females, and is thought to develop at approximately 28 days of gestation. Forebrain development is disrupted, and in its place all that remains is the *area cerebrovasculosa*, a flattened remnant of disorganized brain tissue with admixed ependyma, choroid plexus, and meningothelial cells. The posterior fossa structures are often spared.

An *encephalocele* is a diverticulum of malformed CNS tissue extending through a defect in the cranium. It most often occurs in the occipital region or in the posterior fossa.

The most common forms of NTD in newborns involve the spinal cord with a failure of closure or reopening of the caudal portions of the neural tube. *Spinal dysraphism* or *spina bifida* may be an asymptomatic bony defect (spina bifida occulta) or a severe malformation with a flattened, disorganized segment of spinal cord, associated with an overlying meningeal outpouching. *Myelomeningocele* (or meningomyelocele) refers to extension of CNS tissue through a defect in the vertebral column, while the term *meningocele* applies when there is only a meningeal extrusion. Clinical neurologic dysfunction is most often related to the structural abnormality of the cord itself and to superimposed infection extending from the thin, overlying skin. Myelomeningoceles occur most commonly in the lumbosacral region and present with clinical deficits referable to motor and sensory function in the lower extremities as well as disturbances of the bowel and bladder control.

The etiology of NTDs is unknown; their frequency varies widely among ethnic groups. Antenatal diagnosis has been facilitated by new imaging methods and the screening of maternal blood samples for α-fetoprotein, which is elevated in cases of NTD. The overall recurrence rate for NTD in subsequent pregnancies has been estimated at 4 to 5%. Folate deficiency during the initial weeks of gestation has been implicated as a risk factor.[11]

FOREBRAIN ABNORMALITIES

Polymicrogyria is characterized by a loss of the normal external contour of the convolutions, which on macroscopic examination appear small, unusually numerous, and irregularly formed. The gray matter is composed of four layers (or fewer), with entrapment of apparent meningeal tissue at points of fusion of what would otherwise be the cortical surface. Experimental animal studies suggest that polymicrogyria can be generated by localized tissue injury during the time of neuronal migration.

The volume of brain may be abnormally large *(megalencephaly)* or small *(micrencephaly)*. Micrencephaly, by far the more common of the two, can occur in a wide range of clinical settings, including chromosomal abnormalities, fetal alcohol syndrome, and human immunodeficiency virus 1 (HIV-1) infection acquired *in utero*. A reduction in the number of neurons that reach the neocortex is postulated, and this leads to a simplification of the gyral folding. This can range from a noticeable decrease in the number of gyri to total absence, leaving a smooth-surfaced brain, *lissencephaly (agyria)*.

The migration of neurons from the germinal matrix (the periventricular region of neuronal and glial proliferation), through the deeper structures to reach their final destinations in the cerebral cortex, is a complicated process that can go awry. Stranded clusters of neurons *(neuronal heterotopias)* may then be found strewn along the path of migration, either as large conglomerates or as small clusters within the white matter.

Holoprosencephaly is a spectrum of malformations characterized by incomplete separation of the cerebral hemispheres across the midline (Fig. 29–5). The more extreme forms often occur with midline facial abnormalities, including cyclopia; less serious variants, such as arhinencephaly show absence of the olfactory nerves and related structures. Holoprosencephaly is associated with trisomy 13 and, to a much lesser extent, with trisomy 18. Comparable malformations have been induced in animals with a plant alkaloid.

In *agenesis of the corpus callosum* there is an absence of the white matter bundles that carry cortical projections from one hemisphere to the other (Fig. 29-6). Radiologic imaging studies show misshapen lateral ventricles ("bat-wing" deformity), and, on whole brain histologic sections, bundles of anteroposteriorly oriented white matter can be demonstrated. Agenesis of the corpus callosum can be found in patients with mental retardation or in clinically normal individuals. Unlike patients with surgically-induced callosal section who show clinical evidence of hemispheric disconnection, only minimal deficits can be demonstrated in patients with this malformation even with neuropsychologic testing. The malformation may be complete or partial; in the latter case, the caudal portion of the callosum is absent, and a lipoma sometimes occupies the defect.

POSTERIOR FOSSA ABNORMALITIES

The *Arnold-Chiari malformation* (Chiari type II malformation) consists of a small posterior fossa, a

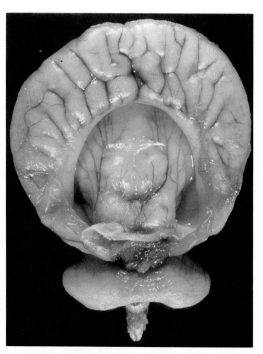

Figure 29–5. Holoprosencephaly. View of the dorsal surface showing a lack of separation of cerebral hemispheres, a single ventricle, and fused basal ganglia.

malformed midline cerebellum with extension of vermis through the foramen magnum (Fig. 29–7), and, almost invariably, hydrocephalus and a lumbar myelomeningocele. Other associated changes include caudal displacement of the medulla (S-shaped deformity), malformation of the tectum, aqueductal stenosis, cerebral heterotopias, and hydromyelia (see below).

In contrast, the *Dandy-Walker malformation* is characterized by an *enlarged* posterior fossa. The

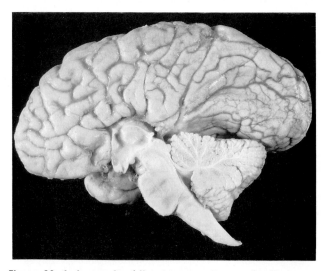

Figure 29–6. Agenesis of the corpus callosum. Sagittal section shows the lack of a corpus callosum above the third ventricle.

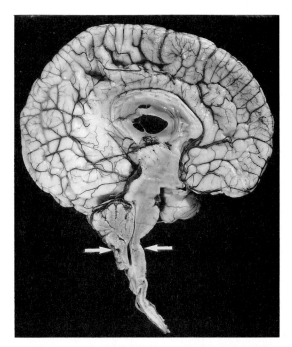

Figure 29-7. Arnold-Chiari malformation. Midsagittal section showing small posterior fossa contents, downward displacement of cerebellar vermis, and S-shaped deformity of medulla (*arrows* indicate approximate level of foramen magnum).

cerebellar vermis is absent or present only in rudimentary form in its anterior portion. In its place is a large midline cyst that is lined by ependyma and is contiguous with leptomeninges on its outer surface. This cyst represents the expanded, roofless fourth ventricle in the absence of a normally formed vermis. Dysplasias of brain stem nuclei are commonly found in association with Dandy-Walker malformation, as are other cerebral and systemic malformations.

SYRINGOMYELIA AND HYDROMYELIA

These are related disorders characterized by a segmental or continuous expansion of the ependymal-lined central canal of the cord *(hydromyelia)* or by the formation of a cleft-like cavity in the inner portion of the cord *(syringomyelia, syrinx)*. These lesions are associated with destruction of the adjacent gray and white matter and are surrounded by a dense feltwork of reactive gliosis. The cervical spinal cord is most often affected, and the slit-like cavity may extend into the brain stem *(syringobulbia)*.

Syrinx cavities can also be found in association with intraspinal tumors (either above or below the tumor mass) or, in adults, as a "degenerative," slowly progressive disorder. In these conditions the

histologic appearance of the lesion is similar to that of maldevelopmental syringomyelia. In all these conditions the etiology and pathogenesis of syringomyelia are unknown. The distinctive initial clinical symptoms and signs of a syrinx are dissociated sensory loss of pain and temperature sensation in the upper extremities, retention of position sense, and absence of motor deficits, due to early involvement of the crossing anterior spinal commissural fibers.

PERINATAL BRAIN INJURY

The term *cerebral palsy* refers to any nonprogressive neurologic motor deficit with onset during the perinatal period, regardless of etiology.

In premature infants, there is an increased risk of *intraparenchymal hemorrhage* within the germinal matrix, near the junction between the thalamus and the caudate nucleus. Hemorrhages may remain localized or extend into the ventricular system and thence to the subarachnoid space, sometimes leading to hydrocephalus.

In the premature newborn, ischemic infarcts may occur in the periventricular white matter *(periventricular leukomalacia, PVL)*. These are chalky-yellow plaques consisting of discrete regions of white matter necrosis and mineralization (Fig. 29-8). Cyst formation may follow in cases where there has been extensive damage; when both gray and white matter are involved, large destructive lesions develop through the hemispheres, *multicystic encephalopathy*.

In perinatal ischemic lesions of the cerebral cortex, the depths of sulci bear the brunt of injury

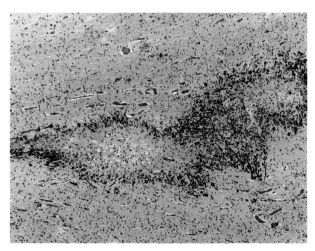

Figure 29-8. Periventricular leukomalacia. Central focus of white matter necrosis with peripheral rim of mineralized axonal processes (staining blue).

and result in thinned-out, gliotic gyri *(ulegyria)*. The basal ganglia and thalamus may also suffer ischemic injury, with patchy neuronal loss and reactive gliosis. Later, with the advent of myelination at about six months of age, aberrant and irregular myelin formation gives rise to a marble-like appearance of the deep nuclei, *status marmoratus.* Clinically, because the lesions are in the caudate, putamen, and thalamus, choreoathetosis and related movement disorders are important sequelae.

TRAUMA

The anatomic location of the lesion and the limited capacity of the brain for functional repair are two factors of great significance in CNS trauma. Necrosis of several cubic centimeters of brain parenchyma may be clinically silent (frontal lobe), severely disabling (spinal cord), or fatal (brain stem).

The magnitude and distribution of a traumatic brain lesion depend on the shape of the object causing the trauma, the force of impact, and whether the head is in motion at the time of injury. A blow to the head may be *penetrating* or *blunt* and may cause either an *open* or a *closed injury.* Severe brain damage can occur in the absence of external signs of head injury, and, conversely, severe lacerations and even skull fractures do not necessarily indicate damage to the underlying brain. Three mechanisms by which physical forces cause their effects can be identified: *skull fractures, parenchymal injuries,* and *vascular injuries;* they are often present in combination.[12]

SKULL FRACTURES

In general, the kinetic energy that causes a fracture is dissipated at a fused suture; fractures that cross sutures are termed *diastatic*. With multiple points of impact or repeated blows to the head, the fracture lines of subsequent injuries do not extend across fracture lines of prior injury. A fracture in which bone is displaced into the cranial cavity by a distance greater than the thickness of the bone is called a *displaced skull fracture*. The thickness of the cranial bones varies, and therefore their resistance to fracture differs greatly. Also, the relative incidence of fractures among skull bones is related to the pattern of falls. Falls while the individual is conscious, such as might occur from a ladder, often lead to an occipital impact; in contrast, a fall that follows a loss of consciousness, such as due to syncope, may result in a frontal impact. Basal skull fractures, which often follow an impact to the occiput or sides of the head rather than the vertex, can be difficult to detect. Symptoms referable to the lower cranial nerves or the cervicomedullary region, or orbital or mastoid hematomas distant from the point of impact, can suggest this fracture; CSF discharge from the nose or ear and infections (meningitis) may follow.

PARENCHYMAL INJURIES

Concussion

Concussion is a clinical syndrome brought about by closed head injury characterized by sudden onset and transient neurologic dysfunction, including loss of consciousness, respiratory arrest, and loss of reflexes. Neurologic recovery is complete, but amnesia for the event persists. The pathogenesis of the sudden disruption of nervous activity is unknown. Although concussive injury, by definition, is reversible and unassociated with permanent structural damage, there is increasing evidence that biochemical abnormalities do occur, such as depletion of mitochondrial adenosine triphosphate (ATP), as well as possibly ultrastructural changes.[1,13]

Direct Parenchymal Injury

Contusion and *laceration*, in contrast to concussion, are conditions in which direct parenchymal injury of the brain has occurred, either through transmission of kinetic energy to the brain and bruising analogous to what is seen in soft tissues (contusion) or via penetration of an object and tearing of tissue (laceration). Since there is a direct relationship between the contusion and the applied force, contusions most often occur on the surface of the brain at sites where the brain makes contact with rough bony surfaces, such as the tips of the temporal lobes, the inferior frontal surfaces, and the occipital poles. As with any other organ, a blow to the surface of the brain, transmitted through the skull, leads to rapid tissue displacement, disruption of vascular channels and subsequent hemorrhage, tissue injury, and edema (Fig. 29–9). The pattern of the lesions reflects the distribution of the applied force: the crests of gyri are most susceptible, whereas sulci are relatively uninvolved. These lesions occur where the direct impact of trauma can reach the brain surface, and thus tend to spare the base of the brain and much of the posterior fossa contents. Contusions, when seen on cross-section, often have a wedge-shaped appearance, with the broad base spanning the surface and centered on the point of impact.

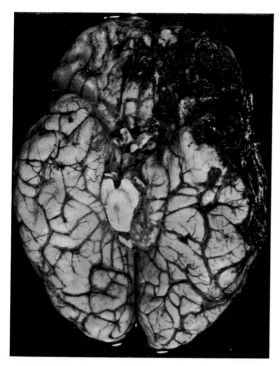

Figure 29-9. Severe contusions of left frontal and temporal lobes. There is also massive left uncal (transtentorial) herniation and compression of right cerebral peduncle.

A patient who suffers a blow with a discrete point of impact may develop only minimal injury underlying the point of contact (a *coup* injury), whereas areas of the brain opposite to it may show extensive damage (a *contrecoup* injury). Both coup and contrecoup lesions are contusions; their histologic appearance is indistinguishable. Coup and contrecoup lesions are the result of sudden deceleration of the head and are not seen when the head is immobile. Whereas the coup lesion is caused by direct impact, the contrecoup contusion is thought to arise from impact of brain with the opposite inner surface of the skull following sudden deceleration.

MORPHOLOGY. The histologic appearance of contusions is independent of the type of trauma. The changes are greatest at the surface of the brain. In the earliest stages, there is evidence of edema and hemorrhage, which is often found in a pericapillary pattern. Over the next few hours, the hemorrhage extends throughout the involved tissue. Morphologic evidence of neuronal injury takes about 24 hours to appear, although functional injury has occurred much earlier. Secondary changes with axonal swellings develop in 24 to 48 hours in the fibers of these neurons as well as in the fibers passing through the lesions. The inflammatory response to the injured tissue follows its usual course, with neutrophils preceding the appearance of macrophages. Old traumatic lesions on the surface of the brain have a characteristic gross appearance: they are depressed, retracted, yellowish-brown patches involving the crests of gyri most commonly located at the sites of contrecoup lesions (inferior frontal cortex, temporal and occipital poles). The term **plaque jaune** (Fig. 29-10) is applied to these lesions; they can be foci of clinical seizure discharges. More extensive hemorrhagic regions of brain trauma give rise to larger cavitated lesions, which can resemble remote infarcts. In sites of old contusions, gliosis and residual hemosiderin-laden macrophages predominate.

White Matter Injury

Another pattern of parenchymal brain injury involves the white matter, often deep within the brain. Microscopic findings include axonal retraction balls indicative of *diffuse axonal injury*, or focal hemorrhagic lesions. It is well demonstrated by silver staining, being found most commonly in the corpus callosum and the dorsal lateral brain stem and less often in the pontine tegmentum. Angular acceleration alone, in the absence of impact, can cause diffuse axonal injury as well as hemorrhage. As many as 50% of patients who develop coma shortly after trauma, even without cerebral contusion, are believed to have white matter damage and diffuse axonal injury.

MORPHOLOGY. The histopathology of diffuse axonal injury is characterized by the wide but often asymmetric distribution of axonal swellings that appear within hours of the injury. Later, there are in-

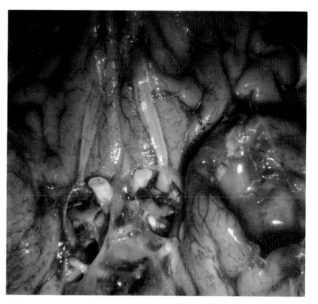

Figure 29-10. Old contusion *(plaque jaune)* in tip of temporal lobe; the lesion is sunken and yellow.

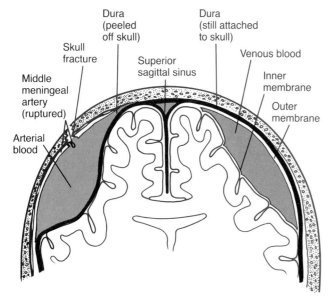

EPIDURAL HEMATOMA   SUBDURAL HEMATOMA

Figure 29–11. Epidural hematoma *(left),* in which rupture of a meningeal artery, usually associated with a skull fracture, leads to accumulation of arterial blood between the dura and the skull. In a subdural hematoma *(right),* damage to bridging veins between the brain and the superior sagittal sinus leads to the accumulation of blood between the dura and the arachnoid.

creased numbers of microglia in related areas of cerebral cortex and, subsequently, degeneration of the involved fiber tracts. Currently, the most widely accepted explanation for diffuse axonal injury is that mechanical forces damage the integrity of the axon at the node of Ranvier, with subsequent alterations in axoplasmic flow.

TRAUMATIC VASCULAR INJURY

Vascular injury is a frequent component of CNS trauma and results from direct trauma and disruption of the vessel wall, leading to hemorrhage. Depending on the anatomic position of the ruptured vessel, hemorrhage will occur in any of several compartments (sometimes in combination): *epidural, subdural, subarachnoid,* and *intraparenchymal* (Fig. 29–11). In the cavernous sinus, a traumatic tear of the carotid artery leads to the formation of an arteriovenous fistula.

Epidural Hematoma

The epidural space is a potential space—the dura is closely applied to the internal surface of the skull and is fused with the periosteum. Vessels that course within the dura—most importantly, the middle meningeal artery—are vulnerable to in-

jury, particularly with skull fractures. Trauma to the skull, especially in the region of the temporal bone, can lead to laceration of this artery if the fracture lines cross the course of the vessel. In children, in whom the skull is deformable, a temporary displacement of the skull bones leading to laceration of a vessel can occur in the absence of a skull fracture.

Once a vessel has been torn, the accumulation of blood, under arterial pressure, can lead to dissection of the dura from the inner surface of the skull. The expanding mass will have a smooth inner contour that compresses the cortical surface. Clinically, patients are often lucid for several hours between the moment of trauma and the development of neurologic signs. An epidural hematoma may expand rapidly and is a neurosurgical emergency requiring prompt drainage.

Subdural Hematoma

The space beneath the inner surface of the dura mater and the arachnoid layer of the leptomeninges is also a potential space. Many *bridging veins* traverse from the surface of the convexities of the cerebral hemispheres through the subarachnoid space and the subdural space to empty with dural vessels into the superior sagittal sinus. Similar anatomic relationships exist with other dural sinuses. These vessels are particularly susceptible to tearing along their course through the subdural space and are the source of bleeding in most cases of subdural hematoma. The most commonly accepted mechanism of damage postulates that the brain, floating freely within the skull in its bath of CSF, can move within the skull, but the venous sinuses are fixed. The displacement of the brain that occurs in trauma can tear the veins at the point where they penetrate the dura. In elderly patients with brain atrophy, the bridging veins are stretched out and the brain has additional space for movement, hence the increased rate of subdural hematomas in these patients, even after relatively minor head trauma.

Subdural hematomas most often become clinically manifest within the first 48 hours after injury. They are most common over the lateral aspects of the cerebral hemispheres and are bilateral in about 10% of cases. Neurologic signs commonly observed are attributable to the pressure exerted on the adjacent brain. There may be focal signs, but often the clinical manifestations are nonlocalizing (e.g., headache, confusion). Over time, there may be slowly progressive neurologic deterioration, but rarely acute decompensation.

MORPHOLOGY. On gross examination, the acute subdural hematoma appears as a collection of

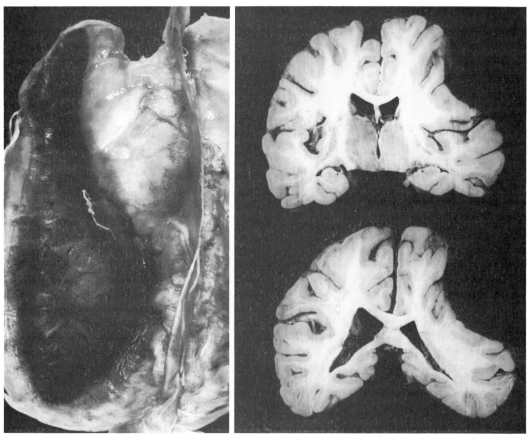

Figure 29–12. *A,* Large organizing subdural hematoma attached to the dura. *B,* Coronal sections of the brain showing compression of the hemisphere underlying the hematoma.

freshly clotted blood apposed along the contour of the brain surface, without extension into the depths of sulci (Fig. 29–12). The underlying brain is flattened, and the subarachnoid space is often clear. Typically, venous bleeding is self-limited; breakdown and organization of the hematoma take place over time. The course of organization of subdural hematomas is (1) lysis of the clot (about 1 week); (2) growth of fibroblasts from the dural surface around the edges of the lesion (2 weeks); and (3) early development of granulation tissue (3 weeks). A remarkable macroscopic characteristic of an organized hematoma is that the lesion is firmly attached by fibrous tissue only to the inner surface of the dura and is not at all adherent to the underlying smooth arachnoid, which does not contribute to its formation. The lesion can eventually retract as the granulation tissue matures. Lesions that evolve to this stage of healing are referred to as chronic subdural hematomas. A common finding in subdural hematomas, however, is the occurrence of multiple episodes of rebleeding, presumably from the thin-walled vessels of the granulation tissue. The risk of rebleeding, in the ab-

sence of repeated trauma, appears to be greatest in the first few months after the initial hemorrhage. Because there are often multiple episodes of hemorrhage and organization within the subdural hematoma, **the age of the lesion is extremely difficult to determine with precision by microscopic examination.** The neurosurgical treatment of subdural hematomas is to remove the organized blood and surrounding reactive connective tissue ("subdural membranes").

Traumatic Subarachnoid Hemorrhage (SAH) and Traumatic Intraparenchymal Hematoma

Subarachnoid and intraparenchymal hemorrhages can occur from a variety of nontraumatic conditions; however, *most cases of traumatic SAH are associated with parenchymal trauma.* Contusion of superficial cerebral tissue or, less frequently, cerebellar cortex is associated with disruption of small vessels within both the brain parenchyma and the overlying leptomeninges. Direct vascular injury, such as laceration of a normal vessel or rupture of a pre-existing aneurysm or malformation, can lead to the accumulation of blood in the subarachnoid space in the absence of parenchymal injury.

SPINAL CORD INJURY

The spinal cord, normally protected within the bony vertebral canal, is vulnerable to trauma from its skeletal encasement. Most injuries that damage the cord are associated with displacement of the spinal column, either rapid and temporary or persistent. The level of cord injury determines the extent of neurologic manifestations; lesions involving the thoracic vertebrae or below can lead to paraplegia, cervical lesions (below C4) result in quadriplegia, and those above C4 can additionally lead to respiratory compromise from paralysis of the diaphragm. Damage to white matter tracts isolates the distal spinal cord from its cortical connections. It is this interruption of white matter tracts that causes the major clinical deficits of spinal cord injury, more so than the neuronal injury at the level of the insult.

MORPHOLOGY. The histologic changes of traumatic injury of the spinal cord are similar to those found at other sites in the CNS. At the level of injury, the acute phase consists of hemorrhage and necrosis surrounded by axonal swellings in the surrounding white matter. The lesion tapers above and below the injured level. Over time, the central necrotic lesion becomes cystic and mildly gliotic, while the surrounding white matter tracts show secondary degenerative changes.

CEREBROVASCULAR DISEASES

Cerebrovascular disease is the third leading cause of death (after heart disease and cancer) in the United States; it is the most prevalent neurologic disorder in terms of both morbidity and mortality. The major categories of vascular disease are (1) hypoxia, ischemia, and infarction; (2) intracranial hemorrhage; and (3) hypertensive cerebrovascular disease.[14]

HYPOXIA, ISCHEMIA, AND INFARCTION

The brain requires a constant supply of glucose and oxygen, which are delivered by the circulation and account for 15% of the resting cardiac output and 20% of the total body oxygen consumption. Cerebral blood flow remains constant over a wide range of blood pressure and intracranial pressure because of autoregulation of vascular resistance, although this protective mechanism may be impaired in ischemic tissue. The brain is a highly aerobic tissue, with oxygen rather than metabolic substrate serving as the limiting substance. Since there is no reserve of oxygen in the brain, normal cerebral function can continue only for 8 to 10 seconds after cerebral ischemia; irreversible damage follows after 6 to 8 minutes. Glucose stores, however, can maintain cerebral function for 30 to 60 minutes after reduction of blood sugar levels to near zero. The brain may be deprived of oxygen by any of several mechanisms: *functional hypoxia* in a setting of a low inspired partial pressure of oxygen (pO_2), impaired oxygen-carrying capacity, or inhibition of oxygen use by tissue; or *ischemia*, either *transient* or *permanent*, following interruption of the normal circulatory flow. Cessation of blood flow can occur as a result of reduction in perfusion pressure, as in hypotension, or secondary to small or large vessel obstruction.

The site and size of the lesion and, consequently, the clinical and pathologic picture it produces are dependent on a large number of modifying factors, including collateral circulation, the duration of ischemia, and the degree and rapidity of the reduction of flow. In clinical practice, two general types of acute ischemic injury are recognized:

- *Ischemic (hypoxic) encephalopathy* occurs when there has been generalized reduction of cerebral perfusion with widespread damage.
- *Cerebral infarction* is the focal ischemic necrosis that follows reduction or cessation of blood flow to a localized area of the brain.

Ischemic (Hypoxic) Encephalopathy

The CNS cells most vulnerable to ischemia are neurons, but if the ischemia is sufficiently severe or prolonged the glial cells also die, producing complete necrosis of the tissue. There is a great variability in the susceptibility of neurons to ischemia from one part of the brain to another, based in part on differences in regional cerebral blood flow. Furthermore, recent evidence suggests that *excitotoxins*, excitatory amino acid neurotransmitters (glutamate and aspartate) whose release increases with ischemia, may cause the death of selected neuronal populations. This occurs perhaps by causing persistent opening of specific membrane channels (*N*-methyl-D-aspartate [NMDA] receptors) and allowing for an uncontrolled influx of calcium ions[15,16] or through activation of the enzyme that synthesizes the transmitter and potential toxin nitric oxide (NO).[17,18] Inhibitors of these ion channels or of this enzyme, NO synthase, have been found to protect against the effects of cerebral ischemia in some model systems and may have therapeutic potential in humans.[19]

Ischemic encephalopathy occurs after episodes of profound systemic hypotension. In mild cases, there may be only a transient postischemic confusional state, with eventual complete recovery. In severe global cerebral ischemia, as in instances of prolonged cerebral hypoperfusion resulting from cardiorespiratory arrest, widespread brain necrosis, irrespective of regional vulnerability, occurs. Patients who survive in this state often remain severely impaired neurologically and deeply comatose (persistent vegetative state). Some other patients meet the current clinical criteria for "brain death," including persistent evidence of diffuse cortical injury (isoelectric—"flat"—electroencephalogram [EEG]) as well as brain stem damage (e.g., absent reflexes, respiratory drive) and absent perfusion. When patients with this pervasive form of injury are maintained on mechanical ventilation, the brain gradually undergoes an autolytic process, leading to soft, purée-like tissue that does not fix or take stain well. This state, which has been termed *respirator brain*, reflects tissue autolysis and is not an effect of the ventilator. Although mechanical ventilation can be maintained, the loss of brain stem function leads to cardiovascular instability.

MORPHOLOGY. Grossly, the brain is swollen, the gyri are widened, and the sulci narrowed. The cut surface shows poor demarcation between gray and white matter. The histopathologic changes that attend ischemic encephalopathy can be grouped into three general categories. Early changes, occurring 12 to 24 hours after the insult, include the acute neuronal cell change (red neurons), characterized at first by microvacuolization, then eosinophilia of the neuronal cytoplasm, and later nuclear pyknosis and karyorrhexis. Similar acute changes occur somewhat later in astrocytes and oligodendroglia. Pyramidal cells of the Sommer's sector (CA1) of the hippocampus, Purkinje cells of the cerebellum, and pyramidal neurons in the neocortex are the most susceptible to irreversible injury. Subacute changes, occurring at 24 hours to 2 weeks, include necrosis of tissue, influx of macrophages, vascular proliferation, and reactive gliosis. Repair, as seen after 2 weeks, is characterized by removal of all necrotic tissue, loss of normally organized CNS structure, and gliosis. In the cerebral cortex, the neuronal loss and gliosis produce an uneven destruction of the neocortex, with preservation of some layers and involvement of others—a pattern termed **(pseudo)laminar necrosis.**
Watershed or **border zone infarcts** are

wedge-shaped areas of coagulation necrosis that occur in those regions of the brain and spinal cord that lie at the most distal fields of arterial irrigation. In the cerebral hemispheres, the border zone between the anterior and the middle cerebral artery distributions seems to be at greatest risk. Damage to this region produces a linear parasagittal lesion.

Cerebral Infarction

"Stroke" is a clinical term that refers to the sudden development of a neurologic deficit caused by abnormalities of the blood supply.[14] The anatomic location of the lesion determines whether the patient develops a hemiplegia, a sensory deficit, blindness, aphasia, or some other symptom.[2] The deficit evolves over time, and the outcome either is fatal or is characterized by some degree of slow improvement over a period of months.

The size, location, and shape of the infarct and the extent of tissue damage that results from focal cerebral ischemia brought about by occlusion of a blood vessel are determined by the size of the vascular bed and the adequacy of blood flow through collateral circulation. The major source of collateral flow is the circle of Willis (supplemented by the external carotid-ophthalmic pathway). Partial and inconstant reinforcement is available over the surface of the brain for the distal branches of the anterior, middle, and posterior cerebral arteries via cortical-leptomeningeal anastomoses. In contrast, there is little, if any, collateral flow for the deep penetrating vessels supplying structures such as the thalamus, basal ganglia, and deep white matter. Occlusive vascular disease of severity sufficient to lead to cerebral infarction can occur from either *in situ thrombosis* or *embolization* from a distant source. In general, thrombosis is more frequent in the extracerebral carotid system, and embolism in the intracranial vessels. The basilar artery, however, is more often occluded by thrombosis than by embolism. Spinal cord infarction may be seen in the setting of widespread hypoperfusion or as a consequence of interruption of the feeding tributaries derived from the aorta. Occlusion of the anterior spinal artery is rarer but may occur as a result of thrombosis or embolism.

The majority of thrombotic occlusions are due to *atherosclerosis*. The most common sites of involvement are the carotid bifurcation, the origin of the middle cerebral artery, and at either end of the basilar artery. The outcome of arterial stenosis varies from progressive narrowing of the lumen and thrombosis, which may be accompanied by anterograde extension to fragmentation and distal embolization. Another important aspect of occlusive vascular disease is its frequent association with other diseases (including hypertension, diabetes, arteriosclerotic heart disease, hypercholesterolemia, and gout).

Arteritis of small and large vessels, in association with syphilis and tuberculosis, formerly accounted for a large proportion of cerebral infarcts but is now of lesser clinical importance. Polyarteritis, temporal arteritis, and lupus erythematosus may result in multiple small infarcts distributed diffusely throughout the brain. Other conditions that may cause thrombosis and infarction include polycythemia, dissecting aneurysm, and trauma.

Embolism to the brain most commonly occurs when a fragment of thrombotic material occludes a vessel. Cardiac mural thrombi are the major offenders; myocardial infarct, valvular disease, and atrial fibrillation are important predisposing factors. Next in importance are fragments of thrombotic material broken off from arterial mural thrombi (mostly carotid), followed by paradoxical emboli (particularly in children with cardiac anomalies), emboli associated with cardiac surgery, or emboli of other material (tumor, fat, or air). Cerebral embolization from pulmonary vein thrombophlebitis associated with pneumonia is rare. The area involved most frequently with emboli is the territory of distribution of the middle cerebral artery; the incidence is about equal in the two hemispheres. Emboli tend to lodge where blood vessels branch or in areas of pre-existing luminal stenosis. In about 50% of cases of presumed cerebral embolization, the site of occlusion cannot be identified at postmortem examination, presumably because the embolus has been lysed. "Shower embolization," as in fat embolism, may occur after fractures; the patient shows generalized cerebral dysfunction with disturbances of mentation and consciousness without localizing signs, thus simulating the clinical presentation of severe metabolic encephalopathy.

A general distinction is made on the basis of the macroscopic, and corresponding radiologic, appearance of infarcts (Fig. 29–13). *Hemorrhagic (red) infarction,* characterized grossly by multiple, sometimes confluent, petechial hemorrhages, is typically associated with embolic events. The hemorrhage is presumed to be secondary to reperfusion of damaged vessels and tissue, either via collaterals or directly following dissolution of intravascular occlusive material. In contrast, *nonhemorrhagic (pale, bland) infarcts* are usually associated with thrombosis. The clinical management of patients with these two types of infarcts differs greatly: anticoagulation is contraindicated in the hemorrhagic infarcts.

MORPHOLOGY. The gross appearance of a nonhemorrhagic infarct changes over time. During the first 6 hours of irreversible injury, little can be observed grossly. By 48 hours, the tissue becomes pale, soft, and swollen, and the corticomedullary junction becomes indistinct. From 2 to 10 days, the brain becomes gelatinous and friable, and the previously ill-defined boundary between normal and abnormal tissue becomes more distinct as edema resolves in the adjacent tissue that has survived. From 10 days to 3 weeks, the tissue liquefies and eventually is removed, leaving a fluid-filled cavity lined by dark gray tissue, which gradually expands as dead tissue is removed (Fig. 29–14).

Microscopically, after the first 12 hours, ischemic neuronal change (red neurons—see above) and edema predominate. There is loss of the usual tinctorial characteristics of white and gray matter structures. Endothelial and glial cells, mainly astrocytes, swell, and myelinated fibers begin to disintegrate. Up to 48 hours, neutrophilic emigration progressively increases and falls off. Phagocytic cells from circulating monocytes, adventitial histiocytes, and activated microglia are evident at 48 hours and become the predominant cell type in the ensuing 2 to 3 weeks. The macrophages become stuffed with the products of myelin breakdown and/or blood and may persist in the lesion for months to years. As the process of liquefaction and phagocytosis proceeds, astrocytes at the edges of the lesion progressively enlarge, divide, and develop an extensive network of protoplasmic extensions. Reactive astrocytes can be seen as early as

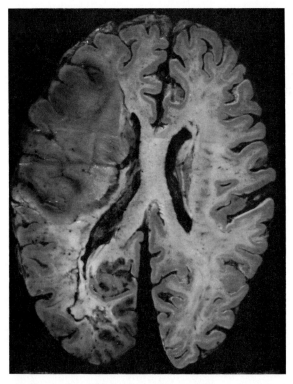

Figure 29–13. Section of the brain showing a large, oval, discolored region (nonhemorrhagic infarct) in the middle of the hemisphere *(upper left)* and a hemorrhagic infarct in the cortex over the posteromedial region of the same hemisphere.

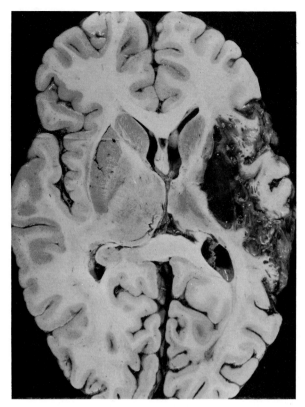

Figure 29-14. Old cystic infarct.

1 week following the insult. After several months, the striking nuclear and cytoplasmic enlargement subsides. In the wall of the cavity astrocyte processes form a dense feltwork of glial fibers admixed with new capillaries and a few perivascular connective tissue fibers. In the cerebral cortex, the cavity is delimited from the meninges and subarachnoid space by a gliotic layer of tissue, derived from the molecular layer of cortex. The pia and arachnoid are not affected and do not contribute to the healing process. Despite this chronology, the signs of ischemic damage to nerve cells and glia and the infiltration of inflammatory cells are more variable than those observed in lower organs (e.g., the heart), making dating of CNS ischemic lesions on histologic grounds quite imprecise.

The microscopic picture and evolution of hemorrhagic infarction parallel ischemic infarction with the addition of blood extravasation and resorption. In anticoagulated patients, hemorrhagic infarcts may be associated with extensive intracerebral hematomas. Venous infarcts are often hemorrhagic and may occur following thrombotic occlusion of the superior sagittal sinus or other sinuses or occlusion of the deep cerebral veins. Carcinoma, localized infections, or other conditions leading to a hypercoagulable state place patients at risk for venous thrombosis and infarction.

NONTRAUMATIC INTRACRANIAL HEMORRHAGE

Brain hemorrhage is often divided into two broad categories, *intraparenchymal* and *subarachnoid*, denoting the site of vascular rupture. They are associated with diverse pathologic conditions. Combinations of the two may occur: intracerebral hemorrhages may rupture into a ventricle and reach the subarachnoid space via the fourth ventricle, or the blood from a ruptured aneurysm in the subarachnoid space may dissect into the adjoining brain. Vascular malformations may be a source of hemorrhage and often induce both subarachnoid and intracerebral bleeding. Traumatic intracranial hemorrhage has been discussed above.

Intraparenchymal Hemorrhage

Although cerebral infarction is a more frequent cause of the stroke syndrome, intracerebral hemorrhage is the leading cause of death (approximately 15% of patients with an intracerebral hemorrhage die with or without treatment). The most important predisposing factor is *arterial hypertension* (80%). Other associated conditions include intracerebral arteriovenous malformations, tumor, hemorrhagic diathesis, and amyloid angiopathy.

Hypertensive intracerebral hemorrhage may originate in the putamen (50 to 60%), thalamus, pontine tegmentum, cerebellar hemispheres (about 10% each), and any other region of the brain in rarer instances (Fig. 29–15). The predilection of these hypertensive lesions for deep gray structures within the cerebral hemispheres has led to the term *ganglionic hemorrhages*, to distinguish them from the more superficial and peripheral hemispheric *lobar hemorrhages*[20] found in association with amyloid angiopathy and hemorrhagic diathesis. The involved areas are most often supplied by branches of the middle, posterior, or basilar arteries that take off at sharp angles from the main vessel. The structural and dynamic changes that directly cause rupture are unknown. The leading pathogenetic theory holds that hypertension damages the vascular wall, leading to wall thickening with fibrinoid change or necrosis and luminal narrowing. Because of the vascular wall injury, there is segmental weakening and dilatation, giving rise to microaneurysms *(Charcot-Bouchard aneurysms)* that may rupture.

The clinical outcome of brain hemorrhage, of course, depends on the size and position of the lesion. A significant increase in intracranial pressure from the mass effect of a supratentorial hematoma, with or without secondary cerebral edema, may lead to transtentorial or subfalcine herniation. In patients who survive, the hematoma is slowly resorbed over a period of months.

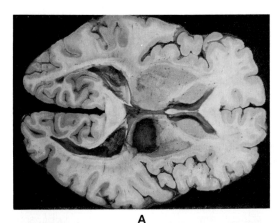

A

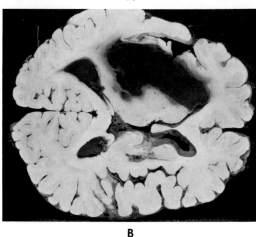

B

Figure 29-15. *A,* Hypertensive hemorrhage, thalamus. *B,* Massive hypertensive hemorrhage, rupturing into a lateral ventricle. (Note the old ganglionic hemorrhage in right hemisphere.)

MORPHOLOGY. Grossly, acute hemorrhages are characterized by extravasation of blood with compression of the adjacent parenchyma. Old hemorrhages show an area of cavitary destruction of brain with a rim of brownish discoloration. Microscopically, the early lesion is characterized by a central core of clotted blood surrounded by a rim of brain tissue showing anoxic neuronal and glial changes as well as edema. Eventually, the edema resolves, pigment-laden and lipid-laden macrophages appear, and proliferation of reactive astrocytes is seen at the periphery, following the same timetable observed after cerebral infarction.

The underlying histologic changes in vessels in hypertensive cerebrovascular disease involve mainly penetrating arteries of the cortex, basal ganglia, and brain stem having a caliber of 75 to 400 μm. They are similar to those seen in other organs.

Lobar hemorrhages do not correlate as well with hypertension.[20] They may arise in the setting of hemorrhagic diathesis, neoplasms, and **amyloid angiopathy.** In amyloid angiopathy, amyloid is deposited within the walls of small arteries within ce-

rebral cortex and leptomeninges, with some predilection for the occipital lobe. Vessels within the white matter and deep nuclei are not affected ordinarily. The amyloid deposited is biochemically identical to that found in Alzheimer's disease.

Subarachnoid Hemorrhage (SAH)

The most frequent cause of SAH of clinical and pathologic importance is rupture of a *berry aneurysm.* SAH may also result from extension of a traumatic hematoma, rupture of a hypertensive intracerebral hemorrhage into the ventricular system, vascular malformation, hematologic disturbances, and tumor. Ruptured berry aneurysm is the fourth most common cerebrovascular disorder, after atherosclerotic thrombosis, embolism, and hypertensive intraparenchymal hemorrhage.

Berry aneurysm *(saccular aneurysm, congenital aneurysm)* is the most frequent type of intracranial aneurysm. Other rarer types of aneurysms include atherosclerotic (fusiform) aneurysms, which mostly affect the basilar artery, as well as mycotic, traumatic, and dissecting aneurysms, all of which involve chiefly the anterior circulation. These ordinarily do not present as subarachnoid hemorrhage.

In a large series, ruptured and unruptured berry aneurysms are found in 1.8% of patients coming to autopsy.[2] There is an increased risk among patients with adult-onset polycystic kidney disease, although the majority occur sporadically. Most aneurysms (90% ± 5) occur in the anterior circulation and are found near branch points (Fig. 29-16).

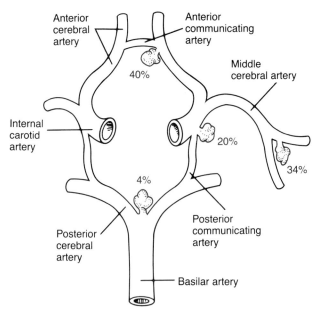

Figure 29-16. Common sites of berry aneurysms in the circle of Willis.

The pathogenesis of berry aneurysms is unknown. Although they are often referred to as *congenital*, they are not identifiable at birth. A congenital defect of the media of involved vessels (internal elastica and muscle wall), particularly at bifurcations, has been demonstrated, which may lead to outpouchings over the course of time. Other disease of the arterial wall brought about by age, hypertension (estimated to be present in 54% of patients), and collagen disorders (Ehlers-Danlos syndrome, pseudoxanthoma elasticum, Marfan syndrome) probably predisposes to the development of berry aneurysms in some patients.

Rupture of the aneurysm is the most frequent complication (74% of patients with autopsy-proven aneurysms have evidence of aneurysmal rupture). Ruptured berry aneurysm with clinically significant subarachnoid hemorrhage is most frequent in the fifth decade (about one-third of patients) and is slightly more frequent in females. When present, aneurysms are multiple in about 20 to 30% based on autopsy series. The probability of rupture increases with the size of the lesion; aneurysms greater than 10 mm have a roughly 50% risk of bleeding per year. Rupture often occurs with acute increases in intracranial pressure, such as with straining at stool or sexual orgasm. Blood under arterial pressure is forced into the subarachnoid space, and patients are stricken with sudden, excruciating headache, typically "the worse headache I've ever had," and may rapidly lose consciousness. Between 25 and 50% of patients die with the first rupture, but most patients who survive improve and recover consciousness in minutes. Rebleeding is common in survivors, and it is currently not possible to predict in which patients rebleeding will occur. The causes of the rebleeding are not understood. With each episode of bleeding, the prognosis is graver. The clinical consequences of blood in the subarachnoid space can be separated into acute events, occurring in the hours to days following the hemorrhage, and late sequelae associated with the healing process. In the early post-SAH period, regardless of the etiology of the hemorrhage, there is an increased risk of vasospastic injury involving vessels other than those originally injured. This vasospasm can lead to additional ischemic injury. This problem is of greatest significance in cases of basal SAH in which vasospasm can involve major vessels of the circle of Willis. Various mediators have been proposed to play a role in this reactive process; some data suggest a contribution from endothelin-1 acting from the adventitial side.[21] In the healing phase of SAH, meningeal fibrosis and scarring occur, sometimes leading to obstruction of CSF flow as well as interruption of the normal pathways of CSF resorption.

MORPHOLOGY. An unruptured berry aneurysm is a thin-walled outpouching at arterial branch points

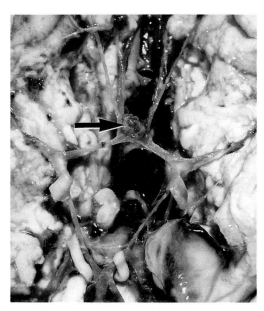

Figure 29–17. View of the base of the brain, dissected to show the circle of Willis with an aneurysm of the anterior communicating artery *(arrow)*. (Courtesy of Dr. E.P. Richardson, Jr., Massachusetts General Hospital, Boston.)

along the circle of Willis or major vessels just beyond. Berry aneurysms measure from a few millimeters to 2 or 3 cm and have a bright, red, shiny surface and a thin translucent wall (Fig. 29–17). The site of rupture is usually readily visible. Atheromatous plaques, calcification, or thrombotic occlusion of the sac may be found. Brownish discoloration of the adjacent brain and meninges is evidence of prior hemorrhage. The neck of the aneurysm may be either wide or narrow. Rupture usually occurs at the apex of the sac. The arterial wall adjacent to the neck of the aneurysm often shows some intimal thickening and gradual attenuation of the medium as it approaches the neck. At the neck of the aneurysm, the muscular wall and intimal elastic lamina are usually absent or fragmentary, and the wall of the sac is made up of thickened hyalinized intima. The adventitia covering the sac is continuous with that of the parent artery.

VASCULAR MALFORMATIONS

Vascular malformations fall into three subgroups based on the characteristics of the component vessels: *arteriovenous malformations (AVMs), cavernous angiomas,* and *capillary telangiectasias.* It is difficult to obtain an accurate assessment of the relative incidence of these lesions.

AVM is the most important type of vascular malformation. The lesion consists of a tangle of numerous, abnormally tortuous, misshapen vessels. Males are affected twice as frequently as females, and the lesion is most often recognized clinically between the ages of 10 and 30, presenting as a seizure disorder, an intracerebral hemorrhage, and/or a subarachnoid hemorrhage. The territory of the middle cerebral artery, particularly its posterior branches, is more commonly affected, but the lesion may occur anywhere along the neuraxis, including the midbrain, cerebellum, or spinal cord. Large AVMs can lead to congestive heart failure in the newborn because of shunt effects, especially if the malformation involves the vein of Galen.

MORPHOLOGY. AVMs involve vessels in the subarachnoid space extending into brain parenchyma, or may occur within the brain. Macroscopically, they resemble a tangled network of worm-like vascular channels. Microscopically, they are composed of greatly enlarged blood vessels separated by gliotic tissue, often with evidence of prior hemorrhage. Some vessels can be recognized as arteries with duplication and fragmentation of the internal elastic lamina, and others with marked thickening and/or partial replacement of the media by hyalinized connective tissue, cannot be further classified.

Cavernous hemangiomas consist of greatly distended, loosely organized vascular channels with thin collagenized walls and are devoid of intervening nervous tissue (thus distinguishing them from capillary telangiectasias). They occur most often in the cerebellum, pons, and subcortical regions, in decreasing order of frequency. Foci of old hemorrhage, infarction, and calcification frequently surround the abnormal vessels. *Capillary telangiectasias* are microscopic foci of dilated, thin-walled vascular channels separated by relatively normal brain parenchyma and occurring most frequently in the pons. *Venous angiomas* (varices) consist of aggregates of ectatic venous channels.

HYPERTENSIVE CEREBROVASCULAR DISEASE

The effects of hypertension on the brain include hypertensive hemorrhage, as discussed previously, lacunes, and hypertensive encephalopathy.

The deep penetrating arterioles that supply the basal ganglia and hemispheric white matter, as well as the brain stem, are involved by *arteriolar sclerosis* which is structurally similar to that described in non-CNS vessels. An important clinical and pathological outcome of these arterial lesions is the *lacune* or *lacunar state* (Fig. 29–18). It consists of small (less than 15 mm) infarcts (often with microscopic evidence of associated hemorrhage) that occur in the lenticular nucleus, thalamus, internal capsule, deep white matter, caudate nucleus, and pons, in descending order of frequency. De-

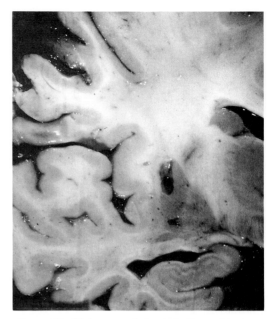

Figure 29–18. Lacunar infarcts in the putamen.

pending on their locations, lacunes can either be clinically silent or cause significant impairment. Lacunar infarcts are often multiple and occur almost invariably in hypertensive patients and in diabetics.

Acute hypertensive encephalopathy is a clinicopathologic syndrome arising in a hypertensive patient characterized by evidence of diffuse cerebral dysfunction (headaches, confusion, vomiting, and convulsions sometimes leading to coma). Rapid therapeutic intervention to reduce the accompanying increased intracranial pressure is required, as the syndrome often does not remit spontaneously. Patients coming to postmortem examination may show an edematous brain weighing more than normal, with or without transtentorial or tonsillar herniation. Petechiae and necrosis of arterioles in the gray and white matter may be seen microscopically.

INFECTIONS

General aspects of the pathogenesis of infections involving the CNS have been discussed in Chapter 8. There are four principal routes of entry for infections of the nervous system. *Hematogenous spread* is the most common means of entry; infectious agents ordinarily enter through the arterial circulation, but retrograde venous spread can occur via anastomotic connections between veins of the face and the cerebral circulation. *Direct implantation* of microorganisms is almost invariably traumatic, or sometimes iatrogenic, such as those introduced with a lumbar puncture needle. *Local extension* can occur secondary to an established infection in an air sinus (most often the mastoid or frontal), an infected tooth, or a surgical site in the cranium or spine causing osteomyelitis, bone erosion, and propagation of the infection into the CNS. Last, the *peripheral nervous system* can be a path of infection into the CNS, as occurs with certain viruses (e.g., rabies and herpes simplex). Damage to nervous tissue may be the consequence of direct injury of neurons or glia by the organism, microbial toxins, the effects of the inflammatory response, or immune-mediated injury.[22]

MENINGITIS

The CSF provides both a culture medium for the infecting organisms and a rapid means of disseminating infection. *Meningitis* refers to an inflammatory process of the leptomeninges and CSF within the subarachnoid space; the increased number of white blood cells in CSF is termed *pleocytosis*. It is usually caused by an infection, but *chemical meningitis* may also occur in response to a nonbacterial irritant introduced into the subarachnoid space. Infiltration of the subarachnoid space by tumor cells has been termed "carcinomatous meningitis," although because this is not an inflammatory disorder, *meningeal carcinomatosis* is a more accurate term. Infectious meningitis can be broadly classified as *acute pyogenic* (usually bacterial), *aseptic* (usually viral), and *chronic* (bacterial or fungal).

Acute Pyogenic (Bacterial) Meningitis

The most commonly encountered causative organisms vary with the age of the patient.[23] In neonates the organisms include *Escherichia coli* and the group B streptococci; in infants and children, *Haemophilus influenzae*; in adolescents and in young adults, *Neisseria meningitidis*; in the elderly, *Streptococcus pneumoniae* and *Listeria monocytogenes*. The typical patient with acute pyogenic meningitis has general signs of infection with the added symptoms and signs of meningeal irritation: headache, photophobia, irritability, clouding of consciousness, and neck stiffness. *A spinal tap yields cloudy or frankly purulent CSF, under increased pressure, with as many as 90,000 neutrophils per mm³, a raised protein level, and a markedly reduced glucose content.* Bacteria may be seen on a smear or may be cultured, sometimes a few hours before the neutrophils appear. In the preantibiotic era, pyogenic meningitis was frequently fatal. In the immunosuppressed patient, purulent meningitis may be caused by other agents, such as *Klebsiella* or an anaerobic organism, and may have an atypical course and uncharacteristic CSF find-

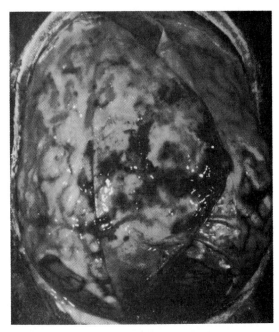

Figure 29–19. Pyogenic meningitis. A thick layer of suppurative exudate is disclosed beneath the retracted dura.

ings, all of which make the diagnosis more difficult.

MORPHOLOGY. Grossly, the normally clear CSF is cloudy and sometimes frankly purulent; the exudate is evident within the leptomeninges over the surface of the brain (Fig. 29–19). The meningeal vessels are engorged and stand out prominently. The location of the exudate varies: in *H. influenzae* meningitis, for example, it is usually basal, whereas in pneumococcal meningitis, it is often densest over the cerebral convexities near the sagittal sinus. From the areas of greatest accumulation, tracts of pus can be followed along blood vessels on the surface of the brain. When the meningitis is fulminant, the inflammation may extend to the ventricles, producing ventriculitis.

Microscopically, neutrophils fill the entire subarachnoid space in severely affected areas and are found predominantly around the leptomeningeal blood vessels in less severe cases. In untreated meningitis, Gram stain reveals varying numbers of the causative organism, although they are frequently not demonstrable in treated cases. In fulminant meningitis, the inflammatory cells infiltrate the walls of the leptomeningeal veins with potential extension of the inflammatory infiltrate into the substance of the brain (focal cerebritis). Phlebitis may also lead to venous occlusion and hemorrhagic infarction of the underlying brain.

Leptomeningeal fibrosis and consequent hydrocephalus may follow pyogenic meningitis, although if it is treated early there may be little remaining evidence of the infection. In some infections, particularly in pneumococcal meningitis, large quantities of the capsular polysaccharide of the organism produce a particularly gelatinous exudate that encourages arachnoid fibrosis, **chronic adhesive arachnoiditis.**

Aseptic (Viral) Meningitis

Nonbacterial, or aseptic, meningitis is a clinically useful term to designate a symptom complex comprising meningeal irritation and alterations of consciousness but with a less fulminant course and CSF findings different from those observed with bacterial meningitis. *There is a lymphocytic pleocytosis, the protein elevation is only moderate, and the sugar content is nearly always normal.* The viral aseptic meningitides are usually self-limiting and are treated symptomatically. In approximately 70% of cases a pathogen can be identified, most commonly an enterovirus (echovirus, coxsackievirus, and nonparalytic poliomyelitis are responsible for up to 80% of these cases). Nonviral aseptic meningitis may develop subsequent to rupture of an epidermoid cyst into the subarachnoid space or the introduction of a chemical irritant therein — "chemical" meningitis. A chronic meningitis may ensue. There is a CSF pleocytosis with neutrophils and a raised protein level, but usually a normal sugar content, and organisms are not present.

MORPHOLOGY. There are no distinctive macroscopic characteristics except for brain swelling, seen in some instances. Pathologic material is limited, however, because recovery of patients is the rule. Microscopically, there is either no abnormality or a mild to moderate infiltration of the leptomeninges with lymphocytes.

BRAIN ABSCESS

Brain abscesses may arise by direct implantation of organisms, local extension from adjacent foci (especially mastoiditis), or hematogenous spread (usually from a primary site in the heart, lungs, or distal bones). Predisposing conditions include *acute bacterial endocarditis*, which tends to produce multiple abscesses; *cyanotic congenital heart disease*, in which there is a right-to-left shunt and loss of pulmonary filtration of organisms; and *chronic pulmonary sepsis* (as can be seen with bronchiectasis). Streptococci and staphylococci are the primary organisms identified.[24]

Clinically, cerebral abscesses are destructive, and patients almost invariably present with progressive focal deficits in addition to the general signs of raised intracranial pressure. *The CSF is*

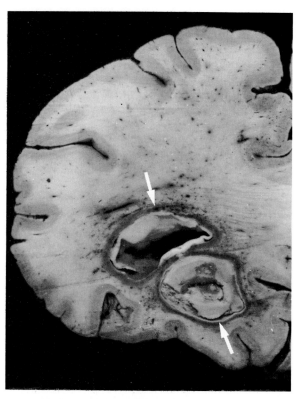

Figure 29–20. Frontal abscesses (arrows).

under increased pressure; the white cell count and protein level are raised, but the sugar content is normal. A systemic or local source of infection may be apparent, or a small systemic focus may have ceased to be symptomatic. The increased intracranial pressure and progressive herniation can be fatal, and abscess rupture can lead to ventriculitis, meningitis, and sinus thrombosis. With surgery and antibiotics, the otherwise high mortality rate can be reduced to less than 20%.

MORPHOLOGY. Abscesses are recognized as discrete lesions with central liquefactive necrosis, a surrounding fibrous, collagenized response, and edema (Fig. 29–20). Microscopically, there is exuberant neovascularization around the necrosis that is responsible for the marked vasogenic edema and formation of granulation tissue. The collagen of the capsule is produced by fibroblasts derived from the walls of blood vessels. Outside the fibrous capsule is a zone of reactive gliosis with numerous gemistocytic astrocytes.

SUBDURAL EMPYEMA

Bacterial or, occasionally, fungal infection of the skull bones or air sinuses can spread to the subdural space and produce a subdural empyema. The underlying arachnoid and subarachnoid spaces are usually unaffected, but a large subdural empyema may produce a mass effect. Further, a thrombophlebitis may develop in the bridging veins that cross the subdural space, resulting in venous occlusion and infarction of the brain. With treatment, including surgical drainage, resolution of the empyema occurs from the dural side, and if it is complete, a thickened dura may be the only residual finding.

Symptoms include those referable to the source of the infection; in addition, most patients are febrile with headache and neck stiffness and, if untreated, may develop focal neurologic signs, lethargy, and coma. The CSF profile is similar to that seen in brain abscesses, because both are parameningeal infective processes. If diagnosis and treatment are prompt, complete recovery is usual. *Extradural abscess*, commonly associated with osteomyelitis, often arises from an adjacent focus of infection, such as sinusitis or a surgical procedure. When the process occurs in the spinal epidural space, it may cause spinal cord compression and constitutes a neurosurgical emergency.

CHRONIC MENINGOENCEPHALITIS

Tuberculous and Chronic Meningitis

Tuberculous meningitis usually manifests as generalized complaints of a headache, malaise, mental confusion, and vomiting. *There is only a moderate CSF pleocytosis made up of mononuclear cells, or a mixture of polymorphonuclear and mononuclear cells; the protein level is elevated, often strikingly so; and the glucose content typically is moderately reduced or normal.*

The most serious complications of chronic meningitis are arachnoid fibrosis, which may produce hydrocephalus, and obliterative endarteritis with arterial occlusion and infarction of underlying brain. Because the process involves the spinal cord subarachnoid space, spinal roots may also be affected.

> **MORPHOLOGY.** Grossly, the subarachnoid space contains a gelatinous or fibrinous exudate, most often at the base of the brain, obliterating the cisterns and encasing cranial nerves. There may be discrete, white granules scattered over the leptomeninges. The most common pattern of involvement is a diffuse meningoencephalitis. Microscopically, the inflammatory reaction is composed of chronic inflammatory cells with mixtures of lymphocytes, plasma cells, and macrophages. Florid cases show well-formed granulomas, often with caseous necrosis and giant cells. Arteries running through the subarachnoid space may show **obliterative endarteritis** with inflammatory infiltrates in their walls and marked intimal thickening. Organisms can often be seen with acid-fast stains. The infectious process may spread to the choroid plexuses and ependymal surface, traveling through the CSF. In cases of long standing, a dense, fibrous adhesive arachnoiditis may develop, most conspicuous around the base of the brain.
>
> Another presentation is as a well-circumscribed intraparenchymal mass **(tuberculoma)**, which may be associated with meningitis. On gross examination, a tuberculoma may be up to several centimeters in diameter, causing significant mass effect. Microscopically, there is usually a central core of caseous necrosis surrounded by a typically tuberculous granulomatous reaction, and calcification may occur in inactive lesions.

Infection by *Mycobacterium tuberculosis* in patients with acquired immunodeficiency syndrome (AIDS) is similar to that in non-AIDS patients. In addition, HIV-positive patients are uniquely at risk for CNS infection by *Mycobacterium avium-intracellulare* (MAI), usually in the setting of disseminated infection. The disease may cause chronic meningitis, brain abscesses, and, rarely, diffuse encephalitis or cranial or peripheral neuropathy. The inflammatory response tends to be less pronounced than in *M. tuberculosis* and consists of foamy macrophages and mononuclear inflammatory cells without the formation of distinctive tubercles. Acid-fast mycobacteria are readily demonstrated by special stains. The response to tuberculosis chemotherapeutic agents has been poor.

Neurosyphilis

Neurosyphilis is a tertiary stage of syphilis, and occurs in only about 10% of patients with untreated infection. Its major forms of expression are meningeal-meningovascular neurosyphilis, paretic neurosyphilis, and tabes dorsalis.

> **MORPHOLOGY. Meningeal neurosyphilis** is a chronic meningitis; there may be an associated obliterative endarteritis accompanied by a distinctive perivascular inflammatory reaction rich in plasma cells.
>
> **Paretic neurosyphilis** is the outcome of invasion of the brain by the treponema, which results in widespread individual cell death and, consequently, brain atrophy, manifested as an insidious but progressive loss of mental and physical functions with mood alterations (including delusions of grandeur) and terminating in severe dementia (general paresis of the insane). Less well explained, but usually present, are Argyll Robertson pupils,

which show accommodation but do not constrict to light. Microscopically, there is loss of cortical neurons with proliferations of microglia (rod cells) and gliosis. The spirochetes can be demonstrated in tissue sections.

Tabes dorsalis is the result of damage by the spirochete to the sensory nerves in the dorsal roots, which produces, among other features, impaired joint position sense and resultant ataxia (locomotor ataxia); loss of pain sensation, leading to skin and joint damage (Charcot joints); other sensory disturbances, particularly the characteristic "lightning pains"; and absence of deep tendon reflexes. Microscopically, there is loss of both axons and myelin in the dorsal roots, with pallor and atrophy in the dorsal columns of the spinal cord. It is not possible to demonstrate organisms in tissue.

Although these three forms of expression of neurosyphilis have been described separately, patients often show incomplete or mixed pictures, notably the combination of tabes dorsalis and general paresis (taboparesis).

Patients with HIV infection are at increased risk for neurosyphilis, and the rate of progression and severity of the disease appear to be accelerated, presumably related to the impaired cell-mediated immunity. CNS involvement by *Treponema pallidum* in this setting may be manifested as asymptomatic infection, acute syphilitic meningitis, meningovascular syphilis, and rarely direct parenchymal invasion of the brain.

Lyme Disease (Neuroborreliosis)

Lyme disease is caused by the spirochete *Borrelia burgdorferi*, transmitted by various species of Ixodes tick. The organism may gain access to the CNS early, but neurologic symptoms occur in later stages of the disease. These include aseptic meningitis, facial nerve palsies, mild encephalopathy, and polyneuropathies.[25]

MORPHOLOGY. The rare cases that have come to autopsy have shown a focal proliferation of microglial cells in the brain as well as scattered organisms (identified by Dieterle stain) in the extracellular spaces. Other findings include granulomas and vasculitis.

VIRAL ENCEPHALITIS

A detailed consideration of pathogenetic mechanisms of viral infection has been given elsewhere (see Chapter 8).

Viral encephalitis (or *encephalomyelitis*) is a parenchymal infection of the brain almost invariably associated with meningeal inflammation, having a very wide spectrum of clinical and pathologic expression.[26] *The most characteristic histologic features of viral encephalitides are perivascular and parenchymal mononuclear cell infiltrates (lymphocytes, plasma cells, and macrophages), glial nodules, and neuronophagia.* However, too much reliance should not be placed on these histologic features alone, because both mononuclear infiltrates and glial nodules can be seen in conditions in which viruses are not thought to be involved. More direct indications of viral involvement are *inclusion bodies* seen in only a minority of viral infections. Furthermore, ultrastructural and molecular methods have greatly contributed to the ability to detect the organisms. The degree of *tropism* exhibited by some viruses is particularly striking in the nervous system. Some viruses infect specific cell types, and others are restricted to particular areas of the brain. The pathogenetic basis of viral tropism is not clear but may reflect a combination of receptor interactions between the host cells and the virus, patterns of access to the nervous system, and the ability of viral genomes to utilize cell type–specific molecular control mechanisms. The capacity of some viruses for *latency* is also particularly important in the nervous system.

There are many indirect effects of viral infection. Systemic viral infections are occasionally followed by an immune-mediated, perivenous demyelinating disorder with no viral penetration of the nervous system (see **ADEM** below). *Congenital malformations* can result from intrauterine viral infection, as occurs with rubella, and *postencephalitic Parkinsonism* followed the presumed viral influenza epidemic during and after the First World War although the specific viral agent for this disease remains unclear.

Arthropod-Borne Viral Encephalitis

These are the typical viral panencephalitides and are responsible for most outbreaks of epidemic viral encephalitis. In the Western Hemisphere the most important types are eastern and western equine, Venezuelan, St. Louis, and California. Types found elsewhere include Japanese B (Far East), Murray Valley (Australia and New Guinea), and tickborne (Russia and Eastern Europe). All have animal hosts and mosquito vectors, except for the tickborne type. Clinically, affected patients develop generalized neurologic deficits, such as seizures, confusion, delirium, and stupor or coma, and often focal signs, such as reflex asymmetry and ocular palsies. *The CSF is usually colorless but with a slightly elevated pressure and, initially, a neutrophilic pleocytosis that rapidly converts to lymphocytes; the protein level is usually raised, but sugar content*

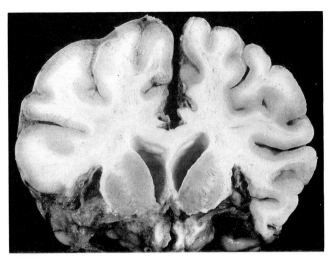

Figure 29-21. Herpes encephalitis showing extensive destruction of inferior frontal and anterior temporal lobes. (Courtesy of Dr. T.W. Smith, University of Massachusetts Medical School, Worcester.)

is normal. Because of the inadequacy of antiviral chemotherapeutic agents, the dominant approach to limiting the spread of these diseases has been through attack on the mosquito vectors.

> **MORPHOLOGY.** The arbovirus encephalitides differ in epidemiology and prognosis, but pathologically their appearance is very similar except for variations in severity. There is a meningoencephalitis with perivascular inflammatory cells, many focal areas of necrosis, and selective neuronal necrosis with neuronophagia. In severe cases there may be a necrotizing vasculitis. Some cases have predominantly cortical involvement, whereas in others the basal ganglia bear the brunt of the disease.

Herpes Simplex Virus Type 1 (HSV-1)

HSV-1 (labialis) produces an encephalitis that occurs in any age group but is most common in children and young adults. Only about 10% of the patients have a history of prior labial herpes. The most commonly observed clinical presenting symptoms are alterations in mood, memory, and behavior. Acyclovir has emerged as the most effective treatment, leading to a significant reduction in the mortality rate.

> **MORPHOLOGY.** The encephalitis starts in, and most severely involves, the inferior and medial regions of the temporal lobes and the orbital gyri of the frontal lobes (Fig. 29-21). The infection is grossly necrotizing and often hemorrhagic in the most severely affected regions. Perivascular inflammatory infiltrates are usually present, and Cowdry intranuclear viral inclusion bodies may be found in both neurons and glia.

HSV-1 may also cause a subacute encephalitis whose clinical manifestations (weakness, lethargy, ataxia, seizures) develop over a more protracted period (4 to 6 weeks) and that is associated with more diffuse involvement of the brain rather than being restricted to the temporal lobes.

Herpes Simplex Virus Type 2 (HSV-2)

HSV-2 (genitalis) also affects the nervous system and is responsible for most cases of *herpetic viral meningitis*. A generalized, and usually severe encephalitis develops in as many as 50% of neonates born by vaginal delivery to women with active *primary* HSV infection. The dependence on route of delivery indicates that the infection is probably acquired during passage through the birth canal rather than transplacentally. HSV-1 causes a similar encephalitis in neonates. In AIDS patients, HSV-2 may rarely cause an acute, hemorrhagic necrotizing encephalitis.

Varicella-Zoster Virus (VZV, Herpes Zoster)

The primary varicella infection presents as one of the childhood exanthems (chickenpox), ordinarily without any evidence of neurologic involvement. Reactivation in adults (commonly called "shingles") usually manifests as a painful, vesicular skin eruption in the distribution of a dermatome (see Chapter 8). Overt CNS involvement with herpes zoster is much rarer but can be more severe. Two types of pathophysiologic processes have been described. First, herpes zoster has been associated with a granulatomatous arteritis. Direct immunocytochemical and electron microscopic evidence of viral involvement has been obtained in a few of these cases. Second, in immunosuppressed patients, herpes zoster may cause an acute *encephalitis* with numerous sharply circumscribed lesions characterized by early demyelination and subsequent necrosis. Inclusion bodies (see Chapter 8) can be found in glia and neurons. VZV infection accounts for about 12% of all systemic herpesvirus infections in patients with AIDS.

Cytomegalovirus (CMV)

This infection of the nervous system occurs in two patient populations: fetuses and the immunosuppressed. The outcome of *in utero* infection is periventricular necrosis that produces severe brain destruction followed later by microcephaly with periventricular calcification. CMV is also the most common opportunistic viral pathogen in patients with AIDS, affecting the CNS in 15 to 20% of cases.[27]

MORPHOLOGY. In the immunosuppressed, the most common pattern of involvement is that of a subacute encephalitis, which may be associated with CMV inclusion-bearing cells (see Fig. 8–36). Although virtually any type of cell within the CNS (neurons, glia, ependyma, endothelium) can be infected by CMV, there is a striking tendency for the virus to localize in the ependymal and subependymal regions of the brain. This results in a severe necrotizing ventriculoencephalitis with massive necrosis, hemorrhage, ventriculitis, and choroid plexitis. Prominent cytomegalic cells with intranuclear and intracytoplasmic inclusions can be readily identified by conventional light microscopy, immunocytochemistry, and *in situ* hybridization. The latter techniques have also shown that normal-appearing, noncytomegalic cells at the edges of the lesions may contain virus.

Poliomyelitis

Poliovirus is an enterovirus that has been controlled by effective immunization. Among the nonimmune, it causes a nonspecific gastroenteritis. In a small fraction of the vulnerable population, however, it secondarily invades the nervous system, where it specifically attacks lower motor neurons. This infection manifests initially with meningeal irritation, which may be its only effect. However, if the motor system is affected, *loss of motor neurons produces a flaccid paralysis with muscle wasting and hyporeflexia in the affected spinal segments that is the permanent neurologic residual of poliomyelitis.* In the acute disease, death can occur from paralysis of the respiratory muscles, and a myocarditis sometimes complicates the clinical course. Permanent cranial nerve (bulbar) weakness is rare, as is any evidence of encephalitis, but severe respiratory compromise is an important cause of long-term morbidity. Coxsackieviruses can cause a somewhat similar paralysis that, although occasionally severe, is usually transitory.

MORPHOLOGY. Acute cases show mononuclear cell perivascular cuffs and neuronophagia of the anterior horn motor neurons of the spinal cord. The inflammatory reaction is usually confined to the anterior horns but may extend into the posterior horns, and the damage is occasionally severe enough to produce cavitation. The motor cranial nuclei may sometimes be involved. Postmortem examination in long-term survivors of symptomatic polio shows loss of neurons and long-standing gliosis in the affected anterior horns of the spinal cord, atrophy of the anterior (motor) spinal roots, and neurogenic atrophy of denervated muscle.

A late neurologic syndrome can develop in patients affected by poliomyelitis who had been stable over intervening years *(postpolio syndrome)*. This syndrome, which typically develops 25 to 35 years after the resolution of the initial illness, is characterized by progressive weakness associated with decreased muscle bulk and pain. There is no evidence, to date, of persistence of polio virus genomes, and there is conflicting evidence regarding the re-emergence of an immune response.[28,29]

Rabies

This disease is transmitted by the bite of a rabid animal, usually a dog although various wild animal populations form natural reservoirs for the disease. It causes a severe encephalitis. The virus enters the CNS by ascent along the peripheral nerves from the wound site. The incubation period varies, depending on the distance between the wound and the brain (commonly between 1 and 3 months). Clinically, the disease manifests with nonspecific symptoms of malaise, headache, and fever, but the conjunction of these symptoms with local paresthesias around the wound is diagnostic. In advanced cases, the patient exhibits extraordinary CNS excitability; the slightest touch is painful, with violent motor responses progressing to convulsions. Contracture of the pharyngeal musculature when swallowing produces foaming at the mouth. The old term for the disease—hydrophobia—describes this phenomenon. There is meningismus and, as the disease progresses, flaccid paralysis. Periods of alternating mania and stupor progress to coma and death from respiratory center failure.

MORPHOLOGY. Grossly, the brain shows intense edema and vascular congestion. Microscopically, there is widespread neuronal degeneration and an inflammatory reaction that is most severe in the basal ganglia, midbrain, and floor of the fourth ventricle, particularly in the medulla. The spinal cord and dorsal root ganglia may also be involved. **Negri bodies,** the pathognomonic microscopic finding, are cytoplasmic, round to oval or bullet-shaped, eosinophilic inclusions and can be found in pyramidal neurons of the hippocampus and Purkinje cells of the cerebellum, sites usually devoid of inflammation.[30]

Human Immunodeficiency Virus 1 (HIV-1)

As many as 60% of patients with AIDS develop neurologic dysfunction during the course of their illness, and in some, it dominates the clinical picture until death[31,32] (see Chapter 6 for a discussion of the epidemiology and pathogenesis of AIDS). Neuropathologic changes have been demonstrated at postmortem examination in as many as 80 to 90% of cases.[33] These include direct or indirect effects of HIV-1, opportunistic infection, and primary CNS lymphoma (see Chapter 8).

HIV-1 Aseptic Meningitis

This occurs within 1 to 2 weeks of seroconversion in about 10% of patients; antibodies to HIV-1 can be demonstrated and the virus can be isolated from the CSF.

MORPHOLOGY. The very few neuropathologic studies of the early and acute phases of symptomatic or asymptomatic HIV-1 invasion of the nervous system have shown only a mild lymphocytic meningitis and some myelin loss in the hemispheres.[34]

HIV-1 Meningoencephalitis (Subacute Encephalitis)

This was recognized as a clinical syndrome well before HIV-1 became identified as the etiologic agent in AIDS. This remarkable neurologic disorder has been called **AIDS dementia** and, more recently, **AIDS-related cognitive-motor complex.** The disorder begins insidiously with mental slowing, memory loss, and mood disturbances, such as apathy and depression. Motor abnormalities, ataxia, bladder and bowel incontinence, and seizures can also be present. Radiologic imaging of the brain may show diffuse cortical atrophy, focal abnormalities of the cerebral white matter, or ventricular dilatation.

MORPHOLOGY. Macroscopic examination of the brain shows clear meninges, some ventricular dilatation, and sulcal widening but normal cortical thickness. Microscopically, the process is best characterized as a chronic inflammatory reaction with widely distributed infiltrates of **microglial nodules,** sometimes with associated foci of tissue necrosis and reactive gliosis (Fig. 29–22). The microglial nodules are also found in the vicinity of small blood vessels, which show abnormally prominent endothelial cells concurrent with perivascular foamy and/or pigment-laden macrophages. These changes occur especially in the subcortical white matter, diencephalon, and brain stem. An important although not invariable component of the microglial nodule is the macrophage-derived **multi-nucleated giant cell.** There is also a disorder of white matter characterized by multifocal or diffuse areas of myelin pallor sometimes associated with axonal swellings and gliosis.

Localization of HIV to the CD4+ mononucleate and multinucleate macrophages and microglia is now well established, as evidenced by ultrastructural studies, immunoperoxidase methods utilizing primarily antisera directed against the HIV-1 envelope glycoproteins, and amplification methods to detect viral nucleic acid sequences. HIV infection has been reported in retinal and cerebral endothelial cells in some studies. There is considerable uncertainty as to whether neurons, astrocytes, or oligodendrocytes are affected directly by HIV-1 (see discussion in Chapter 6).

Vacuolar Myelopathy

This disorder of the spinal cord is found in 20 to 30% of unselected patients with AIDS in the United States, less often in Europe.[35] The pathologic findings show striking resemblance to the lesions of subacute combined degeneration, but vitamin B_{12} levels are normal. Vacuolar myelopathy does not appear to be directly caused by HIV-1; in fact, the organism is often not present within the lesions.[36] Furthermore, vacuolar myelopathy has now been reported in immunosuppressed, non-AIDS patients.

MORPHOLOGY. The disease involves the white matter of the posterior columns extending to the lateral columns and, less often, to other portions of the lower and middle thoracic cord. It is characterized by myelin damage in the form of vacuoles that contain foamy macrophages. Ultrastructural studies indicate both axonal and myelin injury.

Of related interest is the condition known as *tropical spastic paraparesis,* which has been reported in several countries in the Caribbean, along the Indian Ocean, and in South America. Some cases show a severe lymphocytic meningomyelitis quite unlike that seen in vacuolar myelopathy. Virologic studies and polymerase chain reaction data have implicated human T-cell lymphotrophic virus 1 (HTLV-1) in this disorder.

Cranial and Peripheral Neuropathies

Patients with AIDS are susceptible to a wide range of cranial and peripheral neuropathies. The most commonly reported clinical syndromes include acute and chronic inflammatory demyelinating polyneuropathy, distal symmetric polyneuropathy, polyradiculopathy, mononeuritis multiplex, and rarely sensory neuropathy due to ganglioneuronitis. The histopathologic findings observed in most

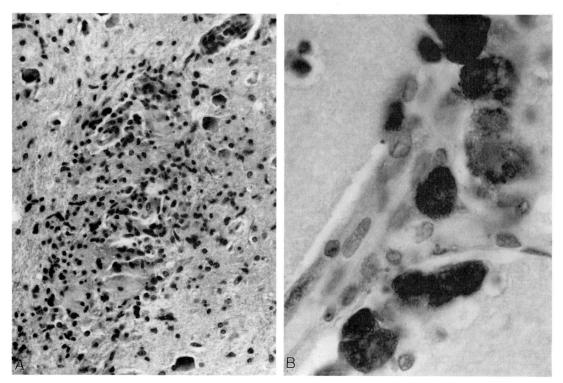

Figure 29–22. HIV-1 encephalitis. *A,* Note microglial nodule and multinucleated giant cells. *B,* Perivascular distribution of HIV-infected macrophages detected by immunoperoxidase to gp41.

of these cases include segmental demyelination, axonal degeneration, and epineurial and endoneurial mononuclear cell inflammation.

Inflammatory myopathy has been the most often described skeletal muscle disorder in patients with HIV-1 infection. The disease is characterized by the subacute onset of proximal weakness, sometimes pain, and elevated levels of serum creatine kinase. The histologic findings in these cases have included muscle fiber necrosis and phagocytosis, interstitial infiltration with HIV-positive macrophages, and in a few cases cytoplasmic bodies and nemaline rods. An acute, toxic, reversible myopathy with "ragged red" fibers and myoglobulinuria may also develop in AIDS patients treated with zidovudine (AZT).

AIDS in Children

Neurologic disease is common in children with congenital AIDS. Clinical manifestations of neurologic dysfunction are evident by the first years of life and include microcephaly with mental retardation and motor developmental delay with long tract signs.

MORPHOLOGY. The most frequently reported abnormality is calcification of the basal ganglia and deep cerebral white matter, involving both large and small vessels and as aggregates with foci of tissue destruction in the gray or white matter. There is also loss of hemispheric myelin or delay in myelination. Opportunistic infections of the CNS, including toxoplasmosis, CMV, PML, and cryptococcal meningitis, are relatively rare in infants and children with AIDS as compared with adults.

Progressive Multifocal Leukoencephalopathy (PML)

PML is a viral infection of oligodendrocytes by a papovavirus (JC virus) that, because it infects and kills the oligodendrocytes that produce myelin, causes demyelination as its principal pathologic effect. The disease appears late in the course of immunosuppression caused by a variety of diseases, including chronic lymphoproliferative, myeloproliferative, immunosuppressive chemotherapy, granulomatous diseases, and AIDS. Although no systemic syndrome has been described, about 65% of normal people have serologic evidence of exposure to JC virus by the age of 14 years. It is not known whether PML results from a primary infection in a susceptible host or from the rekindling of an old infection. Clinically, patients develop focal and relentlessly progressive neurologic symptoms and signs, and both computed tomography (CT) and magnetic resonance imaging (MRI) scans show ex-

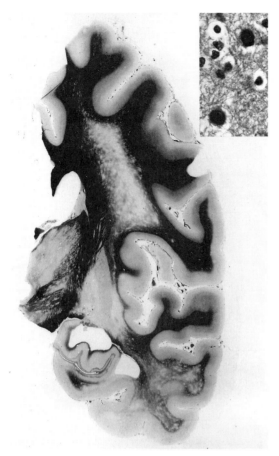

Figure 29–23. Progressive multifocal leukoencephalopathy. Section stained for myelin showing irregular, poorly defined areas of demyelination, which become confluent in places. *Inset,* Enlarged oligodendrocyte nuclei stained for viral antigens.

tensive, often multifocal lesions in the hemispheric or cerebellar white matter.

MORPHOLOGY. The lesions consist of patches of irregular, ill-defined destruction of the white matter ranging in size from millimeters to extensive involvement of an entire lobe of the brain (Fig. 29–23). The cerebrum, brain stem, cerebellum, and, occasionally, the spinal cord all can be involved. Microscopically, the typical lesion consists of a patch of demyelination in the center of which are many lipid-laden macrophages and a few axons. At the edge of the lesion are greatly enlarged oligodendrocyte nuclei whose chromatin is replaced by glassy amphophilic viral inclusion material. These oligodendrocytes can be shown to contain viral antigens by the immunoperoxidase method (see Fig. 29–23, *inset*) and viral genome by *in situ* hybridization. Within the lesions, there are characteristic bizarre giant astrocytes with irregular, hyperchromatic, sometimes multiple nuclei. Reactive fibrillary astrocytes are scattered among the bizarre forms, and there are many foamy macro-

phages containing myelin debris, but strikingly little inflammatory reaction in the brain or meninges. Axons traversing the lesions are conspicuously preserved. Electron microscopy shows numerous papovavirus particles, often in paracrystalline arrays in the oligodendrocyte nuclei, and, sometimes, isolated viral particles in astrocyte nuclei.

The incidence of PML in AIDS patients may range from 1 to 6%. The neuropathologic features of PML in AIDS patients are essentially identical to those observed in non-AIDS immunocompromised individuals except that the extent and severity of lesions may be greater, with an increased tendency toward necrosis and a higher density of papovavirus-infected cells.[37]

SPONGIFORM ENCEPHALOPATHIES

This is a group of diseases that include Creutzfeldt-Jakob disease (CJD) and kuru in humans, scrapie in sheep and goats, transmissible encephalopathy in mink, and bovine spongiform encephalopathy. Microscopically, they all produce a characteristic *spongiform change* in the gray matter. Spongiform encephalopathy occurs in primates following inoculation with kuru and CJD tissue by a variety of parenteral routes, but most easily by intracerebral inoculation. After a long latent period (usually about 18 months), animals develop both clinical and pathologic changes similar to those seen in humans. Some of the human forms of the disease have a heritable variant, linked to specific mutations in a gene encoding a cellular protein.[38]

Attempts to demonstrate nucleic acid, either DNA or RNA, in purified preparations used in transmission experiments have been unsuccessful; instead, a protein has been implicated as the transmitting agent.[39] This protein is termed a *prion;* it is an abnormal form of a normal cellular protein and is relatively resistant to digestion by proteinase K. The gene, on chromosome 20, for this small, 30-kd protein has a single exon coding for the entire open reading frame and shows a high degree of conservation across species. Experiments using transgenic animals have shown that infectious particles derived from one species are highly effective at transmitting disease in any host containing the gene for that species' normal protein. In cases of familial disease, genetic analysis has revealed several different classes of mutations in the prion gene that appear to be tightly linked to the disease phenotype, suggesting that this is the cause of the disease. Tissue preparations from such cases are infectious.

Although the relationship between the abnormal protein and disease remains to be determined, it has been suggested that the disease occurs when the normal cellular prion protein undergoes a conformational change to the abnormal form. This may occur spontaneously at an extremely low rate or at a higher rate if certain amino acid substitutions are present. This abnormal form then facilitates, in a cooperative fashion, comparable transformation of other prion molecules. The infectious nature of abnormal proteins thus comes from their ability to corrupt the integrity of normal cellular components. Studies of the prion gene have found mutations that underline other familial neurodegenerative diseases, which may or may not show spongiform pathology (Gerstmann-Sträussler-Scheinker syndrome [GSS][38] and fatal familial insomnia).

Creutzfeldt-Jakob disease is a rare but well-characterized disease that manifests clinically as a rapidly progressive dementia. Despite the demonstrated transmissibility of its causative agent, it is sporadic in its occurrence, with a worldwide incidence of about one per million and no discernible pattern of exposure. The natural mode of transmission in humans is obscure, but there are a few cases of iatrogenic transmission, notably via corneal transplantation, deep implantation electrodes, and contaminated preparations of human growth hormone. The clinical picture is usually quite typical, with the initial subtle changes in memory and behavior followed by a rapidly progressive dementia,

often with pronounced startle myoclonus. The disease is uniformly fatal, with an average duration of only 7 months, although a few patients survive for several years.

MORPHOLOGY. The progression of the dementia is usually so rapid that there is little, if any, gross atrophy of the brain. Microscopically, the pathognomonic spongiform change is seen in the cortex and sometimes other regions of gray matter, such as caudate and putamen, and consists of a variable vacuolation in the background neuropil (Fig. 29–24A). In more advanced cases there is severe neuronal loss and marked reactive astrocytosis. No inflammatory infiltrate is present. Electron microscopy shows the vacuoles to be intracytoplasmic and membrane-bound in neuronal and glial processes. **Kuru plaques,** which are deposits of aggregate abnormal prion protein, are Congo red–positive as well as PAS-positive and appear in the cerebellum, mostly commonly in GSS (see Fig. 29–24B).

FUNGAL INFECTION

As with the systemic deep mycoses, fungal disease of the CNS is encountered primarily in immunocompromised patients in industrialized nations.

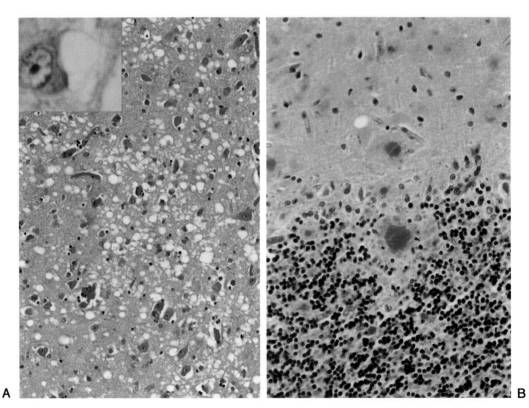

A   B

Figure 29–24. *A,* Creutzfeldt-Jakob disease, showing spongiform change in the cerebral cortex. *Inset,* High magnification of cortical neuropil with vacuoles. *B,* Cerebellar cortex showing kuru plaques, stained with periodic acid–Schiff (PAS) (from a case of Gerstmann-Sträussler-Scheinker disease).

The brain is usually involved only late in the disease, when there is widespread hematogenous dissemination of the fungus, most often *Candida albicans*, *Mucor*, *Aspergillus fumigatus*, and *Cryptococcus neoformans*. In endemic areas, pathogens such as *Histoplasma capsulatum*, *Coccidioides immitis*, and *Blastomyces dermatitidis* may involve the CNS after a primary pulmonary or cutaneous infection; again, this often follows immunosuppression.

There are three basic patterns of fungal infection in the CNS: chronic meningitis, vasculitis, and parenchymal invasion. *Vasculitis* is most frequently seen with Mucor and Aspergillus, both of which have a marked predilection for invasion of blood vessel walls, but occasionally occurs with other organisms, such as Candida. The resultant vascular thrombosis produces infarction that is often strikingly hemorrhagic and that subsequently becomes septic from ingrowth of the causative fungus.

Parenchymal invasion, usually in the form of granulomas or abscesses, can occur with most of the fungi and often coexists with meningitis. The most commonly encountered are Candida and Cryptococcus. Candida usually produces multiple microabscesses, with or without giant cell granuloma formation. Although most fungi invade the brain by hematogenous dissemination, direct extension may also occur, particularly with Mucor, most commonly in diabetics with ketoacidosis.

Cryptococcal meningitis, observed now with increasing frequency in association with AIDS, may be fulminant and fatal in as little as 2 weeks or indolent over months or even years. The CSF may have few cells but a very high level of protein. The mucoid encapsulated yeasts can be visualized in the CSF by India ink preparations and in tissue sections by PAS and mucicarmine as well as fungal silver stains.

> **MORPHOLOGY.** With cryptococcal infection, the brain shows a chronic meningitis affecting the basal leptomeninges, which are opaque and thickened by reactive connective tissue and may obstruct the outflow of CSF from the foramina of Luschka and Magendie, giving rise to hydrocephalus. Sections of the brain disclose a gelatinous material within the subarachnoid space and small cysts within the parenchyma, which are especially prominent in the basal ganglia in the distribution of the lenticulostriate arteries. Parenchymal lesions consist of aggregates of organisms within expanded perivascular (Virchow-Robin) spaces associated with minimal or absent inflammation or gliosis even in the presence of large numbers of organisms. The meningeal infiltrates consist of chronic inflammatory cells and fibroblasts admixed with cryptococci. Well-formed granulomas are not seen ordinarily; in some cases, however, there is a

> marked chronic inflammatory and granulomatous reaction similar to that seen with *M. tuberculosis*, with all the associated complications.

OTHER INFECTIONS

Protozoal diseases (including malaria, toxoplasmosis, amebiasis, and trypanosomiasis), rickettsial infections (such as typhus and Rocky Mountain spotted fever), and metazoal diseases (especially cysticercosis and echinococcosis) may also involve the CNS and are discussed in Chapter 8.

As with cryptococcus, *cerebral toxoplasmosis* has assumed greater importance with the AIDS epidemic.[40] Infection of the brain by *Toxoplasma gondii* is one of the most common causes of neurologic symptomatology and morbidity in patients with AIDS. The average incidence of CNS infection in most clinical and autopsy series ranges from 4 to 30%. The clinical symptoms are subacute, evolving over a 1- or 2-week period, and may be both focal and diffuse. CT and MRI studies may show multiple ring-enhancing lesions; however, this radiographic appearance is not pathognomonic, since similar findings may be associated with CNS lymphoma, tuberculosis, or fungal infections.

> **MORPHOLOGY.** The brain shows abscesses, frequently multiple, most involving the cerebral cortex (near the gray-white junction) and deep gray nuclei, less often the cerebellum and brain stem, and rarely the spinal cord (Fig. 29–25). Acute lesions consist of central foci of necrosis with variable petechiae surrounded by acute and chronic inflammation, macrophage infiltration, and vascular proliferation. Both free tachyzoites and encysted bradyzoites may be found at the periphery of the necrotic foci. The organisms are usually seen on routine hematoxylin and eosin (H&E) or Giemsa stains, but they can be more easily recognized by immunocytochemical methods. The blood vessels in the vicinity of these lesions may show marked intimal proliferation or even frank vasculitis with fibrinoid necrosis and thrombosis. Following treatment, the lesions consist of large, well-demarcated areas of coagulation necrosis surrounded by lipid-laden macrophages. Cysts and free tachyzoites can also be found adjacent to these lesions but may be considerably reduced in number if therapy has been effective. Chronic lesions consist of small cystic spaces containing small numbers of lipid- and hemosiderin-laden macrophages with surrounding gliosis. Organisms are very difficult to detect in these older lesions.

Like CMV encephalitis, toxoplasmosis may also occur in the fetus. Primary maternal infection with toxoplasmosis, particularly if it occurs early in the

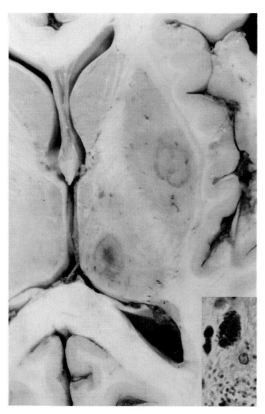

Figure 29–25. Toxoplasma abscesses in putamen and thalamus. *Inset*, Toxoplasma pseudocyst with bradyzoites and free tachyzoites.

pregnancy, may be followed by a cerebritis in the fetus, with the production of multifocal cerebral necrotizing lesions that may calcify, thereby producing severe damage to the developing brain.

A rapidly fatal necrotizing encephalitis is associated with infection with Naegleria species. Another chronic granulomatous meningoencephalitis has been associated with infection with Acanthamoeba. The amebae may sometimes be difficult to distinguish from histiocytes. Methenamine silver or PAS stains are helpful in visualizing the organisms, although definitive identification may ultimately depend on combined immunofluorescence studies, morphology, and culture.

DEMYELINATING DISEASES

Demyelinating diseases are conditions characterized by a preferential damage to myelin, with relative preservation of axons. These can be diseases of either the oligodendrocyte or the myelin sheath. The clinical deficits are due to the effect of myelin loss on the transmission of electrical impulses along axons. The natural history of demyelinating dis-

eases is determined, in part, by the limited capacity of the central nervous system to regenerate normal myelin.

MULTIPLE SCLEROSIS (MS)

MS is defined clinically as a disorder characterized by *distinct episodes of neurologic deficits, separated in time, attributable to white matter lesions that are separated in space.* It is the most common of the demyelinating disorders, having a prevalence of approximately 1 per 1000 persons in most of the United States and Europe. Onset may occur at any age, although onset in childhood or after age 50 is relatively rare. Women are affected more often than men, with an overall ratio of approximately 2:1.

In general, the frequency of MS increases with distance from the equator. However, groups living in relative proximity may have divergent rates. Individuals take on the relative risk of the environment in which they spent their first 15 years.[41] A transmissible agent has been proposed in the pathogenesis of the disorder, but all attempts to identify a well-characterized virus have been unsuccessful.[42] Genetic influences are also clearly evident. The risk of developing MS is 15-fold higher when the disease is present in a first-degree relative. The concordance rate for monozygotic twins is approximately 25%. Linkage studies have indicated that there are associations with several MHC antigens, specifically A3, B7, DR2, DQw1, DQB1, and DQA1, and some studies have claimed association with polymorphisms involving the alpha and beta subunits of the T-cell receptor.

While it is clear that there is an inflammatory component to the lesions of MS, it is uncertain whether the immune system plays a role in initiation of the characteristic white matter damage. There does not appear to be any association of MS with other forms of autoimmune illness, although the data regarding autoimmune thyroid disease are controversial.

CSF examination shows a mildly elevated protein level, and in one-third there is a moderate pleocytosis. The proportion of gamma globulin is increased, and most MS patients show *oligoclonal bands.* This increase in CSF immunoglobulin is the result of proliferation of B cells within the nervous system; the target epitopes of these antibodies are widely variable. These observations suggest that the demyelination is not mediated through an antibody-dependent mechanism.

Cellular immunity directed against myelin components remains a strong candidate mechanism for multiple sclerosis.[43] Both CD4+ and CD8+ lymphocytes are present in the active lesion. Clones reactive with myelin basic protein express a

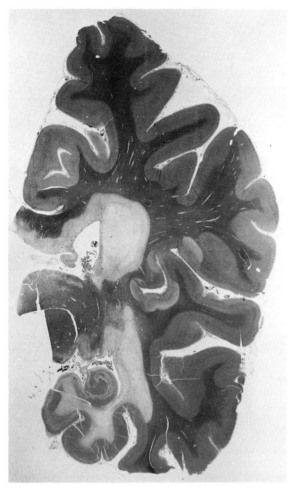

Figure 29–26. Multiple sclerosis. Unstained regions of demyelination (MS plaques) around lateral ventricle and in temporal lobe (Luxol-fast-blue PAS stain for myelin).

range of TCR variable regions, although certain variable regions are over-represented.[44] In addition, antigen-presenting cells, as reflected by the expression of class II molecules on the surface of microglial cells and macrophages, have been found in MS lesions, but there is disagreement as to whether astrocytes express these markers. A potential role for this antigen-presentation can be inferred from the observation that interferon-gamma, which induces the expression of class II molecules, leads to the exacerbation of clinical symptoms in MS patients.

MORPHOLOGY. Since gray matter covers much of the surface of the brain, often the only external evidence of the pathologic process may be the foci of demyelination along the surface of the pons, which appear as glassy, gray lesions. The characteristic multiple lesions of the disease are scattered throughout the white matter and are recognized as sharply circumscribed regions of gray discoloration (plaques) (Fig. 29–26). In the fresh state, these have firmer consistency than the surrounding white matter ("sclerosis"). Plaques may extend into the gray matter, although the recognition of them within these regions is more difficult. Lesions may range in size from microscopic to those that involve nearly all of the white matter of a hemisphere. A common site of occurrence is at the angles of the lateral ventricles, often following the course of a vein.

The lesions have sharply defined borders at the microscopic level (Fig. 29–27). In an **active plaque** there is evidence of active myelin breakdown with abundant macrophages containing lipid-rich, PAS-positive debris. Inflammatory cells, including both lymphocytes and monocytes, are present, mostly as perivascular cuffs. Early lesions are often centered on small veins, especially near the ventricles, and the expansion of growing plaques often tracks along such vessels. Within a plaque, there is relative preservation of axons and depletion of oligodendrocytes. Astrocytic cells remain and show reactive changes. As lesions become quiescent, there is a relative diminution of the inflammatory cell infiltrate and of macrophages. Within the center of an **inactive plaque,** no myelin is found and there are few oligodendrocytes. Instead, astrocytic proliferation and gliosis is evident. Silver stains reveal preservation of axons, although some evidence of fiber loss is not uncommon.

Some MS plaques are less well defined on gross appearance, and this corresponds with partial loss of myelin at the microscopic level. These foci, termed **shadow plaques,** are best characterized by abnormally thinned-out myelin sheaths, especially at the edges of the plaque. These have been variably interpreted as evidence of partial myelin loss as well as of remyelination by oligodendrocytes. Similar abnormally myelinated fibers have been observed at the edges of typical plaques, with comparable interpretations. The finding that some take as evidence of remyelination is the alteration in internode spacing, which is comparable with peripheral nerve remyelination. Remyelination of central axons by Schwann cells has also been described. Although these histologic findings suggest a limited potential for remyelination, most MS plaques and the axons within them remain unmyelinated.

Although the demyelinating lesions can occur anywhere in the central nervous system and, as a consequence, may induce a wide range of symptoms, certain clinical presentations are common. Unilateral visual impairment over the course of a few days, which is due to involvement of the optic nerve (*optic neuritis, retrobulbar neuritis*), is common. However, only some with this initial manifes-

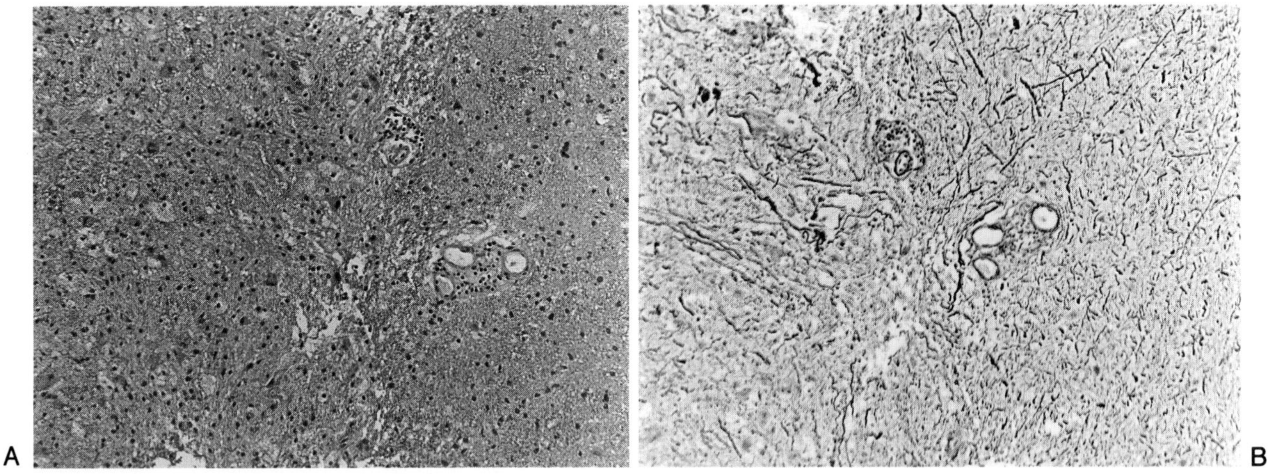

Figure 29-27. Multiple sclerosis. *A,* Myelin-stained section shows the sharp edge of a demyelinated plaque and perivascular lymphocytic cuffs. *B,* The same lesion stained for axons shows relative preservation.

tation will go on to develop MS, with rates ranging from 10 to 50%, depending on the population studied; the remainder do not develop other lesions.

The natural course of multiple sclerosis is variable. In most patients it begins as a relapsing and remitting illness in which episodes of neurologic deficits develop over short periods of time (days to weeks) and show gradual partial remission. The frequency of relapses tends to decrease over the course of time, but in a subset of patients there is a steady neurologic deterioration. The cellular basis for recovery from symptoms is unknown.

The pathologic findings are remarkably similar regardless of the clinical tempo of disease progression. Autopsy studies and radiologic studies using MRI have demonstrated that subclinical forms of the disease exist and that even in symptomatic patients some plaques may be clinically silent.

MULTIPLE SCLEROSIS VARIANTS

Some patients, especially Asians, present with bilateral optic neuritis and spinal cord involvement. This disease is referred to as *neuromyelitis optica* or *Devic's disease.* Patients may have a rapidly progressive course (approximately 20%), a relapsing-remitting course, or a single episode without subsequent relapses. The histologic appearance of lesions in Devic's disease shares characteristics with MS, although lesions are more destructive. Another distinct variant, *acute MS,* tends to occur in young individuals and is characterized clinically by a rapid course over a period of several months. Pathologically, the plaques are large, and there is widespread destruction of myelin with some axonal loss.

ACUTE DISSEMINATED ENCEPHALOMYELITIS (ADEM)

Acute disseminated encephalomyelitis is a monophasic demyelinating disease that follows either a viral infection or, rarely, a viral immunization. Symptoms typically develop a week or two after the antecedent infection and include evidence of diffuse brain involvement with headache, lethargy, and coma rather than focal findings, as in MS. Symptoms progress rapidly, with a fatal outcome in as many as 20% of cases; for the remaining patients, there is complete recovery.

MORPHOLOGY. On gross examination, the brain shows only some grayish discoloration around white matter vessels. Microscopically, however, myelin loss with relative preservation of axons can be found throughout the white matter. The lesions also contain polymorphonuclear leukocytes in the early stages, which gradually give way to a mononuclear infiltrate. The breakdown of myelin is associated with the accumulation of lipid-laden macrophages.

Acute hemorrhagic leukoencephalitis (AHL) shares the perivascular distribution of ADEM but is more fulminant and also includes hemorrhagic necrosis of white and gray matter. These patients, typically young adults, may not have had a prior viral syndrome.

The lesions of ADEM are similar to those induced by immunization of animals with myelin components or with early rabies vaccines that had been prepared from brains of infected animals. This has suggested that ADEM may represent an acute autoimmune reaction to myelin, and that

AHL may represent a hyperacute variant, although no inciting antigens have been identified.

OTHER DEMYELINATING DISEASES

Central pontine myelinolysis (CPM) is characterized by loss of myelin with relative preservation of axons and neuronal cell bodies in a roughly symmetric pattern involving the basis pontis and portions of the pontine tegmentum but sparing the periventricular and subpial regions. Lesions may be found more rostrally, but it is extremely rare for the process to cross the pontomedullary junction. The condition is believed to be caused by rapid correction of hyponatremia.[45] The extent of demyelination is also correlated with the duration of the preceding hyponatremia. The pathogenetic connection between the metabolic disturbance and the disruption of myelin integrity in a localized region of the brain is not understood.

DEGENERATIVE DISEASES

These are diseases of gray matter characterized principally by the *progressive loss of neurons* with associated secondary changes in white matter tracts. Two other general characteristics bring them together as a group. First, the pattern of neuronal loss is *selective, affecting one or more groups of neurons, while leaving others intact.* Second, *the disease arises without any clear inciting event in a patient without previous neurologic deficits.* The neuropathologic findings observed in the degenerative diseases differ greatly; in some there are intracellular abnormalities with some degree of specificity (e.g., Lewy bodies, neurofibrillary tangles), in others there is only loss of the affected neurons. It is empirically convenient to group the degenerative diseases according to the anatomic regions of the brain that are *primarily* affected.

DEGENERATIVE DISEASES AFFECTING THE CEREBRAL CORTEX

The major cortical degenerative diseases are *Alzheimer's disease (AD)* and *Pick's disease,* and their principal clinical manifestation is *dementia,* that is, progressive loss of cognitive function independent of the state of attention. There are many other causes of dementia, including vascular disease (multi-infarct dementia), Creutzfeldt-Jakob disease,

and neurosyphilis. *Dementia is not part of normal aging and always represents a pathologic process.*

Alzheimer's Disease (AD)

This disease usually becomes clinically apparent as insidious impairment of higher intellectual function, with alterations in mood and behavior. Later, progressive disorientation, memory loss, and aphasia indicate severe cortical dysfunction, and eventually, over 5 to 10 years, the patient becomes profoundly disabled, mute, and immobile. Patients rarely become symptomatic before 50 years of age, but the progressive increase in the incidence of the disease in the succeeding decades has given rise to major medical, social, and economic problems in countries with a growing number of elderly individuals. When considered by age groups, the rates are 3% for 65 to 74 years, 19% for 75 to 84 years, and 47% for 85 years or more.[46] Most cases are sporadic in incidence, although at least 5 to 10% of cases (and perhaps more) are familial. Pathologic changes identical to those observed in AD occur in almost all patients with trisomy 21 who survive beyond 45 years, and a decline in cognition can be clinically demonstrated in many. Although pathologic examination of brain tissue remains necessary for the definitive diagnosis of AD, the combination of clinical assessment and modern radiologic methods allows for a diagnostic accuracy of 80 to 90%.

MORPHOLOGY. Gross examination of the brain shows a variable degree of cortical atrophy with widening of the cerebral sulci that is most pronounced in the frontal, temporal, and parietal lobes. With significant atrophy there is compensatory ventricular enlargement secondary to loss of parenchyma (Fig. 29–28). The major microscopic abnormalities of AD are **neurofibrillary tangles, senile (neuritic) plaques, and amyloid angiopathy.** All of these may be present to a lesser extent in the brains of elderly nondemented individuals. However, the diagnosis of AD is based on a clinicopathologic correlation between the patient's neurologic status and the frequency of plaques and tangles. The exact histologic criteria that define AD remain the focus of much controversy.[47]

Neurofibrillary tangles (NFTs) are bundles of filaments in the cytoplasm of the neurons that displace or encircle the nucleus. They often have an elongated "flame" shape; in some cells, the basket weave of fibers around the nucleus takes on a rounded contour (globose tangles). They are visible as basophilic fibrillary structures with H&E staining but are dramatically demonstrated by silver (Bielschowsky) staining (Fig. 29–29A). They are commonly found in cortical neurons, especially in the entorhinal cortex, as well as in other sites such

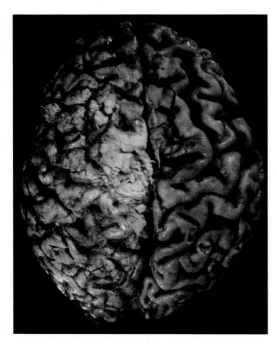

Figure 29-28. Alzheimer's disease with cortical atrophy most evident on the right, where meninges have been removed. (Courtesy of Dr. E.P. Richardson, Jr., Massachusetts General Hospital, Boston.)

as pyramidal cells of the hippocampus, the amygdala, the basal forebrain, and the raphe nuclei. NFT are very insoluble and apparently difficult to proteolyze *in vivo*, thus remaining visible in tissue sections as "ghost" or "tombstone" tangles long after the death of the parent neuron.

Ultrastructurally, they are composed predominantly of paired helical filaments (PHF) along with some straight filaments that appear to have comparable composition. A major component of PHF is abnormally hyperphosphorylated forms of the pro-

tein tau, an axonal protein that enhances microtubule assembly. Other antigens that have been found in PHF include MAP2 (another microtubule-associated protein), ubiquitin, and amyloid beta-peptide (Aβ, see later). PHFs are also found in the dystrophic neurites that form the outer portions of neuritic plaques and in axons coursing through gray matter as neuropil threads.

Although they are characteristic of AD, NFTs are not specific to this condition, being also found in progressive supranuclear palsy, postencephalitic Parkinson's disease, and in the amyotrophic lateral sclerosis–Parkinsonism/dementia complex of Guam. They probably represent the end point of a number of different cellular pathophysiologic processes. The NFT and its major components reflect abnormal organization of cytoskeletal elements in neurons of patients with Alzheimer's disease.

Neuritic plaques are focal, spherical collections of dilated, tortuous, silver-staining neuritic processes (dystrophic neurites) surrounding a central amyloid core, often with a clear halo separating the components (see Fig. 29-29A). Neuritic plaques range in size from 20 to 200 μm in diameter. Microglial cells and reactive astrocytes can be seen around the periphery. Plaques can be found in the hippocampus and amygdala as well as in the neocortex, although there is usually relative sparing of primary motor and sensory cortices (a distinction that holds for NFT as well). Plaques can be found in nondemented older patients, usually in low numbers, and it is the frequency of plaques that supports a diagnosis of AD. Comparable lesions can be found in the corresponding regions of the brains of aged, nonhuman primates as well. The dystrophic neurites contain PHF as well as synaptic vesicles and abnormal mitochondria. The amyloid core, which can be stained by Congo red, by Bielschowsky silver methods, and by thioflavin S,

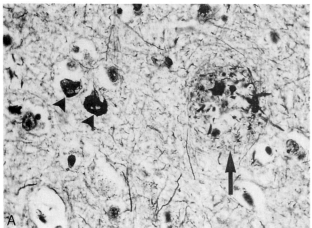

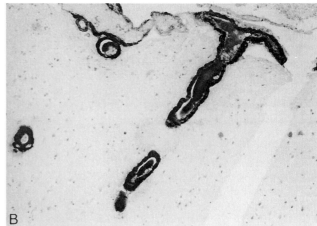

Figure 29-29. Alzheimer's disease. *A,* Neurofibrillary tangles *(arrowheads)* are present within neurons and a neuritic plaque with a rim of dystrophic neurites surrounding an amyloid core *(arrow)*. *B,* Immunohistochemical staining for amyloid beta-peptide (Aβ) showing deposition of amyloid in the wall of the small cortical and subarachnoid vessels.

contains a variety of proteins. The dominant component of the plaque core is Aβ, an approximately 40 to 43 amino acid peptide derived from a larger molecule, amyloid precursor protein (APP).

Although Aβ was originally observed using silver stains, the development of refined immunostaining for Aβ has confirmed the existence, in some patients, of depositions of the amyloid peptide that lack the surrounding neuritic reaction. These lesions, termed **diffuse plaques,** are found in superficial portions of cerebral cortex as well as in basal ganglia and cerebellar cortex. Commonly, when diffuse plaques are found in the cerebral cortex, they appear to be centered on small vessels or on clusters of neurons. These lesions, which can be found in association with clear-cut findings of AD or in isolation, may represent an earlier stage.

Amyloid angiopathy is an almost invariable accompaniment of AD, although it can be found in the absence of other changes of AD (see Fig. 29–29B). This vascular amyloid has the same chemical composition as the amyloid cores of plaques. Amyloid deposition may also be found at sites outside of the nervous system.

Granulovacuolar degeneration is the formation of small (5 μm in diameter), clear intraneuronal cytoplasmic vacuoles, each of which contains an argyrophilic granule. **Hirano bodies,** found in AD as well as other diseases, are elongated, glassy, eosinophilic bodies consisting of paracrystalline arrays of beaded filaments, with actin as a major component. Both are found most commonly in hippocampal pyramidal cells and are of unknown significance.

The pathogenesis of AD is unknown. It is well established that neocortical and hippocampal areas have decreased levels of cholinergic innervation in AD and that there is loss of neurons from the cholinergic nuclei of the basal forebrain. Attention has also focused on Aβ and its precursor protein, APP, as possible etiologic agents.[48,49] The precursor molecule has a large extracellular domain, a single membrane-spanning region, and a short intracellular domain (Fig. 29–30). Aβ corresponds to a region extending from the extracellular portion of the molecule into the transmembrane domain. In some pedigrees with familial AD (FAD), the disease appears to be linked to a point mutation within the coding region of the APP gene. Another point mutation in this gene, found in several Dutch pedigrees, gives rise to the accelerated deposition of amyloid in cerebral vessels with an increased risk of bleeding, a disease termed *hereditary cerebral hemorrhage with amyloidosis* (HCHWA).

Certain isoforms of the protein contain a *Kunitz protease inhibitor (KPI) domain,* and this molecule's role in the regulation of the clotting cascade may be the primary function of APP. Normal processing of APP includes cleavage of a peptide

bond in the middle of the Aβ sequence; the result of this cleavage is to prevent the potential for formation of the insoluble aggregates of Aβ. The development of amyloid deposits has been inferred to arise from abnormal processing of the precursor molecule in such a way that increased amounts of this peptide accumulate. Increased rates of generation of the amyloidogenic Aβ have been found in cells expressing some of the mutations associated with FAD.

Tissue culture studies of neurons have shown both toxic and trophic effects of Aβ as well as interactions with other forms of neuronal injury. The action of the molecule *in vivo* is uncertain.[50] In some families, the FAD locus is separate from the APP gene, either nearby on chromosome 21 or on other chromosomes. One FAD locus, characterized by late-onset disease, has been mapped to chromosome 19, where it is linked to the apolipoprotein E (apoE) gene; one allele of this gene (apoE4) has been associated with increased risk of developing AD and may be a susceptibility factor.[51]

Pick's Disease

Pick's disease occurs far less frequently than Alzheimer's disease but is also clinically manifested as profound dementia over a comparable time course.

MORPHOLOGY. The brain in Pick's disease invariably exhibits a pronounced, although frequently asymmetric atrophy of the frontal and temporal lobes with conspicuous sparing of the posterior two-thirds of the superior temporal gyrus and only rare involvement of either the parietal or occipital lobe. The atrophy can be severe, reducing the gyri to a thin wafer ("knife-edge" appearance). This pattern of **lobar atrophy** is often prominent enough to distinguish Pick's disease from Alzheimer's disease on gross examination. In addition to the localized cortical atrophy, there is also often atrophy of the caudate and putamen. Microscopically, neuronal loss is most severe in the outer three layers of the cortex and may be severe enough to resemble superficially (pseudo)laminar necrosis (see section on cerebrovascular diseases). Some of the surviving neurons may exhibit a characteristic swelling **(Pick cells)** or contain **Pick bodies,** which are cytoplasmic, round to oval, filamentous inclusions that are only weakly eosinophilic but stain strongly with silver methods. Ultrastructurally, they are composed of neurofilaments, vesiculated endoplasmic reticulum, and paired helical filaments that are immunocytochemically similar to those found in Alzheimer's disease. Unlike the NFTs of AD, Pick bodies do not survive the death of their host neuron and do not remain as markers of the disease.

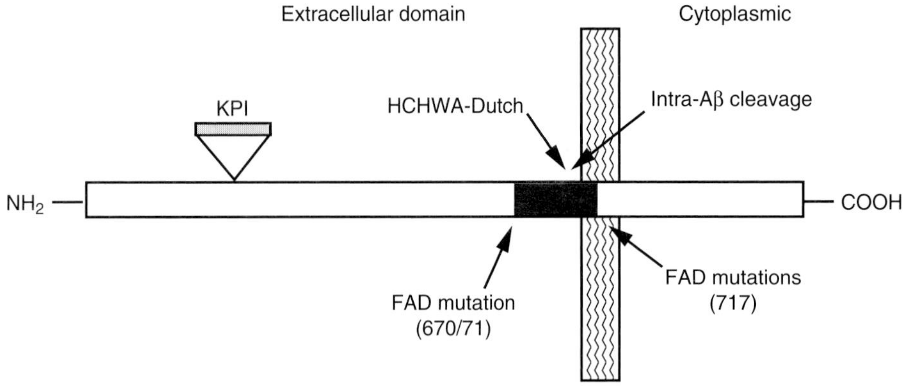

Figure 29–30. Schematic of the structure of amyloid precursor protein. Black bar indicates Aβ peptide. (FAD = familial AD; HCHWA = hereditary cerebral hemorrhage with amyloidosis; KPI = Kunitz protease inhibitor.) (Courtesy of Dr. E. Koo, Brigham and Women's Hospital, Boston.)

DEGENERATIVE DISEASES OF BASAL GANGLIA AND BRAIN STEM

Diseases affecting these regions of the brain frequently are associated with movement disorders, including rigidity, abnormal posturing, and chorea. In general, they can be categorized as manifesting either a reduction of voluntary movement or an abundance of involuntary movement. The nigrostriatal pathway plays an important role in the system of positive and negative regulatory synaptic pathways that serve to modulate feedback from the thalamus to the motor cortex.

Parkinsonism

Parkinsonism is a clinical syndrome characterized by diminished facial expression, stooped posture, slowness of voluntary movement, festinating gait (progressively shortened, accelerated steps), rigidity, and a "pill-rolling" tremor. *This type of motor disturbance is seen in a number of conditions that have in common damage to the nigrostriatal dopaminergic system.* Parkinsonism may also be induced by drugs that affect this system, particularly dopamine antagonists and toxins (notably, 1-methyl-4-phenyl-1,2,3,6-tetrahydropyridine [MPTP]). The principal diseases that involve the nigrostriatal system are *idiopathic Parkinson's disease, striatonigral degeneration, Shy-Drager syndrome,* and *progressive supranuclear palsy.* Postencephalitic parkinsonism was observed in the wake of the influenza pandemic of 1914 to 1918 but is no longer of clinical significance.

Idiopathic Parkinson's Disease (IPD)

This diagnosis is made in patients with progressive parkinsonism in the absence of a toxic or other known etiology. The disease comes on in later life; as in Alzheimer's disease, it is seen with increasing frequency in older age cohorts. Although there is

no evidence for a genetic component to the disease in most cases, some pedigrees have been reported in which IPD is present as an autosomal dominant trait. In addition to the movement disorder, there are other less well-characterized changes in mental function, and a few patients with the pathologic findings of idiopathic Parkinson's disease present with a dementia clinically similar to that of Alzheimer's disease.

MORPHOLOGY. Pathologically, the typical gross findings are **pallor of the substantia nigra** (Fig. 29–31) and locus ceruleus. Microscopically, there is loss of the pigmented, catecholaminergic neurons in these regions associated with gliosis; **Lewy bodies** (see Fig. 29–31C) may be found in some of the remaining neurons. These are intracytoplasmic, eosinophilic, round to elongated inclusions that often have a dense core surrounded by a paler rim. They may occur singly or multiply within neurons. Ultrastructurally, Lewy bodies are composed of fine filaments, densely packed in the core but quite loose at the rim, and antibody studies have shown the presence of neurofilament antigens. Lewy bodies may also be found in the cholinergic cells of the basal nucleus of Meynert, which is depleted of neurons (particularly in patients with abnormal mental function), as well as in other brain stem nuclei. Similar, but less distinct, inclusions are also found in cerebral cortical neurons, especially in the cingulate gyrus and the parahippocampal gyrus. These cortical Lewy bodies, which are best detected by immunohistochemistry for ubiquitin, have been reported to be present in many cases of IPD.

The dopaminergic neurons of the substantia nigra project to the striatum, and their degeneration in Parkinson's disease is associated with a reduction in the striatal dopamine content. The severity of the motor syndrome is proportional to the dopamine deficiency, which can, at least in part, be corrected by replacement therapy with L-dopa

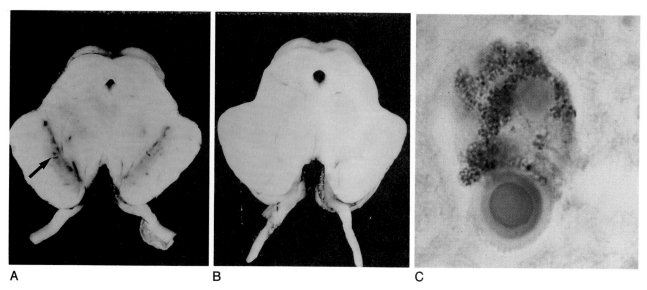

A   B   C

Figure 29–31. Parkinson's disease. *A*, Normal substantia nigra. *B*, Depigmented substantia nigra in IPD. *C*, Lewy body in a substantia nigra neuron stains bright pink.

(the immediate precursor of dopamine); unlike dopamine, L-dopa is able to cross the blood-brain barrier. Treatment does not, however, reverse the morphologic changes or arrest the progress of the disease, and with progression, drug therapy tends to become less effective, and symptoms become more difficult to manage. The ability of L-dopa therapy to influence the symptoms is dependent on the preservation of the striatum.

An acute parkinsonian syndrome and destruction of substantia nigra neurons follows exposure to MPTP, a contaminant in the illicit synthesis of psychoactive meperidine analogues. Action by monoamine oxidase B is required for the toxicity of MPTP. Clinical trials with inhibitors of this enzyme show a slowed rate of clinical progression in patients with early-stage IPD; whether this effect is merely a symptom or truly influences the disease has been the subject of debate.

The most dramatic recent development in the treatment of IPD has been in the field of neural transplantation. Although initial studies using adrenal medullary tissue as the donor source were not promising, clinical improvement has been reported in patients with IPD or MPTP-induced Parkinson's disease treated with stereotactic implants of fetal mesencephalic tissue into the striatum.[52]

Progressive Supranuclear Palsy

Patients with this disorder usually present with loss of vertical gaze progressing to difficulty with all eye movements, associated with truncal rigidity and dysequilibrium, loss of facial expression, and sometimes progressive dementia. The onset of the disease is usually between the fifth and seventh decades; males are affected approximately twice as frequently as females, and death occurs often within 5 to 7 years.

MORPHOLOGY. There is widespread neuronal loss in the globus pallidus, subthalamic nucleus, substantia nigra, colliculi, periaqueductal gray matter, and dentate nucleus of the cerebellum. The cerebral and cerebellar cortices are usually not involved. Neurofibrillary tangles are found in most of the affected regions. Although ultrastructural analysis reveals 15-nm, straight filaments rather than the paired helical filaments found in Alzheimer's disease, some epitopes are shared with the tangles found in Alzheimer's disease.

Multiple System Atrophies

In distinction to the degenerative diseases discussed previously, there is great variation in the pathologic findings in these entities and sometimes a relatively poor correlation between the clinical findings and the distribution of the pathologic changes.

Striatonigral Degeneration

Striatonigral degeneration is clinically similar to IPD in presentation, but the movement disorder is relatively resistant to L-dopa treatment, which can be understood on the basis of the pathologic differences from IPD.

MORPHOLOGY. There is grossly visible atrophy of the caudate nucleus and putamen, and microscopically, both nuclei show severe neuronal loss, particularly of small neurons, and a marked gliosis.

Loss of pigmented neurons also occurs, particularly in the zona compacta of the substantia nigra, but Lewy bodies are not seen. The result of this pattern of neuronal degeneration is that both the dopaminergic projection (from the substantia nigra) and its target neurons (in the striatum) are absent. L-Dopa cannot bolster neurotransmission along this pathway, as happens in the treatment of IPD, in the absence of a target structure. Some of these patients also show evidence of pontocerebellar degeneration or autonomic dysfunction.

Shy-Drager Syndrome

Shy-Drager syndrome describes patients with autonomic system failure, often manifesting as orthostatic hypotension, in addition to parkinsonism. Some cases are similar to IPD with Lewy bodies, while others resemble striatonigral degeneration with widespread neuronal loss. Common to all, and explaining the sympathetic dysfunction, is loss of neurons from the intermediolateral column of the spinal cord.

Huntington's Disease

Huntington's disease (HD) usually appears in persons between 20 and 50 years of age and is characterized by uncontrolled movements and progressive dementia. Affected patients develop chorea, characterized by jerky, hyperkinetic, sometimes dystonic movements affecting all parts of the body; they may later develop parkinsonism with bradykinesia and rigidity. Early signs of higher cortical dysfunction often include forgetfulness and thought and affective disorders. The disease is relentlessly progressive, with an average course of about 15 years to death.

MORPHOLOGY. On gross examination, the brain is small and shows striking atrophy of the caudate nucleus and, less dramatically, the putamen (Fig. 29–32). The globus pallidus may be secondarily atrophied, and the lateral and third ventricles are dilated. Atrophy is frequently seen in the frontal lobe and less often in the parietal lobe, and only occasionally affects the entire cortex.

Microscopically, there is severe loss of striatal neurons; the most severe changes are found in the caudate nucleus, especially in the tail and the portions nearer the ventricle. The putamen is less involved. The nucleus accumbens is the best preserved structure. Both the large and the small neurons are affected, but loss of the small neurons generally precedes that of the larger. The medium-sized, spiny neurons that use gamma-aminobutyric acid (GABA) and enkephalin or GABA and substance P as their neurotransmitters are prominently

affected. Two populations of neurons are relatively spared in the disease: the diaphorase-positive neurons that contain NO synthase and the large cholinesterase-positive neurons. Both appear to serve as local interneurons. There is also fibrillary gliosis that seems much greater than that usually seen in reaction to neuronal loss. The degree of degeneration in the striatum can be related to the severity of clinical symptoms, although neurologic signs may precede pathologic changes.[53]

The functional significance of the loss of striatal neurons is to dysregulate the basal ganglia circuitry that modulates motor output. The loss of the striatal inhibitory output, from the degeneration of GABA-containing neurons, is thought to be the basis of the choreiform movements of the disease. The structural basis of the cognitive changes associated with the disease remains unclear, despite the evidence of cortical atrophy. The neurochemistry of this disease is complex: some transmitter substances, such as GABA, acetylcholine, and substance P, are decreased, and others are either unchanged or even increased (e.g., somatostatin). Excitotoxic amino acids and related compounds can produce pathologic changes similar to those of HD in animals.

The genetic locus for HD was localized to chromosome 4 in one of the early successes of reverse genetics. The apparent HD gene located on 4p16.3 has recently been cloned and encodes a predicted protein of 348-kd molecular weight and unknown function.[54] The coding region of the gene contains a polymorphic trinucleotide repeat, with normal chromosomes containing 11 to 34 copies of the $(CAG)_n$ sequence. In HD the number of triplet repeats is increased, and the larger the number the earlier the onset of disease. Newly occurring mutations are extremely rare, and most apparently "sporadic" cases can be related to nonpaternity or the death of a parent prior to expression of the disease. The combination of autosomal dominant inheritance, the onset of symptoms often in middle life, and the potential for knowing whether one carries the locus for the disease has made Huntington's disease the focal point of discussion of ethical issues of genetic diagnosis.

SPINOCEREBELLAR DEGENERATIONS

This group of diseases affects, to a variable extent, the cerebellar cortex, spinal cord, peripheral nerves, and other regions of the neuraxis. Pathologically, there is degeneration of the neurons in the affected areas, with mild gliosis. Clinically, patients present with a combination of cerebellar and sensory ataxia, spasticity, and peripheral motor and sensory defects that reflect the areas of the nervous system involved.

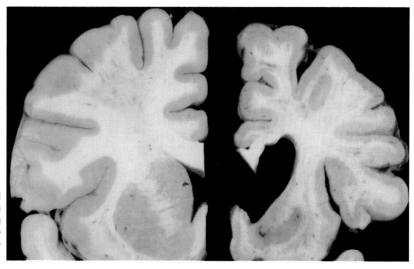

Figure 29–32. Huntington's disease. Normal hemisphere on the left compared with hemisphere with HD on the right showing atrophy of striatum and ventricular dilatation. (Courtesy of Dr. J.-P. Vonsattel, Massachusetts General Hospital, Boston.)

Paraneoplastic cerebellar degeneration is marked by diffuse loss of Purkinje cells possibly related to a circulating antibody that recognizes an antigen on these neurons. Alcoholic cerebellar degeneration also predominantly affects Purkinje cells, especially in the superior vermis.

Olivopontocerebellar Atrophy (OPCA)

Olivopontocerebellar atrophy is characteristically a cerebellar system degeneration that may overlap with the multiple system atrophies. Even in the same family, no two cases are exactly alike. The inheritance is no less varied: most cases are autosomal dominant, but others are autosomal recessive, and still others are clearly nonfamilial. External examination reveals shrinkage of the basis pontis from the loss of the pontine nuclei. The cerebellar cortex shows widespread loss of Purkinje cells, especially in the lateral portions of the hemispheres. Secondary degenerative changes are found in the inferior olives, as in the cerebellar cortical atrophies. Clinically, symptoms and signs include ataxia, eye and somatic movement abnormalities, dysarthria, and rigidity.

Friedreich's Ataxia (FA)

Since FA has a consistent clinical course and pathology, it was long thought to be a single form of spinocerebellar degeneration. Genetic investigations have since shown a previously unrecognized degree of diversity. An autosomal recessive condition with a male preponderance, FA has an average age at onset of about 11 years, although a less common dominantly inherited variant manifests at about 20 years. Initial symptoms include gait ataxia, followed by hand clumsiness and dysarthria.

Deep tendon reflexes are absent, but an extensor plantar reflex is typically present. Joint position and vibratory sense are impaired, and there is sometimes loss of pain and temperature sensation and light touch. Most patients become paralyzed over the course of about 20 years. Some have pes cavus and kyphoscoliosis. There is a high incidence of concomitant diabetes and cardiac disease; the latter manifests as cardiac arrhythmias and congestive heart failure.

MORPHOLOGY. The spinal cord is small, with loss of axons and gliosis in the posterior columns, distal corticospinal tract, and spinocerebellar tracts. Neuronal loss occurs in Clarke's column, cranial nerve nuclei VIII, X, and XII, the dentate nucleus, and the Purkinje cells of the superior vermis. Loss of dorsal root ganglion cells is the cause of the visible degeneration of the dorsal columns as well as of dorsal roots. The heart is enlarged and may have pericardial adhesions. There may be an interstitial myocarditis with focal or diffuse inflammatory infiltrates, and myofiber hypertrophy or, more rarely, necrosis.

Ataxia-Telangiectasia

This apparently autosomal recessive disease presents in childhood with loss of cerebellar function in the setting of recurrent infections. The neurologic signs usually predate the appearance of the numerous telangiectatic lesions in conjunctiva and in other areas. The pathologic findings in the nervous system are predominantly in the cerebellum, with loss of Purkinje and granule cells, although some degeneration of the dorsal columns has been reported. Systemic findings include the absence of a thymus as well as hypoplastic gonads. These patients have a strong tendency for lymphoid malignancy, as is seen with other immunodeficiency syndromes.

DEGENERATIVE DISEASES AFFECTING MOTOR NEURONS

The most common form of this group of degenerative disorders is *amyotrophic lateral sclerosis* (ALS), in which patients have loss of both lower motor neurons (muscular atrophy, fasciculations, weakness) and upper motor neurons (hyperreflexia, spasticity, and a Babinski reflex). The disease affects men slightly more frequently than women and usually presents in the fifth and subsequent decades. Although it may begin with asymmetric weakness, gradually it becomes symmetric and more severe, with death following from respiratory complications. Some patients present with, or develop, bulbar signs from changes in the lower motor neurons of cranial nerves (with sparing of the extraocular muscles). Patients with bulbar disease tend to have a shorter course, probably from a higher rate of complications. Approximately 10% of cases appear to be familial, with an autosomal dominant inheritance pattern linked to chromosome 21 in most pedigrees. Nothing in the clinical course or pathologic findings has allowed these cases to be separated from sporadic ones.

MORPHOLOGY. The distribution of pathologic findings parallels that of symptoms. Lower motor neuron loss is manifested as muscular atrophy and a gray discoloration and atrophy of the anterior (motor) roots of the spinal cord, directly related to the loss of myelinated axons. The areas of devastating lower motor neuron loss show extensive gliosis and, occasionally, neuronophagia. Degeneration of the upper motor neurons results in atrophy and pallor of the corticospinal tracts (Fig. 29–33) and, occasionally, in severe or long-standing cases, atrophy of the precentral gyrus.

The pathogenesis of ALS is unknown. A high prevalence of HLA-A3 and B12 haplotypes has been reported. Neurotoxicologic studies in animals have suggested that a plant-derived, excitotoxic molecule can lead to an ALS-like disease, although its relevance to the human disease is unclear. Other lines of evidence have suggested that abnormalities of the glutaminergic system are present in ALS patients.[55] The genetic locus on chromosome 21 for familial ALS appears to be the Cu/Zn-binding superoxide dismutase gene, with various missense mutations identified in different families.[56]

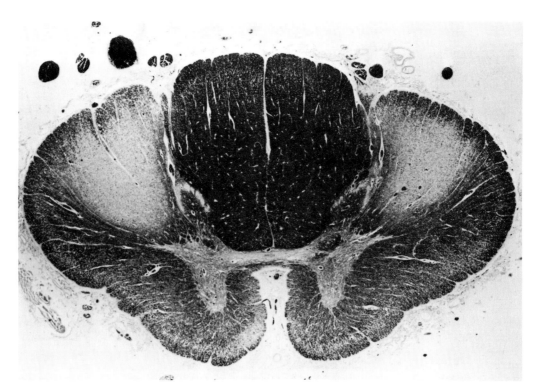

Figure 29–33. Amytrophic lateral sclerosis. Spinal cord showing loss of myelinated fibers (lack of stain) in corticospinal tracts. Anterior roots are smaller than posterior; at higher magnification, loss of anterior horn neurons can also be seen (Woelcke stain for myelin).

Growth factors can prevent the naturally occurring "programmed cell death" of motor neurons as well as support the survival of motor neurons *in vitro* and therefore have also been considered as etiologic candidates. Administration of ciliary neurotrophic factor has been shown to prevent the degeneration of motor neurons in a mouse model.

Other related diseases affect only lower motor neurons. X-linked spinal muscular atrophy has been associated with gynecomastia, testicular atrophy, and oligospermia. It has been linked to amplification of a trinucleotide repeat in the coding sequence of the androgen receptor gene, with severity of the disease related to the number of repeats present.[57]

A severe form of lower motor neuron disease that presents in the neonatal period, often as a "floppy infant," is *Werdnig-Hoffmann disease (infantile progressive spinal muscular atrophy)*, an autosomal recessive condition. In many infants, death ensues within a few months from respiratory failure or aspiration pneumonia. Pathologically, there is severe loss of lower motor neurons, degeneration of the motor axons of the anterior roots, and profound neurogenic atrophy of muscle. The denervated fibers are small but round, rather than having the angulated appearance normally associated with neurogenic atrophy of muscle. Werdnig-Hoffman disease and later-onset forms of spinal muscular atrophy have been linked to a locus on chromosome 5q.

INBORN ERRORS OF METABOLISM

A subset of the characterized genetic diseases of metabolism affect the nervous system. Some have been covered earlier in this book (see Chapter 5), but here their expression in the nervous system will be briefly discussed. Many of the hereditary disorders that affect the nervous system express themselves in children normal at birth but who begin to miss some developmental milestones during infancy and childhood. Some genetic disorders affect neurons predominantly (gray matter diseases, *neuronal storage diseases*), while others affect oligodendrocytes and myelin (white matter diseases, *leukodystrophies*). Cortical neuronal involvement leads to loss of cognitive function and may also cause seizures. In contrast, diffuse involvement of white matter leads to deterioration in motor skills, spasticity, hypotonia, or ataxia.

The neuronal storage disorders are mostly autosomal recessive diseases involving the deficiency of a specific enzyme of sphingolipid, mucopolysaccharide, or mucolipid catabolism. They are characterized by the accumulation of the substrate of the enzyme, often within neuronal lysosomes, leading to neuronal death. The direct relationship between the accumulated material and cell injury and death is usually unclear.

The leukodystrophies generally have no neuronal storage; rather they show a selective involvement of myelin. Although most are autosomal recessive disorders, adrenoleukodystrophy, an X-linked disease, is a notable exception. Subtypes, or variants, are recognized for many of these disorders. These variants may involve separate genetic loci and frequently follow the principle that *the earlier the age at onset, the more severe the deficiency and clinical course.*

LEUKODYSTROPHIES

Krabbe's Disease

This disease is an autosomal recessive leukodystrophy resulting from a deficiency of galactocerebroside β-galactosidase, the enzyme required for the catabolism of galactocerebroside to ceramide and galactose. The recent identification of a similar enzymatic defect and leukodystrophy in mice has allowed new efforts to unravel the details of the biochemistry of Krabbe's disease, and to attempt to identify the gene responsible for this disorder. The deficiency of galactocerebrosidase does *not* cause an identifiable accumulation of galactocerebroside, either in neurons or in white matter. Instead, it appears that an alternative catabolic pathway leads to removal of a fatty acid from this molecule, leading to detectable levels of psychosin (galactosylsphingosine), a cytotoxic compound that could cause oligodendrocyte injury. The clinical course is rapidly progressive, with onset of symptoms often between the ages of three and six months; survival beyond two years of age is uncommon. The clinical symptoms are dominated by motor signs, including stiffness and weakness, with gradually worsening difficulties in feeding. Peripheral nerves are involved, and a biopsy of peripheral nerve may be used to establish the diagnosis. No sites outside the nervous system are involved. Biochemical documentation of the enzyme deficiency is the preferred method of diagnosis.

MORPHOLOGY. There is a gradual loss of myelin and oligodendrocytes in the CNS and a similar process in peripheral nerves. Neurons and axons are relatively spared. A unique feature of Krabbe's disease is the aggregation of macrophages around blood vessels as multinucleated cells **(globoid cells)**. These macrophages contain storage material, which appears in the cytoplasm as linear inclusions by electron microscopy.

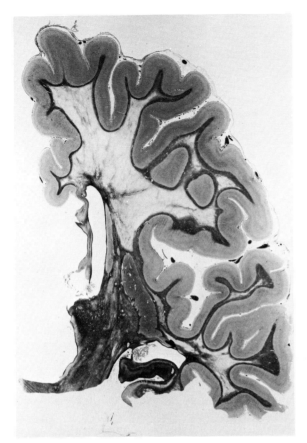

Figure 29–34. Metachromatic leukodystrophy. Demyelination is extensive. Subcortical fibers in cerebral hemisphere are spared (Luxol-fast-blue PAS stain for myelin).

Metachromatic Leukodystrophy

This disorder is transmitted in an autosomal recessive pattern and results from a deficiency of arylsulfatase A. This enzyme, located in a variety of tissues, cleaves the sulfate from sulfate-containing lipids (sulfatides), the first step in their degradation. Deficiency of arylsulfatase A leads to an accumulation of the sulfatides, especially cerebroside sulfate; how this leads to myelin breakdown is not known. Recognized clinical subtypes of the disorder include a congenital form, a late infantile form (the most common), a juvenile form, and an adult form. The gene for arylsulfatase A has been localized to chromosome 22, probably on the long arm near the q13 band. Although there is no known cure, promising results have recently been achieved with bone marrow transplantation.

MORPHOLOGY. Myelin is destroyed in the white matter, with resulting gliosis (Fig. 29–34). Macrophages with vacuolated cytoplasm are scattered throughout the white matter. The membrane-bound vacuoles contain complex crystalloid structures composed of sulfatides. These sulfatides, when bound to certain dyes, shift their absorbance spectrum, causing the dyes to have a different color. Toluidine blue, for example, shifts to a light tan color on binding to the sulfatides. This property is called **metachromasia** and depends on the characteristics of both the dye and the tissue components. Similar changes in peripheral nerve are observed. The detection of metachromatic material in the urine is also a sensitive method of establishing the diagnosis.

Pelizaeus-Merzbacher Disease

An X-linked leukodystrophy, this disorder has a unique clinical presentation and pathologic appearance. Pendular nystagmus stands out as a distinctive sign, although the patients eventually develop the signs and symptoms associated with widespread white matter dysfunction. The disease has recently been shown to arise from a mutation in the gene for proteolipid protein (PLP), a major protein of CNS myelin.[58] Although myelin is nearly completely lost in the cerebral hemispheres, patches may remain, giving a "tigroid" appearance to tissue sections stained for myelin.

Canavan's Disease

This disease results in a spongy degeneration of white matter with Alzheimer type II cells. Aspartoacylase activity has been recognized to be deficient in affected family members and is now thought to be the biochemical basis of this autosomal recessive disease.[59]

Disorders of peroxisomal metabolic processes may also lead to leukodystrophy. Some of these diseases, which often have an associated peripheral neuropathy, are considered in Table 28–3.

MITOCHONDRIAL ENCEPHALOMYOPATHIES

Leigh's Disease

Usually an autosomal recessive disorder, this disease is characterized by an arrest of psychomotor development, feeding problems, seizures, extraocular palsies, and weakness with hypotonia between one and two years of age. The cardinal laboratory finding is lactic acidemia. Death usually occurs within 1 to 2 years of the age at onset. Various biochemical abnormalities have been found, all of which lie in the mitochondrial pathway for converting pyruvate to ATP.

MORPHOLOGY. The brain reveals bilateral regions of destruction with a proliferation of blood vessels, usually symmetric, involving the periventricular gray matter of the midbrain, tegmentum of the pons, and the periventricular regions of the thalamus and hypothalamus.

Other Mitochondrial Encephalomyopathies

Myoclonic epilepsy and ragged-red fibers (MERRF) is a maternally transmitted disease that has been associated with a mutation in the mtDNA gene for a mitochondrial-specific transfer-RNA (tRNA). This appears to result in altered function of several of the oxidative complexes. A similar type of mutation of a tRNA gene has been found in the disease *mitochondrial encephalomyopathy, lactic acidosis, and stroke-like episodes (MELAS)*. A potential etiology for the vascular-based disease in these patients has been suggested from the observation that mitochondrial abnormalities can be found in cerebral vessels.[60] *Leber hereditary optic neuropathy* is an example of an mtDNA-based disease associated with a point mutation in the gene for a single enzyme, although nuclear genes influence the expression of the disease.[61,62]

TOXIC AND ACQUIRED METABOLIC DISEASES

VITAMIN DEFICIENCIES

The vitamin deficiencies are a relatively common cause of neurologic illnesses that, once present, are often permanent. Although vitamin deficiency may occur in otherwise healthy individuals, there is a tendency for it to occur in patients with dietary or digestive problems.

Thiamine (Vitamin B₁) Deficiency

As discussed earlier (Chapter 9), thiamine deficiency may result in the slowly evolving clinical disorder *beriberi*. On the other hand, thiamine deficiency may also lead to the development of psychotic symptoms that begin abruptly, a syndrome termed *Wernicke's encephalopathy*. The acute stages, if unrecognized and untreated, may be followed by a prolonged and largely irreversible condition, *Korsakoff's syndrome, characterized clinically by memory disturbances and confabulation*. Because the two syndromes are so closely linked and may be viewed as different stages of the same

process, the term Wernicke-Korsakoff syndrome is sometimes applied. Although particularly common in the setting of chronic alcoholism, it may also be encountered in patients with thiamine deficiency resulting from gastric problems, including carcinoma, chronic gastritis, or persistent vomiting. The therapy for thiamine deficiency is administration of the vitamin, and while the manifestations of Wernicke's syndrome may clear, the Korsakoff's component persists.

> **MORPHOLOGY.** Wernicke's encephalopathy is characterized by foci of hemorrhage and necrosis, particularly in the mammillary bodies but also present adjacent to the ventricular system, especially the third and fourth ventricles. The early lesions show dilated capillaries in these areas with prominent endothelial cells. Subsequently, the capillaries leak red cells into the interstitium, producing hemorrhagic areas that are easily detectable grossly. With time, these lesions show an infiltration of macrophages that clear the hemorrhage and necrosis, leaving a hemosiderin-laden cystic space as a permanent sign of the process. It is in patients with Korsakoff's syndrome that the chronic hemosiderin-laden lesions predominate. Lesions in the medial dorsal nucleus of the thalamus appear to be the best correlate of memory disturbance.

Vitamin B₁₂ Deficiency

The most severe and potentially irreversible effects of vitamin B₁₂ deficiency are related to its nervous system lesions. The neurologic symptoms may present in a subacute manner, over the course of a few weeks, initially with slight ataxia and numbness and tingling in the lower extremities, and may progress rapidly to include spastic weakness of the lower extremities. Complete paraplegia may occur, but usually only later in the course of the disease. With prompt vitamin replacement therapy, clinical improvement may be expected; however, if complete paraplegia has developed, recovery is poor.

> **MORPHOLOGY.** In the early stages, vitamin B₁₂ deficiency leads to a swelling of myelin layers producing vacuoles, beginning segmentally at the midthoracic level of the spinal cord. With time, axons in both the ascending tracts of the posterior columns and the descending pyramidal tracts degenerate. While isolated involvement of descending or ascending tracts may be observed in a variety of spinal cord diseases, the combined degeneration of both ascending and descending tracts of the spinal cord is characteristic of vitamin B₁₂ deficiency and has led to the designation of the dis-

order as **subacute combined degeneration of the spinal cord.**

NEUROLOGIC SEQUELAE OF METABOLIC DISTURBANCES

Hypoglycemia

Since the brain requires glucose and oxygen for its energy production, the cellular effects of diminished glucose resemble those of oxygen deprivation, as described earlier.

MORPHOLOGY. There is a selective involvement of large pyramidal neurons of the cerebral cortex, which, if severely involved, may result in (pseudo)laminar necrosis of the cortex, predominantly involving layers III to V. The hippocampus is also vulnerable to glucose depletion, as it is to hypoxia, and may show a dramatic loss of the pyramidal neurons in Sommer's sector. Purkinje cells of the cerebellum are also vulnerable to hypoglycemia, and if the level and duration of hypoglycemia is of sufficient severity, there may be global insult to the neurons of the brain.

Hyperglycemia

Hyperglycemia is most commonly found in the setting of inadequately controlled diabetes mellitus and can be associated with either ketoacidosis or hyperosmolar coma. The patient becomes dehydrated and develops confusion, stupor, and eventually coma. The fluid depletion must be corrected gradually, otherwise severe cerebral edema may follow.

Hepatic Encephalopathy

The pathogenesis of hepatic encephalopathy or hepatic coma has been discussed in Chapter 18.

MORPHOLOGY. The cellular response in hepatic coma is predominantly glial. **Alzheimer type II changes** are evident in the cortex and basal ganglia and other subcortical gray matter regions. No structural abnormalities have been identified in neurons.

TOXIC DISORDERS

Human exposures to neurotoxins occur predominantly as a result of industrialization, leading to both isolated cases and epidemics. Defining a toxic agent is difficult, since any agent in sufficient dose is toxic. Thus, water intoxication is a well-defined clinical syndrome, but water is not generally viewed as toxic. Other variables that are important in neurotoxicology include the magnitude of a single dose as well as cumulative effects of repeated exposure.

Carbon Monoxide

MORPHOLOGY. Many of the pathologic findings following acute carbon monoxide exposure are those of hypoxia. Thus, selective injury of the neurons of layers III and V of the cerebral cortex, Sommer's sector of the hippocampus, and Purkinje cells is the recognized consequence of carbon monoxide exposure. Bilateral necrosis of the globus pallidus may also occur and is more common in carbon monoxide–induced hypoxia than in hypoxia from other causes. In contrast to these acute effects, demyelinating lesions of the cerebral white matter may rarely follow exposure to carbon monoxide by several weeks.

Methanol

MORPHOLOGY. The pathologic findings are seen most often in the retina, where degeneration of retinal ganglion cells is the probable basis of the blindness. Selective bilateral putamenal necrosis also occurs when the exposure is severe. The mechanism of methanol retinal injury remains open to investigation, although there is some evidence that formate, a major metabolite of methanol, may play a role in the retinal toxicity.

Ethanol

Although acute effects are reversible and create no long-term neurologic problems, chronic alcohol abuse is associated with a variety of neurologic problems. Since it is accompanied by nutritional deficiencies, it is difficult to determine which of the "toxic" effects of chronic alcohol intake are a direct effect of ethanol and which are due to secondary nutritional deficits. The symptoms of cerebellar dysfunction from chronic alcoholism are well defined; about 1% of patients with a history of long-term high intake of ethanol develop a clinical syndrome of truncal ataxia, unsteady gait, and nystagmus.

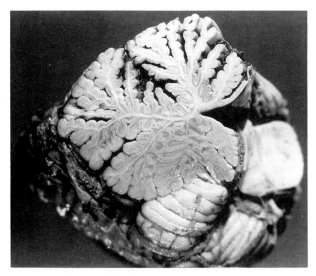

Figure 29-35. Alcoholic cerebellar degeneration. The anterior portion of the vermis *(upper portion of figure)* **is atrophic with widened spaces between folia.**

Methotrexate and Radiation-Induced Injury

Methotrexate toxicity most commonly develops when the drug has been administered in association with radiotherapy, whether delivered synchronously or at separate times. The interval between the inciting events and the onset of symptoms varies considerably but may be as long as months. Symptoms often progress rapidly once they start, beginning with drowsiness, ataxia, and confusion. While some patients recover function after the initial onset of symptoms, others may become comatose, and rarely methotrexate neurotoxicity may be responsible for the patient's death. The precise mechanism of these delayed effects of methotrexate remains to be defined.

> **MORPHOLOGY.** The basis of the symptoms are focal areas of coagulative necrosis within white matter, often adjacent to the lateral ventricles, but at times located in other areas of white matter. They may occasionally be extensively distributed throughout the white matter or may be prominent in the brain stem. Within the lesions, the elements have undergone coagulative necrosis, and surrounding axons are often dilated to form axonal spheroids. Axons and cell bodies in the vicinity of the lesions undergo dystrophic mineralization and there is adjacent gliosis.

> **MORPHOLOGY.** The early changes are atrophy and loss of granule cells predominantly in the anterior vermis (Fig. 29-35). In advanced cases, there is loss of Purkinje cells, which may be complete, and a proliferation of the adjacent astrocytes **(Bergman gliosis)** as a layer between the depleted granular cell layer and the molecular layer of the cerebellum.

Radiation

Ionizing radiation has delayed toxicity independent of methotrexate but it also appears to act synergistically with it. Delayed effects of radiation alone often present with rapidly evolving symptoms of an intracranial mass, including headaches, nausea, vomiting, and papilledema at an interval of months to years following irradiation.[63]

Fetal Alcohol Syndrome

In addition to the effects of ethanol on the mature CNS, the developing nervous system is vulnerable to ethanol toxicity. Alcohol consumption during pregnancy, especially in large amounts, is teratogenic, resulting in the *fetal alcohol syndrome.* The syndrome includes growth retardation (both somatic and cerebral), facial abnormalities (including epicanthal folds), cardiac septal defects, joint abnormalities, and delayed development with mental impairment that may range from mild to severe.

> **MORPHOLOGY.** The pathologic findings in delayed radionecrosis include large areas of coagulative necrosis with adjacent edema. The typical lesion is restricted to white matter, and all elements within the area undergo necrosis, including astrocytes, axons, oligodendrocytes, and blood vessels. Adjacent to the area of coagulative necrosis, proteinaceous spheroids may be identified, and blood vessels have thickened walls with intramural fibrin-like material. The large lesions may be the severe expression of a process that occurs throughout the brain after radiation, since similar vascular changes and small areas of coagulative necrosis may be seen elsewhere in the irradiated brain.

> **MORPHOLOGY.** Microcephaly is a common finding in the fetal alcohol syndrome, and interruption of migration is commonly observed, including heterotopic clusters of neurons (sometimes in the meninges), cerebellar dysplasia, malformations within the brain stem, and agenesis of the corpus callosum. Experimental studies of the effects of ethanol in murine embryogenesis suggest that the effects occur early in embryogenesis, creating abnormalities both in the developing brain and in facial structures. Such findings may bear on the facial features in the human fetal alcohol syndrome as well.

In addition to radiation-induced necrosis, the delayed effects of radiation include tumor induction. These malignancies usually are not seen until years after the therapy and include poorly differentiated sarcomas, gliomas, and meningiomas.

TUMORS

The incidence of tumors of the CNS ranges from 10 to 17 per 100,000 persons for intracranial tumors and 1 to 2 per 100,000 persons for intraspinal tumors. About half are primary tumors and the rest are metastatic. Tumors of the CNS account for as many as 20% of all cancers of childhood. In childhood, 70% of primary tumors arise in the posterior fossa, whereas in adults a corresponding proportion arise above the tentorium.[64-66]

Tumors of the nervous system have several unique characteristics that set them apart from neoplastic processes elsewhere in the body. First, the distinction between benign and malignant lesions is less evident than in other sites. Some glial tumors with the histologic features of a benign neoplasm, including low mitotic rate, cellular uniformity, and slow growth, may infiltrate entire regions of the brain, leading to clinically malignant behavior. Furthermore, the ability to surgically remove the neoplasm is restricted by functional anatomic considerations. Unequivocally benign lesions can have lethal consequences because of their location. The pattern of spread of primary CNS neoplasms also has unusual aspects. Even the most frankly malignant gliomas (glioblastoma multiforme) very rarely metastasize outside of the CNS, except in the setting of surgical intervention. The subarachnoid space provides a pathway for spread of some types of tumor, making cytologic examination of CSF an important procedure in these cases.[67]

GLIOMAS

Gliomas, tumors of glial cells, include *astrocytomas*, *oligodendrogliomas*, and *ependymomas*.

Astrocytoma

Fibrillary Astrocytomas

These account for about 80% of adult primary brain tumors. Usually found in the cerebral hemispheres, fibrillary astrocytomas may also occur in the cerebellum, brain stem, or spinal cord. The tumor is recognized clinically most often in late middle age. The most common presenting signs and symptoms are seizures, headaches, and focal neurologic deficits related to the anatomic site of involvement.

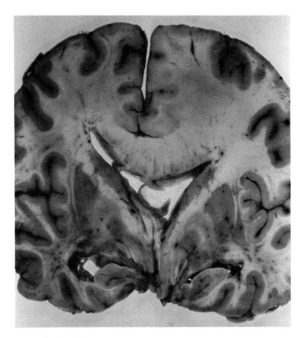

Figure 29–36. Low-grade astrocytoma. Expanded white matter of right cerebral hemisphere and thickened corpus callosum.

MORPHOLOGY. Low-grade astrocytomas are poorly defined, gray-white, infiltrative tumors that expand and distort the underlying brain (Fig. 29–36). They range from a few centimeters in diameter to enormous lesions that replace a cerebral hemisphere and extend into the opposite hemisphere. The highest grade lesions are characterized by a mixture of firm, white areas and softer, yellow foci of necrosis as well as cystic change and hemorrhage (Fig. 29–37); it is this appearance that gives rise to the name **glioblastoma multiforme.**

The unifying histologic feature of these tumors, regardless of grade, is the background of astrocytic processes of varying density and caliber that occurs between the neoplastic astrocytic nuclei. This network of intermingled cell processes replaces or displaces the normal background of myelinated fibers in the white matter or the neuropil in the gray matter and gives the tumor a distinctly abnormal "fibrillary" appearance. Low-grade tumors show hypercellularity and some nuclear pleomorphism. The transition to a higher grade comes with an increased degree of nuclear anaplasia and the presence of mitoses and vascular proliferation. Tufts of proliferated endothelial cells bulge into the vascular lumen, with extreme examples acquiring **glomeruloid** structures (Fig. 29–38). Some recent evidence has suggested that vascular endothelial cell growth factor (VEGF), produced by malignant astrocytes perhaps in response to hypoxia, contributes to this unique form of vascular change associated with malignancy.

The presence of necrosis is the defining histologic feature of glioblastoma multiforme. The ne-

With low-grade astrocytomas, the symptoms may remain static or progress only slowly for a number of years. Eventually, however, patients usually enter a period of more rapid clinical deterioration that is generally correlated with the appearance of anaplastic features and more rapid growth of the tumor. The prognosis for patients with glioblastoma is very poor. With current treatment, comprising resection when feasible together with radiotherapy and chemotherapy, the mean length of survival after diagnosis is only 8 to 10 months, with fewer than 10% of patients alive after 2 years. Survival is substantially shorter in older patients. With anaplastic astrocytomas, the length of survival is more variable, but the presence of a high mitotic rate or vascular cell hyperplasia tends to be associated with a poor prognosis.

Brain Stem Gliomas

A clinical subgroup of astrocytomas, these occur mostly in the first two decades of life and compose about 20% of primary brain tumors in this age group. At autopsy, about 50% of them have progressed to glioblastomas. With current radiotherapy, the 5-year survival rate for the composite group, which includes all grades of astrocytomas, is between 20 and 40%.

Pilocytic Astrocytomas

These astrocytomas are distinguished from the others by their pathologic appearance and almost invariably benign behavior. They typically occur in children and young adults and usually are located in the cerebellum, but may also appear in the floor and walls of the third ventricle, the optic nerves, and, very occasionally, the cerebral hemispheres.

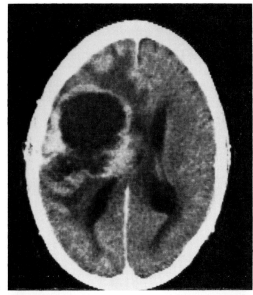

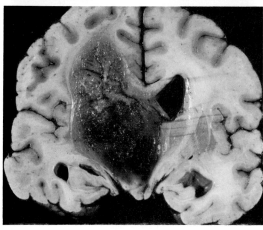

Figure 29–37. *A,* CT scan of a large tumor in cerebral hemisphere showing signal enhancement with contrast material and pronounced peritumoral edema. *B,* Glioblastoma multiforme appearing as a necrotic hemorrhagic infiltrating mass.

crosis, often present in a serpentine pattern, occurs in areas of hypercellularity with highly anaplastic tumor cells crowded along the edges of the necrotic regions, producing so-called **pseudopalisading** (see Fig. 29–38).

Two grading schemes have now received general acceptance. A four-tiered system (I–IV) is based on the features of nuclear pleomorphism, mitosis, endothelial cell proliferation, and necrosis; the alternative three-tiered system recognizes low-grade astrocytoma, anaplastic astrocytoma, and glioblastoma multiforme. The histologic appearance of astrocytoma may be heterogeneous. Thus, a small biopsy taken from a high-grade tumor may give a misleading impression of a lower grade lesion, depending on the area sampled. Astrocytomas have a tendency to become more anaplastic with time.

MORPHOLOGY. Grossly, a pilocytic astrocytoma is often cystic, with a mural nodule in the wall of the cyst (Fig. 29–39); if solid, it may be well circumscribed or, less frequently, infiltrative. Microscopically, the tumor is composed of bipolar cells with long, thin "hair-like" processes; Rosenthal fibers and microcysts are often present. An increase in the number of blood vessels, often with thickened walls, is seen but does not imply an unfavorable prognosis; necrosis, mitoses, and glomeruloid formations are almost never seen. These tumors grow very slowly, and some behave more like hamartomas than true neoplasms. Patients have survived for more than 40 years after incomplete resection.

Oligodendroglioma

These tumors constitute about 5 to 15% of gliomas, depending on the criteria used for diagnosis, and are most common in middle life. Patients may

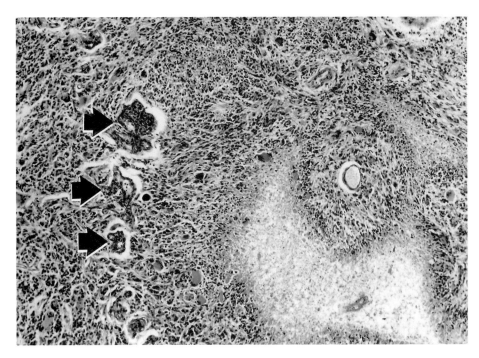

Figure 29-38. Glioblastoma multiforme. Focus of necrosis with pseudopalisading of malignant nuclei and endothelial cell proliferation, leading to a "glomeruloid" structure *(arrowheads)*.

have had several years of neurologic complaints, often including seizures. The lesions are found mostly in the cerebral hemispheres, with a predilection for white matter. In general, patients with oligodendrogliomas have a better prognosis than patients with astrocytomas. Current treatment with surgery and radiotherapy has yielded an average survival of 5 to 10 years. Cases of poorly differentiated tumors with necrosis have a worse prognosis. Current investigations also suggest a possible role

for chemotherapy in the treatment of oligodendroglioma. The term *mixed glioma* has been employed to designate lesions with regions of neoplastic oligodendrocytes and separate regions of other neoplastic glia, most commonly astrocytic.

MORPHOLOGY. Macroscopically, oligodendrogliomas are well-circumscribed, gelatinous, gray masses, often with cysts, focal hemorrhage, and

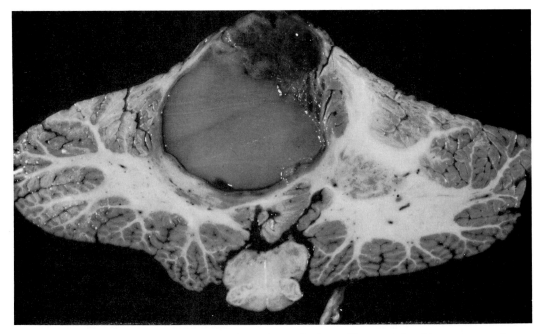

Figure 29-39. Juvenile pilocytic astrocytoma in cerebellum with a nodule of tumor in a cyst.

calcification. Microscopically, the tumor is composed of sheets of regular cells with spherical nuclei containing finely granular chromatin (similar to normal oligodendrocytes) surrounded by a clear halo of cytoplasm. Typically, the tumor contains a delicate network of anastomosing capillaries. The calcification, which is present in as many as 90% of these tumors, ranges from microscopic foci to massive depositions. At present, no diagnostically reliable immunohistochemical markers have been developed for oligodendroglioma; Leu-7, an epitope shared with natural killer cells, has been of some value.

Ependymoma and Related Tumors

Ependymomas often arise next to the ependymal-lined ventricular system, including the oft-obliterated central canal of the spinal cord. In the first two decades of life, they typically occur near the fourth ventricle and constitute 5 to 10% of the primary brain tumors in this age group. In middle life, the spinal cord is their most common location.

Clinically, posterior fossa ependymomas often manifest with hydrocephalus secondary to progressive obstruction of the fourth ventricle rather than invasion of the pons or medulla. Prognosis is poor despite the slow growth of the tumor and the usual lack of histologic evidence of anaplasia. Because of their relationship to the ventricular system, CSF dissemination is a common finding. An average survival of about 4 years following surgery and radiotherapy has been reported.

MORPHOLOGY. In the fourth ventricle, ependymomas are typically solid or papillary masses extending from the floor of the ventricle (Fig. 29–40A). Although often better demarcated from adjacent brain than astrocytomas, their proximity to the vital pontine and medullary nuclei usually makes complete extirpation impossible. In the intraspinal tumors, this sharp demarcation sometimes makes total removal possible. Microscopically, ependymomas are composed of cells with regular, round to oval nuclei with abundant granular chromatin. Between the nuclei, there is a fine fibrillary background that may be very dense. Tumor cells may form gland-like structures that resemble the embryologic ependymal canal with long, delicate processes extending into a lumen; these pathognomonic features are termed **ependymal rosettes.** More frequently present are **perivascular pseudorosettes** (see Fig. 29–40B) in which tumor cells are arranged around vessels with an intervening zone consisting of thin ependymal processes directed toward the wall of the vessel. Immunocytochemi-

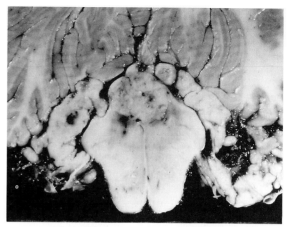

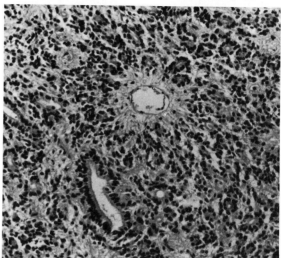

Figure 29–40. Ependymoma. A, Tumor arises from the lining of the floor of the fourth ventricle, fills the ventricle, and extends into the subarachnoid space through the foramina of Luschka. B, Tumor cells align themselves around tubular spaces resembling the ependymal cavity and also around blood vessels.

cally, about 50% of ependymomas can be shown to contain GFAP. Most tumors are well differentiated, but anaplastic forms also occur.

Myxopapillary ependymomas occur in the filum terminale of the spinal cord and, as implied by their name, may contain papillary elements in a myxoid background, admixed with more typical ependymal cells. Cuboidal cells, sometimes with clear cytoplasm, are arranged around papillary cores containing connective tissue and blood vessels. The myxoid areas contain neutral and acidic mucopolysaccharides. Prognosis depends on completeness of surgical resection; if the tumor has extended into the subarachnoid space and surrounded the roots of the cauda equina, recurrence is likely.

Subependymomas are solid, sometimes calcified, very slow-growing nodules attached to the ventricular lining and protruding into the ventricle. They are usually asymptomatic and are incidental findings at autopsy, but if they are sufficiently large or appropriately located, they may cause hydrocephalus or other focal findings. They are most often found in the lateral and fourth ventricles, and in the latter location, as with other fourth ventricular tumors, may be impossible to remove surgically. Microscopically, they have a very characteristic appearance, with clumps of ependymal-appearing nuclei scattered in a very dense, fine, glial fibrillar background.

Choroid plexus papillomas can occur anywhere along the choroid plexus and are most common in children, in whom they are most often found in the lateral ventricles. In adults, they are more often present in the fourth ventricle. These tumors almost exactly recapitulate the structure of the normal choroid plexus and are markedly papillary growths. The papillae have connective tissue stalks covered with a cuboidal or columnar, ciliated epithelium. Clinically, choroid plexus papillomas usually present with hydrocephalus due either to obstruction of the ventricular system by tumor or to overproduction of CSF. An etiologic role for papovavirus has been suggested for these tumors.

There are very rare malignant examples *(choroid plexus carcinomas)* that closely resemble adenocarcinoma. These lesions are usually found in children; when such a lesion occurs in an adult, the possibility of a metastatic carcinoma from elsewhere in the body must be considered.

Colloid cysts of the third ventricle usually occur in young adults. Their precise origin is uncertain. Because of their attachment to the roof of the third ventricle, the tumor can obstruct the foramina of Monro and result in noncommunicating hydrocephalus, sometimes rapidly fatal. Headache, sometime positional, is the major clinical symptom. The cyst has a thin, fibrous capsule, a lining of low to flat cuboidal epithelium, and often contains gelatinous, proteinaceous material.

NEURONAL TUMORS

Several types of CNS tumors contain mature-appearing neurons *(ganglion cells)*; these may constitute the entire population of the lesion *(gangliocytomas)*. More commonly, there is an admixture with a glial neoplasm, and the lesion is termed a *ganglioglioma*. Most of these tumors are slow-growing, but occasionally the glial component becomes frankly anaplastic, and the disease then assumes a much more rapid course.

MORPHOLOGY. Grossly, gangliocytomas are well-circumscribed masses with focal calcification and small cysts usually found in the floor of the third ventricle, the hypothalamus, or the temporal lobe. Microscopically, the neoplastic ganglion cells are present as clumps of cells separated by a not very cellular stroma. The ganglioglioma has a gross appearance that is similar to that of a glioma of comparable grade. They are most commonly found in the temporal lobe and often have a cystic component. The neoplastic ganglion cells are irregularly clustered and have apparently random orientation of neurites. Binucleated forms are frequent. The neoplastic neurons can often be detected with the use of immunohistochemical reactions for neuronal proteins, neurofilaments and synaptophysin.

Cerebral neuroblastomas are extremely rare neoplasms that occur in the hemispheres of children and have a more aggressive behavior. Microscopically, they resemble peripheral neuroblastomas (see Chapter 10), being composed of small undifferentiated cells with characteristic Homer Wright rosettes. *Neurocytoma* is a recently described neuronal neoplasm found principally adjacent to the foramen of Monro, characterized by evenly spaced, round, uniform nuclei resembling those of oligodendroglioma. Ultrastructural and immunohistochemical studies, however, reveal the neuronal origin of these cells.

POORLY DIFFERENTIATED NEOPLASMS

Some tumors, although of neuroectodermal origin, express few, if any, of the phenotypic markers of mature cells of the nervous system and are described as poorly differentiated, or embryonal, meaning that they retain cellular features of primitive, undifferentiated cells. The most common is the *medulloblastoma*, which accounts for 20% of the brain tumors of childhood and occurs in the cerebellum. Other poorly differentiated tumors occur in other locations, and have been collectively termed *primitive neuroectodermal tumors* (PNET) (not to be confused with the peripheral lesion of identical acronym that is closely related to Ewing's sarcoma). Most classification systems continue to recognize the medulloblastoma as a distinct clinicopathologic category and acknowledge the presence of other poorly differentiated tumors that occur predominantly in children.

Primitive neuroectodermal tumor is a highly controversial designation, which has been applied to neoplasms, primarily of childhood, that are histologically similar to medulloblastoma but occur in locations other than the cerebellum, especially the cerebral hemispheres. Many would prefer not to gather all these poorly differentiated tumors into a single category until there is a clearer vision of their biologic behavior; others find the designation useful to evaluate the efficacy of chemotherapeutic protocols. More information is needed to settle this issue.

Medulloblastoma

This tumor occurs predominantly in children and exclusively in the cerebellum. Neuronal markers may be expressed, but often the tumor is largely undifferentiated. Ploidy analysis of the tumor shows that some of the tumors are diploid, and others are aneuploid, with some differences in subsequent clinical course, suggesting that more detailed delineation of the genotype of these tumors may identify subcategories with clinical significance.

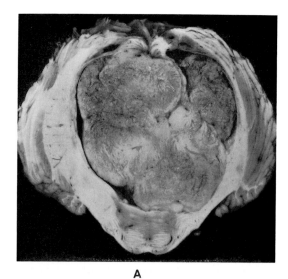

A

MORPHOLOGY. Medulloblastomas are located in the midline of the cerebellum in children (Figure 29–41A); lateral locations are more often found in adults. Rapid growth may occlude the flow of CSF, leading to hydrocephalus. The tumor is often well circumscribed, gray, and friable and may be seen extending to the surface of the cerebellar folia and involving the leptomeninges. Microscopically, the tumor is usually extremely cellular, with sheets of anaplastic cells (see Fig. 29–41B). Individual tumor cells have hyperchromatic nuclei that are often round but are also frequently elongated or crescent shaped. Mitoses are abundant, and markers of cellular proliferation, such as the Ki-67 antigen, are detected in a high percentage of the cells. The cells have little cytoplasm, and the cytoplasm is often devoid of specific markers of differentiation. The tumor has the potential to express divergent neuronal (Homer Wright rosettes, as occur in neuroblastoma [see Chapter 10], or neurosecretory granules) and glial (GFAP) phenotypes. At the edges of the main tumor mass, medulloblastoma cells have a propensity to form linear chains of cells extending through the neuropil, and to extend through the cerebellar cortex to aggregate beneath the pia, penetrate the pia, and seed into the subarachnoid space. Extension into the subarachnoid space may elicit a prominent desmoplastic response. Dissemination through the CSF is a very common complication, presenting as nodular masses throughout the neuraxis, including metastases to the cauda equina that, because of their direct route of dissemination through the CSF, are sometimes termed "drop" metastases.

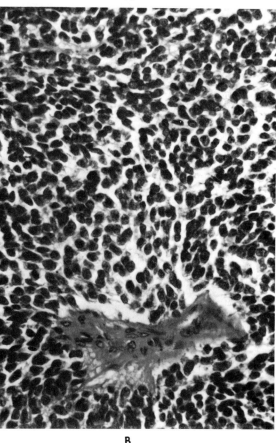

B

Figure 29–41. A, Medulloblastoma growing into fourth ventricle, distorting, compressing, and infiltrating surrounding structures. B, Medulloblastoma.

The tumor is highly malignant, and the prognosis for untreated patients is dismal; however, it is an exquisitely radiosensitive tumor. Prognosis is also related to the amount of tumor resected, with better survival rates following complete resection. In addition, radiation of the entire neuraxis decreases the likelihood of recurrence. With total excision and radiation, the 5-year survival rate has been reported to be as high as 75%.

OTHER PARENCHYMAL TUMORS

Neoplasms arise in the CNS that are derived from cells other than those unique to the CNS. The cells of origin for these tumors are found elsewhere in the body as well, and these lesions are similar to their neoplastic counterparts in other sites.

Primary Brain Lymphoma (PBL)

The CNS accounts for approximately 2% of extranodal lymphomas, and PBL represents approximately 1% of intracranial tumors. In immunosuppressed patients, PBL is a relatively common neoplasm. As a result of the dramatic increase in numbers of AIDS patients, there has been a corresponding increase in the incidence of this neoplasm (see Chapter 6). Apart from this epidemiologic shift, however, there is also evidence of an increase in the incidence of PBL among immunocompetent patients as well. For sporadic cases, the age spectrum is relatively wide, and the frequency increases after 60 years of age.

The term *primary* reflects the distinction between these lesions and secondary involvement of the CNS by non-Hodgkin's lymphoma (NHL) arising elsewhere in the body. Patients with PBL often have multiple tumor masses within the brain parenchyma; nodal, bone marrow, or extranodal involvements outside of the CNS are extremely rare late complications. Conversely, NHL of the nodal or extranodal, non-CNS type rarely involves the brain parenchyma; involvement of the nervous system, when it occurs, is usually manifested by the presence of malignant cells within the CSF and around intradural nerve roots and occasionally by the infiltration of superficial aspects of the cerebrum or spinal cord by lymphoma cells.

The majority of PBL are of B-cell origin, although T-cell lesions are observed on rare occasions. Within the immunosuppressed population, all the neoplasms appear to be of B-cell origin and to contain Epstein-Barr virus genomes within the transformed B cells. Regardless of the clinical context in which it occurs, PBL is an aggressive disease with relatively poor chemotherapeutic response compared with peripheral lymphomas, although it is initially responsive to radiotherapy and steroids.

MORPHOLOGY. PBL lesions, which are frequently multiple, often involve deep gray structures as well as white matter and cortex. Periventricular spread is a common finding. The tumors are relatively well defined compared with glial neoplasms but are not as discrete as metastases and often show extensive areas of central necrosis. The size and appearance of the cells are nearly always those of a high-grade type (Working Formulation, see Chapter 14), most commonly large cell lymphoma, although immunoblastic sarcomas as well as small noncleaved cell patterns are also observed. The malignant cells diffusely involve the parenchyma of the brain. They accumulate around blood vessels, with some vessel walls expanded by multiple layers of malignant cells. Reticulin stains demonstrate that these infiltrating cells are separated from one another by silver staining material; this pattern, which has been referred to as "hooping," is characteristic of PBL. Mild reactive gliosis may be found in the areas at the edge of the lesion; however, the proliferative nature of the lesion outpaces the astrocytic response. A benign mixed T- and B-cell infiltrate, which often contains a plasmacytic component, can also be found in association with lymphoma lesions.

Germ Cell Tumors (GCT)

Primary GCTs occur along the midline, most commonly in the pineal and the suprasellar regions. They account for 0.2 to 1% of brain tumors in people of European descent. Their incidence in Asians is several times higher. Most occur in adolescents and young adults. Tumors in the pineal region show a strong male predominance, which is not seen in suprasellar lesions. It is not clear whether these tumors reflect the transformation of an otherwise normal resident population of germ cells, of a developmentally derived ectopic rest of germ cells, or of germ cells that migrated into the CNS late in development. Regardless of these uncertainties, GCTs—like the lymphomas—share many of the features of their counterparts in the lower organs. In distinction from lymphomas, however, CNS involvement by a gonadal germ cell tumor is not uncommon, and the presence of a non-CNS primary must always be considered. The histologic appearances of GCTs and their classification are the same as those used for lesions elsewhere in the body (see Chapter 22). The lesion called seminoma in the testis goes by the name of germinoma in the CNS, as at other extragonadal sites. The cellular responses to radiotherapy and chemotherapy roughly parallel those of similar histologic lesions at other sites. Despite this, since the tumor frequently extends into the CSF it can disseminate widely along the surface of the brain and within the ventricular system, complicating therapy.

MENINGIOMAS

Meningiomas are predominantly benign tumors of adults. They arise from the meningothelial cell of the arachnoid, although they are most intimately associated with the dura.[68] Because of this histogenesis, meningiomas may be found along any of the external surfaces of the brain as well as within the ventricular system, where they arise from the stromal arachnoid cells of the choroid plexus. Meningiomas are uncommon in the pediatric population and, in general, show a moderate (3 : 2) female predominance. Common sites of tumors include the parasagittal aspect of the convexity, dura over the lateral convexity, the wing of the sphenoid, olfactory groove, the sella turcica, and the foramen magnum. Meningiomas can also be found along the spinal cord; in these patients, there is a female-to-male predominance, approaching 10 : 1.

Meningiomas are usually slow-growing lesions that present either with vague nonlocalizing symptoms or with focal findings referrable to compression of underlying brain. Lesions are usually solitary; their presence at multiple sites, especially in association with acoustic neuromas or glial tumors, suggests a diagnosis of neurofibromatosis type 2. The tumors often express progesterone receptors, and rapid growth during pregnancy has been reported. Cytogenetic investigation of meningiomas has revealed deletions of the long arm of chromosome 22.

MORPHOLOGY. Grossly, meningiomas tend to be rounded masses with a well-defined dural base that compress underlying brain but are easily separated from it (Fig. 29–42A). Extension into the overlying bone is not uncommon. The surface of the mass is usually encapsulated with thin, fibrous tissue and may have a bosselated or polypoid appearance. Another characteristic growth pattern is the **en plaque** variant, in which the tumor spreads in a sheet-like fashion along the surface of the dura. This form is commonly associated with hyperostotic reactive changes in the overlying bone. The lesions may have a finely gritty consistency, reflecting few calcifications, or they may be extremely calcified with psammoma bodies or even contain metaplastic bone. In the absence of these types of changes, the lesions are usually firm to fibrous and lack evidence of necrosis or extensive hemorrhage.

Traditionally, several histologic patterns have been recognized, although it is now felt that most of these carry little prognostic significance. Among the histologic patterns found in meningiomas are **syncytial,** appropriately named for the whorled clusters of cells which sit in tight groups without visible cell membranes; **fibroblastic,** with elongated cells and abundant collagen deposition between them; **transitional,** which shares features of the syncytial and fibroblastic types (see Fig. 29–42B); **psammomatous,** with a dominant pattern of psammoma bodies, apparently forming from calcification of the syncytial nests of meningothelial cells; **secretory,** with PAS-positive intracytoplasmic droplets and intracellular lumina by electron microscopy; and **microcystic,** with a loose, spongy appearance. One histologic pattern is associated with a worse prognosis: the **papillary** variant, which has pleomorphic cells arranged around fibrovascular cores. Tumors may have a mixture of these histologic types as well. Some recognize a group of angioblastic meningiomas; others feel that they constitute a distinct population of neoplasms, as discussed later.

Immunohistochemical studies of meningiomas have revealed them to be positive for epithelial membrane antigen (EMA), in distinction to other tumors arising in this region. Keratin staining is usually restricted to lesions with the secretory pattern, and these tumors are also positive for carcinoembryonic antigen (CEA). Xanthomatous degeneration, metaplasia, and moderate nuclear pleomorphism, are common in meningiomas. These findings are of no prognostic significance. **Malignant meningiomas** are extremely unusual tumors and may be difficult to recognize histologically. Features that support this diagnosis include single cell infiltration of underlying brain and abundant mitoses with atypical forms.

There are also meningeal-based lesions that have the architecture of *hemangiopericytomas.* These tumors show staghorn-like vascular channels lined by benign endothelium but surrounded by a tumor mass of small cells with indistinct cell borders and a whorled architecture. These lesions usually have an aggressive course, similar to that of comparable lesions elsewhere in the body. Cytogenetic studies of these lesions have failed to find loss of heterozygosity on 22q. Other nonmeningothelial neoplasms may also arise in the meninges. True primary sarcomas of the meninges are uncommon but can include fibrosarcomas and malignant fibrous histiocytomas.

METASTATIC LESIONS

Among general hospital patients, metastatic lesions, mostly carcinomas, account for approximately half of intracranial tumors. The five most common primary sites are the lungs, breasts, skin (melanoma), kidneys, and gastrointestinal tract, accounting for about 80% of all metastases. Some rare tumors (e.g., choriocarcinoma) have a high likelihood of

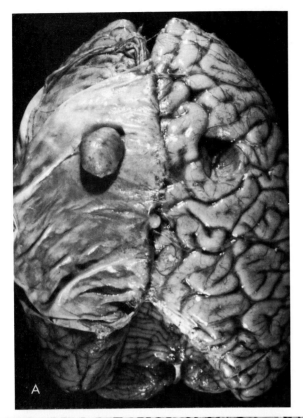

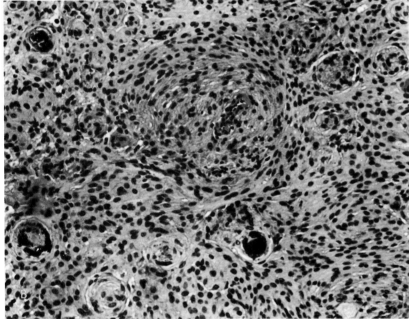

Figure 29–42. *A,* Reflected dura *(on left)* showing one large and one small *(in middle of illustration)* meningioma. Note prominent indentation of right cerebral hemisphere by the larger tumor. *B,* Transitional meningioma with hypercellularity, whorled pattern of cells, and psammoma bodies.

metastasizing to the brain, whereas other more common tumors (e.g., prostate carcinoma) almost never do even when metastatic to adjacent bone. The meninges are also a frequent site of involvement by metastatic disease. Metastatic tumors present as mass lesions and may even occasionally cause the presenting symptoms of a carcinoma. Current treatments including surgical resection of a single brain metastasis, if possible, and radiotherapy have been found to be helpful in some instances.

MORPHOLOGY. Grossly, intraparenchymal metastases form sharply demarcated masses, often at the gray matter–white matter junction, usually surrounded by a zone of edema. Meningeal carcinomatosis, with tumor nodules studding the surface of the brain, spinal cord, and intradural nerve roots, is an occasional complication particularly associated with small cell carcinoma and adenocarcinoma of the lung, and carcinoma of the breast.

In addition to the direct and localized effects produced by metastases, the nervous system can show functional and structural changes in response to systemic effects of malignancy elsewhere in the body. These phenomena, termed *paraneoplastic syndromes*, may precede the clinical recognition of the initiating malignancy.[69] Although a wide variety of tumors have been associated with paraneoplastic syndromes, small cell carcinoma of the lung stands out as a frequent offender. A commonly suggested mechanism for the development of the syndromes is an immunologically mediated attack on nervous system components, presumably following the inappropriate expression of the same or similar antigens on neoplastic tissue. Thus, the neurologic syndrome may improve with plasmapheresis, immunosuppression, or treatment of the neoplasm.

Paraneoplastic cerebellar degeneration is the most common of these expressions of systemic malignancy; the typical findings include destruction of Purkinje cells, gliosis, and a mild inflammatory infiltrate. The process commonly appears to be an antibody-mediated injury of Purkinje cells. Another important site of paraneoplastic degeneration is the spinal cord. Some patients appear to have a relatively selective loss of anterior horn motor neurons. This process usually appears to be self-limited. Other cases show a necrotizing myelopathy usually in the thoracic region. This form of injury is less clearly *para*neoplastic, since radiation therapy along with vascular compromise from tumor bulk may have been of etiologic importance.

Limbic encephalitis is a paraneoplastic syndrome characterized by subacute dementia. The pathologic findings are most striking in the anterior and medial portions of the temporal lobe and resemble an infectious process, with perivascular inflammatory cuffs, microglial nodules, some neuronal loss, and gliosis. Viral or other pathogens have not been demonstrated, and the symptoms are often responsive to treatment of the underlying malignancy. A comparable process involving the brain stem can be seen in isolation or together with limbic system involvement.

PERIPHERAL NERVE SHEATH TUMORS

A large proportion of tumors occurring within the confines of the dura are derived from cellular elements of peripheral nerve. The transition zone between central myelination by oligodendrocytes and peripheral myelination by Schwann cells occurs within several millimeters of the exit of axons from the substance of the brain. Thus, for cranial nerves III through XII as well as for all spinal roots, tumors derived from Schwann cells and other perineurial elements can arise in locations that cause pathologic changes in adjacent brain or spinal cord. In addition, such lesions must be distinguished from other intradural, extraparenchymal lesions (e.g., meningiomas, metastases) as well as from exophytic glial tumors. Tumors of comparable histogenesis and biologic behavior also arise along the peripheral course of nerves. These tumors are composed of cells that express Schwannian characteristics, including the presence of S-100 antigen as well as the potential for melanocytic differentiation.

Schwannoma

These benign tumors arise from the neural crest–derived Schwann cell. Within the cranial vault, the most common location is in the cerebellopontine angle (CPA), where they are attached to the vestibular branch of the eighth nerve: vestibular schwannoma[70] (Fig. 29–43). Patients often present with tinnitus and hearing loss, and the tumor can be referred to as an "acoustic neuroma." The lesion commonly expands the internal auditory meatus, the location of the transition zone for this nerve. In the rare instances that schwannomas are derived from other cranial nerves, sensory nerves are preferentially involved, especially branches of the trigeminal. This association with sensory nerves is also found for spinal tumors, with most arising from dorsal roots. The lesions may extend with the nerve through the vertebral foramen, acquiring a dumbbell configuration. Extension for a short distance into the spinal cord at the root entry zone can be found in a limited number of cases as well. When extradural, schwannomas are most commonly found in association with large nerve trunks, where motor and sensory modalities are intermixed.

MORPHOLOGY. Regardless of site, schwannomas share a gross and microscopic appearance. They are well-circumscribed, encapsulated masses that are attached to the nerve but can be separated from it. Tumors are firm, gray masses but may also have areas of cystic change and a yellow, xanthomatous appearance. Microscopically, tumors show a mixture of two growth patterns (see Fig. 29–43B). Elongated cells with cytoplasmic processes are arranged in fascicles in areas of moderate to high

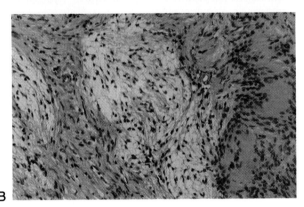

Figure 29–43. Schwannoma. *A,* **Bilateral eighth nerve schwannomas. (Courtesy of Dr. K.M. Earle.)** *B,* **Tumor showing cellular areas (Antoni A), including Verocay bodies *(far right),* as well as looser, myxoid regions (Antoni B).**

cellularity with little stromal matrix **(Antoni A);** the "nuclear-free zones" of processes that lie between the regions of nuclear palisading are termed Verocay bodies. The other major pattern of growth **(Antoni B)** consists of less densely cellular tissue with a loose meshwork of cells similar to those seen in Antoni A areas along with microcysts and myxoid changes. Electron microscopy shows basement membrane deposition encasing single cells and long spacing collagen. Because the lesion displaces the nerve of origin as it grows, silver stains demonstrate that axons are excluded from the tumor, although they may become entrapped in the capsule. The Schwann cell origin of these tumors is borne out by their S-100 immunoreactivity. A variety of degenerative changes may be found in schwannomas, including nuclear pleomorphism, xanthomatous change, and vascular hyalinization; these do not impart a worse prognosis. Malignant change is extremely rare in schwannomas, although local recurrence can follow incomplete resection.

Neurofibroma

Two histologically, and perhaps biologically, distinct lesions have been termed neurofibromas.

Various ultrastructural and immunohistochemical studies have identified the neoplastic cells as showing markers of diverse lineages, including Schwann cells, perineurial cells, and fibroblasts.

The most common form of neurofibroma occurs in the skin *(cutaneous neurofibroma)* or in peripheral nerve *(solitary neurofibroma).* These occur sporadically as well as in association with neurofibromatosis type 1 (NF1). The skin lesions are evident as nodules, sometimes with hyperpigmentation; these lesions may grow quite large and become pedunculated. The risk of malignant transformation from these tumors is extremely small, and cosmetic concerns are their major morbidity.

MORPHOLOGY. Present in the dermis and extending to the subcutaneous fat, cutaneous neurofibromas are well-delineated but unencapsulated masses composed of spindle cells. Although not invasive, the adnexal structures are sometimes enwrapped by the edges of the lesion. The stroma of these tumors is highly collagenized and contains little myxoid material. Lesions within peripheral nerves are of identical histologic appearance.

Plexiform Neurofibroma

In contrast, the *plexiform neurofibroma* is considered by some to be a defining lesion of NF1; by this definition, it does not occur as a sporadic tumor, although the issue remains to be addressed through examination of the genetic locus for NF1. A major concern in the care of these patients is the difficulty of surgical removal of these lesions when they involve major nerve trunks combined with their potential for malignant transformation.

MORPHOLOGY. These tumors may arise anywhere along the extent of a nerve, although the small terminal branches are uncommon sites. They are frequently multiple. At the site of each lesion, the host nerve is irregularly expanded, as each of its fascicles is infiltrated by the neoplasm. Unlike the case with schwannomas, it is not possible to separate the lesion from the nerve. The proximal and distal extremes of the tumor may have poorly defined margins, as fingers of tumor and individual cells insert themselves between the fibers. Microscopically, the lesion has a loose, myxoid background with a low cellularity. A number of cell phenotypes are present, including Schwannian cells with typical elongated nuclei and extensions of pink cytoplasm, larger multipolar fibroblastic cells, and a sprinkling of inflammatory cells often including mast cells. Axons can be demonstrated within the tumor.

Malignant Peripheral Nerve Sheath Tumor (MPNST, Malignant Schwannoma)

These are highly malignant sarcomas that are locally invasive, frequently leading to multiple recurrences and eventual metastatic spread with poor prognosis.[71] Despite their name, these tumors essentially never arise from malignant degeneration of schwannomas. Instead, they arise *de novo* or from transformation of a plexiform neurofibroma. This latter fact provides the basis for their association with NF1. These tumors may also follow radiation therapy. MPNSTs arising from cranial nerve roots are rare and, when they occur, are more commonly associated with cranial nerve V than VIII.

MORPHOLOGY. The lesions are poorly defined tumor masses with frequent infiltration along the axis of the parent nerve as well as invasion of adjacent soft tissues. Associated with the malignant nature of the neoplasm, necrosis is commonly present. Microscopically, a wide range of histologic findings can be encountered. Patterns reminiscent of fibrosarcoma or malignant fibrous histocytoma may be found. In other areas, the tumor cells resemble Schwann cells, with elongated nuclei and prominent bipolar processes. Fascicle formation may be present. Mitoses, necrosis, and extreme nuclear anaplasia are common. Some but not all MPNSTs are immunoreactive for S-100 protein. In addition to the basic appearance of these tumors, a wide variety of "divergent" histologic patterns may be admixed, including epithelial structures, rhabdomyoblastic differentiation (termed **Triton tumors**), cartilage, and even bone. The term **epithelioid malignant schwannoma** has been applied to cases in which aggressive tumors are derived from nerve sheaths and contain tumor cells having visible cell borders, epithelial-type nests, and immunoreactivity for S-100 but not keratin.

NEUROCUTANEOUS SYNDROMES (PHAKOMATOSES)

These are a group of inherited disorders characterized by hamartomas located throughout the body, but most prominently involving the nervous system and skin. Many of the disorders are inherited in an autosomal dominant pattern, and recent studies have reported the genes (within the broad category of tumor suppressor genes) involved in many of them. Symptoms are referable to the hamartomatous tissue or to the development of neoplasms,

which occur with a high incidence in most of the neurocutaneous disorders.

NEUROFIBROMATOSIS TYPE 1 (NF1)

The disorder, discussed in Chapter 5, is characterized by neurofibromas, acoustic nerve schwannomas, gliomas of the optic nerve, meningiomas, pigmented nodules of the iris (*Lisch nodules*), and cutaneous hyperpigmented macules (*café-au-lait spots*). The gene, located at 17q11.2, has been identified and encodes a protein termed neurofibromin. The protein contains a region homologous to one family of GTPase-activating proteins. This activity is presumed to allow neurofibromin to play a role in regulating signal transduction.[72] The NF1 gene product does function as a tumor suppressor gene, based on evidence of loss of heterozygosity in some tumors from NF1 patients, although this has not been found for neurofibromas.[73]

Neurologic manifestations are referable to neoplasms rather than to hamartomas. The tumors that occur in NF1 are, in general, histologically identical to those that occur sporadically. The exception lies in plexiform neurofibromas, which expand each of the fascicles of an entire nerve trunk and are considered by some as pathognomonic of NF1.

The clinical course is as variable as the expression of the disease itself. Some individuals may carry the gene and have no symptoms; others may have a rapidly progressive disease. There is a propensity for the neurofibromas of the peripheral nervous system to undergo malignant degeneration at a higher rate than that observed for comparable tumors in the non-NF population. In the absence of these biologically malignant tumors, many patients suffer the complications of neurofibromas with their potential to create spinal deformity, most commonly kyphoscoliosis. Tumors arising in proximity to the spinal cord or brain stem may also have devastating consequences, independent of their histologic grade.

NEUROFIBROMATOSIS TYPE 2 (NF2)

At one time, this disorder was thought to represent a variant of neurofibromatosis and was termed central neurofibromatosis; however, it is now clear that NF2 is an entirely distinct autosomal dominant disorder whose gene is located on chromosome 22. A candidate gene has been identified; the encoded protein appears to be a member of a group of proteins that interact with both the membrane components and the cytoskeleton.[74] As with NF1, there is a propensity to develop tumors, most commonly bilateral schwannomas of the eighth nerves or multiple meningiomas. The schwannomas seen in NF2 patients are similar in appearance to sporadic lesions but are more likely to have foci of higher cellularity and a lobular growth pattern.[70]

TUBEROUS SCLEROSIS

Tuberous sclerosis is characterized by a triad of findings: angiofibromas, seizures, and mental retardation. Hamartomas within the CNS are a prominent feature of the disease, occurring as *cortical tubers* and subependymal hamartomas. In addition, there may be renal angiomyolipomas, retinal glial hamartomas, and pulmonary and cardiac myomas. Cysts may be found at various sites, including the liver, kidneys, and pancreas. Cutaneous lesions include angiofibromas, leathery thickenings in localized patches (shagreen patches), hypopigmented areas (ash-leaf patches), and subungual fibromas. The disorder is transmitted in an autosomal dominant pattern with variable expressivity and penetrance. Genetic analysis is rendered complex because there are patients who are obligate carriers of the gene but have no evidence of the disease. Linkage studies have shown at least two distinct loci, on chromosomes 9 and 16. The chromosome 16 locus has been identified as encoding a protein (tuberin) with homology to a GTPase-activating protein, although from a family different from that of neurofibromin.[75] Treatment is symptomatic, including anticonvulsant therapy for control of seizures.

> **MORPHOLOGY.** Cortical hamartomas of tuberous sclerosis are firm areas of the cortex that, in contrast to the softer adjacent cortex, have been likened to potatoes, hence the appellation "tubers." These hamartomas are composed of haphazardly arranged neurons that lack the normal laminar organization of neocortex. In addition, some large cells express phenotypes intermediate between glia and neurons, with intermediate filaments of both neuronal (neurofilament) and glial (GFAP) types. These cells have large vesicular nuclei with nucleoli, resembling neurons, and abundant eosinophilic cytoplasm like gemistocytic astrocytes. Similar hamartomatous features are present in the subependymal nodules, where large astrocytic cells cluster beneath the ventricular surface. These multiple drop-like masses that bulge into the ventricular system gave rise to the term "candle-guttering." In these subependymal areas, a tumor unique to tuberous sclerosis (subependymal giant cell astrocytomas) occurs.

VON HIPPEL–LINDAU DISEASE

This disorder is inherited in an autosomal dominant pattern and includes the predilection to develop characteristic tumors within the cerebellar hemispheres (capillary hemangioblastomas), retina, and, less commonly, the brain stem and spinal cord. Patients may also have cysts involving the pancreas, liver, and kidneys and have a strong propensity to develop renal cell carcinoma of the kidney. The gene, a tumor suppressor gene, is located on chromosome 3p25-26 (see discussion in Chapter 20). Therapy is directed at the symptomatic neoplasms, including resection of the cerebellar hemangioblastomas and laser therapy for retinal lesions. Partial nephrectomies may be performed for renal carcinomas when these malignancies are bilateral. Polycythemia is associated with the presence of a hemangioblastoma in about 10% of cases; the tumor has been shown to be a source of erythropoietin in these cases, although the cell origin of the growth factor is not known.

> **MORPHOLOGY.** Capillary hemangioblastomas are the CNS manifestation of the disease, although they may occur as sporadic lesions as well. The identity of the neoplastic cell remains unknown. These tumors commonly present as a cystic lesion with a mural nodule. Microscopically, the lesion is composed of a mixture of variable proportions of delicate capillary vessels with "stromal" cells between them. These cells are of uncertain histogenesis, with abundant vacuolated cytoplasm.

Note: The authors acknowledge with pleasure Drs. James H. Morris and William C. Schoene for generously allowing us to use portions of text and illustrations from previous editions of this chapter and for their review of this draft.

1. Adams, J.H., and Duchen, L.H.: Greenfield's Neuropathology. New York, Oxford University, 1992.
2. Adams, R.D., and Victor, M.: Principles of Neurology. New York, McGraw-Hill, 1993.
3. Peters, A., et al.: The Fine Structure of the Nervous System: Neurons and Their Supporting Cells. Philadelphia, W.B. Saunders Co., 1991.
4. Dickson, D.W., et al.: Microglia in human disease, with a special emphasis on acquired immune deficiency disease. Lab. Invest. 64:135, 1991.
5. Hickey, W.F., and Kimura, H.: Perivascular microglial cells of the CNS are bone–marrow derived and present antigen in vivo. Science 239:290, 1988.
6. Lassman, H., et al.: Inflammation in the nervous system: Basic mechanisms and immunological concepts. Rev. Neurol. 147:763, 1991.
7. Rowland, L.P., et al.: Cerebrospinal fluid: Blood-brain barrier, brain edema, and hydrocephalus. In Kandel, E.R., et al. (eds.): Principles of Neural Science. New York, Elsevier, 1991, pp. 1050–1060.
8. Fishman, R.A.: Cerebrospinal fluid in diseases of the nervous system. Philadelphia, W.B. Saunders Co., 1992.
9. Friede, R.L.: Developmental Neuropathology. Berlin, Springer-Verlag, 1989.
10. Noden, D.M.: Vertebrate craniofacial development:

Novel approaches and new dilemmas. Curr. Opin. Genet. Dev. 2:576, 1992.

11. Czeizel, A., and Dudás, I.: Prevention of the first occurrence of neural-tube defects by periconceptional vitamin supplementation. N. Engl. J. Med. 327:1832, 1992.

12. Leestma, J.E.: Forensic Neuropathology. New York, Raven Press, 1988.

13. Plum, F., and Posner, J.B.: The Diagnosis of Stupor and Coma. Philadelphia, F.A. Davis, 1982.

14. Caplan, L.R.: Stroke. Stoneham, Butterworth-Heinemann, 1993.

15. Beal, M.F.: Mechanism of excitotoxicity in neurologic disease. FASEB J. 6:3338, 1992.

16. Choi, D.W., and Hartley, D.M.: Calcium and glutamate-induced cortical neuronal death. In Waxman, S.G. (ed.): Molecular and Cellular Approaches to the Treatment of Neurological Disease. New York, Raven Press, 1993, pp. 23–34.

17. Dawson, T.M., et al.: A novel neuronal messenger molecule in brain: The free radical, nitric oxide. Ann. Neurol. 32:297, 1992.

18. Lipton, S.A., and Rosenberg, P.A.: Excitatory amino acids as a final common pathway for neurologic disorders. N. Engl. J. Med. 330:613, 1994.

19. Buisson, A., et al.: The neuroprotective effect of a nitric oxide inhibitor in a rat model of focal cerebral ischemia. Br. J. Pharmacol. 106:766, 1992.

20. Molinari, G.F.: Lobar hemorrhages: Where do they come from? How did they get there? Stroke 24:523, 1993.

21. Suzuki, R., et al.: The role of endothelin-1 in the origin of cerebral vasospasm in patients with aneurysmal subarachnoid hemorrhage. J. Neurosurg. 77:96, 1992.

22. Tyler, K.L., and Martin, J.B. (eds.): Infectious Diseases of the Central Nervous System. Philadelphia, F.A. Davis, 1993.

23. Durand, M.L., et al.: Acute bacterial meningitis in adults: Review of 493 episodes. N. Engl. J. Med. 328:21, 1993.

24. Chun, C.H., et al.: Brain abscess: A study of 45 consecutive cases. Medicine 65:415, 1986.

25. Logigian, E.L., et al.: Chronic neurologic manifestations of Lyme disease. N. Engl. J. Med. 323:1438, 1990.

26. Whitley, R.J.: Viral encephalitis. N. Engl. J. Med. 323:242, 1990.

27. Morgello, S., et al.: Cytomegalovirus encephalitis in patients with acquired immunodeficiency syndrome. Hum. Pathol. 18:289, 1987.

28. Melchers, W., et al.: The postpolio syndrome: No evidence for poliovirus persistence. Ann. Neurol. 32:728, 1992.

29. Munsat, T.L.: Poliomyelitis—new problems with an old disease. N. Engl. J. Med. 324:1206, 1991.

30. Mrak, R.E., and Young, L.: Rabies encephalitis in humans: Pathology, pathogenesis and pathophysiology. J. Neuropathol. Exp. Neurol. 41:1, 1994.

31. Epstein, L.G., and Gendelman, H.E.: Human immunodeficiency virus type 1 infection of the nervous system: Pathogenetic mechanisms. Ann. Neurol. 33:429, 1993.

32. Report of a Working Group of the American Academy of Neurology AIDS Task Force: Nomenclature and research case definitions for neurologic manifestations of human immunodeficiency virus-type 1 (HIV-1) infection. Neurology 41:778, 1991.

33. De Girolami, U., and Smith, T.W.: Neuropathology. In Nash, G., and Said, J.W. (eds.): Pathology of AIDS and HIV Infection. Philadelphia, W.B. Saunders Co., 1992, pp. 174–199.

34. Gray, F., et al.: Early brain changes in HIV infection: Neuropathological study of 11 seropositive, non-AIDS cases. J. Neuropathol. Exp. Neurol. 51:177, 1992.

35. Hénin, D., et al.: Neuropathology of the spinal cord in the acquired immunodeficiency syndrome. Hum. Pathol. 23:1106, 1992.

36. Petito, C.K., et al.: HIV antigen and DNA in AIDS spinal cords correlate with macrophage infiltration but not with

vacuolar myelopathy. J. Neuropathol. Exp. Neurol. 53:86, 1994.

37. Schmidbauer, M., et al.: Progressive multifocal leukoencephalopathy (PML) in AIDS and the pre-AIDS era. Acta Neuropathol. 80:375, 1990.

38. Hsiao, K., and Prusiner, S.B.: Inherited human prion diseases. Neurology 40:1820, 1990.

39. Prusiner, S.B.: Molecular biology of prion diseases. Science 252:1515, 1991.

40. Porter, S.B., and Sande, M.A.: Toxoplasmosis of the central nervous system in the acquired immunodeficiency syndrome. N. Engl. J. Med. 327:1643, 1992.

41. Sadovnick, A.D., and Ebers, G.C.: Epidemiology of multiple sclerosis: A critical overview. Can. J. Neurol. Sci. 20:17, 1993.

42. Allen, I., and Brankin, B.: Pathogenesis of multiple sclerosis—the immune diathesis and the role of viruses. J. Neuropathol. Exp. Neurol. 52:95, 1992.

43. ffrench-Constant, C.: Pathogenesis of multiple sclerosis. Lancet 343:271, 1994.

44. Oksenberg, J.R., et al.: Selection for T-cell receptor $V\beta$-$D\beta$-$J\beta$ gene rearrangements with specificity for a myelin basic protein peptide in brain lesions of multiple sclerosis. Nature 362:68, 1993.

45. Kleinschmidt-DeMasters, B.K., and Norenberg, M.D.: Rapid correction of hyponatremeia causes demyelination: Relation to central pontine myelinolysis. Science 211:1068, 1981.

46. Evans, D.A., et al.: Prevalence of Alzheimer's disease in a community population of older persons: Higher than previously reported. J.A.M.A. 262:2551, 1989.

47. Mirra, S.M., et al.: Making the diagnosis of Alzheimer's disease. Arch. Pathol. Lab. Med. 117:131, 1993.

48. Selkoe, D.J.: The molecular pathology of Alzheimer's disease. Neuron 6:487, 1991.

49. Rosenberg, R.N.: A causal role for amyloid in Alzheimer's disease: The end of the beginning. Neurology 43:851, 1993.

50. Price, D.L., et al.: Toxicity of synthetic $A\beta$ peptides and modeling of Alzheimer's disease. Neurobiol. Aging 13:623, 1992.

51. Corder, E.H., et al.: Gene dose of apolipoprotein E type 4 allele and the risk of Alzheimer's disease in late-onset families. Science 261:921, 1993.

52. Ahlskog, J.E.: Cerebral transplantation for Parkinson's disease: Current progress and future prospects. Mayo Clin. Proc. 68:578, 1993.

53. Richardson, E.P., Jr.: Huntington's disease: Some recent neuropathological studies. Neuropathol. Appl. Neurobiol. 16:451, 1990.

54. The Huntington's Disease Collaborative Research Group: A novel gene containing a trinucleotide repeat that is expanded and unstable on Huntington's disease chromosomes. Cell 72:971, 1993.

55. Rothstein, J.D., et al.: Decreased glutamate transport by the brain and spinal cord in amyotrophic lateral sclerosis. N. Engl. J. Med. 326:1464, 1992.

56. Rosen, D.R., et al.: Mutations in Cu/Zn superoxide dismutase gene are associated with familial amyotrophic lateral sclerosis. Nature 362:59, 1993.

57. La Spada, A.R., et al.: Androgen receptor gene mutations in X-linked spinal and bulbar muscular atrophy. Nature 352:77, 1991.

58. Raskind, W.H., et al.: Complete deletion of the proteolipid protein (PLP) gene in a German family with Pelizaeus-Merzbacher disease. Am. J. Hum. Genet. 49:1355, 1991.

59. Bartalini, G., et al.: Biochemical diagnosis of Canavan's disease. Childs Nerv. Syst. 8:468, 1992.

60. Sparaco, M., et al.: Neuropathology of mitochondrial encephalomyopathies due to mitochondrial DNA defects. J. Neuropathol. Exp. Neurol. 52:1, 1993.

61. Bu, X., and Rotter, J.I.: X chromosome–linked and mitochondrial gene control of Leber's hereditary optic neuropathy: Evidence from segregation analysis for depen-

dence on X chromosome inactivation. Proc. Natl. Acad. Sci. U.S.A. *88*:8198, 1991.

62. Wallace, D.C., et al.: Mitochondrial DNA mutation associated with Leber's hereditary optic neuropathy. Science *242*:1427, 1988.

63. Gautin, P.H., et al.: Radiation Injury to the Nervous System. New York, Raven Press, 1991.

64. Russell, D.S., and Rubinstein, L.J.: Pathology of Tumors of the Nervous System, 5th ed. Baltimore, Williams & Wilkins, 1989.

65. Black, P.M.: Brain tumors. Parts 1 and 2. N. Engl. J. Med. *324*:1471–1476, 1555–1564, 1991.

66. Burger, P.C., et al.: Surgical Pathology of the Nervous System and its Coverings. New York, Churchill Livingstone, 1991.

67. Bigner, S.H.: Cerebrospinal fluid (CSF) cytology: Current status and diagnostic applications. J. Neuropathol. Exp. Neurol. *51*:235, 1992.

68. Kepes, J.J.: Meningiomas: Biology, Pathology, and Differential Diagnosis. New York, Masson, 1982.

69. Henson, R.A., and Urich, H.: Cancer and the Nervous System. Oxford, Blackwell, 1982.

70. Sobel, R.A.: Vestibular (acoustic) schwannomas: Histologic features in neurofibromatosis 2 and in unilateral cases. J. Neuropathol. Exp. Neurol. *52*:106, 1993.

71. Wanebo, J.E., et al.: Malignant peripheral nerve sheath tumors. Cancer *71*:1247, 1993.

72. Riccardi, V.M.: The clinical and molecular genetics of neurofibromatosis-1 and neurofibromatosis-2. *In* Rosenberg, R.N., et al. (eds.): The Molecular and Genetic Basis of Neurological Disease. Boston, Butterworth-Heinemann, 1993, pp. 837–853.

73. Viskorhil, D., et al.: The neurofibromatosis type 1 gene. Annu. Rev. Neurosci. *16*:183, 1993.

74. Trofatter, J.A., et al.: A novel moesin-, ezrin-, radixin-like gene is a candidate for the neurofibromatosis-2 tumor suppressor. Cell *72*:791, 1993.

75. The European Chromosome 16 Tuberous Sclerosis Consortium: Identification and characterization of the tuberous sclerosis gene on chromosome 16. Cell *75*:1305, 1993.

Index

Note: Page numbers in *italics* refer to illustrations; page numbers followed by t refer to tables.

Portions of this book, including text and illustrations, have appeared previously in *Basic Pathology*, fifth edition, by Vinay Kumar, Ramzi S. Cotran, and Stanley L. Robbins, published by W.B. Saunders (1992):

Figures:
1–8, 2–3, 2–4, 2–7A, 3–2, 3–4, 3–14, 3–18, 3–20, 3–28, 3–40, 4–1, 4–9, 4–12, 5–25, 5–28, 5–30, 6–1, 6–6, 6–8, 6–16, 6–17, 6–20, 6–36, 6–37, 6–38, 6–39, 6–41, 6–45, 7–9, 7–22, 7–24, 7–25, 7–28, 7–32, 7–38, 7–39, 7–40, 8–3, 8–4, 8–11, 9–8, 9–18, 9–21B, 9–25, 11–10A, 11–14, 11–15, 11–16, 12–18, 13–27, 13–28, 17–9, 17–18, 17–40, 17–47, 17–55, 17–56, 18–3, 18–25, 20–1B, 20–13B, 20–46, 20–56, 24–12, 24–20, 25–14, 25–28, 27–46

Tables:
3–7, 4–3, 7–1, 8–1, 8–6, 9–1, 9–2, 9–4, 9–13, 11–5, 25–7, 27–8